HANDBOOK
of
NUTRITION
and
FOOD

Second Edition

HANDBOOK
of
NUTRITION
and
FOOD

Second Edition

Edited by

CAROLYN D. BERDANIER
JOHANNA DWYER
ELAINE B. FELDMAN

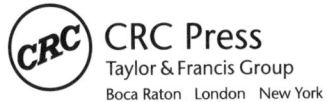

CRC Press
Taylor & Francis Group
Boca Raton   London   New York

CRC Press is an imprint of the
Taylor & Francis Group, an **informa** business

CRC Press
Taylor & Francis Group
6000 Broken Sound Parkway NW, Suite 300
Boca Raton, FL 33487-2742

Library of Congress Cataloging-in-Publication Data

Handbook of nutrition and food / editors, Carolyn D. Berdanier, Johanna Dwyer, and Elaine B. Beldman. -- 2nd ed.
   p. cm.
  Includes bibliographical references and index.
  ISBN-13: 978-0-8493-9218-4 (alk. paper)
  ISBN-10: 0-8493-9218-7 (alk. paper)
  1. Nutrition--Handbooks, manuals, etc. I. Berdanier, Carolyn D. II. Dwyer, Johanna T. III. Beldman, Elaine B. IV. Title.

QP141.H345 2007
612.3--dc22
                                                          2007000892

Visit the Taylor & Francis Web site at
http://www.taylorandfrancis.com

and the CRC Press Web site at
http://www.crcpress.com

Dedication

This book is dedicated to the memory of Dr. Daniel S. Feldman. Dan provided so much support to us in our efforts to produce a high quality handbook. He was responsible for converting all our color photographs into computer-compatible illustrations. He also provided much scientific and editing expertise especially in data management and analysis. Thanks Dan, we miss you.

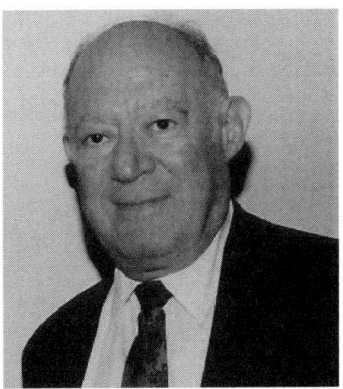

Preface to the Second Edition

Since the first edition was prepared more than 5 years ago, a lot of the large data sets found in that edition have been placed on the web. The reader will note that far more web addresses are given in this edition than in the first edition. By deleting some of the large tables that are now on the web, we then had space to expand this reference text to include a more extensive coverage of basic nutrition concepts. Thus, the reader will note that the book has been reorganized. Part I contains five chapters relating to food. In this section there are web addresses for food composition as well as a broad treatment of food safety, food labeling, and computerized nutrient analysis systems and techniques available for such data analysis.

Part II focuses on nutrition as a science. Basic terminology, intermediary metabolism relevant to the use of nutrients, individual micronutrients, as well as nutrient–nutrient interactions can be found here. In addition, there is a chapter giving web addresses for the nutrient needs of species other than the human. This is particularly useful to the scientists wishing to make interspecies comparisons.

Nutrition need throughout the life cycle and under special circumstances is the focus of Part III. Nutrition during pregnancy and lactation, feeding the preterm and term infant, the toddler, the young child, the adolescent, the healthy adult, and the senior adult is addressed in the chapters of this section. How exercise affects nutrient need and how one can have a healthy well-nourished body consuming a vegetarian diet is also discussed in this section.

Even though we have a large national commitment to provide a wide variety of nutritious food for our population, how do we know whether our people are well nourished? Part IV addresses this question from a variety of perspectives. Education on the national scale through the provision of healthy eating guidelines helps to inform the public of ways to ensure that they are well nourished. Beyond that there are a number of ways to monitor nutritional status of a variety of age groups and cultural groups. These are described in the rest of the chapters in this section.

Lastly, Part V deals with a wide variety of clinical topics with nutritional implications. Starting with medical evaluation techniques and flowing through all the relevant issues awaiting the clinician, nutrition is addressed as these clinical states are described.

Many of the authors of the chapters in the first edition have graciously updated their original contributions and we the editors are very grateful. There are some new chapters as well as some new authors. We hope you will find this multiauthored text an excellent addition to your professional library.

Carolyn D. Berdanier
Elaine B. Feldman
Johanna Dwyer

About the Editors

Carolyn D. Berdanier is a professor emerita, nutrition and cell biology, University of Georgia in Athens. She earned her B.S. from the Pennsylvania State University and her M.S. and Ph.D. from Rutgers University. She has had a long and productive career in nutrition. She began her career as a researcher with U.S. Department of Agriculture in Beltsville, then moved to the University of Nebraska College of Medicine and shortly thereafter moved to the University of Georgia. She served as department head at UGA for 11 years before stepping down to more actively pursue her research interests in nutrient–gene interactions. Her research has been supported by grants from NIH, USDA, the Bly Fund, and several commodity research boards. Her publication record includes 134 research publications in peer-reviewed journals, 16 books (either sole authored, edited or co-edited), 30 invited reviews, 45 chapters in multiauthored scientific books, and numerous short reviews in *Nutrition Reviews*. She has served on a number of editorial boards and contributes regularly to *Nutrition Today*, a lay magazine for the nutrition practitioner. She has received numerous awards for her research accomplishments including the Borden Award, the Lamar Dodd award for creative research, The UGA Research Medal, the National 4H award for alumni, and outstanding alumna awards from both Rutgers and the Pennsylvania State University. She is a member of the American Diabetes Association, The American Society for Nutrition Science, the Society for Experimental Biology and Medicine, and the American Physiological Society. Recently she was elected a fellow of the American Society for Nutrition Science.

Elaine B. Feldman is a professor emerita, medicine, physiology and endocrinology, Medical College of Georgia in Augusta. She is also chief emerita of the section on nutrition and director emerita of the Georgia Institute of Human Nutrition. She was the founding director of the Southeastern Regional Medical Nutrition Education Network of 15 medical schools in the southeast. At the Medical College she was principal investigator of a curriculum development grant from the Department of Health and Human Services and of a clinical nutrition research unit as well as a number of diet and drug studies in hyperlipidemia. She holds an M.D., AB (Magna Cum Laude), and M.S. from New York University where she was elected to Phi Beta Kappa and Alpha Omega Alpha. She trained in internal medicine, metabolism, and nutrition at the Mount Sinai Hospital in New York. She has held research fellowships from the New York Heart Association and the NIH (Career Development Award, Department of Physiological Chemistry, Lund University, Sweden) and served on the faculty of the Department of Medicine, State University of New York Medical School in New York City. She is board certified in internal medicine, clinical lipidology, and clinical nutrition. Dr. Feldman is a noted author and lecturer on nutrition and lipidology. She has published 82 articles in peer-reviewed biomedical journals and 56 invited articles, and has edited or authored 32 books, book chapters, monographs, and a textbook. She has served on numerous review boards and currently serves on the editorial boards of *Nutrition Today* and *Nutrition Update*. She is a fellow of the American Heart Association's Council on Arteriosclerosis, the American College of Physicians, and the American Society for Nutrition Sciences. She serves as a consultant for the American Institute for Cancer Research and the American Medical Women's Association.

Dr. Johanna Dwyer is the director of the Frances Stern Nutrition Center at New England Medical Center, professor of medicine (nutrition) and community health at the Tufts University Medical School, and professor of nutrition at Tufts University School of Nutrition. She is also senior scientist at the Jean Mayer/USDA Human Nutrition Research Center on Aging at Tufts University. Since mid-2003 until the present, Dr. Dwyer is on loan from Tufts University to the Office of Dietary Supplements, National Institutes of Health, where she is responsible for several large projects, including development of an analytically substantiated dietary supplement database and other dietary supplement databases, development of research on the assessment of dietary supplement intake and motivations for their use, and other topics. Dr. Dwyer was the assistant administrator for human nutrition, Agricultural Research Service, U.S. Department of Agriculture from 2001 to 2002. Earlier in her career, Dwyer served in the executive office of the President as staff for the White House Conference on Food Nutrition and Health of 1969, and again in 1976 for the President's Reorganization Project examining the role of nutrition programs in the federal government. As the Robert Wood Johnson Health Policy Fellow (1980 to 1981), she served on the personal staffs of Senator Richard Lugar (R-Indiana) and the Hon. Barbara Mikulski (D-Maryland).

Dwyer received her D.Sc. and M.Sc. from the Harvard School of Public Health, an M.S. from the University of Wisconsin, and completed her undergraduate degree with distinction from Cornell University. She is the author or coauthor of more than 170 research articles and 300 review articles published in scientific journals on topics including preventing diet-related disease in children and adolescents; maximizing quality of life and health in the elderly; vegetarian and other alternative lifestyles; and databases for bioactive substances other than nutrients. She served on the 2000 Dietary Guidelines Committee, was a member of the Food and Nutrition Board of the National Academy of Sciences from 1992 to 2001, was elected a member of the Institute of Medicine National Academy of Sciences in 1998, and served as councilor of the Institute of Medicine from 2001 to 2003.

She is currently secretary of the American Dietetic Association Foundation, and editor of *Nutrition Today*. She is the past president and fellow of the American Institute of Nutrition, past Secretary of the American Society for Clinical Nutrition, and past president and fellow of the Society for Nutrition Education. She received the Conrad V. Elvejhem Award for public service in 2005 from the American Society for Nutrition Sciences, the Alumni Award of Merit from the Harvard School of Public Health in 2004, the Medallion Award of the American Dietetic Association in 2003, and the W.O. Atwater award in 1996.

Contributors

Kelly M. Adams
University of North Carolina at Chapel Hill
Chapel Hill, NC

David B. Allison
Department of Biostatistics
University of Alabama at Birmingham
Birmingham, AL

Ross E. Andersen
Johns Hopkins School of Medicine
Division of Geriatric Medicine
Baltimore, MD

Judith Ashley
Department of Nutrition
University of Nevada at Reno
Reno, NV

Deborah Maddox Bagshaw
Department of Nutritional Sciences
The Pennsylvania State University
University Park, PA

Beth Baisden
Section on Neonatology
Department of Pediatrics
Medical College of Georgia
Augusta, GA

Paule Barbeau
Department of Pediatrics
Medical College of Georgia
Augusta, GA

Richard N. Baumgartner
Department of Epidemiology and
Clinical Investigation Section
University of Louisville
Louisville, KY

Suzanne Domel Baxter
Institute for Families in Society
University of South Carolina
Columbia, SC

Carolyn D. Berdanier
University of Georgia
Deptartment of Nutrition
Athens, GA

Odilia I. Bermudez
New England Medical Center Hospital
Boston, MA

Jatinder Bhatia
Department of Pediatrics
Medical College of Georgia
Augusta, GA

Cynthia A. Blanton
USDA Agricultural Research Service
Western Human Nutrition Research
Center
University of California
Davis, CA

Susan Bowerman
UCLA Center for Human Nutrition
Los Angeles, CA

George A. Bray
The Pennington Biomedical Research
Center
Baton Rouge, LA

Chantrapa Bunyapen
Section on Neonatology
Department of Pediatrics
Medical College of Georgia
Augusta, GA

James Carroll
Department of Neurology
Medical College of Georgia
Augusta, GA

Ronni Chernoff
GRECC
Central Arkansas Veterans Healthcare
System
Little Rock, AR

William Cameron Chumlea
Department of Community Health and
Pediatrics
Lifespan Health Research Center
Wright State University
Boonshoft School of Medicine
Dayton, OH

Gerald R. Cooper
Centers for Disease Control
Atlanta, GA

Richard Cotter
Wyeth Consumer Healthcare
Five Giralda Farms
Madison, NJ

Gail A. Cresci
Department of Surgery
Medical College of Georgia
Augusta, GA

Gary Cutter
Department of Biostatistics
University of Alabama at Birmingham
Birmingham, AL

Cindy D. Davis
Nutritional Science Research Group
Division of Cancer Prevention
National Cancer Institute
Rockville, MD

R. Sue McPherson Day
University of Texas
School of Public Health
Human Nutrition Center
Houston, TX

Mark T. DeMeo
University Gastroenterologists
Rush-Presbyterian-St Luke's
Medical Center, Rush University
Chicago, IL

Dominick P. DePaola
The Forsyth Institute
Boston, MA

Clifford Deveney
Department of General Surgery
Section of Bariatric Surgery
Oregon Health and Science University
Portland, OR

Michael P. Doyle
Department of Food Science and
Technology
University of Georgia
Griffin, GA

Johanna T. Dwyer
Frances Stern Nutrition Center
New England Medical Center Hospital
Boston, MA

Alan R. Dyer
Department of Preventive Medicine
Northwestern University Medical School
Chicago, IL

Carissa A. Eastham
University of Texas
School of Public Health
Human Nutrition Center
Houston, TX

Leon Ellenbogen
Wyeth Consumer Healthcare
Five Giralda Farms, Madison, NJ

Elaine B. Feldman
Medical College of Georgia
Augusta, GA

Claudia S. Plaisted Fernandez
Department of Nutrition
University of North Carolina
Chapel Hill, NC

William P. Flatt
University of Georgia
Department of Nutrition
Athens, GA

John P. Foreyt
Behavioral Medicine Research Center
Baylor College of Medicine
Houston, TX

Gary D. Foster
School of Medicine
Temple University
Philadelphia, PA

Shawn C. Franckowiak
Division of Geriatric Medicine and
Gerontology
Johns Hopkins University
School of Medicine
Baltimore, MD

Naomi K. Fukagawa
Department of Medicine
University of Vermont
College of Medicine
Burlington, VT

Yvette Gamble
Section on Neonatology
Department of Pediatrics
Medical College of Georgia
Augusta, GA

Constance J. Geiger
Geiger & Assoc.
Salt Lake City, UT

Jeanne Goldberg
Tufts University
Friedman School of Nutrition
Boston, MA

Bernard Gutin
Pediatrics, Physiology & Endocrinology
Georgia Prevention Institute
Augusta, GA

James L. Hargrove
Department of Foods and Nutrition
University of Georgia
Athens, GA

David Heber
Division of Clinical Nutrition
Department of Medicine
UCLA School of Medicine
Los Angeles, CA

Linda K. Hendricks
Section of Hematology and Oncology
Department of Medicine
Medical College of Georgia
Augusta, GA

Deanna M. Hoelscher
University of Texas
School of Public Health
Human Nutrition Center
Houston, TX

Mary Horlick
Division of Digestive Diseases and
Nutrition
National Institute of Diabetes and
Digestive and Kidney Diseases
National Institutes of Health
Bethesda, MD

Carolyn H. Jenkins
Division of Endocrinology Research
Medical University of South Carolina
Charleston, SC

Mary Ann Johnson
Department of Foods and Nutrition
University of Georgia, Athens, GA

Craig A. Johnston
Department of Pediatrics-Nutrition
Baylor College of Medicine
Houston, TX

Colin D. Kay
Department of Nutritional Sciences and
Biobehavioral Health
The Pennsylvania State University
University Park, PA

Eileen Kennedy
Tufts University
Friedman School of Medicine
Boston, MA

Nancy L. Keim
USDA Agricultural Research Service
Western Human Nutrition Research
Center
University of California
Davis, CA

Hyunmi Kim
Department of Neurology
Medical College of Georgia
Augusta, GA

Erin M. Koers
University of Texas
School of Public Health
Human Nutrition Center
Houston, TX

Kathryn M. Kolasa
Nutrition Education and Services
Department of Family Medicine
The Brody School of Medicine
East Carolina University
Greenville, NC

Srinadh Komanduri
Section of Gastroenterology and
Nutrition
Rush University Medical Center
Chicago, IL

Ronald M. Krauss
Childrens Hospital
Oakland Research Institute
Oakland, CA

Jessica Krenkel
University of Nevada
School of Medicine
Nutrition Education and Research
Reno, NV

Penny M. Kris-Etherton
Department of Nutrition
The Pennsylvania State University
University Park, PA

Abdullah Kutlar
Medical College of Georgia
Augusta, GA

Emma M. Laing
Department of Foods and Nutrition
University of Georgia
Athens, GA

Michael J. LaMonte
Epidemiology Division
The Cooper Institute
Dallas, TX

Jenny Harris Ledikwe
Oak Ridge Institute for Science and
Education
Department of Nutritional Sciences
The Pennsylvania State University
University Park, PA

Christian R. Lemmon
Eating Disorders Program
Department of Psychiatry & Health
Behavior
Medical College of Georgia
Augusta, GA

Brent H. Limbaugh
Medical College of Georgia
Augusta, GA

Kiang Liu
Department of Preventive Medicine
Northwestern University Medical School
Chicago, IL

Maria F. Lopes-Virella
Division of Endocrinology Research
Medical University of South Carolina
Charleston, SC

Robert G. Martindale
Department of General Surgery
Section of Bariatric Surgery
Oregon Health Sciences University
Portland, OR

Diane C. Mitchell
Diet Assessment Center
Department of Nutritional Sciences
The Pennsylvania State University
University Park, PA

Sohrab Mobarhan
Loyola University Medical Center
Maywood, IL

Connie Mobley
University of Texas Health Science
Center
San Antonio, TX

Judith Moreines
Wyeth Consumer Healthcare
Madison, NJ

Ece A. Mutlu
Division of Gastroenterology
Rush-Presbyterian-St Luke's Medical
Center
Chicago IL

Gökhan M. Mutlu
Division of Respiratory & Critical Care
Medicine
Northwestern University
Chicago, IL

Marian L. Neuhouser
Cancer Prevention Program
Fred Hutchinson Cancer Research
Center
Seattle, WA

Forrest H. Nielsen
USDA, ARS, GFHNRC
University Station
Grand Forks, ND

Scott Owens
Department of Health , Exercise
Science, and Recreational Management
University of Mississippi
University, MS

Patricia W. Pace
Behavioral Medicine Research Center
Baylor College of Medicine
Houston, TX

Sohyun Park
Department of Foods and Nutrition
University of Georgia
Athens, GA

Ruth E. Patterson
Fred Hutchinson Cancer Research
Center
Seattle, WA

Jean Pennington
Division of Nutrition Research
Coordination
National Institute of Health
Bethesda, MD

Suzanne E. Perumean-Chaney
Department of Biostatistics
University of Alabama at Birmingham
Birmingham, AL

Suzanne Phelan
Brown Medical School
The Miriam Hospital
Weight Control and Diabetes Research
Center
Providence, RI

Roxanne Poole
DaVita North Orangeburg Dialysis
Orangeburg, SC

L. Michael Prisant
Hypertension Unit,
Section of Cardiology
Medical College of Georgia
Augusta, GA

Tricia L. Psota
Department of Nutritional Sciences
The Pennsylvania State University
University Park, PA

Diane Rigassio Radler
University of Medicine and Dentistry
of New jersey
School of Health Related Professionals
Newark, NJ

Marsha Read
Department of Nutrition
University of Nevada
Reno, NV

Rebecca S. Reeves
Behavioral Medicine Research Center
Baylor College of Medicine
Houston, TX

Karen E. Remsberg
Department of Social Medicine
Ohio University
College of Osteopathic Medicine
Athens, OH

Richard S. Rivlin
Strang Cancer Research Laboratory
Cornell University Medical College
New York

Barbara J. Scott
University of Nevada School of Medicine
Department of Pediatrics
Reno, NV

Christopher T. Sempos
Center for Scientific Review
Bethesda, MD

Scott H. Sicherer
Allergy & Immunology
Department of Pediatrics
New York

Patty Siri-Tarino
Childrens Hospital
Oakland Research Institute
Oakland, CA

Diane K. Smith
CSRA Partners in Health Inc.
Augusta, GA

Helen Smiciklas-Wright
Diet Assessment Center
Department of Nutritional Sciences
The Pennsylvania State University
University Park, PA

Gwenn Snow
Department of Nutrition
University of Nevada Reno
Reno, NV

Malgorzata Stanczyk
Department of General Surgery
Section of Bariatric Surgery
Oregon Health and Science University
Portland, OR

Lynn Thomas
University of South Carolina
School of Medicine
Department of Medical Education and
Academic Affairs
Columbia, SC

Linda G. Tolstoi
Independent Nutrition Consultants
Uniontown, PA

Riva Touger-Decker
Division of Nutrition
Department of Diagnostic Sciences
New Jersey College of Medicine and
Dentistry
Newark, NJ

Chermaine Tyler
Department of Pediatrics – Nutrition
Baylor College of Medicine
Houston, TX

Marta D. Van Loan
USDA-WHNRC
University of California, Davis, CA

Kumar S. Venkitanarayanan
Department of Animal Science
University of Connecticut, Storrs, CT

Jenifer H. Voeks
Department of Epidemiology
University of Alabama at Birmingham
Birmingham, AL

Stanley Wallach
Hospital for Joint Diseases
New York, NY

Chenxi Wang
Department of Epidemiology and
Clinical Investigation Sciences
University of Louisville
Lousiville, KY

David G. Weismiller
Department of Family Medicine
The Brody School of Medicine
East Carolina University
Greenville, NC

Sheila G. West
Department of Biobehavioral Health
The Pennsylvania State University
University Park, PA

Christine L. Williams
Columbia University
College of Physicians and Surgeons
Institute of Human Nutrition
New York, NY

Winifred Yu
New England Medical Center
Hospital
Boston, MA

Table of Contents

PART V Clinical Nutrition

Part I

Food

1 Food Constituents

Carolyn D. Berdanier

Contents

INTRODUCTION

Humans and animals consume food to obtain the nutrients they need. Throughout the world there are differences in food consumption related to socioeconomic conditions, food availability, and cultural dictates. If a variety of fresh and cooked foods is consumed, in sufficient quantities, to meet the energy needs of the consumer, then the needs for protein and the micronutrients should be met. Having this in mind, it is surprising to learn that some people are poorly nourished and, indeed, may develop one or more nutrition-related diseases. The early years of nutrition research focused on diseases related to inadequate vitamin and mineral intake. An important component of this research was the determination of the vitamin and mineral content of a vast variety of foods. The composition of these foods has been compiled by the United States Department of Agriculture (USDA) and other organizations. Table 1.1 provides Web addresses to access a variety of data sets giving the nutrient content of a variety of foods. Included are some Web addresses for the composition of foods provided by some of the restaurant chains. These are particularly valuable because Americans eat more of their meals away from home than ever before. In addition, the data are from combination foods, that is, the information is for a particular menu item complete with its "fixings."

TABLE 1.1
Web Addresses for Information on the Composition of Food

Data Set	Web Address
Composition of foods, raw, processed, prepared; 6200 foods, 82 nutrients[a]	http://www.nal.usda.gov/fnic/foodcomp/Data/foods,82nutrients
Daidzein, genisten, glycitein, isoflavone content of 128 foods	Use preceding address, click on this file to open
Carotenoid content of 215 foods	Use preceding address, click on this file to open
trans-Fatty acid content of 214 foods	Use preceding address, click on this file to open
Sugar content of 500+ foods	Use preceding address, click on this file to open
Nutritive value of food in common household units; more than 900 items are in this list	Use preceding address, click on Nutritive Value of Foods (HG-72) to open
Vitamin K	Use preceding address, click on vitamin K to open
List of key foods (foods that contribute up to 75% of any one nutrient)	Use preceding address, click on Key Foods to open
Nutrient retention factors: calculations of retention of specific micronutrients	Use preceding address, click on Nutrient Retention Factors, Release 4 (1998)
Primary nutrient data sets (results of USDA surveys)	Use preceding address, click on Primary Nutrient for USDA Nationwide Food Surveys Dataset
Selenium and vitamin D (provisional values)	Use preceding address, click on selenium and vitamin D to open
Food composition (foods from India)	www.unu.edu/unupress/unupbooks/80633e/80633Eoi.htm
European foods	Cost99/EUROFOODS:Inventory of European Food Composition food.ethz.ch/cost99db-inventory.htm
Foods in developing countries	www.fao.org/DOCREP/W0073e/woo73eO6.htm
Other food data	www.arborcom.com/frame/foodc.htm
Soy foods (beneficial compounds)	See preceding entry, isoflavone, etc.
Individual amino acids and fatty acids	http://www.infinite faculty.org/sci/cr/crs/1994
Nutrition Information from Eat'nPark restaurant chain	www.eatnpark.com
Nutrition information from McDonald's	www.mcdonalds.com

[a] A printed format can be obtained from the Superintendent of Documents, U.S. Printing Office, Washington, DC 20402. Request USDA Handbooks 8 through 16. A CD-ROM can also be obtained. None of these are free.

A number of organizations, both governmental and nongovernmental, are interested in providing food intake recommendations to promote good health and reduce the risk of disease. Table 1.2 provides Web sites for these recommendations. Additional information on healthy eating by different age groups is provided in Chapters 8 to 13. Healthy eating focuses on food choices that promote optimal nutrition. Mainly these recommendations address the food needs of adults. However, there are several concerns about food intake that are separate from food choice. The regulation of food intake by internal signals can quantitatively affect what food is consumed and how much. These signals apparently are integrated ones that signal hunger or

TABLE 1.2
Web Sites for Food Intake Recommendations

Recommendation	Web Site
Daily recommended intake (DRI)	www.nap.edu and http://www.nal.usda.gov/fnic/etext/000105.html
Dietary guidelines	www.health.gov/dietary guidelines/
Food pyramid	www.mypyramid.gov/tips resources/menus.html
Cancer risk reduction	www.cancer.org/docroot/PED/content/PED
Food from plants	www.5aday.gov/

TABLE 1.3
Hormones and Drugs that Influence Food Intake

Enhances	Suppresses
Insulin	Estrogen
Testosterone	Phenylethylamines[a]
Thyroxine	Mazindol
Low serotonin levels	Substance P
Glucocorticoids	Glucagon
β-endorphin	Serotonin
Low serotonin levels	Leptin
Dynorphin	Fluoxetine
Neuropeptide Y	"Satietin" (a blood-borne factor)
Galanin	Histidine (precursor of histamine)
Opioid peptides	Pain
Growth-hormone-releasing hormone	Amino acid imbalance in diet
Desacetyl-melanocyte-stimulating hormone	Tryptophan (precursor of serotonin)
Antidepressants[b]	Cholecystokinin (CCK)
Low adiponectin	Calcitonin
	Somatostatin
	Anorectin
	High-fat diet
	Thyrotropin releasing hormone
	Cachectin (tumor necrosis factor)
	Corticotropin-releasing hormone (CRH)
	Neurotensin
	Bombesin
	cyclo-His-Pro
	High-protein diets
	High blood glucose
	Enterostatin

[a] These are drugs, and all except for the drug phenylpropanolamine are controlled substances. Many have serious side effects. They are structurally related to the catecholamines. Most are active as short-term appetite suppressants and act through their effects on the central nervous system, particularly through the b-adrenergic or dopaminergic receptors. This group includes amphetamine, methamphetamine, phenmetrazine, phentermine, diethylpropion, fenfluramine, and phenylpropanolamine. Phenylpropanolamine-induced anorexia is not reversed by the dopamine antagonist haloperidol.

[b] All of these drugs are controlled substances and their use must be carefully monitored. This group includes amitriptyline, buspirone, chlordiazepoxide, chlorpromazine, cisplatin, clozapine, ergotamine, fluphenazine, imipramine, iprindole, and others that block 5-HT receptors.

Source: Berdanier, C.D., *Advanced Nutrition: Macronutrients.* CRC Press, Boca Raton, FL, 2000, p. 122.

the initiation of eating and satiety or the signal to stop eating. Not all of these signals are known, but Table 1.3 provides a list of the ones that have been studied.[1]

Several data sets that may not be available on the Web can be found in this chapter. Table 1.4 provides the tocopherol values for a wide variety of foods.[2] Table 1.5 provides information on the tagatose content of food.[3] Tagatose is a food additive used to reduce the amount of sugar in a food. It has a sweet taste, yet does not have the same energy value as sucrose. Other sugar substitutes are also used in the preparation of reduced-energy foods; however, data on their quantitative occurrence is not as readily available because of the proprietary interests of food producers. A list of sweeteners added to foods is provided in Table 1.6.[4] Following this table is a list of the types of food additives that change the properties of food (Table 1.7; see Reference 4, pp. 11–18). This table describes compounds that increase the shelf life of a class of foods or additives that change

TABLE 1.4
Tocopherols and Tocotrienols in Selected Food Products (mg/100 g)

Product	α-T	γ-T	δ-T	Total	α-Tocopherol Equivalents
Breakfast cereals					
Fortified					
Total King Vitamin	104.50	ND	ND	104.50	104.50
	35.10	ND	ND	35.10	35.10
Nonfortified					
Post natural Raisin Bran	1.50	ND	ND	1.50	1.50
Kellogg's Raisin Bran	1.30	ND	ND	1.30	1.30
Cheese					
American					
Low fat Weight Watchers	1.50	ND	ND	1.50	1.50
Borden Lite Line	0.10	ND	ND	0.10	0.10
Processed					
Kraft	0.40	ND	ND	0.40	0.40
American processed					
Kroger	0.40	ND	ND	0.40	0.40
Cheddar					
Kraft	0.30	ND	ND	0.30	0.30
Kroger	0.20	ND	ND	0.20	0.20
Munster					
Sargento	0.50	ND	ND	0.50	0.50
Kroger	0.30	ND	ND	0.30	0.30
Swiss					
Kraft	0.60	ND	ND	0.60	0.60
Beatrice City Line Old World	0.40	ND	ND	0.40	0.40
Chips					
Potato					
Lay's	1.30	4.60	1.30	7.20	1.80
Wise	7.40	1.20	0.10	8.70	7.52
Tortilla					
Tostitos	1.10	2.40	0.50	4.00	1.36
Tostados	1.50	1.00	0.30	2.80	1.61
					0.00
Fish					
Salmon, waterpack					
Chicken of the Sea	0.70	ND	ND	0.70	0.70
Black Top	0.60	ND	ND	0.60	0.60
Sardines, in tomato sauce					
Spirit of Norway	3.60	0.20	0.10	3.90	3.62
Orleans	3.90	ND	0.10	4.00	3.90
Tuna, canned in oil					0.00
Starkist	1.00	4.80	1.90	7.70	1.54
Chicken of the Sea	0.98	2.60	1.10	4.68	1.27
Fruits and fruit juices					
Grape juice, bottled					
Welch's	ND	ND	ND	0.00	0.00
Seneca	ND	ND	ND	0.00	0.00

Continued

TABLE 1.4
(Continued)

Product	α-T	γ-T	δ-T	Total	α-Tocopherol Equivalents
Orange juice					
Fresh Tropicana	0.20	ND	ND	0.20	0.20
Frozen Minute Maid	0.20	0.10	ND	0.30	0.21
Plums					0.00
Variety 1	0.70	0.10	ND	0.80	0.71
Variety 2	0.50	0.04	ND	0.54	0.50
Milk chocolate, plain	0.50	2.00	ND	2.50	0.70
Nuts					
Brazil nuts					
Health food store	6.60	2.10	1.60	10.30	6.86
Dekalb Farmers Market	11.00	5.10	2.60	18.70	11.59
English walnuts					
Diamond	1.40	9.20	0.60	11.20	2.34
Kroger		6.70	0.50	7.20	0.69
Hazelnuts					
Health food store	21.50	0.10	0.01	21.61	21.51
Dekalb Farmers Market	16.80	0.70	ND	17.50	16.87
Oils					
Margarine, stick					
Mazzola	8.40	24.40	0.40	33.20	10.85
Fleischman	7.90	23.10	0.60	31.60	10.23
Mayonnaise					
Kraft	1.30	6.60	1.00	8.90	1.99
Hellman	1.60	9.80	1.90	13.30	2.64
Shortenings, Crisco	5.60	25.20	5.40	36.20	8.28
Vegetable oil					0.00
Crisco	2.90	33.30	7.00	43.20	6.44
Wesson	2.80	18.30	3.00	24.10	4.72
Protein diet powder					
Slimfast	26.50	ND	ND	26.50	26.50
Herbalife	24.60	ND	ND	24.60	24.60
Salad dressings					
Bleu cheese					
Marie's	4.70	57.50	25.40	87.60	11.21
Kraft	2.80	49.00	14.40	66.20	8.13
French					
Wishbone	3.00	66.90	27.70	97.60	10.52
Kraft	3.10	61.90	18.20	83.20	9.84
Italian					
Wishbone	4.40	60.60	30.00	95.00	11.36
Kraft	4.00	62.70	17.80	84.50	10.80
Tea					
Tea leaves from tea bags					
Tetley	2.40	0.60	ND	3.00	2.46
Lipton	12.30	3.20	ND	15.50	12.62
Tea brewed from tea bags					
Tetley	ND	ND	ND	0.00	0.00
Lipton	ND	ND	ND	0.00	0.00
Tomato products					
Barbecue sauce, Kraft	1.00	0.80	0.10	1.90	1.08
Heinz Catsup	1.10	0.40	0.10	1.60	1.14
Heinz	1.10	0.10	ND	1.20	1.11
Hunt's Tomato chili sauce	1.80	0.20	ND	2.00	1.82

TABLE 1.4
(Continued)

Product	α-T	γ-T	δ-T	Total	α-Tocopherol Equivalents
Del Monte	2.70	0.20	ND	2.90	2.72
Heinz Tomato paste	3.20	0.30	ND	3.50	3.23
Hunt's	4.10	0.30	ND	4.40	4.13
Contadina Tomato sauce	4.50	0.70	ND	5.20	4.57
Hunt's Tomato sauce	1.40	0.10	ND	1.50	1.41
Tomato soup	1.50	0.20	ND	1.70	1.52
Progresso					
Campbell's	0.70	0.30	0.10	1.10	0.73
Kroger	0.60	0.10	ND	0.70	0.61
Tomatoes, stewed Del Monte	0.90	0.20	ND	1.10	0.92
Tomatoes, Stead Stokely's	0.70	0.20	ND	0.90	0.72
Vegetables					
Asparagus					
Sample 1	1.00	0.10	ND	1.10	1.01
Sample 2	1.30	0.10	ND	1.40	1.31
Cabbage					
Sample 1	0.12	ND	ND	0.12	0.12
Sample 2	0.09	ND	ND	0.09	0.09
Cucumbers					
Sample 1	0.04	0.02	ND	0.06	0.04
Sample 2	0.09	0.02	ND	0.11	0.09
Turnip greens					
Sample 1	2.90	0.10	ND	3.00	2.91
Sample 2	2.80	0.20	ND	3.00	2.82

Note: ND, not detectable.

Source: Lentner, C., *Geigy Scientific Tables*, Vol. 1. CIBA-Geigy, West Caldwell, NJ, 1981, pp. 241–266.

the texture of a food. The specific attributes of individual food additives are described in Table 1.8 (see Reference 4, pp. 11–18). This table provides information on how these additives function in particular food products.

A number of food additives and food processing techniques are used to improve the safety of the food. Foods can be contaminated by a wide variety of organisms, some of which are listed in Table 1.9.[5] Some of these contaminants can produce toxins, which, if consumed, can be lethal. Table 1.10 is a list of mycotoxins and bacterial toxins that can occur in food (see Reference 4, pp. 24–36, 1284–1285, 1776–1785, 1790–1803, 2082–2087). The reader should also review Chapter 2 for an extensive description of food-borne illness. Table 1.11 provides a list of antinutrients sometimes found in food.[6]

Antinutritives are compounds that interfere with the use of essential nutrients. They are generally divided into three classes: A, B, and C. Type A antinutritives are substances primarily interfering with the digestion of proteins or the absorption and utilization of amino acids. They are also known as antiproteins. Strict vegetarians, for example, are in danger of nutritional inadequacy by this type of antinutritive. The most important type A antinutritives are protease inhibitors and lectins.

Protease inhibitors, occurring in many plant and animal tissues, are proteins that inhibit proteolytic enzymes by binding to the active sites of the enzymes. Proteolytic enzyme inhibitors were first found in avian eggs around the turn of the century. They were later identified as ovomucoid and ovoinhibitor, both of which inactivate trypsin. Chymotrypsin inhibitors also are found in avian egg whites. Other sources of trypsin or chymotrypsin inhibitors are soybeans and other legumes and pulses, vegetables, milk and colostrum, wheat and other cereal grains, guar gum, and white and sweet potatoes. The protease inhibitors of kidney beans, soybeans, and potatoes can additionally inhibit elastase, a pancreatic enzyme acting on elastin, an insoluble protein in meat. Animals, fed with food containing active inhibitors, show growth depression. This appears to be due to interference in trypsin and chymotrypsin activities and to excessive stimulation of the secretory exocrine pancreatic cells, which become hypertrophic. Valuable proteins may be lost to the feces in this case. *In vitro* experiments with human proteolytic enzymes have been shown that trypsin inhibitors from bovine colostrum, lima beans, soybeans, kidney beans, and quail ovomucoid were active against human trypsin, whereas trypsin inhibitors originating from bovine and porcine pancreas, potatoes, chicken

TABLE 1.5
Occurrence of D-Tagatose in Foods[1]

Food	Result (mg/kg)	Sample Preparation	Apparatus
Sterilized cow's milk	2–3000	Extracted with methanol; prepared trimethylsilyl (TMS) derivatives	Gas chromatography (GC), fused-silica capillary column (18 m × 0.22 mm) coated with AT-1000; carrier gas N2; flame ionization detector (FID)
Hot cocoa (processed with alkali) prepared with milk	140	Extracted with deionized (DI) water	High-performance liquid chromatography (HPLC); used Bio-Rad Aminex® HPX-87C column (300 mm × 7.8 mm) heated to 85°C; mobile phase DI water; flow rate 0.6 ml/min; refractive index (RI) detector
Hot cocoa prepared with milk	190	Extracted with DI water	HPLC; Bio-Rad Aminex® HPX-87C column heated to 85°C; mobile phase DI water; flow rate 0.6 ml/min; RI detector
Powdered cow's milk	800	Extracted three times with distilled water for 3 h at 60°C; column chromatography to remove organic acids and bases; fractionation by partition chromatography	Paper partition chromatography, descending method on Whatman no.1 paper; used three solvent systems
Similac® infant formula	4	Extracted with 90% ethanol; prepared TMS derivatives	GC; DB-5 fused-silica capillary column (15 m × 0.53 mm, 1.5 mm film thickness); carrier gas He; FID detector
Enfamil® infant formula	23	Extracted with 90% aqueous ethanol; prepared TMS derivatives	GC; DB-17 fused-silica capillary column (15 m × 0.53 mm, 1 mm film thickness); carrier gas He; FID detector
Parmesan cheese	10	Extracted with 80% aqueous methanol; prepared TMS derivatives	GC; DB-5 fused-silica capillary column (30 m, 0.25 mm film thickness); carrier gas He; FID detector
Gjetost cheese	15	Extracted with 80% aqueous methanol; prepared TMS derivatives	GC; DB-5 fused-silica capillary column (30 m, 0.25 mm film thickness); carrier gas He; FID detector
Cheddar cheese	2	Extracted with 80% aqueous methanol; prepared TMS derivatives	GC; DB-5 fused-silica capillary column (30 m, 0.25 mm film thickness); carrier gas He; FID detector
Roquefort cheese	20	Extracted with 80% aqueous methanol; prepared TMS derivatives	GC; DB-5 fused-silica capillary column (30 m, 0.25 mm film thickness); carrier gas He; FID detector
Feta cheese	17	Extracted with 80% aqueous methanol; prepared TMS derivatives	GC; DB-5 fused-silica capillary column (30 m, 0.25 mm film thickness); carrier gas He; FID detector
Ultrahigh-temperature milk	~5	Dried under vacuum; water was added, then volatile derivatives extracted with isooctane	GC; Rescom type OV1 capillary column (25 m × 0.25 mm, 0.1 or 0.25 mm film thickness); carrier gas H_2; FID detector
BA Nature® Yogurt	29	Extracted with DI water; passed through a strong cation exchange column followed by an amine column	HPLC; Bio-Rad Aminex® HPX-87C column heated to 85°C; mobile phase DI water; flow rate 0.6 ml/min; RI detector
Cephulac®, an orally ingested medication for treatment of portal-systemic encephalopathy	6500	Deionized with Amberlite IR-120 (H) and Duolite A-561 (free base); diluted to 20 mg/ml with a 50:50 mixture of acetonitrile and water	HPLC; Waters Carbohydrate Analysis Column (300 mm × 3.9 mm); mobile phase water: acetonitrile, 77:23 (w/w); flow rate 2 ml/min; RI detector
Chronulac®, an orally ingested laxative	6500	Deionized with Amberlite IR-120 (H) and Duolite A-561 (free base); diluted to 20 mg/ml with a 50:50 mixture of acetonitrile and water	HPLC; Waters Carbohydrate Analysis Column (300 mm × 3.9 mm); mobile phase-water: acetonitrile, 77:23 (w/w); flow rate 2 ml/min; RI detector

Source: Unpublished data, Lee Zehner, Beltsville, MD, 2000.

ovomucoid, and chicken ovoinhibitor were not. The soybean and lima bean trypsin inhibitors are also active against human chymotrypsin. Many protease inhibitors are heat labile, especially with moist heat. Relatively heat-resistant protease inhibitors include the antitryptic factor in milk, the alcohol-precipitable and nondialyzable trypsin inhibitor in alfalfa, the chymotrypsin inhibitor in potato, the kidney bean inhibitor, and the trypsin inhibitor in lima beans.

Lectin is the general term for plant proteins that have highly specific binding sites for carbohydrates. They are widely distributed among various sources such as soybeans, peanuts, jack beans, mung beans, lima beans, kidney beans, fava beans, vetch, yellow wax beans, hyacinth beans, lentils, peas, potatoes, bananas, mangoes, and wheat germ. Most plant lectins are gly-coproteins, except concanavalin A from jack beans, which is carbohydrate free. The most toxic lectins in food include ricin in castor bean (oral toxic dose in man: 150 to 200 mg; intravenous toxic dose: 20 mg) and the lectins of kidney bean and hyacinth bean. The mode of action of lectins may be related to their ability to bind to specific cell receptors, in a way comparable to that

TABLE 1.6
Sweetening Agents (Sugar Substitutes)

Name	Sweetness	Classification	Uses	Comments
Acesulfame-K (sold under brand Sunette)	130	Nonnutritive; artificial	Tabletop sweetener, chewing gum, dry beverage mixes, puddings	This is actually the potassium salt of the 6-methyl derivative of a group of chemicals called oxathiazinone dioxides; approved by the Food and Drug Administration (FDA) in 1988
Aspartame	180	Nutritive; artificial	In most diet sodas; also used in cold cereals, drink mixes, gelatin, puddings, toppings, dairy products, and at the table by the consumer; not used in cooking due to lack of stability when heated	Composed of the two naturally occurring amino acids, aspartic acid and phenylalanine; sweeter than sugar, therefore less required, hence fewer calories
Cyclamate	30	Nonnutritive; artificial	Tabletop sweetener and in drugs in Canada and 40 other countries	Discovered in 1937; FDA banned all cyclamate-containing beverages in 1969 and all cyclamate-containing foods in 1970; cyclamate safety is now being reevaluated by the FDA
Dulcin (4-ethoxy-phenyl-urea)	250	Nonnutritive; artificial	None	Not approved for food use in the United States; used in some European countries; also called Sucrol and Valzin
Fructose (levulose)	1.7	Nutritive; natural	Beverages, baking, canned goods; anywhere invert sugar or honey may be used	A carbohydrate; a monosaccharide; naturally occurs in fruits; makes up about 50% of the sugar in honey; commercially found in high-fructose syrups and invert sugars; contributes sweetness and prevents crystallization
Glucose (dextrose)	0.7	Nutritive; natural	Primarily in the confection, wine, and canning industries; and in intravenous solutions	Acts synergistically with other sweeteners
Glycine	0.8	Nutritive; natural	Permissible to use to modify taste of some foods	A sweet-tasting amino acid; tryptophan is also a sweet-tasting amino acid
Mannitol	0.7	Nutritive; natural	Candies, chewing gums, confections, and baked goods; dietetic foods	A sugar alcohol or polyhydric alcohol (polyol); occurs naturally in pineapples, olives, asparagus, and carrots; commercially prepared by the hydrogenation of mannose or glucose; slowly and incompletely absorbed from the intestines; only slightly metabolized, most excreted unchanged in the urine; may cause diarrhea
Miraculin	—	Nutritive; natural	None	Actually a taste-modifying protein rather than a sweetener; after exposing tongue to miraculin, sour lemon tastes like sweetened lemon; responsible for the taste-changing properties of miracle fruit, red berries of Synsepalum dulcificum, a native plant of West Africa; first described in 1852; one attempt made to commercialize by a U.S. firm but FDA denied approval and marketing was stopped
Monellin	3000	Nutritive; natural	None; only a potential low-calorie sweetener	Extract of the pulp of the light red berries of the tropical plant *Dioscoreophyllum cumminsii*; also called Serendipity Berry; first protein found to elicit a sweet taste in humans; first extracted in 1969; potential use limited by lack of stability; taste sensation is slow and lingering; everything tastes sweet after monellin
Neohesperidin dihydrochalone (Neo DHC, NDHC)	1250	Nonnutritive; artificial	None approved; potential for chewing gum, mouthwash, and toothpaste	Formed from naringen isolated from citrus fruit; slow to elicit the taste sensation; lingering licorice-like aftertaste; animal studies indicate not toxic
P-4000 (5-nitro-2-pro-poxyaniline)	4100	Nonnutritive; artificial	None approved	Derivative of nitroaniline; used as a sweetener in some European countries but banned in the United States due to toxic effects on rats; no bitter aftertaste; major drawback of P-4000 is powerful local anesthetic effect on the tongue and mouth; used in the Netherlands during German occupation and Berlin blockade

Continued

**TABLE 1.6
(Continued)**

Name	Sweetness	Classification	Uses	Comments
Phyllodulcin	250	Natural	None approved	Isolated from *Hydrangea macrophylla* Seringe in 1916; displays a lagging onset of sweetness with licorice aftertaste; not well studied; possible market for hard candies, chewing gums, and oral hygiene products
Saccharin (0 benzo-sulfimide)	500	Nonnutritive; artificial	Used in beverages, as a tabletop sweetener, and in cosmetics, toothpaste, and cough syrup; used as a sweetener by diabetics	Both sodium and calcium salts of saccharin used; passes through body unchanged; excreted in urine; originally a generally recognized as safe (GRAS) additive; subsequently, saccharin was classed as a carcinogen based on experiments with rats; however, recent experiments indicate that saccharin causes cancer in rats, but not in mice and humans
Sorbitol	0.6	Nutritive; natural	Chewing gum, dairy products, meat products, icing, toppings, and beverages	A sugar alcohol or polyol; occurs naturally in many fruits commercially prepared by the hydrogenation of glucose; many unique properties besides sweetness; on the FDA list of GRAS food additives; the most widely used sugar alcohol; slow intestinal absorption; consumption of large amounts may cause diarrhea
SRI Oxime V (Perilla sugar)	450	Nonnutritive; artificial	None approved	Derived from extract of *Perilla namkinensis*; clean taste; needs research; used as sweetening agent in Japan
Stevioside	300	Nutritive; natural	None approved	Isolated from the leaves of the wild shrub *Stevia rebaudiana* Bertoni; used by the people of Paraguay to sweeten drinks; limited evidence suggests nontoxic to humans; rebaudioside A is isolated from the same plant and is said to taste superior to stevioside; its chemical structure is very similar to stevioside, and it is 190 times sweeter than sugar
Sucrose (brown sugar, liquid sugar, sugar, table sugar, white sugar)	1.0	Nutritive; natural	Many beverages and processed foods; home use in a wide variety of foods	The chemical combination of the sugars fructose and glucose; one of the oldest sweetening agents; most popular and most available sweetening agent; occurs naturally in many fruits; commercially extracted from sugar cane and sugar beets
Splenda (dextrose/ maltodextrin/ sucralose)	4.0	Non nutritive	Used in many beverages and processed foods	Stable to heat
Thaumatins	1600	Nutritive; natural	None	Source of sweetness of the tropical fruit from the plant *Thaumatococcus daniellii*; enjoyed by inhabitants of western Africa; doubtful commercial applications
Xylitol	0.8	Nutritive; natural	Chewing gums and dietetic foods	A sugar alcohol or polyhydric alcohol (polyol); occurs naturally in some fruits and vegetables; produced in the body; commercial production from plant parts (oat hulls, corncobs, and birch wood chips) containing xylans — long chains of the sugar xylose; possible diarrhea; one British study suggests xylitol causes cancer in animals

Source: Ensminger, A.H. et al., *Foods and Nutrition Encyclopedia*, 2nd ed., CRC Press, Boca Raton, FL, 1994, pp. 2082–2087.

of antibodies. Because they are able to agglutinate red blood cells, they are also known as hemaglutinins. The binding of bean lectin on rat intestinal mucosal cells has been demonstrated *in vitro*, and it has been suggested that this action is responsible for the oral toxicity of the lectins. Such bindings may disturb the intestines' absorptive capacity for nutrients and other essential compounds. The lectins, being proteins, can easily be inactivated by moist heat. Germination decreases the hemaglutinating activity in varieties of peas and species of beans.

Type B antinutritives are substances interfering with the absorption or metabolic utilization of minerals and are also known as antiminerals. Although they are toxic per se, the amounts present in foods seldom cause acute intoxication under normal food consumption. However, they may harm the organism under suboptimum nutriture. The most important type B antinutritives are phytic acid, oxalates, and glucosinolates.

TABLE 1.7
Terms Used to Describe the Functions of Food Additives

Term	Function
Anticaking and free-flow agents	Substances added to finely powdered or crystalline food products to prevent caking
Antimicrobial agents	Substances used to preserve food by preventing growth of microorganisms and subsequent spoilage, including fungicides, mold and yeast inhibitors, and bacteriocides
Antioxidants	Substances used to preserve food by retarding deterioration, rancidity, or discoloration due to oxidation
Colors and coloring adjuncts	Substances used to impart, preserve, or enhance the color or shading of a food, including color stabilizers, color fixatives, and color-retention agents
Curing and pickling agents	Substances imparting a unique flavor or color to a food, usually producing an increase in shelf-life stability
Dough strengtheners	Substances used to modify starch and gluten, thereby producing a more stable dough
Drying agents	Substances with moisture-absorbing ability, used to maintain an environment of low moisture
Emulsifiers and emulsifier salts	Substances that modify surface tension of two (or more) immiscible solutions to establish a uniform dispersion of components; called an emulsion
Enzymes	Substances used to improve food processing and the quality of the finished food
Firming agents	Substances added to precipitate residual pectin, thus strengthening the supporting tissue and preventing its collapse during processing
Flavor enhancers	Substances added to supplement, enhance, or modify the original taste or aroma of a food without imparting a characteristic taste or aroma of its own
Flavoring agents and adjuvants	Substances added to impart or help impart a taste or aroma in food
Flour-treating agents	Substances added to milled flour, at the mill, to improve its color or baking qualities, including bleaching and maturing agents
Formulation aids	Substances used to promote or produce a desired physical state or texture in food, including carriers, binders, fillers, plasticizers, film-formers, and tableting aids
Fumigants	Volatile substances used for controlling insects or pests
Humectants	Hygroscopic substances incorporated in food to promote retention of moisture, including moisture-retention agents and antidusting agents
Leavening agents	Substances used to produce or stimulate production of carbon dioxide in baked goods to impart a light texture, including yeast, yeast foods, and calcium salts
Lubricants and release agents	Substances added to food contact surfaces to prevent ingredients and finished products from sticking to them
Nonnutritive sweeteners	Substances having less than 2% of the caloric value of sucrose per equivalent unit of sweetening capacity
Nutrient supplements	Substances that are necessary for the body's nutritional and metabolic processes
Nutritive sweeteners	Substances having greater than 2% equivalent unit of sweetening capacity
Oxidizing and reducing agents	Substances that chemically oxidize or reduce another food ingredient, thereby producing a more stable product
pH-control agents	Substances added to change or maintain active acidity or alkalinity, including buffers, acids, alkalis, and neutralizing agents
Processing aids	Substances used as manufacturing aids to enhance the appeal or utility of a food or food component, including clarifying agents, clouding agents, catalysts, flocculents, filter aids, and crystallization inhibitors
Propellants, aerating agents, and gases	Gases used to supply force to expel a product or used to reduce the amount of oxygen in contact with the food in packaging
Sequestrants	Substances that combine with polyvalent metal ions to form a soluble metal complex in order to improve the quality and stability of products
Solvents and vehicles	Substances used to extract or dissolve another substance
Stabilizers and thickeners	Substances used to produce viscous solutions or dispersions, to impart body, improve consistency, or stabilize emulsions, including suspending and bodying agents, setting agents, gelling agents, and bulking agents
Surface-active agents	Substances used to modify surface properties of liquid food components for a variety of effects, including, other than emulsifiers, solubilizing agents, dispersants, detergents, wetting agents, rehydration enhancers, whipping agents, foaming agents, and defoaming agents
Surface-finishing agents	Substances used to increase palatability, preserve gloss, and inhibit discoloration of foods, including glazes, polishes, waxes, and protective coatings
Synergists	Substances used to act or react with another food ingredient to produce a total effect different or greater than the sum of the effects produced by the individual ingredients
Texturizers	Substances that affect the appearance or feel of the food

Source: Ensminger, A.H. et al., *Foods and Nutrition Encyclopedia*, 2nd ed., CRC Press, Boca Raton, FL, 1994, pp. 11–18.

Phytic acid, or myoinositol hexaphosphate, is a naturally occurring strong acid that binds to many types of bivalent and trivalent heavy metal ions, forming insoluble salts. Consequently, phytic acid reduces the availability of many minerals and essential trace elements. The degree of insolubility of these salts appears to depend on the nature of the metal, the pH of the solution, and, for certain metals, on the presence of another metal. Synergism between two metallic ions in the formation of phytate complexes has also been observed. For instance, zinc–calcium phytate precipitates maximally at pH 6, which is also the pH

TABLE 1.8
Specific Food Additives and Their Functions

Name	Function[a]	Food Use and Comments
Acetic acid	pH control, preservative	Acid of vinegar is acetic acid; miscellaneous or general purposes; many food uses; generally recognized as safe (GRAS) additive
Adipic acid	pH control	Buffer and neutralizing agent; use in confectionery; GRAS additive
Ammonium alginate	Stabilizer and thickener, texturizer	Extracted from seaweed; widespread food use; GRAS additive
Annatto	Color	Extracted from seeds of *Bixa crellana*; butter, cheese, margarine, shortening, and sausage casings; coloring foods in general
Arabinogalactan	Stabilizer and thickener, texturizer	Extracted from western larch; widespread food use; bodying agent in essential oils, nonnutritive sweeteners, flavor bases, nonstandardized dressings, and pudding mixes
Ascorbic acid (vitamin C)	Nutrient, antioxidant, preservative	Widespread use in foods to prevent rancidity or browning; used in meat curing; GRAS additive
Aspartame	Sweetener; sugar substitute	Soft drinks, chewing gum, powdered beverages, whipped toppings, puddings, gelatin; tabletop sweetener
Azodicarbonamide	Flour-treating agent	Aging and bleaching ingredient in cereal flour
Benzoic acid	Preservative	Occurs in nature in free and combined forms; widespread food use; GRAS additive
Benzoyl peroxide	Flour-treating agent	Bleaching agent in flour; may be used in some cheeses
Beta-apo-8'-carotenal	Color	Natural food color; general use not to exceed 30 mg/lb or pt of food
Butylated hydroxyanisole (BHA)	Antioxidant, preservative	Fats, oils, dry yeast, beverages, breakfast cereals, dry mixes, shortening, potato flakes, chewing gum, sausage; often used in combination with butylated hydroxytoluene (BHT); GRAS additive
BHT	Antioxidant, preservative	Rice, fats, oils, potato granules, breakfast cereals, potato flakes, shortening, chewing gum, sausage; often used in combination with BHA; GRAS additive
Biotin	Nutrient	Rich natural sources are liver, kidney, pancreas, yeast, milk; vitamin supplement; GRAS additive
Calcium alginate	Stabilizer and thickener, texturizer	Extracted from seaweed; widespread food use; GRAS additive
Calcium carbonate	Nutrient	Mineral supplement; general purpose additive; GRAS additive
Calcium lactate	Preservative	General purpose or miscellaneous use; GRAS additive
Calcium phosphate	Leavening agent, sequestrant, nutrient	General purpose or miscellaneous use; mineral supplement; GRAS additive
Calcium propionate	Preservative	Bakery products, alone or with sodium propionate; inhibits mold and other microorganisms; GRAS additive
Calcium silicate	Anticaking agent	Used in baking powder and salt; GRAS additive
Canthaxanthin	Color	Widely distributed in nature; color for foods; more red than carotene
Caramel	Color	Miscellaneous or general purpose use in foods for color; GRAS additive
Carob bean gum	Stabilizer and thickener	Extracted from bean of carob tree (locust bean); numerous foods, for example, confections, syrups, cheese spreads, frozen desserts, and salad dressings; GRAS additive
Carrageenan	Emulsifier, stabilizer, and thickener	Extracted from seaweed; a variety of foods, primarily those with a water or milk base
Cellulose	Emulsifier, stabilizer, and thickener	Component of all plants; inert bulking agent in foods; may be used to reduce energy content of food; used in foods that are liquid and foam systems
Citric acid	Preservative, antioxidant, pH-control agent, sequestrant	Widely distributed in nature in both plants and animals; miscellaneous or general purpose food use; used in lard, shortening, sausage, margarine, chili con carne, cured meats, and freeze-dried meats; GRAS additive
Citrus Red No. 2	Color	Coloring skins of oranges
Cochineal	Color	Derived from the dried female insect and coccus cacti; raised in West Indies, Canary Islands, southern Spain, and Algiers; 70,000 insects to 1 lb; provides red color for meat products and beverages
Corn endosperm oil	Color	Source of xanthophyll for yellow color; used in chicken feed to color yolks of eggs and chicken skin
Cornstarch	Anticaking agent, drying agent, formulation aid, processing aid, surface-finishing agent	Digestible polysaccharide used in many foods, often in a modified form; these include baking powder, baby foods, soups, sauces, pie fillings, imitation jellies, custards, and candies

TABLE 1.8
(Continued)

Name	Function[a]	Food Use and Comments
Corn syrup	Flavoring agent, humectant, nutritive sweetener, preservative	Derived from hydrolysis of cornstarch; employed in numerous foods, for example, baby foods, bakery products, toppings, meat products, beverages, condiments, and confections; GRAS additive
Dextrose (glucose)	Flavoring agent, humectant, nutritive sweetener, synergist	Derived from cornstarch; major users of dextrose are confection, wine, and canning industries; used to flavor meat products; used in production of caramel; variety of other uses
Diglycerides	Emulsifiers	Uses include frozen desserts, lard, shortening, and margarine; GRAS additive
Dioctyl sodium sulfosuccinate	Emulsifier, processing aid, surface-active agent	Employed in gelatin dessert, dry beverages, fruit juice drinks, and noncarbonated beverages with cocoa fat; used in production of cane sugar and in canning
Disodium guanylate	Flavor enhancer	Derived from dried fish or seaweed
Disodium inosinate	Flavor adjuvant	Derived from seaweed or dried fish; sodium guanylate is a byproduct
Ethylenediamine-tetraacetic acid (EDTA)	Antioxidant, sequestrant	Calcium disodium and disodium salt of EDTA employed in a variety of foods including soft drinks, alcoholic beverages, dressings, canned vegetables, margarine, pickles, sandwich spreads, and sausage
FD&C colors: Blue No. 1 Red No. 40 Yellow No. 5	Color	Coloring foods in general, including dietary supplements
Gelatin	Stabilizer and thickener, texturizer	Derived from collagen by boiling skin, tendons, ligaments, bones, etc. with water; employed in many foods including confectionery, jellies, and ice cream; GRAS additive
Glycerine (glycerol)	Humectant	Miscellaneous and general purpose additive; GRAS additive
Grape skin extract	Color	Colorings for carbonated drinks, beverage bases, and alcoholic beverages
Guar gum	Stabilizer and thickener, texturizer	Extracted from seeds of the guar plant of India and Pakistan; employed in such foods as cheese, salad dressings, ice cream, and soups
Gum arabic	Stabilizer and thickener, texturizer	Gummy exudate of Acacia plants; used in variety of foods; GRAS additive
Gum ghatti	Stabilizer and thickener, texturizer	Gummy exudate of plant growing in India and Ceylon; a variety of food uses; GRAS additive
Hydrogen peroxide	Bleaching agent	Modification of starch and bleaching tripe; GRAS bleaching agent
Hydrolyzed vegetable (plant) protein	Flavor enhancer	Used to flavor various meat products
Invert sugar	Humectant, nutritive sweetener	Main use in confectionery and brewing industry
Iron	Nutrient	Dietary supplements and food; GRAS additive
Iron–Ammonium citrate	Anticaking agent	Used in salt
Karraya gum	Stabilizer and thickener	Derived from dried extract of *Sterculia urens* found primarily in India; variety of food uses; a substitute for tragacanth gum; GRAS additive
Lactic acid	Preservative, pH control	Normal product of human metabolism; numerous uses in foods and beverages; a miscellaneous general purpose additive; GRAS additive
Lecithin (phosphatidyl-choline)	Emulsifier, surface-active agent	Normal tissue component of the body; edible and digestible additive naturally occurring in eggs; commercially derived from soybeans; margarine, chocolate, and wide variety of other food uses; GRAS additive
Mannitol	Anticaking, nutritive sweetener, stabilizer and thickener, texturizer	Special dietary foods; GRAS additive; supplies half the energy of glucose; classified as a sugar alcohol or polyhydric alcohol (polyol)
Methylparaben	Preservative	Food and beverages; GRAS additive
Modified food starch	Drying agent, formulation aid, processing aid, surface-finishing agent	Digestible polysaccharide used in many foods and stages of food processing; examples include baking powder, puddings, pie fillings, baby foods, soups, sauces, candies, etc.
Monoglycerides	Emulsifiers	Widely used in foods such as frozen desserts, lard, shortening, and margarine; GRAS additive
Monosodium glutamate (MSG)	Flavor enhancer	Enhances the flavor of a variety of foods including various meat products; possible association with the Chinese restaurant syndrome
Papain	Texturizer	Miscellaneous or general purpose additive; GRAS additive; achieves results through enzymatic action; used as meat tenderizer

Continued

**TABLE 1.8
(Continued)**

Name	Function[a]	Food Use and Comments
Paprika	Color, flavoring agent	Provides coloring or flavor to foods; GRAS additive
Pectin	Stabilizer and thickener, texturizer	Richest source of pectin is lemon and orange rind; present in cell walls of all plant tissues; used to prepare jellies and jams; GRAS additive
Phosphoric acid	pH control	Miscellaneous or general purpose additive; used to increase effectiveness of antioxidants in lard and shortening; GRAS additive
Polyphosphates	Nutrient, flavor improver, sequestrant, pH control	Numerous food uses; most polyphosphates and their sodium, calcium, potassium, and ammonium salts; GRAS additive
Polysorbates	Emulsifiers, surface-active agent	Polysorbates designated by numbers such as 60, 65, and 80; variety of food uses including baking mixes, frozen custards, pickles, sherbets, ice creams, and shortenings
Potassium alginate	Stabilizer and thickener, texturizer	Extracted from seaweed; wide usage; GRAS additive
Potassium bromate	Flour treating agent	Employed in flour, whole wheat flour, fermented malt beverages, and to treat malt
Potassium iodide	Nutrient	Added to table salt or used in mineral preparations as a source of dietary iodine
Potassium nitrite	Curing and pickling agent	To fix color in cured products such as meats
Potassium sorbate	Preservative	Inhibits mold and yeast growth in foods such as wines, sausage casings, and margarine; GRAS additive
Propionic acid	Preservative	Mold inhibitor in breads and general fungicide; GRAS additive; used in manufacture of fruit flavors
Propyl gallate	Antioxidant, preservative	Used in products containing oil or fat; employed in chewing gum; used to retard rancidity in frozen fresh pork sausage
Propylene glycol	Emulsifier, humectant, stabilizer and thickener, texturizer	Miscellaneous or general purpose additive; uses include salad dressings, ice cream, ice milk, custards, and a variety of other foods; GRAS additive
Propylparaben	Preservative	Fungicide; controls mold in sausage casings; GRAS additive
Saccharin	Nonnutritive sweetener	Special dietary foods and a variety of beverages; baked products; tabletop sweeteners
Saffron	Color, flavoring agent	Derived from plant of western Asia and southern Europe; all foods except those where standards forbid; to color sausage casings, margarine, or product branding inks
Silicon dioxide	Anticaking agent	Used in feed or feed components, beer production, production of special dietary foods, and ink diluent for marking fruits and vegetables
Sodium acetate	pH control, preservative	Miscellaneous or general purpose use; meat preservation; GRAS additive
Sodium alginate	Stabilizer and thickener, texturizer	Extracted from seaweed; widespread food use; GRAS additive
Sodium aluminum sulfate	Leavening agent	Baking powders, confectionery; sugar refining
Sodium benzoate	Preservative	Variety of food products; margarine to retard flavor reversion; GRAS additive
Sodium bicarbonate	Leavening agent, pH control	Miscellaneous or general purpose uses; separation of fatty acids and glycerol in rendered fats; neutralize excess and clean vegetables in rendered fats, soups, and curing pickles; GRAS additive
Sodium chloride (salt)	Flavor enhancer, formulation acid, preservation	Used widely in many foods; GRAS additive
Sodium citrate	pH control, curing and pickling agent, sequestrant	Evaporated milk; miscellaneous or general purpose food use; accelerate color fixing in cured meats; GRAS additive
Sodium diacetate	Preservative, sequestrant	An inhibitor of molds and rope-forming bacteria in baked products; GRAS additive
Sodium nitrate (Chile saltpeter)	Curing and pickling agent, preservative	Used with or without sodium nitrite in smoked, cured-fish, and cured-meat products
Sodium nitrite	Curing and pickling agent, preservative	May be used with sodium nitrate in smoked- or cured-fish, cured-meat products, and pet foods
Sodium propionate	Preservative	A fungicide and mold preventative in bakery products; GRAS additive
Sorbic acid	Preservative	Fungistatic agent for foods, especially cheeses; other uses include baked goods, beverages, dried fruits, fish, jams, jellies, meats, pickled products, and wines; GRAS additive
Sorbitan monostearate	Emulsifier, stabilizer and thickener	Widespread food usage such as whipped toppings, cakes, cake mixes, confectionery, icings, and shortenings; also many nonfood uses
Sorbitol	Humectant, nutritive sweetener, stabilizer and thickener, sequestrant	A sugar alcohol or polyol; used in chewing gum, meat products, icings, dairy products, beverages, and pet foods
Sucrose	Nutritive sweetener, preservative	The most widely used additive; used in beverages, baked goods, candies, jams and jellies, and other processed foods
Tagetes (Aztec marigold)	Color	Source is flower petals of Aztec marigold; used to enhance yellow color of chicken skin and eggs, incorporated in chicken feed

TABLE 1.8
(Continued)

Name	Function[a]	Food Use and Comments
Tartaric acid	pH control	Occurs free in many fruits, free or combined with calcium, magnesium, or potassium; used in the soft drink industry, confectionery products, bakery products, and gelatin desserts
Titanium dioxide	Color	For coloring foods generally, except standardized foods; used for coloring ingested and applied drugs
Tocopherols (vitamin E)	Antioxidant, nutrient	To retard rancidity in foods containing fat; used in dietary supplements; GRAS additive
Tragacanth gum	Stabilizer and thickener, texturizer	Derived from the plant *Astragalus gummifier* or other Asiatic species of *Astragalus*; general purpose additive
Turmeric	Color	Derived from rhizome of *Curcuma longa*; used to color sausage casings, margarine or shortening, and ink for branding or marking products
Vanilla	Flavoring agent	Used in various bakery products, confectionery, and beverages; natural flavoring extracted from cured, full grown unripe fruit of *Vanilla panifolia*; GRAS additive
Vanillin	Flavoring agent and adjuvant	Widespread confectionery, beverage and food use; synthetic form of vanilla; GRAS additive
Yellow prussiate of soda	Anticaking agent	Employed in salt

[a] Function refers to those defined in Table 1.7.

Source: Ensminger, A.H. et al., *Food and Nutrition Encyclopedia*, 2nd ed., CRC Press, Boca Raton, FL, 1994, pp. 11–18.

TABLE 1.9
Microbial Contaminants of Fresh Food

Foods	Microorganism	Common Contaminants
Fruits and Vegetables	Bacteria	*Erwinia, Pseudomonas, Corynebacterium*
	Fungi	*Aspigillus, Botrytis, Geotrichium, Rhizopus, Penicillium, Cladosporium, Alternaria, Phytopora,* various yeasts
Fresh meat	Bacteria	*Acinetobacter, Aeromonas, Pseudomonas*
Fish Poultry	Bacteria	*Micrococcus, Achromobacter, Flavobacterium, Proteus, Salmonella, Escheria*
	Fungi	*Cladosporium, Mucor, Rhizopus, Penicillium, Geotrichium, Sporotrichium, Candida, Torula, Rhodotorula*
Milk	Bacteria	*Streptococcus, Leuconostoc, Lactococcus, Lactobacillus, Pseudomonas, Proteus*
High-sugar foods	Bacteria	*Clostridium, Bacillus, Flavobacterium*
	Fungi	*Saccharomyces, Torulla, Penicillium*

Source: Lynnes book.

of the duodenum, where mainly calcium and trace metals are absorbed. Phytates occur in a wide variety of foods, such as cereals (e.g., wheat, rye, maize, rice, and barley), legumes and vegetables (e.g., bean, soybean, lentil, pea, and vetch), nuts and seeds (e.g., walnut, hazelnut, almond, peanut, and cocoa bean), and spices and flavoring agents (e.g., caraway, coriander, cumin, mustard, and nutmeg). From several experiments in animals and humans it has been observed that phytates exert negative effects on the availability of calcium, iron, magnesium, zinc, and other trace essential elements. These effects may be minimized considerably, if not eliminated, by increased intake of essential minerals. In the case of calcium, intake of cholecalciferol must also be adequate, as the activity of phytates on calcium absorption is enhanced when this vitamin is inadequate or limiting. In many foodstuffs the phytic acid level can be reduced by phytase, an enzyme occurring in plants that catalyzes the dephosphorylation of phytic acid.

Oxalic acid is a strong acid that forms water-soluble Na^+ and K^+ salts, but is less soluble salts with alkaline earth and other bivalent metals. Calcium oxalate is particularly insoluble at neutral or alkaline pH, whereas it readily dissolves in acid medium. Oxalates mainly exert effects on the absorption of calcium. These effects must be considered in terms of the oxalate-to-calcium ratio (in milliequivalent/milliequivalent): foods having a ratio greater than 1 may have negative effects on calcium availability, whereas foods with a ratio of 1 or below do not. Examples of foodstuffs having a ratio greater than 1 are: rhubarb (8.5), spinach (4.3), beet (2.5 to 5.1), cocoa (2.6), coffee (3.9), tea (1.1), and potato (1.6). Harmful oxalates in food may be removed by soaking in water. Consumption of calcium-rich foods (e.g., dairy products and seafood), as well as augmented cholecalciferol intake, are recommended when large amounts of high-oxalate food are consumed.

TABLE 1.10
Mycotoxins or Bacterial Toxins in Foods

Toxins from bacteria	*Staphylococcus aureus*
	a exotoxin (lethal, dermonecrotic, hemolytic, leucolytic)
	b exotoxin (hemolytic)
	g exotoxin (hemolytic)
	d exotoxin (dermonecrotic, hemolytic)
	leucocidin (leucolytic)
	exfoliative toxin
	enterotoxin
	Clostridium botulinum (four strains)
	Toxins are lettered as A, B, Ca (1, 2, D), Cb, D(C1 and D), E, F, G. All of the toxics are proteolytic and produce NH_3, H_2S, CO_2, and volatile amines. The toxins are hemolytic and neurotoxic
	Escherichi coli (several serotypes)
	Induce diarrhea, vomiting; produce toxins that are heat labile
	Bacillus cereus (several types)
	Produces heat-labile enterotoxins that induce vomiting and diarrhea
Mycotoxins Produced by Fungi	*Aspergillus flavis*
	Claviceps purpura
	Fusarium graminearum
	Aspergillus ochraceus
	Aspergillus parasiticus
	Penicillium viridicatum

Source: Ensminger et al., *Food and Nutrition Encyclopedia*, 2nd ed., CRC Press, Boca Raton, FL, 1994.

TABLE 1.11
Antinutrients in Food

Type of Factors	Effect of Factors	Legumes Containing the Factors
Antivitamin factors	Interfere with the actions of certain vitamins	
Antivitamin A	Lipoxidase oxidizes and destroys carotene (provitamin A)	Soybeans
Antivitamin B_{12}	Increases requirement for Vitamin B_{12}	Soybeans
Antivitamin D	Causes rickets unless extra vitamin D is provided	Soybeans
Antivitamin E	Damage to the liver and muscles	Alfalfa, common beans (*Phaseolus vulgaris*), peas (*Pisum sativum*)
Cyanide-releasing glucosides	Releases hydrocyanic acid. The poison may also be released by an enzyme in *E. coli*, a normal inhabitant of the human intestine	All legumes contain at least small amounts of these factors; however, certain varieties of lima beans (*Phaseolus lunatus*) may contain much larger amounts
Favism factor	Causes the breakdown of red blood cells in susceptible individuals	Fava beans (*Vicia faba*)
Gas-generating carbohydrates	Certain indigestible carbohydrates are acted upon by gas-producing bacteria in the lower intestine	Many species of mature dry legume seeds, but not peanuts; the immature (green) seeds contain much lower amounts
Goitrogens	Interfere with the utilization of iodine by the thyroid gland	Peanuts and soybeans
Inhibitors of trypsin	The inhibitors bind with the digestive enzyme trypsin	All legumes contain trypsin inhibitors; these inhibitors are destroyed by heat
Lathyrogenic neurotoxins	Consumption of large quantities of lathyrogenic legumes for long periods (several months) results in severe neurological disorders	Lathyrus pea (*L. sativus*), which is grown mainly in India Common vetch (*Vicia sativa*) may also be lathyrogenic
Metal binders	Bind copper, iron, manganese, and zinc	Soybeans, Peas (*Pisum sativum*)
Red blood cell clumping agents (hemaglutinins)	The agents cause the red blood cells to clump together	Occurs in all legumes to some extent

Source: Ensminger et al., *Food and Nutrition Encyclopedia*, 2nd ed., CRC Press, Boca Raton, FL, 1994.

A variety of plants contain a third group of type B antinutritives, the glucosinolates, also known as thioglucosides. Many glucosinolates are goitrogenic. They have a general structure, and yield on hydrolysis the active or actual goitrogens, such as thiocyanates, isothiocyanates, cyclic sulfur compounds, and nitriles. Three types of goiter can be identified: (1) cabbage goiter, (2) brassica seed goiter, and (3) legume goiter. Cabbage goiter, also known as struma, is induced by excessive consumption of cabbage. It seems that cabbage goitrogens inhibit iodine uptake by directly affecting the thyroid gland. Cabbage goiter can be treated by iodine supplementation. Brassica seed goiter can result from the consumption of the seeds of brassica plants (e.g., rutabaga, turnip, cabbage, and rape), which contain goitrogens that prevent thyroxine synthesis. This type of goiter can only be treated by administration of the thyroid hormone. Legume goiter is induced by goitrogens in legumes such as soybeans and peanuts. It differs from cabbage goiter in that the thyroid gland does not lose its activity for iodine. Inhibition of the intestinal absorption of iodine or the reabsorption of thyroxine has been shown in this case. Legume goiter can be treated by iodine therapy. Glucosinolates, which have been shown to induce goiter, at least in experimental animals, are found in several foods and feedstuffs: broccoli (buds), brussels sprouts (head), cabbage (head), cauliflower (buds), garden cress (leaves), horseradish (roots), kale (leaves), kohlrabi (head), black and white mustard (seed), radish (root), rape (seed), rutabaga (root), and turnips (root and seed). One of the most potent glucosinolates is progoitrin from the seeds of brassica plants and the roots of rutabaga. Hydrolysis of this compound yields 1-cyano-2-hydroxy-3-butene, 1-cyano-2-hydroxy-3, 4-butylepisulfide, 2-hydroxy-3, 4-butenylisothiocyanate, and (S)-5-vinyl-oxazolidone-2-thione, also known as goitrin. The latter product interferes, together with its R-enantiomer, in the iodination of thyroxine precursors, and so the resulting goiter cannot be treated by iodine therapy.

Type C antinutritives are naturally occurring substances that can inactivate vitamins, form unabsorbable complexes with them, or interfere with their digestive or metabolic utilization. They are also known as antivitamins. The most important type C antinutritives are ascorbic acid oxidase, antithiamine factors, and antipyridoxine factors.

Ascorbic acid oxidase is a copper-containing enzyme that catalyzes the oxidation of free ascorbic acid to diketogluconic acid, oxalic acid, and other oxidation products. It has been reported to occur in many fruits (e.g., peaches and bananas) and vegetables (e.g., cucumbers, pumpkins, lettuce, cress, cauliflowers, spinach, green beans, green peas, carrots, potatoes, tomatoes, beets, and kohlrabi). The enzyme is active between pH 4 and 7 (optimum pH 5.6 to 6.0); its optimum temperature is 38°C. The enzyme is released when plant cells are broken. Therefore, if fruits and vegetables are cut, the vitamin C content decreases gradually. Ascorbic acid oxidase can be inhibited effectively at pH 2 or by blanching at around 100°C. Ascorbic acid can also be protected against ascorbic acid oxidase by substances of plant origin. Flavonoids, such as the flavonols quercetin and kempferol, present in fruits and vegetables, strongly inhibit the enzyme.

A second group of type C antinutritives are the antithiamine factors, which interact with thiamine, also known as vitamin B_1. Antithiamine factors can be grouped as thiaminases, catechols, and tannins. Thiaminases, which are enzymes that split thiamine at the methylene linkage, are found in many freshwater and saltwater fish species and in certain species of crab and clam. They contain a nonprotein coenzyme structurally related to hemin. This coenzyme is the actual antithiamine factor. Thiaminases in fish and other sources can be destroyed by cooking. Antithiamine factors of plant origin include catechols and tannins. The most well-known ortho-catechol is found in bracken fern. In fact, there are two types of heat-stable antithiamine factors in this fern, one of which has been identified as caffeic acid, which can also be hydrolyzed from chlorogenic acid (found in green coffee beans) by intestinal bacteria. Other ortho-catechols, such as methylsinapate occurring in mustard seed and rapeseed, also have antithiamine activity. The mechanism of thiamine inactivation by these compounds requires oxygen and is dependent on temperature and pH. The reaction appears to proceed in two phases: a rapid initial phase, which is reversible by addition of reducing agents (e.g., ascorbic acid), and a slower subsequent phase, which is irreversible. Tannins, occurring in a variety of plants, including tea, similarly possess antithiamine activity. Thiamine is one of the vitamins likely to be deficient in the diet. Thus, persistent consumption of antithiamine factors and the possible presence of thiaminase-producing bacteria in the gastrointestinal tract may compromise the already marginal thiamine intake.

A variety of plants and mushrooms contain pyridoxine antagonists. These compounds interfere with the use of vitamin B_6 and are called antipyridoxine factors. They are hydrazine derivatives. Linseed contains the water-soluble and heat-labile antipyridoxine factor linatine (g-glutamyl-1-amino-D-proline). Hydrolysis of linatine yields the actual antipyridoxine factor 1-amino-proline. Antipyridoxine factors have also been found in wild mushrooms, the common commercial edible mushroom, and the Japanese mushroom shiitake. Commercial and shiitake mushrooms contain agaritine. Hydrolysis of agaritine by g-glutamyl transferase, which is endogenous to the mushroom, yields the active agent 4-hydroxymethylphenylhydrazine. Disruption of the cells of the mushroom can accelerate hydrolysis; careful handling of the mushrooms and immediate blanching after cleaning and cutting can prevent hydrolysis. The mechanism underlying the antipyridoxine activity is believed to be condensation of the hydrazines with the carbonyl compounds pyridoxal and pyridoxal phosphate (the active form of the vitamin), resulting in the formation of inactive hydrazones.

In addition to these antinutritives, foods can contain a variety of toxic substances as shown in Table 1.12 (see Reference 4, pp. 24–36, 1284–1285, 1776–1785, 1790–1803, 2082–2087). Some of these toxic substances are added inadvertently by the food processing methods, but some occur naturally. If consumed in minute quantities, some of these toxic materials are without significant effect, yet other compounds (e.g., arsenic), even in minute amounts, could accumulate and become lethal.

Table 1.13 contains information about plants commonly thought of as weeds.[6] Some of these plants may have toxic components that affect certain consumers. There can be considerable variability among humans with respect to plants that can be tolerated by them. Plants can differ from variety to variety and indeed from one growing condition to another in the content of certain of their herbal or nutritive ingredients. Lastly, Table 1.14 provides a list of toxic plants that should not be consumed under any circumstances (see Reference 4, pp. 24–36, 1284–1285, 1776–1785, 1790–1803, 2082–2087).

TABLE 1.12
Toxic Substances in Food (Toxic if Consumed in Excess)

Poison (Toxin)	Sources	Symptoms and Signs	Distribution	Magnitude	Prevention	Treatment	Remark
Aflatoxins (see Table 1.10)							
Aluminum (Al)	Food additives, mainly presented in such items as baking powder, pickles, and processed cheeses Aluminum-containing antacids	Abnormally large intakes of aluminum irritate the digestive tract. Also, unusual conditions have sometimes resulted in the absorption of sufficient aluminum from antacids, causing brain damage. Aluminum may form nonabsorbable complexes with essential trace elements, thereby creating deficiencies of these elements	Aluminum is widely used throughout the world	The United States uses aluminum more than any other minerals except iron. However, known cases of aluminum toxicity are rare	Based on the evidence presented, no preventative measures are recommended		Aluminum toxicity has been reported in patients receiving renal dialysis
Arsenic (As)	Consumption of contaminated foods and beverages Arsenical insecticides used in vineyards expose the workers (1) when spraying or (2) by inhaling contaminated dusts and plant debris Arsenic in the air is from three major sources: smelting of metals, burning of coal, and use of arsenical pesticides	Burning pain in the throat or stomach, cardiac abnormalities, and the odor of garlic on the breath. Other symptoms may be diarrhea and extreme thirst along with a choking sensation Small doses of arsenic taken into the body over a long period of time may produce hyperkeratosis (irregularities in pigmentation, especially on the trunk); arterial insufficiency; and cancer There is strong evidence that inorganic arsenic is a skin and lung carcinogen in humans	Arsenic is widely distributed, but the amount of the element consumed by humans in food and water, or breathed, is very small and not harmful	Cases of arsenic toxicity in humans are infrequent. Two noteworthy episodes occurred in Japan in 1955. One involved tainted powdered milk; the other contaminated soy sauce. The toxic milk caused 12,131 cases of infant poisoning, with 130 deaths. The soy sauce poisoned 20 people		Induce vomiting, followed by an antidote of egg whites in water or milk. Afterward, give strong coffee or tea, followed by Epsom salts in water or castor oil	Arsenic is known to partially protect against selenium poisoning The highest residues of arsenic are generally in the hair and nails Arsenic in soils may sharply decrease crop growth and yields, but it is not a hazard to people or livestock that eat plants grown in these fields
Chromium (Cr)	Food, water, and air contaminated by chromium compounds in industrialized areas	Inorganic chromium salt reduces the absorption of zinc; hence, zinc deficiency symptoms may become evident in chronic chromium toxicity	Chromium toxicity is not common	Chromium toxicity is not very common	It is unlikely that people will get too much chromium, because (1) only minute amounts of the element are present in most foods, (2) the body utilizes chromium poorly, and (3) the toxic dose is about 10,000 times the lowest effective medical dose		

Copper (Cu)	Diets with excess copper, but low in other minerals that counteract its effects Acid foods or beverages (vinegar, carbonated beverages, or citrus juices) that have been in prolonged contact with copper metal may cause acute gastrointestinal disturbances	Acute copper toxicity: Characterized by headache, dizziness, metallic taste, excessive salivation, nausea, vomiting, stomachache, diarrhea, and weakness. If the disease is allowed to get worse, there may also be racing of the heart, high blood pressure, jaundice, hemolytic anemia, dark-pigmented urine, kidney disorders, and even death Chronic copper toxicity may be contributory to iron-deficiency anemia, mental illness following childbirth (postpartum psychosis), certain types of schizophrenia, and perhaps heart attacks	Copper toxicity may occur wherever there is excess copper intake, especially when accompanied by low iron, molybdenum, sulfur, zinc, and vitamin C	The incidence of copper toxicity is extremely rare in humans. Its occurrence in significant form is almost always limited to (1) suicide attempts by ingestion of large quantities of copper salt, or (2) a genetic defect in copper metabolism inherited as an autosomal recessive, known as Wilson's disease	Avoid foods and beverages that have been in prolonged contact with copper metal	Administration of copper-chelating agents to remove excess copper	Copper is essential to human life and health, but as with all heavy metals, it may be toxic in excess
Ergot	Rye, wheat, barley, oats, and triticale carry this mycotoxin Ergot replaces the seed in the heads of cereal grains, in which it appears as a purplish-black, hard, banana-shaped, dense mass from 1/4 to 3/4 in. (6 to 9 mm) long	When a large amount of ergot is consumed in a short period, convulsive ergotism is observed. The symptoms include itching, numbness, severe muscle cramps, sustained spasms and convulsions, and extreme pain When smaller amounts of ergot are consumed over an extended period, ergotism is characterized by gangrene of the fingertips and toes, caused by blood vessel and muscle contraction stopping blood circulation in the extremities. These symptoms include cramps, swelling, inflammation, alternating burning and freezing sensations ("St. Anthony's fire") and numbness; eventually the hands and feet may turn black, shrink, and fall off Ergotism is a cumulative poison, depending on the amount of ergot eaten and the length of time over which it is eaten	Ergot is found throughout the world wherever rye, wheat, barley, oats, or triticale are grown	There is considerable ergot, especially in rye. But, normally, screening grains before processing alleviates ergotism in people	Consists of an ergot-free diet. Ergot in food and feed grains may be removed by screening the grains before processing. In the United States, wheat and rye containing more than 0.3% ergot are classed as "ergoty." In Canada, government regulations prohibit more than 0.1% ergot in feeds	An ergot-free diet; good nursing; treatment by a doctor	Six different alkaloids are involved in ergot poisoning Ergot is used to aid the uterus to contract after childbirth, to prevent loss of blood. Also, another ergot drug (ergotamine) is widely used in the treatment of migraine headaches

Continued

TABLE 1.12
(Continued)

Poison (Toxin)	Sources	Symptoms and Signs	Distribution	Magnitude	Prevention	Treatment	Remark
Fluorine (F) (fluorosis)	Ingestion of excessive quantities of fluorine through either the food or water, or a combination of these	Acute fluoride poisoning: Abdominal pain, diarrhea, vomiting, excessive salivation, thirst, perspiration, and painful spasms of the limbs	The water in parts of Arkansas, California, South Carolina, and Texas contains excess fluorine. Occasionally, throughout the United States, high-fluorine phosphates are used in mineral mixtures	Generally speaking, fluorosis is limited to high-fluorine areas Only a few instances of health effects in humans have been attributed to airborne fluoride, and they occurred in persons living in the vicinity of fluoride-emitting industries	Avoid the use of food and water containing excessive fluorine	Any damage may be permanent, but people who have not developed severe symptoms may be helped to some extent if the source of excess fluorine is eliminated High dietary levels of calcium and magnesium may reduce the absorption and utilization of fluoride	Fluorine is a cumulative poison The total fluoride in the human body averages 2.57 g Susceptibility to fluoride toxicity is increased by deficiencies of calcium, vitamin C, and protein Virtually all foods contain trace amounts of fluoride
	Except in certain industrial exposures, the intake of fluoride inhaled from the air is only a small fraction of the total fluoride intake in humans	Chronic fluoride poisoning: Abnormal teeth (especially mottled enamel) during the first 8 years of life and brittle bones. Other effects, predicted from animal studies, may include loss of body weight and altered structure and function of the thyroid gland and kidneys					
	Pesticides containing fluorides, including those used to control insects, weeds, and rodents	Water containing 3 to 10 ppm of fluoride may cause mottling of the teeth					
	Although water is the principal source of fluoride in an average human diet in the United States, fluoride is frequently contained in toothpaste, tooth powder, chewing gums, mouthwashes, vitamin supplements, and mineral supplements	An average daily intake of 20 to 80 mg of fluoride over a period of 10 to 20 years will result in crippling fluorosis					
Lead (Pb)	Consuming food or medicinal products (including health food products) contaminated with lead	Develop rapidly in young children, but slowly in mature people Acute lead poisoning: Colic, cramps, diarrhea or constipation, leg cramps, and drowsiness	Predominantly among children who may eat chips of lead-containing paints, peeled off from painted wood	The Centers for Disease Control, Atlanta, GA, estimates that (1) lead poisoning claims the lives of 200 children each year, and (2) 400,000 to 600,000 children have elevated lead levels in the blood Lead poisoning has been reduced significantly with the use of lead-free paint	Avoid inhaling or consuming lead	Acute lead poisoning: An emetic (induce vomiting), followed by drinking plenty of milk and ½ oz (14 g) of Epsom salts in half glass of water	Lead is a cumulative poison When incorporated in the soil, nearly all the lead is converted into forms that are not available to plants. Any lead taken up by plant roots tends to stay in the roots, rather than move up to the top of the plant
	Inhaling the poison as a dust by workers in such industries as painting, lead mining, and refining Inhaling airborne lead discharged into the air from auto exhaust fumes	The most severe form of lead poisoning, encountered in infants and in heavy drinkers of illicitly distilled whiskey is characterized by profound disturbances of the central nervous system and permanent damage to the brain; damage to the kidneys and shortened life span of the erthrocytes					

	Consuming food crops contaminated by lead being deposited on the leaves and other edible portions of the plant by direct fallout. Consuming food or water contaminated by contact with lead pipes or utensils. Old houses in which the interiors were painted with leaded paints prior to 1945 — the chipped wall paint is sometimes eaten by children. Such miscellaneous sources as illicitly distilled whiskey, improperly lead-glazed earthenware, old battery casings used as fuel, and toys containing lead	Chronic lead poisoning: Colic, constipation, lead palsy especially in the forearm and fingers, the symptoms of chronic nephritis, and sometimes mental depression, convulsions, and a blue line at the edge of the gums			Chronic lead poisoning: Remove the source of lead. Sometimes treated by administration of magnesium or lead sulfate solution as a laxative and antidote on the lead in the digestive system, followed by potassium iodide, which cleanses the tracts. Currently, treatment of lead poisoning makes use of chemicals that bind the metal in the body and help in its removal	Lead poisoning can be diagnosed positively by analyzing the blood tissue for lead content; clinical signs of lead poisoning usually are manifested at blood lead concentrations above 80 mg/100 g
Mercury (Hg)	Mercury is discharged into air and water from industrial operations and is used in herbicide and fungicide treatments. Mercury poisoning has occurred where mercury from industrial plants has been discharged into water, then accumulated as methylmercury in fish and shellfish. Accidental consumption of seed grains treated with fungicides that contain mercury, used for the control of fungus diseases of oats, wheat, barley, and flax	The toxic effects of organic and inorganic compounds of mercury are dissimilar. The organic compounds of mercury, such as the various fungicides (1) affect the central nervous system and (2) are not corrosive. The inorganic compounds of mercury include mainly mercuric chloride, a disinfectant; mercurous chloride (calomel), a cathartic; and elemental mercury. Commonly the toxic symptoms are corrosive gastrointestinal effects, such as vomiting, bloody diarrhea, and necrosis of the alimentary mucosa	Wherever mercury is produced in industrial operations or used in herbicide or fungicide treatments.	Limited. But about 1200 cases of mercury poisoning identified in Japan in the 1950s were traced to the consumption of fish and shellfish from Japan's Minamata Bay contaminated with methylmercury. Some of the offspring of exposed mothers were born with birth defects, and many victims suffered central nervous system damage. Another outbreak of mercury toxicity occurred in Iraq, where more than 6000 people were hospitalized after eating bread made from wheat that had been treated with methylmercury	Control mercury pollution from industrial operations	Mercury is a cumulative poison. Food and Drug Administration prohibits use of mercury-treated grain for food or feed. Grain crops produced from mercury-treated seed and crops produced on soils treated with mercury herbicides have not been found to contain harmful concentrations of this element

Continued

**TABLE 1.12
(Continued)**

Poison (Toxin)	Sources	Symptoms and Signs	Distribution	Magnitude	Prevention	Treatment	Remark
Poly-chlorinated biphenyls (PCBs), industrial chemicals; chlorinated hydrocarbons, which may cause cancer when taken into the food supply	Sources of contamination to humans include: 1. Contaminated foods 2. Mammals or birds that have fed on contaminated foods of fish 3. Residues on foods that have been wrapped in papers and plastics containing PCBs 4. Milk from cows that have been fed silage from silos coated with PCB-containing paint; and eggs from layers fed feeds contaminated with PCBs	Clinical effects on people are: An eruption of the skin resembling acne, visual disturbances, jaundice, numbness, and spasms. Newborn infants from mothers who have been poisoned show discoloration of the skin, which regresses after 2 to 5 months. PCBs are fat soluble	PCBs are widespread Their use by industry is declining				PCBs have been widely used in dielectric fluids in capacitors and transformers, hydraulic fluids, and heat-transfer fluids. Also, they have more than 50 minor uses including plasticizers and solvents in adhesives, printing ink, sealants, moisture retardants, paints, and pesticide carriers PCB causes cancer in laboratory animals (rats, mice, and rhesus monkeys). It is not known if it will cause cancer in humans. More study is needed to gauge its effects on the ecological food chain and on human health. When fed Coho salmon from Lake Michigan with 10 to 15 ppm PCB, mink in Wisconsin stopped reproducing or their kits died
Salt (NaCl/ sodium chloride) poisoning	Consumption of high-salt food and beverages	Salt may be toxic (1) when it is fed to infants or others whose kidneys cannot excrete the excess in the urine or (2) when the body is adapted to a chronic low-salt diet	Salt is used all over the world. Hence, the potential for salt poisoning exists everywhere	Salt poisoning is relatively rare	Drink large quantities of fresh water		Even normal salt concentration may be toxic if water intake is low

Selenium (Se)	Consumption of high levels in food or drinking water Presence of malnutrition, parasitic infestation, or other factors, which make people highly susceptible to selenium toxicity	Abnormalities in the hair, nails, and skin Children in a high-selenium area of Venezuela showed loss of hair, discolored skin, and chronic digestive disturbances Normally, people who have consumed large excesses of selenium excrete it as trimethyl selenide in the urine or as dimethyl selenide in the breath. The latter substance has an odor resembling garlic	In certain regions of western United States, especially in South Dakota, Montana, Wyoming, Nebraska, Kansas, and perhaps areas in other states in the Great Plains and Rocky Mountains Also, in Canada	Selenium toxicity in people is relatively rare	Selenium toxicity may be counteracted by arsenic or copper, but such treatment should be carefully monitored	Confirmed cases of selenium poisoning in people are rare, because (1) only traces are present in most foods, (2) foods generally come from a wide area, and (3) the metabolic processes normally convert excess selenium into harmless substances that are excreted in the urine or breath
Tin (Sn)	From acid fruits and vegetables canned in tin cans. The acids in such foods as citrus fruits and tomato products can leach tin from the inside of the can. Then the tin is ingested with the canned food. In the digestive tract tin goes through a methylation process in which nontoxic tin is converted to methylated tin, which is toxic	Methylated tin is a neurotoxin — a toxin that attacks the central nervous system, the symptoms of which are numbness of the fingers and lips followed by a loss of speech and hearing. Eventually, the afflicted person becomes spastic, then coma and death follow	Worldwide	The use of tin in advanced industrial societies has increased 14-fold over the last 10 years	Tin cans are rare. Many tin cans are coated on the inside with enamel or other materials. Most cans are steel	Currently, not much is known about the amount of tin in the human diet

Source: Ensminger et al., *Food and Nutrition Encyclopedia*, 2nd ed., CRC Press, Boca Raton, FL, 1994.

TABLE 1.13
Edible Weeds

Common Name	Scientific Name	Use
Maple tree	Acer (many varieties)	Sap can be collected and reduced by evaporation into syrup
Sweetflag	Acorus calamus	Rootstocks or stems are edible with a sweet taste. Young shoots can be used as salad
Quackgrass	Agropyron repens L. (has many other names)	Rootstocks can be chewed or scorched to use as coffee substitute; seeds can be used for breadstuffs and for beer
Waterplantain	Alisma spp.	Root is starchy and edible; should be dried to reduce acrid taste. Three varieties of this plant can be toxic.
Garlic mustard	Alliaria petiolata	Leaf, stem, flower, and fruit are spicy and hot. If cooked, some of this spiciness is lost. Several plants that resemble this one are not edible
Wild garlic	Allium vineale L.	Used as an herbal seasoning; there are similar plants that are not garlic in aroma; they can be toxic
Pigweed	Amaranthus spp.	Leaves from a young plant can be eaten raw as salad or boiled as is spinach
Serviceberry	Amelanchier spp.	Berries are rich and sweet; pits and leaves contain cyanide; also called shadbush or juneberry
Hog peanut	Amphicarpaea bracteata	Fleshy seedpods found underground are edible
Ground nut	Apios americana Medik	Root can be eaten raw or cooked. Seeds can also be used. Europeans use the term ground nut to refer to peanuts. This is not the same plant
Common burdock	Arctium minus	Young leaves can be eaten as salad; roots are carrot-like in shape and can be cooked (boiled) and eaten. A little baking soda added to the cooking water improves tenderness and flavor. Scorched roots can be used as a coffee substitute
Giant reed	Arundo donax L.	Young shoots and rootstalks are sometimes sweet enough to be used as a substitute for sugar cane. Infusions of the root stocks can have some herbal properties — local weak anesthetic and in some instances either a hypotensive agent or hypertensive agent (depends on dose)
Milkweed	Asclepias syriaca L.	Young shoots, flower buds boiled with at least two changes of water. The plant contains cardiac glycosides and can be toxic
Pawpaw	Asimina triloba L.	The aromatic fruits are quite tasty. Seeds and bark have pesticide properties and should be handled with caution
Wild oat	Avena fatua L.	Seeds are similar to cultivated oats. Useful when dried and ground as a cereal. Seeds can be scorched and used as a coffee substitute
Wintercress/Yellow rocket	Barbarea spp. (B. vema; B. vulgaris)	Young leaves and stems can be used as a salad
Birches	Betula spp. (Betulacea)	Spring sap can be reduced to a syrup; bark can be boiled for tea
Mustard, black or yellow	Brassica nigra	Seeds used to prepare mustard; leaves can be boiled for consumption, as can young stalks
Bromegrass	Bromus japonicus	Seeds can be dried, ground, and used as cereal
Shepherd's purse	Capsella bursa-pastoris	Seeds are used as a spicy pot herb. Tender young shoots can be eaten raw. Has a peppery taste
Bittercress	Cardamme bulbosa	Roots can be ground for a horseradish substitute; leaves and stems can be added to salad. The roots of some species (C. bulbosa) can be toxic
Hornbeam	Carpus caroliniana	Nuts are edible
Hickory	Carya spp.	Nuts are edible
Chestnut	Castanea spp.	Nuts are edible but are covered by a prickly coat. Roasting improves flavor and texture
Sandbur	Cenchrus spp.	Seeds and burrs can be used as cereal grains
Lambsquarter	Chenopodium album L.	Leaves can be eaten raw or cooked as spinach. The Mexican version (Mexicantea, C. ambrosioides) is toxic
Oxeye daisy	Chrysanthemum leucanthemum	Leaves and flowers can be eaten raw or cooked
Chicory	Cichorium intybus L.	Leaves are good salad ingredients
Thistles	Cirsium spp.	The taproot is chewy but tasty
Wandering Jew	Commelina communis	Leaves can be used as potherbs; flowering shoots can be eaten raw
Hawthorn	Crataegus spp.	Berries are edible; thorns can be a problem when gathering the berries. Some species contain heart stimulants
Wild chervil	Cryototaenia canadensis	Roots can be boiled, with a taste like parsnips; young leaves and stems can be eaten as salad; has an herb use in stews and soups
Nutgrass	Cyperus spp.	Tubers can be eaten or ground up to make a beverage called "chufa" or "horchata"

Common name	Scientific name	Description
Queen Anne's lace, also called wild carrot	Daucus carota L.	Root can be eaten after boiling; however, because it looks like poisonous hemlock, one should be cautious
Crabgrass	Digitaria snaguinalis L.	Seeds can be dried and ground for use as a cereal
Persimmon	Diospyros virginiana L.	Fruits when ripe are very sweet
Barnyard grass	Echinochloa crus-galli L.	Seeds can be dried and used as cereal
Russian olive	Elaegnus angustifolia L.	Fruits are edible though astringent
American burnweed	Erechtites hieracifolia	Leaves can be eaten raw as salad or cooked
Redstem filaree	Erodium cicutarium	Tender leaves are eaten as salad; can also be used as potherb
Wild strawberry	Fragaria virginiana	Fruits are small but delicious
Catchweed bedstraw	Galium aparine	Young shoots are good potherbs; leaves and stems can be steamed and eaten as vegetable
Wintergreen	Gaultheria procumbens L.	Berries, foliage, and bark can be used to make tea. Berries can be eaten raw
Huckleberry	Gaylussacia baccata	Berries can be eaten raw or cooked
Honey locust	Gleditsia triacanthos	The pulp around the seeds can be used as a sweetener. (Tender green pods can also be cooked and eaten as a vegetable.) The tree is similar in appearance to the Kentucky coffee tree, and the pods of this tree cannot be eaten
Jerusalem artichoke	Helianthus tuberosus	The tubers are crisp and can be used in place of chinese chestnuts in salads; can also be cooked and mashed
Daylily	Hemerocallis fulva L.	Flower buds can be used in salads. Tubers can be cooked and eaten. Can cause diarrhea in sensitive people
Foxtail barley	Hordeum jubatum	Seeds can be dried and used as cereal
Touch-me-not	Impatients spp.	Leaves can be used for an herbal tea; leaves can be eaten as salad; pods are also edible
Burning bush	Kochia scoparia	Young shoots can be used as a potherb; seeds can be dried and used as cereal
Prickly lettuce	Lactuca scariola L.	Young leaves can be used as salad, but may have a bitter taste
Virginia peppergrass	Lepidium virginicum	Has a pungent mustard-like taste; used as a potherb
Bugleweed	Lycorise spp.	Roots can be eaten raw or cooked
Common mallow	Malva neglecta	Boiled leaves have a slimy consistency much like okra. Flower buds can be pickled; leaves can be used as a thickener for soup
Black medic	Medicago lupulina	Sprouts can be added to salads for texture; leaves can be used as a potherb
Mulberry	Mortis spp.	Berries can be eaten out of hand
Watercress	Nasturtium officinale R.	Leaves can be eaten raw or used as a potherb
American lotus	Nelumbo lutea	Entire plant is edible
Yellow water lily	Nuphar luteum L.	Tubers when cooked are a starch substitute
Fragrant water lily	Nymphaea odorata	Flower buds and young leaves can be boiled and eaten; seeds can be dried and used as cereal
Evening primrose	Oenothera biennis L.	Seeds are a source of g linolenic acid; tap roots can be eaten raw or cooked
Wood sorrel	Oxalis spp.	Leaves can be eaten cooked or raw; seed pods can also be eaten
Perilla mint	Perilla frutescens L.	Leaves can be eaten cooked or raw
Common reed	Phragmites communis	Young shoots are edible. Plant is similar to the poisonous Arundo, so the forager should be very careful to correctly identify the plant
Ground cherry (Chinese lanterns)	Physalis heterophylla	Berries can be eaten cooked or raw
Pokeweed	Phytolacca americana L.	Young shoots can be used as a potherb; berries and roots may be poisonous
Plantain	Plantago major L.	Leaves can be used in salads
Mayapple	Podophyllum peltatum	Fruits are edible raw or cooked; rest of the plant may be poisonous
Japanese knotweed	Polygonum cuspidatum	Young sprouts can be cooked and eaten like asparagus
Purslane	Portulaca oleracea L.	Young leaves can be used as a potherb or salad ingredient
Healall	Prunella vulgaris L.	Boiled and used as a potherb
Wild cherry	Prunus serotina	Fruits are edible

Continued

TABLE 1.13
(Continued)

Common Name	Scientific Name	Use
Kudzu	*Pueraria lobata*	Roots and leaves are edible
Rock chestnut oak	*Quercus prinus* L.	Nuts (acorns) are edible
Sumac	*Rhus glabra* L.	Berries are edible as are the roots; however, some people are allergic to all parts of the plant and will develop skin rash
Multiflora rose	*Rosa multiflora*	The hips are edible in small quantities
Raspberry, blackberry	*Rubus* spp.	Fruits are eaten raw or used to make juice or jam
Red sorrel	*Rumex acetosella* L.	Leaves can be eaten as salad or cooked in water. The leaves contain a lot of oxalic acid, so small quantities would be preferred
Arrowhead	*Sagittaria latifolia* Willd	Roots can be eaten raw or cooked. Plants resemble the poisonous Jack-in-the-pulpit plant, so gatherers should beware
Elderberry	*Sambucus canadensis*	Fruits can be eaten raw or cooked
Hardstem bulrush	*Scrpus acutus* Muhl	Roots can be boiled and eaten
Foxtail grass	*Setaria* spp.	Seed grains can be dried and used as cereal
Tumble mustard	*Sisymbrium altissimum* L.	All parts of the plant are edible but have a strong mustard flavor; better used as a potherb
Roundleaf cabriar	*Smilax rotundiflora* L.	Young tender shoots can be eaten raw. Young leaves can be eaten as salad; roots can be used for tea
Sowthistle	*Sonchus oleraceus* L.	Leaves are prickly and bitter but can be used as a potherb
Johnson grass	*Sorghum halepense* L.	Young shoots can be eaten raw; seeds can be dried and used as cereal; mature stalks can be ground and the liquid extracted for use as syrup
Chickweed	*Stellaria media* L.	Leaves can be eaten raw or cooked
Dandelion	*Taraxacum officinale*	All parts of the plant are edible
Stinkweed	*Thlaspi arvense* L.	All parts of the plant are edible after cooking
Western salsify	*Tragopogon dubius* Scopoli	Roots can be eaten after boiling; leaves, flowers, and stems can be eaten raw
Red clover	*Trifolium pratense* L.	Flowers can be boiled to make a broth; powdered leaves and flowers can be used as seasoning
Coltsfoot	*Tussilago farfara* L.	Can be used as a potherb in small amounts
Cattail	*Typha* spp.	Roots, stalks, and spears are edible
Stinging nettle	*Urtica dioica* L.	Can be eaten cooked or used as a potherb
Bellwort	*Uvularia perfoliata* L.	Young shoots can be cooked and eaten; leaves are bitter
Blueberry, gooseberry	*Vaccinium stamineun*	Berries can be eaten raw or used to make juice, jam, or jelly
Violet	*Viola papilionacea* Purish	Flowers are edible
Wild grapes	*Vitis* spp.	Fruits can be eaten raw or cooked
Spanish bayonnet	*Yucca filimentosa* L.	Flower buds can be eaten raw

Notes

1. Persons using this list should be aware that individuals may differ in their responses to these plants. For some consumers, allergic reactions may be elicited. For others, there may be chemicals in the plants that elicit an undesirable physiological effect. Still other plants, especially the water plants, may harbor parasites that may be injurious. The serious forager should consult a plant taxonomist to be sure that the plant gathered is an edible plant. There are many similar plants that may in fact be poisonous, while others are safe to consume.

2. Weeds are plants that grow in places where we humans do not want them to grow. As such, we may not recognize them as food. The aforementioned plants contain edible portions. Not all parts of these plants may be useful as human food. Some varieties, in fact, may contain toxic chemicals that, if consumed in large quantities, may cause problems. A number of the plants have been identified based on their use by Native Americans. These plants can have many different names as common names.

Source: Duke, J.A., *Handbook of Edible Weeds*, CRC Press, Boca Raton, FL, 1992.

TABLE 1.14
Toxic Plants

Common and Scientific Name	Description	Toxic Parts	Geographical Distribution	Poisoning	Symptoms	Remarks
Baneberry and *Actaea* sp.	Perennial growing to 3 ft (1 m) tall from a thick root; compound leaves; small, white flowers; white or red berries with several seeds borne in short, terminal clusters	All parts, but primarily roots and berries	Native woodlands of North America from Canada south to Georgia, Alabama, Louisiana, Oklahoma, and the northern Rockies; red-fruited western baneberry from Alaska to central California, Arizona, Montana, and South Dakota	Attributed to a glycoside or essential oil, which causes severe inflammation of the digestive tract	Acute stomach cramps, headache, increased pulse, vomiting, delirium, dizziness, and circulatory failure	As few as six berries can cause symptoms persisting for hours. Treatment may be a gastric lavage or vomiting Bright red berries attract children
Buckeye (Horsechestnut) and *Aesculus* sp.	Shrub or tree; deciduous, opposite, palmately, divided leaves with five to nine leaflets on a long stalk; red, yellow, or white flowers; two- to three-valved, capsule fruit; with thick, leathery husk enclosing one to six brown shiny seeds	Leaves, twigs, flowers, and seeds	Various species throughout the United States and Canada; some cultivated as ornamentals, others grow wild	Toxic parts contain the glycoside, esculin	Nervous twitching of muscles, weakness, lack of coordination, dilated pupils, nausea, vomiting, diarrhea, depression, paralysis, and stupor	By making a "tea" from the leaves and twigs or by eating the seeds, children have been poisoned Honey collected from the buckeye flower may also cause poisoning. Roots, branches, and fruits have been used to stupefy fish in ponds. Treatment usually is a gastric lavage or vomiting
Buttercup and *Ranunculus* sp.	Annual or perennial herb growing to 16 – 32 in. (41 – 81 cm) high; leaves alternate entire to compound, and largely basal; yellow flowers borne singly or in clusters on ends of seed stalks; small fruits, single-seeded pods	Entire plant	Widely distributed in woods, meadows, pastures, and along streams throughout temperate and cold locations	The alkaloid protoanemonin, which can injure the digestive system and ulcerate the skin	Burning sensation of the mouth, nervousness, nausea, vomiting, low blood pressure, weak pulse, depression, and convulsions	Sap and leaves may cause dermatitis. Cows poisoned by buttercups produce bitter milk or milk with a reddish color
Castor bean and *Ricinus communis*	Shrub-like herb 4 – 12 ft (1.2 – 3.7 m) tall; simple, alternate, long-stalked leaves with 5 – 11 long lobes, which are toothed on margins; fruits oval, green, or red, and covered with spines; three elliptical, glossy, black, white, or mottled seeds per capsule	Entire plant, especially the seeds	Cultivated as an ornamental or oilseed crop primarily in the southern part of the United States and Hawaii	Seeds, pressed cake, and leaves poisonous when chewed; contain the phytotoxin, ricin	Burning of the mouth and throat, nausea, vomiting, severe stomach pains, bloody diarrhea, excessive thirst, prostration, dullness of vision, and convulsions; kidney failure and death 1 to 12 days later	Fatal dose for a child is one to three seeds, and for an adult two to eight seeds The oil extracted from the seeds is an important commercial product. It is not poisonous and it is used as a medicine (castor oil), for soap, and as a lubricant

Continued

TABLE 1.14 (Continued)

Common and Scientific Name	Description	Toxic Parts	Geographical Distribution	Poisoning	Symptoms	Remarks
Chinaberry and *Melia azedarach*	Deciduous tree 20 – 40 ft (6 – 12 m) tall; twice, pinnately divided leaves and toothed or lobed leaflets; purple flowers borne in clusters; yellow, wrinkled, rounded berries that persist throughout the winter	Berries, bark, flowers, and leaves	A native of Asia introduced as an ornamental in the United States; common in the southern United States and lower altitudes in Hawaii; has become naturalized in old fields, pastures, around buildings, and along fence rows	Most result from eating pulp of berries; toxic principal is a resinoid with narcotic effects	Nausea, vomiting, diarrhea, irregular breathing, and respiratory distress	Six to eight berries can cause the death of a child The berries have been used to make insecticide and flea powder
Death camas and *Zigadenus paniculatus*	Perennial herb resembling wild onions but the onion odor is lacking; long, slender leaves with parallel veins; pale yellow to pink flowers in clusters on slender seed stalks; fruit a three-celled capsule	Entire plant, especially the bulb	Various species occur throughout the United States and Canada; all are more or less poisonous	Due to the alkaloids zygadenine, veratrine, and others	Excessive salivation, muscular weakness, slow heart rate, low blood pressure, subnormal temperature, nausea, vomiting, diarrhea, prostration, coma, and sometimes death	The members of Lewis and Clark Expedition made flour from the bulbs and suffered the symptoms of poisoning. Later some pioneers died when they mistook death camas for wild onions or garlic
Dogbane (Indian hemp) and *Apocynum cannabinum*	Perennial herbs with milky juice and somewhat woody stems; simple, smooth, and oppositely paired leaves; bell-shaped, small, white to pink flowers borne in clusters at ends of axillary stems; paired, long, slender seed pods	Entire plant	Various species growing throughout North America in fields and forests, and along streams and roadsides	Only suspected, as it contains the toxic glycoside, cymarin and is poisonous to animals	In animals, increased temperature and pulse, cold extremities, dilation of the pupils, discoloration of the mouth and nose, sore mouth, sweating, loss of appetite, and death	Compounds extracted from roots of dogbane have been used to make a heart stimulant
Foxglove and *Digitalis purpurea*	Biennial herb with alternate, simple, toothed leaves; terminal, showy raceme of flowers, purple, pink, rose, yellow, or white; dry capsule fruit	Entire plant, especially leaves, flowers, and seeds	Native of Europe commonly planted in gardens of the United States; naturalized and abundant in some parts of the western United States.	Due to digitalis component	Nausea, vomiting, dizziness, irregular heartbeat, tremors, convulsions, and possibly death	Foxglove has long been known as a source of digitalis and steroid glycosides It is an important medicinal plant when used correctly
Henbane and *Hyoscyamus niger*	Erect annual or biennial herb with coarse, hairy stems 1 – 5 ft (30 – 152 cm) high; simple, oblong, alternate leaves with a few, coarse teeth, not stalked; greenish-yellow or yellowish with purple vein flowers; fruit a rounded capsule	Entire plant	Along roads, in waste places across southern Canada and northern United States, particularly common in the Rocky Mountains	Caused by the alkaloids, hyoscyamine hyoscine, and atropine	Increased salivation, headache, nausea, rapid pulse, convulsions, coma, and death	A gastric lavage of 4% tannic acid solution may be used to treat the poisoning

Plant	Description	Distribution	Part involved	Constituents	Symptoms	Comments
Iris (rock mountain iris) and *Iris missouriensis*	Lily-like perennial plants often in dense patches; long, narrow leaves; flowers blue-purple; fruit a three-celled capsule	Wet land of meadows, marshes, and along streams from North Dakota to British Columbia, Canada; south of New Mexico, Arizona, and California; scattered over entire Rocky Mountain area; cultivated species also common	Leaves, but especially the rootstalk	An irritating resinous substance, irisin	Burning, congestion, and severe pain in the digestive tract; nausea and diarrhea	Rootstalks have such an acrid taste that they are unlikely to be eaten
Jasmine and *Gelsemium sempervirens*	A woody, trailing, or climbing evergreen vine; opposite, simple, lance-shaped, glossy leaves; fragrant, yellow flowers; flattened two-celled, beaked capsule fruits	Native to the southeastern United States; commonly grown in the Southwest as an ornamental	Entire plant, but especially the root and flowers.	Alkaloids, geisemine, gelseminine, and gelsemoidine found throughout the plant	Profuse sweating, muscular weakness, convulsions, respiratory depression, paralysis, and death possible	Jasmine has been used as a medicinal herb, but overdoses are dangerous. Children have been poisoned by chewing on the leaves
Jimmyweed (Rayless goldenrod) and *Haplopappus heterophyllus*	Small, bushy, half-shrub with erect stems arising from the woody crown to a height of 2 – 4 ft (61 – 122 cm); narrow, alternate, sticky leaves; clusters of small, yellow flower heads at tips of stems	Common in fields or ranges around watering sites and along streams from Kansas, Oklahoma, and Texas to Colorado, New Mexico, and Arizona	Entire plant	Contains the higher alcohol, tremetol, which accumulates in the milk of cows and causes human poisoning known as "milk sickness"	Other species of *Haplopappus* probably are equally dangerous	White snakeroot also contains tremetol, and causes "milk sickness"
Jimsonwood (Thornapple) and *Datura stramonium*	Coarse, weedy plant with stout stems and foul-smelling foliage; large, oval leaves with wavy margins; fragrant, large, tubular, white to purple flowers; round, nodding or erect prickly capsule	Naturalized throughout North America; common weed of fields, gardens, roadsides, and pastures	Entire plant, particularly the seeds and leaves	Due to the alkaloids hyoscyamine, atropine, and hyoscine (scopolamine)	Dry mouth, thirst, red skin, disturbed vision, pupil dilation, nausea, vomiting, headache, hallucination, rapid pulse, delirium, incoherent speech, convulsion, high blood pressure, coma, and possibly death	Sleeping near the fragrant flowers can cause headache, nausea, dizziness, and weakness. Children using the flowers as trumpets while playing have been poisoned
Lantana (Red Sage) and *Lantana camara*	Perennial shrub with square twigs and a few spines; simple, opposite or whorled oval-shaped leaves with tooth margins; white, yellow, orange, red, or blue flowers occurring in flat-topped clusters; berry-like fruit with a hard, blue-black seed	Native of the dry woods in the southeastern United States; cultivated as an ornamental shrub in pots in the northern United States and Canada; or a lawn shrub in the southeastern coastal plains, Texas, California, and Hawaii	All parts, especially the green berries	Fruit contains high levels of an alkaloid, lantanin or lantadene A	Stomach and intestinal irritation, vomiting, bloody diarrhea, muscular weakness, jaundice, and circulatory collapse; death possible but not common	In Florida, these plants are considered a major cause of human poisoning. The foliage of lantana may also cause dermatitis
Larkspur and *Delphinium* sp.	Annual or perennial herb 2 – 4 ft (61 – 122 cm) high; finely, palmately divided leaves on long stalks; white, pink, rose, blue, or purple flowers each with a spur; fruit a many-seeded, three-celled capsule	Native of rich or dry forest and meadows throughout the United States but common in the West; frequently cultivated in flower gardens	Entire plant	Contains the alkaloids delphinine, delphinidine, ajacine, and others	Burning sensation in the mouth and skin, low blood pressure, nervousness, weakness, prickling of the skin, nausea, vomiting, depression, convulsions, and death within 6 h if eaten in large quantities	Poisoning potential of larkspur decreases as it ages, but alkaloids still concentrated in the seeds. Seeds are used in some commercial lice remedies

Continued

**TABLE 1.14
(Continued)**

Common and Scientific Name	Description	Toxic Parts	Geographical Distribution	Poisoning	Symptoms	Remarks
Laurel (mountain laurel) and *Kalmia latifolia*	Large evergreen shrubs growing to 35 ft (11 m) tall; alternate leaves dark green on top and bright green underneath; white to rose flowers in terminal clusters; fruit in a dry capsule	Leaves, twigs, flowers, and pollen grains	Found in moist woods and along streams in eastern Canada southward in the Appalachian Mountains and Piedmont, and sometimes in the eastern coastal plain	Contains the toxic resinoid, andromedotoxin	Increased salivation, watering of eyes and nose, loss of energy, slow pulse, vomiting, low blood pressure, lack of coordination, convulsions, and progressive paralysis until eventual death	The Mountain laurel is the state flower of Connecticut and Pennsylvania Children making "tea" from the leaves or sucking on the flowers have been poisoned
Locoweed (Crazyweed) and *Oxtropis* sp.	Perennial herb with erect or spreading stems; pea-like flowers and stems — only smaller	Common throughout the south western United States	Contains alkaloid-like substances — a serious threat to livestock	In animals, loss of weight, irregular gait, loss of sense of direction, nervousness, weakness, and loss of muscular control	Locoweeds are seldom eaten by humans, and hence they are not a serious problem	There are more than 100 species of locoweeds
Lupine (Bluebonnet) and *Lupinus* sp.	Annual or perennial herbs; digitately divided, alternate leaves; pear-shaped blue, white, red, or yellow flowers borne in clusters at ends of stems; seeds in flattened pods	Entire plant, particularly the seeds	Wide distribution but most common in western North America; many cultivated as ornamentals	Contains lupinine and related toxic alkaloids	Weak pulse, slowed respiration, convulsions, and paralysis	Rarely have cultivated varieties poisoned children Not all lupines are poisonous
Marijuana (hashish, Mary Jane, pot, grass)	A tall coarse, annual herb; palmately divided and long-stalked leaves; small, green flowers clustered in the leaf axils	Entire plant, especially the leaves, flowers, sap and resinous secretions	Widely naturalized weed in temperate North America; cultivated in warmer areas	Various narcotic resins but mainly tetrahydro-cannabinol (THC) and related compounds	Exhilaration, hallucinations, delusions, mental confusion, dilated pupils, blurred vision, poor coordination, weakness, and stupor; coma and death in large doses	Poisoning results form drinking the extract, chewing the plant parts, or smoking a so-called "reefer" (joint) The hallucinogenic and narcotic effects of marijuana have been known for more than 2000 years. Laws in the United States and Canada restrict the possession of living or dried parts of marijuana
Mescal bean (Frijolito) and *Sophora secundiflora*	Evergreen shrub or small tree growing to 40 ft (12 m) tall; stalked, alternate leaves 4 – 6 in (10 – 15 cm) long, which are pinnately divided and shiny, yellow-green above and silky below when young; violet-blue, pea-like flowers; bright red seeds	Entire plant, particularly the seed	Native to southwestern Texas and southern New Mexico; cultivated as ornamentals in the southwestern United States	Contains cytisine and other poisonous alkaloids	Nausea, vomiting, diarrhea, excitement, delirium, hallucinations, coma, and death; deep sleep lasting 2 to 3 days in nonlethal doses	One seed, if sufficiently chewed, is enough to cause the death of a young child. The Indians of Mexico and the Southwest have used the seeds in medicine as a narcotic and as a hallucinatory drug Necklaces have been made from the seeds

Plant	Description	Toxic parts	Distribution	Toxic constituents	Symptoms	Remarks
Mistletoe and *Phoradendron serotinum*	Parasitic evergreen plants that grow on trees and shrubs; oblong, simple, opposite leaves, which are leathery; small, white berries	All parts, especially the berries	Common on the branches of various trees from New Jersey and southern Indiana southward to Florida and Texas; other species throughout North America	Contains the toxic amines, β-phenylethyl-amine and tyrosamine	Gastrointestinal pain, diarrhea, slow pulse, and collapse; possibly nausea, vomiting, nervousness, difficult breathing, delirium, pupil dilation, and abortion; in sufficient amounts, death within a few hours	Mistletoe is a favorite Christmas decoration. It is the state flower of Oklahoma. Poisonings have occurred when people eat the berries or make "tea" from the berries. Indians chewed the leaves to relieve toothache
Monkshood (Wolfsbane) and *Aconitum columbianum*	Perennial herb about 2 – 5 ft (61 – 152 cm) high; alternate, petioled leaves, which are palmately divided into segments with pointed tips; generally dark blue flowers with a prominent hood; seed in a short-beaked capsule	Entire plant, especially roots and seeds	Rich, moist soil in meadows and along streams from western Canada south to California and New Mexico	Due to several alkaloids, including aconine and aconitine	Burning sensation of the mouth and skin; nausea, vomiting, diarrhea, muscular weakness, and spasms; weak, irregular pulse, paralysis of respiration, dimmed vision, convulsions, and death within a few hours	Small amounts can be lethal. Death in humans reported from eating the plant or extracts made from it. It has been mistaken for horseradish
Mushrooms (toadstools) and *Amanita muscaria, Amanita verna, Chlorophyllum molybdites*	Common types with central stalk, and cap; flat plates (gills) underneath cap; some with deeply ridged, cylindrical top rather than cap	Entire fungus	Various types throughout North America	Depending on type of mushroom; complex polypeptides such as amanitin and possibly phalloidin; a toxic protein in some; the poisons ibotenic acid, muscimol, and related compounds in others	Vary with type of mushroom, but include death-like sleep, manic behavior, delirium, seeing colored visions, feeling of elation, explosive diarrhea, vomiting, severe headache, loss of muscular coordination, abdominal cramps, and coma and death from some types; permanent liver, kidney, and heart damage from other types	Wild mushrooms are extremely difficult to identify and are best avoided. There is no simple rule of thumb for distinguishing between poisonous and nonpoisonous mushrooms — only myths and nonsense. Only one or two bites are necessary for death from some species. During the month of December 1981, three people were killed, and two hospitalized in California after eating poisonous mushrooms
Nightshade and *Solanum nigrum, Solanum eleagnifolium*	Annual herbs or shrub-like plants with simple alternate leaves; small, white, blue, or violet flowers; black berries or yellow to yellow-orange berries depending on species	Primarily the unripe berries	Throughout the United States and southern Canada in waste places, old fields, ditches, roadsides, fence rows, or edges of woods	Contains the alkaloid solanine; possibly saponin, atropine, and perhaps high levels of nitrate	Headache, stomach pain, vomiting, diarrhea, dilated pupils, subnormal temperature, shock, circulatory and respiratory depression, and possible death	Some individuals use the completely ripe berries in pies and jellies. Young shoots and leaves of the plant have been cooked and eaten like spinach
Oleander and *Nerium oleander*	An evergreen shrub or small tree growing to 25 ft (8 m) tall; short-stalked, narrow, leathery leaves, opposite or in whorls of three; white to pink to red flowers at tips of twigs	Entire plant, especially the leaves	A native of southern Europe, but commonly cultivated in the southern United States and California	Contains the poisonous glycosides oleandrin and nerioside, which act similar to digitalis	Nausea, severe vomiting, stomach pain, bloody diarrhea, cold feet and hands, irregular heartbeat, dilation of pupils, drowsiness, unconsciousness, paralysis of respiration, convulsions, coma, and death within a day	One leaf of an oleander is said to contain enough poison to kill an adult. In Florida, severe poisoning resulted when oleander branches were used as skewers. Honey made from oleander flower nectar is poisonous

Continued

**TABLE 1.14
(Continued)**

Common and Scientific Name	Description	Toxic Parts	Geographical Distribution	Poisoning	Symptoms	Remarks
Peyote (Mescal buttons) and *Lophophora williamsii*	Hemispherical, spineless member of the cactus family growing from carrot-shaped roots; low, rounded sections with a tuft of yellow-white hairs on top; flower from the center of the plant, white to rose-pink; pink berry when ripe; black seeds	Entire plant, especially the buttons	Native to southern Texas and northern Mexico; cultivated in other areas	Contains mescaline, lophophorine and other alkaloids	Illusions and hallucinations with vivid color, anxiety, muscular tremors and twitching, vomiting, diarrhea, blurred vision, wakefulness, forgetfulness, muscular relaxation, and dizziness	The effects of chewing fresh or dried "buttons" of peyote are similar to those produced by LSD, only milder In some states, peyote is recognized as a drug Peyote has long been used by the Indians and Mexicans in religious ceremonies
Poison hemlock (poison parsley) and *Conium maculatum*	Biennial herb with a hairless purple-spotted or lined, hollow stem growing up to 8 ft (2.4 m) tall; turnip-like, long, solid taproot; large, alternate, pinnately divided leaves; small, white flowers in umbrella-shaped clusters, dry; ribbed, two-part capsule fruit	Entire plant, primarily seeds and root	A native of Eurasia, now a weed in meadows, and along roads and ditches throughout the United States and southern Canada where moisture is sufficient	The poisonous alkaloid coniine and other related alkaloids	Burning sensation in the mouth and throat, nervousness, dyscoordination, dilated pupils, muscular weakness, weakened and slowed heartbeat, convulsions, coma, and death	Poisoning occurs when the leaves are mistaken for parsley, the roots for turnips, or the seeds for anise Toxic quantities seldom consumed because the plant has such an unpleasant odor and taste Assumed by some to be the poison drunk by Socrates
Poison ivy (poison oak) and *Toxicondendron radicans*	A trailing or climbing vine, shrub, or small tree; alternate leaves with three leaflets; flowers and fruits hanging in clusters; white to yellowish fruit (drupes)	Roots, stems, leaves, pollen, flowers, and fruits	An extremely variable native weed throughout southern Canada and the United States with the exception of the west coast; found on flood plains, along lake shores, edges of woods, stream banks, fences, and around buildings	Skin irritation due to an oil-resin containing urushiol	Contact with skin causes itching, burning, redness, and small blisters; severe gastric disturbance and even death by eating leaves or fruit	Almost half of all persons are allergic to poison ivy Skin irritation may also result from indirect contact such as animals (including dogs and cats), clothing, tools, or sports equipment
Pokeweed (Pokeberry) and *Phytolacca Americana*	Shrub-like herb with a large fleshy taproot; large, simple, entire, oblong or lobed leaves; showy red, white, pink, or purple flowers in clusters at ends of branches; mature fruit a dark purple berry with red juice	Root stalk, leaves, and stems	Native to the eastern United States and southeastern Canada	Highest concentration of poison mainly in roots; contains the bitter glycosides, saponin and glycoprotein	Burning and bitter taste in mouth, stomach cramps, nausea, vomiting, diarrhea, drowsiness, slowed breathing, weakness, tremors, convulsions, spasms, coma, and death if eaten in large amounts	Young tender leaves and stems of pokeweed are often cooked as greens Cooked berries are used for pies without harm It is one of the most dangerous poisonous plants because people prepare it improperly
Poppy (common poppy) and *Papaver somniferum*	An erect annual herb with milky juice, simple, coarsely toothed, or lobed leaves; showy red, white, pink, or purple flowers; fruit an oval, crowned capsule; tiny seeds in capsule	Unripe fruits or their juice	Introduced from Eurasia and widely grown in the United States until cultivation without a license became unlawful	Crude resin from unripe seed capsule source of narcotic opium alkaloids	From unripe fruit, stupor, coma, shallow and slow breathing, depression of the central nervous system; possibly nausea and severe retching (straining to vomit)	The use of poppy extracts is a double-edged sword — addictive narcotics and valuable medicines. Poppy seeds used as toppings on breads are harmless

Plant	Description	Part(s) involved	Distribution	Toxic constituent	Symptoms	Remarks
Rhododendron, azaleas and Rhododendron sp.	Usually evergreen shrubs; mostly entire, simple, leathery leaves in whorls or alternate; snowy white to pink flowers in terminal clusters; fruit a wood capsule	Entire plant	Throughout the temperate parts of the United States as a native and as an introduced ornamental	Contains the toxic resinoid, andromedotoxin	Watering eyes and mouth, nasal discharge, nausea, severe abdominal pain, vomiting, convulsions, lowered blood pressure, lack of coordination, and loss of energy; progressive paralysis of arms and legs until death, in severe cases	Cases of poisoning are rare in this country, but rhododendrons should be suspected of possible danger
Rosary pea (precatory pea) and Abrus precatorius	A twining, more or less woody perennial vine; alternate and divided leaves with small leaflets; red to purple or white flowers; fruit a short pod containing ovoid seeds which are glossy, bright scarlet over three-fourths of their surface, and jet black over the remaining one-fourth	Seeds	Native to the tropics, but naturalized in Florida and the Keys	Contains the phytotoxin abrin and tetanic glycoside, abric acid	Severe stomach pain in 1 to 3 days, nausea, vomiting, severe diarrhea, weakness, cold sweat, drowsiness, weak, fast pulse, coma, circulatory collapse, and death	The beans are made into rosaries, necklaces, bracelets, leis, and various toys, which receive wide distribution. Seeds must be chewed and swallowed to cause poisoning. Whole seeds pass through the digestive tract without causing symptoms. One thoroughly chewed seed is said to be potent enough to kill an adult or child
Snow-on-the-mountain and Euphorbia marginata	A tall annual herb, growing up to 4 ft (122 cm) high; smooth, lance-shaped leaves with conspicuously white margins; whorls of white petal-like leaves border flowers; fruit a three-celled, three-lobed capsule	Leaves, stems, milky sap	Native to the western, dry plains and valleys from Montana to Mexico; sometimes escapes in the eastern United States	Toxins causing dermatitis and severe irritation of the digestive tract	Blistering of the skin, nausea, abdominal pain, fainting, diarrhea, possibly death in severe cases	Milky juice of this plant is very caustic. Outwardly resembles a poinsettia
Skunk cabbage and Veratrum californicum	Tall, broadleaved herbs of the lily family, growing to 6 ft (183 cm) high; large, alternate pleated, clasping, and parallel-veined leaves; numerous whitish to greenish flowers in large terminal clusters; three-lobed, capsule fruit	Entire plant	Various species throughout North America in wet meadows, forests, and along streams	Poisoning; Contains such alkaloids as veradridene and veratrine	Nausea, vomiting, diarrhea, stomach pains, lowered blood pressure, slow pulse, reduced body temperature, shallow breathing, salivation, weakness, nervousness, convulsions, paralysis, and possibly death	These plants have been used for centuries as a source of drugs and as a source of insecticide. As the leaves resemble cabbage, they are often collected as an edible wild plant, but with unpleasant results
Tansy and Tanacetum vulgare	Tall, aromatic herb with simple stems to 3 ft (91 cm) high; alternate, pinnately divided, narrow leaves, flower heads in flat-topped clusters with numerous small, yellow flowers	Leaves, stems, and flowers	Introduced from Eurasia; widely naturalized in North America; sometimes found escaped along roadsides, in pastures, or other wet places; grown for medicinal purposes	Contains an oil, tanacetin, or oil of tansy	Nausea, vomiting, diarrhea, convulsions, violent spasms, dilated pupils, rapid and feeble pulse, and possibly death	Tansys and its oil are employed as an herbal remedy for nervousness, intestinal worms, to promote menstruation, and to induce abortion. Some poisonings have resulted from the use of tansy as a home remedy

Continued

**TABLE 1.14
(Continued)**

Common and Scientific Name	Description	Toxic Parts	Geographical Distribution	Poisoning	Symptoms	Remarks
Water hemlock and *Cicuta* sp.	A perennial with parsley-like leaves; hollow, jointed stems and hollow, pithy roots; flowers in umbrella clusters; stems streaked with purple ridges; 2 to 6 ft (61 to 183 cm) high	Entire plant, primarily the roots and young growth	Wet meadows, pastures, and flood plains of western and eastern United States, generally absent in the plains states	Contains the toxic resin-like higher alcohol, cicutoxin	Frothing at the mouth, spasms, dilated pupils, diarrhea, convulsions, vomiting, delirium, respiratory failure, paralysis, and death	One mouthful of the water hemlock root is reported to contain sufficient poison to kill manna adult Children making whistles and peashooters from the hollow stems have been poisoned The water hemlock is often mistaken for the edible wild artichoke or parsnip. However, it is considered to be one of the poisonous plants of the North Temperate Zone
White snakeroot and *Eupatorium rogosum*	Erect perennial with stems 1 to 5 ft (30 to 152 cm) tall; opposite oval leaves with pointed tips and sharply toothed edges, and dull on the upper surface but shiny on the lower surface; showy, snow white flowers in terminal clusters	Entire plant	From eastern Canada to Saskatchewan and south of Texas, Louisiana, Georgia, and Virginia	Contains the higher alcohol, tremetol and some glycosides	Weakness, nausea, loss of appetite, vomiting, tremors, labored breathing, constipation, dizziness, delirium, convulsions, coma, and death	Recovery from a nonlethal dose is a slow process, due to liver and kidney damage Poison may be in the milk of cows that have eaten white snakeroot — "milk sickness"

Source: Ensminger, A.H. et al., *Food and Nutrition Encyclopedia*, 2nd ed., CRC Press, Boca Raton, FL, 1994.

REFERENCES

1. Berdanier, C.D., *Advanced Nutrition: Macronutrients*. CRC Press, Boca Raton, FL, 2000, p. 122.
2. Lentner, C., *Geigy Scientific Tables*, Vol. 1. CIBA-Geigy, West Caldwell, NJ, 1981, pp. 241–266.
3. Unpublished data, Lee Zehner, Beltsville, MD, 2000.
4. Ensminger, A.H. et al., *Food and Nutrition Encyclopedia*, 2nd ed., CRC Press, Boca Raton, FL, 1994, pp. 2082–2087.
5. Lynnes book.
6. Duke, J.A., *Handbook of Edible Weeds*, CRC Press, Boca Raton, FL, 1992, 246 pages.

2 Microbiological Safety of Foods

Kumar S. Venkitanarayanan and Michael P. Doyle

CONTENTS

INTRODUCTION

The microbiological safety of foods is a major concern to consumers and to the food industry. Despite considerable progress made in technology, consumer education, and regulations, food safety continues to be a major challenge to our public health and economy. During the past two decades, food safety received considerable attention due to the emergence of several new food-borne pathogens and the involvement of foods that traditionally have been considered safe, in many food-borne disease outbreaks. Further, industrialization of the food supply through mass production, distribution, increased globalization, and consumer demands for preservative-free, convenience foods and ready-to-eat meals highlight the significance of the microbial safety of foods. A study published by the U.S. Centers for Disease Control and Prevention (CDC), in 1999, reported an estimated 76 million cases of food-borne illnesses, which resulted in 325,000 hospitalizations and 5,000 deaths in the United States annually.[1] Besides the public health impact, outbreaks of food-borne illness impose major economic losses to both the food industry and society. The annual estimated cost of food-borne illnesses caused by the four most common pathogens alone account for approximately $6.9 billion.[2] The types of microbiological hazards associated with foods can be classified as bacterial, viral, fungal, and parasitic.

BACTERIAL FOOD-BORNE PATHOGENS

Bacteria are the major agents of microbial food-borne illnesses, and account for an estimated 4 million food-borne illnesses annually in the United States (Table 2.1).[1] Bacterial food-borne diseases can be classified into food-borne infections resulting from ingestion of foods containing viable cells of bacterial pathogens, and food-borne intoxications, which result from consumption of foods containing preformed toxins produced by toxigenic bacteria. The primary bacterial pathogens associated with food-borne diseases are discussed below.

ESCHERICHIA COLI O157:H7

Enterohemorrhagic *Escherichia coli* O157:H7 emerged in 1982 as a food-borne pathogen, and is now recognized as a major public health concern in the United States. Many food-associated outbreaks are reported each year, with 217 confirmed cases reported in 2004.[3] Although approximately 50% of the reported outbreaks in the United States have been associated with consumption of undercooked beef burgers, a wide variety of other foods, including raw milk, roast beef, venison jerky, salami, yogurt, lettuce, unpasteurized apple juice, cantaloupe, alfalfa sprouts, and coleslaw, have been implicated as vehicles of *E. coli* O157:H7 infection.[4] In addition, outbreaks involving person-to-person and waterborne transmission have been reported.[4] Cattle have been implicated as one of the principal reservoirs of *E. coli* O157:H7,[5–8] with the terminal rectum being a principal site of colonization in adult animals.[9] *E. coli* O157:H7 can survive in bovine feces for many months,[10] hence potentially contaminating cattle, food, water, and the environment through contact with manure. Although surveys conducted in the 1980s and 1990s generally showed a low fecal prevalence of *E. coli* O157:H7 in cattle,[8,11,12] later studies using improved enrichment and isolation procedures have revealed that the overall prevalence of *E. coli* O157:H7 in cattle may be substantially higher than originally found.[13–16] A study by Elder et al.[13] revealed that, of cattle from 29 feedlots presented for slaughter in the Midwestern United States, 72% had at least one *E. coli* O157-positive fecal sample and 38% had positive hide samples. The study revealed an overall *E. coli* O157 prevalence of 28% (91 out of 327) in feces, and 11% (38 out of 355) on the hide. Studies by others revealed that the prevalence of *E. coli* O157 in feed lots in the United States can be as high as 63%, particularly during the summer, under muddy conditions, or with feeding of barley.[17,18] These results are of particular concern, because high fecal shedding and the presence of *E. coli* O157:H7 on hides can lead to contamination of foods of bovine origin with the pathogen during slaughtering and processing operations.[19] In addition, many *E. coli* O157:H7 outbreaks involving nonbovine foods, such as fruits and vegetables, are often linked to cross contamination of the implicated food with contaminated bovine manure.[20–23] Direct zoonotic and environmental transmission is a more recently recognized mode of *E. coli* O157:H7 spread to humans. Contact with the farm environment, including recreational or occupational visits, has been associated with *E. coli* O157:H7 infections in humans.[24,25] Since reduced fecal shedding of *E. coli* O157:H7 by cattle would potentially decrease food-borne outbreaks of *E. coli* O157:H7, a variety of approaches for reducing its carriage in cattle, including vaccination,[26] feeding cattle with competitive exclusion bacteria,[27] and supplementation of cattle diet with sodium chlorate,[28] have been explored.

Acidification is commonly used in food processing to control growth and survival of spoilage-causing and pathogenic microorganisms in foods. The U.S. Food and Drug Administration (FDA) does not regard foods with pH ≤ 4.6 (high-acid foods) to be microbiologically hazardous. However, *E. coli* O157:H7 has been associated with outbreaks attributed to high-acid foods, including apple juice, mayonnaise, fermented sausage, and yogurt,[29] raising concerns about the safety of these foods. Several studies have revealed that many strains of *E. coli* O157:H7 are highly tolerant to acidic conditions, being able to survive for extended periods of time in synthetic gastric juice and in highly acidic foods.[29,30] Further, exposure of *E. coli* O157:H7 to mild or moderate acidic environments can induce an acid tolerance response, which enables the pathogen to survive extreme acidic conditions. For example, acid-adapted cells of *E. coli* O157:H7 survived longer in apple cider, fermented sausage, and hydrochloric acid than nonacid-adapted cells.[31,32] However, *E. coli* O157:H7 is not unusually heat resistant[33] or salt tolerant[34] unless cells are preexposed to acid to become acid adapted. Acid-adapted *E. coli* O157:H7 cells have been determined to have increased heat tolerance.

In humans, two important manifestations of illness have been reported with *E. coli* O157:H7 infection. These include hemorrhagic colitis and hemolytic uremic syndrome (HUS).[36] Hemorrhagic colitis is characterized by a watery diarrhea that progresses into grossly bloody diarrhea, indicative of significant amounts of gastrointestinal bleeding. Severe abdominal pain is common, but fever is usually not present. The illness typically lasts from 2 to 9 days. HUS is a severe condition, particularly among the very young and the elderly, which involves damage to kidneys, leading to renal failure and death.

TABLE 2.1
Bacterial Food-Borne Pathogens

Microbe	Biochemical and Growth Characteristics	Sources/Reservoirs	Vehicles	Estimated No. of Food-Borne Cases Annually in the United States[1]	Incubation Period, Symptoms, and Duration	Detection Methods	Control/Prevention
Escherichia coli O157:H7	Gram negative, facultative anaerobe, nonsporeforming, optimum growth at 37 to 40°C, inability to grow at $\geq$44.5°C in presence of selective agents, inability to ferment sorbitol within 24 h, does not produce β-glucuronidase, acid tolerance	Cattle, humans	Raw or under-cooked beef, unpasteurized milk and apple juice, lettuce, alfalfa sprouts, and water	62,500	3 – 9 days. Severe abdominal cramps, watery diarrhea that can become bloody, absence of fever, kidney failure, seizures, and coma. Duration is days to weeks	Cultural methods followed by confirmatory biochemical tests[256,257] Latex agglutination assay[258,259] ELISA[260-262] PCR[263-265]	Adequate cooking of beef; pasteurization of milk and apple juice; use of potable water for drinking; avoid eating alfalfa and vegetable sprouts; good personal hygiene
Salmonella spp. (nonthyphoid)	Gram negative, facultative anaerobe, oxidase negative, catalase positive, nonsporeforming, growth at 5 – 47°C, optimum growth at 37°C, metabolize nutrients by respiratory and fermentative pathways	Cattle, swine, poultry, humans	Raw or under-cooked meat, poultry, eggs, and milk and untreated water	1,340,000	6 – 72 h up to 4 days. Abdominal cramps, diarrhea, fever, chills, headache and vomiting. Duration is few days to 1 week, occasionally up to 3 weeks	Cultural methods followed by confirmatory biochemical tests[266-268] Latex agglutination assay[269] ELISA[270] Immunoassay[271] PCR[272-275]	Adequate cooking of food; avoid cross-contamination of raw foods of animal origin with cooked or ready to eat foods; avoid eating raw or undercooked foods of animal origin; use of potable water; good personal hygiene
Salmonella typhi	Gram negative, facultative anaerobe, ferment D-xylose	Humans	Raw milk, shellfish, raw salads, under cooked foods	660 (>70% of cases acquired abroad)	7 – 28 days. Remittent fever with stepwise increments over a period of days, high temperature of 103 to 104 F, abdominal pain, diarrhea, and headache. Duration is up to 3 weeks	Biochemical tests[276] Latex test[277] ELISA[278] PCR[279,280]	Good personal hygiene and food handling practices; proper sewage systems; effective surveillance of known carriers
Campylobacter jejuni and *coli*	Gram negative, microaerophilic, nonsporeforming, optimal growth at 42°C, CO_2 is required for good growth, growth optimal in 3 – 6% O_2, sensitive to dehydration, survives best at refrigeration temperature	Poultry Swine Cattle Sheep Wild birds	Raw or under-cooked, poultry, pork, and beef, and unpasteurized milk	1,960,000	1 – 11 days, usually 2 to 5 days. Abdominal pain, diarrhea, malaise, headache, fever. Duration is up to 10 days	Cultural methods followed by confirmatory biochemical Tests[69, 281] Immunoassay[282,283] PCR[284-289]	Adequate cooking of meat; avoid cross-contamination of raw foods of animal origin with cooked or ready to eat foods; pasteurization of milk
Shigella spp.	Gram negative, facultative anaerobe, nonsporeforming, does not ferment lactose, growth at 10 – 45°C, optimal growth at 37°C	Humans	Raw foods and water contaminated with human feces; prepared salads	89,600	1 – 7 days. Severe abdominal and rectal pain, bloody diarrhea with mucus, fever. Dehydration. Duration is few days to few weeks	Cultural methods followed by confirmatory biochemical tests[290] ELISA[291,292] PCR[293-296]	Good personal hygiene, adequate cooking of food, drinking potable water

Continued

TABLE 2.1
(Continued)

Microbe	Biochemical and Growth Characteristics	Sources/Reservoirs	Vehicles	Estimated No. of Food-Borne Cases Annually in the United States[1]	Incubation Period, Symptoms, and Duration	Detection Methods	Control/Prevention
Yersinia enterocolitica	Gram negative, facultative anaerobe, nonsporeforming, growth at 0 – 44°C, optimal growth at –29°C, growth at pH 4.6 – 9.0, growth in presence of 5% NaCl but not 7% NaCl	Swine is principal reservoir of pathogenic strains. Humans can also act as a source through contaminated blood transfusion	Undercooked or raw pork, especially tongue	86,700	1 – 11 days, usually 24 – 36 h. Severe abdominal pain, nausea, diarrhea, fever, sometimes vomiting. Duration is usually 2 – 3 days but may continue for up to 3 weeks	Cultural methods followed by confirmatory biochemical tests[297]. PCR[298-300]	Adequate cooking of pork, disinfection of drinking water, control of Y. enterocolitica in pigs, prevent cross-contamination of pig viscera, feces, and hair with food and water
Vibrio cholerae	Gram negative, facultative anaerobe, nonsporeforming, growth at 18 – 42°C with optimal growth at 37°C, growth is stimulated in presence of 3% NaCl, pH range for growth is 6 – 11	Humans, marine waters, especially brackish water and estuaries	Undercooked or raw seafoods; vegetables fertilized with contaminated human feces or irrigated with contaminated water; water	49	1 – 3 days. Profuse watery diarrhea, which can lead to severe dehydration, abdominal pain, vomiting. Duration is up to 7 days	Cultural methods followed by confirmatory biochemical tests[301-303]. ELISA[304,305]. Immunoassay[306]. PCR[307-310]	Safe disposal of human sewage, disinfection of drinking water, avoid eating raw seafood, adequate cooking of food
Vibrio parahaemolyticus	Gram negative, facultative anaerobe, nonsporeforming, growth in presence of 8% NaCl, optimal growth at 37°C with rapid generation time (≈10 min), growth at 10°C, sensitive to storage at refrigeration temperature	Coastal seawater, estuarine brackish waters above 15°C, marine fish, shellfish	Raw or under-cooked fish and seafoods	5,100	9 – 25 h, up to 3 days. Profuse watery diarrhea, abdominal pain, vomiting, fever. Duration is up to 8 days	Cultural methods followed by confirmatory biochemical tests[301,302]. ELISA[311]. PCR[312-314]	Adequate cooking of seafood, rapid chilling of seafoods, prevent cross-contamination from raw seafoods to other foods and preparation surfaces
Vibrio vulnificus	Gram negative, nonsporeforming, optimal growth at 37°C	Coastal and estuarine waters	Raw seafood, especially raw oysters	47	12 h to 3 days. Profuse diarrhea with blood in feces, fulminating septicemia, hypotension. Duration is days to weeks	Cultural methods followed by confirmatory biochemical tests[301,302,315]. ELISA[316,317]. PCR[318,319]	Avoid eating raw seafood, especially raw oysters when one has a history of liver disease or alcoholism
Enterobacter sakazakii	Gram negative, Facultative anaerobe, nonsporeforming, α-glucosidase-positive phosphoamidase-negative growth at 5.5 to 37°C, tolerant to high osmotic pressure and desiccation	Not known	Dry, powdered infant formula	Very few	Sepsis, meningitis, meningo-encephalitis, brain abscess, ventriculitis, hydrocephalus, necrotizing enterocolitis largely in preterm infants. Bacteremia, osteomyelitis and pneumonia in elderly adults	Cultural and biochemical methods[320,321]. PCR[322,323]	Proper refrigerated storage of reconstituted infant formula. Avoid feeding formula that has been temperature abused. Prepared infant formula should not be kept warm in bottle heaters for more than 2 h

Organism	Characteristics	Habitat	Foods	Number	Symptoms	Detection methods	Prevention
Aeromonas hydrophila	Gram negative, facultative anaerobe, nonsporeforming, oxidase positive, some strains are psychrotrophic (4°C) optimum growth at ~28°C	Aquatic environment, freshwater fish (especially Salmonids)	Untreated water, Undercooked seafoods, especially fish	Very few	24 to 48 h. Abdominal pain, vomiting, watery stools, mild fever. Duration is days to weeks	Cultural methods followed by confirmatory biochemical tests[324-327] ELISA[328] PCR[329-331]	Avoid consumption of raw seafoods, avoid long-term storage of refrigerated foods, adequate cooking of foods, disinfection of drinking water
Plesiomonas shigelloides	Gram negative, facultative anaerobe, nonsporeforming, oxidase positive, some strains are psychrotrophic	Fresh and estaurine waters, fish, and shellfish	Fish, shellfish, oysters, shrimp, and untreated water	Very few	1 to 2 days. Abdominal pain, nausea, vomiting, diarrhea, chills, headache. Duration is days to weeks	Cultural methods followed by confirmatory biochemical tests[324,325] PCR[332]	Avoid consumption of raw seafoods, disinfection of drinking water
Listeria monocytogenes	Gram positive, facultative anaerobe, nonsporeforming, growth at 2 to 45°C, optimal growth at 30 to 35°C, growth in presence of 10% NaCl	Soil, sewage, vegetation, water, and feces of humans and animals	Raw milk, soft cheese, pâté, ready-to-eat cooked meat products (poultry, hot dogs) and cooked seafoods (smoked fish), and raw vegetables	2,490	Few days to several weeks. Flu-like symptoms such as fever, chills, headache. abdominal pain and diarrhea are present in some cases. In pregnant women, spontaneous abortion and stillbirth. Duration is days to weeks	Cultural methods followed by confirmatory biochemical tests[333-336] Immunoassay[337-339] PCR[340-342]	Proper sanitation of food processing equipment and environments, adequate cooking of meat and meat products, prevent recontamination of cooked products, proper reheating of cooked food, avoid drinking raw milk, avoid certain high-risk foods (e.g., soft cheeses and pâtés) by pregnant women and immunocompromised individuals
Staphylococcus aureus (staphylococcal enterotoxin)	Gram positive, facultative anaerobe, nonsporeforming, coagulase positive, growth at 7 to 48°C, optimal growth at ~37°C, toxin production at a_w of 0.86, toxin is heat stable (can withstand boiling for 1 h)	Humans (nose, throat, and skin) and animals	Ham, chicken and egg salads, cream-filled pastries	185,000	2 to 6 h. Abdominal cramps, nausea, vomiting, diarrhea, headache, chills, and dizziness. Duration is up to 2 days	Cultural methods followed by confirmatory biochemical tests[343,344] PCR[345-347] Immunoassay[348-350] Detection of toxin by microslide gel double diffusion[351]	Good personal hygiene in food preparation and handling, adequate cooking of foods, proper refrigeration of cooked foods
Clostridium botulinum (botulinum neurotoxin)	Gram positive, obligate anaerobe, sporeforming, produce seven potent neurotoxins A to G (only A, B, E and rarely F associated with human illness), proteolytic strains grow at 10 to 50°C, nonproteolytic strains can grow at 3.3°C, spores are resistant to normal cooking temperatures, and survive freezing and drying	Soil, dust, vegetation, animals, birds, insects, and marine and fresh water sediments and the intestinal tracts of fish (type E)	Beef, pork, fish, vegetables, and honey (infant botulism)	58	12 to 36 h, can range from few hours to 8 days. Very severe life-threatening intoxication, headache, fixed and dilated pupils, vertigo, blurred or double vision, lack of muscle coordination, dry mouth, and difficulty in breathing. Gastrointestinal symptoms include abdominal pain, nausea, vomiting, and constipation. Duration is days to months (8 months)	Cultural methods followed by confirmatory biochemical tests[352] PCR[353-357] Detection of toxin by mouse bioassay[358] immunoaffinity chromatograpy[359] mass spectro-photometry[360] immunodetection kit[361]	Boiling of foods will destroy toxin, adequate heat processing of home-canned foods, proper refrigeration of vacuum-packaged fresh or lightly cooked/smoked foods, acid-preserved foods should be below pH 4.6, discard swollen cans, avoid feeding honey to infants

Continued

TABLE 2.1
(Continued)

Microbe	Biochemical and Growth Characteristics	Sources/Reservoirs	Vehicles	Estimated No. of Food-Borne Cases Annually in the United States[1]	Incubation Period, Symptoms, and Duration	Detection Methods	Control/Prevention
Clostridium perfringens	Gram positive, anaerobe, sporeforming, optimum growth at 37 to 47°C, grows slowly below 20°C	Soil, sewage, dust, vegetation, feces of humans and animals	Cooked meat and poultry, especially roast beef, turkey, and gravies	249,000	8 to 24 h. Abdominal pain and diarrhea. Duration is 1 to 2 days	Cultural methods followed by confirmatory biochemical tests[178]. Latex agglutination test[362]. Colony hybridization assay[363]. ELISA[364,365]. PCR[362,366,367]	Adequate cooking of foods; cooked food should be rapidly cooled (<5°C) or held hot (>60°C); proper refrigeration and adequate reheating of stored cooked foods
Bacillus cereus	Gram positive, facultative anaerobe, sporeforming, some strains can grow at 4 to 6°C; optimum growth at 28 to 37°C	Widely distributed in nature, soil, dust, vegetation	Cereals, fried rice, potatoes, cooked meat products, milk and dairy products, spices, dried foods	27,000	*Diarrheal syndrome* (toxic infection): 8 to 16 h. Abdominal pain, and watery diarrhea. Duration is 24 to 36 h. *Emetic syndrome* (preformed, heat-stable toxin): 1 to 5 h. Nausea, vomiting, malaise, and sometimes diarrhea. Duration is 24 to 36 h	Cultural methods followed by confirmatory biochemical tests[368]. ELISA[369,370]. Colony blot immunoassay[371,372]. PCR[373–375]	Adequate cooking of foods; cooked foods should be rapidly cooled (<5°C) or held hot (60°C); avoid leaving cooked foods at room temperature for long period of time
Brucella spp.	Gram negative, aerobe, nonsporeforming, optimal growth at 37°C	Cattle, sheep, pig, goat	Raw milk and products made from unpasteurized milk	780	Acute form: 3 to 21 days, infrequently months. Pyrexia, profuse sweats, chills, constipation, weakness, malaise, body aches, joint pains, weight loss, and anorexia. Chronic form: several months. Long history of fever, inertia, recurrent depression, sexual impotence, and insomnia. Duration is weeks	Cultural methods[376]. ELISA[377–379]. PCR[380–382]	Vaccination of livestock against *Brucella* spp., avoid contact with infected animals, eradication of diseased animals; pasteurization of milk; avoid eating unpasteurized dairy products
Helicobacter pylori	Gram negative, microaerophile to anaerobe	Humans, cats	Untreated water, food-borne transmission of disease has not been proven	Unknown	Gastritis, dyspepsia, peptic ulcer, and gastric carcinoma	Cultural methods[191,383]. ELISA[189]. Immunoassay[384,385]. PCR[386,387]. Rapid paper urease test[388]	Avoid contact with infected animals, use of chlorinated water for cooking and drinking

Two important factors attributed to the pathogenesis of *E. coli* O157:H7 include the ability of the pathogen to adhere to the intestinal mucosa of the host, and production of Shiga toxin I or Shiga toxin II.[35] Retrospective analysis of foods implicated in outbreaks of *E. coli* O157:H7 infection suggests a low infectious dose of the pathogen, probably less than 100 cells.[36]

SALMONELLA SPECIES

Salmonella spp. are facultatively anaerobic, gram-negative, rod-shaped bacteria belonging to the family *Enterobacteriaceae*. Members of the genus *Salmonella* have an optimum growth temperature of 37°C and utilize glucose with the production of acid and gas.[37] *Salmonella* spp. are widely distributed in nature. They colonize the intestinal tract of humans, animals, birds, and reptiles, and are excreted in feces, which contaminate the environment, water, and foods.[38] Many food products, especially foods having contact with animal feces, including beef, pork, poultry, eggs, milk, fruits, and vegetables, have been associated with outbreaks of salmonellosis.[39] *Salmonella* spp. can be divided into host-adapted serovars and those without any host preferences. Most of the food-borne serovars are in the latter group.

The ability of many strains of *Salmonella* to adapt to extreme environmental conditions emphasizes the potential risk of these microorganisms as food-borne pathogens. Although salmonellae optimally grow at 37°C, the genus *Salmonella* consists of strains which are capable of growth from 5 to 47°C.[40] *Salmonella* spp. can grow at pH values ranging from 4.5 to 7.0, with optimum growth observed near neutral pH.[38] Preexposure of *Salmonella* to mild acidic environments (pH 5.5 to 6.0) can induce in some strains an acid tolerance response, which enables the bacteria to survive for extended periods of exposure to acidic and other adverse environmental conditions such as heat and low water activity.[41,42] However, most *Salmonella* spp. possess no unusual tolerance to salt and heat. A concentration of 3 to 4% NaCl can inhibit the growth of *Salmonella*.[43] Most salmonellae are sensitive to heat; hence ordinary pasteurization and cooking temperatures are capable of killing the pathogen.[44]

Salmonellosis is one of the most frequently reported food-borne diseases worldwide.[45] The overall incidence of salmonellosis in the United States has been reported to have declined by approximately 8% during the period from 1996 to 2004.[46] In the United States, food-associated *Salmonella* infections are estimated to cost $0.5 to $2.3 billion annually.[47] The most common serovars of *Salmonella* that cause food-borne salmonellosis in humans are *Salmonella enterica* subsp. *enterica* serovar Typhimurium and *Salmonella enterica* subsp. *enterica* serovar Enteritidis. A wide variety of foods, including beef, pork, milk, chicken, and turkey have been associated with outbreaks caused by *S.* Typhimurium. Although the incidence of *S.* Typhimurium in the United States has decreased by approximately 40% during 1996 to 2004,[46] the emergence of *S.* Typhimurium DT 104, a new phage type in the 1990s in the United States and Europe raised a significant public health concern. This is because *S.* Typhimurium DT 104 is resistant to multiple antibiotics, including ampicillin, chloramphenicol, penicillin, streptomycin, tetracycline, and sulfonamides.[48,49] A major risk factor identified in the acquisition of *S.* Typhimurium DT 104 infection in humans is that the infecting strain is resistant to prior treatment with antimicrobial agents, for the 4 weeks preceding infection.[50] CDC reported that 11% of the total *Salmonella* spp. isolated from humans in 2000 were resistant to at least five different antibiotics, and a few of the multidrug-resistant strains were also resistant to gentamicin and cephalosporins.[51] These aforementioned reports underscore the prudent use of antibiotics in human therapy and animal husbandry.

Salmonella Enteritidis outbreaks are most frequently associated with consumption of poultry products, especially undercooked eggs and chicken. Moreover, international travel, especially to developing countries, has been associated with human infections of *S.* Enteritidis in the United States.[52] CDC reported 677 outbreaks of egg-borne *S.* Enteritidis with 23,366 illnesses, 1,988 hospitalizations, and 33 deaths in the United States during the period of 1990 to 2001.[53] Another report estimated 700,000 cases of egg-borne salmonellosis in the United States, accounting for approximately 47% of total food-borne salmonellosis and costing more than $1 billion annually.[47] Approximately 65 billion shell eggs are sold annually in the United States,[54] with a per capita consumption of approximately 254 eggs per year. Hence, undercooked *Salmonella*-contaminated eggs are a major hazard to human health. Egg contamination with *S.* Enteritidis results by penetration through the eggshell from contaminated chicken feces during or after oviposition.[55–57] Contamination of egg contents (yolk, albumen, and eggshell membranes) may also occur by transmission of the pathogen from infected ovaries or oviducts by the transovarian route before oviposition.[58–60]

Salmonella Typhi is the causative agent of typhoid fever, a serious human disease. Typhoid fever has a long incubation period of 7 to 28 days, and is characterized by prolonged and spiking fever, abdominal pain, diarrhea, and headache.[37] The disease can be diagnosed by isolating the pathogen from urine, blood, or stool specimens of affected persons. In 2003, 356 cases of typhoid fever were reported in the United States.[61] *S.* Typhi is an uncommon cause of food-borne illness in the United States, with approximately 74% of these cases occurring in persons who traveled internationally, especially to South Asia, 6 weeks preceding the disease appearance.[61]

CAMPYLOBACTER SPECIES

The genus *Campylobacter* consists of 14 species; however, *C. jejuni* subsp. *jejuni* and *C. coli* are the dominant food-borne pathogens. *C. jejuni* is a slender, rod-shaped, microaerophilic bacterium that requires approximately 3 to 6% oxygen for growth.

It can be differentiated from *C. coli* by its ability to hydrolyze hippurate.[62] The organism does not survive well in the environment, being sensitive to drying, highly acidic conditions, and freezing. It is also readily killed in foods by adequate cooking.[63]

C. jejuni is the most commonly reported bacterial cause of food-borne infection in the United States,[63–65] with the highest incidence in Hawai.[66] Many animals including poultry, swine, cattle, sheep, horses, and domestic pets, harbor *C. jejuni* in their intestinal tracts, hence serving as sources of human infection. However, chickens serve as the most common reservoir of *C. jejuni*, where the bacterium primarily colonizes the mucus overlying the epithelial cells in the ceca and small intestine. L-Fucose, the major carbohydrate component present in the mucin of chicken cecal mucus is used by *C. jejuni* as a sole substrate for growth.[67,68] Thus, the cecal environment in chickens is favorable for the survival and proliferation of *C. jejuni*,[67] and selects colonization of *C. jejuni* in the birds. Although a number of vehicles such as beef, pork, eggs, and untreated water have been implicated in outbreaks of campylobacter enteritis, chicken and unpasteurized milk are reported as the most commonly involved foods.[69] Epidemiologic investigations have revealed a significant link between human *Campylobacter* infection, and handling or consumption of raw or undercooked poultry meat.[70–74] Since colonization of broiler chickens by *C. jejuni* results in horizontal transmission of the pathogen and carcass contamination during slaughter, a variety of approaches for reducing its cecal carriage by chickens has been undertaken. These approaches include competitive exclusion microorganisms,[75] feeding birds with bacteriophages,[76,77] and acidified feed,[78] and vaccination.[79,80] In the United States, an increasing number of fluoroquinolone-resistant (e.g., ciprofloxacin) human *Campylobacter* infections has been reported,[81] and this is attributed to the use of this antibiotic in poultry production.[82]

Usually *Campylobacter enteritis* in humans is a self-limiting illness characterized by abdominal cramps, diarrhea, headache, and fever lasting up to 4 days. However, severe cases, involving bloody diarrhea and abdominal pain mimicking appendicitis, also occur.[62] Guillain-Barre syndrome (GBS) is an infrequent sequela to *Campylobacter* infection in humans.[83] GBS is characterized by acute neuromuscular paralysis[63] and is estimated to occur in approximately 1 of every 1000 cases of *Campylobacter* enteritis.[84] A few strains of *C. jejuni* reportedly produce a heat-labile enterotoxin similar to that produced by *Vibrio cholerae* and enterotoxigenic *E. coli*.[62] Some strains of *C. jejuni* and *C. coli* can also produce a cytolethal distending toxin, which causes a rapid and specific cell cycle arrest in HeLa and Caco-2 cells.[85]

SHIGELLA SPECIES

Shigella is a common cause of human diarrhea in the United States. The genus *Shigella* is divided into four major groups: *S. dysenteriae* (group A), *S. flexneri* (group B), *S. boydii* (group C), and *S. sonnei* (group D) based on the organism's somatic (O) antigen. Although all four groups have been involved in human infections, *S. sonnei* accounts for more than 75% of shigellosis cases in humans,[86] and has been linked to persistent infections in community and day-care centers.[87–89] Humans are the natural reservoir of *Shigella* spp. The fecal–oral route is the primary mode of transmission of shigellae and proper personal hygiene and sanitary practices of cooks and food handlers can greatly reduce the occurrence of outbreaks of shigellosis. Most food-borne outbreaks of shigellosis are associated with ingestion of foods such as salads and water contaminated with human feces containing the pathogen. Shigellosis is characterized by diarrhea containing bloody mucus, which lasts 1 to 2 weeks. The infectious dose for *Shigella* infection is low. The ID_{50} of *S. flexneri* and *S. sonnei* in humans is approximately 5000 microorganisms and that of *S. dysenteriae* is a few hundred cells, hence secondary transmission of *Shigella* by person-to-person contact frequently occurs in outbreaks of food-borne illness. A new and emerging serotype of *S. boydii*, namely serotype 20 has been reported in the United States.[90]

YERSINIA ENTEROCOLITICA

Yersinia enterocolitica is a gram-negative, rod-shaped, facultative anaerobic bacterium, which was first isolated and described during the 1930s.[91] Swine have been identified as an important reservoir of *Yersinia enterocolitica*, in which the pathogen colonizes primarily the buccal cavity.[92] Although pork and pork products are considered to be the primary vehicles of *Y. enterocolitica*, a variety of other foods, including milk, beef, lamb, seafood, and vegetables, has been identified as vehicles of *Y. enterocolitica* infection.[93] One of the largest outbreaks of yersiniosis in the United States was associated with milk.[94] Water has also been a vehicle of several outbreaks of *Y. enterocolitica* infection.[94] Surveys have revealed that *Y. enterocolitica* is frequently present in foods, having been isolated from 11% of sandwiches, 15% of chilled foods, and 22% of raw milk in Europe.[95] Several serovars of pathogenic *Y. enterocolitica* have been reported, which include O:3, O:5, O:8, and O:9,[96,97] with serovar 0:3 being common in the United States.[98–100] In addition to food-borne outbreaks, reports of blood transfusion-associated *Y. enterocolitica* sepsis indicate another potential mode of transmission of this pathogen.[101,102] Among bacteria, *Y. enterocolitica* has emerged as a significant cause of transfusion-associated bacteremia and mortality (53%), with 49 cases reported since this condition was first documented in 1975.[103] A review of these cases revealed that bacteremia may occur in a subpopulation of individuals with *Y. enterocolitica* gastrointestinal infection.[96] The strains of *Y. enterocolitica* responsible for transfusion-acquired yersiniosis are the same serobiotypes as those associated with enteric infections.

An unusual characteristic of *Y. enterocolitica* that influences food safety is its ability to grow at low temperatures, even as low as $-1°C$.[104] *Y. enterocolitica* readily withstands freezing and can survive in frozen foods for extended periods, even after repeated freezing and thawing.[105] Refrigeration (4°C) is one of the common methods used in food processing to control growth of spoilage and pathogenic microorganisms in foods. However, several studies have revealed growth of *Y. enterocolitica* in foods stored at refrigeration temperature. *Y. enterocolitica* grew on pork, chicken, and beef at 0 to 1°C.[106,107] The psychrotrophic nature of *Y. enterocolitica* also poses problems for the blood transfusion industry, mainly because of its ability to proliferate and release endotoxin in blood products stored at 4°C without manifesting any alterations in their physical appearance. The ability of *Y. enterocolitica* to grow well at refrigeration temperature has been exploited for isolating the pathogen from foods, water, and stool specimens. Such samples are incubated at 4 to 8°C in an enrichment broth for several days to selectively culture *Y. enterocolitica* based on its psychrotrophic nature.

Y. enterocolitica is primarily an intestinal pathogen with a predilection for extra-intestinal spread under appropriate host conditions such as immunosuppression. In the gastrointestinal tract, *Y. enterocolitica* can cause acute enteritis, enterocolitis, mesenteric lymphadenitis, and terminal ileitis often mimicking appendicitis.[96] Infection with *Y. enterocolitica* often leads to secondary, immunologically induced sequelae such as arthritis (most common), erythema nodosum, Reiter's syndrome, glomerulonephritis, and myocarditis.

VIBRIO SPECIES

Seafoods form a vital part of the American diet, and their consumption in the United States has risen steadily over the past few decades from an average of 4.5 kg per person in 1960 to about 7 kg in 2002.[108,109] However, according to a recent report published by the Center for Science in the Public Interest, contaminated seafoods have been recognized as a leading known cause of most food-borne illness outbreaks in the United States.[110] Vibrios, especially *V. parahaemolyticus*, *V. vulnificus*, and *V. cholerae*, which are commonly associated with estuarine and marine waters, represent the major pathogens resulting in disease outbreaks through consumption of seafoods. *V. parahaemolyticus* and *V. vulnificus* are halophilic in nature, requiring the presence of 1 to 3% sodium chloride for optimum growth. *V. cholerae* can grow in media without added salt, although their growth is stimulated by the presence of sodium ions.

Among the three species of *Vibrio*, *V. parahaemolyticus* accounts for the highest number of food-borne diseases outbreaks in the United States. *V. parahaemolyticus* is present in coastal waters of the United States and throughout the world. *V. parahaemolyticus* being an obligate halophile, can multiply in substrates with sodium chloride concentrations ranging from 0.5 to 10%, with 3% being the optimal concentration for growth. The ability of *V. parahaemolyticus* to grow in a wide range of salt concentrations reflects on its existence in aquatic environments with various salinities. *V. parahaemolyticus* has a remarkable ability for rapid growth, and generation times as short as 12 to 18 min in seafoods have been reported at 30°C. Growth rates at lower temperatures are slower, but counts were found to increase from 10^2 to 10^8 CFU/g after 24 h storage at 25°C in homogenized shrimp, and from 10^3 to 10^8 CFU/g after 7 days of storage at 12°C in homogenized oysters.[111] Because of its rapid growth, proper refrigeration of cooked seafoods to prevent regrowth of the bacterium is critical to product safety. A survey by the U.S. FDA revealed that 86% of 635 seafood samples contained *V. parahaemolyticus*, being isolated from clams, oysters, lobsters, scallops, shrimp, fish, and shellfish.[112] A new serotype of *V. parahaemolyticus*, O3:K6 that emerged in Southeast Asia in the 1990s, has been implicated in oyster-related outbreaks in the United States in 1997 and 1998.[113] An important virulence characteristic of pathogenic strains of *V. parahaemolyticus* is their ability to produce a thermostable hemolysin (Kanagawa hemolysin).[114] Studies in humans on the infectious dose of pathogenic *V. parahaemolyticus* strains revealed that ingestion of approximately 10^5 to 10^7 organisms can cause gastroenteritis.[112]

V. cholerae serovars O1 and O139, the causative agents of cholera in humans, are a part of the normal estuarine microflora, and foods such as raw fish, mussels, oysters, and clams have been associated with outbreaks of cholera.[115] Infected humans can serve as short-term carriers, shedding the pathogen in feces. Cholera is characterized by profuse diarrhea, potentially fatal in severe cases, and often described as "rice water" diarrhea due to the presence of prolific amounts of mucus in the stools. Gastroenteritis caused by non-O1 and non-O139 serovars of *V. cholerae* is usually mild in nature. During the period from 1996 to 2005, a total of 64 cases of toxigenic *V. cholerae* O1 were reported in the United States, of which 35 (55%) cases, were acquired during foreign travel and 29 (45%) cases were domestically acquired.[116] Seven (24%) of the 29 domestic cases were attributed to consumption of Gulf Coast seafood (crabs, shrimp, or oysters). Moreover, 7 of the 11 domestic cholera cases in 2005 were reported during October to December, after Hurricanes Katrina and Rita, although no evidence suggests increased risk for cholera among Gulf Coast residents or consumers of Gulf Coast seafood after the hurricanes. In 2003, a total of 111,575 cases of cholera worldwide were reported to the World Health Organization from 45 countries.[117]

V. vulnificus is the most serious of the vibrios and is responsible for most of the seafood-associated deaths in the United States, especially in Florida.[112] *V. vulnificus* results in life threatening bacteremia, septicemia, and necrotizing fasciitis in person with liver disorders and high iron level in blood.[118] Although a number of seafoods has been associated with *V. vulnificus* infection, raw oysters are the most common vehicle associated with cases of illness.[119]

ENTEROBACTER SAKAZAKII

Enterobacter sakazakii is an emerging food-borne pathogen that causes severe meningitis, meningo-encephalitis, sepsis, and necrotizing enterocolitis in neonates and infants.[120–123] The epidemiology and reservoir of this pathogen are still unknown and most strains have been isolated from clinical specimens such as cerebrospinal fluid, blood, skin, wounds, urine, and respiratory and digestive tract samples.[124] The bacterium has also been isolated from foods such as cheese, minced beef, sausage, and vegetables.[125] Recently, Kandhai et al.[126,127] isolated *E. sakazakii* from household and food production facility environmental samples, such as scrapings from dust, vacuum cleaner bags, and spilled product near equipment, and proposed that the bacterium could be more widespread in the environment than previously thought. Although the environmental source of *E. sakazakii* has not been identified, epidemiological studies implicate dried infant formula as the route of transmission to preterm infants.[123,128–130] The bacterium has been isolated from powdered infant formula by numerous investigators.[129,131–133] Muytjens and coworkers[133] isolated the pathogen from powdered infant formula from 35 different countries.

E. sakazakii possesses several characteristics that enable it to grow and survive in infant formula. For example, the bacterium can grow at temperatures as low as 5.5°C,[134] which is within the temperature range of many home refrigerators.[135] A study on the thermal resistance of *E. sakazakii* in reconstituted infant formula indicated that it is one of most thermotolerant bacteria within the family Enterobacteriaceae.[136] A recent study by Breeuwer et al.[137] revealed that *E. sakazakii* also has a high tolerance to osmotic stress and desiccation. In addition, *E. sakazakii* possesses a short lag time and generation time in reconstituted infant formula,[134] whereby improper temperature storage of reconstituted formula may permit its substantial growth. Recently, Iversen and Forsythe[138] reported the isolation of *E. sakazakii* from a variety of foods, including powdered infant formula, dried infant food, and milk powder as well as certain herbs and spices. The first case of neonatal meningitis caused by *E. sakazakii* was reported in 1958,[139] and since then a number of *E. sakazakii* infections in neonates have been reported worldwide, including the United States. In the United States, an outbreak of *E. sakazakii* infection involving four preterm infants occurred in the neonatal intensive care unit of a hospital in Memphis, resulting in sepsis, bloody diarrhea, and intestinal colonization. The source of infection was traced to contaminated infant formula that was termperature abused after reconstitution.[129] In 2002, Himelright et al.[140] reported a case of fatal neonatal meningitis caused by *E. sakazakii* in Tennessee, associated with feeding of contaminated infant formula that was temperature abused following reconstitution. The infection occurred in the neonatal intensive care unit of a hospital and surveillance studies identified two more cases of suspected infection with positive stool or urine in seven more infants. There were many recalls of *E. sakazakii*-contaminated infant formula in the United States. In November 2002, a nationwide recall of more than 1.5 million cans of dry infant formula contaminated with *E. sakazakii* was reported.[141] On April 9, 2002, the FDA issued an alert to U.S. health-care professionals regarding the risk associated with *E. sakazakii* infections among neonates-fed milk-based, powdered-infant formula. The International Commission on Microbiological Specification for Foods classified *E. sakazakii* as a "severe hazard for restricted populations, life threatening or substantial chronic sequelae of long duration," specifically for preterm infants. This places *E. sakazakii* along with other serious food- and water-borne pathogens such as *Listeria monocytogenes*, *Clostridium botulinum* types A and B, and *Cryptosporidium parvum*.[142]

The most common clinical manifestations of infections due to *E. sakazakii* are sepsis and meningitis in neonates. In more than 90% of the cases reported, patients developed meningitis with a very high prevalence for developing brain abscesses, and less frequently ventriculitis and hydrocephalus.[143,144] While the reported mortality rates of *E. sakazakii* infections in neonates has declined over time from 50% or more to less than 20% due to advances in antimicrobial chemotherapy, an increasing incidence of resistance to commonly used antibiotics necessitates a reevaluation of existing treatment strategies.[124] Biering et al.[131] indicated that besides the high rate of mortality, the central nervous system (CNS) infections due to *E. sakazakii* often lead to permanent impairment in mental and physical capabilities in surviving patients. In addition to meningitis, *E. sakazakii* is also reported to cause necrotizing enterocolitis in neonates, and rarely bacteremia, osteomyelitis, and pneumonia in elderly adults.[122,123,145,146]

AEROMONAS HYDROPHILA

Although *Aeromonas* species have been recognized as pathogens of cold-blooded animals, their potential to cause human infections, especially food-borne illness, received attention only recently. *A. hydrophila* has been isolated from drinking water, fresh and saline waters, and sewage.[147] It also has been isolated from a variety of foods such as fish, oyster, shellfish, raw milk, ground beef, chicken, and pork.[147] Although *A. hydrophila* is sensitive to highly acidic conditions and does not possess any unusual thermal resistance, some strains are psychrotrophic and grow at refrigeration temperature.[148] *A. hydrophila* can grow on a variety of refrigerated foods, including pork, asparagus, cauliflower, and broccoli.[149,150] However, considering the widespread occurrence of *A. hydrophila* in water and food and its relatively infrequent association with human illness, it is likely that most strains of this bacterium are not pathogenic for humans. *A. hydrophila* infection in humans is characterized by watery diarrhea and mild fever. Virulent strains of *A. hydrophila* produce a 52-kDa polypeptide, which possesses enterotoxic, cytotoxic, and hemolytic activities.[151]

PLESIOMONAS SHIGELLOIDES

P. shigelloides has been implicated in several cases of sporadic and epidemic gastroenteritis.[152] The pathogen is present in fresh and estuarine waters, and has been isolated from various aquatic animals.[148] Seafoods such as fish, crabs, and oysters have been associated with cases of *P. shigelloides* infection. The most common symptoms of *P. shigelloides* infection include abdominal pain, nausea, chills, fever, and diarrhea. Potential virulence factors of *P. shigelloides* include cytotoxic enterotoxin, invasins, and β-hemolysin.[148] An outbreak of *P. shigelloides* infection linked to well water and involving 30 persons was reported in New York in 1996.[153]

LISTERIA MONOCYTOGENES

Listeria monocytogenes has emerged into a significant food-borne pathogen throughout the world, especially in the United States. There are an estimated 2500 cases of listeriosis annually in the United States, with a mortality rate of ≈25%.[1] Further, *L. monocytogenes* is of economic significance, causing an estimated monetary loss of $2.3 billion annually in the United States.[154] A large outbreak of listeriosis involving more than 100 cases and associated with eating contaminated turkey frankfurters occurred during 1998 to 1999.[155] During this period of time there were more than 35 recalls of a number of different food products contaminated with listeriae.[155] In 2002, a large outbreak of listeriosis in the United States involving 46 people, 7 deaths, and 3 miscarriages, resulted in a recall of 27.4 million pounds of fresh and frozen ready-to-eat chicken and turkey products.[156] In 2003, 696 cases of listeriosis were reported in the United States, with more than 50% of the cases occurring in persons above 60 years of age.[61]

L. monocytogenes is widespread in nature, occurring in soil, vegetation, and untreated water. Humans and a wide variety of farm animals, including cattle, sheep, goat, pig, and poultry, are known sources of *L. monocytogenes*.[157,158] *L. monocytogenes* also occurs frequently in food processing facilities, especially in moist areas such as floor drains, floors, and processing equipment.[159] *L. monocytogenes* can also grow in biofilms attached to a variety of processing plant surfaces such as stainless steel, glass, and rubber.[160] A wide spectrum of foods, including milk, cheese, beef, pork, chicken, seafoods, fruits, and vegetables, has been identified as vehicles of *L. monocytogenes*.[158] However, ready-to-eat cooked foods such as low-acid soft cheese, pâtes, and cooked poultry meat, which can support the growth of listeriae to large populations (>10^6 cells/g) when held at refrigeration temperature for several weeks, have been regarded as high-risk foods.[161,162] *L. monocytogenes* possesses several characteristics which enable the pathogen to successfully contaminate, survive, and grow in foods, thereby resulting in outbreaks. These traits include an ability to grow at refrigeration temperature and in a medium with minimal nutrients, to survive in acidic conditions, for example, pH 4.2, to tolerate up to 10% sodium chloride, to survive incomplete cooking or subminimal pasteurization treatments, and to survive in biofilm on equipment in food processing plants and resist superficial cleaning and disinfection treatments.[155]

Approximately 3 to 10% of humans carry listeriae in their gastrointestinal tract with no symptoms of illness.[163] Human listeriosis is an uncommon illness with a high mortality rate. The infection most frequently occurs in people who are older, pregnant, or immune compromised. Clinical manifestations range from mild influenza-like symptoms to meningitis, and meningoencephalitis. Pregnant females infected with the pathogen may not present symptoms of illness or may exhibit only mild influenza-like symptoms. However, spontaneous abortion, premature birth, or stillbirth are frequent sequela to listeriosis in pregnant females.[162] Although the infective dose of *L. monocytogenes* in not known, published reports indicate that it is likely to be more than 100 CFU/g of food.[162] However, the infective dose depends on the age, condition of health, and immunological status of the host.

L. monocytogenes crosses the intestinal barrier in hosts infected by the oral route. However, before reaching the intestine, the bacterium must withstand the adverse environment of the stomach. Gastric acidity may destroy a substantial number of *L. monocytogenes* ingested with contaminated food. The site at which intestinal translocation of *L. monocytogenes* occurs is not clearly elucidated. However, both epithelial cells and M cells in the Peyer's patches are believed to be the potential sites of entry.[164] The bacteria are then internalized by macrophages where they survive and replicate. This is followed by transport of the pathogen via blood to the mesenteric lymph nodes, spleen, and the liver. The primary site of *L. monocytogenes* replication in the liver is the hepatocyte. In the initial phase of infection, the infected hepatocytes are the target for neutrophils, and subsequently for mononuclear phagocytes, which aid in the control and resolution of the infection.[162] If the immune system fails to contain *L. monocytogenes*, subsequent propagation of pathogen via blood to the brain or uterus takes place.[165] The major virulence factors in *L. monocytogenes* include hemolysin, phospholipases, metalloprotease, Clp proteases and APTases, internalins, surface protein p104, protein p60, listeriolysin O, and the surface protein *ActA*.[162]

STAPHYLOCOCCUS AUREUS

A preformed, heat-stable enterotoxin produced by *S. aureus* that can resist boiling for several minutes is the agent responsible for staphylococcal food poisoning. Humans are the principal reservoir of *S. aureus* strains involved in outbreaks of food-borne illness.

In addition, a recent study revealed that *S. aureus* can be transmitted between healthy, lactating mothers without mastitis and their infants by breast-feeding.[166] Colonized humans can be long-term carriers of *S. aureus*, and thereby contaminate foods and other humans.[167] The bacterium commonly resides in the throat and nasal cavity, and on the skin, especially in boils and carbuncles.[167] Protein-rich foods such as ham, poultry, fish, dairy products, custards, cream-filled bakery products, and salads containing cooked meat, chicken, or potatoes are the vehicles most frequently associated with *S. aureus* food poisoning.[168] *S. aureus* is usually overgrown by competing bacterial flora in raw foods, hence raw foods are not typical vehicles of staphylococcal food poisoning. Cooking eliminates most of the normal bacterial flora of raw foods thereby enabling the growth of *S. aureus*, which can be introduced by infected cooks and food handlers into foods after cooking. The incubation period of staphylococcal food poisoning is very short, with symptoms being observed within 2 to 6 h after eating toxin-contaminated food. Symptoms include nausea, vomiting, diarrhea, and abdominal pain.

S. aureus can grow in media within a wide range of pH values from 4 to 9.3, with optimum growth occurring at pH 6 to 7. *S. aureus* has an exceptional tolerance to sodium chloride being able to grow in foods in the presence of 7 to 10% NaCl, with some strains tolerating up to 20% NaCl.[168] *S. aureus* also has the unique ability to grow at a water activity as low as 0.83 to 0.86.[169] *S. aureus* produces nine different enterotoxins which are quite heat resistant, losing their serological activity at 121°C, but not at 100°C for several minutes.[169]

Besides being a food-borne pathogen, *S. aureus* has emerged as an important pathogen in nosocomial infections and community-acquired diseases, because of its toxin-mediated virulence, invasiveness, and antibiotic resistance.[170] This is especially significant due to the emergence of methicillin-resistant strains of *S. aureus* (MRSA), and 50% of health-care-acquired *S. aureus* isolates in the United States in 1997 were methicillin resistant.[171] Although MRSA is commonly linked to nosocomial infections, the first report of MRSA-associated food-borne disease in a community was reported in 2002.[171]

CLOSTRIDIUM BOTULINUM

Food-borne botulism is an intoxication caused by ingestion of foods containing preformed botulinal toxin, which is produced by *C. botulinum* under anaerobic conditions. Botulinal toxin is a neurotoxin, which causes the neuroparalytic disease called botulism. The toxin binds irreversibly to the presynaptic nerve endings of the nervous system, where it inhibits the release of acetylcholine. Unlike botulism in adults, infant botulism results from the colonization and germination of *C. botulinum* spores in the infant's gastrointestinal tract. The disease usually occurs in infants during the second month of age, and is characterized by constipation, poor feeding or sucking, and decreased muscle tone with a "floppy" head.[172] Although the source of infection is unknown in most cases, the most commonly suspected food in infant botulism is honey.[173]

There are seven types of *C. botulinum* (A, B, C, D, E, F, and G) which are classified on the basis of the antigenic specificity of the neurotoxin they produce.[174] The bacterium is present in soil, vegetation, and sedimentation under water. Type A strains are proteolytic, whereas type E strains are nonproteolytic.[175] Another classification divides *C. botulinum* into four groups: group I (type A strains and proteolytic strains of types B and F), group II (type E strains and nonproteolytic strains of B and F), group III (type C and D strains), and group IV (type G strains). Types A, B, E, and F are associated with botulism in humans. Type A *C. botulinum* occurs frequently in soils of the western United States, whereas type B strains are more often present in the eastern states and in Europe.[175] Type E strains are largely associated with aquatic environments and fish. Foods most often associated with cases of botulism include fish, meat, honey, and home-canned vegetables.[174] Type A cases of botulism in the United States are frequently associated with temperature-abused, home-prepared canned foods. Proteolytic type A, B, and F strains produce heat-resistant spores, which pose a safety concern in low-acid canned foods. In contrast, nonproteolytic type B, E, and F strains produce heat-labile spores, which are of concern in pasteurized or unheated foods.[175] The minimum pH for growth of groups I and II strains is 4.6 and 5, respectively.[174] Group I strains can grow at a minimum water activity of 0.94, whereas group II strains do not grow below a water activity of 0.97.[176] The proteolytic strains of *C. botulinum* are generally more resistant to heat than nonproteolytic strains.

CLOSTRIDIUM PERFRINGENS

C. perfringens is a major bacterial cause of food-borne disease, with 1062 cases reported in the United States in 2004.[3] *C. perfringens* strains are grouped into five types: A, B, C, D, and E, based on the type(s) of toxin(s) produced. *C. perfringens* food-borne illness is almost exclusively associated with type A isolates. *C. perfringens* is commonly present in soil, dust, water, and in the intestinal tract of humans and animals.[177] It is frequently present in foods; about 50% of raw or frozen meat and poultry contain *C. perfringens*.[178] Spores produced by *C. perfringens* are quite heat resistant, and can survive boiling for up to 1 h.[178] *C. perfringens* spores can survive in cooked foods and if not properly cooled before refrigerated storage, the spores will germinate and vegetative cells can grow to large cell numbers during holding at growth temperatures. Large populations of *C. perfringens* cells ($>10^6$/g) ingested with contaminated food will enter the small intestine, multiply and sporulate. During sporulation in the small intestine *C. perfringens* enterotoxin is produced which induces a diarrheal response. The enterotoxin is a 35-kDa heat-labile polypeptide that damages the epithelial cells of the gastrointestinal tract to cause fluid and electrolyte loss.[179,180]

Although vegetative cells of *C. perfringens* are sensitive to cold temperature and freezing, spores tolerate cold temperature well and can survive in refrigerated foods.

BACILLUS CEREUS

Bacillus cereus is a spore-forming pathogen present in soil and on vegetation. It is responsible for a growing number of food-borne illnesses in the industrial countries,[181] with 103 outbreak-associated confirmed cases reported in the United States in 2004.[3] It is frequently isolated from foods such as meat, spices, vegetables, dairy products, and cereal grains, especially fried rice.[182] There are two types of food-borne illness caused by *B. cereus*, that is, a diarrheagenic illness and an emetic syndrome.[181,183] The diarrheal syndrome, caused by heat-labile enterotoxins, is usually mild in its course and is characterized by abdominal cramps, nausea, and watery stools. Types of foods implicated in outbreaks of diarrheal syndrome include cereal food products containing corn and corn starch, mashed potatoes, vegetables, milk, and cooked meat products. The emetic syndrome, caused by a heat-stable peptide toxin,[181] is more severe and acute in its course, characterized by severe vomiting. Refried or rewarmed boiled rice, pasta, noodles, and pastry are frequently implicated vehicles in outbreaks of emetic syndrome.[184] The dose of *B. cereus* required to produce diarrheal illness is estimated at more than 10^5 cells/g.[185]

BRUCELLA SPECIES

Brucella spp. are pathogens in many animals, causing sterility and abortion. In humans, *Brucella* is the etiologic agent of undulant fever. The genus *Brucella* consists of six species, of which those of principal concern are *B. abortus*, *B. suis*, and *B. melitensis*.[186] *B. abortus* causes disease in cattle, *B. suis* in swine, and *B. melitensis* is the primary pathogen of sheep. *B. melitensis* is the most pathogenic species for humans. Human brucellosis is primarily an occupational disease of veterinarians and meat industry workers. Brucellosis can be transmitted by aerosols and dust. Food-borne brucellosis can be transmitted to humans by consumption of meat and milk products from infected farm animals. The most common food vehicle of brucellosis for humans is unpasteurized milk.[186] Meat is a less common source of food-borne brucellosis, because the bacteria are destroyed by cooking. Since the National Brucellosis Education program has almost eradicated *B. abortus* infection from U.S. cattle herds, the risk of food-borne infection of brucellosis through consumption of domestically produced milk and dairy products is minimal.[61]

HELICOBACTER PYLORI

H. pylori is a human pathogen causing chronic gastritis, gastric ulcer, and gastric carcinoma.[187,188] Although, humans are the primary host of *H. pylori*, the bacterium has been isolated from cats.[161] *H. pylori* does not survive well outside its host, but it has been detected in water and vegetables.[189,190] A study on the effect of environmental and substrate factors on the growth of *H. pylori* indicated that the pathogen likely lacks the ability to grow in most foods.[191] However, *H. pylori* may survive for long periods in low-acid environments under refrigerated conditions. *H. pylori* infections spread primarily by person-to-person transmission, especially among children, and contaminated water and food are considered potential vehicles of the pathogen. In the United States, a significant association between *H. pylori* infection and iron deficiency/anemia, regardless of the presence or absence of peptic ulcer, has been reported.[192,193]

VIRAL FOOD-BORNE PATHOGENS

Estimates by the Centers for Disease Control and Prevention of the incidence of food-borne illness in the United States indicate that viruses are responsible for approximately 67% of the total food-borne illnesses of known etiology annually (Table 2.2).[1] Viruses are obligate intracellular microbes and most food-borne viruses contain RNA rather than DNA. Since viruses are intracellular, requiring a host for multiplication, they cannot grow in foods. Therefore, the number of virus particles on foods will not increase during processing, transport, or storage, causing no deterioration in food quality.[194] Food-borne viruses are generally enteric in nature, causing illness through ingestion of foods and water contaminated with human feces. Viruses disseminated through foods also can be spread by person-to-person contact. For example, research with Hepatitis A virus has revealed that a few hundred virus particles can readily be transferred from fecally contaminated fingers to foods and surfaces.[195] Hepatitis A virus, Norovirus (previously known as Norwalk-like viruses) and possibly rotavirus are among the most significant of the viruses that are foodborne.

HEPATITIS A VIRUS

Hepatitis A virus is a member of the family *Picornaviridae* and is transmitted by the fecal-oral route. Raw shellfish harvested from waters contaminated by human sewage is among the foods most frequently associated with outbreaks of hepatitis A virus.[196] Besides shellfish, other foods including sandwiches, dairy products, baked products, salads, fruits, and vegetables have also been implicated in outbreaks of hepatitis A virus infection.[197,198] A large outbreak in Pennsylvania in 2003 involving

TABLE 2.2
Viral Food-Borne Pathogens

Microbe	Significant Characteristics	Sources/Reservoirs	Vehicles	Estimated No. of Food-Borne Cases Annually in the United States[121]	Incubation Period, Symptoms and Duration	Detection Methods	Control/Prevention
Hepatitis A virus	Single-stranded RNA virus, spherical in shape, remains viable for long periods of time in foods stored at refrigeration temperature, virus multiplies in the gut epithelium before being carried by blood to the liver. Virus is shed in feces before symptoms of liver damage become apparent	Humans, sewage-polluted waters	Raw or undercooked shellfish and seafoods harvested from sewage-polluted water, ready-to-eat foods such as salads prepared by infected food handler	4,170	15 to 45 days, usually ~25 days Loss of appetite, nausea, abdominal pain, fever, jaundice, dark urine, and pale stools Duration is a few weeks to months	Cultural methods[389,390] Enzyme immunoassay[391] PCR[392,393]	Avoid consumption of raw seafoods, disinfection of drinking water, good personal hygiene and food handling practices, vaccination of professional food handlers, safe sewage disposal
Norovirus	Single-stranded RNA virus, spherical in shape, does not multiply in any known laboratory host	Humans, sewage-polluted waters	Raw or undercooked shellfish and seafoods harvested from sewage polluted water, drinking water	9,200,000	1 to 2 days Loss of appetite, nausea, abdominal pain, diarrhea, vomiting, and headache Duration is 2 days	Enzyme immunoassay[394,395] PCR[396–398]	Avoid consumption of raw seafoods, disinfection of drinking water, good personal hygiene and food handling practices, hygienic sewage disposal, treatment of wastewater used for irrigation
Rotavirus	Double-stranded RNA virus, icosahedral in shape	Humans	To be determined	39,000	1 to 3 days Vomiting, abdominal pain followed by watery diarrhea Duration is 6 to 8 days	Cultural methods[389,390] ELISA[399,400] PCR[400–402] Flow cytometry[403,404]	Avoid consumption of raw seafoods Avoid drinking of untreated water, Good personal hygiene
Avian influenza virus	Single-stranded RNA virus, medium sized, pleomorphic, enveloped	Chicken, turkey, guinea fowl, and migratory waterfowl	Raw or undercooked contaminated egg and poultry meat	Emerging disease. Not reported in the United States 132 cases worldwide (1997–2005)	Typical flu symptoms such as fever, cough, sore throat, and muscle aches. Also eye infections (conjunctivitis), pneumonia, and acute respiratory distress can be present	Cultural method[204] Rapid antigen detection test[405] PCR[204] Serological test[204]	Properly cook poultry meat and eggs. Use pasteurized eggs for preparing foods that are not cooked Avoid handling infected birds or birds suspected of infection. Use hygienic practices during slaughter and post-slaughter operations. Keep hands away from face and wash hands following exposure to chickens and their feces

more than 500 cases was linked to ingestion of contaminated green onions.[199] Hepatitis A virus is more resistant to heat and drying than other picornaviruses.[196] The incubation period for onset of symptoms of hepatitis A infection ranges from 15 to 45 days, and symptoms include nausea, abdominal pain, jaundice, and fever. The virus is shed in feces by infected humans many days before the onset of symptoms, indicating the importance of good personal hygienic practices of cooks and food handlers who could otherwise contaminate food during the period of asymptomatic fecal shedding. The overall incidence of Hepatitis A virus infection in the United States has decreased since the implementation of routine childhood vaccination against the virus in 1996.[61]

NOROVIRUS

Noroviruses belong to the family *Calciviridae*, and are often referred to as small, round structured viruses. Norovirus is recognized as the most common viral cause of food-borne and waterborne acute gastroenteritis in the United States.[1] The virus has a low infectious dose of less than 100 virus particles.[200] Raw or undercooked shellfish and other seafoods are common vehicles of Norovirus. The incubation period of infection ranges from 24 to 48 h, and symptoms include nausea, vomiting, and diarrhea. Infected humans shed the virus in feces for up to a week after symptoms have subsided. The virus survives freezing, heating to 60°C, and chlorine levels up to 10 ppm.[200] Qualitative studies in human volunteers indicate that the viruses are infective for up to 3 h when exposed to a medium at pH 2.2 at room temperature or for 60 min at pH 7 at 60°C.[201]

ROTAVIRUS

Rotavirus is a nonenveloped, double-shelled virus, with a genome composed of 11 segments of double-stranded RNA. Rotavirus is the most common cause of diarrhea in children worldwide, especially in developing countries. In the United States and other countries with a temperate climate, infection with rotavirus has been reported to peak during the winter season (November to April). In the United States, there is an estimated 3.9 million cases of rotavirus diarrhea each year; however, only 39,000 cases are estimated to be acquired through contaminated foods.[1] Rotavirus infection has an incubation period of 1 to 3 days, and is characterized by fever, vomiting, and diarrhea. The virus is shed in the feces of infected humans and can survive on vegetables at 4 or 20°C for many days.[202] It also can survive the process of making soft cheese.[202] The primary mode of transmission of rotavirus is by the fecal to oral route. In 2006, the U.S. FDA approved a new live, oral vaccine (RotaTeq™) for the prevention of rotavirus gastroenteritis in infants.

AVIAN INFLUENZA VIRUS

Avian influenza (bird flu) is a highly contagious viral infection affecting many species of birds, including chickens, turkeys, guinea fowl, and migratory waterfowl. The disease is of tremendous economic significance to the poultry industry. Recent outbreaks of avian influenza infections in poultry and humans highlight the zoonotic potential of the disease, and its impact on public health.[203] During the period from 1997 to 2005, 132 human cases of avian influenza with 64 deaths have been reported worldwide.[204] Based on virulence, avian influenza virus is classified into the highly pathogenic avian influenza (HPAI) strains that cause a systemic lethal infection, resulting in death of birds as early as 24 h to 1 week post infection, and the low pathogenic avian influenza (LPAI) viruses that rarely result in fatal disease in birds.[205] The HPAI viruses that cause "fowl plague" are restricted to the subtypes H5 and H7; however all the viruses of these subtypes do not cause HPAI. H5N1 is the influenza A virus subtype that occurs mainly in birds, causing fatal disease in chickens and turkeys.

Avian influenza viruses belonging to the family Orthomyxoviridae, are medium sized, pleomorphic, enveloped viruses with glycoprotein projections from the envelope having hemagglutinating (HA) and neuraminidase (NA) activities.[206] The genome of the virus consists of eight segments of single-stranded RNA of a negative sense, which code for ten viral proteins. Antigenically, three distinct types of influenza viruses are reported, namely type A, type B, and type C, with the former type causing natural infections in birds. Based on the antigenic properties of hemagglutinin and neuraminidase surface glycoproteins, type A influenza viruses are divided into various subtypes.[207] Currently, 15 HA and 9 NA subtypes have been reported.[205]

The hemagglutinin glycoproteins play a vital role in the pathogenicity by mediating attachment of the virus to host cell receptors followed by release of viral RNA.[203] The HA glycoprotein precursor (HA0) is post-translationally cleaved into HA1 and HA2 subunits by host proteases, with the HA2 amino terminus mediating fusion between the viral envelope and the endosomal membrane.[208] Klenk and coworkers[209] reported that proteolytic activation of HA glycoprotein is essential for viral infectivity and dissemination, thus highlighting its role in the pathogenesis of avian influenza virus. The HA precursor proteins of LPAI viruses have a single arginine at the cleavage site, hence these viruses are limited to cleavage by host proteases such as trypsin-like enzymes. Therefore replication of LPAI viruses is limited to sites (organs) where such enzymes are found (respiratory and intestinal tracts), thereby resulting in mild infections. However, the HAs of HPAI viruses contain multiple basic amino acids at the cleavage site, which are cleaved by ubiquitous proteases present in a variety of host cells. These viruses therefore are able to replicate throughout the bird, causing lethal systemic infection and death.[210,211]

The source of infection to poultry in most outbreaks is direct or indirect contact with waterbirds. Once the infection is established in birds, the disease is highly contagious. Fecal-to-oral transmission is the most common mode of spread between birds. Contact with infected material is the most important mode of transmission from bird to bird. In infected birds, the virus is excreted in the droppings and nasal and ocular discharges. Fecal shedding of the virus by infected birds has been documented up to 4 weeks postinfection. Contaminated feed, water, rodents, and insects can also play a role in the spread of virus. Movement of infected birds, contaminated equipment, egg flats, feed truck, and service crew can also spread the virus from flock to flock. Airborne transmission of the virus can potentially occur if birds are kept in close proximity and with air movement. Since lesions have been reported in the ovaries and oviducts of infected egg-laying chickens, avian influenza virus could potentially be transmitted via the egg either through viruses in internal egg contents or on the surface of virus-contaminated feces.[212] This could potentially lead to hatching of infected chicks and contamination of the hatchery. Implementation of strict biosecurity measures can greatly reduce the risk of secondary spread after an initial outbreak.

Although humans can contract avian influenza virus by handling infected birds, there is no epidemiologic evidence to suggest transmission of the virus by consumption of properly cooked eggs or other cooked poultry products derived from infected birds. Cooking poultry meat to 160 degrees Fahrenheit (71°C) inactivates the virus.[204] Consumption of raw or partially cooked eggs (runny yolk) or foods containing raw eggs should be avoided.

FUNGAL FOOD-BORNE PATHOGENS

Molds are widely distributed in nature and are an inherent part of the microflora of foods (Table 2.3). Although molds are major spoilage agents of many foods, many molds also produce mycotoxins of which some are carcinogenic and mutagenic. Mycotoxins are secondary metabolites produced by molds usually at the end of their exponential phase of growth. Some of the principal species of molds which produce mycotoxins in foods include the following.

ASPERGILLUS SPECIES

Aspergillus flavus and *A. parasiticus* are the most important toxigenic food-borne aspergilli. A wide variety of foods such as nuts, corn, oil seeds, and sorghum are potential vehicles of these aspergilli. *A. flavus* and *A. parasiticus* produce aflatoxins, which are difuranocoumarin derivatives.[213] The common types of aflatoxins that are produced are B_1, B_2, G_1, and G_2.[214] In addition, two other types of aflatoxins, namely M1 and M2 have also been reported as contaminants of food, especially milk. Aflatoxicosis in animals can be acute or chronic. Acute cases are characterized by severe liver damage, whereas liver cirrhosis, liver cancer, and teratogenesis occur in chronic toxicity. Chronic intake of aflatoxins in animals can lead to poor feed conversion and low weight gain.

In humans, aflatoxins have been reported to cause hepatic cancer. A significant correlation between aflatoxin exposure and stunted growth has been reported in children exposed to aflatoxin during neonatal stages.[215] Additionally, since aflatoxins can cross the placental barrier, they can potentially lead to genetic defects in the fetus.[216] Following intake, aflatoxins are metabolized into a variety of products such as aflatoxicol, aflatoxin Q1, aflatoxin P1, and aflatoxin M1 in the liver by cytochrome p450 group of enzymes. In addition, another metabolite, called aflatoxin 8,9 epoxide, can be formed, which can induce mutations by forming DNA adducts, ultimately leading to hepatic carcinoma.[217–219] Susceptibility of a given species to aflatoxins depends on its liver detoxification systems, genetic make up, age and other nutritional factors.[220]

PENICILLIUM SPECIES

The genus *Penicillium* consists of more than 150 species, of which nearly 100 produce known toxins. Three important food-borne toxigenic *Penicillium* species include *P. verrucosum*, *P. expansum*, and *P. citrinum*. *P. verrucosum* is present on grains grown in temperate zones, and is commonly associated with Scandanavian barley and wheat.[221] *P. verrucosum* produces Ochratoxin A which has immunosuppressive and potential carcinogenic properties.[221] Ochratoxin A also has been associated with nephritis in pigs in Scandanavia.[222] *Pencillium expansum*, a psychrotrophic mold and one of the most common fruit pathogens, causes a condition known as "blue mold rot" on a variety of fruits, including apples, cherries, nectarines, and peaches.[223–226] Besides its economic impact, *P. expansum* is also of potential public health significance because it produces patulin, a mycotoxin known to cause immunological, neurological, and gastrointestinal toxic effects in animal models.[221] Exposure to high levels of patulin also results in vomiting, salivation, anorexia, polyapnea, weight loss, leukocytosis, erythropenia, and necrotic lesions of hemorrhagic enteritis in piglets.[227] Although the toxic effects of patulin in humans have not been proven conclusively, the presence of patulin has been demonstrated in apple juice[228] and grape juice.[229] This is a concern because fruit juices, especially apple juice, are commonly consumed by infants and children. *P. expansum* is commonly present in rotten apples and pears, and to a lesser extent in cereals. Use of moldy fruits contaminated with *P. expansum* greatly increases the risk of patulin contamination in fruit juices. An unusual characteristic of *P. expansum* is its ability to grow at low temperature, that is, −2 to −3°C.[221]

TABLE 2.3
Fungal Food-Borne Pathogens

Microbe/Toxin	Significant Characteristics	Sources/ Reservoirs of Fungi	Vehicles of Toxins	Toxic Effects	Detection Methods	Control/ Prevention
Aspergillus parasiticus and *Aspergillus flavus/* Aflatoxin	Growth at 10 to 43°C, optimal growth at 32°C, produces aflatoxins at 12 to 40°C, growth at pH 3 to 11	Environment, soil, vegetation	Corn, peanuts, cottonseed	Effects of aflatoxin in animals: Acute: hemorrhage in the gastrointestinal tract, liver damage, and death Chronic: cirrhosis of liver, liver tumors, and immunosuppression	Cultural methods[406-409] ELISA[410] Immunoassay[411,412] PCR[413-416]	Proper storage of cereal products
*Penicillium expansum/*Patulin; *Penicillium citrinum/* Citrinin	*P. expansum* is psychrotrophic, capable of growth at −2 to −3°C, optimal growth at 25°C	Environment, soil, vegetation	*P. expansum*: Fruits, especially apples and pears *P. citrinum*: Cereals, especially rice, wheat, corn	Effects of patulin: Gastrointestinal, neurological, and immunological effects in animals Citrinin: Fatty degeneration and renal necrosis in pigs and dogs; significance in human health is unresolved	Cultural methods[407,408,417] PCR[418,419] Detection of mycotoxin by HPLC [420,421] mass spectrometry[422]	Avoid consumption of rotten apples and pears, proper storage of cereal products
Fusarium graminearum/ Deoxynivalernol, nivalenol, zearalenone	Growth at 5°C but not at 37°C, optimal growth at 25°C	Environment, soil, vegetation	Cereals, especially wheat, barley and corn	Effects of deoxynivolenol: Nausea, vomiting, abdominal pain, diarrhea, headache, fever, chills, throat irritation	Cultural methods followed by morphology[423,424] PCR[425-429] Immunoassay[430] ELISA[431]	Proper storage of cereal products

P. citrin is a widely occurring mold commonly present on rice, wheat, and corn. *P. citrin* produces the metabolite citrinin. Although the toxicological effect of citrinin in humans is not known, it has been reported to cause renal toxicity in pigs and cats.[230]

FUSARIUM GRAMINEARUM

Fusarium graminearum is a toxigenic mold commonly present in soil and on cereals such as wheat and corn. It produces a number of mycotoxins, including deoxynevalenol and zearalenone.[231] Ingestion of foods containing deoxynevalenol produces illness termed Scabby grain intoxication, which is characterized by anorexia, nausea, vomiting, diarrhea, dizziness, and convulsions. Foods most frequently implicated as vehicles of deoxynevalenol include cereal grains, wheat, barley, and noodles.

PARASITIC FOOD-BORNE PATHOGENS

Parasitic diseases account for 3% of food-borne illnesses and 21% of food-borne illness-related deaths in the United States (Table 2.4).[1] However, the actual number of parasitic diseases could be higher, because they are often underdiagnosed and underreported in the United States.[232] Parasites constitute more of a food safety concern now than in the past, because of the globalization of our food supply with increased imports of fruits, vegetables, and ethnic foods from countries, where the hygienic and quality control standards in food production may be suboptimal. Foods can be vehicles of several types of parasites, including protozoa, roundworms, and flatworms. Although food-borne transmission of parasites such as *Trichinella spiralis* and *Taenia solium* has been known for many years, the food-borne disease potential of many protozoan parasites such as *Cryptosporidium* and *Cyclospora* has only recently been recognized. Unlike bacteria, parasites do not multiply in foods. Moreover, parasites need at least one specific host to complete their life cycle. Many of the well-recognized parasites that can be transmitted to humans through foods include the following.

GIARDIA LAMBLIA

Giardiasis is the most common parasitic infection reported in the United States, with 21,300 confirmed cases in 1997.[233] *G. lamblia* is a flagellated protozoan parasite that colonizes the intestinal tract of humans and animals. It is commonly present in lakes, rivers, and stagnated waters. The life cycle of *G. lamblia* includes flagellated trophozoites, which become pear-shaped cysts.[234] The cysts contaminate water or food through feces of infected animals or humans. Following ingestion of cyst-contaminated water or food, the trophozoites reach the small intestine where they undergo excystation and multiply by binary fission. New trophozoites subsequently become cysts in the distal small intestine, and the encysted trophozoites are shed in the feces. The symptoms of giardiasis include abdominal pain, abdominal distension, nausea, vomiting, and diarrhea. Although water and foods contaminated with cysts are primary vehicles of giardiasis, little is known about the survival characteristics of the cysts in foods. In most cases of food-borne transmission, infected food handlers transfer the cysts to foods they prepare. Humans can also contract giardiasis through the use of contaminated water for irrigating or washing fruits and vegetables.[235]

ENTAMOEBA HISTOLYTICA

Entamoeba histolytica is a protozoan parasite that causes amoebiasis or amoebic dysentery in humans. Although the parasite survives in the environment and water, humans are the principal source of amoebiasis. In humans, cysts containing the trophozites are released, which in turn multiply, and are subsequently excreted in the feces as cysts.[236] Foods and water contaminated with the cysts transmit the disease. Since the fecal-oral route is the principal route of transmission of amoebiasis, personal hygiene of infected food handlers plays a critical role in preventing food-borne amoebiasis. Human amoebiasis can occur in two forms: intestinal amoebiasis and amoebic liver abscess, which is usually a sequela to the intestinal form. Intestinal amoebiasis is characterized by abdominal pain, vomiting, and watery diarrhea containing mucus and blood. Symptoms of the hepatic form of amoebiasis include wasting, painful and enlarged liver, weight loss, and anemia. Amoebiasis is a common cause of diarrhea in tropical and subtropical countries, and most cases in the United States are reported in immigrants and persons returning from endemic areas.[235]

CRYPTOSPORIDIUM PARVUM

Cryptosporidium parvum is a protozoan parasite that infects a wide range of animals and humans. *C. parvum* is monoexenous in its life cycle, requiring only one host for its development.[234] Infected hosts shed in their feces oocysts of the parasite, sub–sequently contaminating the environment, food, and water. The life cycle of *C. parvum* can be summarized as follows.[234] Upon ingestion of contaminated water or food, or by inhalation of oocysts, sporozoites are released by excystation of oocysts into the gastrointestinal or respiratory tract. The sporozoites enter the epithelial cells and develop into trophozoites, which in turn differentiate into type I and type II meronts. The merzoites from type I meronts invade new tissues and develop into trophozoites to continue the life cycle. The merozoites from type II meronts invade infected cells, and undergo sexual multiplication to

TABLE 2.4
Parasitic Food-Borne Pathogens

Parasite	Significant Characteristics	Sources/Reservoirs	Vehicles	Estimated No. of Food-Borne Cases Annually in the United States[1]	Incubation Period, Symptoms and Duration	Detection Methods	Control/Prevention
Giardia lamblia	Flagellate protozoa, produces oval-shaped cysts ranging from 8 to 20 μm in length and 5 to 12 μm in width, cysts contain four nuclei and are resistant to chlorination used to disinfect water	Humans, animals, especially beavers and muskrats, water	Drinking water, raw fruits and vegetables contaminated with cysts, ready-to-eat foods such as salads contaminated by infected food handlers	200,000	4 to 25 days, usually 7 to 10 days Abdominal cramps, nausea, abdominal distension, diarrhea which can be chronic and relapsing, fatigue, weight loss, and anorexia Duration is weeks to years	Immuno-fluorescence[432] Immunochromatography[433,434] PCR[435-438]	Adequate cooking of foods, filtration of drinking water, good personal hygiene and food handling practices
Entamoeba histolytica	Amoeboid protozoa, anaerobe survives in environment in crypted form, cysts remain viable in feces for several days and in soil for at least 8 days at 30°C and for more than 1 month at 10°C, relatively resistant to chlorine	Humans, dogs, rats	Foods and water contaminated with feces or irrigation water	Unknown	2 to 4 weeks Abdominal pain, fever, vomiting, diarrhea containing blood and mucus, and weight loss Duration is weeks to months	Microscopic examination Line dot hybridization assay[439] ELISA[440,441] PCR[437,442]	Good personal hygiene and food-handling practices, adequate cooking of foods, filtration of water, hygienic disposal of sewage water, treatment of irrigation water
Cryptosporidium parvum	Obligate intracellular coccidian parasite, oocysts are spherical to oval in shape with an average size of 4.5 to 5.0 μm, oocysts are resistant to chlorination used to disinfect water	Humans, wild and domestic animals, especially calves	Contaminated drinking and recreational water, raw milk from infected cattle, fresh vegetables and other foods contaminated with feces from infected humans and animals	30,000	2 to 14 days Profuse, watery diarrhea, abdominal pain, nausea, and vomiting Duration is few days to 3 weeks	Immunofluorescence assay[443] PCR[444-447] Rapid assay[448]	Thorough cooking of food, avoid contact with infected animals, filtration of drinking water, good personal hygiene and food handling practices
Cyclospora cayetanensis	Obligate intracellular coccidian parasite, oocysts are spherical in shape with an average size of 8 to 10 μm	Humans	Water, fruits and vegetables contaminated with oocysts	14,600	1 week Watery diarrhea, abdominal pain, nausea, vomiting, anorexia, myalgia, and weight loss Duration is a few days to 1 month	Staining and microscopic examination[449] Flow cytometry[450] PCR[451-453]	Good personal hygiene, filtration of drinking water

Continued

TABLE 2.4 (Continued)

Parasite	Significant Characteristics	Sources/ Reservoirs	Vehicles	Estimated No. of Food-Borne Cases Annually in the United States[1]	Incubation Period, Symptoms and Duration	Detection Methods	Control/ Prevention
Toxoplasma gondii	Obligate intracellular coccidian protozoa	Cats, farm animals, transplacental transmission from infected mother to fetus	Raw or undercooked meat, raw goat milk, raw vegetables	112,500	5 to 23 days; Fever, rash, headache, muscle pain, swelling of lymph nodes; transplacental infection may cause abortion; Duration is variable	Cell culture and mouse inoculation[454], Immunoassay[455], Serologic assay[456], Immuno fluorescence[457], PCR[458-461]	Prevent environmental contamination with cat feces, avoid consumption of raw meat and milk, safe disposal of cat feces, wash hands after contact with cats
Trichinella spiralis	Nematode with no free living stage in the life cycle, adult female worms are 3 to 4 mm in length, transmissible form is larval cyst, which can occur in pork muscle	Wild and domestic animals, especially swine and horses	Raw or undercooked meat of animals containing encysted larvae such as swine or horses	50	Initial symptoms: 24 to 72 h, Systemic Symptoms: 8 to 21 days; Initial phase: Abdominal pain, fever, nausea, vomiting, and diarrhea; Systemic phase: Periorbital edema, eosinophilia, myalgia, difficulty in breathing, thirst, profuse sweating, chills, weakness, and prostration; Duration is 2 weeks to 3 months	Microscopic examination, ELISA[462-464], Immunoassay[465], PCR[466-468]	Adequate cooking of meat, freezing of meat at −15°C for 30 days or at −35°C, preventing trichinosis in pigs by not feeding swine garbage containing infected meat
Anisakis spp.	Nematode, slender thread-like parasite measuring 1.5 to 1.6 cm in length and 0.1 cm in diameter	Sea mammals	Some undercooked salt water fish, sushi, herring, sashimi, ceviche	Unknown	4 to 12 h; Epigastric pain, nausea, vomiting, sometimes hematemesis; Duration is variable	ELISA[469,470], Immunoblot[471], PCR[472-474]	Adequate cooking of saltwater fish, freezing fish at −23°C for 7 days
Taenia solium Taenia saginata	Tapeworm, dependent on the digestive system of the host for nutrition	Humans, cattle, swine	Raw or undercooked beef or pork	Unknown	Few days to >10 years; Nausea, epigastric pain, nervousness, insomnia, anorexia, weight loss, digestive disturbances, weakness, and dizziness; Duration is weeks to months	Detection of eggs or proglottids in feces, ELISA[475,476], PCR[477-479]	Adequate cooking of beef and pork, proper disposal of sewage and human wastes, freezing of meat at −10°C for 2 weeks
Diphyllobothrium latum	Largest human tapeworm	Saltwater fish, humans	Raw or undercooked saltwater fish	Unknown	Epigastric pain, nausea, abdominal pain, diarrhea, weakness, and pernicious anemia; Duration is months to years	Detection of eggs in feces	Adequate cooking of fish, proper disposal of sewage and human waste

give rise to male and female gametes. The zygotes resulting from fertilized gametes become infectious by sporulation, and the sporulated oocysts are excreted in feces.

Cryptosporidiosis is a self-limiting disease with an incubation period of 1 to 2 weeks, and is characterized by profuse, watery diarrhea, abdominal pain, vomiting, and low-grade fever. During the period from 1993 to 1998, seven major outbreaks of cryptosporidiosis have been reported in the United States.[235] Water is the most common source of *C. parvum* for human infections.[161] The largest outbreak of cryptosporidiosis (waterborne) in the United States occurred in Milwaukee, Wisconsin in 1993, involving more than 400,000 people with 69 deaths.[237,238] In addition to drinking water, water can also potentially contaminate produce when it is used for irrigating plants or washing fruits and vegetables. Oocysts of the pathogen have been detected in fresh vegetables, raw milk, sausage, and apple cider.[161] Infected food handlers can also transfer the oocysts to foods.[239,240] *C. parvum* oocysts are sensitive to freezing and freeze-drying. The oocysts lose infectivity in distilled water stored at 4°C.[241] However, the oocysts are quite resistant to chlorine; no loss in infectivity was observed in water containing 1 to 3% chlorine for up to 18 h.[242] However, the oocysts are sensitive to ozone, losing more than 90% infectivity in the presence of 1 ppm ozone for 5 min.[243]

CYCLOSPORA CAYETANENSIS

Cyclospora cayetanensis is an emerging foodborne, protozoan pathogen, especially in the United States. The parasite was implicated in several food-borne outbreaks in the United States during 1996 and 1997.[244] Water and foods, especially fruits and vegetables containing oocysts, are common vehicles of human infection.[235,245] During the period from 1996 to 2000, eight major outbreaks of cyclosporidiosis were reported, with imported raspberries as the vehicle of infection in 50% of the outbreaks.[235] Humans are the only identified reservoir of *C. cayetanensis*.[245] The symptoms of *C. cayetanensis* infection in humans include watery diarrhea, nausea, abdmonial pain, vomiting, and weight loss. Presently, there is very little information on the effects of heat, freezing, and disinfection agents on *Cyclospora* oocysts. Exposure of oocysts to –20°C for 24 h or 60°C for 1 h prevented oocysts from sporulating. Exposing oocysts to 4 or 37°C for 14 days delayed sporulation.[246]

TOXOPLASMA GONDII

Toxoplasma gondii is an obligate intracellular protozoan parasite for which cats are the definitive host. A survey on the prevalence of *T. gondii* in cats at spay or neuter clinics in Ohio revealed that 48% of the cats were infected with the parasite.[247] In the intestine of cats, the parasite undergoes sexual reproduction to form oocysts, which are excreted in feces.[248] The oocysts undergo maturation and survive in the environment for months, and spread by wind, insects and tapeworms. Toxoplasmosis in humans results following ingestion of food or water contaminated with oocysts. Transmission also occurs from an infected pregnant mother to child by transplacental transmission.[249] In the United States, *T. gondii* has been estimated to cause about 4000 congenital infections annually, potentially resulting in blindness, learning disabilities, and mental retardation in children.[232] *T. gondii* is also attributed as the leading cause of CNS infection in persons with AIDS.[250] Symptoms in healthy adults are usually mild, and include rash, headache, muscle pain, and swelling of lymph nodes. Although the oocysts can survive in refrigerated meat for weeks, they are inactivated by freezing at <12°C.[251] The oocysts are sensitive to irradiation and heat (>67°C). Properly cooked foods are not a vehicle of *T. gondii*.[252]

TRICHINELLA SPIRALIS

Trichinalla spiralis is a round worm that primarily infects wild and domestic animals, especially pigs. Humans contract trichinosis by consumption of raw or undercooked meat containing larvae of the parasite. Pigs are infected by consuming uncooked scraps of infected pork. The encysted larvae upon ingestion are liberated from the cyst in the intestine, where they sexually mature.[253] The mature male and female worms copulate in the lumen of the small intestine, giving rise to a new generation of larvae. The newly born larvae migrate to various tissues in the body. Those larvae that reach the striated muscles penetrate into the sarcolemma of the muscle fibers and develop to maturity as encapsulated cysts.[253] The larvae continue their life cycle when raw or undercooked meat, especially pork containing the larvae, is consumed by humans.

Trichinosis is included under the notifiable diseases in the United States, with its number of cases progressively decreasing since the 1940s.[235] The decline in trichinosis in the United States has been attributed to changes in swine feeding practices and routine inspections at slaughterhouses. The average number of trichinosis cases reported in the United States in 1997 to 2001 was 14/year, down from 400 cases/year in the 1940s.[254] On the other hand, game meat was identified as the most common source of the parasite for humans during 1997 to 2001.[235]

ANISAKIS SPECIES

Anisakiasis in humans is caused by two food-borne roundworms. These include *A. simplex*, whose definitive host is whales, and *Pseudoterranova decipiens*, which primarily inhabits seals. The eggs of these roundworms are excreted in feces by their respective hosts. The eggs then undergo molting in suitable intermediate hosts and subsequently develop into larvae, which are ingested by fish.[255] Humans contract anisakiasis by consumption of raw or undercooked fish and seafoods containing the larvae. In noninvasive anisakiasis, the worms released from ingested foods migrate to the pharynx, resulting in "tingling throat syndrome."[255] The worms are ultimately expelled by coughing. In the invasive form of anisakiasis, the worms penetrate the intestinal mucosa, thereby causing symptoms that include epigastric pain, nausea, vomiting, and diarrhea.

TAENIA SPECIES

The genus *Taenia* includes two meat-borne pathogenic flat worms, *T. saginata* (beef tapeworm) and *T. solium* (pork tapeworm). The eggs of *T. saginata* survive in the environment, including on pastures, and are ingested by cattle in which they hatch into embryos.[253] The embryos migrate to skeletal muscles or the heart, and develop into larvae known as cysticercus bovis. Humans become infected by consuming raw or undercooked beef containing the larvae. Larvae that are released into the small intestine develop into mature, adult worms. The symptoms of *T. saginata* infection in humans include decreased appetite, headache, dizziness, diarrhea, and weight loss.

In the normal life cycle of *T. solium*, pigs serve as the intermediate host. Eggs ingested by pigs develop into embryos in the duodenum, penetrate the intestinal wall, migrate through the blood and the lymphatic system, and finally reach the skeletal muscles and myocardium, where they develop into larvae known as cysticercus cellulose. Humans consuming raw or undercooked pork are infected with the larvae, which develop into adult worms in the small intestine. The symptoms of *T. solium* infection in humans include discomfort, hunger pains, anorexia, and nervous disorders. Worms are passed in the feces. In the abnormal life cycle of *T. solium*, humans serve as intermediate hosts in which the larvae develop in striated muscles and in subcutaneous tissue.

DIPHYLLOBOTHRIUM LATUM

Diphyllobothrium latum is commonly referred to as the broad tapeworm because it is the largest human tapeworm.[255] Humans contract diphyllobothriasis by consuming raw or undercooked fish containing the larval forms called plerocercoids. Upon ingestion, the larvae develop into mature worms in the intestines. Eggs produced by mature worms are excreted in feces. If feces containing the eggs contaminate water, the eggs develop into free-swimming larvae called coricidia. Coricidia are ingested by crustaceans, where they develop into a juvenile stage known as procercoid. Following ingestion of infected crustaceans by fish, procercoids develop into plerocercoids to continue the life cycle. Diphyllobothriasis in humans is characterized by nausea, abdominal pain, diarrhea, weakness, and pernicious anemia.[255] Cases of diphyllobothriasis have been associated with eating foods containing raw salmon such as sushi.

REFERENCES

1. Mead, P. S. et al. *Emerg. Infect. Dis.*, 5, 607, 1999.
2. Centers for Disease Control and Prevention, *Morbid. Mortal. Wkly Rep.*, 47, 782, 1997.
3. Centers for Disease Control and Prevention, Foodborne Outbreak Response and Surveillance Unit, Summary statistics, 2004.
4. Meng, J. and Doyle, M. P. In *Escherichia coli O157:H7 and Other Shiga Toxin-Producing E. coli Strains*, Kaper, J. B. and O'Brien, A. D. (eds.), ASM Press, Washington, D.C. 1998, 92.
5. Laegreid, W. W., Elder, R. O., and Keen, J. E. *Epidemiol. Infect.*, 123, 291, 1999.
6. Shere, J. A., Bartlett, K. J., and Kaspar, C. W. *Appl. Environ. Microbiol.*, 64, 1390, 1998.
7. Zhao, T. et al. *Appl. Environ. Microbiol.*, 61, 1290, 1995.
8. Chapman, P. A. et al. *Epidemiol. Infect.*, 111, 439, 1993.
9. Naylor, S. W. et al. *Infect. Immun.*, 71, 1505, 2003.
10. Wang, G. T., Zhao, T., and Doyle, M. P. *Appl. Environ. Microbiol.*, 62, 2567, 1998.
11. Hancock, D. D. et al. *Epidemiol. Infect.*, 113, 199, 1994.
12. Animal and Plant Inspection Service. 1995. (U.S. Dept. of Agriculture, http://www.aphis.usda.gov/vs/ceah/cahm), National Animal Health Monitoring System Report N182.595.
13. Elder, R. O. et al. *Proc. Natl. Acad. Sci. USA*, 97, 2999, 2000.
14. Gansheroff, L. J. and O'Brien, A. D. *Proc. Natl. Acad. Sci. USA*, 97, 2959, 2000.
15. Heuvelink, A. E. et al. *J. Clin. Microbiol.*, 36, 3480, 1998.
16. Jackson, S. G. et al. *Epidemiol. Infect.*, 120, 17, 1998.
17. Smith, D. et al. *J. Food Prot.*, 64, 1899, 2001.
18. Dargatz, D. A. et al. *J. Food Prot.*, 60, 466, 1997.
19. Brashears, M. M., Jaroni, D., and Trimble, J. *J. Food Prot.*, 66, 355, 2003.
20. Sivapalasingam, S. et al. *J. Food Prot.*, 67, 2342, 2004.
21. Park, G. W. and Diez-Gonzalez, F. *J. Appl. Microbiol.*, 94, 675, 2003.
22. Breuer, T. et al. *Emer. Infect. Dis.*, 7, 977, 2001.

23. McLellan, M. R. and Splittstoesser, D. F. *Food Technol.*, 50, 174, 1994.
24. Crump, J. A. et al. *N. Engl. J. Med.*, 347, 555, 2002.
25. O'Brien, S. J., Adak, G. K., and Gilham, C. *Emerg. Infect Dis.*, 7, 1049, 2001.
26. Potter, A. A. et al. *Vaccine*, 22, 362, 2004.
27. Zhao, T. et al. *J. Clin. Microbiol.*, 36, 641, 1998.
28. Callaway, T. R. et al. *J. Anim. Sci.*, 80, 1683, 2002.
29. Uljas, H. E. and Ingham, S. C. *J. Food Prot.*, 61, 939, 1998.
30. Arnold, K. W. and Kaspar, C. W. *Appl. Environ. Microbiol.*, 61, 2037, 1995.
31. Buchanan, R. L. and Edelson, S. G. *Appl. Environ. Microbiol.*, 62, 4009, 1996.
32. Leyer, G. J., Wang, L. L., and Johnson, E. A. *Appl. Environ. Microbiol.*, 61, 3152, 1995.
33. Doyle, M. P. and Schoeni, J. L. *Appl. Environ. Microbiol.*, 48, 855, 1984.
34. Glass, K. A. et al. *Appl. Environ. Microbiol.*, 58, 2513, 1992.
35. Padhye, N. V. and Doyle, M. P. *J. Food Prot.*, 55, 555, 1992.
36. Doyle, M. P., Zhao, T., Meng, J., and Zhao, S. In *Food Microbiology: Fundamentals and Frontiers*, Doyle, M. P., Beuchat, L. R., and Montville, T. J. (eds.), ASM Press, Washington, D.C. 1997, p. 171.
37. D'Aoust, J.-Y. In *Food Microbiology: Fundamentals and Frontiers*, Doyle, M. P., Beuchat, L. R., and Montville, T. J. (eds.), ASM Press, Washington, D.C. 1997, p. 129.
38. Jay, J. M. *Modern Food Microbiology*, Aspen Publishers, Gaithersburg, MD, 1998, 509.
39. Bean, N. H. et al. *J. Food Prot.*, 53, 711, 1983.
40. D'Aoust, J.-Y. *Int. J. Food Microbiol.*, 13, 207, 1991.
41. Leyer, G. J. and Johnson, E. A. *Appl. Environ. Microbiol.*, 59, 1842, 1993.
42. Leyer, G. J. and Johnson, E. A. *Appl. Environ. Microbiol.*, 58, 2075, 1992.
43. D'Aoust, J.-Y. In *Foodborne Bacterial Pathogens*, Doyle, M. P. (ed.), Marcel Dekker, New York, 1989, p. 336.
44. Flowers, R. S. *Food Technol.* 42, 182, 1988.
45. Schlundt, J. *Int. J. Food Microbiol.*, 78, 3, 2002.
46. Anonymus. *Morb. Mortal. Wkly Rep.*, 54, 352, 2004.
47. Frenzen, P. et al. *Food Rev.*, 22, 10, 1999.
48. Glynn, M. K. et al. *N. Engl. J. Med.*, 338, 1333, 1998.
49. Cody, S. H. et al. *JAMA.*, 281, 1805, 1999.
50. Glynn, M. K. et al., *Clin. Infect. Dis.,* 38, S227, 2004.
51. Anonymous. *Morb. Mortal. Wkly Rep.*, 51, 950, 2002.
52. Kimura, A. C. et al. *Clin. Infect. Dis.,* 38, S244, 2004.
53. Anonymous. *Morb. Mortal. Wkly Rep.*, 51, 1149, 2003.
54. Mishu, B. et al. *Ann. Int. Med.,* 115, 190, 1991.
55. Humphery, T. J. et al. *Epidemiol. Infect.,* 106, 489, 1991.
56. Barrow, P. A., Lovell, M. A., and Berchieri, A. *Vet. Rec.*, 126, 241, 1990.
57. Gast, R. K. and Beard, C. W. *Avian Dis.*, 34, 438, 1990.
58. Shivaprasad, H. L. et al. *Avian Dis.*, 34, 548, 1990.
59. Timoney, J. F. et al. *Vet. Rec.,*125, 600, 1989.
60. Borland, E. D. *Vet. Rec.*, 97, 406, 1975.
61. Hopkins, R. S. et al. *Morb. Mortal. Wkly Rep.*, 52, 1, 2005.
62. Jay, J. M. *Modern Food Microbiology*, Aspen Publishers, Gaithersburg, MD, 1998, 556.
63. Altekruse, S. F. et al. *Emerg. Infect. Dis.*, 5, 28, 1999.
64. Thormar, H., Hilmarsson, H., and Bergsson, G. *Appl. Environ. Microbiol.*, 72, 522, 2006.
65. Anonymous. *Morb. Mortal. Wkly. Rep.*, 54, 352, 2005.
66. Effler, P. et al. *J. Infect. Dis.,* 183, 1152, 2001.
67. Beery, J. T., Hugdahl, M. B., and Doyle, M. P. *Appl. Environ. Microbiol.*, 54, 2365, 1988.
68. Hugdahl, M. B., Beery, J. T., and Doyle, M. P. *Infect. Immun.*, 56, 1560, 1988.
69. Stern, N. J. and Kazmi, S. U. In *Foodborne Bacterial Pathogens*, Doyle, M. P. (ed.), Marcel Dekker, New York, 1989, p. 71.
70. Friedman, C. R. et al. *Clin. Infect. Dis.*, 38, S285, 2004.
71. Samuel, M. C. et al. *Clin. Infect. Dis.*, 38, S165, 2004.
72. Deming, M. S., Tauxe, R. V. and Blake, P. A. *Am. J. Epidemiol.*, 126, 526, 1987.
73. Oosterom, J. et al. *J. Hyg.* (Cambridge), 92, 325, 1984.
74. Hopkins, R. S. and Scott, A. S. *J. Infect. Dis.*, 148, 770, 1983.
75. Stern, N. J. et al. *Poult. Sci.*, 80, 156, 2001.
76. Carillo, C. L. et al. *Appl. Environ. Microbiol.*, 71, 6554, 2005.
77. Wagenaar, J. A. et al. *Vet. Microbiol.*, 109, 275, 2005.
78. Heres, L., B. et al. *Vet. Microbiol.*, 99, 259, 2004.
79. Wyszynska, A. et al. *Vaccine*, 22,1379, 2004.
80. Scott, D. A., Bagar, S., Pazzaglia, G., Guerry, P. and Burr, D. H. In *New Generation vaccines*, 2nd ed., Marcel Dekker, Inc. New York, 1997, p. 885.

81. Kassenborg, H. D. et al. *Clin. Infect. Dis.*, 38, S279, 2004.
82. Smith, K. E., Blender, J. B., and Osterholm, M. T. *Am. Soc. Microbiol.*, 340, 1525, 2000
83. Nachamkin, I., Allos, B. M., and Ho, T. *Clin. Microbiol. Rev.*, 11, 555, 1998.
84. Allos, B. M. *J. Infect. Dis.*, 176, S125, 1997.
85. Whitehouse, C. A. et al. *Infect. Immun.*, 66, 1934, 1998.
86. Gupta, A. et al. *Clin. Infect. Dis.*, 38, 1372, 2004.
87. Sobel, J. et al. *J. Infect. Dis.*, 177, 1405, 1998.
88. Mohle-Boetani, J. C. et al. *Am. J. Public Health*, 85, 812, 1995.
89. Anonymous. *Morb. Mortal. Wkly Rep.*, 39, 509, 1990.
90. Woodward, D. L. et al. *J. Med. Microbiol.*, 54, 741, 2005.
91. Schleifstein, J. and Coleman, M. B. *N. Y. State J. Med.*, 39, 1749, 1939.
92. Robins-Browne, R. M. In *Food Microbiology: Fundamentals and Frontiers*, Doyle, M. P., Beuchat, L. R., and Montville, T. J. (eds.), ASM Press, Washington, D.C. 1997, p. 192.
93. Jay, J. M. *Modern Food Microbiology*, Aspen Publishers, Gaithersburg, MD, 1998, p. 555.
94. Shiemann, D. A. In *Foodborne Bacterial Pathogens*, Doyle, M. P. (ed.), Marcel Dekker, New York, 1989, p. 631.
95. Greenwood, M. *Leatherhead*: Leatherhead Food Research Association, 1990.
96. Bottone, E. J. *Clin. Microbiol. Rev.*, 10, 257, 1997.
97. Schifield, G. M. *J. Appl. Bacteriol.*, 72, 267, 1992.
98. Lee, L. A. et al. *J. Infect. Dis.*, 163, 660, 1991.
99. Lee, L. A. et al. *N. Engl. J. Med.*, 322, 984, 1990.
100. Metchock, B. et al. *J. Clin. Microbiol.*, 29, 2868, 1991.
101. Bottone, J. E. *Microbes Infect.*, 1, 323,1999.
102. Wagner, S. J., Friedman, L. I., and Dodd, R. Y. *Clin. Microbiol. Rev.*, 7, 290, 1994.
103. Bruining, A. and DeWilde-Beekhuizen, C. C. M. *Medilon,* 4, 30, 1975.
104. Mollaret, H. H. and Thal, E. *Bergey's Manual of Determinative Bacteriology*, 8, 330, 1974.
105. Toora, S. et al. *Folia Microbiol. Praha.*, 34, 151, 1989.
106. Hanna, M. O. et al. *J. Food Sci.,* 42, 1180, 1977.
107. Palumbo, S. A. *J. Food Prot.*, 49, 1003, 1986.
108. National Oceanic and Atmospheric Administration. In *Fisheries of the United States.* National Marine Fisheries Service, Fisheries Statistics and Economics Division, Silver Springs, MD, 2003, p. 86.
109. Eastaugh, J. and Shepherd, S. *Arch. Intern. Med.*, 149, 1735, 1989.
110. Anonymous. *Dairy Food Environ. Sanit.*, 22, 38, 2002.
111. Twedt, R. M. In *Foodborne bacterial pathogens*, Doyle, M. P. (ed.). Marcel Dekker, Inc., New York. 1989, p. 395.
112. Oliver, J. D. and Kaper, J. B. In *Food Microbiology: Fundamentals and Frontiers*, Doyle, M. P., Beuchat, L. R., and Montville, T. J. (eds.), ASM Press, Washington, D.C. 1997, p. 228.
113. Daniels, N. A. et al. *J. Am. Med. Assoc.*, 284, 1541, 2000.
114. Miyamato, Y. et al. *Infect. Immun.* 28, 567, 1980.
115. Mintz, E. D., Popovic, T., and Blake, P. A. *Transmission of* Vibrio cholerae *O1,* Vibrio cholerae *and Cholera: Molecular to Global Perspectives*, ASM Press, Washington, D.C. 1994, p. 345.
116. Anonymous. *Morb. Mortal. Wkly Rep.*, 55, 31, 2006.
117. World Health Organization. *Wkly. Epidemiol. Rec.,* 31, 281, 2003.
118. Tauxe, R. V. *Int. J. Food Microbiol.*, 78, 31, 2002.
119. Jay, J. M., *Modern Food Microbiology*, Aspen Publishers, Gaithersburg, MD, 1998, p. 544.
120. Kleiman, M. B. et al. *J. Clin. Microbiol.*, 14, 352, 1981.
121. Nazarowec-White, M. and Farber, J. M. *Int. J. Food Microbiol.*, 34, 103, 1997.
122. Sanders, W. E., Jr. and Sanders, C. C. *Clin. Microbiol. Rev.*, 10, 220, 1997.
123. van Acker, J. et al. *J. Clin. Microbiol.*, 39, 293, 2001.
124. Lai, K. K. *Med.* (Baltimore). 80, 113, 2001.
125. Leclercq, A., Wanegue, C., and Baylac, P. *Appl. Environ. Microbiol.*, 68, 1631, 2002.
126. Kandhai, M. C. et al. *Lancet*, 363, 39, 2004.
127. Kandhai, M. C. et al. *J. Food Prot.*, 67, 1267, 2004
128. Bar-Oz, B. et al. *Acta Paediatr.*, 90, 356, 2002.
129. Simmons, B. P. et al. *Infect. Control Hosp. Epidemiol.*, 10, 398, 1989.
130. Weir, E. *CMAJ*, 166, 1570, 2002.
131. Biering, G. et al. *J. Clin. Microbiol.*, 27, 2054, 1989.
132. Postupa, R. and Aldova, E. *J. Hyg. Epidemiol. Microbiol. Immunol.*, 28, 435, 1984.
133. Muytjens, H. L., Roelofs-Willemse, H., and Jaspar, G. H. *J. Clin. Microbiol.*, 26, 743, 1988.
134. Nazarowec-White, M. and Farber, J. M. *J. Food. Prot.*, 60, 226, 1997.
135. Harris, R. D. *Food Proc.,* 50, 111, 1989.
136. Nazarowec-White, M. and Farber, J. M. *Lett. Appl. Microbiol.*, 24, 9, 1997.
137. Breeuwer, P. et al. *J. Appl. Microbiol.*, 95, 967, 2003.

138. Iversen, C. and Forsythe, S. *Food Microbiol.*, 21, 771, 2004.
139. Urmenyi, A. M. and Franklin, A. W. *Lancet,* 1, 313, 1961.
140. Himelright, I. et al. *Morb. Mortal. Wkly Rep.*, 51, 297, 2002.
141. FSNET. 8, November 2002. Colorado Department of Public Health and Environment Press Release. Available at: http://131.104.232.9/ fsnet/2002/11-2002/fsnet_november_8-2.htm#RECALLED%20BABY.
142. International Commission on Microbiological Specification for Foods. *Micro-organisms in foods*, vol. 7. Microbiolgical testing in food safety management, Chapter 8. Selection of cases and attribute plans. Kluwer Academic/Plenum Publishers, New York, 2002.
143. Gallagher, P. G. and Ball, W. S. *Pediatr. Radiol.*, 21,135, 1991.
144. Kline, M. W. *Infect. Dis. J.*, 7, 891, 1988.
145. Hawkins, R. E., Lissner, C. R., and Sanford, J. P. *South Med. J.*, 84, 793, 1991.
146. Pribyl, C. *Am. J. Med.*, 78, 51, 1985.
147. Beuchat, L. R. *Int. J. Food Microbiol.*, 13, 217, 1991.
148. Kirov, S. M. In *Food Microbiology: Fundamentals and Frontiers*, Doyle, M. P., Beuchat, L. R., and Montville, T. J. (eds.), ASM Press, Washington, D.C. 1997, p. 265.
149. Berrang, M. E., Brackett, R. E., and Beuchat, L. R., *Appl. Environ. Microbiol.*, 55, 2167, 1989.
150. Palumbo, S. A. *Int. J. Food Microbiol.*, 7, 41, 1988.
151. Jay, J. M. *Modern Food Microbiology*, Aspen Publishers, Gaithersburg, MD, 1998, p. 620.
152. Holmberg, S. D. et al. *Ann. Intern. Med.*, 105, 690, 1986.
153. Anonymous. *Morb. Mortal. Wkly Rep.*, 47, 394, 1998.
154. Economic Research Service. 2001. Available at http://www.ers.usda.gov/Emphases/SafeFood/features.htm
155. Nickelson, N. *Food Quality*, April 28, 1999.
156. Anonymous. *Morb. Mortal. Wkly Rep.*, 51, 950, 2002.
157. Nightingale, K. K. et al. *Appl. Environ. Microbiol.*, 70, 4458, 2004.
158. Brackett, R. E. *Food Technol.*, 52, 162, 1998.
159. Cox, L. J. et al. *Food Microbiol.*, 6, 49, 1989.
160. Jeong, D. K. and Frank, J. F. *J. Food Prot.*, 57, 576, 1994.
161. Meng, J. and Doyle, M. P. *Annu. Rev. Nutr.*, 17, 255, 1997.
162. Rocourt, J. and Cossart, P. In *Food Microbiology: Fundamentals and Frontiers*, Doyle, M. P., Beuchat, L. R., and Montville, T. J. (eds.), ASM Press, Washington, D.C. 1997, p. 337.
163. Ryser, E. T. and Marth, E. H. *Listeria, Listeriosis and Food Safety*, Marcel Dekker, Inc., New York, 1999.
164. Vázquez-Boland, J. A. et al. *Clin. Microbiol. Rev.*, 14, 584, 2001.
165. Gaillard, J.-L. *Infect. Immun.*, 55, 2822, 1987.
166. Kwada, M. et al. *J. Hum. Lact.*, 19, 411, 2003.
167. Jablonski, L. M. and Bohac, G. A. In *Food Microbiology: Fundamentals and Frontiers*, Doyle, M. P., Beuchat, L. R., and Montville, T. J. (eds.), ASM Press, Washington, D.C. 1997, p. 353.
168. Newsome, R. L. *Food Technol.*, 42, 182, 1988.
169. Bergdoll, M. L. In *Foodborne Bacterial Pathogens*, Doyle, M. P. (ed.), Marcel Dekker, New York, 1989, p. 463.
170. Le Loir, Y., Baron, F., and Gautier, M. *Genet. Mol. Res.*, 2, 63, 2003.
171. Jones, T. F. et al. *Emerg. Infect. Dis.*, 8, 82, 2002.
172. Wilson, R. et al. *Pediatr. Infect. Dis.*, 1, 148, 1982.
173. Spika, J. S. et al. *Am. J. Dis. Child.*, 143, 828, 1989.
174. Dodds, K. L. and Austin, J. W. In *Food Microbiology: Fundamentals and Frontiers,* Doyle, M. P., Beuchat, L. R., and Montville, T. J. (eds.), ASM Press, Washington, D.C. 1997, 288.
175. Pierson, M. D. and Reddy, N. R. *Food Technol.*, 42, 196, 1988.
176. Jay, J. M. *Modern Food Microbiology*, Aspen Publishers, Gaithersburg, MD, 1998, 462.
177. Hobbs, B. C. In *Clostridium perfringens gastroenteritis, Foodborne Infections and Intoxications*, Riemann, H., and Bryan, F. L. (eds.), Academic Press, New York, 1979, p. 131.
178. Labbe, R. In *Foodborne Bacterial Pathogens*, Doyle, M. P. (ed.), Marcel Dekker, New York, 1989, p. 191.
179. Rood, J. I. et al. *The Clostridia: Molecular Biology and Pathogenesis*. Academic, London, 1997, p. 533.
180. Kokai-Kun, J. F. and McClane, B. A. In: *The Clostridia - molecular Biology and Pathogenesis. The Clostridium perfringens entero-toxin.* Road, IJ., McClane, B. A., Sanger, I. G., and Titball, R. W. (eds) Academic Press, San Diego CA 1997, p. 325.
181. Ehling-Schulz, M., Fricker, M., and Scherer, S. *Mol. Nutr. Food Res.*, 48, 479, 2004.
182. Doyle, M. P. *Food Technol.*, 42, 199, 1988.
183. Kramer, J. M. and Gilbert, R. J. In *Foodborne Bacterial Pathogens*, Doyle, M. P. (ed.), Marcel Dekker, New York, 1989, p. 327.
184. Johnson, K. M. *J. Food Prot.,* 47, 145, 1984.
185. Hobbs, B. C. and Gilbert, R. J. *Proc IV Int. Cong. Food Sci. Technol.*, 3, 159, 1974.
186. Stiles, M. E. In *Foodborne Bacterial Pathogens*, Doyle, M. P. (ed.), Marcel Dekker, New York, 1989, p. 706.
187. Labigne, A. and De Reuse, H. *Infect. Agents Dis.*, 5, 191, 1996.
188. McColl, K. E. L. *J. Infect. Dis.*, 34, 7, 1997.
189. Goodman, K. J. and Correa, P. *Int. J. Epidemiol.*, 24, 875, 1995.
190. Hopkins, R. J. et al. *J. Infect. Dis.*, 168, 222, 1993.

191. Jiang, X. and Doyle, M. P. *J. Food Prot.*, 61, 929, 1998.
192. Baggett, H. C. et al. *Pediatrics,* 117, e396, 2006.
193. Cardenas, V. M. et al. *Am. J. Epidemiol.*, 163, 127, 2006
194. Koopmans, M. and Duizer, E. *Int. J. Food Microbiol.*, 90, 23, 2004.
195. Bidawid, S., Farber, J. M., and Sattar, S. A. *Appl. Environ. Microbiol.*, 66, 2759, 2000.
196. Cromeans, T., Nainan, O. V., Fields, H. A., Favaorov, M O., and Margolis, H. A., Hepatitis A and E viruses. In *Foodborne Diseases Handbook, vol. 2, Diseases Caused by Viruses, Parasites, and Fungi,* Hui, Y. H., Gorham, J. R., Murrel, K. D., and Cliver, D. O. (eds.) Marcel Dekker, New York, 1994, p. 1.
197. Cliver, D. O. *World Health Stat. Q.,* 50, 91, 1997.
198. Feinstone, S. M. *Eur. J. Gastroenterol. Hepatol.*, 8, 300, 1996.
199. Anonymous. *Morb. Mortal. Wkly Rep.*, 52, 1155, 2003.
200. Parashar, U. *Morb. Mortal. Wkly Rep.*, 50, No. RR-9, 2001.
201. Dolin, R. et al. *Proc. Soc. Exp. Biol. Med.,* 140, 578, 1972.
202. Sattar, S. A., Springthorpe, V. S., Ansari, S. A., Hui, Y. H., Gorham, J. R., Murrel, K. D., and Cliver, D. O. *Rotavirus, Foodborne Diseases Handbook, vol. 2, Diseases Caused by Viruses, Parasites, and Fungi,* Marcel Dekker, New York, 1994, p. 81.
203. Horimoto, T. and Kawaoka, Y. *Nat. Rev. Microbiol.*, 3, 591, 2005.
204. World Health Organization, *N. Engl. J. Med.*, 353, 1374, 2005.
205. Webster, R. G. et al. *Microbiol. Rev.*, 56, 152, 1992.
206. Easterday, B. C., Hinshaw, V. S., and Halvorson, D. A. In: *Diseases of Poultry* Calnek, B. W., Barner, H. J., Beard, C. W., McDonald L. R. & Saif, Y. M. (eds) Iowa State Uni Press ames Iowa 1997 p. 583.
207. Lamb, R. A. Genes and proteins of the influenza viruses. In *The Influenza Viruses*, 1st ed., R. M. Krug (ed.), Plenum Press, New York, 1989.
208. White, J., Kartenbeck, J., and Helenius, A. *EMBO J.*, 1, 217, 1982.
209. Klenk, H.-D. et al. *Virology*, 68, 426, 1975.
210. Stieneke-Grober, A. et al. *EMBO J.*, 11, 2407, 1992.
211. Horimoto, T. et al. *J. Virol.*, 68, 6074, 1994.
212. Swayne, D. E. and Beck, J. R. *Avian Pathol.*, 33, 512, 2004.
213. Buchi, G. and Rae, I. D. In *Aflatoxins*, Goldbatt, L. A. (ed.), Academic Press, New York, 1969, p. 55.
214. Hocking, A. D. In *Food Microbiology: Fundamentals and Frontiers,* Doyle, M. P., Beuchat, L. R., and Montville, T. J. (eds.), ASM Press, Washington, D.C. 1997, p. 393.
215. Gong, Y. Y. et al. *BMJ*, 325, 20, 2002.
216. Maxwell, S. M. et al. *J. Toxicol. Toxin Rev.*, 8, 19, 1998.
217. Smela, M. E. and Curier, S. S. *Carcinogenesis*, 22, 535, 2001.
218. Mace, K. et al. *Carcinogensis,* 18, 1291, 1997.
219. Railey, J. et al. *Carcinogensis*, 18, 905, 1997.
220. Ramdell, H. S. and Eaton, D. L. *Cancer Res.*, 50, 615, 1990.
221. Pitt, J. I. In *Food Microbiology: Fundamentals and Frontiers*, Doyle, M. P., Beuchat, L. R., and Montville, T. J. (eds.), ASM Press, Washington, D.C. 1997, p. 406.
222. Krogh, P., Hald, B., and Perdersen, E. J. *Acta Pathol. Microbiol.* Scand. B81, 689, 1977.
223. Karabulut, O. A. et al. *Postharvest Biol. Technol.*, 24, 103, 2002.
224. Karabulut, O. A. and Baykal, N. *Postharvest Biol. Technol.*, 26, 237, 2002.
225. Vero, S. et al. *Postharvest Biol. Technol.*, 26, 91, 2002.
226. Venturini, M. E., Oria, R., and Blanco, D. *Food Microbiol.*, 19, 15, 2002.
227. Krogh, P. et al. *Dansk. vet. Tidsskr.*, 67, 123, 1984.
228. Scott, P. M., Fuleki, T., and Harvig, J. *J. Agric. Food Chem.*, 25, 434, 1977.
229. Moss, M. O. *J. Appl. Microbiol.*, 84, 62S, 1998.
230. Friis, P., Hasselager, E., and Krogh, P. *Acta Pathol. Microbiol. Scand.*, 77, 559, 1969.
231. Bullerman, L. B. In *Food Microbiology: Fundamentals and Frontiers*, Doyle, M. P., Beuchat, L. R., and Montville, T. J. (eds.), ASM Press, Washington, D.C. 1997, p. 419.
232. Jones, J. L. et al. *Clin. Infect. Dis.*, 38, S198, 2004.
233. Hlavsa, M. C., Watson, J. C., and Beach, M. *J. Morb. Mortal. Wkly Rep.*, 54, 9, 2005.
234. Smith, J. *J. Food Prot.*, 56, 451, 1993.
235. Doyle, E. *Foodborne Parasites, A Review of the Scientific Literature*, FRI briefings, 2003.
236. Speer, C. A. In *Food Microbiology: Fundamentals and Frontiers*, Doyle, M. P., Beuchat, L. R., and Montville, T. J. (eds.), ASM Press, Washington, D.C. 1997, p. 478.
237. Fox, K. R. and Lyte, D. A. *J. Am. Water Works Assn.*, 88, 87, 1996.
238. Corso, P. S. et al. *Emerg. Infect. Dis.*, 9, 426,1993.
239. Hoskin, J. C. and Wright, R. E. *J. Food Prot.*, 54, 53, 1991.
240. Petersen, C. *Lancet*, 345, 1128, 1995.
241. Tzipori, S. *Microbiol. Rev.*, 47, 84, 1983.
242. Reduker, D. W. and Speer, C. A. *J. Parasitol.*, 71, 112, 1985.

243. Korich, D. G. et al. *Appl. Environ. Microbiol.*, 56, 1423, 1990.
244. Sterling, C. R. and Ortega, Y. R. *Emerg. Infect. Dis.,* 5, 48, 1999.
245. Rose, J. B. and Slifko, T. R. *J. Food Prot.*, 62, 1059, 2000.
246. Smith, H. V. et al. *Appl. Environ. Microbiol.*, 63, 1631, 1997.
247. Dubey, J. P. et al. *J. Parasitol.*, 32, 99, 2002.
248. Casemore, D. P. *Lancet*, 336, 1427, 1990.
249. Fayer, R. and Dubey, J. P. *Food Technol.*, 39, 57, 1985.
250. Anonymous, *Morb. Mortal. Wkly Rep.,* 48, 1, 1999.
251. Lindsay, D. S., Blagburn, B. L., and Dubey, J. P. *Vet. Parasitol.*, 103, 309, 2002.
252. Fleck, D. G. *PHLS Microbiol. Digest*, 6, 69, 1989.
253. Kim, C. W. In *Food Microbiology: Fundamentals and Frontiers*, Doyle, M. P., Beuchat, L. R., and Montville, T. J. (eds.), ASM Press, Washington, D.C. 1997, p. 449.
254. Centers for disease Control and Prevention, Surveillance summaries, 52, 1, 2003.
255. Hayunga, E. G. In *Food Microbiology: Fundamentals and Frontiers*, Doyle, M. P., Beuchat, L. R., and Montville, T. J. (eds.), ASM Press, Washington, D.C. 1997, p. 463.
256. Kleanthous, H. et al. *Epidemiol. Infect.*, 101, 327, 1988.
257. March, S. B. and Ratnam, S. *J. Clin. Microbiol.*, 23, 869, 1986.
258. Doyle, M. P. and Schoeni, J. L. *Appl. Environ. Microbiol.*, 53, 2394, 1987.
259. March, S. B. and Ratnam, S. *J. Clin. Microbiol.*, 27, 1675, 1989.
260. Okrend, A. J. G., Rose, B. E., and Matner, R. *J. Food Prot.*, 53, 936, 1990.
261. Padhye, N. V. and Doyle, M. P. *Appl. Environ. Microbiol.*, 57, 2693, 1991.
262. Zhao, Z. J. and Liu, X. M. *Biomed. Environ. Sci.*, 18, 254, 2005.
263. Pollard, D. R. et al. *J. Clin. Microbiol.*, 28, 540, 1990.
264. Nguyen, L. T. et al. *Foodborne Pathog. Dis.*, 1, 231, 2004.
265. Johnston, L. M. et al. *J. Food Prot.*, 68, 2256, 2005.
266. Cox, N. A. et al. *Dairy, Food Environ. Sanitat.*, 7, 628, 1987.
267. Cox, N. A. et al. *J. Food Prot.*, 47, 74, 1984.
268. Maciorowski, K. G. et al. *Vet. Res. Commun.*, 30, 127, 2006.
269. Feng, P. *J. Food Prot.*, 55, 927, 1992.
270. Tietjen, M. and Fung, D. Y. C. *Crit. Rev. Microbiol.*, 21, 53, 1995.
271. Kim, U., Su, X. L., and Li, Y. *J. Food Prot.*, 68, 1799, 2005.
272. Nguyen, A. V., Khan. M. I., and Lu, Z. *Avian Dis.*, 38, 119, 1994.
273. Bansal, N. S., Gray, V., and McDonell, F. *J. Food Prot.*, 69, 282, 2006.
274. Seo, K. H. et al. *J. Food Prot.*, 67, 864, 2004.
275. Bolton, L. F. et al. *J. Clin. Microbiol.*, 37, 1348, 1999.
276. Le Minor, L., Craige, J., and Yen, C. H. *Can. Publ. Health J.*, 29, 484, 1938.
277. Lim, P. et al. *J. Clin. Microbiol.*, 36, 2271, 1998.
278. Chaicumpa, W. et al. *J. Clin. Microbiol.*, 30, 2513, 1992.
279. Kumar, S., Balakrishna, K., and Batra, H. V. *Lett. Appl. Microbiol.*, 42, 149, 2006.
280. Farrell, J. J. et al. *Am. J. Clin. Pathol.*, 123, 339, 2005.
281. Park, C. E., Smibert, R. M., Blaser, M. J., Vanderzant, C., and Stern, N. J. In *Compendium of Methods for the Microbiological Examination of Foods*, 2nd ed., Speck, M. L. (ed.), American Public Health Association, Washington D.C. 1984, p. 386.
282. Rice, B. E. et al. *Clin. Diagn. Lab. Immunol.*, 3, 669, 1996.
283. Endtz, H. P. et al. *Eur. J. Clin. Microbiol. Infect. Dis.*, 19, 794, 2000.
284. Linton, D. et al. *J. Clin. Microbiol.*, 35, 2568, 1997.
285. Ng, L. K. et al. *Appl. Environ. Microbiol.*, 63, 4558, 1997.
286. Oliveira, T. C., Barbut, S., and Griffiths, M. W. *Int. J. Food Microbiol.*, 104, 105, 2005.
287. Sails, A. D. et al. *Appl. Environ. Microbiol.*, 69, 1383, 2003.
288. Bolton, F. J. et al. *J. Food Prot.*, 65, 760, 2002.
289. Keramas, G. et al. *J. Clin. Microbiol.*, 42, 3985, 2004.
290. Morris, G. K. In *Compendium of Methods for the Microbiological Examination of Foods*, 2nd ed., Speck, M. L. (ed.), American Public Health Association, Washington D.C. 1984, p. 343.
291. Pal, T. et al. *J. Clin. Microbiol.*, 35, 1757, 1997.
292. Rahman, S. R. and Stimson, W. H. *Hybridoma,* 20, 85, 2001.
293. Lampel, K. A. et al. *Appl. Environ. Microbiol.*, 56, 1536, 1990.
294. Theron, J. et al. *Water Res.*, 35, 869, 2001.
295. Lindqvist, R. *J. Appl. Microbiol.*, 86, 971, 1999.
296. Achi-Berglund, R. and Lindberg, A. A. *Clin. Microbiol. Infect.*, 2, 55, 1996.
297. Restaino, L. et al. *J. Food Prot.*, 42, 120, 1979.
298. Kapperud, G. et al. *Appl. Environ. Microbiol.*, 59, 2938, 1993.
299. Wolffs, P. et al. *J. Clin. Microbiol.*, 42, 1042, 2004.

300. Wannet, W. J. et al. *J. Clin. Microbiol.*, 40, 739, 2002.
301. Farmer, J. J., III., Hickmann-Brenner, F. W., and Kelly, M. T. In *Manual of Clinical Microbiology*, 4th ed., Lennette, E. H., Balows, A., Hausler, W. J., Jr., and Jean-Shadomy, H. (eds.), American Society for Microbiology, Washington, D.C. 1985, p. 282.
302. Twedt, R. M., Madden, J. M., and Colwell, R. R. In *Compendium of Methods for the Microbiological Examination of Foods*, 2nd ed., Speck, M. L. (ed.), American Public Health Association, Washington D.C. 1984, p. 368.
303. Choopun, N. et al. *Appl. Environ. Microbiol.*, 68, 995, 2002.
304. Castillo, L. et al. *Hybridoma*, 14, 271, 1995.
305. Martinez-Govea, A. et al. *Clin. Diagn. Lab. Immunol.*, 8, 768, 2001.
306. Goel, A. K. et al. *Folia Microbiol.* (Praha), 450, 448, 2005.
307. Miyagi, K. et al. *J. Med. Microbiol.*, 48, 883, 199.
308. Varela, P. et al. *J. Clin. Microbiol.*, 32, 1246, 1994.
309. Panicker, G. et al. *Appl. Environ. Microbiol.*, 70, 7436, 2004.
310. Lyon, W. J. *Appl. Environ. Microbiol.*, 67, 4685, 2001.
311. Honda, T. et al. *J. Clin. Microbiol.*, 22, 383, 1985.
312. Kim, Y. B. et al. *J. Clin. Microbiol.*, 37, 1173, 1999.
313. Ward, L. N. and Bej, A. K. *Appl. Environ. Microbiol.*, 72, 2031, 2006.
314. Cai, T. et al. *FEMS Immunol. Med. Microbiol.*, 46, 180, 2006.
315. Cerda-Cuellar, M., Jofre, J., and Blanch, A. R. *Appl. Environ. Microbiol.*, 66, 855, 2000.
316. Parker, R. W. and Lewis, D. H. *Appl. Environ. Microbiol.*, 61, 476, 1995.
317. Marco-Noales, E. et al. *J. Appl. Microbiol.*, 89, 599, 2000.
318. Panicker, G., Myers, M. L., and Bej, A. K. *Appl. Environ. Microbiol.*, 70, 498, 2004.
319. Campbell, M. S. and Wright, A. C. *Appl. Environ. Microbiol.*, 69, 7137, 2003.
320. Guillaume-Gentil, O. et al. *J. Food Prot.*, 68, 64, 2005.
321. U.S. Food and Drug Administration, 2002. Isolation and anumeration of *Enterobacter sakazakii* from dehydrated ordered infant formula available at:http://www.efoan.fda.gov/comm/mmesakaz.html.accessed March 8, 2007.
322. Nair, M. K. M. and Venkitanarayanan, K. *Appl. Environ. Microbiol.*, 72, 2006.
323. Seo, K. H. and Brackett, R. E. *J. Food Prot.*, 68, 59, 2005.
324. Janda, J. M., Abott, S. L., and Carnahan, A. M. In *Manual of Clinical Microbiology*, 6th ed., Murray, P. R., Baron, E. J., Pfaller, M. A., Tenover, F. C., and Yolken, R. H. (eds.), American Society for Microbiology, Washington, D.C. 1995, p. 477.
325. Jeppesen, C. *Int. J. Food Microbiol.*, 26, 25, 1995.
326. Joseph, S. W. and Carnahan, A. *Annu. Rev. Fish Dis.*, 4, 315, 1994.
327. Kannan, S. et al. *Ind. J. Med. Microbiol.*, 19, 190, 2001.
328. Delamare, A. P. et al. *J. Appl. Microbiol.*, 92, 936, 2002.
329. Borrel, N. et al. *J. Clin. Microbiol.*, 35, 1671, 1997.
330. Chu, W. H. and Lu C. P. *J. Fish Dis.*, 28, 437, 2005.
331. Peng, X. et al. *J. Microbiol. Methods*, 49, 335, 2002.
332. Gonzalez-Rey, C. et al. *FEMS Immunol. Med. Microbiol.*, 29, 107, 2000.
333. Jones, G. L. *Isolation and identification of Listeria monocytogenes*, U.S. Department of Health and Human Services, Public Health Service, Centers for Disease Control, 1989.
334. McClain, D. and Lee, W. H. *J. Assoc. Off. Anal Chem.*, 71, 876, 1988.
335. VanNetten, P. et al. *Int. J. Food Microbiol.*, 8, 299, 1989.
336. Gasanov, U., Hughes, D., and Hansbro, P. M. *FEMS Microbiol. Rev.*, 29, 851, 2005.
337. Fliss, I. et al. *Appl. Environ. Microbiol.*, 59, 2698, 1993.
338. Kim, S. H. et al. *J. Vet. Sci.*, 6, 41, 2005.
339. Garrec, N. et al. *J. Microbiol. Methods*, 55, 763, 2003.
340. Amagliani, G. et al. *J. Appl. Microbiol.*, 100, 375, 2006.
341. Oravcova, K. et al. *Lett. Appl. Microbiol.*, 42, 15, 2006.
342. Rodriguez-Lazaro, D. et al. *J. Food Prot.*, 68, 1467, 2005.
343. Bennett, R. W. In *Foodborne Microorganisms and Their Toxins: Developing Methodology*, Pierson, M. D. and Stern, N. J. (eds.), Marcel Dekker, New York, 1986, p. 345.
344. Taitini, S. R., Hoover, D. G., and Lachicha, R. V. F. In *Compendium of Methods for the Microbiological Examination of Foods*, 2nd ed., Speck, M. L. (ed.), American Public Health Association, Washington D.C. 1984, p. 411.
345. Van der Zee, A. et al. *J. Clin. Microbiol.*, 37, 342, 1999.
346. Alarcon, B., Vicedo, B., and Aznar, R. *J. Appl. Microbiol.*, 100, 352, 2006.
347. Cremonesi, P. *Mol. Cell. Probes*, 19, 299, 2005.
348. Sapsford, K. E. et al. *Appl. Environ. Microbiol.*, 71, 5590, 2005.
349. Ruan, C. et al. *Biosens. Bioelectron.*, 20, 585, 2004.
350. Vernozy-Rozand, C. et al. *Lett. Appl. Microbiol.*, 39, 490, 2004.
351. Bennett, R. W. *Bacteriological Analytical Manual*, 6th ed., U.S. Food and Drug Administration, Association of Official Analytical Chemists, Arlington, VA, 1984, p. 15.01.

352. Dowell, V. R., Lombard, G. L., Thompson, F. S., and Armfield, A. Y. *Media for isolation, characterization, and identification of obligate anaerobic bacteria*, Center for Disease Control, Atlanta, GA, 1981.

353. Aranda, E. et al. *Lett. Appl. Microbiol.*, 25, 186, 1997.

354. Fach, P. et al. *Appl. Environ. Microbiol.*, 61, 389, 1995.

355. Braconnier, A. et al. *J. Food Prot.*, 64, 201, 2001.

356. Lindstrom, M. et al. *Appl. Environ. Microbiol.*, 67, 5694, 2001.

357. Dahlenborg, M., Borch, E., and Radstrom, P. *Appl. Environ. Microbiol.*, 67, 4781, 2001.

358. Kautter, D. A., Lynt, R. K., and Solomon, H. M. *Bacteriological Analytical Manual*, 6th ed., U.S. Food and Drug Administration, Association of Official Analytical Chemists, Arlington, VA, 1984, p. 18.01.

359. Gessler, F., Hampe, K., and Bohnel, H. *Appl. Environ. Microbiol.*, 71, 7897, 2005.

360. Barr, J. R. et al. *Emerg. Infect. Dis.*, 11, 1578, 2005.

361. Sharma, S. K. et al. *Appl. Environ. Microbiol.*, 71, 3935, 2005.

362. Fach, P. and Popoff, M. R. *Appl. Environ. Microbiol.*, 63, 4232, 1997.

363. Baez, L. A. and Juneja, V. K. *Appl. Environ. Microbiol.*, 61, 807, 1995.

364. Asha, N. J. and Wilcox, M. H. *J. Med. Microbiol.*, 51, 891, 2002.

365. Hale, M. L. and Stiles, B. G. *Toxicon*, 37, 471, 1999.

366. Wise, M. G. and Siragusa, G. R. *Appl. Environ. Microbiol.*, 71, 3911, 2005.

367. Augustynowicz E., Gzyl, A., and Slusarczyk, J. *J. Med. Microbiol.*, 51, 169, 2002.

368. Harmon, S. M. and Goepfert, J. M. In *Compendium of Methods for the Microbiological Examination of Foods,* 2nd ed., Speck, M. L. (ed.), American Public Health Association, Washington D.C. 1984, 458.

369. Chen, C. H., Ding, H. C., and Chang, T. C. *J. Food Prot.*, 64, 348, 2001.

370. Charni, N. et al. *Appl. Environ. Microbiol.*, 66, 2278, 2000.

371. Chen, C. H. and Ding, H. C. *J. Food Prot.*, 67, 387, 2004.

372. Moravek, M. et al. *FEMS Microbiol. Lett.*, 238, 107, 2004.

373. Mantynen, V. and Lindstrom, K. *Appl. Environ. Microbiol.*, 64, 1634, 1998.

374. Nakano, S. et al. *J. Food Prot.*, 67, 1694, 2004.

375. Hansen, B. J. and Hendriksen, N. B. *Appl. Environ. Microbiol.*, 67, 185, 2001.

376. Ruiz, J. et al. *J. Clin. Microbiol.*, 35, 2417, 1997.

377. Luccero, N. E. et al. *J. Clin. Microibiol.*, 37, 3245, 1999.

378. Romero, C. et al. *J. Clin. Microbiol.*, 33, 3198, 1995.

379. Batra, H. V., Agarwal, G. S., and Rao, P. V. *J. Commun. Dis.*, 35, 71, 2003.

380. Probert, W. S. et al. *J. Clin. Microbiol.*, 42, 1290, 2004.

381. Al Dahouk, S. et al. *Clin. Lab.*, 50, 387, 2004.

382. Tantillo, G. M., Di Pinto, A., and Buonavoglia, C. *J. Dairy Res.*, 70, 245, 2003.

383. Kabir, S. *J. Med. Microbiol.*, 50, 1021, 2001.

384. Hauser, B. et al. *Acta Paediatr.*, 95, 297, 2006.

385. Koletzko, S. et al. *Gut*, 52, 804, 2003.

386. Shahamat, M. et al. *J. Clin. Microbiol.*, 42, 3613, 2004.

387. Smith, S. I. et al. *World J. Gastroenterol.*, 10, 1958, 2004.

388. Mousavi, S. et al. *Med. Sci. Monit.*, 12, PI15, 2006.

389. Smith, E. M. In *Methods in Environmental Virology*, Gerba, C. P. and Goyal, S. M. (eds.), Marcel Dekker, New York, 1982, p. 15.

390. Williams, F. P., Jr., and Fout, G. S. *Environ. Sci. Technol.*, 26, 689, 1992.

391. Polish, L. B. et al. *J. Clin. Microbiol.*, 37, 3615, 1977.

392. Abd el-Galil, K. H. et al. *Appl. Environ. Microbiol.*, 71, 7113, 2005.

393. Sincero, T. C. et al. *Water Res.*, 2006.

394. Herrmann, J. E. et al. *J. Clin. Microbiol.*, 33, 2511, 1995.

395. Dimitriadis, A. and Marshall, J. A. *Eur. J. Clin. Microbiol. Infect. Dis.*, 24, 615, 2005.

396. Jothikumar, N. et al. *Appl. Environ. Microbiol.*, 71, 1870, 2005.

397. Tian, P. and Mandrell, R. *J. Appl. Microbiol.*, 100, 564, 2006.

398. Schmid, M. et al. *BMC Infect. Dis.*, 4, 15, 2004.

399. Tsunemitsu, H., Jiang, B., and Saif, L. J. *J. Clin. Microbiol.*, 30, 2129, 1992.

400. Adler, M. et al. *Biochem. Biophys. Res. Commun.,* 333, 1289, 2005.

401. Kittigul, L. et al. *J. Virol. Methods*, 124, 117, 2005.

402. Reynolds, K. A. *Methods Mol. Biol.*, 268, 69, 2004.

403. Bosch, A. et al. *Methods Mol. Biol.*, 268, 61, 2004.

404. World Health Organization, *N. Engl. J. Med.*, 353, 1374, 2005.

405. Nicholson, K. G., Wood, J. M., and Zambon, M. *Lancet*, 362, 1733, 2003.

406. Pitt, J. I., Hocking, A. D., and Glenn, D. R. *J. Appl. Bacteriol.*, 54, 109, 1983.

407. Pitt, J. I. and Hocking, A. D. *Fungi and Food Spoilage*, Academic Press, Sydney, Australia, 1985.

408. Samson, R. A., Hoekstra, E. S., Frisvad, J. C., and Filtenborg, O. *Introduction to Foodborne Fungi*, 4th ed., Centraalbureau voor Schimmelcultures, Baarn, The Netherlands, 1995.

409. McClenny, N. *Med. Mycol.*, 43, S125, 2005.
410. Shapira, R. et al. *Appl. Environ. Microbiol.*, 63, 990, 1997.
411. Yong, R. K. and Cousin, M. A. *Int. J. Food Microbiol.*, 65, 27, 2001.
412. Fenelon, L. E. et al. *J. Clin. Microbiol.*, 37, 1221, 1999.
413. Shapira, R. et al. *Appl. Environ. Microbiol.*, 62, 3270, 1996.
414. Yang, Z. Y. et al. *J. Food Prot.*, 67, 2622, 2004.
415. Zachova, I. et al. *Folia Microbiol.* (Praha), 48, 817, 2003.
416. Chen, R. S. et al. *J. Food Prot.*, 65, 840, 2002.
417. King, A. D., Pitt, J. I., Beuchat, L. R., and Corry, J. E. L. *Methods for the Mycological Examination of Food*, Plenum Press, New York, 1986.
418. Marek, P., Annamalai, T., and Venkitanarayanan, K. *Int. J. Food Microbiol.*, 89, 139, 2003.
419. Pedersen, L. H. et al. *Int. J. Food Microbiol.*, 35, 169, 1997.
420. Watanabe, M. and Shimizu, H. *J. Food Prot.*, 68, 610, 2005.
421. Franco, C. M. et al. *J. Chromatogr. A.*, 723, 69, 1996.
422. Ito, R. et al. *J Agric. Food Chem.*, 52, 7464, 2004.
423. Nelson, P. E., Tousoun, T. A., and Marasas, W. F. O. *Fusarium Species: An Illustrated Manual for Identification*, The Pennsylvania State University Press, University Park, PA, 1983.
424. Trane, U., Filtenborg, O., Frisvad, F. C., and Lund, F. In *Modern Methods in Food Microbiology*, Hocking, A. D., Pitt, J. I., and King, A. D. (eds.), Elsevier Science Publishers, New York, 1992, p. 285.
425. Demeke, T. et al. *Int. J. Food Microbiol.*, 103, 271, 2005.
426. Jurado, M. et al. *Syst. Appl. Microbiol.*, 28, 562, 2005.
427. Bluhm, B. H., Cousin, M. A., and Woloshuk, C. P. *J. Food Prot.*, 67, 536, 2004.
428. Reischer, G. H. et al. *J. Microbiol. Methods*, 59, 141, 2004.
429. Knoll, S., Vogel, R. F., and Niessen, L. *Lett. Appl. Microbiol.*, 34, 144, 2002.
430. Maragos, C. M. and Plattner, R. D. *J. Agric. Food Chem.*, 50, 1827, 2002.
431. Iyer, M. S. and Cousin, M. A. *J. Food Prot.*, 66, 451, 2003.
432. Deng, M. Q. and Cliver, D. O. *Parasitol. Res.*, 85, 733, 1999.
433. Pillai, D. R. and Kain, K. C. *J. Clin. Microbiol.*, 37, 3017, 1999.
434. Garcia, L. S. et al. *J. Clin. Microbiol.*, 43, 1256, 2003.
435. Ng, C. T. et al. *J. Clin. Microbiol.*, 43, 1256, 2005.
436. Guy, R. A., Xiao, C., and Horgen, P. A. *J. Clin. Microbiol.*, 42, 3317, 2004.
437. Verweij, J. J. et al. *J. Clin. Microbiol.*, 42, 1220, 2004.
438. Guy, R. A. et al. *Appl. Environ. Microbiol.*, 69, 5178, 2003.
439. Verweij, J. J. et al. *J. Clin. Microbiol.*, 41, 5041, 2003.
440. Zengzhu, G. et al. *J. Clin. Microbiol.*, 37, 3034, 1999.
441. Tanyuksel, M. *Exp. Parasitol.*, 110, 322, 2004.
442. Roy, S. *J. Clin. Microbiol.*, 43, 2168, 2005.
443. Sterling, C. R. and Arrowood, M. J. *Pediatr. Infect. Dis.*, 5, 139, 1986.
444. Coupe, S. *J. Clin. Microbiol.*, 43, 1017, 2005.
445. Miller, W. A. et al. *J. Microbiol. Methods*, 65, 367, 2006.
446. Xiao, L., Lal, A. A., and Jiang, J. *Methods Mol. Biol.*, 268, 163, 2004.
447. Ripabelli, G. et al. *Foodborne Pathog. Dis.*, 4, 216, 2004.
448. Muccio, J. L. *J. Am. Vet. Assoc.*, 225, 7, 2004.
449. Eberhard, M. L., Pieniazek, N. J., and Arrowood, M. J. *Arch. Pathol. Lab. Med.*, 121, 792, 1997.
450. Dixon, B. R. et al. *J. Clin. Microbiol.*, 43, 2375, 2005.
451. Chu, D. M. et al. *Am. J. Trop. Med. Hyg.*, 71, 373, 2004.
452. Shields, J. M. and Olson, B. H. *Appl. Environ. Microbiol.*, 69, 4662, 2003.
453. Verma, M. et al. *J. Microbiol. Methods*, 53, 27, 2003.
454. Hitt, J. A. and Filice, G. A. *J. Clin. Microbiol.*, 30, 3181, 1992.
455. Hofgartner, W. T. et al. *J. Clin. Microbiol.*, 35, 3313, 1997.
456. Roux-Buisson, N. et al. *Diagn. Microbiol. Infect. Dis.*, 53, 79, 2005.
457. Abdel Hameed, D. M. and Helmy, H. *J. Egypt Soc. Parasitol.*, 34, 893, 2004.
458. Switaj, K. et al. *Clin. Microbiol. Infect.*, 11, 170, 2005.
459. Kourenti, C. and Karanis, P. *Water Sci. Technol.*, 50, 287, 2004.
460. Matsuo, J. et al. *Southeast Asian J. Trop. Med. Public Health*, 35, 270, 2004.
461. Schwab, K. J. and McDevitt, J. J. *Appl. Environ. Microbiol.*, 69, 5819, 2003.
462. Yopez-Mulia, L. et al. *Vet. Parasitol.*, 81, 57, 1999.
463. Boulos, L. M. et al. *Parasite*, 8, 136, 2001.
464. Yepez-Mulia, L. et al. *Vet. Parasitol.*, 81, 57, 1999.
465. Gamble, H. R. *J. Food Prot.*, 59, 295, 1996.
466. Wu, Z. et al. *Parasitology*, 118, 211, 1999.

467. Sohn, W. et al. *Kor. J. Parasitol.*, 41, 125, 2003.
468. Kapel, C. M. et al. *Parasite*, 8, S39, 2001.
469. Yagihashi, A. et al. *J. Infect. Dis.*, 161, 995, 1990.
470. Campos, M. et al. *Parasitol. Res.*, 93, 433, 2004.
471. Caballero, M. L. and Moneo, I. *Ann. Allergy Asthma Immunol.*, 89, 74, 2002.
472. Zhu, X. et al. *Int. J. Parasitol.*, 28, 1911, 1998.
473. Szostakowska, B., Myjak, P., and Kur J. *Mol. Cell. Probes*, 16, 111, 2002.
474. Kijewska, A. et al. *Mol. Cell. Probes*, 14, 349, 2000.
475. D'Souza, P. E. and Hafeez, M. *Vet. Res. Commun.*, 23, 293, 1999.
476. Dorny, P. et al. *Acta. Trop.*, 87, 79, 2003.
477. Gottstein, B. et al. *Trans. R. Soc. Trop. Hyg.*, 85, 248, 1991.
478. Nunes, C. M. et al. *Exp. Parasitol.*, 104, 67, 2003.
479. Gonzalez, L. M. et al. *J. Clin. Microbiol.*, 38, 737, 2000.

3 Food Labeling: Foods and Dietary Supplements

Constance J. Geiger

CONTENTS

OVERVIEW

DEFINITION OF FOOD LABELING

Food labeling includes all the information present on food packages: Nutrition labeling is one component of the food label. Other components include the principal display panel, the information panel, the identity of the food, the list of ingredients, the name and place of business of the manufacturer, packer, or distributor, and any claims made.[1]

This chapter reviews the regulatory history of food labeling, required sections of the nutrition label, labeling of restaurant and fresh foods, definitions of allowed nutrient content claims, and requirements for allowed health claims and structure/function claims. The chapter also provides additional resources for food labeling.

HISTORY OF FOOD LABELING

MAJOR FOOD AND NUTRITION LABELING LAWS AND REGULATIONS

Food labeling laws have progressed from merely protecting consumers from economic harm (Pure Food and Drug Act of 1906)[2] to reducing consumers' risk of chronic disease (Nutrition Labeling and Education Act [NLEA] of 1990)[3]. NLEA amended the Federal Food, Drug, and Cosmetic Act (FFDCA) of 1938[4] and required nutrition information be conveyed to consumers so they can readily understand the information and its significance in the context of a total daily diet. NLEA[3] mandated major revisions in the Food and Drug Administration's (FDA) food labeling regulations, including requiring nutrition labeling on almost all processed foods, a revised list of nutrients to be labeled, standardized serving sizes, nutrient content claims, and, for the first time, health claims. In the interest of harmony and uniformity, the U.S. Department of Agriculture's (USDA) Food Safety and Information Service (FSIS) issued similar regulations for meat and poultry products.[5] Table 3.1 summarizes the major laws and selected regulations dealing with food labeling (for further details, see References 6 and 7).

REGULATORY OVERSIGHT FOR LABELING

A number of regulatory agencies have jurisdiction over food labeling, including the FDA, Food Safety and Inspection Service (FSIS), Federal Trade Commission (FTC), and Bureau of Alcohol, Tobacco and Firearms (BATF). Table 3.2 shows their responsibilities.

TABLE 3.1
Major Food and Nutrition Labeling Laws/Selected Regulations

Law	Primary Provisions
Pure Food and Drug Act, 1906	Barred false and misleading statements on food and drug labels[2]
FFDCA, 1938	Replaced the Pure Food and Drug Act of 1906. Created distinct food labeling requirements. Required "common and usual name" of food, ingredient declarations, net quantity information, and name and address of manufacturer/distributor. Defined misbranding[4]
Fair Packaging and Labeling Act, 1966	Provided FDA with authority to regulate provision of label information and package size[8]
Regulations for the Enforcement of the FFDCA and the Fair Packaging and Labeling Act, 1972, 1973	Merged existing regulations into one entity. Required nutrition labeling on processed foods that were fortified or that carried claims. Provided for labeling of fat and cholesterol. Established standards for dietary supplements (DS). Established regulations for artificially flavored foods and imitation foods per serving. Disallowed nutrient claims unless food contained 10% or more of the U.S. Recommended Dietary Allowance (RDA). Incorporated label information: number of servings/container; calories, protein, carbohydrate, and fat content; percentage of adult U.S. RDA for protein and seven vitamins and minerals. Provided for sodium labeling without requirement of the full Nutrition Label Panel[9–11]
NLEA, 1990	Provided for mandatory nutrition labeling on almost all food products, expanded required nutrition information in a new format, created standardized serving sizes, provided consistent definitions of nutrient content claims, and delineated permissible health claims[3]
Dietary Supplement Health and Education Act (DSHEA), 1994	Defined DS, provided for nutrition labeling in a new format, required the name and quantity of every active ingredient, provided for structure/functions claims and good manufacturing practices, encouraged research on DS, created two new government entities: Commission on DS Labels and the Office of Dietary Supplements[12]
FDA Modernization Act (FDAMA), 1997	Expanded procedures by which FDA can authorize health claims and nutrient contents; for example, provided for a notification process[13]

TABLE 3.2
Agencies Having Jurisdiction over Food Labeling

Agency	Responsibility
FDA: Department of Health and Human Services	Mandatory labeling of most packaged foods, except products containing certain amounts of meat and poultry and beverages with certain amounts of alcohol. Voluntary labeling of fresh fruits and vegetables, fresh fish, game and restaurant foods, except those containing certain amounts of meat and poultry
FSIS: USDA	Mandatory labeling on most fresh and processed mean and poultry products (e.g., hot dogs and chicken noodle soup)
FTC	Claims made in food advertising
BATF	Voluntary labeling of alcoholic beverages

THE NEW LABEL FORMAT

Product: Plain yogurt

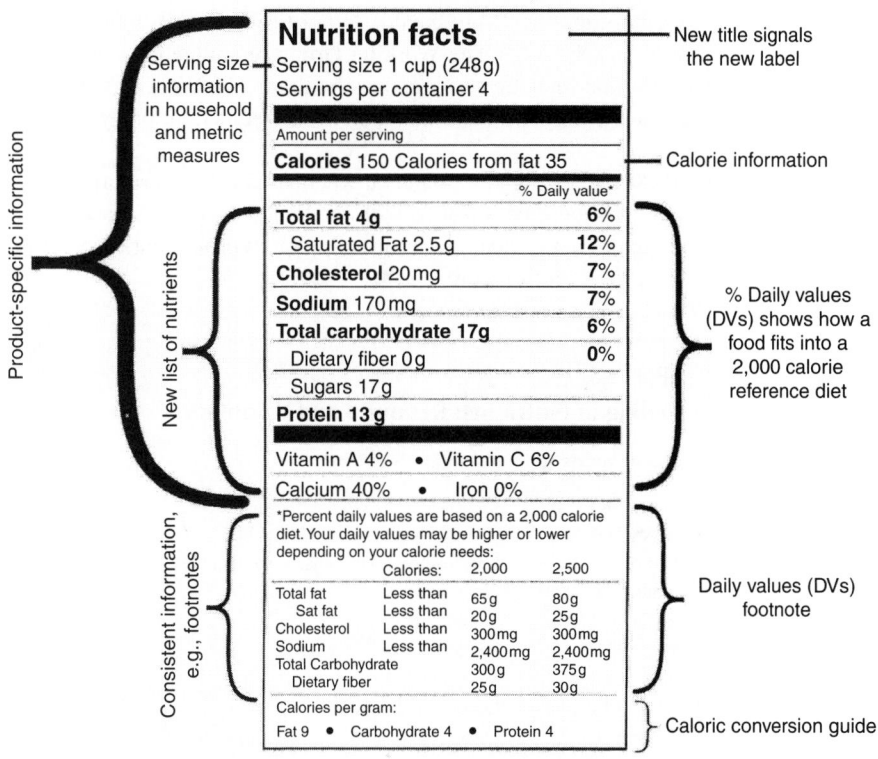

THIS LABEL IS ONLY A SAMPLE. EXACT SPECIFICATIONS ARE IN THE CODE OF FEDERAL REGULATIONS.

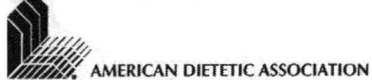

AMERICAN DIETETIC ASSOCIATION

FIGURE 3.1   The Nutrition Facts Panel.

REQUIRED SECTIONS OF THE FOOD LABEL

Those sections of the "Nutrition Facts Panel" that are required are illustrated here (see Figure 3.1). The "Nutrition Facts" information is normally based on a serving of the product as packaged.

REQUIRED NUTRIENTS

The nutrients required to be listed in the Nutrition Facts Panel are listed in Table 3.3. If a product is fortified or a claim is made about a voluntary nutrient, that nutrient also is to be listed. Other nutrients (voluntary nutrients) that may be included in the Nutrition Facts Panel are found in Table 3.3.

SERVING SIZE

Standardized serving sizes, known as Reference Amounts Customarily Consumed (RACCs), are established for many categories of foods. RACCs are based on average amounts people usually eat at one time as determined by the USDA survey data. The basis of using typical consumption data for the standardized serving sizes was mandated by NLEA.[3] The RACCs are based on what people typically consume, not what is recommended by government agencies or health professional associations. These uniform serving sizes help consumers compare products. See Table 3.4 for selected RACCs.

In April 2005, FDA published an Advance Notice of Proposed Rulemaking (ANPRM) entitled: "Food labeling: Serving sizes of products that can reasonably be consumed at one eating occasion; updating of references amounts customarily consumed; approaches for recommending smaller portion sizes."[14] FDA requested comments on serving size information, updating

RACCs, labeling of single-serving containers, and caloric comparisons of foods with different serving amounts. This rule will be finalized with the updating of the Daily Values (DVs) (see the section titled "Daily Values").

CALORIES AND CALORIES FROM FAT

Calories and calories from fat are required because of public health authorities' concern with fat in the diet. In 2004, FDA released the Report of the Working Group on Obesity.[15] The Working Group recommended that the calorie information on the food label be made more prominent and that realistic serving sizes be used. The Working Group also recommended that restaurants be encouraged to display nutrition information and that a consumer education program be launched focusing on a "Calorie Count" message.

In June 2005, FDA published an ANPRM requesting comments on whether calorie information should be more prominent by use of bold print, whether calories from fat should be replaced with % DV from calories, how consumers use calories, and how to reformulate foods or redesign packaging to make calorie information more prominent by other means.[16] An example of the change in calorie information format can be seen in Figure 3.2.

TABLE 3.3
Labeling of Nutrients: Required and Voluntary

Required nutrients	Voluntary Nutrients
Total calories	Calories from saturated fat
Calories from fat	Calories from polyunsaturated fat
Total fat	Calories from monounsaturated fat
Saturated fat	Potassium
trans Fat	Soluble fiber
Cholesterol	Insoluble fiber
Sodium	Sugar alcohol
Total carbohydrate	Other carbohydrates
Dietary fiber	Other essential vitamins and minerals
Sugars	
Protein	
Vitamin A	
Vitamin C	
Calcium	
Iron	

TABLE 3.4
Selected RACCs[a]

Category	RACC
Bakery products: biscuits, bagels, tortillas, soft pretzels	55 g
Beverages: carbonated and noncarbonated beverages, wine coolers, water, coffee or tea (flavored and sweetened), juice, fruit drinks	240 ml
Breads	50 g
Cereals and other grain products	Varies from 25 g for dry pasta to 140 g for prepared rice
Cheese	30 g
Eggs	50 g
Fats and oils	1 tbsp
Fruits: fresh, canned, or frozen, except watermelon	140 g
Meat: entrees without sauce	85 g cooked; 110 g uncooked
Nuts and seeds	30 g
Soups	245 g
Vegetables: fresh, canned, or frozen	85 g fresh or frozen
	95 g for vacuum packed
	130 g for canned in liquid

[a] See Reference 1 (21 CFR 101.12) for further details.

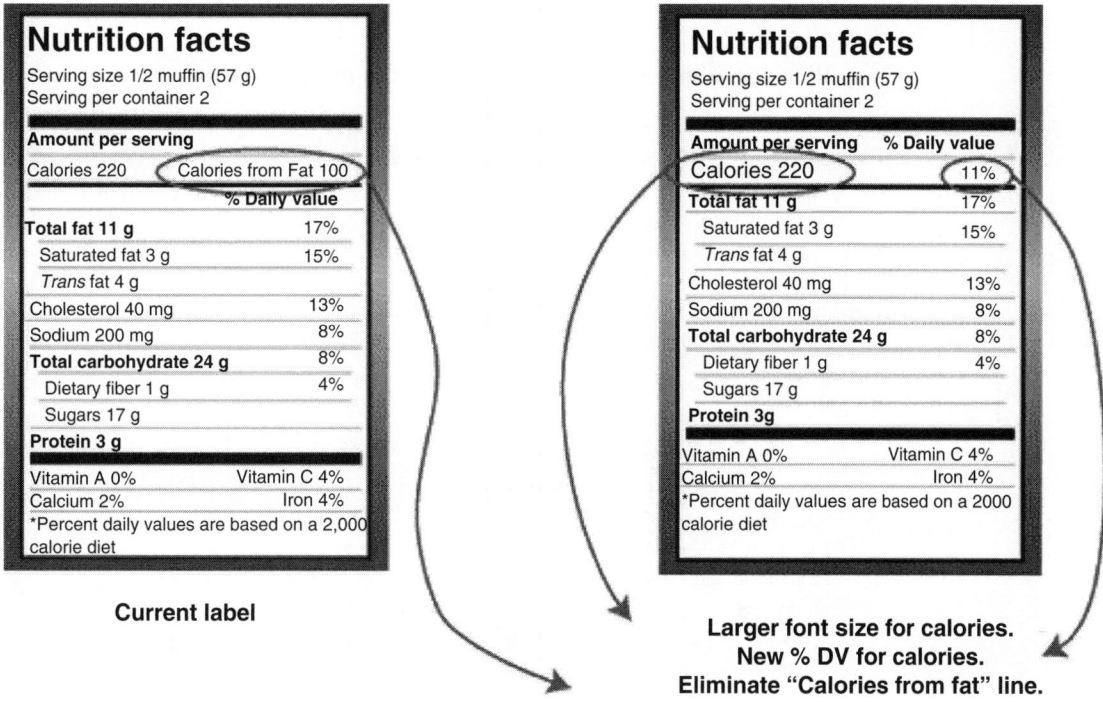

FIGURE 3.2

TABLE 3.5

DRVs for Adults: Calculations and Values[a]

Nutrient	Derivation/Calculation	Label Value
Fat	30% of 2000 cal from fat = 600 cal/9 cal/g	65 g
Saturated fat	10% of calories from saturated fat = 200 cal/9 cal/g	20 g
Carbohydrate	60% of calories from carbohydrate = 1200 cal/4 cal/g	300 g
Protein	10% of calories from protein = 200 cal/4 cal/g	50 g
Fiber	11.5 g per 1000 cal	25 g (rounded up)
Cholesterol[a]	NA	Less than 300 mg
Sodium[a]	NA	Less than 2,400 mg
Potassium[a]	NA	3,500 mg

[a] Based on the 1989 National Research Council's Diet and Health Report.

DAILY VALUES

The standards for labeling of nutrients are known as Daily Values (DVs). The % DV is listed for certain nutrients on the label so that consumers can determine how a serving of a food fits into their total daily diet. The DVs include Daily Reference Values (DRVs) and Reference Daily Intakes (RDIs). DRVs are set for nutrients that previously did not have label standards, such as fat, cholesterol, and saturated fat (see Table 3.5). DRVs are based on a daily intake of 2000 cal, which is a reasonable reference number for adults and children over 4 years, and are calculated based on current nutrition recommendations. The term RDIs replaced the term U.S. Recommended Dietary Allowances (RDAs), but the values are currently the same as the U.S. RDAs, which represent the highest recommended levels of the 1968 RDAs (see Table 3.6).

The DVs for labeling are being updated. The Committee on Use of DRIs in Nutrition Labeling, Food and Nutrition Board, Institute of Medicine, National Academy of Science, developed a report to assist the U.S. FDA, the USDA, and Health Canada by "providing guiding principles for selecting reference values for labeling the nutritive value of foods based on the DRIs and for discretionary fortification of foods including meat and poultry products."[18] The committee's report was published in December 2004.[18] The committee recommended that a population-weighted Estimated Average Requirement (EAR) be used for labeling or, if one does not exist, that the Adequate Intake (AI) be used.

FDA is now finalizing an ANPRM to solicit questions about the values to be used for labeling. Once the ANPRM is published, FDA receives comments, the comments are reviewed, and a proposed rule is published. Comments are again solicited,

TABLE 3.6
RDIs for Adults and Children over 4 Years of Age[a]

Nutrient	RDI
Vitamin A	5000 IU
Vitamin C	60 mg
Calcium	1000 mg
Iron	18 mg
Vitamin D	400 IU
Vitamin E	30 IU
Vitamin K	80 μg
Thiamin	1.5 mg
Riboflavin	1.7 mg
Niacin	20 mg
Vitamin B_6	2.0 mg
Folate	400 μg
Vitamin B_{12}	6 μg
Biotin	300 μg
Pantothenic acid	10 mg
Phosphorus	1000 mg
Iodine	150 μg
Magnesium	400 μg
Zinc	15 mg
Selenium	70 μg
Copper	2 mg
Manganese	2 mg
Chromium	120 μg
Molybdenum	75 μg
Chloride	2400 mg
Choline	

[a] See References 1 (21 CFR 101.9) for further detail.

compiled, and evaluated. Then a final rule implementing the revised DVs is published. The food industry will probably have 2 years to implement these changes. The final rule is not likely to come into effect until 2012 or later.

The DVs, calorie information, and serving-size information will be finalized and implemented together. The change in DVs may affect nutrient content claim and health claim requirements.[19] For example, to carry an "excellent source of folate" claim today, a food would need to provide 20% of the DV for folate, or 80 μg per RACC. If a population-weighted EAR were used for the basis of the claim instead of the RDA, the amount required for a food to carry a health claim could drop to 62 μg. Therefore, using a population-weighted EAR vs. an RDA has important implications for dietary adequacy, educational programs and messaging, and consumer purchase selections.

A footnote is provided at the bottom of the Nutrition Facts Panel to inform consumers of the DVs for both 2000 and 2500 cal levels. The calorie information at the very bottom of the label is voluntary (see Figure 3.1).

SUBSTANCES WITHOUT DVs

Those substances without DVs, such as sugars, *trans* fats, and soluble and insoluble fibers, do not carry a % DV.

LABELING OF RESTAURANT FOODS AND FRESH FOODS

RESTAURANT FOODS

Labeling of restaurant foods is voluntary. Nutrition labeling becomes mandatory if a nutrient content claim or health claim is made. However, the full Nutrition Facts Panel is not required. Only the amount of the nutrient that is the subject of the claim is required to be labeled, for example, "low fat" contains 3 g of fat (21 CFR 101.10).[1] Because Americans spend almost 46% of their food budget on food prepared away from home, FDA commissioned the Keystone Group to hold a forum on Away-From-Home Foods.[20] The group recommended consumers be provided with nutrition information at the point of purchase.

FRESH FRUITS, VEGETABLES, AND SEAFOOD

FDA recommends food retailers provide nutrition information for raw fruits, vegetables, and fish at the point of purchase. Charts, brochures, or signs can be used to depict the nutrition information for the 20 most commonly consumed fruits, vegetables, and raw fish. FDA provides the data for retailers in the Code of Federal Regulations (CFR)[1] (21 CFR 101.45 and Appendix C to Part 101). The data are updated periodically to reflect current analyses.

MEATS AND POULTRY

FSIS recommends food retailers provide point-of-purchase information for meat and poultry.[5] As with fresh produce and fish, charts, brochures, or signs can be used to depict nutrition information. In the near future, fresh meat and poultry labeling will no longer be voluntary. FSIS will be publishing a final rule requiring nutrition labeling on single-ingredient, fresh meat, and poultry products.

NUTRIENT CONTENT CLAIMS ALLOWED FOR FOODS AND DIETARY SUPPLEMENTS

OVERVIEW

FDA and USDA have issued regulations for uniform definitions for nutrient content claims as a result of NLEA.[1,5] Current nutrient content claims have been authorized either by (1) FDA and FSIS as a result of NLEA,[3] which also allowed for petitions for new nutrient content claims or (2) notification of FDA through the FDA Modernization Act (FDAMA).[13] A nutrient content claim characterizes the level of a nutrient in a food (e.g., "high fiber"). Nutrient content claims include two types of claims: absolute (free, low, good source, high, lean, or extra lean) and comparative claims (reduced, light, less, or more). The regulations establish the allowed terms and the criteria/requirements for their use (see Table 3.7). For additional details, see 21 CFR 101.13[1] and 101.54–101.69[1] and 9 CFR 317.360–317.362[5] (Table 3.8). FDA allowed FDAMA nutrition content claims notifications to pass through for choline and omega-3 fatty acids. The labeling page of the FDA's Web site provides detail on the choline notification.[21] The omega-3 fatty acid notifications can be found on the dockets page of FDA's Web site using their docket numbers.[22]

HEALTH CLAIMS ALLOWED FOR FOODS AND DIETARY SUPPLEMENTS

OVERVIEW

NLEA allowed health claims to be carried on qualified food products. Prior to this time, these claims were considered unauthorized drug claims. A health claim describes the relationship between a food, a nutrient, or other substance in a food and the risk of a health-related condition or disease (21 CFR 101.14).[1]

Health claims can be made through third-party references, such as the American Heart Association, and with the use of symbols such as a heart, statements, and vignettes or descriptions. Regardless of the manner of presentation, the requirements for the claim must be met in order for a food or supplement to carry the claim on its product packaging or in its advertising. Health claims carry general and specific requirements. General requirements include not exceeding certain amounts of fat (13 g), saturated fat (1 g), cholesterol (60 mg), and sodium (480 mg). The food must be a "good source" of fiber, protein, vitamin A, vitamin C, calcium, or iron prior to fortification. The specific requirements for each health claim are listed in the CFR (21 CFR 101.72–101.83)[1], except for those authorized through FDAMA[13] or by the courts and enforcement discretion. The requirements for those health claims authorized through FDAMA[13] can be found on FDA's Web site.[21]

Current health claims have been authorized by (1) FDA as a result of NLEA,[3] which also allowed for petitions for new health claims (14 total) (Table 3.9); (2) notification of FDA through FDAMA[13] (Table 3.10); or (3) court action as a result of the Pearson Decision,[23] which provided for qualified health claims (QHCs) for which FDA exercises enforcement discretion (Table 3.11). QHC petitions follow a similar procedure as other health claim petitions.

FDAMA[13] allowed notification of FDA about a health claim. FDAMA health claims, unlike the other claims, allow no opportunity for public comment. A company must compile the data and use an authoritative statement. If FDA takes no action within 120 days of the notification, then the health claim can be made on the foods qualifying for the claim.

The Pearson Decision[23] was brought about by a lawsuit filed by Durk Pearson, Sandy Shaw, and the American Preventive Medical Association to allow four previously denied health claims to be made on dietary supplements (DS). The court decision mandated that FDA (1) reconsider whether to authorize the four previously denied health claims, (2) determine if the weight of the scientific evidence in support of the claims is greater than that against it, and (3) if so, determine if qualifying language would not mislead consumers. FDA was also required to define significant scientific agreement (SSA).

TABLE 3.7
Allowed Nutrient Content Claims with Definitions[a,b]

Claim	Calories	Fat	Saturated Fat	Cholesterol	Sodium	Fiber	Sugar	Protein	Vitamins/Minerals
"Free," "no," "zero," or "without"	Less than 5 cal	0.5 g or less	0.5 g or less	Less than 2 mg cholesterol and 2 g or less saturated fat and *trans* fat	Less than 5 mg	NA	Less than 0.5 g	NA	NA
"Very low"	NA	NA	NA	NA	Less than 35 mg	NA	NA	NA	NA
"Low"	40 cal or less	3 g or less	1 g or less	20 mg or less cholesterol and 2 g or less saturated fat	140 mg or less	NA	NA	NA	NA
"Reduced"	25% lower in calories than the comparable food	25% lower in calories than the comparable food	25% lower in calories than the comparable food	25% lower in calories than the comparable food	25% lower in calories than the comparable food	NA	25% lower in calories than the comparable food	NA	NA
"Light"	1/3 fewer calories than the reference foods, only if the reference food contains less than 50% calories from fat	50% less fat than the reference food	NA	NA	50% less sodium than the reference food; food also is "low fat" and "low calorie"	NA	NA	NA	NA
"Good source," "provides," or "contains"	NA	NA	NA	NA	NA	2.5 to 4.9 g	NA	5 g or more	10% to 19% of the DV
"High," "excellent source of," or "rich in"	NA	NA	NA	NA	NA	5 g or more	NA	10 g or more	20% or more of the DV
"More," "added," "enriched," or "fortified"	NA	NA	NA	NA	NA	NA	NA	10% more of the DV (5 g or more)	10% more of the DV

[a] Definitions vary for meal and main dishes.
[b] Complete definitions are found in Reference 1 (21 CFR 101.13 and 21 CFR 101.54–101.69) and Reference 5 (9 CFR 317.313–317.363).

TABLE 3.8
Other Nutrient Content Claims[a,b]

Claim	Definition
"% Fat free"	Must be "low fat" or "fat free." Must indicate the amount of fat present in 100 g of food.
"Healthy"	Must be "low fat" and "low saturated fat" or "extra lean." Must not exceed disclosure levels for sodium or cholesterol 21 CFR 101.13(h). Must contain 10% DV for vitamin A, vitamin C, iron, calcium, protein, or fiber. (*Exceptions*: fruits and vegetables; frozen or canned single-ingredient fruits and vegetables, except that ingredients whose addition does not change the nutrient profile of the fruit or vegetable may be added; enriched cereal-grain products that conform to a standard of identity.
Lean	Less than 10 g fat, less than 4 g saturated fat, less than 95 mg cholesterol per RACC and per 100 g.
Extra lean	Less than 5 g fat, less than 2 g saturated fat, less than 95 mg cholesterol per RACC and per 100 g.
"High potency"	Food must contain individual vitamins or minerals that are present at 100% or more of the RDI per reference amount or a multi-ingredient food product that contains 100% or more of the RDI for at least $^2/_3$ of the vitamins and minerals with DVs and that are present in the product at 2% or more of the RDI (e.g., "High potency multivitamin, multimineral DS tablets").

[a] Definitions vary for main dish and meal products and may differ for meat, poultry, seafood, and game.
[b] Complete definitions are found in Reference 1 (21 CFR 101.13 and 21 CFR 101.54–101.69) and Reference 5 (9 CFR 3177.313–317.363).

TABLE 3.9
Health Claims Authorized Through the Regulations Implementing NLEA[a]

Health Claim	Model Language	Requirements	Can be Made on Qualified
Cancer			
Fruits and vegetables and cancer	Development of cancer depends on many factors. A diet low in fat and high in fruits and vegetables, such as oranges, which are fat-free and high in vitamin C, vitamin A, and fiber, may reduce the risk of some cancers.	Food product must be or must contain a fruit or vegetable. Product is "low fat" and is a "good source" of at least one of the following: vitamin A, vitamin C, or fiber.	Foods
Fiber-containing grain products, fruits and vegetables and cancer	Low-fat diets rich in fiber-containing grain products, fruits, and vegetables may reduce the risk of some types of cancer, a disease associated with many risk factors.	Food product must be or must contain a grain product, fruit, or vegetable. Food product is "low fat" and is (prior to fortification) a "good source of dietary fiber."	Foods
Fat and cancer	Development of cancer depends on many factors. A diet low in total fat may reduce the risk for some cancers.	Food product is "low fat." Fish and game meats must be "extra lean."	Foods
Coronary heart disease (CHD)			
Fruits, vegetables and grain products that contain fiber, especially soluble fiber, and risk of coronary heart disease	Diets low in saturated fat and cholesterol and rich in fruits, vegetables, and grain products that contain some types of dietary fiber, particularly soluble fiber, may reduce the risk of heart disease, a disease associated with many factors.	Food product contains greater than 0.6 g soluble fiber. Soluble fiber is listed on Nutrition Facts Panel. Food product must be "low fat," "low saturated fat" and "low cholesterol." Food is, or must contain, a vegetable, fruit, or grain product.	Foods
Soluble fiber from certain foods (oats, psyllium, and barley) and coronary heart disease	Diets low in saturated fat and cholesterol that include [ ] g of soluble fiber per day from [name of food] may reduce the risk of heart disease. One serving of [name of food] supplies [ ] g of the [ ] g necessary to have this effect.	*Oats and Barley*: Food contains β-glucan soluble fiber from whole oats or barley. Food contains greater than 0.75 g whole oat soluble fiber or whole grain barley and dry milled barley. Soluble fiber is listed on the Nutrition Facts Panel. Food is "low saturated fat," "low cholesterol," and "low fat" *Psyllium*: Food contains greater than 1.7 g soluble fiber from psyllium husk. Food is "low saturated fat," "low cholesterol," and "low fat." Soluble fiber is listed on the Nutrition Facts Panel.	Foods
Soy protein and coronary heart disease	Diets low in fat and cholesterol that include 25 g of soy protein a day may reduce the risk of heart disease. One serving of [name of food] provides [ ] g of soy protein.	Food contains greater than 6.25 g soy protein. Food is "low saturated fat" and "low cholesterol." Food is "low fat," unless it consists of or is derived from whole soybeans and contains no fat in addition to the fat inherently present in the whole soybeans it contains or from which it is derived.	Foods

Continued

TABLE 3.9
(Continued)

Health Claim	Model Language	Requirements	Can be Made on Qualified
Saturated fat and cholesterol and coronary heart disease	While many factors affect heart disease, diets low in saturated fat and cholesterol may reduce the risk of this disease	Food must be "low saturated fat," "low fat," and "low cholesterol." Fish and game meats must be "extra lean"	Foods
Plant sterols/stanol esters and coronary heart disease	*Plant Stanol Esters*: Diets low in saturated fat and cholesterol that include two servings of foods that provide a daily total of at least 3.4 g of vegetable oil stanol esters in two meals may reduce the risk of heart disease. A serving of [name of food] supplies [ ] g of vegetable oil stanol esters *Plant Sterol Esters*: Foods containing at least 0.65 g per serving of plant sterol esters, eaten twice a day with meals for a daily total intake of at least 1.3 g, as part of a diet low in saturated fat and cholesterol, may reduce the risk of heart disease. A serving of [name of food] supplies [ ] g of vegetable oil sterol esters	Food contains 0.65 g of plant sterol esters/RACC (spreads and salad dressings) or 1.7 g of plant stanol esters/RACC (spreads, salad dressings, snack bars and dietary supplements (DS) in softgel form). Food is "low saturated fat" and "low cholesterol." Food must not exceed the fat disqualifying levels of health claims unless it is a spread or a salad dressing. Those products (spreads or salad dressings) that exceed 13 g of fat must carry a disclosure statement referring consumers to Nutrition Facts Panel for information about fat content. Food contains 10% or more of the DV for vitamin A, vitamin C, iron, calcium, protein, or fiber unless the product is a salad dressing	
Other health claims			
Calcium and osteoporosis	Regular exercise and a healthy diet with enough calcium help teen and young adult White and Asian women maintain good bone health and may reduce their high risk of osteoporosis later in life. Adequate calcium intakes are important, but daily intakes above 2000 mg are not likely to provide any additional benefit	Food or DS must be "high" calcium	Foods and DS
Sodium and hypertension	Diets low in sodium may reduce the risk of high blood pressure, a disease caused by many factors.	Food must be "low sodium"	Foods
Sugar alcohols and dental caries	Frequent eating of foods high in sugars and starches as between-meal snacks can promote tooth decay. The sugar alcohol used to sweeten this food may reduce dental caries	Food must contain less than 0.5 g sugar. Sugar alcohol in the food shall be sorbitol, isomalt, xylitol, lactitol, hydrogenated glucose syrup, hydrogenated starch hydrolysates, or a combination	Foods
Folic acid and neural tube defects	Healthful diets with adequate folate may reduce a woman's risk of having a child with a brain or spinal cord defect	Food or supplements must be a "good source" of folate. Health claim cannot be made on foods that contain more than 100% RDI for vitamin A or D	Foods and DS

[a] See Reference 1 (21 CFR101.14 and 101.72–101.83) for complete requirements.

As a result, FDA now provides enforcement discretion for health claims that are not supported by SSA. A procedure for approving these claims resulted from FDA's Consumer Health Information for Better Nutrition Initiative.[24] In July 2003, FDA published the Task Force Report and Guidance on Qualified Health Claims.[24] Key components included the following:

1. An evidence-based rating system from the Agency for Health Care Research. The strength of the evidence is assigned a rating, and the corresponding language now appears on product packages. The four levels and related qualified statements are as follows:
   "A": SSA (no qualifier).
   "B": "Although there is scientific evidence supporting the claim, the evidence is not conclusive."
   "C": "Some scientific evidence suggests … . However, FDA has determined that this evidence is limited and not conclusive."
   "D": "Very limited and preliminary scientific research suggests … . FDA concludes that there is little scientific evidence supporting this claim."
2. A proposed regulatory framework for QHCs.
3. Consumer studies research agenda.
4. Resources for the review of scientific data.

TABLE 3.10
Health Claims Allowed to Pass Through FDAMA[a]

Health Claim	Model Language	Requirements Per RACC	Can be Made on Qualified
Whole grains and risk of heart disease and certain cancers and coronary heart disease	Diets rich in whole grains and other plant foods and low in total fat, saturated fat and cholesterol, may help reduce the risk of heart disease and certain cancers.	Food contains at least 51% whole grain ingredient(s) by weight, and whole grain is the first ingredient listed. Food must be "low fat, " "low saturated fat," and "low cholesterol." Food must provide at least 16 g of whole grain. Food contains a minimum amount of dietary fiber related to RACC size: 3 g for 55 g RACC, 2.8 g for 50 g RACC, 2.5 g for 45 g RACC, and 1.7 g for 35 g RACC	Foods
Whole grains foods with moderate fat content and CHD and certain cancers	Diets rich in whole grains and other plant foods and low in total fat, saturated fat, and cholesterol may help reduce the risk of heart disease and certain cancers.	Food contains at least 51% whole grain ingredient(s) by weight, and whole grain is the first ingredient listed. Food must be "low saturated fat" and "low cholesterol" and contain less than 6.5 total fat and 0.5 g or less *trans* fat. Food contains a minimum amount of dietary fiber related to RACC size: 3 g for 55 g RACC, 2.8 g for 50 g RACC, 2.5 g for 45 g RACC, and 1.7 g for 35 g RACC Food contains at least 7% of fiber DV if the product does not contain at least 10% DV for protein, calcium, iron, vitamin A or C	Foods
Potassium containing foods and blood pressure and stroke	Diets containing foods that are good sources of potassium and low in sodium may reduce the risk of high blood pressure and stroke.	Food contains at least 10% DV for potassium. Potassium is listed on the Nutrition Facts Panel. Food is "low sodium," "low cholesterol," "low saturated fat," and "low fat"	Foods

[a] See http://www.cfsan.fda.gov/~dms/labfdama.html for further details.

TABLE 3.11
QHC Allowed by the Pearson Decision and FDA Enforcement Discretion[a–d]

Health Claim	Model Language	Requirements Per RACC	Can be Made on Qualified
Cancer Tomatoes or Tomato Sauce and Prostate, Ovarian, Gastric and Pancreatic Cancers: *Docket No. 2004Q-0201*	*Prostate cancer*: Very limited and preliminary scientific research suggests that eating one-half to one cup of tomatoes or tomato sauce a week may reduce the risk of prostate cancer. FDA concludes that there is little scientific evidence supporting this claim *Ovarian cancer*: One study suggests that consumption of tomato sauce two times per week may reduce the risk of ovarian cancer, while this same study shows that consumption of tomatoes or tomato juice had no effect on ovarian cancer risk. FDA concludes that it is highly uncertain that tomato sauce reduces the risk of ovarian cancer *Gastric cancer*: Four studies did not show that tomato intake reduces the risk of gastric cancer, but three studies suggest that tomato intake may reduce this risk. Based on these studies, FDA concludes that it is unlikely that tomatoes reduce the risk of gastric cancer *Pancreatic cancer*: One study suggests that consuming tomatoes does not reduce the risk of pancreatic cancer, but one weaker, more limited study suggests that consuming tomatoes may reduce this risk. Based on these studies, FDA concludes that it is highly unlikely that tomatoes reduce the risk of pancreatic cancer	Food is cooked, raw, dried, or canned tomatoes. Tomato sauces must contain at least 8.37% salt-free tomato solids	Foods

Continued

**TABLE 3.11
(Continued)**

Health Claim	Model Language	Requirements Per RACC	Can be Made on Qualified
Calcium and Colon/ Rectal Cancer and Calcium and Recurrent Colon/ Rectal Polyps: *Docket No. 2004Q-0097*	*Colon/Rectal cancer*: Some evidence suggests that calcium supplements may reduce the risk of colon/ rectal cancer; however, FDA has determined that this evidence is limited and not conclusive *Recurrent colon Polyps*: Very limited and preliminary evidence suggests that calcium supplements may reduce the risk of colon/rectal polyps. FDA concludes that there is little scientific evidence to support this claim	Dietary supplements are "high" calcium. DS contain bioavailable calcium that meets the U.S. Pharmacopeia (USP) standards for disintegration and dissolution applicable to their component calcium salts. For DS for which no USP standards exist, the DS must be bioavailable under conditions of use	DS
Green Tea and Cancer: *Docket No. 2004Q-0083*	*Breast cancer*: Two studies do not show that drinking green tea reduces the risk of breast cancer in women, but one weaker, more limited study suggests that drinking green tea may reduce this risk. Based on these studies, FDA concludes that it is highly unlikely that green tea reduces the risk of breast cancer *Prostrate cancer*: One weak and limited study does not show that drinking green tea reduces the risk of prostate cancer, but another weak and limited study suggests that drinking green tea may reduce this risk. Based on these studies, FDA concludes that it is highly unlikely that green tea reduces the risk of prostate cancer	Food or DS must contain green tea. Food or DS do not need to contain 10% minimum nutrient content requirement	Foods and DS
Selenium and Cancer: *Docket No. 02P-0457*	Selenium may reduce the risk of certain cancers. Some scientific evidence suggests that consumption of selenium may reduce the risk of certain forms of cancer. However, FDA has determined that this evidence is limited and not conclusive	DS must be "high selenium." DS labeling cannot recommend daily intake exceeding 400 g	DS
Antioxidant Vitamins and Cancer: *Docket No. 91N-0101*	Some scientific evidence suggests that consumption of antioxidant vitamins may reduce the risk of certain forms of cancer. However, FDA has determined that this evidence is limited and not conclusive	DS must be "high vitamin C" or "high vitamin E." DS labeling cannot recommend daily intake more than 2000 mg vitamin C or more than 1000 mg vitamin E	DS

Cardiovascular disease risk

Health Claim	Model Language	Requirements Per RACC	Can be Made on Qualified
Omega-3 Fatty Acids and CHD: *Docket No. 2003Q-0401*	Supportive but not conclusive research shows that consumption of EPA and DHA omega-3 fatty acids may reduce the risk of CHD One serving of [Name of the food] provides [ ] gram of EPA and DHA omega-3 fatty acids. (See nutrition information for total fat, saturated fat, and cholesterol content) *Note*: DS may declare the amount of EPA and DHA per serving in "Supplement Facts," instead of making the declaration in the claim	*Fish*: Fish (i.e., "products that are essentially all fish") must have 16 g or less fat per RACC. Fish with fat content greater than 13 g per RACC must include disclosure statement. Fish may not exceed saturated fat disqualifying level and must contain less than 95 mg cholesterol per RACC and per 100 g. If fish contains more than 60 mg, claim must carry disclosure statement *Foods other than fish*: Foods other than fish may not exceed fat disqualifying levels and must be "low saturated fat" and "low cholesterol" *DS*: DS should not recommend daily intake xceeding 2 g of EPA and DHA. DS weighing 5 g or less per RACC are exempted from total fat disqualifying level, but if DS exceed fat disqualifying level must include disclosure statement DS that weigh more than 5 g per RACC must not exceed fat disqualifying level DS must meet the criterion for "low" saturated fat, but not with regard to the no more than 15% calories from saturated fat criterion	Foods and DS

TABLE 3.11
(Continued)

Health Claim	Model Language	Requirements Per RACC	Can be Made on Qualified
		DS that weigh 5 g or less per RACC are exempt from the cholesterol disqualifying level (60 mg per 50 g), but those that exceed cholesterol disqualifying level must include disqualifying statement DS that weigh more than 5 g per RACC must meet the criterion for "low cholesterol"	
Folic Acid, Vitamin B$_6$, and Vitamin B$_{12}$ and Vascular Disease: *Docket No. 99P-3029*	As part of a well-balanced diet that is low in saturated fat and cholesterol, folic acid, vitamin B$_6$, and vitamin B$_{12}$ may reduce the risk of vascular disease. FDA evaluated the above claim and found that, while it is known that diets low in saturated fat and cholesterol reduce the risk of heart disease and other vascular diseases, the evidence in support of the above claim is inconclusive	DS cannot state the daily dietary intake necessary to achieve a claimed effect because the evidence is not definitive. Products greater than 100% DV folic acid must state safe upper limit of 1000 μg. DS containing folic acid must meet USP standards for disintegration and dissolution, except that, if there are no applicable USP standards, folate must be bioavailable under conditions of use	DS
Walnuts and Heart Disease: *Docket No. 02P-0292*	Supportive but not conclusive research shows that eating 1.5 oz per day of walnuts, as part of a low-saturated-fat and low-cholesterol diet and not resulting in increased caloric intake, may reduce the risk of coronary heart disease. See nutrition information for fat (and calorie) content	Food must be whole or chopped walnuts. Food may exceed disqualifying level for fat and is not required to contain 10% minimum nutrient content requirement	Foods
Nuts and Heart Disease: *Docket No. 02P-0505*	Scientific evidence suggests but does not prove that eating 1.5 oz per day of most nuts [such as *name of specific nut*] as part of a diet low in saturated fat and cholesterol may reduce the risk of heart disease. (See nutrition information for fat content). *Notes*: The bracketed phrase naming a specific nut is optional. The bracketed fat content disclosure statement is applicable to a claim made for whole or chopped nuts, but not a claim made for nut-containing products	Food must be whole or chopped nuts or nut-containing products that contain at least 11 g of one or more of almonds, hazelnuts, peanuts, pecans, some pine nuts, pistachio nuts, and walnuts *Nuts*: Nuts must not exceed 4 g saturated fat per 50 g. Nuts may exceed fat disqualifying level. Walnuts do not need to contain 10% minimum nutrient content requirement *Nut-containing products*: Nut-containing products must be "low saturated fat" and " low cholesterol"	Foods
Monounsaturated Fatty Acids from Olive Oil and Coronary Heart Disease: *Docket No. 2003Q-0559*	Limited and not conclusive scientific evidence suggests that eating about two tablespoons (23 g) of olive oil daily may reduce the risk of coronary heart disease due to the monounsaturated fat in olive oil. To achieve this possible benefit, olive oil is to replace a similar amount of saturated fat and not increase the total number of calories you eat in a day. One serving of this product contains [ ] g of olive oil Note: The last sentence of the claim "One serving of this product contains [ ] g of olive oil" is optional when the claim is used on the label or in the labeling of olive oil	*Olive oil*: Food must be pure olive oil *Salad dressing*: Salad dressing must contain at least 6 g olive oil, be "low cholesterol," and not contain more than 4 g of saturated fat per 50 g. *Vegetable oil spreads*: Vegetable oil spreads must contain at least 6 g olive oil, be "low cholesterol," and not contain more than 4 g saturated fat *Olive oil-containing foods*: Olive-oil-containing foods must provide at least 6 g olive oil, be "low cholesterol," and contain 10% DV vitamin A, vitamin C, iron, calcium, protein, or dietary fiber. If the RACC of the olive-oil-containing food is greater than 30 g, the food cannot contain more than 4 g of saturated fat per RACC, and if the RACC of the olive-oil-containing food is 30 g or less, the food cannot contain more than 4 g of saturated fat per 50 g. *Shortenings*: Shortenings must contain at least 6 g olive oil, be "low cholesterol," and not contain more than 4 g of saturated fat per RACC	Foods

Continued

**TABLE 3.11
(Continued)**

Health Claim	Model Language	Requirements Per RACC	Can be Made on Qualified
Calcium and Hypertension, Pregnancy-Induced Hypertension and Preeclampsia: *Docket No. 2004Q-0098*	*Hypertension*: Some scientific evidence suggests that calcium supplements may reduce the risk of hypertension. However, FDA has determined that the evidence is inconsistent and not conclusive *Pregnancy-induced hypertension*: Four studies, including a large clinical trial, do not show that calcium supplements reduce the risk of pregnancy-induced hypertension during pregnancy. However, three other studies suggest that calcium supplements may reduce the risk. Based on these studies, FDA concludes that it is highly unlikely that calcium supplements reduce the risk of pregnancy-induced hypertension *Preeclampsia*: Three studies, including a large clinical trial, do not show that calcium supplements reduce the risk of preeclampsia during pregnancy. However, two other studies suggest that calcium supplements may reduce the risk. Based on these studies, FDA concludes that it is highly unlikely that calcium supplements reduce the risk of preeclampsia	Must be "high calcium." DS calcium content must be bioavailable and must meet USP standards for disintegration and dissolution applicable to their component calcium salts. For DS for which no USP standards exist, the DS must exhibit appropriate assimilability under the conditions of use	DS
Cognitive function Phosphatidylserine and Cognitive Dysfunction and Dementia: *Docket No. 02P-0413*	*Dementia*: Consumption of phosphatidylserine may reduce the risk of dementia in the elderly. Very limited and preliminary scientific research suggests that phosphatidylserine may reduce the risk of dementia in the elderly. FDA concludes that there is little scientific evidence supporting this claim *Cognitive dysfunction*: Consumption of phosphatidylserine may reduce the risk of cognitive dysfunction in the elderly. Very limited and preliminary scientific research suggests that phosphatidylserine may reduce the risk of cognitive dysfunction in the elderly. FDA concludes that there is little scientific evidence supporting this claim	The claim may not suggest level of phosphatidylserine as being useful in achieving the claimed effect. The soy-derived phosphatidylserine must be of very high purity	DS containing soy-derived phosphatidylserine
Diabetes Chromium Picolinate and Diabetes: *Docket No. 2004Q-0144*	One small study suggests that chromium picolinate may reduce the risk of insulin resistance, and therefore possibly may reduce the risk of type 2 diabetes. FDA concludes, however, that the existence of such a relationship between chromium picolinate and either insulin resistance or type 2 diabetes is highly uncertain	DS must be "high chromium"	DS
Neural tube defects 0.8 mg Folic Acid and Neural Tube Birth Defects: *Docket No. 91N-100H*	0.8 mg folic acid in a DS is more effective in reducing the risk of neural tube defects than a lower amount in foods in common form. FDA does not endorse this claim. Public health authorities recommend that women consume 0.4 mg folic acid daily from fortified foods or DS or both to reduce the risk of neural tube defects	There also is a folic acid/neural tube defect health claim authorized by regulation (see 21 CFR 101.79)	DS

[a] For all QHC requirements, the claim meets the general requirements for health claims in Reference 1 (21 CFR 101.14) (unless otherwise noted), *except* for the requirement that the evidence for the claim meet the SSA standard and be made in accordance with an authorizing regulation Reference 1 ([21 CFR 101.14(c)].

[b] All conventional foods must meet the 10% minimum nutrient requirement (vitamin A 5000 IU, vitamin C 6 mg, iron 1.8 mg, calcium 100 mg, protein 5 g, fiber 2.5 g as per RACC), prior to any nutrient addition. The 10% minimum nutrient requirement does not apply to DS [21 CFR 101.14(e)(6)].

[c] If disclosure levels of fat, saturated fat, or cholesterol are exceeded, the appropriate disclosure statements must be included immediately adjacent to the claims, for example, "See nutrition information for total fat content" with the health claim.

[d] Further detail for all claims can be found on the FDA Web site http://www.cfsan.fda.gov/~dms/lab-qhc.html

The final QHC guidance was published in spring 2006.[25] The guidance further details the process for submitting QHC petitions and the language that is used. The process of submitting QHC petitions is similar to that for health claims based on SSA petitions. However, as mentioned, the SSA requirement is not enforced. QHCs need to meet all general health claim requirements unless enforcement discretion is provided. These exceptions are noted in the QHC table (Table 3.11).

FDA authorized 7 claims as a result of NLEA.[3] Since that time, FDA has approved an additional 5 claims submitted as petitions, 3 claims submitted as notifications through FDAMA,[13] and 15 claims as a result of the Pearson Decision and the Consumer Health Information for Better Nutrition Initiative (enforcement discretion). The health claim model language and requirements are indicated in Tables 3.9 to 3.11: those resulting from NLEA[3] and petitions (Table 3.9), those not prohibited by FDA through FDAMA[13] (Table 3.10), and those allowed by court decision[23] (enforcement discretion is applied[24]) and are accompanied by extensive qualifying language (Table 3.11). The qualifying language (an appropriate disclaimer, that is, "some scientific evidence suggests ...") must be placed immediately adjacent to and directly beneath the claim, with no intervening material, and in the same size, typeface, and contrast as the claim itself.

Again, the requirements for the FDAMA[13] and court-mandated health claims[23] or those allowed through enforcement discretion[24] are not published in the CFR.[1] These requirements can be found on FDA's Web site.

Additionally, several QHCs are under review: canola oil and a reduced risk of coronary heart disease, corn oil and corn-oil-containing products and a reduced risk of coronary heart disease, and calcium and vitamin D and a reduced risk of osteoporosis.

STRUCTURE/FUNCTION CLAIMS

OVERVIEW

Structure/function claims can be made on DS.[12] A structure/function claim describes "the role of a nutrient or dietary ingredient intended to affect the structure or function in humans or that characterizes the documented mechanism by which a nutrient or dietary ingredient acts to maintain such structure of function, provided that such statements are not disease claims" (21 CFR 101.93)[1]. "Calcium helps build strong bones" is an example of a structure/function claim.

REQUIREMENTS

The general requirements for structure/function claims include (1) statement be truthful and not misleading, (2) the manufacturer of the DS product carrying the claim notify the FDA within 90 days of entering the product into commerce, and (3) DS carry the following disclaimer:

This product is not meant to prevent, treat, mitigate, or cure any disease.

Specific requirements for structure/function claims are not found in the CFR. Individual claims are not approved by FDA.

RESOURCES

FOOD AND DRUG ASSOCIATION (http://www.fda/gov/)

The FDA Web site provides a wealth of information about FDA labeling activities, regulatory actions and positions, and industry guidance. The site provides FDA organizational structure and a telephone and e-mail directory so that staff contacts can be made. One can check out the "What's New" section for FDA's latest actions. Links are provided to other regulatory agencies such as the FTC and the FSIS.

FOOD SAFETY AND INSPECTION SERVICE (http://www.fsis/gov)

The USDA's FSIS is responsible for overseeing labeling of meat and poultry foods. The agency allows health claims on a case-by-case basis. (FSIS requires label approval prior to use on a product.) The FSIS Web site provides regulatory guidelines and current information.

CFR (http://www.cfsan.fda/gov/~dms/reg-2.html)

The CFR codifies all of the general and permanent rules published in the *Federal Register* by FDA and FSIS, USDA, FTC, and BATF. The CFR is divided into 50 titles, each representing an area of federal regulation, for example, 21 CFR is Food and Drugs, and 9 CFR is USDA. The titles are then divided into chapters that usually bear the name of the responsible agency. Those most pertinent to the food label include 21 CFR 100–169[1] (FDA, food labeling), 21 CFR 170–199[1] (FDA, food additives), and 9 CFR 200 to end[5] (FSIS, food labeling). The CFR can be accessed online through the FDA Web site. The CFR is updated annually.

FEDERAL REGISTER (http://www.cfsan.fda/gov/~dms/reg-2.html)

The federal government, FDA and FSIS, publishes regulations in the *Federal Register* to implement food and DS laws in various forms (notice, proposed rule, and final rule) on a daily basis. Once a final rule is published, it is incorporated into the CFR. The *Federal Register* can be accessed through FDA's Web site. It can be searched by agency, date, date range, or topic.

REFERENCES

1. Food and Drug Administration, U.S. Department of Health and Human Services. Code of Federal Regulations, Title 21, Parts 100–169. Washington, DC: Superintendent of Documents, U.S. Government Printing Office, 2005. http://www.dfsan.fda.gov/~dms/reg-2.html
2. Federal Food and Drug Act of 1906. 34 USC § 768. http://www.fda.gov/opacom/laws/wileyact.htm
3. Nutrition Labeling and Education Act. 1990/ Pub L No. 101-535, 104 Stat 2353. http://thomas.loc.gov/cgi-bin/bdquery/z?d101:HR03562:@@@D&summ2=3&|TOM:/bss/d101query.html|
4. Federal Food, Drug and Cosmetic Act of 1938. 52 USC § 1040. http://www.fda.gov/opacom/laws/fdcact/fdctoc.htm
5. U.S. Department of Agriculture, Food Safety and Information Service. Code of Federal Regulations, Title 9, Parts 200 to end. Washington, DC: Superintendent of Documents, U.S. Government Printing Office, 2005.
6. Geiger, C.J., Parent, C.R.M., Wyse, B.W. *JADA.* 1991; 91: 808.
7. Geiger, C.J. *JADA.* 1998; 98: 1312.
8. Federal Fair Packaging and Labeling Act 1966. 80 USC § 1966. http://www.fda.gov/opacom/laws/fplact.htm
9. Food and Drug Administration. Nutrition labeling: proposed criteria for food label information panel. *Federal Register.* March 30, 1972; 37:6493–6497.
10. Food and Drug Administration. Nutrition labeling. *Federal Register.* January 19, 1973; 38: 2124–2164.
11. Food and Drug Administration. Nutrition labeling. *Federal Register.* March 14, 1973; 38: 6950–6975.
11. Dietary Supplement Health and Education Act of 1994. 108 Stat 4325, 4322. http://www.fda.gov/opacom/laws/dshea.html. Public Law 103–417.
13. Food and Drug Administration Modernization Act of 1997. 21 USC § 301 note. Public Law 105–115. http://www.fda.gov/cder/guidance/105-115.htm
14. Food and Drug Administration. Food labeling: Serving sizes of products that can reasonably be consumed at one eating occasion; Updating of Reference Amounts Customarily Consumed; Approaches for recommending smaller portion sizes: Advance notice of proposed rulemaking. *Federal Register.* 2005; 70: 17010. http://www.fda.gov/OHRMS/DOCKETS/98fr/05-6644.pdf
15. Food and Drug Administration, Working Group on Obesity. Counting Calories: Report of the Working Group on Obesity. 2004. http://www.cfsan.fda.gov/~dms/owg-toc.html
16. Food and Drug Administration. Food labeling; prominence of calories. Advance notice of proposed rulemaking. *Federal Register.* 2005; 70: 1708. http://www.fda.gov/OHRMS/DOCKETS/98fr/05-6643.pdf
17. National Research Council. Diet and Health: Implications for Reducing Chronic Disease Risk. Washington, DC: National Academy Press, 1989.
18. Committee on Use of Dietary Reference Intake in Nutrition Labeling. Dietary Reference Intakes: Guiding Principles for Nutrition Labeling and Fortification. Washington, DC: National Academy Press, 2003.
19. Geiger, C.J., 2006, IFT Annual Meeting Technical Program. Book of Abstracts. No. 103-05, p. 245, 2006.
20. Keystone Center. *Keystone Forum on Away-From-Home Foods: Opportunities for Preventing Weight Gain and Obesity.* Final Report. Washington, DC: The Keystone Center, 2006. ww.keystone.org
21. FDA. *Label claims: FDA Modernization Act of 1997 (FDAMA) Claims.* http://www.cfsan.fda.gov/~dms/labfdama.html.
22. FDA. *FDA Dockets Management.Omega-3 Fatty Acids.* Docket Nos. 2003Q-0401, 2005P-0189 and 2006 P-0137. http://www.fda.gov/ohrms/dockets/default.htm
23. Pearson V. Shalala, 164 F.3d at 661.
24. FDA. *Consumer Health Information for Better Nutrition Initiative: Task Force Final Report.* 2003. http://www.cfsan.fda.gov/~dms/nuttftoc.html
25. FDA. *Guidance for Industry: FDA's Implementation of "Qualified Health Claims": Questions and Answers.* Final Guidance. 2006. http://www.cfsan.fda.gov/~dms/qhcqagui.html
26. FDA. *Label claims: Qualified Health Claims.* http://www.cfsan.fda.gov/~dms/lab-qhc.html

4 Computerized Nutrient Analysis Systems

Judith Ashley and Gwenn Snow

CONTENTS

INTRODUCTION

Since the early 1980s, the incorporation of microcomputer technology into nutrient analysis processes has resulted in the advent of computerized nutrient analysis systems. These systems offer an effective and time-efficient method by which end users can calculate the nutrient composition of foods and beverages for a variety of applications.[1-4] Health professionals can use computerized dietary analyses to provide clients with specific information about their current food/beverage choices and healthful alternatives, with the goal of fostering positive dietary changes. For nutrition educators, the hands-on application of these software programs is an integral part of student education. For researchers and government agencies, nutrient analysis software is an essential tool for analyzing and documenting the usual food intake of individuals, groups, or populations for a variety of uses (e.g., identifying diet–disease relationships). Nutrient analysis software is also important for recipe and menu development by food service managers, chefs, and caterers, and for calculating nutrient information for food labels.

Several companies and organizations offer nutrient analysis software. To be competitive in the market and to stay abreast of changes in scientific knowledge and food production, software vendors must frequently update their programs and the quality and scope of their services. In general, nutrient analysis software provides information about the nutrient composition of foods and beverages selected for analyses. To achieve this end, specific information about foods/beverages (e.g., type or quantity) is entered into the program and assigned a code. The software then uses these codes to locate and store information about the nutrient composition of the specific food items selected and, eventually, to sum across all foods for each nutrient or nutrient component. Programs vary considerably in cost, ease of use, capabilities, size, and available features.[5-7] For the prospective user, the choice of software requires careful consideration of needs and available resources, and financial support for computer hardware and peripherals.

FEATURES OF NUTRIENT ANALYSIS SOFTWARE

Primary features of nutrient analysis software include (1) food descriptions, (2) food portions and weights, (3) nutrients and food components, (4) a user interface, and (5) output options. Commonly, programs include reference standards for evaluating dietary quality (e.g., Dietary Reference Intakes [DRI] and Dietary Guidelines for Americans 2005) and allow users to enter tracking or contact information (e.g., case number, name, address, and telephone number) and data about physiological characteristics (e.g., gender, age, height, and weight; for women, pregnancy or lactation status) specific to individual subjects or clients. This latter feature makes it possible to tailor reference standards to reflect client profiles (e.g., energy needs or targeted weight goals). Refer to Table 4.1 for contact information and details about program applications and database characteristics of several of the larger programs currently available, and Table 4.2 for a comprehensive list of nutrients and food components included in such programs.

Programs vary considerably in the number and types of available output options, with some offering both electronic and printed reports, and textual and graphical data displays (e.g., two- and three-dimensional pie and bar charts). Report contents

TABLE 4.1
Applications and Characteristics of Selected Nutrient Analysis Software Systems

Organization	Axxya Systems	ESHA Research	The CBORD Group, Inc.	The Human Nutrition Center, University of Texas	NutriGenie	The Nutrition Company	Nutrition Coordinating Center, University of Minnesota
Contact Information	www.nutritionist-pro.com 1.800.709.2799	www.esha.com 1.800.659.3742 ext 200	www.cbord.com 1.607.257.2410	www.sph.uth.tmc.edu/hnc/fias/software.htm 1.713.500.9775	nutrigenie.biz Telephone number N/A	www.nutritionco.com 1.888.659.6757	www.ncc.umn.edu 1.612.626.9450
Program Name	Nutritionist Pro™ Nutrition Food Labeling[a]	Food Processor SQL / Genesis SQL	Nutrition Service Suite[®b]	Food Intake Analysis System	NutriGenie[c]	Foodworks 8.0	Nutrition Data System for Research (NDS-R)
Applications							
Nutrition Support		X	X		X	X	
Menu Planning			X		X	X	X
Education		X	X	X	X	X	X
Nutrition Surveys			X	X	X	X	X
Epidemiological Research			X	X	X	X	X
Nutrition Intervention		X	X	X	X	X	X
Recipe Calculations	X	X	X	X	X	X	X
Research and Development	X	X			X	X	X
NLEA Label Values	X	X	X				
Database characteristics							
Number of foods in database	>23,000	32,000	19,082	7,321	8,000	>30,000	18,000
Number of nutrients/food components	90	133	143	52	30	113	139
Database sources							
USDA NDB SR	X	X	X		X	X	X
CSFII/FNDDS	X	X	X	X		X	X
Canadian Nutrient File	X	X					
Other	X	X	X		X	X	X
Demo Available	X	X		X	X	"Delayed Registration"	X

[a] Nutritionist Pro®: Multiple products available; product characteristics vary.

[b] The CBORD Group, Incorporated: Multiple products available; product characteristics vary.

[c] NutriGenie: Multiple products available; product characteristics vary.

Source: 28th National Nutrient Databank Conference, International Nutrient Databank Directory, Software Vendors (2004). Adapted with permission.

TABLE 4.2
Dietary Components Available in Computerized Nutrient Analysis Systems

Energy Sources
Energy (kilocalories)
Energy (kilojoules)
Total protein
Total fat
Total carbohydrate
Alcohol
Animal protein
Vegetable protein
Percentage of calories from
    protein
    fat
    trans fat
    carbohydrate
    alcohol
Fat and Cholesterol
Cholesterol
Total saturated FA[a] (SFA)
Total monounsaturated FA[a]
(MUFA)
Total polyunsaturated FA[a] (PUFA)
Total *trans* FA[a] (TFA)
Total omega-3 FA[a]
    Eicosapentaenoic acid 20:5
    Docosahexaenoic acid 22:6
Total omega-6 FA[a]
    Docosapentaenoic acid 22:5
Percentage of calories from
    SFA
    MUFA
    PUFA
PUFA:SFA
Cholesterol to SFA Index
Fatty Acids
SFA: 4:0 to 22:0
MUFA: 14:1 to 22:1
PUFA: 18:2 to 22:6
Trans FA: 16:1 to 18:2
Carbohydrates
Starch
Total sugar
Added sugar
Fructose
Galactose
Glucose
Lactose
Maltose
Sucrose
Fiber
Total dietary fiber
Soluble fiber
Insoluble fiber
Pectins

Vitamins
Total vitamin A activity
    RE[b]
    IU[c]
        retinol activity equivalents
β-carotene equivalents
Vitamin E, IU[c]
Vitamin E, total α-tocopherol
Natural α-tocopherol
Synthetic α-tocopherol
α-tocopherol equivalents
β-tocopherol
γ-tocopherol
δ-tocopherol
Vitamin C
Vitamin D
    IU[c]
    micrograms
Vitamin K
Thiamin (B$_1$)
Riboflavin (B$_2$)
Niacin (B$_3$)
Niacin equivalents
Folate
Dietary folate equivalents
Natural folate
Synthetic folate (folic acid)
Vitamin B$_6$
Vitamin B$_{12}$
Pantothenic acid
Biotin
Carotenoids
β-carotene (provitamin A carotenoid)
α-carotene (provitamin A carotenoid)
β-cryptoxanthin (provitamin A carotenoid)
Lutein + Zeaxanthin
Lycopene
Minerals
Boron
Calcium
Chloride
Chromium
Copper
Iodine
Iron
Magnesium
Manganese
Molybdenum
Phosphorous
Potassium
Selenium
Sodium
Zinc

Amino Acids
Tryptophan
Threonine
Isoleucine
Leucine
Lysine
Methionine
Cystine
Phenylalanine
Tyrosine
Valine
Arginine
Histidine
Alanine
Aspartic acid
Glutamic acid
Glycine
Proline
Serine
Taurine
Isoflavones
Daidzein
Genestein
Glycitein
Coumestrol
Biochanin A
Formononetein
Other
Ash
Caffeine
Theobromine
Acesulfame Potassium
Aspartame
Saccharin
Sucralose
Sugar alcohols, total
    Glycerol
    Inositol
    Mannitol
    Sorbitol
    Xylitol
Organic acids, total
    Acetic acid
    Citric acid
    Lactic acid
    Malic acid
Oxalic acid
Phytic acid
Sucrose polyester
3-methylhistidine
Choline
Water

[a] FA = Fatty acids.
[b] RE = Retinol equivalents.
[c] IU = International units.

also vary by vendor and may include simple nutrient summaries, lists of foods in descending or ascending order by nutrient contribution, or recommendations for enhancing dietary quality.

Additional software features include mechanisms for comparing food/beverage choices with food exchange lists; assessing nutrient intake by meal, food item, or food category; and classifying foods according to the glycemic index. Programs are also available that allow data to be collected and averaged for individuals or groups or for a specified time period, ranging from a single eating occasion to several days' worth of meals and snacks. Some programs allow users to export data into statistical analysis software packages or word-processing programs or to enter data by scanning questionnaires (e.g., food frequency checklists). The latter would be useful for entering large data sets or calorie-count data for patients who are hospitalized or institutionalized. Alternatively, nutrient analysis software might support multiuser platforms, interface with foodservice management software, provide information about potential food–drug interactions, contain recipe databases, and include nutrient information for nutrition support regimens. Programs are available that allow users to add or modify foods, nutrients, and recipes; scale or cost recipes; plan meals, including meals that must provide one-third of the Recommended Dietary Allowance (RDA) for nutrients; generate sample menus; or customize nutrition support regimens.

BASIC QUESTIONS TO ASK WHEN CONSIDERING DIFFERENT SOFTWARE SYSTEMS

Depending on the projected use of nutrient analysis software, many or all of the following questions may apply when evaluating individual programs:

- What are the operating system and hardware requirements? Are these requirements compatible with existing equipment and peripherals? If not, are funds available to purchase new hardware?
- How many food items are included in the database? What types of foods are included? For example, does the database contain information about baby foods, convenience foods, fast foods, regional specialties, ethnic specialties, fortified/enriched foods, fat-modified foods, sugar-free foods, or nutritional supplements? Can foods, beverages, or recipes be added?
- What specific nutrients and nutritional components are in the database? Does this list include the nutrients and food components or values (e.g., glycemic index) of interest to you? Is the number of nutrients in the database at the low-end, middle, or high-end range of available nutrients? Can information about nutrients and food components be added?
- How complete is the nutrient information? What are the origins of nutrient values? What is the extent of missing values? When data for specific nutrients are missing, are these estimated or left as zero? Are missing nutrient values identified in reports so that findings are not misleading? (Note: Methods for estimating and reporting missing values dramatically affect the accuracy of nutrient reports.)
- What dietary reference standards are available for use? Are these standards up-to-date? Are standards included for subpopulations (e.g., children, pregnant or lactating women)?
- How is the quality of the database maintained? How often is the software upgraded to reflect changes in the market or advances in scientific knowledge?
- How easy or difficult is it to enter dietary information? Do data entry options include numeric code, food name, brand name, and search features? Can users store or copy frequently used food or meal categories for ready access? Is technical support available to assist users in distinguishing among food listings?
- Can data related to portion sizes be entered using weight, volume, dimensions, or all three measures? Can data be entered in common household measures?
- Does the software allow data from standard food frequency forms to be entered? Can data from such forms be scanned? Is this option included in the usual cost of the software or available for a price?
- Are reports available for a variety of criteria such as reference standards (e.g., RDA), dietary recommendations (e.g., MyPyramid Food Guidance System), and meal planning methods (e.g., food exchange lists)? Can reports be customized to reflect specific nutrients?
- Are reports available that summarize intake data from several days or weeks for comprehensive analysis? Are reports available that summarize intake data by eating occasion? Are reports available that summarize intake data by days of the week? Are reports available that compare data from several points in time to allow for longitudinal comparisons?
- Are reports available that identify key sources of nutrients from the data entered? Can lists of food sources of nutrients be generated?
- Are on-screen reports available in a form that is suitable for use with clients? Can dietary choices be manipulated to demonstrate the effects of dietary changes on nutrient intake or dietary quality? Is this feedback provided instantaneously?

- Are printed reports available? How many options for reference criterion and nutrient content are available for printed reports? Can additional information or comments be added to printed reports?
- Are reports available that use easy-to-understand graphics (e.g., bar graphs and pie charts) to compare intake with designated standards? Are these graphical comparisons available for a variety of reference criterion (see above) and nutrients?
- Are reports accurate, descriptive, and attractive? Are key findings or recommendations readily apparent?
- What formulas are used to calculate energy requirements? If healthy or ideal body weights are suggested, how are these determined? Are such recommendations based on current and reasonable standards?
- Can exercise data be incorporated into caloric requirements? Do reports include exercise recommendations?
- Are there system utilities for backing up valuable data and reports? Are there mechanisms in place to maintain the confidentiality of client information?
- What is the quality of software documentation, online help, and tutorials? Are these easy to understand and specific to user needs? Are these comprehensive in scope?
- What is the quality of customer service, product support, and ongoing maintenance? Is there sufficient technical support provided to answer user needs? Is training available or required?
- What does the complete system, with updates and service, cost? Are there additional costs for multiple users or stations?
- How often are upgrades offered? Is there an additional cost for upgrades?
- Who is the target audience of the output? Are appropriate output options available for consumers, health professionals, medical centers or hospitals, or researchers?

IMPORTANCE OF FOOD COMPOSITION DATABASES

Nutrient analysis software relies heavily on existing food composition databases for nutrient information. Importantly, multiple factors affect the accuracy of these databases, such as the sources of nutrient composition information, the number of foods and nutrients in the database, the number of missing values, the methods by which missing values are handled, and the frequency with which databases are updated.[8] Several published reports have compared the accuracy of nutrient calculations among a limited number of database systems.[9–16] When these calculations were compared with a standard[17–19] or tested against chemical analyses from a single source,[20–22] findings indicated that most nutrients were within 15% of reference values. For example, after comparing calculations from four nutrient composition databases with chemically analyzed values for 36 menus, researchers found that the database values for the nutrients examined had relatively good accuracy: Seven nutrients deviated by values < 10%; five, by 10 to 15%; and only one, by 15 to 20%.[23] While these findings are positive, it is important to note that no standardized benchmarks have been established for comparing the different methods used to determine the nutrient content of foods/beverages. In addition to the quality of nutrient composition databases, other factors affect the accuracy of nutrient analyses (e.g., see Table 4.3).

Most nutrient analysis systems in the United States are based on the U.S. Department of Agriculture's (USDA) National Nutrient Database for Standard Reference (NNDSR) and incorporate nutrition information from other scientific sources and food companies.[24,25] The most recent version is NNDSR-Release 18. NNDSR-18 contains data for over 7146 foods and up to 136 nutrients and food components. The following changes were incorporated into SR18: (1) nutrient values for vitamins E and B_{12} for all foods used in the Food and Nutrition Database for Dietary Studies, (2) new and updated food items (e.g., new beef cuts, French fried potatoes, flaxseed, frozen novelties, sweeteners, and noncarbonated or fitness waters), and (3) expanded brand name fast food data.[25] Comprehensive information about NNDSR-18 can be found at USDA's Nutrient Data Laboratory Web site, including details about all of the foods in the database (e.g., scientific name and nutrient content), nutrient lists for selected foods and nutrients, and documentation (e.g., content of files, weights and measures, and data sources).[26] The Nutrient Data Laboratory also provides access to additional data sets that complement NNDSR-18: *Reports by Single Nutrients*, *Nutritive Value of Foods*, special interest databases for some nutrients (i.e., choline and fluoride), and specific dietary components (i.e., flavonoids, isoflavones, oxalic acid, and proanthocyanidins).[27]

TABLE 4.3
Factors That May Affect Consistency of Nutrient Analysis Outputs

- Data entry errors (e.g., misidentification of foods or incorrect food substitutions)
- Nutrient variability in the food supply
- Frequent changes in the nutrient content of processed foods
- Margin of error allowed for nutrient information from food labels
- Estimated or imputed values for missing nutrient information
- Constraints of chemically determined nutrient values used for comparison (e.g., sample collection or assayed values)

TABLE 4.4
Nutrient Analysis Software Reports: Discussion Topics for Patient Counseling

- Comments that explain and clarify results
- Synopsis of the limitations of the analysis
- Suggestions to improve dietary intake (e.g., information about good food sources of specific nutrients)
- Information about dietary supplements (if warranted)
- Information about supplementary resources, as appropriate

TABLE 4.5
Nutrient Analysis Software Systems: Current and Future Trends

- Expansion to include new or revised nutrient standards[4,24] and dietary recommendations
- Standardization of nutrient composition databases to accommodate international differences in nutrient values, food content and preparation methods, units of measure, and recognized food components[28]
- Identification of bioactive components in foods (e.g., phytochemicals, pre- and probiotics, total antioxidant capacity)[3, 29–33]
- Fortification and enrichment of foods[3]
- Adaptation for use with portable and hand-held computerized devices[7]
- Utilization of automated methods for collecting and processing dietary data such as the Automated Multiple Pass Method,[34] smart cards,[35] and bar codes[36]
- Computation of glycemic load values[37] or other, as-yet-unidentified, markers
- Inclusion of food-borne contaminants (e.g., pesticides or heavy metals)[3]
- Addition of bilingual capabilities[38]
- Determination and addition of information about the nutrient composition of dietary supplements[8,32,39]

The development of representative food composition values involves the acquisition, documentation, evaluation, and aggregation of food composition data. These data are compiled from a wide variety of sources, including published (e.g., manuscripts in the scientific and technical literature) and unpublished sources (e.g., food industry and research under restricted USDA Agricultural Research Service contracts).[25,26]

LIMITATIONS OF NUTRIENT ANALYSIS SOFTWARE

Nutrient analysis software programs have unique limitations.[6] For example, calculations of nutrient intakes may lack precision because of the multiple variables involved, including the size and quality of the databases, calculation methods, and extent of missing values. However, these software-related variables are minor when compared with the human challenges to accuracy. Food intake reports from clients and subjects (e.g., food records and food frequencies) may be inaccurate. Data entry errors may occur if operators misinterpret food descriptions or do not select the correct matches from the database.

In other cases, results may be misinterpreted. For example, computer-generated printouts might appear authoritative, giving the impression that reports are extremely precise, but this may not always be the case (e.g., database may contain multiple missing values). Additionally, individuals unfamiliar with DRI/RDA comparisons may misinterpret these values as minimal nutrient needs and assume that intake levels should be over 100% to avoid deficiencies. Even professionals may have difficulty drawing specific conclusions for individuals when using the DRI/RDA as reference standards.

With regard to these and other limitations, health professionals who use nutrient analysis software to evaluate dietary intake of clients and patients are advised to provide counseling along with software-generated reports (see Table 4.4 for suggestions).

TRENDS IN NUTRIENT ANALYSIS SOFTWARE

Continual advances in scientific knowledge and technology, changes in dietary guidance, and variations in the needs and interests of researchers, educators, and health professionals present constant challenges and multiple opportunities for the development and maintenance of and applications for nutrient analysis software (e.g., see Table 4.5).

CONCLUSION

Nutrient analysis software can be a useful tool for individuals, agencies, or organizations interested in assessing the dietary intake of individuals and populations. Output from these programs can be used to provide specific guidance or develop interventions that may ultimately improve dietary intake and health among individuals and populations.

REFERENCES

1. Hoover, L.W., *Clin. Nutr.*, 6: 198; 1987.
2. Feskanich, D., Buzzard, I.M., Welch, B.T. et al., *JADA*, 88: 1263; 1988.
3. Harrison, G.G., *J. Food Compost. Anal.*, 17: 259; 2004.
4. Stumbo, P.J. and Murphy, S.P., *J. Food Compost. Anal.*, 17: 485; 2004.
5. Byers, T. and Thompson, F.E., *J. Nutr.*, 124: 2245S; 1994.
6. Grossbauer, S., in *Communicating as Professionals*, 2nd ed., Chernoff, R., Ed., The American Dietetic Association, Chicago, 11, 1994, 56.
7. Prestwood, E., *Today's Dietitian*, December: 44; 2005.
8. Dwyer, J.T., Picciano, M.F., Betz, J.M. et al., *J. Food Compost. Anal.,* 17: 493; 2004.
9. Adelman, M.O., Dwyer, J.T., Woods, M. et al., *JADA*, 83: 421; 1983.
10. Hoover, L.W., *JADA*, 83: 501; 1983.
11. Frank, G.C., Farris, R.P., Hyg, M.S. et al., *JADA*, 84: 818; 1984.
12. Taylor, M.L., Kozlowski, B.W., and Baer, M.T., *JADA*, 85: 1136; 1985.
13. Shanklin, D., Endres, J.M., and Sawicki, M., *JADA*, 85: 308; 1985.
14. Eck, L.H., Klesges, R.C., Hanson, C.L. et al., *JADA*, 88: 602; 1988.
15. Stumbo, P.J., *JADA*, 92: 57; 1992.
16. LaComb, R.P., Taylor, M.L., and Noble, J.M., *JADA*, 92: 1391; 1992.
17. Nieman, D.C. and Nieman, C.N., *JADA*, 87: 930; 1987.
18. Nieman, D.C., Butterworth, D.E., Nieman, C.N. et al., *JADA*, 92: 48; 1992.
19. Lee, R.D., Nieman, D.C., and Rainwater, M., *JADA*, 95: 858; 1995.
20. Pennington, J.A.T. and Wilson, D.B., *JADA*, 90: 375; 1990.
21. Obarzanek, E., Reed, D.B., Bigelow, C. et al., *Int. J. Food Sci. Nutr.*, 44: 155; 1993.
22. McKeown, N.M., Rasmujssen, H.M., Charnley, J.M. et al., *JADA*, 100: 1201; 2000.
23. McCullough, M.L., Karanja, N.M., Lin, P.H. et al., *JADA*, 99: 545; 1999.
24. Schakel, S.F., Sievert, Y.A., and Buzzard, I.M., *JADA*, 88: 1268; 1988.
25. U.S. Department of Agriculture (USDA), Agricultural Research Service (ARS), *Composition of Foods, Raw, Processed, Prepared, USDA NNDSR-18*. Available online at http://www.ars.usda.gov/Services/docs.htm?docid=8964, *under SR18 documentation*, accessed 060130, 2005.
26. USDA, ARS, *USDA National Nutrient Database for Standard Reference, Release 18*. Available online at http://www.ars.usda.gov/ba/bhnrc/ndl, accessed 050130, 2005.
27. USDA, ARS, *Data Sets Prepared by USDA-ARS's Nutrient Data Laboratory*. Available online at http://www.ars.usda.gov/Services/docs.htm?docid=5121, accessed 060130, 2005.
28. Charrondière, U.R., Vignat, J., and Riboli, E., *IARC Sci. Pub.*, 156: 45; 2002.
29. Spence, J.T., *Research on the Composition of Functional Foods*. Presentation, 28th National Nutrient Databank Conference, Iowa City, IA. Available online at http://www.medicine.uiowa.edu/gcrc/nndc/Conference%20PowerPoint%20Slides.html, accessed 060201, 2004.
30. Pillow, P.C., Duphorne, C.M., Chang, S. et al., *Nutr. Cancer*, 33: 3; 1999.
31. Wu, X., Gu, L., Holden, J. et al., *J. Food Compost. Anal.*, 17: 407; 2004.
32. USDA, ARS, *National Food and Nutrient Analysis Program*. Available online at http://www.ars.usda.gov/Research/docs.htm?docid=9446, accessed 060210, 2006.
33. Zhuo, X.-G. and Watanabe, S., *BioFactors*, 22: 329; 2004.
34. Raper, N., Perloff, B., Ingwersen, L. et al., *J. Food Compost. Anal.*, 17: 545; 2004.
35. Flood, A., *A Method for Adding Glycemic Load Values to a Food Frequency Questionnaire Database*. Presentation, 28th National Nutrient Databank Conference, Iowa City, IA., Available online at http://www.medicine.uiowa.edu/gcrc/nndc/Conference%20Power-Point%20Slides.html, accessed 060201, 2004.
36. Lambert, N., Plumb, J., Looise, B. et al., *J. Hum. Nutr. Diet.*, 18: 243; 2005.
37. Anderson, A.S., Maher, L., Ha, T. et al., *Public Health Nutr.*, 2: 579; 1999.
38. Zoellner, J., Anderson, J., and Gould, S.M., *JADA*, 105: 1205; 2005.
39. Dwyer, J., Picciano, M.F., Raiten, D.J. et al., *J. Nutr.*, 133: 624S; 2003.

5 Nutrient Data Analysis Techniques and Strategies

Alan R. Dyer, Kiang Liu, and Christopher T. Sempos

CONTENTS

OVERVIEW

Analyses of nutrient data pose special challenges to investigators. In such analyses, investigators need to consider:

1. Possible over- or under-reporting of intakes, leading to "impossible" or extreme values in the data set
2. How to adjust for total energy intake
3. How to model nutrients, for example, as continuous or categorical variable
4. How to avoid multicollinearity
5. How to handle dietary supplement data
6. Impact of large day-to-day variability and person-specific biases in self-reported intakes, both of which can lead to misclassification of individuals with respect to usual intake

The objectives of this chapter are to examine various approaches to addressing the aforementioned issues, to briefly describe the common types of observational and experimental studies that collect nutritional data, and to describe the most common methods of analysis used in the types of studies described.

QUALITY CONTROL

Regardless of whether investigators use a validated food frequency questionnaire or single or multiple 24 h recalls to collect dietary data, the importance of quality control in such data collection cannot be overemphasized. The phrase GIGO (garbage in, garbage out) serves as a stark reminder of the importance of ensuring that dietary data are of the highest quality when they are submitted for analysis. No amount of analytic sophistication can make up for poor-quality data.

STEPS TO ENSURE GENERAL STUDY AND INTERVIEWER QUALITY

To improve the quality of collected data, investigators should:

- Develop a "Manual of Operations" for nutrient data collection
- Train and certify dietary interviewers in collection of data and use of the manual
- Tape interviews, after obtaining the consent of the participant
- Immediately review a printout of the data collected, including nutrient totals if the system being used permits
- Develop range limits for important nutrients that result in careful review of the questionnaire or 24 h recall with the participant, if limits are exceeded
- Make inquiries to cooks for clarifying reported information when needed
- Query the participant for a 24 h recall on whether the amount consumed was typical, and if atypical, the reason the amount consumed was unusually low or high, for example, lower than usual due to illness
- Use food composition data to estimate nutrient composition for foods and recipes not found in a database when using 24 h recalls
- Randomly select tape recordings for repeat completion of questionnaires or reentry of data, with assessment of discrepancies and correction of incorrect data
- Develop criteria for recertifying interviewers based on the randomly selected recordings

PLAUSIBILITY OF INTAKES

Interviewers may also be requested to indicate whether they believe the participant has provided reliable data. Persons deemed by the interviewer as not providing reliable data should be excluded from the analyses.

Prior to conducting analyses, investigators may wish to set limits on total caloric intake above or below which persons would be excluded. For example, in the Coronary Artery Risk Development in (young) Adults Study (CARDIA),[1] men who reported intakes of >8000 kcal or <800 kcal and women who reported intakes of >6000 kcal or <600 kcal on food frequency questionnaires were excluded from analyses, because values outside these limits were not considered consistent with a normal lifestyle.[2] The INTERMAP study of macro-/micronutrients and blood pressure excluded from analysis persons who reported energy intakes <500 kcal or >5000 kcal for women or >8000 kcal for men on any of four 24 h recalls.[3,4] Food frequency questionnaires generally have larger standard deviations in total energy intake than 24 h recalls, and thus are more likely to have individuals with "impossible" or extreme values.[5] Hence, investigators using food frequency questionnaires need to be particularly attentive to establishing exclusionary cutoffs for total energy intake, such as those used in CARDIA. Investigators using 24 h recalls should consider whether to exclude persons reporting that their 24 h intakes were unusual as well as whether to establish exclusionary cutoffs similar to those used in INTERMAP.

STATISTICAL ISSUES IN ANALYSIS OF INTAKES

IDENTIFYING OUTLIERS OR EXTREME VALUES

Prior to conducting any analyses, investigators should examine the distribution of each variable of interest for outliers or extreme values. The procedure Proc Univariate in SAS is particularly useful in this regard.[6] In addition to providing the standard descriptive statistics, for example, mean, median, standard deviation, range, interquartile range, etc., this procedure also identifies the five largest and five smallest values for each variable, and the 1st, 5th, 10th, 25th, 75th, 90th, 95th, and 99th percentiles. The user can also request a box plot of the data, which can be very helpful in identifying extreme values. The box plot helps indicate how discrepant the largest and smallest values are from the rest of the data. In the Observing Protein and Energy Nutrition (OPEN) Study,[7] investigators excluded values of dietary variables that fell outside the interval given by the following: 25th percentile minus twice the interquartile range to the 75th percentile plus twice the interquartile range on the logarithmic scale.

The fact that a statistical software package identifies values as large or extreme relative to other values in the distribution should not be taken as prima facie evidence that such values are invalid or that an error was made in data collection or data entry. Values so identified should be examined for such problems. However, if the values are biologically plausible and no error appears to have been made, they should not be arbitrarily excluded from the analysis. Neter et al.[8] suggest that a safe rule is "to discard an outlier only if there is direct evidence that it represents an error in recording, a miscalculation, a malfunctioning piece of equipment, or a similar type of circumstance." When outliers are retained in a data set, the investigator needs to take special steps to assess any influence they may have on the results of the analysis. This can include analyses with and without the outlying value or values, use of nonparametric statistical methods (for example, the Spearman rank correlation instead of the usual Pearson correlation coefficient), transformations of the data that bring the outlying value closer to the other values (for example, the log or square root transformation), specific tests for influential observations,[8] or use of robust regression methods.[9]

ADJUSTMENT FOR TOTAL ENERGY INTAKE

Adjustment for total energy intake is of particular relevance for epidemiologic studies in which investigators use some form of regression models to examine the associations of specific nutrients with an outcome variable, for example, blood pressure or cholesterol in multiple linear regression, case-control status in logistic regression, or coronary heart disease incidence in the Cox proportional hazards regression. Thorough discussions on adjustment for total energy intake can be found in Reference 10 or Reference 11. Only the major issues addressed by these authors are described here. The rationale for adjusting for total energy intake is that most nutrients are correlated with total energy intake. This is because they contribute directly to total energy intake, for example, total fat or carbohydrate, or because persons who consume more kilocalories also eat more, on average, of all nutrients, for example, dietary cholesterol or sodium. For example, in participants of the Multiple Risk Factor Intervention Trial (MRFIT),[12] the baseline correlations of 10 energy energy-contributing nutrients with total energy intake ranged from 0.29 for alcohol intake to 0.87 for total fat intake. Among 24 non-energy-contributing nutrients, the correlations ranged from 0.05 for retinol to 0.78 for phosphorus, with a median of 0.52. No nutrient had a negative correlation with total energy intake. Thus, if total energy intake is positively associated with a dependent variable, almost all specific nutrients will also be positively associated with that variable. Hence, in regression analyses involving specific nutrients, there is a need to adjust associations with specific nutrients for the potential confounding effects of total energy intake.

Data from the OPEN Study[7,13] in which doubly labeled water and urinary nitrogen were used as biomarkers for total energy intake and protein intake, respectively, also strongly reinforce the importance of adjustment for energy intake. In particular, the OPEN investigators found that the attenuation of protein intake–disease associations due to within-person variability and person-specific biases can be expected to be substantially less when protein intake is energy-adjusted than when it is not, particularly if dietary data are obtained from a food frequency questionnaire. For example, based on the OPEN data, a single food frequency questionnaire would be expected to underestimate a regression coefficient relating protein intake in g/day and an outcome in men by 84.4% and in women by 86.3%, while the underestimation with protein intake expressed as percentage of kilocalories would be less at 59.4% and 68.4%, respectively.[13] A true relative risk of disease associated with protein intake in g/day of 2.0 would be estimated as 1.11 and 1.10 for men and women, respectively, while the estimated relative risks would be 1.32 and 1.24 for protein intake in percentage of kilocalories.

The most common methods of adjustment for total energy intake are typically referred to as the nutrient density method, the standard multivariate method, the residual method, and the multivariate nutrient density method.[10,11,14] The nutrient density method has been the traditional method of adjusting for total energy intake. In this approach, nutrient intake is divided by total energy intake, with energy-contributing nutrients expressed as percentage of kilocalories and non-energy-contributing nutrients expressed as intake per 1000 kcal. The strengths of this approach include ease of calculation, familiarity by nutritionists, and use in national guidelines.[10] For example, the Committee on Diet and Health of the National Research Council recommends that total fat intake be less than 30% of the total energy intake and that saturated fat intake be less than 10%.[15] The primary problem with the nutrient density method is that it does not completely eliminate potential confounding with total energy intake, because nutrients expressed as nutrient density often remain correlated with total energy intake. For example, in the MRFIT, the correlations of percentage of kilocalories from protein, fat, and carbohydrate intake with total energy intake at baseline were −0.23, 0.18, and −0.11, respectively.[12] However, with these three nutrients expressed as g/day, the corresponding correlations were 0.73, 0.87, and 0.77.

In the standard multivariate method, total energy intake is included in the multivariate regression model along with the nutrient or nutrients of interest. In this model, the regression coefficient for the nutrient of interest represents the effect of changing the nutrient by one unit while maintaining a constant total energy intake. For energy-containing nutrients, this can only be accomplished by making changes, in other energy-contributing nutrients, that are equal to the amount of energy contained in one unit of the nutrient of interest. Similarly, the regression coefficient for total energy intake does not represent the effect of changing total energy intake by 1 kcal, but the effect of changing energy intake from all other energy-contributing nutrients by 1 kcal. For example, if the nutrient in the model is total protein intake, then the total energy intake represents fat and carbohydrate intakes. In using this approach, estimates of the effect of changing the intake of the nutrient by a specific amount should use variation in the nutrient with total energy intake held constant, that is, the nutrient residual (see later) as the basis for the estimates of effect. Failure to do to so can result in estimates of effect based on unrealistic differences in the intake of the nutrient.

In the residual method, the investigator regresses each nutrient of interest on the total energy intake, and then computes a nutrient residual for each individual by subtracting from the individual's actual intake of that nutrient the amount predicted based on the individual's total energy intake. Because the mean of these residuals is equal to zero, it may be desirable to add a constant to each residual, for example, the mean intake for the nutrient. The resulting value does not, however, represent the individual's actual intake and, in fact, has no "biological" or public policy meaning. The residual method is simply one means by which investigators can adjust for total energy intake. Nutrient residuals are independent of total energy intake. Models that use nutrient residuals can also include total energy intake. The regression coefficient for a nutrient expressed as a nutrient residual is identical to the regression coefficient for the nutrient in the standard multivariate model. However, the regression coefficient for total energy intake will not be identical to that in the standard multivariate model. In the residual model, the association of total energy intake with the dependent variable is not adjusted for intake of the specific nutrient, which could result in an inaccurate estimate of the association of total energy intake with the dependent variable.

In the multivariate nutrient density model, total energy intake is included in the model along with nutrient density. This approach addresses the problem of potential confounding by total energy intake in such analyses. In this model, the regression coefficient for the nutrient estimates the effect of a 1% difference in energy from the nutrient with total caloric intake held constant. As noted by Willett et al.,[10] a major strength of the multivariate nutrient density approach is that it separates diet into two components: composition and total amount.

MODELING NUTRIENT INTAKE

Investigators typically model nutrient intake as a continuous variable or as a series of dummy variables corresponding to quantiles of the nutrient, for example, quartiles or quintiles. The advantages of categorizing nutrient intake include reduction of the potential effects of outlying or extreme values and elimination of the need to assume a linear relation between the nutrient of interest and the dependent variable. Categorization is also more informative to readers since it allows estimation of relative risks in logistic regression and the Cox proportional hazards regression for persons in each exposure category relative to a referent category and, in multiple linear regression, the mean difference in the dependent variable for persons in each exposure category relative to the referent category. The main weakness in categorizing a continuous variable is that, when the relationship is linear, the categorization results in a loss of power. However, regardless of how nutrient intake is modeled in the definitive analysis, categorization is still an extremely useful tool and should be part of any analysis plan. This is because categorization allows the investigator to examine the shape of the relation between the nutrient and the dependent variable, and thus whether or not the relation is sufficiently linear to support inclusion of the nutrient as a continuous variable in the regression model.

When nutrient intake is categorized, one defines $k-1$ dummy variables for each individual for the k categories of the variable. For example, if nutrient intake is divided into quartiles, three dummy variables are defined. In defining the dummy variables, it is necessary to define a referent category. This is the category against which the risks or means for the other exposure categories are compared. If nutrient intake is divided into quartiles and the first quartile is to be the referent category, the three dummy variables corresponding to quartiles 2 to 4 are defined as follows:

$$X_1 = \begin{cases} 1 \text{ if intake in second quartile} \\ 0 \text{ otherwise} \end{cases}$$

$$X_2 = \begin{cases} 1 \text{ if intake in third quartile} \\ 0 \text{ otherwise} \end{cases}$$

$$X_3 = \begin{cases} 1 \text{ if intake in third quartile} \\ 0 \text{ otherwise} \end{cases}$$

These definitions produce the following values on each of the variables for individuals in the first through fourth quartiles:

Quartile of intake	X_1	X_2	X_3
1	0	0	0
2	1	0	0
3	0	1	0
4	0	0	1

In defining categories for a nutrient, investigators should adjust for total energy intake by defining the categories based on nutrient residuals or nutrient densities, rather than absolute intake.[14] While the standard multivariate method and the nutrient residual method provide identical regression coefficients for the nutrient of interest when the nutrient is entered as a continuous variable, this is not the case when nutrient intake is categorized.[14] In this case, the standard multivariate method should be avoided. It is also desirable to model total energy intake as a continuous variable in such analyses rather than as a second categorical variable, particularly if nutrient density is the variable being categorized.[11,14]

MULTICOLLINEARITY

Multicollinearity in a regression model can occur when highly intercorrelated variables are entered simultaneously into the model or when a linear combination of several variables essentially equals a constant. For example, multicollinearity would occur with nutrient data if the model included percentage of kilocalories from total fat, protein, and carbohydrate because the sum of these three variables is often 100 or quite close to 100. Hence, investigators should not attempt to enter more than two of these variables simultaneously into a regression model. Similarly, multicollinearity would also occur if these same three variables were entered into a model as g/day along with total energy intake. In this case, only three of these four variables should be entered simultaneously. In general, investigators need to ensure that they do not include in the same model variables representing total intake for a nutrient and all individual components of that intake, for example, total fat plus saturated fats, polyunsaturated fats, and monounsaturated fats. However, even if investigators are careful to ensure that the types of multi-collinearity described here do not occur, multicollinearity can still be a problem when multiple intercorrelated variables are included in a model, for example, nutrients that come from the same sources. In this situation it may be impossible to determine the separate and independent associations of the multiple variables with the dependent variable. For example, in a study on the associations of potassium, calcium, protein, and milk intakes with blood pressure, the investigators found that, while potassium had a relatively stronger association with blood pressure than the other three dietary factors, the high correlations of potassium intake with intakes of the other three made it impossible to determine the independent association of potassium intake with blood pressure.[16]

The use of nutrient residuals and nutrient densities help to reduce the likelihood of multicollinearity because energy-adjusted nutrients generally have lower intercorrelations than nutrients expressed as absolute amounts.[11] Methods for assessing and detecting multicollinearity, as well as remedial measures, can be found in Neter et al.[8]

Some investigators may believe that procedures that select variables for inclusion in regression models based on whether or not the variable is significantly related to the dependent variable is an appropriate approach for preventing multicollinearity. Such procedures include forward selection or backward elimination of variables, and stepwise regression. In forward selection of variables, variables are entered into the model one at a time, beginning with the variable that has the strongest association with the dependent variable, followed sequentially by those having the strongest residual associations with the dependent variable, that is, after taking into account the association of the entering variable with the variables previously entered and their associations with the dependent variable. Variables are entered into the model until no remaining variable would have a statistically significant association with the dependent variable, if it were to enter the model next. In backward elimination of variables, all available variables are entered into the model, and those with the weakest association are sequentially removed until only variables significantly related to the dependent variable remain. Stepwise regression combines forward selection and backward elimination of variables by removing variables that are no longer significant when a new variable is entered into the model so that the final model only contains variables significantly related to the dependent variable.

These variable selection procedures should be avoided for a number of reasons. First, the final model selected will not necessarily be optimal, for example, maximize R^2. Second, the hypothesis tests used to determine which variables remain in the model are correlated.[9] Third, if a large number of variables is involved, initial entry of all variables may not be possible if one or more is a linear combination of the other variables. Fourth, stepwise procedures may not select possible confounders that should be included whether or not the confounder has a significant association with the dependent variable, for example, age and gender, or total energy intake in the multivariate nutrient density approach. Fifth, the results of these procedures are often not unique, that is, they yield final models that do not include the same variables. For example, in a logistic analysis involving the associations of total energy intake, and intakes of protein, fat, and carbohydrate with coronary heart disease (CHD) incidence, McGee et al.[17] found that only carbohydrate intake had a significant association with CHD incidence if forward selection of variables was used. When backward elimination was used instead, the final model included fat intake and total energy intake as the only variables significantly and independently related to CHD incidence.

In model building, it is appropriate to prespecify variables to be included in models and to carefully build models by sequentially adding variables. For example, in the INTERMAP Study's report on the relationship of protein intake to blood pressure,[18] potential confounders were added sequentially to regression models. First nondiet variables were included, then diet variables were added according to known and putative associations with blood pressure. Models were run both without and with adjustment for height and weight, because of possible overadjustment and because they strongly influenced associations, possibly as a result of their high precision of measurement in comparison with dietary variables. Potential confounders added after adjustment for sample, age, and gender (Model 1) were: reported special diet, history of cardiovascular disease or diabetes, family history of hypertension, physical activity, any reported intake of dietary supplements (Model 2); urinary sodium, potassium, and 7-day alcohol intake (nutrients known to be associated with blood pressure) (Model 3); calcium, saturated fatty acids, polyunsaturated fatty acids, dietary cholesterol (nutrients with putative relationships with blood pressure) (Model 4); and dietary magnesium (Model 5a) or fiber (Model 5b) (also with putative relationship with blood pressure), considered separately to avoid possible distorting effect of multicollinearity given their high intercorrelation with vegetable protein.

It may also be appropriate to conduct additional analyses to assess the sensitivity of findings. For example, in the INTERMAP report on the relationship of protein intake to blood pressure,[18] the following additional analyses were conducted: inclusion of energy intake in all models; nutrient intakes from foods plus dietary supplements; use of g/day adjusted for energy intake (instead of nutrient densities); and exclusions (separately) of those taking antihypertensive or other cardiovascular disease medication, people with a history of cardiovascular disease or diabetes, people on special diet, people with high day-to-day variability of nutrient intakes.

DIETARY SUPPLEMENTS

Dietary supplement use poses substantial complexities for data collection as well as for analyses involving nutrient intake. The primary issue in data collection is whether investigators can obtain accurate estimates of the actual nutrients contained in the supplements. For U.S. participants in INTERMAP,[19] during each of four 24 h recalls, the interviewer asked the participant if he/she had taken vitamins, minerals, tonics, or supplements. Supplements encompassed vitamins/minerals and other products purchased over the counter. Supplements contained in the Nutrition Data System (NDS) (version 29, 1996, Nutrition Coordinating Center, University of Minnesota, Minneapolis) were directly computerized. In NDS version 29, there were 60 nutrient codes encompassing specified quantities of vitamins and minerals generally recognized as important nutritionally and meriting ingestion as supplements. For non-NDS supplements, a separate computerized database was developed with all information from product labels. Non-NDS supplements were often made up of materials of uncertain merit (herbals/botanicals, animal products, phospholipids, enzymes, as well as minerals and vitamins). Often for these supplements no information was obtainable on ingredients and/or their amounts. Twenty-three percent of U.S. INTERMAP participants reported use of non-NDS listed supplements, encompassing 920 products with 1009 specified ingredients. Among these were 294 brand-name products with unknown ingredients or amounts. Some of these products were proprietary formulas with listed ingredients but no amounts; proprietary blends stating "proprietary blend", without ingredients; supplements with no amounts for some ingredients; supplements with ingredients but no specific amounts per serving size; and supplements with unit amounts that were uninterpretable.

For analyses, the first question that must be addressed is whether supplement-based intake should be included or excluded. The approach recommended here is to analyze the data first without inclusion of the supplement-based intake and then with inclusion, because the intake from supplements is likely to be incomplete and of uncertain quality, based on INTERMAP experience.[19] In the INTERMAP report on protein intake and blood pressure,[18] any use of supplements was included as a dichotomous variable in most models, and in sensitivity analyses, intake of vegetable protein based on 24 h recalls was combined with supplemental intake.

For analyses in which food- and supplement-based intakes are combined, the investigator needs to decide whether to simply add the two intakes together as was done in INTERMAP for vegetable protein[18] or to add supplement-based intake to the energy-adjusted intake from foods.[10] It is unclear how, or if, results between these two approaches will differ. If the intake from supplements represents a large proportion of the total intake and thus the correlation between total intake of the nutrient and total energy intake is low, the easiest and probably best approach is to simply combine the supplement-based intake with the food-based intake, and then use the standard multivariate model, whether or not nutrient intake is categorized. If the supplement-based intake does not represent a large proportion of the total intake, it may be worthwhile to examine the associations using both approaches, as it is unclear how the results might differ, of if they will differ in any practical way.

WITHIN-PERSON VARIABILITY AND PERSON-SPECIFIC BIAS

The goal of examining associations of nutrients with an outcome is to estimate the association of usual intake with that outcome. However, information on nutrient intake collected from a single 24 h recall is subject to substantial within-person variability due to day-to-day variability in intake in most individuals. In addition, data from the OPEN Study[13] indicate that self-reported intake from both 24 h recalls and food frequency questionnaires is also subject to person-specific bias. Hence, nutrient intake, whether estimated from a single 24 h recall, multiple 24 h recalls, or a food frequency questionnaire, often does not reflect the individual's average or usual intake. Day-to-day variability and person-specific bias in nutrient intake constitute what is often referred to as "measurement error." Measurement error typically results in underestimation of associations of nutrients with outcomes. For example, in men from the OPEN Study[13] it was estimated that with one 24 h recall, the regression coefficient relating a dependent variable to percentage of calories from protein intake would be underestimated by 77.7% in a simple linear model.

Day-to-day variability in intake represents random error in measurement, while person-specific bias represents systematic error. If the only error present is random, the average of a large number of repeated measurements, for example, multiple 24 h recalls, approaches the true value, or for nutrient intake, the individual's usual intake. While the collection of multiple 24 h recalls can reduce the impact of random variation on observed associations, their use cannot eliminate the impact of person-specific bias or systematic error on associations. For example, in men from the OPEN Study[13] it was estimated that the association between a dependent variable and percentage of kilocalories from protein intake would be underestimated by 50.2% with four 24 h recalls compared with the 77.7% underestimation with one 24 h recall. However, even with an infinite number of recalls, the association would still be underestimated by 19.2%, because of the presence of person-specific bias in estimated intakes.[13]

While methods are available for correcting or adjusting regression coefficients for measurement error,[20–22] their use with nutrient data is problematic. Because of the presence of both random and systematic errors in nutrient data, the ability to correct for these types of error requires that the method of data collection, for example, food frequency questionnaire or multiple 24 h recalls, be validated against a "gold standard" reference method or biomarker.[7,13] Because 24 h recalls are subject to person-specific bias and their errors are generally correlated with those of the food frequency questionnaire and with true intake, multiple 24 h recalls do not meet the criteria for a "gold standard."[23] Currently, the only valid reference measurements or biomarkers appear to be doubly labeled water for total energy intake, urinary nitrogen for protein intake, and urinary sodium for dietary sodium intake.[23] Hence, in the absence of valid "gold standard" reference measures, correction for measurement error in nutrient intakes is not recommended.

APPROACHES TO ANALYSIS OF EPIDEMIOLOGIC STUDIES

TYPES OF EPIDEMIOLOGIC STUDIES

A discussion of the types of epidemiologic studies with particular reference to nutrition can be found in Reference 24, while a more general review of the topic is given in Reference 25. There are generally two types of epidemiologic studies: observational and experimental. The main difference between an experimental and an observational study is the control that the investigator exercises over participants, procedures, and exposures. In an experiment, the investigator controls who enters the study, what drugs or procedures are given to participants, and how the study is carried out. In a nutritional intervention study, the investigator would manipulate or attempt to manipulate some or all participants' dietary intake. An observational study does not involve an intervention or manipulation. In such a study, the investigator does not control who enters the study or the factors or drugs to which participants are exposed. Observational studies of individuals include cross-sectional, case-control, and prospective studies, while studies of groups are referred to as ecologic studies. In nutritional epidemiologic studies, nutrient intake is measured but not manipulated, the frequency and pattern of outcomes are observed, and associations between nutrients and outcomes are estimated using statistical methods.

In a cross-sectional study the question asked is, "What is the correlation or association between nutrient intake and the outcome?" Individuals are included in the study without regard to their status on the outcome or nutrient intake. In these studies, nutrient intake and the outcome are both measured at the same point in time. For example, INTERMAP is a cross-sectional study of the associations of macro-/micronutrients with blood pressure.[3,4] In this study, each participant had blood pressure measured twice on each of four occasions and completed a 24 h recall on each day that blood pressure was measured.

Case-control studies, which are also referred to as retrospective and case-referent studies, are designed to answer the question, "Do persons with disease (cases) have different nutrient intake than persons who have not been diagnosed with the disease (controls)?" For example, do persons with heart disease consume more dietary cholesterol and saturated fatty acids than persons without heart disease? In case-control studies, recently diagnosed persons with the disease and a set of persons without the disease are interviewed concerning their dietary habits. The goal is to determine usual nutrient intake before the onset of disease.

Prospective studies are also referred to as cohort, incidence, follow-up, and longitudinal studies. The question asked in prospective studies when a nutrient is thought to be related to increased risk of disease is, "Do persons with higher intake develop or die from the disease more frequently or sooner than persons with lower intake?" Alternatively, if a nutrient is thought to be related to decreased risk of disease, the question asked is, "Do persons with lower intake develop or die from the disease more frequently or sooner than persons with higher intake?" For example, are persons who consume more than 50 g/day of alcohol more likely to have a stroke than persons who consume less alcohol? Persons found to be disease free at the time of the cross-sectional survey are followed up over time to determine who develops the disease and when the disease occurs.

Ecologic studies compare aggregate data representing entire populations. A common example of this type of study is one in which disease specific mortality rates for different countries are correlated with nutrient measurements based on food disappearance data.[26] The INTERSALT Study included ecologic analyses on associations of urinary electrolytes and other factors with blood pressure, as well as cross-sectional analyses on electrolyte–blood pressure associations within individuals.[27,28]

Experimental studies involving nutritional interventions include feeding or metabolic ward studies and randomized clinical trials. Feeding studies involve feeding groups of individuals precisely measured diets with one or more components varied, with an effect on a biologic variable then measured. The Keys equation for predicting change in total cholesterol from changes in intakes of saturated and polyunsaturated fatty acids and dietary cholesterol was determined from a metabolic ward study.[29] A common design for feeding studies is the crossover design, in which each participant serves as his/her own control. Randomized clinical trial is a prospective study in which individuals are randomly assigned to intervention and control groups. Following randomization, both groups are followed up over time to assess the efficacy and safety of the intervention. For example, the trial on the Primary Prevention of Hypertension was a randomized, controlled clinical trial on the effects of weight loss, reduction in sodium intake, decreased alcohol intake, and increased exercise on the 5-year incidence of hypertension in men and women with high normal blood pressure.[30]

METHODS FOR COMPARING GROUPS IN CROSS-SECTIONAL STUDIES

Table 5.1 lists methods of analysis that can be used to compare nutrient intake between two groups (for example, men and women) or among three or more groups (for example, African-Americans, Hispanics, and Whites). For nutrient intake considered as

TABLE 5.1
Methods for Comparing Nutrient Intake among Groups in Cross-Sectional Studies

Description	Number of Groups (k)	
	$k = 2$	$k > 2$
Nutrient intake continuous		
Usual method	Two-sample t-test	Analysis of variance
Nonparametric alternative	Wilcoxon rank-sum test	Kruskal–Wallis test
Adjustment for other variables		Analysis of covariance or multiple linear regression
Nutrient intake categorical (c categories)		
Usual method	Chi-square test for $2 \times c$ contingency table	Chi-square test for $k \times c$ contingency table

a continuous variable, the goal of the analysis is to determine whether mean or median intake differs significantly between or among groups. For such analyses, the table indicates the usual method of analysis, the nonparametric alternative, and methods that can be used to adjust for potential confounders of differences between groups, for example, age or total energy intake. Nonparametric tests make fewer assumptions about the shape of the distributions of variables than parametric tests such as the two-sample t-test or analysis of variance. In the Wilcoxon rank-sum test and the Kruskal–Wallis test, the actual observations are replaced by their ranks in the combined sample of all observations. If nutrient intake is divided into categories, the goal of the analysis is usually to determine whether the distributions of intake are homogeneous across groups. The methods listed in Table 5.1 can also be used to compare nutrient intake at baseline in an experimental study, for example, to determine whether in a randomized clinical trial randomization has provided comparable groups with respect to intake of specific nutrients.

A useful text on these methods and those described in what follows is that of Rosner.[31]

METHODS FOR COMPARING CASES AND CONTROLS IN CASE-CONTROL STUDIES

Table 5.2 lists methods of analysis that can be used to compare nutrient intake between cases and controls in unmatched and matched case-control studies. Matching is often done in case-control studies to make cases and controls comparable on variables that could confound associations of the variable of interest with disease. For unmatched case-control studies, the methods listed are identical to those for comparing nutrient intake between two groups in cross-sectional studies. For matched case-control studies, the methods of analysis need to take into account the matching. Hence, for a simple comparison of means between cases and controls, the investigator should use a paired t-test rather than a two-sample t-test, or the Wilcoxon signed-rank test rather than the Wilcoxon rank sum test. When multiple regression is used to adjust the mean difference between cases and controls for other variables in matched case-control studies, the investigator needs to ensure that the dependent and independent variables in the model are defined correctly. In such studies, the dependent variable is the difference in nutrient intake for each case-control pair, while the independent variables are the within-pair differences for the potential confounding variables. The test of significance for the adjusted mean difference is the test of the hypothesis that the intercept in the model is equal to zero.

METHODS FOR ASSESSING ASSOCIATIONS IN EPIDEMIOLOGIC STUDIES

Table 5.3 lists methods for assessing associations of nutrient intake with outcome variables in cross-sectional or ecologic studies, matched and unmatched case-control studies, and prospective studies. For each type of study, the table indicates methods that can be used when nutrient intake is modeled as a continuous variable or as a categorical variable. The table also lists the dependent variable for each type of analysis. For example, in the Cox proportional hazards regression, the dependent variable is the time to some event, for example, death from CHD. In unmatched case-control studies, the dependent variable is typically case-control status. As cross-sectional and ecologic studies can have both continuous and dichotomous dependent variables, methods are listed for both types of dependent variables. No dependent variable is listed for conditional logistic regression, as there is no outcome variable that varies from individual to individual in this model. In conditional logistic regression, the independent variables are the case-control difference in each variable, and the model does not include a constant term. Useful texts on logistic and Cox regression methods are those of Kahn and Sempos[32] and Vittinghoff et al.[33]

TABLE 5.2

Methods for Comparing Nutrient Intake between Cases and Controls in Case-Control Studies

Description	Unmatched	Matched
Nutrient intake continuous		
Usual method	Two-sample t-test	Paired t-test
Nonparametric alternative	Wilcoxon rank-sum test	Wilcoxon signed-rank test
Adjustment for other variables	Analysis of covariance or multiple linear regression	Multiple linear regression[a]
Nutrient intake categorical (c categories)		
Usual method	Chi-square test for $2 \times c$ contingency table	McNemar's test for $c = 2$

[a] In this model, differences in each variable for the case-control pair are used, with the difference in the nutrient of interest serving as the dependent variable. The test of significance for the adjusted mean difference is the test of the hypothesis that the intercept of the model is equal to zero.

TABLE 5.3

Methods for Assessing Associations in Epidemiologic Studies

Dependent Variable	Nutrient Intake	Unadjusted	Adjusted for Other Variables
Cross-sectional or ecologic study			
Continuous	Continuous	Pearson correlation Spearman correlation Linear regression	Partial correlation Linear regression
Continuous	Categorical	Linear regression	Linear regression
Dichotomous	Continuous categorical	Logistic regression	Logistic regression
Unmatched case-control study			
Case-control status	Continuous categorical	Logistic regression	Logistic regression
Matched case-control study			
None	Continuous categorical	Conditional logistic regression	Conditional logistic regression
Prospective study			
Time to event	Categorical	Log rank test Cox regression	Cox regression
Time to event	Continuous	Cox regression	Cox regression

The Spearman correlation is listed for use in cross-sectional and ecologic studies as it is the nonparametric alternative to the Pearson product–moment correlation coefficient. The Pearson product–moment correlation coefficient should not be used if either nutrient intake or the second variable has a highly skewed distribution, because the assumption underlying its use is that each variable has a normal distribution for each value of the other variable.

In analyses involving linear regression, interest focuses on the difference in the mean of the dependent variable for a one-unit or greater change in the independent variable. Hence, the focus is on the regression coefficient. In logistic and Cox regression, interest focuses on estimates of relative risk. In logistic regression, the relative risk is given by the odds ratio, and in Cox regression the hazard ratio. In both models, relative risk estimates are obtained by exponentiation of the regression coefficient or the regression coefficient multiplied by some convenient multiplier. For example, if total energy intake is the dietary variable of interest, exponentiation of the regression coefficient gives the relative risk of the outcome for two persons who differ in total energy intake by 1 kcal. Because this is not a particularly meaningful difference for calculating relative risk, an investigator might multiply the regression coefficient by 500 to obtain the relative risk of the outcome for two persons who differ in total energy intake by 500 kcal. When nutrient intake is categorized and dummy variables are included in the regression model, exponentiation of the regression coefficient for a dummy variable gives the risk of the outcome for those in the category corresponding to the dummy variable relative to the referent category, for example, quartile 4 relative to quartile 1.

In analyses based on the Cox regression, true associations between diet and disease may not be found if there are substantial changes in nutrient intake between the baseline assessment of diet and the development of disease, or if there are substantial changes in the rank ordering of study participants with respect to intake over the course of follow-up.

ANALYSES OF INTERVENTION STUDIES WITH CHANGE IN NUTRIENT INTAKE AS OUTCOME

In nutritional intervention studies, investigators often wish to examine the effects of the intervention on intakes of specific nutrients following completion of the intervention. Investigators can use three approaches to determine whether intake of specific nutrients changed in an intervention group relative to a control group or among three or more groups:

1. Compare intake among groups at follow-up, ignoring preintervention intake using the methods for cross-sectional studies in Table 5.1.
2. Compare the change in intake from preintervention to follow-up among groups using the methods for cross-sectional studies.
3. Compare intake among groups at follow-up adjusting for preintervention intake with multiple linear regression or analysis of covariance.

Investigators typically use the second approach for intervention studies, even though it tends to be less powerful than analysis of covariance. Assumptions in regard to the analysis of covariance may or may not be met in an intervention study. The first approach may, however, be preferable to the second if there are no differences in intake among the groups being compared at the preintervention assessment and the correlation between the preintervention and follow-up assessments for the nutrient of interest is less than 0.5. Correlations smaller than 0.5 are not uncommon for many nutrients assessed on two occasions.[12] Hence, for nutrient intake, the best approach may be to ignore preintervention intake. Prior to conducting analyses in nutritional intervention studies, investigators should examine the correlations of the nutrients from preintervention to follow-up and be prepared to ignore preintervention intake in the analyses.

Finally, in conducting analyses of any specific nutrient in relation to an outcome or in relation to disease, it is important to remember that individuals consume foods, not nutrients.

REFERENCES

1. Slattery, ML, et al. *J. Am. Coll. Nutr.* 14: 635; 1995.
2. Goldberg, GR, et al. *Eur. J. Clin. Nutr.* 45: 569; 1991.
3. Stamler, J, et al. *J. Hum. Hypertens.* 17: 591; 2003.
4. Dennis, B, et al. *J. Hum. Hypertens.* 17: 609; 2003.
5. Liu, K. *Am. J. Clin. Nutr.* 59: 262s; 1994.
6. SAS Institute, Inc. *SAS Online Doc®9.1.3.* Cary, NC: SAS Institute, Inc., 2004.
7. Freedman, LS, et al. *J. Nutr.* 134: 1836; 2004.
8. Neter, J, Wasserman, W, and Kutner, MH. *Applied Linear Regression Models.* Homewood, IL: Richard D. Irwin, Inc., 1983.
9. Ryan, TP. *Modern Regression Methods.* New York: John Wiley & Sons, Inc., 1997.
10. Willett, WC, Howe, GR, and Kushi, LH. *Am. J. Clin. Nutr.* 65: 1220s; 1997.
11. Willett, W. *Nutritional Epidemiology.* New York: Oxford University Press, 1990.
12. Grandits, GA, Bartsch, GE, and Stamler, J. In: *Dietary and Nutritional Methods and Findings: The Multiple Risk Factor Intervention Trial (MRFIT).* Stamler J, et al., Eds. *Am. J. Clin. Nutr.* 65: 211s; 1997.
13. Shatzkin, A, et al. *Int. J. Epidemiol.* 32: 1054; 2003.
14. Brown, CC, et al. *Am. J. Epidemiol.* 129: 323; 1994.
15. National Research Council. *Diet and Health: Implications for Reducing Chronic Disease Risk.* Washington, DC: National Academy Press, 1989.
16. Reed, D, McGee, D, Yano, K, and Hankin, J. *Hypertension* 7: 405; 1985.
17. McGee, D, Reed, D, and Yano, K. *J. Chronic Dis.* 37: 713; 1984.
18. Elliott, P, et al. *Arch. Intern. Med.* 166: 79; 2006.
19. Archer, SL, et al. *J. Am. Diet. Assoc.* 105: 1006; 2005.
20. Fuller, WA. *Measurement Error Models.* New York: John Wiley & Sons, 1987.
21. Clayton, D and Gill, C. In: *Design Concepts in Nutritional Epidemiology.* Margetts BM, Nelson M, Eds., Oxford, UK: Oxford University Press, 1991, pp. 79–96.
22. Spiegelman, D, McDermott, A, and Rosner, B. *Am. J. Clin. Nutr.* 65: 1179s; 1997.
23. Kipnis, V, et al. *Am. J. Epidemiol.* 158: 14; 2003.
24. Sempos, CT, Liu, K, and Ernst, N. *Am. J. Clin. Nutr.* 69: 1s; 1999.
25. Hennekens, CH and Buring, JE. *Epidemiology in Medicine.* Mayrent, SL, Ed., Boston, MA: Little, Brown and Company, 1987.
26. Stamler, J and Shekelle, R. *Arch. Pathol. Lab. Med.* 112: 1032; 1988.

27. The INTERSALT Cooperative Research Group. *J. Hypertens.* 4: 781; 1986.
28. The INTERSALT Cooperative Research Group. *Br. Med. J.* 297: 319; 1988.
29. Keys, A, Anderson, JT, and Grande, F. *Metabolism* 65: 776; 1965.
30. Stamler, R, et al. *JAMA* 262: 1801; 1989.
31. Rosner, B. *Fundamentals of Biostatistics*, 6th ed. Belmont, CA: Duxbury Press, 2006.
32. Kahn, HA and Sempos, C. *Statistical Methods in Epidemiology*. New York: Oxford University Press, 1989.
33. Vittinghoff, E, Glidden, DV, Schiboski, SC, and McCulloch, CE. *Regression Methods in Biostatistics. Linear, Logistic, Survival and Repeated Measures Models*. New York: Springer, 2005.

Part II

Nutrition Science

6 Nutrition Terminology

Carolyn D. Berdanier

CONTENTS

As with any discipline, nutrition science has its own vocabulary and terminology. This chapter gives the reader several tables providing this terminology. The first is a table giving the conversion factors for converting the results of laboratory analysis to standard units called SI units. Many scientific journals require the use of these units in manuscripts reporting the results of laboratory investigations. The result, or common component from clinical laboratory assessment, is given in its common form with reference interval and present unit, followed by the conversion factor that is used to convert the result into SI units, its reference intervals, significant digits, and suggested minimum increment. These standard units for expressing biological data are listed in Table 6.1.[1]

Over the years, there has been some confusion over the names of the vitamins. Vitamins were named according to (a) their function; (b) their location; (c) the order in which they were discovered; or (d) combinations of a, b, or c. Some of these names became obsolete as their proposed functions or their isolated structures were found to duplicate already named and described vitamins. Obsolescence also occurred as research showed that certain of these compounds were not needed dietary factors, but were synthesized by the body in needed amounts. Table 6.2 provides a list of vitamin names (both obsolete and current), and it is hoped that the reader will find this useful. Following this is a list (Table 6.3) of all the compounds having vitamin A activity. This is a fairly lengthy list, as this vitamin is found in a variety of foods, both of animal origin and plant origin. The body can convert these forms to its useful and most active form, all *trans*-retinol. These conversions are not 100% efficient, and correction factors must be applied to determine vitamin A activity.

In the area of energy research, there are a number of terms that the workers in this area assume that the reader knows. These are listed with their definitions in Table 6.4.

BODY COMPOSITION ESTIMATION AND TERMINOLOGY

Normal bodies usually consist of 16–20% protein, 3–5% ash (mineral matter), 10–12% fat, and 60–70% water. Age, diet, genetic background, physical activity, hormonal status, and gender can affect not only the proximate composition of the whole body, that is, the magnitude of each of these components, but also their distribution. Body composition can be measured directly or estimated indirectly by using a variety of techniques. Direct measurement involves the analysis of the major body components: fat, water, protein, and ash (mineral matter). Direct measurements are usually impractical for large species, including man. The equations used for the calculation of body components from direct analysis are given in Table 6.5.

Sophisticated techniques using ultrasound, neutron activation analysis, infrared interactance, dual-energy x-ray absorptiometry, computer-assisted tomography, magnetic resonance imaging, or bioelectrical impedance are available for the indirect estimation of body composition. The equations for converting data obtained using these sophisticated techniques are available.[2]

There are locations in the body where subcutaneous fat can be assessed using calipers to measure skin-fold thickness and thereby estimate body fatness. The fold below the upper arm (triceps fold) and the fold at the iliac crest are frequently used locations. Other locations include the abdominal fold and the thigh fold. Equations have been derived (Table 6.6) to calculate body fatness using these measurements.[3] Knowing the composition of the body, particularly its fat content, suggests that there should be ways of estimating body energy need. Some of these equations are shown in Table 6.7.[4]

Perhaps more popular now is the use of body mass index (BMI). This is a useful term, in that it is an index of the body weight (kg) divided by the height (meters) squared (wt/ht^2). BMI correlates with body fatness and with the risk of obesity-related disease or diseases for which obesity is a compounding factor. Overweight is defined as BMI between 25 and 30, and obesity is a BMI over 30. The BMI varies with age. A desirable BMI for people of age 19 to 24 is between 19 and 24, while that for people of age 55 to 64 is between 23 and 28. While simple in concept, this term does not assess body composition per se. It only provides a basis for assessing the health risks associated or presumed to be associated with excess body fatness. BMI applies only to normal individuals, and not the super athlete or the body builder, who may be quite heavy yet have little body fat.

TABLE 6.1
Conversion Factors for Values in Clinical Chemistry (SI Units)

Component Present	Reference Intervals (Examples)	Present Unit	Conversion Factor	SI Reference Intervals	SI Unit	Symbol	Significant Digits	Suggested Minimum Increment
Acetaminophen (P) toxic	>5.0	mg/dl	66.16	>330	mmol/l	XXO	10	mmol/l
Acetoacetate (S)	0.3–3.0	mg/dl	97.95	30–300	mmol/l	XXO	10	mmol/l
Acetone (B,S)	0	mg/dl	172.2	0	mmol/l	XXO	10	mmol/l
Acid phosphatase (S)	0–5.5	U/l	16.67	0–90	nkat/l	XX	2	nkat/l
Adrenocorticotropin [ACTH] (P)	20–100	pg/ml	0.2202	4–22	pmol/l	XX	1	pmol/l
Alanine aminotransferase [ALT] (S)	0–35	U/l	0.01667	0–0.58	mkat/l	X.XX	0.02	mkat/l
Albumin (S)	4.0–6.0	g/dl	10.0	40–60	g/l	XX	1	g/l
Aldolase (S)	0–6	U/l	16.67	0–100	nkat/l	XXO	20	nkat/l
Aldosterone (S)								
Normal salt diet	8.1–15.5	ng/dl	27.74	220–430	pmol/l	XXO	10	pmol/l
Restricted salt diet	20.8–44.4	ng/dl	27.74	580–1240	pmol/l	XXO	10	pmol/l
Aldosterone (U): sodium excretion								
=25 mmol/d	18–85	mg/24 h	2.774	50–235	nmol/d	XXX	5	nmol/d
=75–125 mmol/d	5–26	mg/24 h	2.774	15–70	nmol/d	XXX	5	nmol/d
=200 mmol/d	1.5–12.5	mg/24 h	2.774	5–35	nmol/d	XXX	5	nmol/d
Alkaline phosphatase (S)	0–120	U/l	0.01667	0.5–2.0	mkat/l	X.X	0.1	mkat/l
α_1-Antitrypsin (S)	150–350	mg/dl	0.01	1.5–3.5	g/l	X.X	0.1	g/l
α-Fetoprotein (S)	0–20	ng/ml	1.00	0–20	mg/l	XX	1	mg/l
α-Fetoprotein (Amf)	Depends on gestation	mg/dl	10.0	Depends on gestation	mg/l	XX	1	mg/l
α_2-Macroglobulin (S)	145–410	mg/dl	0.01	1.5–4.1	g/l	X.X	1	mg/l
Aluminum (S)	0–15	mg/l	37.06	0–560	nmol/l	XXO	10	nmol/l
Amino acid fractionation (P)								
Alanine	2.2–4.5	mg/dl	112.2	245–500	mmol/l	XXX	5	mol/l
α-Aminobutyric acid	0.1–0.2	mg/dl	96.97	10–20	mmol/l	XXX	5	mmol/l
Arginine	0.5–2.5	mg/dl	57.40	30–145	mmol/l	XXX	5	mmol/l
Asparagine	0.5–0.6	mg/dl	75.69	35–45	mmol/l	XXX	5	mmol/l
Citrulline	0.2–1.0	mg/dl	75.13	0–20	mmol/l	XXX	5	mmol/l
Cystine	0.2–2.2	mg/dl	57.08	15–55	mmol/l	XXX	5	mmol/l
Glutamic acid	0.2–2.8	mg/dl	67.97	15–190	mmol/l	XXX	5	mmol/l
Glutamine	6.1–10.2	mg/dl	68.42	420–700	mmol/l	XXX	5	mmol/l
Glycine	0.9–4.2	mg/dl	133.2	120–560	mmol/l	XXX	5	mmol/l
Histidine	0.5–1.7	mg/dl	64.45	30–110	mmol/l	XXX	5	mmol/l
Hydroxyproline	0–trace	mg/dl	76.26	0–trace	mmol/l	XXX	5	mmol/l
Isoleucine	0.5–1.3	mg/dl	76.24	40–100	mmol/l	XXX	5	mmol/l
Leucine	1.2–3.5	mg/dl	76.24	75–175	mmol/l	XXX	5	mmol/l
Lysine	1.2–3.5	mg/dl	68.40	80–240	mmol/l	XXX	5	mmol/l
Methionine	0.1–0.6	mg/dl	67.02	5–40	mmol/l	XXX	5	mmol/l
Ornithine	0.4–1.4	mg/dl	75.67	30–400	mmol/l	XXX	5	mmol/l
Phenylalanine	0.6–1.5	mg/dl	60.54	35–90	mmol/l	XXX	5	mmol/l
Proline	1.2–3.9	mg/dl	86.86	105–340	mmol/l	XXX	5	mmol/l
Serine	0.8–1.8	pg/dl	95.16	75–170	pmol/l	XXX	5	mmol/l
Taurine	0.9–2.5	mg/dl	79.91	25–170	mmol/l	XXX	5	mmol/l
Threonine	0.9–2.5	mg/dl	83.95	75–210	mmol/l	XXX	5	mmol/l
Tryptophan	0.5–2.5	mg/dl	48.97	25–125	mmol/l	XXX	5	mmol/l
Tyrosine	0.4–1.6	mg/dl	55.19	20–90	mmol/l	XXX	5	mmol/l
Valine	1.7–3.7	mg/dl	85.36	145–315	mmol/l	XXX	5	mmol/l
Amino acid nitrogen (P)	4.0–6.0	mg/dl	0.7139	2.9–4.3	mmol/l	X.X	0.1	mmol/l
Amino acid nitrogen (U)	50–200	mg/24 h	0.07139	3.6–14.3	mmol/d	X.X	0.1	mmol/d
δ-Aminolevulinate [as levulinic acid] (U)	1.0–7.0	mg/24 h	7.626	8–53	mmol/d	XX	1	mmol/d

TABLE 6.1
(Continued)

Component Present	Reference Intervals (Examples)	Present Unit	Conversion Factor	SI Reference Intervals	SI Unit	Symbol	Significant Digits	Suggested Minimum Increment
Amitriptyline (P,S) therapeutic	50–200	ng/ml	3.605	180–270	mmol/l	XO	10	nmol/l
Ammonia (vP) as								
Ammonia [NH3]	10–80	mg/dl	0.5872	5–50	mmol/l	XXX	5	mmol/l
Ammonium ion [NH4+]	10–85	mg/dl	0.5543	5–50	mmol/l	XXX	5	mmol/l
Nitrogen [N]	10–65	mg/dl	0.7139	5–50	mmol/l	XXX	5	mmol/l
Amylase (S)	0–130	U/l	0.01667	0–2.17	mkat/l	XXX	0.01	mkat/l
Androstenedione (S)								
Male >18 years	0.2–3.0	mg/l	3.492	0.5–10.5	nmol/l	XX.X	0.5	nmol/l
Female >18 years	0.8–3.0	mg/l	3.492	3.0–10.5	nmol/l	XX.X	0.5	nmol/l
Angiotensin converting as								
Enzyme (S)	<40	nmol/ml/min	16.67	<670	nkat/l	XXO	10	nkat/l
Arsenic (H) [as As]	<1	mg/g (ppm)	13.35	<13	nmol/g	XX.X	0.5	nmol/g
Arsenic (U) [as As]	0–5	mg/24 h	13.35	0–67	nmol/d	XX	1 nmol/d	
As$_2$O$_3$	<25	mg/dl	0.05055	<1.3	mmol/l	XX.X	0.1	mmol/l
Ascorbate (P) [as ascorbic acid]	0.6–2.0	mg/dl	56.78	30–110	mmol/l	XO	10	mmol/l
Aspartate amino-transferase [AST] (S)	0–35	U/l	0.0167	0–0.58	mkat/l	O.XX	0.01	mkat/l
Barbiturate (S) overdose total expressed as								
Phenobarbital	Depends on	mg/dl	43.06	—	mmol/l	XX	5	mmol/l
Sodium phenobarbital	composition	mg/dl	39.34	—	mmol/l	XX	5	mmol/l
Barbitone	of mixture usually not known	mg/dl	54.29	—	mmol/l	XX	5	mmol/l
Barbiturate (S) therapeutic	See Phenobarbital, Pentobarbital, Thiopental							
Bile acids, total (S)								
As chenodeoxycholic acid	Trace–3.3	mg/ml	2.547	Trace–8.4	mmol/l	X.X	0.2	mmol/l
Cholic acid	Trace–1.0	mg/ml	2.448	Trace–2.4	mmol/l	X.X	0.2	mmol/l
Chenodeoxycholic acid	Trace–1.3	mg/ml	2.547	Trace–3.4	mmol/l	X.X	0.2	mmol/l
Deoxycholic acid	Trace–1.0	mg/ml	2.547	Trace–2.6	mmol/l	X.X	0.2	mmol/l
Lithocholic acid	Trace	mg/ml	2.656	Trace	mmol/l	X.X	0.2	mmol/l
Bile acids (Df) [after cholcystokinin stimulation] total as								
Chenodeoxycholic acid	14.0–58.0	mg/ml	2.547	35–148	mmol/l	XX.X	0.2	mmol/l
Cholic acid	2.4–33.0	mg/ml	2.448	6.8–81.0	mmol/l	XX.X	0.2	mmol/l
Chenodeoxycholic acid	4.0–24.0	mg/ml	2.547	10.0–61.4	mmol/l	XX.X	0.2	mmol/l
Deoxycholic acid	0.8–6.9	mg/ml	2.547	2–18	mmol/l	XX.X	0.2	mmol/l
Lithocholic acid	0.3–0.8	mg/ml	2.656	0.8–2.0	mmol/l	XX.X	0.2	mmol/l
Bilirubin, total (S)	0.1–1.0	mg/dl	17.10	2–18	mmol/l	XX	2	mmol/l
Bilirubin, conjugated (S)	0–0.2	mg/dl	17.10	0–4	mmol/l	XX	2	mmol/l
Bromide (S) toxic								
As bromide ion	>120	mg/dl	0.1252	>15	mmol/l	XX	1	mmol/l
As sodium bromide	>150	mg/dl	0.09719	>15	mmol/l	XX	1	mmol/l
	>15	mEq/l	1.00	>15	mmol/l	XX	1	mmol/l
Cadmium (S)	<3	mg/dl	0.08897	<0.3	mmol/l	X.X	0.1	mmol/l
Calcitonin (S)	<100	pg/ml	1.00	<100	ng/l	XXX	10	ng/l
Calcium (S)								
Male	8.8–10.3	mg/dl	0.2495	2.20–2.58	mmol/l	X.XX	0.02	mmol/l
Female <50 years	8.8–10.0	mg/dl	0.2495	2.20–2.50	mmol/l	X.XX	0.02	mmol/l
Female >50 years	8.8–10.2	mg/dl	0.2495	2.20–2.56	mmol/l	X.XX	0.02	mmol/l
	4.4–5.1	mEq/l	0.500	2.20–2.56	mmol/l	X.XX	0.02	mmol/l

Continued

TABLE 6.1
(Continued)

Component Present	Reference Intervals (Examples)	Present Unit	Conversion Factor	SI Reference Intervals	SI Unit	SI Unit Symbol	Significant Digits	Suggested Minimum Increment
Calcium ion (S)	2.00–2.30	mEq/l	0.500	1.00–1.15	mmol/l	X.XX	0.01	mmol/l
Calcium (U), normal diet	<250	mg/24 h	0.02495	<6.2	mmol/d	X.X	0.1	mmol/d
Carbamazepine (P) therapeutic	4.0–10.0	mg/l	4.233	17–42	mmol/l	XX	1	mmol/l
Carbon dioxide content (B,P,S) [bicarbonate + CO$_2$]	22–28	mEq/l	1.00	22–28	mmol/l	X	1	mmol/l
Carbon monoxide (B) [proportion of Hb which is COHb]	<15	%	0.01	<0.15	1	O.XX	0.01	
β carotenes (S)	50–250	mg/dl	0.01863	0.9–4.6	mmol/l	X.X	0.1	mmol/l
Catecholamines, total (U) [as norepinephrine]	<120	mg/24 h	5.911	<675	nmol/d	XXO	10	mg/d
Ceruloplasmin (S)	20–35	mg/dl	10.0	200–350	mg/l	XXO	10	mg/l
Chlordiazepoxide (P)								
Therapeutic	0.5–5.0	mg/l	3.336	2–17	mmol/l	XX	1	mmol/l
Toxic	>10.0	mg/l	3.336	>33	mmol/l	XX	1	mmol/l
Chloride (S)	95–105	mEq/l	1.00	95–105	mmol/l	XXX	1	mmol/l
Chlorimipramine (P) [includes desmethyl metabolite]	50–400	ng/ml	3.176	150–1270	nmol/l	XXO	10	nmol/l
Chlorpromazine (P)	50–300	ng/ml	3.136	150–950	nmol/l	XXO	10	nmol/l
Chlorpropamide (P) therapeutic	75–250	mg/l	3.613	270–900	mmol/l	XXO	10	mmol/l
Cholestanol (P) [as a fraction of total cholesterol]	1–3	%	0.01	0.01–0.03	1	O.XX	0.01	
Cholesterol (P)								
<29 years	<200	mg/dl	0.02586	<5.20	mol/l	X.XX	0.05	mmol/l
30–39 years	<225	mg/dl	0.02586	<5.85	mmol/l	X.XX	0.05	mmol/l
40–49 years	<245	mg/dl	0.02586	<6.35	mmol/l	X.XX	0.05	mmol/l
>50 years	<265	mg/dl	0.02586	<6.85	mmol/l	X.XX	0.05	mmol/l
Cholesterol esters (P) [as a fraction of total cholesterol]	60–75	%	0.01	0.60–0.75	1	O.XX	0.01	
Cholinesterase (S)	620–1370	U/l	0.01667	10.3–22.8	mkat/l	XX.X	0.1	mkat/l
Chorionic gonadotropin (P) [βHCG]	0 if not pregnant	mIU/ml	1.00	0 if not pregnant	IU/l	XX	1	IU/l
Citrate (B) [as citric acid]	1.2–3.0	mg/dl	52.05	60–160	mmol/l	XXX	5	mmol/l
Complement, C3 (S)	70–160	mg/dl	0.01	0.7–1.6	g/l	X.X	0.1	g/l
Complement, C4 (S)	20–40	mg/dl	0.01	0.2–0.4	g/l	X.X	0.1	g/l
Copper (S)	70–140	mg/dl	0.1574	11.0–22.0	mmol/l	XX.X	0.2	mmol/l
Copper (U)	<40	mg/24 h	0.01574	<0.6	mmol/d	X.X	0.2	mmol/l
Coproporphyrins (U)	<200	mg/24 h	1.527	<300	nmol/d	XXO	10	nmol/d
Cortisol (S)								
800 h	4–19	mg/dl	27.59	110–520	nmol/l	XXO	10	nmol/l
1600 h	2–15	mg/dl	27.59	50–410	nmol/l	XXO	10	nmol/l
2400 h	5	mg/dl	7.59	140	nmol/l	XXO	10	nmol/l
Cortisol, free (U)	10–110	mg/24 h	2.759	30–300	nmol/d	XXO	10	nmol/d
Creatine (S)								
Male	0.17–0.50	mg/dl	76.25	10–40	mmol/l	XO	10	mmol/l
Female	0.35–0.93	mg/dl	76.25	30–70	mmol/l	XO	10	mmol/l
Creatine (U)								
Male	0–40	mg/24 h	7.625	0–300	mmol/d	XXO	10	mmol/d
Female	0–80	mg/24 h	7.625	0–600	mmol/d	XXO	10	mmol/d

TABLE 6.1
(Continued)

Component Present	Reference Intervals (Examples)	Present Unit	Conversion Factor	SI Reference Intervals	SI Unit	SI Unit Symbol	Significant Digits	Suggested Minimum Increment
Creatine kinase [CK] (S)								
Creatine kinase								
Isoenzymes (S)	0–130	U/l	0.01667	0–2.16	mkat/l	X.XX	0.01	mkat/l
MB fraction	>5 in myocardial infarction	%	0.01	>0.05	1	O.XX	0.01	
Creatinine (S)	0.6–1.2	mg/dl	88.40	50–110	mmol/l	XXO	10	mmol/l
Creatinine (U)	Variable	g/24 h	8.840	Variable	mmol/d	XX.X	0.1	mmol/d
Creatinine clearance (S,U)	75–125	ml/min	0.01667	1.24–2.08	ml/A (where A is the body surface area in square meters [m^2])	X.XX	0.02	ml/s
Cyanide (B)								
Lethal	>0.10	mg/dl	384.3	>40	mmol/l	XXX	5	mmol/l
Cyanocobalamin (S)								
[Vitamin B$_{12}$]	100–200	pg/ml	0.7378	150–750	pmol/l	XXO	10	pmol/l
Cyclic AMP (S)	2.6–6.6	mg/l	3.038	8–20	nmol/l	XXX	1	nmol/l
Cyclic AMP (U)								
Total urinary	2.9–5.6	mmol/g creatinine	113.1	330–630	nmol/mmol creatinine	XXO	10	nmol/mmol creatinine
Renal tubular	<2.5	mmol/g creatinine	113.1	<280	nmol/mmol creatinine	XXO	10	nmol/mmol creatinine
Cyclic GMP (S)	0.6–3.5	mg/l	2.897	1.7–10.1	nmol/l	XX.X	0.1	nmol/l
Cyclic GMP (U)	0.3–1.8	mmol/g creatinine	113.1	30–200	nmol/mmol creatinine	XXO	10	nmol/mmol creatinine
Cystine (U)	10–100	mg/24 h	4.161	40–420	mmol/d	XXO	10	mmol/d
Dehydroepiandrosterone (DHEA) (P,S)								
1–4 years	0.2–0.4	mg/l	3.467	0.6–1.4	nmol/l	XX.X	0.2	nmol/l
4–8 years	0.1–1.9	mg/l	3.467	0.4–6.6	nmol/l	XX.X	0.2	nmol/l
8–10 years	0.2–2.9	mg/l	3.467	0.6–10.0	nmol/l	XX.X	0.2	nmol/l
10–12 years	0.5–9.2	mg/l	3.467	1.8–31.8	nmol/l	XX.X	0.2	nmol/l
12–14 years	0.9–20.0	mg/l	3.467	3.2–69.4	nmol/l	XX.X	0.2	nmol/l
14–16 years	2.5–20.0	mg/l	3.467	8.6–69.4	nmol/l	XX.X	0.2	nmol/l
Premenopausal female	2.0–15.0	mg/l	3.467	7.0–52.0	nmol/l	XX.X	0.2	nmol/l
Male	0.8–10.0	mg/l	3.467	2.8–34.6	nmol/l	XX.X	0.2	nmol/l
DHEA (U)	See steroids	Fractionation						
DHEA sulfate (DHEA-S) (P,S)								
Newborn	1670–3640	ng/ml	0.002714	4.5–9.9	mmol/l	XX.X		mmol/l
Prepubertal children	100–600	ng/ml	0.002714	0.3–1.6	mmol/l	XX.X		mmol/l
Male	2000–3500	ng/ml	0.002714	5.4–9.1	mmol/l	XX.X		mmol/l
Female (premenopausal)	820–3380	ng/ml	0.002714	2.2–9.2	mmol/l	XX.X		mmol/l
Female (postmenopausal)	110–610	ng/ml	0.002714	0.3–1.7	mmol/l	XX.X		mmol/l
Pregnancy [term]	0–1170	ng/ml	0.002714	0.6–3.2	mmol/l	XX.X		mmol/l
11-Deoxycortisol (S)	0–2	mg/dl	28.86	0–60	nmol/l	XXO	10	nmol/l
Desipramine (P) therapeutic	50–200	ng/ml	3.754	170–700	nmol/l	XXO	10	nmol/l
Diazepam (P)								
Therapeutic	0.10–0.25	mg/l	3512	350–900	nmol/l	XXO	10	nmol/l
Toxic	>1.0	mg/l	3512	>3510	nmol/l	XXO	10	nmol/l
Dicoumarol (P) therapeutic	8–30	mg/l	2.974	25–90	mmol/l	XX	5	mmol/l

Continued

TABLE 6.1
(Continued)

Component Present	Reference Intervals (Examples)	Present Unit	Conversion Factor	SI Reference Intervals	SI Unit	SI Unit Symbol	Significant Digits	Suggested Minimum Increment
Digoxin (P)								
Therapeutic	0.5–2.2	ng/ml	1.281	0.6–2.8	nmol/l	X.X	0.1	nmol/l
	0.5–2.2	mg/l	1.281	0.6–2.8	nmol/l	X.X	0.1	nmol/l
Toxic	>2.5	ng/ml	1.281	>3.2	nmol/l	X.X	0.1	nmol/l
Dimethadione (P) therapeutic	<1.00	g/l	7.745	<7.7	mmol/l	X.X	0.1	mmol/l
Disopyramide (P) therapeutic	2.0–6.0	mg/l	2.946	6–18	mmol/l	XX	1	mmol/l
Doxepin (P) therapeutic	50–200	n/ml	3.579	180–720	nmol/l	XO	10	nmol/l
Electrophoresis, protein (S)								
Albumin	60–65	%	0.01	0.60–0.65	1	O.XX	0.01	
α_1-Globulin	1.7–5.0	%	0.01	0.02–0.05	1	O.XX	0.01	
α_2-Globulin	6.7–12.5	%	0.01	0.07–0.13	1	O.XX	0.01	
β-Globulin	8.3–16.3	%	0.01	0.08–0.16	1	O.XX	0.01	
γ-Globulin	10.7–20.0	%	0.01	0.11–0.20	1	O.XX	0.01	
Albumin	3.6–5.2	g/dl	10.0	36–52	g/l	XX	1	g/l
α_1-Globulin	0.1–0.4	g/dl	10.0	1–4	g/l	XX	1	g/l
α_2-Globulin	0.4–1.0	g/dl	10.0	4–10	g/l	XX	1	g/l
β-Globulin	0.5–1.2	g/dl	10.0	5–12	g/l	XX	1	g/l
γ-Globulin	0.6–1.6	g/dl	10.0	6–16	g/l	XX	1	g/l
Epinephrine (P)	31–95 (at rest for 15 min)	pg/ml	5.458	170–520	pmol/l	XXO	10	pmol/l
Epinephrine (U)	<10	mg/24 h	5.458	<55	nmol/d	XX	5	nmol/d
Estradiol (S) male >18 years	15–40	pg/ml	3.671	55–150	pmol/l	XX	1	pmol/l
Estriol (U) [non-pregnant]								
Onset of menstruation	4–25	mg/24 h	3.468	15–85	nmol/d	XXX	5	nmol/d
Ovulation peak	28–99	mg/24 h	3.468	95–345	nmol/d	XXX	5	nmol/d
Luteal peak	22–105	mg/24 h	3.468	75–365	nmol/d	XXX	5	nmol/d
Menopausal woman	1.4–19.6	mg/24 h	3.468	5–70	nmol/d	XXX	5	nmol/d
Male	5–18	mg/24 h	3.468	15–60	nmol/d	XXX	5	nmol/d
Estrogens (S) [as estradiol]								
Female	20–300	pg/ml	3.671	70–1100	pmol/l	XXXO	10	pmol/l
Peak production	200–800	pg/ml	3.671	750–2900	pmol/l	XXXO	10	pmol/l
Male	<50	pg/ml	3.671	<180	pmol/l	XXO	10	pmol/l
Estrogens, placental (U) [as estriol]	Depends on period of gestation	mg/24 h	3.468	Depends on period of gestation	mmol/d	XXX	1	mmol/d
Estrogen receptors (T)								
Negative	0–3	fmol estradiol bound/mg cytosol protein	1.00	0–3	fmol estradiol/ mg cytosol protein	XXX	1	fmol/mg protein
Doubtful	4–10	fmol estradiol bound/mg cytosol protein	1.00	4–10	fmol estradiol/ mg cytosol protein	XXX	1	fmol/mg protein
Positive	>10	fmol estradiol bound/mg cytosol protein	1.00	>10	fmol estradiol/ mg cytosol protein	XXX	1	fmol/mg protein
Estrone (P,S)								
Female 1–10 days of cycle	43–180	pg/ml	3.699	160–665	pmol/l	XXX	5	pmol/l
Female 11–20 days of cycle	75–196	pg/ml	3.699	275–725	pmol/l	XXX	5	pmol/l
Female 20–39 days of cycle	131–201	pg/ml	3.699	485–745	pmol/l	XXX	5	pmol/l
Male	29–75	pg/ml	3.699	105–275	pmol/l	XXX	5	pmol/l
Estrone (U) female	2–25	mg/24 h	3.699	5–90	nmol/d	XXX	5	nmol/d
Ethanol (P)								
Legal limit [driving]	<80	mg/dl	0.2171	<17	mmol/l	XX	1	nmol/l
Toxic	>100	mg/dl	0.2171	>22	mmol/l	XX	1	mmol/l

TABLE 6.1
(Continued)

Component Present	Reference Intervals (Examples)	Present Unit	Conversion Factor	SI Reference Intervals	SI Unit	SI Unit Symbol	Significant Digits	Suggested Minimum Increment
Ethchlorvynol (P) toxic	>40	mg/l	6.915	>280	mmol/l	XXO	10	mmol/l
Ethosuximide (P) therapeutic	40–110	mg/l	7.084	280–780	mmol/l	XXO	10	mmol/l
Ethylene glycol (P) toxic	>30	mg/dl	0.1611	>5	mmol/l	XX	1	mmol/l
Fat (F) [as stearic acid]	2.0–6.0	g/24 h	3.515	7–21	mmol/d	XXX	1	mmol/d
Fatty acids, nonesterified (P)	8–20	mg/dl	10.00	80–200	mg/l	XXO	10	mg/l
Ferritin (S)	18–300	ng/ml	1.00	18–300	mg/l	XXO	10	mg/l
Fibrinogen (P)	200–400	mg/dl	0.01	2.0–4.0	g/l	X.X	0.1	g/l
Fluoride (U)	<1.0	mg/24 h	52.63	<50	mmol/d	XXO	10	mmol/d
Folate (S) [as	2–10	ng/ml	22.66	4–22	nmol/l	XX	2	nmol/l
pteroylglutamic acid]		mg/dl	2.266		nmol/l	XX	2	nmol/l
Folate (Erc)	140–960	ng/ml	2.266	550–2200	nmol/l	XXO	10	nmol/l
Follicle stimulating hormone [FSH] (P)								
Female	2.0–15.0	mIU/ml	1.00	2–15	IU/l	XX	1	IU/l
Peak production	20–50	mIU/ml	1.00	20–50	IU/l	XX	1	IU/l
Male	1.0–10.0	mIU/ml	1.00	1–10	IU/l	XX	1	IU/l
Follicle stimulating hormone [FSH] (U)								
Follicular phase	2–15	IU/24 h	1.00	2–15	IU/d	XXX	1	IU/d
Midcycle	8–40	IU/24 h	1.00	8–40	IU/d	XXX	1	IU/d
Luteal phase	2–10	IU/24 h	1.00	2–10	IU/d	XXX	1	IU/d
Menopausal women	35–100	IU/24 h	1.00	35–100	IU/d	XXX	1	IU/d
Male	2–15	IU/24 h	1.00	2–15	IU/d	XXX	1	IU/d
Fructose (P)	<10	mg/dl	0.05551	<0.6	mmol/l	X.XX	0.1	mmol/l
Galactose (P) [children]	<20	mg/dl	0.05551	<1.1	mmol/l	X.XX	0.1	mmol/l
Gases (aB)								
pO_2 (=Torr)	75–105	mm Hg	0.1333	10.0–14.0	kPa	XX.X	0.1	kPa
pCO_2 (=Torr)	33–44	mm Hg	0.1333	4.4–5.9	kPa	X.X	0.1	kPa
γ-glutamyltransferase [GGT] (S)	0–30	U/l	0.01667	0–0.50	mkat/l	X.XX	0.01	mkat/l
Gastrin (S)	0–180	pg/ml	1.00	0–180	ng/l	XXO	10	ng/l
Globulins (S)	See immuno- globulins							
Glucagon (S)	50–100	pg/ml	1.00	50–100	ng/l	XXO	10	ng/l
Glucose (P) fasting	70–110	mg/dl	0.05551	3.9–6.1	mmol/l	XX.X	0.1	mmol/l
Glucose (Sf)	50–80	mg/dl	0.05551	2.8–4.4	mmol/l	XX.X	0.1	mmol/l
Glutethimide (P)								
Therapeutic	<10	mg/l	4.603	<46	mmol/l	XX	1	mmol/l
Toxic	>20	mg/l	4.603	>92	mmol/l	XX	1	mmol/l
Glycerol, free (S)	<1.5	mg/dl	0.1086	<0.16	mmol/l	X.XX	0.01	mmol/l
Gold (S) therapeutic	300–800	mg/dl	0.05077	15.0–40.0	mmol/l	XX.X	0.1	mmol/l
Gold (U)	<500	mg/24 h	0.005077	<2.5	mmol/d	X.X	0.1	mmol/d
Palmitic acid (Amf)	Depends on gestation	mmol/l	1000	Depends on gestation	mmol/l	XXX	5	mmol/l
Pentobarbital (P)	20–40	mg/l	4.419	90–170	mmol/l	XX	5	mmol/l
Phenobarbital (P) therapeutic	2–5	mg/l	43.06	85–215	mmol/l	XXX	5	mmol/l
Phensuximide (P)	4–8	mg/l	5.285	20–40	mmol/l	XX	5	mmol/l
Phenylbutazone (P) therapeutic	<100	mg/l	3.243	<320	mmol/l	XXO	10	mmol/l
Phenytoin (P)								
Therapeutic	10–20	mg/l	3.964	40–80	mmol/l	XX	5	mmol/l
Toxic	>30	mg/l	3.964	>12	mmol/l	XX	5	mmol/l

Continued

TABLE 6.1
(Continued)

Component Present	Reference Intervals (Examples)	Present Unit	Conversion Factor	SI Reference Intervals	SI Unit	SI Unit Symbol	Significant Digits	Suggested Minimum Increment
Phosphate (S) [as phosphorus, inorganic]	2.5–5.0	mg/dl	0.3229	0.80–1.60	mmol/l	X.XX	0.05	mmol/l
Phosphate (U) [as phosphorus, inorganic]	Diet dependent	g/24 h	32.29	Diet dependent	mmol/d	XXX	1	mmol/d
Phospholipid phosphorus, total (P)	5–12	mg/dl	0.3229	1.60–3.90	mmol/l	X.XX	0.05	mmol/l
Phospholipid phosphorus, total (Erc)	1.2–12.0	mg/dl	0.3229	0.40–3.90	mmol/l	X.XX	0.05	mmol/l
Phospholipids (P) substance fraction of total phospholipid								
Phosphatidyl choline	65–70	%/total	0.01	0.65–0.70	1	O.XX	0.01	
Phosphatidyl ethanolamine	4–5	%/total	0.01	0.04–0.05	1	O.XX	0.01	
Sphingomyelin	15–20	%/total	0.01	0.15–0.20	1	O.XX	0.01	
Lysophosphatidyl choline	3–5	%/total	0.01	0.03–0.05	1	O.XX	0.01	
Phospholipids (Erc) substance fraction of total phospholipid								
Phosphatidyl choline	28–33	%/total	0.01	0.28–0.33	1	O.XX	0.01	
Phosphatidyl ethanolamine	24–31	%/total	0.01	0.24–0.31	1	O.XX	0.01	
Sphingomyelin	22–29	%/total	0.01	0.22–0.29	1	O.XX	0.01	
Phosphatidyl serine + Phosphatidyl inositol	12–20	%/total	0.01	0.12–0.20	1	O.XX	0.01	
Lysophosphatidyl choline	1–2	%/total	0.01	0.01–0.02	1	O.XX	0.01	
Phytanic acid (P)	Trace–0.3	mg/dl	32.00	<10	mmol/l	XX	5	mmol/l
Human Placental lactogen SO [HPL]	>4.0 after 30 wk gestation	mg/ml	46.30	>180	nmol/l	XXO	10	nmol/l
Porphobilinogen (U)	0–2	mg/24 h	4.420	0–9	mmol/d	X.X	0.5	mmol/d
Porphyrins								
Coproporphyrin (U)	45–180	mg/24 h	1.527	68–276	nmol/d	XXX	2	nmol/d
Protoporphyrin (Erc)	15–50	mg/dl	0.0177	0.28–0.90	mmol/l	X.XX	0.02	mmol/l
Uroporphyrin (U)	5–20	mg/24 h	1.204	6–24	nmol/d	XX	2	nmol/d
Uroporphyrinogen								
Synthetase (Erc)	22–42	mmol/mL/h	0.2778	6.0–11.8	mmol/(l.s)	X.X	0.2	mmol/(l.s)
Potassium ion (S)	3.5–5.0	mEq/l	1.00	3.5–5.0	mmol/l	X.X	0.1	mmol/l
		mg/dl	0.2558		mmol/l	X.X	0.1	mmol/l
Potassium ion (U) [diet dependent]	25–100	mEq/24 h	1.00	25–100	mmol/d	XX	1	mmol/d
Pregnaediol (U)								
Normal	1–6	mg/24 h	3.120	3.0–18.5	mmol/d	XX.X	0.5	mmol/d
Pregnancy	Depends on gestation							
Pregnanetriol (U)	0.5–2.0	mg/24 h	2.972	1.5–6.0	mmol/d	XX.X	0.5	mmol/d
Primidone (P)								
Therapeutic	6–10	mg/l	4.582	25–46	mmol/l	XX	1	mmol/l
Toxic	>10	mg/l	4.582	>46	mmol/l	XX	1	mmol/l
Procainamide (P)								
Therapeutic	4–8	mg/l	4.249	17–34	mmol/l	XX	1	mmol/l
Toxic	>12.0	mg/l	4.249	>50	mmol/l	XX	1	mmol/l
N-Acetyl procainamide (P) therapeutic	4–8	mg/l	3.606	14–29	mmol/l	XX	1	mmol/l
Progesterone (P)								
Follicular phase	<2	ng/ml	3.180	<6	nmol/l	XX	2	nmol/l
Luteal phase	2–20	ng/ml	3.180	6–64	nmol/l	XX	2	nmol/l

TABLE 6.1
(Continued)

Component Present	Reference Intervals (Examples)	Present Unit	Conversion Factor	SI Reference Intervals	SI Unit	SI Unit Symbol	Significant Digits	Suggested Minimum Increment
Progesterone receptors (T)								
Negative	0–3	fmol progesterone bound/mg cytosol protein	1.00	0–3	fmol progesterone bound/mg cytosol protein	XX	1	fmol/mg protein
Doubtful	4–10	fmol progesterone bound/mg cytosol protein	1.00	4–10	fmol progesterone bound/mg cytosol protein	XX	1	fmol/mg protein
Positive	>10	fmol progesterone bound/mg cytosol protein	1.00	>10	fmol progesterone bound/mg cytosol protein	XX	1	fmol/mg protein
Prolactin (P)	<20	ng/ml	1.00	<20	mg/l	XX	1	mg/l
Propoxyphene (P) toxic	>2.0	mg/l	2.946	>5.9	mmol/l	X.X	0.1	mmol/l
Propranolol (P) [Inderal] therapeutic	50–200	ng/ml	3.856	190–770	nmol/l	XXO	10	nmol/l
Protein, total (S)	6.0–8.0	g/dl	10.0	60–80	g/l	XX	1	g/l
Protein, total (Sf)	<40	mg/dl	0.01	<0.40	g/l	X.XX	0.1	g/l
Protein, total (U)	<150	mg/24 h	0.001	<0.15	g/d	X.XX	0.01	g/d
Protryptyline (P)	100–300	ng/ml	3.797	380–1140	nmol/l	XXO	10	nmol/l
Pyruvate (B) [as pyruvic acid]	0.30–0.90	mg/dl	113.6	35–100	mmol/l	XXX	1	mmol/l
Quinidine (P)								
Therapeutic	1.5–3.0	mg/l	3.082	4.6–9.2	mmol/l	X.X	0.1	mmol/l
Toxic	>6.0	mg/l	3.082	>18.5	mmol/l	X.X	0.1	mmol/l
Renin (P) normal sodium diet	1.1–4.1	ng/ml/h	0.2778	0.30–1.14	ng/(l.s)	X.XX	0.2	ng/(l.s)
Restricted sodium diet	6.2–12.4	ng/ml/h	0.2778	1.72–3.44	ng/(l.s)	X.XX	0.02	ng/(l.s)
Salicylate (S) [salicylic acid] toxic	>20	mg/dl	0.07240	>1.45	mmol/l	X.XX	0.05	mmol/l
Serotonin (B) [5 hydroxytryptamine]	8–21	mg/dl	0.05675	0.45–1.20	mmoll/l	X.XX	0.05	mmol/l
Sodium ion (S)	135–147	mEq/l	1.00	135–147	mmol/l	XXX	1	mmol/l
Sodium ion (U)	Diet dependent	mEq/24 h	1.00	Diet dependent	mmol/d	XXX	2	mmol/d
Steroids 17-Hydroxy-corticosteroids (U) [as cortisol]								
Female	2.0–8.0	mg/24 h	2.759	5–25	mmol/d	XX	1	mmol/d
Male	3–10	mg/24 h	2.759	10–30	mmol/d	XX	1	mmol/d
17-Ketogenic steroids (U) [as DHEA]								
Female	7–12	mg/24 h	3.467	25–40	mmol/d	XX	1	mmol/d
Male	9–17	mg/24 h	3.467	30–60	mmol/d	XX	1	mmol/d
17-Ketosteroids (U) [as DHEA]								
Female	6–17	mg/24 h	3.467	20–60	mmol/d	XX	1	mmol/d
Male	6–20	mg/24 h	3.467	20–70	mmol/d	XX	1	mmol/d
Ketosteroid fractions (U) androsterone								
Female	0.5–2.0	mg/24 h	3.443	1–10	mmol/d	XX	1	mmol/d
Male	2.0–5.0	mg/24 h	3.443	7–17	mmol/d	XX	1	mmol/d
Dehydroepiandrosterone								
Female	0.2–1.8	mg/24 h	3.467	1–6	mmol/d	XX	1	mmol/d
Male	0.2–2.0	mg/24 h	3.467	1–7	mmol/d	XX	1	mmol/d
Etiocholanolone								
Female	0.8–4.0	mg/24 h	3.443	2–14	mmol/d	XX	1	mmol/d
Male	1.4–5.0	mg/24 h	3.443	4–17	mmol/d	XX	1	mmol/d

Continued

TABLE 6.1
(Continued)

Component Present	Reference Intervals (Examples)	Present Unit	Conversion Factor	SI Reference Intervals	SI Unit	SI Unit Symbol	Significant Digits	Suggested Minimum Increment
Sulfonamides (B) [as sulfanilamide] therapeutic	10–15	mg/dl	58.07	580–870	mmol/l	XXO	10	mmol/l
Testosterone (P)								
Female	0.6	ng/ml	3.467	2.0	nmol/l	XX.X	0.5	nmol/l
Male	4.6–8.0	ng/ml	3.467	14–28	nmol/l	XX.X	0.5	nmol/l
Theophylline (P) therapeutic	10–20	mg/l	5.550	55–110	mmol/l	XX	1	mmol/l
Thiocyanate (P) (nitroprusside toxicity)	10.0	mg/dl	0.1722	1.7	mmol/l	X.XX	0.1	mmol/l
Thiopental (P)	individual	mg/l	4.126	individual	mmol/l	XX	5	mmol/l
Thyroid tests								
Thyroid stimulating hormone [TSH] (S)	2–11	mU/ml	1.00	2–11	mU/l	XX	1	mU/l
Thyroxine [T4] (S)	4–11	mg/dl	12.87	51–142	nmol/l	XXX	1	nmol/l
Thyroxine binding globulin [TGB] (S) [as thyroxine]	12–28	mg/dl	12.87	150–360	nmol/l	XXO	1	nmol/l
Thyroxine, free (S)	0.8–2.8	ng/dl	12.87	10–36	pmol/l	XX	1	pmol/l
Triiodothyronine [T3] (S)	75–220	ng/dl	0.01536	1.2–3.4	nmol/l	X.X	0.1	nmol/l
T3 uptake (S)	25–35	%	0.01	0.25–0.35	1	O.XX	0.01	
Tolbuamide (P) therapeutic	50–120	mg/l	3.699	180–450	mmol/l	XXO	10	mmol/l
Transferrin (S)	170–370	mg/dl	0.01	1.70–3.70	g/l	X.XX	0.01	g/l
Triglycerides (P) [as triolein]	<160	mg/dl	0.01129	<1.80	mmol/l	X.XX	0.02	mmol/l
Trimethadione (P) therapeutic	<50	mg/l	6.986	<350	mmol/l	XXO	10	mmol/l
Trimipramine (P) therapeutic	50–200	ng/ml	3.397	170–680	nmol/l	XXO	10	nmol/l
Urate (S) [as uric acid]	2–7	mg/dl	59.48	120–420	mmol/l	XXO	10	mmol/l
Urate (U) [as uric acid]	Diet dependent	g/24 h	5.948	Diet dependent	mmol/d	XX	1	mmol/d
Urea nitrogen (S)	8–18	mg/dl	0.3570	3.0–6.5	mmol/l UREA	X.X	0.5	mmol/l
Urea nitrogen (U)	2–20 diet dependent	g/24 h	35.700	450–700	mmol/d UREA	XXO	10	mol/d
Urobilinogen (U)	0–4	mg/24 h	1.693	0.0–6.8	mmol/d	X.X	0.1	mmol/d
Valproic acid (P) therapeutic	50–100	mg/l	6.934	350–700	mmol/l	XO	10	mmol/l
Vanillylmandelic acid [VMA], urine	<6.8	mg/24 h	5.046	<35	mmol/d	XX	1	mmol/d
Vitamin A [retinol] (P,S)	10–50	mg/dl	0.03491	0.35–1.75	mmol/l	X.XX	0.05	mmol/l
Vitamin B₁ [thiamine hydrochloride] (U)	60–500	mg/24 h	0.002965	0.18–1.48	mmol/d	ZX.XX	0.01	mmol/d
Vitamin B₂ [riboflavin] (S)	2.6–3.7	mg/dl	26.57	70–100	nmol/l	XXX	5	nmol/l
Vitamin B₆ [pyridoxal] (B)	20–90	ng/ml	5.982	120–540	nmol/l	XXX	5	nmol/l
Vitamin B₁₂ (P,S) [cyanocobalamin]	200–1000	pg/ml	0.7378	150–750	pmol/l	XO	10	pmol/l
Vitamin C	See ascorbate (B,P,S)							
Vitamin D₃								
[cholecalciferol] (P)	24–40	mg/ml	2.599	60–105	nmol/l	XXX	5	nmol/l
25 OH-cholecacliferol	18–36	ng/ml	0.496	45–90	nmol/l	XXX	5	mmol/l
Vitamin E [α-tocopherol] (P,S)	0.78–1.25	mg/dl	23.22	18–29	mmol/l	XX	1	mmol/l
Warfarin (P) therapeutic	1–3	mg/l	3.243	3.3–9.8	mmol/l	XX.X	0.1	mmol/l
Xanthine (U)								
Hypoxanthine	5–30	mg/24	6.574	30–200	mmol/d	XXO	10	mmol/d
		hmg/24 h	7.347		mmol/d	XXO	10	mmol/d
D-xylose (B) [25 g dose]	30–40 (30–60 min)	mg/dl	0.06661	0–2.7 (30–60 min)	mmol/l	X.X	0.1	mmol/l
D-xylose excretion (U) [25 g dose]	21–31	%	0.01	0.21–0.31 (excreted in 5 h)	1	O.XX	0.01	
Xinc (S)	75–120	mg/dl	0.1530	11.5–18.5	mmol/l	XX.X	0.1	mmol/l
Zinc (U)	150–1200	mg/24 h	0.01530	2.3–18.3	mmol/d	XX.X	0.1	mmol/d

TABLE 6.2
Vitamin[a] Terminology

Name	Comment
Vitamin A	A number of compounds have vitamin A activity but differ in biopotency
	All *trans* retinol is the standard, and the activity of other compounds can be stated as retinol equivalents. This includes the aldehyde (retinal), acid (retinoic acid), and provitamin (carotene) forms
Vitamin B	Although originally thought to be a single compound, researchers have found that eight major compounds comprised this "vitamin."
Vitamin B complex	A group of vitamins; includes thiamin, riboflavin, niacin, pyridoxine (3 forms), pantothenic acid, biotin, cyanocobalamin (B_{12}), and folacin
Vitamin B_1	Aneurin; antineuritic factor. Obsolete synonym for thiamin
Vitamin B_2	Lactoflavin, Ovoflavin. Obsolete synonyms for riboflavin
Vitamin B_3	Antipellagra factor. Obsolete synonym for niacin
Vitamin B_4	Not proven to have vitamin activity; thought to be a mixture of arginine, glycine, riboflavin, and pyridoxine
Vitamin B_5	Probably identical to niacin
Vitamin B_6	Synonym for pyridoxine, pyridoxal, pyridoxamine
Vitamin B_7	Not proven to have vitamin activity; sometimes referred to as Vitamin I, a factor that improves food digestibility in pigeons
Vitamin B_8	Not proven to have vitamin activity; found to be adenylic acid
Vitamin B_{10}, B_{11}	An unrefined mixture of folacin and cyanocobalamin; obsolete term
Vitamin B_{12}	Cyanocobalamin; B_{12a} is aquacobalamin; B_{12b} is hydroxocobalamin; B_{12c} is nitritocobalamin
Vitamin B_{13}	Orotic acid; a metabolite of pyrimidine metabolism; not considered a vitamin
Vitamin B_{15}	Synonym for "pangamic acid" a compound of no known biologic value; not a vitamin
Vitamin B_{17}	Synonym for laetrile; a cyanogenic glycoside of no known biologic value; not a vitamin
Vitamin Bc	Obsolete term for pteroylglutamic acid; a component of folacin
Vitamin Bp	A compound that prevents perosis in chicks; can be replaced by choline and manganese
Vitamin Bf	Shown to be carnitine
Vitamin Bx	Probably a mixture of pantothenic acid and p-aminobenzoic acid
Vitamin C	Synonym for ascorbic acid
Vitamin C_2	Unrecognized, unconfirmed compound purported to have antipneumonia activity; also called vitamin J
Vitamin D	Antirachitic factor; a group of sterols (the calciferols) that serve to enhance bone calcification
Vitamin D_2	Ergocalciferol; one of the D vitamins from plant sources
Vitamin D_3	Cholecalciferol; one of the D vitamins from animal sources
Vitamin E	A group of tocopherols that have an important function in the antioxidant system; suppresses free radical formation
Vitamin F	Obsolete term for the essential fatty acids (linoleic and linolenic acids)
Vitamin G	Obsolete term for riboflavin before riboflavin and niacin were recognized as separate vitamins
Vitamin H	Obsolete term for biotin
Vitamin I	Obsolete term for a mixture of B vitamins
Vitamin K	A group of fat soluble compounds that function in the post translational carboxylation of the glutamic acid residues of prothrombin and osteocalcin
Vitamin K_1	Phylloquinone; vitamin K of plant origin
Vitamin K_2	Menaquinone; vitamin K of animal origin
Vitamin K_3	Menadione; synthetic vitamin K
Vitamin L_1	Unrecognized factor that may be related to anthranitic acid and which has been proposed to be important for lactation; not proven to have vitamin activity
Vitamin L_2	See above
Vitamin M	Obsolete term for pteroylglutamic acid (folacin)
Vitamin N	Obsolete term used to designate an anticancer compound mixture; undefined and unrecognized
Vitamin P	Not a vitamin; but is a metabolite of citrin
Vitamin Q	Not a vitamin; but is probably a synonym for coenzyme Q
Vitamin R	Obsolete term for folacin
Vitamin S	Not a vitamin; but does act to enhance chick growth; related to the peptide "streptogenin" and also to biotin
Vitamin T	Not a vitamin; reported to improve protein utilization in rats; an extract from termites
Vitamin U	Not a vitamin; an extract from cabbage that has been reported to suppress gastric acid production; may be important to folacin activity
Vitamin V	Not a vitamin
Bioflavinoids	Not a vitamin
Carnitine	Not a vitamin; except in preterm infants and in severely traumatized persons
Choline	Can be synthesized by the body but some conditions interfere with adequate synthesis

Continued

TABLE 6.2
(Continued)

Name	Comment
Citrovorum factor	Synonym for folacin; a B vitamin
Extrinsic factor	Obsolete term for vitamin B_{12}, cyanocobalamin
Factors U, R, X	Obsolete terms for folacin
Filtrate factor	Obsolete term for riboflavin
Flavin	A general term for the riboflavin containing coenzymes, FMN, and FAD
Hepatoflavin	Obsolete term for riboflavin
Intrinsic factor	Not a vitamin; an endogenous factor needed for vitamin B_{12}, cyanocobalamin, absorption
LLD factor	Obsolete term for vitamin B_{12}, cyanocobalamin
Lipoic acid	Not a vitamin, but does serve as a cofactor in oxidative decarboxylation
Myoinositol	Sometimes a vitamin when endogenous synthesis is inadequate
Norite eluate	Not a vitamin
P–P factor	Obsolete term for niacin
Pyrroloquinoline quinone	Not a vitamin; component of metallo-oxido-reductases
Rhizopterin	Obsolete term for folacin
SLR factor	Obsolete term for folacin
Streptogenin	Not a vitamin
Wills factor	Obsolete term for folacin
Zoopherin	Obsolete term for vitamin B_{12}, cyanocobalamin

[a] A vitamin is an organic compound required in small amounts for the maintenance of normal biochemical and physiological function of the body. These compounds must be present in food and if absent, well defined symptoms of deficiency will develop. An essential nutrient such as a vitamin cannot be synthesized in amounts sufficient to meet needs.

TABLE 6.3
Nomenclature of Compounds with Vitamin A Activity

Recommended Name	Synonyms
Retinol	Vitamin A alcohol
Retinal	Vitamin A aldehyde, retinene, retinaldehyde
Retinoic acid	Vitamin A acid
3-Dehydroretinol	Vitamin A_2 (alcohol)
3-Dehydroretinal	Vitamin A_2 aldehyde, retinene2
3-Dehydroretinoic acid	Vitamin A_2 acid
Anhydroretinol	Anhydrovitamin A
Retro retinal	Rehydrovitamin A
5,6-Epoxyretinol	5,6-Epoxyvitamin A alcohol
Retinyl palmitate	Vitamin A palmitate
Retinyl acetate	Vitamin A acetate
Retinyl β-glucuronide	Vitamin A acid β-glucuronide
11-*cis*-retinaldehyde	11-*cis* or neo γ vitamin A aldehyde
4-Ketoretinol	4-Keto vitamin A alcohol
Retinyl phosphate	Vitamin A phosphate
β-Carotene	Provitamin A
α-Carotene	Provitamin A
γ-Carotene	Provitamin A

TABLE 6.4
Terminology Used in Energy Assessment of Humans and Animals

Anabolism	The totality of reactions that account for the synthesis of the body's macromolecules; heat is a by-product of these reactions
Android obesity	A form of obesity in which fat distribution is mainly in the shoulders and abdomen; sometimes referred to as the "apple" type of obesity
Anthropometry	Measurements of body features, that is, height, weight, skin-fold thickness, etc.
Apparent digestible energy (DE)	Energy of the consumed food (IE) less the energy of the feces (FE); DE = IE − FE
Archimedes principle	An object's volume, when submerged in water, equals the volume of the water displaced. If the mass of the body is known, then the density can be calculated. Less dense bodies have more body fat than very dense bodies
Balance	Intake = expenditure
Body mass index (BMI)	BMI = (Body weight (kg)/Height (cm)^2). Used as a general index of body fatness, however, it does not apply to persons with high muscle mass such as elite athletes.
Basal metabolic rate (BMR)	The minimal amount of energy needed to sustain the body's metabolism. Frequently expressed in terms of the amount of oxygen used to sustain this metabolism, because of the constancy between energy flux and oxygen use
Body cell mass	The metabolically active, energy — requiring mass of the body
Body Density	Mass/unit volume
Calorie	A unit of energy; a calorie is the amount of heat needed to raise the temperature of 1 kg of water 1°C; also referred to as a kilocalorie. Can be converted to kilojoules (kJ): kcal × 4.184 = kJ
Calorimetry	The measurement of heat production by the body. This measurement can be either direct (using a whole body calorimeter) or indirect using measurements of oxygen consumed and carbon dioxide produced
Catabolism	The totality of those reactions that reduce macromolecules to usable metabolites, CO_2 and water. Heat is a by product of these reactions
Digestive energy (DE)	The energy of food after the energy losses of digestion is subtracted. Similar to apparent ingestive energy (see above)
Gaseous products of digestion (GE)	The energy of the combustible gases produced in the digestive tract incident to the fermentation of food by microorganisms. In ruminants, this is a substantial component of the energy balance equation; in humans this is much smaller and perhaps negligible
Gynoid obesity	Excess body fat deposited mainly on the hips, abdomen, and thighs. Sometimes called "pear-shaped" obesity
Heat of activity (HiE)	The heat produced through muscular activity
Heat of digestion and absorption (HdE)	The heat produced in the digestive tract as a result of the activity of the digestive enzymes and the energy of the absorptive processes. Sometimes referred to as diet-induced thermogenesis (DIT)
Heat of fermentation (HfE)	Heat produced in the digestive tract due to the action of microbial action
Heat of product formation (HrE)	The heat produced associated with the production of a product, that is, milk or eggs, etc.
Heat of thermic regulation (HcE)	The heat needed to maintain the body temperature
Heat of waste formation and excretion (HwE)	The heat associated with the production of waste products such as urea in urine, etc.
Heat increment (HI)	The increase in heat production following the consumption of food
IDW	Ideal body weight
Indirect calorimetry	The calculation of energy (heat) production through the measurement of oxygen consumed and carbon dioxide released
Metabolizable energy (ME)	The energy in food minus that is lost through digestion, absorption, and excretion. ME = IE − (FE + UE + GE)
N-corrected metabolizable energy (MnE)	ME adjusted for total nitrogen retained or lost by the body tissue. MnE = ME − (k × TN) where TN = nitrogen retained in the body tissue
NPU	Net protein use
NDp Cal%	Net protein calories percent; the percent of the total energy value of the diet provided by protein
Nutrient density	The nutrient composition of food expressed in terms of nutrient quantity/100 kcal
Nutritional assessment	Measurement of indicators of dietary status and nutrition-related health status of individuals or population groups
Obesity	Excess fat stores
Postprandial	After a meal
Quantitative computed tomography	An imagine technique that allows for the calculation of body fatness and body composition
Respiratory quotient	The ratio of carbon dioxide produced to oxygen consumed
Skin-fold thickness	A double fold of skin and underlying tissue that can be used to estimate body fatness
Thermic effect of food	Same as heat increment
Total heat production (HE)	The energy lost as heat from the body as a result of its metabolism
True digestive energy (TDE)	The intake of energy in food minus that lost through the feces, HfE and digestive gases
True metabolizable energy (TME)	Food energy minus energy lost through feces and urine
Urinary energy	The gross energy of the urine

TABLE 6.5

Equations for Calculating Body Components Using Direct Analysis

$$\% \text{ body fat} = \frac{\text{body weight} - \text{fat solvent extracted body weight}}{\text{body weight}}$$

$$\% \text{ body water} = \frac{\text{body weight} - \text{dried body weight}}{\text{body weight}}$$

$$\% \text{ body ash} = \frac{\text{body weight after complete oxidation in a muffle furnace}}{\text{body weight}}$$

$$\% \text{ body protein} = \frac{\text{nitrogen content} \times 6.25}{\text{body weight}}$$

TABLE 6.6

General Formulas for Calculating Body Fatness from Skin-Fold Measurements[2]

Males $\% \text{ body fat} = 29.288 \times 10^{-2} (X) - 5 \times 10^{-4} (X)^2 + 15.845 \times 10^{-2} (\text{Age})$

Females $\% \text{ body fat} = 29.699 \times 10^{-2} (X) - 43 \times 10^{-5} (X)^2 + 29.63 \times 10^{-3} (\text{Age}) + 1.4072$

where X = sum of abdomen, suprailiac, triceps and thigh skin-folds and age is in years

Other equations for the estimation of body fat

1. $\% \text{ fat} = \dfrac{2.118 - 1.354 - 0.78}{\text{density}} \cdot \dfrac{\% \text{ TBW}}{\text{body weight}}$

where 2.118, 1.354, and 0.78 are constants and the density (g/cc), body weight (kg), and total body weight (TBW) (kg) are determined

2. $\% \text{ fat} = \dfrac{100 (5.548 - 5.044)}{\text{Specific gravity}}$

3. $\% \text{ fat} = \dfrac{100 - \text{TBW}}{0.732}$

Source: Malina, R.M., *Am. J. Human Biol.*, 11: 141; 1999.

TABLE 6.7

Methods and Equations Used for Calculating Basal Energy Need

1.	Heat production, direct measurement (calorimetry)	kcal (kJ)/m^2 (surface area)
2.	Oxygen consumption; indirect	O$_2$ cons/w$^{0.75}$
3.	Heat production; indirect	Insensible Water Loss (IW) = Insensible weight loss (IWL) + (CO$_2$ exhaled − O$_2$ inhaled)
		Heat production = IW × 0.58 (0.58 = kcal to evaporate 1 g water)
4.	Estimate (energy need not measured)	BMR = 66.4730 + 13.751W + 5.0033L − 6.550A (males)
		BMR = 655.0955 + 9.463W + 1.8496L − 4.6756A (females)
5.	Estimate (energy need not measured)	BMR = 71.2W$^{0.75}$ [1 − 0.004(30 − A) + 0.010(L/W$^{0.33}$ − 43.4)] (men)
		BMR = 65.8W$^{0.75}$ [1 + 0.004(30 − A) + 0.018(L/W$^{0.33}$ − 42.1)] (women)

Note: Abbreviations: W: weight in kg; L: height in cm; A: age in years.

REFERENCES

1. Young, D.S., *Ann. Int. Med.*, 106: 20; 1987.
2. Malina, R.M., *Am. J. Human Biol.*, 11: 141; 1999.
3. Jackson, A.S., Pollack, M.L., *Phys. Sport Med.*, 13: 76; 1985.
4. Berdanier, C.D., *Advanced Nutrition: Macronutrients*, 2nd edn, CRC Press, Boca Raton, FL, 2000, p. 69.

7 Nutritional Biochemistry

Carolyn D. Berdanier

CONTENTS

Nutrition science is based on concepts of biochemistry, in particular the pathways that constitute intermediary metabolism. The metabolic use of the dietary macromolecules, proteins, fats, and carbohydrates, the roles for the micronutrients in these pathways, and an understanding of the physiology and endocrinology of the consumer provide the basis for studies in nutritional biochemistry. This chapter reviews these concepts and provides some basic information about the use of the macro- and micronutrients found in food.

The metabolic pathways have been worked out as have the control mechanisms for the reactions within the pathways. Metabolic maps have been drawn to illustrate the flux of nutrients through their use pathways. These pathways are illustrated in Figure 7.1 to Figure 7.30. Detailed maps can be obtained from Boehringer Mannheim (BM) at minimal cost (Boehringer Mannheim, PO Box 31 01 20, D-6800 Mannheim 31, Germany). The maps come complete with citations of the works that provided the critical information for these maps as well as notations on species differences and differences between mammals, plants, and microorganisms.

DIGESTION/ABSORPTION

Before the nutrients in food can be metabolized, they must first be ingested, chewed, swallowed, digested, and absorbed. With each of the macronutrients, the macromolecules must be broken down to their simpler components. In the stomach, the food is mixed with the gastric acid (hydrochloric acid), and moved into the small intestine. The stomach contents that move into the duodenum are called chyme. The movement of chyme into the duodenum stimulates cholesystokinin release. This gut hormone acts on the exocrine pancreas stimulating it to release pancreatic juice into the duodenum and on the gall bladder to release bile. Cholesystokinin is secreted by the epithelial endocrine cells of the small intestine, particularly the duodenum. Its release is stimulated by amino acids in the lumen and by the acid pH of the stomach contents as it passes into the duodenum. The low pH of the chyme also stimulates the release of secretin, which, in turn, stimulates the exocrine pancreas to release bicarbonate and water so as to raise the pH of the chyme. This is necessary to maximize the activity of the digestive enzymes located in and on the surface of the absorptive luminal cell. The digestive enzymes are listed in Table 7.1.

As mentioned, cholesystokinin stimulates the release of bile from the gall bladder. Bile contains the primary bile acids, cholic and chenodeoxycholic acids, that are produced from cholesterol by the liver. They are secreted into the intestine, where they serve as emulsifying agents for the digestion and absorption of fat. Bile that is not immediately used is acted on by the intestinal flora. These flora convert the bile acids to their conjugated forms by dehydroxylating carbon-7. Further metabolism occurs at the far end of the intestinal tract, where lithocholate is sulfated. While the dehydroxylated acids are reabsorbed and sent back to the liver via the portal blood, the sulfated lithocholate is not. It appears in the feces. All four of the bile acids, the primary and dehydroxylated forms, are recirculated via the enterohepatic system such that very little of the bile acids are lost. It has been estimated that the bile acid lost in the feces (~0.8 g/day) equals that newly synthesized by the liver such that the total pool remains between 3 and 5 g. The amount secreted per day is on the order of 16 to 70 g. As the pool size is only 3 to 5 g, this means that these acids are recirculated as many as 14 times a day.

Once a carbohydrate-rich food is consumed, digestion begins. As the food is chewed, it is mixed with saliva, which contains α-amylase. This amylase begins the digestion of starch by attacking the internal α-1,4-glucosidic bonds. It will not attack the branch points having α-1,4- or α-1,6-glucosidic bonds, and hence the salivary α-amylase will produce molecules of glucose, maltose, α-limit dextrin, and maltotriose. The α-amylase in saliva is an isozyme with the same function as that in the pancreatic juice. The salivary α-amylase is denatured in the stomach as the food is mixed and acidified with the gastric hydrochloric acid. The limit dextrins are further hydrolyzed by α-glucosidases on the surface of the luminal cells. The glycosidic bonds of the disaccharides are attacked by the disaccharidases, maltase, lactase, or sucrase (Table 7.1). This results in absorbable monosaccharides, glucose, fructose, and galactose. Carbohydrates having bonds that are not attacked by these glycosidic enzymes are

---

TABLE 7.1
Enzymes of Importance to Digestion

Enzyme	Substrate	Products
α-Amylase	Starch and amylopectin	Glucose, maltose, maltotriose, and α-limit dextrin
α-Glucosidase	α-Limit dextrin	Glucose
Lactase	Lactose	Galactose and glucose
Maltase	Maltose	Glucose
Sucrase	Sucrose	Glucose and fructose
Lipase	Triacylglycerides	Fatty acids, diglycerides (DGs), and monoglycerides (MGs)
Colipase	Triacylglycerides	Fatty acids, DGs, and MGs
Lipid esterase	Cholesterol esters	Cholesterol and fatty acids
	Vitamin A esters	Vitamin A and glycerol
Pepsin	Peptide bonds involving aromatic amino acids	Phenylalanine, tyrosine peptide fragments
Trypsin	Peptide bonds involving arginine and lysine	Arginine, lysine, and peptide fragments
Chymotrypsin	Peptide bonds involving tyrosine, phenylalanine, methionine tryptophan, and leucine	Tyrosine, leucine, tryptophan, phenylalanine, methionine, and peptide fragments
Elastase	Peptide bonds involving alanine, serine, and glycine	Alanine, serine, glycine, and peptide fragments
Carboxypeptidase A	Peptide bonds involving valine, leucine, isoleucine, and alanine	Valine, leucine, isoleucine, alanine, and peptide fragments
Carboxypeptidase B	Peptide bonds involving lysine and arginine	
Endopeptidase	Peptide fragments	Amino acids
Aminopeptidase	Peptide fragments	Amino acids
Dipeptidase	Dipeptides	Amino acids

passed to the lower part of the intestine, where they are attacked by the enzymes of the intestinal flora. Most of the products of this digestion are used by the flora themselves, but some of metabolic products (short-chain fatty acids) may be of use. The flora produces lactate, methane gas, carbon dioxide, water, and hydrogen gas. Gas production (flatus) can be uncomfortable if large amounts of undigestible carbohydrates are consumed. The carbohydrates of legumes typify the substrates these flora use. Raffinose, an α-galactose $1 \rightarrow 6$ glucose $1 \rightarrow 2$ β-fructose, and trehalose, an α-glucose $1 \rightarrow 1$ α-glucose, are the typical substrates from legumes for these flora. The flora will also attack portions of the fibers and celluloses that are the structural elements in fruits and vegetables. Again, some useful products may be produced, but the bulk of these complex polysaccharides having β-linkages and perhaps other substituent groups as part of their structure are largely untouched by both intestinal and bacterial enzymes. These undigested unavailable carbohydrates provide bulk to the diet, which, in turn, helps to regulate the rate of food passage from the mouth to the anus. They also act as adsorbants of noxious or potentially noxious materials in the food, and they assist in the excretion of cholesterol and several minerals, thereby protecting the body from overload. Populations consuming high-fiber diets have a lower incidence of colon cancer, fewer problems with constipation, and lower serum cholesterol levels.

LIPID DIGESTION/ABSORPTION

Food lipids (fats and oils) are digested initially in the mouth and then in the stomach and intestine. The digestion of lipid begins in the mouth with the mastication of food and its mixing with the acid-stable lingual lipase. Digestion can proceed only when the large particles of the food are made smaller through chewing. The action of the tongue and later the churning action of the stomach mix the food particles with the various digestive juices and with hydrochloric acid in the stomach. These actions separate the lipid particles, exposing more surface area for enzyme action and providing the opportunity for emulsion formation. These changes in physical state are essential steps that precede absorption. In the stomach, the proteins of lipid–protein complexes are denatured by gastric hydrochloric acid and attacked by the proteases (pepsin, parapepsin I, and parapepsin II) of the gastric juice with the resultant release of lipid. Little degradation of fat occurs in the stomach except that catalyzed by lingual lipase. Lingual lipase originates from glands in the back of the mouth and under the tongue. This lipase is active in the acid environment of the stomach. However, because of the tendency of lipid to coalesce and form a separate phase, this lipase has limited opportunity to attack triacylglycerols. Those that are attacked release a single fatty acid, usually a short- or medium-chain one. The remaining diacylglycerol is subsequently hydrolyzed in the duodenum. In adults consuming a mixed diet, lingual lipase is relatively unimportant. However, in infants having an immature duodenal lipase, lingual lipase is quite important. In addition, this lipase has its greatest activity on the triacylglycerols commonly present in whole milk. Milk fat has more short- and medium-chain fatty acids than fats from other food sources.

Although the action of lingual lipase is slow relative to lipases found in the duodenum, its action to release diacylglycerol and short- and medium-chain fatty acids serves another function — these fatty acids serve as surfactants. Surfactants spontaneously adsorb to the water–lipid interface, conferring a hydrophilic surface to lipid droplets and thereby provide a stable interface with the aqueous environment. The dietary surfactants are the free fatty acids, lecithin, and phospholipids. The action of acid-stable lingual lipase provides more fatty acids to supplement the dietary supply. All together these surfactants plus the churning action of the stomach produce an emulsion, which is then expelled into the duodenum as chyme.

Once the chyme enters the duodenum, it is mixed with bile. This is an additional surfactant or emulsifying agent and serves to further disperse the lipid droplets at the lipid–aqueous interface, facilitating the hydrolysis of the glycerides (triglycerides [TGs], diglycerides [DGs], and monoglycerides [MGs]) by the pancreatic lipases. Pancreozymin stimulates the exocrine pancreas to release pancreatic juice, which contains three lipases (lipase, lipid esterase, and colipase) that act at the water–lipid interface of the emulsion particles. One lipase acts on the fatty acids esterified at positions 1 and 3 of the glycerol backbone, leaving a fatty acid esterified at carbon 2. This 2 monoacylglyceride can isomerize, and the remaining fatty acid can move to carbon 1 or 3. The pancreatic juice contains another less specific lipase (called a lipid esterase), which cleaves the fatty acid from cholesterol esters, MGs, or esters such as vitamin A ester. Its action requires the presence of the bile salts. The lipase that is specific for the ester linkage at carbons 1 and 3 does not have a requirement for the bile salts and, in fact, is inhibited by them. The inhibition of pancreatic lipase by the bile salts is relieved by the third pancreatic enzyme, colipase. The products of the lipase-catalyzed reaction, a reaction that favors the release of fatty acids having 10 or more carbons, are these fatty acids and MG. The products of the lipid-esterase-catalyzed reaction are cholesterol, vitamins, fatty acids, and glycerol. Phospholipids present in food are attacked by phospholipases specific to each of the phospholipids. The pancreatic juice contains these lipases as prephospholipases, which are activated by the enzyme trypsin.

The bile salts impart a negative charge to the lipids, which in turn attracts the pancreatic enzyme, colipase (see Table 7.1). Colipase binds to both the water–lipid interface and to lipase, thereby anchoring and activating the lipase. As the pH of the chyme rises, aggregates, called micelles, are formed. The micelles are much smaller in size than the emulsified lipid droplets. Micelle sizes vary depending on the ratio of lipids to bile acids but typically range from 40 to 600 Å, and it is from these structures that the products of lipid digestion are absorbed.

CHOLESTEROL ABSORPTION

Only 30 to 40% of the dietary cholesterol is absorbed; it is absorbed by diffusion with the other lipid components of the diet. Absorption requires the emulsification step with the bile acids as emulsifiers. Absorbed cholesterol passes into the lacteals and thence into the thoracic duct. The percentage of cholesterol absorbed depends on a number of factors including the fiber content of the diet, the gut passage time, and the total amount of cholesterol present for absorption. At higher intake levels, less is absorbed, and vice versa at lower intake levels. Compared with fatty acids and the acylglycerides, the rate of cholesterol absorption is very low. It is estimated that the half-life of cholesterol in the enterocyte is 12 h. With high fiber intakes, less cholesterol is absorbed because the fiber (cellulose and lignens) acts as an adsorbent, reducing cholesterol availability. These carbohydrates also shorten the residence time of the ingesta in the intestine. Thus, high-fiber diets reduce gut passage time, which, in turn, results in less time for cholesterol absorption. The mode of action of pectins and gums in lowering cholesterol absorption is different. These carbohydrates increase transit time also, but rather than acting as adsorbants, they lower serum cholesterol levels by giving chyme a gel-like consistency, rendering the cholesterol in the chyme less available for absorption.

LIPID TRANSPORT

Short-chain fatty acids are absorbed directly into the portal blood system and carried by albumin. Longer-chain fatty acids and cholesterol are taken up by the lacteals of the lymphatic system that drains the intestine. They are formed into chylomicrons (a very low-density lipid–protein complex) and then enter the blood via the thoracic duct. Once absorbed, the lipids are transported through the circulatory system by proteins in a complex called lipoprotein. Lipoproteins carry not only the absorbed food lipids but also the lipids synthesized or mobilized from organs and fat depots. Nine different lipid-carrying proteins have been identified, and each plays a specific role in the lipid-transport process. In addition, there are several minor proteins that may be involved in some aspects of lipid cycling and uptake. The proteins involved in lipid transport are listed in Table 7.2. Mutations in the genes that encode these proteins can lead to aberrant lipid transport, and the individual may have either abnormally high or low blood lipid values (see Chapter 54).

The hepatic and intestinal apolipoproteins can be distinguished using electrophoresis, a technique of separating proteins based on their electrophoretic mobility.

The intestinal cell has three apolipoproteins called A-1, A-IV, and B-48. Apolipoprotein B-48 (apo B-48) is unique to the enterocyte and is essential for chylomicron release by the intestinal cell. Apo A-1 is synthesized in the liver. Apo B-48 is actually

TABLE 7.2
Proteins Involved in Lipid Transport

Protein	Function
Apo A-II	Transport protein in high-density lipoprotein (HDL)
Apo B-48	Transport protein for chylomicrons; synthesized in the enterocyte in the human
HDl-binding protein (HDLBP)	Binds HDL and functions in the removal of excess cellular cholesterol
Apo D	Transport protein similar to retinol-binding protein
Apo (a)	Abnormal transport protein for low-density lipoprotein (LDL)
Apo A-I	Transport protein for chylomicrons and HDL; synthesized in the liver and its synthesis is induced by retinoic acid
Apo C-III	Transport protein for very-low-density lipoprotein (VLDL)
Apo A-IV	Transport protein for chylomicrons
CETP	Participates in the transport of cholesterol from peripheral tissue to liver; reduces HDL size
LCAT	Synthesized in the liver and is secreted into the plasma, where it resides on the HDL Participates in the reverse transport of cholesterol from peripheral tissues to the liver; esterifies the HDL cholesterol
Apo E	Mediates high affinity binding of LDLs to the LDL receptor and the putative chylomicron receptor; required for clearance of chylomicron remnant; synthesized primarily in the liver
Apo C-I	Transport protein for VLDL
Apo C-II	Chylomicron-transport protein required cofactor for LPL activity
Apo B-100	Synthesized in the liver and is secreted into the circulation as part of the VLDL. Also serves as the ligand for the LDL-receptor-mediated hepatic endocytosis
Lipoprotein lipase	Catalyzes the hydrolysis of plasma TG into free fatty acids
Hepatic lipase	Catalyzes the hydrolysis of TG and phospholipids of the LDL and HDL. It is bound to the surfaces of both hepatic and nonhepatic tissues

an edited version of the hepatic apo B-100. It is the result of an apo B mRNA editing process that converts codon 2153 to a translational stop codon. Apo B-48 is thus an edited form of apo B-100, and this editing is unique to the intestinal cell.

As chylomicrons circulate, they acquire an additional protein, apo C-II. This additional protein is an essential cofactor for the recognition and hydrolysis of the chylomicron by the capillary endothelial enzyme, lipoprotein lipase (LPL). LPL hydrolyzes most of the core TG in the chylomicron, leaving a remnant that is rich in cholesterol and cholesterol esters. During the LPL-catalyzed hydrolytic process, the excess surface compounds, that is, the phospholipids and apolipoproteins B, A-I, and A-IV are transferred to high-density lipoproteins (HDL) and, in exchange, apo E is transferred from the HDL to the cholesterol-ester-rich chylomicron remnant. These remnants are then cleared from the blood by the liver. On the hepatocyte is a lipoprotein receptor that recognizes apo E, and this receptor plays an important role in remnant clearance.

The chylomicron is a relatively stable way of ensuring the movement, in an aqueous medium (blood), of hydrophobic molecules such as cholesterol and triacylglycerols from their point of origin, the intestine, to their point of use or storage. As mentioned, there are several unique proteins that facilitate this movement. These lipid-transporting proteins determine which cells of the body receive which lipids. At the target cell, the particles lose their lipid through hydrolysis facilitated by an interstitial LPL, which is found in the capillary beds of muscle, fat cells, and other tissues using lipid as a fuel. This LPL is synthesized by these target cells but is anchored on the outside of the cells by a polysaccharide chain on the endothelial wall of the surrounding capillaries.

PROTEIN DIGESTION/ABSORPTION

Upon consumption, food protein is degraded into its component amino acids (Table 7.1). Protein digestion begins in the stomach, where the food is acidified with the gastric hydrochloric acid. Hydrochloric acid also serves to denature the food proteins, thus making them more vulnerable to attack by pepsin, an endopeptidase. Actually, pepsin is not a single enzyme. It consists of pepsin A, which attacks peptide bonds involving phenylalanine or tyrosine, and several other enzymes, which have specific attack points. The pepsins are released into the gastric cavity as pepsinogen. Food entering the stomach stimulates HCl release and the pH of the gastric contents fall below 2. Through the action of the acid environment, the pepsinogen loses a 44-amino-acid sequence. This happens through one of two mechanisms: the first, called autoactivation, occurs when the pH drops below 5. At low pH the bond between the 44th and 45th amino acid residue falls apart and the 44-amino-acid residue (from the amino terminus) is liberated. The liberated residue acts as an inhibitor of pepsin by binding to the catalytic site until pH 2 is achieved. The inhibition is then relieved when this fragment is acid degraded, as happens at pH 2 or below or when it is attacked by pepsin. As the fragment binds at the catalytic site of pepsin, this can happen. The other process is called autocatalysis and occurs when already active pepsin attacks the precursor pepsinogen. This is a self-repeating process and serves to ensure ongoing catalysis of the resident protein. The cleavage of the 44-amino-acid residue, in addition to providing activated pepsin, has another purpose. That is, it serves as a signal peptide for cholecystokinin release in the duodenum. This then sets the stage for the subsequent pancreatic phase of protein digestion. As described in the sections on lipid and carbohydrate digestion, cholecystokinin stimulates both the exocrine pancreas and the intestinal mucosal epithelial cells to release its digestive enzymes. The intestinal cell releases an enzyme, enteropeptidase or enterokinase, which serves to activate the protease, trypsin, released as trypsinogen by the exocrine pancreas. This trypsin not only acts on food proteins but also acts on other preproteases, released by the exocrine pancreas, activating them. Thus, trypsin acts as an endoprotease on chymotrypsinogen, releasing chymotrypsin, on proelastase, releasing elastase, and on procarboxypeptidase, releasing carboxypeptidase. Trypsin, chymotrypsin, and elastase are all endoproteases each having specificity for particular peptide bonds. Each of these three proteases have serine as part of their catalytic site, so any compound that ties up the serine will inhibit the activity of these proteases. Such inhibitors as diisopropylphosphofluoridate react with this serine, and in so doing bring a halt to protein digestion.

The daily protein intake of about 100 g in addition to that protein appearing in the gut as enzymes, sloughed epithelial gut cells, and mucins, is almost completely digested and absorbed. This is a very efficient process that ensures a continuous supply of amino acids to the whole-body amino acid pool. Less than 1% of the total protein that passes through the gastrointestinal tract appears in the feces. If the food contributes between 70 and 100 g of protein and the endogenous protein contributes another 100 g (range: 35 to 200 g), then one might expect to see about 1 to 2 g of nitrogen in the feces. This is equivalent to 6 to 12 g protein. Of the dietary protein, the fecal protein might include the hard-to-chew/digest tough fibrous connective tissue of meat or nitrogen-containing indigestible kernel coats of grains or particles of nuts that are not attacked by the digestive enzymes. Peanuts, for example, eaten whole have a structure that is difficult to broach by the digestive enzymes. Unless chewed very finely, much of the nutritive value of this food may be lost. Peanut butter, on the other hand, is very well digested because the preparation of the peanut butter ensures that its particle size is very small and is thus quite digestible.

The protein hydrolases, called peptidases, fall into two categories. Those that attack internal peptide bonds and liberate large peptide fragments for subsequent attack by other enzymes are called the endopeptidases. Those that attack the terminal peptide bonds and liberate single amino acids from the protein structure are called exopeptidases. The exopeptidases are further subdivided according to whether they attack at the carboxy end of the amino acid chain (carboxypeptidases) or the amino end of the chain (aminopeptidases). The initial attack on an intact protein is catalyzed by endopeptidases, while the final digestive

TABLE 7.3
Carriers for Amino Acids

Carrier	Amino Acids Carried
1	Serine, threonine, alanine
2	Phenylalanine, tyrosine, methionine, valine, leucine, isoleucine
3	Proline, hydroxyproline
4	Taurine, β-alanine
5	Lysine, arginine, cysteine–cysteine
6	Aspartic and glutamic acids

action is catalyzed by the exopeptidases. The final products of digestion are free amino acids and some di- and tripeptides that are absorbed by the intestinal epithelial cells.

AMINO ACID ABSORPTION

Although single amino acids are liberated in the intestinal contents, there is insufficient power in the enzymes of the pancreatic juice to render all the amino acids singly for absorption. The brush border of the absorptive cell therefore not only absorbs the single amino acid but also di- and tripeptides. In the process of absorbing these small peptides, it hydrolyzes them to their amino acid constituents. There is little evidence that peptides enter the blood stream. There are specific transport systems for each group of functionally similar amino acids, di- and tripeptides. These carriers are listed in Table 7.3.

Most of the biologically important L-amino acids are transported by an active carrier system against a concentration gradient. This active transport involves the intracellular potassium ion and the extracellular sodium ion. As the amino acid is carried into the enterocyte, sodium also enters in exchange for potassium. This sodium must be returned (in exchange for potassium) to the extracellular medium. This return uses the sodium–potassium ATP pump. In several instances, the carrier is a shared carrier. That is, the carrier will transport more than one amino acid. Such is the case with the neutral amino acids and those with short or polar side chains (serine, threonine, and alanine). The mechanism whereby these carriers participate in amino acid absorption is similar to that described for glucose uptake. Once amino acids are absorbed and in circulation, they will either be used to synthesize body proteins, essential nitrogenous compounds (thyroxine or epinephrine), or catabolized.

CARBOHYDRATE METABOLISM

GLYCOLYSIS

Once absorbed, glucose travels to the liver and other tissues via the portal blood stream. At the target tissue it enters the glycolytic sequence. The glycolytic pathway for the anaerobic catabolism of glucose can be found in all cells in the body (Figure 7.1). The pathway begins with glucose, a six-carbon unit, and through a series of reactions produces two molecules of ATP and two molecules of pyruvate. The control of glycolysis is vested in several key steps. The first step is the activation of glucose through the formation of glucose-6-phosphate. In the liver and pancreatic β-cells, this step is catalyzed by the enzyme glucokinase. A molecule of ATP is used and magnesium is required. Glucose-6-phosphate is a key metabolite. It can proceed down the glycolytic pathway or move through the hexose monophosphate shunt (see hexose monophosphate shunt) or be used to make glycogen. How much glucose-6-phosphate is oxidized directly to pyruvate depends on the nutritional state of the animal, cell type, the genetics of the animal, and its hormonal state. Some cell types, the brain cell for example, do not make glycogen. Some people do not have shunt activity in the red cell because the code for glucose-6-phosphate dehydrogenase has mutated such that the enzyme is not functional. Insulin-deficient animals likewise have little glycolytic and shunt activity because of the lack of insulin's effect on the synthesis of key enzymes of these pathways. All these factors determine how much glucose-6-phosphate goes in which direction.

Two enzymes are used for the activation of glucose: glucokinase and hexokinase. In the liver, both enzymes are present. While hexokinase activity is product inhibited, glucokinase is not. The hexokinase in the nonhepatic tissues must be product inhibited to prevent the hexokinase from tying up all the inorganic phosphate (Pi) in the cells as glucose-6-phosphate. The Km for glucokinase is greater than that for hexokinase; so the former is the main enzyme for the conversion of glucose to glucose-6-phosphate in the liver. The other enzyme will phosphorylate not only glucose but other six-carbon sugars such as fructose. However, the amount of fructose phosphorylated to fructose-6-phosphate is small in comparison to the phosphorylation of fructose at the carbon 1 position catalyzed by fructokinase. Both kinase reactions require magnesium as a cofactor.

Glucose-6-phosphate is isomerized to fructose-6-phosphate and is then phosphorylated once again to form fructose-1,6-bisphosphate. Another molecule of ATP is used, and again magnesium is an important cofactor. Both kinase reactions are

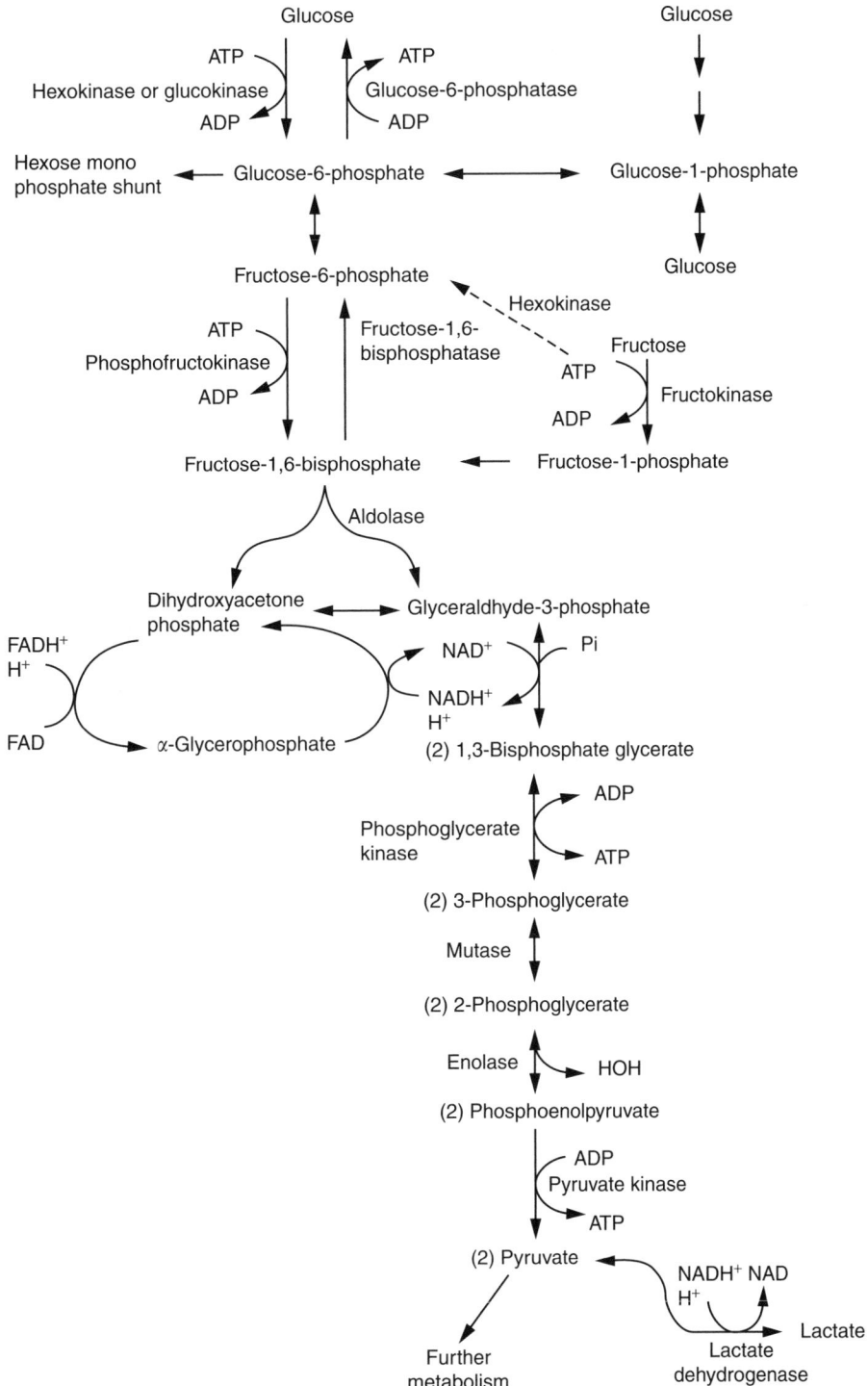

FIGURE 7.1 The glycolytic sequence.

rate-controlling reactions in that their activity determines the rate at which subsequent reactions proceed. The phosphofructo-kinase reaction is unique to the glycolytic sequence, while the glucokinase or hexokinase step provides substrates for either the shunt or the glycogenic sequences. Thus, one could argue that the formation of fructose-1,6-bisphosphate is the first committed step in glycolysis. Glycolysis is inhibited when phosphofructokinase is inhibited. This occurs when levels of fatty acids in the cytosol rise as in the instance of high rates of lipolysis and fatty acid oxidation. Phosphofructokinase activity is increased when levels of fructose-6-phosphate rise or when cAMP levels rise. Stimulation occurs also when fructose-2,6-bisphosphate levels rise. In any event, glycolysis then proceeds with the splitting of fructose-1,6-bisphosphate to dihydroxyacetone phosphate (DHAP) and glyceraldehyde-3-phosphate. At this point another rate-controlling step occurs. This step is one which shuttles reducing equivalents into the mitochondria for use by the respiratory chain. This is the α-glycerophosphate shuttle (Figure 7.2). This shuttle carries reducing equivalents from the cytosol to the mitochondria. DHAP picks up reducing equivalents when it is converted to α-glycerol phosphate. These reducing equivalents are produced when glyceraldehyde-3-phosphate is oxidized in the process of being phosphorylated to 1,3-diphosphate glycerate. The α-glycerophosphate enters the inner mitochondrial membrane, whereupon it is converted back to DHAP, releasing its reducing equivalents to FAD (a riboflavin-containing coenzyme), which in turn transfers the reducing equivalents to the mitochondrial respiratory chain. The reason why this shuttle is rate limiting is the need to regenerate NAD^+. Without NAD^+ the glycolytic pathway ceases. $NADH^+$ (a niacin-containing coenzyme) is produced during glycolysis when reducing equivalents are accepted by NAD^+. $NADH^+$ itself cannot pass through the mitochondrial membrane; so substrate shuttles are necessary. Another means of producing NAD^+ is by converting pyruvate to lactate. This is a nonmitochondrial reaction catalyzed by lactate dehydrogenase. It occurs when an oxygen debt is developed as happens in exercising muscle. In these muscles more oxygen is consumed than can be provided. Glycolysis occurs at a rate higher than can be accommodated by the respiratory chain that joins the reducing equivalents transferred to it by the shuttles to molecular oxygen, making water. If more reducing equivalents are generated than can be used to make water, the excess are added to pyruvate to make lactate. Thus, rising lactate levels are indicative of oxygen debt.

There are other shuttles that also serve to transfer reducing equivalents into the mitosol. These are the malate–aspartate shuttle (Figure 7.3) and the malate–citrate shuttle. Neither of these is rate limiting with respect to glycolysis. The malate–aspartate shuttle has rate-controlling properties with respect to gluconeogenesis, while the malate–citrate shuttle is important to lipogenesis.

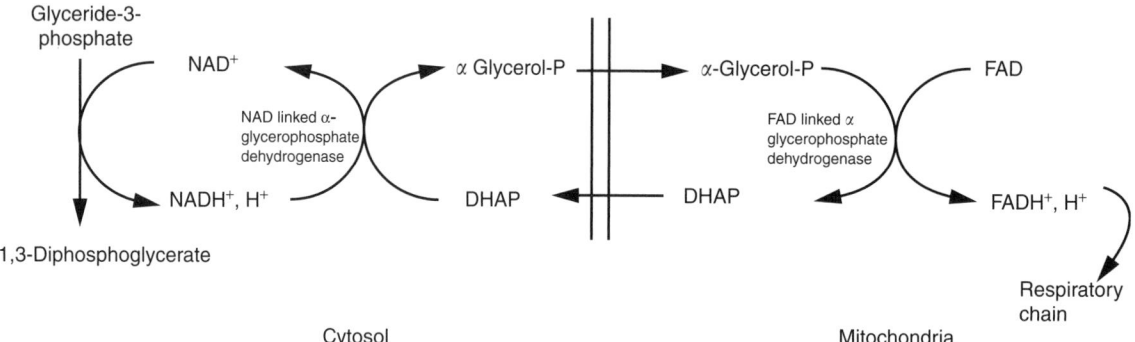

FIGURE 7.2   The α-glycerol phosphate shuttle.

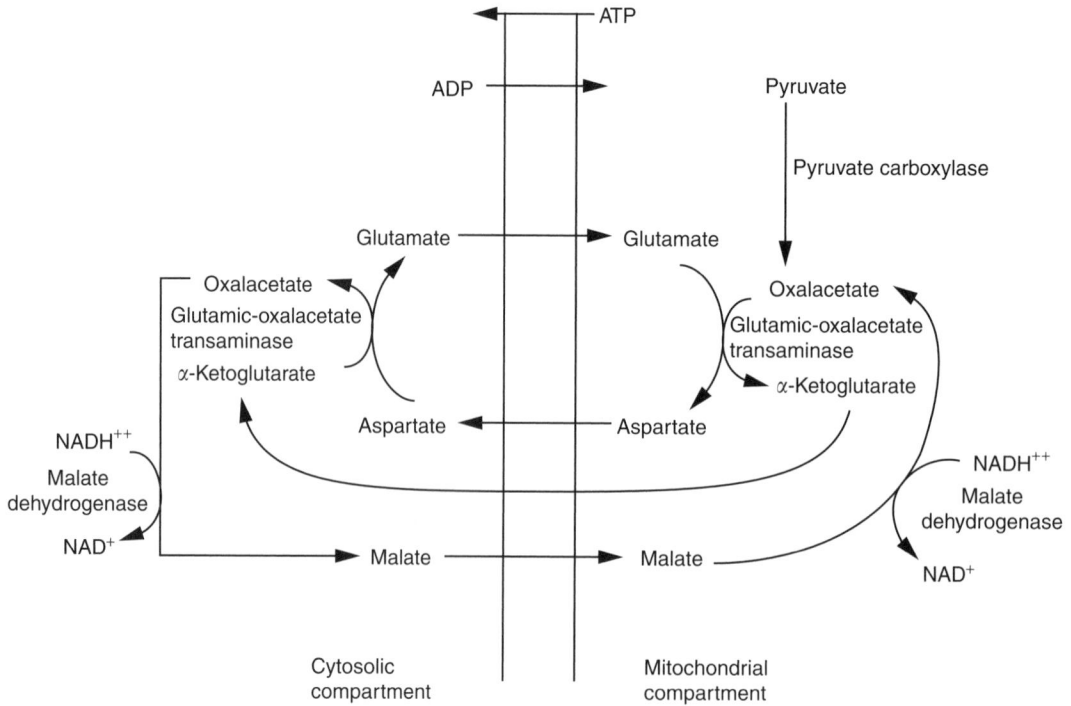

FIGURE 7.3   The malate–aspartate shuttle.

Once 1,3-bisphosphate glycerate is formed it is converted to 3-phosphoglycerate with the formation of one ATP. The 3-phosphoglycerate then goes to 2-phosphoglycerate and then to phosphoenolpyruvate (PEP). These are all bidirectional reactions that are also used in gluconeogenesis. The PEP is dephosphorylated to pyruvate with the formation of another ATP. Because of the great energy lost to ATP formation at this step, this reaction is not reversible. Gluconeogenesis uses another enzyme, phosphoenolpyruvate carboxykinase (PEPCK), to reverse this step. Glycolysis uses pyruvate kinase to catalyze the reaction. At any rate, pyruvate can now be converted to acetyl CoA via pyruvate dehydrogenase or carboxylated to oxalacetate via pyruvate carboxylase. Oxalacetate is the beginning substrate for the citric acid cycle.

The citric acid cycle is the central cycle in intermediary metabolism. All the major macromolecules produce substrates that in one way or another enter the citric acid cycle. This cycle is shown in Figure 7.4. The purpose of this cycle is to produce reducing equivalents that can be used to make water by the respiratory chain (Figure 7.5) and CO_2. In the process of making water substantial energy is released. Some of this is captured in the high-energy bond of ATP, while the majority is released as heat. The citric acid cycle begins with joining of a two-carbon group (acetyl CoA) to oxalacetate to form citrate. The CoA is lost in the reaction and a molecule of water is added. The CoA is a pantothenic-acid-containing reactive group that plays an important role not only in the citric acid cycle but also in the many reactions of lipid metabolism. Citrate then loses a molecule of water, becoming the unstable compound, cis-aconitate. Water is added back, and isocitrate is formed. Reducing equivalents are then lost (picked up by NAD^+) and sent to the respiratory chain at site 1. Another unstable compound is formed, which in turn loses a CO_2 to become α-ketoglutarate. Another CO_2 is lost as are reducing equivalents (again picked up by NAD^+ and again sent to

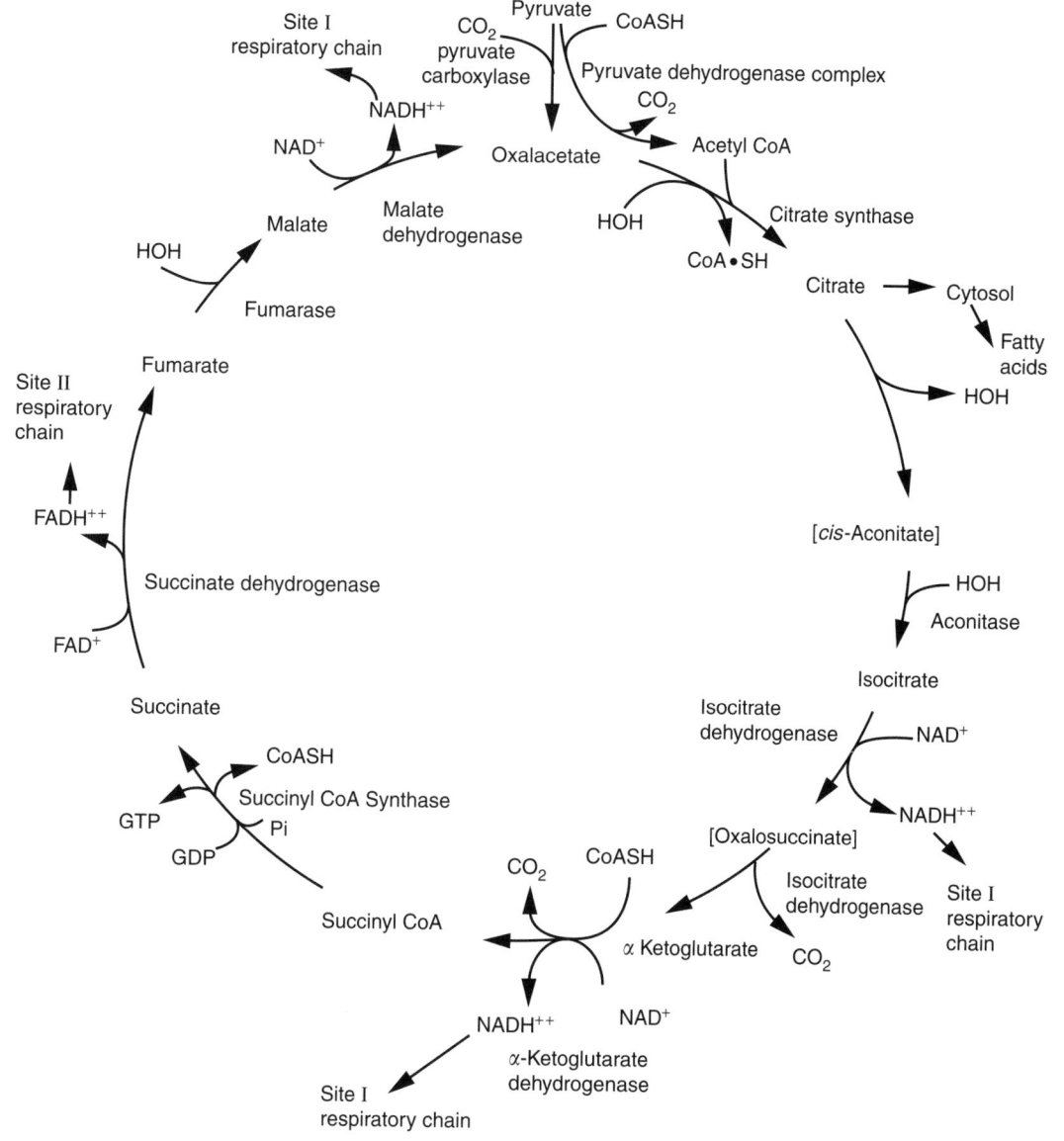

FIGURE 7.4 The citric acid cycle. This cycle is sometimes called the Krebs cycle or the tricarboxylate cycle.

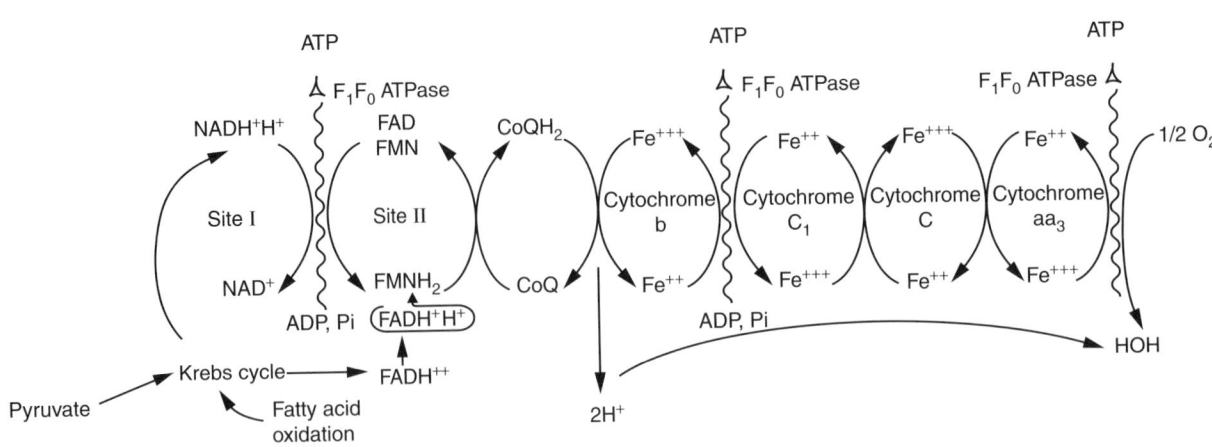

FIGURE 7.5 The respiratory chain showing the points where sufficient energy has been generated to support the synthesis of one molecule of ATP.

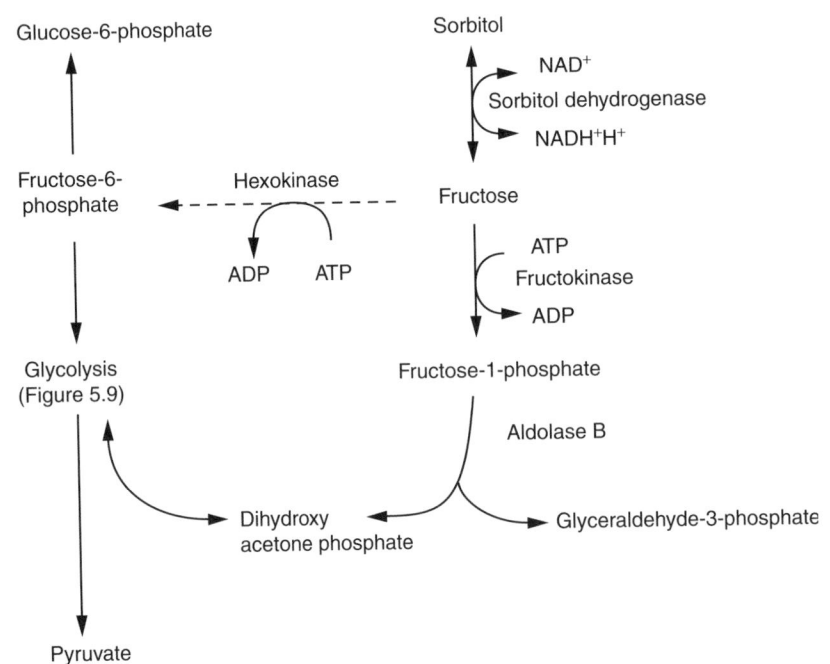

FIGURE 7.6 The metabolism of fructose.

site 1 of the respiratory chain), and succinyl CoA is formed. Succinyl CoA loses its CoA group to become succinate and in turn loses reducing equivalents (picked up by FAD and sent to site 2 of the respiratory chain) to become fumarate. Water is added to fumarate, and malate is produced. This malate can leave the mitochondrial compartment in the malate–citrate shuttle and become oxalacetate, the starting point of gluconeogenesis. In the citric acid cycle, malate loses reducing equivalents (picked up by NAD^+ and sent to site 1 of the respiratory chain), and once again oxalacetate is produced. The cycle has now returned to its starting point.

The glycolytic pathway is dependent on both ATP for the initial steps of the pathway, the formation of glucose-6-phosphate and fructose-1,6-bisphosphate, and on the ratio of ATP to ADP and inorganic phosphate, Pi. In working muscle the continuance of work and the continuance of glycolysis depend on the cycling of the adenine nucleotides and the export of lactate to the liver. ATP must be provided at the beginning of the pathway, and ADP as well as Pi must be provided in the latter steps. If the tissue runs out of ATP, ADP, or Pi, or accumulates lactate and H^+, glycolysis will come to a halt and work cannot continue. This is what happens to the working skeletal muscle. Exhaustion sets in when glycolytic rate is downregulated by an accumulation of lactate.

Many diets contain carbohydrates in addition to starch and glucose. These carbohydrates are metabolized to their primary monosaccharides and used. Of these monosaccharides, two are most important: fructose and galactose. Fructose is converted to glucose after phosphorylation (Figure 7.6). Although two enzymes are available for the phosphorylation of fructose one of these, fructokinase, is present only in the liver. Hexokinase can catalyze the phosphorylation of fructose. However, fructokinase is a much more active enzyme. Its activity is so high that, in fact, most of the dietary fructose whether as the free sugar or as a component of sucrose is metabolized in the liver. This is in contrast to glucose, which is metabolized by all the cells in the body. As a result, fructose- or sucrose-rich diets fed to rats or mice will result in a fatty liver. This occurs because the dietary overload of fructose or sucrose exceeds the capacity of the liver to oxidize it, and so it uses the sugar metabolites as substrate for fatty acid and triacylglyceride synthesis. Until the hepatic lipid export system increases sufficiently to transport this lipid to the storage depots, the lipid accumulates, hence resulting in the fatty liver. Adaptation to a high fructose intake can and does occur in normal individuals, and the fatty liver disappears.

Galactose, a component of the milk sugar, lactose, is converted to glucose and eventually enters the glycolytic sequence as glucose-6-phosphate (Figure 7.7). Galactose is phosphorylated at carbon 1 in the first step of its conversion to glucose. It can be isomerized to glucose-1-phosphate or converted to uridune diphosphate (UDP)-galactose by exchanging its phosphate group for a UDP group. This UDP-galactose can be joined with glucose to form lactose in the adult mammary tissue under the influence of the hormone prolactin. However, usually the UDP-galactose is converted to UDP-glucose and thence used to form glycogen.

PENTOSE PHOSPHATE SHUNT

The pentose phosphate shunt is an alternative pathway for the metabolism of glucose (Figure 7.8). The shunt uses glucose-6-phosphate and generates phosphorylated ribose for use in DNA and RNA synthesis. It also produces reducing equivalents for use by the microsomal P450 enzymes and the lipogenic pathway. It is estimated that approximately 10% of the glucose-6-phosphate generated from glucose is metabolized by the shunt.

The shunt contains two NADP-linked dehydrogenases, glucose-6-phosphate dehydrogenase and 6-phosphogluconate dehydrogenase. These two enzymes catalyze the rate-limiting steps in the reaction sequence. In the instance where there is an active lipogenic state, these reactions provide about 50% of the reducing equivalents needed by the lipogenic process. There is an excellent correlation between this dehydrogenase activity and lipogenesis. The microsomal P450 enzymes also use the reducing equivalents carried by $NADP^+$ as does the red blood cell in the maintenance of glutathione in the reduced state. The glutathione system in the red blood cell maintains the redox state and integrity of the cell membrane. If sufficient reducing equivalents are not produced by the shunt dehydrogenase reactions to reduce glutathione, the red blood cell membrane integrity is lost and hemolytic anemia results. This is important to the red blood cell function of carrying oxygen and exchanging it for carbon dioxide. In any event, glucose-6-phosphate proceeds to 6-phosphogluconolactone, a very unstable metabolite, which is in turn reduced to 6-phosphogluconate. 6-Phosphogluconate is decarboxylated and dehydrogenated to form ribulose 5-phosphate with an unstable intermediate (keto-6-phosphogluconate) forming between the 6-phosphogluconate and ribulose 5-phosphate. Ribulose 5-phosphate can be isomerized to ribose 5-phosphate or epimerized to xylulose 5-phosphate. Xylulose and ribose 5-phosphate can reversibly form sedoheptulose 7-phosphate with release of glyceraldehyde 3-phosphate. If glucose does not proceed down the glycolytic sequence or through the pentose shunt, it can be used to make glycogen.

GLYCOGENESIS

Glycogen synthesis begins with glucose-1-phosphate formation from glucose-6-phosphate through the action of phosphoglucomutase (Figure 7.9). Glucose-1-phosphate then is converted to UDP-glucose, which can then be added to the glycogen already

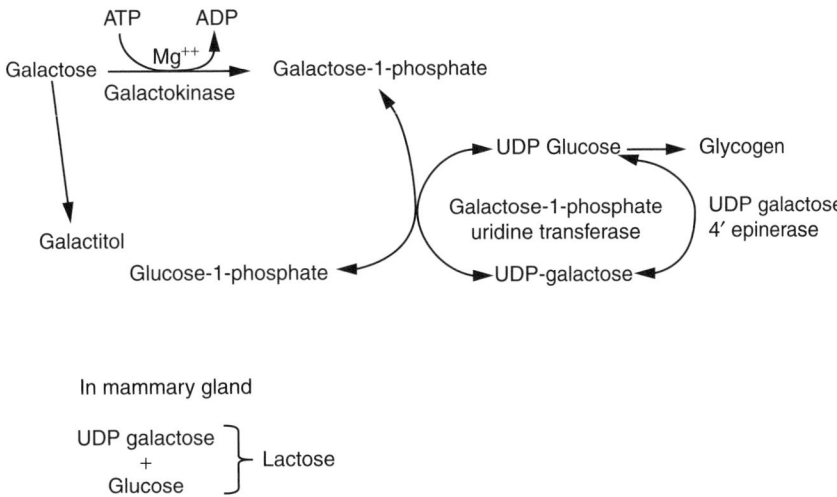

FIGURE 7.7 Conversion of galactose to glucose.

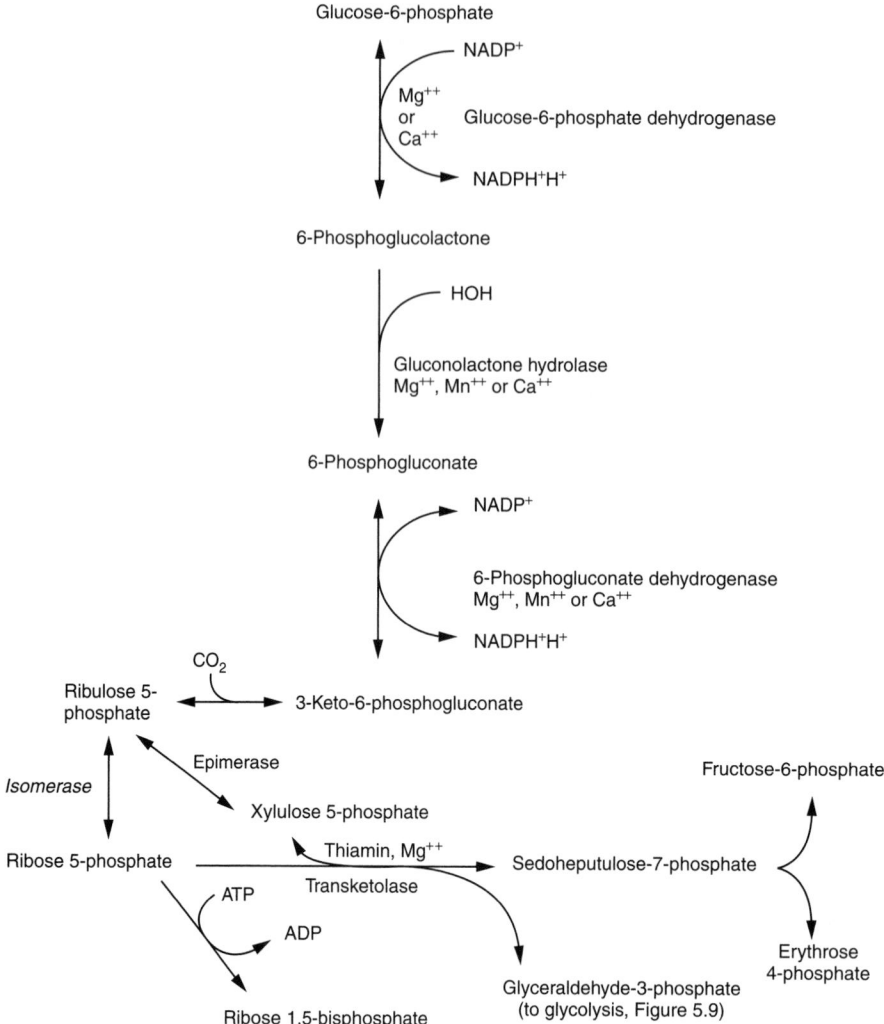

FIGURE 7.8 Reaction sequence of the hexose monophosphate shunt commonly referred to as the "shunt."

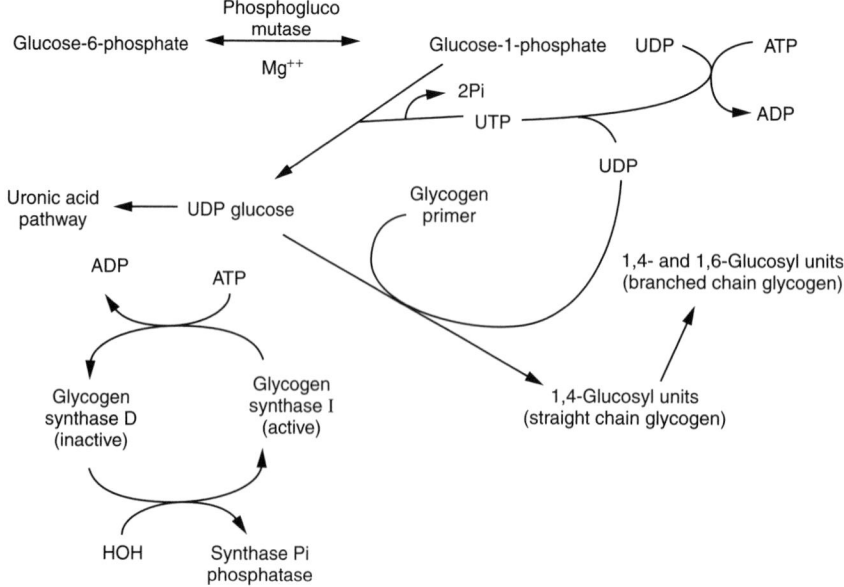

FIGURE 7.9 Glycogen synthesis (Glycogenesis).

in storage (the glycogen primer). UDP-glucose can be added through α 1,6 linkage or α 1,4 linkage. Two high-energy bonds are used to incorporate each molecule of glucose into the glycogen. The straight-chain glucose polymer is comprised of glucoses joined through the 1,4 linkage and is less compact than the branched-chain glycogen, which has both 1,4 and 1,6 linkages. The addition of glucose to the primer glycogen with a 1,4 linkage is catalyzed by the glycogen synthase enzyme, while the 1,6 addition is catalyzed by the so-called glycogen branching enzyme, amylo ($1 \rightarrow 4$, $1 \rightarrow 6$) transglucosidase. Once the liver and muscle cell achieve their full storage capacity, these enzymes are product inhibited and glycogenesis is "turned off." Glycogen synthase is inactivated by a cAMP-dependent kinase and activated by a synthase phosphatase enzyme that is stimulated by changes in the ratio of ATP to ADP. Glycogen synthesis is stimulated by the hormone insulin and suppressed by the catabolic hormones. The process does not fully cease but operates at a very low level. Glycogen does not accumulate appreciably in cells other than liver and muscle although all cells contain a small amount of glycogen. Note that a glycogen primer is required for glycogen synthesis to proceed. This primer is carefully guarded so that some is always available for glycogen synthesis. This means that glycogenolysis never fully depletes the cell of its glycogen content. When glucose is needed by the body, it can generate glucose either from glycogenolysis or through gluconeogenesis.

GLYCOGENOLYSIS

Glycogenolysis is a carefully controlled series of reactions referred to as the glycogen cascade (Figure 7.10). It is called a cascade because of the stepwise changes in activation states of the enzymes involved. To release glucose for oxidation by the glycogenolytic pathway, the glycogen must be phosphorylated. This is accomplished by the enzyme glycogen phosphorylase. Glycogen phosphorylase exists in the cell in an inactive form (glycogen phosphorylase b) and is activated to its active form (glycogen phosphorylase a) by the enzyme phosphorylase b kinase. In turn, this kinase also exists in an inactive form, which is activated by the calcium-dependent enzyme, protein kinase, and active cAMP-dependent protein kinase. These activations each require a molecule of ATP. Lastly, the cAMP-dependent protein kinase must have cAMP for its activation. This cAMP is generated from ATP by the enzyme adenylate cyclase, which, in itself, is inactive unless stimulated by a hormone such as epinephrine, thyroxine, or glucagon. As can be seen, this cascade of activation is energy dependent with three molecules of ATP needed

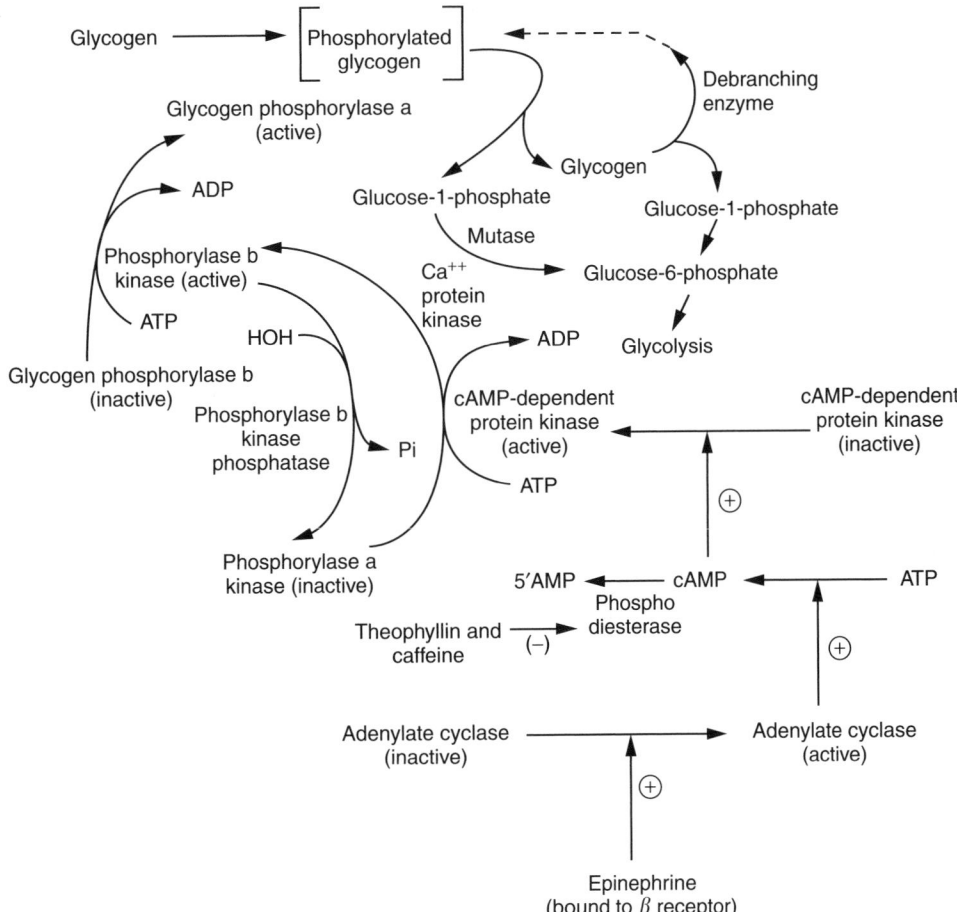

FIGURE 7.10 Stepwise release of glucose from glycogen, the glycogen cascade.

to get the process started. Once started, the glycolytic pathway will replenish the ATP needed initially as well as provide a further supply of ATP to provide needed energy. As mentioned, the liver and muscle differ in the use of glycogen. This also affects how ATP is generated within the glycogen-containing cell and how much is generated by cells that do not store glycogen.

Glycogenolysis is stimulated by the catabolic hormones, glucagon, epinephrine, the glucocorticoids, and thyroxine, and/or by the absence of food in the digestive tract. Because the glycogen molecule has molecules of water as part of its structure, it is a very large molecule and cumbersome to store in large amounts. The average 70 kg man has only an 18 h fuel supply stored as glycogen, while that same individual might have up to a 2-month supply of fuel stored as fat. Muscle and liver glycogen stores have very different functions. Muscle glycogen is used to synthesize ATP for muscle contraction, whereas hepatic glycogen is the glucose reserve for the entire body particularly the central nervous system. The amount of glycogen in the muscle is dependent on the physical activity of the individual. After bouts of strenuous exercise, the glycogen store will be depleted only to be rebuilt during the resting period following exercise. Hepatic glycogen stores are dependent on nutritional status. They are virtually absent in the 24 h starved animal while being replenished within hours of feeding. Clusters of glycogen molecules with an average molecular weight of 2×10^7 form quickly when an abundance of glucose is provided to the liver. The amount of glycogen in the liver is diet and time dependent. There is a 24 h rhythmic change in hepatic glycogen that corresponds to the feeding pattern of the animal. In nocturnal animals such as the rat, the peak hepatic glycogen store will be found in the early morning hours while the nadir will be found in the evening hours just before the nocturnal feeding begins. In humans accustomed to eating during the day, the reverse pattern will be observed.

GLUCONEOGENESIS

Gluconeogenesis occurs primarily in the liver and kidney (Figure 7.11). Except under conditions of prolonged starvation, the kidneys do not contribute appreciable amounts of glucose to the circulation. Most tissues lack the full complement of enzymes needed to run this pathway. In particular, the rate-limiting enzyme PEPCK is not found to be active in tissues other than liver and kidney. The other reactions use the same enzymes as glycolysis and do not have control properties with respect to gluconeogenesis. The rate-limiting enzymes are glucose-6-phosphatase, fructose-1,6-bisphosphatase, and PEPCK. Pyruvate kinase and pyruvate carboxylase are also of interest because their control is a coordinated one with respect to the regulation of PEPCK.

Oxalacetate in the cytosol is essential to gluconeogenesis because it is the substrate for PEPCK that catalyzes its conversion to PEP. This is an energy-dependent conversion that overcomes the irreversible final glycolytic reaction catalyzed by pyruvate kinase. The activity of PEPCK is closely coupled with that of pyruvate carboxylase. Whereas the pyruvate kinase reaction produces one ATP, the formation of PEP uses two ATPs — one in the mitochondria for the pyruvate carboxylase reaction and one in the cytosol for the PEPCK reaction. PEPCK requires guanosine triphosphate (GTP) provided via the nucleoside diphosphate kinase reaction that uses ATP. ATP transfers one high-energy bond to GDP to form ADP and GTP.

In starvation or uncontrolled diabetes, PEPCK activity is elevated as is gluconeogenesis. Starvation elicits a number of catabolic hormones that serve to mobilize tissue energy stores as well as precursors for glucose synthesis. Uncontrolled diabetes elicits similar hormonal responses. In both instances, the synthesis of the PEPCK enzyme protein is increased. Unlike other rate-limiting enzymes, PEPCK is not regulated allosterically or by phosphorylation–dephosphorylation mechanisms. Instead, it is regulated by changes in gene transcription of its single-copy gene from a single promoter site. This regulation is unique because all of the known factors (hormones, vitamins, and metabolites) act in the same place. They either turn on the synthesis of the messenger RNA for PEPCK, or they turn it off. What is also unique is the fact that liver and kidney cells translate this message into sufficient active enzyme protein that catalyzes PEP formation. Other cells and tissues have the code for PEPCK in their nuclear DNA but do not usually synthesize the enzyme. Instead, these cell types synthesize the enzyme that catalyzes glycerol synthesis. In effect then, only the kidney and liver have active gluconeogenic processes.

The next few steps in gluconeogenesis are identical to those of glycolysis but are in the reverse direction. When the step for the dephosphorylation of fructose-1,6-bisphosphate occurs, there is another energy barrier and, instead of a bidirectional reaction catalyzed by a single enzyme, there are separate forward and reverse reactions. In the synthesis of glucose, this reaction is catalyzed by fructose-1,6-bisphosphatase and yields fructose-6-phosphate. No ATP is involved, but a molecule of water and an inorganic phosphate are produced. Rising levels of fructose-2,6-bisphosphatase allosterically inhibits gluconeogenesis while it stimulates glycolysis. AMP likewise inhibits gluconeogenesis at this step.

Lastly, the removal of the phosphate from glucose-6-phosphate via the enzyme complex glucose-6-phosphatase completes the pathway to yield free glucose. This is an irreversible reaction that does not involve ATP. The glucose-6-phosphate moves to the endoplasmic reticulum, where the phosphatase is located and glucose is released for use.

LIPID METABOLISM

FATTY ACID ESTERIFICATION

In course of lipid absorption, the glycerides are hydrolyzed only to be reesterified for transport. This process of hydrolysis and reesterification happens every time a glyceride crosses a membrane. The resultant product of esterification is a MG, DG, or TG.

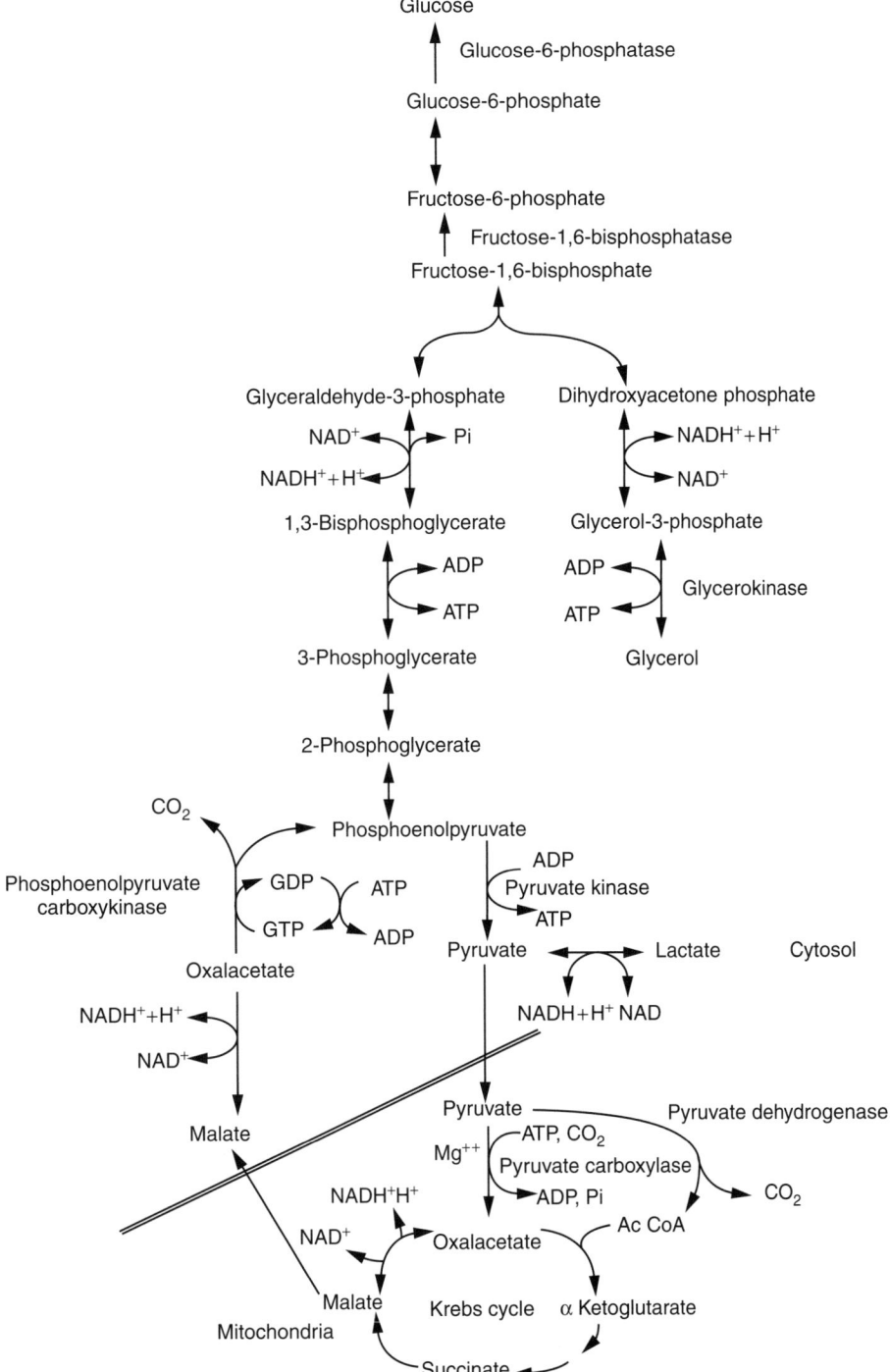

FIGURE 7.11 Gluconeogenesis.

The TG is hydrolyzed by interstitial LPL, and the fatty acids are transported into the target cell and reesterified to glycerol-3-phosphate. In the fat cell, this glycerol-3-phosphate usually is a product of glycolysis rather than the glycerol liberated when stored TG is hydrolyzed. The liberated glycerol usually passes back to the liver, which has a very active glycerokinase to phosphorylate it. In the liver, the phosphorylated glycerol is either used as a substrate for glucose synthesis or recycled into hepatic phospholipids or TG or oxidized to CO_2 and water.

Triacylglycerides are formed in a stepwise fashion (Figure 7.12). First, a fatty acid (usually a saturated fatty acid) is attached at carbon 1 of the glycerophosphate. The phosphate group at carbon 3 is electronegative and because it pulls electrons toward it, it leaves carbon 1 more reactive than carbon 2. The fatty acid (as acyl CoA) is transferred to carbon 1 through the action of a transferase. The attachment uses the carboxy end of the fatty acid chain and makes an ester linkage releasing the CoA.

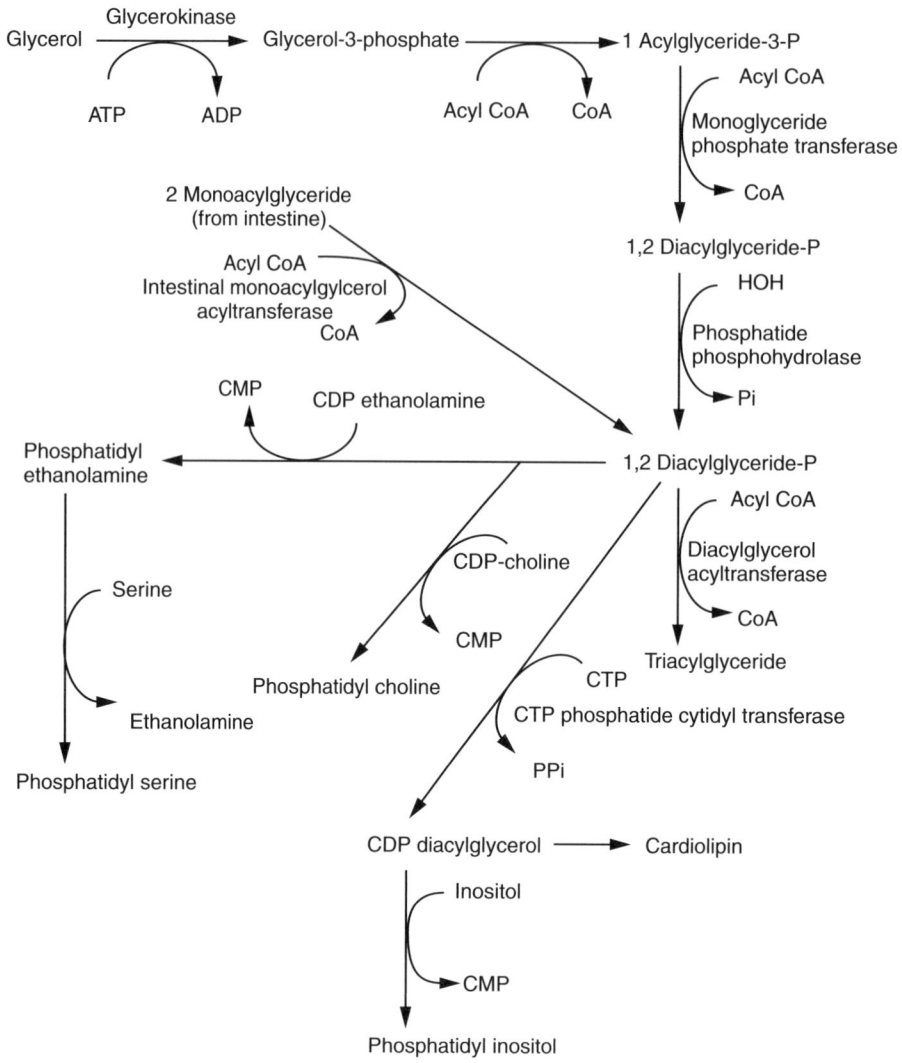

FIGURE 7.12 Fatty acid esterification and phospholipid formation.

Now the molecule has electronegative forces at each end — the phosphate group on carbon 3 and the oxygen plus carbon chain at carbon 1. Now carbon 2 is vulnerable and reactive and another carbon chain can be attached. In this instance the fatty acid is usually an unsaturated fatty acid. At this point, the 1,2 diacylglyceride-phosphate loses its phosphate group so that carbon 3 is now reactive. The 1,2 diacylglyceride can either be esterified with another fatty acid to make triacylglyceride or can be used to make the membrane phospholipids, phosphatidylcholine, phosphatidylethanolamine, phosphatidylinositol, cardiolipin, and phosphatidylserine. In the stored triacylglycerides and in membranes, most unsaturated fatty acids are found at carbon 2. In the membrane phospholipids, the unsaturated fatty acid at carbon 2 is usually arachidonic acid. This arachidonic acid, produced by elongation and desaturation of dietary linoleic acid, is preferentially used in the membrane phospholipid. It can either be attached to the glycerol backbone when the phospholipid is made or exchanged for another fatty acid as the lipids in and around the cells remodel themselves. There is constant hydrolysis and reesterification in the cell and there is a rapid exchange of fatty acids between those in the membranes and those inside the cell.

ENDOGENOUS LIPID TRANSPORT

Fatty acids, TG, cholesterol, cholesterol esters, and phospholipids are synthesized in the body and are transported from sites of synthesis to sites of use and storage. While the transport of these lipids is, in many instances, similar to that of the dietary lipids, there are differences in the processing and in some of the proteins involved. Endogenous fat transport involves the production and secretion of very-low-density lipoproteins (VLDL) by the liver. These lipid–protein complexes are rich in TG and contain cholesterol. The polypeptides that transport these lipids comprise approximately 10% of the weight of the VLDL. They include the polypeptides apo B, B-100, apo C-I, C-II, C-III, and apo E. As mentioned, several of these polypeptides are also involved in exogenous lipid transport (see Chapters 42 & 43). Once the VLDLs are released by the hepatocyte, they are hydrolyzed by the interstitial LPL, and intermediate-density lipoproteins (IDL) are formed. These are cleared from the circulation as they are recognized and bound to hepatic IDL receptors. The hepatic receptors recognize the apo E that is part of the IDL. Any of the IDL that escapes hydrolysis at this stage is available for hydrolysis by the hepatic LPL. This hydrolysis leaves a cholesterol-rich particle of low-density lipoprotein (LDL). The LDL has apo B-100 as its polypeptide carrier, and both hepatic and extrahepatic cells have receptors that recognize this polypeptide. Normally, about 70% of LDL is cleared by the LDL receptors and most of this is cleared by the liver. From the foregoing, it is apparent that considerable lipid recycling occurs in the liver. The VLDLs originate in the liver and the liver is the primary site for LDL disposal. However, other organs and tissues also participate in disposal, but their participation is minor compared with that of the liver.

FATTY ACID OXIDATION

Fatty acids are a source of metabolic fuel. They are available for oxidation once they are released from the glycerides by hydrolysis. This oxidation occurs via the β oxidation pathway and occurs in the mitochondria (Figure 7.13). Prior to oxidation, the fatty acids must be transported into the mitochondria via the acyl-carnitine-transport system (Figure 7.14). The fatty acids are activated by conversion to their CoA thioesters. This activation requires ATP and the enzyme, acyl CoA synthase or thiokinase. There are several thiokinases, which differ with respect to their specificity for the different fatty acids. The activation step is dependent on the release of energy from ATP. Once the fatty acid is activated, it is bound to carnitine with the release of CoA. The acyl carnitine is then translocated through the mitochondrial membranes into the mitochondrial matrix via the carnitine acylcarnitine translocase. As one molecule of acylcarnitine is passed into the matrix, one molecule of carnitine is translocated back to the cytosol and the acylcarnitine is converted back to acyl CoA. The acyl CoA can then enter the β oxidation pathway. Without carnitine, the oxidation of fatty acids, especially the long-chain fatty acids, cannot proceed. Acyl CoA cannot traverse the membrane into the mitochondria and thus requires a translocase for its entry. The translocase requires carnitine. While most of the fatty acids that enter the β oxidation pathway are completely oxidized via the citric acid cycle and respiratory chain to

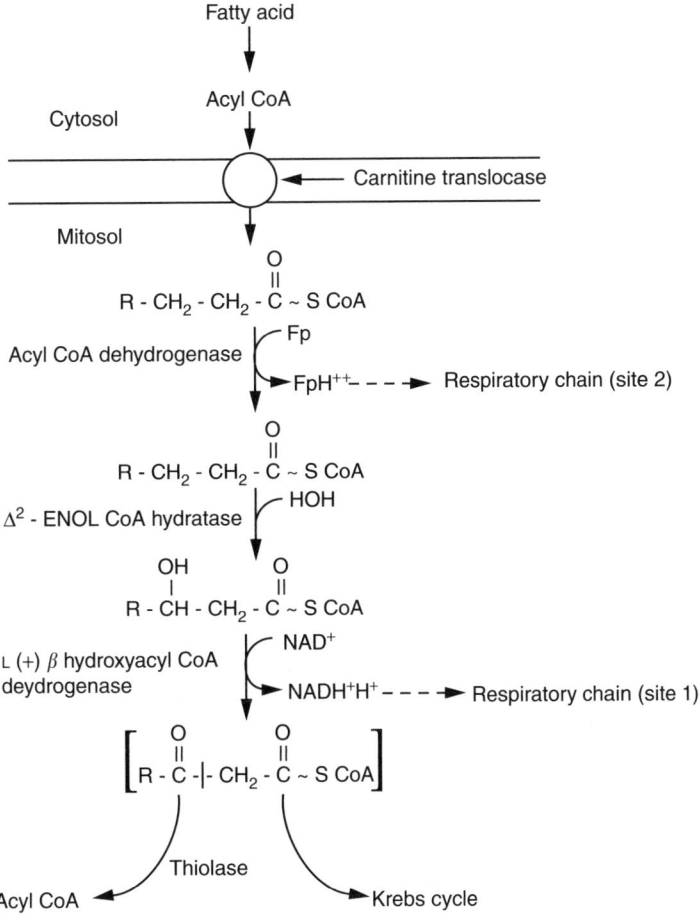

FIGURE 7.13 Fatty acid oxidation.

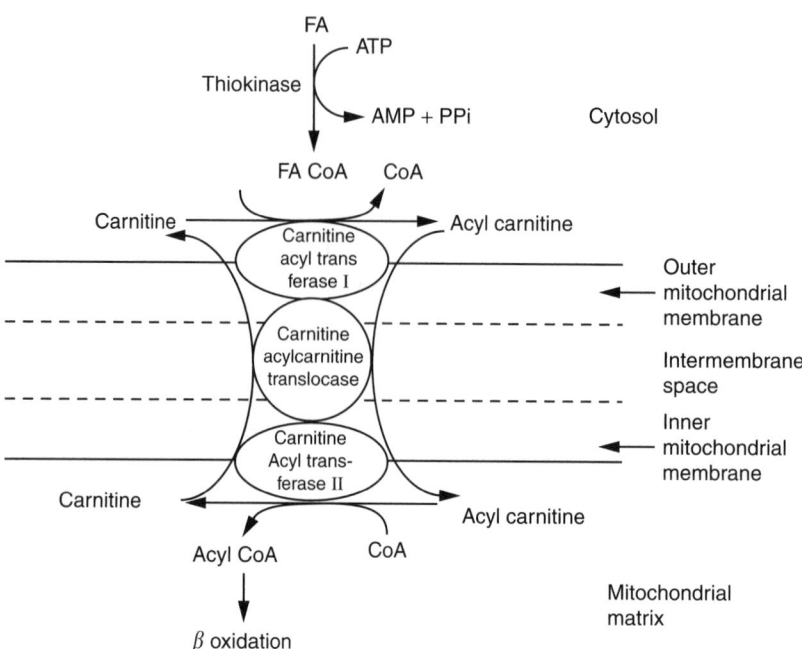

FIGURE 7.14 Mechanism for the entry of fatty acids into the mitochondrial compartment.

CO_2 and HOH, some of the acetyl CoA is converted to the ketones, acetoacetate, and β-hydroxybutyrate. The condensation of two molecules of acetyl CoA to acetoacetyl CoA occurs in the mitochondria via the enzyme β-ketothiolase. Acetoacetyl CoA then condenses with another acetyl CoA to form HMG CoA. At last, the HMG CoA is cleaved into acetoacetic acid and acetyl CoA. The acetoacetic acid is reduced to β-hydroxybutyrate, and this reduction is dependent on the ratio of NAD^+ to $NADH^+H^+$. The enzyme for this reduction, β-hydroxybutyrate dehydrogenase, is tightly bound to the inner aspect of the mitochondrial membrane. Because of its high activity, the product (β-hydroxybutyrate) and substrate (acetoacetate) are in equilibrium.

HMG CoA is also synthesized in the cytosol, where it serves as a starting point for the synthesis of cholesterol. The ketones can ultimately be used as fuel but may appear in the blood, liver, and other tissues at a level of less than 0.2 mM. In starving individuals or in people consuming a high-fat diet, blood and tissue ketone levels may rise above normal (3 to 5 mM). However, unless these levels greatly exceed the body's capacity to use them as fuel (as is the case in uncontrolled diabetes mellitus with levels up to 20 mM) a rise in ketone levels is not a cause for concern. Ketones are choice metabolic fuels for muscle and brain. Although both tissues may prefer to use glucose, the ketones can be used when glucose is in short supply. Ketones are used to spare glucose wherever possible under these conditions.

The oxidation of unsaturated fatty acids follows the same pathway as the saturated fatty acids until the double-bonded carbons are reached (Figure 7.15). At this point, a few side steps must be taken that involve a few additional enzymes. Linoleate has two double bonds in the *cis* configuration. β Oxidation removes three acetyl units, leaving a CoA attached to the terminal carbon just before the first *cis* double bond. At this point an isomerase enzyme, $\Delta 3$ *cis* $\Delta 6$ *trans* enoyl CoA isomerase, acts to convert the first *cis* bond to a *trans* bond. Now, this part of the molecule can once again enter the β oxidation sequence and two more acetyl CoA units are released. The second double bond is then opened and a hydroxyl group is inserted. In turn, this hydroxyl group is rotated to the L position and the remaining product can then reenter the β oxidation pathway. Other unsaturated fatty acids can be similarly oxidized. Each time the double bond is approached, the isomerization and hydroxyl group addition takes place until all of the fatty acid is oxidized.

While β oxidation is the main pathway for the oxidation of fatty acids, some fatty acids undergo α oxidation so as to provide the substrates for the synthesis of sphingolipids. These reactions occur in the endoplasmic reticulum and mitochondria and involve the mixed function oxidases because they require molecular oxygen, reduced NAD, and specific cytochromes. The fatty acid oxidation that occurs in organelles other than the mitochondria are energy-wasteful reactions because these other organelles do not have the citric acid cycle nor do they have the respiratory chain, which takes the reducing equivalents released by the oxidative steps and combines them with oxygen to make water releasing energy that is then trapped in the high-energy bonds of the ATP.

Peroxisomal oxidation in the kidney and liver is an important aspect of drug metabolism. The peroxisomes are a class of subcellular organelles that are important in the protection against oxygen toxicity. They have a high level of catalase activity, which suggests their importance in the antioxidant system. The peroxisomal fatty acid oxidation pathway differs in three important ways from the mitochondrial pathway. First, the initial dehydrogenation is accomplished by a cyanide-insensitive oxidase

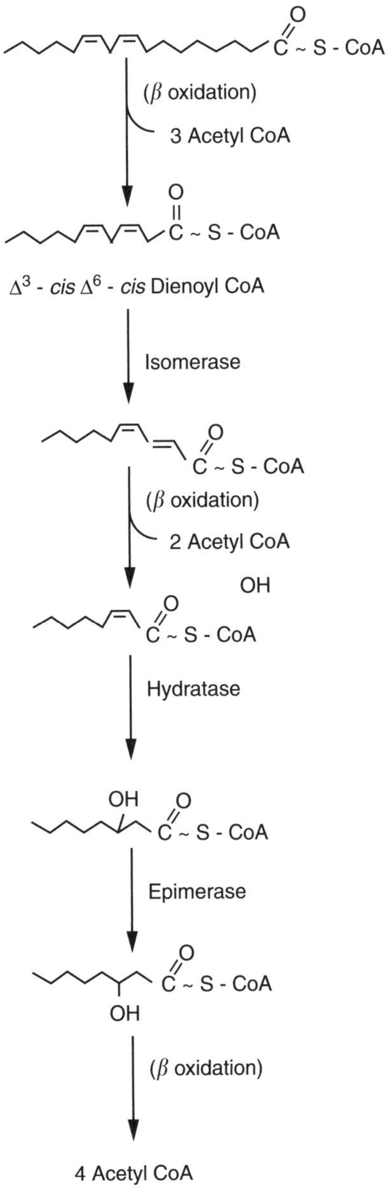

FIGURE 7.15 Unsaturated fatty acid oxidation.

that produces H_2O_2. This H_2O_2 is rapidly extinguished by catalase. Second, the enzymes of the pathway prefer long-chain fatty acids and are slightly different in structure from those (with the same function) of the mitochondrial pathway. Third, β oxidation in the peroxisomes stops at eight carbons rather than proceeding all the way to acetyl CoA. The peroxisomes also serve in the conversion of cholesterol to bile acids and in the formation of ether lipids (plasmalogens).

FATTY ACID SYNTHESIS

Fatty acid synthesis occurs in the cytosol of the living cell using two carbon units (acetyl units) that are the result of glucose oxidation or amino acid degradation (Figure 7.16).

Fatty acid synthesis begins with acetyl CoA. Acetyl CoA arises from the oxidation of glucose or the carbon skeletons of deaminated amino acids. Acetyl CoA is converted to malonyl CoA with the addition of one carbon (from bicarbonate) in the presence of the enzyme acetyl CoA carboxylase. The reaction uses the energy from one molecule of ATP and biotin as a coenzyme. This reaction is the first committed step in the reaction sequence that results in the synthesis of a fatty acid. The activated CO_2 attached to the biotin–enzyme complex is transferred to the methyl end of the substrate. Although most fatty acids synthesized in mammalian cells have an even number of carbons, this first committed step yields a three-carbon product. This results in an asymmetric molecule that becomes vulnerable to attack (addition) at the center of the molecule with the subsequent loss of

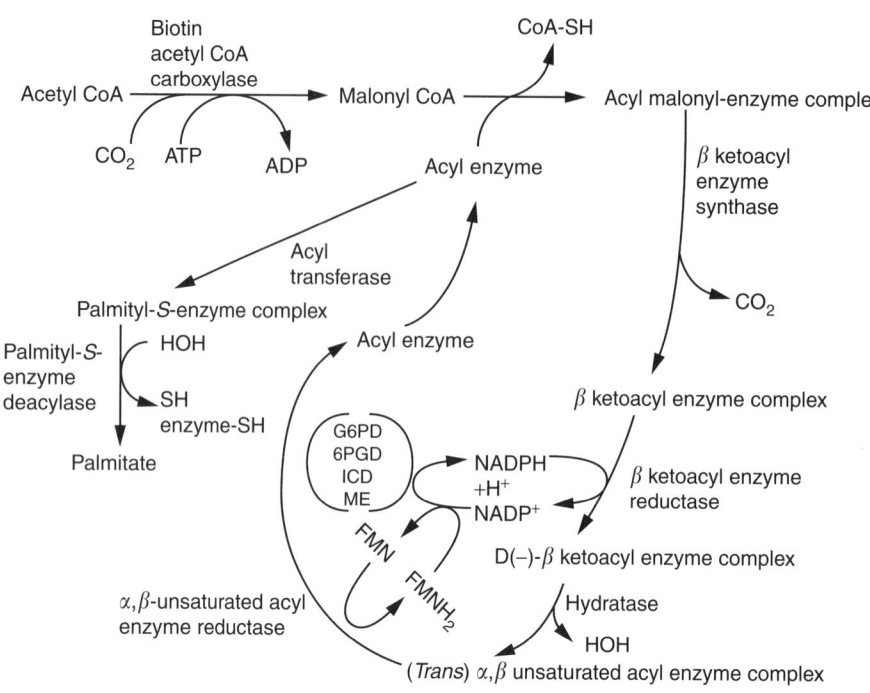

FIGURE 7.16 Fatty acid synthesis.

the terminal carbon. The vulnerability is conferred by the fact that both the carboxyl group at one end and the group at the other end are both powerful attractants of electrons from the hydrogen of the middle carbon. This leaves the carbon in a very reactive state, and a second acetyl group carried by a carrier protein with the help of phosphopantetheine, which has a sulfur group connection can be joined to it through the action of the enzyme, malonyl transferase. Subsequently, the "extra" carbon is released via the enzyme β-ketoacyl enzyme synthase, leaving a four-carbon chain still connected to an SH group at the carboxyl end. This SH group is the docking end for all the enzymes that comprise the fatty acid synthase complex. These enzymes catalyze the addition of two carbon acetyl groups in sequence to the methyl end of the carbon chain until the final product palmityl CoA, and then palmitic acid is produced. Members of this fatty acid synthase complex include the aforementioned malonyl transferase and β-ketoacyl synthase, β-ketoacyl reductase, which catalyzes the addition of reducing equivalents carried by FMN, and an acyl transferase. Upon completion of these six steps, the process is repeated until the chain length is 16 carbons long. At this point, the SH-acyl carrier protein is removed through the action of the enzyme palmityl-S-enzyme deacylase and the palmitic acid is available for esterification to glycerol to form a mono-, di-, or triacylglyceride (see the section titled "Fatty Acid Esterification").

FATTY ACID ELONGATION

Elongation or the lengthening of fatty acids by the addition of two carbon units (acetyl groups), occurs in either the endoplasmic reticulum or the mitochondria (Figure 7.17). The reaction differs depending on where it occurs. In the endoplasmic reticulum, the reaction sequence is similar to that described for the cytosolic fatty acid synthase complex. The source of the two-carbon unit is malonyl CoA, and NADPH+H+ provides the reducing power. The intermediates are CoA esters, not the acyl carrier protein 4′-phosphopantetheine. The reaction sequence produces stearic acid (18:0) in all tissues that make fatty acids except the brain. In the brain, elongation can proceed further producing fatty acids containing up to 24 carbons. In the mitochondria, elongation uses acetyl CoA rather than malonyl CoA as the source of the two-carbon unit. It uses either NADH+H+ or NADPH+H+ as the source of reducing equivalents and uses, as substrate, carbon chains of less than 16 carbons. Mitochondrial elongation is the reversal of fatty acid oxidation, which also occurs in this organelle. Not all species can make all of the fatty acids found in the body tissues. Some of these fatty acids are therefore essential. In mammals the essential fatty acids are linoleic and linolenic acids. In felines the essential fatty acids include these two and arachidonic acid. Table 7.4 gives the structures and names of the important fatty acids.

FATTY ACID DESATURATION

Desaturation occurs in the endoplasmic reticulum and microsomes (Figure 7.17). The enzymes that catalyze this are the Δ4, Δ5, or Δ6 desaturases. Desaturation is species specific. Mammals, for example, lack the ability to desaturate fatty acids in the n-6 or n-3 position. They cannot make linoleic or linolenic acid, and in addition, felines cannot convert linoleic to arachidonic acid.

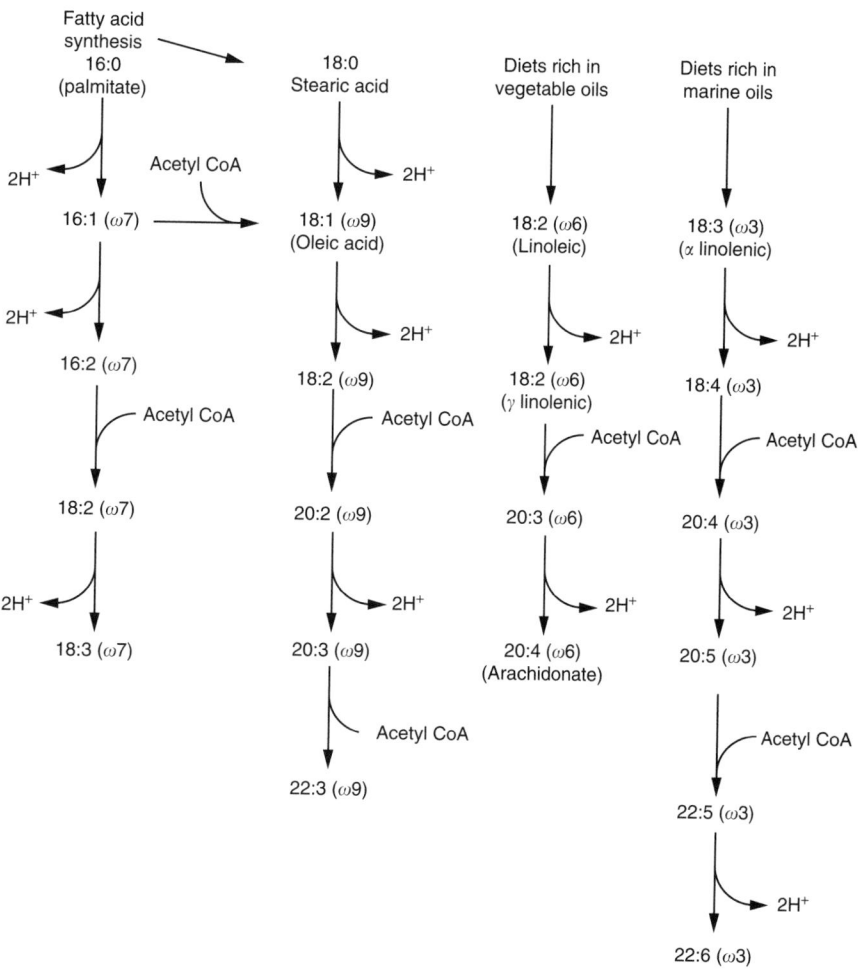

FIGURE 7.17 Fatty acid elongation and desaturation.

TABLE 7.4
Structure and Names of Fatty Acids Found in Food

Structure	Number of Double Bonds	Systematic Name	Trivial Name	Source
Saturated fatty acids				
$CH_3(CH_2)_2COOH$	0	*n*-Butanoic	Butyric	Butter
$CH_3(CH_2)_4COOH$	0	*n*-Hexanoic	Caproic	Butter
$CH_3(CH_2)_6COOH$	0	*n*-Octanoic	Caprylic	Coconut oil
$CH_3(CH_2)_8COOH$	0	*n*-Decanoic	Capric	Palm oil
$CH_3(CH_2)_{10}COOH$	0	*n*-Dodecanoic	Lauric	Coconut oil, butter
$CH_3(CH_2)_{12}COOH$	0	*n*-Tetradecanoic	Myristic	Coconut oil
$CH_3(CH_2)_{14}COOH$	0	*n*-Hexadecanoic	Palmitic	Most fats and oils
$CH_3(CH_2)_{16}COOH$	0	*n*-Octadecanoic	Stearic	Most fats and oils
$CH_3(CH_2)_{18}COOH$	0	*n*-Eicosanoic	Arachidic	Peanut oil, lard
Unsaturated fatty acids				
$CH_3(CH_2)_5CH=CH(CH_2)_7COOH$	1	9-Hexadecenoic	Palmitoleic	Butter and seed oils
$CH_3(CH_2)_7CH=CH(CH_2)_7COOH$	1	9-Octadecenoic	Oleic	Most fats and oils
$CH_3(CH_2)_5CH=CH(CH_2)_9COOH$	1	11-Octadecenoic	Vaccenic	*trans*-Hydrogenated vegetable oils
$CH_3(CH_2)_4CH=CHCH_2CH=CH(CH_2)_7COOH$	2	9,12-Octadecadienoic	Linoleic	Linseed oil, corn oil
$CH_3CH_2(CH=CHCH_2)_3(CH_2)_7COOH$	3	9,12,15-Octadecatrienoic	Linolenic	Soybean and marine oils
$CH_3(CH_2)_4(CH=CHCH_2)_4(CH_2)_2COOH$	4	5,8,11,14-Eicosatetraenoic	Arachidonic	Cottonseed oil

Only plants can do this, and even among plants there are species differences. Cold water plants can desaturate at the n-3 position, while land plants of warmer regions cannot. The cold water plants are consumed by cold water creatures in a food chain that includes fish as well as sea mammals. These, in turn, enter the human food supply and become sources of the n-3, or omega-3, fatty acids in the marine oils. In animals desaturation of *de novo* synthesized fatty acids usually stops with the production of a monounsaturated fatty acid with the double bond in the 9 to 10 position counting from the carboxyl end of the molecule. Hence, palmitic acid (16:0) becomes palmitoleic acid (16:1) and stearic acid (18:0) becomes oleic acid (18:1). In the absence of dietary EFA most mammals will desaturate eicosenoic acid to produce eicosatrienoic acid. Increases in this fatty acid with unsaturations at the n-7 and n-9 positions characterize the tissue lipids of EFA-deficient animals. The enzymes are sometimes called mixed function oxidases because two substrates (fatty acid and NADPH) are oxidized simultaneously. These desaturases prefer substrates with a double bond in the n-6 position but will also act on n-3 fatty acids bonds and on saturated fatty acids. Desaturation of *de novo* synthesized stearic acid to form oleic acid results in the formation of a double bond at the omega-9 position. This is the first committed step of this desaturation/elongation reaction sequence. Oleic acid can also be formed by the desaturation and elongation of palmitic acid. Fatty acid desaturation can be followed by elongation and repeated such that a variety of mono- and polyunsaturated fatty acids can be formed. The body can convert the dietary saturated fatty acids to unsaturated fatty acids, thus maintaining an optimal P:S ratio in the tissues.

AUTOOXIDATION

Unsaturated fatty acids, particularly the polyunsaturated fatty acids, are more reactive than saturated fatty acids. The double bonds can be attacked by oxygen radicals in a process called autooxidation. In food, autooxidation occurs and is responsible for the deterioration of food quality. The discoloration of red meat upon exposure to air at room temperature is an indication of the autooxidation process. The off odor that accompanies this discoloration is the result of the autooxidation of the fatty acids in the meat fat. In living systems, the process of autooxidation is suppressed to a large extent. This is essential because the products of this oxidation, fatty acid peroxides, can be very damaging. Peroxides denature proteins, rendering them inactive, and attack the DNA in the nucleus and mitochondria, resulting in base pair deletions or breaks in the DNA, which, in turn, result in mutations or errors. In the nucleus, these breaks or deletions can be repaired. In the aging animal, the repair mechanism loses its efficiency and one of the characteristics of aged cells is the loss of its DNA repair ability. To prevent widespread damage to cellular proteins and DNA by these radicals, there is a potent antioxidation system. This antioxidation system includes the selenium containing enzyme, glutathione peroxidase, catalase, and superoxide dismutase (SOD). These enzymes are found in the peroxisomes. Superoxide dismutase is also found in the mitochondria. All of these components serve to suppress free radical formation.

The free radical chain reaction occurs when the oxygen atom is excited by a variety of drugs and contaminants or by ultraviolet light. The excited oxygen atom is called singlet oxygen (O_2^-). Pollutants such as the oxides of nitrogen or carbon tetrachloride can provoke this reaction. *In vivo*, the detoxification reactions catalyzed by the cytochrome P450 enzymes generate free radicals. In the respiratory chain of the mitochondria, the possibility of oxygen radical production exists, and it is for this reason the mitochondria possess a particularly potent peroxide suppressor, SOD. SOD in the mitochondria requires the manganese ion as a cofactor. The cytosol also has SOD, but this enzyme requires the copper and zinc ions. Both forms of the enzyme catalyze the reaction,

$$O_2^- + O_2^- + 2H^+ \rightarrow H_2O_2 + O_2.$$

Two superoxides and two hydrogen ions are joined to form one molecule of hydrogen peroxide and a molecule of oxygen. In turn, the peroxide can be converted to water through the action of the enzyme catalase. Peroxides can also be "neutralized" through the action of glutathione-*S*-transferase. This reaction requires 2 *M* of reduced glutathione and produces two molecules of oxidized glutathione and two molecules of water. Fatty acid radicals can also be neutralized by glutathione peroxidase producing a molecule of an alcohol with the same chain length as the fatty acid. Glutathione-*S*-transferase can duplicate the action of glutathione peroxidase. These enzymes and the reactions they catalyze are listed in Table 7.5. In addition to the reactions that counteract the *in vivo* formation of oxygen radicals or fatty acid peroxides, certain of the vitamins have this role as well. Ascorbic acid has antioxidant function as it can donate reducing equivalents to a peroxide converting it to an alcohol. β-Carotene can quench singlet oxygen and thus convert it into O_2. Vitamin E is perhaps the best known antioxidant vitamin and its action is similar to that of ascorbic acid. It donates reducing equivalents to a peroxide converting it to an alcohol.

Although the foregoing has emphasized the negative aspects of the partial reduction products of oxygen, there is some evidence that peroxide formation has some benefit. For example, leukocytes produce peroxides as a means of killing invading bacteria. Other examples, no doubt, will emerge as scientists continue in their efforts to understand the role of peroxidation (and the peroxisomes) in mammalian metabolism.

CHOLESTEROL SYNTHESIS

The body synthesizes nearly 90% of the cholesterol that is in the circulation. The starting point for cholesterol synthesis is the joining of acetyl CoA to acetoacetyl CoA to form HMGCoA (Figure 7.18). HMGCoA through the action of HMGCoA reductase

TABLE 7.5
Free Radical Suppression Enzymes Found in Mammalian Cells

Enzyme	Required Mineral Cofactors	Reaction Catalyzed
Superoxide dismutase	Cu, Zn, Mn	$2O\ 2O_2^- + 2H^+ \rightarrow + H_2O_2$
Glutathione peroxidase	Se	$H_2O_2 + 2GSH \rightarrow GSSG + 2H_2O$ $ROOH + 2GSH \rightarrow GSSG + ROH + H_2O$
Catalase	Fe	$2H_2O_2 \rightarrow 2H_2O + O_2$
Glutathione-S-transferases	—	$ROOH + 2GSH \rightarrow GSSG + ROH + H_2O$

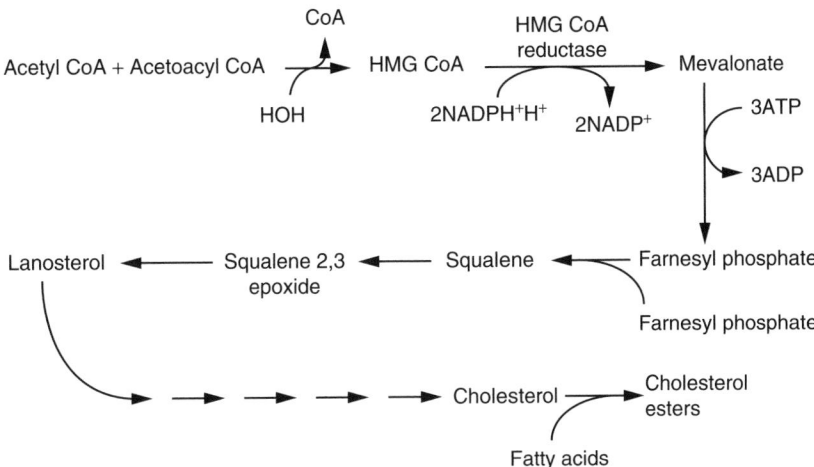

FIGURE 7.18   Cholesterol synthesis.

(the rate-limiting step in this pathway) is converted to mevalonate. Cholesterol-lowering drugs act on this step inhibiting *in vivo* cholesterol synthesis. Mevalonate is phosporylated to farnesyl phosphate, which in turn is converted to squalene and then, through a series of reactions, to cholesterol. Cholesterol serves as the beginning substrate for the synthesis of a variety of hormones, active vitamin D, and the bile acids (Figure 7.19). Cholesterol is also an important component of cellular membranes.

EICOSANOID SYNTHESIS

Eicosanoids are 20 carbon molecules having hormone-like activity. They are produced in their various forms and released by many different mammalian cells. When each of these compounds is produced, their site of action is local. That is, whereas insulin may be transported from the pancreas to peripheral target cells, the eicosanoids are produced, released, and have as their targets the surrounding cells. For this reason, the eicosanoids are called local hormones. They have a variety of actions. Table 7.6 lists the major eicosanoids and their functions.

The eicosanoids fall into three general groups of compounds: the prostaglandins (compounds of the PG series), the thromboxanes (compounds of the TBX series), and the leukotrienes (compounds of the LKT series). All of these compounds arise from a 20-carbon polyunsaturated fatty acid (Figure 7.20). This fatty acid is usually arachidonic acid (20 carbons, 4 double bonds at 5, 8, 11, and 14). However, in instances where the diet is rich in n-3 fatty acids, the precursor may be a twenty-carbon-5 double-bond fatty acid, eicosapentaenoic acid (double bonds at 5, 8, 11, 14, and 17). Other eicosanoids can be synthesized from a 20-carbon fatty acid, dihomo-γ-linoleic acid, which has only three double bonds at carbons 8, 11, and 14. Each of these precursors yields a particular set of eicosanoids. During their synthesis, they take up oxygen and are cyclized. Dihomo-γ-linoleic acid is the precursor of prostaglandin E_1 (PGE$_1$), prostaglandin $E_{1\alpha}$ (PGE$_{1\alpha}$), and subsequent prostaglandins. Arachidonic acid is the precursor of prostaglandins of the 2 series (PGE$_2$, PGF$_{2\alpha}$, etc.), and eicosapentaenoic acid is the precursor of prostaglandins of the 3 series (PGE$_3$, PGF$_{3\alpha}$, etc.).

The cyclization of these 20-carbon fatty acids is accomplished by a complex of enzymes called the prostaglandin synthesis complex. The first step is the cyclooxygenase step, which involves the cyclization of C-9 - C-12 of the precursor to the cyclic

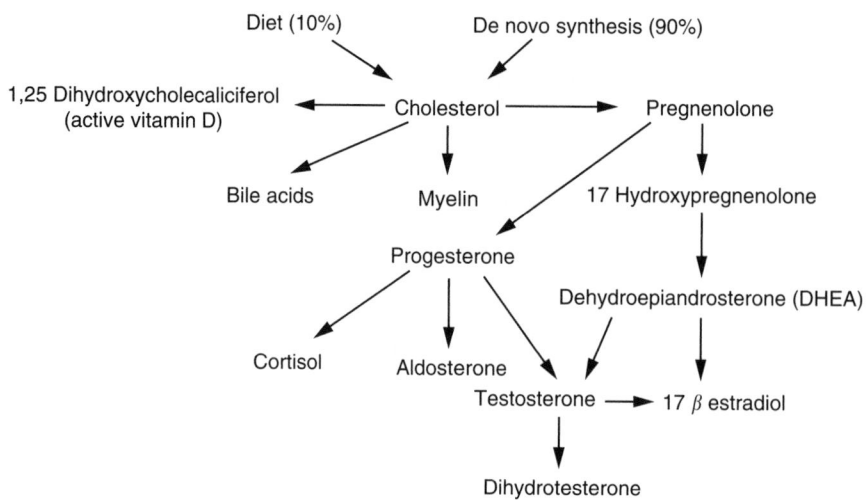

FIGURE 7.19   Uses of cholesterol.

TABLE 7.6
Functions of Eicosanoids

Eicosanoid	Function
PGG_2	Precursor of PGH_2
PGH_2	Precursor of PGD_2, PGE_2, PGI_2, $PGF_{2\alpha}$
PGD_2	Promotes sleeping behavior
	Precursor of PGF_2
PGE_2	Enhances perception of pain when histamine or bradykinin is given
	Induces signs of inflammation
	Promotes wakefulness
	Precursor of $PGF_{2\alpha}$
	Reduces gastric acid secretion, induces partuition
	Vasoconstrictor in some tissues
	Vasodilator in other tissues
	Maintains the patency of the ductus arteriosis prior to birth
$PGF_{2\alpha}$	Bronchial constrictor
	Vasoconstrictor especially in coronary vasculature
	Increases sperm motility
	Induces partuition; stimulates steroidogenesis corpus luteum; induces luteolysis
PGI_2	Inhibits platelet aggregation
PGE_1	Inhibits motility of nonpregnant uterus increases motility of pregnant uterus
	Bronchial dilator
TXA_2	Stimulates platelet aggregation
	Potent vasoconstrictor
TXB_2	Metabolite of TXA_2
LTA_4	Precursor of LTB_4
LTB_4	Potent chemotaxic agent

form 9, 11-endoperoxide 15-hydroperoxide (PGG_2). PGG_2 is then used to form prostaglandin H_2 (PGH_2) through the removal of one oxygen from the carbonyl group at carbon 15. Glutathione peroxidase and prostaglandin H synthase catalyze the reaction shown in Figure 7.20. Prostaglandin H synthase is a very unstable short-lived enzyme with a messenger RNA that is one of the shortest-lived species so far found in mammalian cells. The expression of genes for this enzyme is under the control of polypeptide growth factors such as interleukin-1α, and colony stimulating factor-1. Interferon-α and interferon-β inhibit expression and prostanoid production by the macrophages. Glutathione peroxidase is a selenium-containing enzyme. PGH_2 is then converted through the action of a variety of isomerases to PGD_2, PGE_2, prostacylin I_2 (PGI_2), or prostaglandin $F_{2\alpha}$ ($PGF_{2\alpha}$). These are the primary precursors of the prostaglandins of the D, E, and F series and PGI or thromboxane. The conversion to subsequent prostaglandins is mediated by enzymes that are specific to a certain cell type and tissue. Not all of these subsequent compounds

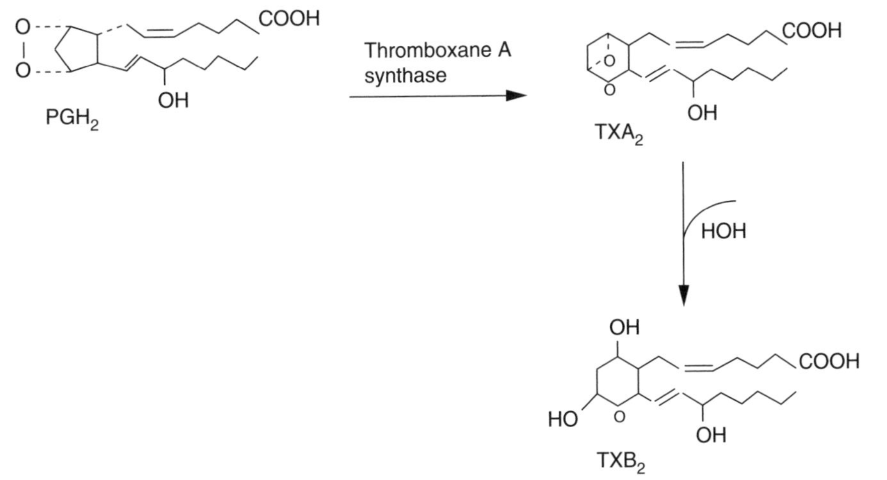

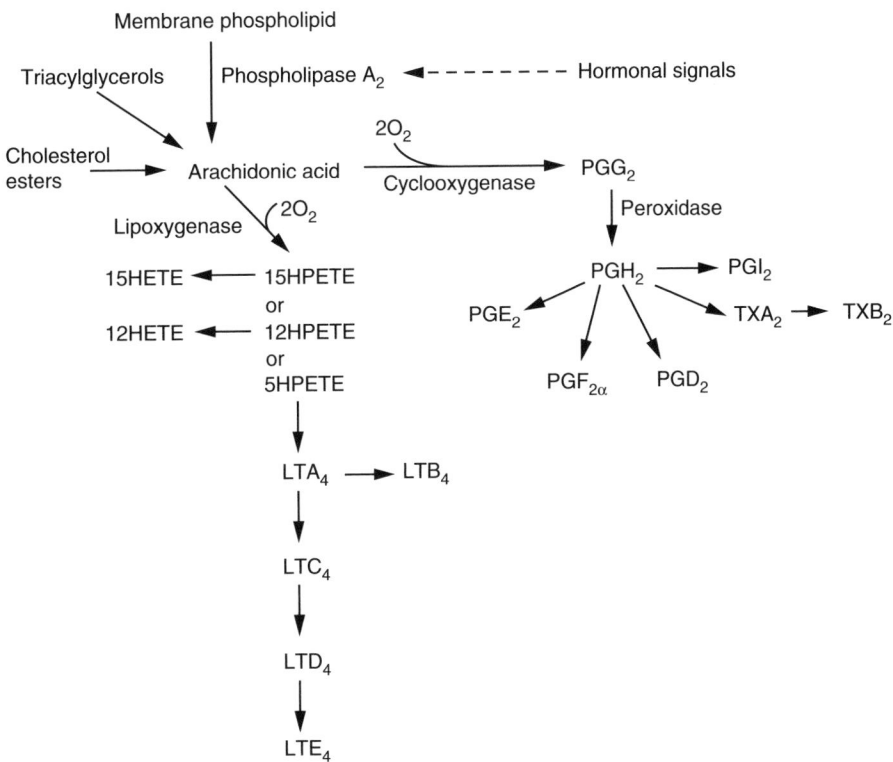

FIGURE 7.20   Eicosanoid synthesis from arachidonic acid.

FIGURE 7.21   Reaction sequence that produces TXA_2 and TXB_2.

are formed in all tissues. Thus, PGE_2 and $PGF_{2\alpha}$ are produced in the kidney and spleen. $PGF_{2\alpha}$ and PGE are also produced in the uterus only when signals from the pituitary induce their production and so stimulate parturition. PGI_2 is primarily produced by endothelial cells lining the blood vessels. This prostaglandin inhibits platelet aggregation and thus is important to maintaining a blood flow free of clots. It is counteracted by thromboxane A_2, which is produced by the platelets when these cells contact a foreign surface. PGE_2, $PGF_{2\alpha}$, and PGI_2 are formed by the heart in about equal amounts. All of these prostaglandins have very short half-lives. No sooner are they released than they are inactivated. The thromboxanes are highly active metabolites of the prostaglandins. As mentioned earlier, they are formed when PGH_2 has it cyclopentane ring replaced by a six-membered oxane ring shown in Figure 7.21. Imidazole is a potent inhibitor of thromboxane A synthase and is used to block TXA_2 production and platelet aggregation.

Thromboxane A_2 has a role in clot formation and the name thromboxane comes from this function (thrombus means clot). The half-life of TXA_2 is less than 1 min. TXB_2 is its metabolic end product and has little biological activity. Measuring TXB_2

levels in blood and tissue can give an indication of how much TXA_2 had been produced. PGD_2 and PGE_2 are involved in the regulation of sleep–wake cycles in a variety of species.

Although the cyclooxygenase pathway is quite important in the production of prostaglandins, equally important is the lipoxygenase pathway. This pathway is catalyzed by a family of enzymes called the lipoxygenase enzymes. These enzymes differ from the cyclooxygenase enzymes in its catalytic site for oxygen addition to the unsaturated fatty acid. One lipoxygenase is active at the double bond at carbon 5, while a second is active at carbon 11 and a third is active at carbon 15. The products of these reactions are monohydroperoxy-eicosatetraenoic acids (HPETEs) and are numbered according to the location of the double bond to which the oxygen is added. 5HPETE is the major lipoxygenase product in basophils, polymorphonuclear leukocytes, macrophages, mast cells, and any organ undergoing an inflammatory response. 12HPETE is the major product in platelets, pancreatic endocrine cells, vascular smooth muscle, and glomerular cells. 15HPETE predominates in reticulocytes, eosinophils, T-lymphocytes, and tracheal epithelial cells. The HPETEs are not in themselves active hormones; rather, they serve as precursors for the leukotrienes. The leukotrienes are the metabolic end products of the lipoxygenase reaction. These compounds contain at least three conjugated double bonds. The unstable 5HPETE is converted to either an analogous alcohol (hydroxy fatty acid) or is reduced by a peroxide or converted to leukotriene. The peroxidative reduction of 5'HPETE to the stable 5HETE (5 hydroxyeicosatetraenoic acid) is similar to that of 12HPETE to 12HETE and of 15HPETE to 15HETE. In each instance the carbon–carbon double bonds are unconjugated and the geometry of the double bonds is *trans* and *cis*, respectively. In contrast to the active thromboxanes, which have very short half-lives, the leukotrienes can persist as long as 4 h. These compounds comprise a group of substances known as the slow-acting anaphylaxis substances. They cause slowly evolving but protracted contractions of smooth muscles in the airways and gastrointestinal tract. Leukotriene C_4 is rapidly converted to LTD_4, which in turn is slowly converted to LTE_4. Enzymes in the plasma are responsible for these conversions.

The products of the lipoxygenase pathway are potent mediators of the response to allergens, tissue damage (inflammation), hormone secretion, cell movement, cell growth, and calcium flux. Within minutes of stimulation, lipoxygenase products are produced. In an allergy attack, for example, an allergen can instigate the release of leukotrienes, which are the immediate mediators of response. The leukotrienes are more potent than histamine in stimulating the contraction of the bronchial nonvascular smooth muscles. In addition, LTD_4 increases the permeability of the microvasculature. The mono-HETEs and LTB_4 stimulate the movement of eosinophils and neutrophils, making them the first line of defense in injury resulting in inflammation.

As mentioned, when dihomo-γ-linoleic acid or eicosapentaenoic acid serve as substrates for eicosanoid production, the products are either of the 1 series or 3 series. The products they form may be less active than those formed from arachidonic acid and this decrease in activity can be of therapeutic value. Hence, ingestion of n-3 fatty acids leads to the decreased production of prostaglandin E_2 and its metabolites, a decrease in the production of thromboxane A_2, a potent platelet aggregator and vasoconstrictor, and a decrease in leukotriene B_4, a potent inflammatory hormone and a powerful inducer of leukocyte hemotaxis and adherence. Counteracting these decreases are an increase in thromboxane A_3 (TXA_3), a weak platelet aggregator and vasoconstrictor, an increase in the production of PGI_3 without an increase in PGI_2, which stimulates vasodilation and inhibits platelet aggregation, and an increase in leukotriene B_5, which is a weak inducer of inflammation and a weak chemotoxic agent.

PROTEIN METABOLISM

The protein in the diet provides the essential and nonessential amino acids that are used to synthesize body proteins. Dietary amino acids fall into two categories: essential and nonessential (Table 7.7). There are species differences in the amino acids that are considered essential. An essential amino acid is one that the body cannot synthesize in sufficient quantities to meets the body's need for that amino acid. Sometimes the physiological state of the animal determines essentiality. Persons with renal disease, for example, have a greater need for arginine than healthy people. People who have been severely burned may need more essential amino acids than healthy people. Felines require taurine in their diets, while other animals do not. Good food proteins are those proteins that provide sufficient quantities of essential amino acids. Poor-quality proteins might have one or two of these essential amino acids in short supply. With careful blending of poor-quality proteins, a good array of amino acids is possible. These proteins must be consumed at or nearly at the same time in order to allow for optimal use.

PROTEIN DENATURATION

One of the most striking characteristics of proteins is the response to heat, alcohol, and other treatments that affect their quaternary, tertiary, and secondary structures. This characteristic response is called denaturation. Denaturation results in the unfolding of a protein molecule, thus breaking its hydrogen bonds and the associations between functional groups; as a result, the three-dimensional structure is lost. Denaturation affects many of the properties of the protein molecule. Its physical shape is changed, its solubility in water is decreased, and its reactivity with other proteins may be lost. When denatured, the protein loses its biological activity. Heating will denature most proteins. As low a temperature as 15°C can denature some proteins, while the

TABLE 7.7
Essential and Nonessential Amino Acids
for Adult Mammals

Essential	Nonessential
Valine	Hydroxyproline
Leucine	Cysteine
Isoleucine	Glycine
Threonine	Alanine
Phenylalanine	Serine
Methionine	Proline
Tryptophan	Glutamic Acid
Lysine	Aspartic Acid
Histidine	Glutamine
Arginine[a]	Asparagine
Taurine[b]	Hydroxylysine. Tyrosine

[a] Not essential for maintenance of most adult mammals.
[b] Felines require taurine, a metabolite of L-cysteine as a component of their diets.

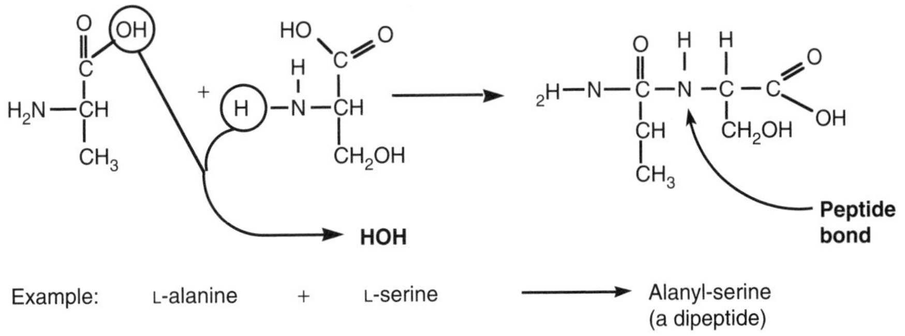

FIGURE 7.22   The formation of a peptide bond.

majority of food proteins are denatured at temperatures in excess of 60°C. Some proteins are very heat stable (those found in thermophillic bacteria for example), while others are quite labile. Heat denaturation, unless extreme, does not affect the amino acid composition of protein, and indeed, may make these amino acids more available to the body because heating provokes the unfolding or uncoiling of the protein and exposes more of the amino acid chain to the action of the proteolytic digestive enzymes. If only mild denaturation occurs, it can be reversed. This process is called renaturation. If a protein is renatured, it will resume its original shape and biological activity.

PROTEIN TURNOVER

Protein turnover consists of two processes: synthesis and degradation. In synthesis, amino acids are joined together to form peptides and proteins. Amino acids in the circulation enter a vast array of cell types, and each cell type has many uses for the amino acids brought to it by the circulation. As mentioned, small, medium, and large molecules can be made. The largest of these molecules are the proteins. Protein synthesis is dependent on the simultaneous presence of all the amino acids necessary for the protein being synthesized and on the provision of energy. If there is an insufficient supply of either, protein biosynthesis will not proceed at its normal pace. Chemically, the polymerization of amino acids into protein is a dehydration reaction between two amino acids that are joined together by a peptide bond.

The peptide bond is the most common amide bond and is formed when two amino acids and joined together as illustrated in Figure 7.22. Two amino acids joined together form a dipeptide, three form a tripeptide, and so on. Each amino acid in a chain is referred to as an amino acid residue. A chain of up to 100 amino acids joined together is called a polypeptide. If many amino acids are involved, then the compound is called a protein. Proteins have been identified that have as many as 300,000 amino acids residues and molecular weights in excess of 4×10^7.

The amino acid sequence of a given peptide or protein can vary, and its variation is controlled genetically. Proteins are complex molecules having characteristic primary, secondary, tertiary, and quaternary structures. The primary structure is determined genetically as the particular sequence of amino acids in a given protein. Protein conformation is usually divided into two categories: secondary and tertiary. The secondary and tertiary structures of a protein result from interactions between the reactive groups on the amino acids in the protein.

The process whereby proteins are synthesized provides the basis for understanding genetic differences. It is also the basis for understanding how the unique properties of each cell type are maintained as the properties that make cells unique are usually conferred by the proteins within them. Some of these proteins are the structural elements of the cell. Others are enzymes that catalyze specific reactions and processes that characterize the cell in question. Still other proteins confer a particular biochemical function on the cell. The amino acid sequence of a particular protein is genetically controlled. This control is exerted through the polynucleotide, deoxyribonucleic acid (DNA). DNA is found in both the nucleus and the mitochondria. The process of protein synthesis using DNA as the template is covered in Chapter 54.

The proteins synthesized by the body have a finite existence. They are subject to a variety of insults and modifications. Some of these modifications have already been described: a prohormone is converted to an active hormone, an enzyme is activated or inactivated with the addition or removal of a substituent, and so forth. Thus, a dynamic state within the body exists with respect to its full complement of peptides and proteins. Some proteins have very short lifetimes and very rapid turnover times; other proteins are quite stable and long lived. Their turnover time is quite long. The estimate of the life of a protein, that is, how long it will exist in the body, is its half-life. A half-life is that time interval that occurs when half of the amount of a compound synthesized at time X will have been degraded. Given the dynamic state of metabolism, some of these time estimates will be very short. Half-lives of biologically active compounds are very difficult to estimate.

Amino Acid Catabolism

Protein degradation results in amino acids that are usually recycled. There are some exceptions to this general rule; histidine in the muscle protein is methylated and excreted as 3-methyl histidine. This 3-methyl histidine cannot be reused and thus is an indication of muscle breakdown. Most of the products of protein degradation (the liberated amino acids) join the body amino acid pool from which the synthetic processes withdraw their needed supply. It is estimated that 75 to 80% of the liberated amino acids are reused.

Different proteins are degraded at different rates, and these rates are determined not only by the physiological status of the individual but also by the amino acid composition of the protein in question. High rates of degradation of the structural proteins mean that considerable structural rearrangement is occurring. Short-lived proteins such as enzymes or receptors have in common regions that are rich in proline, glutamate, serine, and threonine. These amino acids, when clustered, provide a target for rapid degradation.

The process of degradation first reduces the protein to peptides and then reduces these peptides to their constituent amino acids. Two major pathways are used for this process. Extracellular, membrane, and long-lived intracellular proteins are degraded in the lysosomes by an ATP-independent pathway. Short-lived proteins as well as abnormal proteins are degraded in the cytosol using ATP and ubiquitin. This pathway is illustrated in Figure 7.24. Proteins that are degraded via the ubiquitin-dependent pathway are derivatized by several molecules of ubiquitin. The ubiquitin is attached by nonpeptide bonds between the carboxy terminus of ubiquitin and the δ-amino groups of lysyl residues in the protein. This requires ATP.

Although the proteases of digestion are important to the degradation of dietary protein, they have no role in the intracellular protein degradation. Intracellular proteases hydrolyze internal peptides bonds. This is followed by the action of carboxy- and aminopeptidases, which remove single amino acids from the carboxy end or the amino end of the peptides.

Proteins in the extracellular environment are brought into the cell by endocytosis. This is a process similar to pinocytosis, where the cell membrane engulfs and encapsulates the extracellular material. Endocytosis occurs at indentations in the plasma membrane that are internally coated with a protein called clathrin. As in pinocytosis, the extracellular protein is surrounded by the plasma membrane to form an intracellular vesicle, which, in turn, fuses with a lysosome. Degradation then occurs via calcium-dependent proteases called calpains or cathepsin. Both the Golgi and the endoplasmic reticulum are involved in providing proteases that degrade peptide fragments that arise during the maturation of proteins in the secretory pathway.

The rate of degradation varies from protein to protein, and this rate is determined by the amino acid at the amino end of the protein amino acid chain. Proteins with short half-lives have regions rich in proline, glutamate, serine, and threonine. Proteins without these regions are degraded slowly, and therefore have slower turnover times and longer half-lives.

Those amino acids in the body's amino acid pool that are not used for peptide or protein synthesis and that are not used to synthesize metabolically important intermediates are deaminated, and the carbon skeletons are either oxidized or used for the synthesis of glucose or fatty acids. There are three general reactions for the removal of NH_3 from the amino acids: (1) transamination with the amino group transferred to another carbon chain via amino transaminases, (2) oxidative deamination to yield NH_3, or (3) deamination through the activity of an amino acid oxidase.

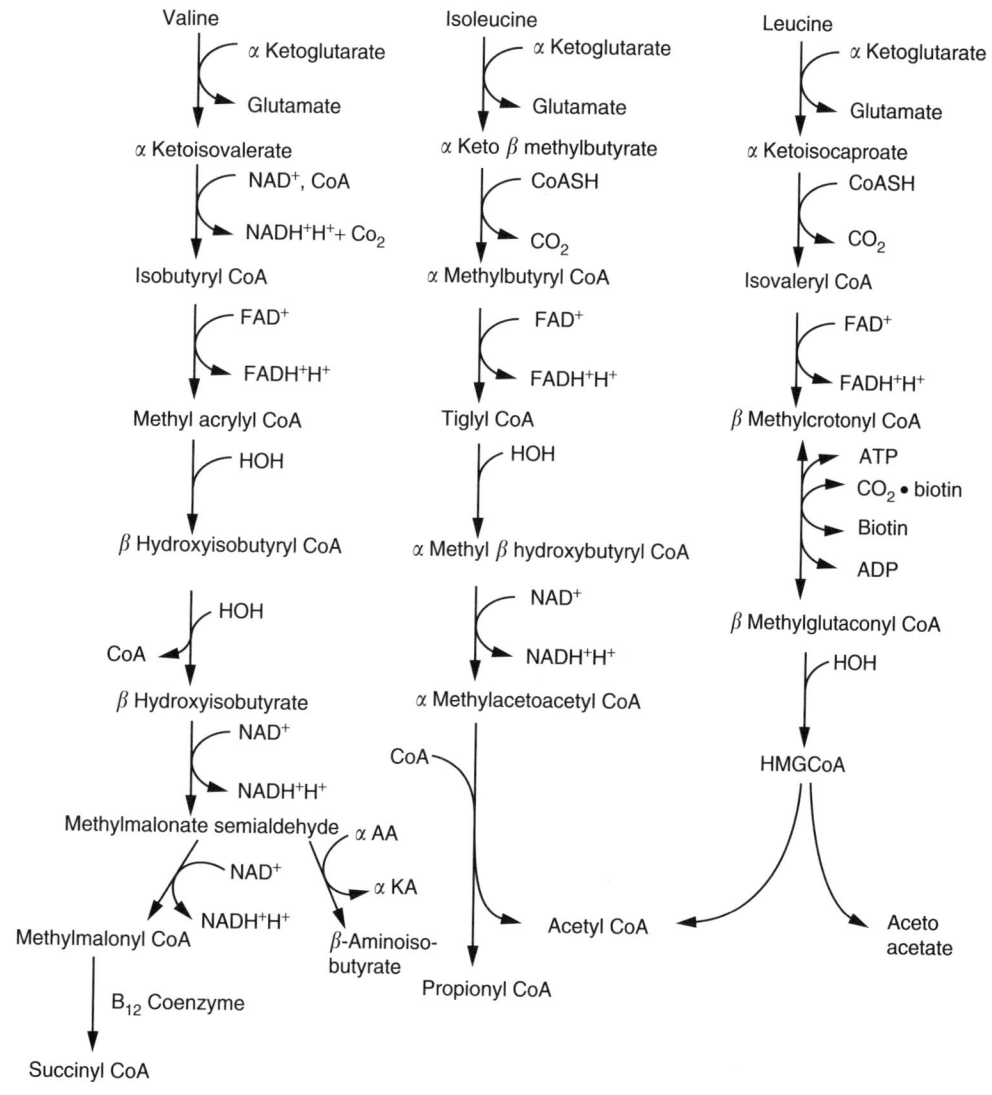

FIGURE 7.23   Degradation of valine, isoleucine and leucine

   The amino acids can be loosely grouped in terms of their catabolism. Valine, leucine, and isoleucine, the branched-chain amino acids, are similar in that each has a methyl group on its carbon chain. They can be transaminated with α-ketoglutarate to form α-keto acids. These acids are considered homologs of pyruvate and are oxidized by a series of enzymes that are similar to those that catalyze the oxidation of α-ketoglutarate and pyruvate. The degradative steps are shown in Figure 7.23. Valine ultimately is converted to succinyl CoA, whereas isoleucine ends up as either acetyl CoA or propionyl CoA, and leucine catabolism results in HMG CoA. HMG CoA is split to acetyl CoA and acetoacetate. The HMG CoA produced in the catabolism of leucine is not used for cholesterol synthesis because it is produced in the mitochondria and does not travel to the cytosol, where cholesterol is synthesized. Instead, HMG CoA is further metabolized to acetoacetate and acetyl CoA.
   Serine, threonine, and glycine are hydroxyamino acids. All three are gluconeogenic precursors. Serine can be deaminated to pyruvate, which then can be transaminated to alanine. Serine can also be demethylated to form glycine, releasing a methyl group useful in one-carbon metabolism. Threonine is degraded to acetyl CoA after deamination as shown in Figure 7.25. Glutamate may be converted to glutamine via the enzyme glutamine synthetase. This enzyme is a mitochondrial enzyme and serves to fix the ammonia released in this compartment. Rat renal tissue is particularly rich in this enzyme; however, human renal tissue is not. In birds and alligators this enzyme is a cytosolic enzyme rather than a mitochondrial enzyme. Although the brain has some urea cycle activity, it uses glutamine formation primarily to reduce its ammonia level. In order to do this, it must also synthesize glutamate from α-ketoglutarate. If it did not also convert pyruvate to oxalacetate, this synthesis of α-ketglutarate would deplete the brain of citric acid cycle intermediates. Fortunately, carboxylation of pyruvate is very active in brain tissue.
   Glutamate is converted to and formed from ornithine and arginine. These two amino acids are essential components of the urea cycle (Figure 7.26). The urea cycle consists of the synthesis of carbamyl phosphate, citrulline, and then arginosuccinate,

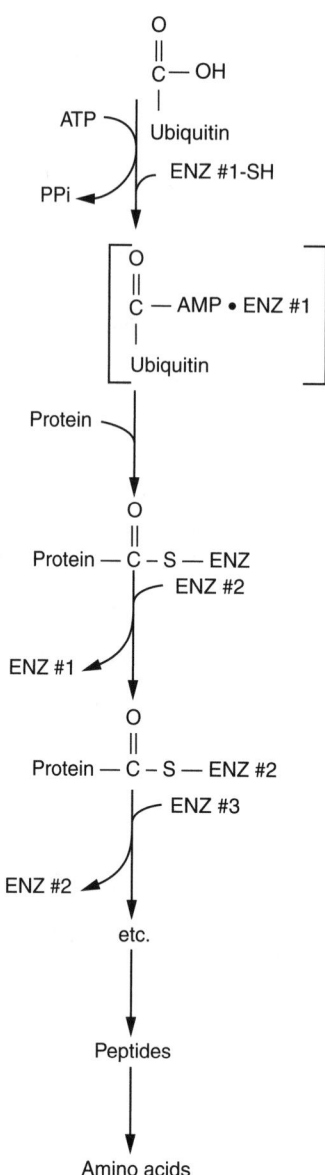

FIGURE 7.24 Protein degradation

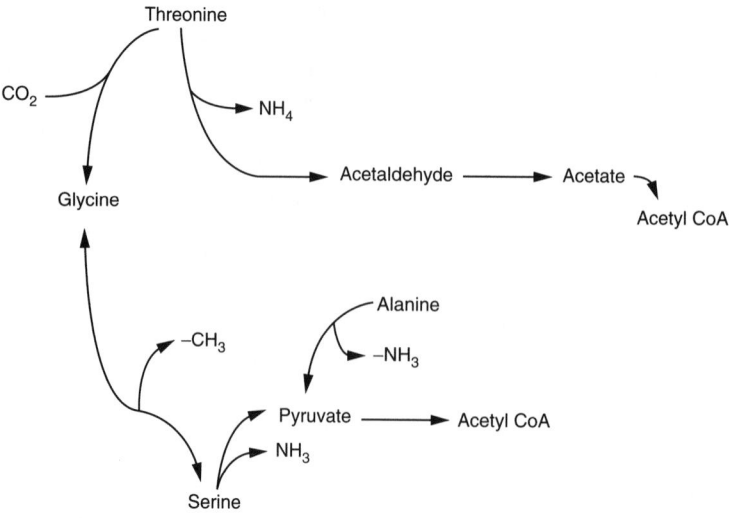

FIGURE 7.25 Serine, threonine, and glycine catabolism.

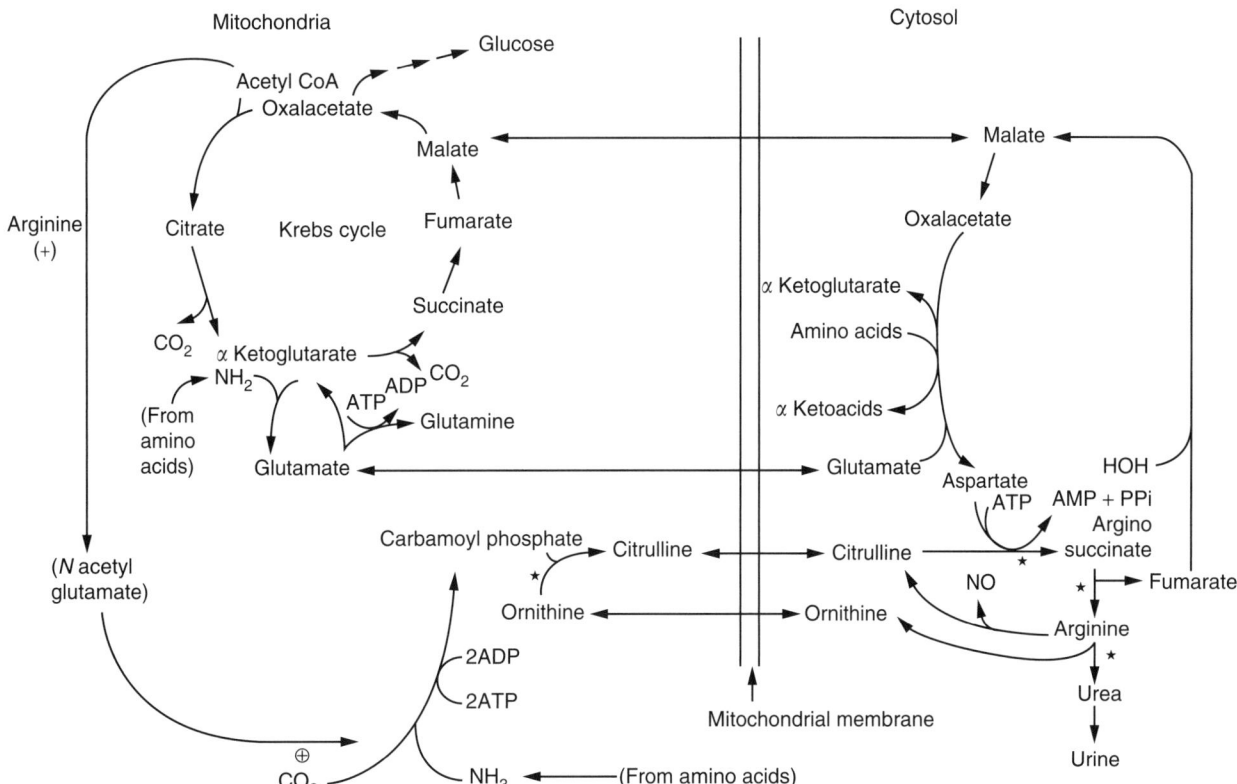

FIGURE 7.26 The urea cycle.

arginine, and finally urea. Ornithine and citrulline are shuttled back and forth as the cycle turns to get rid of the excess ammonia via urea release from arginine. The cycle functions to reduce the potentially toxic amounts of ammonia that arise when the ammonia group is removed from amino acids. Most of the ammonia released reflects the coupled action of the transaminases and L-glutamate dehydrogenase. The glutamate dehydrogenase is a bidirectional enzyme that plays a pivotal role in nitrogen metabolism. It is present in kidney, liver, and brain. It uses either NAD^+ or $NADP^+$ as a reducing equivalent receiver. It operates close to equilibrium using ATP, GTP, NADH, and ADP depending on the direction of the reaction. In catabolism, it channels NH_3 from glutamate to urea. In anabolism, it channels ammonia to α-ketoglutarate to form glutamate. In the brain, glutamate can be decarboxylated to form γ-aminobutyrate (GABA), an important neurotransmitter. The decarboxylation is catalyzed by the enzyme L-glutamate decarboxylase. Putrescine also can serve as a precursor of GABA either by deamination or via N-acetylated intermediates. The urea cycle is, energetically speaking, a very expensive process. The synthesis of urea requires 3 M of ATP for every mole of urea formed. The urea cycle is very elastic. That is, its enzymes are highly conserved, readily activated, and readily deactivated. Adaptation to a new level of activity is quickly achieved. While urea cycle activity can be high when protein rich diets are consumed and low when low protein diets are consumed, the cycle never shuts down completely. The cycle, shown in Figure 7.26, is fine-tuned by the first reaction, the synthesis of carbamoyl phosphate. This reaction, which occurs in the mitochondria, is catalyzed by the enzyme carbamoyl phosphate synthetase. The enzyme is inactive in the absence of its allosteric activator, N-acetylglutamate, a compound synthesized from acetyl CoA and glutamate in the liver. As arginine levels increase in the liver, N-acetylglutamate synthetase is activated, which results in an increase in N-acetylglutamate. The urea cycle is initiated in the hepatic mitochondria and finished in the cytosol. The urea is then liberated from arginine via arginase and released into the circulation, whereupon it is excreted from the kidneys in the urine. Ornithine, the other product of the arginase reaction, is recycled back to the mitochondrion only to be joined once again to carbamyl phosphate to make citrulline. Rising levels of arginine turn on mitochondrial N-acetylglutamate synthetase, which provides the N-acetylglutamate, which, in turn, activates carbamoyl phosphate synthetase, and the cycle goes on.

Arginine has many uses in metabolism. Not only is it an essential component of the urea cycle, it is precursor for nitric oxide (NO), the polyamines, proline, glutamate, and creatine. When citrulline is produced from arginine, NO is produced. This occurs not only in the liver but also in other vital organs and the vascular tree. NO production by endothelial cells is a vasodilator and thus plays a role in the regulation of smooth muscle tone. Many vasodilators such as the widely prescribed drug for angina pain, nitroglycerine, work by increasing the production of NO.

Phenylalanine is the precursor of tyrosine, and tyrosine can be used for the synthesis of thyroxine in the thyroid gland or for the synthesis of epinephrine, norepinephrine, or dopamine (see Figure 7.27). Phenylalanine is converted to tyrosine via

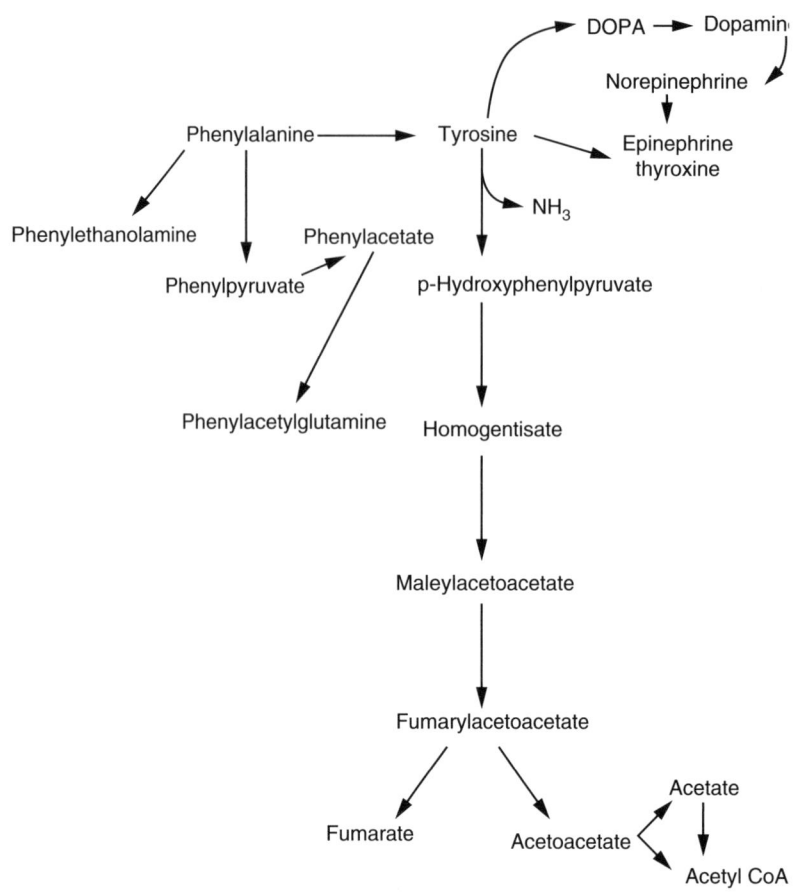

FIGURE 7.27   Phenylalanine and tyrosine catabolism.

the hepatic enzyme, phenylalanine hydroxylase. Tyrosine, if not used to make one of several hormones, is then deaminated and, through a series of reactions, ends up as fumarylacetate, which is split to provide acetoacetate and fumarate. Tryptophan catabolism shows no similarity to the catabolic pathways of any of the other amino acids (Figure 7.28). Tryptophan can be converted to niacin, one of the B vitamins. This conversion is not very efficient. There is considerable product feedback inhibition of this reaction sequence by niacin. The metabolism of tryptophan is dependent on adequate intakes of vitamin B_6, pyridoxine. In pyridoxine deficiency, hydroxyanthranilate formation via the enzyme kynureninase is impaired, resulting in a characteristic increase in urinary levels of xanthurenic acid. This is used as a test of vitamin B_6 sufficiency. If subjects are deficient and are given a load dose of tryptophan, these subjects will excrete abnormal amounts of xanthurenate in their urine. Tryptophan is the precursor of serotonin, an important neurotransmitter, that serves a variety of functions in the regulation of smooth muscle tone especially those smooth muscles of the vascular tree. Histidine, an amino acid especially important for muscle protein biosynthesis, is also of great importance in one-carbon metabolism. The principle pathway of histidine catabolism leads to glutamate formation and is shown in Figure 7.29 (as well as in other figures where glutamate and α-ketoglutarate act in transamination). Glutamate is an important component of the urea cycle (Figure 7.26). The decarboxylation of histidine yields histamine. This amine serves to stimulate gastric hydrochloric acid production and to stimulate vasoconstriction. A number of cold remedies and sinus remedies contain substances known as antihistamines, which interfere with the vasoconstrictor action of histamine. Histidine in muscle can be methylated and the end product 3-methyl histidine can be measured in the urine and used as a measure of muscle protein turnover.

Lysine is one of the two essential amino acids whose amino group does not contribute to the total body amino group pool; the other is threonine. Although lysine can donate its amino group to other carbon chains, the reverse does not occur. Lysine is catabolized to acetoacetyl CoA, which then enters the Krebs cycle as acetyl CoA.

Methionine, cysteine, and cystine are important sulfur group donors. The importance of disulfide bridges in the structure of proteins has been described in the sections on protein structure and synthesis. Methionine is important for carnitine synthesis. The pathway for methionine and cysteine is shown in Figure 7.30. Propionate is also the result of methionine catabolism. Should there be a defect in propionyl CoA carboxylase, propionate will accumulate. This is not the usual situation; for, propionate is usually carboxylated to form succinyl CoA. Accumulations of methyl malonate are characteristic of vitamin B_{12} deficiency. Propionate can serve as the substrate for long-chain odd-numbered fatty acids that are incorporated into myelin, the

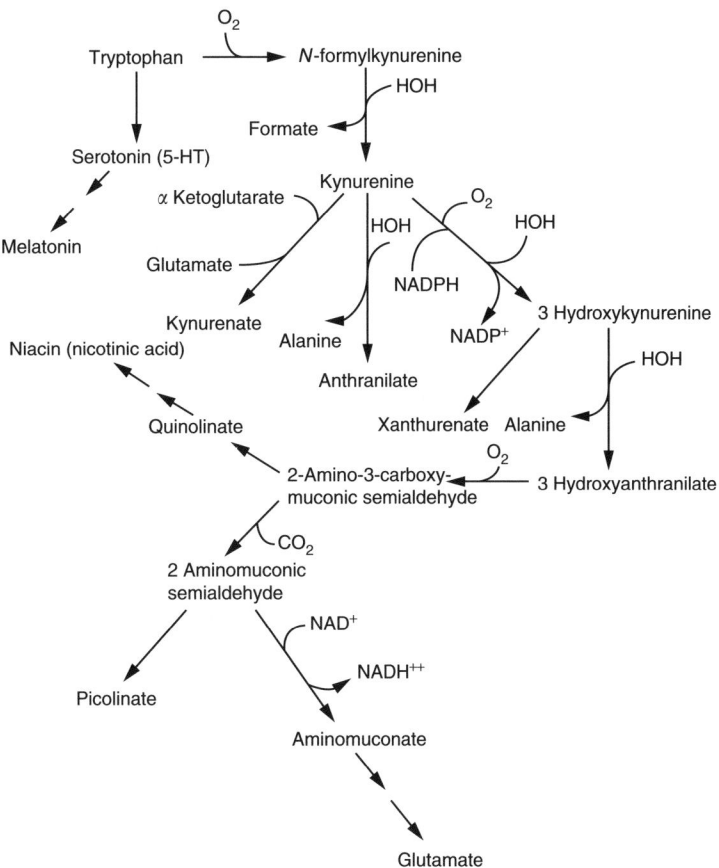

FIGURE 7.28 Tryptophan catabolism.

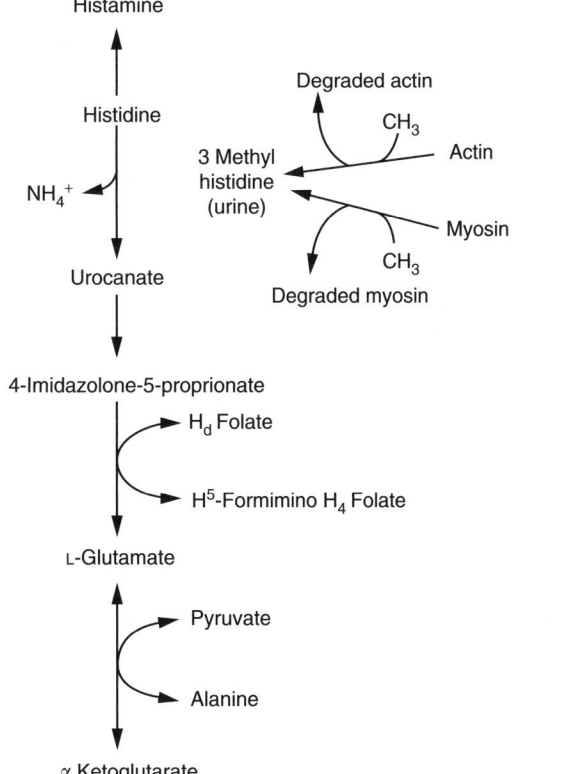

FIGURE 7.29 Histidine catabolism.

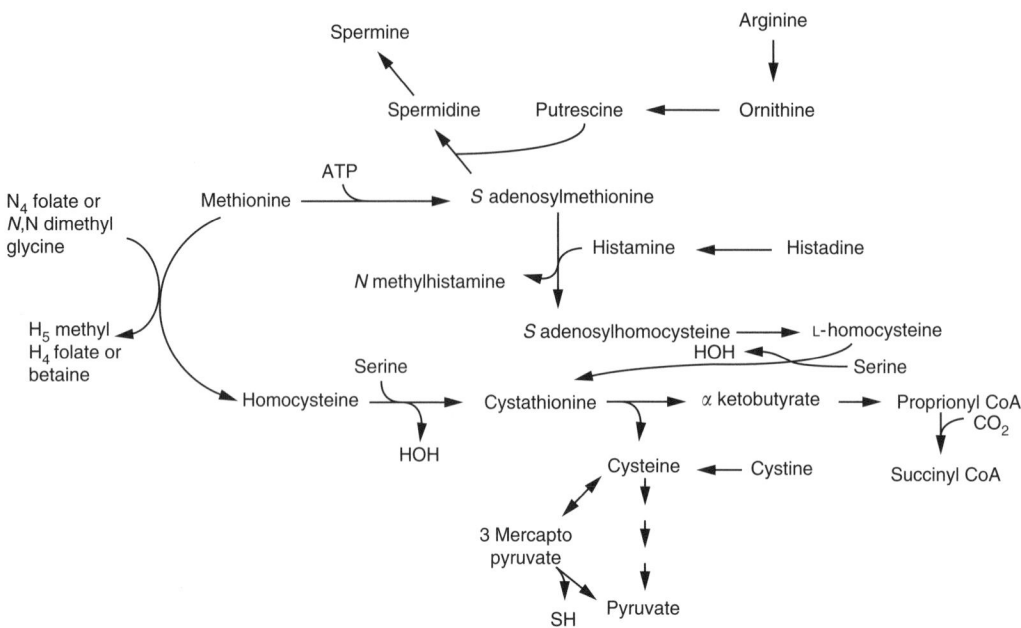

FIGURE 7.30 Methionine catabolism.

fatty covering of nerves. For some unknown reason, this myelin is abnormal in its function and fails to protect the peripheral nerve endings, which then die. This may explain the peripheral paresia that characterizes B_{12} deficiency.

AMINO ACID DERIVATIVES

Creatine phosphate is one of the amino acid derivatives that function in muscle contraction by providing energy for this process. Creatine is formed from glycine, arginine, and S-adenyl methionine in a reaction sequence. The creatine circulates in the blood and can be found in measurable quantities in brain and muscle. The creatine is phosphorylated to form creatine phosphate via the enzyme creatine phosphate. Creatine can be converted to creatinine by irreversible nonenzymatic dehydration. Upon hydrolysis, creatine phosphate will provide sufficient energy for muscle contraction. This hydrolysis yields creatine and inorganic phosphate. Some of the creatine can be rephosphorylated, while the remainder is converted to creatinine that then is excreted in the urine. Creatine phosphate has the same free energy of hydrolysis as ATP. Creatine phosphate is found primarily in the muscle and provides the quick burst of energy needed each time a muscle contracts. Because the muscle activity produces the end product, creatinine, measuring creatinine allows for the estimation of the muscle mass.

Choline is a highly methylated compound synthesized from serine. Choline is an essential component of the neurotransmitter acetylcholine as well as an essential ingredient of the phospholipid, phosphatidylcholine. Certain amino acids can be decarboxylated to form the polyamines. Some polyamines are very-short-lived compounds that are neurotransmitters. They are quickly broken down so as to limit their effects. The catecholamines fall into this category of polyamines. Other polyamines, putrescine and spermine, bind nucleic acids and other polyanions. They have a role in cell division.

ROLE OF VITAMINS AND MINERALS IN INTERMEDIARY METABOLISM

Vitamins (Table 7.8) and minerals (Table 7.9) are essential to life (see chapters 8–10). As described earlier, several of the vitamins as well as minerals are needed for the reaction sequences of intermediary metabolism. Niacin, thiamin, riboflavin, pyridoxine, and pantothenic acid (as part of the CoA molecule) all serve as coenzymes in these reactions. Ascorbic acid, vitamin E, and selenium function in the free radical suppression system. Magnesium, manganese, and other divalent ions serve as cofactors in a variety of reactions. Iron and copper function in the cytochromes and haemoglobin, both of which are essential to the use of oxygen. In the former, oxygen is used to make water by the respiratory chain, and in the latter, oxygen is transported to the cells for exchange for carbon dioxide. The synthesis of the purines and pyrmidines, components of DNA and RNA likewise demand that adequate micronutrients be present for this synthesis.

SYNTHESIS OF PURINES AND PYRIMIDINES

Before pyrimidines and purines can be incorporated into DNA and RNA, they must be synthesized. This synthesis requires a number of micronutrients as well as sufficient energy to support this synthesis. The purines are adenine and guanine, whereas the pyrimidines are cytosine, uracil, and thymine. Uracil is used for RNA synthesis, whereas thymine is used mainly for DNA synthesis. The purines and pyrimidines form glycosidic bonds to ribose. The purine pathway is shown in Figure 7.31. Also shown in Figure 7.31 are the vitamins and minerals needed at each step in the pathway. Where ATP is involved in a reaction step, all of the vitamins that serve as coenzymes in intermediary metabolism are needed. This includes niacin, thiamin, riboflavin, lipoic acid, pantothenic acid, biotin, folacin, vitamin B_{12}, pyridoxine, choline, and inositol. Also needed are the minerals of importance to the redox reactions of oxidative phosphorylation (OXPHOS), that is, iron, copper, and, of course, the iodine-containing hormone thyroxine, which regulates OXPHOS and the selenium-containing enzyme (5'-deiodinase), which converts thyroxine to its active form, triiodothyronine.

MICRONUTRIENTS AS STABILIZERS

Although vitamins and minerals serve in gene expression as just described, certain of the micronutrients have a unique role in assuring that cells and tissues continue to function as intact structures and that these cells continue to produce themselves faithfully. This role is that of protection from insult by peroxides. Peroxides are a normal product of metabolism. They are useful agents in the defense against pathogens. However, peroxides are very reactive substances. They can damage the membranes that are the physical barriers to the cells and the organelles within the cell. They can react with DNA. The DNA, enclosed within the nucleus, can repair itself. Occasionally this is a missense repair, and very occasionally this results in a mutation that is random. That is, the damage and subsequent missense repair can occur anywhere in the nuclear DNA and the resultant gene product could be one of more than a million products encoded by the nuclear genome. Peroxide or free radical damage to the nuclear genome is nowhere as serious on an individual genomic basis as damage to the mitochondrial genome. This genome encodes only 13 products, but these products are important components of the mitochondrial respiratory chain and ATP synthesis. The mitochondrial DNA does not have the repair capacity of the nuclear genome. In fact, its repair capacity is quite limited. When added to the fact that the mitochondria consume about 90% of all the oxygen consumed by the cell, the potential for free radical damage is quite large. Fortunately each cell has many hundred mitochondria, and so the loss of a few has little impact on the overall health and well-being of the cell or organ or whole animal. Nonetheless, should wholesale destruction of the genome occur, the results could be quite devastating.

Fortunately, there is a very active antioxidant system in place that protects against such damage. Some of the vitamins and minerals play an important role in this system. Vitamin E quenches free radicals as they form via the conversion of tocopherol

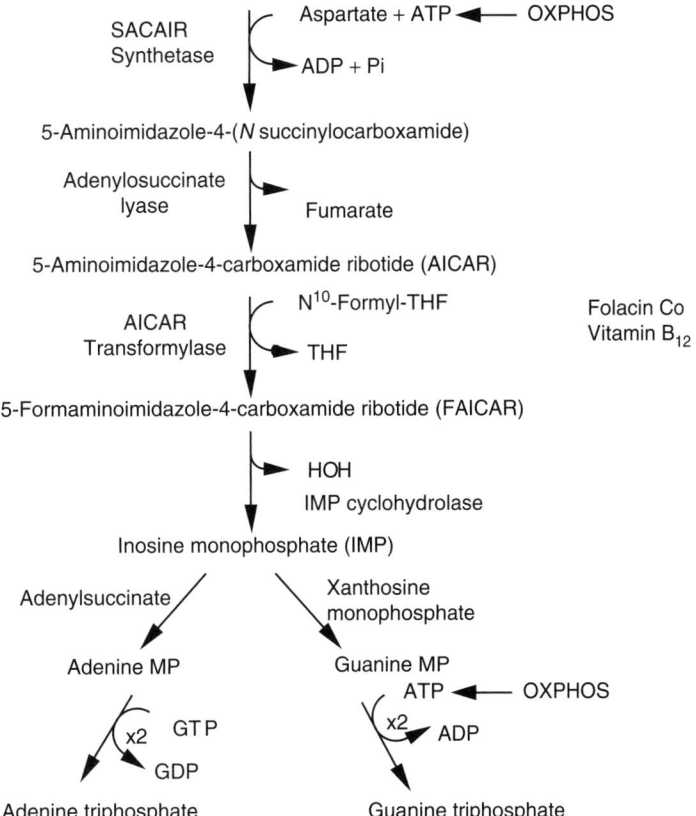

FIGURE 7.31 Roles of the micronutrients in the synthesis of purines.

TABLE 7.8
Summary of Vitamin Function

Vitamin	Functions
Fat-soluble vitamins	
Vitamin A	As retinaldehyde, is essential in the visual cycle
	Essential for body growth
	As retinoic acid, plays an important role in the expression of genes that encode a wide variety of body proteins that play roles in metabolism, growth, and development
	Downregulates uncontrolled cell growth
Vitamin D	Increases calcium and phosphorus absorption from the small intestine, thus promoting the growth and mineralization of bones
	Increases resorption of phosphates from the kidney tubules
	Maintains normal level of citrate in the blood
	Protects against the loss of amino acids through the kidneys
	Serves in gene regulation
Vitamin E	Serves as an antioxidant that protects body cells from free radicals damage
	Has a role in cellular respiration
Vitamin K	Essential for the posttranslational carboxylation of glutamic acid residues in osteocalcin and in four blood-clotting proteins: Factor II, prothrombin; Factor VII, proconvertin; Factor IX, Christmas factor; and Factor X, Stuart-Power. The carboxylation of glutamic acid residues increases calcium-binding activity of these proteins
Water-soluble vitamins	
Biotin	Functions as a coenzyme mainly in decarboxylation-carboxylation and in deamination reactions
Folacin/Folate (Folic Acid)	Serves as a coenzyme in synthesis of purines, pyrmidines, hemoglobin, and in the metabolism of several amino acids and vitamins: Serine to glycine, tyrosine from phenylalanine, glutamic acid from histadine, choline from ethanolamine, N-metylniccotinamide from nicotinamide
Niacin (Nicotinic acid or nicotinamide)	Serves as a coenzyme (NAD and NADP) in intermediary metabolism. These coenzymes function as reducing equivalent (H^+) acceptors or donors
Pantothenic acid	Functions as part of two enzymes — coenzyme A (CoA) and acyl carrier protein (ACP). Both of these are important in intermediary metabolism
Riboflavin	Serves as coenzymes FAD and FMN. These coenzymes accept or donate reducing equivalents.
Thiamin	As a coenzyme in transketolase reactions also has a role in the maintenance of normal appetite, muscle tone, and normal mental function
Vitamin B_6	Serves as a coenzyme (pyridoxal phosphate) in transamination
Pyridoxine; al; amine	Decarboxylation, and *trans*-sulfuration reactions; also is a coenzyme in the conversion of tryptophane to niacin, the absorption of amino acids, glycogenolysis and the elongation of linoleic acid to arachidonic acid
Vitamin B_{12} (cobalamins)	Synthesis or transfer of single carbon units, in the biosynthesis of methyl groups (–CH3), and in reduction reactions such as the conversion of disulfide (S–S) to the sulfhydryl group (–SH)
Vitamin C (ascorbic acid)	Functions in redox systems and aids in the regulation of redox states. This function is due to its interconversion between a reduced an oxidized state; plays a role in collagen synthesis (hydroxylation of proline to hydroxyproline)

See Chapter 9 and Chapter 10 for more information on vitamins and vitamin deficiencies.

to the tocopheroxyl radical, which is then converted to its quinone. Vitamin K, although not truly an antioxidant, does serve as an H^+/e^- donor/acceptor in its role to facilitate the carboxylation of the peptide glutamyl residues of certain proteins to their epoxide form. Vitamin C and vitamin A are both good H^+/e^- donor/acceptors in the suppression of free radical formation. Of course, indirectly, all those vitamins that serve as coenzymes are involved as well. Shown in Table 7.5 is the free radical suppression system. Note that selenium is complimentary to the role of vitamin E in the suppression of free radicals. Some of the antioxidant role for vitamin E could be met if there is a sufficient intake of selenium. This mineral is important to the gluta-thione peroxidase enzyme is an important component of the free radical suppression system. Selenium plays a role in both the synthesis of this enzyme and as a required cofactor. As discussed in Chapter 9, several of minerals and vitamins have roles in gene expression, and these roles have overall importance in the physiological function of the body.

TABLE 7.9

Essential Minerals and Their Functions

Mineral	Function
Macrominerals	
Sodium (Na+)	Participates in the regulation of osmotic pressure
	Functions in nerve conduction (depolarization/repolarization)
	Participates in active transport mechanisms as part of the plasma membrane Na+K+ ATPase
	Is part of the mineral apatite of bones and teeth
Calcium (Ca++)	Is an important part of the mineral apatite of bones and teeth
	Is an important cell signal with respect to metabolic regulation and the transport of metabolites (and some hormones) from one compartment to another or from one cell to the bloodstream
	Is a key mineral in cell death and in muscle contraction
Potassium (K+)	Participates in the regulation of osmotic pressure
	Participates in active transport mechanisms as part of the Na+K+ATPase
	Has a role in muscle contraction
Chloride (Cl+)	Participates in the regulation of osmotic pressure
	Is a part of gastric acid (HCl)
	Is a good oxidizing agent
	Participates in the exchange of oxygen for carbon dioxide
	Important to B_{12} absorption
Phosphorus	As a component of high-energy compounds (ATP, ADP, AMP, UTP [P as PO_4^{3-}], etc.) and phosphorylated metabolites
	Is a component of bones and teeth
	Serves as a component of nucleic acids (RNA and DNA)
Magnesium (Mg++)	Constituent of bones and teeth
	Essential element of cellular metabolism, often as an activator of enzymes involved in phosphorylated compounds and of high-energy phosphate transfer of ADP and ATP
	Involved in activating certain peptidases in protein digestion
	Relaxes nerve impulse, functioning antagonistically to calcium, which is stimulatory
Trace Minerals	
Cobalt (Co+++)	Serves as an integral part of Vitamin B_{12}
Copper (Cu++)	Facilitates the absorption and use of iron
	Essential for the formation of hemoglobin, although it is not a part of hemoglobin as such
	Cofactor for several enzymes
	Important for the development and maintenance of the vascular and skeletal structures (blood vessels, tendons, and bones)
	Structure and function of the central nervous system
	Required for normal pigmentation of hair
	Component of important copper-containing proteins
Fluorine (F-)	Constitutes 0.02 to 0.05% of the bones and teeth
	Necessary for sound bones and teeth
	Assists in the prevention of dental caries
Iodine (I-)	Serves as an important component of the thyroid hormones
Iron (Fe++ and Fe+++)	Iron (heme) combines with protein (globin) to make hemoglobin and the iron–sulfur components of the respiratory chain
Manganese (Mn++)	Formation of bone and the growth of other connective tissues
	Serves as a cofactor for SOD
Molybdenum (Mo)	Cofactor for iron and flavin-containing enzymes
Selenium (Se2+,4+,6+)	Component of the enzyme glutathione peroxidase
Zinc (Zn++)	Component of the zinc fingers of transcription agents
	Serves as a cofactor for more than 70 enzymes

See Chapter 8 for more information on the trace minerals and Chapter 64 for more information on the mineralization of bones.

SUMMARY

From the forgoing brief review of intermediary metabolism, it can be seen that nutrients in the diet function collectively and individually to maintain the health and well-being of the consumer. Subsequent chapters in this book will provide further information on particular aspects of the roles nutrition plays in a variety of situations from conception to death.

FURTHER SOURCES OF INFORMATION

Brody, T. *Nutritional Biochemistry*, Academic Press, San Diego, CA, 1994, 658 pages.

Berdanier, CD. *Advanced Nutrition: Micronutrients*, CRC Press, Boca Raton, FL, 1998, 236 pages.

Berdanier, CD. *Advanced Nutrition: Macronutrients*, 2nd edn, CRC Press, Boca Raton, FL, 2000, 327 pages.

Bender, DA. *Introduction to Nutrition and Metabolism* 3rd ed. CRC Press 2002 450 pages

8 Trace Mineral Deficiencies

Forrest H. Nielsen

CONTENTS

INTRODUCTION

By 1940, the concept of essential nutrients was well established; they were defined as chemical substances found in food, which could not be synthesized by the body to perform functions necessary for life. In the 1960s and 1970s, the standard for essentiality was liberalized for mineral elements that could not be fed at dietary concentrations low enough to cause death or interrupt the life cycle (interfere with growth, development, or maturation such that procreation is prevented). Thus, an essential element, during this time period, was generally defined as one whose dietary deficiency consistently and adversely changed a biological function from optimal, and this change was preventable or reversible by physiological amounts of the element. This definition of essentiality became less acceptable when numerous elements were suggested to be essential, based on small changes in physiological or biochemical variables. Many of these changes were questioned as to whether they were necessarily the result of suboptimal function, and sometimes were suggested to be the consequence of a pharmacologic or toxic action in the body, including an effect on intestinal microorganisms. As a result, if the lack of an element can not be shown to cause death or to interrupt the life cycle, the element is now not generally considered essential, unless it has a defined biochemical function. However, some elements (e.g., chromium) whose essentiality is based on older criteria are still often designated as essential in current literature. Other elements that have defined biochemical functions in lower species (e.g., nickel), or have been found to interrupt the life cycle in only a limited number of vertebrates (e.g., boron) and, only occasionally, are designated as essential. Thus, there is no universally accepted list of essential trace elements. Some elements (e.g., silicon, vanadium, etc.) have beneficial actions when supplemented in supranutritional amounts; these actions may be an indication of an essential function. Thus, because some mineral elements, other than those firmly established as essential, may be of nutritional importance; these possibly essential or beneficial elements are also discussed in this section.

BIOLOGICAL ROLES OF MINERAL ELEMENTS

Trace elements have at least five roles in living organisms. In close association with enzymes, some trace elements are integral parts of catalytic centers at which the reactions necessary for life occur. Working in concert with a protein, and frequently with other organic coenzymes, trace elements are involved in attracting substrate molecules and converting them into specific end products. Some trace elements donate or accept electrons in reactions of reduction or oxidation. In addition to the generation and utilization of metabolic energy, redox reactions frequently involve the chemical transformation of molecules. One trace element, iron, is involved in binding, transporting and releasing oxygen in the body. Some trace elements have structural roles; that is, imparting stability and three-dimensional structure to important biological molecules. Some trace elements have regulatory roles. They control important biological processes through actions such as making hormones active, facilitating the binding of molecules to receptor sites on cell membranes, altering the structure or ionic nature of membranes to prevent or allow specific molecules to enter a cell, and inducing gene expression.

HOMEOSTATIC REGULATION OF MINERAL ELEMENTS

Homeostasis is the term used to describe the ability of the body to maintain the content of a specific substance within a certain range despite varying intakes. Homeostasis involves the processes of absorption, storage, and excretion. The relative importance of these three processes varies among the trace elements. The amount absorbed from the gastrointestinal tract often is a primary controlling factor for trace elements needed in the cationic state such as copper, iron, and zinc. Trace elements absorbed as negatively charged anions such as boron and selenium are usually absorbed quite freely and completely from the gastrointestinal tract. Excretion through the urine, bile, sweat, and breath is, therefore, the primary mechanism for controlling the amount of these trace elements in an organism. By being stored in inactive sites, some trace elements are prevented from causing adverse reactions when present in high quantities. An example of this homeostatic process is the storage of iron as ferritin. Release of a trace element from a storage site also can be important in preventing deficiency.

FACTORS AFFECTING THE MANIFESTATION OF DEFICIENCY SIGNS

Although trace elements play key roles in a variety of processes necessary for life, except for iodine and iron, the occurrence of overt, simple, or uncomplicated deficiency of any trace element in humans is not a common occurrence. The reasons for this are the powerful homeostatic mechanisms for trace elements described above, and the consumption of diets with different types of foods from different sources. However, reductions in health and well-being due to suboptimal status in some trace elements probably are not uncommon, because of other factors affecting their metabolism or utilization. For example, inborn errors of metabolism and diseases that affect absorption, retention, or excretion of a trace element can result in deficiency, even though dietary intake may meet dietary guidelines. Thus, many trace elements become nutritional concerns when their metabolism or utilization is impaired or their need is increased by nutritional, metabolic, hormonal, or physiological stressors. For example, it is difficult to produce signs of simple selenium deficiency in animals or humans. A stressor such as vitamin E deficiency or viral infection is needed to obtain marked pathology such as that seen with Keshan disease, a cardiomyopathy that primarily affects children and women of child-bearing age in some areas of China.

TREATMENT OF MINERAL DEFICIENCIES

Regardless of whether they are essential or not, all mineral elements are toxic when ingested in high amounts. Thus, for most essential and possibly essential trace minerals, the Food and Nutrition Board of the Institute of Medicine[1-3] has set tolerable upper intake levels, which are defined as the maximum level of daily intake likely to pose no risk of adverse effects. The preferred way to treat or prevent trace mineral deficiencies is by consuming a variety of nutrient-dense foods. A diet based on the USDA Food Pyramid[4] is an example of one that is likely to provide trace minerals in adequate amounts. If it is decided that a mineral supplement is needed to overcome a deficiency or for "insurance" to prevent deficiency, consuming those that supply the Recommended Dietary Intake (RDA) or Adequate Intake (AI) of the mineral[1] should be adequate and result in intakes that do not exceed the upper intake level (UL). Higher amounts, however, may be indicated if a deficiency is caused by a factor causing malabsorption or excessive excretion of a mineral. These amounts should be adjusted to intakes that will maintain normal status after indicators of deficiency have abated.

MINERAL ELEMENTS ESSENTIAL FOR HUMANS

ESSENTIAL TRACE ELEMENTS

Trace elements essential for life are ones that generally occur in the body in micrograms per gram of tissue and are usually required by humans in milligrams per day amounts; these elements are copper, iron, manganese, and zinc. The evidence for essentiality for humans is substantial and not controversial for these elements. Specific biochemical functions have been found for each of these minerals. Because magnesium has many characteristics of a trace element, it also will be included in this group of elements. Another element that will be included is boron, because it is required to complete the life cycle of zebrafish[5] and frogs,[6] which suggests that it is essential for higher animals and humans.

Boron

Although it has not been definitively established that boron deficiency interrupts the life cycle of mammals, or has an essential biochemical function in humans, substantial evidence exists for boron being a bioactive food component that is beneficial, if not required, for optimal bone, neurological and immune function in higher animals and humans. Boron deprivation apparently has numerous physiological effects, because it influences the concentration and activity of numerous biochemical substances in tissues and fluids (see Table 8.1). These numerous responses to boron deprivation occur, because boron apparently acts at

TABLE 8.1
Biochemical, Clinical and Nutritional Aspects of Boron

Biological Function

Established	None
Hypothesized	• A metabolic regulator affecting cell membrane function that influences the responses to hormone action, transmembrane signaling, or transmembrane movement of regulatory cations or anions
	• A metabolic regulator, through complexing with a variety of substrate or reactant compounds which contain hydroxyl and amine groups in favorable positions. Regulation is mainly through an inhibitory effect on enzymes

Signs of Deficiency

Biochemical	Because boron apparently has a regulatory role, low dietary boron induces a variety, most likely indirect, of biochemical changes in humans. These include:
	• *Calcium metabolism*: decreased serum 25-hydroxycholecalciferol; increased serum calcitonin
	• *Energy metabolism*: increased serum glucose; decreased serum triglycerides
	• *Nitrogen metabolism*: increased blood urea; increased serum creatinine; decreased urinary hydroxyproline excretion
	• *Reactive oxygen metabolism*: decreased erythrocyte superoxide dismutase; decreased ceruloplasmin
	• *Response to estrogen*: decreased serum 17B-estradiol; decreased plasma copper
Physiological	Because boron can cause a variety of biochemical responses, it is not surprising that boron deprivation also has a variety of physiological effects. These include:
	• Altered electroencephalograms that suggest impaired behavior activation (e.g., more drowsiness) and decreased mental alertness
	• Impaired psychomotor skills
	• Impaired cognitive processes (e.g., attention and memory)
	• Increased platelet and erythrocyte numbers; decreased white blood cells
	A number of physiological signs of deficiency have been found in animals that may have some counterparts in humans. Reported signs include:
	• Impaired bone development and decreased bone strength
	• Impaired inflammatory and immune responses

Pathological Consequences of Deficiency

Established	None
Suggested	• Increased susceptibility to osteoporosis and arthritis
	• Impaired cognitive and psychomotor function
Predisposing Factors for Deficiency	• Stressors that affect hormone action or signal transduction at the cell membrane level including vitamin D deficiency and magnesium deficiency
	• Dietary changes that can increase oxidative stress at the cell membrane level such as high intakes of polyunsaturated fatty acids (e.g., omega-6 fatty acid-rich safflower oil)

Recommended Intakes

Prevention of deficiency	1.0 mg/day has been suggested[14]
Therapeutic or beneficial	Luxuriant intakes (e.g., ≥3 mg/day) *may* be beneficial when stressors are present that lead to osteoporotic or arthritic changes
Food Sources	Food and drink of plant origin, especially noncitrus fruits, leafy vegetables, nuts, pulses, wine, cider

the membrane level to affect the response to hormones, transmembrane signaling, and the movement of regulatory cations and anions. Thus, the numerous reported signs of boron deprivation, shown in Table 8.1, may be mostly secondary responses to an unidentified primary deficient or changed biochemical function at the cell membrane level. Indicators of boron status are still being established. However, plasma boron concentrations lower than 25 ng/ml may be indicative of a low boron status. Most of the information in Table 8.1 can be found in reviews by Nielsen,[7–10] Hunt,[11,12] and Penland.[13]

Copper

Although copper is well established as an essential trace element, its practical nutritional importance for healthy humans, and thus its dietary requirement, still is debated. Well-established consequences of copper deprivation in humans have come mainly from findings from special populations receiving nutrition from limited sources (e.g., parenteral nutrition solutions, milk, or formulas with no supplemental copper), consuming drugs (e.g., penicillamine) or undergoing dialysis resulting in excessive loss of copper, or having a genetic disorder (e.g., Menkes' disease) that results in defective copper metabolism. Other consequences of inadequate copper intakes for humans have been projected or hypothesized from epidemiological, animal, and short-term human copper deprivation studies. Most of the information found in Table 8.2 has been obtained from reviews by Harris,[15] Klevay and Medeiros,[16] Milne,[17] Cordano,[18] Uauy et al.,[19] and Failla et al.[20]

TABLE 8.2
Biochemical, Clinical and Nutritional Aspects of Copper

Biological Function	Copper is a cofactor for several oxidoreductase enzymes that are involved in the generation of oxidative energy, oxidation of ferrous iron, synthesis of neurotransmitters, bestowment of pigment to hair and skin, provision of strength to bones and arteries, assurance of competence of the immune system, and stabilization of the matrices of connective tissues. These enzymes include: amine oxidase, lysyl oxidase, ferroxidase (ceruloplasmin), dopamine B-monooxygenase, tyrosinase, alpha-amidating monooxygenase, cytochrome c oxidase, and superoxide dismutase. Thus, copper is essential for several fundamental processes, including angiogenesis, neuropeptide and neurohormone signaling, iron metabolism, oxygen transport, energy production and the regulation of genetic expression
Signs of Deficiency	
Biochemical	• Decreased plasma copper • Short-term human copper depletion studies have inconsistently resulted in several biochemical changes, including decreased erythrocyte superoxide dismutase • Decreased enzymatic and immunoreactive ceruloplasmin and ratio • Decreased platelet and mononuclear white cell cytochrome c oxidase • Increased plasma cholesterol; and decreased interleukin-2
Physiological	Copper deficiency in premature and malnourished infants and infants with Menkes' disease has established numerous physiological deficiency signs including: • hematologic changes characterized by hypochromic, normocytic, or macrocytic anemia accompanied by reduced reticulocyte count, neutropenia and thrombocytopenia • bone abnormalities that mimic scurvy, for example, osteoporosis, fractures of the long bones and ribs, epiphyseal separation, fraying and cupping of the metaphyses with spur formation, and subperiosteal new bone formation • hypopigmentation of hair • impaired growth • impaired immunity • impaired neurological function
Pathological Consequences of Deficiency	
Established	• *Premature and malnourished infants*: anemia, osteoporosis, bone fractures, poor growth, and increased incidence of infections • *Menkes' disease*: "Kinky-type" steely hair, progressive neurological disorder, death
Suggested	• *Fetus and children*: impaired brain development[21] • *Adults*: Osteoporosis,[22] ischemic heart disease,[23–25] increased susceptibility to infections,[26] and accelerated aging[27]
Predisposing Factors for Deficiency	
Impaired absorption	High intakes of zinc, celiac disease, short bowel syndrome, cystic fibrosis, diarrhea, and jejunoileal bypass surgery
Excessive loss	Peritoneal dialysis, burn trauma, penicilliamine therapy, dexamethasone treatment, and excessive use of antacids
Increased oxidative stress	High iron intake or iron overload and marginal zinc deprivation

Continued

TABLE 8.2
(Continued)

Recommended Intakes	
Prevention of deficiency	RDAs (and AIs) set by the Food and Nutrition Board[3] (mg/day) are: infants age 0–0.5 year, (0.20) and age 0.5–1 year, (0.22); children age 1–3 years, 0.34 and age 4–8 years, 0.44; adolescents age 9–13 years, 0.70 and age 14–18 years, 0.89; adults, 0.90; pregnancy, 1.0; lactation, 1.3
Therapeutic or beneficial	Increased intakes of copper (e.g., 3 mg/day for adults) *may* be beneficial for preventing osteoporosis, overcoming the adverse effects of high zinc intake, and more quickly overcoming the consequences of copper deficiency
Food Sources	Legumes, whole grains, nuts, organ meats (e.g., liver), seafood (e.g., oysters, crab), peanut butter, chocolate, mushrooms, and ready-to-eat cereals

TABLE 8.3
Biochemical, Clinical and Nutritional Aspects of Iron

Biological Function	Iron is involved in oxygen transport and storage, electron transport, and in numerous enzymatic reactions involving substrate oxidation and reduction. The classes of enzymes dependent on iron for activity include the oxidoreductases (e.g., xanthine oxidase/dehydrogenase), monooxygenases (e.g., cytochrome P450), dioxygenases (e.g., amino acid or amine dioxygenases), lipoxygenases, peroxidases, fatty acid desaturases, nitric oxide synthases, and miscellaneous enzymes such as aconitase
Signs and Symptoms of Deficiency	
Biochemical	Decreased tissue and blood iron enzymes, myoglobin, hemoglobin, ferritin, transferrin saturation, and iron, and increased erythrocyte protoporphyrin
Physiological	Anemia, glossitis, angular stomatitis, spoon nails (koiloncychia), blue sclera, lethargy, apathy, listlessness, and fatigue
Pathological Consequences of Deficiency	
Established	Impaired thermoregulation, immune function, mental function and physical performance; complications in pregnancy including increased risk of premature delivery, low birth weight, and infant morbidity
Suggested	Osteoporosis,[30–32] and impaired brain development[33]
Predisposing Factors for Deficiency	Blood loss (e.g., menstruation) and vegetarian diets
Recommended Intakes	
Prevention of deficiency	RDAs (and AIs) set by the Food and Nutrition Board[3] for iron (mg/day) are: infants age 0–0.5 year, (0.27) and age 0.5–1 year, 11; children age 1–3 years, 7, and age 4–8 years, 10; adolescents age 9–13 years, 8, males age 14–18 years, 11, and females age 14–18 years, 15; males age ≥19 years, 8; females age 19–50 years, 18, age >50 years, 8, pregnant, 27, lactating age ≤18 years, 10, and age >19 years, 9
Therapeutic or beneficial	Higher doses than the above can be given to more quickly overcome iron deficiency, usually caused by blood loss; doses used include 50 to 60 mg/day or 120 mg/week.[34,35] However, caution is in order because high intakes of iron have been associated with cardiovascular disease and cancer[3,36]
Food Sources	Red meat, organ meats (e.g., liver), seafood (e.g., oysters, shrimp), fortified cereals, potatoes with skin, tofu; some whole grains and vegetables (e.g., spinach) are high in iron but the bioavailability of this iron may be low

Iron

Among the mineral nutrients, iron has the longest and best-documented history. Despite long and effective intervention activities, iron deficiency is the most prevalent mineral deficiency in the United States and the world. Recently, it has been suggested that high intakes of iron also may be a health concern. Table 8.3 only briefly outlines some of the important aspects of iron nutrition which has been obtained from reviews by Beard and Dawson[28] and Baynes and Stipanuk.[29]

Magnesium

Magnesium is the fourth most abundant cation in the human body, and is second only to potassium in intracellular concentration. This concentration reflects that magnesium is critical for a great number of cellular functions including oxidative phosphorylation, glycolysis, DNA transcription, fatty acid degradation, and protein synthesis. Although it is such a critically important element, surprisingly, reported signs and symptoms of magnesium deficiency in humans through dietary restriction alone are very limited. Described cases of clinical magnesium deficiency have generally been conditioned deficiencies where factors interfering with absorption or promoting excretion were present (see Table 8.4). However, short-term human magnesium depletion experiments suggest that low magnesium intakes similar to those consumed by a significant number of people may induce heart arrhythmias and soft tissue calcium retention that may exacerbate disorders induced by oxidative stress.[37-39] Table 8.4 briefly outlines some of the important aspects of magnesium deficiency, most of which were obtained from reviews by Rude[40] and Shils.[41]

Manganese

The essentiality of manganese for animals has been known for over 50 years. Deficiency causes testicular degeneration (rats), slipped tendons (chicks), osteodystrophy, severe glucose intolerance (guinea pigs), ataxia (mice, mink), depigmentation of hair, and seizures. However, descriptions of signs of manganese deficiency in humans are very limited. The most convincing case of manganese deficiency is that of a child with a postoperative short bowel on long-term parenteral nutrition with low manganese content. The child developed short stature and diffuse bone demineralization resulting in brittle bones.[56] Because manganese deficiency has been so difficult to identify in humans, it is generally not considered to be of great nutritional concern. Most of the information in Table 8.5 has been obtained from reviews by Leach and Harris,[57] Nielsen,[58] and Freeland-Graves and Llanes.[59]

Zinc

Signs of zinc deficiency in humans were first described in the 1960s. However, the prevalence of zinc deficiency is still unknown because of the lack of satisfactory indicators of zinc status. Zinc supplementation studies indicate that a mild zinc deficiency

TABLE 8.4
Biochemical, Clinical and Nutritional Aspects of Magnesium

Biological Function	Magnesium is a cofactor for more than 300 enzymes in the body. This cofactor role is either as a direct allosteric activator of enzymes or as a part of enzyme substrates for some enzyme reactions (e.g., MgATP and MgGTP). Magnesium also has functions that affect membrane properties and thus influences potassium and calcium channels and nerve conduction
Signs and Symptoms of Deficiency	
Biochemical	• Low blood potassium, calcium and magnesium
	• Decreased intracellular potassium
	• Excessive renal potassium excretion
	• Impaired parathyroid hormone secretion and vitamin D metabolism
	• Renal and skeletal resistance to parathyroid hormone
Physiological	• Neuromuscular signs (e.g., positive Trousseau's signs, tremors, fasiculations, gross muscle spasms, muscle cramps and weakness, seizures, dizziness, disequilibrium)
	• Electrocardiographic abnormalities
	• Cardiac arrhythmias (e.g., rapid heart rate, ventricular premature discharges, atrial and ventricular fibrillation)
Pathological Consequences of Deficiency	
Established	Conditioned deficiencies result in cardiac arrhythmias, seizures, cramps, depression, and psychosis
Suggested	Based on numerous epidemiological studies and magnesium supplementation trials, low magnesium status is associated with numerous disorders including coronary heart disease,[42,43] hypertension,[44-46] diabetes,[46,47] various types of headaches,[48-50] pain sensitivity,[51] some cancers,[52] nephrolithiasis,[53] and osteoporosis[54]
Predisposing Factors for Deficiency	Factors interfering with absorption and utilization or promoting excretion including alcoholism, kidney failure, malabsorption syndromes, extensive bowel resection, gastroileal bypass, severe or prolonged diarrhea, protein-calorie malnutrition, acute pancreatitis, hyperaldosteronism, diabetes mellitus, thyroid gland disease, parathyroid gland disease, vitamin D resistance or deficiency, burns, and diuretic therapy
Recommended Intakes	
Prevention of deficiency	RDAs (and AIs) set by the Food and Nutrition Board[1] for magnesium (mg/day) are: infants age 0–0.5 year, (30) and age 0.5–1 year, 75; children age 1–3 years, 80, age 4–8 years, 130 and age 9–13 years, 240; males age 14–18 years, 410, age 19–30 years, 400, and age 31+ years, 420; females age 14–18 years, 360, age 19–30 years, 310, age 31+ years, 320, pregnant, +40
Therapeutic or beneficial	Infusion of magnesium has been indicated as a means to quickly overcome a magnesium deficiency. An effective treatment[55] has been found to be intravenous administration of 24 mmol of magnesium as a 50% solution over 24 h for 3 to 7 days. Patients who are hypomagnesemic and have seizures or an acute dysrhythmia may be given 4 to 8 mmol of magnesium over 5 to 10 min followed by the same regimen
Food Sources	Whole grains, nuts, legumes, green leafy vegetables

TABLE 8.5
Biochemical, Clinical and Nutritional Aspects of Manganese

Biological Function	Manganese is a cofactor for enzymes involved in protein and energy metabolism, antioxidant action, and mucopolysaccharide synthesis. These enzymes include the metalloenzymes manganese-dependent superoxide dismutase, pyruvate carboxylase and arginase, and the manganese-activated enzymes phosphoenolpyruvate carboxykinase, glycosyl transferases, glutamine synthetase and farnesyl pyrophosphate synthetase. Manganese also can activate numerous other enzymes including oxidorectases, lyases, ligases, hydrolases, kinases, decarboxylases, and transferases; these enzymes are activated by other metals, especially magnesium
Signs of Deficiency	
Biochemical	None firmly established
Physiological	Impaired growth and brittle bones (found in one child); another possible sign is a fleeting dermatitis
Pathological Consequences of Deficiency	
Established	Osteoporosis (one case report in a child)[56]
Suggested	Low dietary manganese or low blood and tissue manganese has been associated with osteoporosis, diabetes, epilepsy, atherosclerosis, cataracts, and impaired wound healing[60]
Predisposing Factors for Deficiency	High dietary intakes of calcium, phosphorus, iron, fiber, phytate, and polyphenolic compounds. (Based on human absorption experiments and animal studies)
Recommended Intakes	
Prevention of deficiency	AIs set by the Food and Nutrition Board[3] for manganese (mg/day) are: infants age 0–0.5 year, 0.003, and age 0.5–1 year, 0.6; children age 1–3 years, 1.2, and age 4–8 years, 1.5; males age 9–13 years, 1.9, age 14–18 years, 2.2, and age ≥19 years, 2.3; females age 9–18 years, 1.6, age ≥ 19 years, 1.8, pregnant, 2.0, and lactating, 2.6
Therapeutic or beneficial	Caution is indicated against high intakes of manganese because of potential neurotoxicological effects,[61,62] especially in people with compromised homeostatic mechanisms, or infants whose homeostatic control of manganese is not fully developed
Food Sources	Unrefined grains, nuts, green leafy vegetables, and tea

that results in growth retardation or impaired immune function may be quite prevalent. Unquestionable zinc deficiency has been induced by providing zinc deficient total parenteral nutrition, and by feeding cow's milk to infants who have a genetic inability to absorb zinc from such a source. The information in Table 8.6 primarily comes from reviews by Chesters,[63] Prasad,[64] and Dibley.[65]

ESSENTIAL ULTRA TRACE ELEMENTS

In 1980, the term *ultra trace elements* began to appear in the nutritional literature; the term was defined as an element required by animals in amounts of 50 ng or less per gram of diet. For humans, the term has been used recently to indicate elements with established or estimated requirements quantified by micrograms per day.[58] There are four essential ultra trace elements. The evidence of essentiality for humans is substantial and not controversial for cobalt, iodine, molybdenum, and selenium; specific biochemical functions have been identified for each. Another element, chromium, in the past has been considered an essential ultra trace element, and thus is included in this section. However, it should be noted that a critical review of the findings suggesting essentiality reveal that chromium is unable to meet any definition of essentiality[75–77] and probably belongs in the possibly essential ultra trace element category.

Chromium

Flaws in the early studies of chromium nutrition inhibited the acceptance of chromium as an essential nutrient until 1977. In that year, it was reported that signs of chromium deficiency were found in a patient receiving long-term total parenteral nutrition thought to be low in chromium. This patient developed impaired glucose tolerance and a resistance to insulin, which were reversed by an infusion of chromium.[78] However, skepticism about the nutritional essentiality of chromium began in 1980 when it was found that chromium analyses before then were not valid, and repeated efforts to definitively characterize a chromium-containing glucose tolerance factor were unsuccessful. At present, a clearly defined biochemical function has not been established for chromium. Neither has a chromium deficiency been induced in any animal species that causes death or interrupts the life cycle. Chromium is also unable to meet the older criteria of essentiality, because a consistent reduction in a biological function from optimal that is prevented by physiological amounts of chromium has not been conclusively demonstrated. This inability to fulfill the requirements to be classified as essential does not preclude the possibility that chromium may be found essential in the future. There is no question, however, about chromium being a bioactive beneficial element; supranutritional

TABLE 8.6
Biochemical, Clinical and Nutritional Aspects of Zinc

Biological Function	Zinc has catalytic, structural, and regulatory functions. Zinc is unique in that it is the only trace element with essential actions in all six enzyme classes. Zinc is required for catalytic activity of >300 enzymes. Zinc stabilizes the tertiary structure of some enzymes and also imparts stability to cell membranes. Zinc has a function as a component of transcription factors also known as zinc finger proteins that bind to DNA and activate transcription of a message
Signs of Deficiency	
Biochemical	Decreased plasma, leukocyte, erythrocyte, hair and saliva zinc; plasma metallothionein, thymulin and alkaline phosphatase; extracellular superoxide dismutase; and T-helper cell production of interlukin-2 and interferon-γ.[63–67] Increased plasma 5'-nucleotidase, platelet amyloid precursor protein, and lymphocyte mRNA ZIP1 (a zinc transporter) expression[63–67]
Physiological	Depressed growth; anorexia; parakeratotic skin lesions; diarrhea; and impaired testicular development, immune function, and cognitive function
Pathological Consequences of Deficiency	
Established	Dwarfism, delayed puberty, failure to thrive (acrodermatitis enteropathica infants), mental lethargy, hypogueusia (poor taste), impaired dark adaptation, impaired wound healing, and increased susceptibility to infectious disease
Suggested	Osteoporosis, infertility, impaired neuropsychological function, and increased susceptibility to diabetes, cancer, Alzheimer disease, and rheumatic disease, especially rheumatoid arthritis[64,68–73]
Predisposing Factors for Deficiency	• Factors causing impaired absorption including phytate, vegetarianism, intestinal infestation by bacteria, protozoa and helminthes, gastric and intestinal resection, inflammatory bowel disease, exocrine pancreatic insufficiency, bilary obstruction, and high intakes of zinc, copper and iron • Factors causing excessive loss, including protein-losing enteropathies, renal failure, renal dialysis, chronic blood loss (e.g., sickle cell disease), and exfoliative dermatoses • Factors inducing increased need including rapid tissue synthesis and postcatabolic convalescence
Recommended Intakes	
Prevention of deficiency	RDAs (and AIs) set by the Food and Nutrition Board[3] for zinc (mg/day) are: infants age 0–0.5 year, 2 (AI) and age 0.5–1 year, 3; children age 1–3 years, 3, and age 4–8 years, 5; males age 9–13 years, 8, and age ≥14 years, 11; females age 9–13 years, 8, age 14–18 years, 9, age ≥19 years, 8, pregnant age ≤18 years, 12, and age ≥19 years, 11, lactating age ≤18 years, 13, and age ≥19 years, 12
Therapeutic or beneficial	High zinc intakes have been used for the alleviation and prevention of colds, treatment of macular degeneration, acute diarrhea and Wilson's disease; doses have ranged from 20 mg/day for children with diarrhea to 150 mg/day for treatment of Wilson's disease[64,74]
Food Sources	Red meats, organ meats (e.g., liver), shellfish, nuts, legumes

amounts of chromium enhance insulin sensitivity or action. The information in Table 8.7 comes primarily from reviews by Offenbacher et al.[79] Nielsen,[80] Vincent,[81] and Cefalu and Hu.[82]

Cobalt

Ionic cobalt is not an essential nutrient for humans; however, vitamin B_{12}, in which cobalt is an integral component, is an essential nutrient for humans. In the nineteenth century, a megaloblastic anemia was described that was called pernicious anemia, because it was invariably fatal. The first effective treatment for this disease was 1 lb of raw liver daily. In 1948, the antipernicious anemia factor in liver was isolated and named vitamin B_{12}, and was found to contain 4% cobalt. Vitamin B_{12} deficiency is rarely caused by a dietary insufficiency and most commonly arises from a defect in vitamin B_{12} absorption. People with low vitamin B_{12} status (e.g., vegetarians) can also display signs of deficiency if stressed with a substance such as nitrous oxide (used in dentistry), which destroys vitamin B_{12}. Most of the information in Table 8.8 was obtained from reviews by Smith,[83] Shane,[84] and Stabler.[85]

Iodine

Recognition that iodine is nutritionally important began in the 1920s when it was found that iodine prevented goiter and increased iodine intake was associated with decreased endemic cretinism. The consequences of iodine deficiency, which is common, are so profound that it is one of the largest public health problems in the world today. Iodine deficiency is most prevalent in areas of high new mountains (e.g., Himalayas, Andes, and Alps), areas of frequent flooding, rainfall, and sublimation (e.g., Ganges river plain of northeastern India, Taklamakan desert of western China, and central sub-Saharan Africa), and inland areas of central and Eastern Europe. Most of the information in Table 8.9 has been obtained from reviews by Hetzel and Wellby,[87] Freake,[88] and Stanbury and Dunn.[89]

TABLE 8.7
Biochemical, Clinical and Nutritional Aspects of Chromium

Biological Function	
Established	None
Hypothesized	As part of a low-molecular-weight chromium-binding organic complex (LMWCr), chromium enhances insulin sensitivity or action. A naturally occurring biologically active LMWCr called chromodulin has been described as an oligopeptide of about 1500 Da that binds four chromic ions. *In vitro* findings have resulted in the hypothesis that chromodulin acts in a unique autoamplification system for insulin signaling
Signs of Deficiency	
Biochemical	Based on the response to relatively high amounts of parenteral chromium by some patients, biochemical signs of chromium deficiency *may* be elevated serum glucose, cholesterol, triglycerides and insulin; glycosuria; decreased insulin binding and insulin receptor number
Physiological	Based on the response to relatively high amounts of parenteral chromium by a few patients, physiological signs of chromium deficiency *may* be impaired glucose tolerance, weight loss, neuropathy, and encephalopathy
Pathological Consequences of Deficiency	
Established	None
Suggested	Impaired glucose tolerance, diabetes, and atherosclerosis
Predisposing Factors for Deficiency	Factors that promote urinary excretion including acute strenuous exercise, physical trauma, and high dietary sugar. Factors that inhibit absorption including phytate and drugs that reduce stomach acidity (e.g., antacids)
Recommended Intakes	
Prevention of deficiency	AIs set by the Food and Nutrition Board[3] for chromium (μg/day) are: infants age 0–0.5 year, 0.2, and age 0.5–1 year, 5.5; children age 1–3 years, 11, and age 4–8 years, 15; males age 9–13 years, 25, age 14–50 years, 35, and age $\geq$51 years, 30; females age 9–13 years, 21, age 14–50 years, 25, age $\geq$51 years, 20, pregnant age $\leq$18 years, 29, and age $\geq$19 years, 30, lactating age $\leq$18 years, 44, and age $\geq$19 years, 45
Therapeutic or beneficial	Doses of 200 to 1000 μg/day of chromium, especially as an organic complex (e.g., chromium picolinate), have been shown to enhance the action of low amounts of insulin or improve the efficacy of insulin such that the need for exogenous sources was reduced or eliminated, plasma glucose was decreased, and HbA$_{1c}$ (glycosylated hemoglobin) was decreased in some persons with type I, type II, gestational and steroid-induced diabetes
Food Sources	Whole grains, pulses (e.g., dried beans), some vegetables (including broccoli and mushrooms), liver, processed meats, ready-to-eat cereals, and spices

TABLE 8.8
Biochemical, Clinical and Nutritional Aspects of Cobalt

Biological Function	Vitamin B$_{12}$ is a cofactor for two enzymes, methionine synthase which methylates homocysteine to form methionine, and methyl-malonyl CoA mutase, which converts L-methylmalonyl CoA, formed by the oxidation of odd-chain fatty acids, to succinyl CoA
Signs of Deficiency	
Biochemical	Decreased erythrocyte and plasma folate and plasma vitamin B$_{12}$, and increased plasma homocysteine and urinary formiminogluta-mate and methylmalonate
Physiological	Megaloblastic anemia; spinal cord demyelination and peripheral neuropathy
Pathological Consequences of Deficiency	
Established	Pernicious anemia, memory loss, dementia, irreversible neurological disease called subacute degeneration of the spinal cord, and death.
Suggested	Cardiovascular disease associated with elevated plasma homocysteine
Predisposing Factors for Deficiency	• Factors causing malabsorption including Type A atrophic gastritis, *Helicobacter pylori* infection, GI bacteria overgrowth caused by achlorhydria and intestinal blind loops, total gastrectomy leading to loss of intrinsic factor excretion, pancreatic insufficiency, and celiac disease • Factors inhibiting utilization including drugs such as histamine H$_2$ receptor antagonists, proton pump inhibitors, oral biguanides (used in the treatment of type II diabetes), and nitrous oxide anesthesia • Vegetarian diets
Recommended Intakes	
Prevention of deficiency	RDAs (and AIs) set by the Food and Nutrition Board[86] for vitamin B$_{12}$ (μg/day) are: infants age 0–0.5 year, (0.4) and age 0.5–1 year, (0.5); children age 1–3 years, 0.9, age 4–8 years, 1.2, and age 9–13 years, 1.8; males age $\geq$14 years, 2.4; females age $\geq$14 years, 2.4, pregnant, 2.6, and lactating, 2.8
Therapeutic or beneficial	Milligram doses are used to treat vitamin B$_{12}$ malabsorption and deficiency; a common dose is 1 mg/day of cobalamin
Food Sources	Meat, dairy products, some sea foods, and fortified cereals

TABLE 8.9
Biochemical, Clinical and Nutritional Aspects of Iodine

Biological Function	Iodine has only one function; it is a component of thyroid hormones. However, thyroid hormones have an impact on a wide range of metabolic and developmental functions
Signs of Deficiency	
Biochemical	Decreased plasma or serum thyroxine (T_4) and triiodothyronine (T_3), and urinary iodine, and increased plasma or serum thyroid stimulating hormone (TSH) and cholesterol
Physiological	Decreased basal metabolic rate; increased heart rate, size, stroke volume and output; reduced muscle mass and delayed skeletal maturation; abnormal production of glial cells and myelinogenesis; and goiter
Pathological Consequences of Deficiency	
Established	• The spectrum of iodine deficiency disorders is large and includes fetal congenital anomalies and perinatal mortality • Neurological cretinism characterized by mental deficiency, deaf mutism, spastic diplegia and squint • Psychomotor defects • Fatigue and slowing of bodily and mental functions • Weight increase and cold intolerance caused by slowing of the metabolic rate
Predisposing Factors for Deficiency	Residence in an area with low soil iodine and treatment with lithium
Recommended Intakes	
Prevention of deficiency	RDAs (and AIs) set by the Food and Nutrition Board[3] for iodine (μg/day) are: infants age 0–0.5 year, (110), and age 0.5–1 year, (130); children age 1–8 years, 90, and age 9–13 years, 120; males age $\geq$ 14 years, 150; females $\geq$14 years, 150, pregnant, 220, and lactating, 290
Therapeutic or beneficial	Iodized oil, in which the fatty acids are chemically modified by iodination, slowly releases iodine over a period of months or years in the body. In populations with a high prevalence of severe iodine deficiency disorders (goiter incidence 30% or more), 1 ml of iodized oil containing 480 mg of iodine administered orally or by injection is a therapeutic measure for long term protection against iodine deficiency. An oral iodine dose as potassium iodide or iodate of 30 mg monthly or 8 mg biweekly has been found to be an effective prophylaxis for iodine deficiency
Food Sources	Iodized salt has been the major method for assuring adequate iodine intake since the 1920s. Other sources are sea foods and foods from plants grown on high-iodine soils

Molybdenum

Because molybdenum is a cofactor for some enzymes, its essentiality is well established. However, molybdenum deficiency has not been unequivocally identified in humans other than in an individual nourished by total parenteral nutrition and in individuals with inborn errors of metabolism that affect the synthesis of molybdenum cofactor used in molybdoenzymes. Thus, molybdenum is not of much practical concern in human nutrition. The information in Table 8.10 has been obtained primarily from reviews by Nielsen.[58,80]

Selenium

Although selenium was first suggested to be essential in 1957, it was not firmly established as so until a biochemical role was identified in 1972. The first report of human selenium deficiency appeared in 1979; the subject resided in an area with low-selenium soil and was receiving total parenteral nutrition low in selenium after surgery. Subsequent findings of selenium-responsive disorders in certain populations (e.g., Keshan disease in China) and selenium supplementation reducing the incidence of certain cancers, suggest that a significant number of people may benefit by increasing their intake of selenium. The information in Table 8.11 primarily comes from reviews by Sunde.[91–93]

POSSIBLY ESSENTIAL ULTRA TRACE ELEMENTS

Circumstantial evidence often is used to contend that an element is essential. This evidence generally fits into four categories. These are:

1. Dietary deprivation in some animal model consistently results in a changed biological function, body structure, or tissue composition that is preventable or reversible by an intake of an apparent physiological amount of the element in question.
2. The element fills the need at physiological concentrations for a known *in vivo* biochemical action to proceed *in vitro*.
3. The element is a component of known biologically important molecules in some life form.
4. The element has an essential function in lower forms of life.

TABLE 8.10
Biochemical, Clinical and Nutritional Aspects of Molybdenum

Biological Function	In humans, three molybdoenzymes have been identified; these are aldehyde oxidase, xanthine oxidase/dehydrogenase and sulfite oxidase in which molybdenum exists as a small nonprotein factor containing a pterin nucleus. Molybdoenzymes oxidize and detoxify various pyrimidines, purines and pteridines; catalyze the transformation of hypoxanthine to xanthine and xanthine to uric acid; and catalyze the conversion of sulfite to sulfate
Signs of Deficiency	
Biochemical	• A patient on total parenteral nutrition exhibited hypermethioninemia, hypouricemia, hyperoxypurinemia, hypouricosuria, and low urinary sulfate excretion
	Patients with inborn errors of molybdenum cofactor synthesis exhibited increased plasma and urine sulfite, sulfate, thiosulfate, S-sulfocysteine, taurine, and xanthine; increased serum S-sulfonated transthyretin; and decreased urine and serum uric acid
Physiological	Total parenteral nutrition patient: mental disturbances progressing to coma. Genetic errors patients: seizures, failure to thrive, and brain atrophy/lesions
Pathological Consequences of Deficiency	
Established	Patients with inborn errors of molybdenum cofactor synthesis: mental retardation, dislocated lenses, and death at early age
Suggested	Increased susceptibility to cancer[90]
Predisposing Factors for Deficiency	A high sulfur amino acid intake may increase the need for molybdenum
Recommended Intakes	
Prevention of deficiency	RDAs (and AIs) set by the Food and Nutrition Board[3] for molybdenum (μg/day) are: infants age 0–0.5 year, (2), and age 0.5–1 year, (3); children and adolescents age 1–3 years, 17, age 4–8 years, 22, age 9–13 years, and age 14–18 years, 43; adults, 45; pregnant and lactating females, 50
Therapeutic or beneficial	None have been proposed
Food Sources	Milk and milk products, pulses, organ meats (e.g., liver and kidney), cereals, baked goods

TABLE 8.11
Biochemical, Clinical and Nutritional Aspects of Selenium

Biological Function	Selenium is a component of enzymes that catalyze redox reactions; these enzymes include various types of glutathione peroxidases, iodothyronine 5'-deiodinases, and thioredoxin reductases
Signs and Symptoms of Deficiency	
Biochemical	Decreased plasma and erythrocyte selenium, plasma selenoprotein P and erythrocyte glutathione peroxidase
Physiological	Bilateral muscular discomforts, muscle pain, dry flaky skin, and wasting
Pathological Consequences of Deficiency	
Established	In the presence of other contributing factors, Keshan disease, a multiple focal myocardial necrosis resulting in acute or chronic heart function insufficiency, heart enlargement, arrhythmia, pulmonary edema, and death; other consequences include impaired immune function and increased susceptibility to viral infections
Suggested	Increased susceptibility to certain types of cancer; Kashin-Beck disease, an endemic osteoarthritis; and mood disturbances[93,94]
Recommended Intakes	
Prevention of deficiency	RDAs (and AIs) set by the Food and Nutrition Board[2] for selenium (μg/day) are: infants age 0–0.5 year, (15), and age 0.5–1 year, (20) children age 1–3 years, 20, age 4–8 years, 30; and age 9–13 years, 40; males age ≥14 years, 55; females age ≥14 years, 55, and lactating, 70
Therapeutic or beneficial	A supplement of 200 μg/day of selenium was found to have cancer protective effects
Food Sources	Fish, eggs, and meat from animals fed luxuriant selenium, grains grown on high-selenium soil

An element is considered to have strong circumstantial support for essentiality if all four types of evidences exist for it. There is strong circumstantial evidence for the essentiality of arsenic, nickel, silicon, and vanadium; thus, they are considered possibly essential ultra trace elements.

Arsenic

In addition to the information in Table 8.12, other findings, supporting arsenic essentiality, are that arsenic can activate some enzymes and enhance DNA synthesis by unsensitized and phytohemagglutinin-stimulated human lymphocytes *in vitro*.

TABLE 8.12

Arsenic: Biological Function in Lower Forms of Life, Deficiency Signs in Animals, and Speculated Importance and Postulated Adequate Intake for Humans

Biological Function in Lower Forms of Life	A biochemical function for arsenic has not been identified in lower forms of life. But, the bacterium *Chrysiogenes arsenatis* reduces As^{5+} to As^{3+} to gain energy for growth. There are enzymes in higher animals and humans that methylate arsenic with S-adenosylmethionine as the methyl donor. Arsenite methyltransferase methylates arsenite to monomethylarsenic acid, which is methylated by monomethylarsenic acid methyltransferase to yield dimethylarsinic acid, the major form of arsenic in urine
Possible Biological Function in Humans	Arsenic possibly has a function involving the utilization of labile methyl groups arising from methionine, and thus influencing the function of systems dependent upon or regulated by methyl incorporation
Deficiency Signs in Selected Experimental Animals	
Goat	Depressed growth and serum triglycerides; abnormal reproduction characterized by impaired fertility and elevated perinatal mortality; and death during lactation with myocardial damage
Pig	Depressed growth and abnormal reproduction characterized by impaired fertility and elevated perinatal mortality
Rat	• Depressed growth and hepatic putrescine, spermidine, spermine and S-adenosylmethionine
	• Elevated hepatic S-adenosylhomocysteine
	• Abnormal reproduction
Speculated Importance for Humans	Deficient intakes may increase the risk for some types of cancers
Predisposing Factors for Deficiency	• Stressors that affect the utilization of the labile methyl group including high dietary arginine and taurine, and low dietary methionine and choline
	• Stressors that affect arsenic metabolism including low dietary zinc and high dietary selenium
Postulated Adequate Intake for Humans	Based on the hypothesized requirements for experimental animals, 12–25 μg/day may be beneficial or adequate for humans
Food Sources	Shellfish, fish, grains, and cereal products

Interestingly, although arsenic is considered to be carcinogenic, it has recently been found to be effective in the treatment of acute promyelocytic leukemia[95] and cancer risk is decreased in populations that drink water containing small amounts of arsenic.[96] Hypothesized explanations for the decreased risk range from arsenic having an essential function that protects against oxidative damage and DNA repair inhibition to it having a hormetic effect. Hormesis is a process in which a low dose of a substance stimulates a response that is beneficial, because it protects against adverse actions that are induced by mechanisms similar to toxic doses of the substance. The information in Table 8.12 primarily comes from reviews by Nielsen.[58,97]

Nickel

By 1984, extensive signs of nickel deprivation had been reported for six animal species. Unfortunately, many of the reported signs may have been misinterpreted manifestations of pharmacologic actions, because nickel was provided in relatively high amounts to supplemented controls in some experiments. Thus, many of the early reported nickel deprivation findings are not shown in Table 8.13. Recent animal experiments have shown that nickel is beneficial, if not essential, for optimal reproductive function, bone composition and strength, energy metabolism, and sensory function. Additional evidence supporting the possible essentiality of nickel is that it is essential for some lower forms of life, where it participates in hydrolysis and redox enzyme reactions, regulates gene expression, and stabilizes certain structures. Interestingly, the substrates or products for all the nickel-requiring enzymes are dissolved gases: hydrogen, carbon monoxide, carbon dioxide, methane, oxygen, and ammonia. The gene expression function of nickel also involves the diffusion of oxygen and hydrogen into the cell. The information in Table 8.13 primarily comes from reviews by Nielsen,[58,80,97,98] and Eder and Kirchgessner.[99]

Silicon

In addition to the information in Table 8.14, other findings supporting silicon essentiality include its localization in the active growth areas, or osteoid layer, and within the osteoblasts of bone in young experimental animals; its consistent presence in collagen and glycosaminoglycan fractions from several types of connective tissues; and its increased intake associated with increased cortical bone mineral density in men and premenopausal women. Also, orthosilicic acid at physiological concentrations was found to stimulate collagen type I synthesis in human osteoblast-like cells and enhance osteoblast differentiation in culture. The information in Table 8.14 primarily comes from reviews by Nielsen,[58,80,97,98] and Carlisle.[100]

TABLE 8.13
Nickel: Biological Function in Lower Forms of Life, Deficiency Signs in Animals, and Speculated Importance and Postulated Adequate Intake for Humans

Biological Function in Lower Forms of Life	In lower forms of life, nickel has been identified as an essential component of seven different enzymes: urease, hydrogenase, carbon monoxide dehydrogenase, methyl-S-coenzyme-M reductase, Ni-superoxide dismutase, glyoxalase I, and acireductone dioxygenase. Nickel has been reported to be required for the hydrogenase gene to be expressed in *Bradyrhizobium japonicum*
Possible Functions in Humans	• Nickel may have a function affecting signaling by a gaseous molecule (e.g., carbon monoxide) or regulated by cyclic guanosine monophosphate channels
	• Intracellular calcium ion signaling by affecting a calcium channel or receptor
	• Enzyme reactivity or gene expression requiring a gaseous molecule
Deficiency Signs in Selected Experimental Animals	
Goat	Depressed growth, hematocrits, and reproductive performance
Pig	Depressed growth, and altered distribution and proper functioning of zinc and calcium
Rat	• Depressed growth
	• Altered iron metabolism, brain and erythrocyte fatty acid composition, long bone shape, taste preference to saccharin, and eye mitochondrial morphology
	• Diminished sperm quantity and movement
	• Impaired brightness discrimination
	• Decreased long bone strength and circulating thyroid hormone concentration
	• Increased urinary excretion of nitrate/nitrite and phosphorus
Sheep	• Depressed growth, total serum protein, erythrocyte counts, ruminal urease activity, total hepatic lipids, and cholesterol
	• Altered tissue distribution of copper and iron
Speculated Importance for Humans	Deficient intakes may impair sensory functions and bone strength
Predisposing Factors for Deficiency	• Stressors that affect labile methyl metabolism (e.g., folic acid, vitamin B_6 and vitamin B_{12} deficiencies, low dietary protein, and homocysteine supplementation)
	• Affect iron metabolism (e.g., iron deficiency)
	• Affect signaling (e.g., high dietary sodium chloride)
Postulated Adequate Intake for Humans	Based on hypothesized requirements for animals, 25–35 µg/day may be beneficial or adequate for humans
Food Sources	Nuts, pulses, grains, and chocolate

Vanadium

There is no question that vanadium is a bioactive element. Its ability to selectively inhibit protein tyrosine phosphatases at sub-micromolar concentrations probably explains the broad range of effects that relatively high (supranutritional or pharmacologic) intakes have on cellular regulatory cascades. Protein tyrosine phosphatase inhibition is thought to be the basis for vanadium having insulin-like actions at the cellular level and stimulating cellular proliferation and differentiation. Nutritional intakes may also affect phosphorylation/dephosphorylation such that a regulatory cascade is altered. This may be the basis for the observations that vanadium deprivation altered the response to low and high dietary iodine, impaired reproduction, and induced abnormal bone morphology in experimental animals. The information suggesting vanadium is essential for humans shown in Table 8.15, as well as being essential for some lower forms of life, primarily comes from reviews by Nielsen,[58,80,97,98,101,102] Marzan and McNeill,[103] and Hulley and Davison.[104]

OTHER ELEMENTS WITH BENEFICIAL OR BIOLOGICAL ACTIONS

There are several elements that have limited circumstantial evidence suggesting that they may be essential. This evidence is generally limited to a few gross beneficial effects or apparent signs of deficiency in one or two animal species observed by one or two research groups. Therefore, these elements do not have widespread support for being possibly essential. However, some of these elements have beneficial pharmacological actions (fluoride and lithium), and others may eventually be found to be of some importance from the nutritional point of view. Elements that fit in this category include aluminum, bromine, cadmium, fluorine, germanium, lead, lithium, rubidium, and tin. The information in Table 8.16 comes from reviews by Nielsen[80,97,105] and Anke et al.[106–110]

TABLE 8.14
Silicon: Biological Function in Lower Forms of Life, Deficiency Signs in Animals, and Speculated Importance and Postulated Adequate Intake for Humans

Biological Function in Lower Forms of Life	Silicon has a structural role in some primitive classes of organisms including diatoms (unicellular microscopic plants), radiolarians, and some sponges. Diatoms have an absolute requirement for silicon as monomeric silicic acid for normal cell growth. The diatom, *Cylindrotheca fusiformis*, has five transporter genes that tightly control silicon uptake and use in cell wall formation
Possible Biological Function in Humans	Silicon may be involved in the interaction between a macromolecule and a cell resulting in changes in cell synthetic activity or cytokine secretion such that it affects wound healing, immune function, and cartilage composition and ultimately calcification
Deficiency Signs in Experimental Animals	
Chick	Skulls with a more primitive type of bone and structural abnormalities associated with depressed collagen content; long bone abnormalities characterized by defective endochondral bone growth associated with depressed contents of articular cartilage, water, hexosamine, and collagen
Rat	• Increased humerus hexose; decreased humerus hydroxyproline, femur alkaline and acid phosphatase and plasma ornithine aminotransferase activity (a key enzyme in collagen synthesis)
	• Increased urinary helical peptide (collagen breakdown product) excretion
Speculated Importance for Humans	Deficient intakes may impair bone growth and remodeling, wound healing, and immune function
Predisposing Factors for Deficiency	• Stressors that affect the metabolism of silicon including high dietary fiber and aluminum
	• Stressors that affect the utilization of silicon including wounds (tooth extraction), conditions causing an immune or inflammatory response (e.g., arthritis), and low dietary calcium
Postulated Adequate Intake for Humans	Based on animal findings and human urinary excretion data, suggested beneficial or adequate intakes for humans range from 5 to 25 mg/day. On the basis of weak balance data, a silicon intake of 30 to 35 mg/day was suggested for athletes, which was 5 to 10 mg higher than that suggested for nonathletes
Food Sources	Unrefined grains of high fiber content and cereal products

TABLE 8.15
Vanadium: Biological Function in Lower Forms of Life, Deficiency Signs in Animals, and Speculated Importance and Postulated Adequate Intake for Humans

Biological Function in Lower Forms of Life	Vanadium is an essential cofactor for some nitrogenases that reduce nitrogen gas to ammonia in bacteria, and for bromoperoxidase, iodoperoxidase and chloroperoxidase in algae, lichens and fungi, respectively. The haloperoxidases catalyze the oxidation of halide ions by hydrogen peroxide, thus facilitating the formation of a carbon–halogen bond
Possible Biological Function in Humans	Vanadium may have a role that promotes phosphorylation and/or inhibits dephosphorylation such that a regulatory cascade is altered
Deficiency Signs in Selected Experimental Animals	
Goat	Depressed milk production and life span; increased rate of spontaneous abortion; death, sometimes preceded by convulsions, between ages 7 and 91 days; skeletal deformations in the forelegs; and thickened forefoot tarsal joints
Rat	Increased thyroid weight and thyroid weight/body weight ratio, decreased erythrocyte glucose-6-phosphate dehydrogenase, and altered response to high and low dietary iodide
Speculated Importance for Humans	Low intakes may impair thyroid hormone metabolism and proper bone development
Predisposing Factors for Deficiency	Stressors of thyroid or iodine metabolism and factors that reduce vanadium absorption including high dietary iron, aluminum hydroxide, and chromium
Postulated Adequate Intake for Humans	Based on animal data, a daily dietary intake of 10 μg probably would be adequate for humans. Pharmacologic doses used to experimentally treat diabetes have been in the range of 40 to 50 mg vanadium/day in the form of vanadyl sulfate, sodium orthovanadate, and organic complexes such as bis(maltoalto)oxovanadium (IV). It should be noted that the Food and Nutrition Board[3] has set a tolerable upper intake level (UL) of 1.8 mg vanadium/day for male adults
Food Sources	Shellfish, mushrooms, prepared foods, whole grains

TABLE 8.16

Reported Deficiency Signs in Experimental Animals and Usual Human Dietary Intakes of Apparently Bioactive Beneficial Mineral Elements

Element	Deficiency Signs (Experimental Animals)	Usual Daily Dietary Intake (Humans)	Food Sources
Aluminum	*Chick*: Depressed Growth *Goat*: Depressed growth and insemination success, increased abortions and kid mortality, and uncoordinated and weak hind legs	2–10 mg	Baked goods prepared with chemical leavening agents, grains, vegetables, and tea
Bromine	*Goat*: Depressed feed intake, growth, conception rate, hematocrit and hemoglobin, and increased abortions and kid mortality	2–8 mg	Grains, nuts, and fish
Cadmium	*Goat*: Muscular weakness, degenerative changes in liver and kidney mitochondria, decreased insemination success and milk production, and increased mortality *Rat*: Depressed growth	5–20 μg	Shellfish, grains, and leafy vegetables
Fluorine	*Goat*: Decreased feed efficiency and growth, kid mortality, and skeletal deformities *Rat*: Depressed growth and altered incisor pigmentation	0.4–1.8 mg without fluoridated water	Fish, tea, and fluoridated water
Germanium	*Rat*: Decreased tibial DNA and altered bone and liver mineral composition	0.4–3.4 mg	Vegetables, wheat bran, and leguminous seeds
Lead	*Pig*: Depressed growth and elevated serum cholesterol, phospholipids and bile acids *Rat*: Depressed growth and liver glucose and lipids, increased liver cholesterol and serum ceruloplasmin, and anemia	15–100 μg	Seafood and food from plants grown under high-lead conditions
Lithium	*Goat*: Depressed conception rate, birth weight, milk production, serum citric acid cycle enzyme and liver monoamine oxidase activities, and increased mortality and serum creatine kinase activity *Rat*: Depressed fertility, birth weight, litter size, and weaning weight	100–600 μg	Meat, eggs, fish, milk, milk products, processed meats, potatoes, and vegetables (content varies with geological origin)
Rubidium	*Goat*: Depressed growth, food intake, conception rate, milk production, and plasma progesterone and estradiol, and increased abortions and kid mortality *Rat*: Altered tissue mineral concentrations	1–3 mg	Fruits, vegetables (especially asparagus), poultry, fish, coffee, and tea
Tin	*Rat*: Depressed growth, feed efficiency, and response to sound, altered mineral composition of heart, tibia, muscle, spleen, kidney, and lung	1–5 mg	Canned foods

SUMMARY

Except for iodine and iron, the full extent of the pathological consequences of marginal or deficient intakes of the trace and ultra trace elements has not been established. In addition, it is quite likely that not all the essential mineral elements for humans have been identified, and the mechanisms for the beneficial effects of many bioactive mineral elements have not been clearly defined. Thus, it is difficult to tabulate trace mineral deficiency signs and symptoms for humans. The tables in this section are works in progress, and the presented data can rapidly change because of ongoing research. However, findings to date indicate that many trace and ultra trace minerals are of more practical nutritional concern than currently acknowledged.

REFERENCES

1. Food and Nutrition Board, Institute of Medicine, *Dietary Reference Intakes for Calcium, Phosphorus, Magnesium, Vitamin D, and Fluoride*, National Academy Press, Washington, DC, 1997, Chapters 6 and 8.
2. Food and Nutrition Board, Institute of Medicine, *Dietary Reference Intakes for Vitamin C, Vitamin E, Selenium, and Carotenoids*, National Academy Press, Washington, DC, 2000, Chapter 7.
3. Food and Nutrition Board, Institute of Medicine, *Dietary Reference Intakes for Vitamin A, Vitamin K, Arsenic, Boron, Chromium, Copper, Iodine, Iron, Manganese, Molybdenum, Nickel, Silicon, Vanadium, and Zinc*, National Academy Press, Washington, DC, 2001, Chapters 6–13.
4. <http://www.MyPyramid.gov> accessed 3/16/06
5. Eckhert, C.D., Rowe, R.I., *J. Trace Elem. Exp. Med.*, 12: 213; 1999.
6. Fort, D.J. et al., *Biol. Trace Elem. Res.*, 90: 117; 2002.
7. Nielsen, F.H., *J. Trace Elem. Exp. Med.*, 9: 215; 1996.

8. Nielsen, F.H., *Plant Soil*, 193: 199; 1997.

9. Nielsen, F.H., *Biol. Trace Elem. Res.*, 66: 319; 1998.

10. Nielsen, F.H., in *Boron in Plant and Animal Nutrition*, Goldbach, H.E. et al., Eds., Kluwer Academic/Plenum Publishers, New York, 2002, p. 37.

11. Hunt, C.D., *J. Trace Elem. Exp. Med.*, 9: 185; 1996.

12. Hunt, C.D., in *Boron in Plant and Animal Nutrition*, Goldbach, H.E. et al., Eds., Kluwer Academic/Plenum Publishers, New York, 2002, p. 21.

13. Penland, J.G., *Biol. Trace Elem. Res.*, 66: 299; 1998.

14. World Health Organization, *Trace Elements in Human Nutrition and Health*, World Health Organization, Geneva, 1996, Chapter 13.

15. Harris, E.D., in *Handbook of Nutritionally Essential Mineral Elements*, O'Dell, B.L., Sunde, R.A., Eds., Marcel Dekker, NY, 1997, Chapter 8.

16. Klevay, L.M., Medeiros, D.M., *J. Nutr.*, 126: 2419S; 1996.

17. Milne, D.B., *Am. J. Clin. Nutr.*, 67: 1041S; 1998.

18. Cordano, A., *Am. J. Clin. Nutr.*, 67: 1012S; 1998.

19. Uauy, R., Olivares, M., Gonzalez, M., *Am. J. Clin. Nutr.*, 67: 952S; 1998.

20. Failla, M.L., Johnson, M.A., Prohaska, J.R., in *Present Knowledge in Nutrition*, 8th ed., Bowman, B.A., Russell, R.M., Eds., ILSI Press, Washington, DC, 2001, Chapter 35.

21. Johnson, W.T., in *Nutritional Neuroscience*, Lieberman, H.R., Kanarek, R.B., Prasad, C., Eds., Taylor & Francis, Boca Raton, FL, 2005, Chapter 17.

22. Strain, J.J., in *Copper and Zinc in Inflammatory and Degenerative Diseases*, Rainsford, K.D. et al., Eds., Kluwer, Dordrecht, 1998, Chapter 12.

23. Medeiros, D.M., Wildman, R.E.C., *Proc. Soc. Exp. Biol. Med.*, 215: 299; 1997.

24. Strain, J.J., in *Role of Trace Elements for Health Promotion and Disease Prevention. Bibl. Nutr. Dieta*, Sandstrom, B., Walter, P., Eds., Karger, Basel, 1998, p. 127.

25. Klevay, L.M., in *Clinical Nutrition of the Essential Trace Elements and Minerals: The Guide for Health Professionals*, Bogden, J.D., Klevay, L.M., Eds., Humana Press, Totowa, NJ, 2000, Chapter 15.

26. Percival, S.S., *Am. J. Clin. Nutr.*, 67: 1064S; 1998.

27. Saari, J., *Can. J. Physiol. Pharmacol.*, 78: 848; 2000.

28. Beard, J.L., Dawson, H.D., Iron, in *Handbook of Nutritionally Essential Mineral Elements*, O'Dell, B.L., Sunde, R.A., Eds., Marcel Dekker, New York, 1997, Chapter 9.

29. Baynes, R.D., Stipanuk, M.H., Iron, in *Biochemical and Physiological Aspects of Human Nutrition*, Stipanuk, M.A., Ed., Saunders, Philadelphia, PA, 2000, Chapter 31.

30. Harris, M.M. et al., *J. Nutr.*, 133: 3598; 2003.

31. Medeiros, D.M. et al., *J. Nutr.*, 134: 3061; 2004.

32. Maurer, J. et al., *J. Nutr.*, 135: 863; 2005.

33. Felt, B.T., Lozoff, B., *J. Nutr.*, 126: 693; 1996.

34. Cook, J.D., Reddy, M.B., *Am. J. Clin. Nutr.*, 62: 117; 1995.

35. Viteri, F.E., *Am. J. Clin. Nutr.*, 63: 610; 1996.

36. Yip, R., in *Present Knowledge of Nutrition*, 8th ed., Bowman, B.A., Russell, R.M., Eds., ILSI Press, Washington, DC, 2001, Chapter 30.

37. Klevay, L.M., Milne, D.B., *Am. J. Clin. Nutr.*, 75: 550; 2002.

38. Nielsen, F.H., *Magnesium Res.*, 16: 197; 2004.

39. Nielsen, F.H. et al., *J. Am. Coll. Nutr.*, in press.

40. Rude, R.K., in *Biochemical and Physiological Aspects of Human Nutrition*, Stipanuk, M.H., Ed., Saunders, Philadelphia, PA, 2000, Chapter 29.

41. Shils, M.E., in *Handbook of Nutritionally Essential Mineral Elements*, O'Dell, B.L., Sunde, R.A., Eds., Marcel Dekker, New York, 1997, Chapter 5.

42. Agus, M.S., Agus, Z.S., *Crit. Care Clin.*, 17: 175; 2001.

43. Altura, B.M., Altura, B.T., in *Magnesium: Current Status and New Developments*, Theophanides, T., Anastassopoulou, J., Eds., Kluwer, Dordrecht, 1997, p. 383.

44. Mizushima, S. et al., *J. Human Hypertens.*, 12: 447; 1998.

45. Jee, S.H. et al., *Am. J. Hypertens.*, 15: 691; 2002.

46. Barbagallo, M. et al., *Mol. Aspects Med.*, 24: 39; 2003.

47. Huerta, M.G. et al., *Diabetes Care*, 28: 1175; 2005.

48. Altura, B.M., Altura, B.T., *Med. Hypothesis*, 57: 705; 2001.

49. Boska, M.D. et al., *Neurology*, 58: 1227; 2002.

50. Durlach, J. et al., *Magnesium Res.*, 18: 109; 2005.

51. Alloui, A. et al., *Eur. J. Pharmacol.*, 469: 65; 2003.

52. Chui, H.-F., Chang, C.-C., Yang, C.-Y., *Magnesium Res.*, 17:28; 2004.

53. Massey, L., *Magnesium Res.*, 18: 123; 2005.

54. Rude, R.K., Gruber, H.E., *J. Nutr. Biochem.*, 15: 710; 2004.

55. Tong, G.M., Rude, R.K., *Intensive Care Med.*, 20: 3; 2005.

56. Norose, N., Arai, K., *Jap. J. Parent. Ent. Nutr.*, 9: 978; 1987.

57. Leach, Jr. R.M., Harris, E.D., in *Handbook of Nutritionally Essential Mineral Elements*, O'Dell, B.L., Sunde, R.A., Eds., Marcel Dekker, New York, 1997, Chapter 10.

58. Nielsen, F.H., in *Modern Nutrition in Health and Disease*, 9th ed., Shils, M.E. et al., Eds., Williams and Wilkins, Baltimore, MD, 1999, Chapter 16.

59. Freeland-Graves, J., Llanes, C., in *Manganese in Health and Disease*, Klimis-Tavantzis, D.J., Ed., CRC Press, Boca Raton, FL, 1994, Chapter 3.

60. Klimis-Tavantzis, D.J., Ed., *Manganese in Health and Disease*, CRC Press, Boca Raton, FL, 1994, Chapters 4, 6, 8, 9.

61. Aschner, M., in *Metals and Oxidative Damage in Neurological Disorders*, Connor, J., Ed., Plenum Press, New York, 1997, Chapter 5.

62. Lucchini, R. et al., *NeuroToxicology*, 21: 769; 2000.

63. Chesters, J.K., in *Handbook of Nutritionally Essential Mineral Elements*, O'Dell, B.L., Sunde, R.A., Eds., Marcel Dekker, New York, 1997, Chapter 7.

64. Prasad, A.S., *J. Trace Elem. Exp. Med.*, 11: 63; 1998.

65. Dibley, M.J., in *Present Knowledge in Nutrition*, Bowman, B.A., Russell, R.M., Eds., ILSI Press, Washington, DC, 2001, Chapter 31.

66. Davis, C.D., Milne, D.B., Nielsen, F.H., *Am. J. Clin. Nutr.*, 71: 781; 2000.

67. Andree, K.B. et al., *J. Nutr.*, 134: 1716; 2004.

68. Yamaguchi, M., *J. Trace Elem. Exp. Med.*, 11: 119; 1998.

69. Hadrzynski, C., *J. Trace Elem. Exp. Med.*, 12, 367, 1999.

70. Fernandez-Madrid, F., in *Copper and Zinc in Inflammatory and Degenerative Diseases*, Rainsford, K.D. et al., Eds., Kluwer, London, 1998, Chapter 8.

71. Penland, J.G., *J. Nutr.*, 130: 361S; 2000.

72. Ho, E., Courtemanche, C., Ames, B.N., *J. Nutr.*, 133: 2543; 2003.

73. Tudor, R., Zalewski, P.D., Ratanike, R.N., *J. Nutr. Health, Aging*, 9: 45; 2005.

74. Olson, R.J., DeBry, P., *J. Trace Elem. Exp. Med.*, 11: 137; 1998.

75. Stearns, D.M., *Biofactors*, 11: 149; 2000.

76. Vincent, J.B., *Biol. Trace Elem. Res.*, 99: 1; 2004.

77. Nielsen, F.H., in *New Advances in the Biochemistry of Chromium (III)*, Vincent, J.B., Ed., Elsevier, Chapter 13 (in press).

78. Jeejeebhoy, K.N., *J. Trace Elem. Exp. Med.*, 12: 85; 1999.

79. Offenbacher, E.G., Pi-Sunyer, F.X., Stoecker, B.J., in *Handbook of Nutritionally Essential Mineral Elements*, O'Dell, B.L., Sunde, R.A., Eds., Marcel Dekker, New York, 1997 Chapter 12.

80. Nielsen, F.H., in *Biochemical and Physiological Aspects of Human Nutrition*, Stipanuk, M.H., Ed., W. B. Saunders, Philadelphia, PA, 2000, Chapter 36.

81. Vincent, J.B., *J. Trace Elem. Exp. Med.* 16: 227; 2003.

82. Cefalu, W.T., Hu, F.B., *Diabetes Care*, 27: 2741; 2004.

83. Smith, R.M., in *Handbook of Nutritionally Essential Mineral Elements*, O'Dell, B.L., Sunde, R.A., Eds., Marcel Dekker, New York, 1997, Chapter 11.

84. Shane, B., in *Biochemical and Physiological Aspects of Human Nutrition*, Stipanuk, M.H., Ed., W. B. Saunders, Philadelphia, PA, 2000, Chapter 21.

85. Stabler, S.P., in *Present Knowledge in Nutrition*, 8th ed., ILSI Press, Washington, DC, 2001, Chapter 22.

86. Food and Nutrition Board, Institute of Medicine, *Dietary Reference Intakes: Thiamin, Riboflavin, Niacin, Vitamin B_6, Folate, Vitamin B_{12}, Pantothenic Acid, Biotin, and Choline*, National Academy Press, Washington, DC, 1998, Chapter 9.

87. Hetzel, B.S., Wellby, M.L., in *Handbook of Nutritionally Essential Mineral Elements*, O'Dell, B.L., Sunde, R.A., Eds., Marcel Dekker, New York, 1997, Chapter 19.

88. Freake, H.C., in *Biochemical and Physiological Aspects of Human Nutrition*, Stipanuk, M.H., Ed., W. B. Saunders, Philadelphia, PA, 2000, Chapter 33.

89. Stanbury, J.B., Dunn, J.T., in *Present Knowledge in Nutrition*, 8th ed., Bowman, B.A., Russell, R.M., Eds., ILSI Press, Washington, DC, 2001, Chapter 32.

90. Seaborn, C.D., Yang, S.P., *Biol. Trace Elem. Res.*, 39: 245; 1993.

91. Sunde, R.A., in *Handbook of Nutritionally Essential Mineral Elements*, O'Dell, B.L., Sunde, R.A., Eds., Marcel Dekker, New York, 1997, Chapter 18.

92. Sunde, R.A., in *Biochemical and Physiological Aspects of Human Nutrition*, Stipanuk, M.H., Ed., W. B. Saunders, Philadelphia, PA, 2000, Chapter 34.

93. Sunde, R.A., in *Present Knowledge in Nutrition*, 8th ed., Bowman, B.A., Russell, R.M., Eds., ILSI Press, Washington, DC, 2001, Chapter 33.

94. Finley, J.W., Penland, J.G., *J. Trace Elem. Exp. Med.*, 11: 11; 1998.

95. Kwong, Y.-L., *Expert Opin. Drug Saf.*, 3: 589; 2004.

96. Lamm, S.H. et al., *J. Occup. Environ. Med.*, 46: 298; 2004.

97. Nielsen, F.H., in *Present Knowledge in Nutrition*, 8th ed., Bowman, B.A., Russell, R.M., Eds., ILSI Press, Washington, DC, 2001, Chapter 36.

98. Nielsen, F.H., in *Sports Nutrition — Vitamins and Trace Elements*, 2nd ed., Driskell, J.A., Wolinsky, I., Eds., Taylor & Francis, Boca Raton, FL, 2005, Chapter 20.

99. Eder, K., Kirchgessner, M., in *Handbook of Nutritionally Essential Mineral Elements*, O'Dell, B.L., Sunde, R.A., Eds., Marcel Dekker, New York, 1997, Chapter 14.

100. Carlisle, E.M., in *Handbook of Nutritionally Essential Mineral Elements*, O'Dell, B.L., Sunde, R.A., Eds., Marcel Dekker, New York, 1997, Chapter 21.

101. Nielsen, F.H., in *Handbook of Nutritionally Essential Mineral Elements*, O'Dell, B.L., Sunde, R.A., Eds., Marcel Dekker, New York, 1997, Chapter 22.

102. Nielsen, F.H., in *Vanadium Compounds: Chemistry, Biochemistry, and Therapeutic Applications, ACS Series 711*, Tracey, A.S., Crans, D.C., Eds., American Chemical Society, Washington, DC, 1998, Chapter 23.

103. Marzban, L., McNeill, J.H., *J. Trace Elem. Exp. Med.*, 16: 253; 2003.

104. Hulley, P., Davison, A., *J. Trace Elem. Exp. Med.*, 16: 281; 2003.

105. Nielsen, F.H., in *Clinical Nutrition of the Essential Trace Elements and Minerals, The Guide for Health Professionals*, Bogden, J.D., Klevay, L.M., Eds., Humana Press, Totowa, NJ, 2000, Chapter 2.

106. Anke, M., Müller, M., Hoppe, C., *Biomed. Res. Trace Elem.*, 16: 183; 2005.

107. Anke, M., Groppel, B., Masaoka, T., *Biomed. Res. Trace Elem.*, 16: 177; 2005.

108. Anke, M. et al., *Biomed. Res. Trace Elem.*, 16: 198; 2005.

109. Anke, M. et al., *Biomed. Res. Trace Elem.*, 16: 169; 2005.

110. Anke, M. et al., *Biomed. Res. Trace Elem.*, 16: 203; 2005.

9 Vitamin Deficiencies

Richard S. Rivlin

CONTENTS

In this era of increasing obesity and growing portion sizes, with food fortification well established and nutritional supplements widely consumed by the public, it is important to keep in mind those special circumstances in which vitamin deficiencies still continue to occur. A diet high in calories is not necessarily high in nutrients. In fact, a high-fat diet based to a large degree on "fast foods" may be low in some of the essential vitamins and minerals.

GENERAL COMMENTS ON VITAMIN DEFICIENCIES

In general, vitamin deficiencies arise when the diet is inadequate in its content of one or more nutrients or when the body is unable to utilize dietary nutrients adequately. Impaired intestinal absorption or defects in metabolic processes, storage, or excretion can each result in vitamin deficiency. Single-nutrient deficiencies are rare these days, because a diet that is suboptimal in one vitamin is nearly always suboptimal in others. Thus, a poor diet tends to have multiple inadequacies. Furthermore, some vitamins are involved in the metabolism of other vitamins, and therefore deficiencies may be interconnected.

A number of exogenous factors may serve to intensify the biological effects of a poor diet. For example, excess alcohol consumption has specific and selective effects on vitamin metabolism, interfering with the absorption of some vitamins (e.g., thiamin and riboflavin) and accelerating the metabolic degradation of another (B_6). In addition, a number of medications may affect vitamin metabolism and at multiple sites. From a practical point of view, laxatives and diuretics, often used for minimal indications and prolonged periods by vulnerable elderly patients, are probably among the most common causes of drug-induced vitamin deficiencies.

The concept of risk factors, utilized effectively in the evaluation and prevention of heart disease, needs to be applied to the assessment of vitamin deficiency. Thus, a patient who abuses alcohol, requires several medications chronically, and suffers from malabsorption due to alcohol will have a greatly enhanced risk of becoming grossly vitamin deficient.

A much greater understanding is needed of the effects of herbal products and the so-called alternative/complementary remedies on vitamin metabolism. Many prescription drugs are known to affect vitamin metabolism. With large numbers of people consuming a wide variety of unregulated products about which there is little information, a potential exists for developing significant forms of malnutrition. We urgently need more information on drug–herbal and food–herbal interactions and their implications for vitamin metabolism. Several comments about the patterns of vitamin deficiencies currently emerging in the United States are summarized in Table 9.1.

TABLE 9.1
Some Features of Vitamin Deficiencies at the Present Time

1. Dietary vitamin deficiencies tend to be multiple, not single
2. Clinical evidence of vitamin deficiencies develops gradually, and early symptoms, such as fatigue and weakness, may be vague, ill-defined, and nonspecific
3. The physical examination cannot be relied upon to make a diagnosis of early vitamin deficiency; classic features of vitamin deficiencies, such as the corkscrew hairs of scurvy, are only detectable after a profound deficiency state has been attained
4. The rate of development of vitamin deficiencies is highly variable. In general, most water-soluble vitamins may be depleted within several weeks; longer periods are needed for significant depletion of fat-soluble vitamins. Several years are required for clinical manifestations of vitamin B_{12} deficiency unless there are complicating factors, such as ileal resection or inflammatory bowel disease involving the ileum
5. The impact of dietary deficiencies of vitamins is greatly augmented by the long-term chronic use of certain medications that may affect absorption, utilization, or excretion of vitamins. Chief among these are laxatives and diuretics. These considerations are particularly relevant to older individuals, who use the largest number of drugs and remedies, for the longest duration, and may have marginal diets to begin with
6. The concept of "risk factors" may be helpful in assessing factors, such as drugs and alcohol, that contribute to accelerating the clinical presentation of a given dietary inadequacy

TABLE 9.2
Some Considerations in Correction of Vitamin Deficiencies

1. Approach the clinical setting in its entirety; ask yourself, how could a vitamin deficiency develop in the first place? Ask whether there are complicating conditions, that is, other risk factors, in addition to the poor diet

2. Unless there are specific indications of a single-nutrient deficiency, such as vitamin B_{12} in pernicious anemia, most malnourished patients will have multiple deficiencies and require rehabilitation with multiple nutrients. Repletion is best accomplished primarily with diet, and additionally with specific supplementation, if necessary

3. Simple steps can often improve a diet significantly, such as discarding old produce, avoiding "fast food" meals on a regular basis, and increasing the intake of fresh fruits and vegetables. In modern nutrition, one speaks of "junk diets" rather than single "junk foods," and of the necessity of moderation and variety in one's daily diet

4. Learn how to read a label from a nutritional supplement bottle so that you can properly instruct your patients. The array of choices of nutritional supplements is bewildering, and patients must learn that more is not necessarily better

5. Remember that vitamins may behave like drugs and have a defined toxic: therapeutic ratio. Some vitamins, such as vitamins A and D, have a real potential for causing toxicity. B vitamins may also cause problems, as exemplified by the sensory neuropathy resulting from large doses of vitamin B_6

6. A multivitamin supplement containing all nutrients at the levels of the RDI is safe to take by nearly everyone and may help to alleviate deficiencies and prevent them in the future

While the effects of full-blown vitamin deficiencies are well known and have been thoroughly described, the effects of lesser or marginal deficiencies are not as well appreciated by health professionals. In recent years, both scientists and the general public have been paying more attention to marginal vitamin and mineral deficiencies in attempting to gain maximal benefits from diet for health. Recent findings suggest that the concept of so-called "normal" needs to be carefully reconsidered, inasmuch as there may be different risks for disease within the range considered "normal."

For example, individuals with serum folic acid levels in the lower part of the normal range have been shown to have significantly elevated serum concentrations of homocysteine compared with those whose folic acid concentrations are in the upper range of normal. With elevated serum homocysteine concentrations emerging as a risk factor for heart disease, these observations suggest that perhaps we should set higher standards and more defined expectations for the "normal" range.

In the prevention and treatment of vitamin deficiencies, one must approach the patient in a logical fashion and proceed in an orderly direction. Medical history is of greatest importance and one needs to know details of food intake, portion size supplement use, remedies, and drugs. The physical examination only rarely reveals pathognomonic signs of specific vitamin deficits. Laboratory tests, appropriately utilized, may be helpful in documenting vitamin deficiencies. Long-term compliance with an appropriate diet and the use of supplements, if indicated, is the goal, but may be difficult to achieve. Some of the points regarding correction of vitamin deficiencies are summarized in Table 9.2.

VITAMIN A

FUNCTIONS

Vitamin A has a wide variety of functions, including specific roles in vision, embryogenesis, cellular differentiation, growth, reproduction, immune status, taste sensations, and, increasingly, in disease prevention and treatment.

DEFICIENCY

Deficiency of vitamin A is of crucial importance as a worldwide nutritional problem. The resultant xerophthalmia is a cause of blindness in at least half a million preschool children each year in the developing countries. In these areas, the diet is composed primarily of such items as rice, wheat, maize, and tubers, which contain far from adequate amounts of vitamin A precursors. The World Health Organization (WHO) and other groups have made great efforts to plan programs that identify people at risk and to institute appropriate preventive measures on a broad scale. It is now recognized that dietary deficiency of vitamin A is a clear risk factor for severe cases of measles. Many of the deaths that result from measles in young children could be greatly reduced by large doses of vitamin A given parenterally. The diet prevailing in these areas simply does not contain enough vitamin A precursors or vitamin A itself to prevent a deficient state from developing.

Clinical deficiency of vitamin A may be overt or subclinical. One of the earliest signs of vitamin A deficiency is night blindness, observed in both children and adults. The development of xerophthalmia follows a defined sequence, leading eventually to keratomalacia, in which perforation of the cornea occurs. A characteristic sign that is observed later in advanced vitamin A deficiency is Bitot's spots, collections of degenerated cells in the outer aspects of the conjunctivae that appear white in color.

Vitamin-A-deficiency eye disease in its end stages is irreversible, but if abnormalities are detected earlier and treated vigorously, they may be potentially preventable.

Vitamin A deficiency also causes skin disorders in the form of follicular hyperkeratosis. Although characteristic skin changes occur in response to a deficiency of vitamin A, in practical terms one should remember that skin lesions of some kind may be caused by other nutrient deficiencies such as zinc, biotin, niacin, and riboflavin.

Children significantly deficient in vitamin A manifest increased incidence of serious and life-threatening infections and elevated mortality rates. It has been recognized that deficient vitamin A status is a risk factor for the maternal-to-fetal transmission of human immunodeficiency virus; the relative risk of transmission of the virus is fourfold greater in vitamin-A-deficient than in vitamin-A-sufficient mothers.

Vitamin A deficiency in the United States is identified largely with certain risk groups: the urban poor, elderly persons (particularly those living alone), abusers of alcohol, patients with malabsorption disorders, and persons with poor diets. Vitamin A deficiency is generally found in a setting in which there are multiple vitamin and mineral deficits. Special attention must be paid to deficiency of zinc, a frequent finding in alcoholism, as depletion of zinc interferes with the mobilization of vitamin A from its storage sites in liver. This effect is achieved by blocking the release of holo-retinol-binding protein from the liver. Even in Western countries, severe cases of measles have been found in children with borderline vitamin A stores, suggesting that perhaps parenteral vitamin A should be administered in this setting as well.

Health professionals must keep in mind that deficiency of vitamin A in the United States may develop after the long-term use of several medications. Drug-induced nutritional deficiencies, in general, particularly those involving vitamin A, occur most frequently among elderly persons, because they use medications in the largest number for the most prolonged duration, and they may have borderline nutritional status to begin with. Among the drugs most relevant to compromising vitamin A status are mineral oil, which dissolves this nutrient; other laxatives, which accelerate intestinal transit and may diminish the magnitude of vitamin A absorption; cholestyramine and colestipol, which bind vitamin A; and, under certain conditions, neomycin and colchicines. Olestra may possibly interfere with absorption of a number of vitamins, including A: patients using this agent have been advised to take a multivitamin supplement regularly.

LABORATORY DIAGNOSIS OF DEFICIENCY

The laboratory diagnosis of vitamin A deficiency is based on the finding of a low plasma retinal; levels below 10 μg/dl signify severe or advanced deficiency. Interpretation of plasma retinal concentrations may be confounded, however, by a number of other factors, such as generalized malnutrition and weight loss. Some authorities have preferred to utilize a form of retinal tolerance test, measuring the increment in serum vitamin A levels over 5 h following an oral load of vitamin A.

PREVENTION

Deficiency of vitamin A can be prevented by a diet high in carotenes, which serve as precursors to vitamin A. The carotenes, particularly β-carotene, are derived exclusively from plant sources, the richest of which are palm oil, carrots, sweet potatoes, dark green, leafy vegetables, cantaloupe, oranges, and papaya. Preformed vitamin A is derived only from animal sources, such as dairy products, meat, and fish. The commercial preparations of fish oils are rich, sometimes too rich, as sources of preformed vitamin A.

The nutritional value of dietary sources of vitamin A may be compromised when food items are subject to oxidation, particularly in the presence of light and heat. Antioxidants, such as vitamin E, may prevent the loss of vitamin A activity under these conditions.

TREATMENT

Vitamin A deficiency has been treated worldwide with single intramuscular injections of massive amounts (100,000 to 200,000 IU) of vitamin A, repeated at intervals of approximately 6 months to 1 year. WHO has recommended that doses of 200,000 IU of vitamin A be given initially and at 2 days to children admitted to hospitals in areas of the world where the case fatality rate is very high. Such doses have been effective and are associated with remarkably little toxicity, perhaps because body stores are markedly depleted at the time of therapy. These doses, however, may produce some acute toxic symptoms in well-nourished persons.

Clinical vitamin A deficiency in the United States can be treated with either β-carotene if there is normal body conversion to vitamin A or vitamin A itself. Daily doses in the range of 25,000 IU of β-carotene are being consumed by many healthy individuals. The yellowish discoloration of the skin associated with prolonged use of β-carotene is not believed to be harmful. Vitamin A, in contrast, is quite toxic when ingested in amounts considerably higher than the RDI, especially for prolonged periods. It is probably advisable not to exceed two to three times the RDI for vitamin A when planning a domestic treatment program involving vitamin A administration.

Congenital malformations, a particularly disturbing consequence of vitamin A overdosage, have been reported in women consuming 25,000 to 50,000 IU daily during pregnancy. The lowest dose of vitamin A that would be completely safe as a supplement for pregnant women is not known definitely. Therefore, it is not a good idea for pregnant women to take supplementary vitamin A unless there are specific indications, such as malabsorption, or proven dietary deficiency. Many advisory groups caution that the maximal intake of preformed vitamin A consumed during pregnancy should not exceed 10,000 IU/day.

At present, there is widespread interest in newer therapeutic applications of vitamin A and its derivatives. Certain forms of leukemia have been found to respond to derivatives of vitamin A. The therapeutic potential of this vitamin is being expanded greatly in studies of chemoprevention and treatment of cancer. The toxicity of large doses of vitamin A places important limits on its feasibility in cancer prevention. Attention has turned to β-carotene and related agents, which, in addition to their role as precursors of vitamin A, have strong antioxidant activity and other effects as well. β-Carotene, however, may possibly pose a risk in heavy smokers — two studies in this population have shown an actual increase in prevalence of lung cancer when β-carotene was administered for several years.

Diminished prevalence of certain cancers has been found among people whose intake of fruits and vegetables is high; this finding has been attributable at least in part to the high content of carotenoids in the diet. However, many phytochemicals in addition to carotenoids have been found in fruits and vegetables with potential health benefits. Some data show that a combination of antioxidants (i.e., vitamin E, vitamin C, and β-carotene) may be more effective than any of these single agents, providing more evidence in favor of moderation and variety in the diet.

VITAMIN E

FUNCTIONS

A generally accepted role for vitamin E is as a scavenger of free radicals, and in this capacity it protects cell membranes from damage. The role of vitamin E as an antioxidant in health and disease has attracted wide interest. It has many other properties as well. Vitamin E is essential for the immune system, particularly T-lymphocytes, and has a role in DNA repair. Interest is growing in the effect of vitamin E on inhibiting oxidation of low-density lipoprotein (LDL); oxidized LDL becomes more atherogenic. The neuromuscular system and the retina also require vitamin E for optimal function.

Vitamin E may have additional cellular protective effects. There is evidence that this vitamin may protect sulfhydryl groups in enzymes and other proteins. Similarly, stores of vitamin E may be conserved by the glutathione-S-transferase system, which utilizes reduce glutathione and serves similar antioxidant functions.

DEFICIENCY

Dietary vitamin E deficiency is relatively unusual in the United States under ordinary circumstances, as sources of vitamin E are widely available from the food supply. The recognizable cases of vitamin E deficiency tend to arise in debilitated patients who have had severe and prolonged periods of fat malabsorption. Vitamin E is incorporated into chylomicrons with other products of fat digestion during the process of intestinal absorption. Any illness that interferes with fat digestion, absorption, or metabolism may also impair absorption of vitamin E. Disorders in which symptomatic vitamin E deficiency develops include cystic fibrosis, celiac disease, cholestatic liver disease, and short-bowel syndrome from any cause.

Major abnormalities of neurologic function are observed in a severe and prolonged vitamin E deficiency state. Patients display areflexia, ophthalmoplegia, and disturbances of gait, proprioception, and vibration. In premature infants, vitamin E deficiency results in hemolytic anemia, thrombocytosis, edema, and intraventricular hemorrhage. There is increased risk of retrolental fibroplasia and bronchopulmonary dysplasia under these circumstances.

In hemolytic anemia, such as that caused by glucose-6-phosphate dehydrogenase deficiency and sickle cell anemia, vitamin E levels in blood tend to be decreased. Inborn errors of vitamin metabolism have been identified, but are rare. There are severe neurologic abnormalities in this category. In abetalipoproteinemia, there is a defect in the serum transport of vitamin E. A hallmark of this disease is the finding of extremely low serum cholesterol levels together with very low serum levels of vitamin E.

LABORATORY DIAGNOSIS OF DEFICIENCY

Ideally, the diagnosis of vitamin E deficiency should be made by detailed chromatographic analysis of the various E isomers. In practice, such a procedure is not realistic, and the clinical evaluation usually depends on measurement of total plasma E alone. Plasma concentrations of vitamin E below 0.50 μg/ml are generally regarded as indicative of deficiency. It has been observed that despite a wide range of dietary intake, the serum variations in vitamin E levels often tend to be in a much more limited range.

It is important to keep in mind that vitamin E is transported in blood bound to lipoproteins, particularly LDL. In any condition in which the serum cholesterol is abnormally high or low, the vitamin E level will vary accordingly. Therefore, before concluding that anyone is vitamin-E-deficient or has an excess of vitamin E, the plasma level of this vitamin should be evaluated in relation to the prevailing cholesterol concentrations. Furthermore, an α-tocopherol transport protein has been identified recently; its physiological role is at present under study.

PREVENTION

Deficiency of vitamin E can be avoided by regular consumption of the many sources of this vitamin in the food supply. The richest sources of vitamin E in the U.S. diet are vegetable oils, including corn, cottonseed, safflower and soybean oils, and the margarines and other products made from these oils. Green, leafy vegetables are also good sources of vitamin E. In evaluating the adequacy of any given dietary regimen, one should keep in mind the losses of the vitamin often occur during storage, cooking, and food processing, particularly with exposure to high temperatures and oxygen.

Because vitamin E deficiency frequently occurs as a result of severe intestinal malabsorption, it is essential to identify this condition early and avoid measures that may intensify the degree of malabsorption of vitamin E and other fat-soluble vitamins. Specific supplementation with vitamin E and other vitamins may be needed. The usual multivitamin supplement containing 400 IU should be adequate for this purpose.

There is evidence that dietary zinc is necessary in order for vitamin E to achieve adequate concentrations in peripheral blood. The relationship has been shown in both experimental animals and in patients.

There is a wide margin of safety in the therapeutic administration of the vitamin. Daily doses of vitamin E in the range of 100 to 800 IU can be given safely to nearly all-deficient patients. This dosage is higher than that usually found in multivitamin supplements. This dose range can be used appropriately in those patients with vitamin E deficiency diagnosed in association with celiac disease, inflammatory bowel disease, or other chronic and prolonged forms of intestinal malabsorption. In such instances, many other nutrient deficiencies are likely to be found in association with that of vitamin E, and they, too, necessitate treatment.

In the genetic disorders of vitamin E metabolism, such as isolated vitamin E deficiency, doses in the range of 800 to 1000 IU or higher must be taken. Large doses of vitamin E given therapeutically under these conditions appear to be generally safe. Some investigators have suggested that pharmacologic doses of vitamin E may interfere with the intestinal absorption of vitamins A and K, but there is little data with which to evaluate this potential risk. In addition, there are suggestive reports that doses of vitamin E in excess of 1200 IU/day may possibly interfere with the action of vitamin K and intensify the effects of anticoagulant drugs. Further information is needed on this subject.

The role of vitamin E in prevention of heart disease remains controversial. Some clinical studies have supported this concept while others have not. More research is needed before public health recommendations can be made for the general population.

VITAMIN K

FUNCTIONS

Vitamin K is a cofactor for posttranslational modification in a diverse group of calcium-binding proteins, whereby selective glutamic acid (Glu) residues are transformed into gamma-carboxyglutamic acid (Gla). The vitamin-K-dependent proteins that are best known include the four classic vitamin procoagulants (factors II, VII, IX, and X) and two feedback anticoagulants (proteins C and S), all synthesized by the liver. Therefore, severe liver disease leads to extensive abnormalities in vitamin K metabolism and frequent disturbances in blood coagulation.

Gla proteins also occur in several other tissues besides liver. Actions of vitamin K in bone have assumed greater importance in recent years. Osteocalcin, which contains three Gla residues, is synthesized by the osteoblasts of bone. It is one of the ten most abundant proteins in the body and may play a role in regulating bone turnover. A second protein isolated from bone that is related structurally to osteocalcin is matrix Gla protein. This protein is more widely distributed, and there is now evidence that this protein is an important inhibitor of calcification of arteries and cartilage. Gla residues provide efficient chelating sites for calcium ions that enable vitamin-K-dependent proteins to bind to other surfaces (e.g., procoagulants to platelet and vessel wall phospholipids, and osteocalcin to the hydroxyapatite matrix of bone). The carboxylation reaction is catalyzed by a microtome vitamin-K-dependent gammaglutamyl carboxylase, which requires the dietary quinone form of vitamin K to be first reduced to the active cofactor vitamin K hydroquinone, vitamin KH_2.

In bone, vitamin K achieves gamma-carboxylation of osteocalcin. In addition, vitamin K regulates interleukin-6 production, synthesis of prostaglandin E_2, and urinary excretion of calcium. It is not surprising, therefore, that in patients with long-term low dietary intake of vitamin K, the risk for hip fractures is increased.

DEFICIENCY

Isolated deficiency of vitamin K due entirely to inadequate dietary intake tends to be unusual in adults in the United States, because this vitamin is widely distributed in the food supply. Overt deficiency of vitamin K is more likely to be observed in conditions in which there are significant complicating factors, such as long-term use of broad-spectrum antibiotics, or illnesses and drugs associated with fat malabsorption. It is essential to recognize that vitamin K is synthesized by intestinal bacteria. Antibiotic treatment will largely eliminate these bacterial sources of vitamin K and may have some clinical impact, particularly when treatment is prolonged. One class of antibiotics, the cephalosporins, cause vitamin K deficiency by an entirely different mechanism, namely, by inhibiting the vitamin-K-dependent hydroxylase. The extent to which the bacterial source of vitamin K provides a significant contribution to the bodily supply of the vitamin is a subject of debate among experts.

Fat malabsorption is regularly observed as a feature of severe regional enteritis, nontropical sprue, cystic fibrosis, ulcerative colitis, and a number of other disorders. Following extensive intestinal resection, patients are left with a short-bowel syndrome, in which fat malabsorption is prominent because of the reduction in intestinal surfaces available for absorption and transport. In a recent study of more than 100 patients with cystic fibrosis, evidence of insufficient vitamin K nutrition was found in 70% of the sample. The clinical severity of deficiency was highly individualized.

Vitamin K deficiency with the most serious consequences is that associated with the hemorrhagic disease of the newborn. The pathogenesis of this syndrome derives from (a) the poor placental transport of vitamin K combined with (b) lack of fetal production of vitamin K by intestinal bacteria as the intestinal tract is sterile, and (c) diminished synthesis by an immature liver of prothrombin and its precursors. In adults with vitamin K deficiency, multiple purpuric lesions may be noted (Figure 9.1*).

As noted earlier, dietary sources of vitamin K are widespread in the food supply in the United States. The highest amounts are found in green leafy vegetables, such as broccoli, Brussel sprouts, spinach, turnip greens, and lettuce. Interestingly, the risk of hip fracture is reported to be the highest in women who have the lowest consumption of lettuce, which contributes significantly to vitamin K nutrition. Some vitamin K at lower amounts can be found in meat, dairy products, coffee, and certain teas. Green leafy vegetables contain vitamin K largely as phylloquinone. Meat, cheese and certain fermented foods contain vitamin K in the form of menaquinone.

LABORATORY DIAGNOSIS OF DEFICIENCY

Vitamin K in body fluids and in foods can be measured by biological and chemical methods. The vitamin is light sensitive and must be shielded from light during storage and analysis. In practice, functional vitamin K status is assessed indirectly by measurements of serum prothrombin. Clinical vitamin K deficiency should be suspected wherever there is an unusual hemorrhagic tendency. In assessing vitamin K deficiency clinically, it is important to remember that adequate carboxylation of proteins in bone requires higher doses of vitamin K than the carboxylation of proteins in liver. Thus, in repleting deficient patients, the blood coagulation profile could be normalized early but bone metabolism still compromised.

PREVENTION

For healthy individuals, dietary vitamin K deficiency should be preventable by maintaining a diet high in green, leafy vegetables. When antibiotics are prescribed long-term, they should be kept to the minimal time period and doses necessary. Efforts should be

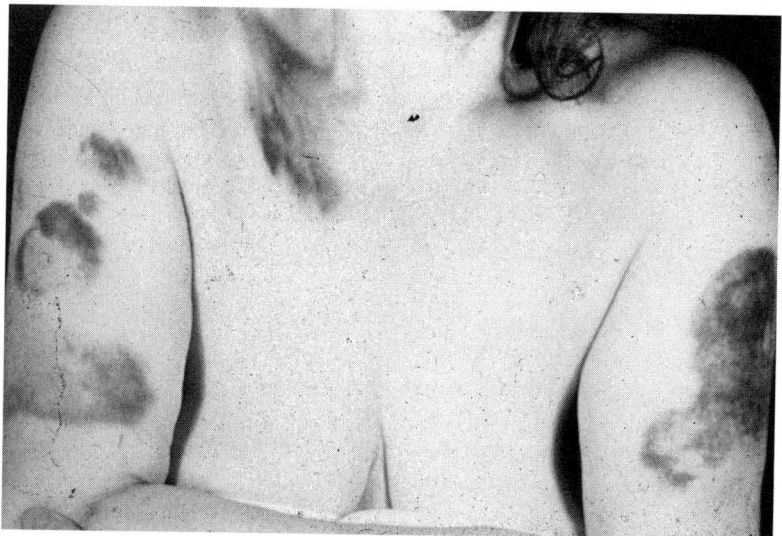

FIGURE 9.1 **(See color insert following page 654.)** Adult female patient with severe vitamin K deficiency illustrating multiple purpuric areas accuring spoentaneously. (Photo courtesy of Elaine B. Feldman.)

initiated early to recolonize the gastrointestinal tract by providing live-culture yogurt or other sources of normal flora. Similar guidelines should be followed in cases in which drugs causing malabsorption of vitamin K are required. Vitamin supplements containing vitamin K may be advisable. Effective treatment of an underlying disorder of the gastrointestinal tract should be undertaken in a specific fashion where possible, such as a gluten-free diet for nontropical sprue. All of these measures should help to prevent vitamin K deficiency.

TREATMENT

Treatment of vitamin K deficiency can be accomplished by oral administration of the purified vitamin, consumption of vitamin-K-rich foods, or parenteral injection of vitamin K. Water-soluble preparations of vitamin K are available. An oral dose of approximately 500 μg/day should correct vitamin K deficiency in terms of the coagulation profile and serum concentration of prothrombin. A poor or inadequate improvement of prothrombin time after vitamin K administration is generally indicative of severe underlying liver disease.

THIAMIN (VITAMIN B$_1$)

FUNCTIONS

Dietary thiamin functions as precursor of the coenzyme thiamin pyrophosphate, which by the process of oxidative decarboxylation converts α-ketoacids to aldehydes. These reactions are an important source of generating energy, and are widely distributed throughout intermediary metabolism. Thiamin pyrophosphate is also the coenzyme for transketolase, which converts xylulose-5-PO_4 and ribose-5-PO_4 to sedoheptulose-7-PO_4 and glyceraldehyde. The efficient generation of energy from oxidation of glucose requires adequate concentrations of thiamin pyrophosphate in the tissues.

More recent evidence suggests that thiamin has a role beyond that of coenzyme in regulating transmission of impulses in peripheral nerves. Some patients with peripheral neuropathy have been improved by thiamin administration. The metabolic role of thiamin in this proposed function is not well understood.

DEFICIENCY

Initial clinical presentations of thiamin deficiency are often subtle and nonspecific, comprising anorexia, general malaise, and weight loss. The typical Western diet is high in carbohydrate and may not be adequately matched in its thiamin content. An increase in carbohydrate content of the diet lowers the plasma and urinary levels of thiamin. Nonspecific symptoms of thiamin deficiency as it progresses are often followed by more intense weakness, peripheral neuropathy, headache, and tachycardia. When thiamin deficiency is far advanced, the patient usually exhibits prominent cardiovascular and neurological features.

Cardiac findings include an enlarged heart, tachycardia, edema, and ST-segment and T-wave changes. There is high-output failure due, at least in part, to peripheral vasodilatation. This clinical syndrome has a number of similarities to that of apathetic hyperthyroidism, with which it is often confused.

The central nervous system findings in advanced thiamin deficiency are those of the Wernicke–Korsakoff syndrome with vomiting, horizontal nystagmus, ataxia, weakness of the extraocular muscles, mental impairment, memory loss, and confabulation. There may be significant peripheral neuropathy as well. It is important to remember that the Wernicke–Korsakoff syndrome is not restricted to alcohol abuse and occurs with severe malnutrition, gastrointestinal disorders, and congestive heart failure. Some investigators have suggested that the reduction of thiamin pyrophosphate concentrations in brains of patients with Alzheimer's disease may have functional significance. Treatment of these patients with thiamin has been reported to be beneficial in some instances.

LABORATORY DIAGNOSIS OF DEFICIENCY

The diagnosis of thiamin deficiency is usually based on the analysis of this vitamin in blood by bioassay or by microbiological, chemical, or functional assays. In practice, urinary thiamin excretion and the erythrocyte transketolase are the most widely utilized assays of thiamin status. One must remember that urinary thiamin excretion reflects recent intake and may be increased after intake of diuretics.

The transketolase assay relies on an indirect measurement of the extent to which the apoenzyme is saturated with its coenzyme, thiamin pyrophosphate. When thiamin stores are depleted, addition of thiamin pyrophosphate *in vitro* to an erythrocyte lysate produces a large increase in measured enzyme activity. When the percentage increase in activity (activity coefficient) exceeds 15% to 20%, significant thiamin deficiency is diagnosed. Well-nourished individuals have much smaller activity coefficients when tested in a similar fashion. Lead intoxication lowers brain thiamin levels, and prompt thiamin treatment helps to restore brain thiamin levels while reducing brain lead levels.

PREVENTION

Thiamin deficiency can best be prevented by a diet consistently high in meat, grains, peas, beans, and nuts. Heating and treating vegetables with baking soda, which is alkaline, a practice often used to preserve the bright green colors, inactivates thiamin.

Intestinal absorption of dietary thiamin is very sensitive to alcohol. Persons who drink alcoholic beverages all day long, but never appear to be intoxicated, are nevertheless at risk for the development of thiamin deficiency. Thiaminases and antithiamin factors in raw fish, seafood, and other food items significantly break down dietary thiamin and may intensify the effects of a dietary deficiency. Polyphenols present in tea and coffee, when consumed excessively, may also inactivate dietary thiamin.

TREATMENT

Large doses of thiamin (50 to 100 mg) may be administered safely by the parenteral route in the acute syndrome, and the results are often dramatic, with rapid resolution of nystagmus. Following several days of treatment with doses at this level, treatment with 5 to 10 mg/day of thiamin is then appropriate. There is little, if any, toxicity when thiamin is given at levels of several times the RDI.

RIBOFLAVIN (VITAMIN B$_2$)

FUNCTIONS

To fulfil its metabolic functions, dietary riboflavin must be converted to its flavin coenzymes, flavin mononucleotide (riboflavin-5'-phosphate; FMN) and flavin adenine dinucleotide (FAD). In addition, several percent of flavins, such as monoamine oxidase, sarcosine dehydrogenase and succinate dehydrogenase, are bound covalently to tissue proteins. The flavin coenzymes as a group catalyze many different types of reactions, particularly oxidation-reduction reactions, dehydrogenations, and oxidative decarboxylation. Most importantly, flavin coenzymes are involved in the respiratory chain, lipid metabolism, the cytochrome P-450 system, and drug metabolism.

Riboflavin has antioxidant activity in its role as precursor to FAD, the coenzyme required by glutathione reductase. The glutathione redox cycle provides major protection against lipid peroxides. Glutathione reductase generates reduced glutathione (GSH) from glutathione (GSSG), which is the substrate required by glutathione peroxidase to inactivate hydrogen peroxide and other lipid peroxides. Thus, increased lipid peroxidation is a feature of riboflavin deficiency, and one that is not widely appreciated.

Some flavoproteins contain both FMN and FAD as coenzymes. Included in this category of biflavin enzymes are microsomal NADPH-cytochrome P450-reductase, nitric oxide synthase, and methionine synthase.

DEFICIENCY

Clinically, patients with advanced riboflavin deficiency exhibit seborrheic dermatitis, severe burning and itching of the eyes, abnormal vascularization of the cornea leading to cataract, cheilosis, angular stomatitits, anemia, and neuropathy. A smooth red tongue is classically observed in riboflavin deficiency (Figure 9.2), but is not pathognomonic of this deficiency.

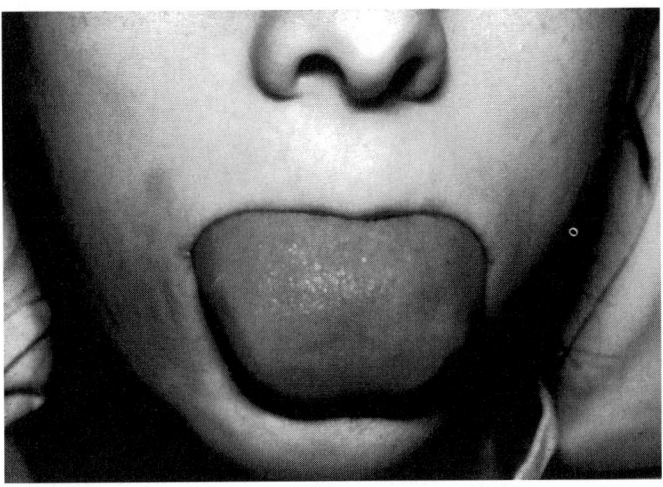

FIGURE 9.2 (See color insert following page 654.) Adult female patient with advanced deficiency of riboflavin (vitamin B$_2$) illustrating large, red, smooth tongue, Paller and Cheelosis. (Photo courtesy of Elaine B. Feldman, MD.)

The clinical features of human riboflavin deficiency are not unique compared with the specificity of some aspects of vitamin C deficiency such as scurvy. The earliest symptoms of riboflavin deficiency include weakness and fatigue, mouth pain, itching eyes, and occasionally personality disorders.

The evolution of dietary riboflavin deficiency may be intensified by diseases, drugs, and endocrine disorders that block riboflavin utilization. The conditions in which such effects are observed include thyroid and adrenal insufficiency, treatment with the psychotropic drugs, chlorpromazine, imipramine, and amitriptyline; the antimalarial, quinacrine; and the cancer chemotherapeutic drug, adriamycin. Alcohol ingestion may be a significant cause of riboflavin deficiency by its interference with both its digestion from food sources and its intestinal absorption.

Riboflavin deficiency seldom occurs as an isolated entity, and is nearly always detected in association with deficiencies of other B vitamins.

LABORATORY DIAGNOSIS OF DEFICIENCY

Riboflavin and its derivatives can be analyzed precisely by high-performance liquid chromatography (HPLC). Other available techniques are not generally utilized in clinical practice. Urinary riboflavin excretion is reduced with long-term dietary deficiency, but may rise abruptly after recent intake of the vitamin. Therefore, the test must be run in the truly basal state. Collections have to be made carefully in subdued light and stored in dark bottles because of the light sensitivity of the vitamin.

A functional test, the erythrocyte glutathione reductase activity coefficiency (EGRAC), measures saturation of the enzyme with its coenzyme (FAD) by the same principle as that developed earlier to assess thiamin status with transketolase. The larger the increase in EGRAC noted after the addition of FAD *in vitro,* the greater the degree of unsaturation of the apoenzyme with its cofactor and the more severe the deficiency of riboflavin.

PREVENTION

Riboflavin deficiency can be prevented by maintaining a diet high in meat and dairy products, the major sources of the vitamin in the United States. Certain green vegetables, including broccoli, asparagus, and spinach, also contain significant quantities of riboflavin, as do fortified cereals. In developing countries, vegetables constitute the major sources of riboflavin.

It should be recalled that because of its heat and light sensitivity, considerable amounts of the vitamin can be lost when liquids are stored in clear bottles, when fruits and vegetables are sun-dried, and when baking soda is added to fresh vegetables to maintain color and texture. Under the latter conditions, riboflavin loss is accelerated by photodegradation.

Riboflavin has been reported to decrease the frequency of migraine attacks, the severity of lactic acidosis in AIDS patients undergoing therapy, and in rare genetic defects of the respiratory chain. The utilization of dietary folate requires adequate FAD, and for this reason, riboflavin (B_2) as well as B_6, B_{12}, and folic acids are needed to regulate homocysteine metabolism optimally.

TREATMENT

Treatment of clinical deficiency can be accomplished by oral intake of the vitamin. Levels greater than 25 mg cannot be completely absorbed as a single dose. This dose level is certainly safe to administer. The parenteral administration of riboflavin is limited by its low solubility. Riboflavin-5'-phosphate is more soluble than riboflavin, but is not usually available for clinical use.

A theoretical risk involved in treatment with riboflavin lies in its photosensitizing properties. *In vitro,* phototherapy results in DNA degradation and increased formation of lipid peroxides. Riboflavin forms an adduct with tryptophan and accelerates its photodegradation. The extent to which these observations have implications for conditions prevailing *in vivo* in humans needs to be elucidated.

NIACIN (SOMETIMES REFERRED TO AS VITAMIN B₃)

FUNCTIONS

Niacin is the dietary precursor of two important coenzymes, nicotinamide adenine dinucleotide (NAD) and nicotinamide adenine dinucleotide phosphate (NADP). Both coenzymes catalyze oxidation-reduction reactions, and are involved in a wide variety of reactions in intermediary metabolism. These reactions include glycolysis and lipid, amino acid, and protein metabolism.

DEFICIENCY

As with the other B vitamins, dietary deficiency of niacin generally occurs together with other vitamin deficiencies. An unusual aspect of niacin compared with other vitamins is that it is not obtained entirely from the diet. Niacin is formed from dietary tryptophan, an essential aromatic amino acid. Thus, high-quality protein sources tend to protect against niacin deficiency, and poor protein sources that are inadequate in tryptophan, such as corn, tend to accelerate niacin deficiency. For this reason, in parts of the world where the diet is based primarily on corn or maize as the dietary staple without other varied sources of protein, pellagra can develop readily.

Alcoholism may result in niacin deficiency, as will drugs, such as isonicotinic acid hydrazide (isoniazid; INH), which interfere with niacin metabolism. The anticancer agent 6-mercoptopurine may produce severe niacin deficiency. One may also find niacin deficiency in the rare inborn error of Hartnup's disease and in the malignant carcinoid syndrome. In this syndrome, dietary tryptophan is diverted to the synthesis of serotonin at the expense of niacin.

Early manifestations of niacin deficiency are generally nonspecific, with anorexia, weight loss, weakness, and irritability. In later stages of deficiency, as pellagra, the patient may develop glossitis, stomatitis, characteristic scaling, and skin lesions, as shown in Figure 9.3 and Figure 9.4. Scaling skin lesions tend to be particularly prominent in sun-exposed areas, such as the arms, legs, and the V of the neck. In advanced disease, one may encounter "the four Ds": dermatitis, diarrhea, dementia, and death.

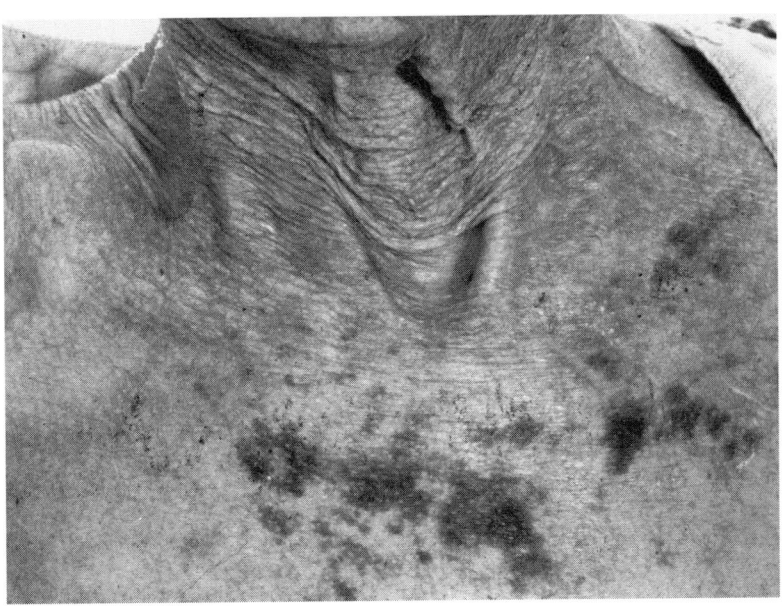

FIGURE 9.3   (See color insert following page 654.) Adult male patient with advanced lesions of pellagra resulting from severe, prolonged main deficiency illustrating a dark scaly, eruptier over the skin particularly the seen exposed areas. (Photo courtesy of Elaine B Feldman MD.)

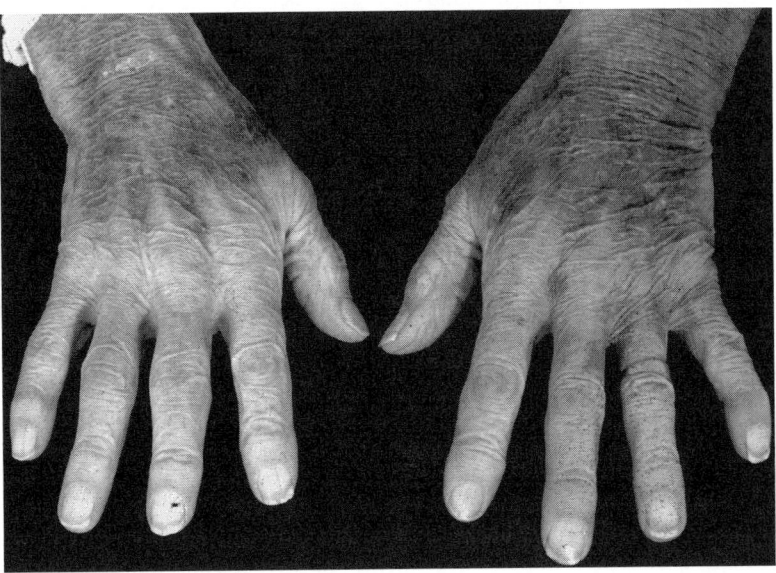

FIGURE 9.4   (See color insert following page 654.) Same patient as in Figure 9.3 showing hands with dark, scaly thickened skin lesions. (Photo courtesy of Elaine B. Feldman MD.)

LABORATORY DIAGNOSIS AND DEFICIENCY

In practice, the diagnosis of niacin deficiency can be established by assay of the urinary excretion of niacin metabolites, specifically *N*-methylnicotinamide, and, less commonly, 2-pyridone. Accurate determinations can be made by high-performance liquid chromatography (HPLC).

PREVENTION

As noted earlier, the diet needs to be adequate in protein of high biological value that contains tryptophan. Intake of meat and dairy products tends to assure adequate intake of tryptophan. A vegetarian diet may contain adequate amounts of niacin if it is sufficiently balanced and varied.

TREATMENT

The syndrome of niacin deficiency can be treated rapidly and effectively with oral administration of the vitamin. Doses in the range of 50 to 150 mg/day of nicotinamide are recommended to treat severe deficiency, and need to be maintained during the initial treatment period. Improvement is usually noted clinically after only a few days of treatment. The patient usually reports relief of pain and pruritis.

Niacin as a drug in the form of nicotinic acid is a first-line agent for the management of an abnormal serum lipid profile. Doses in the range of 1.5 to 6.0 g are administered daily. Niacin may be effective alone and in combination with other agents in lowering LDL-cholesterol, raising HDL-cholesterol, and reducing serum triacylglycerols (triglycerides). There may, however, be significant side effects noted at this dose range, including worsening of diabetes, abnormalities in liver function tests, elevation of the serum uric acid, and ocular abnormalities. Flushing may be troublesome to the patient, but is often transient. In most instances, the flushing can be minimized by taking a tablet of aspirin shortly before the niacin, taking a long-acting preparation of niacin, or taking the niacin at bedtime so that the flushing occurs as the patient sleeps.

The form of niacin selected for the improvement of the serum lipid profile is crucial. Nicotinic acid is the only form that is effective. Often patients choose niacinamide on their own from a health food store because it does not cause a flush. Unfortunately, it also does not benefit the abnormal serum lipid concentrations.

PYRIDOXINE (VITAMIN B$_6$)

FUNCTIONS

The role of vitamin B$_6$ is primarily that of precursor to pyridoxal phosphate. This coenzyme participates in a large number of reactions in intermediary metabolism, particularly transamination and decarboxylation. In addition, pyridoxal phosphate is involved in side-chain cleavage, dehydratase activity, and racemization of amino aids. These reactions relate to gluconeogenesis, lipid metabolism, immune function, cerebral metabolism, nucleic acid synthesis, and steroid hormone action. Deficiency of vitamin B$_6$ can lead to secondary deficiencies of other vitamins because it plays a role in the metabolic pathway leading to synthesis of niacin from tryptophan. Vitamin B$_6$, together with B$_{12}$, folic acid, and probably B$_2$, is involved in synthetic and degradative pathways of homocysteine metabolism.

Although some B$_6$ is present in the diet in the form of pyridoxal, the majority is in other forms. In plants, B$_6$ is present largely as pyridoxine, whereas animal sources comprise pyridoxamine as well as pyridoxal phosphate, and other forms.

DEFICIENCY

As with other B vitamins, isolated pyridoxine deficiency entirely on a dietary basis is seldom found. In some instances a marginal diet may result in overt deficiency if there are other complicating factors, such as the long-term use of specific pyridoxine antagonists. Two common examples of this effect are isoniazid and cycloserine, used to treat tuberculosis and generally prescribed for an extended period to eradicate the organism. In some individuals a genetic trait leads to delays in inactivating isoniazid; as a result, these patients become unusually susceptible to developing B$_6$ deficiency.

Pyridoxine deficiency is a common feature of chronic alcoholism, found in association with overall malnutrition and inadequate intake of many other vitamins and minerals. An unusual feature of the pathogenesis of B$_6$ deficiency in alcoholism is that the major effect of alcohol appears to be that of accelerating the rate of degradation of pyridoxal into its inactive metabolites, particularly pyridoxic acid.

B$_6$ deficiency is not recognizable as a distinct, pathogenomic clinical syndrome. Patients develop degrees of dermatitis, glossitis, cheilosis, and weakness. In more severe deficiency, patients may progress to have dizziness, depression, peripheral neuropathy, and seizures. The risk of kidney stones is increased because of hyperoxaluria. In children, B$_6$ deficiency is an important cause of anemia and seizures. Deficiency of B$_6$ causes a hypochromic, microcytic anemia that resembles the anemia due to iron deficiency.

The diagnosis of B_6-deficiency anemia is suggested when a bone marrow aspiration reveals that stainable iron, instead of being reduced as in iron deficiency, is normal or even increased in amounts.

In a group of rare genetic disorders, called pyridoxine dependency syndromes, large doses of B_6 are required for control of symptoms. Among these disorders are pyridoxine-dependent convulsions, cystathioninuria, and xanthurenicaciduria.

LABORATORY DIAGNOSIS OF DEFICIENCY

Vitamin B_6 can be measured directly in blood, with levels less than 50 ng/ml generally considered to represent deficiency. The measurement needs to be interpreted in the light of the patient's diet, as exceptionally high dietary protein intake depresses plasma pyridoxal phosphate levels, probably because of increased utilization of the coenzyme in protein and amino acid metabolism.

Urinary tests measure the excretion of metabolites of pyridoxine, most commonly 4-pyridoxic acid. Indirect assessments of vitamin B_6 deficiency can be made using functional assays of the enzymes aspartate or alanine aminotransferase with and without the addition of their cofactors *in vitro*. The principle of these assays is similar to that discussed earlier for thiamin and riboflavin deficiency. Activity coefficients greater than 1.2 for alanine aminotransferase and 1.5 for aspartate aminotransferase are generally considered as diagnostic of a deficient state.

At one time, a specific diagnosis of B_6 deficiency was made by measuring xanthurenic acid after a tryptophan load, inasmuch as B_6 is the coenzyme involved in the metabolic transformation. This procedure, although theoretically sound, is very laborious and has largely been abandoned in routine clinical diagnosis.

PREVENTION

Vitamin B_6 is widely available in the food supply and is found in vegetables, beans, (especially soy beans), meat, nuts, seeds, and cereals. A diet that is adequate and diversified in these dietary items will generally prevent vitamin B_6 deficiency. It is evident that this kind of diet will prevent deficiencies of the other B vitamins as well. Certain kinds of food processing, particularly heat sterilization, can result in significant losses of activity of vitamin B_6.

TREATMENT

Once vitamin B_6 deficiency is diagnosed, it can be satisfactorily managed at a level of 2 to 10 mg/day, which represents doses several times those of the RDI. Vitamin B_6 deficiency during pregnancy should be treated with higher doses in the 10 to 20 mg range because of the increased requirement at this time.

Vitamin B_6 is routinely advised during prolonged treatment with isoniazid, which is a pyridoxine antagonist. In doses of 50 to 100 mg/day, vitamin B_6 has been noted to reduce peripheral neuropathy without apparently lessening efficacy of INH against tuberculosis. In patients with Parkinson's disease receiving treatment with L-DOPA, too much pyridoxine will interfere with drug action; therefore, as a general rule, these large doses should not be taken unless there is a specific indication.

It is important not to exceed certain limits in therapeutic administration of vitamin B_6. Cases of sensory neuropathy have been occasionally noted in patients taking 1 to 2 g/day and noted rarely when taking only 500 mg/day. The genetic B_6 dependency syndromes can be managed on doses of 100 to 200 mg/day. There have been some encouraging reports that B_6 supplementation may be beneficial in managing premenopausal young women with depression. These findings require confirmation and extension in larger groups of depressed young women.

VITAMIN C (ASCORBIC ACID)

FUNCTIONS

Ascorbic acid serves in both oxidation and reduction reactions, based on the prevailing environmental conditions. Therefore, depending on circumstances, ascorbic acid may act as either an antioxidant or a prooxidant. An important function of ascorbic acid is that of preventing oxidation of tetrahydrofolate. Ascorbic acid is involved in collagen biosynthesis, wound healing, immune function, and drug metabolism. It enhances the intestinal absorption of nonheme iron. This vitamin is involved in the biosynthesis of neurotransmitters and carnitine.

Ascorbic acid concentrations in plasma are inversely related to markers of inflammation, such as C-reactive protein (CRP). Recent findings suggest that ascorbic acid may have anti-inflammatory effects in addition to its other actions.

DEFICIENCY

Dietary deficiency develops when the diet does not contain adequate amounts of citrus fruits, vegetables, and tomatoes, most commonly among the elderly and the urban poor. Vitamin C deficiency may also arise when there is food faddism or very limited food choices, behaviors that are commonly observed these days. The classical "tea and toast" diet, followed by some elderly people, is particularly deficient in vitamin C. The macrobiotic diet may lead to scurvy both because of poor dietary sources as well as the practice of pressure-cooking food, which destroys ascorbic acid.

In infancy and childhood, a diet composed exclusively of unsupplemented cow's milk is deficient in vitamin C and may lead to scurvy. Chronic alcoholism at any age is associated with poor ascorbic acid intake, and if prolonged, will greatly increase the risk for development of scurvy.

The clinical symptoms of vitamin C deficiency develop slowly, and as with other vitamins, are often vague and nonspecific. Patients complain of weakness and fatigue, progressing to dyspnea and lethargy. The characteristic features of scurvy are not observed until the deficiency syndrome is well advanced. Bone and joint pain may occur because of hemorrhages in the subperiosteum. Perifollicular hemorrhages, especially in relation to hair follicles, are observed, as shown in Figure 9.5. Hairs may show a recognizable corkscrew pattern. Swollen, bleeding gums are observed in advanced deficiency, as shown in Figure 9.6, followed by loss of teeth. Pallor may be due to bleeding or reduced hematopoiesis. Scurvy results in poor wound healing and secondary breakdown of wounds that had healed previously. It is generally believed that clinical features of scurvy become evident after about 3 months without adequate intake of vitamin C, usually because of failure to consume fruits or vegetables.

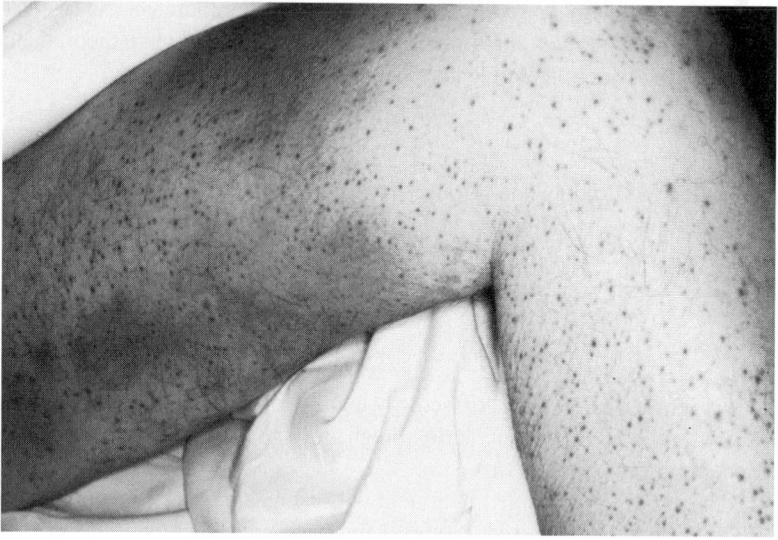

FIGURE 9.5   (See color insert following page 654.) Adult female patient with advanced scurvy resulting from severe deficiency of vitamin C illustrating multiple perifollicular hemorrhages and sore corkscrew hairs. (Photo courtesy of Elaine B Feldman MD.)

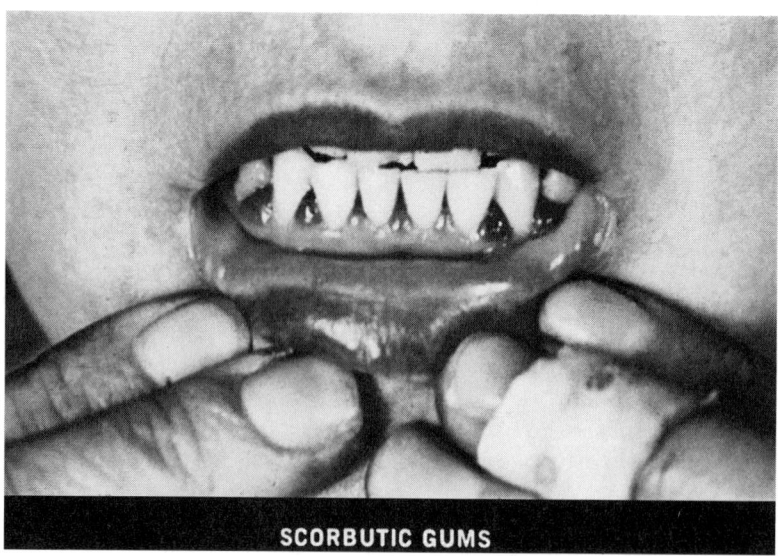

FIGURE 9.6   (See color insert following page 654.) Same patient as in Figure 9.5 showing bleeding, swollen gingeval tissues (Photo courtesy of Elaine B Feldman MD.)

Estimates of the prevalence of vitamin C deficiency in the United States were released in 2004, based upon the results of the Third National Health and Nutrition Examination Survey (HANES), conducted from 1988 to 1994. Evidence of early vitamin C depletion was found in 13% to 23% of the individuals surveyed and evidence of frank ascorbic acid deficiency in 5% to 17% of them. The highest risks for deficiency were found among smokers, non-Hispanic Black males, and persons who did not use nutritional supplements of any kind.

LABORATORY DIAGNOSIS OF DEFICIENCY

Ascorbic acid can be measured directly in the blood serum or plasma by a variety of chemical methods, most commonly spectrophotometric or fluorometric. Levels of 0.1 mg/dl or lower are generally indicative of vitamin C deficiency. Serum levels may be reduced in many chronic digestive disorders in smokers and in some women taking oral contraceptive drugs. Vitamin C concentrations may be measured accurately in leukocytes, but this assay is not commonly available.

Blood levels tend to segregate in a relatively narrow range in the face of very large differences in dietary intake. Megadoses of ascorbic acid remain almost entirely unabsorbed in the gastrointestinal tract, and what little is absorbed is rapidly metabolized by an efficient hepatic drug-metabolizing enzyme system. With its low renal threshold, ascorbic acid is excreted rapidly in the urine.

PREVENTION

Vitamin C deficiency can be prevented simply by consuming a diet adequate in citrus fruits and vegetables. Consuming orange juice with meals may be a healthy habit that increases the intestinal absorption of nonheme iron several-fold. Avoiding heating or prolonged storage of foods containing vitamin C can also help maintain adequate concentrations. Educating people about the potential hazards of a macrobiotic diet, food faddism, and sharply limited food choices should also help to prevent scurvy in the general population.

The prevention of scurvy may be accomplished by ingestion of very small amounts of ascorbic acid. Some authorities believe that doses as low as 10 mg/day may be effective. The maintenance of an adequate vitamin C status has generally been considered to be in the 40 to 60 mg range, as reflected in the RDI.

Recently it has been proposed that the optimal intake of ascorbic acid should be one that not only prevents deficiency but also achieves full concentrations in tissue stores. Based on these assumptions, daily doses of 100 to 200 mg/day may be needed. To achieve this level of intake, major public health efforts will need to be made, particularly to reach the urban poor.

TREATMENT

Doses of ascorbic acid as low as 10 mg/day, as noted earlier, may prevent scurvy and can achieve benefits in treatment. In advanced cases, a dose range of 100 to 200 mg/day orally may be administered safely and effectively, with therapeutic benefit evident within a few days. As noted earlier, it has been proposed that these larger doses need to be maintained to achieve tissue saturation. Meat sources containing heme iron are more bioavailable than the nonheme iron present in vegetables. As noted, the efficiency of absorption of nonheme iron can be greatly improved by simultaneous consumption of orange juice.

Megadoses of vitamin C have been given to patients with advanced cancer, but their anticancer efficacy is unproven. Vitamin C has also been advocated to prevent cancer, because its content in fruits and vegetables may be part of the reason that cancer prevalence is reduced in patients who consume several servings a day. One must keep in mind, however, that fruits and vegetables contain many other beneficial phytochemicals whose full potential is only beginning to be explored. There is also a suggestion from some *in vitro* studies that large amounts of vitamin C may not be advisable in terms of possibly accelerating tumor metabolism.

There is some risk for toxicity in doses greater than 1 to 2 g/day in a highly individual fashion. Gastrointestinal upset may occur. Inasmuch as oxalic acid is a direct metabolite of ascorbic acid, the risk of kidney stones theoretically should be increased with large doses of ascorbic acid. The exact prevalence of symptomatic stone formation after ingestion of variable doses of vitamin C is not known with certainty.

Caution in administering vitamin C should be followed when giving it to individuals with hemochromatosis or those at risk for this disorder, as the intestinal absorption and tissue storage of iron may be increased excessively. As the gene for hemochromatosis is one of the most common genetic abnormalities known, there may be risk associated with indiscriminate use of megadoses of ascorbic acid supplements by the general population.

VITAMIN D

See Chapter 64 on calcium in bone health and Chapter 10 on calcium and vitamin D in dietary supplements.

BIBLIOGRAPHY

1. Adams J, Pepping J. *Am. J. Health Syst. Pharm.* 62:1574; 2005.
2. Agus DB, Vera JC, Golde DW. *Cancer Res.* 59:4555; 1999.
3. Carr A, Frei B. *FASEB J.* 13:1007; 1999.
4. Conway SP, Wolfe SP, Brown Lee KG, et al. *Pediatrics* 115:1325; 2005.
5. D'Souza RM, D'Souza R. *J. Trop. Pediatr.* 48:323; 2002.
6. Fontana M. *Compendium* 15:916; 1994.
7. Hampl JS, Taylor CA, Johnston CS. The Third National Health and Nutrition Examination Survey, 1988 to 1994. *Am J Public Health.* 94:870; 2004.
8. Levine M, Padayatty SJ, Katz A, Kwon O, et al. In: *Vitamin C: Functions and Biochemistry in Animals and Plants*, Asard H, May JM, Smirnoff N, Eds. London, B105 Scientific Publishers, 2004, p. 291.
9. Lonsdale D. *eCAM* 3:49; 2006.
10. Rivlin RS. In: *Present Knowledge in Nutrition*. Russell R, and Bowman B, Eds. Washington DC, ILSI Press, 2007, in press.
11. Rivlin RS. In: *Cecil Textbook of Medicine*, 19th ed., Wyngaarden JH, Smith LH, Jr, Bennett JC, Plum F, Eds. Philadelphia, WB Saunders, 1991; pp. 1170–1183.
12. Sommer A, Davidson FR. *J. Nutr.* 132:2845S; 2002.
13. Standing Committee on the Scientific Evaluation of Dietary References Intakes, Food and Nutrition Board, Institute of Medicine. *Dietary Reference Intakes for Thiamin, Riboflavin, Niacin, Vitamin B_6, Folate, Vitamin B_{12}, Panthothenic Acid, Biotin and Choline.* Washington DC, National Academy Press, 1999.
14. Underwood BA. *J. Nutr.* 134:231S; 2004.
15. Wannamethee SG, Lowe GDO, Rumley A, et al. *Am. J. Clin. Nutr.* 83:567; 2006.
16. Weber P. *Int. J. Vitam. Nutr. Res.* 69:194; 1999.
17. Williams AL, Cotter A, Sabina A, et al. *Fam. Pract.* 5:532; 2005.

10 Potential Benefits for the Use of Vitamin and Mineral Supplements

Richard Cotter, Judith Moreines, and Leon Ellenbogen

CONTENTS

INTRODUCTION

Emerging scientific evidence suggests that vitamins and minerals provide health benefits that may go beyond the repletion of potential nutritional deficiency states. This science indicates that these benefits may be conveyed by intakes at or above recommended daily allowances. For some of these health benefits, the scientific evidence base is convincing, while support for the potential benefits are just emerging for others. In many cases, the association between a particular vitamin and mineral and its beneficial effects is derived from nutritional epidemiological studies. Intervention studies are either underway, or are warranted, in order to demonstrate a casual nutrient benefit link. Additionally, in the case of multivitamin supplementation, further investigation is needed in order to determine and characterize the nutrient or nutrient interactions that may produce a particular beneficial effect. What follows is an up-to-date description of the emerging benefits of vitamins and minerals and the scientific support for each.

As the increasing importance of nutrients and their health benefits become known, the need to update the science surrounding these nutrients became apparent. The U.S. Food and Nutrition Board, Institute of Medicine, National Academy of Sciences undertook such a review between 1997 and 2004, publishing the updated science series, "Dietary Recommended Intakes," in which all of the essential vitamin and minerals were reviewed. In addition, various health agencies and related organizations continue to recognize the importance of good nutrition and issue recommendations for vitamin and mineral supplementation and food fortification. These include the U.S. Public Health Service, Centers for Disease Control, the National Osteoporosis Foundation, and the Department of Health and Human Services, who, in 2005, issued the "Dietary Guidelines for Americans" for 2005. Internationally, many agencies and organizations have, and are, issuing similar guidelines.

VITAMIN A

Dietary antioxidants, including carotenoids and vitamin A, are hypothesized to decrease the risk of age-related cataracts and age-related macular degeneration (AMD) by preventing oxidation of proteins or lipids within the lens.[1,2] Information on the role of vitamins in eye disease is discussed in Chapter 58.

Vitamin A deficiency appears to be common in individuals with HIV infection. Low levels of vitamin A are associated with greater disease severity.[3,4] Transmission of the virus from mothers deficient in vitamin A to their infants has been reported.[5] However, there have been no intervention studies to determine whether vitamin A supplementation is helpful. However, recent studies in HIV infected women have demonstrated a reduction in the progression of this disease as a result of daily multivitamin supplementation.[6]

The potential benefit of vitamin A therapy for measles was first reported in 1932,[7] and a recent study in South African children under 13 years of age showed that large doses (400,000 IU) of vitamin A resulted in lower complication rates and mortality. Low vitamin A levels are associated with the highest mortality in young children with measles.[8] WHO, UNICEF, and the American Academy of Pediatrics recommend that children with measles be examined for vitamin A deficiency.

Large quantities of analogs of vitamin A, on the order of 300,000 IU/day for females and 400,000 to 500,000 IU/day for males, have been used successfully to treat a severe type of acne known as cystic acne.[9] However, such high doses of vitamin A are potentially toxic, and topical retinol therapy is more appropriate.

Vitamin A is needed for the growth and repair of cells that line both the small and large intestines. Over the years, reports have appeared of individuals with Crohn's disease responding to vitamin A therapy at a dose of 50,000 IU/day.[10–12] See Table 10.1 and Table 10.2 for the established and potential benefits of vitamin A.

Although Vitamin A has been shown to have many of the positive benefits indicated above, one should be cautious of the long-term use of vitamin A supplements greater that approximately 6000 IU, since a series of studies indicate such supplementation may result in accelerated bone resorption.[13–15]

β-CAROTENE

Based on the unanimous recommendation by health professionals that diets rich in fruits and vegetables may help reduce the risk of cancer, heart disease, and diabetes, scientists have started to identify the components in these foods that are responsible for the health benefits. Because β-carotene is one of the more abundant carotenoids in fruits and vegetables, it dominated the research on carotenoids in the 1980s, following the report published in *Nature* by Dr. Richard Peto et al., titled "Can dietary β-carotene materially reduce cancer rates?"[16] See Table 10.3 for the established benefits of β-carotene.

In addition to extensive epidemiological data, β-carotene showed strong promise in laboratory studies with cancer cells and animals (see Albanes and Hartman, *Antioxidants and Cancer*,[17] for the long list of epidemiological studies). The results of three

TABLE 10.1
Vitamin A — Established Benefits

Important for normal growth in children
Necessary for wound repair
Involved in RNA synthesis
Helps to form and maintain healthy skin, eyes, teeth, gums,
  hair, mucous membrane, and various glands
Involved in fat metabolism
Important for resisting infectious diseases
Necessary for night and color vision

TABLE 10.2
Vitamin A — Potential Benefits

Use	Findings	Reference
Age-related cataracts	Vitamin A use not related to decreased risk of cataract	2
HIV	High doses may be protective	3–5
Measles	High doses decrease morbidity and mortality	7,8
Acne	High doses may be helpful	9
Crohn's disease	Variable response to high doses	10–12

TABLE 10.3
β-Carotene — Established Benefits

Can be converted into vitamin A
Antioxidant function
Supports the immune system

TABLE 10.4
Important β-Carotene Cancer Trials

α-Tocopherol, β-Carotene Cancer Prevention Study[18] (ATBC Study) — also called the Finnish study	29,133 male smokers, 50 to 69 years of age	50 mg vitamin E, 20 mg β-carotene or both for 5 to 8 years	No evidence of prevention of lung and other cancers. β-carotene group had a 16% greater incidence of lung cancer in smokers
β-Carotene and Retinol Efficacy Trial[19] (CARET)	18,314 men and women smokers and former smokers	25,000 Iu vitamin A, 30 mg β-carotene	Increase of 28% in lung cancer and 17% in cancer mortality
Physicians' Health Study[20] (PHS)	22,071 males, mainly nonsmokers	50 mg β-carotene every other day for 12 years	No effect on cancer rates for prostate, bowel, or lung or for overall incidence of cancer or mortality

major double-blind, randomized, placebo-controlled clinical studies, however, were surprising and perplexing in that not only was there no cancer benefit shown, but in both the ATBC and the CARET study, the data actually indicated potential risk for smokers and asbestos workers.[18,19] The Physicians Health Study (PHS), on the other hand, using higher levels of β-carotene, showed no such risk[20] (see Table 10.4).

The conclusions demonstrating a potentially adverse effect of β-carotene in smokers were questioned because of the evidence from epidemiological and basic biochemical studies whose results were contrary. It has been suggested that the very high doses of β-carotene used in the above studies might have interfered with the absorption of carotenoids other than β-carotene.

Several ongoing intervention studies may help clarify the inconsistency of these findings. The Chinese Cancer Prevention Study[21] evaluated β-carotene (15 mg), vitamin E (30 mg), and selenium (50 μg) and found an insignificant 10% decrease in cerebrovascular mortality in a group receiving treatment compared to that of an untreated group. There was a 13% reduction of borderline significance in total cancer mortality in the treated group and a 21% reduction in gastric cancer, which was significant. Because β-carotene was evaluated in combination with other nutrients, it is not possible to isolate the effect attributable to β-carotene alone. Other nutrients may have had an effect in the poorly nourished group included as study subjects, and results may not be applicable to well-nourished individuals.

Several smaller studies of β-carotene and premalignant lesions have shown interesting preliminary results. A 66% reduction in the frequency of premalignant buccal micronuclei was observed after supplementation of 26 mg of β-carotene for 9 weeks.[22] A 71% reduction was observed in patients with oral leukoplakia after a 6-month intake of 30 mg/day of β-carotene.[23]

Apart from cancer prevention, β-carotene has been studied for its effect in coronary heart disease and cataract. A subgroup of the PHS, which included 333 physicians with unstable angina or a prior coronary revascularization procedure, had a 20 to 30% reduction in vascular disease associated with treatment. High dietary intakes of β-carotene were found to be associated with a decreased risk of myocardial infarction in the Rotterdam study, which investigated the dietary intakes of 4802 elderly men and women over the course of 4 years.[24]

A similar effect was not seen for either vitamins C or E. See Table 10.5 for emerging benefits of β-carotene. The results of several additional important prospective studies are included in Table 10.6.

People with low blood levels of antioxidants and those who eat few antioxidant-rich fruits and vegetables are at high risk for cataract.[28,29] See information in Chapter 58 on eye disease.

Lycopene is an antioxidant carotenoid found commonly in tomatoes. Although not a vitamin per se, or a provitamin (for vitamin A), specific benefits of lycopene are beginning to be elucidated, particularly with respect to certain cancers. Of particular note is an observational finding that high intakes of tomato products containing lycopene are associated with lower rates of prostate cancer. An excellent overview by Giovannucci[30] covers lycopene and the epidemiological evidence supporting its currently known health benefits in the prevention of cancer.

Lycopene has also more recently been associated with cardiac benefits. As the most powerful antioxidant of the carotenoid family, it has naturally aroused interest in the cardiac community. A complete overview of this emerging area can be found in a review by Rao.[31]

Lutein, another carotenoid that is found in large amounts in fruits and vegetables, is as important in eye health for the prevention of both age-related macular degeneration and age-related cataracts. See chapter 58 for further discussion of these benefits.

TABLE 10.5
β-Carotene — Potential Benefits

Cancer — lung, cervix, oral, colorectal, pancreas, prostate
Cardiovascular disease
Cataracts
Restenosis after angioplasty

TABLE 10.6
Important β-Carotene Cardiovascular Trials

Agent	Intake Quintile Highest Daily	Lowest Daily	Relative Risk	P Value
Nurses Health Study[25]				
Antioxidant Vitamins and Risk of Coronary Heart Disease				
β-carotene	>1404 IU	<3850 IU	0.78	.02
Vitamin E	>21.6 mg	<3.5 mg	0.66	<.001
Vitamin C	>359 mg	<93 mg	0.80	.15
Health Professionals Follow-up Study[26]				
Antioxidant Vitamin Intake and Risk of Coronary Heart Disease				
β-carotene			0.71	.03
Vitamin E			0.60	.01
Vitamin C			1.25	.98
Massachusetts Elderly Cohort Study[27]				
β-Carotene Intake and Risk of Cardiovascular Disease				
Endpoint				
CVD death			0.57	.02
Fatal MI			0.32	.02

Further, lutein is found in high concentrations in the skin, where it appears to offer a mild sun protection benefit based on its antioxidant nature.[32]

In conclusion, basic metabolic research, as well as animal and epidemiological studies, all suggests major benefits from carotenoids. These benefits, however, have yet to be confirmed in double-blind intervention studies.

RIBOFLAVIN

Deficiency of riboflavin, a precursor of flavin adenine dinucleotide, has been believed by some to be associated with cataract formation.[33,34] Lenticular reduced glutathione, diminished in all forms of human cataract, requires flavin adenine dinucleotide as a coenzyme for glutathione reductase. Despite this putative connection with riboflavin, clinical results of studies in this area are equivocal, and the degree of riboflavin deficiency encountered in the general population would not be considered to be cataractogenic. Clinically, lower intakes of riboflavin are not found to be a risk factor for cataract.[35,36]

Review of riboflavin requirements associated with exercise in several different study groups yields equivocal results. Aerobic exercise may deplete riboflavin as well as other B-vitamins.[37] However, riboflavin status, assessed using erythrocyte glutathione reductase activity coefficient, shows that while riboflavin requirements of women increase with exercise training, additional riboflavin intake does not enhance or result in improvements in endurance.[38,39] Additionally, riboflavin depletion is not related to the rate or composition of weight loss in overweight women.[40] Interestingly, in a cohort of pregnant women who exercised and took vitamin-mineral supplements, participation in a walking program slightly improved aerobic capacity without affecting riboflavin or thiamin status.[41]

Minimal data are available from one study of high doses (400 mg/day) of riboflavin that successfully treated migraine patients.[42]

Riboflavin has recently emerged as playing a role in the folate one carbon methylation pathways, which, in association with vitamin B_{12} and B_6, may decrease the risk of heart disease. This due to their combined role in reducing the levels of homocysteine,

TABLE 10.7
Riboflavin — Established Benefits

Essential for building and maintaining body tissues
Necessary for healthy skin
Prevents sensitivity of the eyes to light
Necessary for protein, fat, and carbohydrate metabolism
Important for the proper function of the nervous system

TABLE 10.8
Riboflavin — Potential Benefits

Use	Findings	References
Age-related cataract	Riboflavin deficiency associated with higher incidence of cataract	33–36
Exercise	Aerobic exercise may deplete riboflavin. Supplementation with riboflavin does not appear to increase performance	37–40
Pregnancy and exercise	Riboflavin may be helpful	41
Migraine	High doses in a limited trial produced beneficial results	42

TABLE 10.9
Niacin — Established Benefits

Helps prevent pellagra
Helps cells release energy from food
Aids the nervous system
Helps prevent loss of appetite

TABLE 10.10
Niacin — Potential Benefits

Use	Findings	Reference
Hypercholesterolemia	Lowers elevated cholesterol levels	44–47
Hypertriglyceridemia	Lowers elevated triacylglycerol levels	44

an amino acid when present at high levels is associated with increased risk of cardiovascular disease.[43] Riboflavin deficiency has also been reported as playing an important role in overcoming genetic polymorphisms of the folate pathway important in the prevention of birth defects. Further work in this area is needed. See Table 10.7 and Table 10.8 for established and potential benefits of riboflavin.

NIACIN

The body uses niacin in the process of releasing energy from carbohydrates, to form fat from carbohydrates, and to metabolize alcohol. Niacin comes in two basic forms: niacin (also called nicotinic acid) and niacinamide (also called nicotinamide).

High levels of niacin — usually several grams per day — lower cholesterol, triglyceride, and triacylglycerol levels and raise HDL cholesterol levels.[44] The niacinamide form, commonly found in multivitamin preparations, does not decrease elevated cholesterol. See Table 10.9 and Table 10.10 for established and emerging benefits of niacin.

A variation of niacin, called inositol hexaniacinate, has also been used and has not been linked with the flushing seen with high doses of niacin. Physicians in Europe sometimes prescribe it to help lower cholesterol. Dosages used are 500 to 1000 mg, taken three times a day.[45,46] This form of niacin lowers serum cholesterol but appears to have fewer side effects.[47] A form of sustained release niacin (Niaspan®) is available on the U.S. market, by prescription only. It is again aimed at providing the cholesterol benefits of niacin, while reducing the potential of the flushing side effect.

VITAMIN B$_6$

Vitamin B$_6$ has a significant role to play, along with folate and vitamin B$_{12}$, in the reduction of elevated homocysteine levels associated with increased risk of cardiovascular disease — specifically, coronary artery disease and stroke. This topic is covered in the section on folate.

Vitamin B$_6$ also plays a significant role in the immune function of the elderly. *In vitro* indices of cell-mediated immunity in healthy elderly adults indicate that deficiency of vitamin B$_6$ is associated with impairment of immune function. This impairment appears to be reversible with vitamin B$_6$ repletion.[48] The levels of vitamin B$_6$ absorption, phosphorylation, and excretion appear not to be affected by age.[49]

Vitamin B$_6$ has been shown to reduce the preovulatory side effects of estrogen in animals. Since excess estrogen may be responsible in part for premenstrual symptoms (PMS), a number of studies in humans have demonstrated that 200 to 400 mg of vitamin B$_6$ per day for several months can relieve symptoms of PMS.[49–53] In other studies, however, the amount of vitamin B$_6$ used may be too low,[54] or the length of the trial too short,[55] and other studies have not found vitamin B$_6$ so helpful.[56,57]

Many diabetics have low blood levels of vitamin B$_6$.[58,59] Levels of vitamin B$_6$ are even lower in diabetics with nerve damage.[60] Vitamin B$_6$ supplements have been demonstrated to improve glucose tolerance in women with diabetes associated with pregnancy.[61,62] Vitamin B$_6$ is also partially effective for glucose intolerance induced by birth control pills.[63] For some individuals with diabetes, a form of vitamin B$_6$ — pyridoxine α-ketoglutarate — improves glucose tolerance dramatically.[64]

It appears that many people with carpal tunnel syndrome (CTS) have vitamin B$_6$ deficiencies.[67] Some studies show that people with CTS are helped when given 100 mg of vitamin B$_6$ three times per day.[68,69] Although a few researchers have found benefits with lesser amounts,[70–72] the results have not been consistent.[73–75]

Lastly, it is worth noting that vitamin B$_6$ deficiency was found in more than one-third of HIV-positive men, and a deficiency of this vitamin is associated with decreased immune function.[76] See Table 10.11 and Table 10.12 for established and emerging benefits of vitamin B$_6$.

VITAMIN B$_{12}$

Higher blood levels of vitamins B$_6$, B$_{12}$, and folic acid are associated with low levels of homocysteine,[77] and supplementing with these vitamins helps to lower homocysteine levels.[78,79] Preliminary evidence indicates that vitamin B$_{12}$ may be beneficial when included in supplements or in a food-fortification regimen together with folic acid. This topic is discussed further in the section on folate.

The addition of vitamin B$_{12}$ enhances the homocysteine-lowering potential of a folic acid supplement. In one study, female volunteers were given folic acid alone or folic acid combined with one of two supplements containing different doses of vitamin B$_{12}$. Significant reductions in plasma homocysteine were observed in all groups receiving vitamin treatment. The combination of folic acid 400 μg plus 400 μg of vitamin B$_{12}$ resulted in an 18% decrease in homocysteine levels. This was significantly larger than that obtained with a supplement containing folic acid alone (homocysteine decrease of 11%). Folic acid in combination

---

TABLE 10.11
Vitamin B$_6$ — Established Benefits

Important in protein absorption and metabolism

Necessary for red blood cell formation

Necessary for the proper function of the nervous and
   immune systems

Helps maintain healthy teeth and gums

Needed for serotonin and melatonin production

TABLE 10.12
Vitamin B$_6$ — Potential Benefits

Use	Findings	Reference
Immune function	Improves immune function in the elderly	48, 49
Premenstrual symptoms	High doses administered long-term may be helpful	50–57
Diabetes	Low levels are associated with diabetes	58–66
Carpal tunnel syndrome	Inconsistent results	67–75
HIV	Deficiency frequently found and associated with decreased immune function	76

with a low vitamin B_{12} dose (6 μg) affected homocysteine as well (decrease of 15%). These results suggest that the addition of vitamin B_{12} to folic acid supplements or enriched foods helps maximize the reduction of homocysteine and may thus increase the benefits achieved with the use of folic acid in the prevention of vascular disease.[80] The cardiovascular and cerebrovascular intervention trials were B_{12}, B_6, and folate. These nutrients have been shown to reduce homocysteine levels, but not reduce the risk of secondary events.

However, one recent trial reanalyzed the VISP results with respect to association of homocysteine and stroke. A subset of the study population who were initially deficient in B_{12}, then as study participants received 0.4 mg of B_{12} daily for 7 years, showed both a lowering of homocysteine as well as of stroke risk by 23%.[81] Thus, many of the negative trials may need to be reevaluated based on the participants' B_{12} sufficiency and the level of B_{12} that was administered.

Recently, a very important study was published that did not get the attention it deserved. This was a national, population-based, cohort study, conducted by the Centers for Disease Control and Prevention. In this study they compared the stroke occurrence prior to folate fortification of grain (1990 to 1997) in both the United States and Canada to the period after fortification (1998 to 2002).

This was a quasi-experimental intervention, because the entire populations of both of these countries were exposed to folate fortification. These populations were then compared with the populations of England and Wales, who were not exposed to folate fortification. As expected, the folate levels increased and homocysteine levels declined in the fortified populations. The ongoing decline in stroke mortality observed in fortified populations prior to fortification accelerated post fortification with an overall change in the United States from –0.3 to –2.9% (p = .0005) and in Canada from –1 to –5.4% (p = .0001). This is equal to a combined effect of preventing of 15,700 fewer stroke deaths per year. In contrast, the decline in stroke mortality in England and Wales did not change significantly during this period.[82] Thus, many of the negative trials may need to be reevaluated based on their power to detect cardiovascular events and focus on the potential stroke effect that may be easier to demonstrate based on the sufficiency of B_{12} in participants and the level of B_{12} that was administered.

Lastly, vitamin B_{12} has a role in preventing vitamin B_{12} deficiency in the presence of folate use, especially in light of the increased fortification of foods with folic acid. (See rationale by Oakley.[83]) Table 10.13 and Table 10.14 lists the established and potential benefits of vitamin B_{12}.

FOLIC ACID

For the last 40 years, folic acid has almost exclusively been used to treat megaloblastic macrocytic anemia. There is now significant evidence that folate deficiency is associated with increased risk of several diseases. The most convincing is the association of folic acid deficiency with neural tube defects (NTDs) such as spina bifida and anencephaly, a predisposition to occlusive vascular disease associated with hyperhomocysteinemia, and several neoplastic or preneoplastic diseases. In addition, preliminary evidence suggests some association of folate deficiency with neuropsychiatric diseases.

The British Medical Research Council conducted studies on folate and NTDs in 1991.[84] These demonstrated that high-dose folic acid supplements (4.0 mg/day) used by women who had a prior NTD-affected pregnancy reduced the risk of having a subsequent NTD-affected pregnancy by 70%. A conclusive trial conducted in Hungary showed that a multivitamin containing 0.8 mg folic acid protected against a first occurrence of NTD.[85]

TABLE 10.13
Vitamin B_{12} — Established Benefits

Necessary for DNA synthesis
Helps prevent pernicious anemia
Helps to form red blood cells
Enhances utilization of nickel

TABLE 10.14
Vitamin B_{12} — Potential Benefits

Use	Findings	Reference
Hyperhomocysteinemia	Alone and together with folate reduces homocysteine levels	77–80
Folate-induced vitamin B_{12} deficiency	Administration helps unmask vitamin B_{12} deficiency associated with folate use	83

In 1992, the Centers for Disease Control (CDC) in the United States issued a recommendation that all women of childbearing age, capable of becoming pregnant, should consume 0.4 mg of folic acid per day to help prevent NTDs.[86] The U.K. Expert Advisory Group and other countries in Europe made similar recommendations.[87] The U.S. Food and Drug Administration has recently authorized a health claim on food labels and dietary supplements that folic acid contained in these products may help reduce the risk of NTD.[88] More recently, two major studies one in Europe[89] and one in the United States by the CDC[90] have implicated folate in other classes of birth defects. These classes cover a far greater number of birth defects than just neural tube defects. The most interesting findings in these two studies were the similarities in the data; both showed the relationship and magnitude of folate to the same classes of birth defects in both populations studied (Table 10.16).

A large body of evidence reveals that elevated blood homocysteine is a risk factor for cardiovascular disease, including atherosclerotic coronary heart disease and thromboembolic stroke. There is abundant evidence that folate deficiency or a genetic defect in the enzymes involved in homocysteine metabolism give rise to hyperhomocysteinemia. In addition to folate deficiency, vitamin B_6 and B_{12} deficiency has also been associated with elevated homocysteine levels. Patients with higher blood levels of these vitamins are at lower risk for occlusive vascular disease.[91]

Many studies show that folic acid alone or in combination with vitamins B_6 and B_{12} can reduce blood homocysteine levels.[92–101] Observational studies have shown that people who consume multivitamins or cereal fortified with folic acid also have reduced homocysteine levels.[102–106]

Levels of supplemental folic acid as low as 0.4 mg appears to be effective. A meta-analysis of 12 randomized trials confirms that folic acid has the dominant blood-homocysteine-lowering effect.[101] The fortification of enriched grain with folic acid has been shown to increase folate plasma levels and decrease homocysteine levels in middle-aged and older adults.[105] While folic acid fortification was undertaken primarily to reduce the risk of NTDs, it may also have a beneficial effect on vascular disease. This possibility is strongly indicated in the results of recent data on stroke collected by the CDC in both fortified and nonfortified populations .[82]

Based on a meta-analysis of 27 studies relating homocysteine to vascular disease and 11 studies of folic acid effects on homocysteine levels, Boushey and Beresford[92] concluded that an increase of 350 μg/day of folate intake by men and 280 μg/day increase by women could potentially prevent 30,500 and 19,000 vascular deaths annually in men and women, respectively. Recent reports show that a small percentage of children, with or without a positive family history of cardiovascular disease,[107–109] have elevated homocysteine levels. Hyperhomocysteinemia may also be a risk factor for ischemic stroke in children. The data on children suggest that tracking of homocysteine levels from childhood on may be helpful in the planning and evaluation of future initiatives aimed at the prevention of cardiovascular disease.

While it has been shown that higher intake of folate may reduce homocysteine levels and that lower homocysteine levels are associated with reduced cardiovascular mortality, clinical intervention trials are needed to prove unequivocally that higher intakes of folate will help reduce the risk of cardiovascular disease. In a preliminary report, a vitamin mixture of 2.5 mg of folic acid, 25 mg vitamin B_6, and 250 μg vitamin B_{12} stopped the progression of carotid plaques; some regression was also observed.[111] Excellent detailed reviews on homocysteine and vascular disease have been published.[112–116] Hankey and Eikelboomb[110] have published an excellent review of prospective cohort and case-control studies, as well as cross-sectional and retrospective case-control studies concerning the association between homocysteine and cardiovascular risk.

The intervention trials that have been conducted to date Vitamin Intervention for Stroke Prevention (VISP)[117] trial and the recently presented NORVIT and HOPE TWO trials[118,119] have been disappointing. However, as VISP was conducted in a fortified population and NORVIT was are based on treatment of secondary events rather than primary prevention, the question of whether lowering homocysteine prevents cardiovascular disease remains unanswered. The most promising double blind randomized controlled studies in this area are those that have been conducted on patients who have undergone angioplasty and are then studied for their rate of restenosis. A number of studies[120,121] conducted using this human model show a positive effect of folate. In one trial, folate reduced homocysteine and reduced the rate of restenosis by up to 48% in balloon angioplasty only; while in another trial, a trend of 14% reduction was seen in stented lesions with folate supplementation. Further, homocysteine-lowering therapy provided an additional benefit of a 40% relative reduction in major adverse events at six months in these studies. The mechanism of restenosis in balloon angioplasty compared with that in stent restenosis differ; consequently, the failure of folate in one condition may not preclude success in the other. There are currently some large international intervention trials in place to further evaluate the causal relationship of folate, homocysteine, and cardiovascular disease. Hopefully, these trials will help answer the question in the next few years.

Several reports suggest an increased risk of colon, tracheobronchial tree, and cervical cancer, and preneoplastic dysplasia associated with folate deficiency.[122,123] Supplemental folic acid has been shown to partially reverse some cervical dysplasia.[122,124] In some instances, poor folate status may not by itself be carcinogenic, but it may predispose to the carcinogenicity of other agents.[125,126]

Lashner and Heidenreich[126] reported that the rate of colon cancer was 62% lower in patients with ulcerative colitis who were supplemented with folic acid. Giovannucci and Stampfer[127] examined the relationship between the intake of folate, both from supplements and food, and the risk for colon cancer in women in the Nurses Health Study. The results indicate that the use of multivitamin supplements for 15 or more years may decrease the risk for colon cancer by about 75%. The data are consistent with the hypothesis that folate intake is the principal nutritional factor associated with risk reduction. These findings support several recent studies, including the Health Professional Follow-Up Study, which have found a higher risk for colon cancer among persons with low folate. In the Giovannucci report, the association between colon cancer and folate was stronger with supplemental than with dietary folate. This is probably due to the fact that food folate is less bioavailable than supplemental folate. More recently, Zhang and Hunter[128] reported that the excess risk of breast cancer associated with moderate alcohol consumption might be reduced by folate. Alcohol is a known folate antagonist, and this could increase the requirement for folate.

Blount et al.[129] presented data on the possible mechanism by which folate deficiency enhances cancer risk. Folate deficiency results in abnormal DNA synthesis due to misincorporation of uracil into DNA, leading to chromosome breakage. This breakage contributes to the risk of colon cancer.

FOLATE AND DEMENTIA

Prevention and treatment of age-related cognitive impairment and dementia are challenging to the health care system. Products that may help reduce the risk of slow the progression of these disabling events would provide great public health benefits. Several epidemiological studies report that elevated homocysteine levels appear to be correlated with an increased risk of cognitive decline and cerebral atrophy in normal and demented elderly adults.[130–145] Hence, scientists have postulated that lowering homocysteine by supplementation with folic acid, B_6, and B_{12}, may reduce the risk of cognitive decline and dementia, or at least slow the process.[132,146]

Few intervention trials, to determine if lowering homocysteine via B-vitamin supplementation reduces the risk of cognitive decline via B-vitamin supplementation, exist. No studies to date have been conducted in healthy populations. However, two open intervention trials examined supplementation with B-vitamins on cognitive function in the demented elderly. One intervention failed to show an improvement in cognitive function after treatment with folate, B_{12}, and B_6 for approximately nine months in individuals with high homocysteine levels (defined as >13.5 nmol/l).[147] However, another clinical trial found that supplementation with folate and B_{12} for 2 months in individuals with homocysteine levels >19.9 nmol/l could greatly improve cognitive function.[148] This suggests that B-vitamin supplementation may be more effective in treatment of dementia in individuals with higher homocysteine levels (~20 nmol/l). See Table 10.15 and Table 10.16 for the established and potential benefits of folate.

Data to help elucidate the role of folate in Alzheimer's disease and depression are sparse and just emerging. Low blood levels of folate and vitamin B_{12} are often found in individuals with Alzheimer's disease.[149] The role of elevated homocysteine levels has been reported and needs to be expanded further.[150] Low folate blood levels may be associated with the weaker responses of depressed patients to antidepessants.[151] Factor contributing to low serum levels among depressed patients, as well as the circumstances under which folate may have a role in antidepressant therapy, must be further clarified.

VITAMIN C

Vitamin C has many functions in the body, including serving as an antioxidant and as a cofactor for several enzymes involved with biosynthesis.[152] The relationship between vitamin C and total serum cholesterol has been investigated in several studies.[153–158]

TABLE 10.15
Folic Acid — Established Benefits

Necessary for DNA synthesis
Important for cell formation
Prevents certain types of anemias
Neural tube defects
Helps maintain the function of the intestinal tract

TABLE 10.16
Folic Acid — Potential Benefits

Use	Findings	Reference
Neural tube defects	0.4 mg/day prevents neural tube and other common birth defects	84–89
Hyperhomocysteinemia	Lowers homocysteine levels	91–115
Cancer	Deficiency is associated with an increased risk of colon, lung, and cervical cancer	116–128
Cognitive function	Low levels are associated with risk of cognitive decline and dementia	130–145

In one intervention study, consumption of 1000 mg of vitamin C per day for 4 weeks resulted in a reduction in total serum cholesterol.[155] In another study, supplementation with 60 mg/day for 2 weeks had no effect.[153] Two observational studies found an inverse relationship between vitamin C status and total serum cholesterol concentrations.[157,158]

Low concentrations of plasma vitamin C have been associated with hypertension.[157,159–162] Several studies have reported beneficial effects of the administration of high doses of vitamin C on vasodilation.[163–166] One study found a 128% increase in brachial artery dilation in coronary artery disease patients, while a second found an insignificant increase of 27% in chronic heart failure patients.[166] Infusion of 10 mg of vitamin C per minute was observed to effect a 100% reversal of epicardial artery vasoconstriction in coronary spastic angina patients.[167]

Some prospective cohort studies have shown that vitamin C intake is associated with reduced cardiovascular disease risk. A recent analysis from the Nurses Health Study indicates that women in the highest quintile had a 27% lower risk of coronary heart disease, and women taking vitamin C supplements had a 28% lower risk of nonfatal MI and fatal CHD compared with women who took no vitamin C. Table 10.17 (adapted from Carr[185]) lists prospective cohort studies of vitamin C intake associated with reduced cardiovascular disease risk. There is, however, no long-term, controlled-intervention studies using supplemental vitamin C alone which show that supplemental vitamin C prevents heart disease. The recent review from the American College of Cardiology Task Force concludes that vitamin C is not effective in preventing CHD.[168]

As an antioxidant, vitamin C may protect against cancer through several mechanisms, including inhibition of DNA oxidation. One potential mechanism is chemoprotection against mutagenic compounds such as nitrosamines.[169,170] In addition, vitamin C may reduce carcinogenesis through stimulation of the immune system, via a beneficial effect on phagocyte functions, such as chemotaxis,[171–174] or on the activity of natural killer cells and the proliferation of lymphocytes.[175–177]

Two recent prospective studies reported increased total cancer in men but not women with low serum vitamin C levels.[178,179] Recent studies also reported an inverse association between dietary vitamin C and oral cancer,[180] gastric cancer,[181] and premenopausal breast cancer.[182] However, a recent cohort study showed no relationship with vitamin C intakes, and a prospective study showed no association between prediagnostic vitamin C levels and breast cancer risk.[183,184] These are no controlled intervention studies using vitamin C alone that show supplemental vitamin C can prevent cancer (Table 10.18).

TABLE 10.17
Vitamin C Intake Associated with Reduced Cardiovascular Disease Risk (Prospective Cohort Studies)

Reference	Population (Duration in Years)	Endpoint (Events)	Risk and Associated Dietary Intake of Vitamin C
Enstrom[186]	3119 Men and women (10 years)	CVD (127 deaths)	>250 compared with <250 mg/day: no ↓ risk
Enstrom[187,188]	4479 Men (10 y)	CVD (558 deaths)	>50 mg/d + vitamin supplement: ↓ risk by 42%
	6809 Women (10 years)	CVD (371 deaths)	>50 mg/day + vitamin supplement: ↓ risk by 25%
Manson[189,190]	87,245 Female nurses (8 years)	CAD (52 cases)	>359 compared with <93 mg/day: ↓ risk by 20% (NS)
		Stroke (183 cases)	>359 compared with <93 mg/day: ↓ risk by 24%
Rimm[26]	39,910 Male health professionals (4 years)	CAD (667 cases)	392 compared with 92 mg/day median: no ↓ risk
Fehily[191]	2512 Men (5 years)	CVD (148 cases)	>67 compared with <35 mg/d: ↓ risk by 37% (NS)
Knekt[192]	2748 Finnish men (14 years)	CAD (186 deaths)	>85 compared with <60 mg/day: no ↓ risk
	2385 Finnish women (14 years)	CAD (58 deaths)	>91 compared with <61 mg/day: ↓ risk by 51%
Gale[193]	730 U.K. elderly men and women (20 years)	Stroke (125 deaths)	>45 compared with <28 mg/d: ↓ risk by 50% (NS)
		CAD (182 deaths)	>45 compared with <28 mg/day: ↓ risk by 50% (NS)
Kritchevsky[194]	4989 Men (3 years)	Carotid atherosclerosis	>982 compared with <56 mg/day: ↓ intima thickness
	6318 Women (3 years)	Carotid atherosclerosis	>728 compared with <64 mg/day: ↓ intima thickness
Pandey[195]	1556 Men (24 years)	CAD (231 deaths)	>113 compared with <82 mg/day: ↓ risk by 25%
Kushi[196]	34,486 Women (7 years)	CAD (242 deaths)	>391 compared with <112 mg/day (total)2: no ↓ risk,
			>196 compared with <87 mg/day (dietary): no ↓ risk, regular supplement compared with no supplement: no ↓ risk
Losconczy[197]	11,178 Elderly men and women (6 years)	CAD (1101 deaths)	Regular supplement compared with no supplement: no ↓ risk
Sahyoun[198]	725 Elderly men and women (10 years)	CVD (101 deaths)	>388 compared with <90 mg/day: ↓ risk by 62% (NS)
Mark[199]	29,584 Chinese men (5 years)	Stroke	180 mg/d supplement: no ↓ risk (+30 μg Mo/day cosupplement)

Note: CVD = Cardiovascular disease; CAD = Coronary artery disease.

Source: Adapted from Carr AC, Frei B. *Am J Clin Nutr* 69: 1086; 1999.

TABLE 10.18
Vitamin C Intake Associated with Reduced Cancer Risk (Prospective Cohort Studies)

Reference	Population (Duration)	Cancer Site (Events)	Risk and Associated Dietary Intake of Vitamin C
Shekelle[200]	1954 Men (19 years)	Lung (33 cases)	101 mg/d in noncases compared with 92 mg/day in cases (NS)
Enstrom[186]	3119 Men and women (10 year)	All cancers (68 deaths)	>250 compared with <250 mg/day no ↓ risk
Kromhout[201]	870 Dutch men (25 year)	Lung (63 deaths)	83–103 compared with <63 mg/day: ↓ risk by 64%
Knekt[202]	4538 Finnish men (20 year)	Lung (117 cases)	83 mg/d in noncases compared with 81 mg/day in cases (NS)
Enstrom[187]	4479 Men (10 year)	All cancers (228 deaths)	>50 mg/day + regular supplement: ↓ risk by 21% >50 mg/day +
	6869 Women (10 year)	All cancers (169 deaths)	regular supplement: no ↓ risk
Shibata[203]	4277 Men (7 year)	All cancers (645 cases)	>210 compared with <145 mg/day: no ↓ risk, 500 mg/day
	7300 Women (7 year)	All cancers (690 cases)	supplement compared with no supplement: no ↓ risk
			>225 compared with <155 mg/day: ↓ risk by 24%, 500 mg/day
			supplement compared with no supplement: no ↓ risk
Graham[204]	18,586 Women (7 year)	Breast (344 cases)	>79 compared with <34 mg/day: no ↓ risk
Hunter[205]	89,494 U.S. female nurses (8 year)	Breast (1439 cases)	59 compared with <93 mg/day (total): no ↓ risk, regular supplement compared with no supplement: no ↓ risk, supplement >10 years compared with no supplement: no ↓ risk
Bostick[206]	35,215 Women (5 year)	Colon (212 cases)	>392 compared with <112 mg/day (total): ↓ risk (NS), >201 compared with <91 mg/day (diet): no ↓ risk, >60 mg/day supplement compared with no supplement: ↓ risk by 33%
Blot[21]	29,584 Chinese men and women (5 year)	Esophageal-stomach	120 mg/day supplement: no ↓ risk (+30 μg Mo/day cosupplement)
Pandey[195]	1556 Men (24 year)	All cancers (155 deaths)	>113 compared with <82 mg/day: ↓ risk by 39%
Losconczy[197]	11,178 Elderly men and women (6 year)	All cancers (761 deaths)	Regular supplement compared with no supplement: no ↓ risk
Sahyoun[198]	<725 Elderly men and women (10 year)	All cancers (57 deaths)	>388 compared with <90 mg/day: no ↓ risk
Kushi[207]	34,387 Women (5 year)	Breast (879 cases)	>392 compared with <112 mg/day (total): no ↓ risk, >198 compared with <87 mg/day (diet): no ↓ risk, regular supplement compared with no supplement: no ↓ risk
Yong[208]	3968 Men and women (19 years)	6100 Lung (248)	82 mg/day in noncases compared with 64 mg/day in cases

Source: Adapted from Carr AC and Frei B. *Am J Clin Nutr* 69: 1086; 1999.

TABLE 10.19
Vitamin C — Established Benefits

Prevents scurvy
Maintains health of teeth, gums, and blood
  vessels necessary for wound repair
Important for collagen formation
Enhances iron absorption

See under vitamin E Table for the effects of vitamin C in combination with other vitamins on CHD. It remains unclear whether the positive effects in atherosclerosis prevention study (ASAP) and the Cardiac Transplant Study are due to the vitamin C alone or the antioxidant mixture.

Several epidemiologic studies that have investigated the association of vitamin C intake with the incidence of cataract are discussed in Chapter 58. See Table 10.19 for the established benefits of vitamin C.

VITAMIN D

Vitamin D investigations present an exciting area in both research and debate. In 1997, the vitamin D DRI Committee set the adult and elderly vitamin D requirements to approximately 200 and 400 IU/day based on the available science. Now, less than 10 years later, the thought leaders in the field are recommending that every one should receive at least between 600 and 1000 IU of vitamin D per day.[209] Recent data from the National Health and Nutrition Examination Survey (NHANES) database indicate large segments of the population are vitamin D deficient. Recent studies[210] clearly indicate that those living in northern latitude in the United States (North of Boston) are seasonally deficient throughout the winter months. Supplementation in deficient populations especially, during these seasonal periods is necessary to attain and maintain nutritional adequacy. During periods when adequate vitamin D may be obtained from sun exposure, only short periods of sun skin exposure are required (i.e., 5 to 10 min, 2 to 3 times a week).[211] The role of overexposure to sun in stimulating skin cancer is the balancing concern. As to the overall safety intake levels, much debate remains. The DRI safety committee has set the Tolerable Upper Intake Level (UL) at 2000 IU/day. However, several experts suggest that a more reasonable limit should be set at 10,000 IU/day.

Vitamin D is an essential element in the maintenance of healthy bones, because it helps optimize calcium absorption and prevents increased parathyroid hormone (PTH) secretion.[212] High PTH levels stimulate resorption of bone, which may result in a gradual weakening of bones (osteomalacia) leading to an increase in the incidence of fractures.

Increasing evidence suggests that a large portion of the elderly population is vitamin D deficient.[213] Vitamin D deficiency in the elderly may be caused by little exposure to sunlight, a reduced ability of the skin to synthesize cholecalciferol, and decreased dietary intakes.[214] This deficiency leads to hyperparathyroidism, bone loss, and increased incidence of fractures.[215] Vitamin D is synthesized in the skin by the action of ultraviolet light.[1] Vitamin D deficiency was found to be common in the elderly due to lack of mobility, which prevents adequate sun exposure.[216] Various studies have also demonstrated that hypovitaminosis D appears prevalent in the winter months due to a reduction in the number of hours spent outside coupled with the use of more protective clothing.[212,215–220]

The effect of age on vitamin D synthesis in the skin may be due to an age-related decline in the dermal production of 7-dehydrocholesterol, the precursor of previtamin D_3.[221] MacLaughlin and Holick compared the amount of previtamin D_3 produced by the skin of young subjects (8 and 18 years old) with the amount produced by the skin of elderly subjects (77 to 82 years).[222] This study revealed that aging appears to produce a greater than twofold reduction in previtamin D_3 production in subjects over 77 years of age.

Vitamin D deficiency, which can cause osteomalacia, is also important in the pathogenesis of age-related osteoporosis.[214] In a study of 3270 elderly women (mean age 84), 800 IU of vitamin D was given in combination with 1.2 g of elemental calcium to 1634 women, and 1636 women received a placebo. The number of hip fractures was reduced by 43% in the group treated with the combination of vitamin D and calcium after 18 months.[217,223] A recent report based on pooled results of double-blind randomized controlled trials found that oral vitamin D supplementation in doses of 700 to 800 IU/day appears to reduce the risk of hip and nonvertebral factures in ambulatory or institutional elderly persons. An oral vitamin D dose of 400 IU/day is not sufficient for fracture prevention .[209]

Treatment of the elderly with vitamin D may be a cost-effective method of maintaining bone density and reducing the incidence of osteoporotic fractures.[224] Further, it has now been established that vitamin D plays a role in both nerves and muscles and as such appears to be important in reducing fractures by preventing falls.[225]

Vitamin D as 1,25 dihydroxycholecalciferol appears to be potentially useful for people with psoriasis.[224] Topical application has worked well in some,[227–230] but not all, studies.[231,232] Use of vitamin D in psoriatic patients may work by helping skin cells replicate normally. High doses of calcium combined with vitamin D have also been useful in treating cases of migraine[233,234] at a dose of 400 IU of vitamin D combined with 800 mg of calcium per day.

From epidemiological data, Giovannucci[235] reported that high circulating levels of $1,25(OH)_2$ vitamin D, the biologically active form, may decrease the risk of developing prostate cancer, and that diets high in calcium, phosphorus, and sulfur-containing amino acids from animal protein tend to decrease $1,25(OH)_2$ vitamin D. This effect of vitamin D on prostate cancer may be mediated via vitamin D receptors found on prostate cancer cells, and may be genotype specific.[236]

Animal models suggest that low vitamin D and calcium intake, as commonly found in Western-style diets, may be associated with an increased risk of both colon[237] and breast cancer,[238] although a long-term study of serum vitamin D levels and the incidence of breast cancer in humans did not reveal a direct association.[239] The role of vitamin D in cancer prevention has recently received renewed interest, and a series of positive reports reviews[240,241] have appeared. Presently, there is a 5-year, NIH (National Institute of Health)-funded interventional polyp prevention trial underway to look at the effect of vitamin D alone (1000 IU/day) and in combination with calcium. See Table 10.20 and Table 10.21 for the established and potential benefits of vitamin D.

TABLE 10.20

Vitamin D — Established Benefits

Necessary for the proper formation of bones
  and teeth

Important for calcium absorption

Aids in the deposition of calcium and
  phosphorus into bones

TABLE 10.21

Vitamin D — Potential Benefits

Use	Findings	Reference
Osteoporosis	Reduces the incidence of osteoporosis-related fracture	212–224
Psoriasis	Useful in topical application	226–232
Migraine	May be useful	233,239
Cancer	May reduce the risk of prostate cancer	235–239
	Low intake is associated with an increased risk of colon and breast cancer	

TABLE 10.22

Vitamin E — Established Benefits

Essential for the formation of red blood cells, muscle, and other tissues
Necessary for the proper function of the nervous system
Protects the fat in tissues from oxidation

TABLE 10.23

Vitamin E and Coronary Heart Disease — Epidemiological Trials

Stampfer et al.[25]	87,000 Female nurses aged between 34 and 59 years	8-year follow-up	Vitamin E supplements for short periods had little apparent benefit, but those who took them for more than 2 years had a 41% reduction in the risk of major coronary artery disease
Rimm et al.[26]	40,000 U.S. male health professionals aged between 40 and 75 years	4-year follow-up	Men consuming >60 IU/day of Vitamin E had a 36% decreased risk of CHD

VITAMIN E

The potential health benefits of vitamin E are extensive and include reduction in cardiovascular risk, protection against certain forms of cancer, enhanced immunity, and a potential role in the treatment of certain neurological diseases. See Table 10.22 for the established benefits of vitamin E. Early research identified that antioxidant scavengers such as vitamin E may reduce oxidative stress that can affect lipid metabolism, thereby producing oxidized low density lipoprotein (LDL), which is more atherogenic than the unoxidized form.[242,243] Because of this action, vitamin E was investigated to determine its efficacy in reducing the risk of cardiovascular disease.

Vitamin E (tocopherol) is a major lipid antioxidant that inhibits oxidation of low density lipoprotein cholesterol (LDL). Studies *in vitro* have shown that vitamin E inhibits smooth muscle cell proliferation, platelet adhesion, and aggregation, and can improve endothelial function.[244]

Epidemiological studies found a significant inverse correlation between LDL levels, vitamin E concentration, and degree of coronary artery stenosis,[245] or mortality from ischemic heart disease.[246] The Cholesterol Lowering Atherosclerosis Study demonstrated that supplementary vitamin E intake greater than 100 IU/day was associated with a significant reduction in the progression of atherosclerosis in subjects not treated with lipid lowering drugs.[247]

Two major epidemiological studies offer evidence that vitamin E can reduce the incidence and mortality from coronary heart disease. Data from Stampfer et al.[247] and Rimm et al.[26] support the evidence that suggests that antioxidants, especially fat-soluble antioxidants such as vitamin E, may protect against atherosclerosis by reducing the generation of oxidized LDL. Details of the two studies are listed in Table 10.23.

In the past few years, several controlled randomized clinical trials have been completed that investigated the effects of vitamin E and vitamin E in combination with other antioxidants. Some studies showed benefits (see Table 10.24). However, most results failed to show benefits of vitamin E in patients with cardiovascular disease (CVD) or at high risk of cardiovascular disease. See Table 10.25 for a tabulation of the various clinical trials showing no overall benefit in CVD. The Women's Health Study (WHS) was very meaningful due to the very large number (39,876) of apparently healthy persons evaluated for 10 years.[261] Although vitamin E supplementation failed on the primary outcome, that is, overall-reduction in cardiovascular events, there was a 24% reduction in cardiovascular deaths and 26% reduction in major cardiovascular events among the subgroup of women age at least 55 years. The report of the WHS study is indeed surprising as data from some 87,000 women in the Nurses Health Observational Study and 40,000 male health professionals had a 30 to 40% reduction in heart disease (Table 10.23).

TABLE 10.24
Summary of Randomized Clinical Trials of Vitamin E Benefits

Study	Patent Type	Dose Vitamin E – IU	Duration Years	Study Outcome
CHAOS[248]	CHD	400–800	1½	Decreased nonfatal MI
SPACE[249]	Hemodialysis patients	800	1½	Decreased MI stroke and angina
Transplant-associated athrosclerosis[250]	Transplant patients	800 and 1 g vitamin C	1	No increase in intimal thickness compared to placebo
ASAP[251]	CHD	272 and 50 mg vitamin C	6	Progression of intimal thickness reduced — men only, not women
SUVI-MAX[252]	Healthy	30 and 6 mg β-carotene 120 mg vitamin C 100 mg Se 20 mg Zn	7½	Lower cancer incidence and all cause mortality in men, not women.

TABLE 10.25
Summary of Randomized Clinical Trials of Vitamin E —
No Benefits 10.25

Study	Patent Type	Dose (IU)	Duration (Years)
ATBC[253]	Male smokers no history of MI	50 plus 20 mg β-Carotene	5–8
GISSI[254,267]	Post MI	330	3–5
Hope & Hope Too[255,266]	CHD & Diabetes	400	4–7
PPP[256]	CHD	300	3.6
Veap, Kleveled[257]	LOL cholesterol	400	3
Hats[258]	CHD	800 1000 mg vitamin C 25 mg β-carotene	3
Wave[259]	CHD in postmenopausal women	800 plus 1 gm vitamin C	
HPS[260]	CHD	600 250 mg vitamin C 20 mg β-carotene	5
WHS[261a]	Healthy	600 every other day	10

[a] No overall benefit on cardiovascular disease or total cancer. There was, however, a 24% reduction in hemorrhagic stroke and a 26% reduction in major cardiovascular events among the subgroup of women aged at least 65 years.

The discrepancy between observational studies and randomized clinical trials is extremely striking. It may be as Kris-Etherton et al.[262] has stated that the lifelong exposure to an antioxidant may be different than exposure to an antioxidant for 5 to 10 years. Other factors such as type and form of antioxidant or combination of antioxidants may also be important in explaining the discrepancy.

Blumberg[263] recently commented on the failure of some of the clinical trials with vitamin E alone. He stated, "Thus, they ignored the established dynamic relationship within the antioxidant network with its complex arrangement of recycling and sparing and of differential quenching capacities to specific free radicals without various cell compartments." Jialal Devaraj[264] also commented on this subject in a recent review. The results of the SUVIMAX study[252] would indicate that a combination of antioxidants, well balanced, and at low doses together with a well balanced healthy diet, can give positive results.

Many carcinogens create free radicals that damage DNA and cellular structure, and therefore, can promote tumor development. Vitamin E can neutralize these free radicals, thereby preventing cell damage and subsequent malignant tumors. Vitamin E can also prevent cancer by inhibiting cell proliferation and angiogenesis.

Data from a number of epidemiologic studies have shown that individuals with higher intakes of vitamin E have lower risk of cancer. These data are summarized in Table 10.26. There are, however, no controlled intervention studies to confirm that supplemental vitamin E can lower the risk of cancer.

Large intakes of vitamin E are associated with slowing the progression of Alzheimer's disease, according to research from the Alzheimer's Disease Cooperative Study. A 2-year study of 341 individuals with Alzheimer's disease of moderate severity found that 2000 IU/day of vitamin E extended the time patients were able to care for themselves compared with that of those taking a placebo.[265,294]

It has been hypothesized that Parkinson's patients may lack sufficient antioxidant protection and are susceptible to increased attack by free radicals.[288] A small, open trial of patients with early symptoms of Parkinson's disease, conducted in 1989, provided individuals with 400 to 3200 IU of vitamin E per day for up to 7 years. Treated individuals were found to have an increased ability to carry out activities of daily living as compared with age-matched, unsupplemented controls.[289] A larger trial involved 160 patients with early symptoms of Parkinson's disease given 3200 IU of vitamin E and 3000 mg of vitamin C per day for an extended time. Using these two antioxidants prolonged the time to required treatment with levodopa.[290]

The Deprenyl and Tocopherol Antioxidant Therapy of Parkinsonism (DATATOP) study[291,292] was a double-blind, placebo-controlled, multicenter trial involving 800 patients with early Parkinson's disease. Subjects were given deprenyl (a monoamine oxidase inhibitor), or 2000 IU of vitamin E per day. The study showed that deprenyl alone after 9 months of treatment increased the ability to perform activities of daily living; however, there was no effect seen from vitamin E alone or in combination with the deprenyl. An analysis of the results of this trial revealed that a synthetic form of vitamin E was used as opposed to a natural form of vitamin E, which is much more lipid-soluble. This difference in the form of vitamin E may have explained why more positive results were not seen in the antioxidant supplementation group.

The Rotterdam study was a nutritional epidemiological study of 5342 free-living individuals between the ages of 55 and 95, including 31 individuals with pre-existing Parkinson's disease. In examining dietary intakes, there was a significant correlation between the level of daily dietary intake of vitamin E, β-carotene, and vitamin C and protection against development of Parkinson's disease.[293]

TABLE 10.26
Vitamine E Levels and Cancer Incidence

Reference	Cancer Site	Sample Size	Location of Study	Correlation
Stahelin (1984)[270]	Lung, stomach, and colon	4224	Switzerland	Vitamin E levels low in colon and stomach cancer cases
Wald (1984)[271]	Breast	5004	U.K.	Five time greater cancer risk for women with lowest vitamin E level
Salonen (1985)[272]	All sites	12,000	Finland	Risk 11.4 times higher with low vitamin E and selenium levels
Menkes (1986)[273]	Lung	25,802	U.S.	Risk 2.5 times higher with low vitamin E levels
Kok (1987)[274]	Lung, other sites	10,532	Holland	Risk 4.4 times higher for those with low vitamin E levels
Miyamoto (1987)[275]	Lung	55 Cancer cases	Japan	Higher cancer risk with low vitamin E levels
Wald (1987)[276]	All sites	22,000	U.K.	Vitamin E levels lower only in newly diagnosed cancer patients
Knekt (1988)[277]	All sites	21,172	Finland	Lower cancer risk with higher vitamin E levels
Knekt (1988)[278]	Gastrointestinal	36,265	Finland	Higher cancer risk with lower vitamin E levels
Knekt (1988)[279]	Reproductive organs	15,093	Finland	Cancer risk 1.6 times greater with lower vitamin E levels
Verreault (1989)[280]	Cervix	189 Cancer cases	U.S.	Lower risk of cervical cancer associated with higher vitamin E intake
LeGardeur (1990)[281]	Lung	59 Cancer cases	U.S.	Lung cancer patients have lower serum vitamin E levels
Buiatti (1990)[282]	Stomach	1016 Cancer cases	Italy	Risk five times higher with high vitamin E and C intake vs. low
Gridley (1990)[283]	Oropharynx	190 Cancer cases	U.S.	Lower risk associated with increased intake of vitamin E in men
Palan (1991)[284]	Cervix	116 Cancer cases	U.S.	Serum vitamin E levels lower in cervical cancer cases
Comstock (1991)[285]	Nine sites	25,802	U.S.	Vitamin E protective against lung cancer
Harris (1991)[286]	Lung, skin	96 Cancer cases	U.K.	Vitamin E levels lower in cancer patients
Knekt (1991)[203]	Lung	117 Cancer cases	Finland	Risk in nonsmokers associated with lower vitamin C and E intakes
Gridley (1992)[287]	Oropharynx	1103 Cancer cases	U.S.	Use of vitamin E supplements associated with reduced risk

Rationale for Use of Vitamin and Mineral Supplements

VITAMIN K

Vitamin K is the collective name for a group of compounds, all of which contain the 2-methyl-l,4-naphthoquinone moiety. Human tissue contains phylloquinone (vitamin K_1) and several menaquinones (types of vitamin K_2).[295] Phytonadione is the name given to common pharmaceutical preparations,[296] and menadione (vitamin K_3) is the name of a synthetic vitamin K derivative used in animal feed.

Compounds with vitamin K activity are essential for the formation of prothrombin and at least five other proteins involved in the regulation of blood clotting, including Factors VII, IX, and X, as well as protein C and protein S. Although vitamin K is also required for the biosynthesis of several other proteins found in the plasma, bone, and kidney, defective coagulation of the blood is the predominant major known sign initially observed in vitamin K deficiency states.[295,297] Vitamin K deficiency in adults is frequently associated with fat malabsorption syndromes.

Although a wide variation exists, decreased vitamin K levels are generally associated with a decrease in the proportion and absolute amount of carboxylated osteocalcin. Osteocalcin is a vitamin K-dependent protein found in bone matrix, and its levels are a reflection of osteoblastic activity. It has therefore been hypothesized that decreased vitamin K levels might be related to an increased risk for osteoporosis.[298–300]

Vitamin K deficiency has been shown to be associated with decreased bone mass in postmenopausal women with aortic atherosclerosis, but not in a similar group without atherosclerosis.

This may be due to the fact that γ-carboxyglutamate, an amino acid formed by vitamin K action, is known to be involved with regulation of calcification in both bone tissue and atherosclerotic vessel walls, and that abdominal calcification is known to be associated with decreased vitamin K status.[301] Patients treated with warfarin appear to have structural alterations in circulating osteocalcin, which suggest the pathophysiological implication of an association of the use of warfarin with osteoporosis.[302] The use of coumarin (warfarin) therapy in many elderly subjects is often noted as a negative to the intake of vitamin K containing food or supplements. However a recent review[303] of this area concludes that a stable background of vitamin K at the level of 100 mcg would give those undergoing such therapy a nutritionally stable vitamin K background, allowing them the benefits of vitamin K without interfering with there antithrombotic therapy.

Low vitamin K intake is known to be associated with an increased risk of hip fracture in women.[302] Vitamin K supplementation in a group of 20 postmenopausal women with osteoporotic fractures resulted in improved carboxylation of osteocalcin.[304] In summary, these studies suggest a possible link between vitamin K deficiency and osteoporosis. Administration of vitamin K appears to improve a key biochemical parameter that has been associated with decreased bone mass; namely, carboxylated osteocalcin. Additional studies of vitamin K functions and forms active in bone metabolism are warranted. See Table 10.27 and Table 10.28 for established and potential benefits of vitamin K.

CALCIUM

Abundant evidence exists indicating that adequate dietary calcium intake minimizes bone loss in postmenopausal women[305–309] and reduces the increased risk of fracture associated with osteoporosis.[310–313] Additionally, calcium supplementation has been demonstrated to augment the bone-preserving effect of estrogen replacement therapy in postmenopausal women.[306,314] The U.S. Food and Drug Administration permits a health claim for calcium in the prevention and treatment of osteoporosis.

Use of vitamin D in combination with calcium supplementation is particularly important in preventing loss of bone in women who are borderline deficient[315] and reducing the incidence of fractures in the advanced elderly.[316–318] Vitamin D is an essential

TABLE 10.27
Vitamin K — Established Benefits

Necessary for normal blood clotting
Calcium metabolism

TABLE 10.28
Vitamin K — Potential Benefits

Use	Findings	Reference
Osteocalcin formation	Decreased levels are associated with decreased osteocalcin	296–299
Osteoporosis	Possible effect in improving bone mass	300,301

TABLE 10.29
Calcium — Established Benefits

Regulates heart beat
Involved in muscle contraction and nerve transmissions
Assists in blood clotting
Required for bone formation

TABLE 10.30
Calcium — Potential Benefits

Use	Findings	Reference
Osteoporosis and osteoporotic fracture	Increased bone mass, decreased risk of fracture	302, 304–317
Colon cancer, breast cancer	Reduces the incidence of colorectal adenomas	318–321
Premenstrual syndrome	Reduces severity of PMS symptoms	322
Improved hormone replacement therapy	Permits lower dose of HRT to be used	323
Hypertension	May lower high blood pressure in individuals with calcium-poor diet	324, 325

element in the maintenance of healthy bones, because it helps optimize calcium absorption and prevents increased parathyroid (PTH) secretion.[212] High PTH levels stimulate resorption of bone that may result in a gradual weakening of bones leading to an increase in the incidence of fractures.

Calcium supplementation has recently been shown to help prevent colorectal adenomas,[256,257] which are precursors of colon cancer (see also Mobarhan[321] and Lipkin et al.[322] for an excellent review of this subject, and a separate review by Lipkin and Newmark[323] on vitamin D, calcium, and breast cancer) and to effectively reduce premenstrual symptoms associated with the luteal phase.[324]

The administration of 1000 mg of calcium in the presence of normal blood levels of vitamin D has also been demonstrated to permit a lower dose of hormone replacement therapy (HRT) to increase bone density and provide a bone-sparing effect in elderly women similar to or better than that provided by higher dose HRT without calcium and vitamin D supplementation.[325]

A recent study[326] has now indicated that calcium plus vitamin D will prevent the bone loss that accompanies the long-term use of oral contraceptives. This is an important finding as 80% of women of childbearing age in the United States use oral contraceptives.

The value of calcium in control of blood pressure is debatable. Despite conflicting data, meta-analysis of a large number of observational and randomized controlled clinical trials indicates that calcium intake has an impact in reducing blood pressure, particularly in persons regularly consuming low levels of dietary calcium.[327,328] Additional work in this area remains to be done. See Table 10.29 and Table 10.30 for established and potential benefits of calcium. See chapter 64 for additional information on macromineral nutrition.

MAGNESIUM

Magnesium appears to be directly involved in bone metabolism, helping in the formation of bone and indirectly interfacing with hormones regulating bone metabolism. Tranquilli et al.[329] demonstrated that both daily intake and bone mineral content of calcium, phosphorus, and magnesium were significantly reduced in a group of postmenopausal women with osteoporosis compared with nonosteoporotic controls. Additionally, supplementation with magnesium has been shown to help increase bone density in postmenopausal osteoporosis.[330]

Magnesium is a known vasodilator exerting its effect by inhibition of calcium in the vascular smooth cell and through the release of nitric oxide. Magnesium deficiency is found often in diabetics and in people with hypertension.[168] Magnesium deficiency can result in electrocardiographic changes, arrhythmia, and increased sensitivity to cardiac glycosides.[331]

Epidemiological studies suggest that diets high in magnesium as well as magnesium supplements decrease the incidence of cardiovascular disease.[332] A report from the Honolulu Heart Program found a higher risk of CHD among those subjects in the lowest vs. the highest quintile of magnesium intake.[333]

Although not all studies have found that magnesium intake can lower blood pressure, a recent meta-analysis of 20 randomized studies showed blood pressure reduction with magnesium supplementation.[334] The DASH diet (high in magnesium) can cause a reduction in blood pressure in normotensive and hypertensive patients.[335] This reduction, however, could be due to the nutrients in the high fruit and vegetables content of the diet as well as the high calcium content of the diet (dairy products).

TABLE 10.31
Magnesium — Established Benefits

Regulates heart beat, muscle contractions, and nerve
 transmissions
Aids in calcium absorption and the deposition of calcium
 and phosphorus into bones

TABLE 10.32
Magnesium — Potential Benefits

Use	Findings	Reference
Osteoporosis	Helps increase bone mass	327,328
Hypertension	May help lower blood pressure, especially where magnesium has been depleted	329,330,338–340
PMS symptoms	Deficiency is associated with PMS symptoms	341–344
Intermittent claudication	May respond to magnesium	345

Magnesium supplementation decreases the frequency of ventricular arrhythmias in patients with high risk of congestive heart failure, due to magnesium deficiency.[336]

Since the recent NHANES survey data have shown that magnesium intake is suboptimal in U.S. diets, magnesium supplementation can be useful in hypertension and possibly in CVD.[337] Tables 10.31 and 10.32 provide the established and potential benefits of magnesium.

ZINC

Zinc supplementation may be helpful in promoting wound healing in individuals who are zinc deficient. A dose of 220 mg of zinc sulfate (equivalent to 50 mg of elemental zinc) given three times a day for 7 to 8 weeks has been shown to improve wound healing in zinc-deficient patients.[348,349] There is no evidence that zinc supplementation benefits wound healing in individuals whose zinc nutriture is adequate.

Although popular in some countries, the role of zinc supplementation in improving male sexual function is unproven. Studies have shown that zinc is involved in the reproductive process for humans as well as animals. In humans, zinc is thought to be necessary for the formation and maturation of sperm, for ovulation, and for fertilization. High levels of zinc are found in most male reproductive organs, with the highest concentrations located in the prostate. In animal studies, the normal male testis and prostate contain a high concentration of zinc, and zinc deficiency has been shown to lead to defects in sperm along with a depletion of testosterone.[350–353] For men with low testosterone levels, zinc supplementation raises testosterone and increases fertility.[354] For men with low semen zinc levels, zinc supplements may increase both sperm counts and fertility.[355] Most published studies involve infertile men who have taken zinc supplements for at least several months.

Zinc deficiency in humans has been shown to cause retarded growth and slowed skeletal development.[356] Yamaguchi demonstrated that reduced bone growth is sometimes found in conditions associated with zinc deficiency. Additionally, he demonstrated that zinc has a stimulatory effect on bone growth.[357] Other studies have demonstrated a significant correlation between zinc content and bone strength.[358,359] Zinc has an important role in osteogenesis and bone metabolism, although the exact mechanism remains unknown.[356]

Studies have examined the role of zinc in the treatment of anorexia nervosa and in lozenge form to help decrease the duration of symptoms of the common cold. More research is needed to fully characterize the possible benefits of zinc in these conditions. Recent data from cohort epidemiological studies show zinc to be weakly protective against the development of some forms of early age-related macular degeneration (AMD).[360] Zinc was one of the main components in the multivitamin formulation used in the large and successful NIH, Age Related Eye Disease Study (AREDS 1).[361] In this study, the formulation containing zinc at approximately 80 mg/day was shown to prevent the progression of AMD. (See Chapter 58.)

Zinc also helps support immune function. An older comprehensive review of the literature by Good et al.,[363] as well as information from Chandra and McBean[364] and Prasad et al.,[365] suggest that inadequate diet, defective absorption of zinc, disturbances in zinc metabolism, or abnormally increased losses of zinc may be associated with deficits in immune function. Low-dose supplementation of zinc (20 mg) and selenium (100 μg) has been shown to provide significant improvement in elderly patients by increasing humoral response after vaccination.[366] Improved cell-mediated immune response was seen following the

---

TABLE 10.33
Zinc — Established Benefits

Involved protein metabolism
Necessary for insulin synthesis
Important for night vision

TABLE 10.34
Zinc — Potential Benefits

Use	Findings	Reference
Aids in wound repair	Useful in cases of deficiency	346, 347
Male infertility	No proven benefit	348–353
Osteoporosis	May help increase bone strength	354–357
Age-related macular degeneration	Possibly protective	358–362
Immunity	Increases immune response	360, 362–365

administration of zinc 25 mg in an institutionalized elderly population.[367] In this study, a similar effect was not seen for vitamin A 800 μg. See Table 10.33 and Table 10.34 for established and potential benefits of zinc.

SELENIUM

Epidemiological associations between increased selenium intakes and reduced cancer risk, as well as the antioxidant role of selenium in glutathione peroxidase, have provided a basis for research on the potential anticarcinogenic effects of selenium. While the exact mechanism by which selenium exerts its preventative effect against certain types of cancer in humans is unknown, selenium supplementation in animal experiments has been shown to result in enhanced primary immune response in mice, as measured by the plaque-forming cell test and hemagglutination.[368] The addition of supplemental amounts of selenium to the diet has been demonstrated to increase humoral antibody production in swine in response to an antigenic challenge with sheep red blood cells.[369] Selenium deficiency is also known to cause impaired mitogen response in cultures of murine spleen cells.[370]

Two clinical intervention trials published to date have demonstrated that selenium, in combination with other nutrients, may reduce cancer risk. In one study,[21] daily administration of 50 μg of selenium in combination with vitamin E and β-carotene resulted in a moderate reduction in the risk of total mortality, total cancer mortality and stomach cancer mortality. More recently, Clark et al.[371] showed that treatment with 200 μg of selenium per day significantly decreased total mortality and mortality from lung cancer, as well as the incidence of colorectal and prostate cancer.

To test whether supplemental dietary selenium is associated with changes in the incidence of prostate cancer, in another study by Clark, a total of 1312 men with a history of either basal cell or squamous cell carcinoma were randomized to a daily supplement of 200 μg of selenium or a placebo.[372] Patients were treated for a mean of 4.5 years and followed for a mean of 6.4 years. There was no significant change in incidence for the primary endpoints of basal and squamous cell carcinoma of the skin; however, selenium treatment was associated with a significant reduction (63%) in the secondary endpoint of prostate cancer incidence. There were also significant health benefits for other secondary endpoints of total cancer mortality and the incidence of total, lung, and colorectal cancer.

In another study,[373] patients with histories of basal/squamous cell carcinomas of the skin were assigned randomly to either daily oral supplements of selenium-enriched yeast (200 μg Se/day) or a placebo. The results of this study indicate that supplemental selenium intake did not significantly affect the incidence of recurrent basal/squamous cell carcinomas of the skin; however, selenium treatment was associated with reductions in total mortality, mortality from all cancers combined, and the incidence of all cancers combined, lung cancer, colorectal cancer, and prostate cancer.

The consistency of these findings over time strongly suggests that there is an anticancer benefit to selenium supplementation, particularly in reducing the incidence of prostate cancer. An excellent review of selenium and prostate cancer prevention[374] and a review of the mechanisms of the chemopreventive effects of selenium[375,376] have been published.

As emphasized in a recent review by Combs,[377] further randomized clinical trials are needed to confirm and extend previous studies. The Selenium and Vitamin E Cancer Prevention Trial (Select) is currently in progress with an enrollment of 32,400 men. Selenomethionine is the compound that is being tested for the prevention of prostate cancer.

See Table 10.35 for the established and potential benefits of selenium.

TABLE 10.35
Selenium — Established and Emerging Benefits

Established
Needed for proper immune system response
Helps prevent Keshan disease (a cardiomyopathy)
Antioxidant via glutathione peroxidase

Emerging
Prevents certain types of cancer

TABLE 10.36
Chromium — Established and Potential Benefits

Established
Necessary for DNA synthesis
Important for cell formation
Prevents certain types of anemia
Helps maintain the function of the intestinal tract

Emerging
Hyperglycemic control
Increased bone mass
Control of hypertension
Improved lipid profiles

CHROMIUM

Chromium is an essential trace element that is a constituent of glucose tolerance factor and is required for effective insulin action in humans. Data in the literature suggesting a positive benefit of chromium supplementation on glycemic control in diabetes are equivocal, because a consistent beneficial effect of chromium supplementation remains unproven.

The American Diabetes Association (ADA) does not currently recommend supplementation with chromium for individuals with diabetes. The ADA position statement, "Nutrition Recommendations and Principles for People with Diabetes Mellitus,"[378] states:

The only known circumstance in which chromium replacement has any beneficial effect on glycemic control is for people who are chromium deficient as a result of long-term chromium-deficient parenteral nutrition. However, it appears that most people with diabetes are not chromium deficient and, therefore, chromium supplementation has no known benefit.

A great deal of discussion on this topic centers on the chelated form of chromium and chromium picolinate. Several studies[379–391,393,394] indicate that supplementation with chromium may help reduce insulin resistance.

Further studies to assess the effects of dietary chromium supplementation on insulin sensitivity, as well as on other processes such as increased bone mass, improved blood pressure, and lipid profiles in humans are needed.

For further information on this topic, the reader is referred to an excellent review by Schmidt Finney[392] as well as an extensive bibliography of material on this subject.[393–410] See Table 10.36 for the established and potential benefits of chromium.

REFERENCES

1. Olson JA. In: *Modern Nutrition in Health and Disease,* 8th ed., Shils ME, Olson JA, Shike M, Eds. Philadelphia, Lea and Febiger, 1994, chap. 16.
2. Brown L, Rimm EB, Seddon JM et al. *Am J Clin Nutr* 70: 517; 1999.
3. Tang AM, Graham NMH, Kirby AJ et al. *J Acq Immune Def Syn* 6: 949; 1993.
4. Semba RD. *Arch Int Med* 153: 2149; 1993.
5. Semba RD, Miotti PC, Chiphangwi JD. *Lancet* 343: 1593; 1994.
6. Fawzi WW, Msamanga GI, Spiegelman D et al. *N Engl J Med* 351: 23; 2004.
7. Hussey GD, Klein M. *N Engl J Med* 323: 160; 1990.

8. Committee on Infectious Diseases. *Pediatrics* 91: 1014; 1993.

9. Kligman AM et al. *Int J Dermatol* 20: 278; 1981.

10. Dvorak AM. *Lancet* 1: 1303; 1980.

11. Rachet AJ, Busson A. *Paris Medical* 1: 308; 1935.

12. Skogh M, Sundquist T, Tagesson C. *Lancet* 1: 766; 1980.

13. Melhus H, Michaelsson K, Kindmark A et al. *Ann Intern Med* 129: 770; 1998.

14. Feskanich D, Sing V, Willet WC et al. *JAMA* 287: 47; 2002.

15. Michaelsson K, Lithell H, Vessby B et al. *N Engl J Med* 348: 287; 2003.

16. Peto R, Doll R, Buckley JD et al. *Nature* 290: 201; 1981.

17. Albanes D, Hartman TJ. In: *Antioxidant Status, Diet, Nutrition and Health,* Papas AM, Ed. CRC Press, Boca Raton, 1998, p. 497.

18. The α-Tocopherol, β-Carotene Cancer Prevention Study Group. *N Engl J Med* 330: 1029; 1994.

19. Omenn GS, Goodman GE, Thornquist MD et al. *N Engl J Med* 334: 1150; 1996.

20. Hennekens CH, Buring JE, Manson JE et al. *N Engl J Med* 334: 1145; 1996.

21. Blot WJ, Li JY, Taylor PR. *J Natl Cancer Inst* 85: 1483; 1993.

22. Stich HF, Rosin MP, Vallejera MO. *Lancet* 1: 1204; 1984.

23. Garewal HS, Meyske DL, Killen D. *J Clin Oncol* 8: 1715; 1990.

24. Klipstein-Grobusch K, Geleijnse JM, den Breeijen JH et al. *Am J Clin Nutr* 69: 261; 1999.

25. Stampfer MJ, Hennekens CH, Manson JE et al. *N Engl J Med* 328: 1444; 1993.

26. Rimm EB, Stampfer MJ, Ascherio A et al. *N Engl J Med* 328: 1450; 1993.

27. Gaziano JM, Manson JE. *Ann Epidemiol* 5: 255; 1995.

28. Knekt P, Heliovaara M, Rissanen A et al. *Br Med J* 305: 1392; 1992.

29. Taylor A, Jacques PF, Nadler D et al. *Curr Eye Res* 10: 751; 1991.

30. Giovannucci E. *J Natl Cancer Inst* 91: 317; 1999.

31. Rao AO. *Exp Biol Med* 227: 908; 2002

32. Lee EH, Faulhaber D, Hanson KM, *J Invest Dermatol* 122: 510; 2004

33. Bhat KS. *Nutr Rep Int* 36: 685; 1987.

34. Parchal JT, Conrad ME, Skalka HW. *Lancet* 1: 12; 1978.

35. Skalka, HW, Prchal JT. *Am J Clin Nutr* 34: 861; 1981.

36. Jacques PF, Hartz SC, Chylack Jr. LT et al. *Am J Clin Nutr* 48: 152; 1988.

37. Keith R, Alt L. *Nutr Res* 11: 727; 1991.

38. Winters, LR, Yoon JS, Kalkwarf HJ et al. *Am J Clin Nutr* 56: 526; 1992.

39. Belko AZ, Obarzanek E, Kalkwarf HJ et al. *Am J Clin Nutr* 37: 509; 1983.

40. Belko AZ, Obarzanek E, Roach R et al. *Am J Clin Nutr* 40: 553; 1984.

41. Lewis RD, Yates CY, and Driskell JA. *Am J Clin Nutr* 48: 110; 1988.

42. Schoenen J, Lenaerts M, Bastings E. *Cephalalgia* 14: 328; 1994

43. McNulty H, Dowey LRC, Strain JJ et al. *Circulation* 113: 74; 2006

44. Brown WV. *Postgrad Med* 98: 185; 1995.

45. Head KA. *Alt Med Rev* 1: 176; 1996.

46. Murray M. *Am J Nat Med* 2: 9; 1995.

47. Dorner Von G, Fisher FW. *Arzeimittel Forschung* 11: 110; 1961.

48. Meydani, SN, Ribaya-Mercado JD, Russell RM et al. *Am J Clin Nutr* 53: 1275; 1991.

49. Kant AK, Moser-Veillon PB, and Reynolds RD. *Am J Clin Nutr* 48: 1284; 1988.

50. Barr W. *Practitioner* 228: 425; 1984.

51. Gunn ADG. *Int J Vit Nutr Res* 27: 213S; 1985.

52. Kleijnen J, Riet GT, Knipshcild P. *Brit J Obstet Gynaecol* 97: 847; 1990.

53. Williams MJ, Harris RI, Deand BC. *J Int Med Res* 13: 174; 1985.

54. Brush MG, Perry M. *Lancet* 1: 1399; 1985.

55. Dorsey JL, Debruyne LK, Rady SJ. *Fed Proc* 42: 556; 1983.

56. Malgren R, Collings A, Nilsson CG. *Acta Obstet Gynecol Scand* 64: 667; 1985.

57. Collin C. *Rev Med Brux* 3: 605; 1982.

58. Wilson RG, Davis RE. *Pathology* 9: 95; 1977.

59. Davis RE, Calder JS, Curnow DH. *Pathol* 8: 151; 1976.

60. McCann VJ, Davis RE. *Austral NZ Med* 8: 259; 1978.

61. Spellacy WN, Buhi WC, Birk SA. *Am J Obstet Gynecol 127:* 599; 1977.

62. Coelingh HJT, Schreurs WHP. *Br Med J* 3: 13; 1975.

63. Spellacy WN, Buhi WC, Birk SA. *Contraception* 6: 265; 1972.

64. Passariello N, Fici F, Giugliano D et al. *Internat J Clin Pharmacol Ther Toxicol* 21: 252; 1983.

65. Solomon LR, Cohen K. *Diabetes* 38: 881; 1989.

66. Rao RH, Vigg BL, Rao KSJ. *J Clin Endocrinol Metabol* 50: 198; 1980.

67. Fuhr JF, Farrow A, Nelson HS. *Arch Surg* 124: 1329; 1989.

68. Ellis JM, Azuma J, Watanbe T et al. *Res Comm Chem Path Pharm* 17: 165; 1977.

69. Ellis JM. *Res Comm Chem Path Pharm* 13: 743; 1976.
70. D'Souza M. *Lancet* 1: 1104; 1985.
71. Driskell JA, Wesley RL, Hess IE. *Nutr Rep Int.* 34: 1031; 1986.
72. Ellis JM. *Southern Med J* 80: 882; 1987.
73. Smith GP. *Ann Neurol* 15: 104; 1984.
74. Amadio PC. *J Hand Surg* 10A: 237; 1985.
75. Stransky M. *Southern Med J* 82: 841; 1989.
76. Baum MK. *J Acq Immuno Syn* 4: 1122; 1991.
77. Selhub J, Jacques PF, Wilson PW et al. *JAMA* 270: 2693; 1993.
78. Ubbink JB, Hayward WJ, van der Merwe A et al. *J Nutr* 124: 927; 1994.
79. Manson JB, Miller JW. *Ann NY Acad Sci* 669: 197; 1992.
80. Bronstrup A, Hages M, Prinz-Langenohl R et al. *Am J Clin Nutr* 68: 1104; 1998.
81. Spence JD, Bang, H, Chambless, LJ, Stampfer MJ, Stroke 36: 2404; 2005.
82. Yang Q, Botto LD, Erickson JD et al. *Circulation* 113: 1335; 2006.
83. Oakley GP. *Am J Clin Nutr* 65: 1889; 1997.
84. Wald N. *Lancet* 338: 131; 1991.
85. Czeizel AE, Dudas l. *N Engl l Med* 327: 1832; 1992.
86. Centers for Disease Control. *Morb Mortal Wkly Rep* 41: 5; 1992.
87. deBree A, van Dusseldorp M. *Eur J Clin Nutr* 51: 643; 1997.
88. Food Labeling: Health Claims and Label Statements, Folate and Neural Tube Defects, Proposed Rule and Final Rule 2 CFR part 101. *Federal Register* 61: 8752; 1996.
89. Czeizel AE. *Int J Med Sci* 1: 50; 2004.
90. Botto LD, Olney RS, Erickson JD et al. *Am J Med Genet* 1250: 12; 2004.
91. Rimm EB, Willett WC. *JAMA* 279: 359; 1998.
92. Boushey CJ, Beresford SAA. *JAMA* 274: 1049; 1995.
93. Brattstrom LE, Israelsson B. *Scand J Clin Lab Invest* 48: 215; 1988.
94. Brattstrom LE, Israelsson B. *Atherosclerosis* 81: 51; 1990.
95. Jacob RA, Wu MI. *J Nutr* 124: 1072; 1994.
96. Naurath HJ, Joosten E. *Lancet* 346: 85; 1995.
97. O'Keefe CA, Bailey LB. *J Nutr* 125: 2717; 1995.
98. Ubbink JB, Vermaak WJH. *J Nutr* 124: 1927; 1994.
99. Guttormsen AB, Ueland PM. *J Clin Invest* 98: 2174; 1996.
100. Bostom AG, Shemin D. *Kidney Int* 49: 147; 1996.
101. Homocysteine Lowering Trialists' Collaboration. *Br Med J* 316: 894; 1998.
102. Lobo A, Naso A. *Am J Cardiol* 83: 821; 1999.
103. Brouwer IA, Dusseldorp MJ. *Am J Clin Nutr.* 69: 99; 1999.
104. Malinow MR, Nieto FJ. *Arterioscle Thromb Vasc Biol* 17: 1157; 1997.
105. Malinow MR, Duell PB. *N Engl J Med* 338: 1009; 1998.
106. Jacques PF, Selhub J. *N Engl J Med* 340: 1449; 1999.
107. Osdganian J, Stampfer MJ. *JAMA* 281: 1189; 1999.
108. Greenlund KJ, Srinivasan SR. *Circulation* 99: 2144; 1999.
109. Van Beynum IM, Smeitink JAM. *Circulation* 59: 2070; 1999.
110. Hankey GJ, Eikelboom JW. *Lancet* 354: 407; 1999.
111. Peterson JC, Spence JD. *Lancet* 351: 263; 1998.
112. Malinow MR, Bostom AG. *Circulation* 99: 178; 1999.
113. Green R, MIller JW. *Sem Hematol 36:* 47; 1999.
114. Refsum H, Ueland PM. *Ann Rev Med* 49: 31; 1998.
115. Selhub J, D'Angelo A. *Am J Med Sci* 31: 129; 1998.
116. Welch GN, Loscalzo J. *N Engl J Med* 338: 1042; 1998.
117. Toole JF, Malinow MR, Chambless LE et al. *J Am Med Assoc* 291: 565; 2004.
118. Bonaa KH, Njolstad I, Ueland PM. *N Engl J Med* 354: 2006.
119. Lonn E, Arnold MJO, Sheridan P et al. *N Engl J Med* 354: 1; 2006.
120. Schnyder G, Roffi M, Pin R et al. *N Engl J Med* 345: 1593; 2001.
121. Schnyder G, Roffi M, Flammer Y et al. *JAMA* 288: 973; 2002.
122. Mason J. *Nutr Rev* 47: 314; 1989.
123. Butteworth CE. In: *Micronutrients in Health and Disease,* Bendich A, Butteworth CE: Eds., New York: Marcel Dekker, Inc. 1991, p. 165.
124. Butteworth CE, Hatch KD. *JAMA* 267: 528; 1992.
125. Heimburger DC, Alexander CB. *JAMA* 259: 1525; 1998.
126. Lashner BA, Heidenreich PA. *Gastroenterology* 97: 255; 1989.
127. Giovannucci E, Stampfer MJ. *Ann Int Med* 129: 517; 1998.
128. Zhang S, Hunter DJ. *JAMA* 281: 1632; 1999.

129. Blount BC, Mack MM. *Proc Natl Acad Sci USA* 94: 3290; 1997.
130. Adunksky A, Arinzon Z, Fidelman Z et al. *Arch Gerontol Geriatr* 40: 129; 2005.
131. Bottiglieri T, Parnetti L, Arning E et al. *Mech Aging Develop* 122: 2013; 2001.
132. Clark MS, Gunthrie JR, Dennerstein L et al. *Dement Geriatr Cogn Disord* 20: 57; 2005.
133. Gallucci M, Zanardo A, De Valentin L et al. *Arch Gerontol Geriatr* 9: 195; 2004.
134. Mooijaart SP, Gussekloo J, Frolich M et al. *Am J Clin Nutr* 82: 866; 2005.
135. Postiglione A, Milan G, Ruocco A, Gallotta G, Guiotto G, DiMinno G. *Gerontology* 47: 324; 2001.
136. Prins MD, den Heijer T, Hofman A, Koudstaal PJ, Jolles J, Clarke R, Breteler MM. *Neurology* 59: 1375; 2002.
137. Quadri P, Fragiacomo C, Pezzati R et al. *Am J Clin Nutr* 80: 114; 2004.
138. Quadri P, Fragiacomo C, Pezzati R et al. *Clin Chem Lab* 43: 1096; 2005.
139. Ravaglia G, Forti P, Maioli F et al. *Am J Clin Nutr* 82: 636; 2005.
140. Ravaglia G, Forti P, Maioli F, Scali RC, Sacchetti L, Talerico T, Mantovani V, Bianchin M. *Arch Gerontol Geriatr* Suppl 9: 349; 2004.
141. Ravaglia G, Forti P, Maioli F et al. *Mech Ageing Develop* 121: 251; 2000.
142. Sachdev P, Parslow R, Salonikas C, Lux O, Wen WW, Kumar R, Naidoo D, Christensen H, Jorm A. *Arch Neurol* 61: 1369; 2004.
143. Sachdev PS, Wang XL, Looi JCL, Brodaty H. *Neurology* 58: 1539; 2002.
144. Schafer JH, Glass TA, Bolla KI, Mintz M, Jedlicka AE, Schwartz BS. *J Am Geriatr Soc* 53: 381; 2005.
145. Seshadri S, Beiser A, Selhub J et al. *N Engl J Med* 346: 476; 2002.
146. Tucker KL, Ning Q, Scott T et al. *Am J Clin Nutr* 82: 627; 2005.
147. Lehmann M, Regland B, Blennow K et al. *Dement Geriatr Cogn Disord* 16: 145; 2003.
148. Nilsson K, Gustafson L, Hultberg B. *Int J Geriatr Psychiatry* 16: 609; 2001.
149. Smith CR, Jobst KA. *Arch Neurol* 55: 1449; 1998.
150. McCaddon A, Davies G. *Int J Geriatric Psych* 13: 235; 1998.
151. Alpert JE, Fava M. *Nutr Rev* 55: 145; 1997.
152. Burri BJ, Jacob RA. In: *Vitamin C in Health and Disease,* Packer L, Fuchs J, Eds., New York, Marcel Dekker, Inc, 1997, p. 341.
153. Anderson D, Phillips B, Yu T et al. *Environ Mol Mutagen* 30: 161; 1997.
154. Simon JA. *J Am Coll Nutr* 11: 107; 1992.
155. Gatto LM, Hallen GK, Brown AJ et al. *J Am Coll Nutr* 15: 154; 1996.
156. Ness AR, Khaw KT, Bingham S et al. *Eur J Clin Nutr* 50: 724; 1996.
157. Toohey L, Harris MA, Allen KG et al. *J Nutr* 126: 121; 1996.
158. Simon JA, Hudes ES. *J Am Coll Nutr* 17: 250; 1998.
159. Jacques PF. *J Am Coll Nutr* 11: 139; 1992.
160. Moran JP, Cohen L, Greene JM et al. *Am J Clin Nutr* 57: 213; 1993.
161. Jacques PF. *Int J Vitam Nutr Res* 62: 252; 1992.
162. Ness AR, Khaw KT, Bingham S et al. *J Hypertens* 14: 503; 1996.
163. Duffy, SJ, Gokee, N, Holbrook, M, et al. Physiol Heart Circ Physiol 280: H528, 2001.
164. Levine GL, Frei B, Koulouris SN et al. *Circulation* 93: 1107; 1996.
165. Hornig B, Arakawa N, Kohler C et al. *Circulation* 97: 363; 1998.
166. Ito K, Akita H, Kanazawa K et al. *Am J Cardiol* 82: 762; 1998.
167. Kugiyama K, Motoyama T, Hirashima O et al. *J Am Coll Cardiol* 32: 103; 1998.
168. Vogel JH, Bolling SF, Costello RB et al. *J Am Coll Cardiol* 46; 184: 2005.
169. Hecht SS. *Proc Soc Exp Biol Med* 216: 181; 1997.
170. Tannenbaum SR, Wishnok JS. *Ann NY Acad Sci* 498: 354; 1987.
171. Vohra K, Khan AJ, Telang V et al. *J Perinatol* 10: 134; 1990.
172. Johnston CS, Martin LJ, Cai X. *J Am Coll Nutr* 11: 172; 1992.
173. Levy R, Shriker O, Porath A et al. *J Infect Dis* 173: 1502; 1996.
174. Maderazo EG, Woronick CL, Hickingbotham N et al. *J Trauma* 31: 1142; 1991.
175. Hemila H. In: *Vitamin C in health and disease,* Packer L, Fuchs J, Eds., Marcel Dekker Inc, New York, 1997, p. 471.
176. Heuser G, Vojdani A. *Immunopharmacol Immunotoxicol* 19: 291; 1997.
177. Smit MJ, Anderson R. *Agents Actions* 30: 338; 1991.
178. Khaw KT, Bingham S, Welch A et al. *Lancet* 357: 657; 2001.
179. Loria CM, Klag MJ, Caulfield LE et al. *Am J Clin Nutr.* 72: 139; 2000.
180. Negri E, Franceschi S, Bosetti C et al. *Int J Cancer* 86; 122: 2005.
181. You WC, Zhang L, Gail MH et al. *J Natl Cancer Inst* 92: 1607; 2000.
182. Freudenheim JL, Marshall JR, Vena JE et al. *J Natl Cancer Inst* 88: 340; 1996.
183. Michels KB, Holmberg L, Bergkvist L et al. *Int J Cancer* 91: 563; 2001.
184. Wu K, Helzlsouer KJ, Alberg AJ et al. *Cancer Causes Control* 11; 279: 2000.
185. Carr AC, Frei B. *Am J Clin Nutr* 69: 1086; 1999.
186. Enstrom JE, Kanim LE, Breslow L. *Am J Publ Health* 76: 1124; 1986.
187. Enstrom JE, Kanim LE, Klein MA. *Epidemiology* 3: 194; 1992.
188. Enstrom JE. *Nutr Today* 28: 28; 1993.

189. Manson JE, Stampfer MJ, Willett WC et al. *Circulation* 85: 865; 1992.
190. Manson JE, Stampfer MJ, Willett WC el al. *Circulation* 87: 678; 1993.
191. Fehily AM, Yarnell JWG, Sweetnam PM et al. *Br J Nutr* 69: 303; 1993.
192. Knekt P, Reunanen A, Jarvinen R et al. *Am J Epidemiol* 139: 1180; 1994.
193. Gale CR, Martyn CN, Winter PD et al. *Br Med J* 310: 1563; 1995.
194. Kritchevsky SB, Shimakawa T, Tell GS et al. *Circulation* 92: 2142; 1995.
195. Pandey DK, Shekelle R, Selwyn BJ et al. *Am J Epidemiol* 142: 1269; 1995.
196. Kushi LH, Folsom AR, Prineas RJ et al. *N Engl J Med* 334: 1156; 1996.
197. Losonczy KG, Harris TB, Havlik RJ. *Am J Clin Nutr* 64: 190; 1996.
198. Sahyoun NR, Jacques PF, Russell RM. *Am J Epidemiol* l44: 501; 1996.
199. Mark SD, Wang W, Fraumeni JF et al. *Epidemiology* 9: 9; 1998.
200. Shekelle RB, Liu S, Raynor WJ et al. *Lancet* 28: 1185; 1981.
201. Kromhout D. *Am J Clin Nutr* 45: 1361; 1987.
202. Knekt P, Jarvinen R, Seppanen R et al. *Am J Epidemiol* 134: 471; 1991.
203. Shibata A, Paganini-Hill A, Ross RK el al. *Br J Cancer* 66: 673; 1992.
204. Graham S, Zielezny M, Marshall J et al. *Am J Epidemiol* 136: 1327; 1992.
205. Hunter DJ, Manson JE, Colditz GA et al. *N Engl J Med* 329: 234; 1993.
206. Bostick RM, Potter JD, McKenzie DR et al. *Cancer Res* 53: 4230; 1993.
207. Kushi LH, Fee RM, Sellers TA et al. *Am J Epidemiol* 144: 165; 1996.
200. Yong L, Brown CC, Schatzkin A et al. *Am J Epidemiol* 146: 231; 1997.
209. Dawson-Hughes B, Heaney RP, Holick MF et al. *Osteoporos Int* 16: 713; 2005
210. Holick M. *Am J Clin Nutr* 79: 364; 2004.
211. Holick M. *Am J Clin Nutr* 80: 1678S; 2004.
212. Kessenich CR, Rosen CJ. *Orthopaedic Nursing* 15: 67; 1996.
213. Holick MF. *Am J Clin Nutr* 60: 619; 1994.
214. Kinyamu HK, Gallagher JC, Balhorn KE et al. *Am J Clin Nutr* 65: 790; 1997.
215. Goldray D, Mizrahi-Sasson E, Merdler C el al. *J Am Geriatr Soc* 37: 589; 1989.
216. Pogue SJ. *Dermatol Nursing* 7: 103; 1995.
217. Meunier P. *Scan J Rheum* 103: 75S; 1996.
218. McAuley KA, Jones S, Lewis-Barned NJ et al. *NZ Med J* 110: 275; 1997.
219. Compston JE. *Clin Endocrin* 43: 393; 1995.
220. McKenna MJ. *Am J Med* 93: 69; 1992.
221. Ooms ME, Roos JC, Bezemer PD et al. *J Clin Endocrin Metab* 80: 1052; 1995.
222. MacLaughlin J, Holick MF. J *Clin Invest* 76: 1536; 1985.
223. Chapuy MC, Arlot ME, Duboeuf F et al. *N Engl J Med* 327: 1637; 1992.
224. Torgerson DJ, Kanis JA. *QJM* 88: 135; 1995.
225. Bischoff-Ferrari HA, Dawson-Hughes B, Willett WC et al. *JAMA* 291: 1999; 2006.
226. Morimoto S, Yoshikawa K, Kozuka T et al. *Brit J Dermatol* 115: 421; 1986.
227. Morimoto S, Yoshikawa K. *Arch Dermatol* 125: 231; 1989.
228. Kragballe K. *Arch Dermatol* 125: 1647; 1989.
229. Smith EL, Pincus SH, Donovan L et al. *J Am Acad Dermatol* 19: 516; 1988.
230. Kragballe K, Beck HI, Sogaard H. *Brit J Dermatol* 119: 223; 1988.
231. Henderson CA, Papworth-Smith J, Cunliffe WJ et al. *Brit J Dermatol* 121: 493; 1989.
232. Van de Kerkhol PCM, Van Bokhoven M, Zultak M et al. *Brit J Dermatol* 120: 661; 1989.
233. Thys-Jacobs S. *Headache* 34: 544; 1994.
234. Thys-Jacobs S. *Headache* 34: 590; 1994.
235. Giovannucci E. *Cancer Causes Control* 9: 567; 1998.
236. Ma J, Stampfer MJ, Gann PH et al. *Cancer Epidemiol, Biomark Prevent* 7: 385; 1998.
237. Lipkin M, Reddy B, Newmark H et al. *Annu Rev Nutr* 19: 545; 1999.
238. Xue L, Newmark H, Yang K el al. *Nutrition Cancer* 26: 281; 1996.
239. Hiatt RA, Krieger N, Lobaugh B et al. *J Natl Cancer Inst* 90: 6; 1998.
240. Giovannucci E. *Cancer Cause Control* 16: 83; 2005.
241. Garland CF, Garland FC, Gorham ED et al. *Am J Public Health* 96: 9; 2006.
242. Martindale. *The Extra Pharmacopoeia.* 32nd Edition, Reynolds JE, Ed., Pharmaceutical Press, London, 1998.
243. Porkkala-Sarataho E, Nyyssonen K, Salonen JT et al. *Atherosclerosis* 124: 83; 1996.
244. Pyor WP. In: *Present Knowledge in Nutrition.* Bowman BA, Russell RM (Eds.,) ILSL Press, Washington, 2001, p.156.
245. Regnstrom J, Nilsson J, Moldeus P et al. *Am J Clin Nutr* 63: 377; 1996.
246. Azen S. *J Am Heart Assoc* 2369; 1996.
247. Gey KF, Puska P, Jordan P et al. *Am J Clin Nutr* 53: 326S; 1991.
248. Stephens NG, Parsons A, Schofield PM et al. *Lancet* 347; 178: 1996.
249. Boaz M, Smetana S, Weinstein T et al. *Lancet* 356; 1213: 2000.

250. Fang JC, Kimlay S, Hikiti H et al. *Lancet* 359; 1108: 2003.
251. Salonen JT, Nyyssonen K, Salonen R et al. *J Intern Med* 248; 377: 2000.
252. Hercberg S, Galan P, Preziosi P et al. *Arch Intern Med* 164; 2335: 2004.
253. Rapola JM, Virtamo J, Ripatti S et al. *Lancet* 349; 1715: 1997.
254. GISSI Prevention Investigators *Lancet* 354; 447: 1996.
255. Hope and Hope – Too Trial Investigators. *JAMA* 293; 1338: 2005.
256. Collaborative Group of the Primary Prevention Project (PPP) *Lancet* 357; 89: 2001 (Published **erratum** in *Lancet* 357; 1134: 2001).
257. Hodis HN, Mack WJ, LaBree L et al. *Circulation* 106; 1453: 2002.
258. Brown BG, Zhao XQ, Chait A et al. *N Engl J Med* 345; 1583: 2001.
259. Waters DD, Alderman EL, Hsia J et al. *JAMA* 288; 2432: 2002.
260. Heart Protection Study Collaborative Group. *Lancet* 360; 7: 2002.
261. Lee IM, Cook NR, Gaziano JM et al. *JAMA* 294; 56: 2005.
262. Kris-Etherton P, Lichtenstein AH, Howard B et al. *Circulation* 110; 637; 2004 (Leon).
263. Blumberg JB. *Nutr Clin Care* 5; 50: 2002.
264. Jialal I, Devaraj S. *J Nutr* 135; 348: 2005.
265. Petersen RC, Thomas RG, Grundman M et al. *N Engl J Med* 352: 237, 2005.
266. The Heart Outcomes Prevention Evaluation Study Investigators. *N Engl J Med* 342: 154; 2000.
267. GISSI-Prevenzione Investigators. *Lancet* 354: 447; 1999.
268. Jha P, Flather M, Lonn E et al. *Ann Int Med* 123: 860; 1995.
269. DeMaio SJ, King SB, Lembo NJ et al. *J Am Coll Nutr* 11: 68; 1992.
270. Stahelin HB, Rosel F, Buess E et al. *J Natl Cancer Inst* 73: 1463; 1984.
271. Wald NJ, Boreham J, Hayward JL et al. *Br J Cancer* 49: 321; 1984.
272. Salonen IT, Salonen R, Lappetelainen R et al. *Br Med J* 290: 417; 1985.
273. Menkes MS, Comstock GWS, Vuilieumier JP et al. *N Engl J Med* 315: 1250; 1986.
274. Kok FJ, van Duijn CM, Hofman A et al. *N Engl J Med* 316: 1416; 1987.
275. Miyamoto H, Araya Y, Ito M et al. *Cancer* 60: 1159; 1987.
276. Wald NJ, Thompson SG, Densem JW et al. *Br J Cancer* 56: 69; 1987.
277. Knekt P, Aromaa A, Maatela J et al. *Am J Epidemiol* 127: 28; 1988.
278. Knekt P, Aromaa A, Maatela J et al. *Int J Cancer* 42: 846; 1988.
279. Knekl P. *Int J Epidemiol* 17: 281; 1988.
280. Verreault RA, Chu J, Mandelson M et al. *Int J Cancer* 43: 1050; 1989.
281. LeGardeur BY, Lopez A, Johnson WD et al. *Nutr Cancer* 14: 133; 1990.
282. Buiatti E, Palli D, Decarli A et al. *Int J Cancer* 45: 896; 1990.
283. Gridley G, McLaughlin JK, Block G et al. *Nutr Cancer* 14: 219; 1990.
284. Palan PR, Mikhail MS, Basu J et al. *Nutr Cancer* 15: 13; 1991.
285. Comstock GW, Helzlsover KJ, Bush TL. *Am J Clin Nutr* 53: 260S; 1991.
286. Harris RW, Key TJ, Sikocks PB et al. *Nutr Cancer* 15: 63; 1991.
287. Gridley G, McLaughlin JK, Block G et al. *Am J Epidemiol* 135: 1083; 1992.
288. Grimes JD, Hassan MN, Thakar JH. *Prog Neuro-Psychopharmacol Biol Psych* 12: 165; 1988.
289. Factor SA, Weiner WJ. *Ann NY Acad Sci* 570: 441; 1989.
290. Fahn S. *Am J Clin Nutr* 53: 380S; 1991.
291. Parkinson Study Group. *N Engl J Med* 328: 176; 1993.
292. Parksinson Study Group. *Ann Neurol* 39: 29; 1996.
293. de Rijk MC, Breteler MM, den Breeijen JH et al. *Arch Neurol* 54: 762; 1997.
294. Sano M, Ernesto C, Thomas RG et al. *N Engl J Med* 336: 1216; 1997.
295. Suttie JW. In: *The Fat Soluble Vitamins*, Diplock AT, Ed. William Heinemann Ltd., London, 1985, p. 225.
296. USPDI. *Drug Information for the Health Care Professional*, Vol. 1, The United Slates Pharmacopoeial Convention, Rockville, MD, 1997, p. 2995.
297. Olson RE. *Ann Rev Nutr* 4: 281; 1984.
298. Jie KG, Bots ML, Vermeer C et al. *Calcif Tissue Int* 59: 352; 1996.
299. Vermeer C, Gijsbers BIL, Craciun AM et al. *J Nutr* 126: 187S; 1996.
300. Knapen MH, Hamulyak K, Vermeer C. *Ann Intern Med* 111: 1001; 1989.
301. Menon RK, Gill DS, Thomas M et al. *J Clin Endocrinol Metab* 64: 59; 1987.
302. Feskanich D, Wever P, Willett WC et al. *Am J Clin Nutr* 69: 74; 1999.
303. Cotter, R, Booth SL. *Amer Soc Clin Nutr. Thrombosis Res* 117: 211; 2005.
304. Douglas AS, Robins SP, Hutchison JD et al. *Bone* 17: 15; 1995.
305. Prince RL, Smith M, Dick IM et al. *N Engl J Med* 325: 1189; 1991.
306. Aloia JF, Vaswani A, Yeh JK et al. *Ann Int Med* 120: 97; 1994.
307. Dawson-Hughes B, Dallal GE, Krall EA et al. *N Engl J Med* 323: 878; 1990.
308. Skaer TL. *P & T* 20: 88; 1995.
309. Riggs BL, Jowsey J, Kelly PJ et al. *J Clin Endo Metab* 42: 1139; 1976.

310. Riggs BL, Seeman E, Hodgson SF et al. *N Engl J Med* 306: 446; 1982.
311. Birge SJ. *Clinics Geri Med* 9: 69; 1993.
312. Lau EM, Cooper C. *Osteoporosis Internat* 3: 23; 1993.
313. NIH Consensus Development Panel on Optimal Calcium Intake. *JAMA* 272: 1942; 1994.
314. Riis BJ, Christiansen C. *Maturitas* 6: 65; 1984.
315. Dawson-Hughes B, Dallal GE, Krall EA et al. *Ann Int Med* 115: 505; 1991.
316. Chapuy MC, Chapuy P, Meunier PF. *Am J Clin Nutr* 46: 324; 1987.
317. Chapuy MC, Arlot MC, DuBoeuf F et al. *N Engl J Med* 327: 1637; 1992.
318. Sankaran SK. *Drugs Aging* 9: 1; 1996.
319. Baron JA, Beach M, Mandel JS et al. *N Engl J Med* 340: 101; 1999.
320. Whelan RL, Horvath KD, Gleason NR et al. *Dis Colon Rectum* 42: 212; 1999.
321. Mobarhan S. *Nutr Rev* 57: 124; 1999.
322. Lipkin M, Bandaru R, Newmark H et al. *Ann Rev Nutr* 19: 545; 1999.
323. Lipkin M, Newmark HL. *J Am Coll Nutr* 18: 392S; 1999.
324. Thys-Jacobs S, Starkey P, Bernstein D et al. *Am J Obstet Gynecol* 179: 444; 1998.
325. Recker RR, Davies KM, Dowd RM et al. *Ann Intern Med* 130: 897; 1999.
326. Teegarden D, Legowski P, Gunther W et al. *J Clin Endo Met* 90; 5127; 2005.
327. McCarron DA, Reusser ME. *J Am Coll Nutr* 18: 398S; 1999.
328. McCarron DA, Metz JA, Hatton DC. *Am J Clin Nutr* 68: 517; 1998.
329. Tranquilli AL, Lucino E, Garzetti GG et al. *Gynecol Endocrinol* 8: 55; 1994.
330. Stendig-Lindberg G, Tepper R, Leichter I. *Magnesium Res* 6: 155; 1993.
331. Rode RK. *Endocinol Metal Clin North Am* 22: 377; 1993.
332. Aschero A, Rimm EB, Giovannucci EB et al. *Cirrulation* 86: 1475; 1992.
333. Abbott RD, Ando F, Masaki KH et al. *Am J Cardio* 92: 665; 2003.
334. Jee SH, Miller ER III, Guallar E et al. *Am J Hypertens* 15:691; 2002.
335. Appel LJ, Moore TJ, Obarzanek E et al. *N Engl J Med* 336; 1117: 1997.
336. Bashir Y, Sneddon JF, Staunton HA et al. *Am J Cardiol* 72; 1156: 1993.
337. Ford ES, Mokdad AH. *J Nutr* 133; 2879: 2003.
338. Motoyama T, Sano H, Fukuzaki H et al. *Hypertens* 13: 227; 1989.
339. Itoh K, Kawasaka T, Nakamura M. *Br J Nutr* 78: 737; 1997.
340. Patki PS, Singh J, Gokhale SV et al. *Br Med J* 301: 521; 1990.
341. Sacks FM, Willett WC, Smith A et al. *Hypertension* 31: 131; 1998.
342. Dyckner T, Wester PO. *Br Med J* 286: 1847; 1983.
343. Abraham GE, Lubran MM. *Am J Clin Nutr* 34: 2364; 1981.
344. Sherwood RA, Rocks BF, Stewart A et al. *Ann Clin Biochem* 23: 667; 1986.
345. Nicholas A. In: *First International Symposium on Magnesium Deficit in Human Pathology*, J Durlach Ed., Springer-Verlag, Paris, 1973, p. 261.
346. Facchinetti F, Borella P, Sances G et al. *Obstet Gynecol* 78: 177; 1991.
347. Neglen P. *VASA* 14: 285; 1985.
348. Greaves MW. *Lancet* 2: 889; 1970.
349. Serjeant GR. *Lancet* 2: 891; 1970.
350. Favier AE. *Biolog Trace Element Res* 32: 363; 1992.
351. Bedwal RS, Bahuguna A. *Experientia* 50: 626; 1994.
352. Apgar J. *J Nutr Biochem* 3: 266; 1992.
353. Hunt CD, Johnson PE, Herbel JL et al. *Am J Clin Nutr* 56: 148; 1992.
354. Netter A, Hartoma R, Nahoul K. *Arch Androl* 7: 69; 1981.
355. Marmar JL. *Fertil Steril* 26: 1057; 1975.
356. Calhoun NR, Smith JC Jr, Becker KL. *Clin Orthopaedics Related Res* 1: 212; 1974.
357. Yamaguchi M. *J Nutritional Sci Vitaminol* special no. 522, 1992.
358. Alhava EM, Olkkonen H, Puittinen J et al. *Acta Orthopaedica Scand* 48: 1; 1997.
359. Saltman PD, Strause LG. *J Am Coll Nutr* 12: 384; 1993.
360. Mares-Perlman JA, Klein R, Klein BE et al. *Arch Ophthal* 114: 991; 1996.
361. AREDS Report No. 8 *Arch Ophthalmol* 119: 1417; 2001.
362. Smith W, Mitchell P, Webb K et al. *Ophthalmology* 106; 761; 1999.
363. Good RA, Fernandes G, Garofalo JA et al. In: *Clinical, Biochemical and Nutritional Aspects of Trace Elements,* Alan R Liss, NY, 1982, p. 189.
364. Chandra RK, McBean LD. *Nutrition* 10: 79; 1994.
365. Prasad AS, Fitzgerald JT, Hess JW et al. *Nutrition* 9: 218; 1993.
366. Girodon F, Galan P, Monget AI. *Arch Int Med* 159: 748; 1999.
367. Fortes C, Forastiere F, Agabiti N et al. *J Am Geriatr Soc* 46: 19; 1998.
368. Spallholz, JE. In: *Diet and Resistance to Disease,* Phillips M, Baetz A, Eds., Plenum, New York, 1981, p. 43.

369. Peplowski MA, Mahan DC, Murray FA et al. *J An Sci* 51: 344; 1980.
370. Mulhern SA, Taylor GL, Magruder LE et al. *Nutr Res* 5: 201; 1985.
371. Clark LC, Combs GF, Turnbull BW et al. *JAMA* 276: 1957; 1996.
372. Clark LC, Dalkin B, Krongrad A. *Br J Urol* 81: 730; 1998.
373. Combs GF Jr, Clark LC, Turnbull BW. *Medizinische Klinik* 92: 42S; 1997.
374. Nelson MA, Porterfield BW, Jacobs ET et al. *Sem Urologic Oncol* 17: 91; 1999.
375. Combs GF Jr, Gray WP. *Pharmacol Ther* 79: 179; 1998.
376. Ip C. *J Nutr* 128: 1845; 1998.
377. Combs, GF Jr. *J Nutr* 135: 343; 2005.
378. American Diabetes Association. *Diabetes Care* 19: 16S; 1996.
379. Morris BW, Kouta S, Robinson R et al. *Diabetes* 17: 684; 2000.
380. Bahijri SM, Mufti AM. *Biol Trace Elem Res* 85: 97; 2002.
381. Cefalu WT, Bell-farrow AD, Stegner J et al. *J Trace Elements Exp Med* 12: 71; 1999.
382. Offenbacker EG, Pi-Sunyer FX. *Diabetes* 29: 919; 1980.
383. Potter JF, Levin P, Anderson RA et al. *Metabolism* 34: 199; 1985.
384. Rabinovitz H, Friendensohn A, Leibovita A et al. *Int J Vitam Nutr Res* 74: 178; 2004.
385. Racek J, Trefil L, Rajdl D et al. *Biol Trace Elem Res* 109: 215; 2006.
386. Ravina A, Slezak, Mirsky N et al. *Diabet Med* 16: 164; 1999.
387. Riales R, Albrink MJ. *Am J Clin Nutr* 34: 2670; 1981.
388. Vladeva SV, Terzieva DD, Arabadjiiska DT. *Folia Med (Plovidv)* 47: 59; 2005.
389. Wilson BE, Gondy A. *Diabetes Res Clin Pract* 28: 179; 1995.
390. Cheng N, Zhu X, Hongli S et al. *J Trace Elemnts Med Biol* 12: 55; 1999.
391. Jovanovic-Peterson L, Gutierrez M, Peterson CM. *J Trace Elemnts Med Biol* 12: 91; 1999.
392. Schmidt Finney L, Gonzalez-Campoy, JM. *Clin Diabetes* 15: 1; 1997.
393. Anderson, RA. *J Am Coll Nutr* 16: 404; 1997.
394. Anderson RA, Cheng N, Bryden NA et al. *Diabetes* 46: 1786; 1997.
395. Cunningham JJ. *J Am Coll Nutr* 17: 7; 1998.
396. Davies S, McLaren HJ, Hunnisett A et al. *Metabolism* 46: 469; 1997.
397. Davis CM, Vincent JB. *Biochemistry* 36: 4382; 1997.
398. Fox GN, Sabovic Z. *J Fam Pract* 46: 83; 1998.
399. Hahdi GS. *Diabet Med* 13: 389; 1996.
400. Heller RF. *Med Hypotheses* 45: 325; 1995.
401. Jovanovic-Peterson L, Peterson CM. *J Am Coll Nutr* 15: 14; 1996.
402. Lee NA, Reasner CA. *Diabetes Care* 17: 1449; 1994.
403. Linday LA. *Med Hypotheses* 49: 47; 1997.
404. Littlefield D. *J Am Diet Assoc* 94: 1368; 1994.
405. McCarty ME. *Med Hypotheses* 49: 143; 1997.
406. Porter-Field LM. *RN* 59: 71; 1996.
407. Preuss HG. *J Am Coll Nutr* 16: 397; 1997.
408. Romero RA, Salgado O, Rodriguez-lturbe B et al. *Transplant Proc* 28: 3382; 1996.
409. Sampson MJ, Griffith VS, Drury PI. *Diabet Med* 11: 150; 1994.
410. Yurkow EJ, Kim G. *Mol Pharmacol* 47: 686; 1995.

11 Nutrient–Nutrient Interactions

Carolyn D. Berdanier

CONTENTS

No nutrient acts alone. All the nutrients together, when consumed in the appropriate amounts, help to maintain the body in its optimal healthy state. There are however, some nutrient interactions that should be noted. This chapter addresses these interactions and describes their effects within the body.

MINERAL INTERACTIONS

Minerals are found in every cell, tissue, and organ. They are important constituents of essential molecules such as thyroxine (T_4), hemoglobin, and vitamin B_{12}. They serve as critical cofactors in numerous enzymatic reactions (see Chapter 7) and form the hard mineral complexes that comprise bone (see Chapter 64). Minerals serve in the maintenance of pH, osmotic pressure, nerve conductance, muscle contraction, and in almost every aspect of life. Minerals interact such that bioavailability or use is affected.[1,2] The ratios of calcium to phosphorus, iron to copper to zinc, and calcium to magnesium, and other factors are examples of such interactions. Some of these interactions are mutually beneficial while others are antagonistic. Most of these interactions occur at the level of the gut, in that many are concerned with mineral absorption. For example, zinc absorption is impaired by high iron intakes; high zinc intake impairs copper absorption. Molybdenum and sulfur antagonize copper, and tungsten (not an essential nutrient) interferes with molybdenum absorption. These antagonisms contribute to the relative inefficiency of absorption of minerals that are poorly absorbed and just as poorly lost once absorbed.

Many of the trace minerals have more than one charged state; and living cells have preferences for these states. For example, the uptake of iron is much greater when the iron is in the ferrous (+2) state than when in the ferric (+3) state. Minerals that keep iron in the ferric state will interfere with iron absorption and use. Minerals that do the reverse will enhance iron uptake. Such is the beneficial action of copper on iron. The cuprous ion keeps the ferrous ion from losing electrons and becoming the ferric ion. The interactions of essential minerals are best illustrated in Figure 11.1.

The availability of iron from food depends on its source. Soybean protein, for example, contains an inhibitor of iron uptake. Diets such as those in Asia contain numerous soybean products, and iron absorption is adversely affected by this soybean inhibitor. Tannins, phytates, certain fibers (not cellulose), carbonates, phosphates, and low-protein diets also adversely affect the apparent absorption of iron. In contrast, ascorbic acid, fructose, citric acid, high-protein foods, lysine, histidine, cysteine, methionine,

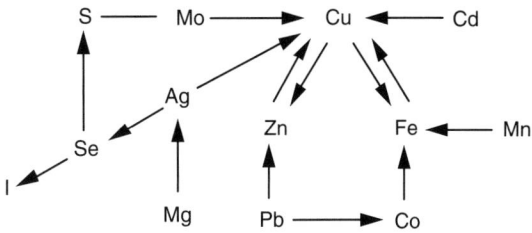

FIGURE 11.1 Trace mineral interaction.

and natural chelates (i.e., heme) all enhance the apparent absorption of iron.[3,4] Zinc and manganese reduce iron uptake by about 30% to 50% and 10% to 40%, respectively. Excess iron reduces zinc uptakes by 13% to 22%. Stearic acid, one of the main fatty acids in meat, enhances iron uptake.

Two types of iron are present in the food, namely, heme iron, which is found principally in animal products, and nonheme iron, which is inorganic iron bound to various proteins in the plant. Most of the iron in the diet, usually greater than 85%, is present in the nonheme form. The absorption of nonheme iron is strongly influenced by its solubility in the upper part of the intestine. Absorption of nonheme iron depends on the composition of the meal and is subject to enhancers of absorption such as animal protein and by reducing agents such as vitamin C. On the other hand, heme iron is absorbed more efficiently. It is not subject to these enhancers. Although heme iron accounts for a smaller proportion of iron in the diet, it provides quantitatively more iron to the body than dietary nonheme iron.

Carcinogenesis can be instigated by some minerals. Nickel subsulfide, for example, is a potent carcinogen, having the renal tissue as its target. In the presence of high to moderate iron levels, the activity of the nickel compound (with respect to carcinogenesis) is increased. In copper excess due to a genetic disorder involving the protein that transports copper, hepatic cancer develops, and this cancer is potentiated by high iron levels. It would appear in these last examples that the role of iron is that of a cancer promoter rather than that of an initiator as described for colon cancer.

Although high iron intakes can be harmful, it should be noted that optimal iron intakes can protect against lead toxicity. Lead competes with iron for uptake by the enterocyte. If the transporter is fully saturated by its preferred mineral, iron, then the lead will be poorly absorbed and get excreted in the feces. Well-nourished individuals with respect to iron nutriture are at lesser risk for lead toxicity than are those whose iron intake is marginal or deficient.

As with iron, zinc absorption is relatively poor. Of the approximately 4 to 14 mg/day consumed, only 10% to 40% is absorbed.[5,6] Absorption is decreased by the presence of binding agents or chelating agents, which bind the mineral making it unavailable. Zinc binds to ligands that contain sulfur, nitrogen, or oxygen. Zinc will form complexes with phosphate groups (PO_4^-), chloride (Cl^-), and carbonate groups (HCO_3^-) as well as with cysteine and histidine. Low zinc status impairs the absorption of calcium.[6]

Zinc can sometimes be displaced on the zinc fingers of DNA-binding proteins (receptors) by other divalent metals.[7] Iron, for example, has been used to displace zinc on the DNA-binding protein that also binds estrogen. This protein binds to the estrogen response element of the DNA promoter region encoding the estrogen responsive gene products. When this occurs in the presence of H_2O_2 and ascorbic acid, damage to the proximate DNA, the estrogen response element, occurs. It has been suggested that, in this circumstance of an iron-substituted zinc finger, free radicals are more readily generated with the consequence of genomic damage. This suggestion has been offered as an explanation of how excess iron (iron toxicity) could instigate the cellular changes that occur in carcinogenesis.

In excess, cadmium can also substitute for zinc in the zinc fingers. In this substitution, the resultant zinc fingers are nonfunctional. Because of the importance of these fingers in cell survival and renewal, a cadmium substitution is lethal. Cadmium toxicity is an acute illness with little lag time needed for the symptom of cell death to manifest itself.

Excess zinc intake can adversely affect copper and iron absorption. Further, excess zinc can interfere with the function of iron as an antioxidant and can interfere with the action of cadmium and calcium as well. Ferritin, the iron storage protein, can also bind zinc. In zinc excess, zinc can replace iron on this protein.[8] Other interactions include a copper–zinc interaction. Copper in excess can interfere with the uptake and binding of zinc by metallothionine in the enterocyte. In humans consuming copper-rich diets, the apparent absorption of zinc is markedly reduced. In part, this is due to a copper–zinc competition for enterocyte transport and in part due to a copper effect on metallothionine gene expression. Metallothionine has a greater affinity for copper than for zinc, and thus zinc is left behind while copper is transported to the serosal side of the enterocyte for export to the plasma, whereupon the copper rather than the zinc is picked up by albumin and transported to the rest of the body. Fortunately, excess copper in the normal diet is not common. Zinc is usually present in far greater amounts, and this interaction is of little import in the overall scheme of zinc metabolism. The metallothionine proteins, in addition to binding zinc and copper, also bind other heavy metals such as mercury and cadmium. This occurs when the individual is acutely exposed to toxic levels of these metals.

Selenium is an integral part of the enzyme, type 1 iodothyronine deiodinase, which catalyzes the deiodination of the iodothyronines notably the deiodination of T_4 to triiodothyronine (T_3), the most active of the thyroid hormones.[9] This deiodination is also catalyzed by type II and type III deiodinases, which are not selenoproteins. While all the deiodinases catalyze the conversion of T_4 to T_3, there are differences in the tissue distribution of these enzymes. The pituitary, brain, central nervous system, and brown adipose tissue contain types II and III, whereas type I is found in liver, kidney, and muscle. These two isozymes (II and III) contribute very little T_3 to the circulation except under conditions (i.e., starvation) that enhance reverse triiodothyronine (rT_3) production. In selenium-deficient animals, type I synthesis is markedly impaired, and this impairment is reversed when selenium is restored to the diet. Under these same conditions, the ratio of T_3 to T_4 is altered. There is more T_4 and less T_3 in selenium-deficient animals, and the ratio of the two is reversed when selenium is restored. Because type II and III deiodinase also exist, these enzymes should increase in activity so as to compensate for the selenium-dependent loss of function. However, they do not do this because their activity is linked to that of the type I. When T_4 levels rise (as in selenium deficiency), this rise feeds back to the pituitary, which in turn alters (reduces) thyroid-stimulating hormone (TSH) release. The conversion of T_4 to T_3 in the pituitary is catalyzed by the type II deiodinase, yet TSH release falls. T_4 levels are high because the type I deiodinase is less active. Whereas the deficient animal might have a T_3/T_4 ratio of 0.01, the selenium-sufficient animal has a ratio of 0.02, a doubling of the conversion of T_4 to T_3. The effect of selenium supplementation on the synthesis and activity of the type I deiodinase probably explains the poor growth of deficient animals. Bermano et al.[10] have reported significant linear growth in deficient rats given a single selenium supplement, and this growth was directly related to the supplement-induced increase in type I deiodinase activity. In turn, the observations of changes in selenium status coincident with changes in thyroid hormone status provided the necessary background for establishing the selenium–iodine interaction that today is taken for granted. The role of selenium in the synthesis of type I deiodinase clearly explains the lack of goiter (enlarged thyroid gland) in cretins who lack both iodine and selenium in their diet. Thus, low selenium intakes impair thyroid hormone activity, and there is a selenium–iodine interaction.

Other trace mineral interactions also exist. Copper-deficient rats and mice have been shown to have reduced glutathione peroxidase activity.[11] Glutathione peroxidase is a selenium-containing enzyme. Copper deficiency increases oxidative stress, yet oxidative stress affects all of the enzymes involved in free radical suppression. Even though glutathione peroxidase does not contain copper, the expression of the genes for this enzyme and for catalase is reduced in the copper-deficient animal. There are numerous nutrient interactions required for the maintenance of the optimal redox state in the cell. This is important not only because it stabilizes the lipid portion of the membranes within and around the cells but also because it optimizes the functional performance of the many cellular proteins. Copper, zinc, magnesium, and manganese are part of the antioxidant system as is $NADPH^+$ and NAD^+ (niacin-containing coenzymes). The NAD^+, although not usually shown as part of the system, is involved because it transfers reducing equivalents via the transhydrogenase cycle to $NADP^+$. Excess selenium intake interferes with zinc absorption and use, reduces tissue iron stores, and increases copper level in heart, liver, and kidney.[12] Manganese and calcium share a uniport mechanism for mitochondrial transport.[13] Manganese can accumulate in this organelle because it is cleared very slowly. Mitochondrial manganese efflux is not sodium dependent, and in fact appears to inhibit both the sodium-dependent and sodium-independent calcium efflux. This manganese effect on calcium is not reciprocal; calcium has no effect on manganese efflux.

As already mentioned, cobalt in excess can block iron absorption. Cobalt together with manganese and iodine are involved in the synthesis of T_4. Whether they interact or are merely essential cofactors in T_4 synthesis has not been satisfactorily resolved.[14]

As ions, minerals react with charged amino acid residues of intact proteins and peptides. Table 11.1 provides a list of minerals and the amino acids with which they react. Depending on their valence state, these electrovalent bonds can be very strong or very weak associations, or anything in between. The marginally charged ion (either an electron acceptor or an electron donor) will be less strongly attracted to its opposite number than will an ion with a strong charge.

The formation of mineral–organic compound bonds is also seen when one examines the roles of minerals in gene expression. Almost every mineral is involved in one or more ways. Zinc–cysteine or zinc–histidine linkages form the zinc fingers that bond with certain base sequences of DNA, thereby affecting transcription. Mineral–protein complexes serve as *cis*- or *trans*-acting elements that enhance or inhibit promoter activity and/or RNA polymerase II activity. Minerals can bond either by themselves or in complexes with proteins to inhibit or enhance translation. Lastly, minerals by themselves or in a complex can influence posttranslation protein modification. Additional information regarding the trace minerals can be found in Chapter 8.

INTERACTIONS OF VITAMINS WITH MINERALS

The uptake of both calcium and phosphorus by bone as well as the regulation of flux of these two minerals by vitamin D is well known. In this instance, vitamin D acts as a hormone in the regulation of calcium homeostasis. Already mentioned is the interaction of ascorbic acid and iron with respect to iron uptake by the intestinal mucosa. There is the interaction of vitamin E and selenium, as well; each of these nutrients plays a role in the maintenance of the free radical suppression system. One can replace the other to a certain extent, and so both are considered partners in this important system. If there is a deficiency of intake of selenium, for example, the effects of this deficiency can be ameliorated to some extent by an adequate intake of vitamin E.

TABLE 11.1
Minerals–Amino Acid Interactions

Minerals	Amino Acid
Calcium	Serine, carboxylated glutamic acid (GLA)
Magnesium	Tyrosine, sulfur containing amino acids
Copper	Histidine
Selenium	Methionine, cysteine
Zinc	Cysteine, histidine

TABLE 11.2
Vitamin–Vitamin Interactions[15]

Vitamins[a]	Effect
B_6–B_{12}	Optimizes absorption of both; together both optimize absorption of thiamin
E–K	One interferes with the absorption of the other
B_6–Niacin	One interferes with the absorption of the other
B_6–Thiamin	B_6 protects against excess thiamin intake
B_{12}–Thiamin	B_{12} deficiency results in increased urinary loss of thiamin
B_{12}–Pantothenic acid	B_{12} spares pantothenic acid
Biotin and Folacin–Pantothenic acid	Biotin and folacin optimize the use of pantothenic acid
Thiamin–Riboflavin	One interferes with the absorption of the other
Riboflavin–B_6–Niacin	One needed for the metabolism of the other
B_6–Niacin	B_6 needed for the synthesis of niacin from tryptophan
C–B_6	C protects B_6 from excess catabolism and urinary excretion
	A deficiency of B_6 reduces blood C levels
E–A	E protects A from oxidative destruction
C–E	C protects E from oxidative destruction
C–A	When A is consumed in excess, tissue C levels fall
A–D	A protects against some of the signs of D excess
A–E	When A is consumed in excess, E requirement is increased
A–K	When A is consumed in excess, K requirement increases
A–C	C can increase the conversion of β-carotene to retinol
E–C	Both are synergistic in maintaining redox state in the cell
Folacin–Thiamin	Folacin optimizes thiamin absorption
Folacin–B_{12}	If B_{12} is deficient, folacin can mask deficiency signs
Riboflavin–Folacin	Riboflavin needed for conversion of folic acid to its coenzyme

[a] Abbreviations used: A, vitamin A (retinal, retinol, retinoic acid); D, vitamin D; E, vitamin E (tocopherols); K, vitamin K; B_6, pyridoxine, pyridoxal, pyridoxamine; C, ascorbic acid.

Although each of these nutrients has a different role in the maintenance of the redox state, their roles are both complementary and substitutive. Additional information on the vitamins can be found in Chapter 9 and Chapter 10.

VITAMIN INTERACTIONS

A number of vitamin interactions have been reported. Table 11.2 summarizes these reports. In the chapter on nutritional biochemistry (Chapter 7), the interacting and complementary roles of the B vitamins were described. These vitamins serve as coenzymes in many reactions of intermediary metabolism. Other interacting and complementary vitamin interactions include that of vitamin C and vitamin E. Both have roles in the regulation of the redox state in the cell. In species that synthesize their own vitamin C (i.e., in rats, mice, etc.), vitamin E deficiency leads to vitamin C deficiency, because the former plays a role in ascorbic acid synthesis from glucose. Vitamin E also interacts with vitamin B_{12} and zinc. Vitamin-E-deficient animals, although furnished with adequate vitamin B_{12}, have been found to have B_{12} deficiency symptoms. Probably this is due to a role of vitamin E on the use of B_{12} as a coenzyme for the enzyme, methylmalonyl-coenzyme A mutase. With respect to zinc, the interaction has to do with the complementary roles of both nutrients as membranes stabilizers.

The fat-soluble vitamins A and D can be toxic if consumed in excess over a period of time. The toxicity of vitamin A can be ameliorated by vitamin E. Vitamin E can downregulate the conversion of the carotenes to retinol and thereby reduce the toxicity of vitamin A. Vitamin E can also ameliorate the cellular responses to excess vitamin A through its actions on membrane stability and its function in the free radical suppression system.

MACRONUTRIENT INTERACTIONS

The need for an adequate energy intake to support growth and development is a long-established principle of nutrition science. The energy intake is primary; for, without sufficient energy, protein synthesis cannot take place at a normal rate. This meets the definition of a nutrient interaction. However, having this as a principle, there are other interactions that are important in intermediary metabolism.

Students of intermediary metabolism have long recognized that these macronutrients share some of the pathways of metabolism. Excess carbohydrate intake results in carbohydrate being converted to lipid. Inadequate energy intake means a depletion of the fat stores, with a subsequent rise in fatty acid oxidation and an increase in glucose production from gluconeogenesis and glycogenolysis (see Chapter 7). The composition of the diet can affect these pathways. Rats fed a 65% sucrose (as compared with those fed starch) have a heightened rate of hepatic lipogenesis. If the fat source is fish oil rather than corn oil or beef tallow, lipogenesis is reduced. If the fat source is coconut oil, lipogenesis is increased.[16–18] In humans, a similar interacting effect of carbohydrate and fat sources has been reported.[19] In this human study, serum cholesterol levels were lower and triglyceride levels were higher in humans fed a sucrose-saturated fat diet vs. a starch-saturated fat diet compared with humans fed a sucrose-unsaturated or starch-saturated fat diet. Thus, there is an interaction between the two energy sources with respect to lipogenesis and overall lipid dynamics.

Amino Acid Interactions

It has long been recognized that interactions and competitions exist between amino acids in the small intestine. The amino acid carriers (carriers that transport amino acids from the lumen into the absorptive cell) will transport more than one amino acid.[20] Neutral amino acids share a common carrier, as do those with short or polar side chains (serine, threonine, and alanine). There is also a carrier for phenylalanine and methionine and a specific one for proline and hydroxyproline. Similarly, there are carriers that transport amino acids across the blood–brain barrier, and there is some competition among amino acids for these carriers. For example, tryptophan competes with tyrosine for entry through the blood–brain barrier. Both tryptophan and the aromatic amino acids (phenylalanine and tyrosine) serve as precursors of neurotransmitters, and a competition between them for transport may have a role in the regulation of the balance of these transmitters in the body. Sulfur-containing amino acids are spared by each other, that is, methionine is spared by cysteine.[21]

In intermediary metabolism, there appears to be an interaction between leucine, isoleucine, and valine.[22] All are branched-chain amino acids and share the same enzymes for their metabolism. All are needed for appropriate rates of protein synthesis. Should one be in short supply, the rate of protein synthesis will fall. Thus, amino acid interactions occur as part of the overall body amino acid economy to ensure appropriate body protein homeostasis.

SUMMARY

Components of the diet can interact sometimes with beneficial and sometimes with deleterious effects. So much depends on the dietary mixture consumed and the physiological status of the consumer. Where the consumer is marginally nourished, the interacting nutrients can have unexpected results. However, in the well-nourished individual consuming a wide variety of foods and not consuming an excess of any one nutrient or class of nutrients, such interactions are probably insignificant. It is only when individuals restrict their food selections and consume unbalanced supplements, should there be concern over deleterious nutrient interactions.

REFERENCES

1. Fairweather-Tait, B., *Food Chem*, 43: 213; 1992
2. Frieden, E.J., *Chem Educ*, 62: 917; 1985
3. Johnson, M.A., *J Nutr*, 120: 1486; 1990
4. Herbert et al., *Stem Cells*, 12: 289; 1994
5. Reyes, J.G., *Am J Physiol*, 270: C401; 1996
6. Emery, M.P., Boyd, B.L., *Proc Soc Exp Biol Med*, 203: 480; 1993
6. Conte, D., Narindrasorasak, S., Sarkar, B., *J Biol Chem*, 271: 5125; 1996
8. Price, D., Joshi, J.G., *Proc Natl Acad Sci (USA)*, 79: 3116; 1982
9. Arthur, J.R., Nicol, F., Beckett, G.J., *Am J Clin Nutr*, 57: 236S; 1993
10. Bermano et al., *Biol Trace Element Res.*, 51: 211; 1996
11. Lai, C.C. et al., *J Nutr Biochem*, 6: 256; 1995
12. Chen, S.Y., Collipp, P.J., Hsu, J.M., *Biol Trace Element Res*, 7: 169; 1985
13. Gavin, C.E., Gunter, K.K., Gunter, T.E., *Biochem J*, 266: 329; 1990
14. Maberly, G.F., *J Nutr*, 124: 1473S; 1994
15. Machlin, L.J., Langseth, L., In: *Nutrient Interactions* (Bodwell, C.E., Erdman, J.W., eds), Marcel Dekker, New York, 1988 pg 287
16. Baltzell, J.K., Berdanier, C.D., *J Nutr*, 115: 104; 1985
17. Berdanier, C.D., In: *Nutrient Interactions* (Bodwell, C.E., Erdman, J.W., eds), Marcel Dekker, New York, 1988 pg 265

18. Berdanier, C.D., Johnson, B.J., Buchanan, M., *Nutri Res*, 9: 1167; 1989
19. Antar, M.A. et al., *Atherosclerosis* 11: 191; 1970
20. Murray, R.K., Granner, D.K., Mayes, P.A., Rodwell, V.W., Harper's Biochemistry Lange MedicaalStamford Conn. pg 643
21. Ball, R.D., Courtney Martin, G., Pencharz, P.B., *J Nutr*, 136: 1682S; 2006
22. Young, V.R., Fukagawa, N.K., In: *Nutrient Interactions* (Bodwell, C.E., Erdman, J.W., eds), Marcel Dekker, New York, 1988, pg 27

12 Comparative Nutrition

William P. Flatt and Carolyn D. Berdanier

CONTENTS

INTRODUCTION

The nutritional requirements for different species of animals, including mammals, birds, and fish, vary markedly. Many factors influence the requirements for specific nutrients. Within species, some of the factors affecting nutritional requirements are age, gender, stage of maturity, level of activity (work), body size, type and level of production (i.e., lean or adipose body tissue, milk, eggs, wool, bone growth, etc.), environment, physiological function (i.e., maintenance, pregnancy, lactation, etc.), health, and endocrinological factors. Between and among species, the type of gastrointestinal tract greatly influences the nutritional requirements of the animal, and the type of food it may eat to provide the nutrients it needs. For example, ruminants (cattle, sheep, goats, and deer), as a result of microbial fermentation in the upper gastrointestinal tract, have quite different nutritional requirements than nonruminants (humans, swine, dogs, cats, nonhuman primates, etc.). Ruminants and other herbivores have extensive microbial fermentation, which allows these species to utilize the cellulose, hemicellulose, and other high-fiber diets that animals without this fermentation cannot use. This fermentation alters the needs for many of the micronutrients, as well as dictates the sources of macronutrients to optimize health, growth, and meat, egg, or milk production.

Other species differences relate to the difference in the basic anatomy and physiology of the animals themselves. For example, humans, swine, cattle, sheep, and chickens store bile from the liver in the gallbladder, whereas rats, horses, deer, elk, moose, and camels have no reservoir to store bile, and this in turn may affect lipid digestion. Another species difference is in nitrogen utilization. For example, mammals excrete excess nitrogen resulting from protein catabolism as urea, whereas birds excrete it as uric acid. Many different species of animals have been used extensively as research models to obtain data on nutrient metabolism and function in humans, and to learn the mode of action of various dietary ingredients. The researcher must be aware of differences in the nutritional requirements of different species, or erroneous conclusions could be drawn. For example, dietary vitamin C is required by humans and other primates, fruit bats, and guinea pigs, but not by swine, mice, and rats. These species are frequently used as animal analogs for human nutrient needs and human health problems (Table 12.1). Animal analogs are useful, because they have a shorter lifespan and are far more uniform with respect to genetic background than are humans. Questions about the efficacy of dietary manipulation, drugs, and environmental conditions have all been answered through the use of such animals. Animals such as rats, guinea pigs, hamsters, gerbils, and mice have been developed (through selective breeding or through biotechnology) to develop human-like diseases such as diabetes mellitus, hyperlipidemia, cardiovascular disease, obesity, and so forth. Many of these special breeds are listed in Table 12.1. The investigator must remember, however, that there can be differences in response between the species and, if dietary variables are being used, the species difference in nutrient need as well as the lifespan difference must be accommodated in the interpretation of the results and the application of these results to humans. The American Society for Nutrition, formerly the American Institute of Nutrition, periodically reviews the diet composition of diets for rodents. It provides guidance for the composition of the standard rodent diet designed to meet rodent needs and to provide baseline data for the investigator using these animals in research. The composition of this basal diet is given in Table 12.2.

The nutrient needs for livestock, poultry, and fish have also been studied, and information is available for food producers, veterinarians, animal caretakers, biomedical research scientists, and others. People involved in caring for and feeding animals need to know what nutrients are required and the amounts of each, the effects of different factors on the efficiency of nutrient utilization, and how best to provide optimal feeds for each of these animals. Because of the economic importance of this knowledge, scientists throughout the world have conducted research with different species of animals, birds, and fish, and feeding standards based on this research have been developed. Diets and rations have been formulated for domestic livestock, poultry, companion animals, laboratory animals, and other species.

During the past century, scientists from many nations have conducted research on the specific nutritional requirements of numerous species of animals, but there are so many interactions among nutrients — and so many factors that influence nutrient utilization by different species — that tables or formulae for calculating nutritional requirements must be modified periodically.

TABLE 12.1
Small Animal Analogs for Human Diseases[1,2]

Type 1 Diabetes Mellitus
Streptozotocin-treated animals of most Species
Alloxan can be substituted for streptozotocin
Pancreatectomy will also produce IDDM
BB rat (autoimmune disease)
db/db mouse
NOD mouse
FAT mouse
NZO mouse
TUBBY mouse
Adipose mouse
Chinese hamster (*Cricetulus griseus*)
South African hamster (*Mystromys albicaudatus*)
Tuco-Tuco (*Clenomys tabarum*)

Type 2 Diabetes Mellitus
ob/ob mouse
KK, yellow KK mouse
Avy, Ay yellow mouse
P, PB13/Ld mouse
db PAS mouse
BHE/Cdb rat
Zucker diabetic rat
SHR/N-cp rat
Spiny mouse
HUS rat
LA/N-cp rat
Wistar Kyoto rat

Obesity
Zucker rat
SHR/N-cp rat
LA/N-cp rat
ob/ob mouse
Ventral hypothalamus lesioned animals
Osborne-Mendel rats fed high-fat diets

Hypertension
SHR rats
JCR:LA rats
WKY rats
Transgenic rats

Gallstones
The rat does not have a gall bladder, nor does it have stones
Gerbil fed a cholesterol-rich, cholic-acid-rich diet
Hamster, prairie dog, squirrel monkey, or tree shrew fed a
  cholesterol-rich diet

Lipemia
Zucker fatty rat
BHE/cdb rat
NZW mouse
Transgenic mice given gene for atherosclerosis

Atherosclerosis
Transgenic mice given gene for atherosclerosis
NZW mouse
JCR:LA cp/cp rat

TABLE 12.2
Composition of the AIN-93 Maintenance (M) and
Growth (G) Diets for Rats[3]

Ingredient	AIN-93M (g/kg)	AIN-93G (g/kg)
Casein	140	200
Cornstarch	465.692	397.486
Dextrose	155	132
Sucrose	100	100
Cellulose	50	50
Soybean oil	40	70
Mineral mix	35	35
Vitamin Mix	10	10
L-cystine	1.8	3
Choline bitartrate	2.5	2.5
t-Butylhydroquinone	0.008	0.014
Energy	~3.8 kcal or ~16 kJ/g	~3.9 kcal or ~16.4 kJ/g

In the United States, the National Academy of Sciences, National Research Council (NRC), Board on Agriculture, Committee on Animal Nutrition has been responsible for developing nutrient intake requirements and feeding recommendations for a variety of animals. These publications are listed in Table 12.3. These recommendations are periodically reviewed and updated as new information becomes available. The information is also available on the web, and the web addresses are listed in Table 12.4. The general address for books published by the National Academy of Sciences is http://books.nap.edu. One can order these books online. In addition to the nutrient requirements, the tables of nutrient composition of the most commonly used feed ingredients that are needed are also given. The 1999 Feedstuffs Reference Issue (Volume 71, Number 31, July 30, 1999, pages 40–84) has

TABLE 12.3
National Academy of Science Publications on the Nutrient Requirements of a Variety of Species

Companion Animals

Cats	*Nutrient Requirements of Cats*, Revised Edition, 1986, 88 pp., 8.5 X 11, 1986 ISBN 0-309-03682-8 (SF 447.6 N88 1986)
Dogs	*Nutrient Requirements of Dogs*, Revised 1985, 79 pp., ISBN 0-309-03496-5 (S 95 .N28 1985)
Mink and Foxes	*Nutrient Requirements of Mink and Foxes*, Second Revised Edition, 1982 (BOA) 72 pp., ISBN 0-309-03325-X
Rabbits	*Nutrient Requirements of Rabbits*, Second Revised Edition, 1977
	Laboratory Animals (Rat, mouse, guinea pigs, hamster, gerbils, voles)
	Nutrient Requirements of Laboratory Animals, Fourth Revised Edition, 1995 (BOA), 173 pages, ISBN 0-309-05126-6
Fish	*Nutrient Requirements of Fish* (BOA) 128 pp., ISBN-04891-5, 1993 (SH 156 .N86 1993)

Avian Species

Poultry (chickens, turkeys, geese, ducks, pheasants, Japanese quail, bobwhite quail)	*Nutrient Requirements of Poultry*, Ninth Revised Edition, 1994 (BOA) 176 pp., ISBN 0-309-04892-3
Domestic Livestock	Nonruminant Species
Swine	*Nutrient Requirements of Swine*, Tenth Edition, 1998 (BOA) 210 pp., ISBN 0-309-05993-3, Computer laser optical disk (4 3/4 in.)
Horses	*Nutrient Requirements of Horses*, Fifth Edition, 1989 (BOA) 112 pp., ISBN 03989-4

Ruminant Species

Beef cattle	*Nutrient Requirements of Beef Cattle*, Seventh Edition, 2000 (BOA) 242 pp., ISBN 0-309-05426-5
Dairy cattle	*Nutrient Requirements of Dairy Cattle*, Sixth Edition, 1989 (BOA) 168 pp., ISBN 0-309-03826-X
Sheep	*Nutrient Requirements of Sheep*, Sixth Edition, 1985 (BOA) 112 pp., ISBN 0-309-03596-1
Goats	*Nutrient Requirements of Goats: Angora, Dairy, and Meat Goats in Temperate and Tropical Countries* (BOA) 84 pp., ISBN 0-309-03185-0
Nonhuman Primates	*Nutrient Requirements of Nonhuman Primates*, 2000, Second Edition, 300 pages, ISBN 0-309-02786-1

TABLE 12.4
Web Addresses for Tables of Nutrient Requirements for a Variety of Animals

National Academy Press. Washington, DC. List of publications with tables of nutrient requirements of each species. http://books.nap.edu. To obtain complete text, including tables, fill in the box labeled SEARCH ALL TITLES with "Nutrient Requirements," and all the following publications with hyperlinks will appear at URL http://books.nap.edu/catalog/910.html.

Cats	http://www.nap.edu/openbook/0309036828/html
Dogs	http://www.nap.edu/openbook/0309034965/html/44.html
Mink and foxes	http://www.nap.edu/openbook/030903325X/html/33.html
Rabbits	http://www.nap.edu/openbook/0309026075/html/14.html
Laboratory animals	http://www.nap.edu/openbook/0309051266/html/11.html
Fish	http://www.nap.edu/openbook/0309048915/html/62.html
Poultry	http://www.nap.edu/openbook/0309048923/html/19.html
Swine	http://www.nap.edu/openbook/0309059933/html/110.html
Horses	http://www.nap.edu/openbook/0309039894/html/39.html
Beef cattle	http://www.nap.edu/openbook/0309069343/html/102.html
Beef cattle	http://stills.nap.edu/readingroom/books/beefmodel/
Dairy cattle	http://www.nap.edu/openbook/030903826X/html/78.html
Sheep	http://www.nap.edu/openbook/0309035961/html/45.html
Goats: Angora, dairy, and meat goats in temperate and tropical countries	http://www.nap.edu/openbook/0309031850/html/10.html
Nonhuman primates	http://books.nap.edu/catalog/34.html

tables based on the NRC publications for swine, beef cattle, dairy cattle, chickens and turkeys, horses, and pets (dogs and cats) (Table 12.5).

It should be remembered that the tables giving the nutrient requirements for each species are different from the recommended intakes for humans. In the latter species, intake recommendations include a very broad (approx. twofold) safety factor and should not be considered as a requirement figure but rather a recommended daily intake figure that should satisfy the need

TABLE 12.5

Publications Providing Information on the Nutrient Needs of Specific Animals

Species	NRC Publication	Year Last Revised	Pages of Tables	Computer Disk	NAP Web Site of Tables
A. Nutrient requirements of companion animals (cats and dogs), rabbits, mink and foxes, and laboratory animals (rats, mice, guinea pigs, hamsters, gerbils, and voles) and rabbits, mink, and foxes. Tables of nutrient requirements from Nutrient Requirements of Domestic Animals: A Series. National Research Council, National Academy Press (http://books.nap.edu)					
Companion Animals					
Cats	*Nutrient Requirements of Cats*	1986	41–44	No	Yes
Dogs	*Nutrient Requirements of Dogs*	1985	44–45	No	Yes
Laboratory Animals	*Nutrient Requirements of Laboratory Animals*	1995	13–105	No	Yes
Rats	*Nutrient Requirements of Laboratory Animals*	1995	13	No	Yes
Mice	*Nutrient Requirements of Laboratory Animals*		82	No	Yes
Guinea pigs	*Nutrient Requirements of Laboratory Animals*		104–105	No	Yes
Hamsters	*Nutrient Requirements of Laboratory Animals*		Text	No	Yes
Gerbils	*Nutrient Requirements of Laboratory Animals*		Text	No	Yes
Voles	*Nutrient Requirements of Laboratory Animals*		Text	No	Yes
Other Small Animals					
Rabbits	*Nutrient Requirements of Rabbits*	1977	14–15	No	Yes
Mink	*Nutrient Requirements of Mink and Foxes*	1982	33–34	No	Yes
Foxes	*Nutrient Requirements of Mink and Foxes*	1982	35–36	No	Yes
B. Nutrient requirements of poultry (chickens, turkeys, geese, ducks, ring-necked pheasants, Japanese quail, and bobwhite quail), fish, nonhuman primates, horses, and swine. Tables of nutrient requirements from Nutrient Requirements of Domestic Animals: A Series. National Research Council, National Academy Press (http://books.nap.edu)					
Avian Species					
Chickens	*Nutrient Requirements of Poultry*	1994	19–45	No	Yes
Chickens	*Nutrient Requirements of Poultry*	1994	19–34	No	Yes
Turkeys	*Nutrient Requirements of Poultry*	1994	35–39	No	Yes
Geese	*Nutrient Requirements of Poultry*	1994	40–41	No	Yes
Ducks	*Nutrient Requirements of Poultry*	1994	42–43	No	Yes
Ring-necked pheasants	*Nutrient Requirements of Poultry*	1994	44	No	Yes
Japanese quail	*Nutrient Requirements of Poultry*	1994	45	No	Yes
Bobwhite quail	*Nutrient Requirements of Poultry*	1994	45	No	Yes
Other Species					
Fish	*Nutrient Requirements of Fish*	1993	62–63	No	Yes
Nonhuman primates	*Nutrient Requirements of Nonhuman Primates*	1978 (2000 in press)	18–19	No	No
Horses	*Nutrient Requirements of Horses*	1989	39–48	Yes (5.25 in.)	Yes
Swine	*Nutrient Requirements of Swine*	1998	110–123	Yes (Laser optical disk) (4.75 in.)	Yes
C. Nutrient requirements of ruminants (beef cattle, dairy cattle, sheep, and goats). Tables of nutrient requirements from Nutrient Requirements of Domestic Animals: A Series. National Research Council, National Academy Press (http://books.nap.edu)					
Ruminant Species					
Beef cattle	*Nutrient Requirements of Beef Cattle*	2000	102–112	Yes (3.5 in.)	Yes
Dairy cattle	*Nutrient Requirements of Dairy Cattle*	1989	78–88	Yes (5.25 in.)	Yes
Sheep	*Nutrient Requirements of Sheep*	1985	45–53	No	Yes
Goats	*Nutrient Requirements of Goats: Angora, Dairy and Meat Goats in Temperate and Tropical Countries*	1981	10–12	No	Yes

for that nutrient by most people. The figures for animals, on the other hand, have a safety factor but it is fairly narrow and should thus be considered closer to the requirement rather than a recommended intake. The reason for this species difference in recommendations is due to the large database for species other than humans and the degree to which nutrient adequacy can be determined in these species. Investigators using rats, for example, can examine in detail particular organs and tissues in the rat, but investigators using humans cannot do these same examinations in humans. Ethical considerations aside, the long life span of humans also makes such investigations difficult. Mice and rats have short life spans by comparison, and so the effects of nutritional manipulation on the long-term responses of these species are possible.

Comparative nutrition studies, therefore, need to remember these differences, and care must be exercised when the results of work with one species is compared to or assumed to be similar to that in another species.

REFERENCES

1. NIH Guide for Animal Resources updated annually; The Jackson Laboratory catalog and a series of books edited by E. Shafrir titled *Lessons in Animal Diabetes* published by Smith Gordon, London.
2. Berdanier, C.D., *Advanced Nutrition: Macronutrients*, 2nd edition, CRC Press, Boca Raton, FL, 2000, p. 15.
3. Berdanier, C.D., *J Nutr*, 123: 1941; 1993.

Part III

Nutrition Throughout Life

13 Nutrition during Pregnancy and Lactation

Kathryn M. Kolasa and David G. Weismiller

CONTENTS

RECOMMENDATIONS FOR WOMEN BEFORE PREGNANCY

It seems logical that the nutritional status of a woman prior to pregnancy as well as maternal nutrition should affect fetal development and subsequent pregnancy outcome. However, many confounding variables are common to the investigation of maternal nutrition and fetal development.[1] This section briefly summarizes recommendations for maternal nutrition.[2–13] It also includes comments about lactation, because maternal diet plays a central role in the transfer of nutriments to the infant. Table 13.1 includes special recommendations for women during childbearing years. Suggestions for counseling and treatment during preconception care office visits are given in Table 13.2.

TABLE 13.1
Special Recommendations for Women before Pregnancy

Maintain a healthy weight
Engage in physical activity regularly
If you need to gain or lose weight, do so gradually (no more than 1 to 2 lb/week)
If trying to become pregnant and ordinarily drink alcoholic beverages, stop drinking or cut back on the amount you drink
If you smoke, quit. Cutting back does not suggest overall improvement in outcomes
To minimize risk of having an infant with a neural tube defect, eat a highly fortified breakfast cereal that provides 100% of the Daily Value (DV) for folate or take a vitamin supplement that provides 600 μg/day of folic acid (4 weeks preconception through 12 weeks postconception). Folic acid, the synthetic form of folate, is obtained only from fortified foods or vitamin supplements. It is not yet known whether naturally occurring folate is as effective folic acid in the prevention of neural tube defects. For secondary prevention, the dosage is 4 mg/day

TABLE 13.2
Nutritional Care at Preconception, Prenatal, and Postnatal Visits

Visit	Assessment	Counseling/Treatment
Preconception care	Determine body mass index (BMI)	If <18 or >25, counsel on appropriate weight
	Evaluate diet/supplement intake	Develop a concrete plan for eating enough food to achieve/maintain a healthy weight
		Begin prenatal vitamin/mineral supplement
		Prescribe calcium supplement if intake <1000 mg
		Prescribe synthetic folic acid supplement of 400 μg/day
	Botanical use	Discontinue those with known or potential toxicities
	Evaluate for anemia	If Hgb <12g/dl, start therapeutic regimen of approximately 60 to 120 mg/day of ferrous iron; give multivitamin/ mineral supplement that contains ~15 mg of zinc and ~2 mg of copper
		When anemia has resolved, discontinue high-dose iron
Prenatal	Use of harmful substances	Reinforcement for any constructive steps already taken; provide assistance with quitting, and refer for further evaluation
	Evaluate diet	Utilize dietary intake questionnaire, for example, Diet Score, and food frequency questionnaires
	Optimal weight gain during pregnancy is controversial	BMI <19.8 28–40 lb
		• 19.8–26.0 25–35 lb
		• 26.1–29.0 15–25 lb
		• >29 ~15 lb
	Optimal weight gain for women carrying twins	Weekly weight gain of 0.75 kg during second and third trimesters to a total of 35 to 44 lbs
	Rate of weight gain, singleton pregnancy	First trimester: 1½ to 5 lb
		Second and third trimester: ½ to 2 lb/week
		Intensive assessment and counseling
		The additional calories needed are 200 to 300 cal/day in patients second and third trimester
	Poor weight gain <2 lb/month <10 lb by midpregnancy	If patient is economically unable to meet nutritional needs — referral to federal food and nutrition programs (Women, Infants, and Children, or WIC)
	Nutritional needs/barriers	Increase knowledge with dietary counseling
	Vitamin/mineral supplementation	No requirement for routine supplementation except folate (400 μg/day) and iron (30 to 60 mg elemental iron/day)
		Dietary supplements should be given if the adequacy of a patient's diet is questionable or if she is at high nutritional risk
		Excessive vitamin and mineral intake (more than twice the Recommended Dietary Allowances [RDA]) should be avoided
	Prophylaxis for iron deficiency	Supplement of ferrous iron is 30 mg elemental iron daily
		Zinc supplements are recommended if taking high doses of iron

Continued

TABLE 13.2
(Continued)

Visit	Assessment	Counseling/Treatment
	Iron-deficiency anemia	60 to 120 mg elemental iron daily
	Calcium supplementation	Recommended for women who have diet deficient in calcium, have prepregnancy hypertension, history of eclampsia or chronic use of heparin or steroids, and adolescents
	Evaluate use of alcohol, tobacco, and drugs	Effects of substance use/abuse on perinatal outcomes
		Abstinence from alcoholic beverages
	Caffeine intake	Consumption of 2 to 3 servings of caffeinated beverages is unlikely to have adverse effects; in general, caffeinated beverages provide few essential nutrients and often crowd out better sources of nutrients
		Moderate intake is <300 mg/day — recently not linked to adverse effects on pregnancy
		5 oz
		• Cup of coffee = 115 mg
		• Iced tea = 40 mg
		• Cola = 15mg
		• Hot Chocolate = 4 mg
		High Intake (>500 mg/day)
		Increased risk (2.2 ×) of first trimester spontaneous abortions
	Lactose intolerance	May result in insufficient calcium intake
		Supplemental calcium necessary if insufficient calcium consumed from food sources
	Gestational diabetes mellitus	Referral for nutrition assessment and counseling. Generally diet is 40% carbohydrate, 30% fat, 30% protein
	Nausea and vomiting during pregnancy	Eat crackers before getting out of bed in the morning; eat frequent small meals; eat low-fat, bland foods; eat ginger (soda, tea, or ginger snaps); suck on hard candy; eat salty/tart foods combined (e.g., potato chips with lemonade); supplement with vitamin B_6 (25 mg three times daily); wear Sea Band® (an elastic band worn on wrists to counter nausea caused by seasickness)
		Strong evidence for taking a multivitamin at the time of conception decreasing the severity Vitamin B_6 with or without doxalamine is safe and effective and should be considered a first-line treatment
		Doxylamine dosage is 12.5 to 25 mg three times daily; lesser evidence for ginger in any form (tea, soda, and tablets [250-mg capsule, four times daily for 4 to 5 days]); antihistamines, phenothiazines, benzamines — safe and effective in refractory cases
		Early treatment may prevent progression to hyperemesis
		Methylprednisolone may be effective in severe cases — treatment of last resort because of potential risk to the fetus
	Constipation	Foods high in dietary fiber, including cereals, bread fruits and vegetables; adequate fluids; moderate exercise; soluble fiber (e.g., Metamucil, Citrucel, or Benefiber); docusate; change brand of iron supplement
		DRI for water is 3.0 l/day
		DRI for dietary fiber is 28 g/day
Postpartum	Diet	Utilize dietary intake questionnaire
		Dietary guidelines are similar to those established during pregnancy
		Continue multiple vitamin–mineral supplements
	Caloric requirement	Balanced, nutritious diet will ensure both the quality and quantity of milk produced without depletion of maternal stores. Increased need of 300 to 500 calories. At least three servings of milk daily. The Adequate Intakes (AI) for water for lactating women is 3.8 l/day
	Vitamin/mineral supplement	Not needed routinely although recommended for the 400 μg/day folic acid; mothers at nutritional risk should be given a multivitamin supplement with particular emphasis on calcium and vitamins B_{12} and D
	Weight retention	The relationship between BMI or total weight gain and weight retention is unclear. It appears that women who gain more than the Institute of Medicine (IOM) guidelines retain twice as much weight as those who gain within the guidelines
	Residual postpartum weight retention	Aging, rather than parity, is the major determinant of increases in a woman's weight over time
		Special attention to lifestyle, including exercise and eating habits

RISK FACTORS FOR PRENATAL NUTRITION RISK AND INDICATIONS FOR REFERRAL

Table 13.2 includes nutrition assessment, counseling, and treatment strategies for women seeking care in both the prenatal and postnatal stages. Fetal growth is affected by the quality and quantity of the maternal diet, the ability of the mother to digest and absorb nutrients, maternal cardiorespiratory function, uterine blood flow, placental transfer, placental blood flow, and appropriate distribution and handling of nutrients and oxygen by the fetus. Factors that put women at nutritional risk for pregnancy are listed in Table 13.3.[5,14–16] Patients at high nutritional risk should be provided professional nutritional counseling and/or referral to a nutrition intervention program (Table 13.4). The Women, Infants, and Children (WIC) Program is a food prescription program designed and proven to reduce poor pregnancy outcomes (Table 13.5).

TABLE 13.3
Risk Factors for Prenatal Nutritional Risk

Risk Factor	Low Risk	High Risk
Is the patient pre- or adolescent or <3 years postmenarche?	No	Yes
Is the patient economically disadvantaged or have limited income for food?	No	Yes
Does the patient have history of anemia or is anemic (hematocrit <32mg/% during pregnancy)?	No	Yes
Is the patient's BMI <19.8 or >26.1?	No	Yes
Does the patient have history of fad dieting or restrictive eating?	No	Yes
Does the patient have illness or medication that will interfere with absorption; is she HIV+?	No	Yes
Does the patient use tobacco, alcohol, or drugs?	No	Yes
Does the patient practice pica (consume ice, starch, clay, or other substances in large amounts)?	No	Yes
Does the patient experience nausea and/or vomiting?	No	Yes
Is the patient lactose intolerant?	No	Yes
Is the weight gain 0.8 to 1.0 lb/week?	No	Yes
Does the patient stay within the weight gain range recommended for her prepregnancy BMI?	Yes	No
Weight gain <15 lbs or >45 lbs?	No	Yes
Prior bariatric surgery	No	Yes

TABLE 13.4
Indications for Referral of Pregnant Patients for Nutrition Assessment and Counseling

Patient has interest in and desire to see a nutritionist
Patient has inappropriate weight gain
Patient has gestational diabetes
Patient has chronic condition managed with diet (e.g., diabetes or hyperlipidemia)
Patient has history of anemia
Patient has inadequate or inappropriate food supply
Patient has history of prepregnancy anorexia or bulimia
Patient has significant discomforts of pregnancy (e.g., heartburn, nausea, or vomiting)
Patient has multiple gestation
Patient is adolescent
Patient is vegetarian
Patient is interested in or undecided about breastfeeding

TABLE 13.5
Characteristics of Women, Infants, and Children (WIC) Program

Target audience	Pregnant women
	Breast-feeding women
	Non-breast-feeding mothers of infants <6 months old
	Infants <1 year old
	Children <5 year old
Purpose	Provide nutritious foods, health checks, referrals, nutrition education, and counseling
Eligibility criteria	Low income: <185%, the U.S. federal poverty level for women and children
Food	Nutrient rich, high in protein, calcium, iron, and vitamins A & C
	Limited brand names
	Patient-purchased food and infant formula from local supermarkets
Nutrition education	Individual and group
	Specific to risk
Health checks	Height, weight, and anemia testing for women, infants children
	1-year-old test for lead

WEIGHT GAIN AND PREGNANCY

PREGNANCY WEIGHT GOALS

There is a lack of consistent findings concerning relationships of birth interval, parity, prepregnancy weight or body mass index (BMI), height, and physical activity to maternal weight or weight gain.[9,17–30] The Cochrane Pregnancy and Childbirth Group[31] summarized the findings on the effects of advising pregnant women to increase their energy and protein intakes, on gestational weight gain, and on the outcome of pregnancy. They found that nutritional advice appears to be effective in increasing pregnant women's energy and protein intakes, but the implications for fetal, infant, or maternal health cannot be judged from the available trials.

Less than 50% of pregnant women gain in the outlined weight ranges. Some researchers question the notion that African-American women gain more weight than Caucasian women, suggesting that the data only showed questionable benefit in reducing risks for low-birth-weight babies.[7] Some experts believe that the weight-gain guidelines are too high for all and that it should be individualized.

Obese women have a greater risk of pregnancy complications, especially excessive weight gain, gestational diabetes, hypertensive disorders, prolonged and difficult labor, postdate pregnancy, meconium, postpartum hemorrhage, operative delivery, and weight retention after pregnancy. Infants of obese women may be at greater risk for perinatal mortality, prematurity, and low birth weight with is associated with diabetes mellitus, hypertension, and heart disease in adulthood.[26,31–32]

The recommendations in Table 13.6 were established by the National Academy of Sciences of the National Institute of Medicine in 1990.[3] They were reviewed and left unchanged by the Maternal Weight Gain Expert Group in 1996.[29] These recommendations remain controversial.[33] Weight-gain goals have been determined to provide optimal risk reduction for delivering a low-birth-weight baby while avoiding adverse effects on the mother's health. The recommendations vary based on pregnancy weight, age, and ethnicity. The weight gain expected is essentially linear, as demonstrated in Figure 13.1.[34] There is no evidence that weight gain in the Institute of Medicine ranges is harmful to the mother or infants of women starting pregnancy at a normal BMI. There is little guidance on appropriate weight gain for women who are not at a normal BMI at the beginning of pregnancy. Women with prepregnant BMIs >35 are at increased risk for gestational diabetes, preeclampsia, placenta abrupta, operative delivery, and endometriosis.[32]

TABLE 13.6
Pregnancy Weight Goals

Optimal Weight Gain (Pounds)	Characteristic
25–35	Most women and normal pregnancy
	Prepregnancy BMI 19.8 to 26.0 or 100% prepregnancy ideal body weight
28–40	Women at higher risk for low-birth-weight babies, including adolescents and African-American women
	Prepregnancy BMI <19.8 (underweight) or 90% ideal body weight
	Twin pregnancy
15–25	Prepregnant BMI >26.1 (overweight or obese) or >120% ideal body weight
15	Prepregnant BMI >29 or >135% ideal body weight
35–44	Women pregnant with twins or 50 to 75% increase based on prepregnant BMI

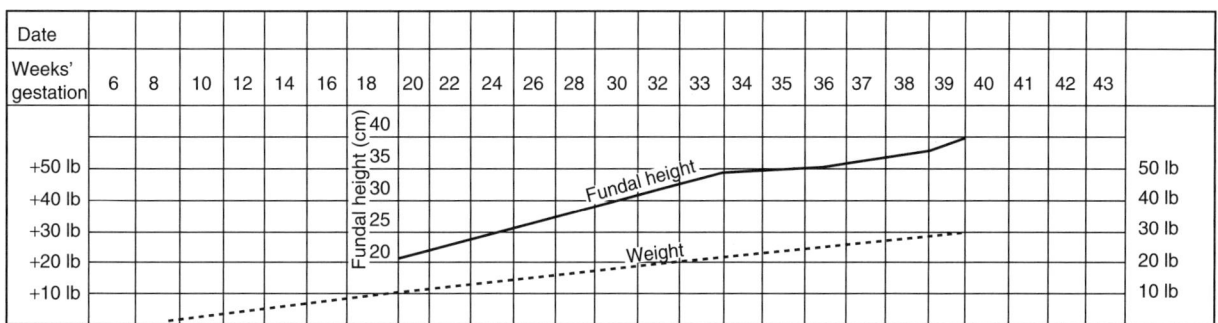

FIGURE 13.1 Graph for tracking weight and fundal height. (With permission from Kolasa, K.M. and Weismiller, D.G. Nutrition during pregnancy, Am Fam Phys. 56(1): 206, July 1995.)

RATE OF WEIGHT GAIN

In 1996, the Maternal and Weight Gain Expert Group[29] suggested a weight gain of 1 lb/week for normal-weight women during the second and third trimester of a singleton pregnancy. Weight gain is the single most reliable indicator of pregnancy outcome.[17,28] Weight status should be routinely assessed for amount and rate. Figure 13.1 depicts an example of a graph for tracking weight.[34] Weight charts should be shown to women and their support partners. Table 13.7 gives recommended weight gains. The optimal weight for a newborn infant of 39 to 41 weeks gestation is 6.6 to 8.8 lb.[15]

Women with inadequate weight gain should eat more frequently, be referred to a dietitian for nutrient assessment and counseling, choose more nutrient-dense foods, avoid alcohol and tobacco use, limit activity, and avoid caffeine or other appetite depressants. Women with excessive gain should reduce portion sizes, limit intake of sweets and foods high in fat, increase activity, and be evaluated by a registered dietitian.

WEIGHT-GAIN DISTRIBUTION DURING PREGNANCY

Weight gain by pregnant women consists of water, protein, and fat. Measurements of maternal water gain may predict birth weight better than measurements of composite weight gain. The total amount of weight gained, the composition of gain, and the rate of energy metabolism all differ among healthy pregnant women. Table 13.8 is a typical teaching tool about weight-gain distribution.

NUTRITION SNACKS

Pregnant women may need suggestions for healthy snacks. Table 13.9 includes snacks of about 100 calories.

DIETARY REQUIREMENTS FOR PREGNANCY AND LACTATION

DIETARY REFERENCE INTAKE (DRI)

Dietary reference Intakes are the levels of intake of essential nutrients considered adequate to meet or exceed known nutritional needs of practically all healthy people. Table 13.10 includes the Recommended Dietary Allowances (RDA) and Adequate Intakes (AI) as available in 2005 for pregnancy and lactation.[35,36] These levels are set by the Food and Nutrition Board of the National Academy of Sciences. Nutrient needs that are increased during pregnancy are for calcium in women at high risk for gestational hypertension — teenagers, previous preeclampsia, women with increased sensitivity to angiotensin II, preexisting hypertension, and in communities with low dietary intake of calcium (<900 mg/day), choline, chromium, copper, folate, magnesium, manganese, molybdenum, niacin, pantothenic acid, riboflavin, selenium, thiamin, vitamin B_6, vitamin B_{12}, vitamin C,

TABLE 13.7
Rate of Weight Gain (Pounds)

Timing (Trimester)	Appropriate	Inadequate	Excessive
First	3–5 Total	Less	More
Second, Third	1/week	Less than 2 lb in a single month for normal-weight women or <1 lb in obese	More than 6.5 lb in a single month

TABLE 13.8
Weight-Gain Distribution during Pregnancy (Pounds)

Source	Pounds
Amniotic Fluid	2–2.6
Baby	7–8.5
Fat/breast tissue stores for breastfeeding	1–4
Increased blood volume	4–5
Increased weight of uterus	2
Maternal fat stores	4–7
Placenta	0.7–1.0
Tissue fluid	3–5
Total	25–35

TABLE 13.9
Nutritious Snacks of 100 kcal or Less

Food Item	Serving Size
Applesauce	$^2/_3$ cup
Bagel	$^1/_2$
Carrot, raw	1 cup or 1 large
Cheese, low-fat	1 oz
Cottage cheese, low-fat	$^1/_3$ cup
Entenmann's fat-free cakes/pastries	1 small slice
Figs, low-fat, or other Newton cookies	1–$^1/_2$ tsp
fruit, dried (like apricots, raisins, prunes)	4 tsp.
Fruit, fresh	1 medium
Graham crackers	2
Grits	1 package
Milk, skim	1 cup
Pretzels	15
Pudding made with skim milk	$^1/_3$ cup
Rice cakes, flavored	2
Tortilla chips, baked, low-fat, and with salsa	12
Tuna	$^1/_2$ cup
Yogurt, frozen	$^1/_2$ cup
Yogurt, low-fat	$^1/_2$ cup

TABLE 13.10
Food and Nutrition Board, National Academy of Sciences — National Research Council Recommended Dietary Allowances, and Dietary Reference Intakes (DRI)
Designed for the Maintenance of Good Nutrition of Practically All Healthy People in the United States

Category	Condition	Protein (g)	Vitamin A (μg RE)[b]	Vitamin E (mg α-TE)[c]	Vitamin K (μg/day)	Vitamin C (mg)	Iron (mg)	Zinc (mg)	Iodine (μg)	Selenium (μg)
Pregnant		71	770	15	90	85	27	11	220	60
Lactating	First 6 months	71	1300	19	90	120	9	12	290	70
	Second 6 months	71	1300	19	90	120	9	12	290	70

[a] The allowances, expressed as average daily intakes over time, are intended to provide for individual variations among most normal persons as they live in the United States under unusual environmental stresses. Diets should be based on a variety of common foods in order to provide other nutrients for which human requirements have been less well defined.

[b] Retinol equivalents. 1 retinol equivalent = 1 μg retinol or 6 μg β-carotene.

[c] α-Tocopherol equivalents. 1 mg d-α tocopherol = α-TE.

Note: Dietary Reference Intakes for calcium, phosphorus, magnesium, vitamin D, and fluoride (1997) and Dietary Reference Intakes for thiamin, riboflavin, niacin, vitamin B, folate, vitamin B$_{12}$, pantothenic acid, biotin, and choline (1998).

and zinc, protein (10% to 35% of calories), carbohydrate (45% to 65% of calories), total fiber, and omega-3 and omega-6 fatty acids. In lactation, requirements for carbohydrates, dietary fiber, water, biotin, choline, chromium, copper, manganese, pantothenic acid, riboflavin, selenium, zinc, vitamin A, vitamin B$_6$, vitamin B$_{12}$, vitamin E, vitamin C, iodine, and potassium are increased over the increased pregnancy needs. In lactation, the iron requirements are reduced. Energy needs are also increased by 340 kcal/day (recommend 200 to 300 kcal/day) in the second trimester of pregnancy and by 452 kcal/day (recommend 200 to 500 kcal/day) during lactation so that adequate breast milk supply is produced.

The 2005 Dietary Guidelines for Americans and MyPryamid[37] include some recommendations for pregnant women but no specific plan. Women are encouraged to obtain adequate nutrients within calorie needs. During the first trimester they should consume adequate synthetic folic acid daily (from fortified foods or supplements) in addition to food forms of folate from a varied diet. They should ensure appropriate weight gain as specified by a health care provider. In the absence of medical or obstetric complications 30 min or more of moderate-intensity physical activity on most, if not all, days of the week should be incorporated. Activities with a high risk of falling or abdominal trauma should be avoided. Alcoholic beverages should not be consumed. Raw (unpasteurized) milk or any products made from unpasteurized milk, raw or partially cooked eggs, foods

TABLE 13.11
Food and Nutrition Board, Institute of Medicine — National Academy of Sciences Designed Reference Intake: Recommended Intakes for Individuals

Life-Stage Group	Calcium (mg/Day)	Phosphorus (mg/Day)	Magnesium (mg/Day)	Vitamin D (μg/Day)[a,b]	Fluoride (mg/Day)	Thiamin (mg/Day)	Riboflavin (mg/Day)	Niacin (mg/Day)[c]	Vitamin B$_6$ (mg/Day)	Folate[d] (μg/Day)	Vitamin B$_{12}$ (μg/Day)	Pantothenic Acid (mg/Day)	Biotin (μg/Day)	Choline[e] (mg/Day)
Pregnancy (in years)														
≤18	1300*	1250	400	5*	3*	1.4	1.4	18	1.9	600[f]	2.6	6*	30*	450*
19–30	1000*	700	350	5*	3*	1.4	1.4	18	1.9	600[f]	2.6	6*	30*	450*
31–50	1000*	700	360	5*	3*	1.4	1.4	18	1.9	600[f]	2.6	6*	30*	450*
Lactation (in years)														
≤18	1300*	1250	360	5*	3*	1.5	1.6	17	2.0	500	2.8	7*	35*	550*
19–30	1000*	700	310	5*	3*	1.5	1.6	17	2.0	500	2.8	7*	35*	550*
31–50	1000*	700	320	5*	3*	1.5	1.6	17	2.0	500	2.8	7*	35*	550*

a As cholecalciferol. 1 μg cholecalciferol = 40 IU vitamin D.

b In the absence of adequate exposure to sunlight.

c As niacin equivalents (NE). 1 mg of niacin = 60 mg of tryptophan; 0–6 months = performed niacin (not NE).

d As dietary folate equivalents (DFE). 1 DFE = 1 μg food folate = 0.6 μg of folic acid (from fortified food or supplement) consumed with food = 0.5 μg of synthesis (supplemental) folic acid taken on an empty stomach

e In view of evidence linking folate intake with neural tube defects in the fetus, it is recommended that all women capable of becoming pregnant consume 400 μg of synthetic folic acid from fortified food or supplements in addition to intake of food folate from a varied diet.

f It is assumed that women will continue consuming 400 μg of folic acid until their pregnancy is confirmed, and they enter prenatal care, which ordinarily occurs after the end of the periconceptual period — the critical time for formation of the neural tube.

Note: This table presents Recommended Dietary Allowances (RDAs) in bold type and Adequate Intakes (AIs) in ordinary type followed by an assessment asterisk (*).

containing raw eggs, raw, or undercooked meat and poultry, raw or undercooked fish or shellfish, unpasteurized juices, and raw sprouts should be avoided. Only deli meats and frankfurters that have been reheated to steaming hot can be eaten. Women are advised to avoid some types of fish and shellfish and to eat fish and shellfish that are lower in mercury. Food and Drug Administration (FDA) maintains toll-free information at 1-888-SAFEFOOD.

There are no specific diet plans for pregnant women. Personalized pyramids showing food groups and amounts of foods from each food group, based on calorie needs, can be downloaded from http://mypyramid.gov. Pregnant women should drink at least 3.0 l of water each day.

DIETARY ASSESSMENT OF THE PREGNANT WOMAN

Individualized nutrition assessment and planning is important because of the strong associations between extremes in prepregnancy BMI, extremes in weight gain, and adverse pregnancy outcomes.[3,7,34,38–40]

There are special nutrition implications for pregnant women who have had bariatric surgery, especially the Roux-en-Y procedure.[41] Adequate weight gain to promote fetal growth is advised. There are no published weight-gain criteria for post-gastric-bypass. Serum iron and TIBC, CBC, folate, and vitamin B_{12} levels should be monitored.

BEHAVIOR-CHANGE TOOL

Assessment relies on the woman's medical record, history, and physical examination. Nutritional factors of importance include previous nutritional challenges, eating disorders, pica, fad dieting, botanicals and teas, strict vegetarian diet, medications, and quantity and quality of current diet. The Institute of Medicine provides a sample dietary history tool (Table 13.12).[3]

What one eats and some of the lifestyle choices one makes can affect nutrition and health now and in the future. One's nutrition can also have an important effect on one's baby's health. Please answer these questions by circling the answers that apply to you in Table 13.12.

Systematic assessment of the diet is preferable to questions such as "How are you eating?" The 24 h dietary recall method is commonly used to recall the types and amounts of foods and beverages consumed during the previous day. The food frequency questionnaire has been demonstrated to detect pregnancy-related changes in diet.

TABLE 13.12
Behavior-Change Dietary Assessment Tool

Eating Behavior

1. Are you frequently bothered by any of the following? (circle all that apply)

    Nausea   Vomiting   Heartburn   Constipation

2. Do you skip meals at least three times a week?   No   Yes
3. Do you try to limit the amount or kind of food you eat to control your weight?   No   Yes
4. Are you on a special diet now?   No   Yes
5. Do you avoid any foods for health or religious reasons?   No   Yes

Food Sources

6. Do you have a working stove?   No   Yes

    Do you have a working refrigerator?   No   Yes

7. Do you sometimes run out of food before you are able to buy more?   No   Yes
8. Can you afford to eat the way you should?   No   Yes
9. Are you receiving any food assistance now? (circle all that apply)

    Food stamps   School breakfast   School lunch

    Donated food   Commodity Supplemental   Food Program

    Food from a food pantry, soup kitchen, or food banks

10. Do you feel you need help in obtaining food?   No   Yes

Food and Drink

11. Which of these did you drink yesterday? (circle all that apply)

    Soft drinks   Coffee   Tea   Fruit drink

    Orange juice   Grapefruit juice   Other juices   Milk

    Kool-Aid   Beer   Wine   Alcoholic drinks

    Water   Other beverages (list)

12. Which of these foods did you eat yesterday? (circle all that apply):

    Cheese   Pizza   Macaroni and cheese

    Yogurt   Cereal with milk

Continued

**TABLE 13.12
(Continued)**

Food and Drink   (Continued)
13. Other foods made with cheese (such as tacos, enchiladas, lasagna, and cheeseburgers)

Corn	Potatoes	Sweet potatoes	Green salad
Carrots	Collard greens	Spinach	Turnip greens
Broccoli	Green beans	Green peas	Other vegetables
Apples	Bananas	Berries	Grapefruit
Melon	Oranges	Peaches	Other fruit
Meat	Fish	Chicken	Eggs
Peanut butter	Nuts	Seeds	Dried beans
Cold cuts	Hot dog	Bacon	Sausage
Cake	Cookies	Doughnut	Pastry
Chips	French fries	Deep fried foods, such as fried chicken or egg rolls	
Bread	Rolls	Rice	Cereal
Noodles	Spaghetti	Tortillas	

Were any of these whole grains?   No   Yes
Is the way you ate yesterday the way you usually eat?   No   Yes

Lifestyle
14. Do you exercise for at least 30 min on a regular basis — three times a week or more?   No   Yes
15. Do you ever smoke cigarettes or use smokeless tobacco?   No   Yes
16. Do you ever drink beer, wine, liquor, or any other alcoholic beverages?   No   Yes
17. Which of these do you take? (circle all that apply)
    Prescribed drugs or medications
    Any over-the-counter products (such as aspirin, acetaminophen, antacids, or vitamins)

Source: Institute of Medicine, 1992.

NUTRITIONAL RISK TOOL

Table 13.13 is an example of a more quantitative method for assessing the diet.[38] The mother's usual intake is determined for each of the food groups (meats and alternatives, dairy, bread and cereal, fruits, and vegetables) and the score is tallied. A patient with fewer than 80 points is at nutritional risk. The evaluator should determine whether the patient has problems such as nausea/vomiting, lactose intolerance, constipation, or cravings for nonfood items. Women with a score of fewer than 50 points should be referred to a registered dietician for counseling.

COMPLICATIONS OF PREGNANCY THAT MAY IMPACT NUTRITIONAL STATUS

A number of complications of pregnancy may impact nutritional status. Some of these include nausea and vomiting, constipation, caffeine intake, and alcohol intake.

NAUSEA AND VOMITING

About 70% of pregnant women report nausea during the first 14 to 16 weeks of pregnancy, and 37% to 58% experience vomiting. The etiology is unknown. The remedies include diet, fluids, and reassurance.[42,43] Table 13.14 is a collection of remedies.

HYPEREMESIS GRAVIDARUM

Vomiting that produces weight loss, dehydration, acidosis from starvation, alkalosis from loss of hydrochloric acid in vomitus, and/or hypokalemia may be treated pharmacologically. Management is to correct dehydration, fluid and electrolyte deficits, acidosis, and alkalosis. Table 13.15 includes some pharmacological approaches.

CONSTIPATION

Constipation is extremely common in pregnancy because of decreased motility of the gastrointestinal (GI) tract. Constipation can be exacerbated by iron supplementation. Constipation is often related to low dietary fiber intake and low fluid intake. Table 13.16 includes foods rich in dietary fiber. The recommended intake is 28 g of dietary fiber daily.

TABLE 13.13
Nutritional Risk Score (Massachusetts Department of Health)

Foods Usually Eaten	Amount
Meat or alternates	
Meats, fish, poultry, (fresh or processed), liver eggs, nuts, peanut butter, legumes	_____servings
1 oz = 5 points	_____oz meat, fish, cheese[a]
Maximum score = 40 points	_____oz alternate
Milk (type) 1 unit = 5 people	_____fluid
1 unit = 8 fl oz	_____cups
Cheese[b] (type) _____	_____oz
Maximum score = 15 points	
Bread and cereal[c] — whole grain, enriched, other maximum	_____servings
Score = 15 points	
Fruits and vegetables	
Citrus and/or vitamin-C-rich vegetables	_____servings
Green and yellow vegetables	_____servings
All other, including potato	_____servings
	Total fruits

Vitamin A	Vitamin C	
1 unit = 5 points	1 unit = 5 points	
2 units = 15 points	2 units = 15 points	_____servings
Supplements[d] (type)		_____amount

Other foods and beverages

Total score: >80 = no risk, less, <80 = risk, <50 = high risk

[a] Cheese in excess of the 3 units scored in milk; 1 oz cheese equals 1 unit.

[b] Maximum of 3 oz scored.

[c] Unit = 1 slice of bread or 1 oz cereal. Less than 3 units = 0, 3 units = 5 points, 4 units = 10 points, 5 units = 15 points.

[d] Not given a score.

Source: From *JADA*: 86(10), 1986, with permission.

TABLE 13.14
Nonpharmacological Remedies for Nausea and Vomiting

Eat small, frequent meals

Eat dry foods/cold foods

Take dietary supplements after meals

Suck on candy

Switch brands of iron supplements

Eat combinations of foods that are salty and tart

Eat vitamin-B_6-rich foods

Try seabands or acupressure bands

Avoid beverages with meat

Avoid caffeine

Avoid spicy, acidic foods, and strong odors

Sniff lemon

Drink ginger root tea, ginger ale; eat ginger snaps; take ginger tablets
(250 mg tablets four times daily for 4 to 5 days)

Drink plenty of fluids to avoid dehydration

CAFFEINE DURING PREGNANCY AND LACTATION

The literature is mixed on the effects of caffeine during pregnancy. The official FDA position advises pregnant women to avoid caffeine or consume it sparingly. Most experts agree that caffeine should be limited to less than two servings per day. Caffeine is known to decrease availability of calcium, iron, and zinc. It is known to exert effects on the fetus. The relationship of caffeine

TABLE 13.15
Hyperemesis Gravidurum

Medication	Dosage
Vitamin B$_6$	25 mg t.i.d. along with doxylamine
Doxylamine	12.5–25 mg t.i.d. along with vitamin B$_6$
Emetrol	5–10 cc in the morning and every 3–4 h as needed
Antiemetic/antinausea medications, for example, trimethobenyamine (Tigan)	200 mg suppository q 8 prn
Promethazine	12.5–25 mg po. Pr or iv q 4–6

TABLE 13.16
Dietary Sources of Fiber

Serving Size	Food	Grams of Fiber
Breads, Cereals, Pastas		
3 cups	Air-popped popcorn	4
1 medium	Bran muffin	3
2/3 cup	Brown rice	3
1 slice	Whole wheat bread	3
1/2 cup	Cooked legumes	5
1/2 cup	Baked beans	10
1/2 cup	Great northern beans	7
1/2 cup	Lima beans	7
1/2 cup	Selected fiber cereals (Read label)	14
Fruit		
1 cup	Raisins	6
3	Dried prunes	5
1 medium	Pear with skin	4
1 medium	Apple with skin	3
1 cup	Strawberries	3
1 medium	Banana	3
1 medium	Orange	3
Vegetables		
1/2 cup	Cooked frozen peas	4
1 medium	Baked potato with skin	4
1/2 cup	Brussels sprouts	3
1/2 cup	Cooked broccoli tops	3
1/2 cup	Cooked carrots	3
1/2 cup	Cooked corn	3

to spontaneous abortion remains controversial. A recent report suggests that risk increases with the consumption in the range of 6 to 18 cups of coffee per day (>450 mg/day of caffeine).[44]

Caffeine does pass into breast milk, and therefore consumption during lactation should be limited. Table 13.17 lists caffeine values for popular beverages.

Some suggestions for reducing caffeine consumption include: (1) switching to decaffeinated coffee or soft drinks, (2) cutting down on caffeinated beverages, (3) mixing caffeinated and decaffeinated coffee grounds together before making coffee, and (4) limiting consumption of caffeinated beverages to a preselected number and then switching to decaffeinated beverages over time.

ALCOHOL

Consumption of alcohol during pregnancy and lactation is controversial.

Pregnancy

A safe lower limit of alcohol during pregnancy is not known. Therefore, the only sure way to avoid the possible harmful effects of alcohol on the fetus is to abstain. Binge drinking or excessive drinking during pregnancy can result in fetal alcohol syndrome. However, even small amounts of alcohol can temporarily alter fetal function. Adverse outcomes have not been found with daily

TABLE 13.17

Caffeine Quiz and Caffeine Values for Popular Beverages

Sound of Caffeine	Column A Number of Servings Per Day		Column B Amount of Caffeine Per Serving (mg)		Column C Total Caffeine (mg)
Coffee (6 oz)					
Automatic drip	_____		180	=	_____
Automatic perk	_____	×	135	=	_____
Instant	_____	×	125	=	_____
Decaffeinated	_____	×	5	=	_____
Coffee Grande, Starbucks (16 oz)			550		
Soft Drinks (12 oz)					
Regular colas	_____	×	37	=	_____
Diet colas	_____	×	50	=	_____
7 Eleven Big Gulp (64 oz)			190		
Cocoa Products					
Chocolate candy (2 oz)	_____	×	45	=	_____
Baking chocolate (1 oz)	_____	×	30	=	_____
Milk chocolate (2 oz)	_____	×	10	=	_____
South American cocoa (6 oz)	_____	×	40	=	_____
Drugs (one tablet or capsule)					
Dexatrim (not caffeine free)	_____	×	200	=	_____
NoDoz	_____	×	100	=	_____
Anacin	_____	×	35	=	_____
Midol	_____	×	30	=	_____
Coricidin	_____	×	30	=	_____
Tea (6 oz)					
Iced tea	_____	×	36	=	_____
Hot tea (moderate steeping time)	_____	×	65	=	_____
Decaf tea			5		
Total				=	_____

TABLE 13.18

Effects of Alcohol, Tobacco, and Drug Use on Nutritional Status and Pregnancy Outcomes and Lactation

Effect	Cause
Increased nutrient requirements/impaired nutrient absorption	Smokers have reduced vitamin C levels Drinkers have reduced serum folate and vitamin C levels
Impaired growth of the fetus/stunted growth of child	Drinkers of one to two alcoholic beverages/day associated with LBW, slow weight gain, and failure to thrive Smokers
Infant sleep disruption/increased arousal	Consumption of one drink/day in the first trimester
Delayed development/mental retardation	Drinkers have children who are more at risk for hyperactivity, poor attention span, language dysfunction
Reduced fertility	Chronic drinking and smoking associated with lower fertility in men and women
Transfer to baby during lactation disrupted sleep pattern of infant	Alcohol is concentrated in breast milk. An occasional small drink is acceptable but breast-feeding should be avoided for 2 h.

consumption of fewer than two standard drinks. The danger from light drinking should not be overstated. This may cause undue stress in some patients who had few drinks before realizing they were pregnant (see Table 13.18).

Lactation

Alcohol does not increase milk volume. Chronic consumption can inhibit milk production. The American Academy of Pediatrics does suggest that an occasional celebratory single, small alcoholic drink is acceptable, but breast-feeding should be avoided for 2 h after the drink as alcohol is concentrated in breast milk.[53,45]

HYPERTENSION

The Seventh Report of the Joint National Committee on Prevention, Detection, Evaluation, and Treatment of High Blood Pressure (JNC 7) outlines five classifications of hypertension in pregnancy. Treatment includes lifestyle modification for women with stage 1 hypertension. Data are sparse but many experts recommend restricting sodium intake to 2.4 g/day. Pharmacological management is described.[45,46]

VITAMIN AND MINERAL REQUIREMENTS, FOOD SOURCES, AND SUPPLEMENTATION

In the United States, vitamin and mineral supplementation is common among pregnant women. During pregnancy, maternal requirements for almost all nutrients increase. Higher RDAs have been defined for calcium in adolescents, choline, chromium, copper, folate, magnesium, manganese, molybdenum, niacin, pantothenic acid, riboflavin, selenium, thiamin, vitamin B_6, vitamin B_{12}, vitamin C, and zinc. For some nutrients, the evidence indicates a direct link between chronic maternal deficiency and poor outcome for the mother and infant. Excessive intake (usually defined as more than twice the RDA) of some nutrients may be harmful to the fetus, especially very early in the pregnancy.[21,36]

Supplementation, with the exception of folic acid, is recommended only after assessment of dietary practices of pregnant women. The Institute of Medicine does not recommend routine use of prenatal vitamins; however, many physicians prescribe them because of the marginal nutritional status of their patients or because it difficult to be completely sure of their patients' nutritional status.[3] Prenatal vitamins and minerals are indicated for high-risk populations and those with an obstetric history of high parity, previous delivery of a low-birth-weight infant, a short interval between births, and smokers, drug or alcohol abusers, and those with multiple pregnancies.

PRENATAL VITAMINS

Indications for vitamin and mineral supplementation are shown in Table 13.19, which lists nutrient dose and indication for use. The contents of typical prenatal vitamin–mineral supplements are shown in Table 13.20, which includes usual formula of an over-the-counter (OTC) and a prescription supplement recommended to pregnant women.

VITAMIN A

Most pregnant women do not need supplemental vitamin A, the teratogenic threshold of which may be lower than previously thought. Vitamin A is essential for embryogenesis, growth and epithelial differentiation. The RDA in pregnancy is only slightly increased to 770 mg/day. Case reports have suggested an association between high doses of vitamin A (>25,000 IU) during pregnancy and birth defects. The American College of Obstetricians and Gynecologists established 10,000 IU (or 3,000 mcg RAE) as the cutoff for supplemental vitamin A (retinol) prior to or during pregnancy. There is no concern about β-carotene intake.

CALCIUM AND MAGNESIUM

About 99% of calcium in pregnant women and their fetus is located in their bones and teeth. Pregnancy and lactation are associated with increased bone turnover to meet needs. If dietary deficiencies occur, maternal bone will supply the calcium to the fetus. Calcium supplementation during pregnancy has been shown to lead to an important reduction in systolic and diastolic blood pressure.[10] Controlled clinical trials to test the hypothesis that calcium supplements during pregnancy reduce the incidence of pregnancy-induced hypertension have had mixed results. Therefore, there is no support for routine supplementation with 2000 mg/day for all pregnant women. In pregnant women who have diets deficient in calcium (<900 mg/day) , are adolescent, have prepregnancy hypertension, history of preeclampsia, or chronic use of heparin and steroids supplemental calcium is recommended.[47]

The fetus absorbs 6 mg of magnesium each day. Maternal magnesium levels remain constant during pregnancy despite reported inadequate intakes. The RDA for most pregnant women is increased to 350 mg/day. Magnesium supplementation has been associated with fewer hospitalizations, fewer preterm births, and more perinatal hemorrhages compared with placebo-supplemented women. Thus, further study is needed before routine supplementation is recommended.

FOLATE AND IRON

The available data from controlled trials provide clear evidence of an improvement in hematological indices in women receiving routine iron and folate supplementation during pregnancy. Iron supplementation with and without folic acid results in substantial reduction of women with hemoglobin levels <100 g/l late in pregnancy, at delivery, and 6 weeks postpartum.[48] The Cochrane Pregnancy and Childbirth Group recommends iron supplementation.[49] Both foliate intake from food and synthetic folic acid should be included in assessing and planning diet. The literature contains a variety of recommendations. The DRI is

TABLE 13.19

Indications for Vitamin and Mineral Supplementation

Indication	Nutrient	Dose
Inadequate diet; during first two trimesters for women at risk for preterm labor or low-birth-weight baby	Prenatal supplements	Read label
Up to 1200 mg/day if dairy or fortified foods not consumed	Calcium	250–300 mg
For women receiving supplemental iron	Copper	2 mg
For all women of child bearing age	Folate	400 μg
Inadequate diet; anemia	Iron[a]	30–60 mg elemental
Inadequate diet	Vitamin B$_6$	2 mg
Inadequate diet	Vitamin C	50 mg
Inadequate diet; no exposure to sunlight	Vitamin D	10 μg
For women receiving supplemental iron	Zinc	15 mg

[a] Supplements containing high levels of folate or iron negatively affect zinc metabolism. Supplementary forms of folic acid are better absorbed than folate occurring in food.

TABLE 13.20

Prenatal Vitamin Mineral Supplements

	Flintstones Complete Chewables	Prenatal Vitamin (PreCare®)
Vitamin A	5000 IU	—
Vitamin C	60 mg	50 mg
Vitamin D	400 IU	6 μg
Thiamin	1.5 mg	—
Riboflavin	1.7 mg	—
Niacin	20 mg	—
Vitamin B$_6$	2 mg	2 mg
Folic acid	400 μg	1 mg
Vitamin B$_{12}$	6 μg	—
Biotin	40 μg	—
Pantothenic acid	10 mg	—
Calcium (as carbonate)	100 mg	250 mg
Iron	18 mg	40 mg
Phosphorus	100 mg	—
Iodine	150 μg	—
Magnesium	20 mg	50 mg
Zinc	15 mg	15 mg
Copper	2 mg	2 mg
Vitamin E	—	3.5 mg

higher than that usually obtained from food. The current recommendation during pregnancy is 600 μg/day of folic acid. It is well established that periconceptional use of folic acid supplementation reduces the risk of first occurrence and recurrence of neural tube defect (NTD) affected pregnancies by 70%. The Center for Disease Control (CDC) recommends supplementation of 400 μg/day for all women of childbearing age. Research is needed to determine effective strategies for disseminating information about the protective effects of folate.[49]

For women with previously affected pregnancy, the recommendation is 4 mg/day starting 1 to 3 months prior to conception and to continue through the first 3 months of pregnancy.

Additional iron is needed by most pregnant women in the United States. A substantial amount of iron is required, given the amount of erythropoiesis. For example, a term infant contains an average of 225 mg of iron and the placenta and cord contain 50 mg of iron through the pregnancy, and the maternal red blood count volume increases by 500 ml. The RDA for iron is increased to 27 mg/day (assuming 75% is heme iron). It is suggested that vegetarians require twice the amount of nonheme iron. Although maternal absorption of iron from the gastrointestinal tract is increased by about 15%, it remains difficult to meet the increased iron need through diet alone. Iron absorption is increased in the presence of ascorbic acid. Adverse pregnancy outcomes are associated with hemoglobin levels below 10.4 g/dl or above 13.2 g/dl. Clinical diagnosis of anemia is made based on hemoglobin below 10.5 g/dl, a low MCV, and a serum ferritin level below 12 μg/dl. Supplementation of 30 to 60 mg/day of elemental iron is usually prescribed, although the benefit of routine iron supplementation for healthy, well-nourished women during pregnancy is unproven, and the USPSTF concludes that there is insufficient evidence to make a recommendation for or against routine iron supplementation.[50] Common side effects include stomach upset, nausea, and constipation. These effects may be relieved by reducing the dosage or switching the brand of iron supplement. Some, but not all, sustained release preparations have been clinically shown to be associated with fewer discomforts. The safety of iron supplementation at dosages <100 mg/day has been questioned. Researchers suggest that excess iron may lead to zinc depletion, which is associated with intrauterine growth retardation.

ZINC

The prevalence and effects of mild zinc deficiency in pregnancy are poorly defined. However, there have been a few case reports of severe human zinc deficiency in pregnancy that led to major obstetric complications and congenital malformation in the fetus. Supplementation studies have yielded mixed results. Iron appears to depress plasma zinc in pregnant women; therefore, zinc supplementation is recommended when >30 mg supplemental iron is taken.[57] Higher birth weights in infants of women with low prepregnancy weight (BMI <26) and low plasma zinc levels have been reported in women who received 25 mg zinc daily. The RDA is increased to 11 mg/day. Vegetarians may need more zinc.

VITAMIN B$_6$

The value of supplementation with Vitamin B$_6$ in pregnancy is controversial. However, it is included in most prenatal vitamins. The RDA is increased to 1.9 mg/day.

VITAMIN C

Taking iron tablets along with a source of vitamin C facilitates iron absorption. The RDA is increased to 75 mg/day.

VITAMIN D

Vitamin D is critical in the absorption, distribution, and storage of calcium. Relatively few foods, except those fortified, are good sources of vitamin D. The RDA is unchanged in pregnancy.

FOOD SOURCES OF SELECTED NUTRIENTS

There are a variety of published recommendations for calcium in pregnancy and lactation. The optimal calcium intake recommended by the National Institutes of Health is 1200 mg/day. This is difficult to meet with a diet containing little dairy or calcium-fortified foods. The DRI for pregnancy and lactation varies, based on age, from 1000 to 1300 mg/day. Meeting usual calcium needs has been demonstrated in reducing pregnancy-induced hypertension in women at high risk for gestational hypertension (teenagers, women with previous preeclampsia, women with increased sensitivity to angiotensin II, and women with preexisting hypertension) and in communities with low dietary calcium intakes (mean intake <900 mg/day). However, no benefit in reducing preeclampsia is seen with supplementing calcium daily. Table 13.21 lists common dietary sources of calcium; Table 13.22, common food sources of folate; Table 13.23, common dietary sources of iron; and Table 13.24, common dietary sources of zinc.

TABLE 13.21
Dietary Sources of Calcium (DRI = 1000–1300 mg/day)

Food item	Serving size
Good > 200 mg	
Broccoli/greens	2 cups
Calcium fortified foods (juice, cereal)	Varies, read label
Canned salmon with bones	3 oz
Canned sardines with bones	3 oz
Cheese (cheddar, edam, Monterey jack, mozzarella, Parmesan, provolone, ricotta)	1 oz
Ice cream	1 cup
Ice milk	1 cup
Milk (skim, 2%, whole, buttermilk)	1 cup
Yogurt	6–8 oz

TABLE 13.22
Dietary Sources of Folate (DRI = 500–600 μg/day of Dietary Folate Equivalents [DFE])

Food item	Serving size
Excellent >100 μg	
Asparagus	½ cup
Baked beans	1 cup
Bean burritos	2
Black-eyed peas	1 cup
Fortified grain and cereal products	Varies, read label
Kidney beans	1 cup
Lentils	1 cup
Liver and other organ meats	
Beef	3.5 oz
Chicken	3.5 oz
Orange juice	1 cup
Peanuts	4 oz
Spinach	½ cup
Good: 15–99 μg	
Almonds	4 oz
Bread, fortified	1 slice
Beets	½ cup
Broccoli, cooked	½ cup
Cantaloupe/Honeydew melon	1 cup
Cauliflower	½ cup
Egg	1 large order
French fries	½ cup
Lettuce (romaine)	
Orange	1 medium
Turnip greens	½ cup

TABLE 13.23
Dietary Sources of Iron (DRI = 15–30 mg/day)

Food item	Serving size
Excellent >4 mg	
Beef liver	3 oz
Clams	½ cup
Figs (dried)	10
Iron-fortified infant cereal	½ cup
Iron-fortified infant cereal	3 tsp
Kidney beans	1 cup
Molasses (blackstrap)	3 tbsp
Peaches (dried)	10 halves
Pinto beans	1 cup
Ready-to-eat, fortified cereals (such as Product 19®, Total®)	¾ cup
Sunflower seeds (dried, hulled)	⅔ cup
Good: 2–4 mg	
Beef	3 oz
Egg yolks	3
Iron-fortified infant formula	4 oz
Lamb	3 oz
Lima beans	½ cup
Oysters	3 oz
Peas	1 cup
Pork	3 oz
Prune juice	1 cup
Raisins	⅔ cup
Soybeans	½ cup

PHYSICAL ACTIVITY DURING PREGNANCY

Several factors influence physical activity during pregnancy, including prepregnancy exercise levels, current levels, personal preferences, risk, limitations, and contraindications.[19] Table 13.25 to Table 13.29 include guidelines for physical activity.

TABLE 13.24
Dietary Sources of Zinc (DRI = 15–19 mg/day)

Food item	Serving Size	mg/Serving
Excellent: >4 mg		
Beef (lean, cooked)	3 oz	5.1
Calves' liver (cooked)	3 oz	5.3
Lamb (lean, cooked)	3 oz	4.0
Oysters, Atlantic	3 oz	63.0
Oysters, Pacific	3 oz	7.6
Good: 0.9–3.4 mg		
Black-eyed peas (cooked)	½ cup	3.4
Chicken	3 oz	2.4
Crabmeat	½ cup	3.4
Green peas (cooked)	½ cup	0.9
Lima beans (cooked)	3 oz	0.9
Milk (whole)	1 cup	0.9
Pork loin (cooked)	3 oz	2.6
Potato (baked with skin)	1 medium	1.0
Shrimp	½ cup	1.4
Tuna (oil-packed, drained)	3 oz	0.9
Whitefish	3 oz	0.9
Yogurt (plain)	1 cup	1.1

TABLE 13.25
Benefits of Physical Activity during Pregnancy and Postpartum

Improvement in circulation

Improved posture

Improved or maintained cardiovascular fitness

Reduced risk of cesarean section, decreased labor time, and decreased use of
  epidural and forceps

Positive effects on mood, energy level

Release of tension and reduction of stress

Prevention of injury

Primary prevention of gestational diabetes, especially in women with BMI > 33

After pregnancy, associated with decreased incidence of postpartum depression

TABLE 13.26
Contraindications to Physical Activity

Active myocardial disease, congestive heart failure,
  and rheumatic heart disease

Thrombophlebitis

Risk of premature labor, incompetent cervix,
  uterine bleeding, and ruptured membranes

Intrauterine growth restriction

Severe hypertensive disease

Suspected fetal intolerance

TABLE 13.27
Warning Signs to Stop Physical Activity

Vaginal bleeding
Uterine contractions
Nausea, vomiting
Dizziness or faintness
Difficulty walking
Decreased fetal activity
Palpitations or rapid heart rate
Numbness in any part of the body
Problems with vision

TABLE 13.28
Guidelines for Physical Activity

Activity	Guideline
Intensity	Reduce the intensity of exercise by 25%
Heart rate	Not to exceed 140 beats/min
Temperature	Not to go above 101°F
Time	Moderate activity of 30 min or more
Position	Avoid supine positions and motionless standing
Frequency	Exercise should be performed on most, if not all days of the week
Duration	Physiological and morphologic changes of pregnancy persist 4 to 6 weeks postpartum

TABLE 13.29
Guidelines for Recreational Activity

Activity	Guideline
General conditioning exercises	Kegal, breathing, calf pumping, abdominal, bridging, lower trunk rotation, tail wagging
Jogging	May be continued moderately, but should not be started as a new activity after pregnancy; watch out for joint pain and decrease overall distance — recommendation is 2 mi or less per day
Aerobics	Avoid high-impact or step aerobics; as for jogging, look out for joint pain or signs of over exertion; avoid exercises that involve lying on the back for more than 5 min
Bicycling	In the third trimester it may be necessary to switch to a stationary bike due to problems with balance
Weight lifting	Can be continued during pregnancy — use light weights and moderate repetitions; avoid heavy resistance
Avoid during pregnancy	Downhill skiing, gymnastics, horseback riding, scuba diving, and any contact sports

POSTPARTUM WEIGHT LOSS

While a great deal of attention is given to counseling women about appropriate weight gain for pregnancy, clinicians have typically given less assistance in achieving postpartum weight loss. Researchers are beginning to link failure to return to prepregnancy weight with increased risks for chronic disease later in life. Table 13.30 includes currently recommended strategies for postpartum weight loss.

Generally, participation in a wide rage of recreational activities appears to be safe; however, each sport should be reviewed for its potential risk and activities.

NUTRITION AND LACTATION

The RDA and AI for lactation are listed in Table 13.10. Suggestions for maternal nutrition to meet the increased energy and nutrient needs are listed in Table 13.31. Until relatively recently, breast-feeding has been considered too imprecise to study.

TABLE 13.30
Strategies for Postpartum Weight Loss

Encourage a healthy diet based on current dietary guidelines
Make energy intake less than energy expenditure
Reduce portion size but do not restrict kilocalories to <1800/day
Determine foods high in fats and calories and substitute with fruits,
  vegetables, lean meats and fish, skinless poultry
Avoid cooking in oil, butter, margarine
Drink 8 to 10 glasses of no/low calorie fluids per day
Discuss feasible physical activity
Monitor women who
    Restrict intake to <1800 kcal/day
    Are vegans (avoid all animal products including dairy, eggs, and meats)
    Avoid foods enriched with vitamin D and have limited exposure to sunlight

TABLE 13.31
Maternal Nutrition during Breast-Feeding

Encourage a healthy diet based on current dietary guidelines
Reinforce that milk quality is generally not affected by the mother's diet
Suggest eating meals and snacks that are easy to prepare
Provide patient with information on normal postpartum weight loss in a breastfeeding woman
Drink enough fluids to keep from getting thirsty
Eat at least 1800 kcal/day
Use appetite as a guide to amount of food eaten in first six weeks
Keep intake of coffee, cola, or other sources of caffeine to two servings or less per day. Caffeine
  accumulates in the infant and use should be discontinued if infant becomes wakeful, hyperactive,
  or has disturbed sleep patterns. This reaction is intensified with a smoking mother

TABLE 13.32
Benefits of Frequent, Early, Unrestricted Nursing

Provides colostrum that the baby needs
Helps decrease newborn jaundice because of the laxative effect of colostrums
Provides a period of practice time before milk volume increases
Stimulates uterine contractions, lessening chances of maternal postpartum hemorrhage
Prevents infant hypoglycemia

TABLE 13.33
Signs of Insufficient Milk Intake in the Newborn

Failure to regain birth weight by 2 to 3 weeks of age; weight loss >7% at
  discharge and >10% at day 3 to 5
Weight gain of <7 oz/week after regaining birth weight and <4 lb in 4 months

A wealth of information is being developed about lactation and breast milk.[51] Table 13.32 lists some of the benefits of unrestricted nursing for the infant. Many women and their clinicians still are concerned about ways to identify whether an infant is obtaining enough nutriture. Table 13.33 lists signs of insufficient milk intake. The social history of infant feeding from the late 1800s to the 1950s in the United States shows a transition from breast-feeding to scientific feeding of infants. As a result of that, much cultural knowledge and support for breast-feeding was lost. Guidebooks are important for women and clinicians.[45,52–54] Table 13.34 and Table 13.35 include common concerns and recommended actions to support breast-feeding.

TABLE 13.34
Breast-Feeding Tips: Common Concerns about the Infant

Concern	Recommended action
Jaundice	Continue to breast-feed at least every 2 h around the clock. Pump breasts to maintain milk supply. Avoid water or formula feeding
Latch-on	Latch-on is necessary for baby to begin sucking at the breasts. Poor latch-on is a major cause of sore nipples. Baby's mouth should be at nipple level. Support the breast by placing the thumb on the top and four fingers underneath. Tickle baby's bottom lip with nipple until baby opens mouth very wide. Center nipple quickly and bring baby very close. Baby's nose and chin should be touching breast. Ear, shoulder, and hip should be in alignment
Leaking	Leaking is a sign of normal letdown in the early weeks of breast-feeding. Use pads in bra between feedings. Avoid pads with plastic lining. During sexual activity, leaking may occur; breast-feed baby first
Duration of breast-feeding: how long and how often?	Frequent (every 2–3 h) and unrestricted breast-feeding for the first weeks. Baby should empty one breast, be burped, and offered the second breast. Watch baby for signs that he or she is full, such as falling asleep, losing interest in feeding, or stopping breast-feeding
Early first feeding	Put baby to breast soon after delivery, within 1 h. Cuddling, licking, and brief sucking are good signs that baby is learning to breast-feed. Offer breast often to let baby practice. Ask a supportive nurse or lactation consultant for help. Offer breast whenever infant shows signs of early hunger. In general there should be 8 to 12 feedings per 24 h
Extra feedings	Healthy breast-fed newborns do not need formula, water, or juice. Breast-feed at least every 2 to 3 h during the first month. Complementary foods should be added at 6 months of age

TABLE 13.35
Breast-Feeding Tips: Common Discomforts that Lead to Breast-Feeding Termination

Concerns	Recommended action
Hospital survival skills	"Rooming in" with the baby is a consumer right. Keep baby with mother as much as possible to facilitate breast-feeding often. Do not give bottles of formula or water. Do not limit feeding time at a breast. Ask a supportive nurse or lactation consultant for help. Do not offer/accept formula gift packs
Mastitis	Mastitis is a swollen, inflamed, or infected area in the breast. Watch for flu-like symptoms such as fever above 101°F, chills and muscle aches, and a reddened, hot, tender, or swollen area in the breasts. Rest, breast-feed often, and drink more fluids. Avoid tight bra or clothing. Apply warm water soaks or cold packs (whichever gives relief). Massage affected area. Antibiotics may be needed. Not a reason to stop breast-feeding
Myths and misconceptions	Breast sagging is not a result of breast-feeding. Breast size does not affect ability to breast-feed. Drinking beer, manzanilla tea, or large amounts of fluids does not make more milk
Nipples, flat or inverted (before birth)	Flat or inverted nipples retract or move in toward the breast. Air-dry nipples if leaking occurs. Breast shells should not be used by women at risk for preterm labor. There is no evidence of harm or benefit for breast shells
Nipples, flat or inverted (after birth)	Begin breast-feeding as soon as possible after birth. Breast-feed frequently to avoid engorgement. Use nipple rolling or stretching before each breast-feeding. Pump breasts for a short period before breast-feeding, or apply ice wrapped in a cloth and place on the nipple before feeding. Breast shells (milk cups) may be used between feedings. Remove the breast shell just before placing baby at breast. Referral to a lactation consultant may be indicated
Engorgement	Engorgement may occur when milk first comes in or when feeding are missed or delayed. Use cold compresses or shower before feedings. Hand-express to soften areola, making it easier for baby to latch on. Breast-feed every 1 to 2 h for 10 to 30 min/breast. Gently massage breast toward nipple. Take nonaspirin pain reliever
Breast care	Nipple pulling, tugging, or rolling during pregnancy is not necessary to prepare for breast-feeding. Avoid soaps or lotions to the nipples. Air dry nipples after breast-feeding
Breast creams	Vitamin E, breast creams, or ointments are not recommended. No evidence exists that they heal the nipple. May make soreness worse by keeping the nipple moist. Use pure lanolin. Can massage drops of breast milk on nipples. Use hydrogel dressings
Breast surgery	Any type of breast surgery can interfere with milk supply. Referral to lactation consultant is appropriate
Operative delivery	Breast-feed baby as soon as possible after delivery, preferably in the recovery room. Hold baby in a comfortable position. Use pillows across abdomen to protect the incision and support baby. Use side lying position

RESOURCE MATERIALS

Agency for Healthcare Research and Quality. Guide to Clinical Preventive Services. http://www.ahrq.gov

American College of Obstetricians and Gynecologists, Office of Public Information, 409 12th Street SW, Washington, DC 20024-2188, 202-638-5577. http://www.acog.org

Best Start Social Marketing, 3500 E. Fletcher Avenue, Suite 519, Tampa FL, 33613; 1-800-277-4975. Best Start is a not-for-profit corporation. One of its largest social marking projects was developed in 1997 for USDA as part of the WIC National Breastfeeding Promotion Project. A wide variety of campaign and professional materials is available. http://www.beststartinc.org/

Erick M. *No More Morning Sickness. A Survival Guide for Pregnant Women.* Plume Book, NJ. http://www.amazon.com

Environmental Protection Agency. Fish advisories. http://www.epa.gov

Food and Nutrition Information Center, National Agricultural Library, ARS, USDA, Beltsville, MD 20705-2351. 301-504-5719 http://www.nal.usda.gov/fnic

La Leche League International, 1400 N. Meacham Rd, PO Box 4079, Schaumburg IL 60168-4079. http://www.lalecheleague.org

Lopes GL. *Gestational Diabetes and You.* NCES, Inc 2001. http://ncescatalog.com

March of Dimes Birth Defects Foundation Resource Center, 1275 Mamoroneck Ave, White Plains, NY 10605. http://modimes.org

National Maternal and Child Health Clearinghouse, 2070 Chain Bridge Road, Suite 450, Vienna, VA 22182-2536, 703-356-1964; fax: 703-821-2098 http://www.ask.hrsa.govcircsol.com/mch

National Center for Nutrition and Dietetics, The American Dietetic Association, 216 W Jackson Blvd. Suite 800, Chicago, IL 60606-6995. http://www.eatright.org

USDA. Is Someone You Know At Risk for Foodborne Illness? Food Safety and Inspection Service, April 1990. http://www.fightbac.org

Womenshealth.gov. Pregnancy and Healthy Diet. http://womenshealth.gov

REFERENCES

1. Am Coll OB-GYN. ACOG Technical Bulletin No. 205, May, 1995.
2. Am Acad Ped. Am Coll OB-GYN. Chapter 4, pages 73–84; Chapter 5, pages 151–158; Chapter 7, pages 221–229. In Guidelines for Perinatal Care 2002.
3. Institute of Medicine, Subcommittee for a Clinical Application Guide. Nutrition During Pregnancy and Lactation: An Implementation Guide, National Academy Press, Washington, DC, 1992.
4. Villar, J., Merialdi, M., and Gulmezoglu. A.M. et al. *J Nutr.* 5: 1606s, 2003.
5. Newton, E. Maternal nutrition. In: Management of High Risk Pregnancy. (Queen, J.T., Ed) Blackwell Science, 4th ed. 1999.
6. Jackson, A.A. and Robinson, S.M. *Public Health Nutr.* 4: 625, 2001.
7. Suitor, CW. Update for Nutrition during Pregnancy and Lactation: An Implementation Guide. National Center for Education in Maternal and Child Health. Maternal and Child Health Bureau, Health Resources and Services Administration, Public Health Service, U.S. Department of Health and Human Services.
8. Kirkham, C., Harris, S., and Grzybowski, S. *Am Fam Physician.* 71: 1307, 2005.
9. Butte, N.F., Wong, W.W., and Treuth, M.S., et al. *Am J Clin Nutr.* 79: 1078, 2004.
10. Atallah, A.N., Hofmeyr, G.J., and Duley, L. (Cochrane Review). In: The Cochrane Library, Issue 4, 2004.
11. Dunstan, J.A., Mor, T.A., and Barden, A. et al. *Eur J Clin Nutr.* 58: 429, 2004.
12. ACOG. Nausea and Vomiting of Pregnancy. ACOG Practice Bulletin No. 52. 2004.
13. Polley, B.A., Wing, R.R., and Sims, C.H. *Intl J Obes.* 26: 1494, 2002.
14. Homan, R.K. and Korenbrot, C.C. *Med Care* 36: 190, 1998.
15. Luke, B. *Clin Obstet Gynecol.* 37: 538, 1994.
16. Matthews, F., Yudkin, P., and Neil, A. *Brit Med J.* 319: 339, 1999.
17. Abrams, B., Carmichael, S., and Selvin, S. *Obstet Gynecol.* 86: 170, 1995.
18. Ananth, C.V., Vintzileos, A.M., and Shen-Schwarz, S. et al. *Obstet Gynecol.* 91: 917, 1998.
19. ACOG. *Clinical Obstetrics and Gyn.* 46: 496, 2003.
20. Cogswell, M.E., Serdula, M.K., Hungerford, D.W., and Yip, R. *Am J Ob-Gyn.* 172: 705, 1995.
21. Keppel, K.G. and Taffel, S.M. *AJPHA* 83: 1100, 1993.
22. King, J.C., Butte, N.F., and Bronstein, M.N. et al. *Am J Clin Nutr.* 59(suppl): 439S, 1994.
23. Luke, B., Hediger, M.L., and Scholl, T.O. *J Mat Fetal Med.* 5: 168, 1996.
24. Parker, J.D. and Abrams, B. *Obstet Gynecol.* 79: 664, 1992.
25. Schieve, L.A., Cogswell, M.E., and Scanlon, K.S. *Obstet Gynecol.* 91: 878, 1998.
26. Scholl, T.O., Hedinger, M.L., and Schall, J.I. et al. *Obstet Gynecol.* 86: 423, 1995.
27. Siega-Riz, A.M., Adair, L.S., and Hobel, C.J. *Nutrition* 126: 146, 1996.
28. Taffel, S.M., Keppel, K.G., and Jones, G.K. *Ann NY Acad Sci.* 678: 293, 1993.
29. Suitor, C.W. Maternal Weight Gain: A Report of an Expert Work Group, National Center for Education in Maternal and Child Health, Arlington, VA, 1997.
30. Rosello-Soberon, M., Fuentes-Chaparro, L., and Casanueva, E. *Nutr Rev.* 63: 295, 2005.
31. Kramer, M.S. and Kakuma, R. Cochrane Pregnancy and Childbirth Group, Cochrane Database of Systematic Reviews, Issue 4, 2005.
32. ACOG. Committee on Obstetric Practice. No. 315, September 2005.
33. Abrams, B., Altman, S.L., and Pickett, K.E. *Am J Clin Nutr.* 71: 1233s, 2000.
34. Kolasa, K.M. and Weismiller, D. *AFP* 56: 205, 1997.
35. Institute of Medicine, Food and Nutrition Board. Dietary Reference Intakes for Thiamin, Riboflavin, Niacin, Vitamin B_6, Folate, Vitamin B_{12}, Pantothenic Acid, Biotin, and Choline. National Academy Press, Washington, DC, 1998.

36. Institute of Medicine, Food and Nutrition Board, Dietary References Intakes for Calcium, Phosphorus, Magnesium, Vitamin D, and Fluoride. National Academy Press, Washington, DC, 1997.

37. US Dept Health and Human Services and USDA. 6th edition. www.healthierus.gov/dietaryguidelines, 2005.

38. Kennedy, E. *JADA* 86: 1372, 1986.

39. Erick, M. *Nutr Rev.* 53: 289, 1995.

40. Stainton, M.C. and Neff, E.J.A. *Health Care Women Intl.* 15: 563, 1994.

41. ACOG. Number 315, September 2005.

42. ACOG. ACOG Practice Bulletin No. 52. 103: 803, 2004.

43. Jewell, D. and Young, G. Cochrane Pregnancy and Childbirth Group. Cochrane Database of Systematic Reviews, Issue 4, 2005.

44. Goldenberg, R., Tamura, T., and Neggers, Y., et al. *JAMA* 274: 463l, 1995.

45. *Am Acad Pediatrics.* Breastfeeding and the use of human milk. *Pediatrics.* 115: 496, 2005.

46. NHLBI. JNC7. NIH Publication No. 04-5230, 2004.

47. Institute of Medicine, Subcommittee on Nutrition During Lactation. Nutrition During Lactation. National Academy Press, Washington, DC, 1991.

48. National Academy of Sciences, Institute of Medicine, Food and Nutrition Board, Committee on Nutritional Status During Pregnancy and Lactation. Nutrition Services in Perinatal Care (2nd ed). National Academy Press, Washington, DC, 1992.

49. Pena-Rosas, J.P., Viteri, F.E., and Mahomed, K. Cochrane Database of Systematic Reviews. 4, 2005.

50. USPSTF. Guide to Clinical Preventive Services, 2nd edition, 1996.

51. Lawrence, R.A. Maternal and Child Health Technical Information Bulletin. National Center for Education in Material and Child Health, Arlington, VA, 1997

52. Lawrence, R.A. and Lawrence, R.M. Breastfeeding: A guide for the Medical Profession. C.V. Mosby, St. Louis, MO, 1998.

53. Mohrbacher, N. and Stock, J. The Breastfeeding Answer Book. La Leche League International. Bartlett, Boston, MA, 1997.

54. Riordan, J. and Auerbach, K.G. Pocket Guide to Breastfeeding and Human Lactation, Jones and Bartlett, Boston, MA, 1997.

14 Feeding the Premature Infant

Beth Baisden, Chantrapa Bunyapen, and Jatinder Bhatia

CONTENTS

With the ever-increasing survival of low-birth-weight and very-low-birth-weight infants, understanding the principles of nutritional therapy becomes all the more important. It is estimated that there are over 4 million births in the United States every year; with an increased estimated prematurity rate of 12%,[1] the number of infants requiring such management is enormous. This review will focus on the nutritional goals, nutrient requirements, and enteral and parenteral routes of nutritional therapy.

NUTRITIONAL GOALS FOR THE PREMATURE INFANT

A premature infant is an infant born before completion of 37 weeks of gestation. A postterm infant is one whose birth occurs from the beginning of the first day of week 43 (>42 weeks). Classifying infants as preterm, term, or postterm assists in establishing the level of risk for neonatal morbidity, nutritional needs, and long-term sequelae. Assessment of gestational age is based on maternal dates, obstetrical dating by ultrasonography, and by physical examination.[2] The Ballard exam, which uses physical and neurological criteria, may overestimate the age of premature infants and, on the other hand, may underestimate that of postterm infants.[3] Because of the error in gestational age assessment, particularly in very-low-birth-weight infants, a new Ballard Score is currently used.[4] This modified examination is particularly suited for the very small premature infant, and the estimated gestational age is accurate to within 1 week. Items of neuromuscular maturity and physical maturity are scored from −1 to 5: a total score obtained and gestational age estimated based on maturity rating score. However, in the case of the very-low-birth weight infant, early estimation of gestational age is more accurately obtained by obstetrical dating vs. the Ballard exam.[5]

Infants are considered low-birth-weight if birth weight is less than 2500 g regardless of gestational age. Very-low-birth weight defines infants with weight less than 1500 g with an additional classification of extremely-low-birth weight describing infants less than 1000 g.

Crown heel length, performed by two examiners, is measured by achieving full extension of the infant on a measuring board with a fixed head piece and movable foot piece. The infant needs to be supine, head held in the Frankfurt plane vertical, legs extended, ankles flexed, and the movable foot piece is brought to rest firmly against the infant's heels. An average of two measurements documents the length. If crown–heel length cannot be measured due to limb anomalies or if there is a discrepancy between weight and length, a crown–rump length is sometimes measured. In preterm infants, this measurement is fraught with error even when performed by a trained team. In addition, measurement in an open bed or on a ventilator or with multiple intravenous lines makes accurate measurements difficult to achieve.

Head circumference measured with a nonstretchable tape is the largest of three measurements around the head with the tape held snugly above the ears.

Weight, length, and head circumference are then plotted on standard curves to classify an infant as appropriate, small, or large for gestational age for each measurement. Most measurements define appropriate for age as measurements that fall within the 10th to 90th percentiles, ideally based on charts constructed for similar race and height above sea level. Infants who are

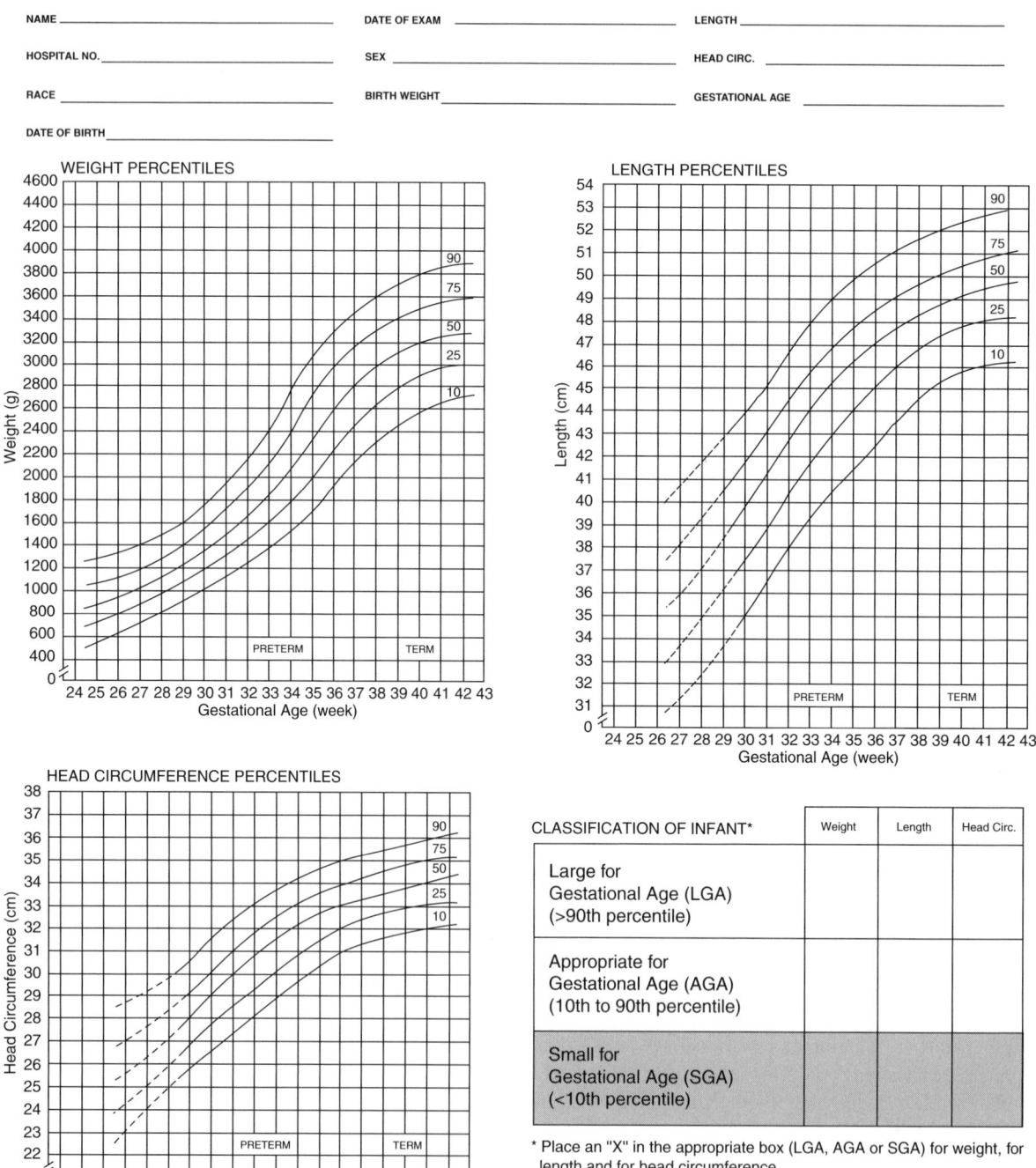

FIGURE 14.1 Classification of newborns (both sexes) by intrauterine growth and gestational age[2,3].

appropriate for age on the three measures are at the lowest risk, within that gestational age grouping, for problems associated with neonatal morbidity and mortality.

An example of growth curves commonly used in neonatal nurseries is depicted in Figure 14.1.

GROWTH AND NUTRIENT REQUIREMENTS

Estimation of nutrient requirements, in premature infants, is based on the goals for growth of this cohort of infants. The common goal has been to achieve growth similar to that of the "reference fetus" as described.[6] These growth standards serve as a reference to judge the adequacy of growth; however, postnatal changes in energy requirements as well as environmental stresses are likely to be different, and the ideal growth of these infants remains to be defined. An alternative approach may be to achieve the best possible growth without adverse metabolic consequences. In a recent NICHD evaluation of more than 1600 preterm infants, most had not achieved the growth rates of the reference fetus of the same postmenstrual age by the time they were discharged.[7]

Nutrient requirements for preterm infants have been estimated by various methods, including the factorial method based on the reference fetus, nitrogen balance studies, and turnover studies or based on nutrient values in the serum. For example, Figure 14.2 depicts the composition of weight gain in normal human fetuses.[8] In a more recent publication, Ziegler[9] provides estimated nutrient intakes needed to achieve fetal weight gain, representing the current best estimates. This approach serves not only as a basis for calculation of nutrient needs, but also as a measure of sufficiency of particular nutrients as discussed above (Table 14.1). The factorial approach is based on the assumption that the requirement for a nutrient is the sum of losses (fecal,

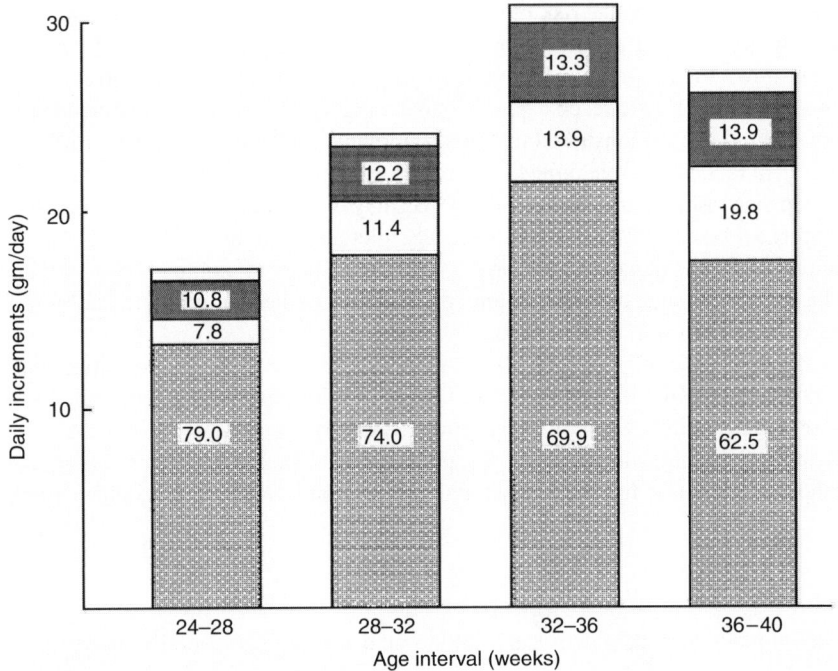

FIGURE 14.2   Composition of weight gain in the human fetus.

TABLE 14.1
Estimated Nutrient Intakes and Fetal Weight Gain

Body Weight (g)	500–700	700–900	900–1200	1200–1500
Fetal weight gain (g/kg/d)	21	20	19	18
Protein intake required, parenteral	3.5	3.5	3.5	3.4
Protein intake required, enteral	4.0	4.0	4.0	3.9
Energy intake required, parenteral	89	92	101	108
Energy intake required, enteral	105	108	119	127

Source: Modified from Ziegler, E.E. *Clin Perinatol* 29: 225; 2002.

urinary, dermal, etc.) and the amount required for growth, that is, incorporation into new tissues. Advisable intakes of protein are obtained by adding 8 to 10% of the estimated requirement.

PROVISION OF NUTRIENTS

Energy Needs

Energy needs are based on basal metabolic rate, cost of growth, and losses in stool and urine. The factorial method cannot be used to estimate energy requirements. It is generally recognized that preterm infants have higher energy requirements compared to their term counterparts.[10] To gain the predicted growth in weight for premature infants (10 to 15 g/kg/d), it is estimated that premature infants would need between 110 and 130 kcal/kg/d, an estimate higher than the usually held notion that infants need 120 kcal/kg/d regardless of size or age. Energy requirements must take into account the route of administration, enteral vs. parenteral, since 90 to 95 kcal/kg/d may satisfy energy requirements by the parenteral route. Disease states such as sepsis, chronic lung disease,[11,12] and concomitant use of corticosteroids will increase energy needs. The mainstay of energy support should be balanced between carbohydrates, fats, and amino acids.

Amino Acid Needs

The factorial approach is commonly used to estimate protein requirements. The protein need will be greater if catch up growth is also to be produced. It is generally accepted that the newborn infant will lose up to 10% of his/her body weight. In sick premature infants, where nutrition cannot be provided or is not tolerated, the amount of catch up growth may be greater. Several studies suggest that endogenous protein losses in the absence of exogenous protein intake are at least 1 g/kg/d.[13] When fed in the conventional manner, premature infants run the risk of undernutrition. Therefore, strategies to optimize amino acid intakes to include provision for catch up growth need to be developed, since early initiation of parenteral nutrition results in positive nitrogen balance and has been shown to be safe.[14–17] The more employed traditional method is to start with 0.5 mg/kg/day of amino acids and slowly increase by 0.5 mg/kg to reach a goal of 3 to 3.5 mg/kg/day. With improvements in amino acid solutions and preterm formulas, recent studies have demonstrated that preterm infants can safely tolerate up to 3.5 mg/kg/day of protein in just a few days after birth.[18,19] In fact, in one randomized controlled trial, infants <1500 g on day of life 1 were given glucose only and protein added in a stepwise fashion, or glucose and 2.4 g/kg/day of amino acid solution from the first day of life, and this trial showed that high amino acid concentrations could be safely tolerated from birth.[20]

Cysteine and tyrosine are provided as cysteine hydrochloride (40 mg/g/amino acid; not to exceed 100 mg/kg/d) and N-acetyl-L-tyrosine (0.24 g%),[21] it has been demonstrated that infants receiving cysteine retain significantly more nitrogen than do infants receiving an isonitrogenous amino acid intake without cysteine.[15]

It is generally accepted that infants receiving between 80 and 90 kcal/kg/d from parenteral nutrition with an adequate amino acid intake should gain weight similar to the intrauterine rate.[22] Most of this energy intake is provided by glucose and lipid. The glucose utilization rate of a preterm infant is 5 to 8 mg/kg/min. Carbohydrates, most readily available as glucose, should provide approximately 35% of the daily kilocalories. However, premature and sick infants may not tolerate increasing glucose concentrations/delivery, without concomitant hyperglycemia making the goal of achieving adequate energy intake difficult in the first week of life.

Lipid Needs

Lipid emulsions are used in conjunction with glucose and amino acid solutions. Generally, lipids are started at 0.5g/kg/d intravenously; increasing by 0.5g/kg to a maximum of 3.0 g/kg/d. The goal is to provide 50% of the daily caloric intake as fat. Infusion rates are maintained between 0.15 and 0.25 g/kg/h in order to avoid hypertriglyceridemia (triglycerides > 175 mg/dl). Essential fatty acid deficiency may be prevented by lipid intakes as low as 0.5 to 1.0 g/kg/d.

Clearance of lipids by premature infants may be limited, thereby requiring frequent assessment of tolerance. Emulsions of 20% are preferred due to lower total phospholipid and liposome content per gram of triglyceride.[23]

Parenteral Nutrition

It is common practice to provide the initial nutrient requirements, especially in a sick neonate, by the parenteral route. A typical parenteral regimen is depicted in Table 14.2. It is generally recommended that parenteral nutrition be started within the first day of life in preterm infants and advanced in a systematic fashion to achieve 3 to 3.5 g/kg/d of amino acids and 90 to 100 kcal/kg/d of energy. Most preterm infants do not achieve these intakes until well into the second week of life because of issues such as glucose and lipid intolerance.

TABLE 14.2
Parenteral Nutrition Regimen

Component	Amount/kg/d	
Amino acids (g)	3–3.5	
Glucose (g)	15–25	
Lipid (g)	0.5–3.0	
Sodium (mEq)[a]	2–5	
Potassium (mEq)[b]	2–4	
Calcium (mg)	80–100	
Magnesium (mg)	3–6	
Chloride (mEq)	2–3	
Phosphorus (mg)[b]	40–60	
Zinc (μg)	200–400	
Copper (μg)	20	
Iron (μg)	100–200	
Other trace minerals[c]	<14 days	>14 days
Manganese (μg)	0.0–0.75	1.0
Chromium (μg)	0.0–0.05	0.2
Selenium (μg)	0.0–1.3	2.0
Iodide (μg)	0.0–1.0	1.0
Molybdenum (μg)	0	0.25
Vitamins[d]		
C (mg)	80	
A (mg)	0.7	
D (μg)	10 (= 400u)	
B_1 (mg)	1.2	
B_2 (mg)	1.4	
B_6 (mg)	1	
Niacin (mg)	17	
Total volume	120–150 ml	

[a] Sodium requirements may vary between infants and within the same infant and should be tailored to serum values.

[b] Phosphorus intakes are maintained in a ratio of 1:2 to 1:2.6 with calcium (mEq:mM) and may be limiting in parenteral nutrition because of insolubility; in general, the more acidic the TPN, the more calcium and phosphorus can be dissolved in the solution without precipitation. Care must be taken to avoid hyperphoshatemia with its resultant hypocalcemia.

[c] amount/kg/d.

[d] Provided as MVI-Pediatric[R]; each 5 ml provides (MVI is to be provided in amounts not exceeding 2.0 ml/kg/d).

Mineral Requirements

Mineral requirements have also been estimated based on body composition of the reference fetus.[6,8] From a practical standpoint, daily needs for sodium, potassium, and chloride are based on serum measurements, while calcium and phosphorus are based on the factorial method.[6,8] Requirements are listed in Table 14.2. In general, it is accepted that sodium is not added to parenteral nutrition regimens until the sodium is below 130 mEq/l. It should be noted that premature infants in general, and very-low-birth-weight infants in particular, receive large amounts of sodium inadvertently.[24] In general, the preterm infant has higher requirements of most minerals compared to term infants. During total parenteral nutrition, requirements for calcium and phosphorus may not be met because of the insolubility of calcium salts. Human milk may not provide adequate amounts of sodium, and hyponatremia has been reported.[25] Calcium and phosphorus needs of preterm infants cannot be met by human milk, whether from mothers delivering preterm or term infants, and will need to be supplemented.[26] Since calcium transfer across the placenta occurs in the third trimester, the very premature infant is relatively "osteopenic," and prolonged parenteral nutrition and or unfortified human milk feedings puts the infant at great risk for further osteopenia and metabolic bone disease.

Iron is accumulated in the fetus in the third trimester with an iron content of 75 mg/kg at term. Gestational age infants, preterm infants, and infants of diabetic mothers have low iron stores at birth. Coupled with the need for frequent blood sampling, the premature infant is at great risk for the development of iron deficiency anemia, and the exact time for supplementation remains controversial. However, given that the criteria for blood transfusion have become more stringent,[26] iron should be supplemented as early as 2 weeks. If recombinant erythropoietin is used to stimulate endogenous iron production,[27] iron requirements may be 6.0 mg/kg/d or higher.

Nutrient Delivery

Delivery of enteral nutrients is based on gestational age. In general, infants of 33 weeks gestation and beyond can be fed orally soon after birth. However, if medical or surgical illness precludes enteral feedings, parenteral nutrition is indicated. Parenteral nutrition can be considered as total (where all nutrients are delivered for example in an infant with a surgical condition precluding enteral nutrition: gastroschisis) or supplemental (to complement enteral nutrition). It can be further described as peripheral parenteral nutrition (provided by a peripheral intravenous line) or central (where the tip of the catheter is in a central location or deep vein). The latter should be the route if long-term parenteral nutrition (e.g., >2 weeks) or the need for >12.5% dextrose in water is anticipated.

A typical nutrition plan for a very-low-birth-weight infant is depicted in Table 14.3.

TABLE 14.3
Initiation and Advancement of Parenteral and Minimal Enteral Feedings in an Infant with a Birthweight of <1000 g

	Parenteral				
Age, Days	Amino Acid (g/kg)	Glucose	Lipids (g/kg)	Electrolytes	Enteral ml/h[a]
1	2.5	D_5W	0.0	0.0	0.0
2	3.0	D_5W	0.5	Add if Na < 130 mEq/l	0.25
3	3.0–3.5	Increments of 2.5%	1.0[b]	Standard	0.25
4	Same	Increase as tolerated	1.5[b]	Standard	0.5
5	Same	Increase as tolerated	2.0[b]	Standard	0.5
6	Same	Increase as tolerated	2.5[b]	Standard	0.75
7	3.0 or higher[c]	Same or higher	3.0[b]	Standard	0.75

[a] In larger infants, studies have demonstrated that feeding of 20 ml/kg/d and advancing at that rate is safe,[28] while other studies have demonstrated an increased incidence of NEC, when feeds are advanced at that rate.[29]

[b] Monitor triglycerides to assess lipid tolerance.

[c] Optional; infants requiring catch up growth, on corticosteroids or demonstrating low BUN despite adequate protein intakes may need higher amino acid intakes at later stages.

Parenteral Nutrition is indicated in the following conditions:

Medical	Inadequate enteral nutrition
	Necrotizing enterocolitis
	Feeding intolerance/difficulty
	Ileus
	Prematurity
Surgical	Omphaolcele
	Gastroschisis
	Tracheo-esophageal fistula
	Atresias
	of the intestine (duodenal/jejunal/ileal)
	Diaphragmatic hernia
	Hirschsprung's disease

Complications of Parenteral Nutrition:

Metabolic	Hypo- or hyperglycemia
	Electrolyte imbalance
	Metabolic bone disease
	Hepatic dysfunction
Infectious	Bacterial sepsis
	Fungal sepsis
Mechanical	Extravasation
	Thrombosis
	Pericardial effusion
	Diaphragmatic palsy
	Pleural effusion

TABLE 14.4

Suggested Monitoring During Parenteral Nutrition

Component	Initial	Later[a]
Weight	Daily	Daily
Length	Weekly	Weekly
Head Circumference	Weekly	Weekly
Na, K, Cl, CO2	Daily until stable	Weekly
Glucose	Daily	PRN
Triglycerides	With every lipid change	Weekly or biweekly
Ca, PO4	Daily until stable	Weekly or biweekly
Alkaline phosphatase	Initial	weekly or biweekly
Bilirubin	Initial	weekly or biweekly
Mg	Initial	weekly or biweekly
Ammonia	PRN	PRN
Gamma GT	Initial	weekly or biweekly
ALT/AST	initial	weekly or biweekly
Complete blood count	Initial	weekly or PRN

[a] A practical way to monitor parenteral nutrition may simply include measurement of direct bilirubin and alkaline phosphatase at 2–4 weeks of age. If they are increased, a comprehensive metabolic panel may be ordered to evaluate the traditional "liver function tests" and calcium and phosphorus. This may achieve the same end point as monitoring the parameters routinely.

The metabolic complications can be avoided by careful assessment of tolerance to the macronutrients as nutrition delivery is advanced. Premature infants do not tolerate high concentrations of glucose or rapid advances in glucose delivery; similarly, rates of fat infusion of greater than 2.0 g/kg/d may result in hypertriglyceridemia, particularly in the small or ill preterm infant (triglycerides >175 mg/dl). A suggested regimen of monitoring parenteral nutrition is depicted in Table 14.4. A multidisciplinary approach with physicians, pharmacists, nutritionists, and nursing staff who are knowledgeable in parenteral nutrition and monitoring should be involved in the care of such infants. Early recognition of metabolic effects (pharmacist/nutritionist) or catheter-related effects (nursing) could assist in minimizing the potential complications of parenteral nutrition. The most common metabolic complications observed are hepatic dysfunction and metabolic bone disease.

Hepatic dysfunction is defined as an increase in serum bile acids, followed by an increase in direct bilirubin, alkaline phosphatase, and gamma-glutamyl transferase. The hepatocellular enzymes, ALT and AST, are late to increase and often seen in the more severe cases. γ-Glutamyl transferase is probably the most sensitive but least specific indicator, whereas elevation in direct bilrubin is the most specific and least sensitive indicator of hepatic dysfunction. The etiology is multi-factorial,[30–32] but the incidence appears to be declining both as a result of specialized amino acid solutions and early provision of enteral nutrients.

Premature infants are at high risk for the development of metabolic bone disease, most commonly due to inadequate intakes of calcium and phosphorus during parenteral nutrition. Infants born before 32 weeks of gestation have some degree of hypomineralization, which is worsened during the subsequent period of hospitalization, especially, coupled with inadequate intakes of calcium and phosphorus. In general, both calcium and phosphorus levels are maintained in serum, while the bones appear more osteopenic on radiographs, and ultimately hypophosphatemia with increasing alkaline phosphatase is observed. Rising alkaline phosphatase in the absence of elevated "liver" enzymes is a strong indicator of metabolic bone disease. Incidence of rickets (metabolic bone disease) is inversely proportional to birth weight and has been reported to be as high as 50 to 60% in very-low-birth-weight infants.[33] Diagnosis is made by routine radiographs that, in the initial stages, would demonstrate bone undermineralization, especially in the ribs and scapula, subsequently showing the classic forms of rickets in the wrists and long bones. Strategies to increase calcium and phosphorus delivery should be considered.

Unfortunately, the very small preterm infant is more often at risk for these complications, given the duration of parenteral nutrition and the coexistence of hepatic dysfunction.

Enteral Nutrition

Even if enteral nutrition is started in the first days after birth, it is suggested that supplemental parenteral nutrition be started because immaturity, feeding intolerance, and GI motility may affect the rate of advancement of enteral nutrition. Further, intakes are also dictated by the feedings used: human milk or formula. Composition of human milk (Table 14.5) from a mother delivering a preterm infant is different from that of mothers delivering at term; further, differences between and within the same woman makes the average content difficult to estimate. Breast milk does appear to provide the best protection from infection and the development of necrotizing enterocolitis. However, it may not provide adequate amounts of calcium, phosphorus, protein, and sodium for the growing premature infant. Various fortifiers are available and appear to enhance short-term weight gain and to be safe. Whether the content is mostly in the form of carbohydrates or fat, the result is increased fat deposition.[34,35]

The route of enteral nutrition is dictated not only by the gestational age of the infant, but also the coexistence or medical or surgical morbidity. Routes and types of delivery are depicted in Table 14.6.

Motor responses to feedings are similar whether feedings are provided by the gastric or transpyloric route.[36] However, when feeds are provided slowly over 120 min as compared to 15 min, gastric emptying is better, suggesting that in the smaller premature infant, slow infusions may be better tolerated.[37,38]

Oral Feeding

Term and preterm infants greater than 33 to 34 weeks gestation may be fed soon after birth by the oral route. This should be attempted in the delivery room in healthy infants or initiated soon after birth. Human milk feedings (i.e., breast feeding) should be encouraged and all steps taken by the medical team and hospital staff to encourage breast feeding once the decision is made. If breast feeding is precluded, due to craniofacial anomalies such as cleft clip or palate, feeding devices are available and speech therapy or feeding teams may need to be involved. Lactation consultation should be sought for mothers who have difficulty in either initiation or maintenance of breast feeding. Hospitals should avoid practices of supplementing breast-fed infants or the use of pacifiers.

Most mothers delivering preterm infants have not made a decision about breast feeding and should be counseled appropriately. All delivery sites should have facilities to pump breast milk if actual breastfeeding is not possible and the mother wishes to breastfeed. Teaching should include appropriate techniques for pumping and storing milk.

Nutrient Delivery

For infants born after 33 to 34 weeks of gestation, enteral feedings may be started *per os*. Although it is recognized that infants at this gestational age can coordinate their suck, swallow, and respiratory activities, thus enabling feedings, not all infants respond in such a fashion, and careful assessment is warranted. In the event of nipple feedings not being achieved, the infant may be fed by the gastric route.

In general, the alternatives to feedings by mouth are delineated as follows: (1) gastric and (2) transpyloric. Gastric feedings can be further described as (1) bolus, provided intermittently every 2 to 3 h or (2) continuous, where the feeds are provided by a pump at a constant hourly rate. Transpyloric feeds are provided continuously with the tip of the feeding tube in the second part of the duodenum. General indications for the latter include failure to tolerate gastric feeding due to delayed gastric emptying, gastric distention due to positive pressure ventilation, or gastroesophageal reflux. In a 2002 review of transpyloric vs. gastric feeds, no difference in the incidence of NEC, aspiration, or perforation was found. There was no difference in weight or head circumference at 3 and 6 months chronological ages. An increased incidence of feeding difficulties was noted with the transpyloric route.[39]

Feedings can also be planned based on birth weight. In general, infants below 1250 g are fed by the continuous, gastric method, whereas bigger infants by the intermittent method.

A further concern with preterm infants is the amount needed to start feedings and how fast to increase feeds. This concern arises from observations that "too much, too soon" can increase the incidence of NEC and feeding intolerance. In neonatal

TABLE 14.5
Composition of Human Milk

	Human milk (2 weeks postpartum)	
	Term	**Preterm**
Volume (ml)	147–161	139–150
Water (ml)	133–145	125–135
Protein		
Content (g)	1.8–2.5	2.4–3.1
% of energy	7–11	9.6–12
Whey/casein ratio	80 : 20	80 : 20
Lipid		
Content (g)	4.4–6	4.9–6.3
% of energy	44–56	42–55
Composition (%)		
Saturated	43	41–47
Monosaturated	42	39–40
Polyunsaturated	15	12–14
Carbohydrate		
Content (g)	9–10.6	8–9.8
% of energy	38–44	31–38
Lactose (%)	100	100
Minerals and Trace Elements		
Calcium (mg)	39–42	31–40
Calcium (mmol)	0.9–1	0.7–1
Chloride (mg)	69–76	76–127
Chloride (mmol)	1.9–2.1	2.1–3.6
Copper (mg)	37–85	107–111
Iodine (μg)	16	—
Iron (mg)	0.04–0.12	0.13–0.14
Magnesium (mg)	3.9–4.5	4.3–4.7
Magnesium (mmol)	0.16–0.18	0.17–0.2
Manganese (μg)	0.9	—
Phosphorus (mg)	22–25	20–23
Phosphorus (mmol)	0.7–0.9	0.6–0.7
Potassium (mg)	90–91	81–93
Potassium (mmol)	2.2–2.4	2.1–2.4
Sodium(mg)	37–43	44–77
Sodium (mmol)	1.6–1.9	1.9–3.3
Zinc(mg)	0.18–0.50	0.61–0.69
Vitamins		
Fat-soluble		
Vitamin A (IU)	155–333	72–357
Vitamin D (IU)	0.7–3.3	0.7–12
Vitamin E (IU)	0.45–0.75	0.42–1.42
Vitamin K (μg)	0.29–3	0.29–3
Water-soluble		
Vitamin B_6 (μg)	15–119	9–129
Vitamin B_{12} (μg)	0.01–1.2	0.01–0.07
Vitamin C (mg)	6.6–7.8	6.3–7.4
Biotin (μg)	0.01–1.2	0.01–1.2
Folic Acid (μg)	7.5–9	5–8.6
Niacin (mg)	0.2–0.25	0.24–0.3
Pantothenic acid (mg)	0.26	0.33
Riboflavin (μg)	15–104	14–79
Thiamin (μg)	3–31	1.4–31
Other (mg)		
Carnitine	1.04	—
Choline	13.4	10–13
Inositol	22.2–83.5	21.3

TABLE 14.6
Routes of Feeding Preterm Infants

Route	<34 weeks	>34 weeks
Per os	No	Yes
Continuous gastric	<1250 g	Failure to tolerate bolus gastric, significant GER
Bolus gastric (every 3 h)	>1250 g; infants <1250 g not tolerating continuous	Failure to tolerate per os
Transpyloric, continuous	Failure to tolerate gastric feeds, gastric distention due to positive pressure, poor gastric emptying	Same as <34 weeks

dogs, as little as 10% of the total daily intake, induced mature gastric motor patterns.[40] Advancement of the feeds by 20 ml/kg/day appears to be well tolerated by most preterm infants. Full-strength formula given slowly (over longer than 15 min) appears to induce the best duodenal motor response.[41]

SPECIAL CONSIDERATIONS

Essential Fatty Acids

Vegetable oils contain the parent essential fatty acids linoleic acid (18:2w-6) and, in most cases, alpha-linolenic acid (18:3w-3). Linoleic and linolenic acids serve as precursors for the synthesis of long-chain polyunsaturated fatty acids (LC-PUFA), including arachdonic (20:4w-6) and docosahexaenoic (22:6w-3) acids. Human milk lipids contain preformed LC-PUFA ; LC-PUFA are essential components of membrane systems and are incorporated in membrane-rich tissues such as the brain during early growth.[42,43] The fetus and the fully breast-fed infant do not depend on active synthesis of LC-PUFA since the placenta and human milk provide LC-PUFA in amounts considered appropriate.[44–47] Preterm birth halts the transfer of DHA and AA — 80% of which is transferred during the third trimester. Preterm infants have high cord blood levels of DHA, AA, and other LC-PUFA, but these levels decline rapidly.[48] Premature infants, fed with formulas without LC-PUFA, develop depletion of LC-PUFA in plasma and red cell membranes, indicating limited endogenous LC-PUFA synthesis.[49]

DHA and AA are important for growth and development and visual acuity. Addition of DHA and AA to preterm formulas leads to levels similar to human milk in North America. This can be achieved with DHA between 0.24 and 0.76% and AA between 0.32 and 1.1%[50] from single oils. Both are required for effective growth and development. Supplementation with DHA alone led to decreased growth in preterm infants in most studies.[51] Supplementation with the precursor ALA did not sustain DHA levels found in breast milk or confer the benefits on growth and visual acuity. Furthermore, ALA supplementation appeared to lower AA levels possibly secondary to competition between AA and DHA for precursor enzymes or the previously mentioned inability of preterm infants to synthesize DHA and AA from precursors.[52–54]

Early trials of DHA and AA supplementation did not show sustained, significant differences in weight, length, or head circumference in larger, healthy preterm infants,[55] but more recent studies including younger, sicker infants have shown improvement in growth.[50,56] DHA is found in large amounts in the retina in the photoreceptor outer segment. In studies of visual acuity, using Teller acuity cards or ERG or VEP, transient improvements in visual acuity were seen in infants fed the supplemented formula, but they were not sustained.[55,57] While some trials showed improvement in Bayley scores of infant development, others did not. A large, randomized, controlled trial by O'Connor et al.[57] in 2001 showed better vocabulary comprehension at 14 months. A recent review by Fleith and Clandinin[58] concurred that there was improvement in development, while a 2004 Cochrane review of the literature did not find benefit in supplementation.[55] DHA and AA supplementation appears to be safe, and blood levels equal to those in breast milk can be achieved. Large differences in numbers of patients studied, birth weights and gestational ages and doses of DHA and AA make comparisons between studies difficult.

Carnitine

Current parenteral nutrition regimens do not contain carnitine. Low plasma concentrations of carnitine and its decline with postnatal age has been demonstrated in infants receiving carnitine-free nutrition.[59,60] Although fatty acid metabolism has not been shown to be impaired in short-term parenteral nutrition, carnitine is an accepted additive for infants requiring parenteral nutrition for longer periods.[61–63] Carnitine is provided at doses of 8.0 to 20 mg/kg/d.

Glutamine

Glutamine is the most abundant amino acid in the human body and is the most important "nitrogen shuttle," accounting for 30 to 35% of all amino acid nitrogen transported in the blood.[64] Glutamine concentrations in blood and tissue fall following starvation, surgery, infection, and trauma.[65,66] In addition, glutamine plays an important role in protein and energy metabolism, nucleotide synthesis, and lymphocyte function.[67] Glutamine is known to be an important fuel for small intestinal enterocytes[68]; however, an absolute need of glutamine for gut growth has not been demonstrated with either detrimental or negligible effects reported in the literature.[69,70] A recent review of six randomized, controlled trials of glutamine supplementation in preterm infants did not show significant decreases in mortality and no significant effect on the incidence of NEC, sepsis, days to full feeds or length of hospitalization.[71]

Taurine

Taurine is considered to be an essential amino acid in preterm infants. Those premature infants fed with formulas enriched with the nutrient had better Bayley scores at 18 months than those fed with term formula without taurine.[72]

Donor Breast Milk

Most women are not able to supply enough breast milk to meet the needs of their growing premature infant, but they still recognize the benefits of human milk, including the prevention of NEC and late-onset sepsis. Donor milk banks grew out of this desire. There are drawbacks to donor human milk. Most of the supply is from women who delivered term infants and, therefore, is not adequate to meet the nutritional needs of a premature infant. In some studies, donor milk use led to slower growth.[39,73] The pasteurization process, while necessary to reduce unwanted bacteria, destroys important bioactive components of breast milk.[74] However, adequate amounts of LC-PUFA and cytokines are still present in pasteurized donor milk. A recent randomized trial using preterm donor milk did not find the expected decrease in NEC and late onset sepsis compared to preterm formula.[22]

POSTNATAL GROWTH

The plotting of growth, as alluded to earlier, facilitates the assessment of trends in growth. The intrauterine charts represent fetal growth; however, as has been described, most small preterm infants fall below the birth percentile and the 10th percentile. Thus, the need to address catch up growth and strategies to minimize postnatal weight loss. The postnatal charts reflect the initial weight loss, which occurs in the first week of life, and growth similar to the in utero counterpart once the infant returns to birth weight has been demonstrated.[7]

Despite the many questions that remain regarding optimal nutritional management of the neonate, it is nonetheless important to develop rational protocols for the management of nutritional issues that arise. This chapter has provided some guidelines and the framework from which these guidelines arose. There are numerous different approaches to feeding a neonate. The ultimate goal should be to optimize nutrition and hence growth and ultimately development in this ever-increasing population of premature infants.

REFERENCES

1. Hoyert, D.L., Mathews, T.J. et al. *Pediatrics* 117: 168; 2006.
2. Ballard, J.L., Novak, K.K. et al. *J Pediatr* 95(5 Pt 1): 769; 1979.
3. Alexander, G.R., de Caunes, F. et al. *Am J Obstet Gynecol* 166: 891; 1992.
4. Ballard, J.L., Khoury, J.C. et al. *J Pediatr* 119: 417; 1991.
5. Jeanty, P. *Fetal Biometry* 1996.
6. Widdowson, E.M. and Spray, C.M. *Arch Dis Child* 26: 205; 1951.
7. Ehrenkranz, R., Younes, A.N. et al. *Pediatrics* 104(2 Pt 1): 280; 1999.
8. Ziegler, E.E., O'Donnell, A.M. et al. *Growth* 40: 329; 1976.
9. Ziegler, E.E. *Clin Perinatol* 29: 225; 2002.
10. Weinstein, M.R., Oh W. *J Pediatr* 99: 958; 1981.
11. Billeaud C., Piedbouef B. et al. *J Pediatr* 120: 461; 1992.
12. Kashyap S., Hierd W.C. NCR (ed.), *Protein Metabolism during Infancy*, Räihä Niels, CR. 1994.
13. Rivera A., Jr., Bell E.F. et al. *J Pediatr* 115: 465; 1989.
14. Saini J., MacMahon P. et al. *Arch Dis Child* 64(10 Spec No): 1362; 1989.
15. Mitton, S.G., Garlick, P.J. *Pediatr Res* 32: 447 ; 1992.
16. van Lingen, R.A., van Goudoever, J.B. et al. *Clin Sci* (Lond) 82:199; 1992.
17. Van Goudoever, J.B., Sulkers, E.J. et al. *JPEN J Parenter Enteral Nutr* 18: 404; 1994.
18. Thureen, P.J., Melara, D. et al. *Pediatr Res* 53: 24; 2003.
19. Ibrahim, H.M., Jeroudi, M.A. et al. *J Perinatol* 24: 482; 2004.
20. te Braake, F.W., van den Akker, C.H. et al. *J Pediatr* 147: 457; 2005.
21. Zlotkin, S.H., Bryan, M.H. et al. *Am J Clin Nutr* 34: 914; 1981.

22. Haumont, D., Deckelbaum, R.J. et al. *J Pediatr* 115(5 Pt 1): 787 ; 1989.
23. Wu, P.Y., Edwards, N. et al. *J Pediatr* 109: 347; 1986.
24. Bartley, J.H., Nagy, S. et al. *J Perinatol* 25: 593; 2004.
25. Schanler, R.J., Lau, C. et al. *Pediatrics* 116: 400; 2005.
26. Widness, J.A., Seward, V.J. et al. *J Pediatr* 129: 680; 1996.
27. Shannon, K.M., Keith, J.F., 3rd et al. *Pediatrics* 95: 1; 1995.
28. Caple, J., Armentrout, D. et al. *Pediatrics* 114: 1597; 2004.
29. Berseth, C.L., Bisquera, J.A. et al. *Pediatrics* 111: 529; 2003.
30. Grant, J.P., Cox, C.E. et al. *Surg Gynecol Obstet* 145: 573; 1977.
31. Balistreri, W.F. Bove, K.E. *Prog Liver Dis* 9: 567; 1990.
32. Bhatia, J., M. Moslen, T. et al. *Pediatr Res* 33: 487; 1993.
33. Greer, F.R. *Acta Paediatr Suppl* 405: 20;1994.
34. Moro, G., Minoli, I. et al. *Acta Paediatr Scand* 73: 49; 1984.
35. Romero, G., Figueras, J. et al. *J Pediatr Gastroenterol Nutr* 38: 407; 2004.
36. Koenig, W.J., Amarnath, A.P. et al. *Pediatr* 95: 203; 1995.
37. Berseth, C.L. *Pediatr* 117: 777; 1990.
38. Berseth, C.L., Ittman, P.I. *J Pediatr Gastroenterol Nutr* 14: 182; 1992.
39. McGuire, W., Anthony, M.Y. *Arch Dis Child Fetal Neonatal Ed* 88: F11; 2003.
40. Owens, L., Burrin, D.G. et al. *J Nutr* 132: 2717; 2002.
41. Baker, J.H., Berseth, C.L. *Pediatr Res* 42: 618; 1997.
42. Clandinin, M.T., Chappell, J.E. et al. *Early Hum Dev* 4: 131; 1980.
43. Martinez, M., Ballabriga, A. *Lipids* 22:133; 1987.
44. Sanders, T.A., Naismith, D.J. *Proc Nutr Soc* 38: 94A; 1979.
45. Putnam, J.C., Carlson, S.E. et al. *Am J Clin Nutr* 36: 106; 1982.
46. Koletzko, B., Thiel, I. et al. *Eur J Clin Nutr* 46: S45; 1992.
47. Jensen, R. *The Lipids of Human Milk. Prog Lipid Res* 35: 53; 1996.
48. Carlson, S.E., Rhodes, P.G. et al. *Am J Clin Nutr* 44: 708; 1986.
49. Koletzko, B., Schmidt, E. et al. *Eur J Pediatr* 148: 669; 1989.
50. Clandinin, M.T., Van Aerde, J.E. et al. *J Pediatr* 146: 461; 2005.
51. Lapillone, A., Clarke, S.D. et al. *J Pediatr* 143(4 suppl): S9; 2003.
52. Jensen, C.L., Prager, T.C. et al. *J Pediatr* 131: 200; 1997.
53. Makrides, M., Neumann M.A. et al. *Am J Clin Nutr* 71: 120; 2000.
54. Udell, T., Gibson, R.A. et al. *Lipids* 40: 1; 2005.
55. Simmer, K., Patole, S. *Cochrane Database Syst Rev* (1): CD000375: 2004.
56. Groh-Wargo, S., Jacobs, J. et al. *Pediatr Res* 57(5 pt1): 712; 2005.
57. O'Connor, D.L., Hall, R. et al. *Pediatr* 108: 359; 2001.
58. Fleith, M., Clandinin, M.T. *Crit Rev Food Sci Nutr* 45: 205; 2005.
59. Penn, D., Schmidt-Summerfield, E. et al. *Early Hum Dev* 4: 23; 1979.
60. Shenai, J.P., Borum, P.R. *Pediatr Res* 18: 679; 1984.
61. Orzali, A., Donzelli, F. et al. *Biol Neonate* 43: 186; 1983.
62. Schmidt-Sommerfeld, E., Penn, D. et al. *J Pediatr* 102: 931; 1983.
63. Orzali, A., Maetzke, G. et al. *J Pediatr* 104: 436; 1984.
64. Souba, W.W. *JPEN J Parent Enteral Nutr* 11: 569; 1987.
65. Askanazi, J., Carpentier, Y.A. et al. *Ann Surg* 192: 78; 1980.
66. Roth, E., Funovics, J. et al. *Clin Nutr* 1: 25; 1982.
67. Neu, J., Shenoy, V. et al. *FASEB J* 10: 829; 1996.
68. Souba, W.W., Herskowitz, K. et al. *JPEN J Parent Enteral Nutr* 14: 458; 1990.
69. Burrin, D.G., Shulam, R.J. et al. *JPEN J Parent Enteral Nutr* 15: 262; 1991.
70. Vanderhoof, J.A., Blackwood, D.J. et al. *J Am Coll Nutr* 11: 223; 1992.
71. Tubman, T.R., Thompson, S.W. et al. *Cochrane Database Syst Rev* (1): CD001457; 2005.
72. Wharton, B.A., Morley, R. et al. *Arch Dis Child Fetal Neonatal Ed* 89: F497; 2004.
73. Wight, N.E. *J Perinatol* 21: 249; 2001.
74. Liebhaber, M., Lewiston, N.J. et al. *J Pediatr* 91: 897; 1977.

15 Feeding the Term Infant

Yvette Gamble, Chantrapa Bunyapen, and Jatinder Bhatia

CONTENTS

Growth, particularly in weight, length, and additional anthropometric measurements, remains a measure of adequacy of nutritional regimens for the growing infant and child. Infant feeding decisions have an impact on lifelong medical illnesses, growth, and developmental abilities well beyond infancy. This chapter will review normal growth and nutrient requirements in healthy term infants.

GROWTH

The average weight of a healthy term infant is 3.5 kg. With an anticipated loss of 10% in body weight in the first week of life, birth weight is regained by two weeks of age in both breast-fed and formula-fed infants, with the formula-fed infants demonstrating a tendency to regain birth weight sooner than their breast-fed counterparts.

Mean weight and selected centiles for weight are summarized in Table 15.1. In clinical practice, however, weight and other anthropometric measurements including length, head circumference, and weight for length are plotted on growth charts (Figure 15.1 and Figure 15.2) adapted from Hamill et al.[1] The plotting of growth on these charts will suffice for monitoring of normal infants; however, a different and more sensitive approach will be needed for infants with faltering growth. The "reference data" provided by Fomon[2] combine data from the University of Iowa and the Fels Longitudinal Study, the latter data used in the growth charts. Current growth charts may be replaced in the future by the World Health Organization (WHO) growth curves generated from an "international" rather than national cross-sectional standard.

A variety of other measures to define growth include skin fold thickness, limb length and circumference, and body mass index (BMI). The latter, BMI, is calculated by dividing the weight in kilograms by the square of the length in meters, replacing weight for length in older children. BMI is becoming an increasingly important parameter to track given the explosion of obesity and/or overweight in the pediatric population, especially among non-Hispanic Black and Mexican-American adolescents.[3]

Normal growth is a strong indicator of nutritional sufficiency and overall health of an infant. Since infancy is a period of rapid growth, particularly early infancy, identifying growth failure is important and requires prompt medical attention. As we

TABLE 15.1
Mean Body Weight and Selected Centiles for Males and Females, 0 to 12 Months of Age

Age (Months)	Mean (g)	5th Centile (g)	50th Centile (g)	95th Centile (g)
Mean body weight and selected centiles for males, 0 to 12 months of age				
Birth	3,350	2,685	3,530	4,225
1	4,445	3,640	4,448	5,238
2	5,519	4,574	5,491	6,475
3	6,326	5,321	6,323	7,393
6	7,927	6,670	7,877	9,146
9	9,087	7,785	9,008	10,448
12	10,059	8,606	9,978	11,676
Mean body weight and selected centiles for females, 0 to 12 months of age				
Birth	3,367	2,750	3,345	4,095
1	4,160	3,548	4,123	4,885
2	5,049	4,301	5,009	5,878
3	5,763	4,837	5,729	6,712
6	7,288	6,063	7,239	8,547
9	8,449	7,072	8,373	9,723
12	9,425	7,942	9,362	10,863

Source: Modified from Fomon, S. J., Nelson, S. E. In *Nutrition of Normal Infants*, (Mosby, C. V., Ed.), 1993, 36, p. 155.

understand more about the complex interactions between genetic, immunologic, metabolic, physiologic, and psychologic factors and their effects on long-term outcomes of infant feeding decisions, defining appropriate growth becomes a very important issue for health care providers of children.

ENERGY

Energy requirements during infancy may be partitioned into basal metabolism, thermic effect of feeding, thermoregulation, physical activity, and growth. The energy requirements for growth relative to maintenance, except in early infancy, are small, and satisfactory growth can be considered a sensitive indicator that energy requirements are being met. Energy balance may be defined as

gross energy intake = energy excreted + energy expended + energy stored.

Gross energy intake, measured by the heat of combustion, is greater than energy available when fed because most foods are not completely digested and protein oxidation is incomplete. Fat absorption varies widely among infants fed various formulas, particularly in infancy. Urea and other nitrogenous compounds are excreted in the urine. Gross energy intake is calculated as 5.7, 9.4, and 4.1 kcal/g obtained from protein, fat, and carbohydrate, respectively, and therefore it varies given the type of diet. The term "digestible energy" refers to gross energy intake minus energy excreted in the feces. Metabolizable energy is defined as digestible energy minus energy lost in urine. The metabolizable energy values for protein, fat, and carbohydrate are close to 4, 9, and 4 kcal/g, respectively. Losses of energy, other than via feces and urine, are negligible and are ignored for practical purposes.

The energy intake of normal infants per unit body weight is much greater than in adult counterparts. Energy requirements for term infants have been estimated by various groups and vary from 100 to 116 kcal/kg/day from 0 to 3 months and decline to about 100 kcal/kg/day by the end of the first year.[4–8] These recommendations are based on the median intake of thriving infants; the intakes of breast-fed infants are lower than that of formula-fed infants, with an average of 3 to 4% lower in the first 3 months and 6 to 7% from 3 to 6 months. As new, more precise estimates of energy expenditure become available, these recommendations are apt to change, given that current recommendations are higher than the "gold" standard — the breast-fed infant. Energy intakes of infants from 6 to 12 months of age have been reported to be between 91 and 100 kcal/kg/day.[9–11]

PROTEIN

Intakes of protein and essential amino acids are generally sufficient in developed countries, in contrast to developing countries, where protein and protein-energy malnutrition are still a frequent occurrence. In appropriately fed infants, protein is not a

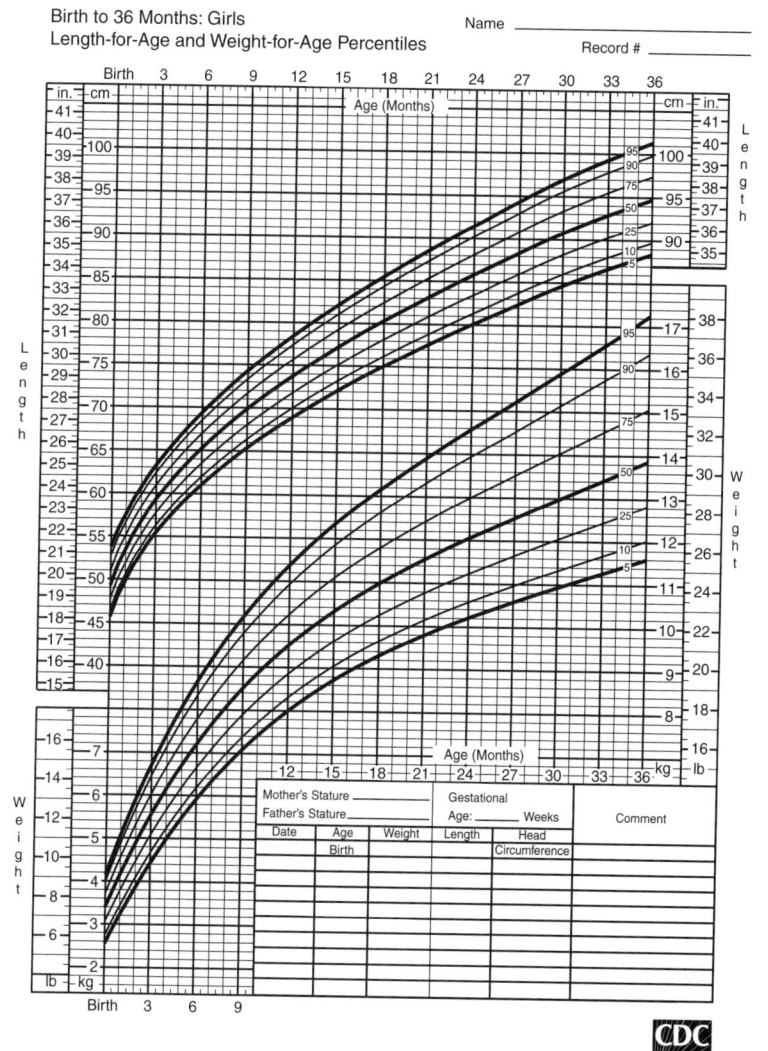

Birth to 36 Months: Girls
Length-for-Age and Weight-for-Age Percentiles

Name _____
Record # _____

FIGURE 15.1 Physical growth of girls, birth to 36 months, according to National Center for Health Statistics percentiles. (Published May 30, 2000 (modified 4/20/01). Developed by the National Center for Health Statics in Collaboration with the National Center for Chronic Disease Prevention and Health Promotion (2000). http://www.cdc.gov/growthcharts

limiting dietary component in infancy and is clearly essential for normal growth and development. For the human infant, histidine, isoleucine, leucine, lysine, methionine, phenylalanine, threonine, tryptophan, and valine are considered essential amino acids. The data for cysteine are conflicting[12,13] for the term infant, although the data are clear for the preterm infant. Conditionally essential amino acids are those that become essential under certain circumstances as they may be produced in inadequate amounts endogenously. An example of this is taurine, which is now added to formulas based on reports of greater concentrations of taurine in the plasma and urine of preterm[14,15] and term[16] infants. The concern about taurine depletion stems from the observations of growth retardation, abnormal retinal findings, and impaired bile acid metabolism in taurine-deficient animals and humans.

Recommended dietary intakes of protein are summarized in Table 15.2. In contrast, intakes recommended by WHO[17] are 2.25, 1.86, 1.65, and 1.48 g/100 kcal from 1 to 2, 3 to 6, 6 to 9, and 9 to 12 months, respectively. Both of these recommendations are generally higher than the intakes observed in human milk-fed infants.

FAT

The importance of dietary fat is underscored by the fact that 35% of the weight gain of an infant in early infancy is accounted for by fat.[18] Most of the dietary fat is in the form of triglyceride formed by three fatty acids esterified to a glycerol backbone. In the body, triglycerides are the main form of storage and transport of fatty acids. Phospholipids and cholesterol are indispensable components of the lipid bilayer of all cell membranes, and the amount of different phospholipids and cholesterol, as well as the

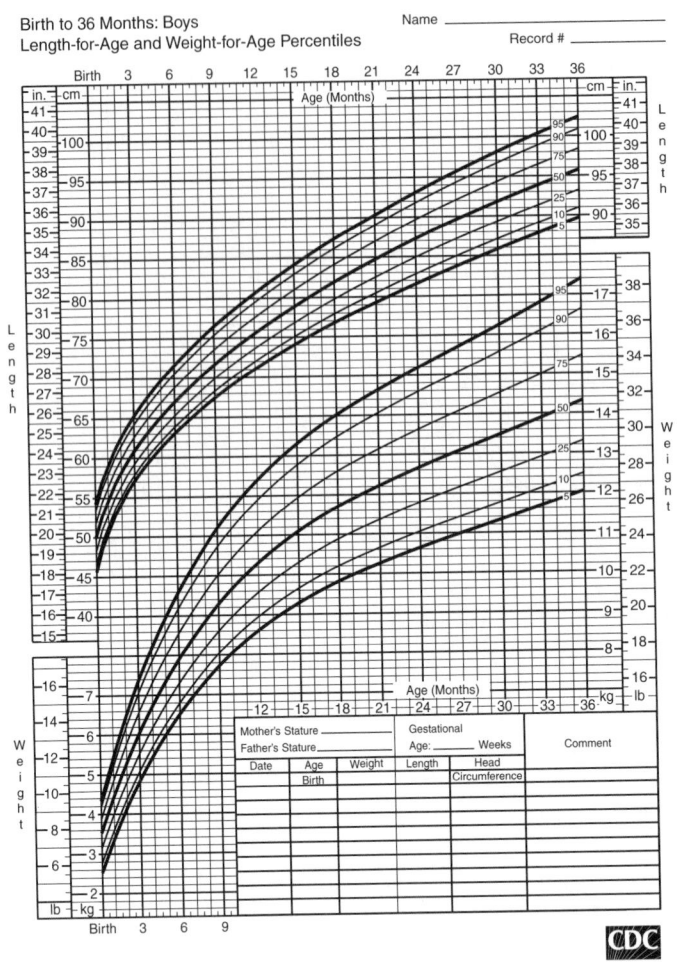

FIGURE 15.2 Physical growth of boys, birth to 36 months, according to National Center for Health Statistics percentiles. (Published May 30, 2000 (modified 4/20/01). Developed by the National Center for Health Statics in Collaboration with the National Center for Chronic Disease Prevention and Health Promotion (2000). http://www.cdc.gov/growthcharts

TABLE 15.2
Recommended Dietary Intakes of Protein

	Recommended Dietary Intake	
Age Interval (Months)	(g/kg/Day)	(g/100 kcal)
0–1	2.6	2.2
1–2	2.2	2.0
2–3	1.8	1.8
3–4	1.5	1.6
4–5	1.4	1.6
5–6	1.4	1.6
6–9	1.4	1.5
9–12	1.3	1.5

Source: Reproduced with permission from Fomon, S. J. *Pediatric Research* 30: 391; 1991.

fatty acid pattern of incorporated phospholipids, modulate membrane fluidity, permeability, enzyme and receptor activity, and signal transduction. Cholesterol is required for the synthesis of steroids and bile acids, although the majority of the cholesterol pool in tissue and plasma is derived from endogenous synthesis; dietary cholesterol contributes to the pool, and diet modifies liver synthesis.[19] Fatty acids (4 to 26 carbon atoms) are either saturated (no double bonds in the carbon chain), monounsaturated (one double bond), or polyunsaturated (two or more double bonds). Double bonds occur in two isomeric forms: *cis* and *trans*; unsaturated fatty acids are folded at the site of each double bond, *cis*- and *trans*-fatty acids have straight carbon chains.

Human milk contains approximately 4% lipids, but the reported variation is between 3.1% and 5.2% [20,21] with 99% of the fat present in the form of triglycerides and the rest in the form of diglycerides, monoglycerides, free fatty acids, phospholipids, and cholesterol. The fat content of human milk increases with duration of lactation.[20,22] During this period, the average size of the fat globules increases and the ratio of phospholipids and cholesterol to triglycerides decreases.[23] The concentration of fat in human milk remains similar regardless of maternal diet or nutritional status, although poor nutrition has been shown to decrease fat content.[24] Fatty acid content of human milk has been reported by numerous investigators and demonstrates a wide range, as summarized by Fomon.[2] Fatty acid content of human milk is also altered by dietary manipulation.[25–28] Human milk fat provides the essential fatty acids linoleic and α-linolenic acids, along with the long-chain polyunsaturated fatty acids such as arachidonic (ARA) and docosahexaenoic (DHA) acids. The latter are now routinely added to all infant formulas but vary in concentration depending on the manufacturer. The decrease of milk phospholipid content during the first few weeks after birth is accompanied by a decrease in ARA and DHA.[29] Fat content of human milk and commonly used formulas is summarized in Table 15.3.

ESSENTIAL FATTY ACID METABOLISM

Human milk lipids contain preformed long-chain polyunsaturated fatty acids (LC-PUFA) in considerable amounts, whereas vegetable oils (with the exception of coconut oil) are also rich in PUFA. The latter has a higher percentage of medium- and short-chain fatty acids.

For the healthy full-term infant, the concerns of the premature infant may not apply given the larger body stores of LC-PUFA at birth and the lower requirements compared with the preterm infant because of slower growth. However, nutritional requirements for PUFAs are not clearly defined for infants, and the issue is complicated by the fact that linoleic acid ($18:2n-6$) and α-linolenic acid ($18:3n-3$) can be converted to both 20- and 22-carbon-length long-chain PUFAs with significant biological activities. The absence of linoleic acid from the diet results in growth retardation and dermatologic manifestations. Intakes of linoleic acid, as low as 0.6% of daily energy intake, can obviate essential fatty acid deficiency as defined by the triene-to-tetraene ratio, and current recommendations[30] specify a minimum level of 0.3 g/100 kcal in infant formulas. During the first postnatal year, there is a rapid accretion of ARA and DHA in the brain, DHA in retina, and ARA in the whole body in infants fed human milk.[31] In order to achieve similar results in formula-fed term infants, both DHA and ARA have to be provided in formulas. SanGiovanni et al.[32] demonstrated a significant overall advantage in visual acuity during the first 2 to 4 months of life for LC-PUFA-supplemented groups of term infants compared with those not supplemented by LC-PUFA. Similar results were observed by Birch et al.,[33] who observed a benefit in visual acuity development for the first year of life in infants fed LC-PUFA formulas compared with infants fed standard formulas. The developmental outcome of these infants also showed significantly better scores on the Bayley Mental Development Index II.[34] However, results of studies assessing development are variable.[35] Improved developmental scores at 18 months of age have been reported, but less than half of the studies reviewed showed beneficial effects on visual, mental, or psychomotor functions.[35] The addition of LC-PUFA to infant formulas is safe with no negative effects reported, and blood LC-PUFA status is similar to that of breast-fed infants.[35]

Fully breast-fed infants have a dietary lipid intake of approximately 50% of their energy intake (3.1 to 5.2 g/dl; see earlier discussion), whereas formulas contain between 3.4 and 3.8 g/dl. Although the importance of limiting the dietary intake of saturated and total fats to prevent cardiovascular disease, obesity, and diabetes is well recognized, adverse effects of limiting fat on weight gain and growth[36,37] should be balanced against providing increased amounts of fat.

CARBOHYDRATE

Carbohydrates generally account for 35% to 42% of the energy intake of breast- or formula-fed infants, and the usual carbohydrates in infants' diets are listed in Table 15.4. Carbohydrates may be classified as monosaccharides, oligosaccharides, and polysaccharides. Monosaccharides can be further defined as aldoses (glucose, galactose, and xylose for example) or ketoses (fructose). Oligosaccharides are consumed in the diet mainly in milk with lactose, maltose, and sucrose being the main sugars present. Polysaccharides are starches, starch hydrolysates, glycogen, or components of fiber. The major carbohydrate in human milk is lactose, although small amounts of glucose and other oligosaccharides are also present. Carbohydrate content of human milk and various formulas is listed in Table 15.3. Carbohydrate malabsorption, apart from genetic causes, is unusual. When the colonic capacity to ferment carbohydrate is exceeded by the unabsorbed load, symptoms of carbohydrate intolerance, usually in the form of diarrhea, occur. The diarrhea improves when dietary carbohydrates are reduced or eliminated from the diet, making the diagnosis of carbohydrate intolerance. Normally, electrolytes in the distal gastrointestinal tract and unabsorbed carbohydrates (fermented to volatile fatty acids) are rapidly absorbed. Inadequate colonic salvage results in diarrhea. In young infants and children with disorders of carbohydrate metabolism, the ultimate goal of carbohydrate digestion and absorption is to render all available carbohydrates into smaller compounds that the body can use — chiefly, glucose and fructose. Lactase deficiency is exceedingly rare in newborn infants. Infants usually develop diet-induced diarrhea following introduction of lactose-containing milk. The disease, thought to be autosomal recessive, is treated with the elimination or limitation of lactose in the diet. More commonly, transient lactose intolerance can occur after acute or repeated bouts of diarrhea. Sucrase-isomaltase deficiency is a rare disease that does not appear until diets containing sucrose, dextrin, or starch are begun. Bouts of diarrhea may be observed

TABLE 15.3
Notification Composition Of Human Milk And Commodity Used Formulas

	Kilocalories/oz	Protein Source gm/dL	Fat Source gm/dL	Carbohydrate Source gm/dL	Na mg/dL	K mg/dL	Phosphorus mg/dL	Calcium mg/dL	Osmolality mOsm/kg Water
Mature Human milk	20	Human milk (1.0)	Human milk (3.9)	Lactose (7.2)	8	52.5	14	32	290
Enfamil Lipil (Mead Johnson)	20	Reduced minerals whey, nonfat milk (1.4)	Plam olein, soy, coconut, high oeic sunflower oils, DHA, ARA (3.6)	Lactose (7.4)	18.3	73	29	53	300
Enfamil AR Lipil (Mead Johnson)	20	Nonfat milk (1.7)	Palm olein, soy, cononut, high oleic sunflower oils, DHA, ARA (3.4)	Lactose, rice starch, maltodextrin (7.4)	27	73	36	53	240
Enfamil Gentlease Lipil (Mead Johnson)	20	Partially Hydrolyzed nonfat milk, whey protein concentrate (1.6)	Palm olein, soy, cononut, high oleic sunflower oils, DHA, ARA (3.6)	Corn syrup solids, lactose (7.3)	22	73	31	55	220
Enfamil Lactofree Lipil (Mead Hohnson)	20	Milk protein isolate (1.4)	Palm olein, soy, coconut, high oleic sunflower oils, DHA, ARA (3.6)	Corn syrup solids (7.4)	20	74	31	55	200
Enfamil Pregestimil Lipil (mead Johnson)	20	Casein hydrolysate with added amino acids (1.9)	MCT, corn, soy, high oleic safflower oils (3.8)	Corn syrup solids, modified cornstarch, dextrose (6.9)	32	74	35	64	230
Enfamil Nutramigen Lipil (Mead Jonson)	20	Casein hydrolysate with added amino acids (1.9)	Palm oein, soy, coconut, high oleic sunflower oils, DHA, ARA (3.6)	Corn syrup solids, modified cornstarch (7)	32	74	35	64	320
Enfamil ProSobee Lipil(Mead Johnson)	20	Soy protein isolate, L-methionine (1.7)	Palm olein, soy, coconut, high oleic sunflower oils, DHA, ARA (3.6)	Corn syrup solids, modified cornstarch (7.2)	24	81	47	71	200
Similac Advance (Ross)	20	Nonfat milk, whey protein concentrate (1.4)	High oleic safflower, soy, coconut oils, DHA, ARA (3.7)	Lactose (7.3)	16.3	71	28	53	300
Similac Lactose Free Advance (Ross)	20	Milk protein isolate (1.4)	High oleic safflower, soy, coconut oils, DHA, ARA (3.7)	Maltodextrin, sucrose (7.2)	20.3	72	38	57	200
Similac Isomil Advance (Ross)	20	Soy protein isolate, L-methionine (1.7)	High oleic safflower, soy, coconut oils, DHA, ARA (3.7)	Corn syrup, sucrose (7.0)	30	73	51	71	200
Similac Isomil DF (Ross)	20	Soy protein isolate, L-methionine (1.8)	Soy, coconut oils (3.7)	Corn syrup, sucrose (6.8)	30	73	51	71	240
Similac Alimentum Advance(Ross)	20	Casein hydrolysate, cystine, tyrosine, tryptophan (1.9)	Safflower, MCT, soy oils, DHA, ARA (3.7)	Sucrose, modified tapioca starch (7.0)	30	80	51	71	370
Carnation Good Start(Nestle)	20	Enzymatically hydrolyzed reduced mineral whey (1.6)	Palm olein, soybean, coconut, high oleic safflower oils (3.4)	Lactose, maltodextrin (7.4)	16	65	24	43	265
Carnation Alsoy (Nestle)	20	Soy protein isolate (1.9)	Palm olein, soy, coconut, high oleic safflower oils (3.4)	Corn, maltodextrins, sucrose (7.5)	23	86	41	71	296

TABLE 15.4
Usual Carbohydrates and
Related Enzymes

Carbohydrate	Enzyme
Lactose	Lactase
Sucrose	Sucrase-isomaltase
Isomaltose	Sucrase-isomaltase
Maltose	Maltase-glucoamylase
Amylose	α-Amylase
Amylopectin	β-Amylase

TABLE 15.5
Commonly Used Formulas and their Indications

Formula	Carbohydrate	Protein	Fat	Indication
Bovine milk based	Lactose	Bovine whey and casein	Vegetable, animal	Normal function
Soy-protein-based	Sucrose, glucose	Soy	Soy	Lactose intolerance, vegetarian, galactosemia (RARE)
Hydrolyzed protein	Sucrose, glucose	Hydrolyzed whey or casein	Medium chain triglycerides	Cow milk and soy protein hypersensitivity, pancreatic insufficiency, history of allergy in sibling and/or parents
Casein-based (modular)	Modified tapioca starch, added carbohydrate	Casein hydrolysate with added amino acids	MCT oil, corn oil	Lactase, sucrose, and maltase deficiency, impaired glucose transport
Elemental	Lactose- and sucrose-free, corn syrup solids, modified corn starch	Hydrolyzed casein	Vegetable	Cow milk allergy
"Metabolic"	Depends on condition	Corn syrup solids/sucrose	Corn oil/coconut oil	Specific metabolic disorders

in infants with this deficiency, and management includes eliminating sucrose and limiting starch in the diet. Older affected children and adults usually tolerate normal quantities of carbohydrates. Glucose-galactose deficiency manifests itself with diet-induced diarrhea soon after birth and responds to withdrawal of these carbohydrates from the diet. The defect appears to be a specific absence of glucose and galactose transport mechanisms, whereas amino acid transport is normal. Fructose transport is normal, and these infants respond to a diet containing fructose with relief from diarrhea. With age, variable amounts of starch and milk may be tolerated. Commonly used formulas for various forms of intolerance are listed in Table 15.5.[38]

IRON

Iron deficiency is the most common nutritional deficiency in the United States and worldwide, with young children being the most susceptible. The increased susceptibility comes from an increased iron requirement for the rapid growth during this period and inadequate amounts of iron in the diet unless adequately supplemented.[39] One of the U.S. Department of Health and Human Services' national health objective is to reduce iron deficiency in infants, children, and adolescents by 3 to 4 percentage points.[40] The estimated prevalence of iron deficiency is greatest among toddlers aged 1 to 2 years (7%).[41] According to the Centers for Disease Control and Prevention, iron deficiency remains 2 to 5 percentage points above the 2010 national health objectives.[41] To prevent iron deficiency, infants and toddlers should eat iron-rich foods and breast-feed or use iron-fortified formulas.[42] The stages of iron nutritional status are listed in Table 15.6.

One should distinguish between anemia and iron deficiency anemia, as the latter occurs when hemoglobin concentration falls below the 90% to 95% range for the same age and sex.[43] A diagnosis of iron deficiency is made when the anemia is accompanied by evidence of iron deficiency or when there is a rise in hemoglobin following treatment with iron. In this regard, serum transferrin receptor may offer an advantage for screening for iron deficiency because it rises with iron deficiency and is not affected by infection or acute liver disease.[44]

Iron deficiency peaks between 6 and 9 months of age and is a consequence of multiple factors: rapid growth, depleted stores, low iron content of the diet, and early feeding of cow's milk.[45,46] Because a milk-based diet is the predominant

TABLE 15.6
Stages of Iron Deficiency

Iron Nutritional Status	Indices
Adequate stores	Normal
Decreased stores	Ferritin (10 to 20 ng/ml) decreased, transferrin normal, erythrocyte protoporphyrin normal, MCV normal, hemoglobin normal, transferrin receptor normal
Iron deficiency	Ferritin decreased, transferrin saturation decreased, erythrocyte protoporphyrin increased, MCV normal, hemoglobin normal, transferrin receptor increased
Iron deficiency anemia	Ferritin decreased, transferrin saturation decreased, erythrocyte protoporphyrin increased, MCV decreased, hemoglobin decreased, transferrin receptor increased

source of energy, at least in the first 6 months of life, the iron content and its bioavailability are strong predictors of iron nutritional status.[47] The estimated requirement of absorbed iron from birth to 1 year is 0.55 to 0.75 mg/day, thereby underscoring the need for adequate iron in the diet to meet these needs. Iron concentration in human milk is low (0.3 to 0.5 mg/l), and although well absorbed, iron content declines between 14 and 183 days of age.[48] Therefore, even given the better absorption as milk intake increases and iron content decreases, it is easy to see that the amount of absorbed iron will be inadequate to meet the estimated requirements. Therefore, breast-fed infants who do not receive iron supplements or iron from other sources are at risk of becoming iron deficient between 6 and 12 months of age.[49] Iron-fortified cow's milk or soy-based formulas are effective in preventing iron deficiency, and the decline in iron deficiency anemia over the past few decades has been attributed to their use.[43] Systemic manifestations of iron deficiency anemia include behavioral and cognitive abnormalities expressed as lower scores on tests of psychomotor development. These effects have to be interpreted keeping the confounding variables of poor nutrition, environment, and poor socioeconomic background that often coexist. Studies suggest that infants with iron deficiency anemia, but not iron deficiency without anemia, have impaired performance of mental and psychomotor development.[50–54] These deficiencies do not improve with iron therapy, and follow-up studies at 5 to 6 years of age still demonstrate poorer scores in the children who were previously anemic.[52,53] Strategies to prevent iron deficiency could include the feeding of iron-fortified formulas, avoidance of non-iron-fortified milks and cow's milk (the latter, at least, till beyond 12 months of age), the feeding of meats and iron-fortified foods, and, if needed, medicinal iron supplementation in the form of ferrous sulfate.

BREAST-FEEDING

The benefits of breast-feeding to the infant, mother, family, and society are numerous and impressive, but they must be put into context when making individual decisions about breast-feeding. These include ready availability, possible enhancement of intestinal development, resistance to infection, and bonding between mother and infant. It is the preferred feeding method for the normal infant. Breast milk, in addition to providing the required nutrients for the healthy infant, has unique constituents, as listed in Table 15.7.

PROTEIN

Approximately 20% of the total nitrogen in human milk is in the form of nonprotein nitrogen compounds, such as free amino acids, and urea, which is considerably greater than the 5% found in bovine milk,[55] although there remains a debate about their contribution to nitrogen utilization.[56] The quality of the protein differs from that of bovine milk as well, with the whey-to-casein-protein ratios being 70:30 and 18:82 in human and bovine milk, respectively. These differences in whey-to-casein ratio are reflected in the plasma amino acid profile of infants and are readily observed within the first 3 days of age.[57] Further, plasma amino acid patterns in human-milk-fed infants has been used as a reference in infant nutrition.[58,59] In addition, specific human whey proteins — lactoferrin, lysozyme, and sIgA — are involved in host defense.[60,61]

LIPIDS

Lipids in human milk provide 40 to 50% of the energy content and are vehicles for fat soluble vitamins. The total fat content varies from 2% in colostrum to 2.5 to 3.0% in transitional milk, and 3.5 to 4.5% in mature human milk.[20] Cholesterol, phospholipids, and essential fatty acids are highest in colostrum, and more than 98% of human milk fat comes from 11 major fatty acids of 10- to 20-carbon length. Human milk lipids can inactivate enveloped viruses including herpes simplex I, measles, and cytomegalovirus, to name a few. Monoglycerides also exert antiviral activity.

TABLE 15.7
Unique Constituents of Breast Milk

Constituent	Function
Docosahexanoic acid	Necessary for growth and development of the brain and retina and for myelinization of nervous tissue
Cholesterol	Enhances myelinization of nervous tissue
Taurine	Second most abundant amino acid in human milk, important for bile acid conjugation
Choline	May enhance memory
Enzymes	Numerous enzymes such as lipases that are important in digestion and absorption of fat
Lactoferrin	Prevents iron from being available to bacteria
Inositol	Enhances synthesis and secretion of surfactant in immature lung tissue
Poly- and oligosaccharides	Inhibit bacterial binding to mucosal surfaces
Protein (α-lactalbumin)	Supply amino acids to the infant, help synthesize lactose in the mammary gland, and bind calcium and zinc
Bifidobacterium species	Predominant bacterial flora in the gastrointestinal tract of breast-fed infants, creates unfavorable pH conditions for the growth of enteric pathogens
Macrophages	Macrophages in human colostrum have high concentrations of sIgA, which is released during phagocytosis
Epidermal growth factor	Promotes cell proliferation in the gastrointestinal mucosa

Fat content of human milk is variable, with the fat content rising throughout lactation but with changes apparent within the course of one day, within feeds, and between women.[62] The effects of these differences in thriving infants is not clear, even given that hind milk has a higher fat content than fore milk. Human milk lipids provide preformed LC-PUFAs in amounts sufficient to meet nutrient needs. In term infants, plasma concentrations of DHA and ARA at 2 and 4 weeks of age were significantly lower in infants fed formula without LC-PUFA compared with breast-fed infants. DHA concentrations were similarly lower at 4 and 8 weeks of age. Neuringer and colleagues showed that visual acuity and learning abilities correlate well with the amount of DHA in the retina and brain phospholipids.[63]

NUCLEOTIDES

Nucleotides represent 2% to 5% of the nonprotein nitrogen in human milk.[64] Nucleotides participate in many biological functions such as forming the basis of genetic information (DNA, RNA) and storing energy (AMP, GMP), and they play roles in immunity as well as cellular activities. Although they can be produced by the liver, the body's requirements vary considerably, especially during infancy.[65] The effect of nucleotides on immune function is not well understood, but infants fed breast milk or nucleotide-supplemented formula have been shown to exhibit increased natural killer cell activity compared with infants fed formulas that are not supplemented.[66] Infants fed nucleotide formulas had enhanced haemophilus influenza type B and diphtheria humoral responses compared with infants fed formulas that are not supplemented.[67] Feeding of human milk resulted in significantly higher neutralizing antibody titers to polio virus at 6 months of age than were found in control or formula-fed cohorts. These data suggest that dietary factors play a role in the antibody response to immunization, and more studies are needed to better understand the mechanisms involved.

INFECTION

There are several enzymes present in human milk that appear to be important in the prevention of infection. These include glutathione peroxidase, alkaline phosphatase, and xanthine oxidase. In addition, other anti-inflammatory agents such as catalase, lactoferrin, immunoglobulins, and lysozyme are also present in human milk. The antimicrobial activities of these are generally found at mucosal surfaces, such as the gastrointestinal, urinary, and respiratory tracts. Specific factors, such as lactoferrin, lysozyme, and sIgA, resist proteolytic degradation and can line the mucosal surfaces, preventing microbial attachment and inhibiting microbial activity. Each of the mammary immune systems is active against a variety of antigens. Prospective studies in developing countries indicate that breast-milk-feeding reduces the incidence or severity of diarrhea,[68] lower-respiratory-tract infection,[69] otitis media,[70] bacteremia,[71] bacterial meningitis,[72] botulism,[73] urinary tract infection,[74] and necrotizing enterocolitis.[75]

Hyperbilirubinemia is more common in breast-fed than formula-fed infants. This is usually transient, and discontinuation of breast-feeding is not recommended unless bilirubin values reach excessively high levels or jaundice persists. Usually, switching to a formula for 1 to 2 days is therapeutic and diagnostic, and breast-feeding can be safely resumed. Other causes of jaundice should be sought before making a firm diagnosis of breast-milk jaundice.

Certain chemicals, drugs, foreign proteins, and viruses may be present in human milk.[76] However, the risk–benefit ratio of artificial milk needs to be weighed, especially if the water sources for mixing the milk are contaminated. Breast-feeding is currently contraindicated in disease states such as active herpes, tuberculosis, and AIDS.

FORMULA FEEDING

A variety of formulas are available for feeding infants (Table 15.3). The most commonly used formulas are from bovine milk, and nutrient specifications for infant formulas are available.[77] Commercially available formulas are recommended when breast-feeding is not chosen. Cow's milk is not recommended in the first year of life because of its nutritional limitations and inappropriate nutrient concentrations. Cow's milk has higher concentrations of protein and phosphorus, a lower calcium-to-phosphorus ratio, limited iron, less essential fatty acids, vitamin C, and zinc than human milk. Increased renal solute load due to cow's milk and increased occult blood loss via the gastrointestinal tract leading to iron deficiency and anemia in infants fed cow's milk not supplemented by other nutrients are additional reasons to discourage the feeding of cow's milk in early infancy.

HYDROLYZED INFANT FORMULAS

Hydrolyzed formulas have been used for the treatment of food allergies and intolerances and for the prevention of atopic disease in high-risk infants. The use of a hydrolyzed infant formula when compared with a cow's milk formula in infants who are not exclusively breast-fed reduces allergies.[78] There is no evidence, however, to support the use of a hydrolyzed formula to prevent allergy in preference to exclusive breast-feeding. Although many infants with atopy do not have a family history,[79–81] a positive family history in one or both parents still remains the most useful method of identifying allergy-prone infants.[82] Hydrolyzed formulas are cow's milk proteins that are subjected to chemical and enzymatic hydrolysis to reduce the molecular weight, the peptide size, and consequently, the allergenicity of the proteins. They are either extensively hydrolyzed casein (molecular weights <3,000 Da) or partially hydrolyzed whey (3,000 to 10,000 Da).

The American Academy of Pediatrics (AAP),[82] the European Society for Paediatric Allergology and Clinical Immunology,[83] and the European Society for Paediatric Gastroenterology, Hepatology and Nutrition[83] recommend extensively hydrolyzed formulas for allergy treatment in high-risk infants — they acknowledge a potential role for partially hydrolyzed formulas in the primary prevention of atopic disease. The German Infant Nutritional Intervention Study[84] found a significantly lower incidence of atopic dermatitis in infants fed partially and extensively hydrolyzed formulas when compared with cow milk formulas at 12 months of age. A recent literature review[85] showed no significant difference in allergy incidence in infancy of partially and extensively hydrolyzed formulas.

SOY-PROTEIN-BASED FORMULAS

The Committee on Nutrition of the AAP reviewed the indications of soy-protein-based formulas.[86] Some of the conclusions include:

1. Isolated soy-protein-based formulas are safe and effective alternatives to provide appropriate nutrition if breast milk or cow-milk-based formulas do not meet the nutritional needs in term infants. However, no advantage is provided over cow-milk-protein-based formulas as a supplement for breast-feeding.
2. Soy-protein-based formulas are appropriate for use in infants with galactosemia and hereditary lactase deficiency.
3. There is no proven value of the routine use of soy-protein-based formula in the prevention or management of infantile colic.
4. There is no proven value of the routine use of soy-protein-based formula in the prevention of atopic disease in healthy or at-risk infants.
5. Infants with documented cow-milk-protein-induced enteropathy or enterocolitis should not be given soy-protein-based formula routinely.

The nutritional needs of infants aged 0 to 6 months can be met by breast milk or infant formulas. Although both groups of infants need to have health surveillance including growth and development, breast-fed infants need to be followed up closely over the first few weeks to assure appropriate feeding practices and resultant growth. Appropriate counseling for common breast-feeding problems needs to be provided, and community support groups can be involved if needed. Beyond 6 months, recommendations for infant feeding are variable, and the recommendations are largely based on extrapolation from data on younger infants. Nutritional composition of "follow-up" formulas is specified with minimum lower limits for energy (60 kcal/dl), higher minimum limits for protein (2.25 to 3.0 g/100 kcal), and lower minimum limits for fat (3.0 to 4.0 g/100 kcal) compared with formulas for younger infants. Nonetheless, iron-fortified formulas designed for younger infants may be safely fed from

6 to 12 months. Infants by this age are physiologically and developmentally ready to accept a variety of dietary items, and feeding practices vary based on ethnic, cultural, and economic reasons. As stated earlier, feeding of bovine milk is discouraged during this period, although a substantial number of infants are indeed fed bovine milk.[87] In addition, there are concerns about the substitution of low-fat or skimmed milks during this period because of higher intakes of protein and sodium and lower intakes of iron and essential fatty acids. However, if infants are being fed nonmilk foods, the actual intake of energy may not be lower than of infants fed bovine milk or formula.[88]

BONE DENSITY

Infants exclusively breast-fed have lower bone accretion and total body bone mineral content than do formula-fed infants.[89] The low vitamin D content in human milk[90] and the decreasing phosphorus concentration with increasing lactation are thought to be the cause.[91,92] Early mineral intake during the first 6 months of age is associated with early bone mass accretion.[89] The Committee on Nutrition and Section of Breast Feeding Medicine of the AAP recommends supplement of 200 IU/day of vitamin D to all breast-fed infants unless weaned to at least 500 ml/day of vitamin-D-fortified formula or milk.[93]

Older-infant studies on soy-based formulas showed a lower radius bone mineral density in infants fed soy-based formulas than did infants fed cow-milk-based formulas.[94,95] Newer formulations of soy formulas have improved both calcium and phosphorus content and availability. Bainbridge et al.[96] showed no difference in bone accretion between these newer formulas and cow-milk-based formulas.

WEANING

The transition from suckling to eating of nonmilk foods occurs during the first year of life based on cultural beliefs and practices, physicians beliefs, mothers' perceptions of their infants' needs, and economic realities. Complementary foods are introduced from before 3 months to nearly 6 months of age, and a variety of foods are offered.[97–99] In the United States, the total transition to beikost usually occurs by the end of the first year of life and continues during the second year.

The weaning process can be considered in three ways. First, it could be the weaning from breast-feeding to other milks that may replace breast-feeding partially or completely. In the second form, weaning could be considered the transition from liquid to nonliquid diet. Health concerns may arise during this period if the added foods are too nutrient dense (protein or energy) or nutrient-deficient (iron or protein), thus altering the protein-to-energy ratio or causing deficiency of specific nutrients. The third aspect of weaning may be the transition from human milk or formula to bovine milk in addition to the provision of beikost. Because weaning typically occurs during a period of rapid growth, attention to both nutritional and developmental issues during this period is warranted. Complementary foods, in addition to providing the required nutrients, are also important in establishing lifelong patterns of eating. The current consensus is to introduce one solid food at a time and wait for several days to a week to assess tolerance before adding a new food. For most babies, it does not matter what the first foods are, but cereals, followed by fruits, strained vegetables and meats are suggested. Teaching good food habits, including offering a variety, will lead to lifelong eating habits. A suggested algorithm for the feeding of term infants and the transition to complementary foods is depicted in Figure 15.3.

FAILURE TO THRIVE

Growth, as assessed by weight, length (and subsequently height), and head circumference, is an important part of anticipatory guidance provided in well-child care. These anthropometric measurements, especially weight, can be used to detect inadequate attained growth or reduced growth velocity. The average birth weight of a full-term infant is 3300 to 3500 g; after a weight loss of ~10%, infants should regain their birth weight by 2 weeks, with formula-fed infants tending to regain their birth weight a little sooner than their breast-fed counterparts. On an average, infants gain about 1 kg/month for the first 3 months, $\frac{1}{2}$ kg/month for the next 3 months, $\frac{1}{3}$ kg/month from 6 to 9 months and $\frac{1}{4}$ kg/month from 9 to 12 months. Full-term infants double their weights by 4 months and triple their weights by 12 months, while doubling their lengths during the same period. Both weight and length gains are slower in the second year of life, underscoring the anticipatory nutritional guidance needed during that period. Growth faltering, or failure to thrive, a descriptive term, is then identified by the following criteria: (1) weight less than 80% to 85% of the 50th percentile on the National Center for Health Statistics (NCHS) growth charts, (2) weight for age less than the 3 to 5 percentile on the NCHS growth charts, (3) drop in weight that crosses two or more percentile categories on standard growth charts from previously established pattern of adequate growth, and (4) a Z-score of −2 SD below the normal 50th percentile. If growth velocity is used, a decrement of 2 SD over a 90-day period and loss of >1 SD Z-score over 90 days is used as a measure of growth faltering.

As decline in rate of weight gain or growth velocity is more sensitive than decline in length or head circumference, serial measurements of weight are an important part of the anticipatory guidance given during well-child checks, and provide an early

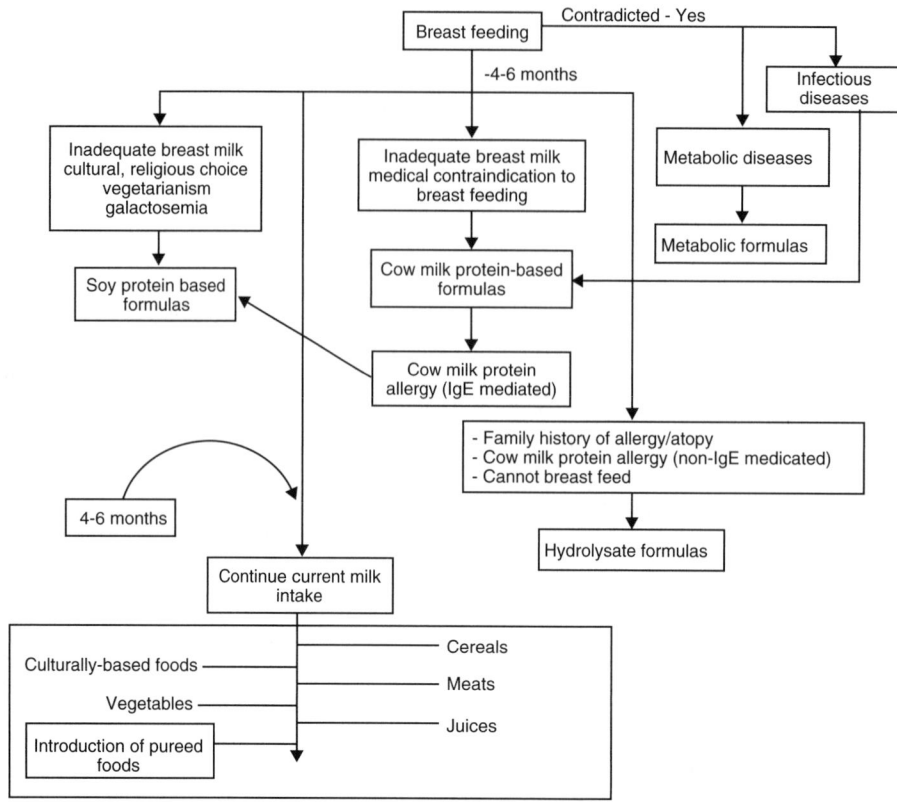

FIGURE 15.3 Birth to 36 months: Boys Head circumference-for-age and weight-for-length percentiles.

TABLE 15.8
Recommendations for Feeding Healthy Full-Term Infants

Breast-feeding is strongly recommended.

Infant formulas that meet AAP guidelines are recommended when breast-feeding is not chosen or breast milk is not available.

Breast milk or infant formula is the preferred feeding in the first year of life.

Adequate intakes of human milk or formula meet all nutrient requirements for the first 6 months of life (exception may be vitamin D in dark-skinned, sun-deprived breast-fed infants). Infant formula or "follow-up" formula may be fed in the second 6 months of life.

Introduction of complementary foods should be based on growth, developmental, cultural, social, psychological, and economic considerations. As a general rule, when an infant is consuming 32 oz of milk per day and appears to want more, supplemental feedings may be indicated. This usually occurs between 4 and 6 months of age.

warning of growth faltering.[100,101] BMI, calculated by dividing weight in kilograms by the square of length/height in meters, has largely replaced weight for stature. It should be recognized that there are growth differences between breast- and formula-fed infants. As reported by Nelson et al.[102] mean gains in both weight (g/day) and length (cm/day) were greater in formula-fed males and females than their breast-fed counterparts from 8 to 122 days of age. As the NCHS growth charts were made from data that was cross-sectional and the infants were fed formulas, attention to growth faltering in the breast-fed infant requires both understanding of the growth of breast-fed infants and the early recognition of decrease in weight or growth velocity.[103] New growth charts from a cross section of breast-fed infants need to be assessed for their use in the United States. There are numerous organic and nonorganic causes of growth failure or faltering that need to be addressed during such an evaluation. It is important to realize that failure to thrive or malnutrition may occur in hospitalized infants and children, as well, and efforts to recognize and nourish these infants and children should be made.

SUMMARY

In summary, the period of infancy is one of rapid changes in growth and attainment of developmental milestones. This period imposes unique nutritional needs and challenges for the health care provider. Understanding nutritional needs, ways of meeting these needs (Table 15.8), deviations in growth and their causes, and providing nutrition in age-appropriate and culturally and ethnically sensitive ways while addressing economic issues is the task of the health care team. Ideally, the infant's nutritional need (expressed as hunger), developmental progress (as observed in attainment of feeding skills), and mother's and care provider's beliefs within the context of the family will guide the infant's feeding experience and transition to the next phase in life.

REFERENCES

1. Hamill, P. V., Drizd, T. A., Johnson, C. L. et al. *Am J Clin Nutr* 32: 607; 1979.
2. Fomon, S. J., Nelson, S. E. In *Nutrition of Normal Infants* (Mosby, C.V., Ed.), Mosby Year books Inc. St Louis Mo 1993, 36, p. 155.
3. Ogden, C. L., Flegal, K. M., Carroll, M. D., Johnson, C. L. *JAMA* 288: 1728; 2002.
4. Butte N. F. *Eur J Clin Nutr* 50: 24S; 1996.
5. Health and Welfare Canada. Nutrition Recommendations. The report of the scientific review committee, Ottawa, Canada: Supply and Services, 1990.
6. Dewey, K. G., Lonnerdal, B. *J Pediatr Gastroenterol Nutr* 2: 497; 1983.
7. Dewey, K. G., Heinig, M. J., Nommsen, L. A. et al. *J Pediatr* 119: 538; 1991.
8. Whitehead, R. G., Paul, A. A., Cole, T. J. *Acta Paediatr Scand* 299: 43S; 1982.
9. Kylberg, H., Hofvander, Y., Sjolin, S. *Acta Paediatr Scand* 75: 932; 1986.
10. Persson, L. A., Johansson, E., Samuelson, G. *Hum Nutr Appl Nutr* 38: 247; 1984.
11. Heinig, M. J., Nommsen, L. A., Peerson, J. M. et al. *Am J Clin Nutr* 58: 152; 1993.
12. Zlotkin, S. H., Anderson, G. H. *Pediatr Res* 16: 65; 1982.
13. Pohlandt, P. *Acta Paediatr Scand* 63: 801; 1974.
14. Gaull, G. E., Rassin, D. K., Raiha, N. C. et al. *J Pediatr* 90: 348; 1977.
15. Rassin, D. K., Gaull, G. E., Jarvenpaa, A. L. et al. *Pediatrics* 71: 179; 1983.
16. Jarvenpaa, A. L., Rassin, D. K., Raiha, N. C. et al. *Pediatrics* 70: 221; 1982.
17. World Health Organization. Energy and protein requirements. WHO Technical Report Series No. 742, Geneva, WHO. 98, 1985.
18. Fomon, S. J., Haschke, F., Ziegler, E. E., Nelson, S. E. *Am J Clin Nutr* 34: 1169S; 1982.
19. Wong, W. W., Hachey, D. L., Insull, W. et al. *J Lipid Res* 34: 1403; 1993.
20. Bitman, J., Wood, L., Hamosh, M. et al. *Am J Clin Nutr* 38: 300; 1983.
21. Harzer, G., Haug, M., Dieterich, I. et al. *Am J Clin Nutr* 37: 612; 1983.
22. Hibberd, C. M., Brooke, O. G., Carter, N. G. et al. *Arch Dis Child* 57: 658; 1982.
23. Jensen, R. G. *The Lipids of Human Milk*. Boca Raton: CRC Press, 1989.
24. Prentice, A., Prentice, A. M., Whitehead, R. G. *Br J Nutr* 45: 495; 1981.
25. Hachey, D. L., Thomas, M. R., Emken, E. A. et al. *J Lipid Res* 28: 1185; 1987.
26. Hachey, D. L., Silber, G. H., Wong, W. W., Garza, C. *Pediatr Res* 25: 63; 1989.
27. Koletzko, B., Thiel, I., Abiodun, P. O. Z. *Ernahrungwiss* 30: 289; 1991.
28. Harris, W. S., Conner, W. E., Lindsey, S. *Am J Clin Nutr* 40: 780; 1984.
29. Genzel-Boroviczeny, O., Wahle, J., Koletzko, B. *Eur J Paediatr* 156: 142; 1997.
30. Joint FAO/WHO Codex Alimentarius Commission, 1984; Food and Drug Administration 1985; Commission of European Communities, 1991.
31. Martinez, M. *J Pediatr* 120: 289; 1992.
32. SanGiovanni, J. P., Berkey, C. S., Dwyer, J. T., Colditz, G. A. *Early Hum Dev* 57: 165; 2000.
33. Birch, E. E., Hoffman, D. R., Uauy, R., Birch, D. G. et al. *Pediatr Res* 44: 201; 1998.
34. Birch, E. E., Garfield, S., Hoffman, D. R., Uauy, R. et al. *Dev Med Child Neurol* 42: 174; 2000.
35. Fleith, M., Clandinin, M. T. *Crit Rev Food Sci Nutr* 45: 205; 2005.
36. Lifshitz, F., Moses, N. *Am J Dis Child* 143: 537; 1989.
37. Michaelsen, K. F., Jorgensen, M. H. *Eur J Clin Nutr* 49: 467; 1995.
38. Bhatia, J., Bucher, C., Bunyapen, C. *Pediatr Ann* 27: 525; 1998.
39. Dallman, P. R., Siimes, M. A., Stekel, A. *Am J Clin Nutr* 33: 86; 1980.
40. U.S. Department of Health and Human Services, 2000. In Healthy people 2010.
41. CDC. Iron Deficiency — United States, 1999–2000. MMWR 51: 897; 2002.
42. CDC. Recommendations to prevent and control iron deficiency in the United States. MMWR 47: (No. RR-3); 1998.
43. Yip, R. In *Dietary Iron: Birth to Two Years* (Filer, L. J., Jr., Ed.), New York: Raven Press, 1989, p. 37.
44. Ferguson, B. J., Skikne, B. S., Simpson, K. M. et al. *J Lab Clin Med* 119: 385; 1992.
45. Ziegler, E. E., Fomon, S. J., Nelson, S. E. et al. *J Pediatr* 116: 11; 1990.
46. Fomon, S. J., Ziegler, E. E., Nelson, S. E. et al. *J Pediatr* 98: 540; 1981.
47. Pizarro, F., Yip, R., Dallman, P. R. et al. *J Pediatr* 118: 687; 1991.
48. Siimes, M. A., Vuori, E., Kuitunen, P. *Acta Paediatr Scand* 68: 29; 1979.
49. Haschke, F., Vanura, H., Male, C. et al. *J Pediatr Gastroenterol Nutr* 16: 151; 1993.
50. Lozoff, B., Brittenham, G. M., Viteri, F. E. et al. *J Pediatr* 100: 351; 1982.
51. Lozoff, B., Brittenham, G. M., Wolf, A. W. et al. *Pediatrics* 79: 981; 1987.
52. Lozoff, B., Jiminez, W., Wolf, A. W. *N Eng J Med* 325: 687; 1991.
53. Walter, T. In *Nutritional Anemias* (Fomon, S. J., Zlotkin, S., Eds.), Nestle Nutrition Workshop Series, 30. New York: Raven Press, 1990, p. 81.

54. Pollitt, E. *Ann Rev Nutr* 13: 521; 1993.
55. Hambraeus, L. *Pediatr Clin N Am* 24: 17; 1977.
56. Fomon, S. J., Bier, D. M., Mathews, D. E. et al. *J Pediatr* 113: 515; 1988.
57. Cho, F., Bhatia, J., Rassin, D. K. *Nutrition* 6: 449; 1990.
58. Lindblad, B. S., Alfven, G., Zetterstrom, R. *Acta Paediatr Scand* 67: 659; 1978.
59. Rassin, D. K. In *Protein Requirements in the Term Infant* (Barness, L., Ed.), Princeton: Excerpta Medica; 1988, p. 3.
60. Goldman, A. S., Cheda, S., Keeny, S. E. et al. *Sem Perinatol* 18: 495; 1994.
61. Hanson, L. A., Ahlstedt, S., Andersson, B. et al. *Pediatrics* 75: 172; 1985.
62. Neville, M. C., Keller, R. P., Seacat, J. et al. *Am J Clin Nutr* 40: 635; 1984.
63. Neuringer, M., Conner, W. E., Van Patten, C. et al. *J Clin Invest* 73: 272; 1984.
64. Uauy, R., Quan, R., Gil, A. *J Nutr* 124: 1436S; 1994.
65. Jyonouchi, H. *J Nutr* 124: 138S; 1994.
66. Carver, J. D. *J Nutr* 124: 144S; 1994.
67. Pickering, L. K., Granoff, D. M., Erickson, J. R. et al. *Pediatrics* 101: 242; 1998.
68. Dewey, K. G., Heinig, M. J., Nommsen-Rivers, L. A. *J Pediatr* 126: 696; 1995.
69. Wright, A. L., Holberg, C. J., Taussig, L. M. et al. *Arch Pediatr Adolesc Med* 149: 758; 1995.
70. Kovar, M. G., Serdula, M. K., Marks, J. S. et al. *Pediatrics* 74: 615; 1984.
71. Takala, A. K., Eskola, J., Palmgren, J. et al. *J Pediatr* 115: 694: 1989.
72. Cochi, S. L., Fleming, D. W., Hightower, A. W. et al. *J Pediatr* 108: 887; 1986.
73. Arnon, S. S. *Rev Infect Dis* 6, 193S.
74. Pisacane, A., Graziano, L., Mazzarella, G. et al. *J Pediatr* 120: 87; 1992.
75. Lucas, A., Cole, T. J. *Lancet* 336: 1519; 1990.
76. Goldfarb, J. *Clin Perinatol* 20: 225; 1985.
77. Food and Drug Administration: Rules and regulations. Nutrient requirements for infant formulas (21 CFR part 107), Fed Reg 50: 45106; 1985.
78. Osborn, D. A., Sinn, J. *Cochrane Database Syst Rev* CD003664; 2003.
79. Bergmann, R. L., Bergmann, K. E., Lau-Schadensdorf, S. et al. *Pediatr Allergy Immunol* 5(Suppl 6): 19; 1994.
80. Sears, M. R., Holdaway, M. D., Flannery, E. M. et al. *Arch Dis Child* 75: 392; 1996.
81. Tariq, S. M., Matthews, S. M., Hakim, E. A. et al. *J Allergy Clin Immunol* 101: 587; 1998.
82. American Academy of Pediatrics, Committee on Nutrition. *Pediatrics* 106: 346; 2000.
83. Host, A., Koletzko, B., Dreborg, S. et al. *Arch Dis Child* 81: 80; 1999.
84. von Berg, A., Koletzko, S., Grubl, A. et al. *J Allergy Clin Immunol* 111: 533; 2003.
85. Hays, T., Wood, R. A. *Arch Pediatr Adolesc Med* 159: 810; 2005.
86. American Academy of Pediatrics, Committee on Nutrition. *Pediatrics* 101: 148; 1998.
87. American Academy of Pediatrics, Committee on Nutrition. *AAP News* 8: 18; 1992.
88. Martinez, G. A., Ryan, A. S., Malec, D. J. *Am J Dis Child* 139: 1010; 1985.
89. Specker, B.L., Beck, A., Kalkwarf, H., Ho, M. *Pediatrics* 99: e12; 1997.
90. Specker, B. L., Tsang, R. C., Hollis, B. W. *Am J Dis Child* 139: 1134; 1985.
91. Oppe, T. E., Redstone, D. *Lancet* 1: 1045; 1968.
92. Tanzer, F., Sunel, S. *Indian Pediatr* 28: 391; 1991.
93. American Academy of Pediatrics, Committee on Nutrition. *Pediatrics* 111: 908; 2003.
94. Chan, G. M., Leeper, L., Book, L. S. *Am J Dis Child* 141: 527; 1987.
95. Steichen, J. J., Tsang, R. C. *J Pediatr* 110: 687; 1987.
96. Bainbridge, R. R., Mimouni, F., Tsang, R. C. *J Pediatr* 113: 205; 1988.
97. Anderson, T. A., Ziegler, E. E. In *Weaning, Why, What and When?* (Ballabriga, A., Ray, J., Eds.), Nestle Nutrition Workshop Series, 10, New York: Raven Press, 1987, p. 153.
98. Ballabriga, A., Schmidt, E. In *Weaning, Why, What and When?* (Ballabriga, A., Ray, J., Eds.), Nestle Nutrition Workshop Series, 10, Raven Press, New York, 1987, p. 129.
99. Ahmad, A. In *Weaning, Why, What and When?* (Ballabriga, A., Ray, J., Eds.), Nestle Nutrition Workshop Series, 10, New York: Raven Press, 1987, p. 197.
100. Zumrawi, F. Y., Min, Y., Marshall, T. *Ann Human Biol* 19: 165; 1992.
101. Healy, M. J. R., Yang, M., Tanner, J. M., Zumrawi, F. Y. In *Linear Growth Retardation in Less Developed Countries* (Waterlow, J. C., Ed.), New York: Raven Press, 41, 1988.
102. Nelson, S. E., Rogers, R. R., Ziegler, E. E. et al. *Early Hum Devel* 19: 223; 1989.
103. Garza, C., Frongillo, E., Dewey, K. G. *Acta Paediatr* 404: 4S; 1994.

16 Nutrition for Healthy Children and Adolescents Aged 2 to 18 Years

Suzanne Domel Baxter

CONTENTS

PHYSICAL GROWTH AND DEVELOPMENT

A child's first year of life is marked by rapid growth, with birth weight tripling and birth length increasing by 50%. After the rapid growth of the first year, physical growth slows down considerably during the preschool and school years, until the pubertal growth spurt of adolescence. Birth weight does not quadruple until 2 years of age, and birth length does not double until 4 years of age. A 1-year-old child has several teeth, and his or her digestive and metabolic systems are functioning at or near adult capacity. By 1 year of age, most children are walking or beginning to walk; with improved coordination over the next few years, activity increases dramatically. Although increased activity in turn increases energy needs, a child's rate of growth decreases. Growth patterns vary in individual children, but each year children from 2 years to puberty gain an average of 4.5 to 6.5 pounds (2 to 3 kg) in weight and 2.5 to 3.5 in. (6 to 8 cm) in height. As the growth rate declines during the preschool years, a child's appetite decreases and food intake may become unpredictable and erratic. Parents and other caregivers need to know that these changes are normal so that they can avoid struggles with children over food and eating.

After the first year of life, more development that is significant occurs in fine and gross motor, cognitive, and social-emotional areas than during the first year of life. During the second year of life, children learn to feed themselves independently. By 15 months of age, children can manage a cup, but with some spilling. At 18 to 24 months of age, children learn to tilt cups by manipulating their fingers. Children are able to transfer food from bowls to their mouths with less spilling by 16 to 17 months of age when well-defined wrist rotation develops. However, 2-year-old children often prefer foods that can be picked up with their fingers without having to chase it across their plates.

The normal events of puberty and the simultaneous growth spurt are the primary influences on nutritional requirements during the second decade of life. During puberty, height and weight increase, many organ systems enlarge, and body composition is altered due to increased lean body mass and changes in the quantity and distribution of fat. The timing of the growth spurt is influenced by genetic as well as environmental factors. Children who weigh more than average for their height tend to mature early, and vice versa. Although stature tends to increase most rapidly during the spring and summer, weight either tends to increase at a fairly steady rate over the entire year or undergoes a more rapid increase during the autumn. The most rapid linear growth spurt for an average American boy occurs between 12 and 15 years of age. For the average American girl, the growth spurt occurs about 2 years earlier, between 10 and 13 years of age. The growth spurt during adolescence contributes about 15% to final adult height, and approximately 50% to adult weight. During adolescence, boys tend to gain more weight than girls do, and to gain it at a faster rate. Furthermore, the skeletal growth of boys continues for a longer time than that of adolescent girls. Adolescent boys deposit more muscle mass, and adolescent girls deposit relatively more total body fat. Menarche, which is closely linked to the growth process, has a lasting impact on nutritional requirements of adolescent girls.

Adolescence is a period of various cognitive challenges. For example, when an adolescent realizes that his or her body is in the process of maturing, he or she may begin to assess changes in his or her own body size and shape, compare them with those of others, and form opinions about any differences. Adolescent girls and boys may be very self-conscious, especially during early and mid-adolescence. According to Piaget's developmental levels, it is usually during adolescence that abstract thinking supersedes concrete thinking. Thus, an adolescent may consider his or her body not just as it is, but also as it *might* be. In addition, an adolescent can contemplate new or different ways of combining or eating food. Furthermore, an adolescent can more easily conceptualize nutrients such as calories and fat, and skillfully manipulate their dietary intake.

ENERGY AND NUTRIENT NEEDS

DIETARY REFERENCE INTAKES

The Dietary Reference Intakes (DRIs)[1] expand and replace reports called *Recommended Dietary Allowances,*[2] published from 1941 to 1989 by the National Academy of Sciences, and *Recommended Nutrient Intakes*, published by the Canadian government. The DRIs include Recommended Dietary Allowance (RDA), Estimated Average Requirement (EAR), Adequate Intake (AI), and Tolerable Upper Intake Level (UL). Within the DRI framework, the RDA serves as a goal for daily intake by individuals; it is the average daily dietary intake level that is sufficient to meet the nutrient needs of almost all (97 to 98%) healthy individuals in a life stage and sex group. The EAR is a nutrient intake value that is estimated to meet the nutrient needs of 50% of the healthy individuals in a life stage and sex group; it is the basis for the RDA and used to assess adequacy of intakes of population groups and to plan intakes of groups. The AI is used instead of an RDA when sufficient scientific evidence is not available to calculate an EAR; the AI is based on observed or experimentally determined approximations of nutrient intake by a life stage and sex group (or groups) of healthy people. The UL is the highest level of nutrient intake per day that is likely to pose no risks of adverse health effects to almost all individuals in the general population. The risk of adverse effects increases as intake increases above the UL.[1] Although the DRIs are based on data, scientific judgment was required in setting all reference values, because data were often scanty or drawn from studies with limitations; this is especially true in deriving DRIs for infants, children, adolescents, the elderly, and pregnant women.[1] The DRIs have been published in a series of 12 reports to date.[1,3–13] Table 16.1 provides new reference heights, weights, and body mass indexes (BMIs) for children and adolescents in the United States. Table 16.2 provides RDAs and AIs for children and adolescents. Table 16.3 provides Acceptable Macronutrient Distribution Ranges (AMDRs) for children and adolescents. Table 16.4 provides additional macronutrient recommendations for children and adolescents. Table 16.5 provides ULs for children and adolescents. Table 16.6 provides EARs for groups of children and adolescents.

ENERGY

Energy is needed to maintain the various functions of the body including respiration, circulation, physical work, and protein synthesis. Energy is supplied in the diet by carbohydrates, proteins, fats, and alcohol. An individual's energy balance depends on his or her intake of dietary energy and expenditure of energy. Within the DRIs, Estimated Energy Requirements (EERs) were established at four levels of energy expenditure, and recommendations were provided for levels of physical activity associated with a normal BMI range.[1] The EER is the average dietary energy intake predicted to maintain energy balance in a healthy individual of a defined age, sex, weight, height, and level of physical activity, consistent with good health.[1] Table 16.7 provides

TABLE 16.1
Dietary Reference Intakes (DRIs): New Reference Heights, Weights, and Body Mass Index (BMIs) for Children and Adolescents in the United States

	Children		Boys		Girls	
	1 to 3 Years	4 to 8 Years	9 to 13 Years	14 to 18 Years	9 to 13 Years	14 to 18 Years
Median Reference Height,[a] cm (in.)	86 (34)	115 (45)	144 (57)	174 (68)	144 (57)	163 (64)
Reference Weight,[b] kg (lb)	12 (27)	20 (44)	36 (79)	61 (134)	37 (81)	54 (119)
Median BMI[a] (kg/m²)	—	15.3	17.2	20.5	17.4	20.4

[a] Taken from height-for-age data and median BMI data for boys and girls from the Centers for Disease Control and Prevention (CDC)/National Center for Health Statistics (NCHS) Growth Charts from Kuczmarski et al., *Adv Data*, 314, 1–28, 2000.
[b] Calculated CDC/NCHS Growth Charts from Kuczmarski et al., *Adv Data*, 314, 1–28, 2000; median BMI and median height for ages 4 through 19 years.

Source: Adapted from: Institute of Medicine, *Dietary Reference Intakes for Energy, Carbohydrate, Fiber, Fat, Fatty Acids, Cholesterol, Protein, and Amino Acids*, National Academies Press, Washington, DC, 2002/2005. This report may be accessed via www.nap.edu.

criteria and DRI values for energy by active children and adolescents by life stage group. In children, the EER includes needs associated with the deposition of tissues. Although equations are provided for estimating four levels of activity, the *active* physical activity level is recommended to maintain health. There is no RDA for energy, because energy intakes above the EER would be expected to result in weight gain. Likewise, the UL concept does not apply to energy, because any energy intake above an individual's requirement would lead to undesirable and potentially hazardous weight gain.[1]

Components of energy expenditure include basal and resting metabolism, thermic effect of food, thermoregulation, physical activity, physical activity level, and total energy requirement.[1] Factors that affect energy expenditure and requirements include body composition and body size (i.e., effects on basal and resting metabolic rate, effects on total energy expenditure, and obesity), physical activity (i.e., effect of exercise on postexercise energy expenditure, spontaneous nonexercise activity), sex, growth, older age, genetics, ethnicity, environment (i.e., climate altitude), and adaptation and accommodation.[1]

TABLE 16.2
Dietary Reference Intakes (DRIs): Recommended Dietary Allowances (RDAs) and Adequate Intakes (AIs) for Children and Adolescents[a]

	Children		Boys		Girls	
	1 to 3 Years	4 to 8 Years	9 to 13 Years	14 to 18 Years	9 to 13 Years	14 to 18 Years
Vitamins						
Vitamin A (µg/day)[b]	300	400	600	900	600	700
Vitamin C (mg/day)	15	25	45	75	45	65
Vitamin D (µg/day)[c,d]	5*	5*	5*	5*	5*	5*
Vitamin E (mg/day)[e]	6	7	11	15	11	15
Vitamin K (µg/day)	30*	55*	60*	75*	60*	75*
Thiamin (mg/day)	0.5	0.6	0.9	1.2	0.9	1.0
Riboflavin (mg/day)	0.5	0.6	0.9	1.3	0.9	1.0
Niacin (mg/day)[f]	6	8	12	16	12	14
Vitamin B$_6$ (mg/day)	0.5	0.6	1.0	1.3	1.0	1.2
Folate (µg/day)[g]	150	200	300	400	300	400[h]
Vitamin B$_{12}$ (µg/day)	0.9	1.2	1.8	2.4	1.8	2.4
Pantothenic Acid (mg/day)	2*	3*	4*	5*	4*	5*
Biotin (µg/day)	8*	12*	20*	25*	20*	25*
Choline (mg/day)[i]	200*	250*	375*	550*	375*	400*
Elements						
Calcium (mg/day)	500*	800*	1300*	1300*	1300*	1300*
Chromium (µg/day)	11*	15*	25*	35*	21*	24*
Copper (µg/day)	340	440	700	890	700	890
Fluoride (mg/day)	0.7*	1*	2*	3*	2*	3*
Iodine (µg/day)	90	90	120	150	120	150
Iron (mg/day)	7	10	8	11	8	15
Magnesium (mg/day)	80	130	240	410	240	360
Manganese (mg/day)	1.2*	1.5*	1.9*	2.2*	1.6*	1.6*
Molybdenum (µg/day)	17	22	34	43	34	43
Phosphorus (mg/day)	460	500	1250	1250	1250	1250
Selenium (µg/day)	20	30	40	55	40	55
Zinc (mg/day)	3	5	8	11	8	9
Potassium (g/day)	3.0*	3.8*	4.5*	4.7*	4.5*	4.7*
Sodium (g/day)	1.0*	1.2*	1.5*	1.5*	1.5*	1.5*
Chloride (g/day)	1.5*	1.9*	2.3*	2.3*	2.3*	2.3*
Total Water and Macronutrients						
Total Water (L/day)[j]	1.3*	1.7*	2.4*	3.3*	2.1*	2.3*
Carbohydrate (g/day)	130	130	130	130	130	130
Total Fiber (g/day)	19*	25*	31*	38*	26*	26*
Fat (g/day)	ND[k]	ND	ND	ND	ND	ND

Continued

TABLE 16.2
(Continued)

	Children		Boys		Girls	
	1 to 3 Years	4 to 8 Years	9 to 13 Years	14 to 18 Years	9 to 13 Years	14 to 18 Years
Linoleic Acid (g/day)	7*	10*	12*	16*	10*	11*
α-Linolenic Acid (g/day)	0.7*	0.9*	1.2*	1.6*	1.0*	1.1*
Protein (g/day)	**13[l]**	**19[m]**	**34[n]**	**52[o]**	**34[n]**	**46[p]**
Protein (g/kg/day)	**1.05**	**0.95**	**0.95**	**0.85**	**0.95**	**0.85**

[a] Recommended Dietary Allowances (RDAs) are presented in **bold type** and Adequate Intakes (AIs) in ordinary type followed by an asterisk (*). RDAs and AIs may both be used as goals for individual intake. RDAs are set to meet the needs of almost all (97 to 98%) healthy individuals in a group. The AI for life stage and sex groups is believed to cover needs of all individuals in the group, but lack of data or uncertainty in the data prevent being able to specify with confidence the percentage of persons covered by this intake.

[b] As retinol activity equivalents (RAEs). 1 RAE = 1 μg retinol, 12 μg β-carotene, 24 μg α-carotene, or 24 μg β-cryptoxanthin. The RAE for dietary provitamin A carotenoids is twofold greater than retinol equivalents (RE), whereas the RAE for preformed vitamin A is the same as RE.

[c] As cholecalciferol. 1 μg cholecalciferol = 40 IU vitamin D.

[d] In the absence of adequate exposure to sunlight.

[e] As α-tocopherol. α-Tocopherol includes *RRR*-α-tocopherol, the only form of α-tocopherol that occurs naturally in foods, and the *2R*-stereoisomeric forms of α-tocopherol (*RRR*-, *RSR*-, *RRS*-, and *RSS*-α-tocopherol) that occur in fortified foods and supplements. It does not include the *2S*-stereoisomeric forms of α-tocopherol (*SRR*-, *SSR*-, *SRS*-, and *SSS*-α-tocopherol), also found in fortified foods and supplements.

[f] As niacin equivalents (NE). 1 mg niacin = 60 mg tryptophan.

[g] As dietary folate equivalents (DFE). 1 DFE = 1 μg food folate = 0.6 μg folic acid from fortified food or as a supplement consumed with food = 0.5 μg of a supplement taken on an empty stomach.

[h] In view of evidence linking folate intake with neural tube defects in the fetus, it is recommended that all women capable of becoming pregnant consume 400 μg from supplements or fortified foods in addition to intake of food folate from a varied diet. It is assumed that females will continue consuming 400 μg from supplements or fortified food until their pregnancy is confirmed and they enter prenatal care.

[i] Although AIs have been set for choline, there are few data to assess whether a dietary supply of choline is needed at all stages of the life cycle, and it may be that the choline requirement can by met by endogenous synthesis at some of these stages.

[j] Total water includes all water contained in drinking water, food, and beverages.

[k] ND = Not determined.

[l] 13 g/day of protein or 1.05 g protein per kg of body weight.

[m] 19 g/day of protein or 0.95 g protein per kg of body weight.

[n] 34 g/day of protein or 0.95 g protein per kg of body weight.

[o] 52 g/day of protein or 0.85 g protein per kg of body weight.

[p] 46 g/day of protein or 0.85 g protein per kg of body weight.

Source: Adapted from: Institute of Medicine, *Dietary Reference Intakes for Calcium, Phosphorus, Magnesium, Vitamin D, and Fluoride*, National Academy Press, Washington, DC, 1997; Institute of Medicine, *Dietary Reference Intakes for Thiamin, Riboflavin, Niacin, Vitamin B₆, Folate, Vitamin B₁₂, Pantothenic Acid, Biotin, and Choline*, National Academy Press, Washington, DC, 1998; Institute of Medicine, *Dietary Reference Intakes for Vitamin C, Vitamin E, Selenium, and Carotenoids*, National Academy Press, Washington, DC, 2000; Institute of Medicine, *Dietary Reference Intakes for Vitamin A, Vitamin K, Arsenic, Boron, Chromium, Copper, Iodine, Iron, Manganese, Molybedenum, Nickel, Silicon, Vanadium, and Zinc*, National Academy Press, Washington, DC, 2001; Institute of Medicine, *Dietary Reference Intakes for Water, Potassium, Sodium, Chloride, and Sulfate*, National Academies Press, Washington, DC, 2005; and Institute of Medicine, *Dietary Reference Intakes for Energy, Carbohydrate, Fiber, Fat, Fatty Acids, Cholesterol, Protein, and Amino Acids*, National Academies Press, Washington, DC, 2002/2005. These reports may be accessed via www.nap.edu.

Physical Activity Level (PAL) is the ratio of total energy expenditure to basal daily energy expenditure (TEE/BEE); it is a convenient comparison used in the DRIs to describe and account for physical activity habits.[1] The PAL categories were defined as sedentary (PAL $\geq$ 1.0 < 1.4), low active (PAL $\geq$ 1.4 < 1.6), active (PAL $\geq$ 1.6 < 1.9), and very active (PAL $\geq$ 1.9 < 2.5).[1]

The EER for boys and girls varies considerably because of variations in growth rate and physical activity. To derive total energy requirements, data from doubly-labeled water studies were utilized to develop equations to predict TEE based on sex, age, height, weight, and PAL category. To obtain the EER, the calculated TEE is increased for estimated energy deposition by an average of 20 kcal/day for ages 3 through 8 years and by 25 kcal/day for ages 9 through 18 years. EER predictions for children and adolescents with reference weights, at yearly intervals by sex, are available and are summarized below for age categories by sex.[1]

For boys age 3 through 8 years,

EER = TEE + energy deposition = 88.5 − (61.9 × age [years]) + PA × (26.7 × weight [kg] + 903 × height [m]) + 20 kcal

For boys age 9 through 18 years,

EER = TEE + energy deposition = 88.5 − (61.9 × age [years]) + PA × (26.7 × weight [kg] + 903 × height [m]) + 25 kcal

Where PA is the physical activity coefficient and, for boys, is 1.00 if PAL is sedentary, 1.13 if PAL is low active, 1.26 if PAL is active and 1.42 if PAL is very active.

For girls age 3 through 8 years,

EER = TEE + energy deposition = 135.3 − (30.8 × age [years]) + PA × (10.0 × weight [kg] + 934 × height [m]) + 20 kcal

For girls age 9 through 18 years,

EER = TEE + energy deposition = 135.3 − (30.8 × age [years]) + PA × (10.0 × weight [kg] + 934 × height [m]) + 25 kcal

Where PA is the physical activity coefficient and, for girls, is 1.00 if PAL is sedentary, 1.16 if PAL is low active, 1.31 if PAL is active and 1.56 if PAL is very active.

TABLE 16.3
Dietary Reference Intakes (DRIs): Acceptable Macronutrient Distribution Ranges (AMDRs) for Children and Adolescents[a]

	Range (Percent of Energy)	
	1 to 3 Years	4 to 18 Years
Macronutrient		
Fat	30–40	25–35
n−6 Polyunsaturated fatty acids[a] (linoleic acid)	5–10	5–10
n−3 Polyunsaturated fatty acids[a] (*α*-linolenic acid)	0.6–1.2	0.6–1.2
Carbohydrate	45–65	45–65
Protein	5–20	10–30

[a] Approximately 10% of the total can come from longer-chain *n*−3 or *n*−6 fatty acids.

Source: Adapted from: Institute of Medicine, *Dietary Reference Intakes for Energy, Carbohydrate, Fiber, Fat, Fatty Acids, Cholesterol, Protein, and Amino Acids,* National Academies Press, Washington, DC, 2002/2005. This report may be accessed via www.nap.edu.

TABLE 16.4
Dietary Reference Intakes (DRIs): Additional Macronutrient Recommendations for Children and Adolescents[a]

Macronutrient	Recommendation
Added sugars	Limit to no more than 25% of total energy
Dietary cholesterol	As low as possible while consuming a nutritionally adequate diet
Saturated fatty acids	As low as possible while consuming a nutritionally adequate diet
Trans fatty acids	As low as possible while consuming a nutritionally adequate diet

Source: Adapted from: Institute of Medicine, *Dietary Reference Intakes for Energy, Carbohydrate, Fiber, Fat, Fatty Acids, Cholesterol, Protein, and Amino Acids,* National Academies Press, Washington, DC, 2002/2005. This report may be accessed via www.nap.edu.

Separate EERs were developed for pregnant and lactating girls aged 14 through 18 years.[1] In addition, separate weight maintenance TEE predictive equations were developed for overweight (i.e., above the 95th percentile for BMI) boys and girls age 3 through 18 years.[1] An accepted and practical method for assessing the adequacy of a child or adolescent's energy intake is to monitor growth by tracking height and weight on growth charts developed by the National Center for Health Statistics; these CDC growth charts may be accessed via http://www.cdc.gov/growthcharts.

PROTEIN

Protein is essential for growth, development, and maintenance of the body; it also provides energy. Protein yields 4 kcal/gram (g). Food sources of protein include meat, fish, poultry, milk, cheese, yogurt, dried beans, peanut butter, nuts, and grain products. Protein from animal sources is called "complete protein," because it contains all nine indispensable amino acids. Protein from plant sources is called "incomplete protein," because it tends to be deficient in one or more of the indispensable amino acids. A vegetable protein may be paired with another vegetable protein or with a small amount of animal protein to provide adequate amounts of all the indispensable amino acids. For example, black-eyed peas can be paired with rice, peanut butter with wheat bread, pasta with cheese, or cereal with milk.

TABLE 16.5
Dietary Reference Intakes (DRIs): Tolerable Upper Intake Levels (ULs) for Children and Adolescents[a]

	1 to 3 Years	4 to 8 Years	9 to 13 Years	14 to 18 Years
Vitamins				
Vitamin A (μg/day)[b]	600	900	1700	2800
Vitamin C (mg/day)	400	650	1200	1800
Vitamin D (μg/day)	50	50	50	50
Vitamin E (mg/day)[c,d]	200	300	600	800
Vitamin K	ND[e]	ND	ND	ND
Thiamin	ND	ND	ND	ND
Riboflavin	ND	ND	ND	ND
Niacin (mg/day)[d]	10	15	20	30
Vitamin B_6 (mg/day)	30	40	60	80
Folate (μg/day)[d]	300	400	600	800
Vitamin B_{12}	ND	ND	ND	ND
Pantothenic Acid	ND	ND	ND	ND
Biotin	ND	ND	ND	ND
Choline (g/day)	1.0	1.0	2.0	3.0
Carotenoids[f]	ND	ND	ND	ND
Elements				
Arsenic[g]	ND	ND	ND	ND
Boron (mg/day)	3	6	11	17
Calcium (g/day)	2.5	2.5	2.5	2.5
Chromium	ND	ND	ND	ND
Copper (μg/day)	1000	3000	5000	8000
Fluoride (mg/day)	1.3	2.2	10	10
Iodine (μg/day)	200	300	600	900
Iron (mg/day)	40	40	40	45
Magnesium (mg/day)[h]	65	110	350	350
Manganese (mg/day)	2	3	6	9
Molybdenum (μg/day)	300	600	1100	1700
Nickel (mg/day)	0.2	0.3	0.6	1.0
Phosphorus (g/day)	3	3	4	4
Potassium	ND	ND	ND	ND
Selenium (μg/day)	90	150	280	400
Silicon[i]	ND	ND	ND	ND
Sulfate	ND	ND	ND	ND
Vanadium (mg/day)[j]	ND	ND	ND	ND

Continued

TABLE 16.5
(Continued)

	1 to 3 Years	4 to 8 Years	9 to 13 Years	14 to 18 Years
Elements (Continued)				
Zinc (mg/day)	7	12	23	34
Sodium (g/day)	1.5	1.9	2.2	2.3
Chloride (g/day)	2.3	2.9	3.4	3.6

[a] UL = The maximum level of daily nutrient intake that is likely to pose no risk of adverse health effects to almost all individuals in the general population. Unless otherwise specified, the UL represents total intake from food, water, and supplements.

[b] As preformed vitamin A only.

[c] As α-tocopherol; applies to any form of supplemental α-tocopherol.

[d] The ULs for vitamin E, niacin, and folate apply to synthetic forms obtained from supplements, fortified foods, or a combination of the two.

[e] ND = Not determinable due to lack of data of adverse effects in these age groups and concern with regard to lack of ability to handle excess amounts. In the absence of ULs, extra caution may be warranted in consuming levels above recommended intakes. Sources of intake should be from food only to prevent high levels of intake.

[f] β-Carotene supplements are advised only to serve as a provitamin A source for individuals at risk of vitamin A deficiency.

[g] Although the UL was not determined for arsenic, there is no justification for adding it to food or supplements.

[h] The ULs for magnesium represent intake from a pharmacological agent only and do not include intake from food and water.

[i] Although silicon has not been shown to cause adverse effects in humans, there is no justification for adding it to supplements.

[j] Although vanadium in food has not been shown to cause adverse effects in humans, there is no justification for adding it to food and vanadium supplements should be used with caution. The UL for adults is 1.8 mg/day of elemental vanadium; the UL for adults is based on adverse effects in laboratory animals, but this data could not be used to set a UL for children and adolescents.

Source: Adapted from: Institute of Medicine, *Dietary Reference Intakes for Calcium, Phosphorus, Magnesium, Vitamin D, and Fluoride,* National Academy Press, Washington, DC, 1997; Institute of Medicine, *Dietary Reference Intakes for Thiamin, Riboflavin, Niacin, Vitamin B₆, Folate, Vitamin B₁₂, Pantothenic Acid, Biotin, and Choline,* National Academy Press, Washington, DC, 1998; Institute of Medicine, *Dietary Reference Intakes for Vitamin C, Vitamin E, Selenium, and Carotenoids,* National Academy Press, Washington, DC, 2000; Institute of Medicine, *Dietary Reference Intakes for Vitamin A, Vitamin K, Arsenic, Boron, Chromium, Copper, Iodine, Iron, Manganese, Molybedenum, Nickel, Silicon, Vanadium, and Zinc,* National Academy Press, Washington, DC, 2001; and Institute of Medicine, *Dietary Reference Intakes for Water, Potassium, Sodium, Chloride, and Sulfate,* National Academies Press, Washington, DC, 2005. These reports may be accessed via www.nap.edu.

Proteins in the body are continuously being degraded and resynthesized. Because the process is not entirely efficient and some amino acids are lost, a continuous supply of amino acids is needed to replace these losses, even after growth has stopped. The primary factor that influences protein needs is energy intake, because when energy intake is insufficient, protein is used for energy. Thus, all protein recommendations are based on the assumption that energy needs are adequately met. In addition, protein recommendations are based on intakes of complete protein; appropriate corrections must be made for diets that customarily provide incomplete proteins.

Three ounces of poultry or lean meat provide about 25 g of protein. Three ounces of fish or 1 cup of soybeans provides about 20 g of protein. One cup of yogurt provides about 8 g of protein. One cup of milk provides about 8 g of protein. One egg provides about 6 g of protein. One ounce of cheese provides about 6 g of protein. One cup of legumes provides about 15 g of protein. Cereals, grains, nuts, and vegetables provide about 2 g of protein per serving.[1]

The RDAs for protein for children and adolescents are provided in Table 16.2 in g/day and g/kg/day. The EARs for protein for children and adolescents are provided in Table 16.6 in g/kg/day. The EARs and RDAs for indispensable amino acids for children and adolescents are provided in Table 16.8. As Table 16.2 indicates, protein requirements slowly decline relative to weight during the preschool to mid-elementary school years, and during the upper elementary to high-school years. A 14-year-old adolescent boy who weighs 61 kilograms (kg) [134 pounds] needs 52 g of protein each day; assuming that energy needs are met, this protein need can be met by eating a hamburger (3-ounce meat patty on a bun for a total of 29 g of protein) and two slices of pizza topped with meat and cheese (for a total of 23 g of protein).

Children aged 1 to 3 years should get 5 to 20% of their daily energy from protein.[1] Children and adolescents aged 4 to 18 years should get 10 to 30% of their daily energy from protein.[1] (See Table 16.3.)

CARBOHYDRATES

Carbohydrates (starches and sugars) provide energy to cells in the body, especially the brain, because it is a carbohydrate-dependent organ. The new RDA for carbohydrate for children, adolescents, and adults is set at 130 g/day based on the average

TABLE 16.6

Dietary Reference Intakes (DRIs): Estimated Average Requirements (EARs) for Groups of Children and Adolescents[a]

	Children		Boys		Girls	
	1 to 3 Years	4 to 8 Years	9 to 13 Years	14 to 18 Years	9 to 13 Years	14 to 18 Years
Carbohydrate (g/day)	100	100	100	100	100	100
Protein (g/kg/day)	0.87	0.76	0.76	0.73	0.76	0.71
Vitamin A (μg/day)[b]	210	275	445	630	420	485
Vitamin C (mg/day)	13	22	39	63	39	56
Vitamin E (mg/day)[c]	5	6	9	12	9	12
Thiamin (mg/day)	0.4	0.5	0.7	1.0	0.7	0.9
Riboflavin (mg/day)	0.4	0.5	0.8	1.1	0.8	0.9
Niacin (mg/day)[d]	5	6	9	12	9	11
Vitamin B_6 (mg/day)	0.4	0.5	0.8	1.1	0.8	1.0
Folate (μg/day)[e]	120	160	250	330	250	330
Vitamin B_{12} (μg/day)	0.7	1.0	1.5	2.0	1.5	2.0
Copper (μg/day)	260	340	540	685	540	685
Iodine (μg/day)	65	65	73	95	73	95
Iron (mg/day)	3.0	4.1	5.9	7.7	5.7	7.9
Magnesium (mg/day)	65	110	200	340	200	300
Molybdenum (μg/day)	13	17	26	33	26	33
Phosphorus (mg/day)	380	405	1055	1055	1055	1055
Selenium (μg/day)	17	23	35	45	35	45
Zinc (mg/day)	2.5	4.0	7.0	8.5	7.0	7.3

[a] EARs serve 2 purposes: for assessing adequacy of population intakes and as the basis for calculating Recommended Dietary Allowances (RDAs) for individuals. EARs have not been established for vitamin D, vitamin K, pantothenic acid, biotin, choline, calcium, chromium, fluoride, manganese, or other nutrients not yet evaluated via the DRI process.

[b] As retinol activity equivalents (RAEs). 1 RAE = 1 μg retinol, 12 μg β-carotene, 24 μg α-carotene, or 24 μg β-cryptoxanthin. The RAE for dietary provitamin A carotenoids is twofold greater than retinol equivalents (RE), whereas the RAE for preformed vitamin A is the same as RE.

[c] As α-tocopherol. α-Tocopherol includes *RRR-α*-tocopherol, the only form of α-tocopherol that occurs naturally in foods, and the *2R*-stereoisomeric forms of α-tocopherol (*RRR-*, *RSR-*, *RRS-*, and *RSS-α*-tocopherol) that occur in fortified foods and supplements. It does not include the *2S*-stereoisomeric forms of α-tocopherol (*SRR-*, *SSR-*, *SRS-*, and *SSS-α*-tocopherol), also found in fortified foods and supplements.

[d] As niacin equivalents (NE). 1 mg niacin = 60 mg tryptophan.

[e] As dietary folate equivalents (DFE). 1 DFE = 1 μg food folate = 0.6 μg folic acid from fortified food or as a supplement consumed with food = 0.5 μg of a supplement taken on an empty stomach.

Source: Adapted from: Institute of Medicine, *Dietary Reference Intakes for Calcium, Phosphorus, Magnesium, Vitamin D, and Fluoride*, National Academy Press, Washington, DC, 1997; Institute of Medicine, *Dietary Reference Intakes for Thiamin, Riboflavin, Niacin, Vitamin B_6, Folate, Vitamin B_{12}, Pantothenic Acid, Biotin, and Choline*, National Academy Press, Washington, DC, 1998; Institute of Medicine, *Dietary Reference Intakes for Vitamin C, Vitamin E, Selenium, and Carotenoids*, National Academy Press, Washington, DC, 2000; Institute of Medicine, *Dietary Reference Intakes for Vitamin A, Vitamin K, Arsenic, Boron, Chromium, Copper, Iodine, Iron, Manganese, Molybedenum, Nickel, Silicon, Vanadium, and Zinc*, National Academy Press, Washington, DC, 2001; and Institute of Medicine, *Dietary Reference Intakes for Energy, Carbohydrate, Fiber, Fat, Fatty Acids, Cholesterol, Protein, and Amino Acids,* National Academies Press, Washington, DC, 2002/2005. These reports may be accessed via www.nap.edu.

amount of glucose utilized by the brain.[1] (See Table 16.2.) However, this level of intake is typically exceeded to meet energy needs while consuming acceptable intake levels of protein and fat.[1] No recommendations based on glycemic index are made due to a lack of sufficient evidence on the prevention of chronic diseases in generally healthy individuals.[1]

Children and adolescents should get 45 to 65% of their daily energy from carbohydrates.[1] (See Table 16.3.) Complex carbohydrates (starchy foods such as pasta, breads, cereals, rice, and legumes) should provide the majority of energy from carbohydrates, and simple carbohydrates (naturally occurring sugars in fruits and vegetables) should provide the rest. The Institute of Medicine recommends that added sugars be limited to no more than 25% of total energy (Table 16.4).[1] Carbohydrate yields 4 kcal/g. An active 6-year-old boy who needs about 1750 kcal/day would need about 788 to 1138 kcal (or 197 to 284 g) from

TABLE 16.7
Criteria and Dietary Reference Intake (DRI) Values for Energy by Active Children and Adolescents by Life Stage Group[a]

Life Stage Group (Years)	Criterion	Active PAL EER[b] (kcal/Day)	
		Boys	Girls
1 through 2	Energy expenditure plus energy deposition	1046	992 (24 months)
3 through 8	Energy expenditure plus energy deposition	1742	1642 (6 years)
9 through 13	Energy expenditure plus energy deposition	2279	2071 (11 years)
14 through 18	Energy expenditure plus energy deposition	3152	2368 (16 years)

[a] For healthy active American and Canadian children and adolescents. Based on the cited age, an active physical activity level, and the reference heights and weights in Table 16.1. Individualized EERs can be determined from the predictive equations in the text for this chapter.

[b] PAL = Physical Activity Level, EER = Estimated Energy Requirement. The intake that meets the average energy expenditure of individuals at the reference age, height, and weight (see Table 16.1).

Source: Adapted from: Institute of Medicine, *Dietary Reference Intakes for Energy, Carbohydrate, Fiber, Fat, Fatty Acids, Cholesterol, Protein, and Amino Acids,* National Academies Press, Washington, DC, 2002/2005. This report may be accessed via www.nap.edu.

TABLE 16.8
Estimated Average Requirements (EARs) and Recommended Dietary Allowances (RDAs) for Amino Acids for Children and Adolescents

	Children		Boys		Girls	
	1 to 3 Years	4 to 8 Years	9 to 13 Years	14 to 18 Years	9 to 13 Years	14 to 18 Years
EAR[a] (mg/kg/day)						
Histidine	16	13	13	12	12	12
Isoleucine	22	18	18	17	17	16
Leucine	48	40	40	38	38	35
Lysine	45	37	37	35	35	32
Methionine + cysteine	22	18	18	17	17	16
Phenylalanine + tyrosine	41	33	33	31	31	28
Threonine	24	19	19	18	18	17
Tryptophan	6	5	5	5	5	4
Valine	28	23	23	22	22	20
RDA[b] (mg/kg/day)						
Histidine	21	16	17	15	15	14
Isoleucine	28	22	22	21	21	19
Leucine	63	49	49	47	47	44
Lysine	58	46	46	43	43	40
Methionine + cysteine	28	22	22	21	21	19
Phenylalanine + tyrosine	54	41	41	38	38	35
Threonine	32	24	24	22	22	21
Tryptophan	8	6	6	6	6	5
Valine	37	28	28	27	27	24

[a] EAR for age 1 through 13 years = maintenance + amino acid deposition × 1.72. EAR for age 14 through 18 years = maintenance + amino acid deposition × 2.13.

[b] RDA for age 1 through 13 years = EAR + 2 × $\sqrt{[(0.12 \times \text{maintenance})^2 + (0.43 \times 2.13 \times \text{mean protein deposition})^2]}$.

Source: Adapted from Institute of Medicine, *Dietary Reference Intakes for Energy, Carbohydrate, Fiber, Fat, Fatty Acids, Cholesterol, Protein, and Amino Acids,* National Academies Press, Washington, DC, 2002/2005. This report may be accessed via www.nap.edu.

carbohydrates daily. An active 11-year-old girl who needs about 2075 kcal/day would need about 934 to 1349 kcal (or 233 to 337 g) from carbohydrates daily.

FAT AND CHOLESTEROL

Fat is a major source of energy for the body and helps in the absorption of fat-soluble vitamins and carotenoids. Neither an AI nor RDA was set for total fat, because there is insufficient data to determine a defined level of fat intake at which risk of inadequacy or prevention of chronic disease occurs.[1] Likewise, a UL was not set for total fat, because there is no defined intake level of fat at which an adverse effect occurs.[1] However, the AMDR for total fat was set at 30 to 40% of energy for children aged 1 to 3 years and 25 to 35% of energy for children and adolescents age 4 to 18 years (Table 16.3).[1] In the 2005 Dietary Guidelines for Americans, the level for total fat intake is between 30 to 35% of energy for children age 2 to 3 years of, and between 25 to 35% of energy for children and adolescents age 4 to 18 years of, with most fats coming from sources of polyunsaturated and monounsaturated fatty acids, such as fish, nuts, and vegetable oils.[14] The levels of total fat intake for children and adolescents found in the 2005 Dietary Guidelines for Americans are recommended by the American Heart Association and the American Academy of Pediatrics.[15,16]

For saturated fatty acids, neither an AI nor RDA was set because they have no known role in preventing chronic diseases and because they are synthesized by the body to provide adequate levels needed for their physiological and structural functions.[1] A UL was not set, because any incremental increase in saturated fatty acid intake increases risk of coronary heart disease.[1] The Institute of Medicine recommends that intake of saturated fatty acids be as low as possible while consuming a nutritionally adequate diet.[1] A key recommendation from the 2005 Dietary Guidelines for Americans is that less than 10% of energy come from saturated fatty acids.[14] The American Heart Association and the American Academy of Pediatrics recommend diets low in saturated fats for children and adolescents.[15,16]

Linoleic acid serves as a precursor to eicosanoids; it is the only $n-6$ polyunsaturated fatty acid that is an essential fatty acid.[1] $n-3$ Polyunsaturated fatty acids (α-linolenic acid) play an important role as structural membrane lipids, especially in nerve tissue and the retina, and are precursors to eicosanoids.[1] AIs and AMDRs are found in Table 16.2 and Table 16.3, respectively, for linoleic acid and α-linolenic acid for children and adolescents. There was insufficient evidence to set a UL for $n-6$ polyunsaturated fatty acids or $n-3$ polyunsaturated fatty acids.[1]

No AI or RDA was set for *trans* fatty acids because they are not essential and provide no known benefit to human health.[1] A UL was not set, because any incremental increase in intake of *trans* fatty acids increases risk of coronary heart disease. The Institute of Medicine and the 2005 Dietary Guidelines for Americans recommend that intake of *trans* fatty acids be as low as possible while consuming a nutritionally adequate diet.[1,14] The American Heart Association and the American Academy of Pediatrics recommend diets low in *trans* fatty acids for children and adolescents.[15,16] Based on data collected in 1994 through 1996, approximately 80% of *trans* fat in the diet is provided by processed foods and oils, and 20% occurs naturally in food from animal sources; however, *trans* fat content of certain processed foods has changed and is likely to continue to change as the industry reformulates products.[14]

Although cholesterol plays an important role in steroid hormone and bile acid biosynthesis and is an integral component of cell membranes, there is no evidence for a biological requirement for dietary cholesterol because all tissues are capable of synthesizing sufficient amounts of cholesterol. Thus, neither an AI nor a RDA was set for dietary cholesterol.[1] An UL was not set, because any incremental increase in intake of dietary cholesterol increases risk of coronary heart disease.[1] The Institute of Medicine recommends that intake of dietary cholesterol be as low as possible while consuming a nutritionally adequate diet.[1] A key recommendation from the 2005 Dietary Guidelines for Americans is to consume less than 300 mg/day of cholesterol.[14]

Dietary recommendations for children and adolescents by the American Heart Association and the American Academy of Pediatrics include a focus on ensuring adequate intakes of omega-3 fatty acids by consuming two servings of fish per week.[15–17] Along with the Food and Drug Administration, they advocate consumption of a wide variety of fish and shellfish and stress that seafood is an important part of a healthy diet. However, young children, women who may become pregnant or are already pregnant, and nursing mothers should avoid shark, swordfish, king mackerel, and tilefish due to high levels of mercury. Commonly eaten varieties of fish that are low in mercury include shrimp, canned light tuna, salmon, pollack, and catfish.[15,16]

Fat yields 9 kcal/g. Dietary sources of fat include oils, margarine, butter, fried foods, egg yolks, mayonnaise, salad dressings, ice cream, hard cheese, cream cheese, nuts, fatty meats, chips, and doughnuts. To keep saturated fat intake low, limit intake of animal fats (e.g., full-fat dairy products such as cheese, milk, butter, and ice cream; fatty meat, bacon, sausage, and poultry skin and fat). To keep *trans* fat intake low, limit intake of foods made with partially hydrogenated vegetable oils. To keep cholesterol intake low, limit egg yolks and organ meats especially, as well as meat, shellfish, and poultry, and dairy products that contain fat. Table 16.9 provides the total fat, saturated fat, and cholesterol content of various foods. Information regarding the safety of low-fat diets for children is provided later in this chapter.

Fiber

Because a variety of definitions of dietary fiber existed worldwide, the Institute of Medicine convened a special panel to develop a proposed definition of fiber.[10] Based on the panel's deliberations, along with consideration of public comments and subsequent modifications, the following definitions were developed[1]:

- *Dietary fiber* consists of nondigestible carbohydrates and lignin that are intrinsic and intact in plants.
- *Functional fiber* consists of isolated, nondigestible carbohydrates that have beneficial physiological effects in humans.
- *Total fiber* is the sum of dietary fiber and functional fiber.[1]

The different properties of fibers result in different physiological effects.[1] For example, viscous fibers may delay gastric emptying; this results in a sensation of fullness, which may contribute to weight control. In addition, delayed gastric emptying may reduce postprandial blood glucose concentrations and potentially have a beneficial effect on insulin sensitivity. Viscous fibers may reduce blood cholesterol concentrations by interfering with the absorption of dietary fat and cholesterol, as well

TABLE 16.9
Total Fat, Saturated Fat, and Cholesterol Content of Various Foods

Food	Amount	Total Fat (g)	Saturated Fat (g)	Cholesterol (mg)	Kcal
Almonds, dry roasted	1 oz (~22 nuts)	15.0	1.1	0	169
Bacon, cured, broiled/pan fried	3 med. slices	9.4	3.3	16	109
Bread, white	0.88 oz slice	0.9	0.1	<1	67
Butter	1 T	11.5	7.2	31	102
Cheese, American processed	1 oz	8.9	5.6	27	106
Cheese, cheddar	1 oz	9.4	6.0	30	114
Chicken breast with skin, roasted	½ breast (3.5 oz)	7.6	2.1	82	193
Chicken breast without skin, roasted	½ breast (3 oz)	3.1	0.9	73	142
Coconut, dried, sweetened, flaked, packaged	1 oz	9.1	8.1	0	134
Corn oil	1 T	13.6	1.7	0	120
Cottonseed oil	1 T	13.6	3.5	0	120
Egg (chicken), boiled, hard/soft	1 large	5.3	1.6	212	78
Egg (chicken), white, raw	1 large	0.0	0.0	0	17
Egg (chicken), yolk, raw	1 large	5.2	1.6	218	61
Finfish, flounder/sole, cooked by dry heat	3 oz	1.3	0.3	58	99
Ground beef, 25% fat, patty, broiled	3 oz patty	15.9	6.1	76	236
Ground beef, 5% fat, patty, broiled	3 oz patty	5.6	2.4	65	145
Ice cream, vanilla, regular (10% fat)	½ c	7.9	4.9	32	145
Lard (pork fat), raw	1 T	12.8	5.0	12	115
Margarine, corn, stick	1 t	3.8	0.7	0	34
Margarine, liquid	1 T	11.4	1.9	0	102
Milk (cow), whole, 3.3 % fat	8 fl oz	8.1	5.1	34	149
Milk (cow), reduced fat, 2% fat	8 fl oz	4.7	2.9	20	122
Milk (cow), low fat, 1% fat	8 fl oz	2.6	1.6	10	102
Milk (cow), nonfat	8 fl oz	0.4	0.3	5	86
Olive oil	1 T	13.5	1.8	0	119
Peanut butter, chunk style/crunchy	2 T	16.0	3.1	0	188
Peanuts, dry roasted	1 oz (~28 nuts)	14.1	2.0	0	166
Pecans, dried	1 oz (20 halves)	20.4	1.8	0	196
Pork, tenderloin, lean, roasted	3 oz	4.1	1.4	67	139
Safflower oil, >70% linoleic acid	1 T	13.6	0.8	0	120
Shrimp, cooked by moist heat	3 oz (15 ½ large)	0.9	0.2	166	84
Soy oil	1 T	13.6	2.0	0	120
Tuna, light, canned in oil, drained	3 oz	7.0	1.3	15	168
Tuna, light, canned in water, drained	3 oz	0.7	0.2	26	99
Turkey, breast with skin, roasted	3 oz	2.7	0.7	77	130
Yogurt, frozen, soft serve, vanilla	½ c	4.0	2.5	1	114

Source: Adapted from Pennington, JAT and Douglass, JS, *Bowes and Church's Food Values of Portions Commonly Used*, 18th edition, Lippincott Williams & Wilkins, Philadelphia, 2005.

as with the enterohepatic recirculation of cholesterol and bile acids. Fecal bulk, laxation, and constipation are improved by consumption of dietary fiber and certain functional fibers, especially those that are poorly fermented. Normal laxation can be a problem for many children. The AIs for total fiber in foods for children and adolescents are found in Table 16.2; ULs were not set for dietary fiber or functional fiber due to insufficient evidence.[1]

The American Health Foundation recommends that children age 2 years and older consume a minimal amount of fiber equal to their age plus 5 g/day, and a maximum amount of age plus 10 g/day, to achieve intakes of a maximum of 35 g/day after the age of 20 years.[18,19] These recommendations were endorsed at a conference held in May 1994 about dietary fiber in childhood.[20] This range is thought to be safe, reasonable, and practical.[21,22] The "age plus 5" recommendation results in a gradual increase in fiber intake over time with a 3-year-old eating 8 g/day and an 18-year-old eating 23 g/day.

Fiber intake should be increased gradually through consumption of a variety of fruits, vegetables, legumes, cereals, and other whole-grain products such as breads and crackers. Fiber supplements for children are not recommended as a means of meeting dietary fiber goals.[18] Increased intakes of dietary fiber should be accompanied by increased intakes of water, because dietary fiber increases water retention in the colon, which leads to bulkier and softer stools.[18] For most children and adolescents, dietary fiber goals can be met if the daily diet includes two servings of vegetables, three servings of fruits, two slices of whole wheat bread, and a serving of breakfast cereal containing three or more grams of fiber.[19] Table 16.10 provides a list of foods containing fiber that most U.S. children and adolescents will eat.

High-fiber diets do have the potential for reduced energy density, reduced kcal intake, and poor growth, especially in very young children. Furthermore, high-fiber diets may reduce the bioavailability of minerals such as iron, calcium, and zinc. However, the potential health benefits of a moderate increase in dietary fiber intake in childhood are thought to outweigh the potential risks significantly, especially in highly industrialized countries such as the United States.[18]

WATER

Water is the largest single constituent of the human body; it is essential for cellular homeostatis and life.[13] A low intake of total water (from drinking water, water in beverages, and food) has been associated with some chronic diseases, but this evidence is

TABLE 16.10
Fiber Content of Foods that Most U.S. Children and Adolescents Will Eat[a]

Food	Serving Size	Approximate Grams of Dietary Fiber
Baked Beans	1 c	13
Chili with beans	1 c	7
Refried beans	4 oz	6
Brown rice	1 c	4
Peanuts (dry roasted)	2 oz	4
Strawberries	1 c	4
Whole-wheat bread	2 slices	4
Potato, baked, with skin	1 medium	3.5
Apple	1 medium	3
Banana	1 large	3
Carrot (raw)	1 medium	3
Corn	½ c	3
Kiwi	1 large	3
Raisins	1/3 c	3
Whole-grain crackers	½ oz	2–3
Cereal	1 c	2–3[a]
Applesauce	½ c	2
Broccoli	½ c	2
Orange	1 medium	2
Peanut butter	2 tbsp	2

[a] Dietary fiber content of cereal varies widely. Best fiber choice for children has 3 + g/cup.

Source: Adapted from Williams, CL, *J Am Diet Assoc*, 95, 1140, 1995.

insufficient to establish water intake recommendations in order to reduce the risk of chronic diseases; thus, an AI for total water (see Table 16.2) was set to prevent deleterious (mainly acute) effects of dehydration, which include metabolic and functional abnormalities.[13]

About 80% of total water intake comes from drinking water and other beverages.[13] Although diuretic effects have been shown in some studies from consumption of caffeinated beverages, available information indicates that this may be transient in nature and thus, such beverages do contribute to total water intake similar to that contributed by noncaffeinated beverages.[13] Deficits in body water can occur over the course of a few hours due to decreased intake or increased water losses from physical activity and environmental factors (e.g., heat, exposure). However, on a daily basis, fluid intake, which is driven by a combination of thirst and consumption of beverages at meals, allows for hydration status and normal levels of total body water to be maintained.[13]

An UL was not set for water, because healthy individuals have considerable ability to excrete excess water and thus maintain water balance.[13] However, there have been reports of acute water toxicity due to rapid consumption of large quantities of fluids that greatly exceeded the kidney's maximal excretion rate of about 0.7 to 1.0 L/h.[13]

Selected Vitamins and Minerals

Vitamin D

Throughout the world, the major source of vitamin D for humans is the exposure of the skin to sunlight; vitamin D that is synthesized in the skin during the summer and fall months can be stored in the body's fat for use in the winter, which minimizes requirements for vitamin D. In nature, very few foods contain vitamin D; thus, children and adolescents who live in far northern latitudes (e.g., northern Canada and Alaska) may need vitamin D supplements. Food sources of vitamin D include some fish liver oils, eggs from hens that have been fed vitamin D, the liver and fat from aquatic mammals such as seals and polar bears, and the flesh of fatty fish. Foods fortified with vitamin D include milk products and other foods such as margarine and breakfast cereals; the majority of human intake of vitamin D is from fortified foods. Fortified milk is supposed to contain 10 μg (400 IU) per quart regardless of the fat content of milk; however, several recent surveys have indicated that many milk samples contained less than 8 μg per quart. Although it is well recognized that vitamin D deficiency causes abnormalities in calcium and bone metabolism, it is premature to suggest that cancer risk is increased by vitamin D deficiency. The AIs for vitamin D for children and adolescents (see Table 16.2) were set to cover the needs of almost all children and adolescents regardless of exposure to sunlight. Currently, there is no scientific evidence that demonstrates an increased requirement for vitamin D during puberty even though metabolism of vitamin D increases during puberty to enhance intestinal calcium absorption to provide adequate calcium for the rapidly growing skeleton. [3]

Calcium

Over 99% of total body calcium is found in teeth and bones. Approximately 45% of adult skeletal mass is accounted for by skeletal growth during adolescence; thus, achieving and maintaining adequate calcium intake during adolescence is necessary for the development of a maximal peak bone mass, which may help reduce the risk of osteoporosis later in adulthood.

The calcium AIs for adolescents are higher than for children because from age 9 through 18 years (see Table 16.2), calcium retention increases to a peak and then declines. However, the calcium AIs remain the same for adolescents from age 9 to 18 years, because calcium absorption efficiency decreases. Thus, during this developmental period, measures of sexual maturity are better predictors of calcium retention than chronological age.[3]

Major food sources of calcium include milk, yogurt, cheese, and green leafy vegetables. Calcium-fortified orange juice is also an excellent source of calcium, as is tofu. Table 16.11 contains the approximate calcium content for one serving of various common foods. Vitamin D (discussed previously in this chapter) is needed for the body to absorb calcium.

The calcium content of food is generally of greater importance than bioavailability when evaluating food sources of calcium. The efficiency of calcium absorption is fairly similar from most foods, including milk and milk products and grains, which are major food sources of calcium in North American diets. Calcium may be poorly absorbed from foods such as spinach, beans, sweet potatoes, and rhubarb which are rich in oxalic acid, and from unleavened bread, raw beans, seeds, nuts, and grains, and soy isolates, which are rich in phytic acid. Calcium absorption is relatively high from soybeans, although they contain large amounts of phytic acid. Compared to calcium absorption from milk, calcium absorption from spinach is about 1/10, and from dried beans is about half.[3]

Children and adolescents (and adults) with lactose intolerance may develop symptoms of diarrhea and bloating after ingesting lactose; however, the likelihood of developing the symptoms depends on the amount of residual lactase activity, the amount of lactose consumed, and the composition of the meal.[23] People who generally are lactose digesters include Northern Europeans, Finns, Hungarians, probably Mongols, the Fulani and Tussi tribes of Africa, and the Punjabis of India; the remainder of the world's population are lactose nondigesters.[24] However, as digesters intermix reproductively with nondigesters, the rate of lactose malabsorption falls. In general, evidence for lactose malabsorption as a clinical problem is not manifest until after

TABLE 16.11
Approximate Calcium Content for One Serving of Various Common Foods[a]

Food	Serving Size	Approximate Calcium Content (mg)
Milk (whole, 1%, 2%, or buttermilk)	8 oz	300
Yogurt	8 oz	300
Cheese (swiss)	1 oz	272
Cheese (cheddar)	1 oz	204
Cheese (mozzarella, part nonfat)	1 oz	183
Cheese (American processed)	1 oz	175
Calcium-fortified orange juice	8 oz	350
Canned salmon (with bones)	3 oz	181
Cooked greens (collards)	1 c	226
Pudding	½ c	150
Spinach (cooked)	1 c	245
Frozen yogurt (vanilla, soft serve)	½ c	103
Ice cream (vanilla, 10% fat)	½ c	92
Cooked greens (mustard, kale)	1 c	100
Cottage cheese	1 c	140
Spinach (raw)	1 c	30
Orange	1 medium	52
Beans, canned (baked)	½ c	60
Sweet potatoes (mashed)	1 c	77
Broccoli (cooked)	1 med. stalk	83

Source: Adapted from Pennington, JAT & Douglass, JS, *Bowes and Church's Food Values of Portions Commonly Used*, 18th edition., Lippincott Williams & Wilkins, Philadelphia, 2005.

5 to 7 years of age, although this age can vary. Individuals with lactose intolerance can increase their tolerance by adding small amounts of lactose-containing foods to their diet.[24] Fermented dairy products, such as yogurt and hard cheese, may be tolerated better than milk; in addition, lactose-free and low-lactose milks are available, and calcium may be obtained by consuming calcium-supplemented foods (such as calcium-fortified soy milk and calcium-fortified juice) and nondairy foods (such as broccoli, collards, and baked beans).[25] Many children with lactose intolerance can drink small amounts of milk without discomfort, especially when they consume other foods with it.[25] Although lactose intolerance may influence intake, lactose-intolerant individuals absorb calcium normally from milk; thus, there is no evidence to suggest that it influences the calcium requirement.[3]

Folate

Folate is important during periods of increased cell replication and growth due to its role in DNA synthesis and the formation of healthy red blood cells; thus, the RDAs for folate are 1.5 times greater for children age 9 to 13 years than for children age 4 to 8 years (see Table 16.2).[4] There is strong evidence that the risk of having a fetus with a neural tube defect decreases with increased intake of folate during the periconceptional period. Therefore, it is recommended that all females capable of becoming pregnant take $400\,\mu g$ of synthetic folic acid daily, from fortified foods or supplements, in addition to consuming food folate from a varied diet. Folate fortification became mandatory for enriched grain products in the United States as of January 1998. Besides fortified grains and cereals, other food sources of folate include leafy green vegetables, orange juice, liver, cantaloupe, yeast, and seeds.[4]

Iron

According to the American Academy of Pediatrics,[26] iron deficiency is the most common nutritional deficiency in the United States. Children aged 1 to 2 years are the most susceptible to iron deficiency due to increased iron needs related to rapid growth during the first 2 years of life and a relatively low iron content in most infant diets when iron is not added by supplementation or fortification. Children aged 3 to 11 years are at less risk for iron deficiency until the rapid growth of puberty. Preadolescent school-age children who consume a strict vegetarian diet are at greater risk for iron deficiency anemia. Adolescent boys are at risk for iron deficiency anemia during their peak growth period when iron stores may not meet the demand of rapid growth;

however, the iron deficiency anemia generally corrects itself after the growth spurt. Adolescent girls are at greater risk for iron deficiency anemia due to blood losses during menstruation. A major consequence of iron deficiency is that significant iron deficiency adversely affects child development and behavior. Furthermore, iron deficiency leads to enhanced lead absorption, and childhood lead poisoning is a well-documented cause of neurological and developmental deficits. These consequences, along with evidence that dietary intake during infancy is a strong determinant of iron status for older infants and younger children, emphasize the importance of prevention. Significant improvements have been made in the iron nutritional status of infants and young children in the United States during the past 2 decades, perhaps because during this same time frame, several changes were made in infant feeding patterns.[26] These changes included increased dietary iron content or iron bioavailability, increased incidence of breastfeeding, increased use of iron-fortified formula, and reduced use of whole milk and low-iron formula during the first year of life.[26]

Dietary iron is classified as "heme" or "non-heme" iron. Heme iron is found in foods from animals such as meat, fish, and poultry. Non-heme iron is provided by plants; good sources include dark-green leafy vegetables, tofu, lentils, white beans, dried fruits, and iron-fortified breads and cereals. On average, healthy people absorb about 5 to 10% of the iron consumed, and people who are iron deficient absorb about 10 to 20%. Heme iron is more easily absorbed than non-heme iron. About 20% of heme iron consumed is absorbed regardless of how it is prepared and served; however, the absorption rate of non-heme iron can be increased by eating foods with non-heme iron with either meat, foods rich in vitamin C, or foods that contain some heme iron at the same meal. Non-heme iron absorption can be hindered by as much as 50% when tannins, phytates, and calcium (which are found in foods such as tea, bran, and milk, respectively) are eaten at the same meal.

The RDAs for iron for children and adolescents are included in Table 16.2.[9] Because the amount of iron available in the American diet is estimated to be about 5 to 7 mg/1000 kcal, it may be difficult for adolescent girls to obtain 15 mg of iron from dietary sources alone if their caloric intake is between 2000 and 2400 kcal/day. Groups of adolescents who are at special risk of iron deficiency include (1) older adolescent girls due to their increased iron need and their low dietary intake, (2) pregnant adolescents, and (3) female athletes such as runners who may lose iron through occult gastrointestinal bleeding.

The Committee on the Prevention, Detection, and Management of Iron Deficiency Anemia Among U.S. Children and Women of Childbearing Age was established under the Food and Nutrition Board of the Institute of Medicine; its recommended guidelines were published in 1993.[27] They concluded that iron enrichment and fortification of the U.S. food supply should remain at current levels rather than increasing or decreasing the levels. Furthermore, they recommended that dietary sources of iron be consumed instead of supplemental sources when possible. Iron supplements should be kept out of reach of children, because iron is a very common cause of poisoning in children.[27]

Zinc

Zinc is needed for protein synthesis, wound healing, and sexual maturation; thus, zinc is especially important during adolescence due to the rapid rate of growth and sexual maturation. (See Table 16.2 for the RDAs for zinc for children and adolescents.[9]) Adolescents undergoing rapid growth are at risk for inadequate zinc levels, and should be encouraged to include zinc-rich foods in their daily diet. Foods high in zinc include red meats, certain seafood, and whole grains; many breakfast cereals are fortified with zinc. The bioavailability of zinc in foods varies widely. Zinc from whole grain products is less available than zinc from meat, liver, eggs, and seafood (especially oysters). Furthermore, consumption of phytate-rich foods limits absorption and maintenance of zinc balance.[9]

Potassium

Potassium is required for normal cellular function. The level of potassium from dietary intake according to the AI (see Table 16.2) should maintain lower blood pressure levels, reduce adverse effects of sodium chloride intake on blood pressure, decrease the risk of recurrent kidney stones, and possibly decrease bone loss.[13] Currently, dietary intake of potassium by all groups in the United States and Canada is much lower than the AI.[13] African Americans would especially benefit from an increased intake of potassium due to their relatively low intake of potassium and a high prevalence of elevated blood pressure and salt sensitivity.[13]

Good sources of potassium are fruits and vegetables. Relatively high amounts of potassium are found in spinach, cantaloupe, dry roasted almonds, Brussels sprouts, mushrooms, bananas, oranges, grapefruit, and potatoes. An UL was not set, because potassium intake from foods above the AI poses no potential for increased risk as excess potassium is readily excreted in the urine in the generally healthy population with normal kidney function.[13]

FOOD GUIDE PYRAMID

In April 2005, USDA released *MyPyramid*[28] as the new food guidance system to replace the original Food Guide Pyramid released in 1992.[29] *MyPyramid* translates the principles of the 2005 Dietary Guidelines for Americans[14] and other nutritional standards to help consumers make healthier food and physical activity choices. The *MyPyramid* symbol was designed to be simple and has no foods pictured on it. Each person has a pyramid that is right for them based on their age, sex, and physical activity level; consumers are encouraged to find out what they need to eat each day and their physical activity level at MyPyramid.gov.[28] The *MyPyramid* Food Guidance System includes a new motivational symbol and slogan, "Steps to a Healthier You," clear and concise nutrition messages for educational materials like posters and brochures that communicate the new food guidance recommendations in ways consumers can more easily understand and put into practice, and interactive activities on the internet at www.mypyramid.gov to help consumers personalize their diet and get more information on topics of interest to them.[28] *MyPyramid* is appropriate for children aged 2 years and older.[28]

MyPyramid includes food intake patterns that identify what and how much food an individual should eat for health based on the individual's age, sex, and activity level. As explained in Table 16.12, there are 12 different calorie levels in increments of 200 from 1000 to 3200 calories. There are food intake pattern calorie levels that identify the calorie level assigned to an individual in the *MyPyramid* plan, based on the individual's sex, age, and activity level. Table 14.13 can be used to help assign children and adolescents to the food intake pattern at a particular energy expenditure. Table 14.4 gives sussgested amounts of

TABLE 16.12
Daily *MyPyramid* Food Intake Patterns

Calorie Level [a]	Fruit Group [b] (Cups)	Vegetable Group [c] (Cups)	Grains Group [d] (oz-eq)	Meats and Beans Group [e] (oz-eq)	Milk Group [f] (Cups)	Oil [g] (tsp)	Discretionary Calorie Allowance [h]
1000	1	1	3	2	2	3	165
1200	1	1.5	4	3	2	4	171
1400	1.5	1.5	5	4	2	4	171
1600	1.5	2	5	5	3	5	132
1800	1.5	2.5	6	5	3	5	195
2000	2	2.5	6	5.5	3	6	267
2200	2	3	7	6	3	6	290
2400	2	3	8	6.5	3	7	362
2600	2	3.5	9	6.5	3	8	410
2800	2.5	3.5	10	7	3	8	426
3000	2.5	4	10	7	3	10	512
3200	2.5	4	10	7	3	11	648

The table provides suggested amounts of food to consume each day from each of the basic food groups, subgroups, and oils to meet recommended nutrient intakes at 12 different calorie levels. Nutrient and energy contributions from each group are calculated according to the nutrient-dense forms of foods in each group (e.g., lean meats and fat-free milk). In addition, the table shows the discretionary calorie allowance that can be accommodated within each calorie level.

[a] **Calorie Levels** are set across a wide range to accommodate the needs of different individuals. Table 16.13 "Estimated Daily Calorie Needs" can be used to help assign children and adolescents to the food-intake pattern at a particular calorie level.

[b] The **Fruit Group** includes all fresh, frozen, canned, and dried fruits and fruit juices. In general, 1 cup of fruit, 1 cup of 100% fruit juice, or ½ cup of dried fruit can be considered as 1 cup from the fruit group.

[c] The **Vegetable Group** includes all fresh, frozen, canned, and dried vegetables and vegetable juices. In general, 1 cup of raw or cooked vegetables or vegetable juice, or 2 cups of raw leafy greens can be considered as 1 cup from the vegetable group. Table 16.14 provides recommended amounts from each of the vegetable subgroups per week.

[d] The **Grains Group** includes all foods made from wheat, rice, oats, cornmeal, or barley, such as bread, pasta, oatmeal, breakfast cereals, tortillas, and grits. In general, 1 slice of bread, 1 cup of ready-to-eat cereal, or ½ cup of cooked rice, pasta, or cooked cereal can be considered as 1 ounce equivalent from the grains groups. *At least half of all grains consumed should be whole grains.*

[e] For the **Meats and Beans Group**, in general, 1 ounce of lean meat, poultry, or fish, 1 egg, 1 tablespoon peanut butter, ¼ cup cooked dry beans, or ½ ounce of nuts or seeds can be considered a 1 ounce equivalent from the meat and beans group.

[f] The **Milk Group** includes all fluid milk products and foods made from milk that retain their calcium content, such as yogurt and cheese. Foods made from milk that have little to no calcium (e.g., cream cheese, cream, butter) are not part of the milk group. Most milk group choices should be fat-free or low-fat. In general, 1 cup of milk or yogurt, 1.5 ounces of natural cheese, or 2 ounces of processed cheese can be considered as 1 cup from the milk group.

[g] **Oils** include fats from different plants and from fish that are liquid at room temperature, such as canola, corn, olive, soybean, and sunflower oil. Some foods are naturally high in oils, like nuts, olives, some fish, and avocados. Foods that are mainly oil include mayonnaise, some salad dressings, and soft margarine.

[h] The **Discretionary Calorie Allowance** is the remaining amount of calories in a food intake pattern after accounting for the calories needed for all food groups — using forms of foods that are fat-free or low-fat and with no added sugars.

Source: Adapted from USDA, Center for Nutrition Policy and Promotion, *MyPyramid Food Intake Patterns*, Washington, D.C. April, 2005. Available at http://www.mypyramid.gov/downloads/MyPyramid_Food_Intake_Patterns.pdf

TABLE 16.13
Estimated Daily Calorie Needs

	Calorie Range	
	Sedentary[a]	Active[b]
Children		
2 to 3 years	1000	1400
Girls		
4 to 8 years	1200	1800
9 to 13 years	1600	2200
14 to 18 years	1800	2400
Boys		
4 to 8 years	1400	2000
9 to 13 years	1800	2600
14 to 18 years	2200	3200

[a] Sedentary means a lifestyle that includes only the light physical activity associated with typical day-to-day life.

[b] Active means a lifestyle that includes physical activity equivalent to walking more than 3 mi/day at 3 to 4 mi/h, in addition to the light physical activity associated with typical day-to-day life.

Source: Adapted from USDA, Center for Nutrition Policy and Promotion, *MyPyramid Food Intake Patterns*, Washington, D.C. April, 2005. Available at http://www.mypyramid.gov/downloads/MyPyramid_Food_Intake_Patterns.pdf

TABLE 16.14
Vegetable Subgroup Amounts Per Week

Calorie Level	Dark Green Vegetables (Cups)	Orange Vegetables (Cups)	Legumes (Cups)	Starchy Vegetables (Cups)	Other Vegetables (Cups)
1000	1	0.5	0.5	1.5	3.5
1200	1.5	1	1	2.5	4.5
1400	1.5	1	1	2.5	4.5
1600	2	1.5	2.5	2.5	5.5
1800	3	2	3	3	6.5
2000	3	2	3	3	6.5
2200	3	2	3	6	7
2400	3	2	3	6	7
2600	3	2.5	3.5	7	8.5
2800	3	2.5	3.5	7	8.5
3000	3	2.5	3.5	9	10
3200	3	2.5	3.5	9	10

Source: Adapted from USDA, Center for Nutrition Policy and Promotion, *MyPyramid Food Intake Patterns*, Washington, D.C. April, 2005. Available at http://www.mypyramid.gov/downloads/MyPyramid_Food_Intake_Patterns.pdf

vegetables for daily consumption from the vegetable group at different energy intake levels. Table 16.15 illustrates these for boys and girls aged 2 to 18 years.

The child-friendly version of the new *MyPyramid* Food Guidance System called *MyPyramid for Kids*[30] was released by USDA in September, 2005 for children age 6 to 11 years.[31] The tagline or slogan on *MyPyramid for Kids* is "Eat Right. Exercise. Have Fun." Illustrations of children involved in a variety of physical activities and of healthy foods from each food

TABLE 16.15

MyPyramid Food Intake Pattern Calorie Levels for Boys and Girls Aged 2 to 18 Years

Age (in Years)	Boys			Girls		
	Sedentary[a]	Moderate[a]	Active[a]	Sedentary[a]	Moderate[a]	Active[a]
2	1000	1000	1000	1000	1000	1000
3	1000	1400	1400	1000	1200	1400
4	1200	1400	1600	1200	1400	1400
5	1200	1400	1600	1200	1400	1600
6	1400	1600	1800	1200	1400	1600
7	1400	1600	1800	1200	1600	1800
8	1400	1600	2000	1400	1600	1800
9	1600	1800	2000	1400	1600	1800
10	1600	1800	2200	1400	1800	2000
11	1800	2000	2200	1600	1800	2000
12	1800	2200	2400	1600	2000	2200
13	2000	2200	2600	1600	2000	2200
14	2000	2400	2800	1800	2000	2400
15	2200	2600	3000	1800	2000	2400
16	2400	2800	3200	1800	2000	2400
17	2400	2800	3200	1800	2000	2400
18	2400	2800	3200	1800	2000	2400

[a] Calorie levels are based on the Estimated Energy Requirements (EER) and activity levels from the Institute of Medicine Dietary Reference Intakes Macronutrients Report, 2002.

Sedentary = less than 30 min a day of moderate physical activity in addition to daily activities.

Moderately Active = at least 30 min up to 60 min a day of moderate physical activity in addition to daily activities.

Active = 60 or more min a day of moderate physical activity in addition to daily activities.

Note: MyPyramid assigns individuals to a calorie level based on their sex, age, and activity level. The chart above identifies the calorie levels for children and adolescents by sex, age, and activity level (sedentary, moderately active, active).

Source: Adapted from: USDA, Center for Nutrition Policy and Promotion, *MyPyramid Food Intake Pattern Calorie Levels*, Washington, DC, April, 2005, CNPP-XX. Available at http://www.mypyramid.gov/downloads/MyPyramid_Calorie_Levels.pdf

group on the graphic encourage schoolchildren to make healthy eating choices and be more physically active.[31] The key messages of *MyPyramid for Kids* are[32]:

- Be physically active every day — the child climbing the steps reminds children that physical activity should be done every day.
- Choose healthier foods from each group — every food group has foods that children should eat more often than others.
- Eat more of some food groups than others — the different-sized stripes suggest how much food children should choose from each group.
- Eat foods from every food group every day — the different colors of the pyramid represent the five different food groups plus oils.
- Make the right choices for you — myPyramid.gov gives everyone in the family personal ideas on how to eat better and exercise more.
- Take it one step at a time — start with one new, good thing a day, and continue to add another new one every day.[32]

The messages of *MyPyramid for Kids* are the same as the messages of *MyPyramid*, but are written in simpler language for children.[31] The graphic, slogan, and messages were developed for and tested with children.[31]

Numerous materials are available from USDA about *MyPyramid for Kids* for children, parents, and families.[30] An interactive computer game called "MyPyramid Blast Off" is available by CD-ROM (or via the internet at http://mypyramid.gov/kids/kids_game.html_game.html). In the game, children can reach Planet Power by fueling their rocket with food and physical activity; "fuel" tanks for each food group help children keep track of how their choices fit into *MyPyramid*. A two-sided poster

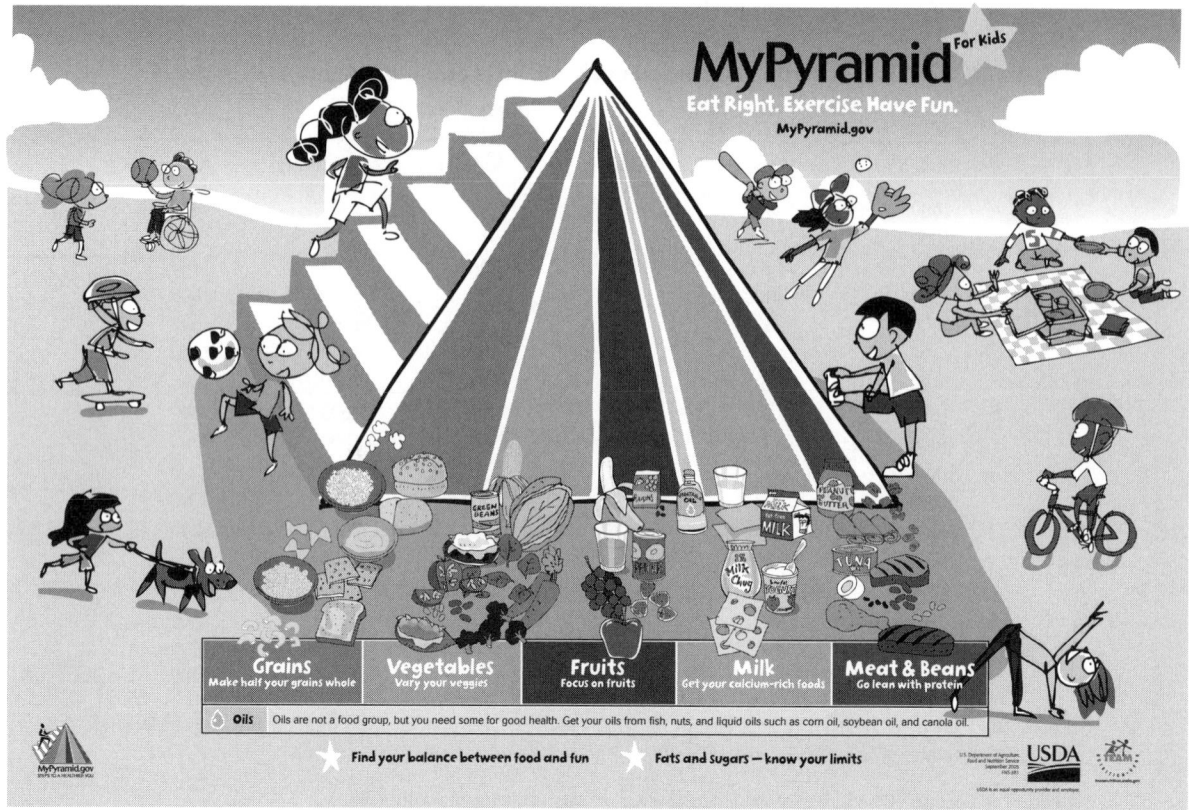

FIGURE 16.1 *MyPyramid* for Kids (simplified graphic). Available at: http://teamnutrition.usda.gov/resources/mpk_poster.pdf

has one side for younger children that features a simplified *MyPyramid for Kids* graphic (see Figure 16.1), and the other side for advanced elementary children that features both the graphic and healthy eating and physical activity messages (see Figure 16.2). A mini-poster for families has the *MyPyramid for Kids* graphic on one side and tips to "eat right" and "exercise" on the other side; Figure 16.3 illustrates the side of this mini-poster with tips for families (available at http://teamnutrition.usda. gov/resources/mpk_tips.pdf). Classroom materials for elementary school educators are available from USDA.[33] Lesson plans integrate nutrition with science, math, health, and language arts; physical activity is emphasized as well. Lessons communicate nutrition concepts through age-appropriate and fun activities, contain handouts to be duplicated, may be taught with minimal preparation, include a link with the school lunch program, and provide an activity to send home to parents.[33]

The USDA food guide (i.e., *MyPyramid*) is one example of an eating pattern that exemplifies the 2005 Dietary Guidelines for Americans which are for Americans over 2 years of age.[14] Another example of an eating pattern that exemplifies the 2005 Dietary Guidelines for Americans is the DASH (Dietary Approaches to Stop Hypertension) eating plan,[14] which was originally developed to study the effects of an eating pattern on the prevention and treatment of hypertension in adults.[34,35] According to the American Heart Association and the American Academy of Pediatrics, although there are no comparable clinical trial data in children, there is no reason to suspect that the DASH diet would not be safe for older children and adolescents.[15,16]

WHAT ARE CHILDREN AND ADOLESCENTS EATING?

1989 TO 1991 CONTINUING SURVEY OF FOOD INTAKES OF INDIVIDUALS (CSFII), UNITED STATES

The 1989 to 1991 CSFII sample consisted of individuals residing in households in the 48 contiguous States (US); a separate survey was conducted in each of the three years and combined to create one large nationally representative data set. Each year, the survey included two independent samples, basic (all income) and low income. Intake information was requested for all household members; for each individual, this included three consecutive days of dietary data, which consisted of one 24-hour recall and a 2-day food record. A knowledgeable adult (usually the primary meal planner/preparer) reported the food intakes of household members younger than 12 years.[36]

Data from the 1989 to 1991 CSFII have been analyzed in numerous ways to provide insight into what children and adolescents are eating. For example, data were analyzed to determine dietary sources of nutrients among 4008 children aged 2 to 18 years.[37] Fortified foods (e.g., ready-to-eat cereals) were influential contributors of many vitamins and minerals; furthermore,

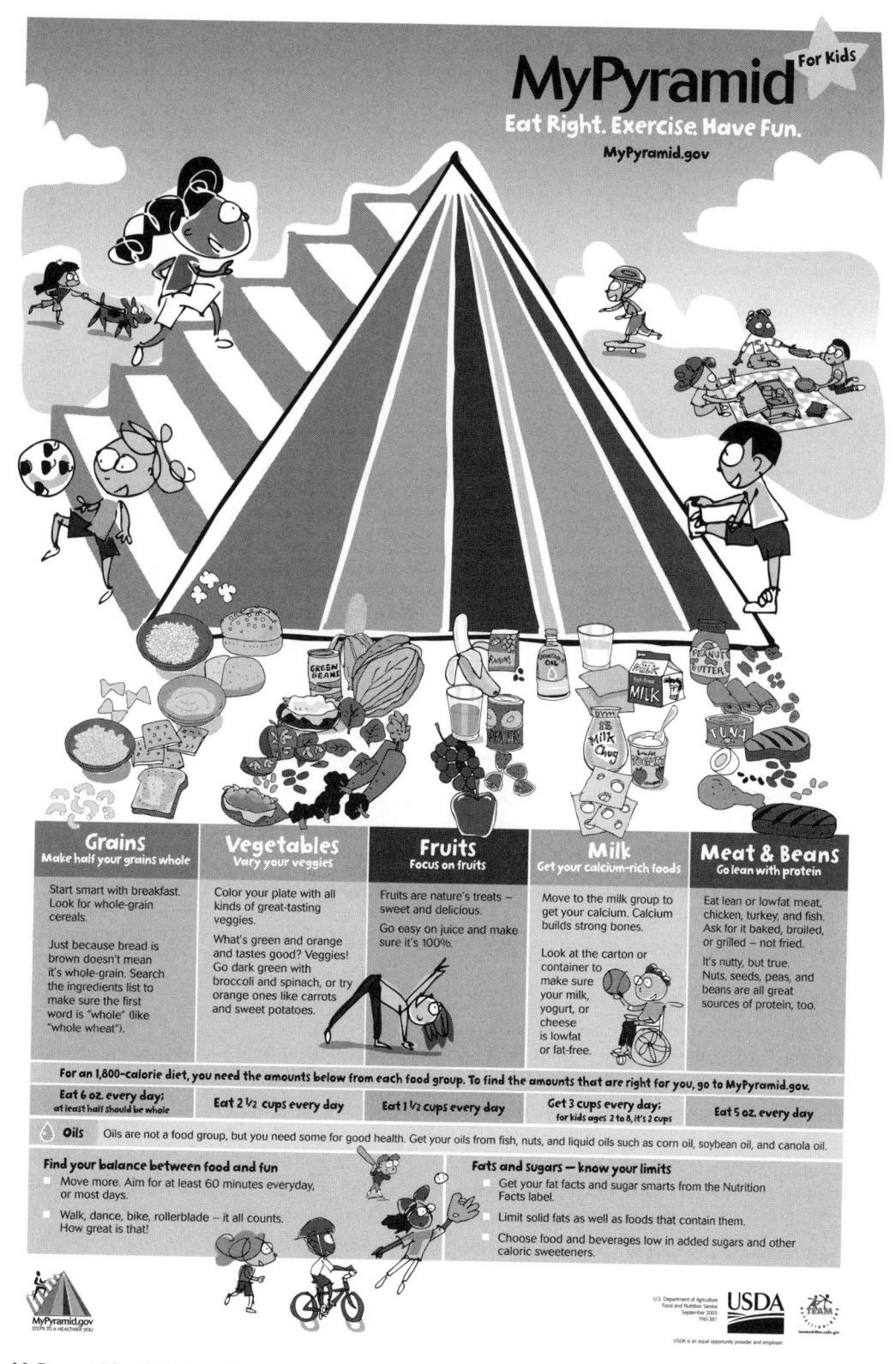

FIGURE 16.2 *MyPyramid* for Kids (graphic with healthy eating and physical activity messages). Available at: http://teamnutrition.usda.gov/resources/mpk_poster2.pdf

low nutrient-dense foods were major contributors of energy, (fats, and carbohydrates,) and these compromise the intakes of more nutrient-dense foods, and may impede compliance with current dietary guidance.[37]

Data from the 1989 to 1991 CSFII were analyzed to determine fruit and vegetable consumption among 3148 children aged 2 to 18 years.[38] Only 1 in 5 children consumed five or more servings of fruits and vegetables per day. Intakes of all fruits and of

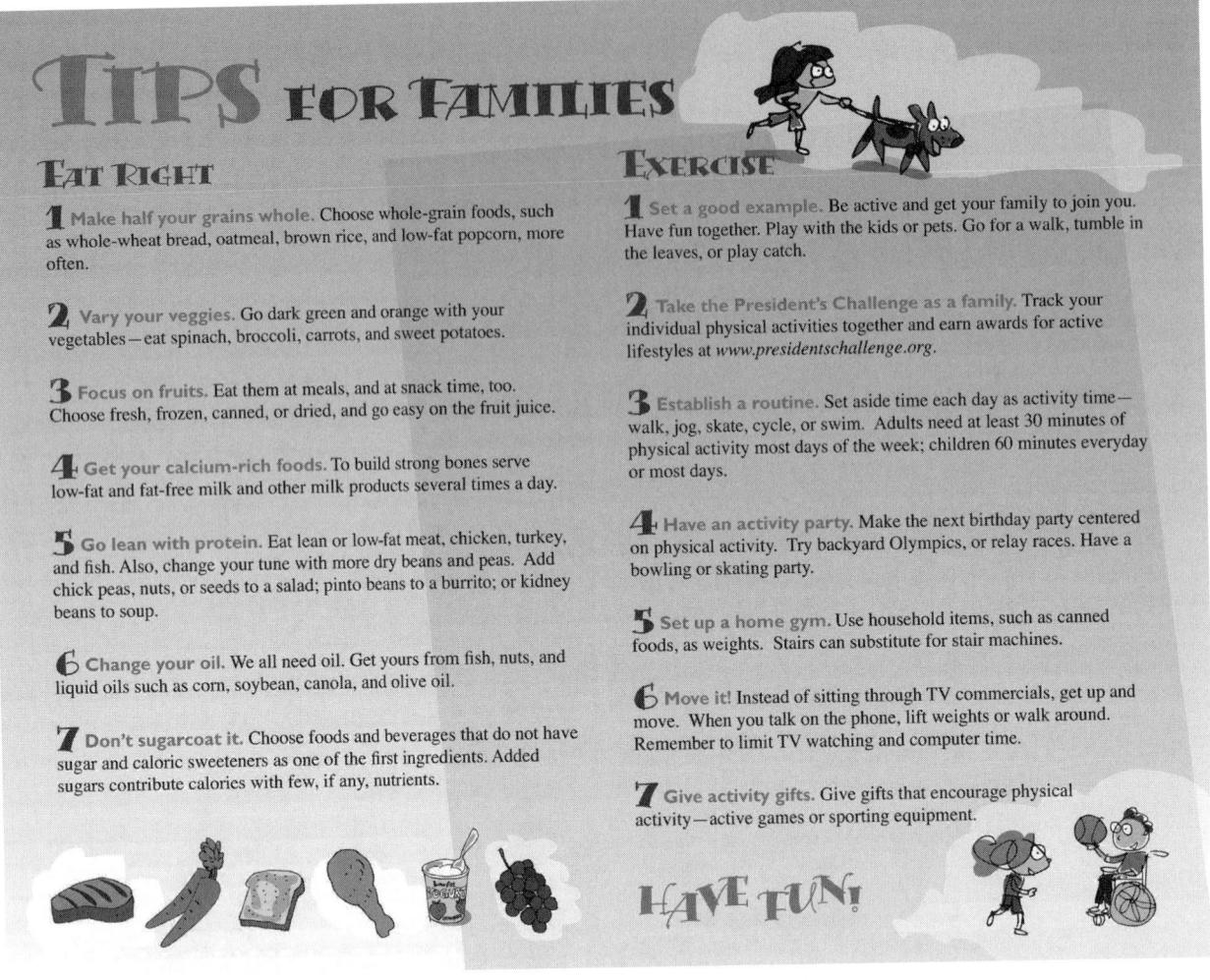

FIGURE 16.3   Tips for Families from *MyPyramid* for Kids. Available at: http://teamnutrition.usda.gov/resources/mpk_tips.pdf

dark green and deep yellow vegetables were very low. Furthermore, almost one-fourth of all vegetables consumed by children and adolescents were french fries.[38]

Data from the 1989 to 1991 CSFII were analyzed to determine what percentage of children aged 4 to 6 years ($n = 603$) and 7 to 10 years ($n = 782$) met the American Health Foundation's age plus 5 recommendation for fiber,[18,19] and what the leading contributors to total dietary fiber intake were.[39] Only 45% of 4- to 6-year-olds and 32% of 7- to 10-year-olds met the age plus 5 rule. Children who met the rule did so by consuming significantly more high- and low-fiber breads and cereals, fruits, vegetables, legumes, nuts, and seeds. Furthermore, children who met the rule had significantly higher energy-adjusted intakes of vitamins A and E, folate, magnesium, and iron compared to children with low fiber intakes who had significantly higher energy-adjusted intakes of fat and cholesterol. Surprisingly, low-fiber breads and cereals provided 21% and 19% of total dietary fiber for 4- to 6-year-olds and 7- to 10-year-olds, respectively, whereas high-fiber breads and cereals provided only 6% of total dietary fiber for both age groups. Conclusions from these results include that substituting high-fiber breads and cereals for low-fiber ones would increase children's fiber intakes and should be relatively easy to accomplish.[39]

1994 to 1996 CSFII, United States

The 1994 to 1996 CSFII sample consisted of individuals residing in households in the 50 states, and included an oversampling of the low-income population. Only selected household members were asked to provide intake information. For each individual, two nonconsecutive days of dietary data were requested using the 24-h recall method through in-person interviews.[36] Proxy interviews were conducted routinely for children under 6 years, and children 6 to 11 years were asked to describe their own food intake assisted by an adult household member (referred to as the assistant). The preferred proxy or assistant was the person responsible for preparing the child's meals.[40]

Data from the 1994 to 1996 CSFII were analyzed to determine whether carbonated soft drink consumption was associated with consumption of milk, fruit juice, and the nutrients concentrated in these beverages among 1810 children and adolescents aged 2 to 18 years.[41] Adolescents (13 to 18 years) were more likely to consume soft drinks than preschool-aged children (2 to

5 years) and school-aged children (6 to 12 years). Among preschool-aged children, school-aged children, and adolescents, 50, 36, and 18%, respectively, did *not* consume any soft drinks during the 2 days of dietary recall; furthermore, the majority of children in each age category were nonconsumers of diet soft drinks (95, 89, and 86%, respectively). White preschool-aged children and adolescents were more likely to consume soft drinks than black preschool-aged children and adolescents. Among adolescents, boys were more likely than girls to consume soft drinks. Among preschool-aged children and adolescents, those who resided in central city metropolitan statistical areas (within a metropolitan area containing the largest population) were more likely to consume soft drinks than those residing in noncentral city metropolitan statistical areas (within a metropolitan area not containing the largest population). No significant differences in soft drink consumption were found by poverty status or region of the country. In general, soft drink consumption was inversely associated with consumption of milk, fruit juice, and the nutrients concentrated in these beverages. For all age groups, energy intake was higher among those in the highest soft drink consumption category compared with nonconsumers. These results indicate that nutrition education messages for children and parents should encourage limited consumption of soft drinks.[41]

Data from the 1994 to 1996 CSFII were analyzed to characterize whole grain consumption among 4802 youth aged 2 to 18 years.[42] Average daily intake of whole grains ranged from 0.8 serving for preschool-aged children to 1.0 serving for adolescents. The major sources of whole grains were ready-to-eat cereals, corn and other chips, and yeast breads, accounting for 31, 22, and 18% of whole grain intake, respectively, among this group of youth. These low levels of intake indicate that interventions are needed to increase the intake of whole-grain foods among youth.[42]

Suitor and Gleason analyzed data from the 1994 to 1996 CSFII by using DRI-based methods to estimate the prevalence of inadequate usual intakes of nutrients by 2692 youth aged 6 to 18 years.[43] Nutrients identified as potential problems for sex/age groups of youth based on comparisons to EARs included vitamin A for teenage girls, vitamin E for all sex/age groups of youth, vitamin C for teenage girls, folate for preteen and teenage boys and girls, phosphorus for preteen and teenage girls, magnesium for teenage boys and for preteen and teenage girls, and zinc for teenage girls. In contrast, most youth had adequate intakes of iron, thiamin, riboflavin, niacin, vitamin B_6, and vitamin B_{12}.[43]

1994 TO 1996 AND 1998 CSFII

The Supplemental Children's Survey to the 1994 to 1996 CSFII (1998 CSFII) was conducted to add intake data from 5559 children age birth through 9 years to the intake data collected from 4253 children of the same age who participated in the 1994 to 1996 CSFII. The 1998 CSFII was designed to be combined with the 1994 to 1996 CSFII, thus, approaches to sample selection, data collection, data file preparation, and weighting were consistent.[44]

Data from the 1994 to 1996 and 1998 CSFII were analyzed to determine the nutritional consequences of flavored-milk consumption by 3888 youth aged 5 to 17 years.[45] Youth who consumed flavored milk had significantly higher total milk intake and lower soft drink and fruit drink intake but similar fruit juice intake compared with youth who were nonconsumers of flavored milk. In addition, youth who consumed flavored milk had higher calcium intakes but similar percentage of energy from total fat and added sugars compared with youth who were nonconsumers of flavored milk.[45]

Data from the 1994 to 1996 and 1998 CSFII were analyzed to determine associations between intakes of the primary food and beverage sources of added sugars and intakes of key nutrients and food pyramid groups among 3038 children and adolescents aged 6 to 17 years.[46] Consumption of sweetened dairy products was positively associated with calcium intakes; furthermore, the consumption of presweetened cereals had a positive impact on meeting recommendations for calcium, folate, and iron. In contrast, consumption of sugar-sweetened beverages, sugars and sweets, and sweetened grains had a negative impact on diet quality.[46]

Data from the 1994 to 1996 and 1998 CSFII were analyzed to quantify the impact of dairy foods on nutrient intakes among 17,959 people over age 2 years, including 8,605 children and adolescents less than 19 years.[47] Although analyses were conducted on the total sample as well as numerous age/sex subgroups, only data for the total sample were reported, because results were consistent for all age/sex groups. Higher intakes of total dairy and milk were associated with significant and often large increase in intakes of essential nutrients including calcium, folate, iron, magnesium, potassium, riboflavin, vitamin A, and zinc. Fat intake generally was not associated with total dairy intake, although fat did increase as cheese intake increased. Dietary cholesterol was lower as intakes of any dairy categories increased, although the opposite was true for saturated fat. Dairy foods contributed an average of 51% of dietary calcium, 19% of total fat, 32% of saturated fat, and 22% of cholesterol. These results reinforce the importance of dairy foods and milk as key calcium sources as well as "packages" of nutrients, and suggest that people who consume more dairy foods and milk also consume other more nutrient-rich foods. Results with saturated fat and cheese suggest the usefulness of continued modification of product composition and education to select lower fat versions.[47]

Data from the 1994 to 1996 and 1998 CSFII were analyzed to examine the dietary profile associated with fast food use among 17,370 people over age 2 years, including 8,550 youth less than 19 years.[48] Results indicated that fast food was consumed by 42% of youth on either of the 2 survey days. Youth with fast food consumption had a significantly lower intake of breads and cereals, dark green vegetables and other vegetables, noncitrus fruits and juices, milk, and legumes, but a higher intake of fried potato, chicken, meat mixture, and carbonated soft drinks. In terms of energy and nutrients, youth with fast food consumption had a significantly lower intake of protein, vitamin A, and β-carotene, and higher intake of total energy and fat compared with youth who did not consume fast food. Fast food consumption may contribute to higher energy and fat intake, and lower intake of healthful nutrients.[48]

Trends in Consumption among Children and Adolescents

Data for children aged 6 to 11 years from the 1977 to 1978 Nationwide Food Consumption Survey ($n = 4107$), 1989 to 1991 CSFII ($n = 1,476$), and 1994 to 96 and 1998 CSFII ($n = 2,000$) were examined to monitor trends in dietary intake.[49] Intakes increased for total grain products, grain mixtures, crackers/popcorn/pretzels/corn chips, fried potatoes, noncitrus juices/nectars, low-fat milk, skim milk, cheese, candy, fruit drinks/fruitades, and soft drinks. Intakes decreased for yeast breads/rolls, corn/green peas/lima beans, green beans, whole milk and total milk, beef, pork, and eggs. Percentages of calories from fat decreased, partly due to increased carbohydrate intakes. Intakes of thiamin and iron increased, but vitamin B_{12} decreased. Despite these shifts in intake, guidance is needed to continue to encourage increased intakes of whole grains, dark-green and deep-yellow vegetables, fruits (both citrus and noncitrus, but emphasizing whole fruits instead of juices), legumes, lean meats and meat alternates, nonfat or low-fat dairy products, and decreased intakes of fat used in cooking and added sugars.[49]

Data for children and adolescents aged 6 to 17 years from the 1977 to 1978 Nationwide Food Consumption Survey ($n = 8908$) and combined 1994 to 1996 and 1998 CSFII ($n = 3177$) were examined to monitor trends in the prevalence, amounts, and sources of soft drink consumption.[50] Among this group, the prevalence of soft drink consumption increased 48%, from 37% in 1977/1978 to 56% in 1994/1998. Mean daily intake of soft drinks more than doubled, from 5 fluid ounces to 12 fluid ounces per day. The home environment remained the largest source of soft drink access for this group; however, an increasing share was obtained from restaurants and fast food establishments, vending machines, and other sources.[50]

Longitudinal data on selected nutrient intake of youth with emphases on differences by sex and race/ethnicity was examined in a sample from the Child and Adolescent Trial for Cardiovascular Health (CATCH) for which nutrient data was provided by 24-h diet recalls from a cohort of third- ($n = 1874$), fifth- ($n = 1360$), and eighth-grade ($n = 1493$) youth.[51] Between the third grade (Fall, 1991) and the eighth grade (Spring, 1994), nutrient consumption differed by sex and race/ethnicity for numerous nutrients. Specifically, relative to boys' intake, girls' intake of energy from total fat, calcium, folic acid, iron, vitamin A, and vitamin D decreased over time, controlling for overall energy intake. African-American youth increased their intake of energy from total fat and saturated fat over time compared with the other ethnic/racial groups.[51]

What We Eat in America

The integration of the Continuing Survey of Food Intakes by Individuals (CSFII) and the National Health and Nutrition Examination Survey (NHANES) has progressed.[52] The dietary portion of the new integrated survey, which is called "What We Eat in America," is collected as part of NHANES. The year 2002 was the first year of full integration of the CSFII (conducted by the USDA) and NHANES (conducted by the U.S. Department of Health and Human Services [HHS]).[53] Data collection for What We Eat in America, will be on a continuous yearly basis; 2 days of data will be collected for all respondents with the Day 2 interview conducted by telephone. Food intake data, from What We Eat in America, can be linked to health status data from other NHANES components to allow researchers to explore relationships between dietary intake and health status. Under the integrated framework, USDA is responsible for the survey's dietary data collection methodology, maintenance of the databases used to code and process the data, and data review and processing HHS is responsible for the sample design and data collection.[52,53] In addition, USDA is funding the collection and processing of the Day 2 data. Each year, the total sample is 5,000.[52] Each annual sample is nationally representative, but the 2-year sample should be used to provide adequate sample sizes for subgroup analyses.[53]

The 2001 to 2002 dataset, which includes NHANES data collected in 2001 along with What We Eat in America data collected in 2002, has recently become available for public use. Table 16.16 through Table 16.18 provide information about the usual nutrient intake from food by children and adolescents who participated in What We Eat in America and NHANES 2001 to 2002, compared to the DRIs.[54]

Table 16.16 provides national estimates of usual nutrient intake from food for 17 nutrients and dietary components by children and adolescents compared to EARs. As discussed previously in this chapter, the EAR is the average daily nutrient intake level estimated to meet the requirement of half of the healthy individuals in a particular life stage and sex group; the EAR is used to estimate the prevalence of inadequate intakes in a population group. As indicated in Table 16.16, based on comparisons to EARs, nutrients identified as potential problems for sex/age groups of youth include vitamin A for teenage boys and for preteen and teenage girls, vitamin E for all sex/age groups of youth, vitamin C for teenage boys and teenage girls, phosphorus for preteen and teenage girls, magnesium for teenage boys and for preteen and teenage girls, and zinc for teenage girls. Most youth had adequate intakes of thiamin, riboflavin, niacin, vitamin B_6, folate, vitamin B_{12}, iron, copper, selenium, carbohydrate, and protein.[54] Many of the results for youth from What We Eat in America and NHANES 2001 to 2002 are similar to results by Suitor and Gleason for youth from 1994 to 1996 CSFII mentioned previously.[43]

Table 16.17 provides national estimates of usual nutrient intake from food for seven nutrients and dietary components by children and adolescents compared to AIs. An AI cannot be used to estimate the prevalence of inadequacy in a population. Table 16.17 provides the percentages of youth with intakes at or greater than the AI (not less than the AI), but this percentage should not be interpreted as a prevalence of "adequacy." If at least 50% of the sex/age group has intakes greater than the AI, then the prevalence of inadequacy should be low; however, if less than 50% have intakes greater than the AI, then no assumption can be made about the prevalence of inadequacy. As indicated in Table 16.17, nutrients for which no EARs have been

TABLE 16.16

What We Eat in America, NHANES 2001–2002: National Estimates of Usual Nutrient Intake from Food for 17 Nutrients and Dietary Components by Children and Adolescents Compared to Estimated Average Requirements (EARs)

	Children		Boys		Girls	
	1 to 3 Years	4 to 8 Years	9 to 13 Years	14 to 18 Years	9 to 13 Years	14 to 18 Years
Number of Children	798	920	574	727	597	677
Vitamin A (RAE)[a]						
Mean (SE)	532 (23.7)	573 (26.3)	670 (49.7)	638 (39.0)	536 (37.5)	513 (35.8)
EAR	210	275	445	630	420	485
% < EAR	< 3	4	13	55	34	54
SE*		1.2	4.6	6.1	6.0	5.7
Vitamin E (mg α-tocopherol)						
Mean (SE)	4.0 (0.14)	5.0 (0.17)	6.0 (0.23)	7.3 (0.31)	5.6 (0.35)	5.6 (0.17)
EAR	5	6	9	12	9	12
% < EAR	80	80	97	>97	95	>97
SE*	3.3	4.1	1.8		3.6	
Thiamin (mg)						
Mean (SE)	1.20 (0.023)	1.45 (0.026)	1.78 (0.088)	1.96 (0.076)	1.44 (0.048)	1.40 (0.052)
EAR	0.4	0.5	0.7	1.0	0.7	0.9
% < EAR	< 3	< 3	< 3	< 3	< 3	12
SE*						2.6
Riboflavin (mg)						
Mean (SE)	1.97 (0.042)	2.10 (0.051)	2.51 (0.131)	2.57 (0.106)	1.94 (0.072)	1.80 (0.079)
EAR	0.4	0.5	0.8	1.1	0.8	0.9
% < EAR	< 3	< 3	< 3	< 3	< 3	6
SE*						1.5
Niacin (mg) [b]						
Mean (SE)	13.5 (0.27)	18.2 (0.48)	22.5 (1.03)	27.0 (1.01)	18.5 (0.55)	18.6 (0.63)
EAR	5	6	9	12	9	11
% < EAR	< 3	< 3	< 3	< 3	< 3	6
SE*						1.4
Vitamin B$_6$ (mg)						
Mean (SE)	1.34 (0.039)	1.50 (0.048)	1.81 (0.105)	2.17 (0.097)	1.52 (0.061)	1.48 (0.049)
EAR	0.4	0.5	0.8	1.1	0.8	1.0
% < EAR	< 3	< 3	< 3	< 3	< 3	16
SE*						2.7
Folate (DFE) [c]						
Mean (SE)	416 (12.4)	528 (18.8)	644 (33.4)	683 (32.4)	512 (25.1)	500 (41.0)
EAR	120	160	250	330	250	330
% < EAR	< 3	< 3	< 3	4	< 3	19
SE*				1.2		4.8
Vitamin B$_{12}$ (µg)						
Mean (SE)	4.51 (0.137)	4.75 (0.175)	6.00 (0.478)	6.69 (0.417)	4.40 (0.164)	4.16 (0.230)
EAR	0.7	1.0	1.5	2.0	1.5	2.0
% < EAR	< 3	< 3	< 3	< 3	< 3	8
SE*						1.7
Vitamin C (mg)						
Mean (SE)	92.1 (3.87)	80.7 (4.27)	80.2 (5.77)	100.0 (8.53)	81.0 (6.09)	75.6 (6.40)
EAR	13	22	39	63	39	56
% < EAR	< 3	< 3	8	26	9	42
SE*			2.9	5.8	2.5	4.8
Phosphorus (mg)						
Mean (SE)	1065 (23.7)	1172 (21.5)	1431 (67.2)	1575 (48.5)	1141 (38.7)	1099 (34.8)
EAR	380	405	1055	1055	1055	1055
% < EAR	< 3	< 3	9	9	42	49
SE*			3.3	2.0	5.5	4.1

Continued

TABLE 16.16
(Continued)

	Children		Boys		Girls	
	1 to 3 Years	4 to 8 Years	9 to 13 Years	14 to 18 Years	9 to 13 Years	14 to 18 Years
Magnesium (mg)						
Mean (SE)	188 (3.7)	212 (5.0)	250 (9.5)	284 (8.1)	215 (8.5)	206 (8.1)
EAR	65	110	200	340	200	300
% < EAR	< 3	< 3	14	78	44	91
SE*			4.2	3.3	6.2	2.6
Iron (mg)[d]						
Mean (SE)	11.0 (0.23)	13.7 (0.39)	17.0 (0.92)	19.1 (0.76)	13.7 (0.45)	13.3 (0.65)
EAR	3.0	4.1	5.9	7.7	5.7	7.9
% < EAR	< 3	< 3	< 3	< 3	< 3	16
SE*						
Zinc (mg)						
Mean (SE)	8.3 (0.22)	10.0 (0.30)	13.0 (0.76)	15.1 (0.63)	9.8 (0.34)	9.5 (0.44)
EAR	2.5	4.0	7.0	8.5	7.0	7.3
% < EAR	< 3	< 3	< 3	4	10	26
SE*				1.2	2.8	4.6
Copper (mg)						
Mean (SE)	0.76 (0.017)	0.95 (0.019)	1.16 (0.041)	1.34 (0.040)	1.00 (0.037)	0.95 (0.034)
EAR	0.260	0.340	0.540	0.685	0.540	0.685
% < EAR	< 3	< 3	< 3	< 3	< 3	16
SE*						2.8
Selenium (µg)						
Mean (SE)	65 (1.7)	82 (1.8)	103 (4.3)	118 (4.5)	82 (2.7)	83 (2.1)
EAR	17	23	35	45	35	45
% < EAR	< 3	< 3	< 3	< 3	< 3	3
SE*						0.9
Carbohydrate (g)						
Mean (SE)	204 (4.2)	257 (4.7)	309 (10.0)	364 (9.8)	262 (8.5)	263 (9.0)
EAR	100	100	100	100	100	100
% < EAR	< 3	< 3	< 3	< 3	< 3	< 3
SE*						
Protein (g/kg body weight)[e]						
Mean (SE)	4.38 (0.100)	2.76 (0.061)	2.00 (0.070)	1.42 (0.051)	1.53 (0.045)	1.13 (0.029)
EAR	0.87	0.76	0.76	0.73	0.76	0.71
% < EAR	< 3	< 3	< 3	< 3	< 3	14
SE*						1.9

* Standard error not displayed when percentage < EAR is < 3 or >97.

[a] Retinol Activity Equivalents. 1 RAE = 1 µg retinol, 12 µg β-carotene, 24 µg α-carotene.

[b] The intake of niacin is for preformed niacin only. However, the EAR for niacin is given as niacin equivalents that include preformed niacin and contributions from tryptophan. Therefore, the estimated percentage less than the EAR may be overestimated.

[c] Dietary Folate Equivalents. 1 DFE = 1 µg food folate = 0.6 µg of folic acid from fortified food. It is recommended that all females capable of becoming pregnant consume 400 µg from supplements or fortified foods in addition to intake of food folate from a varied diet.

[d] Comparison to EAR for iron was determined using a probability approach; standard errors for the estimated percentage less than the EAR were not produced.

[e] For children 1 to 3 years, reference weights were used. For children 4 years and older, actual body weight was used if BMI was in a healthy range; otherwise, the weight that would place the child at the nearest endpoint of the healthy range was used. The sample size excludes children without BMI available from NHANES 2001–2002; thus, the sample sizes for protein were 798 for children 1 to 3 years, 885 for children 4 to 8 years, 566 for boys 9 to 13 years, 717 for boys 14 to 18 years, 587 for girls 9 to 13 years, and 666 for girls 14 to 18 years.

Source: Adapted from Moshfegh A, Goldman J, Cleveland L. *What We Eat in America*, NHANES 2001–2002: Usual Nutrient Intakes from Food Compared to Dietary Reference Intakes. USDA, ARS, 2005. Available at http://www.ars.usda.gov/SP2UserFiles/Place/12355000/pdf/usualintaketables2001-02.pdf (accessed February 13, 2006).

TABLE 16.17

What We Eat in America, NHANES 2001 to 2002: National Estimates of Usual Nutrient Intake from Food for 7 Nutrients and Dietary Components by Children and Adolescents Compared to Adequate Intakes (AIs)

	Children		Boys		Girls	
	1 to 3 Years	**4 to 8 Years**	**9 to 13 Years**	**14 to 18 Years**	**9 to 13 Years**	**14 to 18 Years**
Number of Children	798	920	574	727	597	677
Vitamin K (μg)						
Mean (SE)	33.8 (3.27)	39.2 (2.41)	52.0 (5.11)	56.6 (3.57)	39.9 (2.57)	51.9 (3.78)
AI	30	55	60	75	60	75
% > AI	47	14	27	18	9	13
SE[a]	6.9	4.5	10.5	4.8	4.4	5.4
Calcium (mg)						
Mean (SE)	972 (35.4)	960 (28.7)	1139 (77.9)	1142 (47.1)	865 (36.2)	804 (42.9)
AI	500	800	1300	1300	1300	1300
% > AI	94	69	28	31	6	9
SE[a]	1.5	3.4	10.5	5.3	1.8	2.3
Potassium (mg)						
Mean (SE)	2086 (46.6)	2136 (54.5)	2472 (101.0)	2774 (103.2)	2125 (79.1)	2020 (56.6)
AI	3000	3800	4500	4700	4500	4700
% > AI	6	< 3	< 3	< 3	< 3	< 3
SE[a]	1.1					
Sodium (mg)						
Mean (SE)	2140 (49.7)	2831 (55.7)	3549 (124.0)	4086 (122.2)	2806 (68.6)	2799 (76.3)
AI	1000	1200	1500	1500	1500	1500
% > AI	>97	>97	>97	>97	>97	>97
SE[a]						
Dietary Fiber (g)[b]						
Mean (SE)	9.5 (0.25)	11.6 (0.28)	14.2 (0.51)	15.3 (0.53)	12.3 (0.53)	11.7 (0.41)
AI[c]	19	25	31	38	26	26
% > AI	< 3	< 3	< 3	< 3	< 3	< 3
SE[a]						
Linoleic 18:2 (g)						
Mean (SE)	7.7 (0.21)	11.0 (0.30)	12.8 (0.56)	16.4 (0.79)	12.0 (0.68)	12.1 (0.42)
AI	7	10	12	16	10	11
% > AI	58	61	62	49	66	56
SE[a]	3.4	4.6	9.7	6.9	5.4	4.4
Linolenic 18:3 (g)[d]						
Mean (SE)	0.9 (0.03)	1.1 (0.04)	1.3 (0.06)	1.6 (0.09)	1.1 (0.06)	1.2 (0.05)
AI	0.7	0.9	1.2	1.6	1.0	1.1
% > AI	73	69	58	49	59	55
SE[a]	4.0	4.5	9.8	8.2	6.2	4.5

[a] Standard error not displayed when percentage > AI is < 3 or >97.

[b] The intake of fiber is for dietary fiber only.

[c] AI is for total fiber (dietary + functional). Therefore, the percentage greater than the AI may be underestimated.

[d] The AI is specifically for the α-linolenic isomer (18:3 n–3 c,c,c). Intakes of linolenic 18:3 are for the undifferentiated fatty acid.

Source: Adapted from Moshfegh A, Goldman J, Cleveland L. *What We Eat in America*, NHANES 2001 to 2002: Usual Nutrient Intakes from Food Compared to Dietary Reference Intakes. USDA, ARS, 2005. Available at http://www.ars.usda.gov/SP2UserFiles/Place/12355000/pdf/usualintaketables2001-02.pdf (accessed February 13, 2006).

established that may be of concern among youth include vitamin K, calcium for youth over age 8 years, potassium, and dietary fiber.[54]

Table 16.18 provides the proportion of children and adolescents with usual nutrient intakes (from food only) greater than the ULs. The UL is the maximum level of daily nutrient intake that is likely to pose no risk of adverse health effects for almost all individuals in the general population; as intake increases above the UL, the potential risk of adverse effects may increase. As indicated in Table 16.18, nutrients of concern due to intakes above the UL include zinc for children less than 3 years, and sodium for youth of all ages. The proportions of youth with intakes greater than the ULs, as indicated in Table 16.18, may be

TABLE 16.18
What We Eat in America, NHANES 2001 to 2002: Proportion of Children and Adolescents with Usual Nutrient Intakes, from Food Only, Greater than Upper Tolerable Intake Levels (ULs)

	Children		Boys		Girls	
	1 to 3 Years	4 to 8 Years	9 to 13 Years	14 to 18 Years	9 to 13 Years	14 to 18 Years
Vitamin A [retinol] (μg)						
UL	600	900	1700	2800	1700	2800
% > UL	12	< 3	< 3	< 3	< 3	< 3
SE[a]		3.0				
Folate [folic acid] (μg)						
UL	300	400	600	800	600	800
% > UL	5	4	< 3	< 3	< 3	< 3
SE[a]	1.4	1.6				
Vitamin B$_6$ (mg)						
UL	30	40	60	80	60	80
% > UL	< 3	< 3	< 3	< 3	< 3	< 3
SE[a]						
Vitamin C (mg)						
UL	400	650	1200	1800	1200	1800
% > UL	< 3	< 3	< 3	< 3	< 3	< 3
SE[a]						
Calcium (mg)						
UL	2500	2500	2500	2500	2500	2500
% > UL	< 3	< 3	< 3	< 3	< 3	< 3
SE[a]						
Phosphorus (mg)						
UL	3000	3000	4000	4000	4000	4000
% > UL	< 3	< 3	< 3	< 3	< 3	< 3
SE[a]						
Iron (mg)						
UL	40	40	40	45	40	45
% > UL	< 3	< 3	< 3	< 3	< 3	< 3
SE[a]						
Zinc (mg)						
UL	7	12	23	34	23	34
% > UL	69	22	< 3	< 3	< 3	< 3
SE[a]	3.6	3.8				
Copper (mg)						
UL	1	3	5	8	5	8
% > UL	15	< 3	< 3	< 3	< 3	< 3
SE[a]	2.0					
Selenium (μg)						
UL	90	150	280	400	280	400
% > UL	8	< 3	< 3	< 3	< 3	< 3
SE[a]	1.6					
Sodium (mg)						
UL	1500	1900	2200	2300	2200	2300
% > UL	83	94	>97	>97	88	74
SE[a]	1.9	1.1			2.3	3.5

[a] Standard error not displayed when percentage > UL is < 3 or >97.

Source: Adapted from Moshfegh, A., Goldman, J., Cleveland, L. *What We Eat in America*, NHANES 2001–2002: Usual Nutrient Intakes from Food Compared to Dietary Reference Intakes. USDA, ARS, 2005. Available at http://www.ars.usda.gov/SP2UserFiles/Place/12355000/pdf/usualintaketables2001-02.pdf (accessed February 13, 2006).

underestimated because they do not include intakes from dietary supplements or water (which were not available when the analyses were done).[54]

Researchers nationwide will have numerous opportunities to analyze this dataset for What We Eat in America, and subsequent ones, using the DRIs and updated recommendations in the 2005 Dietary Guidelines for Americans and *MyPyramid*.

HEALTHY EATING INDEX

To assess and monitor the dietary status of Americans, the USDA Center for Nutrition Policy and Promotion developed the Healthy Eating Index (HEI) and first computed the Index by using 1989 CSFII data.[55] The HEI is computed on a regular basis by USDA as a summary measure of people's diet quality. It consists of ten components, each representing different aspects of a healthy diet. Components 1 to 5 measure the degree to which a person's diet conforms to USDA's Food Guide Pyramid serving recommendations for the five major food groups: grains, vegetables, fruits, milk, and meat/meat alternatives. Components six and seven measure total fat and saturated fat consumption, respectively, as percentages of total kcal intake. Components eight and nine measure total cholesterol and sodium intake, respectively. Component ten measures the degree of variety in a person's diet. Each component has a maximum score of 10 and a minimum score of 0. High component scores indicate intakes close to recommended ranges or amounts; low component scores indicate less compliance with recommended ranges or amounts. The maximum combined score for the 10 components is 100. A HEI score above 80 implies a good diet, a score between 51 and 80 implies a diet that needs improvement, and a score less than 51 implies a poor diet.[55]

The HEI was used to examine the diets of 5354 children age 2 to 18 years from the 1994 to 96 CSFII.[56] Most children had a diet that was poor or needed improvement. Furthermore, older children had lower HEI scores than younger children, which were associated with lower fruit and milk component scores of the HEI. Thus, the percentage of children with a diet that needed improvement or was poor was higher for older children than for younger children. For children age 2 to 3 years, 35% had a good diet, and 5% had a poor diet. For children age 4 to 6 years, 16% had a good diet, and 9% had a poor diet. For children age 7 to 10 years, 14% had a good diet, and 10% had a poor diet. For girls age 11 to 18 years, ~7% had a good diet, and ~18% had a poor diet. For boys age 11 to 18 years, ~6% had a good diet, and ~21% had a poor diet. Except for cholesterol and variety to a smaller extent, most children did not meet most recommendations.[56]

The HEI was used to examine the diets of 4,011 children age 2 to 9 years from the 1998 CSFII.[57] Most children age 2 to 9 years had a diet that needed improvement or was poor. Furthermore, older children (age 7 to 9 years) in this age group had lower HEI scores than younger children (age 2 to 3 years), which were associated with lower fruit and sodium component scores of the HEI. The overall HEI score for children age 2 to 9 years did not change significantly from 1989 to 1998, and indicated a diet that needed improvement.[57]

The HEI was used to examine the diets of 7,177 children age 2 to 9 years from 1994 to 1996 and 1998 CSFII.[55] Most children had a diet that needed improvement or was poor; furthermore, the quality of children's diets varied significantly based on age, sex, household income, receipt of food stamps, food sufficiency, and area of residence. Compared with their respective counterparts, diet quality was better for younger children, boys, and children living in suburban areas. Diet quality was worse if children were in households with a low income, that received food stamps, and who categorized themselves as food insufficient.[55]

The HEI was used to examine the diets of 8070 people age 2 to 51+ years from NHANES 1999 to 2000.[58] The diets of most people, including children age 2 to 18 years, need improvement, although children less than 11 years of age had better scores than did most other age groups.[58]

The quality of a child's diet according to the HEI continues to be related to the income of his or her family, with children in families below poverty being less likely than higher-income children to have a diet rated as good.[59] As indicated in Table 16.19, for example, in 1989 to 1990, for children age 2 to 6 years, 9% of those in poverty had a good diet compared with 23% of those living above poverty; the respective percentages were 16 and 22% in 1994 to 1996, and 17 and 22% in 1999 to 2000.[59]

CAVEATS

Assessment of dietary intake is challenging, especially among children who eat several meals and snacks at school or daycare when their parents are not present. Nevertheless, parents are often asked to provide information about their children's intake; unfortunately, several studies underscore concerns that these parents' reports cannot be taken as truth.[60–62] In addition, parents are often asked to provide joint reports with their children about their children's intake. A 1989 study by Eck et al.[63] found that consensus recalls provided by mother, father, and child yielded better estimates of observed intake of a single cafeteria meal by 34 children aged 4 to 9.5 years than did recalls from either the mother or father alone. Unfortunately, the Eck et al.[63] study is often incorrectly cited as the rationale for obtaining joint recalls from parents and children. However, for that study, children by themselves did not provide recalls, so no comparison could be made of the accuracy of child-only recalls, parent-only recalls, and joint parent–child recalls of the child's intake. Furthermore, consensus recalls were always obtained after the mother and father had each provided separate recalls, but having the mother and father provide two back-to-back recalls about the child's intake could have altered reporting accuracy during the second recall, which was always the consensus parent–child recall.

TABLE 16.19

Percentages of Children Aged 2 to 18 by Age, Poverty Status, and Diet Quality as Measured by the Healthy Eating Index, 1989–1990, 1994–1996, and 1999–2000[a]

	Characteristic		
	Good Diet	Needs Improvement	Poor Diet
1989 to 1990			
Ages 2 to 6 years			
At or below poverty	9	74	17
Above poverty	23	74	3
Ages 7 to 12 years			
At or below poverty	11	75	15
Above poverty	11	83	5
Ages 13 to 18 years			
At or below poverty	3	72	25
Above poverty	5	72	23
1994 to 1996			
Ages 2 to 6 years			
At or below poverty	16	72	12
Above poverty	22	69	9
Ages 7 to 12 years			
At or below poverty	7	74	19
Above poverty	10	75	15
Ages 13 to 18 years			
At or below poverty	3	66	31
Above poverty	5	69	26
1999 to 2000			
Ages 2 to 6 years			
At or below poverty	17	78	5
Above poverty	22	72	6
Ages 7 to 12 years			
At or below poverty	7	75	18
Above poverty	8	81	11
Ages 13 to 18 years			
At or below poverty	3	78	19
Above poverty	4	76	20

[a] A Healthy Eating Index (HEI) score above 80 implies a good diet, a score between 51 and 80 implies a diet that needs improvement, and a score less than 51 implies a poor diet. Data for the 3 time periods are not necessarily comparable due to methodological differences in data collection.

Sources:

United States Department of Agriculture, 1989–1990 and 1994–1996 Continuing Survey of Food Intakes by Individuals; Centers for Disease Control and Prevention, 1999 to -2000 National Health and Nutrition Examination Survey.

Adapted from Federal Interagency Forum on Child and Family Statistics, *America's Children: Key National Indicators of Well-Being, 2005.* Federal Interagency Forum on Child and Family Statistics, Washington, DC, U.S. Government Printing Office. The report is also available on the World Wide Web at http://childstats.gov. (accessed March 24, 2006).

Sobo et al.[64,65] provided recommendations to improve the accuracy of data about children's intake obtained during parent-assisted dietary recalls based on a study with 34 children aged 7 to 11 years. Sobo et al. found that parents "*contributed primarily by adding food details and, secondarily, by prompting children;*" in addition, "*children rejected a notable proportion of items added*" by parents, and "*children's knowledge of food details was considerable.*"[64,65] Unfortunately, their study did not validate the children's actual intake, and unassisted children's dietary recalls were not obtained.

Dietary reporting studies with adults have found interesting relationships between reported intake and various characteristics of adults such as BMI, sex, social desirability, body image, and self-esteem. There is some concern that these adult characteristics could affect dietary intake reported during joint parent–child reports about children's intake. Validation studies are needed to determine the impact on accuracy of dietary information obtained from joint parent–child dietary recalls about children's intake.

Children in upper elementary school are able to provide self-reports of dietary intake. Methodological research that has used observations of school meals to validate elementary school children's recalls (obtained without parental assistance) is providing insight into their accuracy; this type of research is needed with adolescents in middle and high school. Among first graders, specific prompting (preference, food category, or visual) after free recall hurt more than helped recall accuracy; in contrast, among fourth graders, prompting for food category after free recall yielded small gains in recall accuracy with minimal losses.[66] When interviewed in the morning about the previous day's intake, individual fourth-grade children were inconsistent in recall accuracy from one interview to the next, but overall accuracy improved slightly between the first and third recalls.[67] Fourth-grade boys were more accurate when prompted to report meals and snacks in reverse order (evening-to-morning), while girls were more accurate in forward order (morning-to-evening).[68] When interviewed in the evening about that day's intake, fourth-grade children's recall accuracy did not depend significantly on whether interviews were conducted in person or by telephone.[69] Accuracy by meal component for school lunch recalls was less when the lunch recalls were obtained in the context of a 24-h dietary recall than as a single meal.[70] Providing meal cues elevated false reports compared to allowing fourth-grade children to report using an open interview format.[71] Fourth-grade children's recall accuracy was significantly better when interviewed about prior 24-h intake (e.g., between 3.00 p.m. on Monday and 3.00 p.m. on Tuesday for an interview on Tuesday at 3.00 p.m.) compared to the previous day's intake (e.g., from midnight to midnight on Monday for an interview anytime on Tuesday).[72] A study that investigated BMI, sex, interview protocol, and fourth-grade children's accuracy for reporting kcal found results consistent with those concerning BMI and sex from studies with adults.[73] Additional validation studies are needed to determine how to obtain more accurate dietary information from youth of various ages.

More information regarding dietary assessment methods with children and adolescents is found in Chapters 29, 33 and 35.

VITAMIN–MINERAL SUPPLEMENTS

A basic premise of the *2005 Dietary Guidelines for Americans* is that nutrient needs should be met primarily through consuming foods, because foods provide an array of nutrients as well as other compounds that may have beneficial effects on health.[14] In certain cases, supplements and fortified foods may be useful sources of one or more nutrients that otherwise might be consumed in less than recommended amounts. Dietary supplements may be recommended in some cases, but they cannot replace a healthful diet.[14]

According to the American Dietetic Association,[74] children can best achieve healthful eating habits by consuming a varied diet in moderation[14] that includes foods from each of the major food groups, as illustrated by *MyPyramid*[75] or *MyPyramid for Kids*.[76] Routine supplementation is not necessary for healthy growing children who consume a varied diet, according to the American Academy of Pediatrics.[77] If parents wish to give supplements to their children, a standard pediatric vitamin–mineral product with nutrients in amounts no larger than the DRI (EAR or RDA) poses no risk; however, megadose levels should be discouraged due to potential toxic effects. Parents should be cautioned to keep vitamin–mineral supplements out of the reach of children, because the taste, shape, and color of most pediatric preparations make them quite appealing to children.[77]

Although the American Academy of Pediatrics advocates that routine vitamin–mineral supplementation is *not* necessary for healthy growing children who eat a varied diet, it does identify groups of children at nutritional risk who may benefit from supplementation;[77] these groups are identified in Table 16.20. Dietary intake over several days should be assessed by a Registered Dietitian to determine if an individual child from one of these groups needs to take a supplement.

LEARNING TO EAT

Widespread evidence indicates that the nutrition guidelines are not being followed by most children. For example, intake for most children is low for fruits, vegetables, fiber, and whole grains,[38,39,42,49,78–80] but high for total fat, saturated fat, and cholesterol.[44,81] Furthermore, the incidence of childhood obesity has increased dramatically during the last three decades.[82–86] To help understand why children eat less of what is recommended by nutrition guidelines and more of what is not recommended, and why the incidence of childhood obesity is increasing, Birch and Fisher[87] recommend that consideration be given to factors that impact children's food preferences and consumption patterns (i.e., what and how much is consumed). Extensive evidence suggests that children's food preferences are shaped by early experience with food and eating, and that family environment and practices used by parents and other adults (e.g., school staff; caregivers, etc.) may permanently affect dietary practices of children.[88] Birch and colleagues[89] have repeatedly found that exposure to novel foods, as well as the social environment in which food is eaten, are crucial in the development of preschool children's food preferences and consumption patterns. Children's food preferences are

TABLE 16.20
Groups of Children at Nutritional Risk Who may Benefit from Vitamin–Mineral Supplementation

- Children from deprived families or who suffer parental neglect or abuse
- Children with anorexia or an inadequate appetite or who consume fad diets
- Children with chronic disease (e.g., cystic fibrosis, inflammatory bowel disease, hepatic disease, etc.)
- Children who participate in a dietary program to manage obesity
- Children who consume a vegetarian diet without adequate dairy products
- Children with failure to thrive
- Children who do not get regular sunlight exposure, who do not ingest at least 500 ml/day of vitamin D-fortified milk, or who do not take a daily multivitamin supplement with at least 200 IU of vitamin D

Source: Adapted from American Academy of Pediatrics (Committee on Nutrition), Feeding the Child, *Pediatric Nutrition Handbook*, 5th edition., Kleinman, R. E., Ed., American Academy of Pediatrics, Elk Grove Village, IL 2004, p 125.

important, because research indicates they are major determinants of consumption;[90–95] therefore, not eating certain items (such as vegetables) is related to low preferences. According to Hill and Trowbridge,[88] insights gained from research concerning children's food preferences and consumption patterns *"can assist in developing interventions to improve child-feeding practices, which may lead to development of healthier eating patterns."* Parents, caregivers, and school staff need to expose children to healthful foods, provide opportunities for children to learn to like rather than dislike healthful foods, encourage children to respect their own feelings of hunger and satiety, and reduce the extent to which learning and experience potentiate children's liking for high-sugar and/or high-fat foods.[96] This section provides an overview of past and continuing research regarding the influence of learning on children's food preferences and consumption patterns.

NEOPHOBIA (REJECTION OF NOVEL FOODS)

During pregnancy, flavors from a pregnant woman's diet are transmitted to amniotic fluid and swallowed by the fetus; thus, the types of food eaten by women during pregnancy and, hence, the flavor principles of their culture may be experienced by infants before birth and well before their first exposure to solid foods.[97] For example, Mennella et al.[97] demonstrated that prenatal and early postnatal exposure to carrot juice enhanced infants' enjoyment of that flavor in cereal during weaning. After birth and during the first years of life, an enormous amount of learning about food and eating occurs as infants transition from consuming only milk (i.e., breast milk or formula) to consuming a variety of foods,[87] and from eating when hungry to eating due to a variety of social, cultural, environmental, or physiological cues.[98] According to Birch and Fisher,[87] this transition from univore to omnivore is shaped by the infant's innate preference for sweet and salty tastes and the rejection of sour and bitter tastes,[99] and by the predisposition of infants and children to be neophobic or to reject novel foods.[100] In addition, a child's experience with food and flavors is shaped by the parents' decision to breastfeed or formula-feed.[87] Research by Sullivan and Birch[101] indicated that infants ate more of novel foods after repeated dietary exposure to the novel foods; furthermore, although they did not differ initially, breastfed infants had greater increases in intake of the novel foods after exposure and an overall greater level of intake than formula-fed infants.

Table 16.21 provides an overview of three studies by Birch and colleagues,[102–104] indicating that preschool children's neophobia or rejection of new foods can be overcome by exposure. Results from these studies indicate that preschool children's food preferences, which are major determinants of consumption, are learned through repeated exposure to foods. Thus, although children may reject novel foods initially, parents and caregivers should continue to make them available to children.

Children's age is a factor when considering exposure to novel foods. For example, results from a study with infants ages 4 to 7 months indicated that exposure dramatically increased infants' intake of a new food and other, similar new foods; however, much of the pre-post increase in intake of the new food actually occurred very early in the sequence of feedings.[105] These rapid increases in intake by infants contrast with the slower changes over repeated exposures seen in young children.[105] Loewen and Pliner[106] found that for older (10- to 12-year-old) children, exposure to novel-good foods increased their willingness to taste novel foods compared to the familiar-good control, but exposure to novel-bad foods had no effect; in contrast, for younger (7- to 9-year-old) children, exposure to both novel-good and novel-bad foods decreased willingness to taste novel foods. Results from a study by Hearn et al.[107] indicated that availability and accessibility to fruits and vegetables (as assessed by telephone interviews with parents) was positively related to upper elementary school children's preferences and consumption.

Reluctance to try novel foods can be decreased by adding the familiar flavor principle (the distinctive combinations of seasonings that characterize many cuisines) to the unfamiliar food. For example, Pliner and Stallberg-White[108] found that 10- to 12-year-old children were more willing to try a novel food when it was accompanied by a familiar flavor principle than when it was served alone.

TABLE 16.21

Research Concerning Exposure to Novel Foods and Preschool Children's Food Preferences and Consumption

Reference #, Authors, & Year	Subjects	Study Design	Results
102, Birch and Marlin, 1982	14 children age 2 years	Each child received 2 to 20 exposures to 5 novel fruits or cheeses over 25 to 26 days	Children ate more of items with higher exposures when given pairs of items, tasted both and picked 1 to consume
103, Birch et al, 1987	43 children in 3 age groups: 26, 38, or 64 months	Each child received 5, 10, or 15 exposures to 7 new fruits, and was asked to taste some and look at others	For all age groups, preferences increased significantly only when foods were tasted
104, Sullivan and Birch, 1990	39 children, age 4 to 5 years	Each child tasted 1 of 3 versions of tofu (sweetened, salty, or plain) 15 times over several weeks	Preferences increased with exposure regardless of added sugar, salt, or plain; 10 exposures were needed

SOCIAL ENVIRONMENT

The social environment of eating is crucial, because children learn about what to eat and why to eat, and receive reinforcements and incentives for eating from their families and the larger environment.[109] Most of this learning occurs during routine mealtime experiences, in the absence of formal teaching.[89] This section provides an overview of several studies that investigated various aspects of the social environment (e.g., rewards, choice offerings, modeling by adults, modeling by peers, class challenges, etc.); Table 16.22 provides details for several of these studies in chronological order by year of publication.

Parents (and researchers) who want young children to eat may offer rewards. Caution is warranted because of the relationship between rewards, children's food preferences, and children's food consumption. For example, a 1980 study by Birch et al.[110] (see Table 16.22) indicated that when specific foods were used as rewards with preschool children, preferences for those "reward" foods were enhanced. In contrast, providing rewards to preschool children for consuming specific foods may result in later decreases in preferences for the foods that had to be consumed to obtain rewards, as illustrated in a 1982 study by Birch et al.,[111] a 1984 study by Birch et al.,[112] and a 1992 study by Newman and Taylor[113] (all described in Table 16.22). In a 1999 study by Hendy[114] (see Table 16.22), modeling by the teacher, insisting that children try one bite, and simple exposure were less effective than choice-offering and reward of a special dessert to encourage acceptance of new fruits and vegetables during preschool lunches. A 2003 study by Wardle et al.[115] indicated that preschool children's preferences for and consumption of vegetables can be enhanced if parents offer children daily tastes for 14 days and keep a daily vegetable "sticker" diary with children.

For elementary school children, research indicates that rewards, if used appropriately, may enhance consumption without negatively affecting preferences. Another 2003 study by Wardle et al.[116] (see Table 16.22) found that exposure increased elementary school children's preferences and consumption more than rewards, but that rewards did not decrease preferences. A 2004 study by Perry et al.[117] (see Table 16.22) found that a 2-year, elementary school, cafeteria-based lunch intervention with daily activities (such as increased availability during lunch and encouragement by food service staff to select foods) and special events (including class competitions) increased fruit but not vegetable intake. A 2005 study by Hendy et al.[118] (see Table 16.22) indicated that token reinforcements provided to elementary school children for eating fruits or vegetables during school lunch did not result in decreased preferences during the program or 2 weeks after it ended. According to Hendy et al.,[118] the token reinforcement used in their program avoided the "overjustification effects" of later decreases in food preferences because it included three recommended components: (1) small and delayed reinforcement, (2) food choice along with the requirement to eat only a small amount, and (3) conditions that encourage peer participation and modeling.

Research studies are providing insight into the effect of modeling by adults and peers on young children's consumption. A series of small studies in 2000 by Hendy and Raudenbush[119] (see Table 16.22) suggest that to encourage preschool children's acceptance of novel foods, teachers should provide enthusiastic modeling (*Mmm! I like mangos!*) rather than silent modeling, and avoid placing competing peer models at the same table with fussy eaters, especially girls. A small 2002 study by Hendy[120] (see Table 16.22) indicated that teachers may train preschool girls as peer models to encourage acceptance of novel foods by other preschool age children during preschool meals; however, the modeling effects on novel food acceptance of observing children may not be present one month later. A small but well-controlled 2005 study by Addessi et al.[121] (see Table 16.22) demonstrated that adult modeling can positively impact preschool children's acceptance of "unusual" and novel foods (e.g., cooked semolina, colored red and flavored with anchovy). Although caregivers may believe they positively influence children's eating behaviors, observed behaviors of caregivers at mealtimes were inconsistent with expert recommendations in a study of influential factors of caregiver behavior at lunch in early child-care programs.[122]

Research indicates that infants are born with the ability to self-regulate their caloric intake by adjusting their formula intake when the caloric level of the formula changes[123] and when solid foods are added.[124] Preschool children are able to adjust the

TABLE 16.22

Research (in Chronological Order by Year of Publication) Concerning the Social Environment and Children's Food Preferences and Consumption

Reference #, authors & Year	Subjects	Description of Study	Results
110, Birch et al., 1980	64 children aged 3 to 4 years; 16 per context	Children given sweet or nonsweet foods (with initially neutral preferences) over several weeks in 1 of 4 contexts: (1) as reward for behavior, (2) paired with adult greeting, (3) as nonsocial behavior (put in child's locker), or (4) at snack time	Preferences increased when foods presented as rewards, or paired with adult greeting; effects lasted longer than 6 weeks after contexts ended. Suggest positive social contexts can be used to increase preferences for foods not liked but more nutritious
111, Birch et al., 1982	12 children aged 3 to 5 years	Children told *if* they drank juice, *then* they could play	Instrumental ("if") use of juice reduced preferences for it
112, Birch et al., 1984	31 children aged 3 to 5 years	Children told *if* they drank milk drink, *then* they received verbal praise or a movie	Instrumental ("if") use of milk beverage reduced preferences for it
113, Newman and Taylor, 1992	86 children aged 4 to 7 years	Children told that *if* they ate 1 snack, *then* they could eat another snack (with both of neutral preference initially)	"If" snacks became *less* preferred and "then" snacks became *more* preferred
114, Hendy, 1999	64 preschool children	To encourage acceptance of 4 new fruits and vegetables during 3 preschool lunches, teachers used 1 of 5 actions: (1) choice-offering ("*Do you want any of this?*"), (2) reward (special dessert), (3) insisting children try 1 bite, (4) modeling by teacher, or (5) simple exposure	Choice-offering and reward were more effective than other actions. Hendy concluded that dessert rewards are *not* needed because the less expensive and more nutritious action of choice-offering works as well
119, Hendy and Raudenbush, 2000	*Study 1:* 58 teachers of preschool children *Study 2:* 18 boys, 16 girls (preschool) *Study 3:* 13 boys, 10 girls (preschool) *Study 4:* 12 boys, 14 girls (preschool) *Study 5:* 6 boys, 8 girls (preschool)	*Study 1:* Teacher questionnaire to rate effectiveness of 5 teacher actions to encourage children's food acceptance *Study 2:* Familiar foods presented under silent teacher modeling or exposure *Study 3:* Novel foods presented under silent teacher modeling or exposure *Study 4:* Novel foods presented under enthusiastic teacher modeling ("*Mmm! I love mangos!*") or exposure *Study 5:* Novel foods presented under enthusiastic teacher modeling versus peer modeling versus exposure Preschool lunch was setting for Studies 2 to 5. Preferences assessed only for Study 5, and after one-month delay	*Study 1:* Teachers rated modeling as most effective over choice-offering, insist, tangible reward, and exposure *Study 2:* Silent teacher modeling ineffective to encourage acceptance of familiar foods *Study 3:* Silent teacher modeling ineffective to encourage acceptance of novel foods *Study 4:* Enthusiastic teacher modeling maintained novel food acceptance across 5 meals *Study 5:* Boys ate and liked novel foods equally under all 3 conditions. Girls ate and liked novel foods most when modeled by peers. Enthusiastic teacher modeling ineffective if peer models were present; peer modeling more effective for girls than boys
120, Hendy, 2002	38 preschool children	Three novel foods presented to 8 tables of 38 children during 5 preschool lunches. After 3 baseline lunches, 16 of 38 children were trained to serve as peer models of food acceptance for 1 novel food in exchange for small toy rewards; each novel food was assigned to either girl model, boy model, or no model conditions for next 2 lunches. Remaining 22 of 38 children were observed and their food bites were recorded during baseline and modeled lunches	For children of either gender, girl models were more effective than boy models at increasing food acceptance by observed children from baseline to modeled lunches. One month later, neither food preferences nor consumption decreased for trained peer models, but both decreased for observed children

Reference	Sample	Description	Results
116, Wardle et al., 2003	49 children age 5 to 7 years	Randomized controlled design with children from 3 primary schools in London assigned to 1 of 2 intervention groups (exposure, reward) or a no-treatment control group for a 2-week period with liking for, and consumption of, red pepper assessed before and after 2-week period. Children in each intervention group had 8 daily, individual sessions with those in exposure group offered a taste of red pepper and told they could eat as much as they liked, and those in reward group shown cartoon stickers and told they could pick 1 if they ate at least 1 piece of pepper	Liking and consumption were increased for the exposure group compared to the control group. For the reward group, the outcomes were intermediate, lying between, and not significantly different from, the exposure and control groups. Contrary to results from previous studies by others, rewards did not decrease liking
115, Wardle et al., 2003	156 children (mean age = 53 months; range from 34 to 82 months) and parents (95% mothers) who had participated in larger study (n=564) of predictors of children's fruit and vegetable intake	Randomized controlled trial with parents of children assigned to 1 of 3 groups: Exposure (offer child taste of target vegetable daily for 14 consecutive days; encourage tasting without offering rewards; keep "vegetable" diary with space for children to record liking using small "face" stickers after each tasting; modeling "taste" was suggested). Information (nutritional advice and leaflet), or Control (no treatment)	Only the Exposure group had significant increases in liking, ranking, and consumption of the target vegetable from pre- to post-intervention. The authors concluded that a parent-led, exposure-based intervention involving daily tasting of a vegetable, along with a daily vegetable "sticker" diary, holds promise for improving children's acceptance of vegetables
117, Perry et al., 2004	Baseline — 1,668 children (in first or third grade); End (2 years later) — 1,168 of same children (in third or fifth grade); 26 schools (13 intervention, 13 delayed-program control); Data collected on ~23 children per grade per school	Randomized controlled trial of school cafeteria-based intervention which lasted two school years and included daily activities (increased availability, appeal, and encouragement of fruits and vegetables in lunch program; changes in lunch line and school snack cart) and special events (2-week kickoff campaign with posters; monthly samplings served at lunch by peers with help from parents; theater production; 2 challenge weeks when students competed to eat 3 fruit and vegetable daily lunch servings and classes rewarded at week's end with frozen fruit yogurt; final meal demonstration)	Students in intervention schools significantly increased total fruit intake by 0.14 to 0.17 servings at lunch with no differences for vegetables. Process measures indicated that verbal encouragement by food service staff was associated with outcomes. Authors concluded that environmental interventions alone may have limited impact without classroom and home (parental) activities, and interventions are needed that focus solely on vegetable intake among children
118, Hendy et al., 2005	188 children in first, second, or fourth grade at baseline	School-cafeteria-based intervention. For 18 lunches (3 per week), children (in classes) randomly assigned to receive token reinforcement for eating either fruits or vegetables. Lunch observers recorded intake and punched holes into nametags each day for children who ate assigned foods. Weekly during lunch, children traded token "punches" for small prizes. Preferences assessed with individual interviews at baseline and follow-up at 2 weeks and 7 months after program	Fruit and vegetable consumption increased for all grades and lasted throughout the program. Preferences increased 2 weeks after the program for both fruits and vegetables, but returned to baseline levels 7 months after the program
121, Addessi et al., 2005	27 children age 2 to 5 years	Children's behaviors towards novel foods (cooked semolina, colored and flavored as yellow cumin, green caper, or red anchovy) were assessed when an adult model (1) was not eating (Presence condition), (2) was eating food of different color (Different color condition), and (3) was eating food of same color (Same color condition). Adult models given same colored semolina but flavored with sugar so they would eat it enthusiastically	Children accepted and ate novel food more in Same color condition than in Different color and in Presence conditions. Children ate less food in first trial than in second and third trials. Authors concluded that "social influences — together with repeated experiences with novelty — are a powerful instrument to promote the acceptance of novel foods in young children"

calories eaten in a snack or meal, based on the calories eaten in a preload snack.[125,126] Furthermore, preschool children are able to adjust the calories eaten at various meals and snacks during the day, so that the number of calories consumed in a 24-h period is relatively constant.[127]

Although children have the ability to self-regulate their caloric intake, well-conducted laboratory studies[128,129] indicate that this ability may be negatively impacted by child-feeding practices that encourage or restrict children's eating. Using observations of family meal times, Klesges and colleagues[130] found that parental prompts, especially encouragements to eat, were highly correlated to preschool children's relative weight, and increased the probability that a child would eat. Furthermore, a child's refusal to eat usually led to a parental prompt to eat more food, whereas a child's food request was not likely to elicit either a parental prompt to eat or subsequent eating by the child. Results from a small but well-controlled study by Fisher and Birch[94] indicated that preschool children's preferences for dietary fat were related to their own triceps' skin-fold measurements, as well as to the composite BMI of their parents. Laboratory experiments with preschool children indicate that restricting access to palatable foods can sensitize children to external rather than internal eating cues, and increase children's desire to obtain and consume the restricted foods.[131] For preschool girls (but not boys), child and maternal reports of restricting access were predictive of girls' snack food intake, with higher levels of snack food intake predicted by higher levels of restriction.[132] Child-feeding practices have been found to be key behavioral variables that explain more of the variance in children's total fat mass than energy intake.[133] Among girls, longitudinal data provide evidence that maternal restriction can promote overeating in the absence of hunger.[134]

Over the past 2 decades, portion sizes have increased significantly (http://hin.nhlbi.nih.gov/portion/index.htm). Young children require fewer calories and smaller amounts of food from each of the food groups compared to adolescents. (See Table 16.12 and Table 16.15 for information from *MyPyramid* about food intake patterns and calorie levels, respectively.) For example, a 4-year-old girl and a 16-year-old girl (each with a moderate activity level), require 1400 and 2000 calories per day, respectively; in terms of amounts of food by food group, this is a difference of one half cup of fruit, 1 cup of vegetables, 1 ounce of grains, 1.5 ounces of meat, 1 cup of milk, 2 teaspoons of oil, and almost 100 discretionary calories.

Research indicates interesting insight into the relationship between portion sizes and young children's intake. In a study by Rolls et al.,[135] 16 younger (3 years) and 16 older (5 years) preschool children participated in three lunches during their usual lunchtime at the day care. Each lunch consisted of macaroni and cheese served in small, medium, or large portion sizes, along with set portion sizes of carrot sticks, applesauce, and milk. Results indicated that older preschoolers consumed more macaroni and cheese, when served the large portion compared to the small portion ($p < .002$). However, portion sizes did not significantly affect food intake among younger preschoolers. These results indicate the important role of portion size in shaping children's dietary intake, and imply that portion size can either promote or prevent the development of overweight among older preschool children. Furthermore, these results indicate the importance of encouraging preschool children to focus on their own internal cues of hunger and satiety instead of "*eating everything to clean the plate.*"[135]

Fisher et al.[136] extended the previous investigation in a study with 30 children aged 3 to 5 years who participated in a series of lunches once a week for 12 weeks during their usual lunchtime at the day care. Each lunch consisted of an entrée of macaroni and cheese served either as an age-appropriate portion, a large portion that was double the size of the age-appropriate one, or a portion self-served by the child, along with standard portion sizes of carrots, applesauce, milk, and sugar cookies. Results indicated that doubling an age-appropriate portion of the entrée increased entrée and total lunch energy intakes by 25 and 15%, respectively. Changes were attributable to increases in children's average bite size of the entrée without compensatory decreases in the intake of other foods served at the lunch. Children's average self-served portion size did not differ significantly from the size of the age-appropriate portion served to them. Furthermore, when the children served their own entrée, they ate 25% less of it than when they were served a large entrée portion. According to the authors, their results "*provide initial evidence that allowing children to self-select portion sizes can affect the amount consumed and may play an important role in reducing the effects of exposure to large portion sizes on children's intake.*"[136]

McConahy et al.[137] analyzed data from 1994 to 1996 and 1998 CFSII for children aged 2 to 5 years to evaluate the relationship of portion size for 10 commonly eaten foods, number of eating occasions per day, and number of foods consumed per day with children's total energy intake. Results indicated that body weight accounted for only 4% of the variability in energy intake in contrast to food portion size, number of eating occasions, and number of foods that accounted for 17–19%, 9%, and 6–8%, respectively. The authors concluded that feeding recommendations for children should focus on moderation in portion sizes as well as frequent feeding.[137]

DIVISION OF FEEDING RESPONSIBILITY

According to Birch,[98] child feeding practices that encourage children to eat in response to external cues instead of internal cues regarding hunger and satiety "*may form the basis for the development of individual differences in styles of intake control that exist among adults. Some of the problems of energy balance seen in adulthood may result from styles of intake control in which hunger and satiety cues are not particularly central.*" According to the American Dietetic Association,[74] "*perhaps some of the best advice regarding child feeding practices continues to be the division of parental and child responsibility advocated by Satter.*" Satter advocates that parents (or adults) are responsible for presenting a variety of nutritious and safe foods to children at regular snack- and mealtimes, as well as the physical and emotional setting of eating; children are responsible for deciding how much, if any, they will eat.[138–140]

Dietary recommendations from the American Heart Association and the American Academy of Pediatrics advocate a similar division of feeding responsibility: Parents choose the time for meals and snacks, provide a wide variety of nutrient-dense foods and beverages, and provide an appropriate social context for eating that include family meals. Children can then choose how much to consume.[15,16] Furthermore, the eating behavior of adults (whether parents, guardians, or caregivers) must provide appropriate role modeling to influence children with "*do as I do*" instead of "*do as I say.*" [15, 16]

CHILDHOOD OBESITY

Overwhelming evidence indicates that the incidence of obesity among children and adolescents has increased dramatically during the last three decades.[82–86] According to Dietz, "*obesity is now the most prevalent nutritional disease of children and adolescents in the United States.*"[141] Critical periods during the childhood years for the development of obesity include the period of adiposity rebound that occurs between 5 and 7 years of age, and adolescence.[141] The causes of childhood obesity are multifactorial, including both genetics and environment. Inactivity appears to play a major role in the increasing rate of childhood obesity, as does television viewing. Results from NHANES III indicated that children aged 8 to 16 years who watched 4 h or more of television each day had greater body fat and greater BMI than children who watched television less than 2 h each day;[142] furthermore, television watching was positively associated with obesity among girls, even after controlling for age, race/ethnicity, family income, weekly physical activity, and energy intake.[143] According to the Youth Behavior Risk Surveillance System, in 2003, 38% of students in grades 9 through 12 watched television for 3 h or more per day on an average school day.[144] With the advances in technology, especially regarding computers, more children are spending more hours in sedentary states.

Preventing childhood obesity is more desirable than trying to treat obesity during adolescence and adulthood. One critical component of obesity prevention is increased physical activity; another is educating parents and caregivers regarding the development of children's food preferences and food consumption patterns. The American Academy of Pediatrics Committee on Nutrition issued a policy statement in 2003 which recommends that parents and caregivers promote healthful eating patterns by offering nutritious snacks, encouraging children's autonomy in self-regulation of food intake, setting appropriate limits on food choices, and modeling healthful food choices, and that television and video time be limited to a maximum of 2 h/day.[145]

In the 2005 Dietary Guidelines for Americans, a key recommendation regarding overweight children is to reduce the rate of weight gain while allowing growth and development.[14] A healthcare provider should be consulted before placing a child on a weight-reduction diet. The topic of childhood obesity is covered thoroughly in Chapter 51 (not so).

LOW-FAT DIETS

Emphasis regarding low-fat, low-cholesterol diets has increased during the past decade, as has the debate over whether low-fat diets are appropriate for children.[146–151] Parental concern about later atherosclerosis or obesity has led to failure to thrive in some infants aged 7 to 22 months who were fed very-low-fat and calorie-restricted diets.[152] However, the safety and efficacy of lower-fat diets in children have been confirmed by results from several studies. The Special Turku Coronary Risk Factor Intervention Project for Babies (STRIP) was a prospective trial for which a total of 1062 healthy infants were randomized at age 7 months into an intervention group ($n = 540$) or usual care control group ($n = 522$). The intervention group received repeated, individualized counseling aimed at promoting a fat intake of 30% of energy, a 1:1:1 ratio of saturated to monounsaturated to polyunsaturated fat intake, and low cholesterol. Growth and development data from the STRIP trial support the safety of a low saturated-fat, low-cholesterol diet administered to infants beginning at age 7 months and continuing through the first several years of life.[153–155] The Dietary Intervention Study in Children (DISC) was a multicenter, randomized controlled trial with preadolescent children;[156] an intervention group ($n = 334$) followed a diet with 28% of kcal from total fat, ~10% of kcal from saturated fat, and 95 mg/day of cholesterol, and a comparable usual care group ($n = 329$) consumed ~33% of kcal from total fat, ~12% of kcal from saturated fat, and 113 mg/day of cholesterol. Results from DISC indicated that dietary fat modifications can be achieved and sustained safely with no adverse effects in pubertal children up to 7 years later, and that children who received the intervention made healthier food choices.[156–159] Further evidence regarding the safety and efficacy of lower fat diets in upper elementary school children (third through fifth grades) was provided by the Child and Adolescent Trial for Cardiovascular Health (CATCH), which is described more fully later in this chapter. Results failed to indicate any evidence of deleterious effects of the 3-year intervention on growth or development of children.[160]

EXCESSIVE FRUIT JUICE CONSUMPTION

Fruit juice is an increasingly common beverage for young children.[77] Although fruit juice is a healthful, low-fat, nutritious beverage, there are health concerns regarding excessive fruit juice consumption by young children. For example, drinking fruit juice helps fulfill nutrition recommendations to eat more fruits and vegetables. However, as children increase their intake of fruit juices, they may decrease their intake of milk,[161] that can decrease their intake of calcium unless the juice is calcium-fortified. Carbohydrate malabsorption is common following the ingestion of several fruit juices in young children with chronic nonspecific diarrhea as well as in healthy young children.[162] Excessive fruit juice consumption may be a contributing factor in nonorganic failure to thrive.[163] Drinking 12 or more fluid ounces of fruit juice per day is associated with short stature and with obesity in young children.[164] In 2001, the Committee on Nutrition of the American Academy of Pediatrics issued a policy statement about the use and misuse of fruit juice, which recommended limiting daily fruit juice intake to 4 to 6 ounces for children aged 1 to 6 years, and to 8 to 12 ounces for children aged 7 to 18 years.[165] In addition, the policy statement recommended that children be encouraged to eat whole fruits (instead of drinking fruit juice) to meet their recommended daily fruit intake, and that unpasteurized juice not be consumed.

CAFFEINE

Caffeine is a stimulant for the central nervous system; it tends to decrease drowsiness and reduce the sense of fatigue, but too much can cause palpitations, stomach upset, insomnia, and anxiety. Its effects vary among individuals, depending on the amount ingested, body size of the individual, and personal tolerance. Some people are able to build up a tolerance to caffeine through regular use; others are more sensitive to it. If someone who has regularly consumed caffeine suddenly stops using it, mild withdrawal symptoms (e.g., headaches, craving for caffeine, etc.) may occur. Substantial amounts of caffeine are found in several soft drinks, coffee, tea, and some pain relievers; smaller amounts are found in chocolate and foods with cocoa.

Consumption of caffeine increases during adolescence with greater intakes of soft drinks, tea, and coffee. This can be a concern, because caffeine has a modest negative impact on calcium retention, yet consumption of foods high in calcium decreases as children get older,[54] especially among girls.[43] Furthermore, the stimulating effect of caffeine may set the stage for needing stimulation; although caffeine is classified as a drug, society is very accepting of this stimulant and has not considered it a nuisance.[166]

NUTRITIVE AND NONNUTRITIVE SWEETENERS

Although there are widespread beliefs that both sugar (i.e., sucrose) and nonnutritive sweeteners (e.g., aspartame) produce hyperactivity and other behavioral problems in children, both dietary challenge and dietary replacement studies have demonstrated that sugar has little if any adverse effects on behavior.[167] For example, Wolraich et al.[168] conducted a double-blind controlled trial with 25 normal preschool children and 23 school-age children who were described by their parents as sensitive to sugar. The different diets that children and their families followed for each of three consecutive 3-week periods were either high in sucrose, aspartame, or saccharin (placebo). Children's behavior and cognitive performance were evaluated weekly. Results strongly indicated that even when intake exceeded typical dietary levels, neither sucrose nor aspartame had discernible cognitive or behavioral effects in normal preschool children or in school-age children who were believed to be sensitive to sugar. Furthermore, the few differences associated with the ingestion of sucrose were more consistent with a slight calming effect than with hyperactivity.[168] Results from a 1995 meta-analytic synthesis of 16 reports containing 23 controlled double-blind challenge studies found that sugar did not affect the behavior or cognitive performance of children; however, a small effect of sugar or effects on subsets of children could not be ruled out.[169]

According to Kanarek,[167] the strong belief of parents, educators, and medical professionals that sugar has adverse effects on children's behavior may be attributed to several factors. First, adults may misconceive the relationship between sugar and behavior. Children in general have difficulty altering their behavior in response to changing environmental conditions, such as shifting from the unstructured nature of a party or snack time at school to the more rigorous demands of class work. If the party or snack included foods with high sugar content, adults may relate the child's sugar intake with behavioral problems as the child tries to adapt from an unstructured activity to one with structure. Second, sugar-containing foods such as candy are often forbidden or given to children in very limited amounts; the prohibited nature of these foods may contribute to the belief that associates them with increased activity. Finally, expectations of both adults and children could promote the idea that sugar leads to hyperactivity. Children hear adults comment that "*too much sugar makes children hyper*" and children believe them and act accordingly to fulfill the prophecy.[167]

Although experimental evidence fails to indicate that sugar affects children's behavior and cognition, children should not have unlimited access to sugar, because undernutrition may occur if foods with essential nutrients are replaced by calories from sugar; furthermore, sugar (and starch) can promote tooth decay. According to *MyPyramid*,[170] the "discretionary calorie allowance" may be used to eat more foods from any food group than the food guide recommends, to select forms of foods that contain solid fats or added sugars (such as sweetened cereal and sweetened yogurt), to add fats or sweeteners (such as sugar) to foods, or to eat or drink items that contain only fats, caloric sweeteners (such as candy and soft drinks), or alcohol. Furthermore, in *MyPyramid*, added sugars are addressed in the overarching theme of "proportionality," which is to eat more of some foods (fruits, vegetables, whole grains, fat-free or low-fat milk products), and less of others (foods high in saturated or *trans* fats, added sugars, cholesterol, salt, and alcohol), and the overarching theme of "moderation," which is to choose forms of foods that limit intake of saturated or *trans* fats, added sugars, cholesterol, salt, and alcohol.[170] According to the 2005 Dietary Guidelines for Americans,[14] key recommendations for carbohydrates include that foods and beverages should be chosen and prepared with little added sugars or caloric sweeteners, and that the incidence of dental caries be reduced by practicing good oral hygiene and consuming sugar- and starch-containing foods and beverages less frequently. According to the DRIs, added sugars should be limited to no more than 25% of total energy, after which dietary quality might be reduced.[1] The position of the American Dietetic Association[171] is that "consumers can safely enjoy a range of nutritive and nonnutritive sweeteners when consumed in a diet that is guided by current federal nutrition recommendations, such as the Dietary Guidelines for Americans and the Dietary Reference Intakes, as well as individual health goals."

MEDIA INFLUENCES

Children's food preferences and consumption patterns can be altered either positively or negatively by media and advertising. Youth are the target of intense and specialized food marketing and advertising efforts via television advertising, in-school marketing, the Internet, toys and products with brand logos, product placements, kids clubs, and youth-targeted promotions.[172] However, foods marketed to youth are predominantly high in fat and sugar, which is inconsistent with dietary recommendations. For example, a 2005 study by Harrison and Marske[173] found that snacks, convenience, fast foods, and sweets dominated food advertisements aired during television programs heavily viewed by children. Furthermore, advertised foods exceeded recommended daily values for total fat, saturated fat, and sodium, but failed to provide recommended daily values for fiber, vitamin A, vitamin C, calcium, and iron.[173] A review by Story and French[172] examines the food advertising and marketing channels used to target youth in the United States, the impact on eating behavior of food advertising, and current regulations and policies. A 2004 Kaiser Family Foundation Issue Brief reviews more than 40 studies and explores what is and is not known about the role of media in the dramatically increasing rates of childhood obesity in the United States.[174] It outlines media-related policy options that have been proposed to help address this important public health problem, such as decreasing the time children spend with media to reducing their exposure to food advertising. In addition, it identifies ways in which media could play a positive role in helping address childhood obesity, such as increasing the number of media messages that promote fitness and sound nutrition.[174]

VEGETARIAN DIETS

There is considerable variation in the eating patterns of vegetarians. For the lacto–ovo–vegetarian, the eating pattern is based on grains, vegetables, fruits, legumes, seeds, nuts, dairy products, and eggs; meat, fish, and fowl are excluded. For the vegan, or total vegetarian, the eating pattern is similar to the lacto–ovo–vegetarian pattern except for the additional exclusion of eggs, dairy, and other animal products. However, considerable variation may exist in the extent to which animal products are avoided within both of this patterns.[175]

The position of the American Dietetic Association and Dietitians of Canada is that "appropriately planned vegetarian diets are healthful, nutritionally adequate, and provide health benefits in the prevention and treatment of certain diseases."[175] Well-planned vegan and other types of vegetarian diets are appropriate for all stages of the life cycle, including childhood and adolescence.[175] Appropriately planned vegan and lacto–ovo–vegetarian diets satisfy nutrient needs of infants, children, and adolescents and promote normal growth.[176] Dietary deficiencies are more common in populations with very restrictive vegetarian diets. Vegan children need a reliable source of vitamin B_{12}; in addition, vitamin D supplements or fortified foods should be used if sun exposure is limited.[175] For vegetarian children, emphasis should be placed on foods rich in calcium, iron, and zinc, along with dietary practices that enhance absorption of iron and zinc from plant foods. Vegetarian children can be helped to meet energy needs through frequent meals and snacks, as well as the use of some refined foods and foods higher in unsaturated fat.[175] Messina and Mangels[177] reviewed research on the growth and nutrient intake of vegan children and provided recommendations for feeding balanced diets to vegan children. Modifications to the vegetarian food guide for children (aged 4 to 8 years) and adolescents (aged 9 to 18 years) are available.[178] During the adolescent years, when there is increased independence and decision making and greater influence by peers and role models, vegetarian diets may be relatively common. Chapter 20 contains additional information regarding vegetarian diets.

FEEDING TODDLERS AND PRESCHOOL CHILDREN

Young children cannot innately choose a well-balanced diet. They depend on adults to offer them a variety of nutritious and developmentally appropriate foods. A child's intake at individual meals may vary considerably, but the total daily caloric intake remains fairly constant.[127] Many parents become anxious about the adequacy of their young child's diet or frustrated with their child's unpredictable eating behavior, which may include refusals to eat certain foods and food jags. Table 16.23 contains suggestions for concerns that parents may commonly encounter when feeding young children.

TABLE 16.23

Suggestions for Concerns Parents Commonly Encounter when Feeding Young Children

If a child refuses to try new foods or refuses to eat what is served …
- Remember, this is normal! Continue to offer each new food 10 to 12 times, twice per week
- Serve a new food with familiar ones
- Ask the child if she or he would like to try some of the new food. Be an effective role model and enthusiastically eat some of the new food yourself; comment to the child about how much you like it
- Involve the child in shopping for and preparing food, and in setting and clearing the table
- Remember, children may have strong likes and dislikes, but this does *not* mean they need to be served different foods than the rest of the family
- Allow the child to choose from the foods available at a meal what she or he will eat, but avoid forcing or bribing him or her to eat
- Include at least one food at each meal that you know your child will eat, but do not cater to a child's likes or dislikes. Avoid becoming a short-order cook. The less attention paid to this behavior, the better
- Avoid pressuring, coaxing, bribing, or nagging the child to eat
- Attempt to have family meals be as pleasant as possible by avoiding arguments and criticism. Use the child's developmental stage to determine expectations for manners and neatness while at the same time setting limits on inappropriate behaviors (such as throwing food)
- Let children determine when they are full and have had enough instead of insisting that they clean their plates
- Schedule meals at regular times. Avoid having a child get too hungry or too tired before mealtime. Snacks should be 1.5 to 2 h before meals

If a child is stuck on a food jag or wants to eat the same food over and over …
- Children may want to eat only one or two foods day after day, meal after meal; common food jags occur with peanut butter and jelly sandwiches, pizza, macaroni, and cheese, and dry cereal with milk
- Relax, and realize this is normal and temporary. Refuse to call attention to the behavior
- Continue to offer regular meals, but do not force or bribe the child to eat them
- Serve the food jag item as you normally would (maybe once or twice a week)

If a child refuses to eat meat …
- Tough meat is often difficult for children to chew. Offer bite-size pieces of tender, moist meat, poultry, or boneless fish
- Use meat in casseroles, meatloaf, soup, spaghetti sauce, pizza, or burritos
- Try other high-protein foods such as eggs, legumes, and peanut butter

If a child refuses to drink milk or drinks too little milk…
- Offer cheese, cottage cheese, yogurt, or pudding either alone or in combination dishes (such as macaroni and cheese, pizza, cheese sauce, banana pudding)
- Use milk when cooking hot cereals, scrambled eggs, macaroni and cheese, soup, and other recipes
- Offer flavored milks
- Use calcium-fortified juices

If a child drinks too much milk or juice …
- Offer water between meals to quench thirst
- Limit milk to one serving with meals or at the end of meals, and offer water for seconds

If a child refuses to eat vegetables and fruits …
- Offer more fruits if a child refuses vegetables, and vice versa
- Avoid overcooking vegetables; serve vegetables steamed or raw (if appropriate). Include dips or sauces (e.g., applesauce with broccoli or carrots)
- Include vegetables in soups, casseroles, and pizza
- Add fresh or dried fruit to cold and hot cereals
- Continue to offer a variety of fruits and vegetables

If a child eats too many sweets …
- Avoid using sweets as a bribe or reward
- Limit the purchase and preparation of sweet foods in the home
- Incorporate sweets into meals instead of snacks for better dental health. Also, by serving desserts (if any) with the meal, they become less important and cannot be used as a reward
- Decrease sugar by half in recipes for muffins, quick breads, cookies, etc.
- Try using fruit as dessert

Source: Adapted from Lucas, B and Ogata, B Normal Nutrition from Infancy through Adolescence, *Handbook of Pediatric Nutrition*, 3rd edition., (Samour, P Q. and, King, K, Eds.), Jones and Bartlett, Boston, 2005, p. 107–130.

SNACKS

Most young children fare best when fed four to six times a day due to their smaller stomach capacities and fluctuating appetites. Snacks should be considered as mini-meals that contribute to the total day's nutrient intake. Snacks generally accepted by many children include fresh fruit, cheese, whole-grain crackers, breads (e.g., bagels, tortilla, etc.), low-fat milk, raw vegetables, 100% fruit juices, sandwiches on whole-grain breads, peanut butter on crackers, or whole-grain bread, and yogurt.

CHOKING

Chewing and swallowing functions are not fully developed until 8 years of age; thus, precautions should be followed to avoid choking.[77] Foods to avoid because they are most likely to cause problems by becoming easily lodged in the esophagus include round candy, nuts, raw carrots, and popcorn. Other potentially problematic foods (e.g., hot dogs, grapes, and string cheese) may be modified by cutting them into small strips. Any food can cause choking if the child is not supervised while eating, if the child runs while eating, or if too much food is stuffed in the mouth. Thus, an adult should always be present when children are eating, children should sit down while eating, and the mealtime environment ideally should be free of distractions such as television, loud music, and activities. Allowing children to eat in the car is discouraged, because it can be difficult to help a choking child if the only adult present is driving.[77]

FEEDING SCHOOL-AGE CHILDREN AND ADOLESCENTS

During the school-age years (ages 6 to 12), steady growth is paralleled by increased food intake. Although children tend to eat fewer times a day, after-school snacks are common.

Studies indicate that eating breakfast is related positively to children's cognitive function and school performance, especially for undernourished children (for a review, see Pollitt[179]). Specifically, schoolchildren who had fasted both overnight and in the morning, particularly children who were nutritionally at risk, demonstrated slower stimulus discrimination, increased errors, and slower memory recall.[180] According to Grantham-McGregor, "*studies to date have provided insufficient evidence to determine whether children's long-term scholastic achievement is improved by eating breakfast daily.*"[181]

Although eating breakfast is important, research indicates that between 6 and 16% of elementary school children skip breakfast.[182–184] Furthermore, between 1965 and 1991, breakfast consumption declined significantly for each age group of children (1 to 4 years, 5 to 7 years, 8 to 10 years) and adolescents (11 to 14 years and 15 to 18 years), especially for older adolescents aged 15 to 18 years; breakfast was consumed by 90% of boys and 84% of girls in 1965, and by 75 and 65%, respectively, in 1991.[185] Children who skip breakfast tend to have a lower kcal intake and consume fewer nutrients than children who eat breakfast.[182,183] When breakfast nutrient consumption patterns of third graders were examined using 1991 baseline data from CATCH, a surprisingly large percentage of the sample (94% of the 1872 children from 96 public schools in four states) reported eating breakfast on the day of the survey;[182] of the 94% who ate breakfast, 80% ate at home, 13% ate at school, 3% ate at both home and school, and 4% ate breakfast elsewhere. During the second decade of life, breakfast skipping tends to increase, perhaps due to time constraints or lack of appetite in the morning.

Adolescents often experience newly found independence, busy schedules, searches for self-identification, dissatisfaction with body image, difficulty accepting existing values, and a desire for peer acceptance.[186] Each of these events may help explain changes in food habits of adolescents. Common characteristics of food habits of adolescents include an increased tendency to skip meals (especially breakfast and lunch), eating more meals outside the home, increased snacking (especially on candy), consumption of fast foods, and dieting.[186]

Insight regarding adolescents' perceptions about factors influencing their food choices and eating behaviors was provided from a 1999 study for which focus groups were conducted with 141 seventh or tenth graders (40% white, 25% Asian American, 21% African American, 7% multiracial, 6% Hispanic, 1% Native American) from two urban schools in St. Paul, Minnesota.[187] Factors identified by the adolescents as being most influential on their food choices included hunger and food cravings, appeal of food (primarily taste), time considerations of themselves and their parents, and convenience of food. Factors identified by the adolescents to be of secondary importance included food availability, parental influences on eating behavior (including the family's culture or religion), perceived benefits of food (e.g., for health, energy, body shape), and situational factors (e.g., place, time). Additional factors discussed included mood, body image concerns, habit, cost, media influences, and vegetarian lifestyle choices. A sense of urgency about personal health in relation to other concerns, and taste preferences for other foods were major barriers to eating more fruits, vegetables, and dairy products and eating fewer high-fat foods. Suggestions provided by the adolescents to help adolescents eat a more healthful diet included making healthful food taste and look better, making healthful food more available and convenient, limiting the availability of unhealthful options, teaching them good eating habits at an early age, and changing social norms to make it "cool" to eat healthfully. These results suggest that if interventions to improve adolescent nutrition are to be effective, they need to have adolescent input and address a broad range of factors, especially environmental factors (e.g., increased availability and promotion of appealing, convenient foods in homes, schools, and restaurants).[187]

Evidence of a strong positive association between frequency of family meals and quality of dietary intake among adolescents was provided by a 2003 study that included 4746 middle and high-school students of diverse racial and socioeconomic backgrounds who attended public schools in Minneapolis/St. Paul.[188] Variability in the frequency of family meals during the previous week was wide and ranged from never (14%), 1 or 2 times (19%), 3 or 4 times (21%), 5 or 6 times (19%), 7 times (9%), and more than 7 times (18%). Sociodemographic characteristics associated with more frequent family meals included socioeconomic status (high), mother's employment status (not employed), race (Asian American), school level (middle), and sex (boy). Frequency of family meals was negatively associated with soft drink consumption and positively associated with intake of calcium-rich foods, grains, fruits, and vegetables. Because of the important role family meals appear to play in promoting healthful dietary intake among adolescents, feasible ways of increasing the frequency of family meals need to be explored with adolescents and their families.[188]

The Minnesota Adolescent Health Survey (MAHS) was completed by more than 30,000 adolescents from 1986 through 1987. The MAHS was a comprehensive assessment of adolescent health status, health behaviors, and psychosocial factors; although it included relatively few nutrition-related items, a wealth of knowledge about adolescent nutrition was gained. Neumark-Sztainer et al. summarized the knowledge gained from a decade of subsequent analyses of data collected in the MAHS, as well as implications for working with youth.[189] Major concerns identified included overweight status, unhealthful weight-control practices, and high prevalence rates of inadequate intakes of fruits, vegetables, and dairy products. Risk factors for inadequate food intake patterns or unhealthful weight-control practices included low socioeconomic status, minority status, chronic illness, poor school achievement, low family connectedness, weight dissatisfaction, overweight, homosexual orientation among boys, and use of health-compromising behaviors. The results suggest a need for innovative outreach strategies that include educational and environmental approaches to improve adolescent eating behaviors. A critical issue that needs to be addressed is the validity of adolescents' self-reported behaviors.[189]

Story et al.[190] proposed an ecological model to help understand and explain the numerous and interacting influences on adolescent eating behavior. Four levels of influence described include individual or intrapersonal (such as biological and psychosocial), social environmental or interpersonal (such as peers and family), physical environmental or community settings (such as school, fast food restaurants, and convenience stores), and macrosystem or societal (such as social and cultural norms, mass media, marketing, and advertising). Interventions that address factors at these different levels of influence, as well as complement and build on each other, are needed to improve eating behaviors of youth.[190]

YOUTH RISK BEHAVIOR SURVEILLANCE — UNITED STATES, 2003 (YRBS 2003)

The Youth Risk Behavior Surveillance System (YRBSS) monitors six categories of priority health-risk behaviors among high-school youth in grades 9 through 12.[144] The YRBSS includes a national school-based survey conducted by the Centers for Disease Control and Prevention as well as state and local school-based surveys conducted by education and health agencies. A report was published in 2004 with results from the national survey, 32 state surveys, and 18 local surveys conducted in 2003; a total of 15,214 questionnaires completed by youth in 158 schools in 43 states and 22 large cities were usable.[144] Table 16.24 provides an overview of YRBS 2003 results overall and those with significant differences for the risk behaviors regarding fruit and vegetable consumption, milk consumption, at risk of overweight, overweight, perceived overweight, and attempts to lose weight or keep from gaining it; significant differences were evident by sex, race/ethnicity, grade level, and/or their interactions for each risk behavior included in the table.[144]

Data from YRBSS are being used to measure progress toward achievement of numerous national health objectives for 2010 as well as several of the leading health indicators.[144] Furthermore, YRBSS data are used by education and health officials at the national, state, and local levels to improve policies and programs to decrease priority health-risk behaviors among youth.[144]

HEALTH BEHAVIOUR IN SCHOOL-AGED CHILDREN STUDY: INTERNATIONAL REPORT FROM THE 2001/2002 SURVEY

The Health Behaviour in School-Aged Children Study is a unique cross-national research study conducted by an international network of research teams in collaboration with the World Health Organization (WHO) Regional Office for Europe.[191] The first survey was carried out in 1983 to 1984; since 1985, surveys have been conducted at 4-year intervals in an increasing number of countries. The target population for the study is young people attending school ages 11, 13, and 15. The aim was to increase understanding of young people's health, well-being, health behavior, and social context. The 2001/2002 survey was the sixth in the series and the most recent; it was conducted in 35 countries and regions including the United States, with approximately 1500 youth in each of the three age groups targeted in every country.[191] Youth were selected using a clustered sampling design, where the initial sampling unit was either the school class or the school. Results regarding eating habits indicated that the percentage of youth on average who eat breakfast every morning on school days was higher for boys at 69% than for girls at 60%, and decreased as age increased respectively from 11 to 13 to 15 years for both sexes (boys at 73, 68, and 64%; girls at 69, 57, and

TABLE 16.24
Results (Overall and those with Statistically Significant Differences) Regarding Dietary Behaviors, Overweight and Weight Control from the Youth Risk Behavior Survey, United States, 2003

Ate fruits and vegetables (defined as 100% fruit juice, fruit, green salad, potatoes [excluding French fries, fried potatoes, or potato chips], carrots, or other vegetables) ≥ 5 times/day during the 7 days preceding the survey:
Overall (22%)
Boys (24%) vs. Girls (20%)
Black boys (26%) vs. Black girls (20%)
Ninth-grade boys (25%) vs. ninth-grade girls (21%)
Eleventh-grade boys (25%) vs. eleventh-grade girls (18%)
Hispanics (24%) vs. Whites (21%)
Black boys (26%) and Hispanic boys (27%) vs. White boys (21%)
Ninth graders (23%) and tenth graders (23%) vs. twelfth graders (20%)
Drank ≥ 3 glasses/day of milk during the 7 days preceding the survey:
Overall (17%)
Boys (23%) vs. Girls (11%)
White boys (27%) vs. White girls (13%)
Black boys (16%) vs. Black girls (8%)
Hispanic boys (17%) vs. Hispanic girls (9%)
Ninth-grade boys (25%) vs. ninth-grade girls (14%)
Tenth-grade boys (24%) vs. tenth-grade girls (12%)
Eleventh-grade boys (23%) vs. eleventh-grade girls (10%)
Twelfth-grade boys (18%) vs. twelfth-grade girls (9%)
Whites (20%) vs. Blacks (12%) and Hispanic (13%)
White girls (13%) vs. Black girls (8%)
White boys (27%) and Black boys (16%) vs. Hispanic boys (17%)
Ninth graders (20%) vs. twelfth graders (14%)
Ninth-grade girls (14%) vs. twelfth-grade girls (9%)
Ninth-grade boys (25%) vs. twelfth-grade boys (18%)
At risk for becoming overweight (defined as ≥ 85th percentile but < 95th percentile for BMI, by age and sex, based on reference data) using self-reported height and weight:
Overall (15%)
Blacks (18%) and Hispanics (17%) vs. Whites (13%)
Black girls (21%) vs. White girls (12%) and Hispanic girls (16%)
Hispanic boys (19%) vs. White boys (14%)
Eleventh graders (17%) vs. twelfth graders (14%)
Eleventh-grade girls (16%) vs. twelfth-grade girls (12%)
Overweight (defined as ≥ 95th percentile for BMI, by age and sex, based on reference data) using self-reported height and weight:
Overall (12%)
Boys (16%) vs. Girls (8%)
White boys (14%) vs. White girls (7%)
Hispanic boys (21%) vs. Hispanic girls (12%)
Ninth-grade boys (18%) vs. ninth-grade girls (11%)
Tenth-grade boys (16%) vs. tenth-grade girls (8%)
Eleventh-grade boys (15%) vs. eleventh-grade girls (7%)
Twelfth-grade boys (13%) vs. twelfth-grade girls (7%)
Blacks (16%) and Hispanics (16%) vs. Whites (10%)
Black girls (14%) and Hispanic girls (12%) vs. White girls (7%)
Black boys (18%) and Hispanic boys (21%) vs. White boys (14%)
Ninth graders (14%) and tenth graders (12%) vs. twelfth graders (10%)
Ninth graders (14%) vs. eleventh graders (12%)
Ninth-grade girls (11%) vs. eleventh-grade girls (7%) and twelfth-grade girls (7%)
Ninth-grade boys (18%) vs. twelfth-grade boys (13%)

Considered themselves as slightly or very overweight:
Overall (30%)
Girls (36%) vs. boys (24%)
White girls (39%) vs. White boys (24%)
Black girls (26%) vs. Black boys (18%)
Hispanic girls (36%) vs. Hispanic boys (27%)
Ninth-grade girls (33%) vs. ninth-grade boys (23%)
Tenth-grade girls (36%) vs. tenth-grade boys (23%)
Eleventh-grade girls (37%) vs. eleventh-grade boys (24%)
Twelfth-grade girls (39%) vs. twelfth-grade boys (24%)
Whites (31%) and Hispanics (32%) vs. Blacks (22%)
White girls (39%) and Hispanic girls (36%) vs. Black girls (26%)
White boys (24%) and Hispanic boys (27%) vs. Black boys (18%)
Twelfth graders (31%) vs. ninth graders (28%)
Twelfth-grade girls (39%) vs. ninth-grade girls (33%)
Trying to lose weight:
Overall (44%)
Girls (59%) vs. Boys (29%)
White girls (63%) vs. White boys (28%)
Black girls (47%) vs. Black boys (23%)
Hispanic girls (62%) vs. Hispanic boys (37%)
Ninth-grade girls (54%) vs. ninth-grade boys (31%)
Tenth-grade girls (62%) vs. tenth-grade boys (28%)
Eleventh-grade girls (60%) vs. eleventh-grade boys (28%)
Twelfth-grade girls (62%) vs. twelfth-grade boys (28%)
Whites (45%) and Hispanics (49%) vs. Blacks (35%)
White girls (63%) and Hispanic girls (62%) vs. Black girls (47%)
White boys (28%) and Hispanic boys (37%) vs. Black boys (23%)
Tenth-grade girls (62%) and twelfth-grade girls (62%) vs. ninth-grade girls (54%)
Ate less food, fewer calories, or foods low in fat during the 30 days preceding the survey to lose weight or to keep from gaining weight:
Overall (42%)
Girls (56%) vs. boys (29%)
White girls (61%) vs. White boys (29%)
Black girls (39%) vs. Black boys (22%)
Hispanic girls (55%) vs. Hispanic boys (34%)
Ninth-grade girls (53%) vs. ninth-grade boys (29%)
Tenth-grade girls (58%) vs. nenth-grade boys (28%)
Eleventh-grade girls (56%) vs. eleventh-grade boys (29%)
Twelfth-grade girls (58%) vs. twelfth-grade boys (30%)
Whites (45%) and Hispanics (44%) vs. Blacks (31%)
White girls (61%) and Hispanic girls (55%) vs. Black girls (39%)
White girls (61%) vs. Hispanic girls (55%)
White boys (29%) and Hispanic boys (34%) vs. Black boys (22%)
Twelfth graders (44%) vs. ninth-graders (40%)
Twelfth-grade girls (58%) vs. ninth-grade girls (53%)

Continued

TABLE 16.24
(Continued)

Exercised during the 30 days preceding the survey to lose weight or to keep
  from gaining weight:
  Overall (57%)
  Girls (66%) vs. boys (49%)
  White girls (70%) vs. White boys (48%)
  Hispanic girls (64%) vs. Hispanic boys (54%)
  Ninth-grade girls (66%) vs. ninth-grade boys (50%)
  Tenth-grade girls (69%) vs. tenth-grade boys (50%)
  Eleventh-grade girls (65%) vs. eleventh-grade boys (49%)
  Twelfth-grade girls (63%) vs. twelfth-grade boys (46%)
  Whites (59%) and Hispanics (59%) vs. Blacks (48%)
  White girls (70%) and Hispanic girls (64%) vs. Black girls (49%)
  Hispanic boys (54%) vs. Black boys (46%)
Went without eating for ≥ 24 h during the 30 days preceding the survey to
  lose weight or to keep from gaining weight:
  Overall (13%)
  Girls (18%) vs. Boys (9%)
  White girls (18%) vs. White boys (7%)
  Black girls (15%) vs. Black boys (11%)
  Hispanic girls (18%) vs. Hispanic boys (9%)
  Ninth-grade girls (19%) vs. ninth-grade boys (11%)
  Tenth-grade girls (19%) vs. tenth-grade boys (7%)
  Eleventh-grade girls (20%) vs. eleventh-grade boys (8%)
  Twelfth-grade girls (16%) vs. twelfth-grade boys (7%)
  White girls (18%) and Hispanic girls (18%) vs. Black girls (15%)
  Black boys (11%) vs. White boys (7%)
  Ninth graders (15%) vs. twelfth graders (11%)
  Eleventh-grade girls (20%) vs. twelfth-grade girls (16%)
  Ninth-grade boys (11%) vs. tenth-grade boys (7%) and
    twelfth-grade boys (7%)

Took diet pills, powders, or liquids during the 30 days preceding the survey
  to lose weight or to keep from gaining it:
  Overall (9%)
  Girls (11%) vs. boys (7%)
  White girls (13%) vs. White boys (7%)
  Tenth-grade girls (11%) vs. tenth-grade boys (6%)
  Eleventh-grade girls (13%) vs. eleventh-grade boys (8%)
  Twelfth-grade girls (13%) vs. twelfth-grade boys (9%)
  Whites (10%) and Hispanics (11%) vs. Blacks (5%)
  White girls (13%) and Hispanic girls (12%) than Black girls (5%)
Vomited or took laxatives during the 30 days preceding the survey to lose
  weight or to keep from gaining weight:
  Overall (6%)
  Girls (8%) vs. boys (4%)
  White girls (9%) vs. White boys (3%)
  Tenth-grade girls (9%) vs. tenth-grade boys (4%)
  Eleventh-grade girls (9%) vs. eleventh-grade boys (3%)
  Twelfth-grade girls (7%) vs. twelfth-grade boys (4%)
  White girls (9%) and Hispanic girls (10%) vs. Black girls (6%)

Source: Adapted from Grunbaum, J, Kann, L, Kinchen, S. et al, *Youth Risk Behavior Surveillance — United States*, 2003, In CDC Surveillance Summaries,
MMWR 53 (No. SS-2), 2004; available at http://www.cdc.gov/mmwr/PDF/SS/SS5302.pdf (accessed March 7, 2006).

52%); the respective percentages of U.S. youth by age followed a similar pattern but were among the lowest across all countries
at 65, 55, and 41% for boys, and 54, 40, and 29% for girls. On average, the percentages of youth who eat fruit every day was
lower for boys at 30% than for girls at 37%, and decreased as age increased respectively for both sexes (boys at 36, 30, and
25%; girls at 41, 36, and 33%); the respective percentages of U.S. youth by age followed a similar pattern at 34, 29, and 21%
for boys, and 33, 28, and 22% for girls. On average, the percentages of youth who eat vegetables every day was lower for boys
at 28% than for girls at 34%, and decreased slightly as age increased for both sexes (boys at 31, 28, and 26%; girls at 36, 33,
and 32%); the respective percentages of U.S. youth were similar at 29, 26, and 25% for boys, and 34, 33, and 31% for girls.
On average, the percentages of youth who drink soft drinks every day was higher for boys at 32% than for girls at 25%, and
increased slightly as age increased for both sexes (boys at 29, 33, and 35%; girls at 23, 27, and 26%); unfortunately, U.S. youth
were among the leaders for daily soft drink consumption with percentages by age of 41, 48, and 47% for boys, and 38, 41, and
40% for girls. On average, approximately one-third of the youth eat sweets every day; however, the age and sex differences
were negligible compared to those for the other food and drink items presented. Although results varied substantially across
countries and regions, they indicate the need to improve the eating habits of youth, because on a daily basis, large percentages
of youth worldwide skip breakfast, drink soft drinks, consume sweets, and do not eat fruits or vegetables.[191]

EATING DISORDERS

Increases in the incidence and prevalence of eating disorders in youth have made it increasingly important for health professionals to be familiar with the early detection and appropriate management of eating disorders.[192] Eating disorders are a common chronic illness in adolescent girls; the average onset of bulimia nervosa occurs between mid-adolescence and the late 20s,
with a great diversity of socioeconomic status.[193] Optimal assessment and ongoing management of eating disorders requires an
interdisciplinary team with professionals from medicine, nursing, nutrition, and mental health.[193] According to the YRBS 2003,

44% of adolescents in grades 9 to 12 reported trying to lose weight; furthermore, to lose weight or to keep from gaining weight, during the 30 days preceding the survey, risky behaviors were reported by 13% of adolescents in grades 9 to 12 who had gone without eating for ≥ 24 h, 9% who had taken diet pills, powders, or liquids; and 6% who had vomited or taken laxatives.[144] As indicated in Table 16.24, these risky behaviors were more commonly reported by adolescent girls than by adolescent boys in the YRBS 2003.[144] More information regarding eating disorders may be found in Chapter 56.

TEEN PREGNANCY

Per year, about 500,000 live births are reported for teenage girls, with more than one-tenth of the girls aged 15 years or younger.[186] The adolescent growth spurt is not complete until a few years after menarche; thus, fetal demand for nutrients could jeopardize maternal growth, especially in girls who mature early and in girls whose nutritional status is unsatisfactory prior to pregnancy.[186] Eating habits of adolescents (e.g., skipped meals, increased snacking, consumption of fast foods, and dieting) create a health risk for pregnant adolescents, because during pregnancy, nutritional needs for the fetus are met before needs of the mother are met.[166] However, pregnancy may provide a unique opportunity to help the adolescent girl understand and improve her eating habits. Adolescents who are pregnant should be cautioned against skipping meals, especially breakfast, because skipping meals may increase the risk of ketosis.[186] More information regarding teen pregnancy may be found in Chapter 13.

GROUP FEEDING

Many young children spend some or most days away from home in childcare centers, preschools, Head Start programs, or home childcare centers where they may eat up to two meals and two snacks daily. Federal and state regulations or guidelines exist for food service in childcare centers, Head Start programs, and preschool programs in public schools. Some centers participate in USDA-sponsored child nutrition programs. When choosing a childcare center or preschool, parents should be encouraged to consider the feeding program, including food variety, quality, safety, cultural aspects, and developmental appropriateness. A report by the American Dietetic Association provides guidance for nutrition professionals, health care practitioners, childcare providers, and parents regarding meal plans, food preparation and service, physical and social environment, and nutrition training and consultation for childcare settings.[194]

Children have acquired knowledge about eating and have developed food preferences by the time they enter school; however, their food preferences and consumption patterns are continually modified, because they eat daily.[195] More than 95% of children in the United States are enrolled in school, where they may eat one or two meals per school day.[196] One in ten children gets two of their three major meals in school, and more than half get one of their three major meals in school.[197] Thus, schools play a critical role in shaping children's food acceptance patterns and can, therefore, help improve their diet.[198] No other public institution has as much continuous and intensive contact with children during their first two decades of life than public schools.[199] School staff have a greater potential influence on a child's health than any other group outside of the home.[200] School-based programs offer a systematic and efficient means to improve the health of youth in America by promoting positive lifestyles.[201] Health promotion programs in schools have the potential to help prevent chronic diseases in U.S. adults.[200] Although school-based health programs may promote healthful lifestyles, classroom lessons are not sufficient to produce lasting changes in students' eating behaviors.[109] In fact, curriculum-based nutrition education in schools has had minimal effects on student's eating behavior.[202] Children's food preferences and consumption are influenced by the school environment through familiarity and reinforcement.[203] Students of public schools generally attend for 7 h a day, 180 days a year. Although students have options for obtaining food in schools, the most prominent federally supported programs are the National School Lunch Program and the School Breakfast Program.

NATIONAL SCHOOL LUNCH PROGRAM AND SCHOOL BREAKFAST PROGRAM

The National School Lunch Program (NSLP) is a federally assisted meal program that operates in approximately 100,000 public and nonprofit private schools and residential childcare institutions; it provides nutritionally balanced, free, low-cost, or full-price lunches to more than 28 million children each school day.[204] In 1998, Congress expanded the NSLP to include reimbursement for snacks served to children in afterschool educational and enrichment programs.[204]

The School Breakfast Program (SBP) is a federally assisted meal program that operates in nearly 80,000 public and nonprofit private schools and residential childcare institutions.[205] It provides nutritionally balanced, free, low-cost, or full-price breakfasts to more than 8 million children each school day.[205]

Regulations stipulate that NSLP lunches and SBP breakfasts meet the applicable recommendations of the Dietary Guidelines for Americans, which recommend no more than 30% of energy from fat, and less than 10% of energy from saturated fat.[204,205] In addition, regulations stipulate that a NSLP lunch provide one-third, and that a SBP breakfast provide a quarter, of the RDAs for energy, protein, iron, calcium, and vitamins A and C.[204,205] Although NSLP lunches and SBP breakfasts must meet federal nutrition requirements, decisions about what specific foods to serve and how they are prepared are made by local school food authorities.[204,205]

Any child at a participating school may purchase a NSLP lunch or a SBP breakfast.[204,205] Children from families with incomes at or below 130% of the poverty level are eligible for free breakfasts and lunches. Children from families with incomes between 130% and 185% of the poverty level are eligible for reduced-price breakfasts and lunches, for which students can be charged no more than 40 cents. Children from families with incomes over 185% of the poverty level pay a full price, but their meals are still subsidized to some extent. Although local school food authorities set their own prices for full-price meals, they must operate their meal services as nonprofit programs. The majority of the support provided by the USDA to schools in the NSLP and SPB comes in the form of a cash reimbursement for each lunch or breakfast served that meets NSLP and SBP requirements, respectively; in addition, schools participating in the NSLP receive donated commodities from the USDA for each meal served.[204,205]

USDA School Meals Initiative (SMI) for Healthy Children and Team Nutrition

The USDA issued the final *School Meals Initiative* (SMI) *for Healthy Children* regulations in 1995 after the *Healthy Meals for Healthy Americans Act of 1994* (P. L. No. 103-448, sec. 106, 1994) was passed; the SMI requires that meals in the NSLP and SBP meet the Dietary Guidelines for Americans, and thus SMI regulations define how the Dietary Guidelines are applied to school meals.[206]

Team Nutrition is USDA's integrated, behavior-based, comprehensive plan for improving school meals and promoting the nutritional health and education of school children in the United States; the goal of Team Nutrition is "*to improve children's lifelong eating and physical activity habits by using the principles of the Dietary Guidelines for Americans and MyPyramid.*"[207] The focal point for Team Nutrition is schools, and three strategies are used to change behavior — training and technical assistance, nutrition education, and school and community support. Training and technical assistance are provided to Child Nutrition food service professionals (e.g., NSLP, SBP) to help them serve meals that look good, taste good, and meet nutrition standards. Nutrition education for children and their parents encourages children to eat a variety of foods; eat more fruits, vegetables, and grains; eat lower-fat foods more often; get calcium-rich foods; and be physically active. Support for schools and communities focuses on behavioral outcomes for school and community leaders to adopt and implement school policies that promote healthy eating and physical activity, provide school resources adequate to achieve success, and foster school and community environments that support healthy eating and physical activity. Six communication channels utilized include food service initiatives, classroom activities, school-wide events, home activities, community programs and events, and media events and coverage. A network of public and private organizations is used to promote Team Nutrition, develop and disseminate materials, leverage resources, expand the reach of messages, and build a broad base of support; the network includes private sector companies and nonprofit and advocacy organizations including nutrition, health, education, industry, and entertainment groups.[207]

Team Nutrition has developed resources to help foster healthy school nutrition environments. For example, *Changing the Scene — Improving the School Nutrition Environment* is a tool kit that addresses the entire school nutrition environment from a commitment to nutrition and physical activity, pleasant eating experiences, quality school meals, other healthy food options, nutrition education, and marketing the issue to the public.[208]

School Nutrition Dietary Assessment Study (SNDAS) and SNDAS-II

During the 1991 to 1992 school year, the School Nutrition Dietary Assessment Study (SNDAS) collected information on school meals from a nationally representative sample of schools ($n = 545$) and 24-h recalls from approximately 3350 students from these schools.[209] Results from the SNDAS regarding dietary intakes of NSLP participants and nonparticipants[210] indicated that (1) NSLP participants had higher lunch intakes of vitamin A, calcium, and zinc, and lower intakes of vitamin C than nonparticipants who ate lunch; (2) NSLP participants' lunches provided a higher percentage of kcal from fat and saturated fat, and a lower percentage of carbohydrate than nonparticipants' lunches; (3) NSLP participants were more than twice as likely as nonparticipants to consume milk and milk products at lunch; and (4) NSLP participants also consumed more meat, poultry, fish, and meat mixtures than nonparticipants.

Results from the SNDAS regarding dietary intakes of SBP participants and nonparticipants[210] indicated that (1) SBP participants had higher average breakfast intakes of kcal, protein, and calcium, and derived a greater proportion of kcal from fat and saturated fat than nonparticipants; (2) SBP participants were three times more likely than nonparticipants to consume meat, poultry, fish, or meat mixtures at breakfast; and (3) SBP participants were also more likely than nonparticipants to consume milk or milk products at breakfast. The most surprising finding from the SNDAS was that the presence of the SBP in schools did not affect the likelihood that a student ate breakfast before starting school. Research is needed to determine the best ways to encourage elementary school students to consume healthful breakfasts. Universal school breakfast, which allows all students to eat school breakfast for free, has been advocated by some as a means to increase the percentage of children who eat breakfast. However, results from the SNDAS indicated that approximately 42% of children who were eligible for free or reduced price school breakfast did not eat it.[184] Perhaps scheduling the SBP for classes to eat as a part of regular school hours (similar to the NSLP) is what is needed to increase the percentage of children who eat breakfast.

During the 1998 to 1999 school year, SNDAS-II was conducted to provide information about how schools are progressing toward meeting nutrition standards of the *School Meals Initiative* (SMI) *for Healthy Children* (discussed previously in this chapter), and to provide information about menu planning practices used in school food service programs.[211] Data collection was primarily a mail survey completed by 1075 cafeteria managers who each provided data for meals served during a single week; in addition, a telephone interview was completed by 430 school food service directors, who provided supplementary information about district and school characteristics.[211] Results from SNDAS-II indicated that more than 1 in 5 elementary schools served lunches which met the SMI standard for ≤30% of calories from fat, and about 1 in 7 met the SMI standard for <10% of calories from saturated fat; for secondary schools, about 1 in 7 schools met each of the SMI standards. Even when the average lunch served to (i.e., selected by) students did not meet the SMI standards for fat and saturated fat, 82% of elementary schools and 91% of secondary schools offered options that were consistent with these SMI standards. Lunches served in elementary and secondary schools provided more than a third of the recommended levels for all targeted nutrients, except in secondary schools where they fell short of providing one third of the recommended level for calories. Breakfasts served were consistent with the SMI standard for calories from fat, and came very close to meeting the SMI standard for calories from saturated fat. Breakfasts served in both elementary and secondary schools provided one-fourth or more of the recommended levels for all targeted nutrients, but fell short of providing one-fourth of the recommended level of calories.[212] Results from SNDAS-II confirm the important role that school meals have towards helping youth achieve nutritional recommendations, and that more research is needed to determine how to encourage more youth to actually select the healthful options available in schools.

FEEDING CHILDREN AND ADOLESCENTS IN ELEMENTARY, MIDDLE, AND HIGH SCHOOLS

Research with upper elementary school children indicates that they prefer vegetables less than fruits.[92,213,214] Results from studies in the mid-1990s that conducted focus groups with ~600 fourth and fifth graders from Georgia, Alabama, and Minnesota indicate that children predominantly believe that vegetables taste "*nasty*"[214] and "*if it's good for you, then it must taste bad,*"[213,214] *which are related to statements made by adults such as "I don't care if they don't taste good; eat your vegetables because they're good for you."*[214] Research concerning the influence of a variety of psychological and social factors on children's fruit and vegetable consumption indicates that preferences are the strongest predictors.[93,215] This suggests that interventions that alter children's preferences for fruits and vegetables may be more effective in increasing their consumption than other strategies pursued to date. However, intensive, school-based interventions designed to specifically increase children's *preferences* for fruits and vegetables have had limited success.[79,216,217] Furthermore, although some elementary school programs have helped children to improve their dietary intake,[218] intensive interventions specifically designed to increase children's *consumption* of fruits and vegetables have had only limited success.[79,117,216,217,219–221] Changes in fruit consumption were better than changes in vegetable consumption in several of these studies,[79,117,220] which suggests that future interventions should focus solely on vegetables. Finally, schools may represent a potentially useful setting for preventing childhood obesity, but comprehensive elementary school programs in the United States such as CATCH and Know Your Body have not had major effects on children's body weight.[199,218,222]

School breakfast and lunch menus typically follow a cycle that repeats several times during the school year; thus, youth are provided with repeated exposures to healthful foods (e.g., fruits and vegetables).[223] However, schools also provide youth with repeated exposures to other foods (e.g., candy and pizza) which are used by school staff as rewards.[224] Unfortunately, some of the social contexts in which vegetables are available at school (e.g., "*If you eat your peas, then you can eat your cookie*") probably negatively affects preferences for them, thereby potentially decreasing their consumption.[223] In contrast, the social context in which candy and pizza are offered probably positively affects preferences for them, thereby potentially increasing their consumption.[223] These repeated exposures to vegetables and foods such as candy and pizza in negative and positive social contexts, respectively, may enhance the associative learning that help youth develop food consumption patterns that are inconsistent with nutrition guidelines[89] which recommend increased intake of vegetables but decreased sugar and fat intake. In addition, school staff may encourage youth to finish all of their food, regardless of whether or not they are still hungry,[225] which encourages them to disregard their own feelings of hunger and satiety.

Nevertheless, research also indicates the positive role schools can have in promoting healthful dietary intake by youth. For example, a 1997 study by Baranowski et al.[226] indicated the important contribution that school lunch makes in increasing children's consumption of fruits and vegetables. Differences in children's consumption of fruits and vegetables by meal and day of the week were assessed using 7-day food records completed by third graders (*n* = 2984) from 48 elementary schools in the Atlanta, Georgia area. Fruits and vegetables were most frequently consumed at weekday lunch, and participation in school lunch accounted for a substantial proportion of fruits and vegetables consumed at lunch. Few fruits and vegetables were consumed at breakfast or snack.[226]

Verbal encouragement by school food service staff during school lunch was associated with increased total fruit intake by children during school lunch according to process measures obtained during the elementary school cafeteria-based intervention in a 2004 study by Perry et al.[117] mentioned previously (see Table 16.22). Perry et al. concluded that school food service staff should be encouraged to play an active role in promoting fruit and vegetable consumption among children during lunch.[117]

The perceptions that adolescents have about school food service and nutrition programs were assessed in a 2000 study that surveyed 2566 adolescents in grades 6 through 8 (which covers ages 10 to 15 years).[227] Results indicated that the top predictors of satisfaction were school menus which include food that students like, quality of the food choices, and prices that are acceptable for what students get. Girls were more satisfied with school-prepared foods than boys, perhaps, because girls mature faster than boys during these years, which may be reflected as willingness to try new foods at an earlier age. Sixth-grade students were more satisfied than either seventh- or eighth-grade students. This may be because as adolescents move into the early teenage years, they become more independent from their parents and begin making their own decisions instead of eating school meals because their parents want or expect them to do so.[227]

In a 2002 study, a survey completed by 235 food service staff members from 16 high schools in Minneapolis/St. Paul and observations of 210 staff–student interactions, indicated that food service staff members could play an important role in encouraging healthful food choices by high-school students during school meals.[228] Although the majority of food service staff members indicated they were comfortable giving recommendations to students about which foods to purchase, only about one-fourth believed their suggestions were influential with students. Observations of staff–student interactions indicated that none of the staff spontaneously made food product recommendations to students to purchase. Only 16 students (8%) asked for a recommendation about their purchase; in each case, the staff person recommended a product, and the student purchased the product recommended by the staff person in 15 of these 16 interactions. The authors concluded that food service staff could be trained to encourage students to make healthful food choices at the point of purchase and thus enhance the dietary intake of adolescents.[228]

The effects of pricing strategies on sales of fruits and vegetables with adolescents in two high schools (1431 students at an urban school and 1935 students at a suburban school) were examined in a 1997 study by French et al.[229] Fruit, carrot, and salad purchases were monitored in each school cafeteria during an initial baseline period. Next, prices for these items were reduced by 50%, and sales were monitored. Finally, prices were returned to baseline, and sales were monitored for an additional 3 weeks. Results indicated that even though promotion was minimal, lower pricing significantly increased sales for fruit and carrots but not salads among high-school students. However, the magnitude of the intervention effects differed by school, which suggests that contextual factors (e.g., packaging, display) may modify pricing effects. These results imply that adolescents can be encouraged to select fruits and vegetables when the prices of these items are lowered, and that this may occur without measurable changes in the overall a la carte sales revenue or the number of meal pattern customers, which are both important considerations for school food service operations.[229]

The effects of pricing and promotion strategies on purchases of low-fat snacks from 55 vending machines in 12 secondary schools and 12 diverse worksites were examined in a 2001 study by French et al.[230] Low-fat snacks were added to vending machines, and four pricing levels (equal price, 10% price decrease, 25% price decrease, 50% price decrease) were crossed with three promotional conditions (none, low-fat label, low-fat label plus promotional sign). Throughout the 12-month intervention, sales of low-fat vending snacks were measured continuously. Results indicated that significant increases in low-fat snack sales by 9, 39, and 93% were associated with price reductions on low-fat snacks of 10, 25, and 50%, respectively, at both worksites and secondary schools. Promotional condition was independently but weakly associated with increases in low-fat snack sales. Average profits per vending machine were not affected by the intervention. These results indicate that lowering prices is a very effective method for promoting lower-fat snack purchases from vending machines in both adolescent and adult populations.[230]

LOCAL WELLNESS POLICIES IN SCHOOL DISTRICTS

Concern about food rewards as well as issues regarding competitive foods, vending machines, "pouring rights" issues, scheduling of meals and recess, time allowed for meals, and physical education programs, along with growing concern about childhood obesity have increased momentum for addressing school-based nutrition issues legislatively.[231] Congress now requires each local education agency participating in USDA Child Nutrition Programs to develop local wellness policies beginning in the 2006 to 2007 school year.[231] The USDA has reviewed and compiled web-based resources to help schools and communities develop and implement local wellness policies that promote healthy eating and physical activity; the USDA's local wellness policy website was placed on the Team Nutrition website (http://teamnutrition.usda.gov/Healthy/wellnesspolicy.html).[231,232] The dietary recommendations for children and adolescents from the American Heart Association and the American Academy of Pediatrics summarizes some strategies being implemented in many schools, as well as types of legislation under consideration to improve children's nutrition.[15,16]

The position of the American Dietetic Association is that "Educational goals, including the nutrition goals of the National School Lunch Program and School Breakfast Program, should be supported and extended through school district wellness policies that create overall school environments that promote access to healthful school meals and physical activity and provide learning experiences that enable students to develop lifelong healthful eating habits."[231] That position statement includes a summary of selected resources for changing school nutrition environments as well as a sample of web-based resources to help with developing local wellness policies.[231]

The joint position of the American Dietetic Association, Society for Nutrition Education, and the American School Food Service Association is that *"comprehensive nutrition services must be provided to all of the nation's preschool through twelfth-grade students. These nutrition services shall be integrated with a coordinated, comprehensive school health program and implemented through a school nutrition policy. The policy should link comprehensive sequential nutrition education; access to and promotion of child nutrition programs providing nutritious meals and snacks in the school environment; and family, community, and health services' partnerships supporting positive health outcomes for all children."*[233] According to the Centers for Disease Control and Prevention 1996 document titled *"Guidelines for School Health Programs to Promote Lifelong Healthy Eating,"*[198] students need exposure to healthful foods as well as the support of people around them, and teachers need to be discouraged from using food for disciplining or rewarding students.

In 2004, the American Academy of Pediatrics Committee on Nutrition issued a policy statement about nutrition concerns regarding soft drink consumption in schools.[234] Potential health problems associated with high intake of soft drinks include overweight or obesity because of the additional calories, displacement of milk consumption which results in calcium deficiency with an increased risk of osteoporosis and fractures, and dental caries and enamel erosion.[234]

CHILD AND ADOLESCENT TRIAL FOR CARDIOVASCULAR HEALTH (CATCH)

CATCH was a four-center, randomized field trial that evaluated the effectiveness of a school-based cardiovascular health promotion program.[235] A total of 5106 ethnically diverse students (who were third graders at baseline in the fall of 1991 and fifth graders at the end of the intervention in the spring of 1994) participated in 56 intervention and 40 control public schools in California, Louisiana, Minnesota, and Texas. Of the 56 intervention schools, 28 schools participated in a third-through-fifth-grade intervention, which included school food service modifications, enhanced physical education, and classroom health curricula; the other 28 schools received these components plus family education. Results at the end of the 3-year intervention indicated that the percentage of energy from fat in intervention school lunches fell significantly more (from 39 to 32%) than in control school lunches (from 39 to 36%) ($p < .001$). The intensity of physical activity in physical education classes increased significantly in intervention schools compared with control schools ($p < .02$). The percentage of energy from fat from 24-h recalls among intervention school students was significantly reduced (from 33 to 30%) compared with that among control school students (from 33% to 32%) ($p < .001$). Intervention students reported significantly more daily vigorous activity than controls (59 min vs. 47 min, $p < .003$). However, no significant differences were detected in blood pressure, body size, and cholesterol measures for students at the intervention schools compared to those at the control schools.[160]

A 3-year follow-up was conducted with 3714 students (73%) of the initial CATCH cohort of 5106 students.[236] End-point comparisons were made between students from intervention and control schools to determine whether changes at the end of intervention in grade five were maintained through grade eight. Results for eighth graders indicated that self-reported daily energy intake from fat remained lower for intervention than control students (31 vs. 32%, $p = .01$). Intervention students maintained significantly higher daily vigorous physical activity than controls ($p = .001$), although differences narrowed over time. Significant differences in favor of intervention students persisted at grade eight for dietary knowledge and dietary intentions, but not for social support for physical activity. No significant differences were noted for BMI, blood pressure, or serum lipid and cholesterol levels. In summary, follow-up of the CATCH cohort suggests that behavior changes from the intervention were sufficient to produce effects detectable 3 years later. However, differences between the intervention and control groups were narrowing in magnitude over time. Additional research is needed to determine how best to maintain the intervention effects long-term.[236]

A previous section titled "Trends in Consumption among Children and Adolescents" in this chapter provided results from longitudinal data on selected nutrient intake for a cohort of third, fifth, and eighth graders in CATCH.[51] Those results suggest that the diets of youth change over time, with negative trends more common in girls and in African American students.[51]

The CATCH Institutionalization Study provided insight into maintenance of CATCH school-level goals regarding the amount of total and saturated fat in school lunches 5 years post-intervention in former intervention schools ($n = 56$) and comparison schools ($n = 20$); 12 new schools with no exposure to CATCH during the previous 5 years served as controls.[237] Assessment of 5 consecutive days of school lunch menus from Spring 1999 indicated that the guideline for total fat ($\leq 30\%$ of energy) was met by 50% of former intervention schools compared to 10% of former comparison schools and 17% of unexposed control schools ($p < .005$). However, there were no significant differences in the percentage of schools meeting the guideline for saturated fat ($\leq 10\%$ of energy) with 45% of former intervention schools compared to 30% of former comparison schools and 17% of unexposed control schools ($p = 0.11$), and none of the schools met the guideline for sodium (≤ 1000 mg). The authors commented that the maintenance effect for total fat was probably due in part to policy changes from the SMI (discussed previously in this chapter) that occurred at the end of CATCH. Participation in the full CATCH program appeared to ensure that schools had trained food service staff who were better prepared to comply with federal standards for school meals.[237]

HEALTH PROMOTION AND DISEASE PREVENTION

HEALTHY PEOPLE 2010 NUTRITION OBJECTIVES FOR CHILDREN AND ADOLESCENTS

Table 16.25 includes Healthy People 2010[238] nutrition objectives, as well as dental objectives related to nutrition, for children and adolescents, along with progress reviews[239] available for these objectives. The nutrition objectives address reducing weight, reducing growth retardation, improving eating behavior (e.g., increasing consumption of fruit, vegetables, grain products, and calcium products; decreasing consumption of fat, saturated fat, and sodium), reducing iron deficiency, and improving meals

TABLE 16.25
Healthy People 2010 Nutrition Objectives for Children and Adolescents with Progress Review

		Baseline 1988 to 1994	Progress Review 1999 to 2000	Target 2010
19-3	Reduce the proportion of children and adolescents who are overweight or obese. Reduction in overweight or obese children and adolescents[a] Children and adolescents age			
19-3a	6 to 11 years	11%	15%	5%
19-3b	12 to 19 years	11%	16%	5%
19-3c	6 to 19 years	11%	15%	5%
19-4	Reduce growth retardation (defined as height-for age below the 5th percentile in the age–sex appropriate population) among low-income children under age 5 years.[b]	6% (in 1997)	6% (in 2002)	5%
19-5	Increase the proportion of persons aged 2 years and older who consume at least two daily servings of fruit. [c]	28% (in 1994 to 1996)	—	75%
19-5(1)[c]	Fruit intake — average number of daily servings (age adjusted, ages 2 years and older).	1.6 (in 1994 to 1996)	1.5	NA
19-6	Increase the proportion of persons aged 2 years and older who consume at least three daily servings of vegetables, with at least 1/3 being dark green or orange vegetables.[d]	3 (in 1994 to 1996)	—	50
19-6(1a)[c]	Vegetable intake — proportion who consume ≥ 3 daily servings (age adjusted, ages 2 year and over)	49 (in 1994 to 1996)	—	—
19-6(1b)[c]	Vegetable intake — proportion who consume 1/3 or more servings from dark green or orange vegetables (age adjusted, ages 2 year and over)	8 (in 1994 to 1996)	—	—
19-6(2a)[c]	Vegetable intake — average number of daily servings (age adjusted, ages 2 years and over).	3.4 (in 1994 to 1996)	3.3	—
19-6(2b)[c]	Vegetable intake — average number of daily servings that are dark green or orange vegetables.	0.3 (in 1994 to 1996)	0.3	—
19-7	Increase the proportion of persons aged 2 years and older who consume at least six daily servings of grain products, with at least being whole grains.[d]	7% (in 1994 to 1996)	—	50%
19-7(1a)[c]	Grain intake — proportion who consume ≥ 6 daily servings (age adjusted, ages 2 years and over)	51% (in 1994 to 1996)	—	—
19-7(1b)[c]	Grain intake — proportion who consume ≥ 3 daily whole grain servings (age adjusted, ages 2 years and over)	7% (in 1994 to 1996)	—	—
19-7(2a)[c]	Grain intake — average number of daily servings (age adjusted, ages 2 years and over).	6.8 (in 1994 to 1996)	6.8	—
19-7(2b)[c]	Grain intake — average number of daily whole grain servings (age adjusted, ages 2 years and over).	1.0 (in 1994 to 1996)	0.9	—
19-8	Increase the proportion of persons aged 2 year and older who consume < 10% of calories from saturated fat.[d]	36% (in 1994 to 1996)	—	75%
19-8(1)[c]	Saturated fat intake — average percent of calories from saturated fat.	11% (in 1994 to 1996)	11%	—
19-9	Increase the proportion of persons aged 2 year and older who consume ≤30% of calories from total fat.[d]	33% (in 1994 to 1996)	—	75%
19-9(1)[a]	Total fat intake — average percent of calories from total fat.	33% (in 1994 to 1996)	33%	—

Continued

TABLE 16.25
(Continued)

		Baseline 1988 to 1994	Progress Review 1999 to 2000	Target 2010
19-10	Increase the proportion of persons aged 2 years and older who consume ≤2,400 mg of sodium daily.[d]			
		21%	—	65%
19-10(1)[c]	Total sodium intake — average daily intake, mg (age adjusted, ages 2 years and over).			
		—	3,574 (in 2000)	—
19-11	Increase the proportion of persons aged 2 years and older who meet dietary recommendation for calcium. [d,e]			
		45%	—	75%
19-12	Reduce iron deficiency among young children and females of childbearing age. Reduction in iron deficiency[f]			
19-12a	Children aged 1 to 2 years	9%	7%	5%
19-12b	Children aged 3 to 4 years	4%	DSU	1%
19-12c	Nonpregnant females aged 12 to 49 years	11%	12%	7%
19-15	(Developmental) Increase the proportion of children and adolescents aged 6 to 19 years whose intake of meals and snacks at school contributes proportionally to good overall dietary quality.			
21-1	Reduce the proportion of children and adolescents who have dental caries experience in their primary or permanent teeth. Dental Carries Experience			
21-1a	Young children (aged 2 to 4 years), primary teeth	18%	23%	11%
21-1b	Children (age 6 to 8 years), primary and permanent teeth	52%	50%	42%
21-1c	Adolescent (age 15 years), permanent teeth	61%	59%	51%
21-2	Reduce the proportion of children and adolescents with untreated dental decay. Untreated Dental Decay			
21-2a	Young children (ages 2 to 4 years), primary teeth	16%	20%	9%
21-2b	Children (ages 6 to 8 years), primary and permanent teeth[g]	28%	26%	21%
21-2c	Adolescent (ages 15 years), permanent teeth	20%	16%	15%
21-13	(Developmental) Increase the proportion of school-based health centers with an oral health component.			

Notes:

— means data are not available for progress review.

DSU means data do not meet the criteria for statistical reliability, data quality, or confidentiality.

[a] Defined as at or above the sex- and age-specific 95th percentile of BMI based on the revised CDC Growth Charts for the United States.

[b] Baseline has been revised according to the 2000 CDC Growth Chart.

[c] Objective measures with numbers in parentheses show supplemental data that were either included in the reporting of the baseline estimates or were recommended by an interagency group.

[d] The reporting of update estimates for Healthy People 2010 objectives 19-5 through 19-11 is pending the availability of additional days of dietary data from NHANES. However, mean intake estimates are shown as supplemental data for these objectives using 1-day diet recall data.

[e] Baseline has been revised according to a new algorithm on the contribution of antacids to total calcium intake.

[f] Defined as having abnormal results for two or more of the following tests: serum ferritin concentration, erythrocyte protoporphyrin, or transferrin saturation.

[g] Baseline has been revised.

Source: Adapted from: U.S. Department of Health and Human Services, *Healthy People 2010,* 2nd edition., With Understanding and Improving Health and Objectives for Improving Health, 2 vols, Washington, DC: U.S. Government Printing Office, November, 2000, available online at http://www.health.gov/healthypeople (accessed March 25, 2006); U.S. Department of Health and Human Services, Healthy People 2010 Progress Review: Nutrition and Overweight, January, 2004, available online at http://www.healthypeople.gov/Data/2010prog/focus19/Nutrition_Overweight.pdf and www.cdc.gov/nchs/about/otheract/hpdata2010/focusareas/fa19-nutrition.htm (accessed March 12, 2006); and U.S. Department of Health and Human Services, Healthy People 2010 Progress Review: Oral Health, March, 2004, available online at http://www.healthypeople.gov/Data/2010prog/focus21/OralHealthPR.pdf and www.cdc.gov/nchs/about/otheract/hpdata2010/focusareas/fa21-oral.htm (accessed March 12, 2006).

and snacks at school. The dental objectives that are related to nutrition address dental caries, untreated dental decay, and school-based health centers with an oral health component. The progress reviews provide a venue for Federal agencies to report progress towards achieving the Healthy People 2010 goals and objectives for each of the 28 focus areas; two rounds of reviews are planned for the decade for each of the focus areas, with the first one held in June, 2002 and others following, usually in alphabetical order.[239] The first progress review for nutrition and overweight (focus area 19) was held in January 2004.[240] The first progress review for oral health (focus area 21) was held in March 2004.[241] As indicated in Table 16.25, the progress reviews for nutrition and overweight, as well as for oral health, indicate that considerable work will be needed to achieve the Healthy People 2010 objectives.

5-A DAY FOR BETTER HEALTH PROGRAM

The *5-A Day for Better Health* program was instituted in 1991 to encourage Americans to eat five or more servings of fruits and vegetables every day. It originated as a public-private partnership between the National Cancer Institute (NCI) and the Produce for Better Health Foundation (which is a nonprofit foundation representing the fruit and vegetable industry), and included retail, media, community, and research components.[242] At the beginning of the program in 1991, a baseline survey with adults indicated that only 23% reported consuming five or more daily servings of fruits and vegetables.[243] The NCI funded nine studies in the spring of 1993 to develop, implement, and evaluate interventions in specific community channels to increase the consumption of fruits and vegetables in specific target populations; four of the nine projects used school-based programs to target children or adolescents.[244] Of these four projects, one targeted fourth graders and their parents,[221] two targeted fourth and fifth graders,[216,220] and one targeted high-school students.[219] Although all four interventions increased daily consumption of fruits and vegetables, the increases were small for three interventions and ranged from 0.2 servings for "*Gimme 5 Fruit, Juice, and Vegetables for Fun and Health*" in Georgia,[216] 0.4 servings for "*Gimme 5: A Fresh Nutrition Concept for Students*" in New Orleans,[219] and 0.6 servings for "5 A Day Power Plus" in Minnesota.[220] Increases were larger at 1.4 servings for "High Five" in Alabama, possibly because classroom lessons were delivered by trained curriculum coordinators instead of classroom teachers.[221]

In 2000, the *5 A Day for Better Health* program went under review by the NCI.[245] In response to recommendations in the Evaluation Report that resulted from this review, the National 5 A Day Partnership was established in 2001 to guide the 5 A Day program into the future with an expanded base of health-oriented government agencies, businesses, and nonprofits willing to commit significant resources to the 5 A Day effort. The *5 A Day for Better Health* program is the nation's largest public–private nutrition education initiative with 5 A Day coordinators in each state, territory, and the military. The goal of the partnership is to increase fruit and vegetable consumption to five servings a day for 75% of Americans by 2010. The partnership's steering committee is chaired by the president of the Produce for Better Health Foundation and includes representatives from the NCI, USDA, Centers for Disease Control and Prevention, American Cancer Society, Produce Marketing Association, United Fresh Fruit and Vegetable Association, National Alliance for Nutrition and Activity, Directors of Health Promotion and Education, American Heart Association, and Council of 5 A Day Coordinators.[245] More information is available at www.5aday.org.

3-A-DAY OF DAIRY

The *3-A-Day of Dairy* campaign was launched in January 2003 to help make people aware of the health benefits of including three servings of dairy in their daily diet.[246] The nutrition-based marketing and consumer education campaign is managed by the American Dairy Association/National Dairy Council, with monetary support from the dairy industry and professional support from the American Academy of Family Physicians, American Academy of Pediatrics, American Dietetic Association, and the National Medical Association.[247] The 3-A-Day logo may be found on packages of milk, cheese, and yogurt to indicate they are excellent sources of calcium.[246] More information is available at www.3aday.org.

FOOD SAFETY

The *2005 Dietary Guidelines for Americans* include a focus area regarding food safety, because it is estimated that about 76 million people in the United States each year become ill from pathogens in food.[14] Furthermore, a key recommendation in the food safety focus area is that young children (as well as infants, pregnant women, older adults, and people who are immunocompromised) avoid eating or drinking raw or partially cooked eggs or foods containing raw eggs; raw (unpasteurized) milk or any products made from unpasteurized milk; unpasteurized juices; raw or undercooked meat, poultry, fish, or shellfish; and raw sprouts.[14] Food safety messages are woven into appropriate sections of the consumer materials developed for *MyPyramid*.[170]

Fight Bac!® is a food safety education campaign of the Partnership for Food Safety Education that combines resources of the federal government, industry, and consumer organizations to conduct broad-based food safety education.[248] The multi-faceted Fight Bac!® campaign has materials for educators, the media, and consumers. The goal of Fight Bac!® is to educate consumers about four simple steps (clean, separate, cook, and chill) to take to fight foodborne bacteria and reduce the risk of foodborne illnesses.[248] Table 16.26 provides details regarding these four steps.

Children, adolescents, and adults of all ages need to understand the important role they play in decreasing the incidence of foodborne illnesses through proper hand-washing as well as safe food preparation and storage. According to the Hospitality Institute of Technology and Management,[249,250] hands should be washed with soap, a fingernail brush with soft bristles, and a large volume of flowing water to ensure adequate removal of pathogenic microorganisms (e.g., those from fecal sources) from fingertips and under fingernails. Fingernails should be neatly trimmed to less than 1/16 in. to make them easier to clean.

TABLE 16.26
Details Regarding the Four Steps of the Fight Bac!® Campaign

Clean: Wash hands and surfaces often
- Wash hands with hot soapy water before preparing food
- Wash hands with hot soapy water after using the bathroom, changing diapers, and touching animals
- For best results, use warm water to moisten hands and then apply soap; rub hands together for 20 s before rinsing thoroughly
- Wash dishes, utensils, cutting boards, and countertops in hot soapy water after preparing each food item and before preparing the next food item
- Use plastic or other nonporous cutting boards. Always wash cutting boards in the dishwasher or with hot soapy water after use
- Use paper towels to dry hands and clean kitchen surfaces. If cloth towels are used, wash them often in the hot cycle of the washing machine

Separate: Do not cross-contaminate
- Keep raw meat, poultry, and seafood separate from other foods in grocery carts when shopping, and grocery bags when bringing food home
- In the refrigerator, store raw meat, poultry, and seafood in sealed containers or plastic bags to prevent juices from dripping onto other foods
- Use one cutting board for raw meats and another cutting board for salads and other foods ready to be eaten
- Wash hands, cutting boards, dishes, and utensils with hot soapy water after they come in contact with raw meat, poultry, or seafood
- Do not place cooked food on a plate or serving dish that previously held raw meat, poultry, or seafood
- Sauce used to marinate raw meat, poultry, or seafood should not be used on cooked foods unless it is boiled before applying

Cook: Cook to proper temperatures
- Use a meat thermometer to measure the internal temperature of cooked meat and poultry to make sure the meat is cooked all the way through
- Cook roasts and steaks to at least 145° F (62.7°C); cook whole poultry to 180° F (82.2°C)
- Cook ground meat to at least 160° F (71.1°C). Do not eat ground beef that is still pink inside
- Cook eggs until the white and yolk are firm, not runny
- Do not use recipes or eat foods in which eggs remain raw or only partially cooked
- Cook fish until it is opaque and flakes easily with a fork
- When microwaving foods, make sure there are no cold spots by stirring and rotating food for even heating
- Reheat sauce, soup, and gravy to a boil. Heat other leftovers thoroughly to at least 165° F (73.8°C)

Chill: Refrigerate properly and promptly
- Use a refrigerator thermometer to be sure the temperature is consistently 40° F (4.4°C) or below
- Refrigerate or freeze prepared foods, perishables, and leftovers within 2 h or sooner of purchase or use
- Defrost food in the refrigerator, in an airtight package in cold water, or in the microwave, but never at room temperature
- Marinate foods in the refrigerator
- Divide large amounts of leftovers into small, shallow containers for quick cooling in the refrigerator
- Avoid packing the refrigerator because cold air must circulate to keep food safe

Source: Adapted from *Fight Bac!®* Partnership for Food Safety Education, www.fightbac.org (accessed on March 5, 2006).

When working with food, hand washing without the fingernail brush is sufficient, because the pathogen count is much lower. Table 16.27 describes the double and single methods of hand washing. Although young children may be encouraged to wash their hands long enough for them to sing their "A, B, Cs" slowly, the amount of lathering and the volume of water used to wash off the lathering appear to be more important than the length of time spent washing or the temperature of the water.[249,250]

DENTAL HEALTH

Nutrition is an integral component of oral health.[251] Nutrition and diet may affect the development and progression of diseases of the oral cavity. Likewise, oral infectious diseases, and acute, chronic, and terminal systemic diseases with oral manifestations, affect ability to eat and diet and nutritional status. When determining the cariogenic, cariostatic, and anticariogenic properties of the diet, the primary factors to be considered include the form of the food (liquid, solid or sticky, long-lasting), frequency of consumption of sugar and other fermentable carbohydrates, potential to stimulate saliva, nutrient composition, sequence of food intake, and combinations of foods.[251] One of the key recommendations regarding the focus area for carbohydrates in the *2005 Dietary Guidelines for Americans* is to "*reduce the incidence of dental caries by practicing good oral hygiene and consuming sugar- and starch-containing foods and beverages less frequently.*"[14] In 2005, the American Dietetic Association reaffirmed that "*fluoride is an important element for all mineralized tissues in the body. Appropriate fluoride exposure and usage is beneficial to bone and tooth integrity and, as such, has an important, positive impact on health throughout life.*"[252]

Because children of all ages eat frequently, snacks should emphasize foods that are low in sucrose, are not sticky, and that stimulate saliva flow, which helps limit acid production in the mouth.[253] Protein foods such as nuts and cheese may provide nutritional and dental benefits, because some protein foods are thought to have a protective effect against caries. When desserts are consumed, it is best if they are eaten with meals. Fruits, juices, and most bread/cereal products contain fermentable carbohydrate, so try to limit these foods to one serving in a snack, and other servings eaten with meals. Chewing sugarless gum after snacks containing

TABLE 16.27
Two Methods of Hand Washing

Double Wash Procedure (to be used to remove fecal pathogens and other pathogenic microorganisms from skin surfaces when entering the kitchen, after using the toilet, after cleaning up vomitus or fecal material, or after touching sores or bandages):

First wash using the fingernail brush:
- Turn on water so it flows rapidly at 2 gallons/min. (Flowing water, not the temperature of the water, removes the pathogens.) Place hands, lower arms, and fingernail brush under flowing water and thoroughly wet them
- Apply half to one teaspoon of hand soap or detergent (enough to produce a good lather) to fingernail brush
- Brush and lather hand surfaces gently with tips of bristles on fingernail brush under flowing water, especially fingertips and around and under fingernails. (Gently brush means without bending the bristles.) Build a good lather
- Continue to use fingernail brush under water until there is no more soapy lather on hands, lower arms, or nail brush. This takes about 10 s. Hazardous microorganisms in the lather are only removed to a safe level when all the soap is rinsed off the hands, arms, and fingertips with flowing water
- Place nailbrush on holder with bristles up so bristles can dry

Second wash without the nailbrush (~10 s required to complete):
- Apply half to one teaspoon of hand soap or detergent (enough to produce a good lather) to hands
- Under flowing water, massage the hands, fingertips, between the fingers, and lower arms to produce a good lather
- After lathering, rinse all of lather from hands, fingertips, hands, and lower arms in flowing water. This takes about 10 s. The volume of water used for rinsing hands, not the time of the wash or temperature of the water, is the critical factor
- Thoroughly dry hands and arms using disposable paper towels. Discard paper towels in waste container without touching container

Single Wash Procedure (to be used to remove normal low levels of pathogens before and after eating and drinking; after handling garbage; after handling dirty dishes or utensils; between handling raw and cooked foods; after blowing or wiping nose; after touching skin, hair, or soiled clothes; and as often as necessary to keep hands clean after they become soiled):
- Turn on water so it flows rapidly at 2 gallons/min. Place hands and lower arms under flowing water and thoroughly wet them
- Follow directions above for "Second wash without the nailbrush"

Source: Adapted from Snyder, O P, Hospitality Institute of Technology and Management, 1998, http://www.hi-tm.com/Documents/Safehands.html (accessed March 5, 2006) and http://www.hi-tm.com/Documents/handflow-PDF.pdf 2005 edition (accessed March 5, 2006).

---

fermentable carbohydrate may benefit school-age children and adolescents. The efforts of dietary control are complemented by good oral hygiene. A fluoride supplement is recommended into the teen years if the water supply is not fluoridated.[253]

Early childhood caries (ECC), previously referred to as baby bottle tooth decay or maxillary anterior caries, is the major nutrition-related dental disease found in young children; ECC is defined as rampant dental caries in infants and toddlers.[251] The risk of ECC is increased by a combination of infant/child feeding practices and repeated sequential consumption of fermentable carbohydrates.[251] The primary cause of ECC is prolonged exposure of the teeth to a sweetened liquid such as milk, formula, juice, soft drinks, or other sweetened drinks.[253] This often occurs when a child is routinely given a bottle at bedtime or naptime; the liquid pools around the teeth during sleep, saliva flow decreases, and the child may continue to suck liquid over an extended period of time. Toddlers are also at high risk if they hold their own bottles or sippy cups and have access to them throughout the day. The primary strategy to prevent ECC is education. Parents and childcare providers should be encouraged to avoid putting infants or young children to sleep with bottles, and to use regular cups to offer juices and liquids other than breastmilk or formula.[253] Chapter 59 provides additional information regarding the prevention of dental caries in children and adolescents.

ACKNOWLEDGMENTS

Grateful appreciation is expressed to Julie A. Royer, MSPH (for helping to prepare the text and tables, managing citations, and obtaining references), Caroline H. Guinn, RD (for helpful feedback provided on an earlier version of this chapter), and Christina M. Devlin, RD (for helping to prepare several tables).

REFERENCES

1. Institute of Medicine, *Dietary Reference Intakes for Energy, Carbohydrate, Fiber, Fat, Fatty Acids, Cholesterol, Protein, and Amino Acids*, National Academies Press, Washington, DC, 2002/2005. Available online at www.nap.edu.
2. Food and Nutrition Board and National Research Council, *Recommended Dietary Allowances*, 10th edition., National Academy Press, Washington, DC, 1989.
3. Institute of Medicine, *Dietary Reference Intakes for Calcium, Phosphorus, Magnesium, Vitamin D, and Fluoride*, National Academy Press, Washington, DC, 1997. Available online at www.nap.edu.

4. Institute of Medicine, *Dietary Reference Intakes for Thiamin, Riboflavin, Niacin, Vitamin B$_6$, Folate, Vitamin B$_{12}$, Pantothenic Acid, Biotin, and Choline*, National Academy Press, Washington, DC, 1998. Available online at www.nap.edu.

5. Institute of Medicine, *Dietary Reference Intakes: Proposed Definition Plan for Review of Dietary Antioxidants and Related Compounds*, National Academy Press, Washington, DC, 1998. Available online at www.nap.edu.

6. Institute of Medicine, *Dietary Reference Intakes: A Risk Assessment Model Establishing Upper Intake Levels for Nutrients*, National Academy Press, Washington, DC, 1998. Available online at www.nap.edu.

7. Institute of Medicine, *Dietary Reference Intakes for Vitamin C, Vitamin E, Selenium, and Carotenoids*, National Academy Press, Washington, DC, 2000. Available online at www.nap.edu.

8. Institute of Medicine, *Dietary Reference Intakes: Applications in Dietary Assessment*, National Academy Press, Washington, DC, 2000. Available online at www.nap.edu.

9. Institute of Medicine, *Dietary Reference Intakes for Vitamin A, Vitamin K, Arsenic, Boron, Chromium, Copper, Iodine, Iron, Manganese, Molybdenum, Nickel, Silicon, Vanadium, and Zinc*, National Academy Press, Washington, DC, 2001. Available online at www.nap.edu.

10. Institute of Medicine, *Dietary Reference Intakes: Proposed Definition of Dietary Fiber*, National Academy Press, Washington, DC, 2001. Available online at www.nap.edu.

11. Institute of Medicine, *Dietary Reference Intakes: Guiding Principles for Nutrition Labeling and Fortification*, National Academies Press, Washington, DC, 2003. Available online at www.nap.edu.

12. Institute of Medicine, *Dietary Reference Intakes: Applications in Dietary Planning*, 2003. Nat. Gcad. Press Washington DC. available online at. www.map. edu

13. Institute of Medicine, Dietary Reference Intakes for Water, Potassium, Sodium, Chloride, and Sulfate, National Academies Press, Washington, DC, 2005. Available online at www.nap.edu.

14. U.S. Department of Health and Human Services and U.S. Department of Agriculture, Dietary Guidelines for Americans, 2005. 6th edition, Washington, DC, U.S. Government Printing Office, 2005. Available online at www.healthierus.gov/dietaryguidelines. (accessed January 19, 2006).

15. American Heart Association, et al., *Pediatrics*, 117: 544; 2006.

16. Gidding, S.S. et al., *Circulation*, 112: 2061; 2005.

17. Kris-Etherton, P.M. et al., *Circulation*, 106: 2747; 2002.

18. Williams, C.L., Bollella, M., and Wynder, E.L., *Pediatrics*, 96: 985; 1995.

19. Williams, C.L., *JADA*, 95: 1140; 1995.

20. American Academy of Pediatrics, *Pediatrics*, 96: 1023; 1995.

21. Dwyer, J.T., *Pediatrics*, 96: 1019; 1995.

22. Williams, C.L. and Bollella, M., *Pediatrics*, 96: 1014; 1995.

23. American Academy of Pediatrics (Committee on Nutrition), Carbohydrate and Dietary Fiber, in Pediatric Nutrition Handbook, 5th edition, Kleinman, R.E., Ed., American Academy of Pediatrics, Elk Grove Village, IL, 2004, 247.

24. American Academy of Pediatrics (Committee on Nutrition), *Pediatrics*, 86: 643; 1990 (reaffirmed 4/00).

25. Greer, F.R., Krebs, N.F., and Committee on Nutrition, *Pediatrics*, 117: 578; 2006.

26. American Academy of Pediatrics (Committee on Nutrition), Iron Deficiency, in Pediatric Nutrition Handbook, 5th edition, Kleinman, R.E., Ed., American Academy of Pediatrics, Elk Grove Village, IL, 2004, 299.

27. Earl, R. et al., Iron Deficiency Anemia: Recommended Guidelines for the Prevention, Detection, and Management Among U.S. Children and Women of Childbearing Age, National Academy Press, Washington, DC, 1993. http://www.nap.edu/catalog/2251.html.

28. U.S. Department of Agriculture, Frequently Asked Questions — Food Guidance System, http://www.mypyramid.gov/global_nav/media_questions.html. (accessed January 30, 2006).

29. U.S. Department of Agriculture (Human Nutrition Service), *Food Guide Pyramid: A Guide to Daily Food Choice*, Washington, DC, Home and Garden Bulletin No. 252, 1992.

30. U.S. Department of Agriculture, MyPyramid.gov For Kids, http://mypyramid.gov/kids/index_print.html. (accessed January 30, 2006).

31. U.S. Department of Agriculture, Frequently Asked Questions — MyPyramid for Kids, http://www.mypyramid.gov/global_nav/media_kids_questions.html. (accessed January 30, 2006).

32. U.S. Department of Agriculture, Johanns unveils *MyPyramid for Kids*, http://www.mypyramid.gov/global_nav/media_kids_press_release.html. (accessed January 30, 2006).

33. U.S. Department of Agriculture (Food and Nutrition Service), *MyPyramid for Kids* Classroom Materials, http://teamnutrition.usda.gov/resources/mypyramidclassroom.html. (accessed January 30, 2006).

34. Karanja, N.M. et al., *JADA*, 99: 19S; 1999.

35. U.S. Department of Health and Human Services, National Institutes of Health, and National Heart, L., and Blood Institute, *Facts about the DASH Eating Plan (NIH Publication No. 03-4082)*, 1998 (originally printed), 1999 (reprinted), 2003 (revised) http://www.nhlbi.nih.gov/health/public/heart/hbp/dash/new_dash.pdf.

36. Borrud, L.G., Introduction and Overview, Design and Operation: The Continuing Survey of Food Intakes by Individuals and the Diet and Health Knowledge Survey, 1994–96, in USDA, Agricultural Research Service, NFS Report No. 96-1, Tippett, K.S. and Cypel, Y.S., Ed., 1997, 1. available at http://www.aro.usda.goo/SP2 userfeleo/place/1235500/pdf/Dor9496.pdf

37. Subar, A.F. et al., *Pediatrics*, 102: 913; 1998.

38. Krebs-Smith, S.M. et al., *Arch. Pediatr. Adolesc. Med.*, 150: 81; 1996.

39. Hampl, J.S., Betts, N.M., and Benes, B.A., *JADA*, 98: 1418; 1998.
40. Guenther, P.M., Cleveland, L.E., and Ingwersen, L.A., Questionnaire Development and Data Collection Procedures, Design and Operation: The Continuing Survey of Food Intakes by Individuals and the Diet and Health Knowledge Survey, 1994–96, in USDA, Agricultural Research Service, NFS Report No. 96-1, Tippett, K.S. and Cypel, Y.S., Ed., 1997, 42. available online at www. ers.usda. gov/SP User Files/Place/12355000/pdf/Dor 9496.pdf.
41. Harnack, L., Stang, J., and Story, M., *JADA*, 99: 436; 1999.
42. Harnack, L., Walters, S.H., and Jacobs, D.R., *JADA*, 103: 1015; 2003.
43. Suitor, C.W. and Gleason, P.M., *JADA*, 102: 530; 2002.
44. U.S. Department of Agriculture (Agricultural Research Service), *Food and Nutrient Intakes by Children 1994–96, 1998*, ARS Food Surveys Research Group, 1999. Available Online on the "Products" page at http://www.barc.usda.gov/bhnrc/foodsurvey/home.htm. (accessed March 23, 2006).
45. Johnson, R.K., Frary, C.D., and Wang, M.Q., *JADA*, 102: 853; 2002.
46. Frary, C.D., Johnson, R.K., and Wang, M.Q., *J. Adolesc. Health*, 34: 56; 2004.
47. Weinberg, L.G., Berner, L.A., and Groves, J.E., *JADA*, 104: 895; 2004.
48. Paeratakul, S. et al., *JADA*, 103: 1332; 2003.
49. Enns, C.W., Mickle, S.J., and Goldman, J.D., *Fam. Econ. Nutr. Rev.*, 14: 56; 2002.
50. French, S.A., Lin, B., and Guthrie, J.F., *JADA*, 103: 1326; 2003.
51. Lytle, L.A. et al., *Public Health Nutr.*, 5: 319; 2002.
52. Dwyer, J. et al., *JADA*, 101: 1142; 2001.
53. U.S. Department of Agriculture (Agricultural Research Service), What We Eat in America, NHANES 2001–2002, http://www.ars. usda.gov/Services/docs.htm?docid=7674&pf=1&cg_id=0. (accessed February 20, 2006).
54. Moshfegh, A., Goldman, J., and Cleveland, L., *What We Eat in America, NHANES 2001–2002: Usual Nutrient Intakes from Food Compared to Dietary Reference Intakes*, U.S. Department of Agriculture, Agricultural Research Service, 2005. Available at http:// www.ars.usda.gov/SP2UserFiles/Place/12355000/pdf/usualintaketables2001-02.pdf. (accessed February 13, 2006).
55. Lino, M. et al., *Fam. Econ. Nutr. Rev.*, 14: 52; 2002.
56. U.S. Department of Agriculture (Center for Nutrition Policy and Promotion), *Nutrition Insights, Insight 9*, 1998. http://www.cnpp. usda.gov/Publications/nutrition insights/consight 9.pdf (accessed March 24, 2006).
57. Carlson, A. et al., *Fam. Econ. Nutr. Rev.*, 15: 52; 2003.
58. Basiotis, P.P. et al., *Fam. Econ. Nutr. Rev.*, 16: 66; 2004.
59. Federal Interagency Forum on Child and Family Statistics, *America's Children: Key National Indicators of Well-Being, 2005*, Federal Interagency Forum on Child and Family Statistics, Washington, DC, U.S. Government Printing Office, 2005. Available online at http://childstats.gov. (accessed on March 24, 2006).
60. Emmons, L. and Hayes, M., *JADA*, 62: 409; 1973.
61. Mack, K., Blair, J., and Presser, S., *Health Survey Research Methods Conference Proceedings*, Warnecke, R, Ed., DHHS Publication No. (PHS) 96-1013, 51, 1996.
62. Presser, S. et al., Final Report on the University of Maryland-USDA Cooperative Agreement to Improve Reporting for Children in the Continuing Survey of Food Intakes by Individuals, Survey Research Center, University of Maryland, 1993.
63. Eck, L., Klesges, R., and Hanson, C., *JADA*, 89: 784; 1989.
64. Sobo, E. and Rock, C., *Med. Anthropol. Q.*, 15: 222; 2001.
65. Sobo, E. et al., *JADA*, 100: 428; 2000.
66. Baxter, S.D., Thompson, W.O., and Davis, H.C., *JADA*, 100: 911; 2000.
67. Baxter, S.D. et al., *JADA*, 102: 386; 2002.
68. Baxter, S.D. et al., *Prev. Med.*, 36: 601; 2003.
69. Baxter, S.D. et al., *J. Nutr. Educ. Behav.*, 35: 124; 2003.
70. Baxter, S.D. and Thompson, W.O., *Nutr. Res.*, 22: 679; 2002.
71. Baxter, S.D. et al., *Nutr. Res.*, 23: 1537; 2003.
72. Baxter, S.D. et al., *Ann. Epidemiol.*, 14: 385; 2004.
73. Baxter, S.D. et al., *JADA*, 104: 1654; 2004.
74. American Dietetic Association, *JADA*, 104: 660; 2004.
75. U.S. Department of Agriculture, MyPyramid, Available at http://www.mypyramid.gov. (accessed January 30, 2006).
76. U.S. Department of Agriculture (Food and Nutrition Service), *MyPyramid for Kids*, www.mypyramid.gov. (accessed January 30, 2006).
77. American Academy of Pediatrics (Committee on Nutrition), Feeding the Child, in Pediatric Nutrition Handbook, 5th edition, Kleinman, R.E., Ed., American Academy of Pediatrics, Elk Grove Village, IL, 2004, 119.
78. Domel, S.B. et al., *J. Am. Coll. Nutr.*, 13: 33; 1994.
79. Domel, S.B. et al., *J. Nutr. Educ.*, 25: 345; 1993.
80. Wolfe, W.S. and Campbell, C.C., *JADA*, 93: 1280; 1993.
81. Nicklas, T.A., *JADA*, 95: 1127; 1995.
82. Ogden, C.L. et al., *JAMA*, 288: 1728; 2002.
83. National Center for Health Statistics, Prevalence of Overweight among Children and Adolescents: United States 1999–2002, available at http://www.cdc.gov/nchs/products/pubs/pubd/hestats/overwght99.htm. (accessed March 2, 2006).
84. Freedman, D.S. et al., *Pediatrics*, 99: 420; 1997.

85. Troiano, R.P. and Flegal, K.M., *Pediatrics*, 101: 497; 1998.
86. Hedley, A.A. et al., *JAMA*, 291: 2847; 2004.
87. Birch, L.L. and Fisher, J.O., *Pediatrics*, 101: 539; 1998.
88. Hill, J.O. and Trowbridge, F.L., *Pediatrics*, 101: 570; 1998.
89. Birch, L.L., Johnson, S.L., and Fisher, J.A., *Young Child.*, 50: 71; 1995.
90. Birch, L.L., *J. Nutr. Educ.*, 11: 189; 1979.
91. Calfas, K.J., Sallis, J.F., and Nader, P.R., *J. Dev. Behav. Pediatr.*, 12: 185; 1991.
92. Domel, S.B. et al., *Prev. Med.*, 22: 866; 1993.
93. Domel, S.B., et al., *Health Educ. Res.*, 11: 299; 1996.
94. Fisher, J.O. and Birch, L.L., *JADA*, 95: 759; 1995.
95. Baxter, S.D., Thompson, W.O., and Davis, H.C., *Nutr. Res.*, 20: 439; 2000.
96. Birch, L.L., *Nutr. Rev.*, 50: 249; 1992.
97. Mennella, J.A., Jagnow, C.P., and Beauchamp, G.K., *Pediatrics*, 107: e88; 2001.
98. Birch, L.L., *Bull. Psychon. Soc.*, 29: 265; 1991.
99. Cowart, B.J., *Psychol. Bull.*, 90: 43; 1981.
100. Birch, L.L., *JADA*, 87: 36S; 1987.
101. Sullivan, S.A. and Birch, L.L., *Pediatrics*, 93: 271; 1994.
102. Birch, L.L. and Marlin, D.W., *Appetite*, 3: 353; 1982.
103. Birch, L.L. et al., *Appetite*, 9: 171; 1987.
104. Sullivan, S.A. and Birch, L.L., *Dev. Psychol.*, 26: 546; 1990.
105. Birch, L.L. et al., *Appetite*, 30: 283; 1998.
106. Loewen, R. and Pliner, P., *Appetite*, 32: 351; 1999.
107. Hearn, M.D. et al., *J. Health Educ.*, 29: 26; 1988.
108. Pliner, P. and Stallberg-White, C., *Appetite*, 34: 95; 2000.
109. Lytle, L. and Achterberg, C., *J. Nutr. Educ.*, 27: 250; 1995.
110. Birch, L.L., Zimmerman, S.I., and Hind, H., *Child Dev.*, 51: 856; 1980.
111. Birch, L.L. et al., *Appetite*, 3: 125; 1982.
112. Birch, L.L., Marlin, D.W., and Rotter, J., *Child Dev.*, 55: 431; 1984.
113. Newman, J. and Taylor, A., *J. Exp. Child Psychol.*, 53: 200; 1992.
114. Hendy, H.M., *Ann. Behav. Med.*, 21: 20; 1999.
115. Wardle, J. et al., *Appetite*, 40: 155; 2003.
116. Wardle, J. et al., *Eur. J. Clin. Nutr.*, 57: 341; 2003.
117. Perry, C.L. et al., *Health Educ. Behav.*, 31: 65; 2004.
118. Hendy, H.M., Williams, K.E., and Camise, T.S., *Appetite*, 45: 250; 2005.
119. Hendy, H.M. and Raudenbush, B., *Appetite*, 34: 61; 2000.
120. Hendy, H.M., *Appetite*, 39: 217; 2002.
121. Addessi, E. et al., *Appetite*, 45: 264; 2005.
122. Nahikian-Nelms, M., *JADA*, 97: 505; 1997.
123. Fomon, S.J., *Nutrition of Normal Infants*, Mosby-Yearbook, St. Louis, MO, 1993, 114.
124. Adair, L.S., *JADA*, 84: 543; 1984.
125. Birch, L.L. and Deysher, M., *Learn. Motiv.*, 16: 341; 1985.
126. Birch, L.L. and Deysher, M., *Appetite*, 7: 323; 1986.
127. Birch, L.L. et al., *N. Engl. J. Med.*, 324: 232 1991.
128. Birch, L.L. et al., *Learn. Motiv.*, 18: 301; 1987.
129. Johnson, S.L. and Birch, L.L., *Pediatrics*, 94: 653; 1994.
130. Klesges, R.C. et al., *J. Appl. Behav. Anal.*, 16: 371 1983.
131. Fisher, J.O. and Birch, L.L., *Am. J. Clin. Nutr.*, 69: 1264; 1999.
132. Fisher, J.O. and Birch, L.L., *Appetite*, 32: 405; 1999.
133. Spruijt-Metz, D. et al., *Am. J. Clin. Nutr.*, 75: 581; 2002.
134. Birch, L.L., Fisher, J.O., and Davison, K.K., *Am. J. Clin. Nutr.*, 78: 125; 2003.
135. Rolls, B.J., Engell, D., and Birch, L.L., *JADA*, 100: 232; 2000.
136. Fisher, J.O., Rolls, B.J., and Birch, L.L., *Am. J. Clin. Nutr.*, 77: 1164; 2003.
137. McConahy, K.L. et al., *JADA*, 104: 975; 2004.
138. Satter, E., *How to Get Your Kids to Eat But Not Too Much*, Bull Publishing, Palo Alto, CA, 1987.
139. Satter, E., *Child of Mine: Feeding with Love and Good Sense*, Bull Publishing, Palo Alto, CA, 2000.
140. Satter, E.M., *JADA*, 86: 352; 1986.
141. Dietz, W.H., *Pediatrics*, 101: 518; 1998.
142. Andersen, R.E. et al., *JAMA*, 279: 938; 1998.
143. Crespo, C.J. et al., *Arch. Pediatr. Adolesc. Med.*, 155: 360; 2001.
144. Grunbaum, J. et al., Youth Risk Behavior Surveillance — United States, 2003, In CDC Surveillance Summaries, MMWR 53 (No. SS-2), 2004. http://www.cdc.gov/mmwr/PDF/SS/SS5302.pdf. (accessed March 7, 2006).

145. American Academy of Pediatrics (Committee on Nutrition), *Pediatrics*, 112: 424; 2003.

146. Olson, R.E., *JADA*, 100: 28; 2000.

147. Satter, E., *JADA*, 100: 32; 2000.

148. Dwyer, J., *JADA*, 100: 36; 2000.

149. Krebs, N.F. and Johnson, S.L., *JADA*, 100: 37; 2000.

150. Lytle, L.A., *JADA*, 100: 39; 2000.

151. Van Horn, L., *JADA*, 100: 41; 2000.

152. Pugliese, M.T. et al., *Pediatrics*, 80: 175; 1987.

153. Niinikoski, H. et al., *Pediatrics*, 99: 687; 1997.

154. Niinikoski, H. et al., *Pediatrics*, 100: 810; 1997.

155. Simmell, O. et al., *Am. J. Clin. Nutr.*, 72: 1316S; 2000.

156. The Writing Group for the DISC Collaborative Research Group, *JAMA*, 273: 1429, 1995.

157. Obarzanek, E. et al., *Pediatrics*, 100: 51; 1997.

158. Obarzanek, E. et al., *Pediatrics*, 107: 256; 2001.

159. Van Horn, L. et al., *Pediatrics*, 115: 1723; 2005.

160. Luepker, R.V. et al., *JAMA*, 275: 768; 1996.

161. Dennison, B.A., *J. Am. Coll. Nutr.*, 15: 4S; 1996.

162. Hyams, J.S. et al., *Pediatrics*, 82: 64; 1988.

163. Smith, M.M. and Lifshitz, F., *Pediatrics*, 93: 438; 1994.

164. Dennison, B.A., Rockwell, H.L., and Baker, S.L., *Pediatrics*, 99: 15; 1997.

165. American Academy of Pediatrics (Committee on Nutrition), *Pediatrics*, 107: 1210; 2001.

166. Frank, G., Nutrition for Teens, in Promoting Teen Health: Linking Schools, Health Organizations and Community, Henderson, A., Champlin, S., and Evashwick, W., Ed., Sage Publications, Thousand Oaks, CA, 1998, 28.

167. Kanarek, R.B., *Nutr. Rev.*, 52: 173; 1994.

168. Wolraich, M.L. et al., *N. Engl. J. Med.*, 330: 301; 1994.

169. Wolraich, M.L., Wilson, D.B., and White, J.W., *JAMA*, 274: 1617 1995.

170. U.S. Department of Agriculture, MyPyramid Food Guidance System Education Framework, http://www.mypyramid.gov/downloads/MyPyramid_education_framework.pdf. (accessed January 30, 2006).

171. American Dietetic Association, *JADA*, 104: 255; 2004.

172. Story, M. and French, S., *Int. J. Behav. Nutr. Phys. Activity*, 1: 3; 2004.

173. Harrison, K. and Marske, A.L., *Am. J. Public Health*, 95: 1568; 2005.

174. Henry J. Kaiser Family Foundation, *The Role of Media in Childhood Obesity* (Issue Brief; publication #7030), http://www.kff.org/entmedia/7030.cfm. (accessed March 11, 2006).

175. American Dietetic Association, *JADA*, 103: 748; 2003.

176. Sanders, T.A. and Reddy, S., *Am. J. Clin. Nutr.*, 59: 1176S; 1994.

177. Messina, V. and Mangels, A.R., *JADA*, 101: 661; 2001.

178. Messina, V., Melina, V., and Mangels, A.R., *JADA*, 103: 771; 2003.

179. Pollitt, E., *JADA*, 95: 1134; 1995.

180. Pollitt, E., Cueto, S., and Jacoby, E.R., *Am. J. Clin. Nutr.*, 67: 779S; 1998.

181. Grantham-McGregor, S.M., Chang, S., and Walker, S.P., *Am. J. Clin. Nutr.*, 67: 785S; 1998.

182. Dwyer, J.T. et al., *Fam. Econ. Nutr. Rev.*, 11: 3; 1998.

183. Nicklas, T.A. et al., *JADA*, 93: 886; 1993.

184. Gleason, P.M., *Am. J. Clin. Nutr.*, 61: 213S; 1995.

185. Siega-Riz, A.M., Popkin, B.M., and Carson, T., *Am. J. Clin. Nutr.*, 67: 748S, 1998.

186. American Academy of Pediatrics (Committee on Nutrition), Adolescent Nutrition, in Pediatric Nutrition Handbook, 5th edition, Kleinman, R.E., Ed., American Academy of Pediatrics, Elk Grove Village, IL, 2004, 149.

187. Neumark-Sztainer, D. et al., *JADA*, 99: 929; 1999.

188. Neumark-Sztainer, D. et al., *JADA*, 103: 317; 2003.

189. Neumark-Sztainer, D. et al., *JADA*, 98: 1449; 1998.

190. Story, M., Neumark-Sztainer, D., and French, S.A., *JADA*, 102: 40S; 2002.

191. World Health Organization, Young People's Health in Context. Health Behaviour in School-aged Children (HBSC) Study: International Report from the 2001/2002 Survey, Health Policy for Children and Adolescents, No. 4, Denmark, 2004. http://www.euro.who.int/Document/e82923.pdf. (accessed March 8, 2006).

192. American Academy of Pediatrics (Committee on Adolescence), *Pediatrics*, 111: 204; 2003.

193. American Dietetic Association, *JADA*, 101: 810; 2001.

194. American Dietetic Association, *JADA*, 105: 979; 2005.

195. Birch, L.L., *Dev. Psychol.*, 26: 515; 1990.

196. Kennedy, E., *Prev. Med.*, 25: 56; 1996.

197. Dwyer, J., *Am. J. Clin. Nutr.*, 61: 173S; 1995.

198. Centers for Disease Control and Prevention, *Guidelines for School Health Programs to Promote Lifelong Healthy Eating*. MMWR, No.RR-9, 1, 1996.

199. Resnicow, K., *Ann. N. Y. Acad. Sci.*, 699: 154; 1993.
200. Berenson, G.S. et al., *Ann. N. Y. Acad. Sci.*, 623: 299; 1991.
201. Kolbe, L.J., *Prev. Med.*, 22: 544; 1993.
202. Contento, I.R., Manning, A.D., and Shannon, B., *J. Nutr. Educ.*, 24: 247; 1992.
203. Contento, I.R. et al., *J. Nutr. Educ.*, 27: 298; 1995.
204. U.S. Department of Agriculture (Food and Nutrition Service), National School Lunch Program — Nutrition Program Facts, http://www.fns.usda.gov/cnd/lunch/AboutLunch/NSLPFactSheet.pdf. (accessed March 9, 2006).
205. U.S. Department of Agriculture (Food and Nutrition Service), School Breakfast Program — Nutrition Program Facts, http://www.fns.usda.gov/cnd/breakfast/AboutBFast/FactSheet.pdf. (accessed March 9, 2006).
206. U.S. Department of Agriculture (Food and Nutrition Service), Road to SMI Success — A Guide for School Foodservice Directors, http://www.fns.usda.gov/tn/Resources/roadtosuccess.html. (accessed March 6, 2006).
207. U.S. Department of Agriculture (Food and Nutrition Service), Team Nutrition, http://www.fns.usda.gov/tn. (accessed March 6, 2006).
208. U.S. Department of Agriculture (Food and Nutrition Service), Changing the Scene — Improving the School Nutrition Environment, http://teamnutrition.usda.gov/Resources/changing.html. (accessed March 6, 2006).
209. Burghardt, J.A., *Am. J. Clin. Nutr.*, 61: 182S; 1995.
210. Burghardt, J.A., Devaney, B.L., and Gordon, A.R., *Am. J. Clin. Nutr.*, 61: 252S; 1995.
211. U.S. Department of Agriculture, Food and Nutrition Service, and Office of Analysis Nutrition and Evaluation, *School Nutrition Dietary Assessment Study-II Final Report*, Alexandria, VA, 2001. http://www.fns.usda.gov/oane/menu/Published/CNP/FILES/sndaII.pdf. (accessed March 11, 2006).
212. U.S. Department of Agriculture, Food and Nutrition Service, and Office of Analysis Nutrition and Evaluation, *School Nutrition Dietary Assessment Study-II Summary of Findings*, Alexandria, VA, 2001. http://www.fns.usda.gov/oane/menu/Published/CNP/FILES/SNDAIIfind.sum.htm (accessed March 9, 2006).
213. Baranowski, T. et al., *J. Nutr. Educ.*, 25: 114; 1993.
214. Kirby, S.D. et al., *J. Nutr. Educ.*, 27: 261; 1995.
215. Resnicow, K. et al., *Health Psychol.*, 16: 272; 1997.
216. Baranowski, T. et al., *Health Educ. Behav.*, 27: 96; 2000.
217. Resnicow, K. et al., *Am. J. Public Health*, 88: 250; 1998.
218. Luepker, R.V. et al., *J. Nutr. Biochem.*, 9: 525; 1998.
219. Nicklas, T.A. et al., *J. Sch. Health*, 68: 248; 1998.
220. Perry, C.L. et al., *Am. J. Public Health*, 88: 603; 1998.
221. Reynolds, K.D. et al., *Prev. Med.*, 30: 309; 2000.
222. Donnelly, J.E. et al., *Obes. Res.*, 4: 229; 1996.
223. Baxter, S.D. *J. Sch. Health*, 68: 111; 1998.
224. Molnar, A., and Garcia, D.R., *Empty Calories: Commercializing Activities in America's Schools (Executive Summary)*. Education Policy Studies Laboratory (Commercialism in Education Research Unit [CERU]), Arizona State University, 2005. Available at http://www.asu.edu/educ/epsl/CERU/Annual%20reports/EPSL-0511-103-CERU-exec.pdf. (accessed March 24, 2006).
225. Gittelsohn, J. et al., *Am. J. Clin. Nutr.*, 69: 767S; 1999.
226. Baranowski, T. et al., *J. Am. Coll. Nutr.*, 16: 216; 1997.
227. Meyer, M.K., *JADA*, 100: 100; 2000.
228. Fulkerson, J.A. et al., *JADA*, 102: 97; 2002.
229. French, S.A. et al., *JADA*, 97: 1008; 1997.
230. French, S.A. et al., *Am. J. Public Health*, 91: 112; 2001.
231. American Dietetic Association, *JADA*, 106: 122; 2006.
232. U.S. Department of Agriculture (Food and Nutrition Service), Healthy Schools, http://teamnutrition.usda.gov/healthy-schools.html. (accessed March 6, 2006).
233. American Dietetic Association, Society for Nutrition Education, and American School Food Service Association, *JADA*, 103: 505; 2003.
234. American Academy of Pediatrics (Committee on Nutrition), *Pediatrics*, 113: 152; 2004.
235. Perry, C.L. et al., *J. Sch. Health*, 60: 406; 1990.
236. Nader, P.R. et al., *Arch. Pediatr. Adolesc. Med.*, 153: 695; 1999.
237. Hoelscher, D.M. et al., *Prev. Med.*, 38: 594; 2004.
238. U.S. Department of Health and Human Services, *Healthy People 2010*. 2nd edition. *With Understanding and Improving Health and Objectives for Improving Health. 2 volumes*, Washington, DC: U.S. Government Printing Office, November 2000. Available online at http://www.health.gov/healthypeople. (accessed March 25, 2006).
239. U.S. Department of Health and Human Services, Healthy People 2010 Progress Reviews, http://www.healthypeople.gov/Data/PROGRVW/default.htm. (accessed March 12, 2006).
240. U.S. Department of Health and Human Services, Healthy People 2010 Progress Review: Nutrition and Overweight, January 2004. Available online at http://www.healthypeople.gov/Data/2010prog/focus19/Nutrition_Overweight.pdf. (accessed March 12, 2006).
241. U.S. Department of Health and Human Services, Healthy People 2010 Progress Review: Oral Health, March 2004. Available online at http://www.healthypeople.gov/Data/2010prog/focus21/OralHealthPR.pdf. (accessed March 12, 2006).
242. Havas, S. et al., *JADA*, 94: 32; 1994.
243. Subar, A.F. et al., *Am. J. Health Promot.*, 9: 352; 1995.

244. Havas, S. et al., *Public Health Rep.*, 110: 68; 1995.
245. Produce for Better Health Foundation, 5 a Day — Background, Mission, & History, http://www.5aday.org/html/background/mission. php. (accessed March 13, 2006).
246. Dairy Management Inc., 3-A-Day of Dairy Fact Sheet, http://www.3aday.org/3aDay/about/pdf/3AD_Backrounder.pdf. (accessed March 6, 2006).
247. Dairy Management Inc., 3-A-Day of Dairy Frequently Asked Questions, http://www.3aday.org/3aDay/about/pdf/FAQs.pdf. (accessed March 6, 2006).
248. Partnership for Food Safety Education, Fight Bac! http://www.fightbac.org. (accessed March 5, 2006).
249. Hospitality Institute of Technology and Management, Double hand washing with a fingernail brush HACCP, http://www.hi-tm.com/ Documents/handflow-PDF.pdf. (accessed March 5, 2006).
250. Snyder, O.P., Hospitality Institute of Technology and Management, http://www.hi-tm.com/Documents/Safehands.html. (accessed March 5, 2006).
251. American Dietetic Association, *JADA*, 103: 615; 2003.
252. American Dietetic Association, *JADA*, 105: 1620; 2005.
253. Lucas, B. and Ogata, B., Normal Nutrition from Infancy through Adolescence, in *Handbook of Pediatric Nutrition*, Samour, P.Q. and King, K., Ed., Jones and Bartlett Publishers, Inc., Sudbury, MA, 2005, 107.

17 Health-Promoting Diet for Adults

Marsha Read

CONTENTS

INTRODUCTION

The normal diet for adults is based on the need to provide sufficient nutrients to sustain life and an appropriate balance of nutrient intake to support optimal health. The first *Surgeon General's Report on Nutrition and Health* in 1988[1] brought together a substantial body of research that documented that diet, aside from providing the essential nutrients for daily functioning, was a key factor with respect to chronic diseases such as coronary heart disease, cancer, diabetes, and obesity. The underlying premise of the various dietary guidelines/recommendations that have been developed has been to provide adequate nutrient intake while avoiding dietary patterns that might place an individual at greater risk for chronic disease. The following subsections describe the most commonly used dietary guidelines/recommendations, guidelines for counseling healthy adults, information on current food and nutrient consumption patterns of adults, and current research with respect to health implications of inappropriate macronutrient intake.

DIETARY RECOMMENDATIONS AND GUIDELINES

DIETARY GUIDELINES

Dietary guidelines have undergone several revisions from the late 1970s to the recently released Dietary Guidelines for Americans 2005.[2] The 1970s Dietary Goals provided recommendations with respect to energy intake, carbohydrate, fat, and sodium intakes.

Specific percentage of calories from carbohydrate and fat were put forth, 48% and 30% respectively. Cholesterol intake was recommended at 300 mg/day and sodium intake was recommended not to exceed 5 g/day.[3] The first set of the U.S. Dietary Guidelines was published in 1980[4]. The most recent version is the 2005 Dietary Guidelines for Americans. (See chapter 21 for details on these guidelines)

From the first edition of the guidelines to the current, the focus has been on a variety of foods to supply adequate nutrient intake, increase complex carbohydrate consumption, moderate fat intake, and moderate alcohol consumption if one drinks. The 2005 guidelines add emphasis on "Weight Management," as well as a section on "Food Groups to Encourage." Another new feature to the 2005 guidelines, in contrast to earlier versions, are recommendations for specific population groups under each major guideline and a glossary of terms and appendices and tables for more detailed information. As with previous versions, the guidelines continue to be based on current research.[5] A review of all iterations, including the 2005 Dietary Guidelines, is provided at: www.health.gov/dietaryguidelines/

THE FOOD GUIDE PYRAMID

The 1992 Food Guide Pyramid set forth recommendations for a pattern of daily food choices based on servings from five major food groups — bread, cereal, rice, and pasta; fruit; vegetable; milk, yogurt, and cheese; and meat, poultry, fish, dry beans, eggs, and nuts. The visual presentation as a pyramid was meant to convey that, from the five food groups, emphasis should be placed on those shown in the lower three levels/sections of the pyramid. The Food Guide Pyramid was also meant to be used in concert with the dietary guidelines, that is, to eat a variety of foods and balance the foods eaten with physical activity and either maintain or improve weight. Each food group suggests a range of servings. Selecting the lower number of recommended servings is estimated to provide approximately 1600 kcal, with the midrange providing approximately 2200 kcal, and 2800 kcal at the upper range.[6]

Cited advantages and disadvantages of the 1992 Food Guide Pyramid according to Kant et al.[7] include:

Advantages:
- The Pyramid depicted foods, rather than nutrients and numbers such as Recommended Dietary Intakes (RDAs) or Daily Reference Intakes (DRIs), which made it easier for consumers to relate to.
- The Pyramid was relatively simple, easy to read, and remember.
- The Pyramid food groups and recommended servings from each food group were likely to represent a variety of foods that can provide adequate nutrient intake.
- The Pyramid food groups allowed for personal choice within a food group and thus allowed for individual food choices.

Disadvantages:
- Applicability of the food groups within the Pyramid to alternate dietary patterns such as vegetarianism and ethnic food patterns was unclear.
- The Food Guide Pyramid did not address the dietary guideline regarding alcohol intake.
- The Pyramid did not address the consumption of combination foods such as pizza or stew. Lastly, dietary adequacy might not be obtained if individuals made poor choices within the Pyramid food groups.

The most recent version is titled "My Pyramid" (http://www.mypyramid.gov/tips_resources/menus.html). It is designed to reflect the diversity of nutrient needs and food patterns and to address the disadvantages noted for the 1992 edition. The latest version is intended to allow individuals to formulate a dietary pattern that is consistent with their age, gender, activity levels, etc. The pyramid shows six-color-coded grids that correspond to the food groups of grains, vegetables, fruit, milk, meat, beans, and oils. A chart is provided to give guidance as to amounts (by gender and age) recommended daily. In addition, a serving size is defined; lists of the variety of foods within each category are provided. The importance of physical activity to overall energy intake and healthy weight is depicted by the figure climbing the side of the pyramid. The food Pyramid Web site provides sample menus and provides for the inclusion of mixed dishes as part of the Pyramid serving recommendations. There is also information about vegetarian diets.

RECOMMENDED DIETARY ALLOWANCES, ESTIMATED SAFE AND ADEQUATE DAILY DIETARY INTAKES, DAILY REFERENCE INTAKE, AND DAILY VALUES

The most common reference standard for nutrient intake has been the RDA. This standard was first established by the Food and Nutrition Board in 1941, with the most recent edition in 1989.[8] The original intent was to review and revise the RDAs every four to five years, taking into account current research. The constructs used in formulating a specific RDA were: (1) an estimation of how much of each essential nutrient the average healthy person requires to maintain health, and how those requirements vary among people; (2) an increase in the average requirement to cover the needs of almost all members of the population, based on a bell curve distribution; (3) an increase in the RDA again to cover cooking losses and inefficient body utilization, as well as provide for cases of greater nutrient need such as in pregnancy and infancy; and (4) use of scientific judgment in establishing the RDA. The following three central premises underlie the RDAs:

- The RDA is an amount intended to be consumed as part of a normal diet.
- The RDA is neither a minimal requirement nor an optimal level of intake, but instead it represents a safe and adequate level of intake based on current scientific knowledge.
- The RDA is most appropriately used as a nutrient intake guide applied to subgroups of the population, but can be used to estimate the probable risk of nutrient deficiency for an individual.

For nutrients that have scientific evidence providing support for their essentiality, but are insufficient to establish an RDA, there are Estimated Safe and Adequate Daily Dietary Intakes (ESADDIs). Most ESADDIs are shown as a range of intake values that represent the upper and lower limits of safe intake. ESADDIs are established for biotin, copper, manganese, and molybdenum.[8]

The current iteration of recommended intakes includes the DRI, which, in essence, replaces the RDA. DRI encompasses four types of nutrient recommendations for healthy individuals: Adequate Intake (AI), Estimated Average Intake (EAR), RDA, and tolerable Upper Intake Levels (UL).[9,10] AI is a nutrient recommendation based on observed or experimentally determined approximation of nutrient intake by a group (or groups) of healthy people when sufficient scientific evidence is not available to calculate an RDA or an EAR. The EAR is the average requirement of a nutrient for healthy individuals in which a functional or clinical assessment has been conducted and measures of adequacy have been made at a specified level of dietary intake. The EAR is an amount of intake of a nutrient at which approximately 50% of subjects would have their needs met and 50% would not. The EAR is intended to be used for assessing nutrient adequacy of populations and not individuals. The new RDA is the amount of a nutrient needed to meet the requirements of nearly all (97% to 98%) of the healthy population of individuals for whom it was developed.

An RDA for a nutrient should serve as an intake goal for individuals and not as a standard of adequacy for diets of populations. This is different than the previous or old RDA. UL values are established in cases where there is adequate scientific evidence to suggest an upper level of intake that is consistent with adverse or toxic reactions. The UL represents the maximum level of intake for a nutrient that will not cause adverse effects in most of the population ingesting that amount. The DRI can be found at: http://www.nal.usda.gov/fnic/etext/000105.html.

One other indication of dietary quality is the Health Eating Index (HEI). The HEI is intended to take into consideration compliance with the Dietary Guidelines for Americans as well as intake data to create a "score" that reflects how well American dietary patterns conform to the recommendations. The HEI score of American diets was 63.8, and can be interpreted as "needing improvement." [11]

WORLD HEALTH ORGANIZATION RECOMMENDATIONS

The World Health Organization (WHO) has also published diet recommendations with the goal of reducing risk for chronic disease.[12] WHO recommendations are expressed as a range of average daily intakes from lower to upper limits (Table 17.1).

FOOD LABELS

Food labeling became mandatory in 1993 with the enactment of the Nutrition Labeling and Education Act (NLEA).[13] The legislation required food labeling on most foods with the exceptions of low-nutrient-dense foods such as coffee, spices, and

---

TABLE 17.1
WHO Dietary Recommendations

Total Energy: sufficient to support normal growth, physical activity, and
  body weight (body mass index = 20–22)
Total Fat: 15%–30% of total energy
Saturated fatty acids: 0%–10% total energy
Polyunsaturated fatty acids: 3%–7% total energy
Dietary cholesterol: 0–300 mg/day
Total carbohydrate: 55%–75% total energy
Complex carbohydrates: 50%–75% total energy
Dietary fiber: 27–40 g/day
Refined sugars: 0%–10% total energy
Protein: 10%–15% total energy
Salt: upper limit of 6 g/day (no lower limit set)

TABLE 17.2
Nutrition Facts Panel Information

Serving size (based on amounts commonly used)

Number of servings per container

Kilocalories per serving

Kilocalories from fat

Percentage Daily Value of total fat, saturated fat, cholesterol, sodium, total
  carbohydrate, dietary fiber, sugars, protein, vitamin A, vitamin C, calcium, and iron

Reference values for total fat, saturated fat, cholesterol, sodium, total carbohydrate,
  and fiber

Kilocaloric conversion guide for protein, fat, and carbohydrates

A more complete description of food labels can be accessed at:
http://www.fda.gov/opacom/backgrounders/foodlabel/newlabel.html

ready-to-eat foods prepared on site. Nutrition information remains voluntary on many raw foods. The nutrition facts panel on food labels provides information to help the consumer make more informed choices, including information on calories per serving, calories from fat, saturated fat and cholesterol, and protein among other nutrients (Table 17.2).

Daily Values (DVs) are used as standards in food labeling. DVs provide reference intake standards for nutrients that have an RDA, in which case they are referred to as reference daily intakes (RDIs), and for nutrients for which no RDA exists, in this case referred to as daily reference values (DRVs). DRVs are established for fat, saturated fat, cholesterol, carbohydrate, dietary fiber, sodium, and potassium. As a rule, the RDIs are greater than the RDA for specific nutrients and provide a large margin of safety. The term RDI replaces the term U.S. Recommended Daily Allowances (USRDAs), used earlier on food labels.[13]

AMERICAN CANCER SOCIETY AND NATIONAL CANCER INSTITUTE GUIDELINES

In the 1980s the American Cancer Society issued the following dietary guidelines aimed at reducing cancer risk within the populace[14] (http://www.cancer.org/docroot/PED/content/PED_3_2X_Diet_and_Activity_Factors_That_Affect_Risks.asp?sitearea=PED):

- Choose most of the foods you eat from plant sources.
- Eat five or more servings of fruits and vegetables every day (http://5aday.gov/).
- Eat foods from plant sources, such as breads, cereals, grain products, rice, pasta, or beans several times each day.
- Limit your intake of high-fat foods, particularly from animal sources.
- Choose foods low in fat.
- Limit consumption of meats, especially high-fat meats.
- Be physically active: achieve and maintain a healthy weight.
- Be at least moderately active for 30 min or more on most days of the week.
- Stay within your healthy weight range.
- Limit consumption of alcoholic beverages, if you drink at all.

The National Cancer Institute endorses the following guidelines, which reflect in large part the recommendations of the American Cancer Society:[15]

- Avoid obesity.
- Reduce fat intake to 30% of total energy intake as a start.
- Then consider a reduction closer to 20% of total energy intake if at high risk, such as a family history of cancer.
- Eat more higher-fiber foods, such as fruits, vegetables, and whole-grain cereals.
- Include foods rich in vitamins A, E, and C, as well as carotenoids, in the daily diet.
- If alcohol is consumed, do not drink excessively.
- Use moderation when consuming salt-cured, smoked, and nitrite-cured foods.

There are also guidelines set forth by the National Cholesterol Education Program and the American Heart Association (refer to the section on cardiovascular disease).

NUTRITION COUNSELING FOR ADULTS

DETERMINING ENERGY REQUIREMENTS

To plan a diet consistent with dietary guidelines, the nutrition professional should first determine the caloric requirements of a client. The total energy requirements will be the sum of the resting energy requirement, energy needs for physical activity, and the energy needed for the thermic effect of foods. To determine the total energy requirement:

Step 1: Estimating Appropriate Body Weight. The Hamwi method is a common tool to estimate appropriate body weight. For females, the estimation is 100 lb for the first 5 ft of height and 5 lb/in. over 5 ft; for example, a 5'6" woman would be calculated as: (100 lb for the first 5 ft) + (5 lb/in. over 5 ft = $5 \times 6 = 30$) = 130 lb. For men the estimation is 106 lb for the first 5 ft of height and 6 lbs/in. over 5 ft; for example, a 6'0" man's desirable weight would be calculated as: (106 lb for the first 5 ft) + (6 lb/in. over 5 ft = $6 \times 12 = 72$) = 178 lb.

Adjustments are made for a large frame (+10%) or a small frame (−10%).

Step 2: Estimating Energy Needs Based on Body Weight. To estimate energy needs, the first step is to determine resting energy requirements (REE). Although several methods exist to calculate energy requirements based on weight, the abbreviated or quick method is probably useful for normal adults. The abbreviated method is as follows:

For adults:

$$\text{Women} \quad \text{weight in kg} \times 23$$
$$\text{Men} \quad \text{weight in kg} \times 24$$

Step 3: Estimating Energy Required for Physical Activity.

- Once the REEs is determined, an estimate of the energy needs for physical activity must be made. Again, there are several alternatives to use to estimate caloric needs for physical activity. The Physical Activity Levels (PALs)[16] method is shown in the following text:
  - Seated work with no option of moving around and little or no strenuous leisure activity (PAL factor = 1.4 to $1.5 \times$ REE)
  - Seated work with ability or requirement to move around but little or no strenuous leisure activity (PAL factor = 1.6 to $1.7 \times$ REE)
  - Standing work (housework, shop clerks) (PAL factor = 1.8 to $1.9 \times$ REE)
  - Significant amounts of sport or strenuous leisure activity (30–60 min 4–5/week) (PAL factor + 0.3 increment over 1.8 to $1.9 \times$ REE)
  - Strenuous work or highly active leisure (PAL factor = 2.0 to 2.4)

Step 4: Add REE (Step 2) and Physical Activity (Step 3).

Step 5: Calculate Thermic Effect of Food.

- To estimate the thermic effect of food, multiply the sum of the REE and physical activity by 10% and add that amount to the total.
- Determining protein, fat, and carbohydrate requirements.
- After the total energy requirements are determined, the contributions from protein, fat, and carbohydrate need to be determined.
  - Protein: by converting grams of protein into its caloric equivalent, the percentage of protein from total calories can be derived.
  - Fat: the recommendation for fat is 30% or less of the total energy requirements.
  - Carbohydrate: the percentage of calories that will come from carbohydrate will be the difference between total energy requirements and the percentage of kilocalories from protein and fat.
- Estimates of Actual Intakes of Adults for Macronutrients

Nutrition monitoring has been going on since the early 1900s in the United States, when the USDA's Food Supply Series was initiated.[17] Currently, the National Nutrition Monitoring and Related Research Program (NNMRRP) is the umbrella for activities that provide regular information about the contribution that diet and nutritional status make to health.[18]

ENERGY INTAKE

With respect to total energy intake, caloric consumption of adult men consistently exceeds that of adult women by approximately 400 kcal. With one age group exception (ages >70 years), men consumed in excess of 2000 kcal on average, whereas women consistently averaged less than 2000 kcal/day. Fat was contributing slightly above the recommended 30% of kcal for

TABLE 17.3

Total Energy Intake and Sources of Energy for Adult Men and Women

| | | | Sources of Energy Intake (Percentage of Total Kilocalories) | | | | | | | |
| | Total Energy Intake | | Protein | | Fat | | Carbohydrate | | Alcohol | |
Age	M	F	M	F	M	F	M	F	M	F
20–29	2821	1841	15.2	14.7	32.4	31.8	49.8	63.0	3.4	1.9
30–39	2665	1710	15.9	15.7	34.0	32.4	48.8	61.8	2.4	1.5
40–49	2435	1682	16.0	15.6	33.1	33.4	49.2	51.1	2.8	1.4
50–59	2270	1600	16.3	16.5	33.8	32.4	48.7	51.2	2.5	1.6
60–69	2072	1489	16.6	16.7	33.5	32.6	49.3	61.2	2.1	1.3
>70	1834	1384	16.3	16.7	33.0	31.4	50.9	63.3	1.6	1.5
<20	2455	1646	16.0	15.9	33.3	32.4	49.3	51.9	2.6	1.4

M = males, F = females

TABLE 17.4

Contribution (Percentage of Kilocalories) of Breakfast, Snacks, and Foods Consumed Away from Home to Total Energy Intake (1 Day) 1994–1996[a]

| | Breakfast | | Snacks | | Foods Away from Home | |
Age (Years)	M	F	M	F	M	F
20–29	14.2	16.0	18.2	17.0	40.0	34.3
30–39	15.5	16.9	15.5	16.9	31.4	26.6
40–49	16.3	16.9	15.5	17.1	29.4	25.4
50–59	18.2	19.1	15.4	15.2	26.7	23.0
60–69	20.9	19.9	15.0	15.1	20.0	17.6
70 >	23.8	23.0	12.2	12.3	14.2	12.5
20 <	17.1	18.2	15.7	15.9	29.4	24.5

M = males; F = females
[a] http://www.ars.usda.gov/SP2UserFiles/Place/12355000/pdf/Tbs1995.PDF

both men and women. Adult men derive somewhat more kilocalories from alcohol compared with women, but women are considerably higher in their carbohydrate intake than men. Men consumed not quite a third of their total energy intake from foods consumed away from home. The contribution of energy from foods eaten away from home is one-fourth of the total energy intake of women.

Men were more likely than women to consume a diet that met 100% of the RDA. Table 17.3 provides energy intake data on age cohorts for adult men and women based on the 1994 to 1996 Continuing Survey of Food Intake for Individuals (CSFII). Foods eaten away from home are contributing approximately 30% to 40% of total kilocalories consumed by young adults. The percentage of kilocalories derived from foods eaten away from home decreases with age (Table 17.4).

TOTAL PROTEIN, CARBOHYDRATE, AND FAT INTAKES

Protein intake is higher for adult men compared with adult women, yet the mean protein intake for both men and women exceeds the 1989 RDA (Table 17.5). With their higher mean protein intake, more men (80.2%) than women (69.2%) met 100% of the 1989 RDA for protein. As with total energy intake, foods consumed away from home contribute at least 25% of the overall protein intake. For men, 29% of the total protein intake was derived from foods eaten away from home. For women, this was 24.6%.

Total carbohydrate intake is higher for men than women, consistent with their higher total energy intake. The mean intake of carbohydrate for adult men was roughly 50 to 60 g/day higher than the adult female intake (Table 17.5).

The mean fiber intake per day for both men and women is below even the lower level of the recommended 24 to 70 g/day (Table 17.6).

TABLE 17.5
Percentage of Individuals Meeting 100% of the 1989 RDA for Energy (Two-Day Average)

Age (Years)	Males	Females
20–29	35.4	20.5
30–39	32.5	17.4
40–49	26.4	14.0
50–59	39.0	21.4
60–69	32.5	15.2
70>	19.5	12.4
20>	31.5	17.0

http://www.ars.usda.gov/SP2UserFiles/Place/12355000/pdf/Tbs1995.PDF

TABLE 17.6
Total Protein, Carbohydrate, and Fat Intakes (g/Day)[a]

Age (Years)	Protein		Carbohydrate		Fat	
	M	F	M	F	M	F
20–29	104.1	65.9	344.9	241.6	103.3	65.9
30–39	102.7	65.3	322.3	218.8	102.7	63.2
40–49	95.3	63.5	294.7	213.8	95.3	63.5
50–59	90.3	64.1	273.1	201.5	90.3	59.4
60–69	83.5	60.4	252.5	188.7	83.5	56.2
70 >	72.9	56.6	239.2	183.5	72.9	49.2
20 <	94.9	63.8	298.8	211.7	94.9	50.5

M = males, F = females
http://www.ars.usda.gov/SP2UserFiles/Place/12355000/pdf/Tbs1995.PDF

Fat intake for adult men and women, as with protein and carbohydrate intakes, reflects the gender differences in total energy intake pattern, that is, men consume more than women. The majority of adult men and women exceed the recommended 30% of energy from fat. Only 29.4% of adult men and 36.8% of adult women maintained a diet within the 30% recommendation. Foods eaten away from home contributed 30.9% of the total fat intake for men and 26.2% for women (Table 17.7). Cholesterol intake is considerably lesser in women than men. Women of all age groups consumed under 300 mg/day, whereas adult men generally consumed slightly more than 300 mg/day on average (Table 17.8 and Table 17.9). More adults consumed a diet consistent with the recommended cholesterol intake (55.1% of men; 79.4% of women) than that for total fat, where only 29.4% of adult men and 36.8% of adult women maintained a diet within 30% of the total energy intake. The intake of the types of fat — saturated, polyunsaturated, monounsaturated, and cholesterol — is presented in Table 17.8.

ENERGY AND OBESITY ISSUES

Overweight is associated with several chronic diseases — coronary heart disease, hypertension, non-insulin-dependent diabetes mellitus, and some forms of cancer.[19,20] WHO declared overweight as one of the current top ten health risks.[21] An estimated 300,000 Americans die every year from obesity-related conditions.[20] Obesity is also an associated risk factor for joint disease, gallstones, and obstructive sleep apnea.[22] In 1995, the economic cost associated with obesity was estimated at $62.3 billion.[23] The seriousness of obesity was further emphasized by the *Surgeon General*'s "Call to Action."[24]

From 1976–1980 and 1988–1994, the Centers for Disease Control and Prevention (CDC) reported an increase of 10% in the incidence of overweight in the American population.[25] Data from the CSFII, 1994 (http://www.ars.usda.gov/SP2UserFiles/

TABLE 17.7
Fiber Intake (g/Day)[a]

Age (Years)	M	F
20–29	18.3	13.2
30–39	19.4	13.6
40–49	18.3	14.0
50–59	18.5	14.5
60–69	18.5	14.2
70 >	17.7	14.2
20 <	18.6	13.9

M = males, F = females
A http://www.ars.usda.gov/SP2UserFiles/Place/
12355000/pdf/Tbs1995.PDF

TABLE 17.8
Daily Intake of SFA, MUFA, PUFA, and Cholesterol

	SFA		MUFA		PUFA		CHOL	
Age	M	F	M	F	M	F	M	F
20–29	35.4	22.3	40.1	25.2	19.6	13.5	348	219
30–39	35.3	21.3	39.4	24.1	20.1	12.8	362	217
40–49	30.6	21.0	35.6	24.0	18.3	13.6	331	222
50–59	28.6	19.1	33.9	22.6	18.1	13.1	332	200
60–69	25.9	17.9	30.1	20.8	16.5	12.1	307	218
>70	22.8	15.9	26.4	18.7	13.9	10.6	270	188
<20	31.3	20.0	36.8	23.0	18.4	12.8	331	213

SFA = Saturated fatty acids; MUFA = Monounsaturated fatty acids; PUFA =
Polyunsaturated fatty acids; CHOL = Cholesterol.

TABLE 17.9
**Percentage of Individuals Meeting the Recommendations
for Daily Total Fat, Saturated Fat, and Cholesterol Intakes**

	Total Fat (g)		SFA (g)		CHOL (mg)	
Age (Years)	M	F	M	F	M	F
20–29	29.3	40.1	34.1	42.3	63.1	77.0
30–39	28.1	35.9	30.7	39.7	62.6	80.9
40–49	27.4	30.5	31.7	38.5	53.5	76.0
50–59	28.0	36.5	36.2	46.0	54.2	80.7
60–69	33.9	38.0	42.1	46.1	58.1	78.7
>70	34.4	42.2	41.6	47.9	67.1	84.5
<20	29.4	36.8	34.5	42.7	55.1	79.4

M = males, F = females; SFA = Saturated fatty acids, CHOL = Cholersterol.
http://www.ars.usda.gov/SP2UserFiles/Place/12355000/pdf/Tbs1995.PDF

Place/12355000/pdf/Tbs1995.PDF), indicate that among adults, both men and women, the incidence of overweight is approximately 30% (Table 17.10). If the incidence of obesity continues to rise at current rates, it is predicted that, by 2230, every adult in the United States will be overweight.[26] Recent Behavioral Risk Factor Surveillance System (BRFSS) data indicate an increase in overweight in all demographic and geographic segments of the U.S. population.[27]

TABLE 17.10
Incidence of Overweight (%)[a]

Age (Years)	Men	Women
20–29	21.5	22.1
30–39	32.3	27.4
40–49	37.0	36.1
50–59	39.9	37.8
>60	40.7	33.4
<20	31.8	31.7

[a] http://www.ars.usda.gov/SP2UserFiles/
Place/12355000/pdf/Tbs1995.PDF

The prevalence of overweight/obesity among Americans is at odds with the perceptions of the importance of maintaining an appropriate body weight. When Americans were surveyed as part of the 1994 to 1996 USDA Diet and Health Knowledge survey, 68.1% of adult males over 20 years of age reported that "maintaining a healthy weight" was very important. For that same survey, 77% of the adult women over 20 years of age reported maintenance of a healthy body weight as very important. Given the importance Americans place on maintaining healthy body weight and given the high incidence of overweight/obesity, it is little wonder that Americans are forecast to spend some $54 billion on weight-loss products in 2009.[28] In addition, there are the myriad of weight-loss diets that appear on the market every year. In 1992, 33% to 40% of American women and 20% to 24% of American men reported being on a diet.[29]

FAD DIETS USED FOR WEIGHT-LOSS PROMOTION

While numerous fad diets come and go, several categories tend to remain fairly common. These include high-protein/low-carbohydrate diet regimens, low-fat diets, and very-low-calorie diets.

HIGH-PROTEIN/LOW-CARBOHYDRATE DIETS

These diets generally restrict the carbohydrate intake to 100 g/day or less. Restriction of carbohydrate leads to an initial mobilization of glycogen and then to gluconeogenesis and ketosis, all of which promote water loss and some lean tissue loss, which constitute a significant portion of the weight loss. Some of the low-carbohydrate diets promote high protein and consequently a higher animal fat intake, which is inconsistent with the dietary guidelines for fat intake.[30] Examples of high-protein/low-carbohydrate diets are Atkins' Diet Revolution, Calories Don't Count, and The Doctor's Quick Weight Loss Diet (Stillman's).

LOW-FAT DIETS

Generally these diets restrict fat intake to 20% or less of the total energy intake. Examples of these types of diets include the T-factor Diet, the Pasta Diet, the Pritikin Diet, and Fit or Fat. The average weight loss on these types of diets is 0.1 to 0.2 kg/week. With the limited fat intake, one drawback is the low-satiety factor, which may prompt noncompliant diet behavior.[31]

VERY-LOW-CALORIE DIETS

These diets arose during the 1970s and were known as protein-sparing modified fasts or liquid protein diets. These diet plans generally rely on liquid supplements to substitute for food intake and restrict the overall caloric level to less than 800 kcal/day. These diets may be indicated for moderately to highly obese patients (body mass index >30). The severe caloric restriction does lead to weight loss, but generally this level of caloric intake cannot be sustained, and weight regain is a potential problem. These diets may also lead to weight loss from lean tissue mass.[26,32]

THE ZONE DIET

The Zone Diet is a modified approach to the low-carbohydrate/high-protein type of diet. The diet promotes a macronutrient intake of 30% protein, 30% fat, and 40% carbohydrate. At this ratio of protein, fat, and carbohydrate, the author contends that insulin levels will remain stable, and this, in turn, dampens insulin's potential to promote the conversion of carbohydrates into fat and thereby to promote weight gain. The Zone Diet claims go beyond the promise of weight loss via insulin regulation into the realms of disease prevention. The Zone Diet author argues that a high-carbohydrate/low-fat diet promotes an imbalance in "bad" eicosanoid production, which can lead to the development of such diseases as arthritis and coronary heart disease. However, there is no significant body of evidence to support the author's claims.[33,34]

Putting fad diets aside, an approach to weight management that recognizes overweight or obesity as a chronic condition and incorporates the elements of a healthy diet, exercise, and behavior modification is more likely to be successful over time, particularly in the maintenance of weight loss.[35]

The Weight Control Information Network (WIN) provides research-based educational resources to Americans on weight-loss strategies, etc. [36]

PROTEIN INTAKE — HEALTH ISSUES

The average American diet is very liberal with respect to protein intake. The RDA for protein for women aged 19 to 24 years is 46 g, and for men of the same age the RDA is 58 g.[7] In contrast, the average protein intake in grams for adults over 20 years in the United States is 63.8 g for women and 94.9 g for men. Some concern has been expressed over the long-term health consequences of excessive protein intake. There is some evidence in humans that a lifetime on a high-animal-protein diet (typical American diet pattern) can aggravate existing renal problems,[37] may increase the risk for cancer of the kidney,[38] and can accelerate adult bone loss.[39, 40] Lastly, higher animal protein intake is associated with higher-than-desirable levels of total fat and saturated fat intake.

A primary, although not exclusive, source of protein in the American diet is meat. The U.S. Food Guide Pyramid recommends between 5 and 7 oz of cooked lean meat or equivalent in meat alternatives per day. To be consistent with the Dietary Guidelines to reduce total fat and saturated fat in the diet, it would be helpful to consume lower-fat types of meat and perhaps a greater amount of some forms of meat alternatives such as soybean products. However, Americans derive the majority of their protein from meat. The 1994 to 1996 CSFII indicated that, for adult males over 20 years of age, the average daily intake of meat and meat alternatives was 6.4 oz, and for women the total was 3.9 oz. With respect to total intake, men were consuming sufficient amounts of meat and meat alternatives when compared with the recommended 5 to 7 oz. Women, on the other hand, fell below the minimum 5 oz recommended in the U.S. Food Guide Pyramid. With that in mind, data from the CSFII indicate that, regardless of meat servings, protein intake is meeting RDA requirements. Consequently, the source of protein may be an important consideration. The ratio of meat to meat alternatives is skewed heavily in favor of meat (beef, pork, lamb, and veal). In men, of the average 6.4 oz of lean meat and meat alternatives consumed daily, 2.7 oz are derived from lean meat and another 1.0 oz from the higher fat-sources of frankfurter and lunch meat. Consequently, 3.7 of the 6.4 oz, or 58%, were from meat. Only 1.5 and 0.5 oz, respectively, were contributed by poultry and fish. Among women, 1.4 oz of meat and 0.5 oz of frankfurter and lunch meat were consumed on a daily average. This accounts for 49% of the total meat or meat-alternative consumption. In women, poultry contributed 1.1 oz and fish 0.4 oz toward the total meat and meat-alternative intake. Some data suggest that an increase in fish and consequently in omega-3 fatty acid intake may be warranted from a cancer prevention perspective.[41]

PROTEIN SUPPLEMENTS

Protein supplements are quite common among athletes and physically active adults as part of their strength training regimens.[42] Bucci[42] argues that, although there is very little research that documents the benefits of protein supplementation, high-protein diets are safe. However, the amount recommended for endurance athletes is 70 g/day, and for strength athletes 112 to 178 g. The lower range of these recommendations is clearly within the normal intake of American men. This argues against the need for further protein supplementation.

AMINO ACID SUPPLEMENTS

Individual amino acid supplements have periodically been promoted on the market periodically. Again, a target audience has often been the athlete or physically active adult, with promises of enhanced performance. There is a dearth of research that can support such claims.[42] In addition, in 1992 a scientific panel convened to address the safety of amino acid supplements concluded that there is little research on which to support making amino acid supplement recommendations, and some amino acid supplementation (serine and proline) can have adverse health effects. Consequently, the panel concluded that no level of amino acid supplementation may be considered safe at this time.[43]

FAT INTAKE ISSUES — AMOUNT AND TYPE OF FAT

The fat intake in the adult American diet is slightly over the recommended 30% of the total energy. Data from the 1994 to 1996 CSFII reveals that approximately 25% of the total energy intake is contributed by discretionary fats such as cream, butter, margarine, cream cheese, oil, lard, meat drippings, cocoa, and chocolate. Based on the average energy intake of adult males, discretionary fat contributes 614 kcal/day and, in females, 412 kcal/day. By cutting back on discretionary fat intake, American adults could conceivably lose 0.8 to 1.0 lb/week. This would be helpful in dealing with the adult obesity rates in the United States. Simple changes in discretionary fat intake could be helpful. For example, substituting mustard for mayonnaise on sandwiches gives 5 g (45 kcal) fat savings; ordering a hamburger instead of a cheeseburger gives 9 g(81 kcal) fat savings; using salt and pepper instead of sour cream on a baked potato gives 3 g (27 kcals) fat savings. Americans consume more saturated fat than is generally considered desirable. In addition, approximately 5% of the total fat intake in the American diet is contributed from *trans*-fatty acids.[44]

Biochemically, *trans*-fatty acids act similarly to saturated fatty acids, raising low-density lipoprotein (LDL) levels and decreasing high-density lipoprotein (HDL) levels.[45] Although their effect is not as great as saturated fat, they may contribute to a lipid intake pattern that raises the risk for coronary heart disease.[46] *trans*-Fatty acids are formed as a result of the hydrogenation process and are found in such food items as margarine, shortening, commercial frying fats, and many high-fat baked and snack foods. *trans*-Fatty acids also occur naturally in milk and butter because of the fatty acids synthesized by rumen flora in the rumen. Concern over *trans*-fatty acid intake has led some consumers to question whether they should forgo margarine and return to butter. Research suggests that saturated fat, as in butter, still exerts a greater negative effect on a person's lipid profile than do *trans*-fatty acids. However, use of less-hydrogenated forms such as tub rather than stick margarine may be beneficial.

However, some controversy has recently arisen with respect to the efficacy of low-fat diets with respect to breast cancer, colorectal cancer, and cardiovascular disease. Data from the Women's Health Initiative randomized, controlled dietary modification trial failed to demonstrate that low-fat diets could significantly reduce the risk for these conditions.[47-49]

CARBOHYDRATE INTAKE ISSUES

Two issues arise with respect to the carbohydrate intake of American adults — low-fiber intake and high-sugar intake. Low-fiber intake is associated with a higher incidence of such chronic diseases as heart disease,[50] cancer,[51] and diabetes.[52] At least partial explanation for the low-fiber intake is related to the low fruit and vegetable intake associated with the typical American diet. Data from the 1994 to 1996 CSFII indicated that for adult males the average total servings (based on the Food Guide Pyramid serving recommendations) of vegetables per day was four. For females, the average was three servings. For both men and women, one-third of the vegetable servings were accounted for by white potatoes. Average serving of fruit per day for both men and women was 1.5. This is just under the minimum Food Guide Pyramid recommendation for two servings per day. Another contributing factor to the low-fiber intake is the lack of whole-grain foods in the diet. Adult men consumed on average 8 servings of grain products per day, which is approximately midrange of the 6 to 11 servings of grain products recommended by the Food Guide Pyramid. Women averaged 6 servings from grain products. However, for both men and women, only one of these servings was from whole-grain products. The health benefits of a higher-fiber diet are addressed in other relevant sections of this handbook.

The other carbohydrate intake issue is the consumption of refined sugar, which contributes calories but little other nutritive value to the diet. The 1994 to 1996 CSFII data revealed that approximately 14% of the average energy intake for adult males was from added sugars. For women, the caloric contribution from added sugars was slightly higher at approximately 15%. Foods such as breads, cakes, soft drinks, jam, and ice cream were contributing to the discretionary sugar intake. In 1994 to 1996, soft drink consumption outpaced milk and coffee, and approximately 75% of the soft drink consumption is of the sugar-sweetened variety.[53]

During the last decade, consumption of snack foods such as cakes, cookies, pastries, and pies has increased 15%, likely contributing to the high intake of discretionary sugar.[52] These data are in contrast to the importance consumer's report they place on a diet moderate in sugar intake. A majority (slightly over 50%) of adults surveyed in the 1994 to 1996 CSFII indicated that it was very important to consume a diet moderate in sugar.

SUMMARY

Counseling the normal healthy American adult should focus on dietary intake patterns that promote health and reduce risk for chronic disease, that is, diet recommendations should follow the U.S. Dietary Guidelines. Therefore, consistent with the 2005 version of the U.S. Dietary Guidelines, the focus on nutrition counseling should be:

Adequate nutrients within calorie needs:
- Consume a nutrient-dense diet and adopt a healthy eating pattern as recommended in the USDA Food Guide or the DASH eating pattern.

Weight management:
- Calculate the appropriate weight for the individual.
- Consider the fat distribution pattern and take a more aggressive posture with individuals whose body fat distribution is more "apple" than "pear" shaped as that places them at higher health risk.

For individuals whose body weight is inappropriate, initiate counseling to assist in weight reduction. This may include calculation of appropriate caloric intake, recommendations of sources of caloric intake from the macronutrients of protein, fat, and carbohydrate, appropriate portion sizes to control caloric intake, and increases in physical activity.

Be physically active each day (see following guideline):

- *Physical Activity*: To reduce risk of chronic disease in adulthood, engage in 30 min of moderate intensity activity most days of the week. To manage body weight and prevent gradual weight loss, engage in 60 min of moderate intensity activity most days of the week. To sustain weight loss, participate in 60 to 90 min of moderate intensity activity daily.
- *Fats*: Keep total fat to 20% to 35% of total calories with less than 10% from saturated fats and a minimum of *trans*-fatty acids, as well as 300 mg of cholesterol or less per day.
- *Carbohydrates*: Choose fiber-rich sources of carbohydrates, and select and/or prepare foods with little added sugar or caloric sweeteners.
- *Sodium and Potassium*: Consume less than 2300 mg of sodium per day (< 1 teaspoon of salt). Choose and prepare foods with low sodium content/added sodium/salt. Consume more potassium-rich foods such as fruits and vegetables.
- *Alcoholic Beverages*: For those who drink, do so in moderation (defined as one drink per day for women and two drinks per day for men). Alcohol should not be consumed by those at risk for addiction to alcohol, pregnant or lactating women, children and adolescents, and those whose medication contraindicates alcohol consumption.
- *Food Safety*: Practice safe food preparation methods — washing of hands, clean contact surfaces in the preparation of foods, cooking to the appropriate temperature, refrigeration/freezing of food for proper storage, and the avoidance of raw eggs, poultry, sprouts, unpasteurized milk, and juices.

REFERENCES

1. U.S. Department of Health and Human Services, Public Health Service, No. 88-50210, *Surgeon General's Report on Nutrition and Health.* U.S. Government Printing Office, Washington, DC, 1988.
2. Dietary Guidelines for Americans, 2005. www.health.gov/dietaryguidelines
3. U.S. Senate, Select Committee on Nutrition and Human Needs, U.S. Senate, December 1977, 95th Congress — 1st Session.
4. U.S. Department of Agriculture, U.S. Department of Health and Human Services, *Nutrition and Your Health. Dietary Guidelines for Americans.* Home and Garden Bulletin No. 232, Washington, DC, 1980.
5. Kant, A.K., Graubard, B.I., Schatzkin, A., *J Nutr,* 134: 1793; 2004.
6. U.S. Department of Agriculture, *The Food Guide Pyramid.* Home and Garden Bulletin No. 252.a, U.S. Printing Office, Washington, DC, 1992.
7. Kant, A.K., Block, G., Schatzkin, A. et al., *JADA,* 91: 1526; 1991.
8. Food and Nutrition Board, National Research Council, *Recommended Dietary Allowances,* 10th ed. National Academy Press, Washington, DC, 1989.
9. Food and Nutrition Board, Institute of Medicine, *Dietary Reference Intakes for Calcium, Phosphorus, Magnesium, Vitamin D and Fluoride.* National Academy Press, Washington, DC, 1997.
10. Food and Nutrition Board, Institute of Medicine, *Dietary Reference Intakes for Thiamin, Riboflavin, Niacin, Vitamin B_6, Folate, Vitamin B_{12}, Pantothenic Acid, Biotin, and Choline.* National Academy Press, Washington, DC, 1998.
11. Bowman, S.A. et al., *The Healthy Eating Index: 1994–1996,* Publication CNPP-5, Center for Nutrition Policy and Promotion, U.S. Department of Agriculture, U.S. Government Printing Office, Washington, DC, 1998.
12. Bowman, S.A. et al., *Nutr Rev,* 49: 291; 1991.
13. Food and Drug Administration, Focus on Food Labeling. Special Issue of FDA Consumer Magazine, May 1993, DHHS Publication No. (FDA) 93-2262, U.S. Government Printing Office, Washington, DC, 1993.
14. American Cancer Society, Nutrition and Prevention, www2.cancer.org/Prevention/index.cfm?prevention=importance.
15. Wardlaw, G. *Contemporary Nutrition: Issues and Insights,* 3rd ed. Brown and Benchmark, Madison, WI, 1997.
16. Shetty, P.S., Henry, C.J.K., Black, A.E., Prentice, A.M., *Eur J Clin Nutr,* 1006: 11S; 1996.
17. Boyle, M.A., Morris, D.H., *Community Nutrition in Action: An Entrepreneurial Approach,* 2nd ed., Wadsworth Publishing, Belmont, CA, 1999, p. 112.
18. Federation of American Societies for Experimental Biology, Third Report on Nutrition Monitoring in the United States, Vol. 1, U.S. Government Printing Office, Washington, DC, 1995.
19. Centers for Disease Control and Prevention, National Diabetes Fact Sheet: National Estimate and General Information on Diabetes in the United States, U.S. Department of Health and Human Services, Centers for Disease Control and Prevention, Atlanta, GA, Nov. 1, 1977.
20. McGinnis, J.M., Foege, W.H., *JAMA,* 270: 2207; 1993.
21. World Health Organization (WHO), World Health Report, 2002: Reducing Risks, Promoting Healthy Lifestyle. World Health Organization, Geneva, Switzerland, 2002.

22. National Institutes of Health, National Heart, Lung and Blood Institute, Clinical guidelines on the identification, evaluation, and treatment of overweight and obesity in adults — the evidence report, Ob Res, 6: 51S; 1998.

23. Colditz, G.A., Wolf, A.M., In: *Progress in Obesity Research* (Anderson, A.H. et al., eds.) 7th International Congress on Obesity, John Libbey & Co., London 1996.

24. U.S. Department of Health and Human Services. *The Surgeon General's Call to Action to prevent and decrease overweight and obesity.* U.S. Department of Health and Human Services, Public Health Service, Office of the Surgeon General, Rockville, MD, 2001.

25. Centers for Disease Control and Prevention, Update: prevalence of overweight among children, adolescents and adults, United States, 1988–1994, Mortality and Morbidity Weekly Report, 46: 199; 1997b.

26. Foreyt, J., Goodrick, K., *Lancet*, 346: 134; 1995.

27. Center for Disease Control. Behavioral Risk Factor Surveillance System. www.cdc.gov/brfss/

28. http://www.foodnavigator.com/news/ng.asp?n=65804-obesity-weight-low-fat

29. National Institutes of Health, *Methods for voluntary weight loss and control*, Technology Assessment Conference, Bethesda, MD, 1992.

30. The Low-Carb, High-Protein Craze, *Am Inst Cancer Res Newslett*, 67, Spring 2000. p. 1.

31. American Dietetic Association, Position of the American Dietetic Association: Very-low-calorie weight loss diets, *JADA*, 90: 722; 1990.

32. Kendall, A., Levitski, D.A., Strupp, B.J., Lissner, L., *Am J Clin Nutr*, 53: 1124; 1991.

33. U.C. Berkeley Wellness Letter, June, 1998. p. 1.

34. Liebman, B., *Nutr Action Health Lett*, July/August, 1996. p. 1.

35. Rippe, J.M., Crossley, S., Ringer, R., Obesity as a chronic disease: modern medical and lifestyle management, *JADA*, 98: S9; 1998.

36. National Institute of Health. National Institute of Diabetes and Digestive and Kidney Diseases. Weight Control Information Network. www.niddk.nih.gove/health/nutrit/WIN.htm

37. Ahmed, F.E., *JADA*, 91: 1266; 1991.

38. Chow, W.H., Gridley, G., McLaughlin, J.K. et al., *J Natl Cancer Inst*, 86: 1131; 1994.

39. Hu, J., Zhao, X.H., Parpia, B., *Am J Clin Nutr*, 58: 398; 1993.

40. Heaney, R.P., *JADA*, 93: 1259; 1993.

41. Simopoulos, A.P., Kim, Y., Mason, J.B., *Nutr Rev*, 54: 259; 1996.

42. Bucci, L., *Nutrients as Ergogenic Aids for Sports and Exercise*, CRC Press, Boca Raton, 1993.

43. Anderson, S.A., Raiten, D.J., Eds, *Safety of Amino Acids Used as Supplements*, Federation of American Societies for Experimental Biology, Bethesda, MD, 1992.

44. Emken, E.A., *Am J Clin Nutr*, 62: 659S; 1995.

45. Katan, M.B., Zock, P.L., *Ann Rev Nutr*, 15: 473; 1995.

46. Shapiro, S., *Am J Clin Nutr*, 66: 1011S; 1997.

47. Prentice, R.L. et al., *JAMA*, 295: 629. 2006.

48. Beresford, S.A.A. et al., *JAMA*, 295: 643. 2006.

49. Howard, B.V., *JAMA*, 295: 655; 2006.

50. Jenkins, D.J.A., *New Eng J Med*, 329: 21; 1993.

51. Munster, I.P., de Boer, H.M., Jansen, M.C. et al., *Am J Clin Nutr*, 59: 626; 1994.

52. Salmeron, J., Manson, J.E., Stampfer, M.J. et al., *JAMA*, 277: 472; 1997.

53. Frazao, E., Ed., *America's Eating Habits, Economic Research Service Report*. Agriculture Information Bulletin No. 750. Washington, DC, 1999.

18 Nutrition in Later Years

Mary Ann Johnson and Sohyun Park

CONTENTS

INTRODUCTION

Older adults are a diverse and growing population. They range in age from 65 to more than 100 years and include the very fit and the very frail. Older adults vary in ethnicity and culture, income, mobility, knowledge of nutrition and health, health behaviors, and health status. The main nutritional problems are poor food patterns and nutrient intake, as well as an increasing prevalence of overweight and obesity. The requirements for most essential vitamins and minerals do not change with advanced age, with only a few exceptions. Requirements for calcium and vitamin D are increased, and the recommended chemical form of vitamin B_{12} changes to crystalline. Decreased lean body mass and low physical activities are the main determinants of the low energy requirements of older people. Paradoxically, older adults are at increased risk for both overnutrition (overweight and obesity) and undernutrition, with the accompanying problems of nutritional deficiencies and weight loss. This chapter will review the primary nutritional problems associated with aging and recommend ways to improve the nutritional status of older people.

DEMOGRAPHICS OF AGING

The growth rate of elderly population (over 65 years) has rapidly increased during the last few decades and will continue to increase for the next 50 years in the United States.[1] The number of people over 65 was 36 million in 2003 and is expected to increase to nearly 55 million in 2020 and to 87 million in 2050.[1,2] About 88% of older adults were aged 65 to 84, and 12% were aged 85 and older in 2000 (Figure 18.1).[1] The majority of people aged 65 and more are white, followed by black and Hispanic (Figure 18.2).[2] Over 96% of older adults live in the community rather than in long-term care facilities.[2] Human life expectancy has increased dramatically during the last decades. Those who are 65 years old today can expect to live more than 18 additional years, and 85 year olds can expect more than 6 additional years.[2]

Aging is an inevitable process. The efficiencies of cell function and homeostatic mechanisms decrease with advanced age. In some organs, new cells replace old cells.[3] However, during each replication; the telomeres are shortened in chromosomes.

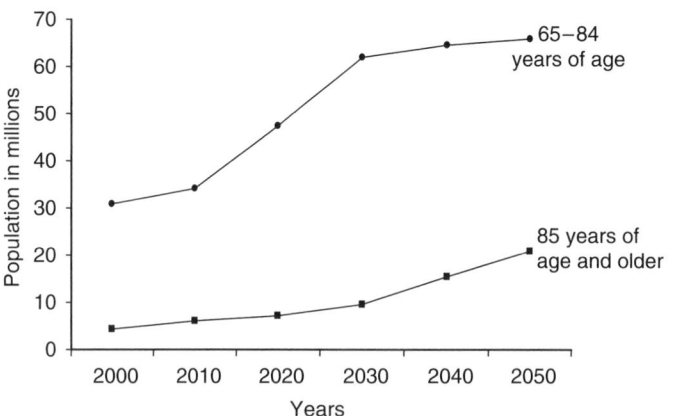

FIGURE 18.1 Projected population over 65 years of age in the United States: 2000 to 2050. (From U.S. Census Bureau, U.S. Interim projection by age, sex, race, and Hispanic origin, 2004.)

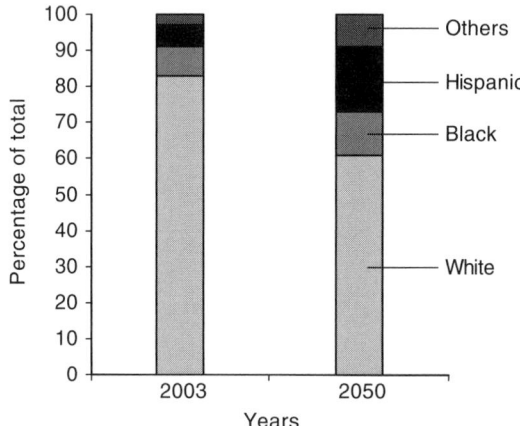

FIGURE 18.2 Projected population aged 65 and older in the United States by race: 2003 and 2050. (From Federal Interagency Forum on Aging and Related Statistics, Older Americans 2004: Key Indicators of well being, 2004.)

This incomplete replication is a part of the aging process and results in diminished cell functions.[4] Cells in some organs (e.g., reproductive organs) are not replaced by new cells. The numbers of cells are decreased as part of the natural aging process. However, aging itself may not cause visible diminished cell function. For example, physically and emotionally active older adults have better body function than less-active older adults.[3]

Most older adults have one or more age-related diseases. Common diseases are memory loss, cognitive impairment, depression, chronic disability, hearing impairment, visual impairment, osteopenia, Parkinson's disease, dental and oral health problems, gastrointestinal disorders, neoplasms, kidney disease, and paralysis (Table 18.1). Nutrition is a component in the prevention or management of most of this health conditions.[5] With increased human longevity, healthy aging, and well-being are important issues. Although certain age-related diseases are common in older adults, healthy diet, and lifestyle may delay the onset of diseases and diminish the severity of symptoms.[4,6]

NUTRITION ASSESSMENT

As will be discussed throughout this chapter, overnutrition and undernutrition are serious and prevalent problems in older people. Undernutrition and overnutrition can impair many aspects of the quality of life.[7] However, nutrition assessment is not routinely considered in geriatric assessments.[6] Nutrition assessment helps to prevent or improve health risks caused by malnutrition.[8] Most tools are questionnaires that collect information about food intake, ingestion and digestion, alcohol intake, mobility, age, presence of diseases, medical history, mental condition, family history, anthropometric measures, biochemical measures, and functional impairment.[9] Some tools are developed for hospital patients or for fragile older adults[9] and may not provide useful information for healthy, community-dwelling older adults who may have different nutrition problems and goals than frail individuals.[10] Nutritional assessment tools that meet criteria for reliability, validity, sensitivity, and specificity are recommended and are described elsewhere.[9]

TALBE 18.1

Selected Chronic Health Conditions in Adults 65 and Older (2001 to 2002)

	Men (%)	Women (%)
Hypertension	47	52
Heart disease	37	27
Arthritis symptoms	31	39
Any cancer	25	18
Diabetes	18	14
Stroke	10	8
Asthma	7	9
Chronic bronchitis	5	7
Emphysema	7	4

Source: From Federal Interagency Forum on Aging and Related Statistics, Older Americans 2004: Key Indicators of Well-being, 2004.

DIET, LIFESTYLE, MORBIDITY, AND MORTALITY

Similar to other age groups, the older adult population does not consume the recommended amounts of key nutrients and food groups such as fruits, vegetables, whole grains, and milk products (Table 18.2). Healthy diets and body weight, along with other healthy lifestyle practices, delay disability, improve quality of life, and compress morbidity — that is, shorten the period of poor health and disability prior to death.[22–25] Abundant intakes of fruits, vegetables, and whole grains with adequate protein and essential fats are associated with the lowest risk of chronic diseases.[19,25–28] In midlife, for example, controlling body weight and cardiovascular disease risk factors, both of which are profoundly affected by food patterns and portion sizes, leads to better quality of life in the domains of physical and mental limitations, bodily pain, energy and fatigue, social functioning, and mental health later in life.[22,23] The combination of a healthy lifestyle and a "Mediterranean diet" reduced mortality from cardiovascular diseases, coronary heart disease, and cancer[25] and lowered blood pressure.[29] Men in the Baltimore Longitudinal Study of Aging who consumed ≥ 5 servings and fruits and vegetables daily and $\leq 12\%$ of energy from saturated fat were 76% less likely to die of cardiovascular disease and 31% less likely to die of any cause.[30]

Increasing health care costs and the personal burdens of chronic diseases caused by the global obesity epidemic are prompting serious evaluation of the roles of nutrition and other lifestyle factors in preventing and managing chronic diseases.[31] The Institute of Medicine (IOM) evaluated the role of nutrition in maintaining health for the Medicare population.[32] They emphasized that poor nutrition, inadequate nutrient intakes, and obesity are major problems, and the vast majority (86%) of older Americans have chronic conditions in which nutrition interventions have been shown to improve both health and quality of life. As part of a comprehensive management and treatment approach, nutrition therapy was recommended for dyslipidemia (high blood cholesterol and triglycerides), hypertension, heart failure, diabetes, and kidney failure. The IOM recognized the Registered Dietitian (RD) as the most qualified health professional to provide medical nutrition therapy, which includes individualized nutrition services and procedures to treat an illness, injury, or condition.

RISK FACTORS FOR POOR NUTRITIONAL STATUS

Many social, mental, physical, economical, and individual choice factors contribute to poor nutritional status (Table 18.3).[10,33] Hearing and visual impairments may cause social segregation due to difficulty in communicating with others. Physical disability may decrease mobility and limit daily activities, such as shopping for groceries and cooking meals.[6,34] Low income,[35,36] taking several medications,[37] eating alone, loneliness, bereavement, depression, and cognitive impairment,[38,39] cause poor nutritional status in the elderly. Oral health disorders may limit food intakes and choices because of chewing and swallowing difficulties. Therefore, diminished quantity and quality of food are concerns.[40–43] In addition to being homebound, residing in a nursing home or being hospitalized may also impair nutrition status.[33] Although older adults are less likely to be in poverty than children, poverty rates are high among older adults (10 vs. 17% in 2002).[2] Poverty increases the risk of having inadequate income for food, housing, health care, and other needs. Some older adults may have difficulty with transportation,[44] which could impair access to food.

HUNGER AND FOOD SECURITY

Incomes below poverty line increase the risk of food insufficiency, food insecurity, hunger, low intakes of calories, vitamins, and minerals, and low body weight.[35,36,45,46] For example, compared to older adults with sufficient food, those experiencing

TABLE 18.2
Nutrient and Food Recommendations versus Intake among Older Adults

Nutrients	Recommendations	Intakes from Diet (not Including Supplements)
Calcium (mg/day)		
Men	1200[11]	797[12]
Women	1200	660
Vitamin D (IU/day)		
Men	1000[11]	212[13]
Women	1000	188
Vitamin B$_{12}$ (μg of crystalline/day)		
Men	2.4[14]	5.3[15] (crystalline unknown)
Women	2.4	3.9 (crystalline unknown)
Sodium (mg/day)		
Men	< 1300[16]	3447[12]
Women	< 1300	2532
Potassium (mg/day)		
Men	4700[16]	3059[12]
Women	4700	2367
Protein (g/day)		
Men	56[17]	79.7[17]
Women	46	59.1
Fiber (g/day)		
Men	30[17]	18.0[17]
Women	21	14.2
Saturated fat (% energy)		
Men	10[17]	10.8[18]
Women	10	10.6
Food groups		
Milk and milk products as a source of calcium and other key nutrients (cups of milk/day)	3[19]	~1[13]
Whole grains (servings/day)	3[19]	~1[20]
Fruits and vegetables (servings/day)		
Men, sedentary, 2000 calories/day		
Women, sedentary, 1600 calories/day	> 9[19]	5.7[21]
	> 7	4.7

Source: From USDHHS & USDA, 2005. *2005 Dietary Guidelines for Americans.* Institute of Medicine, *Dietary Reference Intakes for Calcium, Phosphorus, Magnesium, Vitamin D, and Fluoride.* National Academy of Sciences. Washington DC, National Academy Press, 1997. Ervin, R.B. et al, *Advanced data from vital and health statistics,* no. 341, 2004. Moore, C.E., Murphy, M.M., and Holick, M.F. *J. Nutr.,* 135:2478, 2005. Institute of Medicine, *Dietary Reference Intakes for Thiamin, Riboflavin, Niacin, Vitamin B$_6$, Folate, Vitamin B$_{12}$, Pantothenic Acid, Biotin, and Choline.* National Academy of Sciences, Washington DC, National Academy Press, 1998. Ervin, R.B. et al, *Advanced data from vital and health statistics,* no. 339, 2004. Food and Nutrition Board. *Dietary Reference Intakes for Water, Potassium, Sodium, Chloride, and Sulfate, National Academy of Sciences.* Washington DC, National Academy Press, 2004. Food and Nutrition Board, *Dietary Reference Intakes for Energy, Carbohydrate, Fiber, Fat, Fatty Acids, Cholesterol, Protein, and Amino Acids (Macronutrients),* National Academy of Sciences. Washington DC, National Academy Press, 2005. Wright, J.D. et al, *Advanced data from vital and health statistics,* no. 334, 2003. Cleveland, L.E. et al, J. Am. College. Nutr., 19(3), 331S, 2000. Produce for Better Health Foundation, 2005.

food insufficiency were four times more likely to have a low body weight, consumed nearly 300 fewer calories each day, and consumed less protein, meat, and vegetables.[36] Older adults have low participation rates in food stamp programs and other federal, state, and local assistance programs.[35] Reasons include a lack of awareness of the programs, perception that the benefits are too low to be worth the effort of applying, reluctance to accept food assistance because of stigma associated with receiving public assistance, and a lack of transportation or physical mobility to reach the site of the program.[35] Residence in rural and urban areas can present problems related to food access. Older adults may not have transportation to the grocery store or may have physical impairments in their ability to shop, cook, or eat. Elder abuse or neglect also can interfere with the ability to obtain adequate food.

TABLE 18.3

Lifestyle and Socioeconomic Changes Affecting the Nutritional Status of the Elderly

Changes with aging include:
- Reduced income with retirement
- Insufficient funds for purchase of food
- Skipping meals
- Illness and increased medical expenses
- Loss of mobility
- Diminished acuity in sensory perceptions (hearing, vision, and taste)
- Inability to drive to doctor's appointments or to the grocery store
- Inability to prepare or store food
- Loss of balance
- Diminished self-esteem
- Social isolation

Diseases that are common in the elderly and impact on their nutritional status include:
- Senile dementia of Alzheimer's type, with cognitive impairment and memory
- Arthritis, with fractures and deformities
- Parkinson's disease, with rigidity and tremor
- Dental and oral health problems — problems with chewing
- Gastrointestinal disorders — swallowing difficulties
- Neoplasms, with hypercatabolism, anorexia, and cachexia
- Diabetes mellitus, with restrictive diets and medication interactions
- Renal insufficiency, with restrictive diets and dialysis treatment
- Paralysis, limiting mobility
- Depression, leading to anorexia

Source: From Feldman, E.B., in *Handbook of Nutrition and Food*, Berdanier, C.D., Ed. CRC Press. Boca Raton, FL, 2002.

There are several ways to address the problem of food security.[45] Screening for food insecurity with tools that assess all the dimensions of food insecurity in older adults will improve identification of those in need. Screening and information about local food resources and food budgeting can be provided in many settings such as senior centers, public health programs, faith-based organizations, physician's offices, and hospitals.

UNDERNUTRITION, POOR APPETITE, AND WEIGHT LOSS

A physiological decrease in food intake called "anorexia of aging" occurs even in healthy older adults.[39,42] Weight loss is common and is associated with frailty, functional impairment, immune disorders, pressure ulcers, hip fractures, cognitive impairment, low quality of life, and increased mortality. Weight loss results in loss of muscle mass, which decreases energy needs. Physical activity helps maintain muscle mass, so physically active older people experience fewer declines in muscle mass. The digestion process in the stomach diminishes with advanced age, which leads to faster feelings of satiety and lower food intake. Also, changes in some hormones that sense satiety and changes in energy expenditure contribute to decreased food intake. The ability to adjust subsequent food intake after under- or overeating is impaired with advanced age. Sensing and responding to thirst is impaired, increasing the risk of dehydration.

Some chronic diseases are associated with negative energy balance (e.g., more energy is expended than is taken in) and weight loss.[42] Weight loss associated with low food intake is common in Alzheimer's disease. Energy needs are increased with congestive heart failure, chronic obstructive pulmonary disease, Parkinson's disease, and infections. Infectious diseases can increase energy needs and at the same time interfere with appetite. Low income,[35,36] taking several medications,[37] poor oral health and dysphagia (swallowing difficulties),[6,41,42] alcoholism,[39,47] eating alone, loneliness, social isolation, bereavement, depression, and cognitive impairment[38,39] are also risk factors for poor appetite, low food intake, malnutrition, and weight loss. Changes in taste and smell associated with aging, chronic health problems, and medications can interfere with appetite and the ability to enjoy food.[42]

Treatment for poor appetite, weight loss, and undernutrition is guided by a medical evaluation and recommendations and should involve the older adult, as well as their family members and caregivers.[38,39,48,49] Poor appetite and eating habits are not a normal part of aging. The goal is to improve oral intake, which can be facilitated by honoring food preferences at meals and snacks, using stronger flavorings and seasonings, or substituting higher-calorie versions of familiar foods. Taste tests by the older individual can help identify nutritional supplements, such as liquids and bars that are most palatable and best tolerated in addressing poor appetite, weight loss, and undernutrition.

Families, caregivers, and the health care team needs to find a balance between the benefits and risks of therapeutic diets for older people experiencing poor appetite and weight loss. When medically appropriate, therapeutic diets should be liberalized for the undernourished older adult. Overly restrictive diets, such as those low in cholesterol, fat, salt, and sugar, may take much of the enjoyment out of eating. Therefore, these restrictions should be used with caution in those with poor appetite and unintentional weight loss. To maintain muscle mass and energy levels, it is vitally important that those with poor appetite and weight loss ingest adequate proteins, vitamins, and minerals from a variety of foods insofar as possible. Failure to consume protein will result in further deterioration of muscle mass, loss of strength, and poor recovery from illness.

BODY COMPOSITION, OBESITY, OVERWEIGHT AND CHRONIC DISEASE

Older adults are affected by the obesity epidemic.[48,50–55] The prevalence of overweight (BMI ≥ 25 to <30 kg/m^2) and obesity (BMI ≥ 30 kg/m^2) among those aged ≥ 60 is 73.9% in men and 68.4% in women (National Health and Nutrition Examination Survey, NHANES, 1999–2000).[51] The prevalence of obesity among those aged ≥ 60 in men is 30.5% and in women is 34.7%.

In addition to weight gain, aging is associated with marked increases in total body fat and visceral fat increases and decreases in skeletal muscle.[55,56] This loss of skeletal muscle is called sarcopenia, and may be caused by low physical activity, changes in hormone function, resistance to insulin, and perhaps increased dietary protein needs.[56] The process of sarcopenia is accelerated by low physical activity, weight loss, and low protein intake. "Sarcopenic obesity" is a condition in which low muscle mass and high-fat mass coexist.[57] High-fat mass promotes a biochemical imbalance that promotes insulin resistance and further muscle loss, eventually leading to disability and obesity-related disorders (Figure 18.3).[57]

Overweight and obesity are associated with increased health care costs and numerous chronic disorders in older adults including hypertension, diabetes mellitus, metabolic syndrome, dyslipidemia, coronary artery disease, respiratory disease, and some types of cancers.[48,50,55,59,60] Depressive symptoms may accompany obesity. Of particular significance are the physical

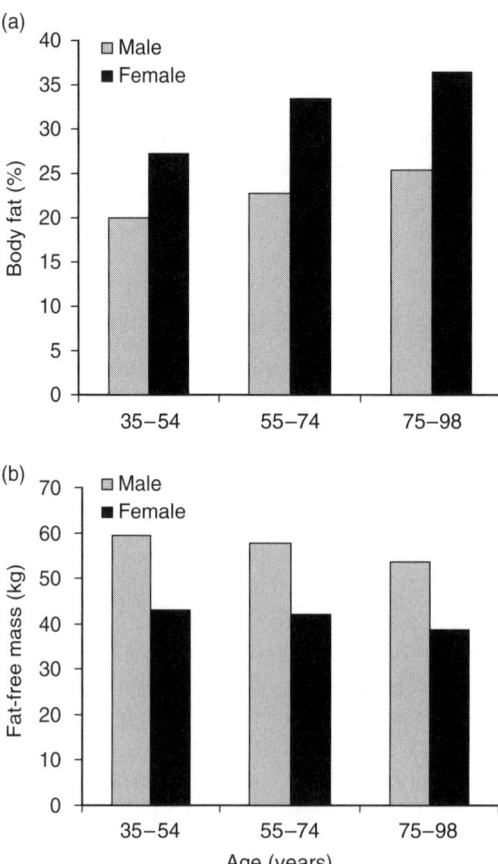

FIGURE 18.3   (a) Changes in percentage of body fat by age and gender. (b) Changes in fat-free mass (kg) by age and gender. (From Schutz, Y. et al., *Int. J. Obes.*, 26: 953; 2002.)[58]

disabilities associated with overweight and obesity, such as impaired walking, traveling, shopping, and preparing food. Obesity may cause premature aging. For example, the prevalence of severe disability (having three or more impairments in activities of daily living) was 6% in those aged 51 to 60, which was similar to nonobese people aged 70 and older (7%).[50]

Although genetic predisposition is related to obesity, there are several modifiable risk factors for obesity such as environment, lifestyle, and behavioral issues. During middle age, many people experience weight gain that is associated, at least in part, with a sedentary lifestyle. Weight gain and a sedentary lifestyle might be accepted as a normal part of the aging process, which might cause older adults to make few efforts toward prevention.[48]

In the older adult, obesity appears to be associated with poor food choices, high intakes of fat and saturated fat, low intakes of fiber and micronutrients, and low blood levels of micronutrients.[61,62] Obesity also has been associated with poor vitamin D status, perhaps because of low vitamin D intakes or redistribution of vitamin D into the fat mass.[63] Thus, obese older adults are at risk for nutrient excesses (energy, fat, and carbohydrate) as well as nutrient deficiencies (protein, vitamins, and minerals).[61–63]

The American Society for Nutrition (ASN) and NAASO, The Obesity Society provided a technical review and position statement regarding obesity in older adults.[55] They noted that appropriate treatment for obesity in older adults is controversial, but current research shows that weight-loss therapy in obese older people improves physical function, quality of life, and the medical complications associated with obesity. Of the three treatment options, lifestyle intervention is the primary approach, while pharmacotherapy and surgery appear to have less support and higher complication rates. It is widely agreed that overweight or obese older adults should not gain additional weight, but weight loss cannot be broadly recommended or attempted without medical evaluation and supervision.[48,53,54,64] Thus, ASN and NAASO emphasize the importance of a thorough medical history, physical examination, medication review, and assessment of readiness to lose weight before initiating weight loss therapy.[55]

The value of medically supervised lifestyle intervention has been demonstrated.[55,64] For example, a medically supervised 3-month weight loss program was conducted in obese older women ($N = 18$, 16 non-Hispanic white, 2 African Americans, 60 to 75 years).[64] At baseline, there was an average of 3.2 comorbidities per participant, 72% had a history of hypertension, 39% had a history of dyslipidemia, 6% had a history of diabetes, 11% had elevated glucose, and 39% presented with a history of the metabolic syndrome. Participants took an average of more than seven medications. Women met with a bariatric physician at the beginning and end of the intervention and had eight 30-min counseling sessions with a dietitian. This intervention emphasized prudent diet, behavior modification, and physical activity (primarily walking). Participants were advised to take multivitamins, as well as calcium and vitamin D supplements to help prevent the bone loss that may accompany weight loss. After the intervention, these women had decreased body weight (4.3 kg), BMI, fat-free mass (muscle), fat mass, diastolic blood pressure, total cholesterol, triglycerides, improved physical performance and vitality, and increased step counts.[64] Given the overall disease history of these obese women, it is clear that medical supervision is required. In agreement with others,[53–55] Jensen et al.[64] emphasized that management of weight loss in older adults should be guided by an evaluation of the potential risks and benefits for each individual. It was also emphasized that the preservation of strength and flexibility, rather than weight reduction, might be a better goal than weight reduction in the obese and frail older adult.

NUTRIENT REQUIREMENTS AND INTAKES

The authoritative sources of nutrient recommendations for older adults are the Dietary Reference Intakes[65] and the Dietary Guidelines for Americans.[19] Recommended intakes vary with age and gender (Table 18.2 and Table 18.4). The low intake of several key nutrients and food groups shows a great need for nutrition education and health promotion targeted to older adults (Table 18.2). Compared to younger people, nutrient requirements are not uniformly increased or decreased. Aging decreases energy needs because of the loss of muscle mass and low physical activity. Iron needs are decreased in women because of the cessation of menstruation. The increased need for calcium is related to decreased absorption efficiency, and the increased recommendation for vitamin D is related to decreased sun exposure and skin synthesis.

DIETARY SUPPLEMENTS

Dietary supplements include vitamins, minerals, herbs and other botanicals, amino acids, and other substances. Dietary supplement use is high among older adults — about 40% in women and 52% in older men.[66] Non-Hispanic black and Mexican Americans are less likely to use dietary supplements than non-Hispanic whites.[66]

Some nutrient-containing dietary supplements are recommended for older adults by the Dietary Guidelines and other reliable sources.[67] Recommended supplements include vitamin B_{12}[19] and vitamin D[19,67] from fortified foods or supplements, and calcium supplements for those not consuming adequate calcium from dietary sources.[67] While typical foods can be consumed to meet the dietary requirements for vitamin B_{12} and calcium, it is unlikely that those foods will be fortified to the high levels needed to meet the recommendation of 1000 IU of vitamin D daily. It has been recognized for several years that older adults are particularly vulnerable to deficiencies of vitamin B_{12}, vitamin D, and calcium,[68] so these three nutrients will be discussed in the next sections.

TABLE 18.4
Vitamin and Mineral Recommendations for the Elderly (Recommended Dietary Allowances, Adequate Intakes or Dietary Guidelines for Americans)

	Males (Age in Years)		Females (Age in Years)	
	51 to 70	> 70	51 to 70	> 70
Vitamin A, retinol (μg/d)	900	900	700	700
Vitamin C (mg/d)	90	90	75	75
Vitamin D (μg/d)	25	25	25	25
Vitamin E (mg/d)	15	15	15	15
Vitamin K (μg/d)	120	120	90	90
Thiamin (mg/d)	1.2	1.2	1.1	1.1
Riboflavin (mg/d)	1.3	1.3	1.1	1.1
Niacin (mg/d)	16	16	14	14
Vitamin B_6 (mg/d)	1.7	1.7	1.5	1.5
Folate (μg/d)	400	400	400	400
Vitamin B_{12}, crystalline (μg/d)	2.4	2.4	2.4	2.4
Pantothenic (mg/d)	5	5	5	5
Biotin (μg/d)	30	30	30	30
Choline (mg/d)	550	550	425	425
Calcium (mg/d)	1200	1200	1200	1200
Chromium (μg/d)	30	30	20	20
Copper (μg/d)	900	900	900	900
Fluoride (mg/d)	4	4	3	3
Iodine (μg/d)	150	150	150	150
Iron (mg/d)	8	8	8	8
Magnesium (mg/d)	420	420	320	320
Manganese (mg/d)	2.3	2.3	1.8	1.8
Molybdenum (μg/d)	45	45	45	45
Phosphorus (mg/d)	700	700	700	700
Selenium (μg/d)	55	55	55	55
Zinc (mg/d)	11	11	8	8

Source: From Food and Nutrition Board, Institute of Medicine, National Academies. *Dietary Reference Intakes (DRIs): Recommended Intakes for Individuals, Vitamins, Elements.* National Academy of Sciences. Washington DC, National Academy Press, 2004. USDHHS & USDA, 2005. *2005 Dietary Guidelines for Americans.*

VITAMIN B_{12}

Vitamin B_{12} is essential for cognition, the nervous system, vascular health, and red blood cell synthesis.[69] Poor vitamin B_{12} status has been linked to depression in some studies.[70] Poor vitamin B_{12} status is prevalent among older adults (5% to 20%)[69] and is particularly high among recipients of home delivered or congregate meals.[71] Vitamin B_{12} deficiency among these vulnerable elders was associated with poor cognition.[71,72] The prevalence of vitamin B_{12} deficiency increases with age, mainly because of decreased ability to digest the natural chemical form of vitamin B_{12} found in meat, poultry, fish, and dairy foods.[69] About 10 to 30% of older adults have atrophic gastritis, which is caused by infection of the stomach with *Helicobacter pylori* and subsequent atrophy of the cells in the stomach that secrete acid and digestive enzymes needed for the digestion and absorption of vitamin B_{12}.[69] Protein-bound vitamin B_{12} from animal foods requires these digestive enzymes, while the crystalline form does not. Crystalline vitamin B_{12} from fortified foods and dietary supplements is believed to be normally absorbed in those with atrophic gastritis. About 1 to 2% of older adults have pernicious anemia, which is a loss of the intrinsic factor needed for intestinal absorption of vitamin B_{12}. Under medical supervision, vitamin B_{12} status in these individuals is maintained by monthly injections of vitamin B_{12} or daily oral doses of 500 to 2000 μg.[73]

Similar to the Dietary Reference Intakes, the Dietary Guidelines recommends that the RDA for vitamin B_{12} (2.4 μg/day) be met from crystalline sources such as a vitamin B_{12}-containing fortified foods or supplements. Crystalline vitamin B_{12} is in many, but not all, fortified breakfast cereals and multivitamin supplements. The Daily Value for vitamin B_{12} is 6 μg;[74] therefore, a single serving of a vitamin B_{12}-containing food and supplement with at least 40% of the Daily Value would meet the RDA for vitamin B_{12}. Several studies show that older adults consuming between 9 and 50 μg of vitamin B_{12} daily, often found in multivitamins marketed to older adults, have improved vitamin B_{12} status.[46] There is no Upper Level for vitamin B_{12}, and it is generally considered nontoxic.

VITAMIN D

The 2005 Dietary Guidelines for Americans recommends that older adults consume 1000 IU (25 μg) daily of vitamin D, which is a substantial increase above the Adequate Intake (50 to 70 years: 400 IU; >70 years: 600 IU).[11] There is considerable interest in vitamin D, which was the subject of two recent symposia.[75,76] Adequate vitamin D status is needed for optimal calcium absorption,[19] and poor vitamin D status has been linked to numerous health conditions.[75,76] There is evidence from randomized control trials that vitamin D or calcium supplements decrease the risk of falls and bone fractures.[77–82]

Vitamin D comes from diet, supplements, and skin synthesis. Older adults, as well as people with dark pigmented skin or people who use sunscreen properly, have low synthesis of vitamin D precursors in the skin, even in sunny areas of the United States such as southern Florida.[83,84] People living at higher altitudes in the northern United States are particularly at risk for vitamin D deficiency. In addition to low skin synthesis, darker skinned ethnic/racial groups may be at increased risk of poor vitamin D status because of lower intakes of dairy foods and vitamin D containing supplements, as well as from obesity which may lead to less time spent in the sun or sequestration of vitamin D in the fat mass.[84]

The best marker of vitamin D status from oral intake and skin synthesis is serum 25-hydroxyvitamin D. Optimal serum 25-hydroxyvitamin D may be as high as 80 nmol/L based on randomized control trials of vitamin D supplementation and bone fractures and minimization of parathyroid hormone.[85] Mean concentrations of serum 25-hydroxyvitamin D are well below 80 nmol/L, particularly in darker-skinned older individuals.[86] In NHANES III, concentrations among older non-Hispanic whites, Hispanics, and non-Hispanic blacks in men were 76, 66, and 53 nmol/L, respectively, and in women were 64, 59, and 47.[86]

It is very difficult to meet vitamin D recommendations from food alone, so supplements are needed. The amount of supplement needed depends on the dietary intake of vitamin D. Salmon has about 324 to 624 IU vitamin D per 100 g, and canned tuna has 236 IU vitamin D per 100 g, and the average among the 26 fish products was about 300 IU per 100 g.[87] Milk has 100 IU per cup. Most other vitamin-D-fortified foods have less than 40 IU of vitamin D per serving. The Upper Level of vitamin D is 2000 IU daily, so older adults should carefully read the labels on supplements to ensure staying below the Upper Level. This will be particularly important if the supplement industry markets higher potency vitamin D supplements than those currently available.

CALCIUM

Calcium is most well-known for its role in bone health and is required for many other essential functions.[11,19] Diet provides only 55 to 66% of the recommended amounts of calcium (Table 18.2). The Dietary Guidelines recommend food sources of calcium, but does not mention calcium supplements. The Surgeon General's report on bone health and osteoporosis provides an algorithm to calculate calcium intake from the diet,[67] which can then be used to determine the amount of calcium, if any, needed from supplements. For older adults, they suggest starting with a baseline amount of calcium of 290 mg, which is the average of amount of calcium from non-calcium-rich foods, then adding 300 mg for each 8-ounce serving of milk or equivalent serving of other calcium-rich foods (e.g., yogurt, cheese, calcium-fortified juice). The shortfall can be obtained from supplements. Careful labeling reading should ensure that the Upper Level for calcium 2500 mg daily is not exceeded.

ANTIOXIDANT SUPPLEMENTS

The United States Preventive Services Task Force (USPSTF)[88] concluded that there is insufficient evidence to recommend for or against the use of vitamin A, C, or E supplements, multivitamins with folic acid, or antioxidant combinations for prevention of cancer or cardiovascular disease. The USPSTF did recommend against using supplements of β-carotene for prevention of cancer or cardiovascular disease because of adverse outcomes in some people such as heavy smokers.

NONNUTRIENT SUPPLEMENTS

The top ten nonnutrient supplements in order of use are Echinacea, ginseng, ginkgo biloba, garlic supplements, glucosamine, St. John's wort, peppermint, fish oils/omega-3 fatty acids, ginger supplements and soy supplements.[89] Very few of these supplements have been systematically reviewed for safety and efficacy, such as by the Agency for Healthcare Research and Quality or the Cochrane Review system. Such reviews have shown that glucosamine is both effective and safe for relieving some symptoms of osteoarthritis.[90] St. John's wort may be effective for short-term treatment of mild to moderately severe depressive disorders.[91] Some studies show that ginkgo biloba modestly improves cognition and function in those with cognitive impairment or dementia.[92] Garlic modestly improves blood lipid profiles, but has little effect on other indices of cardiovascular health or cancer.[93] Fish or fish oils containing omega-3 fatty acids reduce all cause mortality and some cardiovascular disease outcomes.[94]

CAUTIONS ABOUT DIETARY SUPPLEMENTS

Older adults must use dietary supplements carefully (see Chapters 70 – 75), treat them like any other medication, and inform their physicians about the products they are using.[95] Most supplements contain active ingredients that may interfere with several medications, making them stronger or weaker. For example, garlic, ginkgo, Echinacea, ginseng, St. John's wort, and kava are all suspected of interacting with medications, especially anticancer drugs and blood thinners.[96–98] Some supplements promote bleeding or interfere with other aspects of surgery and recovery.

FOOD SAFETY

Although the most important food safety problem is microbial foodborne illness from bacteria and viruses, there are also food safety risks from parasites, toxins, and chemical and physical contaminants in foods. The food safety recommendations in the 2005 Dietary Guidelines are based on the FightBAC principles of safe food handling practices (clean, separate, cook, and chill). Two specific recommendations for older people are to (1) avoid raw animal products, raw sprouts, and unpasteurized juices[19] and (2) reheat certain deli meats and frankfurters to steaming hot. Other reliable sources of information on food safety and foodborne illness are the FightBAC Partnership for Food Safety Education (www.fightbac.org), the American Dietetic Association,[99,100] and the medical profession.[101] Risk of foodborne illness may be decreased by education targeted to older adults, caregivers, and foodservice staff in nursing homes, cafeterias, restaurants, assisted living facilities, congregate meal sites, and home-delivered meals programs.[100–102]

Foodborne illness can cause mild to fatal reactions involving diarrhea, vomiting, and other symptoms. The Centers for Disease Control and Prevention reported that, compared to younger people, older adults have safer food handling and food consumption behaviors and lower rates of infection from several foodborne illnesses.[102] However, along with children and immune-compromised people, older adults are at high risk for severe complications from foodborne illness, such as death from gastroenteritis. These high complication rates may result from poor nutritional status, age-related decreases in stomach acid which allow more microorganisms to survive in the gastrointestinal tract, dehydration related to impaired sense of thirst, increased intestinal transit time, age-related impairments in immunity, and surgery or other illnesses that may also impair immunity.

People in nursing homes are particularly vulnerable to foodborne illness, with fatality rates 10 to 100 times higher than the general population.[102] Risk factors include illness, impaired immunity, and close confinement with others. Proactive steps that nursing homes take in preventing foodborne illness include cooking eggs and meat thoroughly, and using pasteurized eggs and irradiated meats with decreased bacterial loads. Older adults living in assisted living facilities, receiving home-delivered meals, or receiving meals at congregate meal sites may also be at higher risk for foodborne illness than other older adults because of their advanced age and higher prevalence of frailty.

PHYSICAL ACTIVITY

Along with a healthy diet, physical activity can extend years of active life, help maintain a healthy body weight, decrease risk of cardiovascular disease and other chronic diseases, reduce disability, relieve symptoms of depression, help maintain independent living, and enhance the overall quality of life.[19,52,103] An alarming 75% of older Americans do not engage in at least 30 min of daily physical activity.[104] The Best Practices Statement from the American College of Sports Medicine recommends a well-rounded physical activity program encompassing strength, endurance, balance and flexibility for overall health, fitness, and well being.[103] Strength training can reverse and slow the progression of sarcopenia. However, only 12% of older people reported engaging in strengthening exercises in 2001 to 2002.[105] Flexibility training increases the range of motion around the joint. Endurance training may provide the greatest protection against the deleterious effects of chronic diseases associated with aging. Balance exercises improve the body's base of support to decrease the risk of falling. Balance training, static or dynamic, improves the ability to maintain standing balance and balance while moving. Physical activity programs targeted at older adults are available in hospitals, senior centers, and other community-based organizations.

CONCLUSION

A growing body of evidence shows that nutrition promotes health and quality of life as people age. To reap the full benefits, nutrition needs to be integrated into all aspects of health promotion, disease prevention, and disease management. This can be accomplished in a variety of ways, including nutrition screening, assessment and referral to registered dietitians and other appropriate health professionals in routine physician visits, as well as community-based nutrition education programs that target older adults, families, caregivers, and health professionals. Key recommendations from the 2005 White House Conference on Aging that are relevant to nutrition include reauthorizing the Older Americans Act; supporting geriatric education and training for all healthcare professionals, paraprofessionals, health profession students, and direct care workers; attaining adequate numbers of health care personnel in all professions who are skilled, culturally competent, and specialized in geriatrics; and improving state- and local-based integrated delivery systems to meet 21st century needs of seniors.[106] Such strategies will improve the quality and availability of nutrition services for older people.

REFERENCES

1. U.S. Census Bureau, U.S. Interim projection by age, sex, race, and Hispanic origin, 2004.
2. Federal Interagency Forum on Aging and Related Statistics, Older Americans 2004: Key Indicators of Well-being, 2004.
3. Beers, M.H. et al., *The Merck Manual of Health & Aging*, Merck Research Laboratories, Whitehouse Station, NJ, 2004.
4. Norman, R.A. and Henderson, J.N., *Dermatol. Ther.*, 16: 181; 2003.
5. American Dietetic Association, *JADA*, 105: 616; 2005.
6. Sahyoun, N.R., *Nutr. Clin. Care*, 2: 155; 1999.
7. Amarantos, E., Martinez, A., and Dwyer, J. Geron., 56A: 54; 2001.
8. Green, S. and McDougall, T., *Nurs. Older People*, 14: 31; 2002.
9. Green, S.M. and Watson, R., *J. Adv. Nurs.*, 50: 69; 2005.
10. Callen, B.L. and Wells, T.J., *Public Health Nursing*, 22: 138; 2005.
11. Institute of Medicine, *Dietary Reference Intakes for Calcium, Phosphorus, Magnesium, Vitamin D, and Fluoride*, National Academy of Sciences, Washington DC, National Academy Press, 1997.
12. Daviglus, M.L. et al., *Arch. Intern. Med.*, 163: 2460; 2003.
13. Ervin, R.B. et al., *Adv. Data*, 27: 1; 2004.
14. Moore, C.E., Murphy, M.M., and Holick, M.F., *J. Nutr.*, 135: 2478; 2005.
15. Institute of Medicine, *Dietary Reference Intakes for Thiamin, Riboflavin, Niacin, Vitamin B_6, Folate, Vitamin B_{12}, Pantothenic Acid, Biotin, and Choline*, National Academy of Sciences, Washington DC, National Academy Press, 1998.
16. Ervin, R.B. et al., *Adv. Data*, 12: 1; 2004.
17. Food and Nutrition Board, *Dietary Reference Intakes for Water, Potassium, Sodium, Chloride, and Sulfate*, National Academy of Sciences, Washington DC, National Academy Press, 2004.
18. Food and Nutrition Board, *Dietary Reference Intakes for Energy, Carbohydrate, Fiber, Fat, Fatty Acids, Cholesterol, Protein, and Amino Acids (Macronutrients)*, National Academy of Sciences, Washington DC, National Academy Press, 2005.
19. Wright, J.D. et al., *Adv. Data*, 17: 1; 2003.
20. U.S. Department of Health and Human Services and U.S. Department of Agriculture, Dietary Guidelines for Americans, 2005.
21. Cleveland, L.E. et al., *J. Am. College. Nutr.*, 19: 331S; 2000.
22. Produce for Better Health Foundation, Consumption statistics, 2005.
23. Daviglus, M.L. et al., *Arch. Intern. Med.*, 163: 2448; 2003.
24. Fries, J.F., *Ann. Intern. Med.*, 139(5 Pt 2): 455; 2003.
25. Knoops, K.T. et al., *JAMA.*, 292: 1433; 2004.
26. Cerhan, J.R. et al., *Cancer Epidemiol. Biomarkers Prev.*, 13: 1114; 2004.
27. Hu, F.B., *Am. J. Clin. Nutr.*, 78: 544S; 2003.
28. Kant, A.K., *J. Am. Diet. Assoc.*, 104: 615; 2004.
29. Writing Group of the PREMIER, Collaborative Research Group, *JAMA*, 289: 2083; 2003.
30. Tucker, K.L. et al., *J. Nutr.*, 153: 556; 2005.
31. Yach, D. et al., *JAMA*, 291: 2616; 2004.
32. Institute of Medicine, *The Role of Nutrition in Maintaining Health in the Nation's Elderly: Evaluating Coverage of Nutrition Services for the Medicare Population*, National Academy of Sciences, Washington DC, National Academy Press, 2000.
33. Feldman, E.B., in *Handbook of Nutrition and Food*, Berdanier, C.D., Ed. CRC Press. Boca Raton, FL, 2002, pp. 319–336.
34. Holmes, S., *Nurs. Standard*, 15: 42; 2000.
35. Food Security Institute, Center on Hunger and Poverty, the Heller Graduate School for Social Policy and Management, Brandeis University, *Hunger Issue Brief*, February 2003.
36. Sahyoun, N.R. and Basiotis, P.P., *Nutrition Insights*, United States Department of Agriculture, Center for Nutrition Policy and Promotion, 2000.
37. Fick, D.M. et al., *Arch. Intern. Med.*, 163: 2716; 2003.
38. Elsner, R.J.F., *Eat. Behav.*, 3: 15; 2002.
39. Morley, J.E., *Nutr.*, 17: 660; 2001.
40. Sheiham, A. et al., *Community Dent. Oral. Epidemiol.*, 29: 195; 2001.
41. Bailey, R.L. et al., *JADA*, 104, 1273: 1276; 2004.
42. Wilson, M.M. and Morley, J.E., *J. Appl. Physiol.*, 95: 1728; 2003.
43. Sahyoun, N.R., Pratt, C.A., and Anderson, A., *JADA*, 104: 58; 2004.
44. American Association for Retired Persons, *The Impact of Federal Programs on Transportation for Older Adults*, Koffman, D., Raphael, D., Weiner, R., Nelson/Nygaard Consulting Associates, San Francisco, CA, December 2004.
45. Frongillo, E.A. and Horan, C.M., *Generations*, 28: 28; 2004.
46. Johnson, M.A., *Generations*, 28: 45; 2004.

47. Knauer, C., *Geriatr. Nurs.,* 24: 152; 2003.
48. Callahan, E. and Jensen, G.L., *Generations,* 28: 39; 2004.
49. Johnson, M.A. and Fischer, J.G., *Generations,* 28: 11; 2004.
50. Center on an Aging Society, Obesity among older Americans, 2003.
51. Hedley, A.A. et al., *JAMA,* 291: 2847; 2004.
52. Kennedy, R.L., Chokkalingham, K., and Srinivasan, R., *Curr. Opin. Clin. Nutr. Metab. Care,* 7: 3; 2004.
53. National Institutes of Health, *Clinical Guidelines on the Identification, Evaluation, and Treatment of Obesity in Adults: The Evidence Report,* NIH Publication Number 98-4083, 1998.
54. National Institutes of Health, *The Practical Guide: Identification, Evaluation, and Treatment of Overweight and Obesity in Adults,* NIH Publication Number 00-4084, 2000.
55. Villareal, D.T. et al., *Obes. Res.,* 13: 1849; 2005.
56. Evans, W.J., *J. Am. Coll. Nutr.,* 23: 601S; 2004.
57. Roubenoff, R., *Obes. Res.,* 12: 887; 2004.
58. Schutz, Y., Kyle, U.U.G., and Pichard, C., *Int. J. Obes.,* 26: 953; 2002.
59. Finkelstein, E.A., Fiebelkorn, I.C., and Wang, G., *Health Aff. (Millwood),* Suppl Web Exclusives:W3-219-26; 2003.
60. Finkelstein, E.A., Fiebelkorn, I.C., and Wang, G., *Obes. Res.,* 12: 18; 2004.
61. Ledikwe, J.H. et al., *Am. J. Clin. Nutr.,* 77: 551; 2003.
62. Ledikwe, J.H. et al., *J. Am. Geriatr. Soc.,* 52: 589; 2004.
63. Jacques, P.F. et al., *Am. J. Clin. Nutr.,* 66: 929; 1997.
64. Jensen, G.L. et al., *Obes. Res.,* 12: 1814; 2004.
65. Food and Nutrition Board, Institute of Medicine, National Academies, *Dietary Reference Intakes (DRIs): Recommended Intakes for Individuals, Vitamins, Elements,* National Academy of Sciences, Washington DC, National Academy Press, 2004.
66. Radimer, K. et al., *Am. J. Epidemiol.,* 160: 339; 2004.
67. United States Department of Health and Human Services, *Bone Health and Osteoporosis: A Report of the Surgeon General.* Rockville, MD: U.S. Department of Health and Human Services, Office of the Surgeon General, 2004.
68. Russell, R.M., Rasmussen, H., and Lichtenstein, A.H., *J. Nutr.,* 129: 751; 1999.
69. Baik, H.W. and Russell, R.M., *Ann. Rev. Nutr.,* 19: 357; 1999.
70. Coppen, A. and Bolander-Gouaille, C., *J. Psychopharmacol.,* 19: 59; 2005.
71. Johnson, M.A. et al., *Am. J. Clin. Nutr.,* 77: 211; 2003.
72. Lewis, M.S. et al., *J. Nutr. Elder.,* 24: 47; 2005.
73. Kuzminski, A.M. et al., *Blood,* 92: 1191; 1998.
74. Code of Federal Regulations, Title 21. Volume 2, Part 101, 2003.
75. Calvo, M.S. and Whiting, S.J., *J. Nutr.,* 135: 301; 2005.
76. Raiten, D.J. and Picciano, M.F., *Am. J. Clin. Nutr.,* 80: 1673S; 2004.
77. Chapuy, M.C. et al., *N. Engl. J. Med.,* 327: 1637; 1992.
78. Bischoff-Ferrari, H.A. et al., *JAMA.,* 291: 1999; 2004.
79. Bischoff-Ferrari, H.A. et al., *JAMA.,* 293: 2257; 2005.
80. Dawson-Hughes, B. et al., *N. Engl. J. Med.,* 337: 670; 1997.
81. Papadimitropoulos, E. et al., *Endocr. Rev.,* 23: 560; 2002.
82. Shea, B. et al., *Endocr. Rev.,* 23: 552; 2002.
83. Levis, S. et al., *J. Clin. Endocrinol. Metabol.,* 90: 1557; 2005.
84. Park, S. and Johnson, M.A., *Nutr. Rev.,* 63: 203; 2005.
85. Dawson-Hughes, B., *Am. J. Clin. Nutr.,* 80: 1763S; 2004.
86. Looker, A.C. et al., *Bone,* 30: 771; 2002.
87. Weihrauch, J.L. and Tamaki, J., Provisional table on the vitamin D content of foods, USDA, HNIS, PT-108, 1991.
88. U.S. Preventive Services Task Force, *Ann. Intern. Med.,* 139: 51; 2003.
89. National Center for Complementary and Alternative Medicine at the NIH, A New Portrait of CAM Use in the United States, *Newsletter,* XI: 1; 2004.
90. Towheed, T.E. et al., *The Cochrane Database of Systematic Reviews,* Issue 2. Art. No. CD002946.pub2. DOI: 10.1002/14651858. CD002946.pub2. 2005.
91. Linde, K. et al., *The Cochrane Database of Systematic Reviews,* Issue 3. Art. No. CD000448.pub2. DOI: 10.1002/14651858. CD000448.pub2. 2005.
92. Birks, J. and Grimley Evans, J., *The Cochrane Database of Systematic Reviews,* Issue 4, Art, No. CD003120. DOI: 10.1002/14651858. CD003120. 2002.
93. Agency for Healthcare Research and Quality, Summary, Evidence Report/Technology Assessment: Number 20, AHRQ Publication No. 01-E022, Rockville, MD, 2000.
94. Agency for Healthcare Research and Quality, Summary, Evidence Report/Technology Assessment: Number 94, AHRQ Publication No. 04-E009-1, 2004.
95. U.S. Food and Drug Administration, Center for Food Safety and Applied Nutrition, Office of Nutritional Products, Labeling, and Dietary Supplements, Dietary Supplements, Tips for Older Dietary Supplement Users, 2003.
96. Ernst, E., *Complement. Altern. Med. Ser.,* 136: 42; 2002.

97. Sparreboom, A. et al., *J. Clin. Oncol.,* 22: 2489; 2004.

98. Memorial Sloan-Kettering Cancer Center, Information Resource: About Herbs, Botanicals & Other Products.

99. Kendall, P. et al., *JADA,* 103: 1646; 2003.

100. McCabe-Sellers, B.J. and Beattie, S.E., *JADA,* 104: 1708; 2004.

101. Mao, Y., Zhu, C., and Boedeker, E.C., *Curr. Opin. Gastroenterol.,* 19: 11; 2003.

102. Buzby, J.C., *Food Rev.,* 25: 30; 2002.

103. Cress, M.E. et al., *J. Aging Phys. Act.,* 13: 61; 2005.

104. National Institute on Aging, *Portfolio for Progress*, 2001.

105. Older Americans 2004: Key Indicators of Well-Being, Federal Interagency Forum on Aging-Related Statistics.

106. White House Conference on Aging, 50 Resolutions, As Voted by 2005 WHCoA Delegates, 2005.

19 Exercise and Nutrient Need

Emma M. Laing

CONTENTS

INTRODUCTION

Nutrition is fundamental to exercise performance, whether the goal is to attain health and fitness or a desired peak competition level. Achieving the appropriate combination of energy, macronutrient, micronutrient, and hydration needs will support the regulation of metabolism, maintenance of normal endocrine function, and the provision of adequate fuel during exercise participation. Together, these factors impact body weight and composition, level of fatigue, recovery from exercise, and overall health.

According to the most recent (2000) Nutrition and Athletic Performance Position Statement[1] issued by the American Dietetic Association, Dietitians of Canada, and the American College of Sports Medicine, the individual seeking to optimize exercise performance should "follow good nutrition and hydration practices, use supplements and ergogenic aids carefully, minimize severe weight-loss practices, and eat a variety of foods in adequate amounts." This chapter highlights the basic principles outlined in the Nutrition and Athletic Performance Position Statement[1] while integrating national recommendations for healthy adults such as those from the Institute of Medicine's Dietary Reference Intakes (DRIs)[2-7] and the 2005 Dietary Guidelines for Americans.[8] "Nutrient/Exercise Considerations" are presented for each nutrient (in Table 19.2 and Table 19.3) to provide additional recommendations based on the most contemporary information supporting the role of nutrition in exercise performance (e.g., nutrient functions in the metabolic processes of exercise, nutrient recommendations for physically active individuals, groups at risk for nutrient deficiency, and possible effects of dietary/supplemental interventions on exercise performance). At present, available data are not sufficient to develop specific nutrient reference values for recreational, modestly competitive, and elite athlete categories. Therefore, national recommendations should be considered appropriate for all athletic individuals, unless otherwise stated. Whereas exercising vs. inactive persons generally require higher caloric and fluid intakes, the needs of most nutrients to support exercise participation can be met by consuming an adequate, well-balanced diet, while considering the timing and frequency of food intake to optimize nutrient metabolism and availability.

This chapter begins by summarizing energy intake requirements for Americans, categorized by physical activity level (PAL; shown in Table 19.1). Table 19.2 and Table 19.3 outline the recommendations for macronutrients and micronutrients, respectively. Table 19.4 lists the number of daily servings within each food group according to varying levels of caloric need. Table 19.5 highlights recommendations for the timing of foods and fluids, including water and electrolytes, for optimal exercise performance. Finally, Table 19.6 lists some of the more popular nutritional supplements touted to enhance physical performance. The recommendations presented here should be specially modified by nutritional professionals to target variations in age, sex, fitness level, mode of activity, intensity and duration of training, time between exercise sessions, as well as body weight and composition goals. The content of this chapter reflects data collected from adults, rather than children, and does not center on any particular type of athlete or sporting event. Nutrition guidelines tailored to specific sports, as well as to child and adolescent athletes, are summarized elsewhere.[9-11] For individualized nutrient assessment, MyPyramid, recently developed by the U.S. Department of Agriculture, provides useful dietary and physical activity assessment tools, which are available online at http://www.mypyramid.gov/. Importantly, this program provides higher "discretionary calories" to meet the energy needs of physically active individuals.

ENERGY INTAKE

Meeting energy intake requirements is essential for achieving optimal physical performance. Energy balance (energy intake = energy expenditure) in most healthy adults occurs at an energy availability of 45 kcal/kg fat-free mass.[12] The types of physical activities performed can have an impact on energy intake regulation.[13] For example, participation in strenuous endurance activities (that use predominantly oxidative phosphorylation as the main energy source) produces an increase in overall energy turnover and leads to either a loss of body weight or to a compensatory increase in food intake. In order to achieve the health benefits of an active lifestyle, 30 to 60 min/day of moderately intense activity is currently recommended by national authorities.[7,8,14–16] According to the 2005 *Dietary Guidelines for Americans*,[8] 60 min of moderately intense physical activity is required

TABLE 19.1
Energy Intake Recommendations Based on the Position on Nutrition and Athletic Performance, the Dietary Reference Intakes, and the Dietary Guidelines for Americans

Position on Nutrition and Athletic Performance[1]	Dietary Reference Intakes[7] Estimated Energy Requirement (EER)[a–c]			Dietary Guidelines for Americans[8] Estimated Kilocalorie Requirements[d]		
	Height (m)/ Activity Level	EER Males BMI 18.5–24.99	EER Females BMI 18.5–24.99	Age (Years)/ Activity Level	Males Average BMI 21.5	Females Average BMI 22.5
2200 kcal/day for females and 2900 kcal/day for males 19 to 50 years of age who are slightly to moderately active	1.50 Sedentary Low Active Active Very Active	1848–2080 2009–2267 2215–2506 2554–2898	1625–1762 1803–1956 2025–2198 2291–2489	19–30 Sedentary Moderate Active	2400 2600–2800 3000	2000 2000–2200 2400
1.5 to 1.7 times resting energy expenditure or at a rate of 37 to 41 kcal/kg body weight/day	1.65 Sedentary Low Active Active	2068–2349 2254–2566 2490–2842	1816–1982 2016–2202 2267–2477	31–50 Sedentary Moderate Active	2200 2400–2600 2800–3000	1800 2000 2200
44 to 50 kcal/kg body weight/day for strength athletes	Very Active 1.80 Sedentary	2880–3296 2301–2635	2567–2807 2015–2211	51+ Sedentary	2000	1600
>50 kcal/kg body weight/day for those in more serious training	Low Active Active Very Active	2513–2884 2782–3200 3225–3720	2239–2459 2519–2769 2855–3141	Moderate Active	2200–2400 2400–2800	1800 2000–2200

[a] *Dietary Reference Intake* values represent requirements for males and females 30 years of age; for each year below/above 30, add/subtract 7 kcal/day for females and add/subtract 10 kcal/day for males, respectively.

[b] EER= the average energy intake that is predicted to maintain energy balance in healthy, normal weight individuals of a defined age, sex, weight, height, and level of physical activity consistent with good health (based on body mass index [BMI; kg/m^2] values of 18.5 and 24.99).

[c] Regression equations based on doubly labeled water data:
- Female EER= $354 - 6.91 \times$ age (years) + PA × [$9.36 \times$ weight (kg) + $726 \times$ height (m)]
- Male EER= $662 - 9.53 \times$ age (years) + PA × [$15.91 \times$ weight (kg) + $539.6 \times$ height (m)]

PA represents physical activity, which differs depending on PAL (physical activity level; the ratio of total energy expenditure/basal energy expenditure):
- PA= 1.0 for both males and females if PAL 1.0–1.39; *Sedentary* (Typical daily living activities)
- PA= 1.11 (males) 1.12 (females) if PAL 1.4–1.59; *Low Active* (Typical daily living activities + 30 to 60 min of daily moderate activity)
- PA= 1.25 (males) 1.27 (females) if PAL 1.6–1.89; *Active* (Typical daily living activities + at least 60 min of daily moderate activity)
- PA= 1.48 (males) 1.45 (females) if PAL 1.9–2.5; *Very Active* (Typical daily living activities + at least 60 min of daily moderate activity + 60 min of vigorous activity; or 120 min of moderate activity)

[d] Values are based on EER and the reference size of median height and weight for that height to give a BMI of 21.5 for adult females and 22.5 for adult males:
- *Sedentary* = a lifestyle that includes only the light physical activity associated with typical day-to-day life
- *Moderate* = a lifestyle that includes physical activity equivalent to walking ~1.5 to 3 mi/day at 3 to 4 miles/h, in addition to the light physical activity associated with typical day-to-day life
- *Active* = a lifestyle that includes physical activity equivalent to walking more than 3 mi/day at 3 to 4 mi/h, in addition to the light physical activity associated with typical day-to-day life
- The kilocalorie ranges shown are to accommodate the needs of different ages within the group; fewer calories are needed at older ages

to maintain a healthy weight, by increasing energy expenditure to approximately 150 to 200 kcal/day. Various levels of physical activities and their associated energy requirements are described in Table 19.1.

Consistent overconsumption of calories can hinder athletic performance because of increases in body weight or changes in body composition. By contrast, low-energy intakes (<1800 to 2000 kcal/day) can lead to such declines in exercise performance as muscle and bone mass losses and increased risk of fatigue, injury, and illness.[1,17,18] The overt practice of energy restriction is common among both men and women who are driven to achieve a body weight/composition goal believed to be desirable for peak exercise performance; however, disordered eating among women has escalated considerably in recent years (reported to occur in up to 78% of female athletes).[19,20] Likewise, menstrual dysfunction is quite common in female athletes (up to 79%),[21] resulting mostly from an energy deficit vs. a low proportion of body fat or excessive exercise.[17,22] When energy availability is below 30 kcal/kg fat-free mass/day, luteinizing hormone pulsatility, glucoregulatory hormones, and bone formation are disrupted. In most amenorrheic females, normal menstrual function can return after additional energy is supplied in the diet. However, in prolonged cases of menstrual disturbances where bone resorption exceeds that of bone formation, the rate of bone mass accretion can be slowed (in adolescents) or bone loss can occur (in adults).[19,23] In 1997, the syndrome describing the phenomenon of disordered eating, coupled with amenorrhea and osteoporosis, was termed the "female athlete triad."[23] As stated in the International Olympic Committee Medical Commission Position Statement,[24] "[a]lthough any one of these [triad] problems can occur in isolation, inadequate nutrition for a woman's level of physical activity often begins a cycle in which all three occur in sequence." The most recent evidence to date on this topic estimates that up to 27% of elite athletes and up to 15% of nonelite recreational athletes have at least two components of this triad syndrome.[25,26] As further evidence of the importance of meeting energy needs with exercise, a negative energy balance has also been shown to result in poor macro- and micronutrient intakes, loss of strength and endurance (due to the use of lean tissue by the body for fuel), as well as early fatigue, frequent injuries, irritability, an increased susceptibility to infection, and overall poor athletic performance.[27,28]

Table 19.1 summarizes energy intake recommendations based on the Position on Nutrition and Athletic Performance.[1] These recommendations (as well as those provided in Table 19.2 and Table 19.3) are presented alongside those contained in the DRI reports, to allow for comparison with target intakes for the general population. Table 19.1 also includes recommendations from the recently published Dietary Guidelines for Americans,[8] although energy intake values in this publication are derived from the DRIs.[7] The DRI recommendations for energy (i.e., the Estimated Energy Requirement [EER]) should meet the needs of most active individuals; however, data from competitive elite athletes who participate in high-intensity training for several hours per day (e.g., PAL values >2.5) were not included in establishing the predictive equations for energy need.[7,29] Therefore, the EER should be modified according to macronutrient recommendations (i.e., the Acceptable Macronutrient Distribution Range [AMDR]) addressed later to meet the energy needs of highly trained elite athletes.[29]

MACRONUTRIENTS

Macronutrients supply the energy required by the body, as well as important dietary constituents for varying physiological functions. The macronutrient needs of individuals who exercise regularly are influenced by total caloric intake; the ratio, timing and quality of macronutrients in the diet; intensity, duration and type of activity; as well as training history, sex, and age.[30] Table 19.2 summarizes the carbohydrate, protein, and fat intake recommendations based on the Position on Nutrition and Athletic Performance[1] and the current DRI.[7] New to this DRI report[7] is the AMDR, which represents a range of intakes (as percentage of energy) associated with reduced risk of chronic disease, within the context of suggested intakes for each macronutrient. The macronutrient needs for physically active individuals should fit within these ranges; however, specific nutrient guidelines presented as Recommended Dietary Allowance (RDA) and/or Adequate Intake (AI) reference standards should also be adhered to.[29]

Carbohydrate is the primary energy source used by the body during endurance-type activities. When suboptimal levels of endogenous sources (i.e., muscle and liver glycogen) occur, usually after 60 to 90 min of exercise, there may be deleterious effects on physical performance. Carbohydrate loading to elevate glycogen stores prior to exercise does not appear to delay fatigue in activities that are <90 min in duration.[31] Numerous studies, however, support the efficacy of consuming carbohydrates during endurance-type exercise for the purpose of delaying fatigue, improving feelings of perceived exertion, and enhancing overall physiologic performance.[32,33] Carbohydrate supplementation has also demonstrated glycogen-sparing effects during shorter bouts of intermittent, high-intensity exercise (e.g., in sports such as tennis and soccer),[34] and has been shown to suppress the release of cortisol and promote muscle glycogen resynthesis following resistance training exercise.[35,36]

Proteins serve to repair exercise-induced microdamage to muscle fibers and improve energy utilization during endurance activities. With an increase in exercise duration, maintenance of blood glucose may occur through gluconeogenesis in the liver.[30,37,38] In general, proteins should not be consumed in excess of the DRI[7] to enhance exercise performance. However, some physically active individuals may need slightly more protein than the current DRI recommendations, depending on the type, frequency, and duration of the exercise (Table 19.2). Although it has often been suggested that supplementation with macronutrient molecules (e.g., fatty acids and amino acids) is not necessary for improved athletic performance unless intakes of energy or particular food groups are restricted,[29,30,38] recent evidence in the area of amino acid supplementation in both highly trained

TABLE 19.2
Macronutrient Recommendations Based on the Dietary Reference Intakes and the Position on Nutrition and Athletic Performance

Macronutrient/Function	Dietary Reference Intakes[7] Recommendations	Position on Nutrition and Athletic Performance[1] Recommendations and other Nutrient/Exercise Considerations
Carbohydrate: Important for maintaining normal levels of glucose in the brain and in circulation; conpler carbohydrates are needed to supply fiber, a key nutrient to reducing blood cholesterol and maintaining blood glucose levels; excess amounts can result in low intakes of essential fatty acids and indispensable amino acids, and could lead to surplus body fat storage, body weight gain, and associated chronic diseases	*AMDR[a] (% of Energy)* Adults aged 19 to >70 years: 45–65 *Carbohydrate RDA[b] (g/day)* Males aged 19 to >70 years: 130 Females aged 19 to >70 years: 130 *Total Fiber AI[c,d] (g/day)* Males aged 19 to 50 years: 38 Females aged 19 to 50 years: 25 Males aged 51 to >70 years: 30 Females aged 51 to >70 years: 21 *Added Sugars[e]* Limit to no more than 25% of energy	*Position Stand Recommendation:* • Range for exercising adults: 6–10 g/kg body weight/day *Nutrient/Exercise Considerations:* • Carbohydrates serve as the most efficient fuel for exercise (producing more adenosine triphosphate per unit of oxygen) compared with other macronutrients; they are essential for maintaining blood glucose levels and muscle glycogen stores; their availability for muscle contraction during exercise is inversely related to the rate of protein catabolism[30,43] • As intensity and length of exercise increases, the source of carbohydrate shifts from muscle glycogen to circulating blood glucose; an ingestion rate of 1g carbohydrate/min (0.04 oz/min in beverage form) maintains optimal carbohydrate metabolism during endurance exercise[44,45] • Glycemic index and glycemic load were not considered in current carbohydrate recommendations for exercise;[1,7] however, recent data suggest that consumption of low-glycemic-index foods may be beneficial in increasing fat oxidation[46,47]
Protein: Needed to maintain body nitrogen and supply indispensable amino acids for the synthesis of protein (during growth, repair of damaged tissues, muscle hypertrophy, and enzyme synthesis); provides indispensable amino acids, which are found in high-quality-protein foods in the diet; excess protein can interfere with maintaining sufficient dietary carbohydrates to replenish muscle glycogen as well as maintaining proper hydration; excess protein ingestion could lead to the progression of renal function impairments, surplus body fat storage, and associated chronic diseases	*AMDR (% of Energy)* Adults aged 19 to >70 years: 10–35 *Protein RDA[f] (g/day)* Males aged 19 to >70 years: 56 Females aged 19 to >70 years: 46 *Indispensable Amino Acids RDA (mg/kg/day)* Adult Males and Females: Histidine: 14 Isoleucine: 19 Leucine: 42 Lysine: 38 Methionine + cysteine: 19 Phenylalanine + tyrosine: 33 Threonine: 20 Tryptophan: 5 Valine: 24	*Position Stand Recommendations:* • Range for endurance exercisers: 1.2–1.4 g/kg body weight/day • Range for strength-trained exercisers: 1.6–1.7 g/kg body weight/day • Range for vegetarian exercisers: 1.3–1.8 g/kg body weight/day • The use of branched-chain amino acid supplements cannot be advocated *Nutrient/Exercise Considerations:* • Skeletal muscle oxidizes up to 6% of total energy from amino acids during endurance exercise[48] • Protein needs are increased depending on exercise level, in order to maintain a greater protein synthetic rate to accommodate augmented lean tissue mass (strength training) or enzyme (endurance training) levels[30,49] • Increasing dietary protein beyond the recommended levels is unlikely to result in endurance benefits or additional increases in lean mass because there is a limit to the rate at which protein tissue can be accrued[37,49,50] • Prolonged intakes of excess protein are associated with increased urea production and excretion,[51] blood urea nitrogen and urine-specific gravity,[52] and may affect the hydration status of exercising individuals • Branched-chain amino acids (isoleucine, leucine and valine) are preferentially oxidized during exercise compared to other amino acids[48,53] • The effects of amino acid supplementation with exercise, particularly in conjunction with carbohydrates, may be useful for improving short-term training efficiency and recovery; however, confirming research is needed[39–42]

Fat: Provides energy, essential fatty acids, and fat-soluble vitamins; assists in the absorption of these vitamins; serves as a structural component for the development of tissues and as a precursor to numerous compounds; excess dietary fat could lead to alterations in carbohydrate and protein intakes and ultimately body weight gain; linoleic acid is an essential component of structural membrane lipids; α-linolenic acid is involved in neurological development and growth; both fatty acids are precursors of eicosanoids

AMDR (% of Energy) for Fat[g]
Adults aged 19 to >70 years: 20–35
AMDR (% of Energy) for n-6 Polyunsaturated Fatty Acids[h]
Adults aged 19 to >70 years: 5–10
AMDR (% of Energy) for n–3 Polyunsaturated Fatty Acids[i]
Adults aged 19 to >70 years: 0.6–1.2
Linoleic Acid AI (g/day)
Males aged 19 to 50 years: 17
Females aged 19 to 50 years: 12
Males aged 51 to >70 years: 14
Females aged 51 to >70 years: 11
α-Linolenic Acid AI (g/day)
Males aged 19 to >70 years: 1.6
Females aged 19 to >70 years: 1.1

Position Stand Recommendations:
• Total fat intake should be >15% and <25% of total energy intake
• Fat composition should be 10% saturated, 10% polyunsaturated and 10% monounsaturated

Nutrient/Exercise Considerations:
• Lipids are transported to the site of oxidation in the exercising muscle where they are used in the oxidative process to supply energy and spare carbohydrate stores[7]
• There is no physical performance benefit in consuming a fat-restricted diet (less than 15% of energy from fat) *vs.* a diet containing 20%–25% energy from fat[1]
• The practice of "fat loading" (i.e., consumption of a high-fat diet (65%–70% of total energy) to increase fat oxidation and spare the use of muscle glycogen during exercise has been shown to either have no effect or impair high-intensity training efficiency[54,55]
• Supplementation with essential fatty acids in well-trained athletes has no beneficial effect on body composition, muscle strength, exercise fatigue, immune function, or exercise-induced elevation of pro- or anti-inflammatory cytokines[56-58]

a AMDR = Acceptable Macronutrient Distribution Range; a range of intakes associated with reduced risk of chronic diseases while providing adequate intakes of essential nutrients; values are expressed as percentages of total energy intake.

b RDA = Recommended Dietary Allowances; values are set to meet the needs of almost all (97% to 98%) individuals in a group.

c AI = Adequate Intake; values are set to cover the needs of all individuals in a group, but lack of data or uncertainty in the data prevent being able to specify with confidence the percentage of individuals covered by this intake.

d AI for fiber is based on 14 g total fiber/1000 kcal.

e Added sugars are defined as sugars and syrups that are added to food during processing and preparation.

f RDA for protein is based on 0.8 g protein/kg body weight/day.

g No RDA or AI was set due to insufficient data linking a defined level of dietary fat to prevention of chronic disease; however, the recommendation states that intakes of dietary cholesterol, *trans*-fatty acids and saturated fatty acids should be "as low as possible while consuming a nutritionally adequate diet."

h Linoleic acid.

i α-Linolenic acid, eicosapentaenoic acid, and docosahexaenoic acid.

and untrained individuals shows promise for improving training effectiveness and recovery from exercise.[39–42] But, advocating amino acid supplementation for improved performance in physically active individuals is rather premature since the long-term effectiveness of such practices, given varying training conditions and combinations with other nutrients, have not yet been elucidated.

Dietary fat provides the free fatty acids needed to supply energy for mild to moderate intensity endurance exercise. Physically active individuals should consume dietary fat in amounts similar to what is recommended in the DRI report[7] (Table 19.2). Supplementation with free fatty acids is generally not recommended to improve exercise performance. Consultation with a registered dietitian, particularly in the case of elite athletes who have increased energy requirements, should be encouraged to ensure a balanced macronutrient intake and to assess the need for supplementation on an individual basis.

MICRONUTRIENTS

Vitamins and minerals facilitate the use of macronutrients for all physiologic processes, including exercise-related energy metabolism, immune response, growth and maintenance of bone mineral, as well as the protection of body tissues from oxidative stress. Table 19.3 outlines the micronutrient intake recommendations, categorized as B-complex vitamins, antioxidants, and other vitamins and minerals, based on the Position on Nutrition and Athletic Performance[1] and the current DRI report.[7] Physical activity was examined as a key factor in approximately one-third of the micronutrients considered for the RDA and AI guidelines (i.e., vitamins B_6, C, E, choline, and thiamin, as well as calcium, iron, magnesium, and sodium); however, no specific recommendations within the DRI reports were made with regard to micronutrient needs during exercise.[59] The recommendations issued by the DRI panel for micronutrients should be appropriate for most physically active individuals unless otherwise indicated.

During prolonged, high-intensity exercise, micronutrient requirements are expected to increase relative to inactive individuals.[59] Since caloric requirements also increase with exercise intensity and duration, micronutrient needs should easily be met with appropriate energy consumption, and supplementation above what is achieved through a well-balanced diet may not be necessary. As stated in the Position on Nutrition and Athletic Performance,[1] "[s]upplementation with single micronutrients is discouraged unless clear medical, nutritional, or public health reasons are present." In cases where energy intake is restricted or food groups omitted, there is a greater probability for poor micronutrient status in exercising individuals.[1,27] In these cases, consumption of a multivitamin/mineral supplement may be warranted.

Because of their increased energy needs, it may be challenging for more highly active individuals (particularly elite athletes) to balance the recommended intakes of vitamins and minerals. That is, there may be a risk for overconsumption of micronutrients, either with food intake alone or with supplement use. The risk may be further exacerbated if one erroneously perceives that consuming "more" of a nutrient marketed to improve exercise performance is actually "better." Most micronutrients in the DRI reports have an assigned Tolerable Upper Intake Level (UL), defined as the maximum level of daily nutrient intake that is likely to pose no risk of adverse effects. The UL represents total intake from food, water, and supplements.[109] It would be prudent for exercising individuals to consider the ULs before making decisions about altering their intake of micronutrients. Further discussions concerning UL recommendations are available in detail elsewhere.[109-112]

Table 19.4 provides an example from The Dietary Guidelines for Americans report[8] indicating how the macronutrient- and micronutrient-focused recommendations summarized in the preceding text can be expressed in terms of whole food serving sizes. This example outlines the number of daily servings within each food group to meet recommended nutrient intakes presented across a range of calorie levels. The exact numbers of servings in this eating plan are not intended to be consumed every day, but on average, over time. Table 19.1 should serve as a tool to help identify an individual's caloric requirement based on sex, age, and PAL, which can then be applied to the recommendations presented in Table 19.4.

TIMING OF FOODS AND FLUIDS

The nutrition status of an individual prior to exercise training or event competition can have a considerable impact on athletic performance. Dietary recommendations should focus primarily on adequate hydration and maximizing liver and muscle glycogen stores with sufficient carbohydrates. The timing of meals and snacks depends on the intensity of the exercise and an individual's gastrointestinal ability to tolerate varying amounts of foods and fluids. Therefore, strategies typically include consuming meals that are composed of familiar foods, moderate in protein, and low in fat and fiber to facilitate gastric emptying and to minimize gastrointestinal distress. Table 19.5 summarizes the recommendations for the timing of meals and fluids to promote optimal exercise performance.

Maintaining proper hydration status is critical both to overall health and physiological performance with exercise. Optimal exercise performance can occur if the rates of fluid ingestion/absorption are equal to the rate of fluid loss through sweat and/or urination.[1] Dehydration and associated health risks result from a fluid imbalance, in which fluid losses exceed fluid intakes and exercise performance becomes impaired.[112] Dehydration can be further exacerbated in temperature/humidity extremes, where hot/humid conditions produce increased fluid losses through evaporation, and cold environments result in reduced rates of

TABLE 19.3
Micronutrient Recommendations Based on the Dietary Reference Intakes and the Position on Nutrition and Athletic Performance

B-Complex Vitamins

Overall Function	The B-complex vitamins are involved in energy production during exercise and are required for the production of red blood cells, protein synthesis, as well as for tissue repair and maintenance.	
Position on Nutrition and Athletic Performance[1] Recommendation	Exercise may increase the need for the B-complex vitamins, perhaps up to twice the current recommended amounts. These increased needs can generally be met via the higher energy intakes required by exercising individuals to maintain body weight.	
Micronutrient Function	**Dietary Reference Intakes[3] Recommendations**	**Nutrient/Exercise Considerations**
Thiamin: plays a role in carbohydrate and amino acid metabolism; acts as a coenzyme in the conversion of pyruvate to acetyl CoA and α-ketoglutarate to succinyl CoA; participates in the decarboxylation of branched-chain amino acids	*RDA[a] (mg/day)* Males age 19 to >70 years: 1.2 Females age 19 to >70 years: 1.1	• Individuals who consume low-energy diets or low-nutrient-dense foods may be at risk for inadequate thiamin status[59] • 0.5 mg thiamin/1000 kcal has been recommended for physically active individuals who have increased energy needs[3,59] • Short-term variations in dietary thiamin do not appear to have direct effects on strength or performance indices; however, a temporary thiamin insufficiency can lead to pyruvate accumulation and an increase in circulating lactate during exercise, which may result in muscle fatigue[60] • Thiamin supplementation has been shown to improve perceived recovery from exercise fatigue but has not been shown to alter metabolic or other physical performance indices[61,62]
Riboflavin: required for oxidative energy production; functions specifically in the mitochondrial electron transport system as the coenzymes flavin mononucleotide and flavin adenine dinucleotide	*RDA (mg/day)* Males age 19 to >70 years: 1.3 Females age 19 to >70 years: 1.1	• Riboflavin needs increase during the initiation of strenuous physical activities; however, performance is generally not affected with variations in dietary intake[63] • 0.6 mg riboflavin/1000 kcal has been recommended for physically active individuals who have increased energy needs[3] • For exercising women who may be restricting energy intake or choosing to omit certain food groups, 1.4 to 1.6 mg riboflavin/day has been suggested for those engaging in moderate exercise and 2 to 3 mg riboflavin/day for those participating in high-intensity competitive activities[27,59,64] • For older competitive adults (aged 50+ years), increases to 1.7 mg riboflavin/day for males and 1.3 mg riboflavin/day for females have been suggested[65,66] • Marginal riboflavin deficiency, in combination with other B-complex vitamin deficiencies, has been shown to negatively impact measures of exercise performance[67]
Niacin: an electron carrier in many oxidative reactions; a precursor of electron (nicotinamide adenine nucleotide) and proton (nicotinamide adenine dinucleotide) acceptors	*RDA (as NE;[b] mg/day)* Males age 19 to >70 years: 16 Females age 19 to >70 years: 14	• Individuals who consume low-energy, low-nutrient-dense, or strict vegetarian diets may be at risk for inadequate niacin status[59,64] • While niacin supplementation has been shown to decrease circulating free fatty acid concentrations and reduce excess postexercise oxygen consumption, supplementation does not appear to improve overall performance outcomes during exercise[68–70]
Vitamin B₆: a cofactor for transferases, transaminases, decarboxylases, and cleavage enzymes used in transformations of amino acids; needed for gluconeogenesis and glyconeogenesis processes	*RDA (mg/day)* Males age 19 to 50 years: 1.3 Females age 19 to 50 years: 1.3 Males age 51 to >70 years: 1.7 Females age 51 to >70 years: 1.5	• Individuals who consume low-energy/low-protein diets or low-nutrient-dense foods may be at risk for inadequate vitamin B₆ status[71,72] • Because vitamin B₆ is involved in the process of muscle glycogen breakdown, exercise may increase the turnover and urinary losses of vitamin B₆[71,73,74] • Physically active females may need up to 2–3 mg vitamin B₆/day, in proportion to increased energy needs[27] • 2.0 mg vitamin B₆/day has been recommended for older (aged 50+ years), competitive males and females[75]

Continued

TABLE 19.3
(Continued)

Micronutrient/Function	RDA / AI	Position on Nutrition and Athletic Performance[1] Recommendation
B-Complex Vitamins (Continued)		
Vitamin B₁₂: a coenzyme for the reaction that converts homocysteine to methionine; required for normal erythrocyte production and neurologic function	RDA (*μg/day*)[c] Males aged 19 to >70 years: 2.4 Females aged 19 to >70 years: 2.4	• Individuals consuming low-energy or strict vegetarian diets may be at risk for vitamin B₁₂ deficiency[59,64,76] • 2.8 μg vitamin B₁₂/day has been recommended for older male and female competitive athletes, aged 50+ years[75] • Vitamin B₁₂ supplementation has not been shown to demonstrate positive effects on physical performance[77,78]
Choline: a constituent of lecithin; essential in the metabolism of fat; a precursor of the neurotransmitter, acetylcholine	AI[d] (*mg/day*) Males aged 19 to >70 years: 550 Females aged 19 to >70 years: 425	• Strenuous physical activity has been shown to reduce plasma choline concentrations[3] • Choline supplementation appears to lower lipid peroxidation following mild exercise[79] • No effect of choline supplementation during prolonged exercise has been demonstrated on physical performance measures or in delaying fatigue[80–82]
Antioxidants		
Overall Function		Vitamins A, C, E, and selenium may protect cell membranes from oxidative damage. Because exercise can increase oxygen consumption 10- to 15-fold, chronic exercise produces a constant "oxidative stress" on the muscles and other cells. Muscle tissue damage caused by intense exercise can lead to lipid peroxidation of membranes. Increased exercise duration and intensity appear to elevate levels of lipid peroxide by-products,[83,84] and may necessitate increases in dietary antioxidants; however, the evidence to date on this topic is conflicting[85,86] and remains uncertain
Position on Nutrition and Athletic Performance[1] Recommendation		There is no clear consensus on whether supplementation of antioxidant nutrients is necessary. Habitual exercise has been shown to result in an augmented antioxidant system and a reduction of lipid peroxidation. Thus, a well-trained athlete may have a more developed endogenous antioxidant system than a sedentary person. Active individuals at greatest risk for poor antioxidant intakes are those who follow a low-energy, low-fat diet, or those with limited dietary intakes of fruits and vegetables
Micronutrient/Function	Dietary Reference Intakes[4,5]	Recommendations Nutrient Exercise Considerations
Vitamin A: a fat-soluble antioxidant; essential for vision, gene expression, immune function, and growth; β-carotene, a precursor of vitamin A, also has antioxidant properties	RDA (*as RAE;*[e] *μg/day*) Males aged 19 to >70 years: 900 Females aged 19 to >70 years: 700	• The risk for vitamin A insufficiency is increased if total energy and/or fruit and vegetable intakes are restricted[59] • Evidence is lacking to suggest that exercise increases vitamin A needs, since competitive athletes have improved β-carotene status compared to non-athletes[87] • Supplementation with vitamin A, in combination with vitamins C and E has been shown to prevent exercise-induced oxidative stress[88]
Vitamin C: a water-soluble antioxidant; participates in bone formation and scar tissue repair; needed for synthesis of carnitine for fatty acid transport; serves to regenerate vitamin E from its oxidized by-product	RDA (*mg/day*) Males aged 19 to >70 years: 90 Females aged 19 to >70 years: 75	• The requirement for vitamin C may be increased during physical activity due to its roles in immune and antioxidant function and in collagen repair[59] • Vitamin C supplementation, in combination with vitamin E, has been shown to prevent endurance exercise-induced lipid peroxidation[89] • Vitamin C supplementation alone, or in combination with vitamin E or carbohydrate, does not appear to have a beneficial effect on exercise-induced increases in muscle damage or recovery, on the hormonal, or immune response after prolonged exercise[90,91]
Vitamin E: a fat-soluble antioxidant; acts on polyunsaturated fatty acids in cell membranes; essential for maintaining erythrocyte and neurological function	RDA (*mg/day*)[f] Males aged 19 to >70 years: 15 Females aged 19 to >70 years: 15	• Vitamin E deficiency results in oxidative stress and muscle degeneration[59] • Older, competitive athletes (aged 50+ years) may require supplementation of vitamin E (100–200 mg/day)[75] • Vitamin E supplementation in younger adults has little beneficial effect on performance related parameters, other than reducing lipid membrane peroxidation[90,92] • Those who are unaccustomed to exercise training are likely to gain more benefit from supplementation vs. trained exercisers[93] • Large doses of α-tocopherol supplementation may actually exhibit prooxidant effects during high-intensity exercise[94]

Micronutrient/Function	Dietary Reference Intakes[2,5] Recommendations	Position on Nutrition and Athletic Performance[1] Recommendations and other Nutrient/Exercise Considerations
Selenium: an essential element in the glutathione peroxidase enzyme system; involved in DNA repair, enzyme activation, and immune system function	*RDA (μg/day)* Males aged 19 to >70 years: 55; Females aged 19 to >70 years: 55	• The risk for selenium insufficiency is increased if total energy and/or fruit and vegetable intakes are restricted • Selenium supplementation, in combination with several other antioxidants, has not been shown to protect against DNA damage or plasma cytokine concentrations following aerobic exercise[95,96] • Selenium supplementation for exercise performance is generally not recommended due to potential toxic effects of overconsumption

Other Micronutrients

Micronutrient/Function	Dietary Reference Intakes[2,5] Recommendations	Position on Nutrition and Athletic Performance[1] Recommendations and other Nutrient/Exercise Considerations
Calcium: needed for growth and repair of bone tissue and the maintenance of blood calcium levels; required for blood clotting, muscle contraction, nerve transmission and overall bone health	*AI (mg/day)* Males age 19–50 years: 1000; Females age 19–50 years: 1000; Males age 51 to >70 years: 1200; Females age 51 to >70 years: 1200	**Position Stand Recommendations:** • Exercising individuals should strive to meet the recommended intakes for calcium because inadequate dietary calcium increases the risk of osteopenia and stress fractures.[27] Females are at greatest risk for low bone mineral density if energy intakes are low, dairy products are eliminated or restricted in the diet and menstrual dysfunction is present Nutrient/Exercise Considerations: • The amount of calcium in the diet has been shown to modify the musculoskeletal response to exercise; where the combination of dietary calcium and moderate physical activity produces a dose-response effect on bone mineral density in both older and younger females[97,98]
Vitamin D: promotes growth and mineralization of bone by maintaining calcium and phosphorus homeostasis; enhances absorption of calcium; has a role in the modulation of immune cells	*AI (μg/day)[g,h]* Males age 19 to 50 years: 5; Females age 19 to 50 years: 5; Males age 51 to 70 years: 10; Females age 51 to 70 years: 10; Males age >70 years: 15; Females age >70 years: 15	Position Stand Recommendations: • Exercising individuals living at northern latitudes or who train primarily indoors throughout the year (e.g., gymnasts and figure skaters) may be at risk for poor vitamin D status, especially if foods fortified with vitamin D are not consumed. These individuals would benefit from vitamin D supplementation at the level of the DRI[2,8] Nutrient/Exercise Considerations: • Among both active and inactive elderly persons (aged 60+ years), higher circulating 25(OH)D concentrations (due to diet and/or sunlight exposure) have been associated with improved musculoskeletal function and strength[99,100]
Magnesium: involved in numerous enzymatic reactions such as glycolysis, fat and protein metabolism, adenosine triphosphate hydrolysis, and the second messenger system; regulates neuromuscular, cardiovascular, immune and hormonal functions	*RDA (mg/day)* Males age 19 to 30 years: 400; Females age 19 to 30 years: 310; Males age 31 to >70 years: 420; Females age 31 to >70 years: 320	Position Stand Recommendations: N/A Nutrient/Exercise Considerations: • The risk for magnesium insufficiency is increased if energy intakes are restricted[27] • Magnesium depletion has been directly related to impairments in exercise performance[59] • Supplementation with magnesium in physically active, magnesium-replete individuals has not consistently shown to aid in the recovery of muscle function or improve immune cell function[101-103]
Iron: required for the formation of hemoglobin, myoglobin, cytochromes, and for enzymes involved in energy production	*RDA (mg/day)* Males age 19 to 50 years: 8; Females age 19 to 50 years: 18; Females age 19 to 50 years who use oral contraceptives:[i] 11; Males age 51 to >70 years: 8; Females age 51 to >70 years: 8	Position Stand Recommendations: • As iron depletion is one of the most prevalent nutrient deficiencies observed in athletic females (up to 36%), there is an increased risk for impaired physical performance associated with symptoms of iron deficiency.[104-106] • Assessment of iron status in physically active females should be done routinely, especially in amenorrheic cases; these individuals may benefit from iron supplementation.[27] Nutrient/Exercise Considerations: • For those who perform regular endurance or intense exercises, the iron requirement is higher (30 to 70%) than what is recommended for inactive individuals.[5] • Other considerations for iron and athletic performance include blood donation, which adds 0.65 to basal losses, and practicing vegetarianism, which reduces iron absorption from 18% to 10%.[5] • Older female endurance exercisers (particularly those who are vegetarian), aged 50+ years, and training in extreme temperatures, may need up to 15 mg iron/day.[75]

Continued

TABLE 19.3
(Continued)

	RDA (mg/day)
Zinc: important for growth and repair of muscle and skeletal tissues, maturation and reproduction, wound healing and energy production; functions in a number of metallic enzymes including carbonic anhydrase, alkaline phosphatases and RNA polymerases; required to maintain the structure of nucleic acid protein	Males aged 19 to >70 years: 11 Females aged 19 to >70 years: 8

Antioxidants

Position Stand Recommendations:

- Exercising individuals should strive to meet the recommended intakes for zinc, because athletic females, particularly those who are vegetarian, have been shown to have diets low in zinc

Nutrient/Exercise Considerations:

- The training ability of athletic females who avoid animal products and limit intakes of whole or fortified cereals and grains may be enhanced with zinc supplementation[27]
- Supplementation with zinc has been shown to improve measures of muscle strength and endurance in healthy women[107]
- Zinc supplementation, in combination with several antioxidants, has not been shown to protect against oxidative stress following aerobic exercise[108]

---

[a] RDA= Recommended Dietary Allowances; values are set to meet the needs of almost all (97–98%) individuals in a group.

[b] NE= niacin equivalents; 1 mg niacin = 60 mg tryptophan.

[c] People over age 50 years are advised to consume vitamin B_{12} in its crystalline form from fortified foods and/or supplements[8].

[d] AI= Adequate Intake; values are set to cover the needs of all individuals in a group, but lack of data or uncertainty in the data prevent being able to specify with confidence the percentage of individuals covered by this intake.

[e] RAE= Retinol Activity Equivalents; 1 RAE = 1 µg retinol, 12 µg β-carotene, 24 µg α-carotene, 24 µg β-cryptoxanthin.

[f] As α-tocopherol.

[g] As cholecalciferol; 1 µg cholecalciferol = 40 IU vitamin D; values are in the absence of adequate exposure to sunlight.

[h] For older adults, people with dark skin, and people exposed to insufficient ultraviolet band radiation (i.e., from sunlight), the recommendation is to consume 25 µg or 1000 IU vitamin D/day via vitamin-D-fortified foods and/or supplements[8].

[i] The RDA for iron is reduced for women who use oral contraceptives, because of their lower menstrual iron losses.

TABLE 19.4

The Number of Daily Servings in a Food Group Based on Caloric Need

Food Group	1600 Calories	2000 Calories	2600 Calories	3100 Calories
Grains[a]	6	7–8	10–11	12–13
Vegetables[b]	3–4	4–5	5–6	6
Fruits[c]	4	4–5	5–6	6
Low-fat or fat-free dairy foods[d]	2–3	2–3	3	3–4
Meat, poultry, fish[e]	1–2	2 or less	2	2–3
Nuts, seeds, legumes[f]	3–4/week	4–5/week	1	1
Fats and oils[g]	2	2–3	3	4
Sweets[h]	0	5/week	2	2

Source: Adapted from the 2005 Dietary Guidelines for Americans[8] and the U.S. Department of Agriculture MyPyramid Food Intake Patterns: http://www.mypyramid.gov/

Values are number of servings.

Serving sizes:

[a] 1 slice bread; 1 oz dry cereal; ½ cup cooked rice, pasta or cooked cereal.

[b] 1 cup raw leafy vegetable; ½ cup cooked vegetable; 6 oz vegetable juice.

[c] 6 oz fruit juice; 1 medium fruit; ¼ cup dried fruit; ½ cup fresh, frozen or canned fruit.

[d] 8 oz milk; 1 cup yogurt; 1 ½ oz cheese.

[e] 3 oz cooked meats, poultry or fish.

[f] ⅓ cup or 1 ½ oz nuts; 2 tablespoons or ½ oz seeds; ½ cup cooked dry beans or peas.

[g] 1 teaspoon soft margarine; 1 tablespoon low-fat mayonnaise; 2 tablespoons light salad dressing; 1 teaspoon vegetable oil.

[h] 1 tablespoon sugar, 1 tablespoon jelly or jam; ½ oz jelly beans; 8 oz lemonade.

fluid ingestion.[113] In higher altitudes (higher than 2500 m), diuresis and respiratory fluid losses increase the recommendation for fluid intake up to 3 to 4 l/day to sustain optimal kidney function.[1] According to the DRI report concerning hydration,[6] the AI recommendation for total water (including drinking water, water in beverages, and water that is part of food) is 2.7 and 3.7 l/day for adult females and males, respectively. Both reports from the DRI and Dietary Guidelines for Americans recommend that drinking according to thirst and consuming beverages with meals are adequate to achieve these recommendations and maintain the hydration status of most Americans.[6,8] Furthermore, the AI guidelines for water consumption were established for individuals participating in light/moderate activities in relatively mild temperatures (~20°C). For more physically active individuals who may exercise in warmer climates, these recommendations would need to be adjusted accordingly.[59,113,115]

Elite athletes or individuals who engage in higher-intensity, endurance-type exercises may be at risk of developing hyponatremia.[116,117] Exercise-associated hyponatremia (EAH) is defined as "the occurrence of hyponatremia in individuals engaged in prolonged physical activity (>4 h) defined by a serum or plasma sodium concentration below the normal reference range (usually 135 mmol/l)."[117] According to the (2005) EAH Position Statement,[117] women, novice athletes, slow-paced runners, and athletes with relatively low body weight, exercising in extreme hot/cold environments or have excessive drinking behaviors (either water or sports drinks), are at risk for hyponatremia. Therefore, it is the recommendation of the EAH Position Statement panel[117] that any individual participating in endurance exercise should avoid overconsumption of fluids, by either drinking according to thirst or to their estimated hourly sweat rate. The panel[117] recommended using a method such as the U.S. Track and Field Self-Testing Program for Optimal Hydration formula (summarized as follows)[118] for estimating fluid needs according to hourly sweat rate:

Fluid needs per h of exercise (oz) = [(preexercise body weight; lb) – (postexercise body weight following 1 h of typical intensity exercise; lb)] × [15.3 (conversion factor for body weight to fluid ounces)] + [(fluid intake; oz) – (urine volume; ml)]

To eliminate urine volume from the preceding equation, the individual should be weighed before and after a typical 1 h exercise bout and should not be permitted to urinate during this session. The following indices of hydration status, based on percent body weight change,[45] could also help guide individuals in maintaining proper hydration and avoiding serious dehydration during exercise: well hydrated (+1% to –1%); minimal dehydration (–1% to –3%); significant dehydration (–3% to –5%); and (>5%) serious dehydration.

NUTRITIONAL NEEDS FOR THE AGING ATHLETE

Among U.S. adults over the age of 55 years, 29.9% of men and 26.5% of women routinely participate in regular leisure time or competitive physical activities.[119] Dietary recommendations within the Position on Nutrition and Athletic Performance[1]

TABLE 19.5
Timing of Foods and Fluids for Optimal Exercise Performance

Timing and Recommendations

Preexercise
- Sufficient fluid in the 24 h before an exercise session
- 400–600 ml of fluid 2–3 h before exercise
- 200–300 ml of fluid 10–20 min before exercise
- 200–300 g carbohydrate in food or fluid consumed 3–4 h before exercise
- Moderate amounts of low-glycemic-index carbohydrates (may promote the availability of the sustained carbohydrate)
- Limited or no caffeine, alcohol (both increase urine output) or carbonated beverages (may promote stomach fullness)

During Exercise
Goal: consume sufficient fluids to maintain fluid balance and carbohydrates (fluid, solid or gel) to maintain blood glucose levels and muscle glycogen stores that are easily tolerated and are sufficient in calories to prevent hunger during the exercise session. The nutrition plan should include:
- 150–350 ml of fluid at 15–20 min intervals during exercise
- Plain water or fluids/foods containing carbohydrate in concentrations of 4%–8% for activities lasting <1 h
- Fluids containing carbohydrate in concentrations of 4%–8% for activities lasting >1 h; or 0.7 g carbohydrate/kg/h (~ 30–60 g/h) for activities >1 h
- Carbohydrates that yield primarily glucose and no more than 2%–3% (2–3 g/100 ml) fructose; or fructose in amounts that do not cause gastrointestinal discomfort/diarrhea
- 0.5–0.7 g sodium/l for exercise lasting >1 h (to increase the drive to drink fluids)[a]
- Adjusting fluid intake not to exceed sweat rate (to decrease risk of hyponatremia)
- Limited or no caffeine or alcohol

Postexercise
Goal: if completed exercise session was long enough in duration to deplete glycogen stores (usually >90 min), consume sufficient fluids/foods to replenish these stores before next exercise session. The nutrition plan should include:
- Consuming fluids up to 150% of the weight lost during an exercise session
- A meal containing carbohydrates alone (yielding primarily glucose or sucrose) or carbohydrates + protein and fat, in close proximity to the end of exercise
- 1.5 g carbohydrate/kg at 2 h intervals following intense training sessions (only applies if exercise sessions are <1–2 days apart)
- Moderate amounts of high glycemic index carbohydrates (may promote greater insulin and glucose responses)
- Modest amounts of sodium may be consumed in fluids and/or meals following high-intensity/duration exercise[a]
- Limited or no caffeine or alcohol

[a] Sodium intake recommendations from the Dietary Guidelines for Americans report:[8]
- Consume less than 2300 mg (~1 tsp of salt) sodium/day
- Individuals with hypertension, people with dark skin, and middle-aged and older adults should aim to consume no more than 500 mg sodium/day and meet the potassium recommendation (4700 mg/day) with food

Note: Recommendations are targeted toward individuals who perform exercise at a moderate- to high-intensity, and are based on the Position on Nutrition and Athletic Performance,[1] the ACSM Position Stand on Exercise and Fluid Replacement,[113] and the National Athletic Trainers' Association Position Statement: Fluid Replacement for Athletes.[45]

do not distinguish between the nutrient needs of younger vs. older physically active persons. The following section highlights nutritional areas of concern for the older athlete, which are addressed in more detail in the papers by Campbell and Geik[120] and Larkin[121]:

1. *Energy*: Identifying nutrient needs for peak performance in the aging athlete can be complicated by weight gain, decreases in the level of physical activity, changes in hormonal status, and losses in muscle mass; older athletes have a lower energy requirement compared with younger athletes, but higher than what is recommended for aged-matched sedentary controls;[122] the goal should be to balance energy intake with expenditure and maintain desired body weight and composition.
2. *Macronutrients*: Older athletes should aim for meeting goals set within the nutrient-specific DRIs, appropriate for their age group, and the Position on Nutrition and Athletic Performance[1] recommended ranges for macronutrients; a diet low in energy intake (<2000 kcal/day) may pose a risk for insufficient macronutrient intakes.
3. *Micronutrients*: Older athletes who have a reduced energy requirement and are unable to at least meet the recommended DRIs may require supplementation with select micronutrients.
4. *Fluids*: Older competitors may have an increased risk for dehydration due to a blunting of the thirst mechanism and changes in kidney function and sweat responses that occur with increased age.[123–126]

ERGOGENIC AIDS

Supplementation with ergogenic aids (products claiming to enhance exercise performance) is a widespread practice among exercising individuals and deserves consideration when evaluating one's dietary and supplemental habits.[127] Regulation of these substances is not performed by the Food and Drug Administration; rather, the Dietary Supplement Health and Education Act (1994) has permitted supplement manufacturers to make claims of improved exercise performance, as long as there are no claims on the packaging to "diagnose, mitigate, treat, cure, or prevent" disease. The Position on Nutrition and Athletic Performance[1] reports the following criteria for assessing the validity of such claims:

- Evaluate the scientific validity of an ergogenic claim
- Evaluate the quality of the supportive evidence for using the ergogenic aid
- Evaluate the safety and legality of the ergogenic aid

Discretion is advised when using any nutritional supplement in an attempt to enhance physical performance. The consumption of improper amounts of certain ergogenic aids may cause a wide range of health problems, from diarrhea to more serious illnesses and fatalities. The recommendation by the Position on Nutrition and Athletic Performance[1] states that ergogenic products should be "used with caution and only after careful examination of the product [by a nutritional professional] for safety,

---

TABLE 19.6
Popular Nutritional Ergogenic Supplements Categorized by Performance-Enhancing Claim

Performance-Enhancing Claim

Increase energy supply/delay fatigue
Alkaline salts (e.g., sodium bicarbonate)[a]
Bee Pollen[b]
Caffeine[a,c,d]
Carnitine[b]
Coenzyme Q10 (ubiquinone)[b]
Creatine (methylguanidine-acetic acid)[a]
Dihydroxyacetone pyruvate[b]
Ephedrine (ephedra, ma huang)[b,c]
Ginseng[b]
Glycerol[b]
Phosphates[b]
Ribose[b]

Promote immune system function
Bee Pollen[b]
Coenzyme Q10 (ubiquinone)[b]
Echinacea[a]
Ginseng[b]

Achieve neuromuscular relaxation;
 decrease anxiety
Alcohol[b,c]

Maintain joint/cartilage health
Boron[b]
Glucosamine[a]
Chondroitin[a]
Collagen[b]

Enhance muscle anabolism and strength; reduce muscle catabolism
Androstenediol[b,c]
Androstenedione[b,c]
Bee Pollen[b]
Boron[b]
Chromium[b]
Chrysin[b]
Colostrum[b]
Creatine (methylguanidine-acetic acid)[a]
Dehydroepiandrosterone (DHEA)[b,c]
Dihydroxyacetone pyruvate[b]
Ginseng[b]
β-hydroxy-β-methylbutyrate (HMB)[a]
Mummio[b]
Norandrostenedione[b,c]
Ornithine alphaketoglutarate (OKG)[b]
Saw palmetto[b]
Smilax[b]
Tribulus terrestris[b]
Vanadium[b]
Yohimbine[b]

Increase fatty acid oxidation; promote weight loss
Caffeine[a,c,d]
Carnitine[b]
Collagen[b]
Ephedrine (ephedra, ma huang)[b,c]

Strength of Evidence (refers to individual supplements taken alone):

[a] Available studies generally support effectiveness for some individuals in some circumstances; confirming research is needed.

[b] Modest, inconclusive, or no positive data available to support effectiveness.

[c] Refers to substances that are currently banned by the Federal Drug Administration, International Olympic Committee, National Collegiate Athletic Association, National Football League, National Basketball Association, and/or Major League Baseball.

[d] Substance is prohibited in competition by most sports-governing organizations if urine concentrations >12 to 15 μg/ml.

Note: Information in this table was obtained from the National Center for Drug Free Sport, Inc.: http://www.drugfreesport.com/, the National Institutes of Health Office of Dietary Supplements: http://dietary-supplements.info.nih.gov/, and the President's Council on Physical Fitness and Sports Research Digest: Nutritional Ergogenics & Sports Performance: http://www.fitness.gov/

efficacy, potency, and legality." A detailed review of available ergogenic aids is beyond the focus of this chapter; however, some of the more popular nutritional supplements touted to improve physical performance not featured in earlier sections are listed in Table 19.6. Organizations such as the International Olympic Committee, the National Collegiate Athletic Association, and several sport-specific authorities (e.g., the National Football League, the National Basketball Association, and Major League Baseball) maintain updated lists of available performance-enhancing products and strive to enforce the prohibition of unsafe substances for use in competitive sport. Comprehensive examinations of the basic science, side effects, and efficacy of presently existing ergogenic supplements are published elsewhere.[127,128]

SUMMARY AND PRACTICAL APPLICATIONS

Appropriate intakes of energy, macronutrients, micronutrients, and water are necessary to ensure optimal performance with exercise. If any nutrient associated with the production of energy is limited in the diet, physical functioning during exercise could also be limited. A key strategy to meeting nutrient needs of almost all exercising individuals is to maintain variety in the diet; that is, consume the appropriate number of servings for a given caloric requirement, such as those reported in the 2005 Dietary Guidelines for Americans. If energy intakes are appropriate for energy expenditure, the specific nutrient needs for the exercising individual should not differ considerably from the foremost recommendations targeted at the general population (e.g., as outlined in the DRI reports). Activities of moderate to vigorous intensity typically require additional energy, primarily in the form of carbohydrates, and fluids in order to maintain glycogen stores and optimize physical performance. Special considerations related to vigorous activity place several nutrient recommendations for elite and/or endurance athletes above the DRI guidelines, which are most often required in proportion to individual caloric needs.

There is insufficient scientific evidence to recommend supplementing with individual micronutrients, unless intakes from major food groups, such as fruits and vegetables, are inadequate. For individuals on energy-restricted diets, vitamin/mineral supplements may be necessary to improve exercise performance (and at the very least, help achieve the AI/RDA recommendations), whereas such supplements may not be as effective in well-nourished individuals. Similarly, the level of training proficiency can impact the metabolic response to nutrients with exercise, where the presence of nutrients (or supplements) in the diet may elicit more pronounced effects on physiological responses in the inexperienced vs. the experienced exerciser.

As supplementation with certain nutrients above the DRI may actually have a negative impact on exercise performance and overall health, consumption of megadoses of vitamins and minerals is not advised. Furthermore, supplementation with any ergogenic aid is discouraged unless the product has been evaluated for safety, efficacy, potency, and legality. Physically active individuals should be encouraged to seek advice from a registered dietition to provide advice with regard to food, fluid, and supplement intakes based on personalized nutrient needs.

ACKNOWLEDGMENTS

Sincere appreciation is expressed to Ruth A. Gildea, Katy H. Yurman, Norman K. Pollock, Richard D. Lewis, and Donald C. Monkhouse for their technical and editorial expertise in reviewing this chapter.

REFERENCES

1. American Dietetic Association, Dietitians of Canada, and the American College of Sports Medicine *J Am Diet Assoc* 100, 1543, 2000.
2. Institute of Medicine, *Dietary Reference Intakes For Calcium, Phosphorus, Magnesium, Vitamin D, and Flouride*, National Academies Press, Washington, DC, 1997.
3. Institute of Medicine, *Dietary Reference Intakes for Thiamin, Riboflavin, Niacin, Vitamin B_6, Folate, Vitamin B_{12}, Pantothenic Acid, Biotin, and Choline*, National Academies Press, Washington, DC, 1998.
4. Institute of Medicine, *Dietary Reference Intakes for Vitamin C, Vitamin E, Selenium, and Carotenoids*, National Academies Press, Washington, DC, 2000.
5. Institute of Medicine, *Dietary Reference Intakes for Vitamin A, Vitamin K, Arsenic, Boron, Chromium, Copper, Iodine, Iron, Manganese, Molybdenum, Nickel, Silicon, Vanadium, and Zinc*, National Academies Press, Washington, DC, 2000.
6. Institute of Medicine, *Dietary Reference Intakes for Water, Potassium, Sodium, Chloride, and Sulfate*, National Academies Press, Washington, DC, 2004.
7. Institute of Medicine, *Dietary Reference Intakes for Energy, Carbohydrate, Fiber, Fat, Fatty acids, Cholesterol, Protein, and Amino acids (Macronutrients)*, National Academies Press, Washington, DC, 2005.
8. U.S. Department of Agriculture, Dietary Guidelines Committee report, Available at: http://www.health.gov/dietaryguidelines/dga2005/report/, 2005, Accessed May 2006.
9. Vickery, C.E., Cotunga, N., and McBee, S. *J Sch Nurs* 21, 323, 2005.
10. Calfee, R. and Fadale, P. *Pediatrics* 117, e577, 2006.

11. Fink, H., Mikesky A., and Burgoon, L. *Practical Applications in Sports Nutrition*, Jones and Bartlett Publishers, Inc., Sudbury, MA, 2006.
12. Swinburn, B. and Ravussin, E. *Am J Clin Nutr* 57, 766S, 1993.
13. Melzer, K. et al. *Clin Nutr* 24, 885, 2005.
14. American College of Sports Medicine, *Med Sci Sports Exerc* 30, 975, 1998.
15. U.S. Department of Health and Human Services, The Surgeon General's Call to Action to Prevent and Decrease Overweight and Obesity, Available at: http://www.surgeongeneral.gov/topics/obesity/, 2001, 2003, Accessed May 2006.
16. U.S. Department of Health and Human Services, *Nasnewsletter* 15, 3, 2000.
17. Dueck, C.A., Manore, M.M., and Matt, K.S. *Int J Sport Nutr* 6, 165, 1996.
18. Loucks, A.B. et al. *Med Sci Sports Exerc* 24, S288, 1992.
19. Loucks, A.B. and Nattiv, A. *Lancet* 366, S49, 2005.
20. Byrne, S. and McLean, N. *J Sci Med Sport* 4, 145, 2001.
21. Warren, M.P. and Perlroth, N.E. *J Endocrinol* 170, 3, 2001.
22. Harber, V.J. *Exerc Sport Sci Rev* 28, 19, 2000.
23. Otis, C.L. et al. *Med Sci Sports Exerc* 29, i, 1997.
24. International Olympic Committee Medical Commission Working Group on "Women in Sport," Position Stand on the Female Athlete Triad, Available at: http://www.olympic.org/uk/organisation/commissions/medical/full_story_uk.asp?id=1540, 2005, Accessed May 2006.
25. Torstveit, M.K. and Sundgot-Borgen, J. *Med Sci Sports Exerc* 37, 1449, 2005.
26. Beals, K.A. and Hill, A.K. *Int J Sport Nutr Exerc Metab* 16, 1, 2006.
27. Manore, M.M. *Sports Med* 32, 887, 2002.
28. Beals, K.A. and Manore, M.M. *Int J Sport Nutr Exerc Metab* 12, 281, 2002.
29. Zello, G.A. *Appl Physiol Nutr Metab* 31, 74, 2006.
30. Lemon, P.W. *J Am Coll Nutr* 19, 513S, 2000.
31. Hawley J.A. and Burke, L.M. *Br J Nutr* 77, S91, 1997.
32. Hargreaves, M. *Nutr Rev* 54, S136, 1996.
33. Backhouse, S.H. et al. *Med Sci Sports Exerc* 37, 1768, 2005.
34. Nicholas, C.W. et al. *Med Sci Sports Exerc* 31, 1280, 1999.
35. Bird, S.P., Tarpenning, K.M., and Marino, F.E. *Metabolism* 55, 570, 2006.
36. Roy, B.D. and Tarnopolsky, M.A. *J Appl Physiol* 84, 890, 1998.
37. Butterfield, G.E. *Med Sci Sports Exerc* 19, S157, 1987.
38. Lemon, P.W. *Int J Sport Nutr* 8, 426, 1998.
39. Bird, S.P., Tarpenning, K.M., and Marino, F.E. *Eur J Appl Physiol* 97, 225, 2006.
40. Ratamess, N.A. et al. *J Strength Cond Res* 17, 250, 2003.
41. Ohtani, M., Sugita, M., and Maruyama, K. *J Nutr* 136, 538S, 2006.
42. Shimomura, Y. et al. *J Nutr* 134, 1583S, 2004.
43. Lemon, P.W. and Mullin, J.P. *J Appl Physiol* 48, 624, 1980.
44. Coyle, E.F. *Am J Clin Nutr* 61, 968S, 1995.
45. Casa, D.J. et al. *J Athl Train* 35, 212, 2000.
46. Stevenson, E. et al. *Int J Sport Nutr Exerc Metab* 15, 333, 2005.
47. Wu, C.L. et al. *Br J Nutr* 90, 1049, 2003.
48. McKenzie, S. et al. *Am J Physiol Endocrinol Metab* 278, E580, 2000.
49. Gaine, P.C. et al. *Metabolism* 55, 501, 2006.
50. Metges, C.C. and Barth, C.A. *J Nutr* 130, 886, 2000.
51. Young, V.R. et al. *J Nutr* 130, 761, 2000.
52. Martin, W.F. et al. *J Am Diet Assoc* 106, 587, 2006.
53. Tarnopolsky, M. *Nutrition* 20, 662, 2004.
54. Havemann, L. et al. *J Appl Physiol* 100, 194, 2006.
55. Burke, L.M. and Kiens, B. *J Appl Physiol* 100, 7, 2006.
56. Kreider, R.B. et al. *J Strength Cond Res* 16, 325, 2002.
57. Toft, A.D. et al. *J Appl Physiol* 89, 2401, 2000.
58. Huffman, D.M. et al. *Eur J Appl Physiol* 92, 584, 2004.
59. Whiting, S.J. and Barabash, W.A. *Appl Physiol Nutr Metab* 31, 80, 2006.
60. Lukaski, H.C. *Nutrition* 20, 632, 2004.
61. Chen, J.D. et al. *Am J Clin Nutr* 49, 1084, 1989.
62. Webster, M.J. *Eur J Appl Physiol Occup Physiol* 77, 486, 1998.
63. Suzuki, M. and Itokawa, Y. *Metab Brain Dis* 11, 95, 1996.
64. Belko, A.Z. et al. *Am J Clin Nutr* 37, 509 (1983).
65. Janelle, K.C. and Barr, S.I. *J Am Diet Assoc* 95, 180, 1995.
66. Russell, R.M. and Suter, P.M. *Am J Clin Nutr* 58, 4, 1993.
67. Winters, L.R. et al. *Am J Clin Nutr* 56, 526, 1992.
68. van der Beek, E.J. et al. *J Am Coll Nutr* 13, 629, 1994.

69. Manore, M.M. *Int J Sport Nutr* 4, 89, 1994.
70. Manore, M.M. *Am J Clin Nutr* 72, 598S, 2000.
71. Manore, M.M., Leklem, K.E., and Walter, M.C. *Am J Clin Nutr* 46, 995, 1987.
72. Crozier, P.G., Cordain, L., and Sampson, D.A. *Am J Clin Nutr* 60, 552, 1994.
73. Sacheck, J.M. and Roubenoff, R. *Clin Sports Med* 18, 565, 1999.
74. Heath, E.M., Wilcox, A.R., and Quinn, C.M. *Med Sci Sports Exerc* 25, 1018, 1993.
75. Murray, R. et al. *Med Sci Sports Exerc* 27, 1057, 1995.
76. Trost, S. Wilcox, A., and Gillis, D. *Int J Sports Med* 18, 83, 1997.
77. Venderley A.M. and Campbell, W.W. *Sports Med* 36, 293, 2006.
78. Montoye, H.J. et al. *J Appl Physiol* 7, 589, 1955.
79. Tin May, T. et al. *Br J Nutr* 40, 269, 1978.
80. Sachan, D.S., Hongu, N., and Johnsen, M. *J Am Coll Nutr* 24, 172, 2005.
81. Spector, S.A. et al. *Med Sci Sports Exerc* 27, 668, 1995.
82. Warber, J.P. et al. *Int J Sport Nutr Exerc Metab* 10, 170, 2000.
83. Deuster, P.A. et al. *Mil Med* 167, 1020, 2002.
84. Quindry, J.C. et al. *Med Sci Sports Exerc* 35, 1139, 2003.
85. Hessel, E. et al. *Clin Chim Acta* 298, 145, 2000.
86. Schneider, C.D. et al. *Can J Appl Physiol* 30, 723, 2005.
87. Powers, S.K. et al. *J Sports Sci* 22, 81, 2004.
88. Watson, T.A., MacDonald-Wicks, L.K., and Garg, M.L. *Int J Sport Nutr Exerc Metab* 15, 131, 2005.
89. Senturk, U.K. et al. *J Appl Physiol* 99, 1434, 2005.
90. Mastaloudis, A. et al. *Free Radic Biol Med* 36, 1329, 2004.
91. Mastaloudis, A. et al. *Med Sci Sports Exerc* 38, 72, 2006.
92. Davison, G. and Gleeson, M. *Int J Sport Nutr Exerc Metab* 15, 465, 2005.
93. Sumida, S. et al. *Int J Biochem* 21, 835, 1989.
94. Evans, W.J. *Am J Clin Nutr* 72, 647S, 2000.
95. McAnulty, S.R. et al. *J Nutr Biochem* 16, 530, 2005.
96. Davison, G.W., Hughes, C.M., and Bell, R.A. *Int J Sport Nutr Exerc Metab* 15, 480, 2005.
97. Hagobian, T.A. et al. *Med Sci Sports Exerc* 38, 276, 2006.
98. Devine, A. et al. *J Bone Miner Res* 19, 1634, 2004.
99. Stear, S.J. et al. *Am J Clin Nutr* 77, 985, 2003.
100. Bischoff-Ferrari, H.A. et al. *Am J Clin Nutr* 80, 752, 2004.
101. Bischoff, H.A. et al. *Z Rheumatol* 59, 39, 2000.
102. Terblanche, S. et al. *Int J Sport Nutr* 2, 154, 1992.
103. Mooren, F.C. et al. *Life Sci* 77, 1211, 2005.
104. Finstad, E.W. et al. *Med Sci Sports Exerc* 33, 493, 2001.
105. Barr, S.I. and Rideout, C.A. *Nutrition* 20, 696, 2004.
106. Sinclair, L.M. and Hinton, P.S. *J Am Diet Assoc* 105, 975, 2005.
107. Chatard, J.C. et al. *Sports Med* 27, 229, 1999.
108. Krotkiewski, M. et al. *Acta Physiol Scand* 116, 309, 1982.
109. Subudhi, A.W. et al. *Aviat Space Environ Med* 75, 881, 2004.
110. Barr, S.I. *Appl Physiol Nutr Metab* 31, 61, 2006.
111. Barr, S.I. *Appl Physiol Nutr Metab* 31, 66, 2006.
112. Noakes, T.D. *Exerc Sport Sci Rev* 21, 297 (1993).
113. Convertino, V.A. et al. *Med Sci Sports Exerc* 28, i, 1996.
114. Millard-Stafford, M.L. et al. *Int J Sport Nutr Exerc Metab* 15, 117, 2005.
115. Von Duvillard, S.P. et al. *Nutrition* 20, 651, 2004.
116. Noakes, T.D. et al. *Proc Natl Acad Sci USA* 102, 18550, 2005.
117. Hew-Butler, T. et al. *Clin J Sport Med* 15, 208, 2005.
118. Casa, D.J. USATF self-testing program for optimal hydration, Available at: http://www.usatf.org/groups/coaches/library/hydration/USATFSelfTestingProgramForOptimalHydration.pdf, 2003, 2006, Accessed May 2006.
119. Schoenborn, C.A., Vickerie, J.L., and Powell-Griner, E. *Adv Data* 370, 1, 2006.
120. Campbell, W.W. and Geik, R.A. *Nutrition* 20, 603, 2004.
121. Larkin, M. *Lancet* 366, S27, 2005.
122. Butterworth, D.E. et al. *J Am Diet Assoc* 93, 653, 1993.
123. Rolls, B.J. and Phillips, P.A. *Nutr Rev* 48, 137, 1990.
124. Kenney, W.L. and Fowler, S.R. *J Appl Physiol* 65, 1082, 1988.
125. Kenney, W.L. and Chiu, P. *Med Sci Sports Exerc* 33, 1524, 2001.
126. Ainslie, P.N. et al. *J Appl Physiol* 93, 714, 2002.
127. Tokish, J.M., Kocher, M.S., and Hawkins, R.J. *Am J Sports Med* 32, 1543, 2004.
128. Maughan, R.J., King, D.S., and Lea, T. *J Sports Sci* 22, 95, 2004.

20 Vegetarian Diets in Health Promotion and Disease Prevention

Claudia S. Plaisted Fernandez and Kelly M. Adams

CONTENTS

OVERVIEW/INTRODUCTION

Vegetarianism is rapidly growing in popularity. Technically defined, vegetarians are individuals who do not eat any meat, poultry, or seafood.[1,2] Estimates on the number of vegetarians in the United States vary greatly according to the definition of vegetarianism provided in the survey. True vegetarians make up about 2.8% of the population representing approximately 5.7 million adults according to a 2003 poll.[3] A higher percentage of teenagers than adults follow a vegetarian diet.[3]

Vegetarian dietary patterns can represent an exceptionally healthy way of eating. They are typically rich in vitamins, minerals, phytochemicals, and fiber while often also low in fat, saturated fat, and cholesterol.[1,4] However, each individual diet will need to be assessed for its nutritional adequacy. This chapter provides some guidance in characterizing vegetarian dietary patterns, health benefits, and concerns as well as in identifying sources of various nutrients that may be marginal in many vegetarian diets.

CHARACTERISTICS OF VEGETARIAN EATING STYLES

When working with someone who follows a vegetarian diet, it is important to ask them a variety of questions about their usual dietary patterns. Many people consider themselves to be vegetarian when they eat nonflesh foods several days a week. Others will claim to be vegetarians when they consume fish or poultry. Table 20.1 lists the types of vegetarian diets and describes what foods fall into or out of those categories.

In popular culture, there are many diets that incorporate principles of vegetarianism and may represent more restrictive ways of eating as described in Table 20.2. For the purposes of this chapter, "vegetarian" will refer to an individual following a lacto and/or ovo pattern or a vegan dietary pattern.

A more restrictive diet makes the individual following it more susceptible to dietary deficiencies and imbalances.[1,2] Table 20.3 describes the nutrients that may be of concern in many vegetarian diets.

HEALTH BENEFITS AND RISKS OF VEGETARIANISM

Most health risks associated with a vegetarian diet are found with strict vegetarianism (veganism) only, not with the more liberal forms of intake found in lacto-vegetarians, ovo-vegetarians, or lacto-ovo vegetarians.[1,10,11] Table 20.4 lists the health risks of vegetarianism, most of which are related to the potential for nutrient deficiencies found with this type of diet. These health risks are not unique to vegetarians, however, as they can be quite common in people following an imbalanced omnivorous diet.

TABLE 20.1
Types of Vegetarian Diets

Vegan	Consumes nuts, fruits, grains, legumes, and vegetables. Does not consume animal-based food products, including eggs, dairy products, red meats, poultry, or seafood. Some vegetarians may avoid foods with animal processing (honey, sugar, vinegar, wine, beer, etc.)
Lacto-vegetarian	Consumes milk and other dairy products, nuts, fruits, grains, legumes, and vegetables. Does not consume eggs, red meats, poultry, or seafood
Ovo-vegetarian	Consumes eggs, nuts, fruits, grains, legumes, and vegetables. Does not consume milk or dairy, red meats, poultry, or seafood
Lacto-ovo vegetarian	Consumes milk and other dairy products, eggs, nuts, fruits, grains, legumes, and vegetables. Does not consume red meats, poultry, or seafood
Pollo-vegetarian[a]	Not technically considered a vegetarian type of diet, although often referred to as "vegetarian" in popular culture. Consumes milk and other dairy products, eggs, nuts, fruits, grains, legumes, vegetables, and poultry
Peche-vegetarian, also called pesco- and pecto-vegetarian[a]	Not technically considered a vegetarian type of diet, although often referred to as "vegetarian" in popular culture. Consumes milk and other dairy products, eggs, nuts, fruits, grains, legumes, vegetables, and seafood
Omnivore	Consumes from a wide variety of foods, including meats, grains, fruits, vegetables, legumes, and dairy products. Individuals who consume red meats (beef, pork, lamb, etc), poultry, seafood, or any still or once living nonplant based matter are not vegetarians

[a] This is not technically a vegetarian diet, although it is often referred to as such.

TABLE 20.2
Types of Popular Diets[a] Incorporating Various Principles of Vegetarianism

Fad diets	Popular weight loss diets often incorporate various principles of vegetarianism, although not generally in nutritious, balanced ways. The cabbage soup diet is an example, which is based on consuming only a vegetable soup based on cabbage as a weight-loss technique
Fruitarian	Consumes botanical fruits (including nuts and seeds), avoids meats, poultry, seafood, dairy, eggs, and vegetables. May avoid legumes
Macrobiotic	Largely based on grains and in-season foods, including vegetables (except those of the nightshade family), sea vegetables, soups, and beans. Nuts and seeds are not consumed on a daily basis, along with fruits, which are included with the exception of tropical ones. Seafood is sometimes included as well. Asian foods contribute significantly to food choices
	This is an example of a diet following a food-combining philosophy
Natural hygiene or raw foods diet	Generally raw vegetables, fruits, whole grains or sprouted grains (in some cases may be cooked), sprouted or nonsprouted legumes, nuts, and seeds. Some consumers may consume raw dairy products. There is great variation in this diet plan: many followers do consume cooked foods and some consume meat as well
	This is an example of a diet following a food-combining philosophy, but has many variations among followers

[a] Many variations exist on each of these types of diets. This is not intended as a comprehensive listing.

Many vegetarians follow a dietary pattern that reduces their risks for common chronic diseases as noted in Table 20.5 and Table 20.6.[4] New vegetarians, in particular, however, may rely heavily on high fat dairy products, which may actually increase risk for cardiovascular disease. Other practical concerns for new vegetarians are found in Table 20.7.

Table 20.8 compares the typical dietary intake of vegans and lacto-ovo vegetarians with omnivores while the health risks/outcomes associated with specific kinds of vegetarian diets are mentioned in Table 20.9. The nutrients of special concern will vary depending on the type of vegetarian diet followed. As discussed in Table 20.10, some nutrients are more critical during specific developmental phases; deficiency of that particular nutrient at that stage of the lifecycle can have dramatic consequences.[10,12,29,30]

ENERGY AND MACRONUTRIENTS IN THE VEGETARIAN DIET

A common misconception about a vegetarian diet concerns protein. Many new vegetarians are frequently confronted with the question: "So how do you get your protein?" Individuals following a lacto-ovo vegetarian diet rarely have to worry about protein. Even vegans eating a reasonably balanced diet with adequate calories can easily meet their protein needs.[1,4] In reality, it is much more likely that the individual is suffering from a dietary deficiency of a micronutrient, such as calcium or zinc, than a protein deficiency. Energy and protein can be of concern in some adult vegetarian diets, particularly if the individual follows severe dietary restrictions, and in children.[29]

TABLE 20.3

Nutrients Potentially at Risk in Vegetarian Diets, Dietary Reference Intakes (DRIs), Functions, and Sources [2,5–7]

Vitamin/Mineral	RDA (Unless otherwise Noted): Adult Value 31–50 Year Old, Nonpregnant, per Day	Function	Good Sources in Vegetarian Diet
Vitamins			
Vitamin B$_{12}$	M: 2.4 mcg F: 2.4 mcg	Works with folic acid to make red blood cells; important in maintaining healthy nerve fibers; helps the body use fat and protein	Dairy products, eggs, fortified cereals, fortified soy products/meat substitutes, and fortified nutritional yeast
Vitamin D	Adequate Intake (AI): M: 5 mcg F: 5 mcg	Promotes absorption of calcium and phosphorus and helps deposit them in bones and teeth	Fortified milk; made in body when skin is exposed to sunlight
Riboflavin (B$_2$)	M: 1.3 mg F: 1.1 mg	Helps the body release energy from protein, fat, and carbohydrates	Fortified dairy products, fortified breads and cereals, tomatoes, lima beans, raisins, avocado, beans, and legumes
Minerals			
Calcium	AI: M: 1000 mg F: 1000 mg	Used to build bones and teeth and keep them strong; important in muscle contraction and blood clotting	Dairy products, broccoli, mustard, and turnip greens
Iron[a]	M: 8 mg F: 18 mg	Carries oxygen in the body, both as a part of hemoglobin (in the blood), and myoglobin (in the muscles)	Whole-grain and enriched cereals, some dried fruits, and soybeans
Zinc	M: 11 mg F: 8 mg	Assists in wound healing, blood formation, and general growth and maintenance of all tissues; component of many enzymes	Plant and animal proteins
Manganese[b]	AI: M: 2.3 mg F: 1.8 mg	Found in most of body's organs and tissues, particularly in bones, liver, and kidneys. Serves as a cofactor in many metabolic processes. Deficiency not seen in human populations	Whole grains, cereal products, tea, some fruits, and vegetables
Iodine	150 mcg	Constituent of thyroid hormones (regulation of metabolic rate, body temperature, growth, reproduction, making body cells, muscle function, and nerve growth).	Fortified in salt, found widely in processed foods and grains where soil concentration is adequate.
Copper[c]	AI: M: 900 mcg F: 900 mcg	Necessary for the formation of hemoglobin; keeps bones, blood vessels, and nerves healthy	Nuts, legumes, and whole grains
Selenium	Males: 55 mcg Females: 55 mcg	Antioxidant functions, role in eicosanoid metabolism, regulation of arachadonic acid and lipid peroxidation, and some hormone conversions	Eggs, whole grains, legumes, and brazil nuts
Macronutrients and other dietary components			
Protein	Male: 56 g or .8g/kg Female: 46 g or .8 gm/kg	Building of nearly all body tissues, particularly muscle tissue, energy	Dairy products, legumes, meat analog products often made from soy; whole grains and vegetables are poorer sources
Omega-3 fatty acids	AI: M: 1.6 g F: 1.1 g	Energy source, cell wall structure, may play a role in disease prevention. Fats also play a role in the absorption and transport of fat-soluble vitamins. Linolenic acid cannot be made by the body, omega-3 series fatty acids can be found in grains, seeds, nuts, and soybeans and the body can manufacture eicosapentaenoic acid (EPA) and docosahexaenoic acid (DHA) from these precursors, but conversion is inefficient	Fats and oils (bean, nut, and grain oils), nuts, and seeds (butternuts, walnuts, and soybean kernels), soybeans, flax seeds, and flax seed oil

[a] There is some evidence that vegetarian diets tend to be quite high in iron and that iron deficiency anemia is no more common among vegetarians than in meat eaters.[1]

[b] Manganese is not necessarily at risk for deficiency in vegetarians. Some research has indicated that vegetarians have a higher intake of this nutrient; however, bioavailability may be a concern.[8,9]

[c] Copper is not necessarily at risk for deficiency in vegetarians. Some research has indicated that vegetarians have a higher intake of this nutrient; however, bioavailability may be a concern.[8,9]

TABLE 20.4
Health Risks of Vegetarianism[1,10,12–20]

Dietary Factor	Risk
Calcium	Low calcium intake in vegan or macrobiotic diet can lead to low bone mineral density.
Iodine	A strict vegan consuming no iodized salt or processed food products can develop goiter.
Vitamin B_{12}	In strict vegans or in the offspring of vegan mothers only, deficiency can lead to anemia or in far more severe cases, neuropathy.
Energy	Impaired growth can result in infants and children with inadequate energy intake or those weaned to "homemade" formulas.
Docosahexaenoic acid (DHA)	Greatest concern for fetus and young infants. DHA is needed for neural and retinal development.
Dairy products	Iron deficiency with excessive consumption of dairy products in young children. Limited evidence exists linking high consumption of dairy products to diabetes (type 1).

TABLE 20.5
Health Benefits of Vegetarianism[1,2,4,13,21–26]

Lower risk of:
    Cancer (particularly colon and lung)
    Obesity
    Heart disease
    Type 2 Diabetes
    Hypertension
    Constipation and Hemorrhoids
    Kidney stones
    Gallstones
Potential lower risk for (limited evidence suggesting):
    Arthritis
    Gout
    Dementia
    Tooth decay
    Duodenal ulcers

TABLE 20.6
Protective Factors in the Typical
Lacto-Ovo Vegetarian Diet[1,4,21,27,28]

Higher fiber
Lower fat, saturated fat, and cholesterol
Higher folate intake
Higher intake of antioxidants
Higher intake of phytochemicals
Lower intake of total and animal protein

TABLE 20.7
Practical Concerns about Vegetarianism

New vegetarians or those who are vegetarian for philosophical (as opposed to health) reasons may rely heavily on the use of dairy products and eggs.
Whole-milk cheeses, 2% and higher-fat-content milk, eggs, and whole-milk yogurts are rich in fat, saturated fat and, in some cases, cholesterol as well. These can contribute to higher risks for cardiovascular disease in particular and should be evaluated.
Some adolescents with eating disorders may use vegetarianism as a rationalization for avoiding foods or entire food groups.

TABLE 20.8

Nutrient Differences between Omnivore, Lacto-Ovo, and Vegan Dietary Patterns[1,2]

Dietary Component	Vegan	Lacto-Ovo	Omnivore
Total fat (% of total energy)	25–30	28–34	34
Saturated Fat	Generally low saturated fat intake	Generally moderate saturated fat intake	Generally higher saturated fat intake
P/S ratio	High P/S	Mod P/S	Poor P/S
Fiber (g/d range)	25–50	20–35	15–20
Carbohydrate (% total calories)	50–65	50–55	<50
Protein (% of total calories)	10–12 (none from animal sources)	12–14 (~1/2 from animal sources)	14–18 (~2/3 from animal sources)
Folate (mcg/d ranges)	170–385	214–455	252–471
Cholesterol (mg dietary intake)	0	150–300	300
Cholesterol serum levels (mmol/L)	4.29	4.88	5.31
Blood pressure (mm HG systolic/diastolic)	112.5/65.3	111.8/68.8	120.8/76.4

TABLE 20.9

Health Risks of Individuals Following Various Types of Vegetarian Diets[1,2]

Type of Vegetarian Diet	Health Risk Profile	Nutrients at Greatest Risk
Vegan	Low risk of obesity, heart disease, cancer, hypertension, and diabetes. Vegans may have a lower health risk than lacto-ovo vegetarians due to the typical lower fat and higher fiber content than either lacto-ovo or nonvegetarians	Vitamin B_{12} Vitamin D Calcium Zinc Energy Potentially Iron
Lacto-vegetarian	Generally low risk of obesity, heart disease, cancer, hypertension, and diabetes. Unskilled or new vegetarian may rely heavily on whole-milk-based products, thus consuming high fat, saturated fat and cholesterol intakes, which could increase the risk of cardiovascular-related diseases	Zinc Potentially Iron
Ovo-vegetarian	Generally low risk of obesity, heart disease, cancer, hypertension, and diabetes. Unskilled or new vegetarian may rely heavily on eggs and egg-based products, thus consuming high fat, saturated fat, and cholesterol intakes, which could increase the risk of cardiovascular-related diseases	Zinc Potentially Iron
Lacto-ovo Vegetarian	Generally low risk of obesity, heart disease, cancer, hypertension, and diabetes. Unskilled or new vegetarian may rely heavily on whole-milk- or egg-based products, thus consuming high fat, saturated fat and cholesterol intakes, which could increase the risk of cardiovascular-related diseases	Zinc Potentially Iron

Table 20.11 through Table 20.13 provides information about essential and nonessential amino acids and protein complementation. In the 1970s, carefully complementing proteins at each meal was thought to be the only way that vegetarians could avoid protein deficiency. We now know that it is not necessary to combine proteins at each meal,[1,4] yet it is important to understand the terminology related to the body's protein needs and the principles of complementation.

Table 20.14 compares average protein intakes in the United States, while Table 20.15 and Table 20.16 provide information about protein and nutrient dense/energy dense food sources. As an arbitrary guideline, foods with 2 g or less of protein were not included. The information about nutrient- and energy-dense foods can be useful for young children who may fill up quickly on a bulky vegetarian diet without meeting their calorie and nutrient needs.[30]

TABLE 20.10
Critical Periods of Importance for Selected Nutrients[2,5,17]

Nutrient	Critical Periods During Lifecycle
Vitamin B_{12}	Throughout, particularly critical during pregnancy, infancy, and childhood
Riboflavin (B_2)	Pregnancy, periods of growth
Vitamin D	Childhood and prepuberty, pregnancy, and elderly
Calcium	Childhood and prepuberty, elderly
Iron	Infancy, childhood, adolescence, pregnancy, and adulthood (women particularly)
Zinc	Puberty, pregnancy, and elderly
Iodine	Adolescence, pregnancy, and lactation
Protein	Infancy, childhood, adolescence, and pregnancy
Omega-3 fatty acids (especially DHA)	Pregnancy and infancy
Energy	Periods of growth, especially toddlers/preschoolers, due to small stomach capacity

TABLE 20.11
Definitions Related to Protein Complementation[2]

Complete protein	Contains all essential amino acids in ample amounts; amino acid pattern is very similar to humans
Incomplete protein	May be low in one or more amino acids; amino acid pattern is very different from humans
Limiting amino acid	The essential amino acid(s) that are in the smallest supply in the food
Essential amino acid	Cannot be synthesized by the human body. Include: Arginine, Histidine, Isoleucine, Leucine, Lysine, Methionine, Phenylalanine, Threonine, Tryptophan, and Valine

TABLE 20.12
Limiting Essential Amino Acids and Vegan Sources[1,2]

Food	Limiting Amino Acids	Vegan Sources of the Limiting Amino Acids
Legumes	Methionine, cysteine	Grains, nuts, seeds, and soybeans
Cereals/grains	Lysine and threonine	Legumes
Nuts and seeds	Lysine	Legumes
Peanuts	Methionine, lysine, and threonine	Legumes, grains, nuts, seeds, and soybeans
Vegetables	Methionine	Grains, nuts, and seeds, and soybeans
Corn	Tryptophan, lysine, and threonine	Legumes, sesame and sunflower seeds, and soybeans

TABLE 20.13
Guidelines for Protein Complementation[1,2]

Type of Vegetarian Diet	Guidelines for Complementation[a]
Lacto-ovo	Dairy products and eggs provide complete protein, as do other animal products
Vegan	A vegan diet that contains a variety of grains, legumes, vegetables, seeds, and nuts over the course of a day in amounts to meet a person's calorie needs will provide adequate amino acids in appropriate amounts. Soybeans match human needs for essential amino acids as precisely as animal foods and are, thus, a complete protein.
Any	It is not necessary to combine proteins in each meal. Young children, however, may need to have the complementary proteins consumed within a few hours of each other.

[a] All proteins except gelatin provide all of the amino acids. Some protein sources have relatively low levels of some amino acids, so large amount of that food would need to be consumed if it were the only source of those "limiting" amino acids.[1]

TABLE 20.14

Protein Intakes in United States[1]

Type of Diet	Percentage of Calories from Protein	Sufficient to Meet RDA?
Typical U.S. diet	14–18	Yes
Lacto-ovo vegetarians	12–14	Yes, provided adequate calories are consumed
Vegans	10–12	Yes, provided adequate calories are consumed

TABLE 20.15

Protein: Vegetarian Sources and Amounts[5,31,32]

Food	Portion Size	Protein (g)	Kcal
Cereals/Grains			
Quinoa	0.5 cup	11.1	318
Millet, cooked	1 cup	8.4	286
Wheat germ, toasted	0.25 cup	8.4	111
Bagel, plain	1 bagel	7.5	195
Couscous, cooked	1 cup	6.8	200
Macaroni, enriched, cooked	1 cup	6.7	197
Pita, whole wheat	1 pita	6.3	170
Grape-Nuts, Post	0.5 cup	6.0	200
Oatmeal Crisp, almond, and General Mills	1 cup	6.0	220
Oatmeal, old fashioned, and Quaker	0.5 cup dry	5.5	148
Oat bran, raw	0.33 cup	5.4	76
Brown rice, medium grain, cooked	1 cup	4.5	218
English muffin, plain	1 muffin	4.4	134
Barley, pearled, cooked	1 cup	3.5	193
Whole wheat bread	1 slice	2.7	69
Corn grits, instant, white, enriched	1 oz. packet dry	2.4	96
Vegetables			
Peas, green, canned	0.5 cup	3.8	59
Corn, yellow, boiled	0.5 cup	2.7	89
Broccoli, boiled	0.5 cup	2.3	22
Fruits			
Prunes, dried	10 prunes	2.2	201
Dairy/Soymilk			
Cottage cheese, 1% fat	1 cup	28.0	164
Yogurt, low fat (1.5% milk fat), plain, Breyers	1 cup	11.0	130
Simple Pleasures, chocolate	0.5 cup	8.9	134
Gruyere cheese	1 oz.	8.5	117
Milk, low fat (1%)	1 cup	8.0	102
Cheddar cheese	1 oz.	7.1	114
Soymilk	1 cup	6.6	79
American processed cheese	1 oz.	6.3	106
Pudding, all flavors, from instant mix Jell-O Brand	0.5 cup	4.0	155
Frozen yogurt, soft serve	0.5 cup	2.9	115
Ice cream, vanilla, regular (10% fat)	0.5 cup	2.3	133
Beans/Legumes			
Soybean nuts, roasted	0.5 cup	30.3	405
Lentils, boiled	1 cup	17.9	230
Lima beans, boiled	1 cup	14.7	216
Kidney beans, canned	1 cup	13.3	207
Garbanzo beans, canned	1 cup	11.9	286

Continued

TABLE 20.15
(Continued)

Food	Portion Size	Protein (g)	Kcal
Soy Products/Meat Substitutes			
Tofu, raw, firm	0.5 cup	19.9	183
Tempeh	0.5 cup	15.7	165
Pepperoni from meat substitute	16 slices	14	70
Better 'n Burger, Morningstar Farms	1 patty	11.3	75
Soybeans, green, boiled	0.5 cup	11.1	127
Ground Meatless, frozen, Morningstar Farms	0.5 cup	10.3	60
Meatless deli turkey	3 slices	9	40
Nuts/Seeds			
Peanut butter, chunk style/crunchy	2 T	7.7	188
Sunflower seeds, dried	1 oz.	6.2	160
Almonds, blanched	1 oz.	6.0	174
Sesame butter (tahini)	2 T	5.0	174
Cashews, dry roasted	1 oz.	4.3	163
Eggs			
Egg substitute, frozen	0.25 cup	6.8	96
Egg, chicken, whole, fresh/frozen	1 large	6.2	75
Egg, chicken, yolk fresh	1 large	2.8	61
Mixed Foods			
Frozen french bread pizza, vegetarian	6 oz. pizza	17.0	270
Shells and cheese, from mix	1 cup	16.0	360
Burritos with beans	2 burritos	14.1	447
Biscuit with egg	1 item	11.1	316
Potato, baked, with sour cream and chives	1 potato	6.7	393

Adult RDA: Males 56 g/day Females 46 g/day; taking into account the lower digestibility and amino acid profile, a reasonable RDA for vegans is approximately 10% more protein than omnivores.

TABLE 20.16
Vegetarian Sources of Energy-Dense, Nutrient-Dense Foods[31,32]

Food	Portion Size	Kcal
Cereals/Grains		
Granola, low-fat	1 cup	422
Quinoa	0.5 cup	318
Millet, cooked	1 cup	286
Pancakes, Bisquick, and blueberry	3 each	220
Oatmeal Crisp	1 cup	210
Grape-Nuts, Post	0.5 cup	200
Macaroni, enriched, cooked	1 cup	197
Bagel, plain	1 bagel	195
Raisin bran, dry	1 cup	175
Corn muffin (2.5 × 2.25 in.)	1 muffin	174
Pita, whole wheat	1 pita (6.5 in diameter)	170
Banana nut muffin, from mix	1 muffin	160
Oat bran muffin	1 muffin	154
Vegetables		
Tater Tots, frozen, heated	4 oz.	204
Potatoes, mashed from granules	1 cup	166

Continued

TABLE 20.16
(Continued)

Food	Portion Size	Kcal
Fruits		
Avocado, California, raw	0.5 medium	153
Raisins, golden, seedless	0.66 cup	302
Mixed fruit, dried, diced, Delmonte	0.66 cup	220
Dairy/Soymilk		
Milkshake, thick vanilla	1 cup	256
Yogurt, flavored, low-fat, 1% milk-fat, Breyers	1 cup	251
Ricotta cheese, part-skim	0.5 cup	171
Cottage cheese (1% fat)	1 cup	164
Pudding, all flavors, from instant mix Jell-O)	0.5 cup	155
Milk, whole	1 cup	150
Yogurt, low-fat (1.5 % milk fat), plain, Breyers	1 cup	130
Cheddar cheese	1 oz.	114
Milk, low fat (1%)	1 cup	102
Soymilk	1 cup	79
Beans/Legumes		
Soybean, dried, boiled, mature	1 cup	298
Garbanzo beans, canned	1 cup	286
Lentils, boiled	1 cup	230
Soy Products/Meat Substitutes		
Soybean nuts (roasted)	0.5 cup	405
Tempeh	1 cup	330
Soyburger with cheese	1 each	316
Chicken nuggets, meatless	5 pieces	245
Frankfurter, meatless	1 each	102
Nuts/Seeds		
Peanut butter, chunky style	2 T	188
Almonds, blanched	1 oz.	174
Sesame butter (tahini)	2 T	174
Sunflower seeds, dried	1 oz.	160
Mixed Foods		
Egg salad	1 cup	586
Burritos, with beans	2 burritos	447
Potato, baked, with sour cream and chives	1 potato	393
Shells and cheese, from mix	1 cup	360
Peanut butter and jam sandwich on wheat	1 each	344
Cheese enchilada	1 item	320
Biscuit with egg	1 item	316
Lasagna, no meat, recipe	1 piece	298
Chili, meatless, canned	0.66 cup	190
Trail mix, regular	0.25 cup	150
Vegetable soup	1 cup	145
Pizza, cheese	1/8 of 12-in.	140
Pasta with marinara sauce	1 cup	180–450

MICRONUTRIENTS IN THE VEGETARIAN DIET

Although vegetarian dietary patterns can be extremely healthful,[1,13,21–23] certain micronutrients can be challenging to obtain in sufficient quantities depending on the specific dietary restrictions the individual follows. Table 20.17 through Table 20.28 provide information about sources of micronutrients that can be of concern for some vegetarian individuals.[1,4,8–13,22,37,38] As a guideline, foods with less than 5 to 10% of the recommended amount of that particular nutrient per serving were not included in the table.

Bioavailability of minerals can influence the amount available for absorption. Table 20.24 and Table 20.28 list factors that may enhance or inhibit the absorption of iron and zinc.

TABLE 20.17
Riboflavin[a]: Vegetarian Sources and Amounts[5,6,31,32]

Food	Portion Size	Riboflavin (mg)	Kcal
Cereals[b,c]/Grains			
Raisin bran	1 cup (2.1 oz.)	0.678	175
Bran flakes	0.66 cup (1 oz.)	0.43	91.5
Corn flakes, Kellogg's	1 cup (1 oz.)	0.375	90
Bagel, plain	1 bagel (3.5 in.)	0.22	195
Sesame breadsticks	2 sticks	0.22	120
Pita, white	1 pita (6.5 in. diameter)	0.20	165
Lasagna noodles	2 oz. dry	0.20	210
Cornbread, homemade from low-fat milk	1 slice	0.19	173
Corn muffin (2.5 × 2.25 in.)	1 muffin	0.19	174
English muffin, wheat	1 muffin	0.17	127
English muffin, plain	1 muffin	0.16	134
Muffin, blueberry, homemade (2.75 × 2 in.)	1 muffin	0.16	163.5
Macaroni, enriched and cooked	1 cup	0.14	197
Wild rice, cooked	1 cup	0.14	166
Rye bread	1 slice	0.11	83
Vegetables			
Mushrooms, boiled	0.5 cup	0.23	21
Tomato puree, canned	1 cup	0.14	100
Sweet potatoes, baked, with skin	1 medium	0.14	117
Tomato, red, sun-dried	0.5 cup	0.13	69.5
Garden cress, boiled	0.5 cup	0.11	16
Fruits			
Raisins, golden seedless	0.66 cup	0.19	302
Banana	1 medium	0.11	105
Raspberries, raw	1 cup	0.11	60
Avocado, Calif. raw	0.5 medium	0.105	153
Dairy/Soymilk			
Yogurt, plain, low fat	1 cup	0.493	209
Milk, whole	1 cup	0.395	150
Cottage cheese, 1% fat	1 cup	0.37	164
Milk, nonfat	1 cup	0.34	86
Feta cheese	1 oz.	0.24	75
Ricotta cheese, part-skim	0.5 cup	0.23	171
Soymilk	1 cup	0.17	79
Cheddar cheese, reduced fat	1 oz.	0.14	80
Cheddar cheese	1 oz.	0.11	114
Goat cheese, soft	1 oz.	0.11	76
Beans/Legumes			
Soybeans, boiled	1 cup	0.49	298
Kidney beans, canned	1 cup	0.18	207
Great northern beans, canned	1 cup	0.16	299
Pinto beans, boiled	1 cup	0.16	234
Lentils, boiled	1 cup	0.14	230
Soy Products/Meat Substitutes			
Chicken nuggets, meatless	5 pieces	0.30	245
Vegetarian burger, grilled, Morningstar Farms	1 patty	0.24	140
Breakfast links, Morningstar Farms	2 links	0.22	63
Tofu, raw, firm	0.5 cup	0.13	183
Nuts/Seeds			
Almonds, dry roasted	1 oz.	0.17	166
Eggs			
Egg, chicken, boiled	1 large	0.298	89.9
Egg substitute, frozen	0.25 cup	0.188	52.8

Continued

TABLE 20.17
(Continued)

Food	Portion Size	Riboflavin (mg)	Kcal
Mixed Foods			
Bean burrito	2 each	0.61	447
Cheese enchilada	1 each	0.42	319
Egg omelet with onion, pepper, tomato, and mushroom	1 each	0.344	125
Vegetarian chili, fat-free with black beans, Health Valley	5 oz.	0.255	70
Beverages			
Coffee substitute with milk	0.75 cup	0.298	120
Miscellaneous			
Brewers yeast	1 T	0.342	22.6

Adult RDA: Males 1.3 mg/day; females 1.1 mg/day.

[a] Also called vitamin B_2.
[b] Most fortified breakfast cereals contain 0.43–0.51 mg per serving.
[c] Many "100% Natural" breakfast cereals are not enriched and contain 0.03–0.12 mg per serving.

TABLE 20.18
Vitamin B_{12}: Vegetarian Sources and Amounts[5,6,31,32]

Food	Portion Size	Vitamin B_{12} (mcg)	Kcal
Cereals[a]/Grains			
Total, wheat	1 cup	7.00	116
Waffle, whole grain	2 each	3.11	154
Bran flakes	1 cup	2.49	152
Granola, low-fat	0.33 cup	1.50	120
Kix	1.5 cup	1.50	110
Corn flakes, dry	1 cup	1.27	92.9
Waffle, frozen, toasted	1 each	0.882	92.4
Dairy/Soy milk[b]			
Soymilk, Edensoy Extra	1 cup	3.0	130
Cottage cheese, 1% fat	1 cup	1.43	164
Milk, skim	1 cup	0.93	86
Yogurt, flavored, low-fat 1% milk-fat, Breyers	1 cup	0.90	251
Milk, whole	1 cup	0.87	150
Yogurt, whole, plain	1 cup	0.84	139
Yogurt, nonfat, flavored with aspartame, Light 'n Lively Free 70 Cal	1 cup	0.60	70
Buttermilk, cultured	1 cup	0.54	99
Feta cheese	1 oz.	0.479	74.8
Swiss cheese	1 oz.	0.476	107
Ricotta cheese, part-skim	0.5 cup	0.36	171
Havarti cheese	1 oz.	0.357	105
American processed cheese food	1 oz.	0.235	68.9
Cheddar cheese	1 oz.	0.23	114
Soy Products/Meat Substitutes[c]			
Breakfast links	2 each	3.41	63
Soyburger with cheese	1 each	1.72	316
Soyburger	1 each	1.70	142
Tempeh	1 cup	1.66	330
Breakfast patties	1 each	1.49	68
Chicken, meatless, breaded, fried patty	1 piece	0.95	177

Continued

TABLE 20.18
(Continued)

Food	Portion Size	Vitamin B$_{12}$ (mcg)	Kcal
Eggs			
Egg, chicken, boiled	1 large	0.56	78
Mixed Foods			
Spinach soufflé	1 cup	1.37	219
Cheese pizza	1 piece (1/8 of a 15-in. pie)	0.53	223
Miscellaneous			
Fortified nutritional yeast (Red Star T6635)	1 T	4.0	40

Adult RDA: 2.4 mcg/day.

[a] Some commercial cereals are not fortified with vitamin B$_{12}$, check labels carefully.

[b] Subject to fortification; unfortified soymilk contains no vitamin B$_{12}$.

[c] Subject of fortification; check labels of individual product carefully.

TABLE 20.19
Vitamin D: vegetarian sources and amounts[5,6,31–33]

Food	Portion Size	Vitamin D (IU)[a]	Kcal
Cereals/Grains			
Raisin bran	1 cup (2.1 oz.)	56	175
Corn Pops	1 cup	50	110
Lucky Charms	1 cup	44.8	125
Corn flakes	1 cup (1 oz.)	44	90
Granola, low-fat	0.33 cup	39.9	120
Wheat bran muffin from recipe with 2% milk	1 muffin (57 g)	25.1	161
Waffles, plain, recipe	1 each (75 g)	23.5	218
Vegetables			
Mushrooms, boiled	0.5 cup	59.3	21.1
Dairy/Soymilk			
Soymilk, Soy Moo, fat free, Health Valley	1 cup	100	110
Milk, nonfat	1 cup	98	85.5
Milk, whole	1 cup	97.6	150
Pudding, vanilla, instant, with whole milk	0.5 cup	49.0	162
Eggs			
Egg, chicken, boiled	1 large	26	78
Egg yolk, cooked	1 each	24.6	59.2
Mixed Foods			
Soup, tomato bisque, with milk	1 cup	49.2	198
Egg salad	0.5 cup	38.5	293
Egg omelet with mushroom	1 each (69 g)	36.4	91.2
Fats/Oils/Dressings			
Margarine, hard, hydrogenated soybean[b]	1 tsp.	19.9	29.8
Desserts			
Egg custard pie, frozen, baked	1 piece (105 g)	40.1	221
Chocolate-filled crepe	1 each (78 g)	28.1	119
Coffee cake, from mix	1 piece (72 g)	22.2	229

Adult Adequate Intake: 5 mg cholecalciferol (200 IU/day).

[a] 1 IU vitamin D = 0.025 μg cholecalciferol.

[b] Subject to fortification; check labels.

TABLE 20.20
Calcium: Vegetarian Sources and Amounts[5,6,19,31,32]

Food	Portion Size	Calcium (mg)	Kcal
Cereals/Grains			
Calcium fortified cereal bars	1 bar (37 g)	200	140
Vegetables			
Collards, frozen, boiled	0.5 cup	179	31
Kale, frozen, boiled	1 cup	179	39
Turnip greens, canned	0.5 cup	138	16
Squash, acorn, baked	1 cup	90.2	115
Okra, boiled	0.5 cup	88	34
Squash, butternut, baked	1 cup	84	82
Broccoli, cooked	1 cup	72	44
Peas, green, cooked, from frozen	0.5 cup	19.2	62.4
Fruits			
Calcium-fortified orange juice	8 oz	300	120
Dairy/Soymilk			
Soy milk, fortified	8 oz (1 cup)	400	110
Malted milk, chocolate (Ovaltine)	8 oz	384	225
Evaporated milk, skim	4 oz	372	100
Evaporated milk, whole	4 oz	329	169
Goat's milk	8 oz (1 cup)	327	168
Yogurt, tofu yogurt, frozen	8 oz	309	254
Cow's Milk, skim	8 oz (1 cup)	302	86
Cow's Milk, 1/2%	8 oz (1 cup)	300	90
Cow's Milk, 1%	8 oz (1 cup)	300	102
Yogurt, fat-free	8 oz	300	100
Yogurt, low-fat	8 oz	300	200
Yogurt, regular	8 oz	300	250
Cow's Milk, 2%	8 oz (1 cup)	297	121
Cow's Milk, whole		290	150
Swiss cheese	1 oz	272	107
Cheddar cheese	1 oz	204	114
American cheese	1 oz	174	106
Mozzarella cheese, part skim	1 oz	183	72
Feta cheese	1 oz	140	75
Soy milk, nonfortified	8 oz (1 cup)	79.3	150
Cottage cheese, 1% fat	0.5 cup	69	82
Beans/Legumes			
Great Northern Beans	0.5 cup	60	105
Soy Products/Meat Substitutes			
Tofu, raw, firm	0.5 cup	258	183
Tempeh	1 cup	154	330
Nuts/Seeds			
Almonds, dried	1 oz (about 24 nuts)	75	167
Desserts			
Custard, 2% milk	1 cup	394	298
Sherbet, orange	1 cup	264	104
Soft serve ice cream, French vanilla	1 cup	226	370
Frozen yogurt, soft serve	1 cup	212	230
Ice cream, vanilla, regular, 10% fat	1 cup	168	226
Miscellaneous			
Blackstrap Molasses	1 tbsp	172	47

Adult AI: Males 1000 mg/day; females: 1000 mg/day.

TABLE 20.21
Copper[a]: Vegetarian Sources[b] and Amounts [5,31,32]

Food	Portion Size	Copper (mg)	Kcal
Cereals/Grains			
100% Bran	1 c	1.04	178
Granola, low-fat, Kellogg's	0.5 c	0.655	211
Vegetables			
Potatoes, baked, stuffed with cheese	1 ea (254 g)	0.671	373
Vegetable juice cocktail, V-8	1 c	0.484	46.0
Potatoes, baked, with skin	1 ea (122 g)	0.372	133
Fruits			
Avocado, California	1 ea	0.460	306
Prunes, dehydrated, cooked	0.5 c	0.286	158
Dairy/Soy milk			
Soy milk	1 c	0.288	79.2
Beans/legumes			
Beans, adzuki, canned, sweetened	0.5 c	0.384	344
Garbanzo beans, boiled	0.5 c	0.289	135
Soy Products/Meat Substitutes			
Tempeh	1 c	1.11	330
Scallops, meatless, breaded, fried	0.5 c	0.819	257
Luncheon slice, meatless	1 piece (67 g)	0.608	188
Soyburger with cheese	1 ea	0.559	316
Tofu, raw, firm, calcium sulfate	0.5 c	0.476	183
Nuts & Seeds			
Cashew, dry roasted	0.25 c	0.76	197
Sunflower seeds, toasted	0.25 c	0.61	208

Adult RDA: Males 900 mcg/day Females: 900 mcg/day.

[a] Severe copper deficiency is rare in humans with no dietary deficiency documented. Generally this is only seen with extended supplemental feeding/total nutrition through manufactured nutrition such as total parenteral nutrition or impaired utilization. [32]
[b] High zinc intake (from supplements) can cause copper deficiency.[2]

TABLE 20.22
Iodine: Vegetarian Sources and Amounts [5,31,32]

Food	Portion Size	Iodine (mcg)	Kcal
Cereals/Grains			
Rice, white, enriched, cooked, long grain	0.5 c (82.5 g)	52	81
Bread, cornbread, homemade	1 piece (65 g)	44.2	176
Fruit-flavored, sweetened	1.1 oz (32 g)	41	120
Roll, white	2 rolls (38 g)	31	100
Muffin, blueberry/plain	1 ea (50 g)	28.5	150
Tortilla, flour, 7–8 in. diameter	1 ea (35 g)	26.3	114
Corn flakes	1 oz (28 g)	26	102
Bread, white	1 slice (28.4 g)	25.8	76.4
Pancakes, from mix, 4"	1 ea (38 g)	21	74
Crisped rice	1 oz (28 g)	18.5	111
Noodles, egg, enriched, boiled	1 c (160 g)	17.6	213
Bread, whole wheat	1 slice (28 g)	17.6	69
Bread, rye, American	1 slice (32 g)	15.7	83

Continued

TABLE 20.22
(Continued)

Food	Portion Size	Iodine (mcg)	Kcal
Vegetables			
Potato, boiled with peel	1 ea (202g)	62.6	220
Fruit cocktail, heavy syrup, canned	0.5 c (128 g)	42.24	93
Potato, scalloped, homemade	0.5 c (122 g)	37.8	105
Navy beans, boiled	0.5 c (91 g)	35.5	129
Lima beans, baby, frozen, boiled	0.5 c (90 g)	27.9	95
Orange breakfast drink (from dry)	1 cup	27.3	114
Prunes, heavy syrup	5 ea (86 g)	25.8	90
Cowpeas/blackeye peas	0.5 c (85 g)	22.1	112
Dairy/Soymilk			
Yogurt, low-fat, plain	1 cup	87.2	155
Buttermilk, skim, cultured	1 cup	60.0	99.0
2% fat milk	1 cup	56.6	137
Cottage cheese 1% fat	1 cup	56.5	164
Nonfat milk	1 cup	56.4	85.5
Whole milk, 3.3%	1 cup	56.1	150
Fruit yogurt, low-fat	1 cup	45.3	250
Eggs			
Fried in margarine	1 ea (46 g)	29	91.5
Scrambled, with milk, in margarine	1 large, (61 g)	25.6	101
Soft-boiled	1 ea (50 g)	24	78
Mixed Foods			
Grilled cheese on wheat	1 ea (118 g)	28.9	392
Macaroni and cheese, box mix	0.5 c	17.3	199
Condiments/seasonings			
Salt, Morton light salt mixture	1 tsp	119	0

Adult RDA 150 mcg males and females.

TABLE 20.23
Iron: Nonheme Sources in the Vegetarian Diet[5,31,32,34]

Food	Portion Size	Total Iron (mg)	Available Iron (mg) (Where Info Available)	Kcal
Cereals/grains				
Raisin bran, dry	0.75 cup	Range: 18.54 to 3.7	0.19	200
Quinoa	1 cup	13.4	—	576
Corn flakes, dry	0.75 cup	6.5	0.32	90
Oatmeal, instant, fortified	0.5 cup	4.2	0.21	145
Special K	0.75 cup	3.4	—	75
Bran muffin,	1 med	2.4	0.12	
Oatmeal, instant, regular	1 cup	1.59	—	145
Shredded Wheat, dry	1 oz	1.2	0.06	102
Bagel, enriched	1/2, 3.5″ diameter	1.2	0.06	154
Vegetables				
Potato, baked, skin	1 med	2.8	0.14	220
Asparagus, pieces, canned	0.5 cup	2.21	—	23
Peas, cooked	0.5 cup	1.3	0.06	59
Spinach, boiled	0.5 cup	3.21	—	21

Continued

TABLE 20.23
(Continued)

Food	Portion Size	Total Iron (mg)	Available Iron (mg) (Where Info Available)	Kcal
Fruits				
Prune juice	8 oz	3.02	—	182
Figs, dried	5 ea (93.5 g)	2.1	—	239
Raisins	2/3 c (100 g)	2.08	—	300
Prunes, dried	5 ea (42 g)	1.04	—	100
Beans/Legumes				
Split pea & carrot soup	7.5 oz	4.5	—	90
Lentil and carrot soup	7.5 oz	4.5	—	90
Black bean and carrot soup	7.5 oz	4.5	—	70
Kidney beans, boiled	0.5 cup	2.6	0.13	112
Navy beans, canned	0.5 cup	2.44	—	148
Chickpeas, boiled	0.5 cup	2.4	0.12	134
Soybeans, green, boiled	0.5 cup	2.25	—	127
Pinto beans, boiled	0.5 cup	2.23	—	117
Lima Beans, cooked	0.5 cup	2.09	—	104
Pinto beans, canned	0.5 cup	1.94	—	93.6
Kidney beans, canned	0.5 cup	1.6	0.08	103
Chickpeas, canned	0.5 cup	1.6	0.08	143
Soy Products/Meat Substitutes				
Tofu, raw, regular,	~4 oz	6.65	0.32	94
Chili, made with meat substitute	0.67 cup	5.59	—	186
Garden burger	3.4 oz	2.89	—	186
Scallops, meatless, breaded, and fried	.5 cup	1.77	—	257
Soy burger	1 each	1.49	—	142
Breakfast patties	1 each	1.42	—	97.3
Nuts/Seeds				
Pumpkin seed kernel, roasted	.25 cup	8.45	—	296
Sunflower seeds, kernels, dry	.25 cup	2.44	—	205
Cashew, dry roasted	.25 cup	2.1	—	197
Coconut milk, canned	.25 cup	1.9	—	111
Almonds, dried, whole	.25 cup	1.3	—	209
Mixed nuts, dry roasted with peanuts	.25 cup	1.27	—	204
Miscellaneous				
Molasses, blackstrap	1 Tbsp	3.5	—	47

Adult RDA: Male 8 mg/day; female: 18 mg/day.

NONNUTRITIVE AND OTHER IMPORTANT FACTORS IN THE VEGETARIAN DIET

Typical vegetarian diets are rich in many beneficial nonnutritive factors such as dietary fiber and phytochemicals.[24,27,28] Table 20.29 and Table 20.30 provide information about sources of these beneficial but nonnutritive factors.

Omega-3 fatty acids are a type of polyunsaturated fatty acid that are thought to reduce the risk of cardiovascular disease through their effects on triglyceride levels and platelet aggregation.[2,39] One type of omega-3 fatty acid, alpha-linolenic acid, is an essential fatty acid and must be consumed in the diet to prevent deficiency. Two other types of omega-3 fatty acids are eicosapentaenoic acid (EPA) and docosahexaenoic acid (DHA). Omega-3 fatty acids may be of concern to vegetarians, because although alpha-linolenic acid is found in many plant foods, EPA and DHA are not.[1] For healthy adults, this is not usually a concern, because the body has the ability to manufacture EPA and DHA from alpha-linolenic acid although vegetarians still have lower levels of blood DHA.[1,14] The fetus and young infant have a dramatically reduced ability to perform this conversion.[15] Because DHA is needed for brain and retinal development, some pregnant or breastfeeding vegetarian women may need to reduce their intake of linoleic acid (an omega-6 fatty acid) relative to their intake of alpha-linolenic acid to increase DHA levels, or they may choose to try DHA-enriched eggs or DHA supplements derived from microalgae although the safety of this has not

TABLE 20.24
Iron: Absorption Enhancers and Inhibitors[1,2,34]

Class of Inhibitors	Examples	Found in	Effect on Iron Absorption
Polyphenols	Tannic acid, gallic acid and catechin	Coffee, tea, red wines, certain spices, fruits and vegetables	Coffee: 35–40% Tea: 60% Red wine: 50%
Phytates	Substances that form insoluble complexes with nonheme iron	Whole grains, bran, soy products	
EDTA (ethylenediamine-tetraacetic acid)	Food additive used as sodium EDTA, calcium EDTA (prevents color changes and oxidation in foods)	Used broadly	Possibly up to 50% in some cases
Calcium	Calcium chloride (naturally occurring sources of calcium in self selected diets did not show an inhibitory effect, however there is a potential effect of other forms of calcium)	Additive to bread products, potential effect of other forms of calcium	Possibly up to 30–50% in some cases found with calcium chloride fortification
Fiber	Insoluble fibers, Phytate content may be responsible	Whole grains	Possibly 30–50%

Class of enhancers	Examples	Found in	Effect on Iron Absorption
Organic acids[a]	Malic, ascorbic, citric, and bile acids	Found widely in foods	Enhances absorption
Amino acids	Some amino acids such as cysteine	Protein foods, also found widely in vegetables and grains	Enhances absorption
Vitamin A and β-carotene	Retinol, retinaldehyde, retinoic acid, β-carotene	Spinach, carrots, squash, sweet potatoes, greens, cantaloupe, and mango	Enhances absorption, possibly by forming a complex with iron

[a] The presence of these acids with a meal will significantly improve iron absorption and in some cases potentially overcome the inhibitory effects of other components in foods.

TABLE 20.25
Manganese: Vegetarian Sources and Amounts[5,31,32]

Food	Portion Size	Manganese (mg)	Kcal
Cereals/Grains			
100% Bran	1 c	5.96	178
Most Cereal	1 c	3.63	175
Grape Nuts	1 c	2.65	389
Bran Chex	1 c	2.53	156
All Bran	0.33 c	2.39	70.7
Raisin Bran	1 c	2.16	175
Noodles, cooked, Spinach	1 c	2.1	182
Noodles, cooked, Macaroni, whole wheat	1 c	1.93	174
Rice flour, brown	0.25 c	1.59	144
Noodles, cooked, Lasagna, whole wheat	2 ea	1.52	136
Wheat Chex	1 c	1.34	169
Vegetables			
Lima bean, boiled	0.5 c	1.07	105
Fruits			
Pineapple, chunks	1 c	2.56	76.0
Blackberries	1 c	1.86	74.9
Soy products/meat substitutes			
Tofu, raw, firm, with Nigari	0.5 c	1.49	181
Tempeh	0.5 c	1.19	165

AI: Males: 2.3 mg/day; female: 1.8 mg/day.

Manganese is not necessarily at risk for deficiency in vegetarians. Some research has indicated that vegetarians have higher intake of this nutrient, however, bioavailability may be a concern. [8,9]

TABLE 20.26
Selenium[a]: Vegetarian Sources and Amounts[5,31,32,35]

Food	Portion Size	Selenium (mcg)	kcal
Cereals/Grains			
Special K, Kellogg's	1 cup	54.9	100
Bagel, plain, toasted	1 each	22.7	195
Granola, low-fat	1 cup	22.5	422
Pita pocket, 100% whole wheat, toasted	1 each	20.2	120
Barley, whole, cooked	0.5 cup	18.2	135
Pita pocket, white	1 each	18	165
Egg noodles, cooked	0.5 cup	17.4	107
Spaghetti/macaroni, enriched, cooked	0.5 cup	14.9	98.5
Puffed wheat	1 cup	14.8	44.4
Whole wheat bread	1 slice	12.8	86.1
Oatmeal, instant, prepared	0.5 cup	12.68	159
Buns, hamburger-style	1 each	12.5	129
English muffin, plain	1 each	11.5	134
Cheerios	1.25 cup	10.6	111
Matzo, whole wheat	1 each	9.89	99.5
Brown rice, long grain	0.5 cup	9.6	108.5
Vegetables			
Brussels sprouts, boiled	1 cup	21.1	60.8
Cucumbers, slices with peel	0.5 cup	6.19	6.76
Mushrooms, raw	5 pieces	14.3	32.4
Fruits			
Grapes, Thompson seedless	0.5 cup	7.7	57
Applesauce, canned	0.5 cup	6.5	52.5
Dairy/Soymilk			
Cottage cheese, 1%	1 cup	13.6	164
Yogurt, fruit, low-fat (12 g protein/8 oz.)	1 cup	8.09	155
Milk, nonfat	1 cup	5.15	85.5
Frozen yogurt, chocolate, nonfat	1 cup	5.02	208
Beans/Legumes			
Black beans, dry, boiled	1 cup	13.7	227
Lima Beans, cooked	1 cup	8.19	229
Great northern beans, cooked	1 cup	7.26	209
Chickpeas, boiled	1 cup	6.10	269
Soy Products/Meat Substitutes			
Tofu	0.5	1.79	94.2
Nuts/Seeds			
Brazil nuts, dried	0.25 cup	1036	230
Sunflower seeds, kernels, dry	0.25 cup	21.4	205
Cashew, dry roasted, unsalted	0.25 cup	8	197
Eggs			
Egg, hard cooked	1 each	10.7	77.5
Egg yolk, cooked	1 each	7.50	59.2
Egg white, cooked	1 each	5.88	16.6
Mixed Foods			
Lasagna, no meat, recipe	1 piece (218 g)	29.9	298
Avocado and cheese sandwich on wheat bread	1 each	25.2	456
Peanut butter and jam sandwich on wheat	1 each	24.3	344
Pizza, cheese	1/8 of 15-in. (120 g)	20.0	268
Bean burrito	1 each	14.1	223.5
Cucumber and vinegar salad	1 cup	11.1	47.8
Desserts			
Coffee cake, from mix	1 piece (72 g)	11.0	229
Carrot, with cream cheese icing, recipe	1 piece (112 g)	9.91	488

Adult RDA: Males 55 mcg/day; females 55 mcg/day.

[a] Selenium content of food can vary widely, according to the selenium content of the soil.[35]

TABLE 20.27
Zinc: Vegetarian Sources and Amounts[5,31,32,36]

Food	Portion Size	Zinc (mg)[a,b]	Kcal
Cereals/Grains			
Just Right	1 cup	22.8	152
Product 19, Kellogg's	1 cup	15	100
Complete bran	1 cup	8.07	195
100% Bran	1 cup	5.74	178
Raisin bran, dry	1 cup	5.71	175
Bran flakes	1 cup	5.15	127
Cap'n Crunch	1 cup	4.00	156
Granola, low-fat	0.33 cup	3.74	120
Quinoa	1 cup	3.4	576
Muffin, wheat bran, from recipe with 2% milk	1 each (57 g)	1.57	161
Noodle, spaghetti, spinach, cooked	1 cup	1.53	182
Bagel, oat bran	1 each	1.42	173
Pancakes, Aunt Jemima, blueberry	3 each (106 g)	1	246
Vegetables			
Palm hearts, cooked	1 cup	5.45	150
Dairy/soymilk			
Soymilk	1 cup	2.90	150
Frozen, nonfat, chocolate yogurt	1 cup	2.18	208
Ricotta cheese, part-skim	0.5 cup	1.66	170
Edam/ball cheese	1 oz.	1.07	101
Buttermilk, cultured	1 cup	1.03	99
Beans/legumes			
Adzuki, cooked	1 cup	4.07	294
Lentils, cooked	1 cup	2.52	230
Blackeye peas, boiled from dry	1 cup	2.22	198
Soybean, dried, boiled	1 cup	2.0	298
Kidney beans, red, cooked	1 cup	1.89	225
Chickpeas, canned	0.5 cup	1.28	143
Soy products/meat substitutes			
Natto	1 cup	5.32	371
Miso	0.5 cup	4.60	284
Tempeh	1 cup	3.02	330
Tofu, raw, firm	0.5 cup	1.98	183
Chili with meat substitute	0.66 cup	1.67	186
Meatless scallops, breaded, fried	0.5 cup	1.24	257
Luncheon slice, meatless	1 piece	1.07	188
Nuts/Seeds			
Pumpkin seeds, kernel, dry roasted	0.25 cup	2.58	187
Cashew, dry roasted,	0.25 cup	1.9	197
Almonds, dry roasted	0.25 cup	1.7	203
Sunflower seeds, kernels, dry roasted	0.25 cup	1.7	186
Sesame butter/tahini from nonroasted kernels	1 T	1.58	91.1
Peanuts, dry roasted	0.25 cup	1.2	214
Peanut butter, natural	2 T	1.06	187
Eggs			
Egg substitute	0.5 cup	1.6	74
Mixed Foods			
Cheese enchilada	1 each	2.51	319
Avocado and cheese sandwich on wheat bread	1 each	1.83	456
Pizza, cheese	1/8 of 15-in.	1.56	268

Continued

TABLE 20.27
Zinc: Vegetarian Sources and Amounts[5,31,32,36]

Food	Portion Size	Zinc (mg)[a,b]	Kcal
Desserts			
Nutrigrain bar, fruit filled	1 each	1.5	150
Pecan pie, 1/8 of a 9" pie	1 piece (122 g)	1.26	503
Trail mix, regular	0.25 cup	1.21	173
Doughnut, egg-less, carob-coated, raised	1 piece (78 g)	1.14	285

Adult RDA: Males 11 mg; females 8 mg.

[a] Zinc content of food is influenced by genetic breeding and fertilizer and soil conditions.

[b] Bioavailability is greater from animal than plant sources.

TABLE 20.28
Zinc: Absorption Enhancers and Inhibitors[1,2,36]

Possible Absorption Enhancers[a]	Sources	Possible Absorption Inhibitors[b]	Sources
Yeast (acts by reducing phytates)	Fermented bread dough	Phytates	Whole grains (rye, barley, oatmeal, and wheat), soy products
Animal proteins	Animal products	Oxalate	Spinach, Swiss chard, leek, kale, collard greens, okra, rhubarb, raspberries, coffee, chocolate, tea, peanuts, and pecans
Histidine	Amino acid widely distributed in foods containing protein	Fiber	Whole grains, fruits, vegetables, and legumes
Albumin	Widely distributed in foods containing protein, egg white	Nonheme iron	Legumes, fortified cereals, and leafy greens
Organic acids	Found widely in foods	Copper	Legumes, whole grains, nuts, seeds, and vegetables
		Calcium supplements	Over-the-counter supplements, multivitamins, some antacids
		Iron supplements	
		Casein	Milk

[a] Yeast and animal proteins are the only noncontroversial zinc absorption enhancers.

[b] Phytates is the only noncontroversial zinc absorption inhibitors.

TABLE 20.29
Fiber: Types, Functions and Sources[1,2,5,32]

Type of Fiber	Fiber Type	Food Sources	Function
Cellulose	Incompletely fermented	Whole wheat flour, bran, cabbage, peas, green beans, broccoli, cucumbers, peppers, apples, and carrots	Increases stool bulk and water absorption, decreases transit time through the GI system
Hemicellulose	Incompletely fermented	Bran cereals, whole grains, brussels sprouts, greens, and beet root	,,
Lignin	Incompletely fermented	Breakfast cereals, bran, older vegetables, strawberries, eggplant, pears, green beans, and radishes	,,
Gums	Viscous	Oatmeal, oat products, dried beans, oat bran, and barley	Binds to bile acids and certain lipids to help lower blood cholesterol levels, metabolized to short-chain fatty acids in the gut, which may play a role in signaling hepatic slowed cholesterol production
Pectin	Viscous	Squash, apples, citrus fruits, cauliflower, cabbage, dried peas and beans, carrots, and strawberries	

AI: Male: 38 g/day; female: 25 g/day.

been established.[14–18] Due to the increased interest in the health benefits of DHA, food companies are exploring incorporating it into products such as cereals. DHA has been developed from *Crypthecodinium cohnii* and *schizochytrium* microalgae strains. Martek Biosciences Corporation markets this vegetarian DHA source, and products containing it must display the MARTEK DHA™ logo.[40] Vegetarians can also include two daily servings of foods such as flaxseed (or flaxseed oil), canola or soybean oil, walnuts, or hempseed products (such as a veggie burger), to promote healthy intakes of alpha linolemic acid, but the longer chanin omega 3 fatty acids, DHA and EPA are absent from a vegetarian diet without supplementation. Table 20.31 lists vegetarian dietary sources of the omega-3 fatty acid alpha-linolenic acid.

TABLE 20.30
Common Phytochemicals[a] in Foods[27]

Chemical Names	Sources	Proposed Mechanism of Action
Sulforaphane	Isothiocyanates found in broccoli, cauliflower, cress, cabbages, and radishes	Activates phase II enzymes in liver (removes carcinogens from cells)
Flavonoids	Citrus fruits and berries	Blocks the cancer-promotion process
Monoterpenes (polyphenols)	Perillyl alcohol in cherries	May inhibit the growth of early cancers
	Limonene in citrus	
	Ellagic acid in strawberries and blueberries	
Genistein	Soybeans, tofu	Prevents the formation of capillaries required to nourish tumors
Indoles	Cruciferous vegetables (broccoli, cauliflower, cress, cabbages, and radishes)	Increase immunity, facilitate excretion of toxins
Saponins	Kidney beans, chickpeas, soybeans, and lentils	May prevent cancer cells from multiplying.
Lycopene	Tomatoes	May fight lung and prostate cancer

[a] More than 10,000 phytochemicals are thought to exist. This table represents only a partial listing.

TABLE 20.31
Omega-3 Fatty Acids: Vegetarian Sources and Amounts[2,5,7,41]

Food	Portion Size	Alpha-Linolenic Acid (18:3) (mg)	Kcal
Cereals/Grains			
Oats, germ	0.25 cup	0.4	119
Wheat germ	0.25 cup	0.2	104
Barley, bran	0.25 cup	0.1	115
Vegetables			
Soybeans, green, raw	0.5 cup	4.1	188
Kale, raw, chopped	1 cup	0.13	21
Broccoli, raw, chopped	1 cup	0.1	24
Cauliflower, raw	1 cup	0.1	26
Fruits			
Avocados, California, raw	1 medium	0.173	306
Dairy/Soymilk			
Cheese, Roquefort	1 oz.	0.2	105
Beans/Legumes			
Soybeans, dry	0.5 cup	1.5	387
Beans, pinto, boiled	1 cup	0.2	234
Nuts/Seeds			
Butternuts (dried)	1 oz.	2.4	174
Walnuts, dried, English/Persian	1 oz.	1.9	182
Fats/Oils/Dressings			
Linseed oil	1 T	7.5	124
Flax seed	1 T	2.2	124
Canola oil (rapeseed oil)	1 T	1.6	124
Walnut oil	1 T	1.5	124
Salad dressing, comm., mayonnaise, soybean	2 T	1.38	116
Soybean oil	1 T	1.0	124
Wheat germ oil	1 T	1.0	124
Salad dressing, comm., Italian, regular	2 T	1.0	140

AI: Males: 1.6 g/day; females: 1.1 g/day.

THE EFFECTS OF COOKING, STORAGE, AND PROCESSING ON THE CRITICAL NUTRIENTS

Cooking, storage, and processing methods can influence the amount of a nutrient present in a food. Table 20.32 presents the effects of cooking, storage, and processing on the nutrients that may be of concern in a vegetarian diet.

GENERAL VITAMIN AND MINERAL DEFICIENCY AND TOXICITY SYMPTOMS

It is important for practitioners to be aware of the symptoms of nutrient deficiencies in any patient. As a group, vegetarians tend to be more health-conscious and knowledgeable about nutrition than the general public.[1] Some vegetarians choose megadoses of vitamins or minerals to combat real or perceived threats to their health. Therefore, toxicity may be more of a risk than a nutrient deficiency. Table 20.33 presents deficiency and toxicity symptoms of the nutrients potentially at risk in a vegetarian diet.

SAMPLE MEAL PLANS

Table 20.34 through Table 20.37 present sample meal plans for adults and children following a lacto-ovo or vegan diet. These menus provide the Recommended Dietary Allowances (RDA) for energy and protein while presenting an appropriate macro-nutrient breakdown.

TABLE 20.32
Effects of Cooking, Storage, and Processing on the Critical Nutrients[2]

Nutrient	Cooking	Storage	Processing
Riboflavin	Stable to heat	Destroyed by light and irradiation	—
Vitamin B$_{12}$	Some losses (30%)	Stable	Small losses (10%)
Copper	Increased content using water from copper pipes	Canning with copper adds content to the food	—
Iron	Cooking in iron vessels increases iron content of foods	—	—
Omega-3 fatty acids (a polyunsaturated fatty acid)	Stable in baking; unstable if smoking point is reached	May go rancid with prolonged storage	—

TABLE 20.33
General Vitamin and Mineral Deficiency and Toxicity Symptoms[2,5,8,33]

Vitamin/Mineral[a]	Deficiency Symptoms[b]	Toxicity Symptoms[c]
Vitamins		
Vitamin D	Children — rickets Adults — osteomalacia	Excessive bone and soft tissue calcification (lung, kidney, kidney stones, and tympanic membrane) Hypercalcemia with symptoms of headache, weakness, nausea and vomiting, constipation, polyuria, and polydipsia In infants: retarded growth, gastrointestinal upsets, and mental retardation
Vitamin B$_{12}$	Pernicious (megaloblastic) anemia Smooth red tongue Fatigue Skin hypersensitivity (numbness, tingling and burning of the feet, and stiffness and generalized weakness of the legs) Degeneration of peripheral nerves progressing to paralysis Other (glossitis and hypospermia)	Physiological stores substantial (~2000 mcg). Stores and enterohepatic recycling may prevent deficiency symptoms for several years (~5) in the absence of intake None known up to 100 mcg/d. No known benefit to high doses
Riboflavin (vitamin B$_2$)	Anemia (normocytic and normochromic) Neuropathy Purple/magenta tongue General B-vitamin deficiency symptoms (soreness and burning of lips, mouth, and tongue) Cheilosis, glossitis, angular stomatitis, seborrheic dermatitis of nasolabial fold, vestibule of the nose, and sometimes the ears and eyelids, scrotum and vulva	None known

Continued

TABLE 20.33
Continued

Vitamin/Mineral[a]	Deficiency Symptoms[b]	Toxicity Symptoms[c]
Minerals		
Calcium	Bone deformities including osteoporosis, tetany, and hypertension	Hypercalcemia of soft tissues and bone (children and adults)
Iron	Hypochromic, microcytic anemia	Poor iron and zinc absorption (of particular concern during pregnancy)
	Seen across populations, particularly in women, children, and those from low socioeconomic status	Seen at >45 mg intake
	Fatigue	Constipation
	Spoon-shaped nails	Liver toxicity
		Infections
		Hemochromatosis
		Potential increased risk for heart disease and myocardial infarction
Zinc	Growth retardation resulting in short stature, mild anemia, low plasma zinc levels, and delayed sexual maturation.	Toxicity is rare (300 mg/d)
		Tolerable Upper Intake Level is 40 mg/day
	Possible in diets very rich in fiber and phytate, which chelates the zinc in the intestine, thus preventing absorption	Continuous supplementation with high dose zinc can interfere with copper absorption
	Poor taste acuity, poor wound healing, night blindness, baldness and skin lesions have also been reported	Excessive supplementation may decrease HDL and can result in nausea, vomiting, diarrhea, and dizziness
		Iron and copper losses in urine with doses as low as 25 mg/day and if large doses (10–15 × the RDA) are taken for even short periods of time
Copper	Severe copper deficiency: rare in humans	Gastrointestinal distress, liver damage
	Adults: neutropenia and microcytic anemia	Seen in genetic diseases such as Wilson's disease (genetic deficiency in liver synthesis of ceruloplasmin)
	Children: neutropenia and leukopenia	
	Decrease in serum copper and ceruloplasmin levels followed by failure of iron absorption leading to microcytic, hemochromic anemia	
	Neutropenia, leukopenia and bone demineralization are later symptoms	
	Deficiencies have not been reported in otherwise healthy humans consuming a varied diet	

[a] Absorption of some nutrients is affected by concentration of others; intestinal absorption of some nutrients is competitive.
[b] Deficiency can result from inadequate provision in the diet or via inadequate absorption.
[c] Toxicity is typically from overuse of nutritional supplements, although in some cases can be the cause of improper food fortification procedures (such as milk vitamin D fortification problems that arose in 1992).

TABLE 20.34
Sample Meal Plan for Lacto-Ovo Vegetarian Adult[31,32]

Breakfast
Raisin bran (1 cup, 2.15 oz)
Milk, 1% fat, 0.75 cup (for cereal)
Milk, 1% fat, 1 cup (beverage)
Orange juice, 1 cup
Banana, 1 med

Lunch
Whole wheat bread, 2 slices
Griller veg. Burger patty, 1 each
Mustard
Tomato, sliced, 1/2 tomato
Jack cheese, 1 oz
Apple, 1 med

Dinner
Bean Burrito
Black beans, 1 cup
Corn tortilla, 2 each, 6"
Rice, brown, 1 cup
Salsa, 2 tbsp
Sour Cream, 1 tbsp
Cheddar cheese, 1 oz
Green salad, 2 cups
Vinegar and oil dressing (1 tsp olive oil)
Broccoli, 1 cup
Milk, 1% fat, 1 cup

Snack
Cereal bar, raspberry
Dried apricots, 10 halves

Kcals: 2218; Carbohydrate: 374 g (67.35%); Protein: 100 g (18.%); Fat: 55 g (22.29%).

TABLE 20.35
Sample Meal Plan for Vegan Adult[31,32]

Breakfast
Raisin bran (1 cup, 2.15 oz)
Soy milk, 1% fat, 1 cup (for cereal)
Soy milk, 1% fat, 1 cup (beverage)
Orange juice, 1 cup, Ca fortified
Banana, 1 med

Lunch
Whole wheat bread, 2 slices
Griller veg. Burger patty (Morningstar
 Farms), 1 each, cooked
Mustard
Tomato, sliced, 1/2 tomato
Almonds, slivered, blanched, 1 oz
Apple, 1 med

Dinner
Bean Burrito
 Black beans, e cup
 Corn tortilla, 2 each, 6"
 Rice, brown, 1 cup
 Salsa, 2 Tbsp
 Walnuts, ground, .5 oz
 Green salad, 2 cups
 Vinegar and Oil dressing
  (1 tsp olive oil)
 Broccoli, 1 cup
 Soy milk, 1 cup

Snack
Cereal bar, raspberry
Dried apricots, 10 halves

Kcals: 2217; Carbohydrate: 350g (63%); Protein: 90g (16%); Fat: 62g (25%).

TABLE 20.36
Sample Meal Plan for Vegan Child Age 4 to 6[31,32]

Breakfast
1 packet instant oatmeal
8 oz soymilk fortified with calcium
 and vitamin B_{12}
1 banana

Lunch
0.5 cup hummus spread made from
 chickpeas and sesame butter
2 slices whole wheat bread
6 oz. 100% orange pineapple banana
 juice
Carrot sticks
2 molasses cookies

Dinner
Veggie hot dog on bun
0.5 cup mashed potatoes
0.5 cup cooked "creamed" spinach
0.5 cup applesauce
8 oz soymilk

Snack
4 oz fortified soymilk
4 graham crackers

Snack
1.5 oz (~0.25 cup) trail mix
4 oz fortified soy milk

Kcals: 1864; Carbohydrate: 283 g (60.8%); Protein: 68 g (14.5%); Fat: 62 g (30%).

TABLE 20.37
Sample Meal Plan for Lacto-Ovo Vegetarian Child Age 4 to 6[31,32]

Breakfast
1 cup Honey Nut Cheerios with 4 oz
 milk on cereal
4 oz 1% milk to drink
Orange slices

Lunch
0.5 cup homemade macaroni and cheese
celery sticks and 2 Tbsp peanut butter
2 fruit cookies

Dinner
Burrito with salsa and sour cream,
 made with vegetarian chili
0.5 cup rice
4 oz 1% milk
0.5 cup green salad with broccoli
0.5 cup applesauce

Snack
1.5 oz cheese
5 Ritz crackers
4 oz 1% milk

Snack
Fruit smoothie made with juice,
 frozen yogurt, and fruit

Kcal: 1794; Carbohydrate: 255 g (57%); protein: 63 g (14%); fat: 63 g (31.5%).

SUMMARY

In summary, the term "vegetarianism" may mean different things to different people. Before making or accepting generalizations about vegetarianism, it is important to define the term. A person following a vegetarian lifestyle can have significantly lower risks of many chronic diseases, such as heart disease or cancer, than an omnivore does. However, some nutrients are more difficult to easily obtain from a vegetarian diet and may be a concern for deficiency, especially in children or during other critical lifecycle periods.

REFERENCES

1. Messina, M. and Messina, V. *The Dietitian's Guide to Vegetarian Diets: issues and applications*, 2nd edition. Jones and Bartlett Publishers, Sudbury, MA, 2004.
2. Mahan, L.K. and Escott-Stump, S. *Krause's Food, Nutrition, and Diet Therapy*, 11th Edition, W.B. Saunders Co., Philadelphia, 2004.
3. Vegetarian Resource Group. How many vegetarians are there? *Vegetarian J,* 3: 8; 2003.
4. Messina, V.K. and Burke, K.I. *JADA,* 97: 1317; 1997.
5. Dietary Reference Intakes (series), Institute of Medicine, National Academy Press, Washington, DC 1997–2005. Available at. www.nap.edu.
6. Yates, A.A., Schlicker, S.A., and Suitor, C.W. *JADA,* 98: 699; 1998.
7. Health and Welfare Canada. *Nutrition Recommendations: The Report of the Scientific Review Committee*, Authority of the Minister of Health and Welfare, Ottawa, 1990.
8. Gibson, R.S. *Am J Clin Nutr,* 59: 1223S; 1994.
9. Kadrabova, J. et al. *Biol Trace Element Res,* 50: 13; 1995.
10. Parsons, T.J. et al. *J Bone Min Res,* 12: 1486; 1997.
11. Draper, A. et al. *Br J Nutr,* 69: 3; 1993.
12. Remer, T., Neubert, A., and Manz, F. *Br J Nutr,* 81: 45; 1999.
13. Harman, S.K. and Parnell, W.R., *N Z Med J,* 111: 91; 1998.
14. Sanders, T.A.B. *Am J Clin Nutr,* 70: 555S; 1999.
15. Gordon, N. *Brain Dev,* 19: 165; 1997.
16. Gibson, R.A., Neumann, M.A., and Makrides, M. *Lipids,* 31:177S; 1996.
17. Kretchmer, N., Beard, J.L., and Carlson, S., *Am J Clin Nutr,* 63: 997S; 1996.
18. Conquer, J.A. and Holub, B.J., *Vegetarian Nutr Int J,* 1–2: 42; 1997.
19. Drezner, M.K. and Hoben, K.P., *Eating Well, Living Well with Osteoporosis.* Viking Press, New York, 1996.
20. Thaler, S.M., Teitelbaum, I., and Berl, T. *Am J Kidney Dis,* 31: 1028; 1998.
21. Alexander, H. et al. *J. Am Coll. Nutr,* 18: 127; 1999.
22. Craig, W.J. *Am J Clin Nutr,* 59: 1233S; 1994.
23. Burr, M.L. and Butland, B.K. *Am J Clin Nutr,* 48: 840; 1988.
24. Tham, D.M., Gardner, C.D., and Haskell, W.L. *J Clin Endocrinol Metab,* 83: 2223; 1998.
25. Toohey, M.L. et al. *J. Am Coll Nutr,* 17: 407; 1998.
26. Key, T.J.A. et al. *Br Med J,* 313: 775; 1996.
27. Craig, W.J. *JADA,* 97: 199S; 1997.
28. Bingham, S.A. et al. *Br J. Nutr,* 79: 393; 1998.
29. Sanders, T.A. *Ped Clin N Am,* 42: 955; 1995.
30. Sanders, T.A. and Reddy, S., *Am J Clin Nutr,* 59: 1176S; 1994.
31. Pennington, J.A.T. *Bowes & Church's Food Values of Portions Commonly Used*, 17th Edition, Lippincott-Raven, Philadelphia, 1998.
32. Hands, E.S. *Food Finder: Food Sources of Vitamins & Minerals*, ESHA Research, Salem, 1995.
33. Holick, M.F. et al. *N Engl J Med,* 326: 1178; 1992.
34. Morris, D.H. *Iron in Human Nutrition*, 2nd Edition, National Cattlemen's Beef Association, Chicago, 1998.
35. Holben, D.H. and Smith, A.M. *JADA,* 99: 836; 1999.
36. McBean, L.D. *Zinc in Human Nutrition*, National Cattlemen's Beef Association, Chicago, 1997.
37. Nieman, D.C. et al. *JADA,* 89: 1763; 1989.
38. Donovan, U.M. and Gibson, R.S. *J Adolesc Health,* 18: 292; 1996.
39. Uauy-Dagach, R. and Valenzuela, A. *Nutr Rev,* 54: 102S; 1996.
40. Mangels, R. Nutrition Hotline. *Vegetarian J,* 2005:3.
41. United States Department of Agriculture, Agricultural Research Service, Nutrient Data Laboratory, *USDA Nutrient Database for Standard Reference, Release 13*, www.nal.usda.gov/fnic/foodcomp/

Part IV

Nutrition Assessment

21 Dietary Guidelines, Food Guidance, and Dietary Quality

Eileen Kennedy and Jeanne Goldberg

CONTENTS

DIETARY GUIDELINES

The Dietary Guidelines for Americans have served as the cornerstone of federal nutrition policy in the United States since the first edition was released in 1980. While many factors may have contributed to the development of that document, two earlier efforts were of particular importance. One was the 1969 White House Conference on Food, Nutrition, and Health,[1] which recommended that the government examine the links between diet and chronic disease. The second was the U.S. Senate Dietary Goals, released in 1977[2]; that document, the product of several years of hearings before the Senate Select Committee on Nutrition and Human Needs, for the first time, summarized specific recommendations for diet-related goals for the American public.

The Dietary Guidelines that came 3 years later have served as the basis of nutrition standards for all government food programs. Programs such as Food Stamps, School Lunch/School Breakfast, and Women, Infants, and Children (WIC) use them to develop program services; nutrition education programs at the federal level must have messages consistent with the Dietary Guidelines. An estimated one out of every five Americans participates in at least one federal nutrition program. As a result, the impact of the Dietary Guidelines is broad.

HISTORY OF THE DIETARY GUIDELINES FOR AMERICANS

The Dietary Guidelines attempt to answer the question, "What should Americans eat to stay healthy?" Specifically, the Guidelines provide advice for healthy Americans aged 2 years and over about food choices that promote health and reduce the risk of disease.

Since the first edition was released in 1980[3] they have been updated every 5 years in 1985, 1990, 1995, 2000, and most recently in 2005.[4-8] It was not until the passage of the National Nutrition Monitoring and Related Research Act of 1990,[9] however, that the Secretary of Agriculture and the Secretary of Health and Human Services were required by law to jointly publish a report every 5 years entitled "The Dietary Guidelines for Americans." The 1995 edition was the first to be statutorily mandated by the U.S. Congress. The report must (1) contain nutrition and dietary information and guidelines for the general public, (2) be based on the preponderance of scientific and medical knowledge current at the time of publication, and (3) be promoted by each federal agency in carrying out federal food, nutrition, or health programs.

Since 1985, the United States Department of Agriculture (USDA) and the Department of Health and Human Services (HHS) have used essentially the same process to prepare the Dietary Guidelines. An external Dietary Guidelines Advisory Committee (DGAC) that includes widely recognized nutrition and medical experts is appointed by the secretaries of the two agencies to review and revise the Guidelines where indicated by newer evidence. The Committee holds a series of open public meetings to review and discuss the guidelines and then prepares a technical report, which they transmit to the two secretaries for review within the two departments. In addition, in 1995, 2000, and 2005 consumer research was conducted[10–11] to test reactions to specific design and content elements of the technical report. The consumer research is also used as one element in promoting the Guidelines.

DIETARY GUIDELINES FOR AMERICANS

The 1995 Dietary Guidelines

For the first three editions, the Dietary Guidelines were relatively stable (Table 21.1), maintaining seven guidelines. However, the 1995 guidelines reflected some exciting and important changes. More than ever before, the emphasis was on total diet. The wording moved away from individual foods in the direction of a total diet based on variety, moderation, and proportionality. The concept of total diet is reflected symbolically through the graphic of the 1995 Dietary Guidelines bulletin that links all seven guidelines together, anchored around "Eat a Variety of Food."

Each edition has been accompanied by a bulletin for consumers that describe the Guidelines in some detail. In the 1995 guideline on variety, the bulletin[6] stresses a total diet rather than an individual foods approach to healthy eating. The recommendation is to choose foods from each of the five major food groups in the Food Guide Pyramid. Also, there is an emphasis on foods from the base of the pyramid (grains) to form the center of the plate, accompanied by food from other food groups.

For the first time, the 1995 document recognized that, with careful planning, a vegetarian diet can be consistent with the both the Dietary Guidelines and the Recommended Dietary Allowances (RDAs).[11] The guidelines also present a clear message that food sources of nutrients are preferred to supplements. This "food first" strategy is reinforced by a discussion of other healthful substances present in food but not in dietary supplements. However, the 1995 guidelines do provide specific examples of situations in which dietary supplements may be needed.

The 1995 guidelines provided a more direct discussion of the link between diet and health. Weight gain with age was discouraged for adults. Weight maintenance is encouraged as a first step to achieving a healthy weight. The benefits of physical activity are emphasized, and for the first time, the Guidelines included a statement on the benefits of moderate alcohol consumption in reducing the risk of heart disease. On this point, both HHS and USDA were clear that the alcohol guideline was not intended to recommend that people start drinking.

The 1995 Guidelines included a direct reference to nutrition education tools that could be used to promote them. They explain how consumers can use the "three crown jewels" of consumer nutrition education to build a healthy diet — the Dietary Guidelines, the Food Guide Pyramid,[12] and the Nutrition Facts Label.

TABLE 21.1
Dietary Guidelines for Americans, 1980–1995

1980	1985	1990	1995
Eat a variety of foods	Eat a variety of foods	Eat a variety of foods	Eat a variety of foods
Maintain ideal weight	Maintain desirable weight	Maintain healthy weight	Balance the food you eat with physical activity — maintain or improve your weight
Avoid too much fat, saturated fat, and cholesterol	Avoid too much fat, saturated fat, and cholesterol	Choose a diet low in fat, saturated fat, and cholesterol	Choose a diet low in fat, saturated fat, and cholesterol
Eat foods with adequate starch and fiber	Eat foods with adequate starch and fiber	Choose a diet with plenty of grain products, vegetables, and fruits	Choose a diet with plenty of grain products, vegetables, and fruits
Avoid too much sugar	Avoid too much sugar	Use sugars only in moderation	Choose a diet moderate in sugars
Avoid too much sodium	Avoid too much sodium	Use salt and sodium only in moderation	Choose a diet moderate in salt and sodium
If you drink alcohol, do so in moderation	If you drink alcoholic beverages, do so in moderation	If you drink alcoholic beverages, do so in moderation	If you drink alcoholic beverages, do so in moderation

---

TABLE 21.2
Dietary Guidelines for Americans, 2000

Let the Pyramid guide your food choices
Aim for a healthy weight
Be physically active each day
Choose a diet that is low in saturated fat and cholesterol, and
  moderate in total fat
Choose a variety of grains daily, especially whole grains
Choose a variety of fruits and vegetables daily
Choose beverages and foods to moderate your intake of sugars
Choose and prepare foods with less salt
If you drink alcoholic beverages, do so in moderation
Keep food safe to eat

The 2000 Dietary Guidelines

The Dietary Guidelines 2000, released by President Clinton in May 2000,[7] broke the tradition of seven guidelines and included ten guidelines. Not only did the Guidelines continue to emphasize a total diet approach, they also emphasized a healthy lifestyle. This is reflected clearly in three concepts that are used as organizing principals for the 2000 Guidelines: aim for fitness, build a healthy base, and choose sensibly. Three new guidelines were added in the 2000 edition (Table 21.2). For the first time, Dietary Guidelines 2000 included a guideline on physical activity: "Be physically active every day." In addition to help in maintaining a healthy weight, this guideline discusses other health benefits of physical activity. Specific quantitative recommendations are given for amount of physical activity for adults (30 min or more) and children (60 min or more) per day. In addition, for the first time, there is a guideline on food safety. Again, this reinforces components of a healthy diet and healthy lifestyle. Finally, there is a separate guideline for fruits and vegetables.

Consumer research conducted as part of the Dietary Guidelines 2000 process[11] influenced the development of the guidelines. One clear message from that research was that consumers preferred simple, action-oriented guidelines. Thus, the 2000 guidelines are much more direct and action oriented as evidenced by "aim for a healthy weight" and "keep foods safe to eat." The 2000 guidelines are also more consumer friendly, and emphasize practical ways for consumers to put the concepts into practice. To that end, a section entitled "Advice for Today" at the end of each guideline includes suggestions on key ways to operationalize it. Consumer research on the 2000 Dietary Guidelines indicated that consumers particularly appreciated sections such as "Advice for Today."

Dietary Guidelines 2005

The Dietary Guidelines 2005 are even more of a departure from earlier editions. Since the first edition, it has been clear that the guidelines needed to be based on the preponderance of scientific evidence. For the 2005 edition, it was clearly specified that conclusions from the Dietary Guidelines Advisory Committee must rest on an evidence-based rating system in order to minimize the potential for individual bias to influence decisions. It was further specified that the task of the advisory committee would be limited to the preparation of a set of evidence-based recommendations. The Committee was not to concern itself with how these recommendations would be communicated to the public.[13] An internal group from USDA/DHHS would assume the task of translating the guidelines into a set of recommendations for policymakers, nutrition educators, nutritionists, and health care providers. These guidelines would then serve as the basis for the development of communications to the public. The brochure, "Finding Your Way to a Healthier You," released on the same day as the guidelines, was a first attempt at this approach to consumer communications.[14]

What emerged from the 2005 Dietary Guidelines Advisory Committee was a set of nine key messages (Table 21.3). Notably, the wording for just three of them — physical activity, food safety, and alcohol is exactly the same as that in the 2000 guidelines. The internal USDA/DHHS committee translated the messages into a total of 41 key recommendations, including 23 for the general public and 18 for specific population groups (Table 21.4). These recommendations are designed to take into account nutrients that are in short supply in the diets of significant numbers of individuals in the population. They include Vitamin E, calcium, magnesium, potassium, as well as fiber in children and adults, and Vitamins A and C in adults.

In sum, modification of the approach to developing the 2005 Dietary Guidelines for Americans finally appears to address one of the frustrations of earlier committees. It divides the process into two distinct components, one focusing solely on the science that drives the recommendations and the other on the translation of those recommendations.

TABLE 21.3
Nine Key Messages, Dietary Guidelines for Americans, 2005

Consume a variety of foods within and among the basic food groups while staying
    within energy needs
Control calorie intake to manage body weight
Be physically active every day
Increase daily intake of fruits and vegetables, whole grains, and nonfat or low-fat
    milk and milk products
Choose fats wisely for good health
Choose carbohydrates wisely for good health
Choose and prepare foods with little salt
If you drink alcoholic beverages, do so in moderation
Keep food safe to eat

TABLE 21.4
Key Recommendations, Dietary Guidelines for Americans, 2005

Adequate Nutrients within Calorie Needs
- Consume a variety of nutrient-dense foods and beverages within and among the basic food groups while choosing foods that limit the intake of saturated and *trans*-fats, cholesterol, added sugars, salt, and alcohol
- Meet recommended intakes within energy needs by adopting a balanced eating pattern, such as the U.S. Department of Agriculture (USDA) Food Guide or the Dietary Approaches to Stop Hypertension (DASH) Eating Plan

Weight Management
- To maintain body weight in a healthy range, balance calories from foods and beverages with calories expended
- To prevent gradual weight gain over time, make small decreases in food and beverage calories and increase physical activity

Physical Activity
- Engage in regular physical activity and reduce sedentary activities to promote health, psychological well-being, and a healthy body weight
- To reduce the risk of chronic disease in adulthood: Engage in at least 30 min of moderate-intensity physical activity, above usual activity, at work or home on most days of the week
- For most people, greater health benefits can be obtained by engaging in physical activity of more vigorous intensity or longer duration
- To help manage body weight and prevent gradual, unhealthy body weight gain in adulthood: Engage in approximately 60 min of moderate- to vigorous-intensity activity on most days of the week while not exceeding caloric intake requirements
- To sustain weight loss in adulthood: Participate in at least 60 to 90 min of daily moderate-intensity physical activity while not exceeding caloric intake requirements. Some people may need to consult with a health care provider before participating in this level of activity
- Achieve physical fitness by including cardiovascular conditioning, stretching exercises for flexibility, and resistance exercises or calisthenics for muscle strength and endurance

Food Groups to Encourage
- Consume a sufficient amount of fruits and vegetables while staying within energy needs. Two cups of fruit and two-and-half cups of vegetables per day are recommended for a reference 2000 cal intake, with higher or lower amounts depending on the calorie level
- Choose a variety of fruits and vegetables each day. In particular, select from all five vegetable subgroups (dark green, orange, legumes, starchy vegetables, and other vegetables) several times a week
- Consume three or more ounce-equivalents of whole-grain products per day, with the rest of the recommended grains coming from enriched or whole-grain products. In general, at least half the grains should come from whole grains
- Consume three cups per day of fat-free or low-fat milk or equivalent milk products

Fats
- Consume less than 10% of calories from saturated fatty acids and less than 300 mg/day of cholesterol, and keep *trans*-fatty acid consumption as low as possible
- Keep total fat intake between 20% to 35% of calories, with most fats coming from sources of polyunsaturated and monounsaturated fatty acids, such as fish, nuts, and vegetable oils
- When selecting and preparing meat, poultry, dry beans, and milk or milk products, make choices that are lean, low-fat, or fat-free
- Limit intake of fats and oils high in saturated or *trans*-fatty acids, and choose products low in such fats and oils

Continued

**TABLE 21.4
(Continued)**

Carbohydrates

- Choose fiber-rich fruits, vegetables, and whole grains often
- Choose and prepare foods and beverages with little added sugars or caloric sweeteners, such as amounts suggested by the USDA Food Guide and the DASH Eating Plan
- Reduce the incidence of dental caries by practicing good oral hygiene and consuming sugar- and starch-containing foods and beverages less frequently

Sodium and Potassium

- Consume less than 2300 mg (approximately 1 teaspoon of salt) of sodium per day
- Choose and prepare foods with little salt. At the same time, consume potassium-rich foods, such as fruits and vegetables

Alcoholic Beverages

- Those who choose to drink alcoholic beverages should do so sensibly and in moderation — defined as the consumption of up to one drink per day for women and up to two drinks per day for men
- Alcoholic beverages should not be consumed by some individuals, including those who cannot restrict their alcohol intake, women of childbearing age who may become pregnant, pregnant and lactating women, children and adolescents, individuals taking medications that can interact with alcohol, and those with specific medical conditions
- Alcoholic beverages should be avoided by individuals engaging in activities that require attention, skill, or coordination, such as driving or operating machinery

Food Safety

- To avoid microbial food-borne illness:
  - Clean hands, food contact surfaces, and fruits and vegetables. Meat and poultry should not be washed or rinsed
  - Separate raw, cooked, and ready-to-eat foods while shopping, preparing, or storing foods
  - Cook foods to a safe temperature to kill microorganisms
  - Chill (refrigerate) perishable food promptly and defrost foods properly
  - Avoid raw (unpasteurized) milk or any products made from unpasteurized milk, raw or partially cooked eggs or foods containing raw eggs, raw or undercooked meat and poultry, unpasteurized juices, and raw sprouts

**TABLE 21.5
U.S. Dietary Guidelines 2000 and Countries Having Similar Guidelines**

U.S. Dietary Guidelines 2000[7]	Countries Having Similar Guidelines[1]
Aim for a healthy weight	Australia, Canada, China, Japan, Korea, Malaysia, The Netherlands, New Zealand, Philippines, Singapore, Thailand, United Kingdom
Let the Pyramid guide your food choices	Variety: Australia, Canada, China, France, Germany, Hungary, Indonesia, Korea, Malaysia, New Zealand, Philippines, Singapore, South Africa, Sri Lanka, Thailand, United Kingdom, Japan Five Steps to Healthy Eating: India
Eat a variety of grains daily, especially whole grains	Australia, Canada, Denmark, Germany, Hungary (choose potatoes over rice), India, Malaysia, Norway, Singapore, South Africa (starchy foods), Thailand
Choose a diet that is low in saturated fat, and cholesterol, and moderate in total fat	Australia (but low fat diets not suitable for children), Canada, Japan, The Netherlands, New Zealand, Singapore, South Africa
Choose and prepare foods with less salt	Australia, Canada, China, Denmark, Germany, Hungary, India, Japan, Korea, Malaysia, The Netherlands, Singapore, South Africa, Thailand
If you drink alcoholic beverages, do so in moderation	Canada, China, France, Germany, Indonesia (avoid), Hungary (forbidden for pregnant women and children), Korea, The Netherlands, New Zealand, Singapore, South Africa, United Kingdom

COMPARISON OF DIETARY GUIDELINES FOR AMERICANS WITH OTHER DIETARY GUIDELINES

Many countries — both industrialized and developing — have authoritative sets of dietary guidelines.[15] Despite vastly different geographical and sociocultural contexts, there are six fairly consistent elements (Table 21.5).

A guideline on variety is common; it is often the core element of the different sets of dietary guidelines, and is used to reflect the concepts of dietary diversity. The variety guidelines range from general statements such as, "Eat a variety of foods" to very specific quantifications, such as that as found in the Japanese guideline: "Obtain well-balanced nutrition with a variety of foods; eat 30 foodstuffs a day."

Many of the country-specific dietary guidelines emphasize limiting or moderating total fat and saturated fat intake. Where an amount is quantified, this is most commonly specified as a diet containing no more than 30% of total energy from fat and less than 10% of energy from saturated fat.

Countries typically also include weight guidelines, clearly emphasizing maintaining or achieving a healthy weight; in the French guideline this is more specific, indicating that individuals should weigh themselves monthly.[15] Most of the dietary guidelines worldwide promote a plant-based diet as the building block of healthful eating. To that end, many countries emphasize grains as the basis of a good diet. Reduction of salt or sodium is emphasized in a number of the sets of dietary guidelines.

Finally, the issue of alcohol consumption is addressed in many sets of dietary guidelines. There is always a level of caution related to the role of alcohol as part of a healthy diet. The most recent 2005 Dietary Guidelines for Americans, for example, indicates that there are many strategies, other than alcohol, to reduce the risk of heart disease: maintaining a healthy weight, cessation of smoking, increasing physical activity, and reducing the level of fat and saturated fat in the diet. The report specifies further that it is not recommended that anyone begin drinking or drink more frequently on the basis of health considerations. Indeed, countries such as Venezuela go so far as to specify that "alcoholic beverages are not part of a healthy diet."[16]

FUTURE DIRECTIONS

Many countries have been successful in developing and promoting food-based Dietary Guidelines. Typically they apply to individuals aged two and older. That has been the case in the United States since the first Dietary Guidelines were released in 1980. There is a clear gap in addressing the needs of younger children.

A limited number of countries do address that group in their food-based guidelines. In most cases the advice relates to a discussion of breast-feeding. Australia, for example, has a guideline that states: "encourage and support breast-feeding." Similar wording is found in guidelines from the Philippines and Singapore.

Most industrialized countries rely on national pediatric associations to guide the broad policy recommendations for infant feeding and/or feeding practices for the first 2 years of life. In almost all cases, advice from pediatric associations stresses that human milk is the preferred form of infant feeding.[17]

If food-based dietary guidelines for children under two were to be developed, it would be necessary to segment by age groups based upon the relevant dietary issues of three groups: birth to 6 months, 6–12 months, and 13–24 months.

OTHER DIETARY GUIDANCE

The previous section traced the development of the U.S. Dietary Guidelines. USDA has a long, rich history of providing science-based nutrition information and education for the general public. The Organic Act of 1862 not only created USDA but also mandated that the Department "acquire and diffuse among people useful information on subjects connected to agriculture." This led to some of the pioneering work of W.O. Atwater, who in the 1890s began "identifying the links between food composition, dietary intake, and health." This seminal science led to the development of the USDA food guides. Dissemination of the food guides was facilitated by the 1914 Smith-Lever Act, which created the Cooperative Extension Service and specified that the Extension Service provide people with, "useful and practical information on subjects relating to agriculture and home economics."

THRIFTY FOOD PLAN

In the 1930s the USDA began developing family food plans at four separate cost levels. These food plans have been used ever since.

The best known of these, the Thrifty Food Plan, served as the nutritional basis that were used to establish the benefits package of the Food Stamp Program. Even among upper-income people there was a lack of understanding of the elements of good nutrition. Former Secretary of Agriculture Henry Wallace once commented, "The lack of commonsense knowledge of nutrition even among the many well-to-do people in the U.S. is appalling."

In 1941 the first set of RDAs was released at the National Nutrition Conference for Defense; at this conference USDA scientists noted that consumers spent enough money on food but did not obtain an adequate diet. As a result, the USDA was urged to develop nutrition education and media-type materials to promote good nutrition for the American public. This emphasis on nutrition education continued in the 1950s and 1960s, culminating with the 1969 White House Conference on Food, Nutrition, and Health.[18–19] The 1969 conference reinforced the need for aggressive nutrition promotion activities for all Americans, with a special emphasis on reaching low-income populations.

Throughout the 1970s, federal agencies increased funding for nutrition programs and nutrition education activities. New programs were created, including the Special Supplemental Food Program for Women, Infants, and Children (WIC), School Breakfast; other programs such as Food Stamps and School Lunch were expanded nationwide.

The 1977 Food and Agriculture Act named USDA as the lead agency for nutrition research, extension, and teaching. Throughout the 1980s and into the 1990s USDA placed a renewed emphasis on developing comprehensive, coordinated efforts to promote nutrition for all Americans.

USDA Food Guide Pyramid

The release of the 1980 Dietary Guidelines for Americans provided the impetus for the development of a new food guide that would allow consumers to put the dietary guidelines into action. Work throughout the 1980s and into the early 1990s culminated in the now well-known 1992 USDA Food Guide Pyramid.[12] The Pyramid has been a popular success, recognized by the majority of Americans. It reflects the extensive experience with food guidance systems within USDA. The three essential concepts underlying the Food Guide Pyramid are variety, balance, and moderation. Different visuals were tested with consumers to assess which graphic portrayal most effectively communicated the underlying concepts of balance, variety, and moderation. The graphics were tested first with adults with at least a high school education; consumer testing was expanded later to include children and low-literacy and low-income adults. The Pyramid shape emerged as the most effective graphic, communicating the concepts of variety, balance, and moderation (Figure 21.1).

1992 Food Guide Pyramid

The USDA 1992 Pyramid communicated a wealth of information with little accompanying text. A more detailed publication explains the complex information provided in the visual. This publication discusses the differing energy needs of individuals illustrated at 1600, 2200, and 2800 kcal. The Food Guide Pyramid Bulletin[12] includes an in-depth discussion of "How to Make the Pyramid Work for You." Topics such as what constitutes serving, different types of fats, and how to use the Pyramid to make low-fat selections are also included.

The Pyramid graphic shown in Figure 21.1 communicates not only balance, variety, and moderation but also provides the basis of a healthful diet. The number and amounts of foods recommended in the Pyramid are based on three factors:

- RDAs for age and gender groups
- Dietary Guidelines for Americans
- Typical consumption patterns of Americans

The advice provided in the Food Guide Pyramid was designed to provide dietary guidance that ensures nutritional adequacy — defined as the RDAs and Dietary Guidelines — within the framework of typical consumption patterns. Thus, while ostensibly an infinite number of food combinations could be used to ensure nutritional adequacy, the five major food groups emphasized in the USDA Pyramid anchor the food selections to current consumption patterns.

A proliferation of pyramids has emerged since the USDA version was published in 1992. However, all of them, whether Asian, Mediterranean, or vegetarian, are based on the same building blocks — grains, vegetables, and fruits. The similarities in the various pyramids are more dominant than the differences.

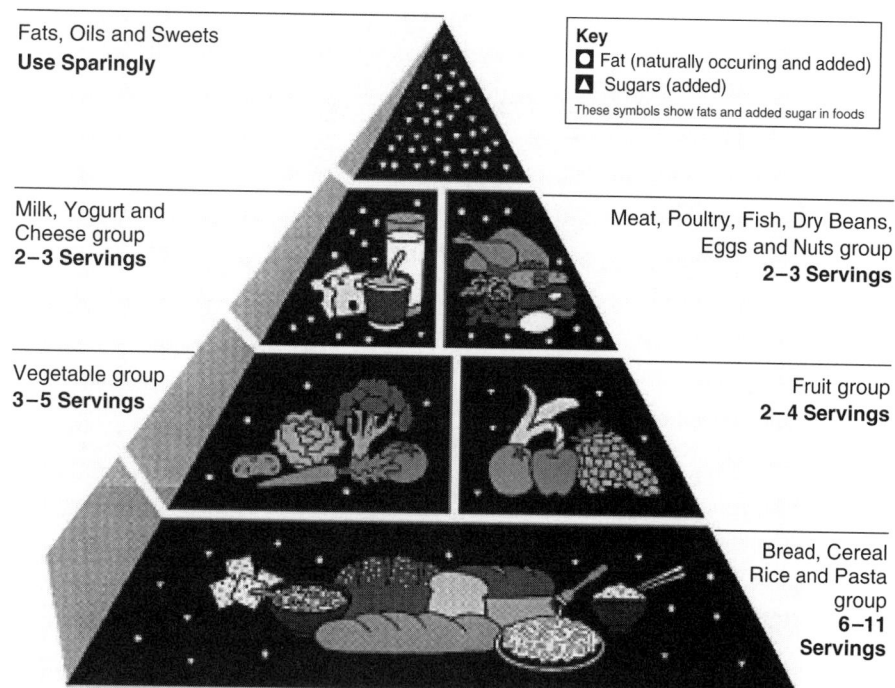

FIGURE 21.1 1992 Food Guide Pyramid.

In addition, in 1999, USDA released a children's version of the Food Guide Pyramid targeted at children aged 2 to 6 years. Here again, the concepts of balance, variety, and moderation underpin the graphic (Figure 21.2). The specific icons used in the food groups are based on foods typically consumed by children. Worth noting are the age-specific recommendations for serving sizes at the bottom of the graphic as well as the deliberate inclusion of exercise icons.

The 2000 Dietary Guidelines for Americans[7] for the first time included the Food Guide Pyramid as part of a specific guideline; "Let the Pyramid Guide Your Food Choices." Including it as a direct part of the Dietary Guidelines reflects the wide-ranging familiarity of consumers with the Pyramid and the messages embedded within. The USDA Food Guide Pyramid (and more recently, MyPyramid) and the Children's Food Guide Pyramid will continue to be essential parts of the nutrition education and nutrition promotion efforts within the USDA.

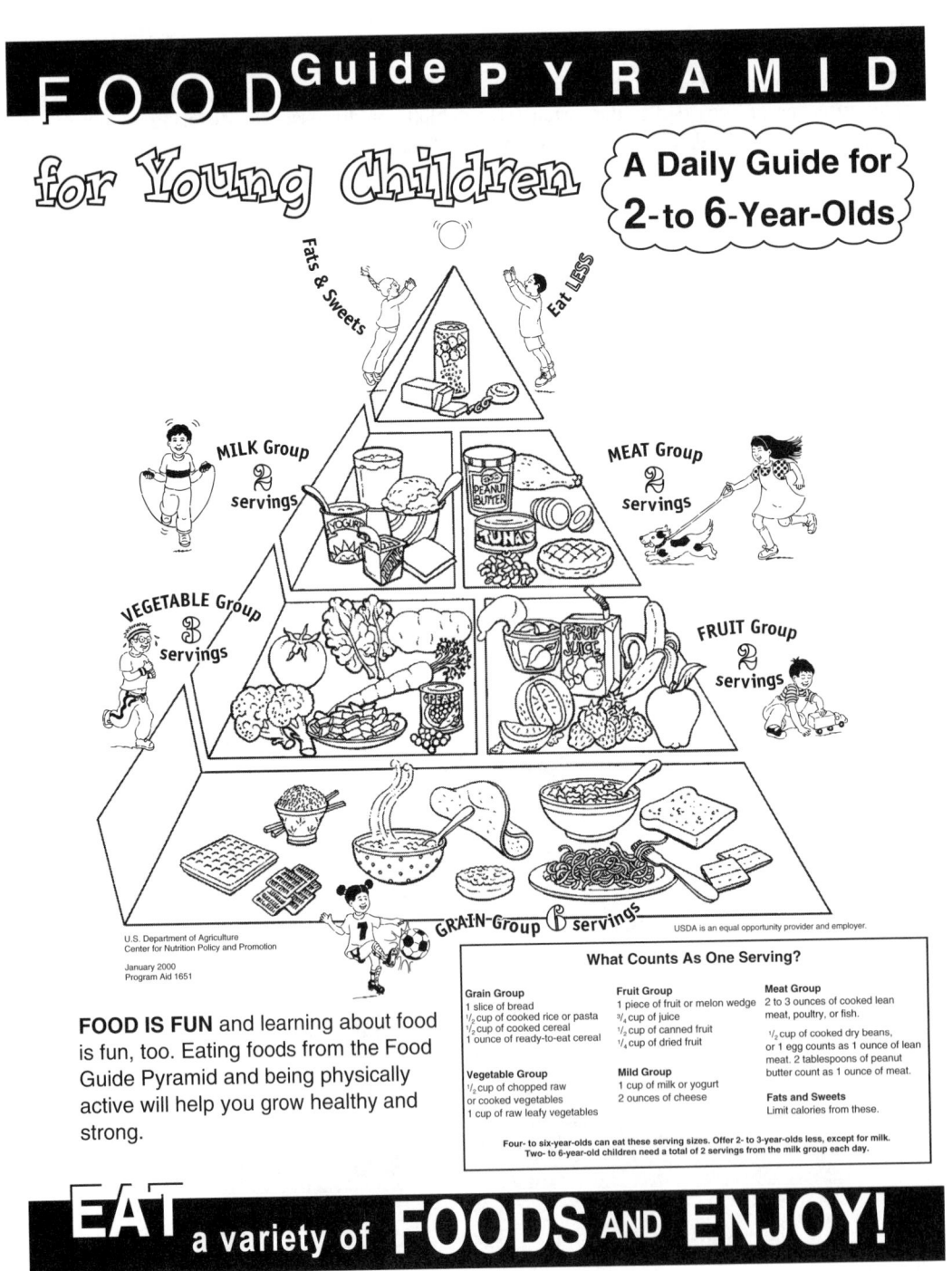

FIGURE 21.2   1999 Children's Food Guide Pyramid.

USDA's MyPyramid, 2005

MyPyramid, the first revision to the Food Guide Pyramid, was released on April 19, 2005, almost 13 years to the day after the original graphic made its appearance and just 4 months after the release of the 2005 Dietary Guidelines for Americans (Figure 21.3). According to the USDA/DHHS the rationale for the revision was "to motivate consumers to make healthier choices and to ensure that USDA's food guidance system reflects the latest nutrition science." Extensive qualitative research was conducted by USDA to provide information about the development of the new graphic. This included a series of focus groups in 2002 to assess the understanding and clarity of messages embedded in the graphic. Consumers recognized the pyramid but had difficulty understanding the specific messages.

A second series of eight focus groups was designed to identify alternative ways to describe the food recommendations so that consumers would understand them. These focus groups also explored consumers' ability to understand nutrition language and messaging about grains, vegetables, types of fats, sugars and added sugars, and physical activity levels. This research documented the fact that consumers did not understand the intended meaning of servings and serving sizes and, more broadly, that their understanding of nutrition terms was limited.

In July 2004, USDA's Center on Nutrition Policy and Promotion (CNPP) solicited public comments on the proposed Food Guidance System and it graphic representation and educational materials through a notice in the Federal Register. Over 1200 comments were received. CNPP also requested a synthesis of previous research that could inform further revisions to the Food Guidance System. In October 2004, ten 2 h focus groups explored participants' awareness of healthy-eating messages and the information conveyed in those messages. This was the first series that explored different concepts for the new graphic. Two months later 200 adults participated in a Web–TV survey to provide feedback to further refine the elements of the graphic. This phase also included testing of actionable messages.

Publicity on the day that MyPyramid was released was extensive and obtained as many as 15 million hits to the Web site within the first 6 h. As reported in the media, many members of the academic community reacted negatively, pointing out that the new materials do not provide messages about which specific foods to eat more of and which to eat in lesser quantities. Some complained more specifically that the new materials cater to the food industry.

DIET QUALITY MEASURES

Since the early 1900s, the major areas of concern in public health nutrition have shifted from problems of nutritional deficiency to problems of excesses and imbalances. Problems of relative overconsumption are, on average, more prevalent today than problems of underconsumption. The successive sets of U.S. Dietary Guidelines that have emerged since 1980 have emphasized the links between diet and a range of chronic diseases. An extensive body of scientific literature documents the association between diets high in total and saturated fat and low in fiber and complex carbohydrate with coronary heart disease, stroke, diabetes, and certain forms of cancer.

While extensive research links the typical American diet to a range of chronic diseases, there has been considerably less progress in improving approaches and techniques that measure diet quality. Until recently, most diet quality measures focused on individual nutrients; most often these measures were based on standards such as mean percentage of the RDAs.[20] Despite the U.S. Dietary Guidelines' emphasis on total diet, indices based on the dietary guidelines have tended to be selective in the components included.[21–22] Few indices have been developed to assess overall diet quality. In an effort to measure how well American diets conform to recommended healthy eating patterns, USDA developed the Healthy Eating Index (HEI) in 1995.

HEI STRUCTURE

HEI was designed to measure various aspects of a healthful diet.[23] As shown in Table 21.6; the HEI is a ten-component index; components 1 through 5 measure the degree to which a person's diet conforms to the Food Guide Pyramid's serving recommendations for the five major food groups of grains, vegetables, fruits, milk, and meat. The number of recommended servings for each food group varies with the individual's age, gender, physiological status, and energy requirements. The use of food groups rather than nutrients was meant to provide consumers with an easier standard against which to judge their dietary patterns. In addition, there may be as-yet-unknown components in foods that would not be picked up by measuring only the nutrients in foods.

Components 6 to 9 measure various aspects of the Dietary Guidelines, including total fat, saturated fat, cholesterol, and sodium, respectively. Component 10 provides a measure of dietary variety. Despite general agreement that dietary variety is important, it is surprising how few studies have attempted to quantify the concept of variety.[24] The HEI counted the total number of different foods that contribute substantially to meeting one or more of the five food group requirements. Foods were counted only if they were eaten in amounts sufficient to contribute at least a half serving in any of the food groups. Identical foods eaten on separate occasions were aggregated before imposing the one-half serving cutoff point. Foods that were similar, such as different forms of potatoes or two different forms of white bread, were counted only once in the variety category.

TABLE 21.6
Components of the Healthy Eating Index

Component	Range of Score	Criteria for Perfect Score of 10	Criteria for Minimum Score of Zero
Food Group			
1. Grains	0–10	6–11 servings	0 servings
2. Vegetables	0–10	3–5 servings	0 servings
3. Fruits	0–10	2–4 servings	0 servings
4. Milk	0–10	2–3 servings	0 servings
5. Meat	0–10	2–3 servings	0 servings
Dietary Guidelines			
6. Total Fat	0–10	30% or less energy from fat	45% or greater energy from fat
7. Saturated fat	0–10	Less than 10% energy from saturated fat	15% or greater energy from saturated fat
8. Cholesterol	0–10	Less than 300 mg	Greater than or equal to 450 mg
9. Sodium	0–10	Less than 2400 mg	Greater than or equal to 4800 mg
10. Variety	0–10	16 different kinds of food over a 3-day period	6 or fewer food items over a 3-day period

Each of the ten components has a score ranging from 0 to 10; cutoffs for scoring the minimum and maximum scores are shown in Table 21.6. Thus, the HEI can vary from 1 to 100.

HEI APPLIED: WHAT ARE AMERICANS EATING?

The HEI was applied to nationally representative data derived from the Continuing Survey of Food Intake by Individuals (CSFII) for two time periods, 1989 to 1990 and 1994 to 1996. The combined score for 1989 to 1990 was 63.9, which contrasted with 63.6, 63.5, and 63.8 for 1994, 1995, and 1996, respectively.[25] Clearly there were not wide variations in the average HEI across this 7-year period.

In addition, the distribution of the average HEI scores did not vary dramatically over the period of 1989 to 1996. Throughout this time period, the majority of individual scores fell in the 51% to 80% range, a category defined as "needs improvement." No more than 12% of individuals fell in the "good diet" category at any point in time; conversely, approximately 18% of individuals were classified in the "poor diet" category. Scores for the individual HEI components varied with the average score. The fruit category was consistently the lowest, and the cholesterol score was the best.

The HEI score varied with some economic and demographic factors.[25] Females had slightly higher scores than males, and persons in the younger and older groups scored higher than adults in the 19 to 50 age category. Children aged 2 to 3 years had the highest HEI score. Children in this age category scored particularly high on the fruit and dairy component of the HEI when compared with older children, suggesting changes in dietary habits as children age.

Throughout the 7-year period there is a pattern of increasing HEI with increased income. The effect of increased education on HEI is even more dramatic, however. One interpretation is that higher education may enable individuals to translate dietary guidance into improved food patterns.

The scientific rigor of the HEI depends on its ability to accurately measure diet quality. Research has documented that the average HEI in 1989 and 1990 correlated with a range of nutrients and energy intake. For most nutrients, the likelihood of falling below 75% of the RDA for a selected nutrient decreased as the HEI score increased. For example, only 47% of persons with an HEI of 50 or less had vitamin C intake greater than 75% of the RDA, compared with approximately 91% of people scoring 80 or more on the HEI. The data would suggest that as the HEI increases, levels of nutrient intake also increase. Interestingly, the correlation of the HEI with overall energy intake was modest, suggesting that simply consuming larger quantities of food will not by itself result in a better diet.

Finally, the HEI was compared with individuals' self-rating of their diets. Persons who rated their diets as excellent or good had a significantly higher probability of having an HEI classified as a "good diet." Conversely, individuals who self-rated their diet as fair or poor had an HEI more likely to be classified as "needs improvement."

The most recent data from the National Health and Nutrition Examination Survey from 1999 to 2000 show similar trends.[26] The average HEI score during 1999 to 2000 was 63.8, indicating again that the typical American diet "needs improvement."[27]

POLICY IMPLICATIONS

The Food Guide Pyramid/MyPyramid and the Dietary Guidelines for Americans provide a standard against which to evaluate the total diet. However, neither the Pyramid nor the Dietary Guidelines provide a method for easily assessing total diet. The development of the USDA HEI provided an easy to use, single summary measure of diet quality. The HEI also provides a method for monitoring diet quality over time using national survey data. In addition, it has the potential to serve as a tool for individuals to self-evaluate diet quality.

The data from both 1989 to 1990 and 1994 to 1996 and most recently in 1999 to 2000 indicate that the dietary patterns of most Americans need improvement. The data obtained from applying the HEI to nationally representative surveys can continue to be one tool to help focus our national nutrition promotion interventions.

SUMMARY

Major improvements worldwide in public health will be accomplished by improvement in dietary patterns. Food-based dietary guidelines have been developed in a broad range of countries. A move toward consensus on food-based dietary guidelines is a practical way to develop core elements of global dietary guidelines that can be effectively promoted by individual countries as well as international health organizations.

REFERENCES

1. Office of the President, Proceedings of White House Conference on Food, Nutrition and Health. White House, Washington, DC, 1970.
2. U.S. Senate Select Committee on Nutrition and Human Needs. Dietary Coals for tin' United States (2nd ed.), W7. 1977
3. U.S. Department of Agriculture and U.S. Department of Health and Human Services. *Nutrition Hint Your Health: Dietary Guidelines far American**. Home and Garden Bulletin No. 232, 1980.
4. U.S. Department of Agriculture and U.S. Department of Health and Human Services. *Nutrition and Your Health: Dietary Guidelines for Americans* (2nd ed.). Home and Garden Bulletin No. 232, 1985.
5. U.S. Department of Agriculture and U.S. Department of Health and Human Services. *Nutrition and Your Health: Dietary Guidelines for Americans* (3rd ed.). Home and Garden Bulletin No. 232, 1990.
6. U.S. Department of Agriculture and U.S. Department of Health and Human Services. *Nutrition and Your Health: Dietary Guideline** *for Americans* (4th ed.). Home and Garden Bulletin No. 232, 1995.
7. U.S. Department of Agriculture, U.S. Department of Health and Human Services, *Nutrition and Your Health: Dietary Guidelines for Americans* (5th ed.). Home and Garden Bulletin No. 232, 39 pp, May 2000.
8. U.S. department of Health and Human Services *Finding Your Way to a Healthier You: Based on Dietary Guidelines for Americans*. U.S. department of Health and Human Services; U.S. Department of Agriculture, Washington, DC, 2005.
9. U.S. Congress, Public Law Wl-445, 7U.S.C53-J1, Library of Congress, Washington, DC, 1990.
10. Prospect Associates. Dietary Guidelines Focus Group Report, Final Report, Washington, DC, Nov 1995.
11. Systems Assessment & Research, Inc. Report to USDA of the Initial Focus Groups on *Nutrition and Your Health: Dietary Guidelines for Americans* (4th ed.), Lanham, MD, September 1999.
12. U.S. Dept of Agriculture, *Food Guide Pyramid*, Human Nutrition Information Service, Washington, DC, Home and Garden Bulletin No. 252, 1992.
13. Goldberg, J, Dietary Guidelines 2005 In *The Nations Nutrition*, E. Kennedy and R. Deckelbaum, eds. ILSI Press: Washington, DC, 2006.
14. USDA. *Finding Your Way to a Healthier You*. Government Printing Office, Washington, DC, 2005.
15. March of Dimes. 2001. *Nutrition Today Matters Tomorrow*. MOD, New York.
16. Pan American Health Organization. *Dietary Guidelines for the Americas*. PAHO, Washington, DC, 1996.
17. American Academy of Pediatrics Breastfeeding and the use of Human Milk, *Pediatrics* 100: 1035, 2003.
18. White House. Proceedings of the White House Conference on Food, Nutrition and Health. Government Printing Office, Washington, DC, 1970.
19. The Surgeon General's Report MI Nutrition and Health, U.S. Dept of Health and Human Services Washington, DC, DHHS (PHS) publication 88-50210, 1988.
20. National Research Council, National Academy of Sciences. *Recommended Dietary Allowances* (10th ed.), Washington, DC, National Academy Press, 1989.
21. Patterson, RE, Haines, RS, Popkin, BM. *JADA* 94: 57; 1994.

22. Kent, AK, Schatzkin, A, Harris, TU et al. *Am J Clin Nutr* 57: 434; 1993.
23. Kennedy, E, Ohls, J, Carlson, S, Fleming, K. *JADA* 95: 1103; 1995.
24. Krebs-Smith, S, Smieiklas-Wright, H, Guthrie HAKrubs-Smith, J. *JADA* 87: 807; 1987
25. Kennedy, E. Family Economics Review 11: 183; 1998.
26. Basiotis, PP, Carlson, A, Gerrior, SA et al. *Family Econom Nutr Rev* 16: 39; 2004.
27. Basiotis, PP, Carlson, A, Gerrior, SA, Juan, WY, and Lino, M. The Healthy Eating Index: 1999–2000. U.S. Department of Agriculture, Center for Nutrition Policy and Promotion. CNPP-12, 2002.

22 Dietary Guidelines around the World: An Update

Odilia I. Bermudez, Johanna T. Dwyer, Winifred Yu, and Linda G. Tolstoi

CONTENTS

INTRODUCTION AND OVERVIEW

Dietary guidelines are "recommendations for achieving appropriate diets, and healthy lifestyles."[1] In this chapter, we examine the similarities and differences as well as strengths and weaknesses of examples of dietary guidelines in five regions of the world. Dietary guidelines from many other countries are also available at the Food and Agricultural Organization's website http://www.fao.org/ag/agn/nutrition/education_guidelines_country_en.stm

The chapter concludes with some recommendations for crafting dietary guidelines in the future.

Effective dietary guidelines have several elements in common. They are designed to address and mitigate the major diet-related nutrition problems of the population to which they are addressed. Health problems change over time and, therefore, the recommendations cannot be static but must also shift when the problems demand, as guidelines in the United States of America have done.[1,2] Effective guidelines are evidence-based, and the strength of supportive evidence underlying them is strong. Eating habits, cultural beliefs, and available food supplies are considered. The dietary guideline messages conveyed are tested prior to their finalization to ensure that the guidelines can be communicated effectively. Successful guidelines are also integrated with other nutritional guidance of a public health nature. Effective guidelines are also recognized as only one of a group of essential components of effective food and nutrition policies. Other factors include access to a variety of safe and affordable foods from available resources and sustainability. Ideally, successful guidelines are promulgated simultaneously with ways to evaluate their effectiveness.

This material is based on work supported by the U.S. Department of Agriculture, under agreement No. 58-1950-9-001. Any opinions, findings, conclusions, or recommendations expressed in this publication are those of the authors and do not necessarily reflect the views of the U.S. Department of Agriculture.

In this chapter we draw examples of guidelines from regions representing different health realities, culinary approaches, dietary practices, food ways, and economies. The European, American, Canadian, Japanese, Taiwanese, and Australian/ New Zealand guidelines are directed to highly industrialized, affluent populations. The Indian, Latin American, and African guidelines are tailored to populations that are often in the nutrition transition, with both highly affluent and very poor populations differing in degree of urbanization and standards of living all within the same country.

In English-speaking North America and Oceania, diseases of affluence (i.e., obesity, heart disease, and certain cancers) are common, and these issues are therefore given attention. All of these affluent countries share similar dietary patterns and nutrition-related problems, including a diet excessive in calories, fat, salt, sugars, and alcohol, and diets too low in fruits, vegetables, and whole grains. Their guidelines have addressed excessive as well as inadequate food consumption, weight, and physical activity since they were first formulated in the late 1970s and early 1980s.

Each of these countries has an ethnically diverse population. In the United States, according to 2000 census data, 12% of the population was African American and 9% was of Hispanic origin.[3] The Aboriginal and Torres Strait Islander people comprise only about 2% of the Australian population, but they often live under impoverished, overcrowded conditions that put them at nutritional risk,[4] and have a high prevalence of android pattern obesity, which is associated with many health problems.[5] In New Zealand, 13% of the population belongs to the rapidly growing Maori minority, and another 5% of the population is Pacific Islanders.[6] Some of these minority groups have increased risks of chronic degenerative diseases as they move away from traditional customs to modern diets and lifestyles. The information accompanying the Australian and New Zealand dietary guidelines refers to these special problems of minority populations, although the dietary guidelines are targeted to the general population.

NORTH AMERICA AND OCEANIA

FORMULATION

Table 22.1 shows the approaches used in the development of the dietary guidelines in these countries and their key characteristics. In guideline development, all of these countries used nutrition experts and scientists, and all of the guidelines were endorsed by a relevant government agency. In the United States, the National Nutrition Monitoring and Related Research Act of 1990 required that the Dietary Guidelines for Americans be updated every 5 years and reviewed by the Departments of Health and Human Services and Agriculture. The latest Dietary Guidelines for Americans were issued in 2005, and are summarized in Table 22.2.

TABLE 22.1
Development of Dietary Guidelines in the United States, Canada, Australia, and New Zealand

Country	United States	Canada	Australia	New Zealand
Title of Guidelines	Dietary Guidelines for Americans	Canada's Guidelines for Healthy Eating	Dietary Guidelines for All Australians	Food and Nutrition Guidelines
Year	2000, 2005	2002	2003	1991
Endorsing Unit	U.S. Department of Agriculture and U.S. Department of Health and Human Services	Department of National Health and Welfare	National Health and Medical Research Council	Nutrition Task Force at the Ministry of Health
Approaches[a]	1–5, 7	1–5, 7	1–5	1–5
Number of Guidelines	27	5	13	6
Target audiences[b]	G, H, P, N	G, H, P, N	G, H, P	G, H, P
Major Nutrition Problems Addressed in Guidelines[c]	C, E, I, O	C, E, I, O	C, E, I, O	C, E, I, O
Graphic representation	My Pyramid	Rainbow	Pyramid	none
Other Dietary Guidelines	National Cancer Institute, American Institute of Cancer Research and American Heart Association		National Physical Activity Guidelines	Dietary Guidelines for: • Healthy Children • Healthy Adolescents • Healthy Breast-feeding women • Healthy Pregnant women • Older People

[a] 1 = Nutrition experts, nutrition scientists views; 2 = Review of former guidelines; 3 = From food groups; 4 = From consumption/nutrition survey; 5 = Definition of nutritional objectives; 6 = Economic data; 7 = Consumer focus groups.

[b] G = general population; H = health professionals; P = policy makers; N= nutrition education of school children.

[c] C = diet-related chronic degenerative diseases; I = dietary inadequacy; E = dietary excess (other nutrients); O = overnutrition (energy); PEM = protein-energy malnutrition.

TABLE 22.2
2005 Dietary Guidelines for Americans: Main Areas and Key Recommendations

Adequate Nutrients within Calorie Needs

Key Recommendations

Consume a variety of nutrient-dense foods and beverages within and among the basic food groups while choosing foods that limit the intake of saturated and *trans* fats, cholesterol, added sugars, salt, and alcohol

Meet recommended intakes within energy needs by adopting a balanced eating pattern, such as the USDA Food Guide or the DASH Eating Plan

Key Recommendations for Specific Population Groups

People above age 50: Consume vitamin B_{12} in its crystalline form (i.e., fortified foods or supplements)

Women of childbearing age who may become pregnant: Eat foods high in heme-iron or consume iron-rich plant foods or iron-fortified foods with an enhancer of iron absorption, such as vitamin C-rich foods

Women of childbearing age who may become pregnant and those in the first trimester of pregnancy: Consume adequate synthetic folic acid daily (from fortified foods or supplements) in addition to food forms of folate from a varied diet

Older adults, people with dark skin, and people exposed to insufficient ultraviolet band radiation (i.e., sunlight): Consume extra vitamin D from vitamin D-fortified foods or supplements

Weight Management

Key Recommendations

To maintain body weight in a healthy range, balance calories from foods and beverages with calories expended

To prevent gradual weight gain over time, make small decreases in food and beverage calories and increase physical activity

Key Recommendations for Specific Population Groups

Those who need to lose weight: Aim for a slow, steady weight loss by decreasing caloric intake while maintaining an adequate nutrient intake and increasing physical activity

Overweight children: Reduce the rate of body weight gain while allowing growth and development. Consult a healthcare provider before placing a child on a weight-reduction diet

Pregnant women: Ensure appropriate weight gain as specified by a healthcare provider

Breast-feeding women: Moderate weight reduction is safe and does not compromise weight gain of the nursing infant

Overweight adults and overweight children with chronic diseases or on medication: Consult a healthcare provider about weight loss strategies prior to starting a weight-reduction program to ensure appropriate management of other health conditions

Physical Activity

Key Recommendations

Engage in regular physical activity and reduce sedentary activities to promote health, psychological well-being, and a healthy body weight

To reduce the risk of chronic disease in adulthood: Engage in at least 30 min of moderate-intensity physical activity, above usual activity, at work or home on most days of the week

For most people, greater health benefits can be obtained by engaging in physical activity of more vigorous intensity or longer duration

To help manage body weight and prevent gradual, unhealthy body weight gain in adulthood: Engage in approximately 60 min of moderate- to vigorous-intensity activity on most days of the week while not exceeding caloric intake requirements

To sustain weight loss in adulthood: Participate in at least 60 to 90 min of daily moderate-intensity physical activity while not exceeding caloric intake requirements. Some people may need to consult with a healthcare provider before participating in this level of activity

Achieve physical fitness by including cardiovascular conditioning, stretching exercises for flexibility, and resistance exercises or calisthenics for muscle strength and endurance

Key Recommendations for Specific Population Groups

Children and adolescents: Engage in at least 60 min of physical activity on most, preferably all, days of the week

Pregnant women: In the absence of medical or obstetric complications, incorporate 30 min or more of moderate-intensity physical activity on most, if not all, days of the week: Avoid activities with a high risk of falling or abdominal trauma

Breast-feeding women: Be aware that neither acute nor regular exercise adversely affects the mother's ability to successfully breast-feed

Older adults: Participate in regular physical activity to reduce functional declines associated with aging and to achieve the other benefits of physical activity identified for all adults

Food Groups to Encourage

Key Recommendations

Consume a sufficient amount of fruits and vegetables while staying within energy needs. Two cups of fruit and 2½ cups of vegetables per day are recommended for a reference 2000-calorie intake, with higher or lower amounts depending on the calorie level

Choose a variety of fruits and vegetables each day. In particular, select from all five vegetable subgroups (dark green, orange, legumes, starchy vegetables, and other vegetables) several times a week

Consume 3 or more ounce-equivalents of whole-grain products per day, with the rest of the recommended grains coming from enriched or whole-grain products. In general, at least half the grains should come from whole grains

Consume 3 cups per day of fat-free or low-fat milk or equivalent milk products

Continued

TABLE 22.2
Continued

Food Groups to Encourage (*Continued*)
Key Recommendations for Specific Population Groups
Children and adolescents. Consume whole-grain products often; at least half the grains should be whole grains. Children 2 to 8 years should consume 2 cups per day of fat-free or low-fat milk or equivalent milk products. Children 9 years of age and older should consume 3 cups per day of fat-free or low-fat milk or equivalent milk products

Fats
Key Recommendations
Consume less than 10% of calories from saturated fatty acids and less than 300 mg/day of cholesterol, and keep *trans* fatty acid consumption as low as possible
Keep total fat intake between 20 to 35% of calories, with most fats coming from sources of polyunsaturated and monounsaturated fatty acids, such as fish, nuts, and vegetable oils
When selecting and preparing meat, poultry, dry beans, and milk or milk products, make choices that are lean, low-fat, or fat-free
Limit intake of fats and oils high in saturated or *trans* fatty acids, and choose products low in such fats and oils

Key Recommendations for Specific Population Groups
Children and adolescents. Keep total fat intake between 30 to 35% of calories for children 2 to 3 years of age and between 25 to 35% of calories for children and adolescents 4 to 18 years of age, with most fats coming from sources of polyunsaturated and monounsaturated fatty acids, such as fish, nuts, and vegetable oils

Carbohydrates
Key Recommendations
Choose fiber-rich fruits, vegetables, and whole grains often
Choose and prepare foods and beverages with little added sugars or caloric sweeteners, such as amounts suggested by the USDA Food Guide and the DASH Eating Plan
Reduce the incidence of dental caries by practicing good oral hygiene and consuming sugar- and starch-containing foods and beverages less frequently

Sodium and Potassium
Key Recommendations
Consume less than 2300 mg (approximately 1 tsp of salt) of sodium per day
Choose and prepare foods with little salt. At the same time, consume potassium-rich foods, such as fruits and vegetables

Key Recommendations for Specific Population Groups
Individuals with hypertension, blacks, and middle-aged and older adults: Aim to consume no more than 1500 mg of sodium per day, and meet the potassium recommendation (4700 mg/day) with food

Alcoholic Beverages
Key Recommendations
Those who choose to drink alcoholic beverages should do so sensibly and in moderation—defined as the consumption of up to one drink per day for women and up to two drinks per day for men
Alcoholic beverages should not be consumed by some individuals, including those who cannot restrict their alcohol intake, women of childbearing age who may become pregnant, pregnant and lactating women, children and adolescents, individuals taking medications that can interact with alcohol, and those with specific medical conditions
Alcoholic beverages should be avoided by individuals engaging in activities that require attention, skill, or coordination, such as driving or operating machinery

Food Safety
Key Recommendations
To avoid microbial foodborne illness:
  Clean hands, food contact surfaces, and fruits and vegetables. Meat and poultry should not be washed or rinsed
  Separate raw, cooked, and ready-to-eat foods while shopping, preparing, or storing foods
  Cook foods to a safe temperature to kill microorganisms
  Chill (refrigerate) perishable food promptly and defrost foods properly
  Avoid raw (unpasteurized) milk or any products made from unpasteurized milk, raw or partially cooked eggs or foods containing raw eggs, raw or undercooked meat and poultry, unpasteurized juices, and raw sprouts

Key Recommendations for Specific Population Groups
Infants and young children, pregnant women, older adults, and those who are immunocompromised. Do not eat or drink raw (unpasteurized) milk or any products made from unpasteurized milk, raw or partially cooked eggs or foods containing raw eggs, raw or undercooked meat and poultry, raw or undercooked fish or shellfish, unpasteurized juices, and raw sprouts
Pregnant women, older adults, and those who are immunocompromised: Only eat certain deli meats and frankfurters that have been reheated to steaming hot

TABLE 22.3

Dietary Guidelines of Canada, Australia, and New Zealand

Canada	Australia	New Zealand
1. Enjoy a variety of foods	1. Prevent excess weight gain	1. Eat a variety of foods from each of the four major food groups each day
2. Emphasize cereals, breads, other grain products, vegetables, and fruits	2. Enjoy a wide variety of nutritious foods	2. Prepare meals with minimal added fat (especially saturated fat), salt, and sugar
3. Choose lower-fat dairy products, leaner meats, and foods prepared with little or no fat	3. Eat plenty of vegetables, legumes, and fruits	3. Choose prepared foods, drinks and snacks that are low in fat (especially saturated fat), salt, and sugar
4. Achieve and maintain a healthy body weight by enjoying regular physical activity and healthy eating	4. Eat plenty of cereals, preferably wholegrain	4. Maintain a healthy body weight by regular physical activity and by healthy eating
5. Limit salt, alcohol, and caffeine	5. Include lean meats, fish, poultry or alternatives	5. Drink plenty of liquids each day
	6. Include milk, yoghurt, cheese or alternatives	6. If drinking alcohol, do each day so in moderation
	7. Drink plenty of water	
	8. Limit saturated fats and moderate total fat intake	
	9. Choose foods low in salt	
	10. Limit your alcohol intake if you choose to drink	
	11. Consume only moderate amounts of sugars and foods containing added sugars	
	12. Care for your food; prepare and store it safely	
	13. Encourage and support breast-feeding	

Other U.S. federal food guidance for the general public is now being modified to be consistent with these guidelines.[1,2] In the United States, several professional associations have also promulgated guidelines for those at risk or already suffering from chronic degenerative diseases such as cancer or heart disease.[1,2]

All four countries address their guidelines to either the general population and health professionals or other policy makers. New guidelines usually follow the precedents established in earlier versions. Some changes simply involve a change in wording. For example, the American guideline regarding sugar is evolved from "Avoid too much sugar" in 1980[7] to "Use sugars only in moderation" in 1990[8] and "Choose a diet moderate in sugars" in 1995[9] to the 2000 "Choose beverages and foods that limit your intake of sugars"[10] and the current one "Choose and prepare foods and beverages with little added sugars or caloric sweeteners"[11]. Other changes are more innovative. The United States added new guidelines on food safety in 2000 and expanded them in 2005. It also included recommendations for specific population groups at high nutritional risk with the guidelines.

Table 22.3 shows that in 2003 Australia continued to have a hybrid of food-based and nutrient-based recommendations. Australia and New Zealand both have specific guidelines for infants, toddlers, school-age children, adolescents, and the elderly that also address other health recommendations related to nutrition, such as breast-feeding of infants and physical activity for everyone. New Zealand also has dietary guidelines for pregnant and breast-feeding women.

As described in Table 22.1, the United States, Canada, and Australia all have pictorial representations or graphics for their dietary recommendations. The United States updated its food pyramid with a set of personalized interactive pyramids entitled MyPyramid (www.Mypyramid.gov).[12] Canada uses a rainbow graphic to depict the components of a healthy diet. Australia has two graphics; a pyramid and also used a circular plate in the past.

SIMILARITIES AND DIFFERENCES

All these countries have recommendations for certain nutrients and also for groups of foods, such as fruits/vegetables, grains, dairy, and meats. Food-based guidelines are easier for consumers to implement than nutrient-based guidelines since human beings eat foods, and not specific nutrients. In all of these countries, heart disease, hypertension, diabetes with its complications, and cancer are the leading causes of death.[5,11,13–15] Obesity is prevalent and increases the severity and adverse outcomes from many of these diseases.[15,16]

Although the core messages in all of these dietary guidelines are similar — eat a variety of foods and include physical activity to achieve/maintain a healthy weight (Table 22.3) — the American dietary guidelines (Table 22.2) have adopted a particularly strong emphasis on weight control through diet and physical activity. They note that major causes of illness and death are related to poor diet and a sedentary lifestyle, both associated with the epidemic of obesity in that country, and this is the reason for the stress on weight control.

The report of the 2005 Dietary Guidelines for Americans committee[11] is now oriented toward policy makers and health professionals, rather than to the general public, since its intent is to summarize current knowledge regarding individual nutrients and food components into recommendations for a pattern of eating that can be adopted by the public. A simplified booklet for consumers has also been prepared by communications experts.[17]

All these countries have recommendations on limiting fat, salt, and alcohol, and increasing fruits, vegetables, and whole grains. The United States, Canada, and New Zealand, all suggest limiting alcoholic beverages to less than 2 drinks per day for men and one for women. Australia has a higher limit; less than four drinks for men and two for women per day.

The background and supporting information accompanying the Dietary Guidelines provides the rationale for quantitative suggestions for intakes of specific nutrients.[5,11,18,19] All these countries suggest that 50 to 55% of total calories should come from carbohydrates. The United States, Canada, and Australia recommend less than 10% from saturated fat but vary in the amount of total fat from 30 to 35% of calories. New Zealand is more liberal, suggesting no more than 12% from saturated fat.

There are some differences in the guidelines of these highly industrialized countries. In the 2000 edition of the U.S. guidelines, food safety was addressed and it continues to be included in 2005. Australia includes a guideline specifically to encourage and support breast-feeding.[18] Most of the guidelines for the United States and Canada are for all healthy individuals over age 2 years. However, the fat guideline in Canada is not applicable until a child reaches age 5 years.

Other health recommendations that are included in New Zealand's guidelines are nonsmoking, especially for adolescents, pregnant, and breast-feeding women. The elderly, who may suffer from isolation and therefore poor nutrition, are encouraged to "make mealtime a social time." Australia encourages its elderly to eat at least three meals per day. Elderly people and pregnant women are especially vulnerable to risks associated with food-borne illnesses. Australia's food safety guidelines specifically address food safety in the elderly (care for your food: prepare and store it correctly) and the New Zealand guidelines discuss *Listeria* in the information specifically directed to pregnant women.

CONCLUSIONS

The guidelines for these English-speaking countries in different parts of the world are very similar, reflecting the affluent lifestyles and common food ways that they share.

LATIN AMERICA

Dietary guidelines were first formulated in Latin America in the late 1980s.[20] Guidelines from Chile, Guatemala, Mexico, Panama, and Venezuela are provided as examples of dietary guidelines in the region.

Latin America is a region with great inequalities in the distribution of welfare and also large variations in the nutritional health of its population groups. There has been a shift from dietary deficiency disease to problems of dietary excess in many countries of the region over the past two decades. In Chile, the prevalence of protein–calorie malnutrition in children is declining rapidly. However, the prevalence of chronic degenerative diseases associated with imbalances in food intake and sedentary lifestyles is rising.[21] In contrast, in Guatemala, Mexico, and Panama, poverty-related undernutrition and dietary deficiency diseases are still prevalent, especially among children and women of reproductive age in rural areas. At the same time, the prevalence of diet-related chronic diseases is rising. Venezuela is an oil-exporting country, but still has large economic inequalities and grapples with poverty-related malnutrition as well as dietary excess.

In most Latin American countries, food consumption patterns are influenced by those of the United States. Changing cultural and economic influences, rural–urban migration, greater availability of processed foods, and advertising are also affecting food consumption,[22] resulting in both over- and undernutrition.[23] The development of poor ghettos in metropolitan areas, short lactation periods, low wages, and low maternal educational levels is associated with undernutrition in young children. The interactions of urbanization, sedentary lifestyles, lack of nutrition education, and excessive consumption of cheap foods low in nutritional value lead to diseases of overconsumption, such as obesity, diabetes, and cardiovascular disease.[23] Other countries in Latin America, including Argentina, Brazil, Cuba, Peru, Colombia, Costa Rica, Honduras, and El Salvador are either formulating or have completed country-specific dietary guidelines.

FORMULATION

Most of the Latin American countries are in the implementation stage in formulating dietary guidelines.[24] The dietary guidelines for the Mexican population were issued by the Mexican Institute of Nutrition.[25] Venezuela issued dietary guidelines in the late 1980s that were later revised and updated.[26] The dietary guidelines have been implemented in many ways. For example, they have been incorporated into Venezuelan kindergarten, elementary, and secondary school curricula.[26–28]

Table 22.4 contains details about the dietary guidelines development process in selected Latin American countries: Chile, Guatemala, Mexico, Panama, and Venezuela.[21,26,29–31] All have dietary guidelines for the general population. Some also have guidelines for specific population groups (Chile, Panama, and Venezuela) or target certain groups on specific concerns (Guatemala for food safety among the poor). Governmental or quasi-governmental organizations develop and promulgate the guidelines based on the views and opinions of experts and scientists. Some also use background data on food consumption surveys (Chile, Mexico, and Panama) and economic data (Venezuela and Mexico). Most of the countries also refer to food groups in their dietary guidelines.[21,26,32]

TABLE 22.4
Development of Dietary Guidelines in Latin American Countries

Country:	Chile	Guatemala	Mexico	Panama	Venezuela
Title of Guidelines	Food Guidelines for Chile	Food Guidelines for Guatemala	Food Guidelines - Mexico	Food Guidelines for Panama	Food Guidelines for Venezuela
Year	1997	1998	1993	1995	2003
Endorsing Unit	Ministry of Health, Food Technology and Nutrition Institute, and University of Chile	Food Guidelines National Committee	National Nutrition Institute	Ministry of Health	CAVENDES Foundation, National Institute of Nutrition, and several universities
Approaches[a]	1, 3, 4	1, 3, 6	1, 3, 4, 5, 6	1, 3, 4, 5	1, 2, 5, 6
Target audiences[b]	G, P, N	G	G	G, P	G, P, N
Graphic representation	Pyramid	Family pot	Pyramid	Pyramid	none
Other Guidelines	For school age children and for the elderly	Food safety	None	For the first year of age	For the preschooler, school age children, and for the elderly

[a] 1 = Nutrition experts, nutrition scientists views; 2 = Review of former guidelines; 3 = From food groups; 4 = From consumption / nutrition survey; 5 = Definition of nutritional objectives; 6 = Economic data.

[b] G = general population; H = health professionals; P = policy makers; N= nutrition education of school children.

Four of the countries also use graphic representations of food groups and supporting messages (see Table 22.4). Chile and Panama adapted the food guide pyramid used in the United States. Mexico now uses a plate rather than the pyramid it formerly employed. Guatemala summarized its food groups and dietary guidelines in a family pot or "crock pot" graphic. Venezuela has no graphic, but the government has produced an extensive set of educational materials directed to different target groups.[27,28]

SIMILARITIES AND DIFFERENCES

Table 22.5 summarizes the dietary guidelines for certain Latin American countries. The number of guidelines range from five in Panama to ten in Mexico; Venezuela has issued nine guidelines and also 40 educational messages to facilitate the implementation of the guidelines. Mexico has 10 dietary guidelines, but each guideline contains several additional messages.

In general, the guidelines are focused on foods and provide general guidance. Variety is mentioned in all guidelines. Guatemala, Mexico, and Venezuela discuss economic disparities in supporting documents. For example, Guatemala recommends to those with limited resources to eat meats, eggs, and dairy products at least once or twice a week, while Venezuela urges prudence in the management of financial resources (see Table 22.5).

Some countries incorporate specific concerns about food consumption (Table 22.5). Guatemala emphasizes the importance of washing hands, and keeping food and water well covered in its graphic. Venezuela has a guideline emphasizing good hygiene in handling food.

Guidelines directed to overconsumption are included by all the countries. These include specific recommendations to increase physical activity (Mexico), maintain a healthy weight (Mexico and Panama) or to moderate or reduce the use of fats and sugars (Chile, Mexico, Panama, and Venezuela). Chronic disease risks are also addressed. These include recommendations to moderate use of salt (Chile and Venezuela) or sodium (Panama), limiting consumption of fats and sugars (Chile, Mexico, Panama, and Venezuela), saturated fats (Mexico and Panama), cholesterol (Mexico and Panama). Other guidelines are directed to limiting specific foods or nutrients, or to increase other more nutrient-rich foods (fruits, vegetables, and whole grains) (see Table 22.5).

The Latin American guidelines focus mostly on foods, not specific nutrients (Table 22.5). However, Panama recommends moderation in the use of sodium and salt. Guatemala, a country with low literacy rates, also emphasizes nutrients but in simple, short messages; it singles out energy, protein (both animal and vegetable), vitamins A and C, calcium, iron, and zinc, as well as fiber. This emphasis reflects Guatemala's goals of preventing both dietary deficiencies and excesses. Venezuela's guidelines have little emphasis on specific foods and focus on salt, alcohol, and sugar, and also stress economical choices of foods (Table 22.5). Mexico and Venezuela share an emphasis on nutrition-related healthy behaviors such as physical activity and breast-feeding.

All of the Latin American countries include advice on consuming fruits, vegetables, and grains daily. Guatemala specifically mentions beans and tortillas. Other countries (Chile, Mexico, and Venezuela) mention the need for limiting fat. Salt restriction is mentioned in Mexico, Venezuela, and Panama. Both Mexico and Venezuela have a guideline limiting alcohol. Chile and Guatemala include a guideline on use of dairy products; Chile focuses on low-fat milk products; Guatemala urges at least 1 to 2 servings of whole-fat milk products, since many members of the population are poor and do not consume milk. Mexico and

TABLE 22.5
Dietary Guidelines of Selected Latin American Countries

Chile	Guatemala	Mexico	Panama	Venezuela
1. Eat different types of foods throughout the day.	1. Include, at each meal, grains, cereals, or potatoes, because they are nutritious, tasty, and have low cost	1. Avoid monotony by consuming a wide variety of foods	1. Eat a variety of foods	1. Eat food from all food groups
2. Increase your consumption of fruits, vegetables, and green vegetables	2. Eat every day vegetables and greens to benefit your body	2. Include, at every meal, at least two servings of fruits and vegetables	2. Eat sufficient grains, roots, vegetables, and fruits	2. Daily, do 30 minutes of physical activity
3. Prefer vegetable oil and limit animal fats	3. Every day, eat some type of fruit, because they are healthy, easy to digest, and nutritious	3. Eat, at every meal, a variety of grains and grain products, preferably whole grains, mixing cereals and legumes	3. Select a diet low in saturated fat, cholesterol, and oil	3. Practice hygienic habits in your food preparation
4. For meat, prefer fish and poultry	4. If you eat tortilla and beans every day, eat one spoonful of beans with each tortilla to make it more nutritious	4. Include, at every meal, a moderate serving of animal products, choosing those with the least fat	4. Eat sugar and sweets in moderation	4. Use your money wisely in your food selection and expenditures
5. Increase your consumption of low-fat milk	5. At least twice a week, eat one egg, or one piece of cheese, or drink one glass of milk, to complement your diet	5. Limit your consumption of fats, including cooking oils and fatty foods (to less than 30% of daily energy intake). Also, limit saturated fats, of animal origin (to lees than 10% of total energy). And, reduce cholesterol intake to less than 300 mg per day	5. Eat salt and sodium in moderation	5. Breast milk is the only food without substitute for infants below 6 months of age
6. Reduce salt intake	6. At least once per week, eat a serving of liver (beef) or meat to strengthen your body	6. Reduce the consumption of salt and sugar, starting by not using salt at the table and reducing sugars in your liquids (coffee, tea, drinks, or juices)	6. Maintain a healthy weight	6. Increase your consumption of fruit, vegetables, legumes and cereals
7. Moderate the consumption of sugar	7. To stay healthy, eat a variety of foods as indicate in the household pot	7. Restrict the consumption of products with excess of additives (colorants, flavorings, etc. Avoid alcohol and do not smoke		7. Use moderation in the consumption of sugar, salt, and alcoholic beverages
		8. Breast-feed children from birth and start comple mentary food at the fourth month of age		8. Consume animal products in moderate amounts
		9. Avoid obesity by monitoring your weight according to the suggested weight for your stature		9. Water is indispensable for life and its consumption helps to maintain your help
		10. Increase your physical activity, walk briskly or practice any other type of aerobic exercise for about 20 to 30 minutes 4 or 5 times a week		

Venezuela have specific guidelines stressing the importance of breast-feeding. Panama has special dietary guidelines for infants that recommend exclusive breast-feeding during the first 6 months of life and for complementary feeding thereafter.

CONCLUSIONS

Dietary guidelines for Latin American countries reflect the diversity in socioeconomic situations and nutritional problems in the region and each country's unique perspectives. They offer the general public, service providers, and policy maker's actionable recommendations for improving nutrition and health status. Some of these countries have already identified barriers that limit the use of the dietary guidelines (Chile, Venezuela). Others, such as Mexico, still need to evaluate the applicability of their guidelines to the eating practices of the diverse Mexican population. Dietary guidelines in Guatemala were directed to the poor; problems associated with overconsumption of foods and sedentary lifestyles still need to be addressed.

ASIAN COUNTRIES

Asia's diversity is reflected in the many nutritional problems that were evident in the ten countries we reviewed: China, India, Indonesia, Japan, Korea, Malaysia, Philippines, Singapore, Taiwan, and Thailand.[33–43,44] Until the mid-1950s, poverty-related malnutrition was the major problem. The primary concern was to ensure adequate energy intakes and prevention or control of dietary deficiency diseases.[32,45] Today, nutrition problems in Asia cover the entire spectrum from deficiency disease to excess. Some countries are experiencing new affluence, and increasingly issues of chronic degenerative disease also have to be addressed.

Asian dietary guidelines focus on reducing or preventing both chronic deficiency and chronic degenerative diseases since both problems are often prevalent.[46–48] Presently, India still has high rates of protein-energy malnutrition among some groups as well as very affluent population groups with chronic disease problems. The national guidelines address both groups. In countries such as Korea, Japan, Taiwan, and Singapore, deficiency diseases have declined dramatically in the past three decades.[45,48,49] Countries such as Thailand and China have low rates of protein-energy malnutrition, but micronutrient deficiencies (iron, iodine, vitamin A, and riboflavin) are still common.[33,37,43,50] Indonesia and the Philippines face both persistent problems of undernutrition and deficiency disease among the poor, coupled with emerging problems of overnutrition and increased chronic degenerative disease rates, particularly among the affluent.[32,35,37] Filipino guidelines for more affluent populations focus on chronic degenerative diseases and avoiding excess,[51] whereas Filipino guidelines for less affluent population groups emphasize achieving sufficiency of nutrient intakes.[35]

FORMULATION

Table 22.6 shows the various approaches used in developing dietary guidelines in Asia. The guidelines are all intended to provide nutrition education and dietary guidance to the general public in terms that are understandable to most consumers. They are also often used to help officials in the health, agricultural, and education sectors in program planning. All of the countries surveyed rely on government agencies or professional societies to develop and endorse their official guidelines.[35] Some countries (Philippines, Korea, and Japan) formulate guidelines based on findings from national nutrition or food consumption surveys. Others develop their dietary guidelines based on what experts deem to be appropriate.

Graphics have been adopted by many Asian countries to help the public visualize these dietary guidelines and food guides. These include pyramids (Malaysia and Singapore), stairs (India), pagodas (Korea and China), a flag (Thailand), a plum flower (Taiwan), the "big 6" for the six food groups (Japan), and a six-sided star (Philippines). A pyramid is also available for more affluent Filipinos.[51]

SIMILARITIES AND DIFFERENCES

Table 22.7 presents information on representative dietary guidelines from the Asian region. Most of the guidelines are general, and are food rather than nutrient-based. The exception is Singapore, which has guidelines that are quantitative and nutrient-specific.[52] There are common core food-based messages in all the guidelines, these include: choose a diet composed of a wide variety of foods; eat enough food to meet bodily needs and maintain or improve body weight; select foods that are safe to eat; and enjoy your food.

The guidelines also vary with respect to number and in relative emphasis given on balance, adequacy, moderation, and restriction. Although all the Asian dietary guidelines recommend eating a variety of foods, they differ on how they suggest achieving a varied pattern (see Table 22.7). Some include recommendations for frequency of consumption. Eating breakfast daily is recommended in the Indonesian guidelines, and having regular meals is recommended in the Korean guidelines.[37,38] Other guidelines recommend specific amounts of different kinds of foods. For example, to assure a well-balanced diet, the Japanese guidelines

TABLE 22.6
Development of Dietary Guidelines in Asian Countries

Country	Title of Guidelines	Year	Endorsing Unit	Approaches[a]	Target Audiences[b]	Graphic Representation
China	Chinese Dietary Guidelines for Chinese Residents	1997	Chinese Nutrition Society	1	G	Pagoda
India	Dietary Guideline for Indians Foundation to Nutrition and Health	1998	National Institute of Nutrition	1–6	N	Stairs
Indonesia	13 Core Messages for a Balanced Diet	1995	National Development and Planning Coordinating Board	1	G	None
Japan	Guidelines for Health Promotion: Dietary Guidelines	1985	Ministry of Health and Welfare	1, 2, 3, 5	G, H	Numeral 6
Korea	National Dietary Guidelines	1990	Korean Nutrition Society/ Ministry of Health and Welfare	1, 2, 4	G	Pagoda
Malaysia	Proposed Dietary Guidelines for Malaysia	1996	Ministry of Health	1, 2, 3	G, H	Pyramid
Philippines	Nutritional Guidelines for Filipinos	1990	Department of Science and Technology (National Guidelines Committee)	1–5	G, H	Pyramid, 6-sided star
Singapore	Guidelines for a Healthy Diet	1993	National Advisory Committee on Food and Nutrition, Ministry of Health	1	G	Pyramid
Taiwan	Dietary Guidelines for the Population	1995	Department of Health	1	G	Plum flower
Thailand	The Thai Dietary Guidelines for Better Health	1995	The Division of Nutrition, Department of Health, Ministry of Public Health	1	G	None

[a] 1 = Nutrition experts and nutrition scientists views. 2 = Review of former guidelines. 3 = From food groups. 4 = From consumption/nutrition survey. 5 = Definition of nutritional objectives. 6 = Economic data.

[b] G = General population. H = Health professionals. P = Policy makers. N = Nutrition education of school children.

recommend eating 30 or more different kinds of foods daily.[41] Japanese guidelines also suggest balancing main and side dishes around staple foods. Malaysia recommends choosing foods from each of the food group's daily.[42] The Filipino and Chinese guidelines also focus on achieving dietary adequacy, emphasizing food rather than nutrient-based interventions.

Virtually all examined Asian countries emphasize ensuring adequacy of energy/calorie intake (see Table 22.7). Korea mentions achieving and maintaining energy balance by balancing intakes and expenditure.[37] Most guidelines stress getting enough food with increased intakes of fruits, vegetables, cereal, and dairy food to promote fiber, vitamins, and minerals intakes. Some also indicate the proportion of foods that should be consumed in relation to total energy intake. The national Indian guidelines are very general emphasizing: variety, food safety, moderation with respect to sugar and salt, adequate diets especially by children and adolescents, and a nutrient-rich diet for elders. They represent a change from the older guidelines that focused on specific population groups by economic status.[34]

In countries in which deficiencies of vitamins and minerals have been identified as public health problems, the guidelines reflect this, and emphasize food sources rich in those nutrients (see Table 22.7). For example, calcium is mentioned specifically in some guidelines. A specific calcium-rich food (milk) is mentioned in the Taiwanese, Chinese, Filipino, and Korean guidelines, and fish and seaweed in the Japanese guidelines. In Indonesia, people are advised to "consume iron-rich foods, and to use only iodized salt."[38] The Filipino guidelines recommend "choosing foods fortified with nutrients."[35] The guidelines for poor Indonesians recommend eating enough food.[34,38]

The more affluent countries such as Taiwan, Singapore, Korea, and Japan, (and also the guidelines for the more affluent members of the population in Indonesia) emphasize moderation in fat, saturated fat, or simple sugars. The major difference between the various guidelines in Asia is in the amounts and the relative balance suggested between dietary constituents. The Asian guidelines on moderation in fat and salt intake vary greatly. Some simply say to avoid excess, or to limit/restrict the use of fat (see guidelines for India, Malaysia, Taiwan, China), others specify the type of fat to be consumed. For example, the Japanese guidelines recommend use of vegetable oil instead of animal fat.

China, Taiwan, and Singapore are three countries with similar ethnic origins and dietary patterns that share similar dietary guidelines recommending reducing intake of salt and salt-cured foods. Singapore is the most specific, recommending eating less than 5 g of salt or 2000 mg of sodium per day.[52] General recommendations on limiting salt intake are present in other guidelines throughout the region. The Japanese guidelines recommend eating less than 10 g of salt per day. Neither Malaysia nor the Philippines mentions salt.[52]

TABLE 22.7
Dietary Guidelines of Selected Asian Countries

China
1. Eat a variety of foods
2. Eat appropriate quantity of foods
3. Moderate oil and fat
4. Eat moderately polished cereals
5. Limit salt intake
6. Eat fewer sweets
7. Limit alcohol balance food distribution through three meals

India
1. Nutritionally adequate diet should be consumed through a mix: choice from a variety of foods
2. Additional food and extra care are required during pregnancy and lactation
3. Exclusive breast-feeding should be practiced for 4–6 months. Breast-feeding can be continued up to 2 years
4. Food supplements should be introduced to infants by 4–6 months
5. Adequate and appropriate diet should be taken by children and adolescents, both in health and disease
6. Green leafy vegetables, other vegetables and fruits should be used in plenty
7. Cooking oils and animal foods should be used in moderation, and vanaspati/ghee/butter should be used only sparingly
8. Overeating should be avoided to prevent overweight and obesity Proper physical activity is essential to maintain desirable body weight
9. Salt should be used in moderation
10. Foods consumed should be safe and clean
11. Healthy and positive food concepts and cooking practices should be adopted
12. Water should be taken in adequate amounts and beverages should be consumed in moderation
13. Processed and ready-to-eat foods should be used judiciously. Sugar should be used sparingly
14. The elderly should eat a nutrient-rich diet to keep fit and active

Indonesia
1. Eat a wide variety of foods
2. Consume foods that provide sufficient energy
3. Obtain about half of total energy requirements from complex CHO-rich foods
4. Obtain not more than a quarter of total energy intake from fats or oils
5. Use only iodized salt
6. Consume iron-rich foods
7. Breast-feed your baby exclusively for four months
8. Have breakfast everyday
9. Drink adequate quantities of fluids that are free of contaminants
10. Take adequate exercise
11. Avoid drinking alcoholic drinks
12. Consume foods prepared hygienically
13. Read the labels of packaged foods

Japan
1. Obtain well-balanced nutrition with a variety of foods (30 foods a day); take staple food, main dish, and side dishes together
2. Take energy corresponding to daily activity
3. Consider the amount and the quality of the fats and oils you eat: avoid too much; eat more vegetable oils than animal fat
4. Avoid too much salt, not more than 10 g a day
5. Happy eating makes for happy family life; sit down and eat together and talk; treasure family taste and home cooking

Korea
1. Eat a variety of grains, vegetables and fruits, fish, meat, poultry, and dairy products
2. Choose less salt-preserved foods and prepare foods with less salt
3. Increase physical activity for a healthy weight and balance what you eat with your activity
4. Enjoy every meal, and do not skip breakfast
5. If you drink alcoholic beverages, do so in moderation
6. Prepare foods properly and order sensible amounts
7. Enjoy our rice-based diet

Malaysia
1. Enjoy a variety of foods
2. Maintain healthy body weight by balancing food intake with regular physical activity
3. Eat more rice and other cereal products, legumes, fruit, and vegetables
4. Minimize fat in food preparation and choose foods that are low in fat and cholesterol
5. Use a small amount of salt and choose foods low in salt
6. Drink plenty of water daily
7. Practice and promote breast-feeding

Philippines
1. Eat a variety of foods every day
2. Breast-feed infants exclusively from birth to 6 months, and then, give appropriate foods while continuing breast-feeding
3. Maintain children's normal growth through proper diet and monitor their growth regularly
4. Consume fish, lean meat, poultry, or dried beans
5. Eat more vegetables, fruits, and root crops
6. Eat foods cooked in edible/cooking oil in your daily meals
7. Consume milk, milk products, and other calcium-rich foods
8. Use iodized salt, but avoid excessive intake of salty foods

Singapore
1. Eat a variety of foods
2. Maintain desirable body weight
3. Restrict total fat intake to 20 to 30% of total energy intake
4. Modify composition of fat in the diet to one-third polyunsaturated, one-third monounsaturated, and one-third saturated
5. Reduce cholesterol intake to less than 300 mg/day
6. Maintain intakes of complex carbohydrates at about 50% total energy intake
7. Reduce salt intake to less than 5 g a day (2000 mg Na)
8. Reduce intake of salt-cured, preserved, and smoked foods
9. Reduce intake of refined and processed sugar to less than 10% of energy
10. Increase intake of fruit and vegetables and whole-grain cereal products
11. For those who drink, have not more than two standard drinks (about 30 g alcohol) per day
12. Encourage breast-feeding in infants until at least 6 months of age

Thailand
1. Eat a variety of foods from each of the five food groups and maintain proper weight
2. Eat adequate amount of rice or alternative carbohydrate sources
3. Eat plenty of vegetables and fruits regularly
4. Eat fish, lean meat, eggs, legumes, and pulses regularly
5. Drink milk in appropriate quality and quantity for one's age
6. Eat a diet containing appropriate amounts of fat
7. Avoid sweet and salty foods
8. Eat clean and safe food
9. Avoid or reduce the consumption of alcoholic beverages

The majority of the guidelines stress common nonfood-related healthy behaviors such as not smoking, dental hygiene, stress management, weight control, and physical activity. Asian dietary guidelines also specify the settings (places or environments) or other circumstances surrounding food and eating (Table 22.7). Most countries in this region also acknowledge the impacts of lifestyle changes on health, and emphasize attaining a healthy body weight to prevent diet-related disease. The Indonesian guideline recommends "consuming foods to provide sufficient energy."[38] Some of these differences in emphasis reflect the vastly different levels of affluence, within and between countries in Asia. For many years, India had two sets of guidelines. One was for the poor and emphasized nutrient adequacy and avoidance of dietary deficiency diseases. The other Indian guidelines were for affluent individuals and emphasized energy balance, restricting energy intakes to levels "commensurate with sedentary occupation, so that obesity is avoided," coupled with moderation and restriction of fat, saturated fat, and sugar to reduce chronic degenerative disease.[34] The 2003 Indian guidelines are 14 in number and are national guidelines rather than specific recommendations by economic group.

Asian guidelines also recognize that eating is more than just "refueling" or nourishment from the physiological standpoint. They recognize that food provides pleasure and has strong links to family, tradition, and culture. Therefore, enjoyment of meals is a concern in all countries, but it is especially evident in the Japanese and Korean guidelines. In Japan, dietary guidelines that promote family values are included; citizens are advised to "make all activities pertaining to food pleasurable ones." Another Japanese guideline also advises to "enjoy cooking and use mealtimes as occasions for family communication."[36,53] In Korea, eating is viewed as a way to keep harmony between diet and other aspects of daily life, and this is stated in the guidelines.[37]

CONCLUSIONS

Dietary guidelines for the Asian countries are all directed to the general population. Many countries, including Malaysia, Indonesia, China, and Japan, also have specific guidelines focusing on those of different ages, sexes, and conditions, such as infants, pregnant and lactating women.[33,36,52,53] Specific foods are recommended for these population groups. For example, breast-feeding in early infancy is a common recommendation in the dietary guidelines of many Asian countries. Human breast milk is recognized as the best food for infants. Encouragement of breast-feeding and recognition of breast milk's unique properties are included in the guidelines.[53] The duration of exclusive breast-feeding, ranges from 4 months (Indonesia) to 4–6 months (Philippines), and to 6 months in Singapore. Another difference is age of weaning, introduction of other foods in addition to breast milk. For example, it is at 4 to 6 months in the Philippines, but weaning is recommended at no earlier than 5 to 6 months in the Malaysian guidelines, with breast-feeding continuing for up to 2 years.

Some dietary guidelines are common to all Asian countries. One is to eat clean and safe foods; such recommendations are especially important in areas where the climate is very hot and foods are easily spoiled. The hygienic messages range from "consume food that is hygienically prepared" in Malaysia, to "eat clean and safe food to prevent food-borne disease in the family" in the Philippines. Similar guidelines are provided in both the Taiwan and the People's Republic of China's guidelines. "Drink more boiled water" is mentioned in Taiwan, and the guidelines for Mainland China are "avoiding unsanitary and spoiled foods."[38,54,55]

AFRICA

Africa consists of more than 50 nations, most of which are developing countries. Food insecurity is a prominent phenomenon in the majority of this continent. Protein–energy malnutrition, nutrient deficiencies, infectious diseases such as HIV, tuberculosis, and malaria are prevalent especially in central Africa, while diseases of affluence raise concerns in more wealthy and developed southern African countries. Dietary guidelines for South Africa, Nigeria, and Republic of Namibia are summarized here.[56–58]

FORMULATION

South Africa Guidelines for Healthy Eating were revised by Department of Health of South Africa in 2004. The guidelines aim to improve health as well as to relieve chronic diseases, overweight, nutrient deficiencies, and malnutrition. In the process of dietary guidelines formulation, scientific findings, dietary recommendations from other countries, WHO guidelines, and health status surveys were reviewed. Dietary guidelines for Nigeria, published in four languages spoken in the country, were established collaboratively by several ministries, WHO, and other professional organizations in 2001[56] (see Table 22.8).

The Food and Nutrition Guidelines for Namibia were prepared by the National Food Security and Nutrition Council in 2000 (see Table 22.8). However, there is limited information related to the development process that was involved in the Nigerian and Namibian guidelines. South Africa published brochures with detailed illustration and suggested applications on each guideline. South Africa recommends specific numbers of servings on each food group, but similar feature from Namibia and Nigeria is not found. No graphic representation of dietary guidelines was designed in African countries.

While South African guidelines target all adults and children older than 7 years of age, Nigerian guidelines were presented in ten age categories, and Namibian guidelines were not age-specific.

TABLE 22.8
Development of Dietary Guidelines in African Countries

Country	South Africa	Republic of Namibia	Nigeria
Title of Guidelines	South African Guidelines For Healthy Eating	Food and Nutrition Guidelines for Namibia Food Choices For A Healthy Life	Food Guidelines for Nigeria
Year	2001	2000	2001
Endorsing Unit	Department of Health, Association for dietetics in South Africa, and Nutrition Society of South Africa	National Food Security and Nutrition Council	Ministries of Health, Agriculture and Rural Development and other Organizations
Approaches[a]	1, 2, 3, 4, 5	1, 2, 4	1, 2, 4
Number of Guidelines	11	10	
Target audiences [b]	G, H, P	G, H, P	G, H, P
Major Nutrition Problems Addressed in Guidelines[c]	O, C, PEM, I	O, C, PEM, I	O, C, PEM, I
Graphic representation			
Other Guidelines			

[a] 1 = Nutrition experts and nutrition scientists views. 2 = Review of former guidelines. 3 = From food groups. 4 = From consumption/nutrition survey. 5 = Definition of nutritional objectives.

[b] G = General population. H = Health professionals. P = Policy makers.

[c] C = Diet-related chronic degenerative diseases. I = Dietary inadequacy; O = Overnutrition (energy). PEM = Protein-energy malnutrition.

TABLE 22.9
Dietary Guidelines for South Africa and the Republic of Namibia

South Africa	Republic of Namibia
1. Enjoy a variety of foods	1. Eat a variety of foods
2. Be active	2. Eat vegetables and fruit every day
3. Make starchy foods the basis of most meals	3. Eat more fish
4. Eat dry beans, split peas, lentils, and soy regularly	4. Eat beans or meat regularly
5. Chicken, fish, milk, meat, or eggs can be eaten daily	5. Use whole-grain products
6. Drink lots of clean, safe water	6. Use only iodized salt, but use less salt
7. Eat plenty of vegetables and fruits every day	7. Eat at least three meals a day
8. Eat fats sparingly	8. Avoid drinking alcohol. Consume clean and safe water and food
9. Use salt sparingly	9. Achieve and maintain a healthy body weight
10. Use food and drinks containing sugar sparingly and not between meals	

SIMILARITIES AND DIFFERENCES

Dietary guidelines for South Africa and Namibia are summarized in Table 22.9, and those for Nigeria in Table 22.10. Dietary guidelines from all three African countries are food-based instead of nutrient-based. While South Africa has 11 dietary guidelines and Namibia has 10, Nigeria presents over 40 recommendations in three general sections — Good Nutrition, Physical Activity, and Healthy Lifestyle.

All the African dietary guidelines are similar in several ways (see Table 22.9 and Table 22.10). All three guidelines recommend choosing a variety of foods, and at the same time emphasize vegetables and fruits intake. Similarly, all of African guidelines suggest consuming beans, meat, and fish regularly or daily. Additionally, advice on reducing salt intakes as well as avoiding or limiting alcohol intake is found in all guidelines. Furthermore, South Africa and Nigeria recommend limitation on sugar and fat intake. However, only Namibia advocates consuming whole grain products. Only South Africa alone suggests daily milk intake.

All African guidelines recognize the importance of maintaining a healthy body weight with physical activities. South Africa, but not Nigeria and Namibia, further defines healthy body weight in terms of body mass index and provides specific guidelines on the duration and ways to be physically active (see Table 22.9 and Table 22.10).

TABLE 22.10
Dietary Guidelines for the Nigerian Population

1. Good Nutrition

No single food by itself (except breast milk) provides all the nutrients in the right amounts that will promote growth and maintain life. To achieve good nutrition, therefore, it is necessary to consume as wide a variety of foods as possible from the age of 6 months

1.1. Infants (0–6 months)
- Start exclusive breast-feeding immediately after birth and continue for 6 months
- There should be no bottle-feeding

1.2. Infants (7–12 months)
- Continue breast-feeding
- Introduce complementary feeds made from a variety of cereals, tubers, legumes, fruits, animal foods and give with cup and spoon

1.3. Toddlers (13–24 months)
- Continue to breast-feed until child is 2 years
- Give enriched pap or mashed foods twice daily
- Give family diet made soft with less pepper and spices
- Give fruits and vegetables in season

1.4. Children (25–60 months)
- Give diet that contains a variety of foods in adequate amounts.
- Add palm oil or vegetable oil to raise the energy level of complementary foods
- Gradually increase food intake to 4–5 times daily as baby gets older
- Provide dark green leafy vegetables, yellow/orange colored fruits, citrus fruits, cereals, legumes, tubers and foods of animal origin.
  – Limit the consumption of sugary food
- Continue feeding even when child is ill

1.5. School-aged children (6–11 years)
- Give diet that contains a variety of foods in adequate amounts
- Encourage consumption of good quality snacks, but limit the consumption of sugary snacks

1.6. Adolescents (12–18 years)
- Consume diet containing a variety of foods
- Most of the energy should be delivered from roots/tubers, legumes, cereals, vegetables, and less from animal foods
- An increase in total food intake is very important at this stage, so is the need to enjoy family meals
- Snacks especially pastry and carbonate drinks should not replace main meals. If you must eat out, make wise food choices
- Liberal consumption of whatever fruits that is in season should be encouraged
- Females need to eat more iron-containing foods like meat, fish, poultry, legumes, cereals as well as citrus fruits to enhance body's use of iron

1.7. Adults (male and female)

Total food intake should take into consideration the level of physical activity. Individuals who do manual work need to consume more food than those who do sedentary work
- Limit the fat intake from animal foods
- Diet should consist of as wide a variety of foods as possible for example, cereals, legumes, roots/tubers, fruits, vegetables, fish, lean meat, local cheese (wara)
- Limit intake of salt, bullion cubes, and sugar
- Liberal consumption of whatever fruits that is in season is encouraged

1.8. Pregnant women
- Eat diet that contains a variety of foods in adequate amounts
- Consume enough food to ensure adequate weight gain
- Eat more of cereals, legumes, fruits, vegetables, dairy products, and animal foods
- Take iron and folic acid supplements as prescribed
- Avoid alcohol, addictive substances, and smoking

1.9. Breast-feeding mothers
- Eat diet that contains a variety of available food items like cereals, tubers, legumes, meat, fish, milk, fruits, vegetables, etc.
- Consume more of foods rich in iron such as liver, fish, beef, etc.
- Eat fruits in season at every meal
- Consume fluids as needed to quench thirst
- Avoid alcohol, addictive substances and smoking

1.10. The elderly
- Eat diets that are prepared from a variety of available foods for example cereals, tubers, fruits, vegetables, etc.
- Increase consumption of fish and fish-based diets
- Eat more of fruits and vegetables
- Eat more frequently

2. Physical Activity/Exercise

Physical activity both as short periods of intense exercise or prolonged periods of modest activity on a daily basis generally has beneficial effects.
- Children and adolescents should engage in leisure time exercise
- Adults should undertake some form of exercise as recommended by their doctors

3. Healthy Lifestyle

Some habits and lifestyles for example tobacco use and excessive alcohol consumption have been found to be bad for health

Prolonged indulgence in these lifestyles predisposes to noncommunicable diseases like cancer, diabetes, heart problems, and hypertension

3.1. Alcohol

Too much alcohol consumption can lead to risk of hypertension, liver damage, malnutrition, and various cancers. There is also the problem of alcohol abuse
- If you must drink, take alcohol in moderation
- Avoid drinking alcohol when driving a vehicle or operating any machinery

3.2. Tobacco

Tobacco use is associated with lung cancers and other chronic disorders. Smoking during pregnancy can harm the developing baby and can result in low birth weight babies
- Avoid the use of tobacco in any form

South Africa and Namibia include food safety guidelines by suggesting drinking clean and safe water only. Both South Africa and Nigeria emphasize enjoyment of meals. Nigeria developed different guidelines on food intake along the life cycle, categorizing the lifespan into infants of 0 to 6 months, infants of 7 to 12 months, toddlers, preschool children, school-aged children, adolescents, adults, and elderly. Guidelines for pregnant and lactating women are also available. Breast-feeding is suggested to be the sole nutrition for infants under 6 months of age, and to be continued till 2 years old. Such age-specific division is not observed in South African and Namibian dietary guidelines.

CONCLUSIONS

Dietary guidelines for Africa reflect the large economic differences among African countries. South Africa, being a more wealthy country, emphasizes on promotion of balanced diet and prevention of diseases of affluence. In contrast, others, such as Namibia and Nigeria, aim to advocate food safety and adequacy of nutrition intake. Education and literacy level also affect the content and complexity of dietary guidelines in these countries. Many African countries have yet to develop their own dietary guidelines.

EUROPE

With a rich and varied history, Europe demonstrates a variety of economic, political, and healthcare conditions. European countries have numerous differences in culture and dietary habits. In 2000, the WHO Regional Office for Europe developed a Countrywide Integrated Noncommunicable Disease Intervention (CINDI) effort that included a section on "Twelve Steps to Healthy Eating" (see Table 22.11), which serve as the basis for formulating country-specific dietary guidelines in European countries. Most countries in the Nordic, western, southern, and central eastern regions of Europe have their national dietary guidelines in various stages of development and, as seen in Table 22.11, have incorporated some of the 12 steps to healthy eating in their own national guidelines. The heterogeneous nature within Europe makes the review of these guidelines interesting and complex.

Beginning in the late 1990s, European countries started a regional process of development and implementation of Food-based Dietary Guidelines (FBDG),[59] following the recommendations issued by the World Health Organization in 1996.[60] The evolution of the process is a regional enterprise coordinated by regional groups who work closely with the national sectors involved in the establishment of their FBDG.

TABLE 22.11

WHO Food-Based Dietary Guidelines and Number of European Countries, by Region, that Incorporated them into Their National Dietary Guidelines

	Southeast Europe and Central Asia	Central and Eastern Europe	Western Europe	Southern Europe	Nordic Countries	Other European Countries[a]
Total number of countries in region	11	6	9	10	5	10
Number of countries that adopted the WHO food-based dietary guidelines						
1. A varied diet, consisting mainly of plant foods	4	5	7	7	5	5
2. Daily intake of bread, grains, rice, potatoes, or pasta	4	4	5	6	5	6
3. Daily intake of fresh and local vegetables and fruits	6	4	6	6	5	3
4a. Healthy Body Mass Index (BMI) range	3	3	5	5	4	5
4b. Physical Activity	2	3	4	3	4	3
5a. Low fat intake (total fat)	3	6	7	7	5	6
5b. Low fat intake (saturated fat)	3	6	5	6	5	6
6. Intake of lean meat, poultry, fish, and legumes	3	5	6	7	4	6
7. Intake of low-fat milk and low-fat dairy products	2	5	6	5	5	6
8. Low sugar intake	3	4	5	7	5	6
9. Low salt intake	3	5	7	6	5	6
10. Limited alcohol intake	3	5	6	4	4	5
11. Hygienic preparation of food[b]	3	0	4	0	1	4
12. Exclusive breast-feeding[b]	3	4	2	3	5	5

[a] Include Baltic countries and Commonwealth of Independent States.

[b] Many countries include guidelines on these areas in separate guidelines.

The efforts in developing FBDG are continuing and are changing rapidly, because the European countries are at different stages in guidelines development. The process of developing guidelines in Europe is dynamic, and well integrated into other regional efforts as well nutrient recommendations which are also based on the deliberations of the WHO/FAO joint expert consultation group's report.[61]

FORMULATION

To develop this section, we selected arbitrarily a group of European countries: United Kingdom, Germany, Spain, Greece, Finland, and Portugal with enough literature in English, Spanish, or Portuguese, and analyzed their process for the establishment and implementation of their FBDG (see Table 22.12). All of these dietary guidelines are based on scientific reviews and what was in the former guidelines of the countries. All of the countries chosen as examples use national government bodies for defining and formulating them.

SIMILARITIES AND DIFFERENCES

Tables 22.13 and 22.14 present the dietary guidelines for the selected European countries. WHO advocates the use of food-based dietary guidelines for better comprehension and application by the general public. All of the European dietary guidelines examined present their key recommendations in terms of food. Among the European dietary guidelines reviewed, Finland and Portugal offered the most detailed nutrient-based recommendations that they present in addition to the food-based guidelines. Finnish guidelines include all macro- and micronutrients. Portugal, on the other hand, focuses only on carbohydrates, fiber, fats, saturated fats, cholesterol, and calcium. Portugal has one set of 9 nutrient-based guidelines and a separate set of 11 food-based dietary recommendations that are available for different purposes (planning for nutrients, and communications to the public for the food based guidelines).

The United Kingdom, Germany, and Spain display their guidelines in short, bulleted sentences (with 9, 10, and 10 points, respectively). In contrast, the Greek and Finnish guidelines are presented in narrative form (data not shown). Virtually all of the European guidelines categorize food into different groups, but the classifications of food are slightly different from country to country. For example, most countries consider potatoes in the starch group but Finland and Greece discuss potatoes separately and classify them in neither the vegetable nor the starch groups.

Virtually all of the European countries include a variety guideline, emphasize fruit, vegetables and whole grains, and all have some guideline for the amount of alcohol and fat in the diet. All except Spain have a guideline on salt, and all but Germany have guidelines about sweets. Countries differ to the extent they are nutrient-based and which nutrients they concentrate upon; for example, Finland and Portugal are more quantitative in terms of nutrient recommendations, whereas Spain and Greece are more food-based. For example, Finland recommends 5% or less of food energy from alcohol.

European guidelines are consistent in that variety in food choices is encouraged but the message is conveyed in various ways. Germany promotes the idea that there is no "forbidden food" and that people should pay attention to the quantity of food intake.

TABLE 22.12
Development of Dietary Guidelines in Selected European Countries

	United Kingdom	Germany	Spain	Greece	Finland	Portugal
Title of Guidelines	Guidelines for a Healthier Diet	10 Guidelines of the German Nutrition Society for a Wholesome Diet	The Bilbao Declaration (2000)	Dietary Guidelines for Adults in Greece	Finnish Nutrition Recommendations	
Year			2000	1999	1999	1997
Number of Guidelines	9	10	10	(Not listed in bullets)	(Not listed in bullets)	9 & 11
Endorsing Unit	Institute of Food Research	German Nutrition Society	Spanish Society of Community Nutrition	Ministry of Health and Welfare and Supreme Scientific Health Council	National Nutrition Council	National Council of Food and Nutrition
Other Guidelines	Vegetarian Diet Guidelines					
Graphic representation	Food plate	Food plate	Pyramid	Pyramid	Food pyramid, food plate, and food circle	Food wheel

TABLE 22.13
Dietary Guidelines for the Populations of Selected European Countries

United Kingdom

1. Eat a wide variety of different foods
2. Eat the right amount to be a healthy weight
3. Eat plenty of fruit and vegetables
4. Eat plenty of foods rich in starch and fiber
5. Try to limit fat intake
6. Choose fruit or bread rather than chocolate or sweets
7. Look after the vitamins and minerals in your food
8. If you drink, keep within sensible limits
9. Taste your food before adding salt

Germany

1. Choose from among many different foods
2. Cereal products several times per day and plenty of potatoes
3. Fruit and vegetables - take "5 a day"
4. Milk and dairy products daily, fish once a week, meat, sausages, and eggs in moderation
5. Low-fat diet
6. Sugar and salt in moderation
7. Plenty of liquid
8. Make sure your dishes are prepared gently and taste well
9. Take your time and enjoy eating
10. Watch your weight and stay active

Spain

1. To adjust energy intake to energy output in order to achieve an energy balance conductive to maintain body mass index (BMI) within the desirable range
2. To harmonize the percentage contribution of macronutrients to energy intake
3. To achieve a healthier lipid profile in the diet by enhancing a relevant contribution of monounsaturated fatty acids (MUFAs), mostly from olive oil
4. To stimulate changes in carbohydrate profile, through a higher proportion of complex carbohydrates
5. To adjust daily frequency of consumption of sugary foods to less than four occasions per day
6. A daily consumption of vegetables equal to or greater than 250 g is recommended, including at least one portion as fresh raw vegetables in a salad. A consumption of 400 g or more of fruit per person per day is also recommended
7. Moderation in the consumption of alcoholic beverages is advised, within the Mediterranean consumption pattern, i.e., small amounts of wine with meals
8. Introducing moderate physical exercise for at least 30 minutes within daily practices is highly recommended
9. It would be advisable that public administrations and institutions stimulate, support, and implement programs at developing individual skills contributing to food choices and preparations conductive to a healthy food pattern. Actions targeted to socially deprived environments should be a priority
10. The need to draw global strategies to protect and recover traditional cooking styles is also notices (gastronomic heritage) as a source of cultural and health wellness

TABLE 22.14
Dietary Guidelines for the Portuguese Population

Nutrient-Based Guidelines

1. Total carbohydrates should contribute a total daily energy value of 50–70%
2. Fiber intake should vary between 27 and 40 g/day
3. Total lipids consumption ≤ 30% of total daily energy
4. Consumption of saturated fatty acids < 10% of total daily energy
5. Cholesterol consumption < 300 mg/day
6. Total saccharose < 20–30 g/day
7. Salt < 6 g/day
8. Reduce alcohol consumption
9. Calcium — total daily intake of 800 mg

Food-Based Guidelines

1. Breast-feeding in the first months of a baby's life, especially during the first 6 months
2. Adequate consumption of cereals and cereal products
3. Increase of the consumption of vegetable products and fresh fruit
4. Reduction of the consumption of fats, especially solid and overheated fats; preference giving to olive-oil consumption
5. Increase of fish consumption
6. Reduction of sugar and sugar-like products consumption
7. Reduction of salt consumption
8. Moderate consumption of alcoholic drinks. Pregnant women, children and those younger than 17 should not drink alcohol
9. Adequate consumption of milk and dairy products
10. Weight control kept through a balanced diet and physical activity
11. A balanced meal first thing in the morning

European guidelines also agree in promoting fruit and vegetable intakes. Although most countries do not specify the appropriate amounts of fruits and vegetables, Spain recommends consumption of at least 250 g of vegetables and 400 g of fruits daily and Germany advocates "5 a day" for five portions of fruits and vegetables on each day. The majority of European countries suggest daily consumption of dairy products and an increase in fish intake, but there is no consensus concerning the optimal amount of intake.

All countries suggest moderation in eggs, meats, and poultry reflecting the fact that these protein-rich foods are abundant in current diets these countries. All European dietary guidelines urge limiting sugar and consumption of sweets, but the recommended numbers of servings from these guidelines vary. Greece suggests half a serving of sweets per day, while Spanish recommends having sweets on no more than "4 occasions" per day. United Kingdom, Finland, and Spain relate sugar intake to dental problems and obesity.

All countries except for Greece recommend limiting fat intake to 30–35% of total food energy. In Mediterranean countries such as Greece, Portugal, and Spain, use of olive oil is encouraged over other types of lipids. Greece, Finland, and Spain also mention the negative effect of trans-fatty acids on health.

All countries but Spain advice reducing salt intake. Greece and Germany suggest using more herbs to substitute salt. Recommended salt intakes range from 3 g in United Kingdom to 6 g in Portugal.

Recommendations on alcohol intake differ among European countries. Portugal, Spain, Greece, and Finland advise moderate consumption of alcohol, while Germany and United Kingdom recommend limiting ethanol intake. Greece proposes 1.5 servings for women and 3 servings for men of wine for more beneficial health effects, whereas Finland suggests that energy from alcohol should not exceed 5% of total energy intake.

Body weight is mentioned in most of the European guidelines. Although some guidelines simply advise for a "healthy" or "desirable" weight, the Portuguese and Spanish guidelines discuss energy balance. Spain and Finland offer specific physical activity guidelines on duration and frequency. Virtually all of the countries with the exception of the United Kingdom have physical activity guidelines, but all countries address weight control.

Interestingly, Finland and Germany encourage the leisurely enjoyment of meals and avoiding stress and haste in eating. Germany mentions that food should be appetizing and processed as little as possible. Germany has an interesting and unique guideline that refers to protecting and recovering traditional cooking styles.

In addition to written documents, graphic presentations of dietary guidelines are available in most European countries. The icons used to represent the guideline are usually a pyramid (Spain and Greece), circle (Finland), a wheel with slices representing the amounts of recommended foods (Portugal) or a food plate (United Kingdom and Germany). Finland also has a pyramid and plate.

CONCLUSIONS

In contrast to many parts of the world, most European countries have developed dietary guidelines. Many of these guidelines were developed using the WHO CINDI dietary guidelines as a template. The dietary guidelines from different European countries are quite similar in their main ideas. Key common recommendations are food-based, and they encourage the public to increase fruits and vegetables intake, to decrease fat and sugar usage, to moderate meat, dairy, and egg consumption, and to increase physical activities. Despite the similarity among European dietary guidelines, there are variations between each of the country to cater the unique cultural and health concerns of each country.

Some European countries offer additional guidelines for children and elderly. The Finns prepared nutrient recommendations for ages between 1 month and above 75 years while Portugal encouraged breast-feeding for at least the first 6 months. Other countries like Greece referred to other publications like the "European Union Project on Promotion of Breast-feeding in Europe" for specific breast-feeding guidelines.

SUMMARY AND CONCLUSIONS

Dietary guidelines in the future must continue to take into account local dietary patterns, cultural traditions, and food availability. They are most effective when they indicate what aspects of diet need to be addressed to promote nutritional health in both the poor and rich. In some countries where disparities in incomes are very large, two sets of guidelines may be necessary.

Dietary guidelines should be flexible so that they can be used by people with different lifestyles, as well as by people of different ages, and with different population groups (pregnant, lactating, infant, children, and elderly persons). Different guidelines may be needed for urban and rural populations or for other special groups such as ethnic minorities in some countries.

Messages delivered to the public in dietary guidelines should provide advice on the selection of a nutritionally balanced diet and encourage other suitable lifestyle behaviors to promote health in such target group. It is difficult to include all without making the guidelines so long that their communicability is compromised. Therefore, other ancillary forms of nutrition education are also needed. Graphics allow people to put dietary guidelines and other recommendations about food consumption into action.

Nutrition education using dietary guidelines is only one ingredient for ensuring that knowledge is sufficient to choose a healthful diet. Motivation and opportunities for people to change their nutrition and health behaviors in favorable directions are also necessary. Knowledge, science, technology, culture, and food sources all change with the times, and so do food ways. Therefore, it is necessary to review guidelines periodically and make appropriate modifications (i.e., every 5 or 10 years).

In conclusion, dietary guidelines can and do serve multiple purposes. These include providing useful information to the public policy maker; serving as communication tools to nutrition and health professionals, as guides to the food industry in product formulation and as instructional objectives for those involved in the provision of food, nutrition, and health education. Food is not the only factor that can influence health. Most health problems in modern society are multifactorial in origin. However, people can help themselves by establishing healthy dietary habits and paying attention to other factors (such as physical activity, not smoking, decreasing stress, and improving their work environments). Such measures increase their chances for a long and active life. It is what individuals and families understand, accept, and do in their living from day-to-day that matters the most in implementing healthy lifestyles. The Dietary Guidelines help them to ensure the nutritional health of the population, and represent a useful advance in the public health.

REFERENCES

1. Dwyer JT. Dietary Guidelines. In: al MSe, ed. *Modern Nutrition in Health and Disease.* Philadelphia: Lippincott, Williams & Wilkins, 2005.
2. Dwyer JT. Dietary Guidelines for Cancer Prevention. In: Heber D, ed. *Nutritional Oncology,* Ch 47. New York: Elsevier, 2006; 757–778.
3. U.S. Census Bureau. *Overview of Race and Hispanic Origin.* Census 2000 Brief. Washington DC: U.S. Census Bureau. Report prepared by EM Grieco and RC Cassidy, 2001;11.
4. Australian Bureau of Statistics. Population Distribution, Indigenous Australians (2001). Australian Bureau of Statistics. At: http://www.abs.gov.au/Ausstats/abs@.nsf/0/14e7a4a075d53a6cca2569450007e46c?OpenDocument, Accessed December 8, 2005.
5. National Health and Medical Research Council. *Dietary Guidelines for Australians.* Canberra, Australia: Australian Government Publishing Service, 1992.
6. Thompson CD. Dietary Guidelines: The New Zealand experience. In: Florencio CA, ed. *Dietary Guidelines in Asia-Pacific.* Philippines, Quezon City: ASEAN-New Zealand IILP Project 5, 1997;69.
7. U.S. Department of Agriculture, U.S. Department of Health, Dietary Guidelines Advisory Committee. *Report of the Dietary Guidelines Advisory Committee on the Dietary Guidelines for Americans, 1980.* Springfield, IL: National Technical Information Service, 1980.
8. U.S. Department of Agriculture, U.S. Department of Health, Dietary Guidelines Advisory Committee. *Report of the Dietary Guidelines Advisory Committee on the Dietary Guidelines for Americans, 1990.* Springfield: National Technical Information Service, 1990.
9. U.S. Department of Agriculture, U.S. Department of Human Health. *Nutrition and your health: Dietary Guidelines for Americans.* 1995. US Government Printing Office, Wash DC
10. U.S. Department of Agriculture, Dietary Guidelines Advisory Committee. *Dietary Guidelines for Americans, 1980 to 2000.* Department of Agriculture, U.S. Department of Health. At: http://www.usda.gov/cnpp/Pubs/DG2000/Dgover.PDF, Accessed November 26, 2001.
11. U.S. Department of Health and Human Services, U.S. Department of Agriculture. Dietary *Guidelines for Americans, 2005.* 6th Edition, Washington, DC: U.S. Government Printing Office, 2005.
12. U.S. Department of Agriculture. *MyPyramid: Steps to a Healthier You* (2005). At: http://www.mypyramid.gov/, Accessed on February 15, 2006.
13. Centers for Disease Control and Prevention. Cancer prevention and control. At: http://www.cdc.gov/cancer/nper/register.htm. Washington, DC: CDC. Accessed March 22, 2000.
14. Centers for Disease Control and Prevention. *Chronic Disease Conditions.* At: http://www.cdc.gov/nccdphp/major.htm. Washington, DC: CDC. Accessed March 22, 2000.
15. Mokdad AH, Serdula MK, Dietz WH, Bowman BA, Marks JS, Koplan JP. The spread of the obesity epidemic in the United States, 1991–1998. *JAMA* 1999;282:1519–1522.
16. Health Canada on-line. Nature and dimensions of nutrition-related problems. At: http://www.hc-sc.gc.ca. Accessed March 15, 2000. Minister of Public Works and Government Services Canada., 1999.
17. U.S. Department of Health and Human Services, U.S. Department of Agriculture. *Finding Your Way to a Healthier You: Based on the Dietary Guidelines for Americans.* Consumer's brochure. At: www.healthierus.gov/dietaryguidelines. Accessed February 15, 2006. Washington, DC: U.S. Government Printing Office, 2005.
18. Department of National Health and Welfare. *Canada's Guidelines for Healthy Eating.* Ottawa, Canada: Department of Health and Welfare. 1990.
19. Nutrition Taskforce. *Food for Health (pamphlet).* Wellington, England: Department of Health, 1991.
20. Bengoa J, Torun B, Behar M, Scrimshaw N. Nutritional goals and food guides in Latin America. Basis for their development. *Arch Latinoam Nutr* 1988;38:373–426.
21. Chilean Ministry of Health, Institute of Nutrition and Food Technology, Nutrition Center at the University of Chile. Dietary Guidelines for the Chilean population. Santiago, Chile: Ministry of Health, 1997.
22. Tagle MA. Cambios en los patrones de consumo alimentario en America Latina. *Arch Latinoam Nutr* 1988;38:750–765.
23. Valiente S, Abala C, Avila B, Monckeberg F. Patologia nutricional en America Latina y el Caribe. *Arch Latinoam Nutr* 1988;38:445–465.
24. Peña M, Molina V. Food based dietary guidelines and health promotion in Latin America. Washington, DC: Pan American Health Organization and Institute of Nutrition of Central America and Panama, 1999.
25. Chavez MM, Chavez A, Rios E, Madrigal H. Guias de alimentacion: Consejos practicos para alcanzar y mantener un buen estado de nutricion y salud. Mexico, D.F.: Salvador Zubiran National Institute of Nutrition, 1993.
26. Instituto Nacional de Nutrición, Fundación Cavendes. Guías de Alimentación para Venezuela. Caracas, Venezuela: Fundación Cavendes, 1991;88.

27. Ministerio de la Familia, Fundación Cavendes. Guías de Alimentación para Venezuela del Niño menor de seis Años. Manual para hogares y multihogares de cuidado diario. Caracas, Venezuela: Fundación Cavendes, 1996;131.

28. Ministerio de la Familia, Fundación Cavendes. Guías de Alimentación en el Niño menor de 6 Años. Orientacion Normativa. Caracas, Venezuela: Fundación Cavendes, 1997;44.

29. Chavez VA, Ledesma SA. Recomendaciones de nutrimentos para México. Recomendaciones de energía y proteínas por día (Nutrient recommendations for Mexico. Daily energy and protein recommendations). At: www.nutripac.com.mx/software/rec-mex.pdf., Accessed February 20, 2001.

30. Comisión Nacional de Guías Alimentarias de Guatemala. *Guías alimentarias para Guatemala: Los siete pasos para una alimentación sana.* Guatemala: Comisión Nacional de Guías Alimentarias, 1998;44.

31. Ministerio de Salud de Panama. *Guias alimentarias para Panama.* Ciudad de Panama, Panama: Ministerio de Salud, 1995;1–40.

32. Florentino RF. Micronutrients of concerns in the formulation of dietary guidelines. In: Florentino RF, ed. *Proceedings of the workshop on Meeting national needs of Asian Countries in the 21st Century.* Singapore, Singapore, International Life Sciences Institution Press, 1996; p. 32.

33. Chinese Nutrition Society. Dietary Guidelines and the food guide pagoda for Chinese residents: balanced diet, rational nutrition, and health promotion. *Nutr Today* 1999;34:106–115.

34. Devadas RP. Dietary Guidelines for India. In: Florencio CA, ed. *Dietary Guidelines in Asia-Pacific.* Quezon City, Philippines: ASEAN-New Zealand IILP Project 5, 1997; 28 pages.

35. Florencio CA. Nutritional Guidelines for the Philippines. In: Florencio CA, ed. *Dietary Guidelines in Asia-Pacific.* Quezon City, Philippines: ASEAN-New Zealand IILP Project 5, 1997;1–77.

36. Ge K. Diet and dietary guidelines in China. In: Florencio CA, ed. *Dietary guidelines in Asia-Pacific.* Quezon City, Philippines: ASEAN-New Zealand IILP Project 5, 1997;17.

37. Kim SH, Jang YA, Lee HS. Nutritional (Dietary) guidelines of Korea. In: Florencio CA, ed. *Dietary Guidelines in Asia-Pacific.* Quezon City, Philippines: ASEAN-New Zealand IILP Project 5, 1997;1–52.

38. Kusharto CM, Hardinsyah, Rimbawan. Nutritional guidelines for Indonesia. In: Florencio CA, ed. *Dietary Guidelines in Asia-Pacific.* Quezon City, Philippines: ASEAN-New Zealand IILP Project 5, 1997; 52 pages.

39. Lian LS. Dietary Guidelines in Asian countries: Towards a food based approach. In: Florentino RF, ed. *Proceedings of the Workshop on Meeting National Needs of Asian Countries in the 21st Century.* Singapore, Singapore, International Life Sciences Institution Press, 1996.

40. Ministry of Health. Recommended Dietary Allowances for Koreans. Korean Ministry of Health, 1995.

41. Sakamoto M. Dietary guidelines of Japan. In: Florencio CA, ed. *Dietary guidelines in Asia-Pacific.* Quezon City, Philippines: ASEAN-New Zealand IILP Project 5, 1997;1–43.

42. Siong TE, Yusof AM. Development of Dietary Guidelines for Malaysians. In: Florencio CA, ed. *Dietary Guidelines in Asia-Pacific.* Quezon City, Philippines: ASEAN-New Zealand IILP Project 5, 1997;1–59.

43. Tanphaichitr V, Leelahagul P. Dietary Guidelines for Thais: Implications for reducing nutritional risk. In: Florencio CA, ed. *Dietray Guidelines in Asia-Pacific.* Philippines, Quezon City: ASEAN-New Zealand IILP Project 5, 1997; page 97.

44. Asian Food Information Center. The Dietary Guidelines. Online access to Dietary Guidelines in Asia. At: http://www.afic.org/index-old.htm, Accessed February 13, 2006.

45. Karyadi D, Karyadi E. Addressing Asian nutritional issues through dietary guidelines: co-existence of over and undernutrition. In: Florentino RF, ed. *Proceedings of the workshop on Meeting national needs of Asian countries in the 21st century.* Singapore, Singapore, International Life Sciences Institution Press, 1996;1–28.

46. Department of Health Taiwan ROC. Changes in ten leading causes of death, Taiwan area (1999). At: http://www.doh.gov.tw, Accessed March 23, 2000.

47. Tontisirin K, Kosulwat V. National Dietary Guidelines: Current status and application in Asian countries. In: Florentino RF, ed. *Proceedings of the workshop on Meeting national needs of Asian Countries in the 21st Century.* Singapore, Singapore, International Life Sciences Institution Press, 1996; page 15.

48. WHO. Malnutrition — The Global Picture. At: http://www.who.int/nut/malnutrition_worldwide.htm, Accessed March 15, 2000.

49. WHO. Obesity epidemic puts millions at risk from related diseases, press release WHO/46. 1996. At: http://www.who.int/dsg/justpub/obesity.htm., Accessed March 15, 2000.

50. Japan Dietetic Association. Recommended dietary allowances for Japanese Fifth revision (1994). Newsletter the Japan Dietetic Association. Tokyo, 1995;2.

51. Orbeta SS. The Filipino pyramid food guide-the perfect food match for the Philippines. *Nutrition Today* 1998;33:210.

52. National Dietary Guidelines. Dietary guidelines in Asian countries: Towards a food-based approach. In: Florentino RF, ed. *Proceedings of the workshop on Meeting national needs of Asian countries in the 21st century.* Singapore, Singapore: International Life Sciences Institution Press, 1996.

53. Sakamoto M. Nutrient needs through the life cycle. In: Florentino RF, ed. *Proceedings of the workshop on Meeting national needs of Asian countries in the 21st century.* Singapore, Singapore: International Life Sciences Institution Press, 1996;1–43.

54. Department of Health Taiwan ROC. Daily Food Guide. 1999. At: http://health99.doh.gov.tw/Query/ShowPic.pl?p048.htm, Accessed March 23, 2000.

55. Department of Health Taiwan ROC. Daily Dietary Guidelines for all population. 1999. At: http://health99.doh.gov.tw/Query/ShowPic.pl?t106.htm., Accessed March 23, 2000.

56. Vorster HH, Love P, Browne C. Development of food-based dietary guidelines for South Africa — The process. *South African J Clin Nutr* 2001;14:S3–S6 (Suppl).

57. FAO. Dietary Guidelines for Nigeria. Food guidelines by country. FAO Nutrition Information, Communication and Education. At: http://www.fao.org/ag/agn/nutrition/education_guidelines_nga_en.stm, Accessed February 13, 2006.

58. FAO. Dietary Guidelines for Namibia. Food guidelines by country. FAO Nutrition Information, Communication and Education. At: http://www.fao.org/ag/agn/nutrition/education_guidelines_nam_en.stm, Accessed February 13, 2006.

59. International Life Sciences Institute. National food-based dietary guidelines: Experiences, implications and future directions. Summary report of a workshop on "National Food-Based Dietary Guidelines" ILSI Europe. Budapest, Hungary, 2004.

60. World Health Organization, Food and Agriculture Organization. Preparation and use of food-based dietary guidelines. In: WHO/NUT/96.6, ed. Report of a joint FAO/WHO consultation Nicosia, Cyprus. Geneva, Switzerland: Nutrition Programme — WHO, 1996.

61. FAO/WHO. Human Vitamin and Mineral Requirements, 2001. Report of a Joint FAO/WHO expert consultation on human vitamin and mineral requirements, September 1998. At: www.fao.org/es/esn/vitrni/pdf/TOTAL.PDF. Bangkok, Thailand. FAO/WHO, Food and Nutrition Division, Accessed February 24, 2002;Technical Report Series No. 724.

23 Nutrition Monitoring in the United States

Jean Pennington

CONTENTS

INTRODUCTION

Most descriptions of nutrition monitoring use the comprehensive definition developed by Mason et al. in 1984, "an ongoing description of nutrition conditions in the population, with particular attention to subgroups defined in socioeconomic terms, for purposes of planning and analyzing the effects of policies and programs on nutrition problems, and predicting future trends."[1] In the United States, nutrition monitoring refers to the many federal and state surveys and surveillance activities that provide information about food composition, food consumption, nutrition status, or health status. These surveys and activities were first identified as the U.S. National Nutrition Monitoring System in 1978, and were renamed as the National Nutrition Monitoring and Related Research Program (NNMRRP) with the passage of the National Nutrition Monitoring and Related Research Act of 1990.[2] Although the act expired in 2002 and has not been reauthorized, many of the surveys and activities of the NNMRRP are still ongoing, and federal and state agencies continue to work together to produce and disseminate information about food composition and consumption and about nutrition and health status.

The five measurement areas of the NNMRRP were identified as nutrition and related health measurements; food and nutrient consumption; consumer knowledge, attitudes, and behavior assessments; food composition and nutrient databases; and food-supply determinations.[2] Previous reports, publications, and book chapters have covered the topic of nutrition monitoring and described the NNMRRP surveys and activities.[3–9] This chapter provides a brief history of the development of the U.S. nutrition monitoring program from 1977 to 2005, a summary of ongoing nutrition monitoring surveys and surveillance activities, an overview of the uses of nutrition monitoring data, and a discussion of future challenges.

HISTORY OF NUTRITION MONITORING

BEGINNINGS

A 1977 act of Congress required that the U.S. Department of Agriculture (USDA) and the U.S. Department of Health, Education, and Welfare (now the Department of Health and Human Services [DHHS]) develop plans to coordinate the DHHS National Health and Nutrition Examination Survey (NHANES) and USDA Nationwide Food Consumption Survey (NFCS).[10] This act mandated the development of a reporting system to translate the findings from these two national surveys and other monitoring activities into periodic reports to Congress on the nutritional status of the American population. A proposal for a comprehensive nutrition monitoring system was submitted to Congress in 1978, and the NHANES and NFCS became the cornerstones for the beginning of the National Nutrition Monitoring System.

In 1983, the Joint DHHS/USDA Nutrition Monitoring Evaluation Committee was formed, and in 1986 this Committee provided an overview of the dietary and nutritional status of the population and recommendations for improvements in the *First Progress Report on Nutrition Monitoring in the United States.*[11] Several papers on nutrition monitoring were published in 1984.[12–14] In 1987, the Operational Plan for the National Nutrition Monitoring System was developed, and in 1988, the Interagency Committee on Nutrition Monitoring was established to improve the planning, coordination, and communication of nutrition monitoring activities among agencies.[15] In 1989, An updated *Report on Nutrition Monitoring* (the *Second Progress Report on Nutrition Monitoring in the United States*) was prepared by an expert panel, and the *Directory of Federal Nutrition Monitoring Activities* was published.[16,17]

THE 1990 ACT AND BEYOND

The National Nutrition Monitoring and Related Research Act of 1990 established the National Nutrition Monitoring and Related Research Program (NNMRRP) and helped establish the collaboration and coordination of federal, state, and local government agencies involved in nutrition monitoring.[2] Under this act, the secretaries of DHHS and USDA had joint responsibility for implementing the Program and transmitting the required reports to Congress.

In 1991, the previous Interagency Committee on Nutrition Monitoring became the Interagency Board for Nutrition Monitoring and Related Research (IBNMRR) and included 22 agencies that contributed or used national nutrition monitoring data. The IBNMRR served through 2002 as the central focus for federal nutrition monitoring activities. The Board coordinated the preparation of an annual budget report on nutrition monitoring, biennial reports on progress and policy implications of scientific findings to the President and Congress, and the periodic scientific reports that described the nutritional and related health status of the population to Congress.

The 1990 act also established the National Nutrition Monitoring Advisory Council to provide scientific and technical guidance to the IBNMRR. The council was formed in 1992 and included nine members (five appointed by the president and four by Congress) with expertise in the areas of public health, nutrition, monitoring research, and food production and distribution. Also in 1992, the *Directory of Federal Nutrition Monitoring Activities* was updated and expanded to include state surveillance efforts.[18]

The 1990 act called for the development of a Ten-Year Comprehensive Plan to guide federal actions for nutrition monitoring. The proposed DHHS/USDA Ten-Year Comprehensive Plan was published in 1991 and finalized in 1993.[3,19] The primary goal of this plan was "to establish a comprehensive nutrition monitoring and related research program by collecting quality data that are continuous, coordinated, timely, and reliable; using comparable methods for data collection and reporting of results; conducting relevant research; and efficiently and effectively disseminating and exchanging information with data users."[3]

Three federal working groups were established by the Board to improve communication and coordination among member agencies. The Survey Comparability group was led by DHHS National Center for Health Statistics (NCHS), and USDA's Agriculture Research Service (ARS) assisted the IBNMRR in working toward close communication and coordination on federal surveys and surveillance activities, including continued efforts to address the development of a common automated dietary assessment system. The group also assisted in the determination of resource needs and options for developing the dietary system in a timely manner for the next round of surveys. The Federal-State Relations and Information Dissemination and Exchange Group was led by ARS and the Centers for Disease Control and Prevention (CDC) and assisted the IBNMRR in the identification of measures, methodologies, and interpretive criteria for nutrition indicators that would improve the capacity of states and localities to conduct nutrition monitoring. The Food Composition Group, led by ARS, continued to assess progress in meeting the nutrition monitoring program needs for food composition data and assisted in identification of future needs. After the enactment of the welfare reform law in 1996, the Welfare Reform, Nutrition, and Data Needs Working Group, with both federal and nonfederal members, was established to determine if federal surveys and surveillance activities could capture the effects of welfare reform on nutrition, hunger, and health status and to foster collaborative research on nutrition and welfare reform.

In 1993, the IBNMRR published *Chartbook I: Selected Findings from the National Nutrition Monitoring and Related Research Program.*[20] In 1995, the IBNMRR published *Third Report on Nutrition Monitoring in the United States*, which identified food components (energy, total fat, saturated fatty acids, cholesterol, alcohol, iron, calcium, and sodium) that were of public health concern in the U.S. population.[4] The report also included a range of health issues of concern for low-income, high-risk populations including anemia, low birth weight, overweight, high serum total cholesterol, hypertension, osteoporosis, low intakes of a number of nutrients (including folate, calcium, and iron), and food insufficiency.

The major nutrition monitoring issue during 1997 to 2002 was the integration of NHANES and the Continuing Survey of the Food Intakes of Individuals (CSFII).[21] NCHS (responsible for NHANES) and the ARS (responsible for CSFII) signed a memorandum of understanding in 1998 to integrate these two national food consumption surveys. An Expert Panel on Survey Integration was convened in 1998 to review the scope of the proposed merger and provide recommendations to the two agencies to strengthen the overall integration plan and the dietary research and evaluation component. The survey integration was completed in 2002 when the ARS What We Eat in America survey became the dietary data collection component of the NHANES.[21,22] In 2002, a workshop was held with nutrition monitoring stakeholders to develop recommendations on how best to meet data needs for policy and research with the integrated survey.[23]

CURRENT STATUS

In December 1999, the National Academy of Sciences (NAS) organized a public symposium entitled "Nutrition Monitoring in the US: Preparing for the Next Millennium to draw attention to the federal, research, industry, media, and consumer uses of monitoring data, to discuss future challenges for the NNMRRP, and to encourage reauthorization of the 1990 act. This symposium convened nutrition scientists from industry, academia, government, and the public sector along with policymakers to discuss efforts to streamline and integrate the monitoring program and to identify and highlight future diet, nutrition, and health data needs. The participants discussed ways to optimize the utility and relevance of the nutrition monitoring program for organizations whose activities depend on the availability and reliability of the data obtained from the program.

DHHS and USDA sponsored the National Nutrition Summit during May 30–31 2000, in Washington, D.C., to provide an opportunity to highlight accomplishments in food, nutrition, and health; identify continuing challenges and emerging opportunities; and focus on nutrition and lifestyle issues, especially those related to overweight and obesity.[24] Also in 2000, the *Directory of Federal Nutrition Monitoring Activities* was updated.[25] The American Society for Nutritional Sciences convened a Working Group on Nutrition Monitoring, and a report from this group was published in 2002.[26]

In 2004, an Institute of Medicine (IOM) panel made recommendations to improve the data infrastructure on food consumption to support food and nutrition programs and policies within the USDA.[27,28] In 2005, the IOM published a review of the infrastructure to support food and nutrition programs, research, and decision making and provided recommendations to improve the data for such purposes.[28]

NUTRITION MONITORING SURVEYS AND SURVEILLANCE ACTIVITIES

As noted earlier, the nutrition monitoring legislation was not renewed in 2002. Many of the nutrition monitoring surveys and surveillance activities are continuing, but without the coordinated guidance of an interagency board or legislative mandate. Descriptions of the surveys and surveillance activities within the five measurement components of the NNMRRP have been described elsewhere.[3,4,17–20,25,29] Bialostosky et al.[7] summarized the major activities through 1999, and Briefel[9] provided a similar summary focusing on surveys and activities from the mid-1990s through 2005. Some of the ongoing surveys and surveillance activities are described in the following sections, and Table 23.1 provides a list of those that have Web sites for easy reference.

NUTRITION AND RELATED HEALTH MEASUREMENTS

1. *NHANES.* The NCHS NHANES provides national data on nutrition and related health measurements as well as data on food and nutrient consumption.[30] It also provides national population reference distributions, prevalence rates of disease and risk factors, and trends in nutritional and health status over time. NHANES includes a household interview followed by a physical examination and personal interviews in a mobile examination center. It includes body measurements, blood pressure, dental examinations, and biochemical and hematological tests. NHANES became a yearly survey in 1999 and has a nationally representative sample design of Black, White, and Mexican-American persons for all income and low-income households. There is oversampling of Mexican-Americans, Blacks, older persons, adolescents, pregnant women, and low-income Whites to allow for comparisons of differences in health conditions and prevalence of risk factors for these groups.

2. *NHANES I Epidemiologic Follow-up Study (NHEFS).* The NCHS NHANES I NHEFS allows for epidemiologic investigations of the relationships of nutrition and health to risk of death and disability.[31] The NHEFS is a longitudinal

TABLE 23.1
Nutrition Monitoring Surveys and Surveillance Activities Listed by Measurement Component

Agency	Survey/Surveillance Activity	Web Sites	Reference(s)
MEASURE: Nutrition/Health Status			
NCHS	National Health and Nutrition Examination Survey (NHANES)	http://cdc/gov/nchs/nhanes/htm	30
NCHS	NHANES III Mortality Follow-up Survey (NHEFS)	http://www.cdc.gov/nchs/r&d?nchs_datalinkage/nhefs_nhefs_data>kubjage_activities.htm	31
NCSH	National Health Interview Survey (NHIS)	http://www.cdc.gov/nchs.nhis/htm	32
NCHS	State and Local Area Integrated Telephone Survey (SLAITS)	http://www.cdc.gov/nchs/slaits.htm	33
CDC	Pediatric Nutrition Surveillance System (PedNSS)	http://www.cdc.gov/pednss/	34, 35
CDC	Pregnancy Nutrition Surveillance System (PNSS)	http://www.cdc.gov/pednss/	34
NCHS	National Health Care Survey (NHCS)	http://www.cdc.gov/nchs.nchs.htm	36
NCHS	National Survey of Family Growth (NSFG)	http://www.cdc.gov/nchs.nsfg.htm	37
NCHS	National Vital Statistics System (NVSS)	http://www.cdc.gov/cnhs/nvss.htm	38
MEASURE: Food/Nutrient Intake			
NCHS	National Health and Nutrition Examination Survey (NHANES)	http://cdc/gov/nchs/nhanes/htm	30
FDA	Total Diet Study	http://www.cfsan.fda.gov/~comm/tds-toc.html	53
FNS	Study of WIC Program	http://www.fns.usda.gov/win/resources/wicstudies.htm; http://www.fns.usda.gov/wic/aboutwic/default.htm	55, 56
CDC	School Health Policies and Programs Study (SHIPPS)	http://www.cdc.gov/healthyyouth/obesity/index.htm	60
CB	Current Population Survey (CPS)	http://www.bls.census.gov/cps/overmain.htm	61
ERS	Food Security Efforts	http://www.ers.usda.gov/Briefing/FoodSecurity/; http://www.fns.usda.gov/fsec/measurement.htm; www.ers.usda.gov/publications/err11	65, 66, 67
CDC/FDA/FSIS	FoodNet-Foodborne Disease Active Surveillance Network	http://www.cdc.gov/foodnet/surveillance.htm	68
MEASURE: Knowledge/Attitudes/Behavior			
CDC	Behavioral Risk Factor Surveillance System (BRFSS)	http://www.cdc.gov/nccdphp/aag_brfss.htm	69, 70
CDC	Youth Risk Behavior Surveillance System (YRBSS)	http://www.cdc.gov/nccdphp/bb_brfss_yrbss/index.htm	72, 75
CDC	Youth Risk Behavior Survey (YRBS)	http://www.cdc.gov/healthyyouth/obesity/facts.htm	
CDC	Pregnancy Risk Assessment Monitoring System (PRAMS)	http://www.cdc.gov/reporductivehealth/PRAMS/index.html	76
FDA	Consumer Surveys	http://vm.cfsan.fda.gov/~lrd/ab-nutri.html; http://www.cfsan.fda.gov/~lrd/ab-foodb.html	77, 80
ARS	Diet and Health Knowledge Survey (DHKS)	http://www.ars.usda.gov/Services/docs.htm?docid=7776	82
MEASURE: Food Composition			
ARS	National Nutrient Database for Standard Reference (NNDSR)	http://www.nal.usda.gov/fnic.foodcomp/	84
ARS	Food and Nutrient Database for Dietary Studies (FNDDS)	http://www.ars.usda.gov/Services/docs/htm?docid-7673; http://www.ars.usda.gov/foodsearch	90, 92
ODS, NIH	Dietary Supplement Database Activities	http://dietarysupplements.infonih.gov/Health_Information/Dietary_Supplement_Ingredient_and_Labeling_Databases.aaspx	97

TABLE 23.1
Continued

Agency	Survey/surveillance Activity	Web sites	Reference(s)
MEASURE: Food Composition (*Continued*)			
FDA	Food Label and Package Survey (FLAPS)	http://www.cfsan.fda.gov/~dms/lab-flap.html	104
ARS/NIH/ Other	National Food and Nutrient Analysis Program (NFNAP)	http://www.ars.usda.gov/Research/docs.htm?docid=9446	105
MEASURE: Food Supply Determinations			
ERS/CNPP	U.S. Food and Nutrition Supply Series	http://www.ers.usda.gov/Data/FoodConsumption/; http://209.48.219.54/FoodAvailability.htm http://209.48.219.54/	112, 113, 114
NMFS	Fisheries of the U.S. Survey	http://www.st.nmfs.noaa.govst1/mission.htm; http://www.st.nmfs.gov/st1/publications.htm; http://www.st.nmfs.noaa.gov/st1/fus/fus03/index.html	116
	AC Nielsen SCANTRACK Services	http://www.acnielsen.com/products/reports/scantrack/	117

Acronyms used in this table:

ARS: Agricultural Research Service, USDA; CB: Census Bureau, DOC; CDC: Centers for Disease Control and Prevention, DHHS; CNPP: Center for Nutrition Policy and Promotion, USDA; DOC: Department of Commerce; FDA: Food and Drug Administration, DHHS; ERS: Economic Research Service, USDA; FNS: Food and Nutrition Service, USDA; FSIS: Food Safety and Inspection Service, USDA; DHHS: Department of Health and Human Services; NCHS: National Center for Health Statistics, CDC, DHHS; NIH: National Institutes of Health, DHHS; NMFS: National Marine Fisheries Service, NOAA, DOC; NOAA: National Oceanic and Atmospheric Administration; ODS: Office of Dietary Supplements, NIH, DHHS; USDA: U.S. Department of Agriculture.

follow-up study, which includes 14,407 participants, 25 to 74 years of age, who completed a medical examination during the NHANES I survey period (1971 to 1975). NCHS conducted a mortality linkage of NHEFS with the NCHS National Death Index to investigate the association of a variety of health factors with mortality. The current version of the NHEFS linked mortality file includes information for all deaths including those previously identified during the NHEFS periods of 1982–1984, 1986, 1987, and 1992.

3. *National Health Interview Survey (NHIS).* The NCHS NHIS provides annual information about self-reported health conditions and periodic information about special nutrition and health topics such as dietary supplement use, youth risk behavior, food program participation, diet and nutrition knowledge, cancer and disability, and food preparation.[32] In 2004, NHIS collected data on self-reported height and weight, diagnosed diabetes, and alcohol consumption. The large sample numbers of NHIS allow the data to be reported by race/ethnicity, age, sex, and income.

4. *State and Local Area Integrated Telephone Survey (SLAITS).* The NCHS SLAITS was developed as a telephone survey to supplement national data on identified topics with state and regional data.[33] Previous topics were a child well-being and welfare survey module and a national study on early childhood health.

5. *Pediatric Nutrition Surveillance System (PedNSS).* The CDC PedNSS has been used since 1973 to monitor indicators of nutritional status among low-income, high-risk infants and children who participate in health, nutrition, and food assistance programs.[34,35] Information on anemia, weight, birth weight, breast-feeding, and television/video watching are collected primarily from children in the Special Supplemental Nutrition Program for Women, Infants, and Children's (WIC). The data can be evaluated at individual, clinic, county, state, and national levels.

6. *Pregnancy Nutrition Surveillance System (PNSS).* Since 1978, the CDC PNSS has monitored nutrition-related problems and behavioral risk factors associated with low birth weight among high-risk prenatal women.[34] The PNSS sample is drawn primarily from the WIC Program. PNSS data are used to identify preventable nutrition-related problems and behavioral risk factors to target interventions.

7. *National Health Care Survey (NHCS).* The NCHS NHCS collects nutrition-related information on physician-reported hypertension and obesity and on counseling services for diet, weight reduction, and cholesterol reduction for hospital outpatient department visits.[36]

8. *National Survey of Family Growth (NSFG).* The NCHS NSFG collects information on maternal and child health such as breast-feeding and prenatal care.[37] The information is obtained with personal in-home interviews with a probability sample of subjects 15 to 44 years of age.

9. *National Vital Statistics System (NVSS).* The NVSS is the mechanism by which NCHS collects and disseminates national vital statistics.[38] The data are provided to NCHS through contracts in jurisdictions responsible for the registration of births, deaths, marriages, divorces, and fetal deaths. In the United States, legal authority for the registration of these events resides within the 50 states, 2 cities (Washington, D.C., and New York City), and 5 territories (Puerto Rico, the Virgin Islands, Guam, American Samoa, and the Commonwealth of the Northern Mariana Islands). These jurisdictions are responsible for maintaining registries of vital events and for issuing copies of birth, marriage, divorce, and death certificates. Standard forms for the collection of the data and model procedures for the uniform registration of the events have been developed for nationwide use.

FOOD AND NUTRIENT CONSUMPTION

1. *NHANES.* The dietary component of NHANES, What We Eat in America, is an automated multiple-pass 24 h dietary recall that was developed by ARS.[22,39–42] The first day's interview is conducted in person and the second day's is conducted by telephone. In 2002, NHANES included a food propensity questionnaire along the 2 days of dietary.[40,41,43] The food propensity questionnaire was developed by the National Cancer Institute to assess infrequently consumed foods and thus augment the two dietary recalls.[41,44] A recent report from the ARS Food Surveys Research Group compares dietary data from 2001 to 2002 with Dietary Reference Intakes.[45]
Progress continues to be made in research regarding dietary intake assessment. Doubly labeled water studies have been used to validate energy intakes assessed with 24 h recalls and other dietary methods, such as food frequency instruments.[46] The 24 h recall method, which is used in NHANES, has a systematic bias and underestimates total energy intake.[46–48] The doubly labeled water technique provides a noninvasive method of assessing energy expenditures that allows for interpreting energy intakes derived from dietary survey methods.
The National Cancer Institute's Observing Protein and Energy Nutrition Study (OPEN) assessed measurement error using two self-reported dietary methods — one 24 h recall and a food frequency questionnaire (FFQ) and two unbiased methods (doubly-labeled water and urinary nitrogen) — and found that men and women underreported energy and protein on both instruments.[49] About 9% of men and 7% of women underreported energy intake based on the 24 h recall compared with 35% and 23%, respectively, based on the FFQ. Protein intake was underreported by 11% to 12% by the 24 h recall and 30 to 34% by the FFQ. Underreporting of energy and protein was even higher when compared with total energy expenditure.
Research and information about techniques for dietary assessment are shared at the International Dietary Assessment Conference (IDAC), which is held every 2 years. The first IDAC was held in 1995 in Boston, Massachusetts; the fifth IDAC was held in Chiang Rai, Thailand, in 2004; and the sixth IDAC was held in Copenhagen, Denmark, in 2006.[50]
2. *Total Diet Study.* The Food and Drug Administration (FDA) Total Diet Study provides annual analytical data on the levels of dietary minerals, folic acid, heavy metals, radionuclides, pesticide residues, industrial chemicals, and other chemical contaminants in the core foods of the U.S. food supply and assesses dietary intakes of these food components for eight age/sex group diets on an annual basis.[51–53] The core foods of the U.S. food supply are identified based on data from NHANES. The foods are purchased from retail markets, prepared for consumption, and analyzed individually for nutrients and other food components at the FDA Total Diet Laboratory in Missouri. Yearly results are available from the Total Diet Study Web site.[53]
3. *Infant Feeding Studies.* The FDA Infant Feeding Study II assessed the diets of pregnant women and new mothers and their infant-feeding practices.[54] FDA plans to conduct a second Infant Feeding Practices Survey to assess the diets of pregnant and new mothers and to track breast-feeding and other infant-feeding practices.[54]
4. *WIC.* The USDA Food and Nutrition Service (FNS) WIC Program provides supplemental foods, information on healthy eating, and referrals to health care to low-income women, infants, and children up to age five who are at nutritional risk. A number of studies have been conducted to evaluate the nutrition and health effects of participation in WIC and to provide current participant and program characteristics of the WIC program.[55–57]
5. *School Nutrition Dietary Assessment Study (SNDAS).* The USDA FNS SNDAS assessed the diets of American school children and the contribution of the National School Lunch Program to overall nutrient intake in 1992.[58] A second study was conducted from 1998 to 1999 to compare changes in the food and nutrient content of USDA school meals and food service operations.[59] The study reported that schools had made substantial improvements in the nutritional quality of the meals they were providing, especially with regard to total fat and saturated fat content, and were meeting one-third of the daily nutrient recommendations. A third study was conducted in 2005 and measured school children's heights and weights, usual nutrient intake and food intake, and collected information on school food service operations, the quality of meals offered, and food and beverages available in vending machines, school stores, and *a la carte* lines.

6. *School Health Policies and Programs Study (SHIPPS).* The CDC SHIPPS is a national survey conducted periodically to assess school health policies and programs at the state, district, school, and classroom levels, including those related to nutrition and physical activity.[60] Fact sheets available from the Web site provide information on foods sold outside the school meal programs, food service, health services, nutrition services, and physical educations and activities.[60]

7. *Current Population Survey (CPS).* CPS is a monthly survey of about 50,000 households conducted by the Bureau of the Census for the Bureau of Labor Statistics.[61] The CPS is the primary source of information on the labor force characteristics of the U.S. population; respondents are interviewed to obtain information about the employment status of each member of the household 15 years of age and older. Estimates obtained from the CPS include employment, unemployment, earnings, hours of work, and other indicators. Supplemental questions on a variety of topics including school enrollment, income, previous work experience, health, employee benefits, and work schedules are also often added to the regular CPS questionnaire. Since 1995, the yearly CPS supplement has been devoted to measuring the extent of food insecurity and hunger among people living in low-income households.[62–64]

8. *Food Security Efforts.* The USDA Economic Research Service (ERS) plays a leading role in federal research on food security and hunger in U.S. households and communities.[65–67] The ERS annual publication, *Household Food Security in the United States*, provides data on food security, the amount U.S. households spend on food, and the extent to which food-insecure households participated in federal and community food assistance programs.[67]

9. *FoodNet.* FoodNet-Foodborne Disease Active Surveillance Network is a cooperative surveillance effort of the CDC Emerging Infections Program, FDA, and the USDA Food Safety and Inspection Service to monitor food-borne illness and to conduct epidemiologic research on illnesses attributable to food-borne pathogens.[68] The core of FoodNet is laboratory-based active surveillance at over 650 clinical laboratories that test stools samples in the ten FoodNet sites. Population surveys are conducted to assess diarrhea disease and exposure to food-borne illness.

KNOWLEDGE, ATTITUDES, AND BEHAVIOR ASSESSMENTS

National surveys that measure knowledge, attitudes, and behavior about diet and nutrition and how these relate to health were added to the nutrition monitoring program in 1982. The focus of these surveys is on consumer awareness of relationships between diet and risk for chronic disease and on health-related knowledge and attitudes.

1. *Behavioral Risk Factor Surveillance System (BRFSS).* The CDC BRFSS is a telephone survey of adults that focuses on personal health practices such as food intake, physical activity, weight-control practices, and health-screening practices.[69,70] BRFSS has been used by state health departments to plan, initiate, and guide health promotion and disease prevention programs, and to monitor their progress over time.[69,70] BRFSS collects self-reported height and weight for estimates of overweight and includes modules on dietary habits that states can collect periodically. Topics have included the consumption of fruits and vegetables and high-fat and high-cholesterol foods, binge drinking, physical activity, and the use of supplements, particularly folic acid. Since 2002, BRFSS data have been used for prevalence estimates for metropolitan and smaller statistical areas, allowing CDC to make estimates for counties to assist local public health planners and program evaluators.[71]

2. *Youth Risk Behavior Surveillance System (YRBSS).* The CDC YRBSS includes national school-based surveys of high school students as well as state, territorial, and local school-based surveys conducted by health and education agencies.[72–74] Information is collected on students' health risk behaviors such as smoking, dietary intake, weight-loss practices, and physical activity.[72,73] Every 2 years, CDC conducts a national YRBSS to produce data representative of students in grades 9 to 12 in the 50 states and the District of Columbia. The CDC Youth Risk Behavior Survey identifies the percentage of high school students who are overweight, engage in unhealthy dietary behaviors, or are physically inactive by selected states and cities.[75]

3. *Pregnancy Risk Assessment Monitoring System (PRAMS).* The CDC PRAMS is used by 29 states to monitor selected maternal attitudes, behaviors, and experiences related to adverse maternal and infant outcomes.[76]

4. *FDA Consumer Surveys.* The focus of the FDA Health and Diet Survey is on consumer awareness of relationships between diet and risk for chronic disease and on health-related knowledge and attitudes.[77] The survey has studied consumer use of food labels and weight-loss practices.[78,79] The FDA Food Safety Survey tracks consumers' knowledge, behaviors, and perceptions about food safety and consumption of potentially risky foods.[80] FDA conducted a study to assess consumer food-handling practices and awareness of microbiological hazards and several studies to evaluate the usefulness of shelf-labeling for consumers.[80,81]

5. *Diet and Health Knowledge Survey (DHKS).* The ARS DHKS was initiated in 1989 as a telephone follow-up to the CSFII and focused on the relationship of knowledge and attitudes about dietary guidance, food safety, food choices, and nutrient intakes.[82] The DHKS was last conducted in 1994 to 1996, and there are plans to collect similar information via a future NHANES module.[83]

FOOD COMPOSITION AND NUTRIENT DATABASES

1. *National Nutrient Database for Standard Reference (NNDSR).* ARS, USDA, maintains the NNDSR, which currently contains up to 140 food components for approximately 7000 foods.[84] Data are obtained from the food industry, USDA-initiated analytical contracts, and the scientific literature. The NNDSR is updated periodically to incorporate data from new analyses (from foods not previously analyzed and from newer analytical methods).[85,86] The NNDSR nutrient data are used as the core of most nutrient databases developed in the Unites States, such as those used in colleges, universities, medical facilities, hospitals, clinics, and commercial dietary analysis programs.[87] ARS also produces special interest databases (e.g., fluoride, choline, oxalic acid, flavonoids, isoflavones, and proanthocyanidins) as requested and supported by other agencies.[84,88] As the information in the special databases increases in quantity and quality, it may be added to the NDDSR in new data fields.

2. *Food and Nutrient Database for Dietary Studies (FNDDS).* ARS also produces the FNDDS, which contains data for energy and 60 food components for foods reported as being consumed in the NHANES dietary component What We Eat in America.[89,90] The FNDDS is periodically updated with current information from the NNDSR. Revised and new food composition data are retroactively applied to earlier versions of the FNDDS to allow for tracking nutrient consumption patterns.[86] ARS uses the Food Databases Management System software to manage the NDDS.[91] This software is used to update the database files with new information, to integrate time-related changes, and to replace older data values in the database (with start and end dates for time-specific changes). An online search tool, "What's In the Foods You Eat," provides access to nutritional information for 13,000 foods in the FNDDS.[92]

3. *Dietary Supplement Databases.* Because of the extensive use of dietary supplements in the United States, it is necessary to have a national dietary supplement database to estimate total nutrient intakes from both foods and supplements and to determine the impact of dietary supplements on nutrition and health.[93–96] NCHS and NIH have developed a database on dietary supplements for use with NHANES.[93,94] The NIH Office of Dietary Supplements (ODS) is planning to undertake the project of developing a Dietary Supplement Database using label data for use in national surveys.[97] ODS has several other initiatives regarding dietary supplements. They maintain the International Bibliographic Information on Dietary Supplements (IBIDS), which provides access to bibliographic citations and abstracts from published, international, and scientific literature on dietary supplements as well as Computer Access to Research on Dietary Supplements (CARDS), a database of federally funded research projects pertaining to dietary supplements.[98–100]

4. *Food Label and Package Survey (FLAPS).* The FDA FLAPS monitors the labeling practices of U.S. food manufacturers.[101–104] The FLAPS database includes the ingredient list, Nutrition Facts Panel information, nutrition and health claims, and food safety and other statements about the product. FLAPS also includes a surveillance program to identify the accuracy of selected nutrient declarations compared with values obtained form nutrient analyses. FDA uses FLAPS data to provide weighted estimates of the percentage of products sold with nutrition labeling, health or nutrient content claims, and food safety statements.

PROGRESS IN FOOD COMPOSITION DATA AND DATABASES

1. *National Food and Nutrient Analysis Program (NFNAP).* Nutrient data are lacking for some foods and food components in the NNDSR primarily because of the high cost and secondarily because of the lack of reliable analytical methods for certain food components. NFNAP was initiated in 1997 to help ARS produce accurate and current food composition data characterizing the U.S. national food supply.[105] NFNAP provides for stratified random sample collection and analysis of commonly eaten foods. The data obtained through NFNAP are incorporated into the NNDSR. The activities of NFNAP are: evaluation of existing data for scientific quality, identification of key foods and nutrients for sampling and analysis, development and implementation of nationally-based sampling plans for foods selected for analyses, and analyses of sampled foods under USDA-supervised laboratory contracts.[85,86] NFNAP is funded primarily by NIH Institutes and Centers and also by other government agencies.[88,105]

2. *National Nutrient Databank Conference (NNDC).* The NNDC meets yearly as a forum for food composition database developers and users.[106] ARS activities with regard to the NNDSR, Food and Nutrient Database for Dietary Studies (FNDDB), dietary supplement database, special databases, and analytical methods are presented at these meetings, and other researchers share their work on food analysis, database development, and software development. The 27th NNDC was held in Washington, D.C., in conjunction with the 5th International Food Data Conference (IFDC).[107] The focus of the meeting was data quality, and papers from the conference are available.[107] The 28th NNDC focused on the practical application of quality food composition data, and papers from this conference are available.[108] The 30th NNDC will be held as a Workshop to the American Dietetic Association Food and Nutrition Conference and

Exposition in Honolulu, Hawaii, in September 2006.[106] The theme for this meeting was the importance of food composition data for dietitians.

3. *International Food Data Conference (IFDC).* The IFDC was initiated in the International Network of Food Data Systems (INFOODS) in 1995 and are held every 2 years.[109] The 6th IFDC was held in Pretoria, South Africa in September 2005.[110] As noted earlier, papers from the 5th IFDC, which was held in conjunction with the 27th NNDC in 2003, are available.[107]

4. *Journal of Food Composition and Analysis (JFCA). JFCA* is the publication of INFOODS and is cosponsored by The United Nations University and the Food and Agriculture Organization of the United Nations.[111] Papers in the journal focus on the composition of human foods and emphasize new methods of analysis; the production, compilation, and dissemination of food composition data; and data use, including nutritional epidemiology, clinical research, agro-biodiversity, food security, and food trade.

FOOD-SUPPLY DETERMINATIONS

1. *U.S. Food and Nutrient Supply Series.* Since the early 1900s, USDA has provided food-supply estimates for foods and food components available to the population for per capita consumption for about 400 foods.[112–115] These data, which are published annually by USDA as the U.S. Food and Nutrient Supply Series, are used to assess the potential of the U.S. food supply to meet the nutritional needs of the population and to track changes in the food supply over time. They are also used to evaluate the effects of technological and marketing changes of the food supply over time; to study the relationships between food and nutrient availability and nutrient–disease associations; and to facilitate management of federal food assistance, nutrition education, and food fortification policies. Food-supply data indicate trends in food available for consumption rather than actual food consumption estimates. Food-supply data overestimate actual consumption because they include food wastage, food fed to pets, and other nonhuman use of food.

2. *Fisheries of the U.S. Survey.* The Fisheries of the U.S. Survey has been conducted by the National Marine Fisheries Service (NMFS), National Oceanic and Atmospheric Administration, Department of Commerce, since 1909 to provide annual per capita estimates of fish and shellfish availability in the United States.[116]

3. *AC Nielsen SCANTRACK Services.* Since 1985, monthly and annual proprietary sales data have been purchased by USDA ERS and USDA Center for Nutrition Policy and Promotion (CNPP) from AC Nielsen Company to measure grocery store sales of scannable packaged food products.[117] Households participating in the Homescan Consumer Panel transmit data on scanned purchases, including fresh packaged foods, weekly through a telephone line. These supermarket scanner data (SCANTRACK) do not reflect all fruits and vegetables or prepared foods from supermarkets, nor do they include foods obtained from restaurants or other food outlets.

USES OF NUTRITION MONITORING DATA

The NNMRRP surveys and surveillance activities were designed for the primary goals of each initiating agency, and these goals relate specifically to each agency mission. These primary goals were identified earlier for each survey/surveillance activity. In general, they include:

- Assessment of the nutrient intake of population groups compared with reference standards
- Monitoring of the nutrient and contaminant/toxin content of the food supply and identification of at-risk groups
- Assessment of the nutrition and health status of population groups and attempts to relate this to food/nutrient intake
- Tracking trends in food/nutrient intake and in nutrition/health status

In addition to these primary goals, nutrition monitoring data have additional uses when they are evaluated in greater detail and/or when data from several surveys/surveillance activities are combined. Some of these additional data uses include establishing national health objectives, tracking progress to reach national health objectives, development of nutrition education programs, policy decisions (i.e., regulations regarding food labeling, fortification, and safety), development of dietary and physiological reference standards and distributions, and identification of research opportunities. For example, monitoring and surveillance data are used to identify high-risk population groups to plan public health intervention programs and target food assistance awareness efforts and to evaluate progress towards achieving the Healthy People national health objectives[118,119]; establish guidelines for the prevention, detection, and management of nutritional conditions[120–126]; and evaluate the impact of nutrition initiatives for military feeding systems.[127,128] Specific examples of the use of nutrition monitoring data are mentioned in the following text for tracking national progress, nutrition education, food assistance/security, dietary/nutrition standards, regulatory activities, and research opportunities.

TRACKING NATIONAL PROGRESS

1. *Healthy People Year 2010 Health Objectives.* Nutrition monitoring data are essential to track progress in meeting the Healthy People 2010 agenda for the nation.[119] The major research questions currently under consideration include the role of diet and lifestyle with regard to overweight and obesity; diet-related chronic diseases (diabetes, cardiovascular disease); health disparities with regard to gender, race/ethnicity, and income; food insecurity; behavior modification of consumer habits; biomarkers for nutrition/health status; and genetic differences in food component actions/needs.

2. *Overweight/Obesity.* Overweight and obesity are likely the top priority of national and state nutrition monitoring efforts. Data on dietary intake; physical activity patterns; weight-loss efforts; and consumer knowledge, attitudes, and behaviors are important for public health education and research efforts to reduce the prevalence of overweight and obesity in the United States. Trends in energy and food and nutrient intake based on national dietary data have been used to understand the relationship between changes in dietary intake and the population's increase in over-weight and health status.[4,119,129,130] For men and women aged 20 to 74 years, the prevalence of overweight (body mass index [BMI] ≥ 25) was 59% and obesity (BMI ≥ 30) was 20% in NHANES III (1988 to 1994), compared with 51% and 12%, respectively, in NHANES II (1976 to 1980).[119,131] This increasing trend has also been observed for adolescents, children, and preschoolers.[132,133] Using the 95th percentile of BMI from NHANES II as the definition of overweight and the 85th to 95th percentile as the definition of risk for overweight, 11% of children and adolescents were overweight and another 14% were at risk for overweight during 1988 to 1994.[132] The prevalence of overweight in children and adolescents increased from about 5% in the 1960s and 1970s.[132]

NHANES III anthropometry data serve as the baseline measure for the Healthy People 2010 weight objectives.[119] Future NHANES data will be used to track progress in reducing the prevalence of overweight and obesity. NIH published *Clinical Guidelines on the Identification, Evaluation and Treatment of Overweight and Obesity in Adults — The Evidence Report* in 1998.[122] NIH continues to fund research related to the etiology and prevention of overweight and obesity and supports public health efforts to educate the public about overweight and obesity.[134–136]

NUTRITION EDUCATION

1. *Nutrition Education Programs.* Nutrition monitoring data are used to develop nutrition education programs such as the NIH 5 A Day for Better Health (now a CDC program),[137,138] the National Cholesterol Education Program,[120] the National High Blood Pressure Education Program,[121] and the Weight-Control Information Network (WIN).[134] The DHHS initiative, HealthierUS focuses on physical fitness, nutrition, prevention (i.e., screenings), and healthy choices (i.e., avoiding risky behaviors), and offers various Web sites relating to these topics as well as sponsoring the National Prevention Summits and Steps to a HealthierUS.[139–141]

2. *Nutrition Education Materials.* Consumers and practitioners are beneficiaries of national nutrition data as the infor-mation is translated into nutrition education materials so that consumers and practitioners can learn about diet and health. Monitoring data are used to develop nutrition education materials such as the *Dietary Guidelines for Americans*[142] and the Dietary Guidelines Report upon which they are based.[143] Other government nutrition education materials include the USDA MyPyramid[144] and the FDA nutrition labels.[145,146] Many government agencies provide nutrition education materials for the public. For example, a listing of materials developed by NIH Institutes and Centers is available at the NIH Division of Nutrition Research Coordination (DNRC) Web site.[147]

3. *Review of Nutrition Education Materials.* Title III of the National Nutrition Monitoring and Research Act of 1990 requires joint review by the DHHS and USDA of any dietary guidance materials developed by any federal agency for the general population or identified subpopulation.[2] This joint review process is carried out by the DHHS Nutrition Policy Board Committee on Dietary Guidance and the USDA Dietary Guidance Working Group.[148] The DHHS group is chaired by the ODPHP and consists of members representing DHHS agencies; the USDA group is chaired by CNPP and consists of members from USDA agencies. Each submitted document is reviewed by members of each group, and comments are summarized by the two chairs. The comments are then forwarded to the authors, who revise the document in accordance with the comments. Issues of concern are addressed through conference calls or meetings. This review process has continued despite the lack of reauthorization of the 1990 act.

FOOD ASSISTANCE/SECURITY

1. *Food Assistance Programs.* Evaluations of the USDA nutrition and food assistance programs are routinely conducted.[149,150] Monitoring data are used to develop federally supported food assistance programs[27,28,150] such

as the National School Lunch Program,[151] Food Stamp Program,[152] WIC,[55,153] and the US food Plans,[154] as well as programs to provide foods and meals for older Americans[155] and Native Americans.[156] NHANES III data have also been used to assess the usual nutrient intake of the low-income population, school-age children, older adults, and participants in WIC and the Food Stamp Program for USDA.[30,57]

2. *Food Security.* Food Security refers to assured access to nutritionally adequate and safe foods "without resorting to emergency food supplies, scavenging, stealing, and other coping strategies."[157] National surveys such as NHANES and the USDA food consumption surveys used questions related to food security as early as 1977.[63,158–161] Efforts by the private sector and academia paved the way toward a scientific basis for defining and measuring food insecurity and hunger in the mid-1980s.[162–164]

The Ten-Year comprehensive Plan for the NNMRR Program called for the development of a standard measure of food insecurity.[3] An 18-item food security measure was developed to track the prevalence of hunger and food insecurity in the population and high-risk subgroups and was first included as a supplement to the 1995 CPS.[63] Using the scale, it was estimated that the prevalence of food security in U.S. households was approximately 88%.[64] The 18-item food security scale developed in the 1990s was used in NHANES and several other surveys and is under review by an expert IOM panel.[165] A short form (6 items derived from the 18 items) was developed to meet state and local needs to assess food insecurity.[166] Policy documents such as Healthy People 2010[119] and the U.S. Action Plan on Food Security[167] use the food security measure to assess progress, and the scale can also be used as a yardstick by which to evaluate federal food and nutrition assistance programs with respect to welfare reform. Logan et al.[149] summarized the types of data available from national surveys and surveillance systems that can be used to assess the relationship between food assistance program participation and nutrition and health outcomes.

DIETARY/NUTRITION STANDARDS

1. *U.S. Growth Charts.* Data from NHANES III were used to develop the revised U.S. Growth Charts, which were released in 2000.[168] The revised standards include charts for infants through 19 years of age, as well as a chart for BMI by age.
2. *Dietary Reference Intakes (DRIs).* National data on dietary intakes and serum nutrient levels have been used for the investigation of nutrient requirements for age and sex groups for the development of the DRIs by the NAS.[169,170]

REGULATORY ACTIVITIES

1. *Food Fortification.* Dietary intake and serum data collected in NHANES III were used to assess folate status and the relationships between serum determinations, diet, and other nutrition and health variables prior to, and following, folate food fortification rulemaking by FDA.[171–174]
2. *Contaminants/Toxin Intakes.* NHANES data have been used to assess levels of metals, including lead, cadmium, and mercury.[175] The Environmental Protection Agency (EPA) has used monitoring data to provide dietary exposure estimates for nutrient and nonnutrient food components.[176,177] CSFII 1994 to 1996 and 1998 data were used to assess the exposure of children to pesticides in the diet for EPA,[178] and NHANES III data were used to prepare methyl mercury intake estimates for an EPA report to Congress assessing human exposure to mercury from fish and shellfish intake.[177]

RESEARCH OPPORTUNITIES

Nutrition monitoring data have been used to identify food and nutrition research priorities of significance to public health.[118, 119,125,126,178–180] Much of the data generated by the NNMRRP are available from published government and peer-reviewed reports, CD-ROMs, and/or the Internet, along with documentation on sampling methods, survey design, sample sizes, and survey instruments and questionnaires. The Web sites for the major surveys and surveillance systems are listed in Table 23.1. NHANES data are available on the Internet,[30] and ARS posts food composition data on its Web site.[84] NCHS releases short reports and Health-E Stats,[181] and CDC publishes the *Morbidity and Mortality Weekly Report* online.[182] Thus, government survey and surveillance data are widely available for academics and graduate student to test new hypothesis and discover new diet–health relationships.

Nutrition research that is done with federal funds is tracked through the Human Nutrition Research and Information (HNRIM) System, which is housed at NIH.[183] The HNRIM database provides information for each research project including an abstract, principal investigator and organization, nutrition classification categories, percent nutrition related, and fiscal year and start date.

FUTURE CHALLENGES

Nutrition monitoring, research, and policy are interrelated. Nutrition monitoring provides data needed for public policy decisions and for establishing research priorities. Nutrition research provides data for policymaking and for identifying nutrition monitoring data needs. Continuous collection of diet- and nutrition-related data in cross-sectional and longitudinal surveys and surveillance systems are used to assess the health of the U.S. population and to plan nutrition services and educational programs.

Current U.S. nutrition monitoring surveys and surveillance activities are firmly grounded in NHANES and the other surveys and surveillance activities identified in Table 23.1. The future of nutrition monitoring will be based on the nutrition issues and needs of the population. The focus may shift as past health problems are resolved through nutrition education and public policy changes and as new diet-related health concerns emerge. The surveys and surveillance activities will be adapted to meet changing needs, and new studies will be added as resources permit.

Improvements to the nutrition monitoring surveys and surveillance activities may result from research that develops new methodologies and improves existing ones to assess nutrition and health status. New and improved methods may allow more accurate and efficient assessment of food and nutrient intake, assessment of physiological measures of nutrient status, and techniques to relate food and nutrient intake to health status. Newer data from NHANES and other surveys/activities may shift the focus of the nutrition monitoring. Availability of monitoring data may prompt researchers to do unique analysis, and the development of biomarkers may spur refinements to the surveys. Biochemical measures of long-term nutritional status or exposure are not subject to the same inaccuracies or bias as the reporting of long-term dietary intake, but the sensitivity and specificity of biomarkers need to be evaluated for their role in assessing exposure to foods and nutrients and for identifying high-risk population groups.[184]

Speculation about the future of the nutrition monitoring requires consideration of the factors that may change the health concerns of the population. Some of the factors are changes in the food supply, in the demographics of the U.S. population, and in individual dietary and other lifestyle behaviors.

CHANGES IN THE FOOD SUPPLY

The U.S. food supply is in a constant state of flux with new products and alterations of the food supply. Recent examples include the introduction of sports beverages, traditional foods with nutrients and phytochemicals added, and new formulations to reduce levels of *trans*-fats. The nutrient intake of the population or of specific population groups may change as these altered or new foods are consumed. Changes in the food supply may also result from genetic engineering of plants or animals, changes in agricultural practices, and new manufacturing processes or technologies. Over the past several decades there has been increased consumption of food from fast food chains and other restaurants, increased availability of prepared foods from grocery stores that require only microwave heating prior to consumption, and increased consumption of ethnic dishes. Such changes towards convenience, food diversity, and complexity of the food system are likely to continue.

There is also considerable activity within the United States toward a more sustainable food supply with the introduction of gardens in schools and emphasis on use of local foods to reduce food miles.[185,186] This may also affect food consumption as well as the nutrient content of foods consumed.

DEMOGRAPHICS OF THE UNITED STATES

Alternations in the demographics of the U.S. population may affect the mean food and nutrient intakes from national surveys because the surveys reflect the food preferences, patterns, and practices of the population. The number of Hispanics and Blacks in the U.S. population is increasing at a rate faster than the White, non-Hispanic population. The population is also becoming older as post–World War II "boomers" and their children age. Income disparities among racial/ethnic and age groups will continue to be important in identifying population groups that are more vulnerable to diet- and health-related problems.

DIETARY AND LIFESTYLE BEHAVIORS

Modification in individual dietary and other lifestyle behavior may lead to changes in health. Consumers are encouraged to follow the Dietary Guidelines for Americans[142] with regard to diet and physical activity and the MyPyramid food guide,[144] and to use Nutrition Facts Labels[145,146] for comparison shopping. These nutrition education efforts may help consumers improve their health. Consumers may become increasing knowledgeable of the health effects of overweight and obesity and make attempts to alter their eating patterns and physical activity to lose weight. People are also influenced by the nutrition information they receive from other sources (the Internet, TV, radio, books, magazines, and advertisements). They may begin to take (or alter their intake of) dietary supplements, increase intake of functional foods, or become interested in organic produce, herbal products, or botanicals. Such behavior changes could affect health. Hopefully, consumers will adopt behaviors that will improve their health; however, it is possible that poor dietary advice may have the opposite effects. It is also possible that continued sedentary lifestyles and wide access to food will maintain the current problems of overweight and obesity in the United States and the health problems related to them.

CONCLUSIONS

Recent progress in nutrition monitoring has included the development of the ARS multiple-pass 24 h dietary intake methodology[22] and integration and merging of NHANES and CSFII into one national dietary data collection effort.[21,22] Recent uses of nutrition monitoring data include development of the DRIs,[169,170] the *2005 Dietary Guidelines Report*,[143] the 2005 edition of the Dietary Guidelines for Americans, [142] the HealthierUS Initiative,[139] and the USDA development and release of the MyPyramid food guide.[144] Communication among federal and state agencies helps improve the quality of these efforts and also helps prevent duplication of effort and efficient use of available resources. Reinstitution of the IBNMRR and reauthorization of the 1990 act would result in a more focused, comprehensive nutrition monitoring program to help improve methodologies for the collection and interpretation of data, timely processing and release of data, adequate coverage of population subgroups, and research that addresses current nutrition and public health issues.

ACRONYMS USED IN TEXT

ARS: Agriculture Research Service
BMI: Body Mass Index
BRFSS: Behavioral Risk Factor Surveillance System
CARDS: Computer Access to Research on Dietary Supplements
CDC: Centers for Disease Control and Prevention
CNPP: Center for Nutrition Policy and Promotion
CPS: Current Population Survey
CSFII: Continuing Survey of the Food Intake of Individuals
DHHS: Department of Health and Human Services
DHKS: Diet and Health Knowledge Survey
DNRC: Division of Nutrition Research Coordination
EPA: Environmental Protection Agency
ERS: Economic Research Service
FDA: Food and Drug Administration
FFQ: Food Frequency Questionnaire
FLAPS: Food Labeling and Packaging Survey
FNDDB: Food and Nutrient Database for Dietary Studies
FNS: Food and Nutrition Service
HNRIM: Human Nutrition Research Information Management
IBIDS: International Bibliographic Information on Dietary Supplements
IBNMRR: Interagency Board for Nutrition Monitoring and Related Research
IDAC: International Dietary Assessment Conference
IFDC: International Food Data Conference
INFOODS: International Network of Food Data Systems
IOM: Institute of Medicine
JFCA: Journal of Food Composition and Analysis
NAS: National Academy of Sciences
NCHS: National Center for Health Statistics
NFCS: Nationwide Food Consumption Survey
NFNAP: National Food and Nutrient Analysis Program
NHANES: National Health and Nutrition Examination Survey
NHCS: National Health Care Survey
NMFS: National Marine Fisheries Service
NNDC: National Nutrient Databank Conference
NNDSR: National Nutrient Database for Standard Reference
NNMRRP: National Nutrition Monitoring and Related Research Program
NHEFS: National NHANES I Epidemiologic Followup Study
NHIS: National Health Interview Survey
NSFG: National Survey of Family Growth

NVSS: National Vital Statistics System
ODS: Office of Dietary Supplements
PedNSS: Pediatric Nutrition Surveillance System
PNSS: Pregnancy Nutrition Surveillance System
SHIPPS: School Health Policies and Programs Study
SLAITS: State and Local Area Integrated Telephone Survey
SNDAS: School Nutrition Dietary Assessment Study
US: United States
USDA: U.S. Department of Agriculture
WIC: Women, Infants, and Children
YRBSS: Youth Risk Behavior Surveillance System

REFERENCES

1   Mason, J.B. et al., *Nutritional Surveillance*, World Health Organization, Geneva, 1984.
2. U.S. Congress, Pub. L. 101-445. *National Nutrition Monitoring and Related Research Act of 1990*, 101st Congress, Washington, DC, October 22, 1990.
3. U.S. Department of Health and Human Services and U.S. Department of Agriculture, Ten-year comprehensive plan for the national nutrition monitoring and related research program, *Fed Reg* 58, 32752, June 11, 1993.
4. Life Sciences Research Office, Federation of American Societies for Experimental Biology, *Third Report on Nutrition Monitoring in the United States: Volumes 1 and 2*, U.S. Government Printing Office, Washington, DC, 1995.
5. Kuczmarski, M.F., Moshfegh, A.J., and Briefel, R.R., *JADA* 94: 753; 1994.
6. Kuczmarski, M.F. and Kuczmarski, R.J., in *Modern Nutrition in Health and Disease*, 8th ed, Shils, M.E., Olson, J.A., and Shike, M., eds, Lea & Febiger, Philadelphia, 1994, 1506.
7. Bialostosky, K., Briefel, R.R., and Pennington, J. in *Handbook of Nutrition and Food*, Berdanier, C.D., ed., CRC Press, Washington, DC, 2001, 407.
8. Briefel, R.R. and Bialostosky, K., in *Research. Successful Approaches*, 2nd edition. Monsen, E.R., ed., American Dietetic Association, Chicago, IL, 2003, 185.
9. Briefel, R., in *Present Knowledge in Nutrition*, 9th edition, Bowman, B. and Russell, R., eds., ILSI Press, Washington, DC, 2006.
10. Food and Agriculture Act of 1977 (P: 95-113). Sec. 1428., *Cong Rec* 123, September 29, 1977.
11. U.S. Department of Health and Human Services and U.S. Department of Agriculture, *Nutrition Monitoring in the United States: A Progress Report from the Joint Nutrition Monitoring Evaluation Committee*. DHHS Pub No (PHS) 86-1255, U.S. Government Printing Office, Washington, DC, 1986.
12. Calloway, W., *JADA* 84: 1179; 1984.
13. Ostenso, G.L., *JADA* 84: 1181; 1984.
14. Brown Jr, G.E., *JADA* 84: 1185; 1984.
15. U.S. Department of Health and Human Services, Interagency Committee on Nutrition Monitoring, Announcement of committee formation, *Fed Reg* 53-26505(134), 1988.
16. Life Sciences Research Office, *Nutrition Monitoring in the United States: An Update Report on Nutrition Monitoring*, DHHS Pub No (PHS) 89-1255, U.S. Government Printing Office, Washington, DC, 1989.
17. Interagency Committee on Nutrition Monitoring, *Nutrition Monitoring in the United States: The Directory of Federal Nutrition Monitoring Activities*, DHHS Pub No (PHS) 89-1255-1, Public Health Service, Washington, DC, 1989.
18. Interagency Board for Nutrition Monitoring and Related Research, Wright, J., ed., *Nutrition Monitoring in the United States: The Directory of Federal and State Nutrition Monitoring Activities*, DHHS Pub No (PHS) 92-1255-1, Public Health Service, Hyattsville, MD, 1992.
19. U.S. Department of Health and Human Services and Department of Agriculture, Proposed Ten-Year Comprehensive Plan for the National Nutrition Monitoring and Related Research Program, *Fed Reg* 91-25967:SS716-55767, October 29, 1991.
20. Interagency Board for Nutrition Monitoring and Related Research. Nutrition Monitoring in the United States, *Chartbook I: Selected Findings from the National Nutrition Monitoring and Related Research Program*, Ervin, B. and Reed, D., eds., DHHS Pub No (PHS) 93-1255-2, Public Health Service, Hyattsville, MD, 1993.
21. National Center for Health Statistics, CDC, DHHS, *DHHS-USDA Dietary Survey Integration – What we eat in America*, http://www.cdc.gov/nchs/about/major/nhanes/faqs.htm. Accessed October 13, 2005.
22. Agricultural Research Service, USDA, What We Eat in America, NHANES 2001–2002, http://www.ars.usda.gov/Services/docs/htm?docid=7674. Accessed October 13, 2005]
23. Dwyer, J., Picciano, M.F., and Raiten, D.J., *J Nutr* 133: 576S; 2003.
24. National Nutrition Summit 2000, http://www.nns.nih.gov/2000/background/background.htm. Accessed October 26, 2005.
25. Interagency Board on Nutrition Monitoring and Related Research, Bialostosky, K., ed. *Nutrition Monitoring in the United States. The Directory of Federal and State Nutrition Monitoring and Related Research Activities*, DHHS Pub No (PHS) 00-1255, National Center for Health Statistics, Hyattsville, MD, 2000. (http://www.cdc.gov/nchs/pressroon/00facts/nutrit.htm and http://www.cdc.gov/nchs/about/otheract/nutrishn/nutrishn.htm. Accessed October 13, 2005.)

26. Woteki, C.E. et al., *J Nutr* 132: 3782; 2002. (Data supplement available at http://www.nutrition.org/cgi/data/132/12/3782/DC1/1. Accessed October 13, 2005.)

27. National Research Council, Institute of Medicine, Committee on National Statistics, in *Summary of Workshop on Food and Nutrition Data Needs.* Casey, J. and Scholz, J.K., eds., National Academies Press, Washington, DC, 2004.

28. National Research Council, Institute of Medicine, Panel on Enhancing the Data Infrastructure in Support of Food and Nutrition Programs, Research, and Decision Making, *Improving Data to Analyze Food and Nutrition Policies,* National Academies Press, Washington, DC, 2005.

29. Woteki, C.E. and Wong, F.L., in *Research. Successful Approaches,* Monsen, E.R., ed., American Dietetic Association, Chicago, IL, 204, 1992.

30. National Center for Health Statistics, CDC, DHHS, National Health and Nutrition Examination Survey, http://www.cdc.gov/nchs/nhanes/htm. Accessed October 12, 2005.

31. National Center for Health Statistics, CDC, DHHS. NHANES I Epidemiologic Followup Study (NHEFS), http://www.cdc.gov/nchs/r&d/nchs_datalinkage/nhefs_data_linkage_activities.htm. Accessed October 13, 2005.

32. National Center for Health Statistics, CDC, DHHS, National Health Interview Survey (NHIS), http://www.cdc.gov/nchs/nhis/htm. Accessed October 13, 2005.

33. National Center for Health Statistics, CDC, DHHS, State and Local Area Integrated Telephone Survey, http://www.cdc.gov/nchs/slaits.htm. Accessed October 13, 2005.

34. Centers for Disease Control and Prevention, DHHS. Pediatric and Pregnancy Nutrition Surveillance System, http://www.cdc.gov/pednss/. Accessed October 13, 2005.

35. Polhamus, B. et al., *Pediatric Nutrition Surveillance 2003 Report,* Centers for Disease Control and Prevention, Atlanta, GA, 2004. (Available at http://www.cdc.gov/pednss/pdfs/PedNSS_2003_Summary.pdf. Accessed May 17, 2005.)

36. National Center for Health Statistics, CDC, DHHS, National Health Care Survey, http://www.cdc.gov/nchs/nchs.htm. Accessed October 13, 2005.

37. National Center for Health Statistics, CDC, DHHS, National Survey of Family Growth, http://www.nichd.nih.gov/about/cpr/dbs/res_national5.htm; http://www.cdc.gov/nchs/about/major/nsfg/nsfgback.htm; http://www.cdc.gov/nchs.nsfg.htm. Accessed October 31, 2005.

38. National Center for Health Statistics, CDC, DHHS, National Vital Statistics System, http://www.cdc.gov/nchs/nvss.htm. Accessed October 27, 2005.

39. What We Eat in America Automated Multiple-Pass Method, (http://www.ars.usda.gov/Services/docs/htm?docid=7710). Accessed October 13, 2005.

40. Dwyer, J., Picciano, M.F., and Raiten, D.J., *J Nutr* 133: 590S; 2003.

41. Dwyer, J., Picciano, M.F., Raiten, D.J., *J Nutr* 133: 609S; 2003.

42. Raper, N. et al., *J Food Comp Anal* 17: 545; 2004.

43. Carriquiry, A.L., *J Nutr* 133: 601S; 2003.

44. National Cancer Institute (NCI), NIH, DHHS, *How is NCI supporting the NHANES?* http://www.riskfactor.cancer.gov/studies/nhanes/. Accessed October 13, 2005.

45. Food Surveys Research Group, ARS, USDA, What We Eat in American, NHANES 2001–2002: Usual Nutrient Intakes from Food Compared to Dietary Reference Intakes, http://ww.ars.usda.gov/foodsurvey. Accessed October 13, 2005.

46. Schoeller, D.A., *J Nutr* 129: 1765; 1999.

47. Bingham, S.A., *Nutr Abst Rev* 57: 705; 1987.

48. Johnson, R.K. and Hankin, J.H., in *Research. Successful Approaches*, 2nd ed., Monsen, E.R., ed., American Dietetic Association, Chicago, IL, 2003, 227.

49. Subar, A.F. et al., *Am J Epidemiol* 158: 1; 2003.

50. Sixth International Dietary Assessment Conference (IDAC), http://www.icdam6.dk/main.htm. Accessed October 13, 2005.

51. Pennington, J.A.T. and Gunderson, E.L., *J Assoc Off Anal Chem* 70: 772; 1987.

52. Pennington, J.A.T. et al., *J AOAC Int* 79: 163; 1996.

53. Food and Drug Administration, Total Diet Study, http://www.cfsan.fda.gov/~comm/tds-toc.html. Accessed October 13, 2005.

54. Food and Drug Administration, Submission for Office of Management and Budget Review, Infant Feeding Practices Study II, *Fed Reg* 69(190): 58915; 2004.

55. Food and Nutrition Service, USDA, Resources. Status of Recent and Ongoing Studies Funded by WIC, http://www.fns.usda.gov/win/resources/wicstudies.htm. Accessed October 13, 2005.

56. Food and Nutrition Service, USDA, About WIC, http://www.fns.usda.gov/wic/aboutwic/default.htm. Accessed October 27, 2005.

57. Fox, M.K. and Cole, N., *Nutrition and Health Characteristics of Low-Income Populations: Volume III, School-Age Children,* Economic Research Service, USDA, Washington, DC, 2004.

58. Burghardt, J.A., Devaney, B.L., and Gordon, A.R., *Am J Clin Nutr* 61: 252S; 1995.

59. Fox, M.K. et al., *School Nutrition Dietary Assessment Study- II. Final Report,* Food and Nutrition Service, USDA, Alexandria, VA, 2001.

60. Centers for Disease Control and Prevention, DHHS, School Health Policies and Programs Study (SHPPS), http://www.cdc.gov/healthyyouth/obesity/index.htm. Accessed October 3, 2005.

61. Bureau of the Census, for the Bureau of labor Statistics, Current Population Survey (CPS), http://www.bls.census.gov/cps/overmain.htm. Accessed October 27, 2005.

62. Hamilton, W.L. et al., *Measures of Food Security, Food Insecurity, and Hunger in the United States in 1995: Technical Report of the Food Security Measurement Study,* Food and Consumer Service, USDA, Alexandria, VA, July 1997.

63. Hamilton, W.L. et al., *Household Food Security in the United States in 1995: Summary Report of the Food Security Measurement Project,* Food and Consumer Service, USDA, Alexandria, VA, September 1997.

64. Carlson, S.J., Andrews, M.S., and Bickel, G.W., *J Nutr* 129: 510S; 1999.

65. Economic Research Service, USDA, Briefing Room. Food Security in the United States, http://www.ers.usda.gov/Briefing/FoodSecurity/. Accessed October 13, 2005.

66. Economic Research Service, USDA, Food Security Measurement, http://www.fns.usda.gov/fsec/measurement.htm. Accessed November 10, 2005.

67. Economic Research Service, USDA, Household Food Security in the United States, 2004, www.ers.usda.gov/publications/err11. Accessed October 31, 2005.

68. Centers for Disease Control and Prevention, DHHS, FoodNet Surveillance, http://www.cdc.gov/foodnet/surveillance.htm. Accessed October 13, 2005.

69. Centers for Disease Control and Prevention, DHHS, Health Risks in the United States: Behavioral Risk Factor Surveillance System. At A Glance 2005, http://www.cdc.gov/uc/aag/aag_brfss.htm. Accessed October 13, 2005.

70. Centers for Disease Control and Prevention, DHHS, Behavioral Risk Factor Surveillance System (BRFSS), http://www.cdc.gov/brfss/. Accessed October 13, 2005.

71. Serdula, M.K. et al., *Am J Public Health* 84: 1821; 1994.

72. Centers for Disease Control and Prevention, DHHS, Healthy Youth! YRBSS: Youth Risk Behavior Surveillance System, http://www.cdc.gov/HealthyYouth/yrbs/index.htm. Accessed October 13, 2005.

73. Youth Risk Behavior Surveillance — United States, 1997, *Morb Mort Wkly Rpt* 47(SS-3); 1998.

74. Centers for Disease Control and Prevention, DHHS, *Morb Mort Wkly Rpt* 53(RR-12); 1: 2004.

75. Centers for Disease Control and Prevention, DHHS, Youth Risk Behavior Survey Childhood Obesity Fact Sheets, (http://www.cdc.gov/healthyyouth/obesity/facts.htm). Accessed October 3, 2005.

76. Centers for Disease Control and Prevention, DHHS, Pregnancy Risk Assessment Monitoring System (PRAMS), http://www.cdc.gov/reproductivehealth/PRAMS/index.html. Accessed October 13, 2005.

77. Food and Drug Administration, DHHS, Consumer Research on Nutrition, Diet, and Health. The FDA Health and Diet Survey: A Data Resource, http://vm.cfsan.fda.gov/~lrd/ab-nutri.html. Accessed October 13, 2005.

78. Heaton, A.W. and Levy, A.S., *J Nutr Educ* 27: 182; 1995.

79. Levy, A.S. and Heaton, A.W., *Ann Intern Med* 119: 661; 1993.

80. Food and Drug Administration, DHHS, Consumer Research on Foodborne Illness. Consumer Research Studies, http://www.cfsan.fda.gov/~lrd/ab-foodb.html. Accessed October 13, 2005.

81. Schucker, R.E. et al., *J Nutr Educ* 24: 75; 1992.

82. Agriculture Research Service (ARS), USDA, Diet and Health Knowledge Survey (DHKS) Variable List, http://www.ars.usda.gov/Services/docs.htm?docid=7776. Accessed October 13, 2005.

83. Tippett, S., Enns, C.W., and Moshfegh, A., *Nutr Today* 34: 33; 1999.

84. Agricultural Research Service (ARS), USDA, Nutrient Data Laboratory, http://www.nal.usda.gov/fnic.foodcomp/. Accessed October 13, 2005.

85. Haytowitz, D.B. et al., *J Food Comp Anal* 9: 331; 1996.

86. Anderson, E. et al., *J Food Comp Anal* 13: 287; 2001.

87. National Nutrient Databank Conference (NNDB), International Nutrient Databank Directory, http://www.nal.usda.gov/fnic/foodcomp/conf.index.html. (Follow link for PDF file.) Accessed October 13, 2005.

88. Pennington, J.A.T., *J Food Comp Anal* 16: 359; 2003.

89. Perloff, B.P. et al., *J Nutr* 120: 1530; 1990.

90. Agricultural Research Service (ARS), USDA, USDA Food and Nutrient Database for Dietary Studies (FNDDS), http://www.ars.usda.gov/Services/docs.htm?docid-7673. Accessed October 13, 2005.

91. Anderson, E., Steinfeldt, L.C., and Ahuja, J.K.C., *J Food Comp Anal* 17: 557; 2004.

92. Food Survey Research Group (FSRG), ARS, USDA, What's In the Foods You Eat, http://www.ars.usda.gov/foodsearch. Accessed October 31, 2005.

93. Ervin, R.B., Wright, J.D., and Kennedy-Stephenson, J., *Vital Health Stat* 244(i–iii), 1, June 11, 1999.

94. Dwyer, J., Picciano, M.F., and Raiten, D.J., *J Nutr* 133: 624S; 2003.

95. Commission on Dietary Supplements Labels, *Report of the Commission on Dietary Supplements Labels*, Office of Disease Prevention and Health Promotion, Washington, DC, November, 1997.

96. Heimbach, J.T., *J Nutr* 131: 1335S; 2001.

97. Office of Dietary Supplements, NIH, DHHS, Dietary Supplement Database, http://dietary-supplements.info.nih.gov/Health_Information/Dietary_Supplement_Ingredient_and_Labeling_Databases.aspx. Accessed November 3, 2005.

98. Office of Dietary Supplements, NIH, DHHS, International Bibliographic Information on Dietary Supplements (BIDS), http://dietary-supplements.info.nih.gov/Health_Information/Health_Information.aspx. Accessed November 3, 2005.

99. Office of Dietary Supplements, NIH, DHHS, Computer Access to Research on Dietary Supplements (CARDS), http://dietary-supplements.info.nih.gov/research/cards_database.aspx. Accessed November 3, 2005.

100. Haggans, C.J. et al., *J Nutr* 135: 1796; 2005.

101. LeGault, L. et al., *J Am Diet Assoc* 104: 952; 2004.

102. Brandt, M. et al., *Food Protection Trends* 23: 870; 2003.
103. Brecher, S. et al., *J A D A* 100: 1057; 2000.
104. Food and Drug Administration, DHHS, Food Label and Package Survey 2000–2001, http://www.cfsan.fda.gov/~dms/lab-flap.html. Accessed October 27, 2005.
105. Agriculture Research Service, USDA, National Food and Nutrient Analysis Program (NFNAP), http://www.ars.usda.gov/Research/docs.htm?docid=9446. Accessed October 13, 2005.
106. National Nutrient Databank Conference, http://www.nal.usda.gov/fnic/foodcomp/conf.indes.html. Accessed October 13, 2005.
107. Papers from the Joint Meeting of the 5th International Food Data Conference and the 27th U.S. National Nutrient Databank Conference, Pennington, J.A.T. and Stumbo, P.J., guest eds., *J Food Comp Anal* 17: 247; 2004.
108. Papers from the 28th National Nutrient Databank Conference, Pennington, J.A.T. and Stumbo, P.J., guest eds., *J Food Comp Anal.* in press.
109. International Network of Food Data Systems, http://www.iuns.org/features/INFOODS%20progress%20report%202003-2005.htm. Accessed November 3, 2005.
110. The International Network of Food Data Systems, International Food Data Conference (IFDC), http://www.fao.org/infoods/food_data_conf_en.stm. Accessed October 13, 2005.
111. *Journal of Food Composition and Analysis*, http://www.elsevier.com/wps/find/journaldescription.cws_home/622878/description. Accessed October 13, 2005.
112. Economic Research Service, USDA, Food Consumption (per capita) Data System, http://www.ers.usda.gov/Data/FoodConsumption/. Accessed November 3, 2005.
113. Economic Research Service, USDA, Food Availability, http://209.48.219.54/FoodAvailability.htm. Accessed November 3, 2005.
114. Center for Nutrition Policy and Promotion, USDA, Nutrient Content of the U.S. Food Supply, http://209.48.219.54/. Accessed October 13, 2005
115. Gerrior, S. and Bente, L., *Nutrient Content of the US Food Supply 1909–99. A Summary Report,* Center for Nutrition Policy and Promotion (CNPP), USDA, Home Economics Research Report No. 55, 2002.
116. NOAA Fisheries, Office of Science and Technology, http://www.st.nmfs.noaa.govst1/mission.html. Publications http://www.st.nmfs.noaa.gov/st1/publications.html (follow link for "2003"). Fisheries of the United States — 2003. http://www.st.nmfs.noaa.gov/st1/fus/fus03/index.html (follow link to "Per Capita" for pdf file on Per Capita Consumption.) Accessed October 31, 2005.
117. A.C. Nielsen Scantrack Services, http://www.acnielsen.com/products/reports/scantrack/. Accessed October 13, 2005.
118. U.S. Department of Health and Human Service, *Healthy People 2000: National Health Promotion and Disease Prevention Objectives.* DHHS Pub No (PHS) 91-50212, U.S. Government Printing Office, Washington, DC, 1991.
119. U.S. Department of Health and Human Services, *Healthy People 2010.* Conference Edition in Two Volumes, U.S. Department of Health and Human Services, Washington, DC, January 2000.
120. National Cholesterol Education Program, *Third Report of the National Cholesterol Education Program (NCEP) Expert Panel on Detection, Evaluation, and Treatment of High Blood Cholesterol in Adults (Adult Treatment Panel III),* NIH Pub No 02-5215, National Heart, Lung, and Blood Institute, Bethesda, MD, 2002.
121. National Heart, Lung, and Blood Institute (NHLBI), NIH, DHHS, *Seventh Report of the Joint National Committee on Prevention, Detection, Evaluation, and Treatment of High Blood Pressure (JNC 7),* DHHS Pub No 04-5230, U.S. Department of Health and Human Services, Washington, DC, 2004.
122. National Institutes of Health (NIH), DHHS, *Obesity Research* 6 (suppl 2): 51S: 1998.
123. Centers for Disease Control and Prevention, DHHS, *Morb Mort Wkly Rpt* 47(RR-3), 1, 1998.
124. National Institutes of Health (NIH), DHHS, *NIH Consensus Statement: Optimal Calcium Intake,* National Institutes of Health, Bethesda, MD, June 6–8, 1994.
125. U.S. Department of Health and Human Services, *The Surgeon General's Report on Nutrition and Health.* PHS Pub No 88-50210, U.S. Department of Health and Human Services, Washington, DC, 1988.
126. National Research Council (NRS), *Diet and Health. Implications for Reducing Chronic Disease Risk.* National Academy Press, Washington, DC, 1989.
127. Committee on Military Nutrition Research, Food and Nutrition Board, Institute of Medicine, *Military Nutrition Initiatives,* IOM Report 91-05, Institute of Medicine, Washington, DC, February 25, 1991.
128. Poos, M., Costello, R., and Carlson-Newberry, S.J., *Committee on Military Nutrition Research Activity Report 1994-1999.* National Academy Press, Washington, DC, 1999.
129. Briefel, R.R. and Johnson, C.L., *Annu Rev Nutr* 24: 401; 2004.
130. Nielsen, S.J., Siega-Riz, A.M., and Popkin B.M., *Obesity Res* 10: 370; 2002.
131. Pamuk, E. et al., *Socioeconomic Status and Health Chartbook. Health, United States, 1998,* National Center for Health Statistics, Hyattsville, MD, 1998.
132. Troiano, R.P. et al., *Arch Pediatr Adolesc Med* 149: 1085; 1995.
133. Ogden, C.L. et al., *Pediatrics* 99: 1; 1997.
134. National Institute of Diabetes and Digestive and Kidney Diseases, National Institutes of Health, DHHS, Weight-control Information Network (WIN), http://www.win.niddk.nih.gov/. Accessed November 10, 2005.
135. National Institute of Diabetes and Digestive and Kidney Diseases, National Institutes of Health, DHHS, Obesity-Related Research Activities Supported by NIH and NIDDK, Obesity Research Plan and Advisory Groups, http://win.niddk.nih.gov/research/index.htm. Accessed November 10, 2005.
136. National Heart, Lung, and Blood Institute, National Institutes of Health, DHHS, Obesity Education Initiative, http://www.nhlbi.nih.gov/about/oei/index.htm. Accessed November 10, 2005.

137. Subar, A.S. et al., *5 A Day for Better Health: A Baseline Study of American's Fruit and Vegetable Consumption*, National Cancer Institute, Rockville, MD, 1992.
138. National Cancer Institute, National Institutes of Health, DHHS, Eat 5 to 9 A Day for Better Health. About the Program, http://www.5aday.gov/about/index/html. Accessed October 13, 2005.
139. DHHS HealthierUS Initiative, http://www.healthierus.gov/index.htm. Accessed October 18, 2005.
140. Office of Disease Prevention and Health Promotion, DHHS, Steps To A HealthierUS Initiative. 3rd National Prevention Summit. Innovations in Community Prevention, http://www.healthierus.gov/steps/summit.html. Accessed November 10, 2005.
141. DHHS Steps to a HealthierUS Initiative, http://www.healthierus.gov/steps/. Accessed October 13, 2005.
142. DHHS and USDA, *Dietary Guidelines for Americans, 2005*, HHS Pub No HHS-ODPHP-2005-01-DGA-A. USDA Home and Garden Bulletin No 232, U.S. Government Printing Office, Washington, DC, 2005. (also available at http://www.health.gov/dietary-guidelines/. Accessed November 14, 2005; http://www.healthierus.gov/dietaryguidelines/index.thml. Accessed November 14, 2005; and http://www.usda.gov/cnpp/dietary_guidelines.html. Accessed November 14, 2005.)
143. Dietary Guidelines Advisory Committee, *Report of the Dietary Guidelines Advisory Committee on the Dietary Guidelines for Americans, 2005*, National Technical Information Service, August 2004.
144. USDA, MyPyramid, http://www.mypyramid.gov/. Accessed October 13, 2005.
145. Food and Drug Administration, DHHS, How to Understand and use the Nutrition Facts label, http://www.cfsan.fda.gov/~dms/food-lab.html. Accessed October 13, 2005.
146. Food and Drug Administration, DHHS, Examples of revised Nutrition Facts panel listing *trans* fat, http://www.cfsan.fda.gov/~dms/labtr.html. Accessed October 13, 2005.
147. Division of Nutrition Research Coordination, National Institutes of Health, NIH Nutrition Educational Materials, http://www.dnrc.nih.gov/nutrition_education/index.htm. Accessed November 10, 2005.
148. Pennington, J.A.T. and Hubbard, V.S., *J Nutr Ed Behavior* 34: 53; 2002.
149. Logan, C., Fox, M.K., and Lin, B.H., *Effects of Food Assistance and Nutrition Programs on Nutrition and Health, Volume 2*, Food Assistance and Nutrition Research Report Number 19-2, U.S. Department of Agriculture, Washington, DC, 2002.
150. Fox, M.K., Hamilton, W., and Biing-Hwan, L., *Effects of Food Assistance and Nutrition Programs on Nutrition and Health. Volume 4. Executive Summary of the Literature Review*, Food Assistance and Nutrition Research Report No 19-4, Economic Research Service, USDA, Washington, DC, 2004.
151. Carlson, A. et al. The Low-Coast, Moderate cost, and Liberal Food Plans: 2003 administrative Report, Center for Nutrition Policy and Promotion, USDA, CN PP-13, 2003 Alexandria.
152. Devaney, B. and Fraker, T.M., *J Policy Anal Management* 5: 725; 1986.
153. Centers for Disease Control and Prevention, DHHS, *Morb Mortal Wkly Rpt* 45(3): 65; 1995.
154. Carlson, A., Kinsey, J., and Nadav, C., *USDA Family Economics Nutr Rev.* Spring, 2003.
155. Administration on Aging, DHHS, http://www.aoa.dhhs.gov/prof/aoaprog/nutrition/program_info/program_info.asp. Follow link to The Elderly Nutrition Program. Accessed November 10, 2005.
156. Indian Health Service, DHHS, Public Health Nutrition, http://www.ihs.gov/NonMedicalPrograms/PlanningEvaluation/rrm-ch-public-health-nutrition.asp. Accessed November 17, 2005. Food Services. http://www.ihs.gov/nonmedicalprograms/planningevaluation/rrm-gsfo-food-services.asp. Accessed November 17, 2005.
157. Life Sciences Research Office, Federation of American Societies for Experimental Biology. *J Nutr* 120: 1559S; 1990.
158. Briefel, R.R. and Woteki, C.E., *J Nutr Ed* 24: 24S; 1992.
159. Alaimo, K. et al., *Am J Public Health* 88: 419; 1998.
160. Basiotis, P.P., in *American Council on Consumer Interests 38th Annual Conference: The Proceedings*, Halderman, V.A., ed., Columbia, MO, 1992.
161. Rose, D. and Oliveira, V., *Am J Public Health* 87: 1956; 1997.
162. Wehler, C.A., *Community Childhood Hunger Identification Project: New Haven Risk Factor Study*, Connecticut Association for Human Services, Hartford, CT, 1986.
163. Radimer, K.L., Olson, C.M., and Campbell, C.C., *J Nutr* 120: 1544; 1990.
164. Guyer, B. et al., *Mass J Community Health*, Fall/Winter 1985–1986, 3.
165. National Research Council, Panel to Review U.S. Department of Agriculture's Measurement of Food Insecurity and Hunger, *Measuring Food Insecurity and Hunger: Phase 1 Report*, National Academies Press, Washington, DC, 2005.
166. Blumberg, S.J. et al., *Am J Public Health* 89: 1231; 1999.
167. U.S. Department of Agriculture, *U.S. Action Plan on Food Security: Solutions to Hunger*, USDA, Washington, DC, March 1999.
168. Kuczmarski, R.J. et al., *Advance Data from Vital and Health Statistics*. no 314, National Center for Health Statistics, Hyattsville, MD, 2000.
169. Institute of Medicine, Food and Nutrition Board, National Academy of Sciences, Dietary Reference Intakes, http://www.iom.edu/project.asp?id=4574. Accessed October 13, 2005.
170. Institute of Medicine, *Dietary Reference Intakes: Applications in Dietary Assessment*, National Academy Press, Washington, DC, 2000.
171. Crane, N.T. et al., *Am J Public Health* 85: 660; 1995.
172. Lewis, C.J. et al., *Am J Clin Nutr* 70: 198; 1999.
173. Wright, J.W. et al., *Vital Health Stat* 11(243), 1998.
174. Centers for Disease Control and Prevention (CDC), DHHS, *Morb Mort Wkly Rpt* 49: 962; 2000.

175. Centers for Disease Control and Prevention, DHHS, Third National Report on Human Exposure to Environmental Chemicals, http://www.cdc.gov/exposurereport/3rd/. Accessed October 13, 2005.

176. Life Sciences Research Office. *Estimation of Exposure to Substances in the Food Supply.* Anderson, S.A., ed, Life Sciences Research Office, Bethesda, MD, 1988.

177. U.S. Environmental Protection Agency (EPA), Office of Air Quality Planning & Standards and Office of Research and Development, *Mercury Study Report to Congress,* EPA-452/R-97-003, Environmental Protection Agency, Washington, DC, December 1997.

178. Woteki, C.E., *J Nutr* 133: 582S; 2003.

179. Sims, L.S., in *The Research Agenda for Dietetics Conference Proceedings,* American Dietetic Association, Chicago, IL, 1993, 25.

180. Office of Science and Technology Policy, Executive Office of the President, *Meeting the Challenge. A Research Agenda for America's Health, Safety, and Food,* Government Printing Office, Washington, DC, February, 1996.

181. National Center for Health Statistics (NCHS), CDC, DHHS, Health-E Stats, http://www.cdc.gov/nchs/products/pubs/pubd/hestats/hestats.htm. Accessed October 13, 2005.

182. Centers for Disease Control and Prevention, DHHS, MMWR. Morbidity and Mortality Weekly Report, http://www.cdc.gov/mmwr/. Accessed October 26, 2005.

183. Human Nutrition Research Information Management (HNRIM) System, http://hnrim.nih.gov/. Accessed October 13, 2005.

184. Byers, T. and Lyle, B., *Am J Clin Nutr* 69: 1365S; 1999.

185. Sustainable Communities Network, http://www.sustainable.org/economy/agriculture.html. Accessed November 13, 2005.

186. Sustainable Agriculture and Food Systems Funders Group, http://www.safsf.org/. Accessed October 13, 2005.

24 Nutrition Monitoring and Research Studies: Observational Studies

Jenifer H. Voeks, Suzanne E. Perumean-Chaney, and Gary Cutter

CONTENTS

INTRODUCTION

The purpose of this chapter is to give an overview and to provide current examples of observational studies. Specifically, cohort observational studies that incorporate nutritional assessment are the primary focus of this chapter. After a brief review of the types and purposes of observational studies, a detailed description of the characteristics, advantages, and disadvantages of a cohort study is provided. Next, several cohort studies, which utilized nutritional assessments, are discussed to demonstrate the use of the cohort design in the area of nutrition. Finally, selected nutrition-related publications from these cohort studies are referenced along with the corresponding measured nutritional variables.

OBSERVATIONAL STUDIES

Epidemiology is classically known as the study of the distribution of disease in human populations; however, the definition expands and often overlaps with other areas of research. Observational studies in epidemiology include natural history studies, case-control studies, prevalence (cross-sectional or population) studies, and cohort (incidence) studies. The research question of interest would generally dictate which type of observational study would be used (see Table 24.1). For example, the diagnosis or frequency of a disease would be facilitated by using the prevalence study design. Cohort studies provide the opportunity to observe populations prospectively, thereby enabling the observation of incidence rates as well as prevalence rates. Risk factors and prognosis of a disease can be identified through several different types of observational studies.

OBSERVATIONAL STUDIES AND CLINICAL TRIALS

In this section we are primarily concerned with observational studies, but will briefly discuss the relationship between observational studies and randomized clinical trials. The primary difference between these two types of research is the randomization of subjects into study groups. Clinical trials allow for the randomization of subjects into various treatment or control groups,

TABLE 24.1
The Question and Appropriate Design

Question	Observational Studies
Diagnosis	Prevalence
Prevalence	Prevalence
Incidence	Cohort
Risk factors	Cohort, case/control, nested case-control, prevalence
Prognosis	Cohort, natural history

whereas observational studies examine the subjects according to their natural selection into groups.[1] In many instances, the results from randomized clinical trials and cohort studies do not always agree. For example, observational studies have consistently found an association between low β-carotene levels and elevated risk of lung cancer in smokers; however, clinical trials have failed to find beneficial effects of supplementary β-carotene, and indeed there is some evidence of harm.[2–4] Similarly, observational studies have shown hormone replacement therapy to have a protective effect on myocardial infarction, but randomized trials have shown a slight increase in risk.[5–8] These two recent examples have raised many questions about when observational studies will be as convincing as randomized trials.

A major reason for the discrepancy in results between randomized trials and cohort studies is related to measurement error of the exposure variable of interest, or, stated another way, selection biases. This measurement error, known as residual confounding, can result from confounding from unmeasured variables and confounding from measurement error in variables. In the smoking and β-carotene studies mentioned above, it has been suggested that residual confounding occurred in the observational studies due to imperfect measurement of smoking status.[9] If smoking exposure is imperfectly measured, and β-carotene is related to true smoking exposure but β-carotene is not related to decreased risk of lung cancer then there will still be an apparent protective effect of β-carotene on lung cancer even after controlling for smoking exposure.

A number of statistical methods exist to address this potential confounding after the fact; however, taking preventive measures to reduce the problem in the design of the cohort study may be a better and ultimately a more convincing strategy. Restricting the research topics, design, and analysis may help observational research to attain some of the desired benefits of randomization.[10] Other suggested approaches are for cohort studies to utilize biomarkers to more accurately measure the exposure of interest.

COHORT STUDIES

As noted in Table 24.1, the purpose of cohort studies is to identify the risk factors associated with a disease of interest, obtain the incidence of disease, or the prognosis of disease.[11] Cohort studies allow the development of a disease to be described and, as such, are often considered to be a preferred type of observational study.[12]

Some of the defining characteristics of a cohort study are given in Table 24.2. The first characteristic is the identification of a study cohort that currently does not have the disease of interest. Any group of individuals who have either been exposed to the same occurrence, live in a defined geographic area or have the same risk factors may be identified as a cohort.[1,12,13] When similar risk factors identify a cohort, a second, similar cohort without the identified risk factors and the disease of interest must also be obtained for comparison purposes[12].

A second characteristic is that the study cohort(s) is followed over time. Because the study cohort(s) is disease free, the cohort(s) is followed over time to see which individuals in the cohort(s) actually develop the disease of interest.[1,12,13] The new cases of the particular disease which developed within a specified time period are then measured to obtain the incidence and absolute risk of the particular disease. Finally, a comparison between the incidence in those individuals who had the risk factors and those who did not have the risk factors produce a relative risk and attributable risk of these factors on the development of the disease of interest.

Some argue that placebo groups from clinical trials offer excellent opportunities for cohort studies. This may or may not be true and depend heavily on the entrance criteria for the trial. For example, a prevention study in the general population may provide useful data as a cohort study, while one that attempts to prevent prostate cancer, for example, would be deficient because of the all male gender and the likelihood of self selection for participation by the "healthy' at risk participants.

ADVANTAGES AND DISADVANTAGES OF COHORT STUDIES

There are several advantages and disadvantages of using cohort studies over other types of observational studies (see Table 24.3). With respect to the advantages, cohort studies make it easier to distinguish cause from simply an association. Because the risk

---

TABLE 24.2
Characteristics of a Cohort or Incidence Study

1. Selection of a study cohort WITHOUT disease.
2. Follow study cohort over time (prospective).
3. Measurement of incidence and/or absolute risk (new cases developed in a time period).
4. Comparison of incidence in those with and without the risk factor (relative risk and attributable risk).

TABLE 24.3
Advantages and Disadvantages of a Cohort Study

Advantages	Disadvantages
1. Easier to distinguish cause from association	1. Results are delayed for low incidence or long incubation
2. Incidence can be obtained	2. Large N may be needed
3. Multiple outcomes can be studied	3. Expensive in resources
4. Standard questions and measurements can be used	4. Losses may bias results
5. May lead to identification of variables that can be experimentally examined.	5. Methods, criteria, and exposure status may change over time

---

TABLE 24.4
Factors Associated with Causality

1. The magnitude of the association's strength
2. The ability to show the association's consistency through replication
3. The association's identification of one risk factor to one outcome
4. The risk factor must precede the outcome
5. The outcome is sensitive to different levels of the risk factor
6. The association's logical adherence to current theory
7. The association's consistency with other information about the outcome
8. The association's correspondence to other causal associations

---

factors are measured prior to the development of the disease of interest, temporal order is established. Temporal order is one of eight factors classically associated with causality (see Table 24.4)[14] and strengthens a causal conclusion instead of simply describing a relationship between risk factors and outcome that is often found in other study designs.[1,11,14] To compare different cohorts based on risk factors assumes that both cohorts are similar except for the suspected risk factor. Because this assumption can rarely be completely supported, causal implications are restricted.[11]

Another important advantage to cohort studies is that the incidence of a disease can be useful to provide estimates of the impact that preventive programs might have, and can be used to identify programmatic needs and support budgetary plans for achievable reductions over specified time periods.[14] Further, multiple outcomes can be studied, and standard questions and measurements can be used to compare results found in this study to previously completed studies. For example, the Framingham study has provided important information on blood pressure, cholesterol, diet, eye disease, and a number of other risk factors and outcome measures.[15–21] Other studies, such as the Coronary Artery Risk Factor Development in Young Adults (CARDIA) study have emulated Framingham. In this study,[22] variables were selected for inclusion in the baseline examination because of their known or suspected relationships to cardiovascular disease and as such can be compared to Framingham results. The availability of multiple and often related endpoints in the same populations further enables one to study the temporal development and to study their inter-relationships. Finally, cohort studies may permit the identification of additional variables related to specific outcome measures, which can then be further examined experimentally.[13]

One of the most obvious disadvantages of the cohort studies is that the study's length has to be adequate enough to allow for the development of the disease or a surrogate of the disease of interest.[11,14] For example, consider blood pressure and cardiovascular disease. Cardiovascular disease is the ultimate outcome of interest, but the surrogate development of blood pressure is sufficiently linked to the outcome to make it a reasonable outcome in its own right. For those diseases or surrogates with low incidence or long incubation periods, the results are delayed. With low disease incidence rates, the sample size for each study cohort may need to be extremely large in order to make the necessary comparisons.[11,14] From a statistical perspective, power is directly related to the number of events and not just the sample size. With both a lengthy process and large sample size being usually necessary, another disadvantage is the expense associated with conducting the study.[4] The length of the study may also influence the ability to recapture all the individuals at the end of the study. This ability to recapture the study participants depends on their geographic mobility, interest in continuing the study, and their mortality rates.[14] The inability to capture all study participants and take account of their experience may bias the results[11,12] by so-called informative censoring and even if the biases are not there, low follow-up rates leave a suspicion of bias that is often difficult to overcome. The length of the study dictates other potential concerns. Methods, criteria, and exposure status may change over time. For example, environmental, cultural, or technological changes may influence the risk factors identified and the measurement of the variables under study, and this is especially true of biological risk factors such as weight.[12,14]

One modification of the basic cohort study design, known as a nested case-control study, inserts a case-control study into a retrospective or prospective cohort study.[1] In a nested case-control design, the baseline risk factor data is collected for the entire cohort, and all participants are followed for development of the disease. Once an adequate number of cases are identified, the risk factor is analyzed for the cases and a comparison group of controls. This type of study design can often be conducted at a fraction of the cost of conducting a cohort study. These studies cannot estimate the relative risk of occurrences, but can, because of the cohort from whom the nested case-control study comes, offer more information than a stand-alone case-control study.

SUMMARY OF OBSERVATIONAL STUDIES

Observational studies are an important part of epidemiological research, in that diseases are studied in their natural environment. Of the various types of observational studies, cohort studies provide the most valuable approach for identifying temporal relationships between risk factors and outcomes. The primary characteristic of cohort studies is that it enables the cohort (or a subgroup of it) to be identified disease-free at the beginning of the study, facilitating the study of the incidence of disease. The development of the disease of interest can then be measured and compared across cohorts. Like all observational studies, cohort studies have both advantages and disadvantages. The primary advantage is the cohort study's ability to distinguish cause from association while the primary disadvantage is the cost in time, money, large sample size, and loss of subjects, which can lead to substantive biases in the inferences.

EXAMPLES OF COHORT STUDIES UTILIZING NUTRITION ASSESSMENT

The remainder of this chapter focuses on eight selected examples of cohort studies that utilized some form of nutritional assessment (see Table 24.5). Although there are many cohort studies available and additional cohort studies that include nutritional assessments, the following examples were selected to provide a wide range of nationally recognized studies, unique uses of the cohort design, and, most importantly, different methods of collecting nutritional data. The selected examples include the following studies:

1. Framingham Study: Heart and Vascular Disease Program
2. The Nurses' Health Study
3. Coronary Artery Risk Development in Young Adults (CARDIA)
4. The RENO (Relationship of Energy and Nutrition to Obesity) Diet-Heart Study
5. The Health Professionals Follow-up Study
6. The Atherosclerosis Risk in Communities (ARIC) study
7. Women's Health Initiative Observational Study
8. Reasons for Geographic and Racial Differences in Stroke (REGARDS) Study.

FRAMINGHAM STUDY: HEART AND VASCULAR DISEASE PROGRAM

The purpose of the Framingham Study was to provide a population-based prospective examination of the development of cardiovascular disease and its risk factors.[23] The sample consisted of 5209 primarily white men and women between the ages of 30 and 62 years who lived in Framingham, Massachusetts.[23,24] Measurements were taken biennially from 1949 through 1989, representing one of the first prospective observational studies of its kind. Measurements included blood labs, medical history,

TABLE 24.5
Examples of Cohort Studies Utilizing Nutrition Assessments

Cohort Study	Years Conducted	Sample Studied	Outcome	Nutrition Intake Measurement
Framingham Study: Heart and Vascular Disease Program	1949–1989	5209 men and women, primarily whites, 30 to 62 years old	Cardiovascular risk factors	Semi-Quantitative Food Frequency Questionnaire (Willet)
The Nurses' Study	1976–1996	121,700 female registered nurses, primarily whites, 30 to 55 years old	Cancer risk factors	Semi-Quantitative Food Frequency Questionnaire (Willet)
Coronary Artery Risk Development in Young Adults (CARDIA)	Baseline: 1985–1986 Year 2: 1987–1988	5116 men and women, blacks and whites, 18 to 30 years old	Coronary heart disease risk factors	Baseline: Diet History Questionnaire (Interview Administered) Year 2: NCI (Block) Food Frequency Questionnaire
The RENO (Relationship of Energy and Nutrition to Obesity) Diet-Heart Study	1985–1993	508 men and women, primarily whites, 20 to 69 years old, normal/overweight	Cardiovascular risk factors	1. 24-h Dietary Recall 2. 7-Day Food Record 3. NCI (Block) Food Frequency Questionnaire
The Health Professionals Follow-Up Study	1986–1994	51,529 male health professionals, primarily whites, 40 to 75 years old	Heart disease and cancer risk factors	Semi-Quantitative Food Frequency Questionnaire (Willet)
Atherosclerosis Risk in Communities (ARIC)	1987–1998	15,792 men and women	Coronary heart disease risk factors and atherosclerosis and CHD events	Semi-Quantitative Food Frequency Questionnaire (Willet)
Women's Health Initiative Observational Study	1993–1998	93,721 women, primarily whites 50–79 years old	Causes of morbidity and mortality in postmenopausal women	WHI Food Frequency Questionnaire
REGARDS	2003–Ongoing	21,734 (to date) with in-home interview, Equal number of whites and African-Americans, 45 and older	Underlying causes for the geographic and racial differences in stroke mortality	NCI (Block 98) self-administered food frequency questionnaire completed after in-home interview

and a physical examination.[23] Additional assessments of stress, nutrition intake, and physical activity were added to the study at a later time. The latest nutrition intake was assessed through the Willet Semi-Quantitative Food Frequency Questionnaire.[24]

The Nurses' Health Study

Initially, the purpose of the Nurses' Health Study was to examine the relationship between oral contraceptives and breast cancer.[25] The study was then expanded to examine other female-related cancers, lung cancer, and life-style factors such as diet and exercise.[26] The sample consisted of 121,700 registered female nurses who were 30 to 55 years of age. Nurses, selected from 11 states, were chosen because they were expected to be more accurate in the reporting of the incidence of diseases and life-style factors and, in addition, were expected to have higher participation and retention rates.[25,27]

Measurements were requested biennially from 1976 to 1996. Unique to this study, researchers did not have personal contact with the nurse participants; instead, all contact was maintained through the mail. That is, study participants were required to mail in their bodily samples, anthropometric information and the various questionnaires.[25–29] Only when a participant was nonresponsive to mailing in the measurements were telephone interviews conducted. Measurements included basic demographics, medical history including the use of medications, blood and toenail samples, anthropometrics, lifestyle factors such as diet, exercise, and cigarette smoking, quality of life, and social support questionnaires.[25,26] In order to confirm the presence of a specified outcome (e.g., cancer, myocardial infarction, diabetes, or fractures), medical chart reviews were conducted when participants indicated an outcome's existence.[25,27,29] Nutrition intake was measured with Willett's semi-quantitative food frequency questionnaire, which assessed the consumption frequency of specified portions of food within the last year.[25,27–29] In 1980, the food frequency questionnaire identified only 61 common foods,[25] while the 1984, 1986, 1990, and 1994 measures were expanded to include 120 common foods and both vitamin and mineral supplementations.[26]

CORONARY ARTERY RISK DEVELOPMENT IN YOUNG ADULTS

The purpose of the CARDIA study was to identify risk factors that either contributed to or protected young adults from coronary heart disease.[22] The sample consisted of 5116 black and white men and women from four cities, who were 18 to 30 years of age.[22,30] Measurements were taken at baseline (1985 through 1986) and at two years (1987 through 1988) and biannually thereafter.[30–32] Baseline measurements included a sociodemographic questionnaire, medical (family history, current medical history, and use of medications), anthropometrics (weight, height, skinfolds, and various circumferences), lab work (lipids, apolipoprotein, insulin, and cotinine), blood pressure, lifestyle (treadmill test, questions on tobacco and marijuana use, and nutrition intake) and psychosocial questionnaires (type A/B personality, life satisfaction, hostility, social support, and job demand or latitude).[22]

Dietary intake was assessed with an interview-administered Diet History Questionnaire at baseline and the NCI (Block) Food Frequency Questionnaire at year two.[30,32] Reliability and validity of the Diet History Questionnaire were assessed in a preliminary study prior to its use in the main study. Reliability was measured through the simple correlation between a one-month test, and retest methods of the Diet History Questionnaire.[31,33] Accuracy was compared to 24-h recalls.

The nutrient intakes and mean caloric intakes of the Diet History Questionnaire were compared to the same variables derived from 24-h recalls,[31,33] NCI (Block) Food Frequency Questionnaire,[32] NHANES II,[31] and RDA's Body Mass Index[31] as an assessment of concurrent validity. For both reliability and validity, the Diet History Questionnaire appears to be more applicable for whites than for blacks. The relationship between diet and disease will await the results for this cohort, now entering their 20th year of observation and disease development.

THE RENO (RELATIONSHIP OF ENERGY AND NUTRITION TO OBESITY) DIET-HEART STUDY

The purpose of the RENO Diet-Heart Study was to examine prospectively over a 5-year period the behavioral patterns with respect to weight between normal-weight and mild-to-severe obese individuals.[34] The sample consisted of 508 healthy primarily white men and women between the ages of 20 and 69. Subjects were stratified by gender, weight (overweight and normal weight), and five age decades. Measurements were taken over an 8-year period (1985 through 1993). Measurements included history questionnaires (weight, activity, health, and demographics), anthropometrics, energy expenditure, laboratory analyses, blood pressure, pulse, weight and dieting measures, activity data (Caltrac Monitors and activity diary), nutrition intake and attitudes, cancer questionnaire, and psychosocial questionnaires (general well-being, depression, cohesion, locus of control, hostility inventory, social support, and perceived stress).[35]

Dietary intake was assessed through several measures. The first nutrition assessment was the 24-h dietary recalls measured at years one and five.[36] The NCI (Block) Food Frequency Questionnaire[37] was used to measure nutrient intake at years two, three, and five. Finally, a 7-day food record that collected information about the day, time, location, and the amount and type of food eaten was measured at years one, three, and five.[38,39]

THE HEALTH PROFESSIONALS FOLLOW-UP STUDY

The purpose of the Health Professionals Follow-Up Study was to examine the relationship between diet and two types of chronic diseases: heart disease and cancer.[40] The sample consisted of 51,529 primarily white male health professionals who were 40 to 75 years of age.[29,40,41] The health professions included dentists, optometrists, osteopaths, pharmacists, podiatrists, and veterinarians.

Measurements were taken biennially from 1986 through 1994.[29,40,41] Similar to the Nurses' Health Study, the measures were all self-administered, mailed, and the outcome identifications were verified through medical chart reviews.[29,41–43] The measurements included demographics, medical history, anthropometrics (height, weight, and body mass index), chronic disease risk factors (heart disease and cancer in particular), and lifestyle factors such as diet, physical activity, cigarette smoking, and alcohol use.[40–44]

Dietary intake was assessed with Willett's 131-item semi-quantitative food frequency questionnaire used as the expanded version in the Nurse's Health Study.[29,42] As in the Nurse's Health Study, the food frequency questionnaire assessed the consumption frequency of specified portions of food within the last year.[29,42,44] Dietary intake was assessed in 1986 and 1990.[41]

THE ATHEROSCLEROSIS RISK IN COMMUNITIES (ARIC) STUDY

The purpose of ARIC, a complementary study to CARDIA, was to measure associations of established and suspected coronary heart disease risk factors with both atherosclerosis and new coronary heart disease (CHD) events in men and women from four geographically diverse communities.[45] The project had two components: community surveillance of morbidity and mortality and a cohort component with repeated examinations of men and women from the selected communities. The cohorts were comprised of randomly selected samples of 4000 individuals aged 45 to 64 from a defined population in each of the four communities. A total of 15,792 participants received an extensive examination at which time medical, social, and demographic data were collected. All cohort participants were examined four times at 3-year intervals (baseline occurring in 1987–1989, the second in 1990–1992, the third in 1993–1995, and the final exam in 1996–1998) and then contacted annually to update their medical histories. Atherosclerosis was measured by carotid ultrasonography. Some of the risk factor data collected included: blood lipids and lipoprotein cholesterols, plasma haemostatic factors, blood chemistries and hematology, blood pressures, anthropometry, fasting blood glucose and insulin levels, electrocardiography findings, physical activity levels, dietary aspects, cigarette and alcohol use, and family history.[45] Diet was assessed using a semi-quantitative food frequency questionnaire adapted from the questionnaire developed by Willett.[46–48] The questionnaire was asked at baseline and then at each of 3-year follow-up visits.

WOMEN'S HEALTH INITIATIVE OBSERVATIONAL STUDY

The purpose of the Women's Health Initiative (WHI) Observational Study (OS) was to explore predictors and natural history of causes of morbidity and mortality in postmenopausal women and also to serve as a secular control for the WHI Trial.[49] The sample consisted of 93,676 women aged 50 to 79, enrolled from 40 centers throughout the United States between October 1, 1993, and December 31, 1998. These women met exclusion criteria for the various randomized trial components of the WHI (including not wanting to be randomized), but were willing to be followed. The follow-up interval for the OS was approximately 7 years. All OS women had a physical examination at baseline and 3 years. Additional data (risk exposures, health behaviors, and other less common diseases) were obtained with annual mailed questionnaires. Demographic, family, and medical history data, as well as risk exposure, were collected by self-report through standardized questionnaires. Physical measurements including blood pressure, height and weight, as well as blood samples, were collected at the clinic visits. Nutrition intake was assessed using the WHI Food Frequency Questionnaire,[49] which was derived from survey instruments used in previous studies.[50–53] The WHI food frequency questionnaire was composed of three sections including 19 adjustment questions used to calculate nutrient content of specific food items, 122 foods or food groups with questions on portion size and usual frequency of intake, and several summary questions on usual intake of fruits, vegetables, and fat.[54] The reference time for all questions was "in the past 3 months."

REASONS FOR GEOGRAPHIC AND RACIAL DIFFERENCES IN STROKE (REGARDS) STUDY

The purpose of the REGARDS study is to understand the underlying causes for the geographic and racial differences in stroke mortality.[55] REGARDS is an ongoing population-based longitudinal cohort study. The goal of the study is to recruit 30,000 individuals over the age of 45 with equal representation of men and women and whites and African Americans. Participants are randomly sampled with recruitment by mail, and then by telephone. Data on stroke risk factors, sociodemographic, lifestyle, and psychosocial characteristics are collected at the initial telephone interview. Physical and physiological measures, in addition to fasting samples, are collected during a subsequent in-home visit.[55] The NCI (Block 98) semi-quantitative food frequency questionnaire is used to collect dietary information. Participants are given this questionnaire at their in-home visit and are asked to return it by mail. Patients are then followed via telephone at 6-month intervals for up to 4 years for identification of stroke-like symptoms and events.

Selected nutrition-related publications from the aforementioned studies and their respective measured nutrient variables are shown in Table 24.6.

TABLE 24.6
Selected Nutrition-Related Publications From the Six Cohort Examples

Reference	Nutrition Variables
Tucker, KL, Selhub, J, Wilson, PWF, Rosenberg, IH. Dietary Intake Pattern Relates to Plasma Folate and Homocysteine Concentrations in the **Framingham Heart Study**. *Human and Clinical Nutrition*, 126:3025–3031; 1996	Folate intake, Ranking of dietary contributors to folate intake by gender and age (67 to 95 years old). Folate intake through supplements and breakfast cereals, orange juice, and green leafy vegetables
Colditz, GA. The **Nurses' Health Study**: A Cohort of US Women Followed Since 1976. *JAMWA*, 50:40–63; 1995	Selected Macronutrients and selected Micronutrients by breast cancer, CHD/stroke, colon cancer, fracture, diabetes, and other diseases. Fruits and vegetables by CHD/stroke, red meat by colon cancer, and caffeine by fractures
The Nurses' Health Study Hu, FB, Stampfer, MJ, Manson, JE, Ascherio, A, Colditz, GA, Speizer, FE, Hennekens, CH, Willett, WC. Dietary Saturated Fats and Their Food Sources in Relation to the Risk of Coronary Heart Disease in Women. *Am J Clin Nutr*, 70:1001–1008; 1999	Saturated fat consumption over 10 years. Saturated fat top five contributors. Saturated fat consumption by coronary heart disease risk factors. Red meat, white meat, high-fat, and low-fat dairy consumption by coronary heart disease

Continued

TABLE 24.6
(Continued)

Reference	Nutrition Variables
The Nurses' Health Study	
Liu, S, Willett, WC, Stampfer, MJ, Hu, FB, Franz, M, Sampson, L, Hennekens, CH, Manson, JE. A Prospective Study of Dietary Glycemic Load, Carbohydrate Intake, and Risk of Coronary Heart Disease in US Women. *Am J Clin Nutr*, 71:1455–1461; 2000	Selected macronutrients, selected micronutrients, and selected food sources by glycemic load. Energy-adjusted dietary glycemic load by CHD. Energy-adjusted total carbohydrate, type of carbohydrate and glycemic index by CHD
The Nurses' Health Study and The Health Professionals' Follow-Up Study	
Michels, KB, Giovannucci, E, Joshipura, KJ, Rosner, BA, Stampfer, MJ, Fuchs, CS, Colditz, GA, Speizer, FE, Willett, WC. Prospective Study of Fruit and Vegetable Consumption and Incidence of Colon and Rectal Cancers. *J Natl Cancer Inst*, 92:1740–1752; 2000	Frequency of fruit and vegetable intake by colorectal cancer age-standardized risk factors. Selected categories of fruit and vegetables by relative risk of colon cancer and rectal cancer. Selected categories of fruits and vegetables stratified by vitamin supplement usage by relative risk of colon cancer
Slattery, ML, Dyer, A, Jacobs, DR, Jr., Hilner, JE, Cann, BJ, Bild, DE, Liu, K, McDonald, A, Van Horn, L, Hardin, MA. Comparison of Two Methods to Ascertain Dietary Intake: The **CARDIA** Study. *J Clin Epidemiol*, 47:701–711; 1994	Total kcal, macronutrients, and selected micronutrients by gender and race
Liu, K, Slattery, M, Jacobs, D Jr., Cutter, G, McDonald, A, Van Horn, L, Hilner, JE, Caan, B, Bragg, C, Dyer, A, Havlik, R. A Study of the Reliability and Comparative Validity of the **CARDIA** Dietary History. *Ethn Dis*, 4:15–27; 1994	Total kcal, macronutrients, and selected micronutrients by gender and race
Bild, DE, Sholinsky, P, Smith, DE, Lewis, CE, Hardin, JM, Burke, GL. Correlates and Predictors of Weight Loss in Young Adults: The **CARDIA** Study. *Int J Obes*, 20:47–55; 1996	Baseline caloric and fat intake; change in caloric and fat intake at year 2 by gender and race
RENO Diet-Heart Study	
Dodds, MP, Silverstein, LJ. "The 24-Hour Dietary Recall." In *Obesity Assessment: Tools, Methods, Interpretations* (St. Jeor, S, Ed.). New York: Chapman and Hall, 1997	Total kcal, macronutrients, and selected micronutrients by gender and weight status. Total kcal, macronutrients and selected micronutrients by BMI and age
RENO Diet-Heart Study	
Scott, BJ, Reeves, RB. "Seven Day Food Records." In *Obesity Assessment: Tools, Methods, Interpretations* (St. Jeor, S, Ed.). New York: Chapman and Hall, 1997	Total kcal, macronutrients, and selected micronutrients by gender and weight status
RENO Diet-Heart Study	
Benedict, JA, Block, G. "Food Frequency Questionnaires." In *Obesity Assessment: Tools, Methods, Interpretations* (St. Jeor, S, Ed.). New York: Chapman and Hall, 1997	Total kcal, macronutrients, and selected micronutrients by gender and weight status. Total kcal, macronutrients, and selected micronutrients by BMI and age
RENO Diet-Heart Study	
Silverstein, LJ, Scott, BJ, St. Jeor, ST. "Eating Patterns." In *Obesity Assessment: Tools, Methods, Interpretations* (St. Jeor, S, Ed.). New York: Chapman and Hall, 1997	Number of foods per day, caloric density, number of meals per day and number of eating incidents per day by age group. Number of foods per day, caloric density, eating incidents per day, calories per eating incident, percent fat and total calories by gender and weight status. Breakfast eating variables by gender and weight status
The Health Professionals' Follow-Up Study	
Van Dam, RM, Huang, Z, Giovannucci, E, Rimm, EB, Hunter, DJ, Colditz, GA, Stampfer, MJ, Willett, WC. Diet and Basal Cell Carcinoma of the Skin in a Prospective Cohort of Men. *Am J Clin Nutr*, 71:135–141; 2000	Demographics related to nutrient intake, energy-adjusted dietary fat intake by relative risk of basal cell carcinoma of the skin, energy-adjusted intake of select micronutrients and relative risk of basal cell carcinoma of the skin
The Health Professionals' Follow-Up Study	
Platz, EA, Willett, WC, Colditz, GA, Rimm, EB. Proportion of Colon Cancer Risk That Might be Preventable in a Cohort of Middle-Aged US Men. *Cancer Causes Control*, 11:579–588; 2000	Mean alcohol intake, mean red meat intake, mean folic acid intake by colon cancer risk factors
The Health Professionals' Follow-Up Study	
Giovannucci, E, Rimm, EB, Colditz, GA, Stampfer, MJ, Ascherio, A, Chute, CC, Willett, WC. A Prospective Study of Dietary Fat and Risk of Prostate Cancer. *J Natl Cancer Inst*, 85:1571–1579; 1993	Fat intake by cancer-free members and by relative risk of prostate cancer. Levels of fat from various animal sources by relative risk of advanced prostate cancer
The Health Professionals' Follow-Up Study	
Giovannucci, E, Rimm, EB, Wolk, A, Ascherio, A, Stampfer, MJ, Colditz, GA, Willett, WC. Calcium and Fructose Intake in Relation to Risk of Prostate Cancer. *Cancer Res*, 58:442–447; 1998	Low and high intake of total calcium, total fructose, fruit fructose, and nonfruit fructose by age-standardized selected characteristics. Total calcium intake and total fructose intake by total, advanced, and metastatic prostate cancer

Continued

TABLE 24.6
(Continued)

Reference	Nutrition Variables
WHI OS	
Hsia J, Rodabough R, Rosal MC, Cochrane B, Howard BV, Snetselaar L et al. Compliance with National Cholesterol Education Program dietary and lifestyle guidelines among older women with self-reported hypercholesterolemia. The Women's Health Initiative. *Am J Med* 113:384–392; 2002	Total calories from fat, calories from saturated fat, daily dietary cholesterol among women with self-reported high cholesterol. Factors associated with compliance with National Cholesterol Education Program dietary recommendations
ARIC	
Houston DK, Stevens J, Cai J, Haines PS. Dairy, fruit, and vegetable intakes and functional limitations and disability in a biracial cohort: the Atherosclerosis Risk in Communities Study. *Am J Clin Nutr* 81:515–522; 2005	Dairy, fruit, and vegetable intake stratified by race and gender. Combined baseline intakes of fruit and vegetables associated with functional limitations and disability
ARIC	
Steffen LM, Jacobs DR, Jr., Stevens J, Shahar E, Carithers T, Folsom AR. Associations of whole-grain, refined-grain, and fruit and vegetable consumption with risks of all-cause mortality and incident coronary artery disease and ischemic stroke: the Atherosclerosis Risk in Communities (ARIC) Study. *Am J Clin Nutr* 78:383–390; 2003	Whole-grain, refined-grain, and fruit and vegetable intake related to risk of death and the incidence of CAD and ischemic stroke, with adjustment for age, sex, ethnicity, energy intake, and cardiovascular disease risk factors
ARIC	
Diez-Roux AV, Nieto FJ, Caulfield L, Tyroler HA, Watson RL, Szklo M. Neighbourhood differences in diet: the Atherosclerosis Risk in Communities (ARIC) Study. *J Epidemiol Community Health* 53:55–63; 1999	Neighborhood median household income and food and nutrient intakes, before and after adjustment for individual level variables Relationship between energy adjusted intake of fruits, vegetables, fish, and meat and living in lower income neighborhoods

SUMMARY

In summary, this chapter briefly describes the benefits of the cohort study and has provided examples of several studies that have used this form of design. There are certainly other forms that can be utilized to assess the impact of diet on disease or health. The value of prospective observational studies relative to cross-sectional studies, the necessary must be weighed against the real difficulty in obtaining, funding for them. Many such studies today are either directly sponsored by the government through direct funding via a contract or as add-ons to multicenter clinical trials. It is difficult to convince funding sources that observational studies, especially in disease areas where a good deal of information already exists, are worth the investment. Thus, adding components to existing studies such as a clinical trial can sometimes be done to gather prospective information. However, in this type of observation add-on, care must be taken to consider generalizability due to the eligibility criteria in the primary study.

REFERENCES

1. Hennekens, CH, Burning, JE. *Epidemiology in Medicine*. Boston/Toronto: Little, Brown and Company, 1987.
2. Hirvonen, T, Virtamo, J, Korhonen, P et al. *Cancer Causes Control* 12:789; 2001
3. Holick, CN, Michaud, DS, Stolzenberg-Solomon, R et al. *Am J Epidemiol* 156:536; 2002.
4. Woodson, K, Tangrea, JA, Barrett, MJ et al. *J Natl Cancer Inst* 91:1738; 1999.
5. Beral, V, Banks, E, Reeves, G. *Lancet* 360:942; 2002.
6. Hu, FB, Grodstein, F. *Am J Cardiol* 90:26F; 2002.
7. Lawlor, DA, Davey, SG, Ebrahim, S. *Int J Epidemiol* 33:464; 2004.
8. Vandenbroucke, JP. *Int J Epidemiol* 33:456; 2004.
9. Stram, DO, Huberman, M, Wu, AH. *Am J Epidemiol* 155:622; 2002.
10. Vandenbroucke, JP. *Lancet* 363:1728; 2004.
11. Monsen, ER, Cheney, CL. *JADA* 88:1047; 1988.
12. Friedman, GD. *Primer of Epidemiology*. New York: McGraw-Hill Book Company, 1987.
13. Zolman, JF. *Biostatistics: Experimental Design and Statistical Inference*. New York: Oxford University Press, 1993.
14. Slome, T. et al. *Basic Epidemiological Methods and Biostatistics: A workbook*. Monterey: Wadsworth Health Sciences Division, 1982.
15. Atwood, LD, Wolf, PA, Heard-Costa, NL et al. *Stroke* 35:1609; 2004.

16. Dhingra, R, Pencina, MJ, Benjamin, EJ et al. *Am J Hypertens* 17:891; 2004.
17. Fox, CS, Coady, S, Sorlie, PD et al. *JAMA* 292:2495; 2004.
18. Fox, CS, Cupples, LA, Chazaro, I et al. *Am J Hum Genet* 74:253; 2004.
19. Massaro, JM, D'Agostino, RB, Sr., Sullivan, LM et al. *Stat Med* 23:351; 2004.
20. Peeters, A, Bonneux, L, Nusselder, WJ et al. *Obes Res* 12:1145; 2004.
21. Weiner, DE, Tighiouart, H, Stark, PC et al. *Am J Kidney Dis* 44:198; 2004.
22. Friedman, GD, Cutter, GR, Donahue, RP et al. *J Clin Epidemiol* 41:1105; 1988.
23. Dawber, TR. *The Framingham Study: The Epidemiology of Atherosclerotic Disease.* Cambridge: Harvard University Press, 1980.
24. Tucker, KL, Selhub, J, Wilson, PW, Rosenberg, IH. *J Nutr* 126:3025; 1996.
25. Colditz, GA. *J Am Med Womens Assoc* 50:40; 1995.
26. Colditz, GA, Coakley, E. *Int J Sports Med* 18 Suppl 3:162S; 1997.
27. Hu, FB, Stampfer, MJ, Manson, JE et al. *Am J Clin Nutr* 70:1001; 1999.
28. Liu, S, Manson, JE, Stampfer, MJ et al. *Am J Public Health* 90:1409; 2000.
29. Michels, KB, Edward, G, Joshipura, KJ et al. *J Natl Cancer Inst* 92:1740; 2000.
30. Bild, DE, Sholinsky, P, Smith, DE et al. *Int J Obes Relat Metab Disord* 20:47; 1996.
31. McDonald, A, Van Horn, L, Slattery, M et al. *J Am Diet Assoc* 91:1104; 1991.
32. Slattery, ML, Dyer, A, Jacobs, DR, Jr. et al. *J Clin Epidemiol* 47:701; 1994.
33. Liu, K, Slattery, M, Jacobs, D, Jr. et al. *Ethn Dis* 4:15; 1994.
34. St. Jeor, ST, Dyer, AR. In: *Obesity Assessment: Tools, Methods, Interpretations* (St. Jeor, S, ed.) New York: Chapman and Hall, 1997.
35. Voeks, J. In: *Obesity Assessment: Tools, Methods, Intepretations.* New York: Chapman and Hall, 1997.
36. Dodds, MP, Siverstein, LJ. In: *Obesity Assessment: Tools, Methods, Intepretations* (St. Jeor S, ed.). New York: Chapman and Hall, 1997.
37. Benedict, JA, Block, G. In: *Obesity Assessment: Tools, Methods, Intepretations* (St. Jeor S, ed.). New York: Chapman and Hall, 1997.
38. Scott, BJ, Reeves, RB. In: *Obesity Assessment: Tools, Methods, Intepretations* (St. Jeor S, ed.). New York: Chapman and Hall, 1997.
39. Siverstein, LJ, Scott, BJ, St. Jeor, S. In: *Obesity Assessment: Tools, Methods, Intepretations* (St. Jeor S, ed.) New York: Chapman and Hall, 1997.
40. Rimm, EB, Giovannucci, EL, Willett, WC et al. *Lancet* 338:464; 1991.
41. van Dam RM, Huang Z, Giovannucci E et al. *Am J Clin Nutr* 71:135; 2000.
42. Giovannucci, E, Rimm, EB, Colditz, GA et al. *J Natl Cancer Inst* 85:1571; 1993.
43. Platz, EA, Willett, WC, Colditz, GA et al. *Cancer Causes Control* 11:579; 2000.
44. Giovannucci, E, Rimm, EB, Wolk, A et al. *Cancer Res* 58:442; 1998.
45. Atherosclerosis Risk in Communities (ARIC).http://www.cscc.unc.edu/aric/2006.
46. Diez-Roux, AV, Nieto, FJ, Caulfield, L et al. *J Epidemiol Community Health* 53:55; 1999.
47. Houston, DK, Stevens, J, Cai, J, Haines, PS. *Am J Clin Nutr* 81:515; 2005.
48. Steffen, LM, Jacobs, DR, Jr., Stevens, J et al. *Am J Clin Nutr* 78:383; 2003.
49. Langer, RD, White, E, Lewis, CE et al. *Ann Epidemiol* 13:107S; 2003.
50. Henderson, MM, Kushi, LH, Thompson, DJ et al. *Prev Med* 19:115; 1990.
51. Kristal, AR, Patterson, RE, Glanz, K et al. *Prev Med* 24:221; 1995.
52. Kristal, AR, Feng, Z, Coates, RJ et al. *Am J Epidemiol* 146:856; 1997.
53. White, E, Shattuck, AL, Kristal, AR et al. *Cancer Epidemiol Biomarkers Prev* 1:315; 1992.
54. Hsia, J, Rodabough, R, Rosal, MC et al. *Am J Med* 113:384; 2002.
55. Howard, VJ, Cushman, M, Pulley, L et al. *Neuroepidemiology* 2005; 25:135; 2005.

25 Nutrition Screening and Monitoring Tools

Ronni Chernoff

CONTENTS

INTRODUCTION

Malnutrition is not a condition that occurs rapidly; it is a chronic condition that develops slowly over time. It is widely accepted that malnutrition from any etiology is not a positive factor in health status, and may have a negative impact on other health conditions. There have been many reports of the health consequences of malnutrition, particularly in hospitalized individuals where poor nutritional status has been associated with increased lengths of hospital stay, poor wound healing, other comorbidities, complications, incomplete rehabilitation, readmissions, and mortality.[1–6] This is particularly important because it has been estimated that 85% of noninstitutionalized older adults have one or more chronic conditions, many of which are related to nutritional status.[7] If it is possible to identify indicators of risk for the development of malnutrition, and these factors are reversible conditions, then interventions that will alleviate risk can be instituted before malnutrition becomes overt and worsens chronic conditions.[8]

SCREENING FOR MALNUTRITION

Nutritional screening is of value if it: (1) reliably identifies the existence of risk factors for malnutrition, (2) recognizes the existence of poor nutritional status, (3) contributes to the avoidance of malnutrition, (4) minimizes suffering, and (5) the condition causing the malnutrition can be reversed.[7,9] Reuben et al.[7] describe criteria necessary to define the potential effectiveness of interventions; these criteria are whether or not identification of malnutrition can be achieved more accurately with screening than without it, and whether or not individuals who have malnutrition detected early have a better outcome than those who have malnutrition detected later in the course of their illness. Rush[10] defines the role of nutrition screening in older adults in different terms. He describes another criteria set for screening including specificity, sensitivity, inexpensive screening devices, and interventions in which health benefit is not sacrificed by not treating those who are at moderate or low risk. He indicates that screening is appropriate where there is a relatively small but important proportion of the population that is affected, where those who are affected can be identified by an easily applied tool, and where there is an effective intervention.

Subjective Global Assessment (SGA)

One of the first tools developed for screening was the Subjective Global Assessment (SGA). Devised by a group of clinicians in Canada, the SGA uses a brief set of history and physical assessment items to make an evaluation of nutritional status.[11] The SGA includes an analysis of weight changes, dietary change, gastrointestinal symptoms, functional capacity, medical status, and physical assessment (Figure 25.1). This tool relies on a subjective rating by using clinical judgment on weight loss, dietary intake, loss of subcutaneous tissue, functional capacity, fluid retention, and apparent muscle wasting.[8,11] This tool has been successfully adopted and used by physicians and nurses in clinical settings. The SGA has been tested in the clinical setting with different assessors with a high degree of interrater reliability (0.91).[12,13] Most of validity reports of the SGA were conducted on hospitalized subjects with a mean age of 50 years or older, which may contribute to some questions about its general applicability. In a recent report by a group of German investigators, the SGA was able to identify malnutrition-related muscle dysfunction, validated by using a measure of grip strength.[14] However, the addition of laboratory values to the SGA did not improve its validity.[12]

Nursal and colleagues[15,16] explored different approaches to increasing the reliability of the SGA in predicting malnutrition in hospitalized patients. In a series of 2211 patients, they examined two approaches to evaluating malnutrition and found that the issue of unintended weight loss and loss of subcutaneous fat on the SGA predicted malnutrition with 93% accuracy. In a subsequent study,[16] these investigators found that weighting several items on the SGA (MQ-SGA) outperformed the usual SGA in predictive value. The most important factor was loss of subcutaneous fat, whereas the least effective item on the SGA was weight loss during the previous 6 months. The sensitivity and specificity were derived from statistical tests conducted on their data from a sample of 2167 patients and those among them who had a score of 18 on the MQ-SGA, which is highly predictive of malnutrition. The most heavily weighted items were the loss of subcutaneous fat (10 points), sacral edema (6 points), and ascites (3 points).

Although the SGA is a short tool that can be used successfully by health practitioners, there are limitations as to its use as a screening tool. It requires a trained clinician to administer it because there is some clinical judgment involved, which would not be expected in someone who is not a health professional. It requires that the individual being assessed is undressed, which does not lend itself to community-based assessment programs, and able to be turned, which may not be possible for extremely ill patients.

A. History
1. Weight change
Overall loss in past 6 months: amount = # ________ kg; % loss = # ________
Change in past 2 weeks: ________ Increase
________ no change
________ decrease
2. Dietary intake change (relative to normal
________ No change
________ Change Duration = # ________ weeks
Type: ________ suboptimal solid diet ________ full liquid diet
________ htoicakiruc kuqyuds ________anorexia
3. Gastrointestinal symptoms (that persisted for >2 weeks)
________ none ________ nausea________ vomiting ________ diarrhea ________ anorexia
4. Functional capacity
________ No dysfunction (e.g., full capacity)
________ Dysfunction Duration = # ________ weeks
Type:________ working suboptimally
________ ambulatory
________ bedridden
5. Disease and its relation to nutritional requirements ________
Primary diagnosis (specify(________
Metabolic demand (stress): ________ no stress ________ low stress
________ moderate stress________ high stress

B. Physical (for each trait specify: 0 = normal, 1+ = mild, 2+ = moderate, 3+ = severe)
________ loss of subcutaneous fat (triceps, chest)
________ muscle wasting (quadriceps, deltoids)
________ ankle edema
________ sacral edema
________ ascites

C. SGA rating (select one)
________ A = Well nourished
________ B = Moderately (or suspected of being) malnourished
________ C = Severely malnourished

FIGURE 25.1 Features of the SGA.

THE NUTRITION SCREENING INITIATIVE

Keeping these criteria in mind, and looking for a way to make both professional and volunteer care providers more attentive to the malnutrition risks encountered by older adults, the Nutrition Screening Initiative (NSI) was established as a public awareness initiative with tools that could easily be used by community and health care workers who have regular contact with older adults. The tools included a checklist to identify risk factors — level I and level II nutrition assessment instruments. These tools were developed as a joint venture project, begun in 1990, of The American Dietetic Association, the American Academy of Family Physicians, and the National Council on the Aging. The premise of the NSI is that, if factors associated with malnutrition risk are identified early, interventions can be instituted that may delay or avoid the progression of the risk factors towards overt malnutrition.[17,18]

The NSI was developed as a nested set of tools that serve to identify risk factors for poor nutritional status and then to diagnose malnutrition. The items on the tools were developed by reviewing the literature and consensus among a technical advisory committee of experts. The checklist was tested using a follow-up sample from a previous study of nutritional status in older people.[19]

The Checklist

The checklist was created as a public awareness screening tool for use by health care and social services personnel and other providers who work in community-based programs in which older adults participate. The checklist was conceived and designed to bring awareness to nutritional issues that may impact on the health status of elderly clients. It is widely available for reproduction and information collection.

The checklist was titled "DETERMINE Your Nutritional Health" based on a mnemonic that contains the risk factors for malnutrition listed on the reverse side of the checklist. (Figure 25.2a and 25.2b) The checklist is a one-page questionnaire that can be used in community, long-term care, or acute health settings by volunteers, health aides, or health professionals. The objective of awareness of potential nutritional problems in older people was easily achieved; those who have been critical have built their criticisms on the basis of assumptions that have gone further than the original intent of the tool or the Nutritional Screening Initiative campaign.[20]

The items on the checklist were developed using the reference literature, expert opinion, existing databases, and pilot testing.[17–19] Using biochemical or laboratory parameters to define nutritional status may be misleading because the most commonly used measures, such as serum proteins, are affected by so many different factors that are independent of diet or nutritional status.[21]

Implementation Strategies

Screening can be conducted in many settings and by health professionals as well as health care workers or lay volunteers. Involving interested participants (nurses, aides, admission clerks, etc.) will increase the likelihood that data collection (weights, heights, completion of screening instruments) being more complete.

Modifications that allow the screening tools to be used in different settings and for unique purposes make this approach and instrument user friendly, applicable, and relevant. A tool that is flexible, valid and reliable, and allows different applications in diverse settings is very valuable. The easier and less time consuming it is to collect data that give insights into an individual's nutrition and health status, the more valuable the information. One example is the slight modifications made to the NSI Checklist for use in a dental office (Figure 25.3).[22,23] Dental professionals are in a unique position to monitor their patients' nutritional status as many of the consequences of poor nutrition manifest themselves in the oral cavity (bleeding or swollen gums; pain in mouth, teeth, and gums; angular cheilosis; alterations in the surface of the tongue). Additionally, oral health problems may contribute to the development of inadequate nutritional status because of lesions, loose or missing teeth, poorly fitting dentures, dry mouth, tooth decay or disease, and difficulty in chewing or swallowing.

The checklist can also be modified for use in specialized community or clinical settings. One example is the use of the checklist in a rural community setting as reported by Jensen et al.[24] They found that the checklist items indicating poor appetite, eating problems, low income, eating alone, and depression were associated with functional limitation.

Implementation Partners

The NSI was designed to be a project that included many health professionals working in partnership to identify nutritional problems in older adults. It is important to include any professional who has direct patient contact. Therefore, nurses are essential partners and participants in nutrition screening. They are the best individuals to gather anthropometric data and health history information; they are well-positioned to evaluate individuals' functional status by assessing ability to engage in activities of daily living (ADL) (self-care) and instrumental activities of daily living (IADL) (managing independence). Clinical nurse specialists (CNS) are uniquely positioned to conduct health and nutrition screenings in clinic settings, particularly to identify

(a)

The warning signs of poor nutritional health are often overlooked. Use this checklist to find out if you or someone you know is at risk.

Determine Your Nutritional Health

Read the statements below. Circle the number in the yes column for those that apply to you or someone you know. For each yes answer, score the number in the box. Total your nutritional score.

	YES
I have an illness or condition that made me change the kind and/or amount of food I eat.	2
I eat fewer than 2 meals per day.	3
I eat few fruits or vegetables, or milk products.	2
I have 3 or more drinks of beer, liquor, or wine almost every day.	2
I have tooth or mouth problems that make it hard for me to eat.	2
I don't always have enough money to buy the food I need.	4
I eat alone most of the time.	1
I take 3 or more different prescribed or over-the-counter drugs a day.	1
Without wanting to, I have lost or gained 10 pounds in the last 6 months.	2
I am not always physically able to shop, cook, and/or feed myself.	2
TOTAL	

Total Your Nutritional Score. If it's -

0-2 Good! Recheck your nutritional score in 6 months.

3-5 You are at moderate nutritional risk.
See what can be done to improve your eating habits and lifestyle. Your office on aging, senior nutrition program, senior citizens counter, or health department can help. Recheck your nutritional score in 3 months.

6 or more You are at high nutritional risk.
Bring this checklist the next time you see your doctor, dietitian, or other qualified health or social service professional. Talk with them about any problem you may have. Ask for help to improve your nutrition health.

These materials developed and distributed by the Nutrition Screening Initiative, a project of:

 AMERICAN ACADEMY OF FAMILY PHYSICIANS

 THE AMERICAN DIETETIC ASSOCIATION

 NATIONAL COUNCIL ON THE AGING

Remember that warning signs suggest risk, but do not represent diagnosis of any condition. Turn this page to learn more about the warning signs of poor nutritional health.

FIGURE 25.2 DETERMINE Your Nutritional Health.

risk factors that are modifiable before nutritional status begins a slippery slope downward. The advantage of implementing health promotion programs before or concurrently with the emergence of risk-associated conditions should be apparent.[25]

Other health practitioners (dentists, social workers, physical therapists, speech pathologists, etc.) may also use the screening tool for clients who may have risk factors for the development of malnutrition. Community workers who run senior centers, senior meal programs, home health agencies, etc. can also use the checklist to help identify those clients who may require more attention to their dietary intake, social circumstance, and chronic disease management.

The NSI contributed a unique approach to addressing the issues of malnutrition in older adults. It also opened the creativity of others to develop and test new tools in nutrition screening and assessment.

(b)

The Nutrition Checklist is based on the Warning Signs described below. Use the word DETERMINE to remind you of the Warning Signs.

DISEASE

Any disease, illness, or chronic condition which causes you to change the way you eat, or makes it hard for you to eat, puts your nutritional health at risk. Four out of five adults have chronic diseases that are affected by diet. Confusion or memory loss that keep getting worse is estimated to affect one out of five or more older adults. This can make it hard to remember what, when, or if you've eaten. Feeling sad or depressed which happens to about one in eight older adults, can cause big changes in appetite, digestion, energy level, weight, and well-being.

EATING POORLY

Eating too little and eating too much both lead to poor health. Eating the same foods day after day or not eating fruit, vegetables, and milk products daily will also cause poor nutritional health. One in five adults skips meals daily. Only 13% of adults eat the minimum amount of fruit and vegetables needed. One in four older adults drinks too much alcohol. Many health problems become worse if you drink more than one or two alcoholic beverages per day.

TOOTH LOSS/MOUTH PAIN

A healthy mouth, teeth, and gums are needed to eat. Missing, loose, or rotten teeth, or dentures which don't fit well or cause mouth sores make it hard to eat.

ECONOMIC HARDSHIP

As many as 40% of older Americans have incomes of less that $6000 per year. Having less - or choosing to spend less - than $25 to 30 per week for food makes it very hard to get the foods you need to stay healthy.

REDUCED SOCIAL CONTACT

One-third of all older people live alone. Being with people daily has a positive effect on morale, well-being, and eating.

MULTIPLE MEDICINES

Many older Americans must take medicines for health problems. Almost half of older Americans take multiple medicines daily. Growing old may change the way we respond to drugs. The more medicines you take, the greater the chance for side effects such as increased or decreased appetite, change in taste, constipation, weakness, drowsiness, diarrhea, nausea, and others. Vitamins or minerals when taken in large doses act like drugs and can cause harm. Alert your doctor to everything you take.

INVOLUNTARY WEIGHT LOSS/GAIN

Losing or gaining a lot of weight when you are not trying to is an important warning sign that must not be ignored. Being overweight or underweight also increases your chance of poor health.

NEEDS ASSISTANCE IN SELF CARE

Although most older people are able to eat, one of every five has trouble with walking, shopping, and buying and cooking food, especially as they get older.

ELDER YEARS ABOVE AGE 80

Most older people lead full and productive lives, but as age increases, risk of frailty and health problems increase. Checking your nutritional health regularly makes good sense.

 The Nutrition Screening Initiative, 1010 Wisconsin Avenue, NW, Suite 800, Washington, D.C. 20007
The Nutrition Screening Initiative is funded in part by a grant from Ross Laboratories, a division of Abbott Laboratories.

FIGURE 25.2 (Continued).

MINI-NUTRITIONAL ASSESSMENT

The Mini-Nutritional Assessment (MNA) is a tool that was developed to be used easily to evaluate the nutritional status of frail elderly individuals.[26,27] This instrument was developed to meet a perceived need to go beyond the DETERMINE checklist developed by the NSI, which was designed to raise the awareness of potential malnutrition risks, and the SGA, which was designed for use with hospitalized individuals. The MNA, therefore, was created to complement the screening tools already described.

The objectives for the MNA were to meet the criteria of: (1) a reliable instrument, (2) defined thresholds, (3) ability to be used with minimal training, (4) ability to be free of rater bias, (5) ability to be minimally intrusive to patients, and (6) ability to be inexpensive. The tool was designed to collect 18 items that combine objective and subjective data. These data include simple anthropometric measures (height, weight, arm and calf circumferences, and weight loss), general geriatric assessment items, a brief general dietary assessment, and self-assessment of health and nutrition perception. (Figure 25.4)

This tool has been validated in many clinical studies by comparing the scores with the judgments of trained nutrition clinicians, the NSI instruments, and a comprehensive nutritional assessment that collected in-depth data about the nutritional status

The warning signs of poor nutritional health are often overlooked. A checklist can help determine if someone is a nutritional risk:

Read the statements below. Circle the number in the yes column for those that apply to you. For each yes answer, score the number in the box. Total your nutritional score.

	YES
An illness or condition makes me change the kind and/or amount of food I eat.	2
I avoid eating a food group, i.e., meat, dairy, vegetables, and/or fruit.	2
I have two or more drinks of beer, liquor, or wine almost every day	2
I have tooth pain or mouth sores that make it hard to eat or make me avoid certain foods.	2
I snack or drink sweetened beverages two or more times per day between meals.	2
I had three or more new cavities at a recent dental check-up	2
I don't always have enough money to buy the food I need.	4
I eat alone most of the time.	1
I have a dry mouth, which makes me drink or use gum, hard candy, cough drops, or mints to moisten my mouth two or more times per day.	1
I take three or more different prescription or over-the-counter drugs daily.	1
Without wanting to, I have lost or gained 10 pounds in the last six months.	2
I am not always physically able to shop, cook, and/or feed myself.	2
Total	

Totaly your nutritional score, if it is:

0–2	Good! recheck your nutritional score in 6 months.
3–5	You are at moderate nutritional risk. Try to improve your eating habits and lifestyle.
6 or more	You are at high nutritional risk. take with your doctor, dental hygienist, or dietitian about any problems you may have. Ask for help to improve your nutritional health.

FIGURE 25.3   Nutritional assessement form modified for use in dental office.

of the subjects.[28] The MNA has also been tested in a variety of populations including cognitively impaired elderly[29] linked to other conditions common in older adults such as osteoporosis,[30] long-term care residents, and elderly individuals in different populations throughout the world.[29–38] These studies found that the threshold for the well-nourished on this instrument with a 30-point scale was 22 to 24 points; the threshold for malnutrition was 16 to 18 points on this scale. A short form with only six items[39] has been used with some success as a quick screening tool.[40]

The MNA meets its objectives of being a practical, noninvasive tool that contributes to the rapid evaluation of an elderly subject's nutritional status, contributing early intervention to correct nutritional deficits. This tool is easily used in a variety of settings including hospital, nursing home, home care settings, or physician offices or clinics.

UNIQUE NUTRITIONAL SCREENING TOOLS

Investigators from around the world have developed tools, using validated nutrition screening instruments such as the MNA as a starting point but modified for their unique populations. One example is the Chinese nutrition screen that uses the MNA as a base and adjusts for Chinese eating patterns, health care system, and culture. Using physicians' physical examinations as a method of validation, this tool had a 60% chance of correctly identifying people at nutrition risk.[41]

Another instrument using the MNA as a base was tested for use with elderly South Africans and validated using measures of ADL and IADL. The investigators[42] reported a sensitivity of 87.5% and a specificity of 95%.

Another group in Iceland, using the MNA as a base along with a screening sheet for malnutrition and a full nutrition assessment as validation, identified four items predictive of malnutrition (body mass index [BMI], unintended weight loss, recent surgery, and loss of appetite). The investigators suggest validation of this screening tool in other populations.[43]

The British Association for Parenteral and Enteral Nutrition (BASPEN) developed a nutrition screening tool based on four parameters (weight, height, recent unintentional weight loss, and appetite).[44] Another screening tool was developed and validated using interrater reliability between dietitians and nurses for the South Manchester University Hospitals Trust; this instrument used BMI, mid-upper-arm circumference, percentage of weight loss, and energy intake using the patients' first full hospital day intake.[45]

MINI NUTRITIONAL ASSESSMENT
MNA™

ID# _____

Last Name: _____ First Name: _____ M.I. _____ Sex: _____ Date: _____

Age: _____ Weight,kg: _____ Height, cm: _____ Knee Height, cm: _____

Complete the form by writing the numbers in the boxes. Add the numbers in the boxes and compare the total assessment to the Malnutrition Indicator Score.

ANTHROPOMETRIC ASSESSMENT

	Points
1. Body Mass Index (BMI) (weight in kg) / (height in m)² a. BMI < 19 = 0 points b. BMI 19 to < 21 = 1 points c. BMI 21 to < 23 = 2 points d. BMI ≥ 23 = 3 points	☐
2. Mid-arm circumference (MAC) in cm a. MAC < 21 = 0.0 points b. MAC 21 ≤ 22 = 0.5 points c. MAC > 22 = 1.0 points	☐.☐
3. Calf circumference (CC) in cm a.CC < 31 = 0 points b. CC ≥ 31 = 1 point	☐
4. Weight loss during last 3 months a. weight loss greater than 3kg (6.6 lbs) = 0 points b. does not know = 1 point c. weight loss between 1and 3 kg (2.2 and 6.6 lbs) = 2 points d. no weight loss = 3 points	☐

GENERAL ASSESSMENT

5. Lives independently (not in a nursing home or hospital) a. no = 0 points b. yes = 1 point	☐
6. Takes more than 3 prescription drugs per day a. yes = 0 points b. no = 1 point	☐
7. Has suffered psychological stress or acute disease in the past 3 months a. yes = 0 points b. no = 2 points	☐
8. Mobility a. bed or chair bound = 0 points b. able to get out of bed/chair but does not go out = 1 point c. goes out = 2 points	☐
9. Neuropsychological problems a. severe dementia or depression = 0 points b. mild dementia = 1 point c. no psychological problems = 2 points	☐
10. Pressure sores or skin ulcers a. yes = 0 points b. no = 1 point	☐

DIETARY ASSESSMENT

11. How many full meals does the patient eat daily? a. 1 meal = 0 points b. 2 meals = 1 point c. 3 meals = 2 points	☐

	Points
12. Selected consumption markers for protein intake • At least one serving of dairy products (milk, cheese, yogurt) per day? yes ☐ no ☐ • Two or more servings of legumes or eggs per week? yes ☐ no ☐ • Meat, fish, or poultry every day? yes ☐ no ☐ a. if 0 or 1 yes = 0.0 points b. if 2 yes = 0.5 points c. if 3 yes = 1.0 points	☐.☐
13. Consumes two or more servings of fruits or vegetables per day? a. no = 0 points b. yes = 1 point	☐
14. Has food intake declined over the past three months due to loss of appetite, digestive problems, chewing or swallowing difficulties? a. severe loss of appetite = 0 points b. moderate loss of appetite = 1 point c. no loss of appetite = 2 points	☐
15. How much fluid (water, juice, coffee, tea, milk,...) is consumed per day? (1 cup = 8 oz.) a. less than 3 cups = 0.0 points b. 3 to 5 cups = 0.5 points c. more than 5 cups = 1.0 points	☐.☐
16. Mode of feeding a. Unable to eat without assistance = 0 points b. self-fed with some difficulty = 1 point c. self-fed without any problem = 2 points	☐

SELF ASSESSMENT

17. Do they view themselves as having nutritional problems? a. major malnutrition = 0 points b. does not know or moderate malnutrition = 1 point c. no nutritional problem = 2 points	☐
18. In comparison with other people of the same age. how do they consider their health status? a. not as good = 0.0 points b. does not know = 0.5 points c. as good = 1.0 points d. better = 2.0 points	☐.☐

ASSESSMENT TOTAL (max.30 points):   ☐☐.☐

MALNUTRITION INDICATOR SCORE		
≥ 24 points	well-nourished	☐
17 to 23.5 points	at risk of malnutrition	☐
< 17 points	malnourished	☐

FIGURE 25.4 MNA form.

Investigators in the Netherlands developed and validated a short nutritional assessment questionnaire (SNAQ) for early detection and screening for malnutrition in hospital patients.[46] The questions most predictive of malnutrition focused on unintentional weight loss, a decrease in appetite, and use of supplemental drinks or tube feedings. Another group in the Netherlands focused on community interventions for elderly people in a randomized controlled trial[47] of an EASYcare instrument that includes IADLs, cognition evaluation, mood, and a goal-setting item, which were assessed in follow-up visits at 3 and 6 months after inclusion in this validation study.

It is evident that adjustments and refinements will continue to be made to nutrition screening tools so that the available validated, reliable instruments can meet the needs of unique populations. Although there are screening instruments that are widely used, adapting these tools to make them more useful in different settings with different racial or ethnic groups is important.

NUTRITIONAL ASSESSMENT IN OLDER ADULTS

The descriptions of the screening tools used to define nutritional status among elderly people highlight the fact that one of the more difficult determinations in elderly people is the accurate assessment of their nutritional status. This evaluation is more challenging in older adults because of the physiologic changes that occur with normal aging. Many of the commonly used assessment standards are not reliable in this population for a variety of reasons, one being the lack of validated standards.[48]

ANTHROPOMETRIC MEASURES

Anthropometric measures, including height, weight, and skin-fold measures, are usually important components of a nutritional assessment. These parameters are the ones most affected by the aging process.[49] The most apparent age-related change occurs in height. Height decreases as people get older because of changes in skeletal integrity, most noticeably affecting the spinal column. Loss of height may be due to thinning of the vertebrae, compression of the vertebral discs, development of kyphosis, and the effects of osteomalacia and osteoporosis.[50] Loss of height occurs in both males and females, although it may occur more rapidly in elderly women with osteoporosis. Therefore, stature changes and body appearance may be altered.

Height is difficult to measure in individuals who are unable to stand erect, cannot stand unaided, cannot stand at all owing to neuromuscular disorders, paralysis or loss of lower limbs, or are bed-bound due to other medical problems. One estimate of stature in these individuals is to measure their recumbent height or the bone lengths of extremities.[51] This estimate of stature may not be very reliable but it provides some estimate of height to help determine whether body weight is appropriate for height.

Weight is another important anthropometric measure that is altered with advancing age. Weight changes occur at different rates among elderly people. Use of most standard height and weight tables is not valid in older people as most reference tables do not include elderly people in their subject pool, and most are not age-adjusted.

BMI is a commonly used measure to evaluate relative weight for height using a mathematical ratio of weight (in kilograms) divided by height (meters squared).

$$Wt \ (kg)/Ht \ (m^2)$$

This formula yields a whole number that should be greater than 21 and less than approximately 35.[17] (*Note*: The upper healthy limit in older people is a matter of current dispute, but most experts consider that the limit is somewhat higher than in younger persons.) Nomograms and tables are available that minimize the need for calculation. Use of the BMI depends on accurate height and weight measures. It is used frequently to evaluate weight for height, but standards are not available for an elderly population.[52]

Skin-fold measurements (triceps, biceps, subscapular, suprailiac, and thigh) are often included in a thorough nutritional assessment. However, loss of muscle mass, shifts in body fat compartments, changes in skin compressibility and elasticity, and lack of age-adjusted references serve to decrease the reliability of skin-fold measures in the assessment of nutritional status in elderly people.[53]

BIOCHEMICAL MEASURES

Biochemical assessment parameters are also affected by advancing age.[54] Laboratory measures may reflect an age-related decline in renal function, fluid imbalances or hydration status, or the effects of long-term chronic illnesses. Among the commonly used biochemical markers of nutritional status, serum transferrin is one that is markedly affected by advancing age. As tissue iron stores increase with age, circulating serum transferrin levels are reduced. A lower-than-normal serum transferrin should be evaluated in relation to other biochemical measures and serum iron levels, if obtainable.[55]

The most commonly used predictor of nutritional status in elderly people is serum albumin. Serum albumin below 4.0 g/dl (depending on local laboratory normal ranges) is not usual in an older person unless the subject is overhydrated, has cancer, renal or hepatic disease, or is taking medications that may interfere with hepatic function. Recent evidence suggests that serum albumin is also altered when there is an inflammatory response, common with the presence of chronic disease, infection, or injury.[21] A depressed serum albumin level seems to be a primary prognostic indicator of rehospitalization, extended lengths of stay, and other complications associated with protein energy malnutrition in elderly people.[56,57] However, this malnutrition may be secondary to other causes and not correctable by increasing food intake. Unless there are medical reasons, most biochemical measures should remain within normal limits.

Serum cholesterol has been considered a risk factor for coronary heart disease, but a depressed serum cholesterol level is also associated with poor health status in older people.[57] It may be predictive of impending mortality[58] and should be evaluated carefully within the context of other health measures.

IMMUNOLOGIC ASSESSMENT

Tests for immunocompetence are often included as part of a nutritional assessment because malnutrition results in compromised host-defense mechanisms. However, the incidence of anergy is reported to increase with advanced age and the response to skin test antigens appears to peak after longer intervals in older people.[59] The value of these tests is limited in elderly people.

SOCIOECONOMIC STATUS

Social history, economic status, drug history, oral health condition, family and living situations, and alcohol use should be evaluated along with the physical and physiologic measures usually assessed.[48] It is also useful to assess elderly individuals using instruments that evaluate how well elderly people perform the ADL. Available tools assess the capability of an individual in managing the activities necessary for independence; these tools add another valuable dimension to the assessment of elderly people (Table 25.1 and Table 25.2).[60,61]

SUMMARY

Nutrition monitoring, screening, and assessment in the older adult population pose challenges to health care professionals because of the heterogeneity of this group and the wide range of their health status. The difficulty in using the tools discussed here is that people age at different rates and in different ways related to their health status, their lifestyle, and their genetic inheritance. Particularly in long-term care, the available instruments, particularly the Minimum Data Set (MDS 2.0), are not sensitive or specific for malnutrition risk.[62] Although there are a variety of reasonable approaches to nutrition assessment and

---

TABLE 25.1
Activities of Daily Living

Toileting
Cares for self; no incontinence
Needs to be reminded or needs help with cleanliness; accidents rare
Soiling or wetting at least once a week
No control of bladder or bowels

Feeding
Eats without assistance
Eats with minor assistance or with help with cleanliness
Feeds with assistance or is messy
Requires extensive assistance with feeding
Relies on being fed

Dressing
Independent in dressing and selecting clothing
Dresses and undresses with minor assistance
Requires moderate assistance with dressing and undressing
Needs major assistance with dressing but is helpful
Completely unable to dress and undress oneself

Grooming
Always neatly dressed and well groomed
Grooming adequate; may need minor assistance
Requires assistance in grooming
Needs grooming care but is able to maintain groomed state
Resists grooming

Ambulation
Totally independent
Ambulates in limited geographical area
Ambulates with assistance (cane, wheelchair, walker, railing)
Sits unsupported in chair or wheelchair but needs help with motion
Bedridden

Bathing
Bathes independently
Bathes self with help getting into bath or shower\
Washes hands and face but needs help with bathing
Can be bathed with cooperation
Does not bathe and is combative with those trying to help

Adapted from Lawton, M.P. *J Am Geriatr Soc*, 19: 4465; 1971.

TABLE 25.2
Instrumental Activities of Daily Living

Ability to use telephone
Shopping
Food preparation
Housekeeping
Laundry
Mode of transportation
Responsibility for own medications
Ability to handle finances

Adapted from Lawton, M.P. *J Am Geriatr Soc*, 19: 4465; 1971.

---

monitoring in the older population, it is wise for the clinician to understand that the definitive tool or definition of malnutrition in older people has yet to be reported and that there are vast opportunities for research in this area.

REFERENCES

1. Bienia, R., Ratcliff, S., Barbour, G.L., et al. *J Am Geriatrics Soc*, 30: 433; 1982.
2. Herrmann, F.R., Safran, C., Levkoff, S.E., et al. *Arch Internal Med*, 152: 125; 1992.
3. Galanos, A.N., Pieper, C.F., Cornoni-Hunt, J.C., et al. *J Am Geriatrics Soc*, 42: 368; 1994.
4. Harris, C.L., Fraser C. *Ostomy Wound Manage*, 50: 10; 2004.
5. Donini, L.M., De Bernardini, L., De Felice, M.R., et al. *Aging Clin Exp Res*, 16: 132; 2004.
6. O'Flynn, J., Peake, H., Hickson, M., et al. *Clin Nutr*, 24: 1078; 2005.
7. Reuben, D.B., Greendale, G.A., Harrison, G.G. *J Am Geriatrics Soc*, 43: 415; 1995.
8. Chernoff, R. in Chernoff, R. (ed). *Geriatric Nutrition: A Health Professional's Handbook*, 3rd edition, Gaithersburg, MD: Aspen Publishers, 2006.
9. MacLellan, D.L., Van Til, L.D. *Can J Pub Health*, 89: 342; 1998.
10. Rush D. *Ann Rev Nutr*, 17: 101; 1997.
11. Detsky, A.S., McLaughlin, J.R., Baker, J.P., et al. *J P E Nutr*, 11: 8; 1987.
12. Detsky, A.S., Baker, J.P., Mendelson, R.A., et al. *J P E Nutr*, 8: 153; 1984.
13. Baker, J.P., Detsky, A.S., Wesson, D., et al. *N Eng J Med*, 306: 969; 1982.
14. Norman, K., Schütz, T., Kemps, M., et al. *Clin Nutr*, 24: 143; 2005.
15. Nursal, T.Z., Noyan, T., Atalay, B.G., et al. *Nutrition*, 21: 659; 2005.
16. Nursal, T.Z., Noyan, T., Tarim, A., et al. *Nutrition*, 21: 666; 2005.
17. Lipschitz, D.A., Ham, R.J., White, J.V. *Am Family Phys*, 45: 601; 1992.
18. Wellman, N.S. *Nutrition Today* II, 44S: 1994.
19. Posner, B.M., Jette, A.M., Smith, K.W., Miller, D.R. *Am J Pub Health*, 83: 972; 1993.
20. Rush, D. *Am J Pub Health*, 83: 944; 1993.
21. Sullivan, D.H. *J Gerontology*, 56A: M71; 2001.
22. Boyd, L.D., Dwyer, J.T. *J Dental Hygiene*, 72: 31; 1998.
23. Saunders, M.J. *Spec Care Dentist*, 15: 26; 1995.
24. Jensen, G.L., Kita, K., Fish, J., et al. *Am J Clin Nutr*, 66: 819; 1997.
25. Curl, P.E., Warren, J.J. *Clin Nurse Spec*, 11: 153; 1997.
26. Guigoz, Y., Vellas, B., Garry, P.J. *Nutr Rev*, 54: 59S; 1996.
27. Guigoz, Y., Vellas, B., Garry, P.J. *Facts ResGerontol*, 4(suppl 2): 15; 1994.
28. Vellas, B., Guigoz, Y., Baumgartner, M., et al. *J Am Geriatrics Soc*, 48: 1300; 2000.
29. Arellano, M., Garcia-Caselles, M.P., Pi-Figueras, M., et al. *Arch Gerontol Geriatr Suppl*, 9: 27; 2004.
30. Gerber, V., Krieg, M.A., Cornuz, J., et al. *J Nutr Health Aging*, 7: 140; 2003.
31. Saletti, A., Lindgren, E.Y., Johansson, L., et al. *Gerontology*, 46: 139; 2000.
32. Cohendy, R., Gros, T., Arnaud-Battandier, F., et al. *Clin Nutr*, 18: 345; 1999.
33. de Rezende, C.H.A., Cunha, T.M., Júnior, V.A., et al. *Gerontol*, 51: 316; 2005.
34. Kuzuya, M., Kanda, S., Koike, T., et al. *Nutrition*, 21: 498; 2005.
35. Kucukerdonmez, O., Koksal, E., Rakicioglu, N., et al. *Saudi Med J*, 26: 1611; 2005.
36. Soini, H., Routasalo, P., Lagstrom, H. *Eur J Clin Nutr*, 58: 64; 2004.
37. Ruiz-Lopez, M.D., Artacho, R., Olivia, P., et al. *Nutrition*, 19: 767; 2003.
38. Chubb, P.E. *Asia Pac J Clin Nutr*, 14: 70S; 2005.

39. Guigoz, Y., Lauque S., Vellas, B.J. *Clin Geriatr Med*, 18: 737; 2002.
40. Ranhoff, A.H., Gjoen, A.U., Mowe, M. *J Nutr Health Aging*, 9: 221; 2005.
41. Woo, J., Chumlea, W.C., Sun, S.S., et al. *J Nutr Health Aging*, 9: 203; 2005.
42. Charlton, K.E., Kolbe-Alexander, T.L., Nel, J.H. *Pub Health Nutr*, 8: 468; 2005.
43. Thorsdottir, I., Jonsson, P.V., Asgeirsdottir, A.E., et al. *J Hum Nutr Diet*, 18: 53; 2005.
44. Weekes, C.E., Elia, M., Emery, P.W. *Clin Nutr*, 23: 1104; 2004.
45. Burden, S.T., Bodey, S., Bradburn, Y.J., et al. *J Hum Nutr Diet*, 14: 269; 2001.
46. Kruizenga, H.M., Seidell, J.C., de Vet, H.C.W., et al. *Clin Nutr*, 24: 75; 2005.
47. Melis, R.J.F., van Eijken, M.I.J., Borm, G.F., et al. *BMC Health Serv Res*, 5: 65; 2005.
48. Mitchell, C.O., Chernoff, R. in Chernoff, R. (ed). *Geriatric Nutrition: The Health Professional's Handbook*, 3rd edition, Boston, MA: Jones & Bartlett Publishers, 2006.
49. Mitchell, C.O., Lipschitz, D.A. *Am J Clin Nutr*, 35: 398; 1982.
50. Chumlea, W.C., Garry, P.J., Hunt, W.C., et al. *Human Biol*, 60: 918; 1988.
51. Martin, A.D., Carter, J.E.L., Hendy, K.C., et al. in Lohman, T.G., Roche, A.F., Martorell, R. (eds). *Anthropometric Standardization Reference Manual*, Champaign, IL: Human Kinetics Publishers Inc., 1988.
52. Cook, Z., Kirk, S., Lawrenson, S., et al. *Proc Nutr Soc*, 64: 313; 2005.
53. Chumlea, W.C., Guo, S.S., Glasser, R.M., et al. *Nutr Health Aging*, 1: 7; 1997.
54. Fleming, D.J., Jacques, P.F., Dallal, G.E., et al. *Am J Clin Nutr*, 67: 722; 1998.
55. Ferguson, R.P., O'Connor, P., Crabtree, B., et al. *J Am Geriatrics Soc*, 41: 545; 1993.
56. Sullivan, D.H., Walls, R.C., Lipschitz, D.A. *Am J Clin Nutr*, 53: 599; 1991.
57. Wilson, P.W.F., Anderson, K.M., Harris, T., et al. *J Gerontol Med Sci*, 49: M252; 1994.
58. Rudman, D., Mattson, D.E., Nagraj, H.S., et al. *J P E Nutr*, 12: 155; 1988.
59. Cohn, J.R., Buckley, C.E., Hohl, C.A., et al. *J Am Geriatrics Soc*, 31: 261; 1983.
60. Katz, S. *J Am Geriatrics Soc*, 31: 721; 1983.
61. Spector, W.D. in Spilker, B. (ed). *Quality of Life Assessments in Clinical Trials*, New York: Raven Press Ltd, 1990.
62. Bowman, J.J., Keller, H.H. *Can J Diet Pract Res*, 66: 155; 2005.

26 Dietary Intake Assessment: Methods for Adults

Helen Smiciklas-Wright, Diane C. Mitchell, and Jenny Harris Ledikwe

CONTENTS

INTRODUCTION

> One of the most difficult tasks in nutrition research is documenting the actual or habitual food and nutrient intake of individuals or groups.
>
> National Research Council[1]

There has been long-standing interest in assessing diets of individuals. Early in the twentieth century, nutritionists studied food and nutrient intakes in order to provide guidance in food selection,[2] to interpret clinical and laboratory findings,[3] and to establish dietary requirements.[4] In the latter part of the century, interest in dietary assessment was stimulated with the increasing evidence for the role of diet in promoting health and reducing chronic disease risk.[1,5]

Early investigators were concerned with many of the issues that continue to be important for dietary assessment: (1) selecting appropriate methods for collecting dietary data,[6,7] (2) assessing the day-to-day variability of intakes by individuals,[8–10] (3) establishing procedures for data analysis,[11,12] and (4) estimating food/food group and nutrient intake.[3]

We should not be surprised that assessment of dietary intake is a challenging undertaking. Food intake can be a complex behavior.[13] on any day, an individual may consume many different foods, on different occasions, both at home and away from home. Willingness and ability to report what is consumed can be influenced by social, environmental, and cognitive events.[14–16] Furthermore, food composition databases must continuously be updated to reflect an expanding food market place and an increasing number of dietary components associated with health.[17]

This chapter is organized to review the methods that are most commonly used to assess intakes by individuals. Attention is given to methodological validity as well as to the current emphasis on indexes of dietary quality, dietary supplements, and functional foods.

METHODS OF DIETARY ASSESSMENT

The common methods for assessing intakes by individuals are food records, recalls, and food frequency questionnaires. Several reviews of dietary assessment methods have considered appropriate uses, modes of administration and sources of error.[18–23] These are generally characterized either by the reference period in which respondents are asked to provide information (i.e., retrospective and prospective methods)[23] or by the time frame for which data are collected (i.e., quantitative daily and food frequency methods).[20]

There is no single, optimal dietary assessment method. The objectives of an assessment should be used as a guide in selecting the most appropriate method. Some 30 years ago, Christakis advised that the assessment method selected should be no more detailed, no more cumbersome, and no more expensive than necessary.[24] This advice is still sound. Assessment protocols, regardless of method, may need to provide highly quantitative and detailed data on food consumption. This would be the case for research studies such as clinical trials.[25] More qualitative data is likely to be appropriate when food intake information is used for dietary guidance and counseling.

FOOD RECORDS

Food records, also known as food diaries, provide a prospective account of foods and beverages consumed in a defined period of time. Generally, records are kept for brief time periods (1 to 7 days), but they have been kept for up to a month[26] and even a year.[27] To be representative of usual intake, multiple days of records are needed.[28]

Food records may be used to meet a variety of objectives. Records are useful for detecting imbalances in food intake and making dietary change recommendations.[29] They are used as self-management tools in weight loss interventions and may be valuable in predicting successful weight loss.[30] Food records have been used extensively to calibrate other dietary assessment methods.[31–33] Records are also useful for documenting compliance of an individual's food intake with a feeding protocol in studies where adherence to a specific diet regimen is important.[34] Intervention studies may use food records to document effectiveness.[35]

Food portions may be either weighed or estimated depending on the subjects and the purposes of the assessment.[36] While weighing foods will increase the accuracy of the portion size recorded, it can also increase respondent burden. Sophisticated scales that do not disclose food weights to subjects are available, decreasing respondent recording burden,[37] but increasing cost. A variety of portion size aids, listed in Table 26.1, are available when portion sizes are to be estimated.

While records are usually kept by respondents, they may also be kept by observers. When food intake is recorded by observation, trained personnel visually estimate dietary intake.[43] Observation is particularly useful when circumstances preclude self-reporting of food intake. Thus, observation has been used in assessing intake of nursing home residents. The Omnibus Budget Reconciliation Act[44] requires that all Medicare- and Medicaid-certified nursing facilities implement a standardized comprehensive assessment, including a measure of nutrient intake, for all residents. Observers visually estimate the portion of served items consumed (i.e., from all to none) by a resident.[45]

When using food records, consideration should be given to the record forms to be used as well as instructions and training for subjects, particularly regarding portion size. Instructions should include guidance on completing the record form as well as

TABLE 26.1
Tools for Portion Size Estimation

Type	Examples
Household measures	• Measuring cups and spoons[38]
	• Rulers[38]
Food models	• Food replicas[39]
	• Graduated food models[40]
	• Thickness sticks[38]
Pictures	• 2-Dimensional portion shape drawings[41]
	• Portion photos of popular foods[42]
	• Portion drawings of popular foods[38]
Food labels	• Nutrition facts label
	• Food package weights

TABLE 26.2

Sample Instructions for the Administration of a Food Record

To help us do the best analysis of your food intake, please follow these instructions

1. *Maintain your usual eating pattern.* Try not to modify your food intake, because you are keeping a record
2. *Record everything you eat or drink.* Be sure to include all snacks and drinks. Also include any vitamin or mineral supplements and the dosage for each day
3. *Write foods down as soon as you eat them.* Three daily record pages are provided for each day; however, you may not need to use all three. Try to write clearly

Details are Important!

Completing the food record form

1. *Date.* Please record the date at the top of each form
2. *Name.* Please write your name in the space at the top of the form
3. *Time of Day.* Record the time of the day you ate each meal, including AM or PM
4. *Meal/where prepared?* Record the name of the meal eaten (i.e., breakfast, lunch, dinner, supper, or snack) and where the meal was prepared (i.e., at home or at a restaurant)
5. *Food item.* Write the name of each food item eaten
6. *Description/preparation.* Include information on how each food was prepared
7. *Amount.* Record the amount of each food either by using the poster provided or common household measures

---

directives encouraging subjects to record foods at the time of consumption and not to alter normal eating patterns. Table 26.2 provides sample instructions for the administration of a food record.

After records have been completed, they should be reviewed to ensure completion. If reviewed with the subject, probing questions may be used to clear up ambiguities and ensure the completeness of the record. These are termed interviewer-assisted food records. When data from food records are to be compiled and analyzed, records will need to be coded using a standard method.

As subject burden can be high for food records, participant willingness and abilities are to be considered when using this method. Literacy is required for completion of records; therefore, the method may not be appropriate for all individuals. The act of keeping food records can affect dietary intake,[46] which may be critical for estimates of usual intake. Cost is an additional consideration, as reviewing records for completeness, data entry, and data analysis can be expensive.[23]

RECALLS

Dietary recall provides a retrospective record of intake over a defined time period. While dietary recall may be for any length of time, this method is almost always administered to cover a 24-h time period and is generally termed the 24-h recall. Data can be collected either for the previous day or for the 24-h preceding the interview. To estimate the usual intake of individuals, multiple recalls are needed, preferably on random, nonconsecutive days, including weekends and weekdays.[21,27] Typically, an individual is asked to recall all foods eaten during the reference time period, describe the foods, and estimate the quantities consumed.

The 24-h recall has become a favored way of collecting dietary data[47] as recalls can be administered easily and quickly with low respondent burden. Depending on the objectives of the recall, the amount and depth of information collected will vary. This method is becoming the gold standard; particularly as methodological improvements[48–52] and technological capabilities[53] increase validity. With the emergence of technological aids in dietary assessment, it is becoming more common for interviewers to collect intake data using interactive software, entering intake data directly into a computer as it is collected.

Recalls may be obtained either in-person or by telephone-administered interviews. Because recalls by telephone interview have been shown to be practical, valid, and cost-effective,[53–55] they are becoming an increasingly popular mode of data collection, especially for research and population-monitoring purposes.

Prior to conducting recalls, training of interviewers is important. This is particularly relevant when more quantitative data are required, increasing the need to use multiple pass and probing techniques. Figure 26.1 provides a sample probing sequence to elicit detailed information regarding one specific food (i.e., macaroni and cheese). The complexity of this probing sequence exemplifies the potentially complex nature of probing questions and need for good interviewer training. More qualitative food intake data can be achieved with more limited questions.

The 24-h recall has been criticized because of accuracy related to portion size estimation and subject memory. Portion size estimation aids are available to facilitate quantity estimation (Table 26.1). While 24-h recalls are not designed to affect the "encoding" of food information, they can incorporate strategies to facilitate memory retrieval. Those strategies include

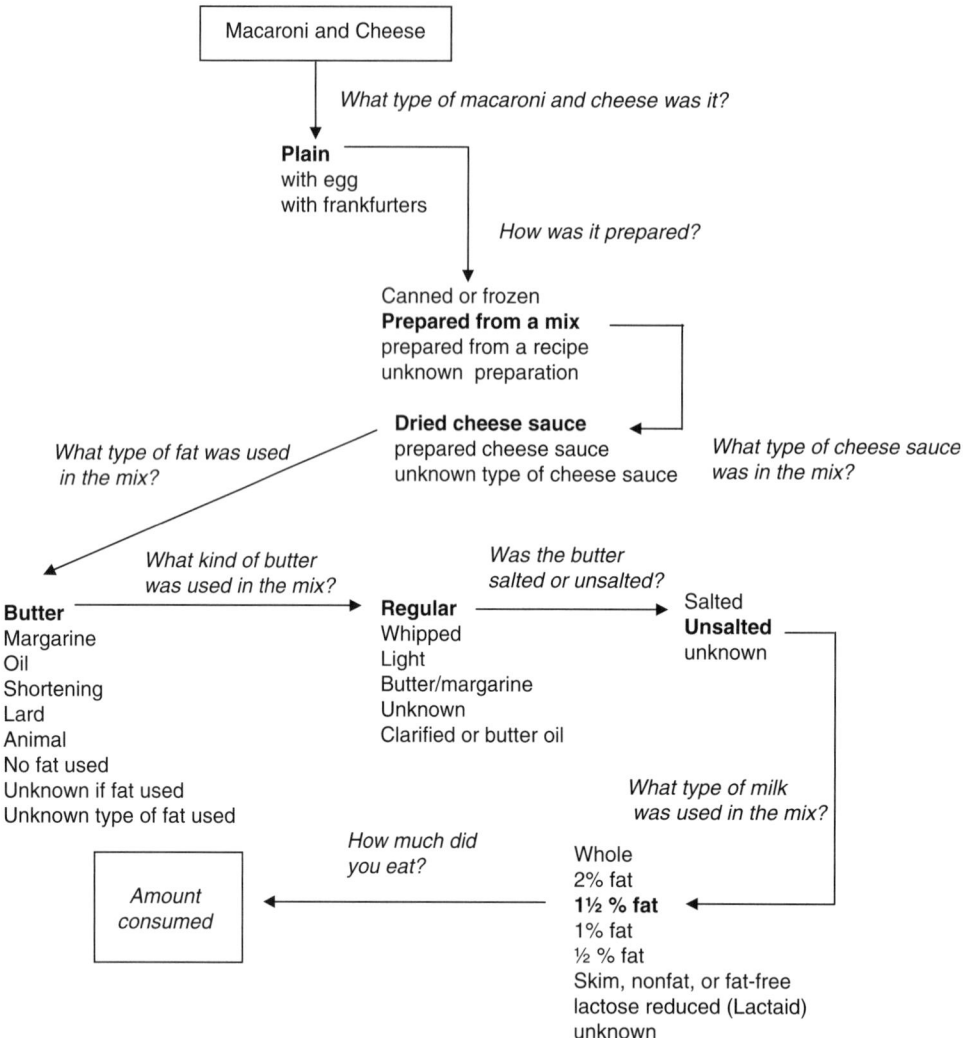

FIGURE 26.1   A sample probing scheme. This scheme could be used with recalls to elicit more information from a respondent that consumed macaroni and cheese. Bold print indicates respondent's reply. Probing questions, which are specific for each response, are italicized. (Adapted from Nutrition Data System for Research [NDS-R] software, developed by the Nutrition Coordination Center [NCC], University of Minnesota, Minneapolis, MN.)

standardized data collection protocols, structured probes to ensure standardized collection and interactive interview systems.[47] The multiple-pass technique, which will be discussed in "Current Issues in Assessment and Analysis," has also been designed to facilitate memory retrieval.

FOOD FREQUENCY METHODS

Food frequency methods are designed to obtain information about usual long-term food consumption patterns. The methods evolved from the dietary history method originally developed by Burke.[56] The dietary history interview included a 24-h recall, a 3-day food record, and a check-list of foods with questions about likes, dislikes, and consumption over the previous month. It was time consuming to administer and process the dietary information. However, the checklist with its list of foods and consumption options was the basis of food frequency questionnaires (FFQ) widely used in epidemiologic studies. The use of FFQ in large epidemiologic studies assumes the importance of usual dietary exposures to morbidity and mortality.[22] The use in epidemiologic studies also reflects the feasibility of administration.

FFQs consist of a list of foods, frequency-of-use response categories and may also include portion size response categories. Food lists may be extensive in order to provide estimates of total intake. Commonly used FFQs are The Nurses' Health Study Dietary Questionnaire[22] and the NCI FFQ developed by Block et al.[31]

Food frequency questionnaires may be abbreviated when used to screen for nutritional risk or when the focus is on specific foods (e.g., fruits and vegetables[57] and soy foods[58]) or nutrients (e.g., fats[59] and folate[60]). While not necessarily appropriate for identifying precise nutrient intake, these instruments can provide a rapid, cost-effective way to estimate usual intake. Very abbreviated instruments may not be representative of true intake.[61]

Subar has provided a succinct but thorough summary of considerations in selecting an FFQ.[62] A basic question is whether to select or adapt a commonly used questionnaire, or to develop and validate a new instrument. Willett[22] and others[63,64] have described the very intensive processes involved with the development of new FFQs. An example of the development process and the use of cognitive interviewing are described for the new National Cancer Institute Diet History Questionnaire.[64] Validating a new instrument or administration of a standard instrument on a specific population is also challenging. FFQs are commonly validated by calibrations with other dietary assessment method.[33,65,66] Kipnis and colleagues used biomarkers for energy and protein validation in the Observing Protein and Energy Nutrition (OPEN) study.[67]

FFQs without portion size information generally provide qualitative data. If portion size information is included, nutrient intakes may be estimated to enable relative ranking of intakes. Several investigators have studied the use of standard versus reported portion intakes. Laus and colleagues[68] found little difference in nutrient estimates when a standard (medium-size) portion was substituted for reported sizes. However, others have indicated that the use of standard portion size data may attenuate relationships between diet and disease.[69]

SUMMARY

Several methods have been listed that can be used to assess the dietary intake of adults. Well-designed quality control procedures are particularly important in research studies to ensure consistency of data across time and subjects. Additionally, the advantages and disadvantages of data collection modes (i.e., self- or interviewer-completed) should be considered (see Table 26.3). The success of any assessment method is based on a partnership between the individual respondent and the assessment staff. Care should be taken to ensure the appropriateness of the method and the level of detail collected. Respecting participants' abilities and ensuring their dignity is not compromised is salient in establishing a successful partnership.

ISSUES AFFECTING VALIDITY

In his address at the First International Conference on Dietary Assessment Methods, Beaton stated, "There has been a great deal published about the errors in dietary data ... this is understandable, but unfortunate because it can easily leave the impression that dietary data are worthless."[70] He reminded his audience that, while dietary intake data cannot and never will be estimated without error, a serious limitation is not the errors themselves, but failure to understand the nature of the errors and the consequent impact on data analysis and interpretation. Several reviews have delineated potential sources of error for different assessment methods.[21,22,37] Issues for consideration include: (1) accuracy with which individuals can or are willing to report food items eaten as well as portion sizes, (2) representation of usual intake and (3) adequacy of diet calculation systems, both data entry and food composition bases, to reflect composition of foods eaten.[22] Food composition database issues are covered in Chapter 1. In this chapter, we include potential error sources that can affect validity. Consideration of strategies to minimize error is pertinent in yielding accurate intake data, regardless of assessment method (see Table 26.4).

TABLE 26.3
Self-Completed and Interviewer Completed Data Collection

Collection mode	Advantages	Disadvantages
Self	• Interviewer training not needed • Sense of privacy • Data collection time may be reduced	• Response rate may be low • Respondent burden may be high • Tasks may be misinterpreted • Respondent training needed for more complete data • Data preparation and entry time may be high
Interviewer by phone	• Good Response rate • Opportunities for probing • Low Respondent Burden • Relatively quick • Interviewer anonymity	• Contact times may be inconvenient • Hearing problems for some subjects • Availability of portion aids • Data collection may be more expensive for toll calls • Potential for interviewer bias
Interviewer in person	• Good response rate • Opportunities for probing • Low respondent burden • Respondent interviewer rapport	• Contact times may be inconvenient • Potential for interviewer bias

TABLE 26.4
Benefits Derived from Minimizing Assessment Error

Clinical setting	Research Setting
• Improve ability to detect inadequate, imbalanced, or excessive dietary intake	• Improve accuracy of nutrient intake estimations
• Provide a better basis for nutrition counseling and interventions	• Decrease attenuation between intake data and biomarkers
• Improve ability to monitor dietary changes	• Provide a better basis for nutrition education program
	• Provide a better basis for elucidation of diet-disease relationships

MEMORY

Recalls and FFQs require that respondents remember intakes, albeit for different time frames. Our understanding of memory for diet assessment has been developed from advances in cognitive psychology as described by Dwyer and colleagues.[14] Critical memory processes include: encoding information, transmission to long-term memory, and retrieval.[71–73] Early studies described strategies for encoding information as well as strategies for retrieving memories, such as free recall, recognition, and cued recall.

The memory model of cognitive psychology is applicable to dietary recall.[74] To accurately report intake, people must be able to remember what foods were consumed, how the foods were prepared and the quantities of foods eaten. This requires the acquisition of specific food memories and the ability to retrieve the memories. Individuals that pay little attention to foods consumed as well as people that have difficulty storing information in memory, and those that lack the cognitive ability to retrieve food memories may have difficulty in recalling dietary intake.

Several techniques have been developed to reduce memory-related error in dietary data. For the 24-h recall, techniques such as probing (See Figure 26.1),[75] encoding strategies,[74] memory retrieval cues,[25] and multiple pass[48,51,52,63] have been employed to improve memory. Campbell and Dodd's[75] classic paper showed that probing elicited additional information with significant impact on total caloric intake. Ervin and Smiciklas-Wright found that older adults were able to remember more foods when a deeper processing strategy was used during encoding and a recognition task was used for memory retrieval.[74] Record assisted recalls may be used to help reduce memory-related errors in food records.[76,77]

Recent work suggest that 24-h recalls which incorporate a multiple-pass technique into a standardized interview protocol with structured probes can reduce the commonly observed underestimation of intake for groups of individuals. A multiple-pass technique provides respondents several opportunities (i.e., passes) to recall foods eaten using both free recall and cued (probed recall) strategies.[48,50–52] Historically, the strategy involves three recall passes: an introductory opening sequence in which a respondent is asked to recall all items eaten; an interactive, structural probe sequence to elicit detailed food descriptions and amounts; and a final review of the recall. The multiple-pass technique is theoretically sound and when incorporated into a well-structured interactive interview process may decrease underreporting for groups of individuals.[48,50] More recently, Conway et al. have developed and tested newer multiple pass methodologies that include five passes: (1) a quick list or uninterrupted listing of all foods and beverages; (2) a forgotten foods list or questions about nine food categories that are often forgotten; (3) time of day foods were consumed and the eating occasion; (4) detailed questions about each food including preparation and amounts consumed; (5) a final review and probe of all foods consumed. Research using these newer methods has demonstrated in an experimental setting that individuals are able to accurately report intakes within 10% of actual intake for obese and normal weight men and women.[51,52] While these studies are encouraging for the presentation of group data, there is room for improvement in assessing individuals' intakes.[48] There is little data, however, comparing alternative modes of administering a multiple pass strategy and the "gains" at each pass.

A multiple-pass technique can be facilitated by the use of interactive software.[78] This allows for a greater level of detail and facilitates data collection, but the technology is generally expensive and is not used commonly in clinical settings. However, written tools, such as probing guides, may be used to mimic this process when quantitative analysis is critical.

PORTION SIZES

Many individuals have difficulty estimating amounts of foods and beverages.[79–81] Errors may occur because the visual memory is not retained or knowledge is lacking to estimate amounts.[74] There is a tendency toward overestimation of smaller portion sizes and underestimation of larger portion sizes. Portion size estimation aids (Table 26.1) may reduce portion size estimation error.[82]

Estimation aids vary in sophistication and cost. Choice of tools is dictated partially by feasibility. In a clinical setting, aids such as food replicas, real foods, and food picture books may be appropriate. For interviews conducted by phone, tools that are compact for mailing, such as a chart with two-dimensional portions,[83,84] would be more appropriate. Commonly used food models and portion estimation aids may not adequately depict the increased portion sizes customarily consumed by many persons.[85] Harnack and coworkers[86] reported that typically used models resulted in underreporting of several foods served in a restaurant. With larger-sized modes, reported amounts more closely matched amounts actually consumed. This is consistent with cognitive studies that support respondents' preferences for aids more similar to portions eaten.[87] Cognitive psychologists have recommended aids such as moldable objects or modifiable computer images to assist in portion estimation.[87]

A number of investigators have investigated whether training subjects to "judge" portion sizes improves quantity estimates.[88–90] These studies suggest that training effects may be retained for some days after training and may have significant impact on some, but not all foods. For example, amorphous foods (e.g., salads) are more resistant to training effects. Methods such as digital photography have been shown to reduce reported portion size errors and may be useful in settings allowing for direct observation of food selection.[91]

CONSUMPTION FREQUENCY

Accurate estimation of how often foods are consumed is important for accurate estimations by food frequency methods. The cognitive demands required to estimate consumption frequency contribute to the error involved with these methods. For food frequency questionnaires, frequency of consumption estimates may contribute more error than portion size estimates.[92] Willett[22] considers the challenges to selecting proper response format. Options include multiple-choice versus open-ended responses. It has been suggested that the precision of food frequency questionnaires can be increased by not using predefined consumption frequency categories (i.e., multiple choice), instead allowing participants to simply enter a number to reflect intake (i.e., open-ended).[92] However, multiple-choice categories may lead to fewer errors than open-ended categories. Decisions about number of response options may also affect ease of recall and precision of responses. Not surprisingly, Willett alludes to FFQ formats as appearing simple but providing opportunities for pitfalls.[22]

RESPONSE BIAS

All assessment methods are subject to response bias. Social desirability may lead some individuals to selectively omit foods that may be regarded as unacceptable (e.g., alcohol and high-fat foods),[23] while others may report eating a healthier diet than was actually consumed.[93,94] Self-reported assessment data may also be biased by participation in a dietary intervention.[95]

For both interviewer-assisted and self-completed assessments, questions should be reviewed for face validity to help ensure that the participant's comprehension of the questions is appropriate. When using interviewers to collect data, training to avoid leading questions and verbal and nonverbal cues that may appear to be judgmental can decrease response bias. Quality control procedures can ensure that interviewer questioning is consistent and nonbiasing.[96,97] Conducting interviews by telephone may reduce bias as compared to face-to-face interviews.[48]

In regard to particular assessment methods, food frequency questionnaires may be subject to response bias as current diet may influence recall of dietary intake in the past,[98] especially, for individuals with a diet-related illness.[99] Response bias can also be induced by methods with a high participant burden. For example, the burden of keeping food records may lead subjects to submit incomplete records, introducing a response bias.[100] Techniques that reduce respondent burden, such as interviewer-assisted food records, can reduce this effect and may improve the quality of data collected.

VARIABILITY OF INTAKE

Day-to-day variation of food intake has been well documented in the literature.[27,101,102] Accordingly, assessment of an individual's total dietary intake, particularly by quantitative daily methods, at any one time may not yield an accurate measure of usual intake.[27] Basiotis et al.[103] found that over 100 days of dietary data may be needed to accurately estimate an individual's typical intake for certain nutrients, such as vitamin A. To lessen the effect of day-to-day dietary variation when using 24-h recalls, assessment should be done on multiple, random, nonconsecutive days[27,104] that include both weekend and weekdays. For food records and 24-h recalls, increasing the number of assessment days will decrease error related to variation in food intake; however, this must be balanced with subject tolerability and assessment objectives.

Several statistical approaches have been developed for estimating usual dietary intake distributions at the population level when intake data are collected by 24-h recalls. A method developed at Iowa State University, the ISU method, based its estimates from distributions available for two independent days from a subsample of individuals.[105,106] Freedman and colleagues[107] adjusted 24-h recall energy intake estimates in the OPEN study using doubly labeled water (DLW) as the reference biomarker.

DATA ENTRY

Data entry is the link between the information that is provided by a respondent and the analysis of the data. Data entry often requires decisions by coders to adjust information provided to meet the demands of a specific data analysis program.[108] If the respondent provides incomplete data or the database does not include all diet items, coders must decide on reasonable substitutions for portion size or food items. Thus, the quality of the data provided by respondents, the quality of the database, and the default assumptions by coders can all contribute to variability in the final food and nutrient data descriptions.[108]

Decisions about amounts of foods eaten may be guided by U.S. Department of Agriculture (USDA) publications on portions commonly consumed in the United States. The USDA has published several reports on foods commonly eaten and the quantities consumed at an eating occasion.[109,110] These reports provide data on amounts reported as eaten by participants in nationwide food consumption surveys.

SUMMARY

Dietary assessment is a dynamic field, with novel approaches being developed, such as computer-assisted self-interviews.[111] Various techniques to improve validity have been developed (see Table 26.5); but much work still needs to be done to decrease both systematic and random errors. Refinement of current methods and the development of new, innovative techniques will further confidence in the accuracy of dietary data.

CURRENT ISSUES IN ASSESSMENT AND ANALYSIS

REPORTING ACCURACY

Recent attention to the accuracy of dietary intake data has focused on the underreporting of energy by 10 to almost 40%.[48,64,112–115] These findings are based on an extensive literature comparing intakes to energy needs estimated using doubly labeled water,[63,67,116,117] weight maintenance data,[48] or age- and sex-specific equations to estimate energy requirements.[112,118] Although DLW is considered an unbiased biomarker of energy expenditure, the procedure is costly and not feasible for many studies. Prediction equations are widely used as an alternative to DLW to estimate energy requirements. The prediction equations based on DLW studies consider estimated basal metabolic rate and physical activity level (PAL) in determining the total energy expenditure.[118–120] Cutoff limits are used to establish minimum energy to sustain life. Limits are used to determine both implausibly low and high self-reported intakes. The cutoffs developed by Goldberg[118] have been updated with new assumption about PAL. Recent updates have been based on U.S. population data.[121,122] Correlates between energy intake and weight are much stronger for plausible reporters than all reporters.[123]

TABLE 26.5
Considerations to Reduce Error when Collecting Assessment Data

Potential Error Sources	24-h Recalls	Food Records	Food Frequency Questionnaire
Memory	• Multiple-Pass Technique • Probing Questions • Encoding Strategies	• Interviewer-Assisted Records • Encouraging Adherence to Appropriate Instructions	• Memory Retrieval Techniques
Portion size	• Portion Size Estimation Aids • Subject Training • Interviewer Training	• Portion Size Estimation Aids • Weighing Scale • Subject Training	• Portion Size Estimation Aids • Subject Training
Day-to-day variability	• Multiple Recall Days • Nonconsecutive Days of Data • Include Weekdays and Weekends • Collect Data in Different Seasons	• Multiple Days of Records • Include Weekdays and Weekends • Collect Data in Different Seasons	N/A
Response bias	• Interviewer Training • Clearly Worded, Open-ended Questions • Objective Interviewer Responses • Recalls on Unannounced, Random Days	• Objective Instructions • Reduce Respondent Burden • Limit Days of Data Collection	• Objective Responses for Interviewer Mode
Data Entry	• Documentation of Decisions • Interactive Software with Detailed Probes and Automatic Coding	• Strict Coding and Data Entry Rules • Interviewer Assisted Records • Detailed Probing Guides and Instructions	• Strict Coding and Data Entry Rules • Computer Scannable Forms for Automatic Coding

Underreporting has been found to be more common among women and older persons[124,125] as well as overweight,[126] postobese,[112] and weight-conscious individuals. Low literacy,[127] depression,[128] and diet-related social desirability[129] have been associated with underreporting. Underreporting may be more prevalent in participants assigned to an intervention group in clinical trials.[130,131] Selective underreporting has also been associated for certain food types such as fats and sweets[123,132] and bias toward underreporting of fat and carbohydrate over protein.[63]

While underreporting of energy is common in groups of individuals,[48,98,99,133–135] both underreporting and overreporting can occur.[48,125] Black and Cole reviewed studies with repeated dietary assessment, by more than one method and over time and found evidence for subject-specific bias. Thus, underreporters by one method were likely to be underreporters when tested by other methods and were likely to be so when reporting data over time.[136]

Reporting inaccuracies occur with all methods. In their review of dietary misreporting in the OPEN Study, and using DLW as reference, Subar and colleagues[63] reported more underreporting with a FFQ than 24-h recalls. They also indicated that accuracy declines the more respondents consume, suggesting that more foods and larger portion sizes present a challenge to accurate reporting.

DIET QUALITY

Indexes

Many indexes have been developed to assess diet quality. Kant summarized the three major categories as follows: indexes derived from nutrients only; indexes based on foods/food groups; and indexes based on combinations of nutrients and foods.[137]

Individual nutrient scores have been a method of interpreting nutrient intakes of an individual by comparison with a dietary standard such as the Recommended Dietary Allowances and the Dietary Reference Intakes or relative to energy intake. The nutrient adequacy ratio (NAR), which is the amount of a particular nutrient in the diet divided by the dietary standard, is an example of a single nutrient score.[138] A mean adequacy ratio (MAR) can also be calculated and represents the mean of NARs for several nutrients of interest.[138] Recently Drewnowski[139] reviewed various nutrient density scores and proposed a "naturally nutrient rich" score based on a nutrients-to-calorie ratio.

Food-based assessment indexes of quality vary from estimates of food diversity/variety to intakes of designated food groups. Kant[137] described such indexes as promising, because they "retain the complexity of foods and permit an indirect assessment of nonnutrient constituents" as well as nutrients.

A commonly used food-based approach is to calculate the number of servings from each food group and compare this with food grouping standards such as the USDA Food Guide Pyramid.[140] Another approach is to group intakes (e.g., low, medium, and high) for analysis with health outcomes.[141] However, depending on the food group scheme used, serving sizes and placement of foods into groups may vary considerably. Approaches to food group analyses also differ.[142] For individuals, a behavioral approach, in which food group changes are based on nutrition education strategies, is more appropriate. This approach usually defines specific nutritional education programs for health promotion, such as the National Cancer Institute's 5-a-day program.

Increasingly, diet pattern analyses are applied in studies of diet and health outcomes.[141,143–146] Kant recently provided a comprehensive review of diet patterns and health outcomes.[146] A number of multivariate statistical techniques is used for diet pattern analyses, including factor and cluster analyses. With these methods, a number of foods or nutrients are combined into composite variables or patterns that are reasonably homogenous. Across many studies, diet patterns identified as "prudent," "healthy," or "nutrient dense" are associated with more favorable micronutrient intakes, and reduced morbidity. Fruits, vegetables, fish, and whole grains are characteristics of such patterns.

A few global nutrition indexes (i.e., nutrient and food combination) have been developed. The Healthy Eating Index (HEI) score, created by the USDA,[147] as well as others such as the Diet Quality Index (DQI)[148] represent indexes of overall diet quality. They are based on the premise that diets are not comprised of single nutrients or foods but combinations of nutrients and nonnutrient components. The interactions of all these dietary components make it difficult to determine the effects of single dietary components. Additionally, dietary behaviors are complex, and many different patterns of intake may be occurring simultaneously such as decreasing fat intake while increasing fruits and vegetables.

Energy Density

Energy density is another way dietary quality can be addressed. Energy density refers to the amount of energy in a particular weight of food. It is generally presented as the number of calories in a gram. Foods with a low energy density provide less energy relative to their weight than foods with a high energy density. Energy density values, which are influenced by the moisture content and macronutrient composition of foods, range from 0 to 9 kcal/g. The component of food with the greatest impact on energy density is water.[149] Water has an energy density of 0 kcal/g as it contributes weight but not energy to foods. Foods with high water content, such as fruits and vegetables, have a relatively low energy density. Fiber also has a relatively low energy density, providing 1.5 to 2.5 kcal/g and can lower the energy density of foods. However, the influence of fiber on energy density is more modest than that of water since only a limited amount can be added to foods. On the opposite end of the energy density spectrum, fat is the most energy-dense component of food. Fat increases the energy content of foods, providing 9 kcal/g, more than twice as many as carbohydrates or protein, which provide 4 kcal/g.

Energy density values reported in the literature have been calculated by a variety of different methods that include only food, as well as food and various combinations of beverages, such as all beverages, all beverages excluding water, energy-containing beverages, milk, juice, and so forth.[150–152] Since energy density values vary widely depending on the beverage inclusion method,[150,153] studies investigating energy density should clearly define the treatment of beverages. Although insufficient data are available to state definitively which beverage calculation method is superior, calculations based on food, excluding all beverages, are becoming increasingly common. This method lacks some of the controversies associated with other methods. For example, values based on food and all beverages (including water) are rarely reported in the literature, as water intake is not commonly collected in research studies. Calculations based on food and all beverages excluding water may not provide meaningful measures of dietary energy density because noncaloric beverages such as diet cola, coffee, and tea, are not excluded. Additionally, values based on food- and energy-containing beverages may lead to increased within-person variance values, which may diminish associations with outcome variables.[153]

While calculating dietary energy density can be challenging due to the data coding and manipulations necessary to appropriately deal with beverages, recent evidence indicating that energy density is associated with weight status[151,154,155] necessitates additional energy density investigations in a variety of populations. Furthermore, given that low-energy-dense diets have been associated with high intakes of fruits and vegetables, high intakes of fiber, high intakes of a variety of vitamins and minerals, and good overall diet quality,[152] dietary energy density values appear to a marker for a healthy diet pattern.

Glycemic Index/Glycemic Load

Because of the considerable attention given to low-carbohydrate-diet approaches and the new Dietary Guidelines emphasis on whole grains, interest in carbohydrate quality as assessed by glycemic index and glycemic load is increasing.[156] International of tables of glycemic index values[157] are quickly becoming integrated into nutrient databases used to enter, collect, and analyze dietary data.

Glycemic index is the scale used to classify the quality of carbohydrates by their potential to increase blood glucose independent of its carbohydrate content, whereas the glycemic load of the diet reflects the total glycemic effect of the diet and is the product of the carbohydrate content that each food and its glycemic index value.[157] Carbohydrate-containing foods vary widely with respect to their glycemic response. Many dietary factors such as grain size and structure, fiber content, cooking methods, amylose content, previous meal, and satiety all play a role in the total glycemic effect of the diet.[158] Glycemic index is measured *in vivo* by comparing the glucose responses of a test food with an amount of carbohydrate equivalent to a reference food (usually 25 or 50 g of glucose or starch). Because of the differences in methodology and the wide variety of factors affecting glycemic response, the glycemic values of foods vary considerably and, for this reason, assessing glycemic is still somewhat controversial. Databases are still somewhat incomplete, and they are subject to errors in measurement and interpolation, not unlike nutrient databases and other food component databases.

Lower dietary glycemic index and glycemic load of the diet has, never-the-less, been shown to have beneficial health effects by altering metabolic endpoints such as improved blood glucose, insulin, and lipid levels, improved glycemic control in diabetes, decreased fat mass, and reduced colon cancer risk.[159–164] Recently, Davis et al.[156] studied the glycemic load of older adults, finding that a healthier dietary pattern was associated with a lower glycemic index and glycemic load.

Any method of assessing an individual's dietary intake is dependent on the methods of interpretation. More comprehensive methods of interpretation may facilitate the identification of more specific patterns of intake and their relationship to disease.

DIETARY SUPPLEMENTS

Increased nutrient intakes from supplements have been related to certain disease risk such as cardiovascular disease (vitamin E), neural tube defects (folate), osteoporosis (calcium), and cancer (antioxidants such as vitamin C and beta carotene). Approximately 40–50% of the general population over the age of 2 years in the United States takes a dietary supplement (see Table 26.6).[165,166] These numbers continue to rise especially for more nontraditional or complementary therapies such as herbal or botanical supplements. Supplement use is higher in non-Hispanic white females and increases with age in some segments of the population.[165,167] The supplement intake of special populations such as those individuals with cancer diagnosis is much high, as high as 80% in some studies.[167,168] Knowledge of dietary supplements as well as an understanding of assessment methods is critical to the overall assessment of nutrient and other dietary components.

Supplement intake data can be assessed in a variety of ways and is usually collected by questionnaire, including food frequency questionnaires, or as part of intake data such as by 24-h dietary recall or by food records. When collected by the latter methods, it is important to recognize that the intake of supplements for the day of data collection may not reflect the pattern of intake over an extended period of time. Detailed questionnaires, which are better for capturing long-term intake and frequency of intake, are used frequently in research studies, clinical practice, and in nutrition monitoring and surveys.[169]

TABLE 26.6
Categories of Supplements

Category	Examples
Vitamins (single or multiple formulations)	Vitamin C, E, D, B-6
Minerals (single or multiple formulations)	Iron, calcium, chromium, and zinc
Vitamins with minerals	Calcium with vitamin D; vitamin E with selenium
Herbs and other botanicals	St. John's Wort, ginkgo biloba, ginseng, saw palmetto
Flavonoids	Quercetin, rutin, hesperidin, diadzin
Carotenoids	Lycopene, zeaxanthin, lutein, dried carrot extract, and other vegetable extracts
Fatty acids/fish oils, other oils	Linoleic acid, omega 3 fatty acids, and DHA EPA
Amino acids/nucleic acids/proteins including coenzymes, enzymes, and hormones	L-glutamine, coenzyme Q-10, bromelain, tryptophan
Microbial preparations/probiotics	*Lactobacillus acidophilus, B. bifidus, L. bulgaris*
Glandular and other organ preparations	Desiccated glands such thyroid and adrenal
Miscellaneous	Shark cartilage, pycogenol, chrondoitin sulfate

Quantifying supplement intake is a difficult and tedious process. When collecting supplement information, it is important to identify what level of detail is needed to describe or quantify dietary intakes with dietary supplements. Strategies may include having those individuals bring in their supplement labels, or photocopy the labels. Other strategies include having the participants respond to questionnaires that provide lists of single vitamins and minerals as well as common brand names for multiple formulations. For herbal and botanical ingredients and other components not typically found in common formulations, it might be necessary to identify the active components and, above all else, to obtain brand name and label information.

FUNCTIONAL FOODS

A *functional food* has been defined as "any food or food ingredient that may provide a health benefit beyond the traditional nutrients it contains."[170] Functional foods are both natural or formulated (designed) foods with components in addition to nutrients that prevent or treat diseases. Potential mechanisms of action for physiologically active compounds include antioxidants, antimutagens, antiinflammatory agents, neuroregulatory substances, to cite a few.[171] Physiologically active components may occur naturally in foods, may be enhanced with biotechnological techniques, or may be added to fortified foods. Excellent reviews of physiologically active substances' potential mechanisms of action and functional food products have been published in recent years.[171–173]

Since many of the phytochemicals in foods are still under investigation, it is premature to emphasize quantification of single functional food components in dietary assessment. However, improvements in individual assessment methods will make it possible to quantify and link these components in functional foods with their potential health benefits. Examples of where individual assessment plays a significant role in providing this linkage can be found in the literature examining fruit and vegetable intakes. There are now databases that can accurately quantify the carotenoid content of foods.[174] As cooking methods, storage, and exposure to air and water are known to affect the carotenoid content of fruits and vegetables, the development of these databases has been a challenge. In the case of assessing carotenoids, for example, it is important to distinguish between pink and white grapefruit (i.e., pink grapefruit has 3740 mg lycopene, whereas white grapefruit has 0 mg). This one simple observation in assessing an individual's intake can have a significant impact on determining the relationship between dietary carotenoids and blood carotenoids and the potential role they may have in cancer risk in groups of individuals.

In assessing diets for research purposes, it is important to consider the level of detail required for other components in foods as well. The assessment issues outlined in the chapter are the same for assessing functional foods. As more components are identified and quantification is possible, databases need to be developed that make analysis of functional foods and their components possible. The knowledge gained in the study of functional foods will drive the type and level of detail in methodology and database development.

REFERENCES

1. National Research Council, *Diet and Health: Implications for Reducing Chronic Disease Risk*, National Academy Press, Washington, DC, 1989, 46.
2. Mudge, G.G. *JADA*, 1: 166; 1926.
3. Turner, D. *JADA*, 16: 875; 1940.

4. Widdowson, E.M. *J. Hygiene*, 36: 269; 1936.
5. U.S. Department of Health and Human Services, *Healthy People 2010: Understanding and Improving Health*, 2nd edition. Washington, DC, 2000.
6. Huenemann, R.L. and Turner, D. *JADA*, 18: 562; 1942.
7. Young, C. et al. *JADA*, 28: 124; 1952.
8. Leverton, R.M. and Marsh, A.G. *J. Home Econ.*, 31: 111; 1939.
9. Wait, B. and Roberts, L.J. *JADA*, 8: 323; 1932.
10. Yudkin, J. *Br. J. Nutr.*, 5: 177; 1951.
11. Burke, B.S. and Stuart, H.C. *J. Pediatr.*, 12: 493; 1938.
12. Donelson, E.G. and Leichsenring, J.M. *JADA*, 18: 429; 1942.
13. Blundell, J.E. *Am. J. Clin. Nutr.*, 71: 3; 2000.
14. Dwyer, J.T., Krall, E.A., and Coleman, K.A. *JADA*, 87: 1509; 1987.
15. Smith, A.F. *Eur. J. Clin. Nutr.*, 47: 6S; 1993.
16. Quandt, S.A. In *Modern Nutrition in Health and Disease*, 10th edition, Shils, M.E., Shike, M., and Ross, A.C., Eds., Lippincott Williams & Wilkins, Philadelphia, 1741, 2005.
17. Caballero, B., Cousins, R.J., Bidlack, W.R., and Wang, W. In *Modern Nutrition in Health and Disease*, 10th edition, Shils, M.E., Shike, M., and Ross, A.C., Eds., Lippincott Williams & Wilkins, Philadelphia, 582, 2005.
18. Bingham, S. *Nutr. Abstr. Rev. (Series A)*, 57: 705; 1987.
19. Smiciklas-Wright, H. and Guthrie, H.A. In *Nutrition Assessment A Comprehensive Guide for Planning Intervention*, 2nd edition, Simko, M.D., Cowell, C., and Gilbride, J.A., Eds., Aspen Publishers, Inc., Gaithersburg, MD, 165, 1995.
20. Life Sciences Research Office, *Guidelines for Use of Dietary Intake Data*, Federation of American Societies for Experimental Biology, Bethesda, MD, 1996.
21. Gibson, R.S. *Principles of Nutrition Assessment*, 2nd edition, Oxford University Press, New York, 2005.
22. Willett, W. *Nutritional Epidemiology*, 2nd edition, Oxford University Press, New York, 1998.
23. Dwyer, J. In *Modern Nutrition in Health and Disease*, 9th edition, Shils, M.E., Olson, J.A., Shike, M., and Ross, A.C., Eds., Williams & Wilkins, Philadelphia, 937, 1999.
24. Christakis, G. *Am. J. Public Health*, 63: 1S; 1973.
25. Copeland, T. et al. *JADA*, 100: 1186; 2000.
26. St. Jeor, S.T., Guthrie, H.A., and Jones, M.B. *JADA*, 83: 155; 1983.
27. Tarasuk, V. and Beaton, G.H. *Am. J. Clin. Nutr.*, 54: 464; 1991.
28. Craig, M.R. et al. *JADA*, 100: 421; 2000.
29. Tian, H.G. et al. *Eur. J. Clin. Nutr.*, 49: 26; 1995.
30. Streit, K.J. et al. *JADA*, 91: 213; 1991.
31. Block, G., Hartman, A.M., and Naughton, D. *Epidemiology*, 1: 58; 1990.
32. Kristal, A.R. et al. *Am. J. Epidemiol.*, 146: 856; 1997.
33. Kumanyika, S. et al. *Ann. Epidemiol.*, 13: 111; 2003.
34. Jackson, B. et al. *JADA*, 86: 1531; 1986.
35. Gorbach, S.L. et al. *JADA*, 90: 802; 1990.
36. Moulin, C.C. et al. *Am. J. Clin. Nutr.*, 67: 853; 1998.
37. Bingham, S.A. *Ann. Nutr. Metab.*, 35: 117; 1991.
38. Tippett, K.S. and Cypel, Y.S., Eds. *Design and Operation: The Continuing Survey of Food Intakes by Individuals and the Diet and Health Knowledge Survey*, 1994–96, Nationwide Food Survey Report No. 91-1. US Department of Agriculture, Agricultural Research Service; 1998.
39. NASCO, *Nasco Nutrition Teaching Aids, 1999–2000 Catalog*, Number 437, NASCO, Fort Atkinson, WI, 1999.
40. National Center for Health Statistics, *Dietary Intake Source Data: United States, 1976–80 (DHHS publication no. PHS 83-1681)*, Series 11, No. 231, US Department of Health and Human Services, Washington, DC, 1983.
41. Nutrition Consulting Enterprises, *Food Portion Visual*, Nutrition Consulting Enterprises, Framingham, MA, 1981.
42. Hess, M.A., *Portion Photos of Popular Foods*, Ed. American Dietetic Association and Center for Nutrition Education, University of Wisconsin, Stout, 1997.
43. Gittelsohn, J. et al. *JADA*, 94: 1273; 1994.
44. Omnibus Budget Reconciliation Act of 1990, Public Law 101-508, 1990.
45. Andrews, Y.N. and Castellanos, V.H. *JADA*, 103: 873; 2003.
46. Rebro, S.M. et al. *JADA*, 98: 1163; 1998.
47. Buzzard, I.M. et al. *JADA*, 96: 574; 1996.
48. Jonnalagadda, S.S. et al. *JADA*, 100: 303; 2000.
49. Lyons, G.K. et al. *JADA*, 96: 1276; 1996.
50. Johnson, R.K., Driscoll, P. and Goran, M.I. *JADA*, 96: 1140; 1996.
51. Conway , J.M. et al. *Am. J. Clin. Nutr.*, 77: 1171; 2003.
52. Conway, J.M. et al. *JADA*, 104: 595; 2004.
53. Fox, T.A., Heimendinger, J., and Block, G. *JADA*, 92: 729; 1992.
54. Derr, J.A. et al. *Am. J. Epidemiol.*, 136: 1386; 1992.

55. Casey, P.H. et al. *J. Am. Diet. Assoc.*, 99: 1406; 1999.
56. Burke, B.S. *JADA*, 23: 1041; 1947.
57. Thompson, F.E. et al. *JADA*, 102: 1764; 2002.
58. Frankenfeld, C.L. et al. *JADA*, 102: 1407; 2002.
59. Kris-Etherton, P. et al. *JADA*, 101: 81; 2001.
60. Yen, J. et al. *JADA*, 103: 991; 2003.
61. Mitchell, D.C. et al. *JADA*, 102: 842; 2002.
62. Subar, A.F. *JADA*, 104: 769; 2004.
63. Subar, A.F. et al. *Am. J. Epidemiol.*, 158: 1; 2003
64. Subar, A.F. et al. *JADA*, 95: 781; 1995.
65. Potischman, N. et al. *Nutr. Cancer*, 34: 70; 1999.
66. Lund, S.M., Brown, J., and Harnack, L. *Eur. J. Clin. Nutr.*, 52: 53S; 1998.
67. Kipnis, V. et al. *Am. J. Epidemiol.*, 158: 14; 2003.
68. Laus, M.J. et al. *J. Nutr. Elder.*, 18: 1; 1999.
69. Clapy, J.A. et al. *JADA*, 91: 316 1991.
70. Beaton, G.H. *Am. J. Clin. Nutr.*, 59: 253S; 1994.
71. Wessells, M.G., *Cognitive Psychology*, Harper & Row Publishers, New York, 1982.
72. Craik, F.I.M. *Phil. Trans. R. Soc. Lond. B Biol. Sci.*, 302: 341; 1993.
73. Schaie, K.W. and Willis, S.L. In *Adult Development and Aging*, 2nd edition, Schaie, K.W., and Willis, S.L., Eds., Little, Brown and Company, Boston, MA, 1986, 324.
74. Ervin, R.B. and Smiciklas-Wright, H. *JADA*, 98: 984; 1998.
75. Campbell, V.A. and Dodds, M.L. *JADA*, 51: 29; 1967.
76. Lytle, L.A. et al. *JADA*, 93: 1431; 1993.
77. Eldridge, A.L. et al. *JADA*, 98: 777; 1998.
78. Nutrition Coordinating Center, *Nutrient Data System for Research (NDS-R) Software*, University of Minnesota, Minneapolis, MN.
79. Blake, A.J., Guthrie, H.A., and Smiciklas-Wright, H., *JADA*, 89: 962; 1989.
80. Guthrie, H. *JADA*, 84: 1441; 1984.
81. Young, L.R.N. and Marion, *Nutr. Rev.*, 53: 149; 1995.
82. Cypel, Y.S., Guenther, P.M., and Petot, G.J. *JADA*, 97: 289; 1997.
83. Posner et al. *JADA*, 92: 738; 1992.
84. Godwin, S.L. et al. *JADA*, 104: 585; 2004.
85. Smiciklas-Wright, H. et al. *JADA*, 103: 41; 2003.
86. Harnack, L. et al. *JADA*, 104: 804; 2004.
87. Chambers, E. et al. *JADA*, 100: 891; 2000.
88. Bolland, J.E., Ward, J.Y., and Bolland, T.W. *JADA*, 90: 1402; 1990.
89. Weber, J.L. et al. *JADA*, 97: 176; 1997.
90. Slawson, D.L. and Eck, L.H. *JADA*, 97: 295; 1997.
91. Williamson, D.A. et al. *J. Am. Diet. Assoc.*, 103, 1139, 2003.
92. Flegal, K.M. et al. *Am. J. Epidemiol.*, 128: 749; 1988.
93. Hebert, J.R. et al. *Int. J. Epidemiol.*, 24: 389; 1995.
94. Hebert, J.R. et al. *Am. J. Epidemiol.*, 146: 1046; 1997.
95. Kristal, A.R. et al. *J. Am. Diet. Assoc.*, 98: 40; 1998.
96. Edwards, S. et al. *Am. J. Epidemiol.*, 140: 1020; 1994.
97. Smiciklas-Wright, H. et al. *JADA*, 81: 28S, 1991.
98. Dwyer, J.T. and Coleman, K.A. *Am. J. Clin. Nutr.*, 65: 1153S; 1997.
99. Malila, N. et al. *Nutr. Cancer*, 32: 146; 1998.
100. Gersovitz, M., Madden, J.P., and Smiciklas-Wright, H. *JADA*, 73: 48; 1978.
101. Guthrie, H.A. and Crocetti, A.F. *JADA*, 85: 325; 1985.
102. McAvay, G. and Rodin, J. *Appetite*, 11: 97; 1988.
103. Basiotis, P.P. et al. *J. Nutr.*, 117: 1638; 1987.
104. Hartman, A.M. et al. *Am. J. Epidemiol.*, 132: 999; 1990.
105. Nusser, S.M. et al. *J. Am. Stat. Assoc.*, 91: 1440; 1996.
106. Guenther, P.M., Kott, P.S., and Carriquiry, A.L. *J. Nutr.*, 127: 1106; 1996.
107. Freedman, L.S. et al. *J. Nutr.*, 134: 1836; 2004.
108. Lacey, J.M. et al., *Coder Variability in Computerized Dietary Analysis*, Research Bulletin Number 729, Massachusetts Agricultural Experiment Station, MA, 1990.
109. Krebs-Smith, S.M. et al. *Foods Commonly Eaten in the United States: Quantities Consumed Per Eating Occasion and in a Day, 1989–1991*, NFS Report No. 91-3, US Department of Agriculture, Agriculture Research Service, Washington, DC, 1997.
110. Smiciklas-Wright H, et al. *Foods Commonly Eaten in the United States: Quantities Consumed Per Eating Occasion and in a Day, 1994–96.* Available at:http://www.barc.usda.gov/bhnrc.foodsurvey/home.htm accessed December 5, 2005.
111. Kohlmeier, L. et al. *Am. J. Clin. Nutr.*, 65: 1275S; 1997.

112. Black, A.E. et al. *Eur. J. Clin. Nutr.*, 51: 405; 1997.

113. Champagne, C.M. et al. *JADA*, 98: 426; 1998.

114. Schoeller, D.A. *Metabolism*, 44: 18; 1995.

115. Goris, A.H., Westerterp-Plantenga, M.S., and Westerterp, K.R. *Am. J. Clin. Nutr.*, 71: 130; 2000.

116. Seale, J.L. et al. *Nutrition*, 18: 568; 2002.

117. Schoeller, D.A. and Fjeld, C.R. *Annu. Rev. Nutr.*, 11: 355; 1991.

118. Goldberg, G.R. et al. *Eur. J. Clin. Nutr.*, 45: 569; 1991.

119. Black, A.E. et al. *Eur. J. Clin. Nutr.*, 45: 583; 1991.

120. Black, A.E. *Eur. J. Clin. Nutr.*, 54: 395; 2002.

121. McCrory, M.A., Hajduk, C.L., and Roberts, S.B. *Public Health Nutr.*, 5: 873; 2002.

122. Huang, T.T. et al. *Obes. Res.*, 12: 1875; 2004.

123. Scagliusi, F.B. et al. *JADA*, 103: 1306; 2003.

124. Briefel, R.R. et al. *Am. J. Clin. Nutr.*, 65: 1203S; 1997.

125. Johansson, L. et al. *Am. J. Clin. Nutr.*, 68: 266; 1998.

126. Stallone, D.D. et al. *Eur. J. Clin. Nutr.*, 51: 815; 1997.

127. Johnson, R.K., Soultanakis, R.P., and Matthews, D.E. *JADA*, 98: 1136; 1998.

128. Smiciklas-Wright, H. et al. *FASEB J.*, 13: 263A; 1999.

129. Novotry, J.A. et al. *JADA*, 103: 1146; 2003.

130. Caan, B. et al. *JADA*, 104: 355; 2004.

131. Mitchell, D.C. et al. *FASEB J.*, 19: 63A; 2005.

132. Bingham, S. *Am. J. Clin. Nutr.*, 59: 227S; 1994.

133. Champagne, C.M. et al. *JADA*, 96: 707; 1996.

134. Kortzinger, I. et al. *Ann. Nutr. Metab.*, 41: 37; 1997.

135. Mertz, W. et al. *Am. J. Clin. Nutr.*, 54: 291; 1991.

136. Black, A.E. and Cole, T.J. *JADA*, 101: 70; 2004.

137. Kant, A.K. *JADA*, 96: 785; 1996.

138. Guthrie, H.A. and Scheer, J.C. *JADA*, 78: 240; 1981.

139. Drewnowski, A. *Am. J. Clin. Nutr.*, 82: 721; 2005.

140. http://www.mypyramid.gov. Accessed December 5, 2005.

141. Daviglius, M.L. et al. *JADA*, 105: 1735; 2005.

142. Cullen, K.W. et al. *JADA*, 99: 849 1999.

143. Millen, B. et al. *JADA*, 105: 1723: 2005.

144. Smiciklas-Wright, H., Mitchell, D.C., and Tucker, K.L. *Top. Clin. Nutr.*, 19: 193; 2004.

145. Newby, P.K. et al. *Am. J. Clin. Nutr.*, 77: 1417; 2003.

146. Kant, A.K. *JADA*, 104: 615; 2004.

147. Bowman, S.A. et al., *The Healthy Eating Index: 1994–96*, *CNPP-5*, U.S. Department of Agriculture, Center for Nutrition Policy and Promotion, 1998.

148. Haines, P.S., Siega-Riz, A.M., and Popkin, B.M. *JADA*, 99: 697; 1999.

149. Rolls, B.J. and Bell, E.A. In *Medical Clinics of North America*, Jensen, M.D., Ed., W.B. Saunders Company, Philadelphia, 84, 401, 2000.

150. Ledikwe, J.H., et al. *J Nutr.*, 135: 273; 2005.

151. Ledikwe, J.H., Blanck, H.M., Kettel-Khan, L. et al. *Am. J. Clin. Nutr.* (in Press).

152. Ledikwe, J.H., Blanck, H.M., Kettel-Khan, L. et al. *JADA,* (in press).

153. Cox, D.N. and Mela, D.J. *Int. J. Obes. Relat. Metab. Disord.*, 24: 49; 2000.

154. Kant and Graubard. *Int. J. Obes.*, 29: 950; 2005.

155. Rolls, B.J. et al. *Obes. Res.*, 13: 1052; 2005.

156. Davis, M.S., et al. *JADA*, 104: 1828; 2004.

157. Foster-Powell, K. et al. *Am. J. Clin. Nutr.*, 76: 5; 2002.

158. Venn, B.J. et al. *Eur. J. Clin. Nutr.*, 58: 1443; 2004.

159. Giacco, R. et al. *Diabetes Care*, 23: 1461; 2000.

160. Jarvi, A.E. et al. *Diabetes Care*, 22: 10; 1999.

161. Jenkins, D.J.A. et al. *Am. J. Clin. Nutr.*, 76: 266S; 2002.

162. Jenkins, D.J.A. et al. *J. Am. Coll. Nutr.*, 6: 609; 1998.

163. Salmeron, J. et al. *JAMA*, 277: 472; 1997.

164. Bouche, C. et al. *Diabetes Care*, 25: 822; 2002.

165. Ervin, R.B., Wright, J.D., and Kennedy-Stephenson, J., *Use of Dietary Supplements in the United States*, *1988–94*, Series 11, No. 244, Department of Health and Human Services, National Center for Health Statistics, Hyattsville, MD, 1999.

166. Slesinski, M.J., Subar, A.F., and Kahle, L.L. *J. Nutr.*, 126: 3001; 1996.

167. Newman, V. et al. *JADA*, 98: 285; 1998.

168. Winters, B.L. et al. *FASEB J.*, 13: 253A; 1999.

169. Dwyer, J. et al. *J. Nutr.*, 133: 590S; 2003.

170. Milner, J.A. *J. Nutr.*, 129: 1395S; 1999.
171. Bidlack, W.R. and Wang, W. In *Modern Nutrition in Health and Disease*, 10th edition, Shils, M.E. et al., Eds., Lippincott Williams & Wilkins, Philadelphia, 2789, 2005.
172. Prior, R.L. In *Modern Nutrition in Health and Disease*, 10th edition, Shils, M.E. et al., Eds., Lippincott Williams & Wilkins, Philadelphia, 582, 2005.
173. Hasler, C. et al. *JADA*, 104: 814; 2004.
174. U.S. Department of Agriculture, *USDA-NCC Carotenoid Database for U. S. Foods*, 1998–1999.

27 Use of Food Frequency Questionnaires in Minority Populations

Rebecca S. Reeves and Patricia W. Pace

CONTENTS

INTRODUCTION

Food frequency questionnaires (FFQ) are selected by investigators to assess the usual food or nutrient intakes of groups or individuals because they are relatively easy to administer, less expensive than other dietary assessment methods, and can be adapted to all racial and ethnic populations in the United States.[1] Investigators can also modify these dietary instruments for telephone interviews or a self-administered mailed survey. FFQs are commonly used in epidemiologic studies on diet and disease, and are also chosen by investigators as the dietary assessment instrument in clinical intervention studies. The use of these questionnaires in minority populations in the United States is increasing for several reasons: the country is becoming more racially and ethnically diverse,[2] government agencies have placed emphasis on including minority population in health-related research,[3] and variations in disease incidence and dietary practices within and across ethnic minorities offer important opportunities for examining the role of diet in relation to risk of chronic disease.[4]

This chapter reviews 16 published studies evaluating the validity or reliability of FFQs used in measuring dietary intakes in adult minority populations in the United States over the last 25 years. Also included in this chapter are selected samples of FFQs and information on obtaining copies of them. Recommendations on the use of these FFQs are discussed.

VALIDITY AND RELIABILITY OF QUESTIONNAIRES

A search of the National Library of Medicine's (Bethesda, MD) MEDLINE system was conducted using various terms such as validity, reliability, reproducibility, diet, FFQ, minority, Hispanic, black, Asian, pacific-islander, and native American to identify articles published between 1980 and 2005. These searches were supplemented by cross-referencing from author reference lists. Articles were selected that described the evaluation of any FFQ that assessed the usual daily diet and provided data on the validity or reliability of the instrument in a specific U.S. ethnic minority population or a diverse population representing at least 40% minority persons. The degree of reliability or validity of the instrument reported was not considered an inclusion factor. Validity and reliability studies that were reported in the same article were considered separately and are referenced in different tables. The measures of performance that were chosen were reliability, comparison of means (when available), and validity because these are usually reported to describe the results of the evaluation of the FFQ. Correlation coefficients were selected as indicators of reliability and validity because they are commonly used and are more easily summarized. Factors that can influence correlation coefficients are the number of days between the times the questionnaire is administered (reliability coefficients) and the number of days of food records or 24 h recalls used for the referent period (validity coefficients). Adjusted and unadjusted correlation coefficients are reported in the tables. The methods for adjusting the coefficients are discussed in each article.

Terms used to describe FFQs in the tables are as follows:

Quantitative: Quantity of food consumed was estimated using weights, measures, or food models. Responses were open ended.

Semiquantitative: Quantity of food consumed was estimated using a standard portion size, serving, or a predetermined amount, and the respondent was asked about the number of portions consumed.

Nonquantitative: Quantity of food was not assessed.

Self-administered: An adult completed the dietary assessment without assistance.

Interviewer administered: A trained interviewer collected the dietary information from the adult in a one-on-one setting.

Diverse Studies: Publications that include various combinations of racial or ethnic groups.

Minority Studies: Publications that include only one racial or ethnic group.

The 16 studies reviewed for this chapter were divided into two groups based on ethnic participation. Within the group labeled "Minority" studies, three consisted of only Black subjects,[5–7] one of Asian,[8] and one of Hispanic subjects.[9] In the group labeled "Diverse," five studies included Black and White subjects,[10–14] one study Black and Hispanic,[15] two studies Black, Hispanic, and White subjects,[16,17] one study Hispanic and White,[18] one study Asian and White[19] and one recruited Asian, Black, Hispanic and White subjects.[20]

The review of the validation studies on FFQs was not conclusive. The median correlations (Table 27.1) between questionnaire-based estimates of nutrient intakes and estimates derived from referent methods were not consistent for ethnic groups, but trends were suggested. The median correlations for Black males and females across validations studies were in the range of 0.23 to 0.42; for Hispanic females, 0.32 to 0.49 except for one study conducted in Starr County, Texas, which reported a median correlation of 0.75; for White males and females, 0.53, and Asian males and females, 0.53. If it is considered that a measure of ≥0.05 is satisfactory or good, 0.30 to 0.49 is fair, and <0.30 is poor,[19] then these median correlations suggest that Black and Hispanic groups do not perform well on FFQs.

The validation correlations for total energy, total fat, and vitamin A were inconsistent and in some cases very low across studies. In Table 27.2 the correlation coefficients for total fat ranged from 0.23 to 0.65 with the higher correlations usually found in the Asian or White populations. A similar trend was found for energy among the various groups. The correlation coefficients for Hispanic and Black populations were commonly in the range of 0.24 to 0.43, but in the White and Asian groups the coefficients ranged from 0.41 to 0.61. Values for vitamin A were more inconsistent ranging from 0.15 to 0.67 across all groups. The number of days of food records and recalls that are compared against FFQs can explain some of these low correlations especially for vitamin A. Many days are required to provide a precise estimate of vitamin A intake, and in these studies the greatest number of daily recalls or records collected over 1 year was 28. Even in this study, certain subgroups correlations for vitamin A were still 0.23 and 0.29.

The study[5] that reported serum nutrient concentrations of carotenoids, vitamin E, lycopene and lutein as a referent reported correlations that were much lower for smokers (<0.02) than for nonsmokers (<0.40). The investigators concluded that their FFQ is reasonably valid for use in a southern, urban, low-income Black population except for the analysis of lutein and lycopene. Another study comparing adipose tissue fatty acids and dietary fat intake collected from eight different 24 h recalls and a 200-item FFQ confirmed previous findings that 24 h recalls are valid for assessing dietary intake of different types of fat. The correlation of FFQ values for fat intake and adipose tissue fatty acids resulted in correlations on the order of 0.4 to 0.6.[14]

In most of the studies reviewed, the FFQ overestimated the mean of the referent recall or records and in some cases by non-trivial amounts. One explanation for this difference was again the number of days of recalls or records collected for comparison to the FFQ. Depending on which nutrient is of interest in the study and the time period the participant is asked to recall on the FFQ, more than 4 to 7 days may be required to capture the actual intake of the individual.

The reliability coefficients across all diverse and minority studies were much higher than the validity coefficients (Table 27.3). The median correlations for Black males and females across studies were in the range of 0.51 to 0.88; for Hispanic females, 0.51 to 0.58 except for one study conducted in Starr County, Texas, which reported a median correlation of 0.85; for White males and females, 0.64 to 0.71. These coefficients would suggest that, within minority and diverse populations, the FFQ can usually describe, with some consistently, the food or nutrient intakes of individuals when administered at two points in time.

In most of the studies reviewed, the investigators made suggestions and recommendations for improving the performance of the FFQ in minority populations. It was repeatedly mentioned that a "gold standard" referent method was not available, so collecting valid dietary intake data remains challenging. The need to identify a complete food list on the FFQ that captures all of the foods in the usual diet of the study population was highly recommended. Depending on the study, the food list should

TABLE 27.1

Median and Reported Range of Correlation Coefficients

	Median and Reported Range	
Study	**Validity Coefficients**	**Reliability Coefficients**
Diverse Groups		
Baumgartner et al.[18]	0.50 (0.21–0.57) HF + WF (adjusted value)	0.62 (0.40–0.71) unadjusted
Hankin et al.[19]	0.63 (0.58–0.67) Chinese females	
	0.46 (0.38–0.64) White females	
	0.56 (0.49–0.60) Filipino females	
	0.38 (0.29–0.41) Hawaiian females	
	0.60 (0.23–0.68) Japanese females	
	0.58 (0.38–0.68) Chinese males	
	0.45 (0.34–0.64) White males	
	0.57 (0.21–0.84) Filipino males	
	0.36 (0.26–0.62) Hawaiian males	
	0.55 (0.46–0.77) Japanese males	
Knutsen et al.[14]	0.41 (0.51–0.13) SFA black M&F	
	0.435 (0.68–0.34) MonoFA black M&F	
	0.61 (0.77–0.23) polyFA black M&F	
	0.31 (0.57–0.08) SFA white M&F	
	0.27 (0.48–0.13) MonoFA white M&F	
	0.31 (71–0.05) PolyFA white M&F	
Kristal et al.[15]	Baseline	
	0.31 (0.26–0.46) Black females	0.51(0.37–0.60) Black females
	0.35 (0.25–0.48) Hispanic females	0.51(0.19–0.75) Hispanic females
	6 months (control group)	
	0.40 (0.29–0.49) Black females	
	0.37 (–0.01–0.48) Hispanic females	
Larkin et al.[11]	0.43 (0.26–62) White males	
	0.23 (0.09–0.41) Black males	
	0.44 (0.27–0.57) White females	
	0.32 (0.24–0.43) Black females	
Liu et al.[12]	0.64 (0.50–0.86) White males	0.70 (0.60–0.91) White males and females
	0.53 (0.13–0.68) White females	0.58 (0.45–0.85) Black males and females
	0.42 (0.23–0.67) Black males	
	0.27 (0.04–0.53) Black females	
Mayer-Davis et al.[16]	0.58 (0.30–0.77) White females, urban	0.71 (0.43–0.82) White females
	0.38 (0.22–0.62) Black females, urban	0.62 (0.26–0.69) Black females
	0.57 (0.24–0.68) White females, rural	0.64 (0.25–0.88) White females, rural
	0.32 (0.21–0.44) Hispanic females, rural	0.58 (0.33–0.66) Hispanic females, rural
Morris et al.[13]	0.47 (0.67–0.31) black + white males and females	0.60 (0.70–0.50) black + white males and females
Stram et al.[20]	Average correlation for amount	
	0.30 (0.16–0.41) Black males and females	
	0.43 (0.27–0.62) Hispanic males and females	
	0.57 (0.48–0.64) White males and females	
	0.48 (0.31–0.67) Japanese males and females	
Forsythe et al.[10]		0.88 (0.69–0.98) females
Suitor et al.[17]	0.32 (0.12–0.52) all females combined	0.88 (0.80–0.94) all females
Minority Groups		
Coates et al.[5]	0.34 (–0.02–0.45) nonsmokers	
	0.08 (–0.02–0.20) smokers	
Kumanyika et al.[6]	0.33 (0.51–0.15) black females	
Lee et al.[8]	0.46 (0.21–0.66) Chinese females	
McPherson et al.[9]	0.75 (0.53–0.77) Hispanic males and females	0.85 (0.84–0.90) Hispanic males and females
Resnicow et al.[7]	0.31 (0.35–0.02) black males M + F	

TABLE 27.2
FFQ Validity Studies among Minority Adult Populations in the United States

References	Sample	Instrument	Response Categories	Validation Standard	Design	Results
Baumgartner et al.[18]	43 HF (Hispanic) 89 NHF	140-items; interviewer administered; open-ended; referent period was previous 4 weeks	Included per month, week, or day	4-day food records	Compared subject's report of past month's food intake against four randomly selected nonconsecutive day food records; third FFQ taken 6 months after first FFQ to recall original month and then compared against subject's 4-day FR	Pearson's correlation coefficients (log-transformed and energy-adjusted); nutrients that differed significantly by ethnicity between FFQ2 + FFQ3 and food records: *Protein (g):* HF 0.40 NHF 0.35 *Vitamin A:* HF 0.67 NHF 0.38 *Vitamin C:* HF 0.34 NHF 0.64 *Calcium:* HF 0.49 NHF 0.58
Hankin et al.[19]	Japanese: 29 M + 29 F Chinese: 29 M + 26 F Filipino: 22 M + 25 F Hawaiian: 19 M + 28 F Caucasian: 29 M + 26 F	Hawaiian Cancer Research Center: 47 items, semiquantitative; administered; covers past 12 months; color photographs showing S, M, L portion sizes were used by subjects to estimate intake on FFQ and FR	8 (never or hardly ever to 2 or more times/day)	4, 1 week FR at approximately 3-month intervals	Compared subject's report of nutrient intake (FFQ) against average of 4, 1 week FR collected at 3-month intervals during a 1-year period. FFQ collected at end of 12-month period	Intraclass correlations (log-transformed) between the subjects' reports on FFQs and average 7-day FR: *Total fat:* JapM 0.55, WM 0.34, ChinM 0.39, FilM 0.60 HawM 0.26, JapF 0.65, WF 0.44, ChinF 0.61, FilF 0.55, HawF 0.40 *Vitamin A:* JapM 0.74, WM 0.38, ChinM 0.65, FilM 0.53, HawM 0.35 and JapF 0.23, WF 0.40, ChinF 0.64, FilF 0.53, HawF 0.29 Intraclass correlation for total fat for all males was 0.48 and for all females 0.60. FFQ overestimated means of FR by large amounts but results on the agreement of the FFQ with FR were generally satisfactory

| Kristal et al.[15] | 555 WF, 271 black F, 159 Hispanic F recruited at three clinical centers. Because Hispanics were recruited at Miami clinic only, their data was compared with WF from same clinic; data for WF and BF at two other centers were collapsed and compared | 100 items, self-administered, semiquantitative; covering last 3 months; portion sizes were S, M, L. FFQ collected at screening, baseline, and 6 months. Printed in both English and Spanish | 9 (never or <once/month to 2 or more times/day for foods and 6+/day for beverages) | 4-day FR collected at baseline and 6 months | Compared subjects recall of baseline FFQs with the baseline food records and at 6 months, the 6-month FFQ with the 6-month FR | FFQ overestimated percentage of energy from fat compared with FR. Pearson's correlations (log-transformed) between FFQ and 4-day FR:
Baseline:
Fat (percentage of energy, adjusted):
BF: 0.26
WF: 0.49
HF: 0.35 (Miami Clinic)
WF: 0.35
Saturated fat (percentage of energy adjusted):
BF: 0.32
WF: 0.50
HF: 0.37
WF: 0.56
β-Carotene (unadjusted)
BF: 0.42
WF: 0.32
HF: 0.26
WF: 0.30
Correlations at baseline were significantly larger among Whites than Blacks and tended to be larger for Whites than Hispanics.
6 months (control group)
Fat (percentage of energy):
BF: 0.49
WF: 0.52
HF: 0.48 (Miami)
WF: 0.61
Saturated fat (percentage of energy):
BF: 0.47
WF: 0.53
HF: 0.48 (Miami)
WF: 0.68
β-Carotene (unadjusted):
BF: 0.34
WF: 0.23
HF: 0.27(Miami)
WF: 0.57
Educational level associated with poor validity of FFQ and/or FR measures |

Continued

TABLE 27.2 (Continued)

References	Sample	Instrument	Response Categories	Validation Standard	Design	Results
Kumanyika et al.[6]	408 BF	NCi FFQ (short form) 11 items added to short resulting in food list of 68 items; semiquantitative; Collected at basline	9 (never or <1/month through 2 + times/day)	3 telephone, 24 hr. recalls obtained during a different season; 1 written 3 day food record; all data collected over a one year period	Compare dietary data over a one year period to baseline FFQ data for 12 dietary constituents with relevence to chronic disease including fat, sat fat, protein, carbohydrate, fiber, calcium, iron, B-carotene.folate and vitamine E.	Pearson correlation coefficients (energy adjusted) between FFQ and mean of combined recall and diary data: Fat 0.32 Saturated Fat 0.37 Protein 0.31 Carbohydrate 0.30 Dietary Fiber 0.51 Calcium 0.28 Iron 0.33 Vitamin C 0.43 Folate 0.47 Beta-Carotene 0.40 Vitamin E 0.15
Knutsen et al.[14]	17 BM 32 BF 27 WM 45 WF	FFQ designed to include vegetarian dietary patterns	Simple portion size segment	One adipose tissue biopsy; valid measure collected from 49 Black and 72 White subjects. 4 – 24 hour recalls completed twice during a 6 month period; collected at random by telephone	Proportion of total dietary fat for the intake of individual fatty acids was calculated from the 24-hr recalls. Total poly-mono-saturated fat, linoleic and linolenic acid were calculated from both the 24 hr recalls and FFQ. Pearson's correlation compared the proportions as assessed by the two different dietary methods to the fat biopsies.	Correlation of FFQ data with adipose tissue data is of the order 0.4 to 0.6. Correlation between 24 hr FR data and different fatty acids varied. Corrected 24 hr Correlation coefficient and total fatty acids for BM&F Total SFA 0.46 (sig) Total MUF 0.29 (sig) Total PUF. 0.78 (sig) Crude Correlation coefficient for FFQ and total fatty acids for BM&F. Total SFA 0.21 (ns) Total MUF 0.07 (ns) Total PUF 0.78 (sig) Corrected 24 hr Correlation coefficient and total fatty acids for WM&F. Total SFA 0.56 (sig) Total MUF 0.04 (ns) Total PUF 0.70 (sig) Crude Correlation coefficient for FFQ and total fatty acids for WM&F. Total SFA 0.31 (sig) Total MUF 0.31 (sig) Total PUF 0.70 (sig)

Larkin et al.[11]

43 BM
48 BF
64 WM
73 WF
(40% subjects Black)

Un Michigan FFQ:
113 food items
based on data from
NFCS 77 to 78;
semiquantitative;
collected food
intake over past
12 months

9 (not in past year to more
than once a day)

1-24 h recall + 3-day food
record collected four times/
year about 3 months apart.
FR's administered and
reviewed in subject's home.
FFQ administered in
subject's home about
3 months after fourth set of
records had been completed

Compared by sex and ethnic group
(BM, BF, WM, WF) report of food
intake (4 sets of FR) against
the FFQ

Pearson correlation (nonadjusted)
values between FFQ and 16 days of
FR:
Energy:
BM: 0.23
BF: 0.26
WM: 0.41
WF: 0.43
Protein (g):
BM: 0.23,
BF: 0.40
WM: 0.41
WF: 0.36
Total fat (g):
BM: 0.23
BF: 0.35
WM: 0.44
WF: 0.39
Vitamin A(IU):
BM: 0.15
BF: 0.28
WM: 0.26
WF: 0.27
FFQ showed larger mean nutrient
intakes compared with FR. Black
M + F had lower coefficients
between FFQ and FR than white
M + F

Liu et al.[12]

33 BM
32 BF
30 WM
33 WF

About 300 items in
20 categories;
Interviewer-
administered
quantitative FFQ
based on the
Western Electric
dietary history;
referent period is
past month

Open ended

7 – 24 h food recalls collected
by phone

Compared subject's recall of last
30 days against 7 to 24 h food
recalls

Mean nutrient values for WM are
similar between two methods; for
WF values from FFQ are generally
higher than recalls (Vitamin A
significantly different); for BM +
BF values from history are much
higher than recalls (vitamin A + kcal
significantly different);
Pearson's correlations
(log-transformed)
Total calories:
WM: 0.64
WF: 0.47
BM: 0.43
BF: 0.21
Total Fat:
WM: 0.65
WF: 0.37

Continued

TABLE 27.2 (Continued)

References	Sample	Instrument	Response categories	Validation Standard	Design	Results
Liu et al.[12] (Continued)						BM: 0.36 BF: 0.23 *Vitamin A:* WM: 0.67 WF: 0.62 BM: 0.62 BF: 0.32
Mayer-Davis et al.[16]	32 WF (Urban) 63 BF (Urban) 30 WF (Rural) 61 HF (Rural)	114-item, interviewer-administered FFQ; modified from NCI-HHHQ to include regional and ethnic food choices; past year	9 (never or <1/month to 2 or more times/day)	8 – 24 h recalls over course of 1 year (randomly selected days, about every 6 weeks)	Compared subject's report of frequency of intake from FFQ2 to average of 8 to 24 h recalls	Pearson correlations (log-transformed) between FFQ2/FR: *Energy:* WF (urban): 0.61 BF (urban): 0.37 WF (rural): 0.56 HF (rural): 0.27 *Total fat:* WF (urban): 0.66 BF (urban): 0.59 WF (rural): 0.58 HF (rural): 0.40 *Vitamin A:* WF (urban): 0.38 BF (urban): 0.28 WF (rural): 0.62 HF (rural): 0.43 Correlations by educational status: *Total fat:* <12 grade: 0.05 12 grade: 0.59 *Total CHO:* <12 grade: 0.19 12 grade: 0.53 *Saturated fat:* <12 grade: 0.07 12 grade: 0.63 *Vitamin A:* <12 grade: 0.31 12 grade: 0.21

Morris et al.[13]	60 BF 58 BM 65 WF 49 WM	NA	Modified, semi-quantitative Harvard FFQ, measured food intake over 1 year; 139 food items and vitamin and mineral supplements; self administered	6-24 hour dietary recall interviews conducted at 2 month intervals over one year (Avg. no. RC/person was 3.6)	Compared analysis of 15 nutrients from the 3.6 avg FR/person with 1 FFQ covering food intake over 1 year	Pearson's correlation between a 12 month SFFQ and avg. 24 hour dietary recalls for total sample of 232 participants: Protein – 0.31 Carbohydrate- 0.42 Saturated fat – 0.47 Poly fat – 0.36 Mono fat – 0.40 Cholesterol – 0.39 Vitamin E – 0.67 Vitamin C – 0.60 Vitamin D 0.51 Calcium – 0.56 Folate – 0.50 Vitamin B6 – 0.51 Vitamin B12 – 0.38
Resnicow et al.[8]	African American M&F recruited from 14 churches:	Varied by instrument	1) 7-item fruit and vegetable (F&V) FFQ based on intake of last month 2) 2-item F&V measure asking servings consumed each day 3) 36-item FFQ of F&V intake based on Health Habits and History Questionnaire, version 2.1. Asked consumption of F&V in last week. Portion size was fixed at medium 4) One 24 hour recall by telephone 5) 3 24 hour recalls by telephone	Serum Carotenoid levels (lycopene, lutein, cryptoxan-thin. Alpha carotene, and beta carotene)	Comparison of four methods of assessing fruit and vegetable intake with a serum carotenoid levels	Validity correlations based on transformed values for the 36-item FFQ which proved generally as strong as both 1 and 3 days of dietary recalls are provided: Lycopene: 0.02 Lutein: 0.21 Cryptoxanthin: 0.26 Alpha carotene: 0.34 Beta carotene: 0.31 Total carotenoids: 0.32 Caroteniods without lycopene: 0.35

Continued

TABLE 27.2 (Continued)

References	Sample	Instrument	Validation Standard	Response categories	Design	Results
Stram et al.[20]	African-American 151 BM, 186 BF Japanese 224 JM, 222 JF Hispanics 136 HM, 123 HF Caucasians 264 WM, 264 WF	Based on Hawaiian Cancer Research Center FFQ; quantitative by placing serving size photos beside the amount category; eight frequency categories for food and nine for beverages	Three random, 24 h recalls conducted by phone	Unknown; highest response for food is >2 times/day; for beverages, 4 times/day	An initial FFQ was mailed to random sample of prospective subjects; 3 – 24 h recalls were collected by phone after the initial contact; a second FFQ was sent 4 to 6 weeks after the recalls were completed; the subjects' responses on the second FFQ were compared against the 24 h recall values	Corrected correlations for the regression of mean 24 h recalls on the second FFQ by ethnic sex/group for following nutrients: *Total kilocalories:* BM 0.16 BF 0.17 JM 0.34 JF 0.19 HM 0.33 HF 0.40 WM 0.48 WF 0.28 *Total Protein:* BM 0.17 BF 0.22 JM 0.31 JF 0.25 HM 0.27 HF 0.35 WM 0.51 WF 0.38 *Total Fat:* BM 0.29 BF 0.24 JM 0.41 JF 0.32 HM 0.33 HF 0.57 WM 0.57 WF 0.39 *Vitamin A:* BM 0.30 BF 0.22 JM 0.45 JF 0.49 HM 0.62 HF 0.52 WM 0.59 WF 0.58
Suitor et al.[17]	Initially who provided three diet recalls: WF: 54 BF: 20 HF: 18 Subjects who provided FFQ2 and FR = 62 but no ethnic breakdown	Willett (Harvard Un.) 111 items, self-administered (edited foods, portion size information deleted); developed as a prenatal FFQ	3 – 24 h recalls conducted by phone	Unknown (recall of past 2 weeks)	Compared female's report of food intake between food recalls and FFQ2 which were mailed.	Pearson correlation (unadjusted, log transformed values) between FFQ2's and recalls: *Energy:* 0.41 *Protein:* 0.33 *Vitamin A:* 0.12 *Calcium:* 0.52
Coates et al.[5]	91 BF	HHHQ: original 98 item FFQ revised to include 19 ethnic/regional foods resulting in 117 item FFQ; past year	Serum carotenoids, α-tocopherol, lycopene, crytoxanthin, lutein/xeaxanthin	4 (times/day, week, month or year)	Compared female's FFQ responses to 15 ml nonfasting venous blood sample	Pearson's correlations (log-transformed, unadjusted) between FFQ and serum for nonsmokers: *α-Tocopherol (food only):* 0.19 *Provitamin A carotenoids:* 0.37 *β-Carotene:* 0.34 *Cryptoxanthin:* 0.37 *Lycopene:* -0.02 *Lutein:* 0.12

Pearson's correlations (log-transformed, unadjusted) for smokers were:

α-Tocopherol: −0.12
Provitamin A carotenoids: 0.07
β-Carotene: 0.11
Cryptoxanthin: 0.18
Lycopene: −0.02
Lutein: 0.11

Results suggest that FFQ was reasonably valid for black females. Analysis of lycopene and lutein may not reflect validity of the assessment of these nutrients.

| Forsythe et al.[10] | 80 BF ethnic mix of African blacks, Asian Indians, Caribbean whites, Guyanese Amerindians, and Caribbean Chinese | FFQ: 82 items compiled from Caribbean food tables, Willett FFQ, Stower prenatal food guide, and regional recipes | Unknown (weekly intake patterns) | 3, 24-h recalls | Compared female's report of intake against 3, 24-h recalls, one recall at prenatal visit and two others by phone during next 7 days. Second FFQ administered 3 weeks later | Paired *t*-tests examined differences between the food recall means and the means of the FFQ at time 1. Most of the 14 nutrients were significantly different using the two instruments, with the exception of saturated fat, vitamin A and caffeine. The percentage of energy from protein, CHO, and fat showed no significant differences on either method of assessment. Mean difference scores were computed between food recalls and time two FFQ responses in the subsample. Significant differences were found for energy, CHO and vitamin C and the percentage of energy from CHO The 24 h recalls did not fully support the responses provided on the FFQ's |

Continued

TABLE 27.2 (Continued)

References	Sample	Instrument	Response Categories	Validation Standard	Design	Results
Lee et al.[8]	74 ChinW	84 items; interviewer administered; past year; portion size asked for foods eaten >1/week; three-dimensional actual size food models used; type of fat used in cooking asked.	5 (day, week, month, year or not at all)	1 – 24 h recall (typical day during past month)	Compared female's report of frequency of intake against the 1 – 24 recall	Pearson correlations between the FFQ and the food recall: *Total kilocalories:* 0.05 *Total fat:* 0.21 *Protein:* 0.56 *Vitamin A:* 0.46 Nutrient intakes by FFQ that were significantly higher than 24 h recall were total kcal, total fat, vitamin A, saturated fat, cholesterol and β-carotene. Use of only 1 – 24 h recall could explain the modest correlations
McPherson et al.[9]	33 HM + F	38 mutually exclusive food types; interviewer administered; referent period last 4 weeks;	Unknown	3, random nonconsecutive food records	Compared subject's report of past month's food intake against 3 – 24 h food records	Pearson's correlation coefficients (unadjusted) between FFQ and records *Energy:* 0.77 *Total fat:* 0.76 *Cholesterol:* 0.61 None of the differences between nutrients on FFQ1 and FR were significant

TABLE 27.3

FFQ Reliability Studies among Adult Minority Populations in the United States

References	Sample	Instrument	Response Categories (Range)	Design	Results
Baumgartner et al[18]	43 HF (Hispanic) 89 WF	140-items; interviewer administered; semiquantitative; referent period was previous 4 weeks	Included per month, week, or day	Compared 6-month test–retest reproducibility of nutrient estimates from FFQ2 and FFQ3. Reproducibility coefficients were not reported by ethnic group except for two nutrients	Pearson's coefficients (log-transformed, adjusted) by ethnic group between the two FFQ's for two nutrients: *Saturated fat:* HF: 0.57 WF: 0.77 *Retinol:* HF: 0.50 WF: 0.80
Forsythe et al[10]	80 BF ethnic mix of African blacks, Asian Indians, Caribbean whites, Guyanese Amerindians, and Caribbean Chinese	FFQ: 82 items compiled from Caribbean food tables, Willett FFQ, Stower prenatal food guide, and regional recipes	Unknown (weekly intake patterns)	Compared 3-week test–retest reproducibility of nutrient estimates from FFQs and food recalls	Paired t-tests examined differences between the food recall means and the means of the FFQ at time 1. Most of the 14 nutrients were significantly different using the two instruments, with the exception of saturated fat, vitamin A, and caffeine. The percentage of energy from protein, CHO, and fat showed no significant differences on either method of assessment. Mean difference scores were computed between food recalls and time 2 FFQ responses in the subsample. Significant differences were found for energy, CHO and vitamin C and the percentage of energy from CHO Pearson's correlations between the two FFQs were: *Energy:* 0.91 *Protein:* 0.97 *Total fat:* 0.89 *Vitamin A:* 0.73
Kristal et al[15]	555 WF 271 BF 159 HF recruited at three clinical centers. Because Hispanics recruited at Miami clinic only, their data was compared with WF from same clinic; data for WF and BF at two other centers were collapsed and compared	100 items, self-administered, semiquantitative; last 3 months; portion sizes were S, M, L. FFQ collected at screening, baseline and six months	9 (never or <once/month to 2 or more times/day)	Compared 6-month test–retest reproducibility of selected nutrient estimates from baseline and 6-month FFQ's in the control group only. Analyses were also stratified on level of education	Pearson's coefficients (log-transformed) between the two FFQ's were: *Fat (percentage of energy):* BF: 0.37 WF: 0.51 HF: 0.45 (Miami Center) WF: 0.34 *Vitamin C (unadjusted):* BF: 0.60 WF: 0.67 HF: 0.75 (Miami Center) WF: 0.44 *β-Carotene (unadjusted):* BF: 0.54 WF: 0.61 HF: 0.62 (Miami Center) WF: 0.46 Little evidence that reliability was affected by poor education

Continued

TABLE 27.3 (Continued)

References	Sample	Instrument	Response Categories (Range)	Design	Results
Liu et al.[12]	33 BM, 32 black F, 30 WM, 33 WF	About 300 items in 20 categories; interviewer-administered quantitative history based on the Western Electric dietary history; referent period is past month	Open ended	Compared subject's history of last 30 days against baseline history	Sex-adjusted partial correlation coefficients (log-transformed, not calorie-adjusted) between the first and last histories *Energy:* WM + F: 0.76 BM + F: 0.50 *Total fat:* WM + F: 0.73 BM + F: 0.56 *Protein:* WM + F: 0.70 BM + F: 0.57 *Vitamin A:* WM + F: 0.77 BM + F: 0.74
Morris et al.[13]	97 Black Adults 95 White Adults	Modified, Semi-Quantitative Harvard FFQ: self-administered; referent period is past 12 months	NA	Comparison of 15 nutrients between 2 self-administered FFQ's at the beginning and end of a 12 month period.	Intraclass correlations between 2 SFFQ's 12 months apart for total sample for following nutrients Protein – 0.57 Carbohydrate – 0.65 Saturated – fat 0.60 Poly fat – 0.54 Mono fat – 0.61 Cholesterol – 0.57 Vitamin E – 0.67 Vitamin C – 0.62 Vitamin D – 0.60 Clacium – 0.51 Folate – 0.70 Vitamin B6 – 0.58 Vitamin B12 – 0.50
McPherson et al.[10]	20 HM + F	38 mutually exclusive food types; interviewer administered; referent period last 4 weeks	Unknown	Compared 1 month test–retest reproducibility of nutrient estimates between FFQ2 and FFQ3 and FFQ2 and FFQ4	Absolute nutrient intakes from FFQ2 were greater than those of FFQ3 and FFQ4. Pearson's coefficients (unadjusted) between FFQ2 and FFQ3: *Energy:* 0.90 *Total fat:* 0.85 *Cholesterol:* 0.85 Coefficients (unadjusted) between FFQ2 and FFQ4 were *Energy:* 0.84 *Total fat:* 0.70 *Cholesterol:* 0.79

Reference	Subjects	FFQ description	Response categories	Study comparison	Results
Mayer-Davis et al.[16]	32 WF (urban) 63 BF (urban) 30 WF (rural) 61 HF (rural)	114-item, first FFQ interviewer administered and second was conducted over phone; modified from NCI-HHHQ to include regional and ethnic food choices; past year	9 (never or <1/ month to 2 or more times/day)	Compared 2 to 4 year test–retest reproducibility of baseline FFQ1 with FFQ2	Pearson's coefficients (log-transformed, unadjusted) between two FFQs were: *Energy:* WF (urban): 0.81 BF (urban): 0.64 HF (rural): 0.83 WF (rural): 0.61 *Total fat (g):* WF (urban): 0.81 BF (urban): 0.69 HF (rural): 0.87 WF (rural): 0.63 *Vitamin A (IU):* WF (urban): 0.67 BF (urban): 0.26 HF (rural): 0.63 WF (rural): 0.53 Reproducibility of FFQs was similar across all subgroups evaluated including educational attainment
Suitor et al.[17]	Initially who provided three diet recalls: WF: 54 BF: 20 HF: 18 Subjects who provided FFQ1 and FFQ2 = 43 but no ethnic breakdown	Willett (Harvard Un.) 111 items, self-administered (edited foods, portion size information deleted); developed as a prenatal FFQ	Unknown (recall of past 2 weeks)	Compared female's report of food intake between baseline FFQ1, which was completed in the clinic and FFQ2 which was mailed. Those returning FFQ2 were unrepresentative of the original sample	Pearson's correlation (unadjusted, log-transformed values) between FFQ1 and FFQ2: *Energy:* 0.92 *Protein:* 0.87 *Vitamin A:* 0.89 *Calcium:* 0.80

include foods that will contribute substantially to the nutrients under investigation. This importance of a food list capturing the usual intake of study participants was demonstrated in the study conducted in Starr County, Texas. Because of the limited number of overall foods that the participants consumed, the food list of the FFQ was able to reflect the major sources of food and nutrient intake of these individuals. Because of this unique situation, the nutrient values from the FFQ were more likely to agree with the values from the food records.

Several suggestions were made regarding the administration of the dietary assessment forms in minority populations. It is recommended that any staff person who is responsible for interviewing a subject for any dietary assessment measure should be of the same ethnic background of the subject irrespective of whether the conversation takes place in person or over the phone.

Educational attainment of participants appeared to be a major determinant of the validity of the dietary assessment measures in several studies. Agreement between the food frequency and the criterion measure of 24 h dietary recalls was substantially compromised among individuals with less than a high school education. This was particularly true within a Hispanic group of one study. In another study, it was found that increasing validity with increased education suggested that poor education is a barrier to accurate completion of the FFQ, the food record, or both. In this same study, low educational levels did not affect reliability measures. These findings would suggest that special efforts are needed when using dietary assessment tools with participants of low educational status or culturally diverse dietary habits. Small group instruction and practice in using the dietary tools could improve the dietary information collected. Instructing participants by videotape on completing dietary forms is another method to help improve the accuracy of information.

EXAMPLES OF FFQS

This section includes examples of the FFQs that have been used or adapted for studies of minority populations. This is not intended to be a complete list of all the questionnaires that were used in the 16 studies reviewed, nor is inclusion in this set of examples an implied endorsement of one instrument. The FFQs included are those that are widely available. The FFQs in this set were originally selected by an investigator for modification to his or her population or are the actual instrument used to assess dietary intake. Readers who are interested in using or adapting these dietary assessment tools should contact the resource persons listed with each tool.

In selecting a FFQ, the reader should consider several points:

1. What is the primary purpose of the project or study you are planning to conduct and how does the food intake data relate to the outcome?
2. For what length of time are you interested in assessing food intake? 12 months, 3 months?
3. How current is the food list? Does it reflect the current food supply?
4. Does the food list contain foods that contribute significantly to the nutrients you are interested in assessing?
5. Does the food list reflect the traditional or cultural foods eaten by your population?
6. Is the nutrient software analysis program updated on a regular basis to reflect the changing composition of our food supply?
7. Can you individualize the food list of the FFQ to your specific population? How much latitude do you have to modify the existing questionnaire? Can the existing software be modified to reflect the changes you wish to make?
8. Request a list of the validity and reliability studies that investigators have conducted using the FFQ you are considering. Were these studies conducted with populations similar to the groups of persons you wish to recruit into your study?

Diet History Questionnaire

Investigators at the National Cancer Institute have developed a new self-administered, scannable FFQ, the Diet History Questionnaire (DHQ). This instrument was designed with particular attention to cognitive ease and has been updated with respect to the food list and nutrient database using national dietary data (USDA's 1994–1996 Continuing Survey of Food II). This instrument is available on the Internet and can be downloaded from the site http://appliedresearch.cancer.gov. The data analysis program that accompanies this questionnaire became available for downloading from this site in November, 2005. Validity studies have been completed but not within minority populations.

Harvard University FFQ ("Willett Questionnaire")

Several FFQs are available from the Harvard School of Public Health including this current version designed for use in African-American populations. This is a scannable, self-administered FFQ and is referred to as the "green version." This questionnaire contains a section on the assessment of vitamin and mineral intake, which is followed by approximately 174 food items. The assessment period of the FFQ is the past 12 months, and respondents are asked to average seasonal use of foods over the entire year. This tool is designed to enhance an individual's ability to respond more appropriately to the food items. For example, the response categories are individualized for each item ranging from "never" to "six or more times/day" and probing questions are asked regarding specific characteristics of foods consumed. Information can be found at https://wchanning.bwh.harvard.edu/KIDS/files.

Resource:
Laura Sampson, M.S., R.D.
HSPH — Nutrition
Bldg. #2, Room 335
665 Huntington Ave.
Boston, MA 02115
E-mail: nhlas@channing.harvard.com

FRED HUTCHINSON CANCER RESEARCH CENTER FFQ ("KRISTAL QUESTIONNAIRE")

This questionnaire links answers from an extensive list of food questions to specific food frequency items to derive more precise nutrient estimates for those items. The FFQ is machine-readable and is accompanied by a software system to process the questionnaire. The format has nine frequency categories and a small, medium, and large portion size. The food list is composed of 122 foods and is preceded by 19 behavioral questions related to preparation techniques and types of food selected. Answers to these questions are used directly in the program to choose more appropriate nutrient composition values for certain foods in the food list. This questionnaire is available in Spanish.

Resource:
Dr. Alan R. Kristal, P.H.
Fred Hutchinson Cancer Research Center
Cancer Prevention Research Program
1100 Fairview Ave. N
MP-702
Seattle, WA 98109-1024
Phone: 206 667 4686
Fax: 206 667 5977
E-mail: akristal@fhcrc.org

CANCER RESEARCH CENTER OF HAWAII'S DIETARY QUESTIONNAIRE
(THE HAWAII CANCER RESEARCH SURVEY)

The Cancer Research Center of Hawaii, part of the University of Hawaii, has developed a variety of quantitative FFQs for use with the multiethnic population of Hawaii. Recently a questionnaire was developed to assess the diets of the five main ethnic groups in the Hawaii-Los Angeles Multiethnic Cohort Study: Hispanics, African-Americans, Japanese, Hawaiians, and Caucasians. Unlike previous questionnaires, the cohort questionnaire was designed to be self-administered. Three-day measured food records were collected from all ethnic groups in advance and were used to identify food items for inclusion in the questionnaire. To ensure more accurate specifications of amounts usually consumed, photographs showing three portion sizes were printed on the questionnaire. A customized, and in part ethnic-specific, food composition table was developed for the cohort questionnaire. A calibration study, comparing questionnaire responses to three 24 h recalls for the same subjects showed highly satisfactory correlations, particularly after energy adjustment.

Resource:
Donna Au, M.P.H, R.D.
Research Dietitian Supervisor
Cancer Research Center of Hawaii
University of Hawaii
1236 Lauhala St.
Honolulu, HI 96813
Phone: 808 564 5950
Fax: 808 586 2982
E-mail: dtakemor@crch.hawaii.edu

New Mexico Women's Health Study, Epidemiology, and Cancer Control Program, University of New Mexico Health Sciences Center

This FFQ was developed for an adjunct trial to the New Mexico Women's Health Study, a population-based case-control study of breast cancer in non-Hispanic and Hispanic women. The 140-item FFQ was a modified version of a questionnaire developed by the Human Nutrition Center, University of Texas School of Public Health, Houston, for a Texas Hispanic population. The FFQ was revised to include important food sources of energy, macronutrients, and vitamins that were identified following an analysis of food intake recalls. Emphasis was placed on specific rather than grouped food items because recall is considered better for specific items. Usual portion size, based on two-dimensional food models, included data on number of servings, the type of food model, and thickness of food. Common serving descriptions were included for each food item and were based either on food models or a defined portion size. This FFQ was translated into Spanish.

Resource:
R. Sue Day, Ph.D.
Director Human Nutrition Center
Associate Professor of Epidemiology and Nutrition
University of Texas — Houston School of Public Health
1200 Herman Pressler
Houston, TX 77030
Phone: 713 500 9317
Fax: 713 500 9329
E-mail: rena.s.day@uth.tmc.edu

Insulin Resistance Atherosclerosis Study Food Frequency Questionnaire, School of Public Health, University of South Carolina

The Insulin Resistance Atherosclerosis Study (IRAS) provided the opportunity to evaluate the comparative validity and reproducibility of a FFQ within and across subgroups of non-Hispanic White, Hispanic, and African-American individuals. The 114-item questionnaire was modified from the National Cancer Institute — Health Habits and History Questionnaire, which was originally created by Gladys Block, Ph.D. This interviewer-administered FFQ was modified to include regional and ethnic food choices that were commonly consumed by the participants of the study. The FFQ contains nine categories of possible responses ranging from "never or less than once a month" to "two or more times a day." Portion sizes are determined as "small, medium, or large compared to other men/women about your age." At the end of the FFQ an open-ended question is asked to describe foods that are usually eaten "at least once a week" and were not asked on the FFQ. Also, nine additional questions probe for information regarding common food preparation methods, specific fats used in cooking, and frequency of consumption of fruits and vegetables.

Resource:
Dr. Mara Z. Vitolins, P.H., R.D., L.D.N.,
Wake Forest University School of Medicine
Department of Public Health Sciences
Medical Center Blvd.
Piedmont Plaza 2, Suite 512
Winston-Salem, NC 27157-1063
Phone: 336 716 2886
Fax: 336 716 4300
E-mail: mvitolin@wfubmc.edu

REFERENCES

1. Coates, R.J. and Monteilh, C.P. *A J Clin Nutr* 65: 1108S; 1997.
2. Spencer, G. *Projections of the Hispanic population: 1983–2089.* US Department of Commerce, Bureau of Census, (Series P-25), Washington, DC, 1989.
3. National Institutes of Health, NIH guidelines on the inclusion of women and minorities as subjects in clinical research, *Federal Registry*, 59: 14508; 1994.
4. Hankin, J.H. and Wilkens, L.R. *A J Clin Nutr* 59: 198S; 1994.
5. Coates, R.J., Eley, J.W., Block, G., Gunter, E.W., Sowell, A.L., Grossman, C., and Greenberg, R.S. *A J Epidemiol* 15: 658; 1991.

6. Kumanyika, S.K., Manger, D., Mitchell, D.C., et al. *Ann Epidemiol* 13: 111; 2003.
7. Resnicow, K., Odom, E., Wang. T., et al. *A J Epidemiol* 152: 1072; 2000.
8. Lee, M.M., Lee, F., Ladenla, S.W., and Miike, R. *Ann Epidemiol* 4: 188; 1994.
9. McPherson, R.S., Kohl, H.W., Garcia, G., et al. *Ann Epidemiol* 5: 378; 1995.
10. Forsythe, H.E. and Gage, B. *A J Clin Nutr* 59: 203S; 1994.
11. Larkin, F.A., Metzner, H.L., Thompson, F.E., et al. *JADA* 89: 215; 1989.
12. Liu, K., Slattery, M., Jacobs, D., et al. *Ethnicity Dis* 4:15; 1994.
13. Morris, M.C., Tangney, C.C., Bienias, J.L., et al. *A J Epidemiol* 158: 1213; 2003.
14. Knutsen, S.F., Fraser, G.E., Beeson, W.L., et al. *Ann Epidemiol* 13: 119; 2003.
15. Kristal, A.R., Feng, Z., Coates, R.J., et al. *A J Epidemiol* 146: 856; 1997.
16. Mayer-Davis, J.E., Vitolins, M.Z., Carmichael, S.L., et al. *Ann Epidemiol* 9: 314; 1999.
17. Suitor, C., Gardner, J., Willett, W.C. *JADA* 89: 1786; 1989.
18. Baumgartner, K.B., Gilliland F.D., Nicholson, C.S., et al. *Ethnicity and Dis* 8: 81; 1998.
19. Hankin, J.H., Wilkens, L.R., Kolonel, L.N., Yoshizawa, C.N. *A J Epidemiol* 15: 616; 1991.
20. Stram, D.O., Hankin, J.H., Wilkens, L.R., et al. *A J Epidemiol* 15: 358; 2000.

28 Methods and Tools for Dietary Intake Assessment in Individuals vs. Groups

Marian L. Neuhouser and Ruth E. Patterson

CONTENTS

INTRODUCTION

Dietary intake is an important, modifiable determinant of health and longevity. Comprehensive reviews of the literature have consistently concluded that there are clear causal links between food intake and major causes of morbidity and mortality, such as coronary heart disease, cancer, diabetes, and obesity.[1–3] In addition, undernutrition contributes to substantial health problems, particularly in resource-poor countries.[4]

Given the importance of diet in human health, assessment of dietary intake plays a pivotal role in efforts to improve the health of individuals and populations throughout the world. Dietary intake data are used for three major purposes:

1. At the individual level, assessment of dietary intake is necessary for determining a person's dietary adequacy or risk, assessing adherence to recommended dietary patterns, and tailoring education and counseling efforts.
2. Dietary intake assessment is an integral part of research studies investigating how diet determines the health of individuals and populations. Etiologic studies assess dietary intake as an exposure for association with disease outcomes. Behavioral research assesses dietary intake (or change in intake) as an outcome in studies designed to develop and test strategies to encourage adoption of healthful eating patterns.

3. Finally, at the population level, assessment of dietary intake is necessary to identify national health priorities and develop public health dietary recommendations. These data are used to determine the success of public health interventions to improve dietary patterns and for identification of population subgroups at risk or in need of special assistance. Nutrition monitoring also serves as a key role in food assistance programs, fortification initiatives, food safety evaluations, and food labeling programs.

It is clear that dietary assessment is a cornerstone of efforts to improve the health of individuals and groups. However, there are significant concerns about the accuracy and usefulness of self-reported dietary data. The challenges associated with assessing dietary intake are well known and have to do with day-to-day variation in intake, respondent reporting errors and biases, limitations of the assessment instruments, and error in food composition databases.[5] Several different assessment methods and tools have been developed to address these difficulties, and each method has different strengths and weaknesses with regard to the type and quality of data produced. In addition, there are significant differences among these assessment methods in practical matters of respondent burden and cost. Therefore, it is necessary to carefully consider the specific objectives of the dietary assessment as a precursor to choosing the best or most appropriate method. Perhaps the first and most important question is whether the data will be used for assessing intake in individuals or groups.

Here, we describe the three major types of dietary assessment methods: (1) food records and 24-h dietary recalls, (2) food frequency questionnaires (FFQs), and (3) brief assessment instruments. We summarize both the scientific and practical advantages and disadvantages of each of these methods. Then, we consider the use of these three dietary assessment methods for assessing diet in individuals vs. groups. More specifically, we discuss these three assessment methods when used for: (1) determination of an individual's dietary adequacy for purposes of counseling, (2) research studies of dietary intake and disease risk, and (3) nutrition monitoring of populations. Additional information on dietary assessment can be found in the Chapters 26 and 29.

A DESCRIPTION OF THE THREE MAJOR DIETARY ASSESSMENT METHODS

FOOD RECORDS AND DIETARY RECALLS (RECORDS/RECALLS)

For many years, food records were considered the "gold standard" of dietary assessment methods. Briefly, food records or diaries require individuals to record everything consumed over a specified period of time, usually 1 to 7 days. Participants are typically asked to carry the record with them and to record foods as eaten. Some protocols require participants to weigh or measure foods before eating, while less stringent protocols use models and other aids to instruct respondents on estimating serving sizes. While most protocols specify that the food record be reviewed by a dietitian to confirm portion sizes of foods, fats added in cooking and at the table, and other food details, a recent study showed when detailed instructions about completion of the food record are given to participants, the review and documentation by a dietitian may not be necessary.[6] Regardless of the data collection protocol, ultimately the food consumption information from records/diaries is entered into a specialized software program for calculation of nutrient intakes. This data-entry step is a time-consuming task and requires trained data technicians or nutritionists.

Food records are somewhat burdensome for clients or study-participants to complete. In the foreseeable future, the use of personal digital assistants (PDAs), digital cameras, mobile telephones, and other electronic devices both to record and transmit food record data will likely alleviate some of the participant burden.[7,8] In a crossover intervention study, diabetic patients were asked to record their diet and blood glucose values using either traditional methods or a hand-held electronic device that would transmit the data to medical staff. The digital device was much preferred by the patients; the ease of operation reported by 95% of patients is likely to result in better quality food recording than a burdensome paper and pencil record.[9]

A dietary recall is a 20 to 30 min interview in which the respondent is asked to recall all foods and beverages consumed over the previous 24 h. Dietary supplement use may be included in the recall although methods for doing so are still under development (Dr. Lisa Harnack, personal communication, 2005). Dietary recall-interviews can be conducted in person or by telephone. In some settings, this information is captured on paper forms and subsequently entered into a software program for nutrient analysis. However, ideally the interview will be conducted simultaneously with direct data entry into the software program. It is very important that the interviewer be well-trained; tone of voice, body posture (when in-person), and reactions to participant descriptions of foods consumed can influence the quality of the data.

The use of portion size estimate aids increases the reliability of the recall data.[10,11] Recalls conducted in person utilize three-dimensional food models while those conducted over the telephone use two-dimensional booklets. For the latter approach, the portion size aids should be sent to clients or study participants in advance of the recall. Before the recall begins the interviewer should ask the participant to retrieve the portion size aid to use during the course of the interview. In some special population groups, in-person training in the proper use of the portion size estimators may improve the quality of the data.[12] Among older adults with poor memory, additional memory cues such as recall of the previous day's activities may be needed to stimulate recollection of food intake.[13]

One of the most widely used approaches to collect standardized dietary recall data is the USDA Automated Multiple Pass method that is currently in use in the integrated NHANES–CSFII survey, "What We Eat in America." [14–16] This five-step method includes the following sequence of queries:

1. *Quick list*: Trained interviewers first ask participants to list all foods and beverages consumed during the previous 24 h.
2. *Forgotten food list*: Interviewers probe for details about foods or additions to foods that are frequently forgotten. Examples of foods that are often added to this list are milk on cereal, sugar in coffee, and between meal snacks and beverages.
3. *Time and place*: The interviewer asks the participant to recall the time of day and the location (e.g., home, school, restaurant, etc.) of the food consumption. This time and place memory probe frequently helps participants to better recall the foods consumed.
4. *Detail cycle*: The interviewer probes for details about each food named in the quick list and forgotten list, including cooking methods, portion size, brand names, type, and amount of fat added during cooking and at the table. These details include the collection of information on mixed dishes and recipes. The questions in the detail cycle are highly standardized with computerized prompts to ensure uniform data collection.
5. *Final review*: The interviewer does a final review of the foods and beverages consumed and queries participants about any additional items that may have been omitted.

Advantages and Disadvantages of Records/Recalls

Both records and recalls provide the same type of data: detailed information on all foods and beverages consumed on specified days. In theory, a food record provides a "perfect" snapshot of intake. In practice, there are significant limitations associated with this method for assessing food intake. The principal problems are the large respondent burden of recording food intake and the impact on usual food consumption caused by record keeping. Respondents may alter their normal food choices merely to simplify record keeping because they are sensitized to food choices. The latter reason appears more likely among women,[17] restrained eaters,[18] obese respondents,[19] or participants in a dietary intervention.[20–23] Other sources of error by respondents include mistakes or omissions in describing foods and assessing portion sizes.

Unannounced, interviewer administered 24-h dietary recalls are often recommended because respondents cannot change what they ate retrospectively.[24] One major disadvantage of dietary recalls is that they rely on the respondent's memory and ability to estimate portion sizes, although the latter limitation can be alleviated by the use of portion size aids. In addition, it cannot be verified that social desirability does not influence self-report of the previous day's intake.[25] A noteworthy benefit of recalls is that they are appropriate for low literacy populations and children.[26,27]

Both records and recalls are expensive and time-consuming methods of assessing dietary intake. However, the major scientific issue with records/recalls concerns the issue of day-to-day variability in intake, which means that several days of records/recalls are required to characterize usual intake. Using data on variability in intake from food records completed by 194 participants in the Nurses Health Study,[28] the number of days needed to estimate the mean intakes for individuals within 10% of "true" means would be 57 days for fat, 117 days for vitamin C, and 67 days for calcium. For estimating food consumption for individuals, variability can be even greater. For example, the number of days needed to estimate the following foods within 10% of "true" means would be 55 days for white fish and 217 days for carrots. Unfortunately, research has shown that reported energy intake, nutrient intake, and recorded numbers of foods decreases with as few as 4 days of recording dietary intake.[29] These changes may reflect reduced accuracy and completeness of recording intake or actual changes in dietary intake to reduce the burden of recording intake. In either case, there are considerable limitations on the usefulness of this methodology for characterizing usual intake in individuals.

Food Frequency Questionnaires

FFQs were developed for conducting research on dietary intake and chronic diseases, such as heart disease and cancer. Because these diseases develop over 10 or more years, the biologically relevant exposure is long-term diet consumed many years prior to disease diagnosis. Therefore, instruments that only capture data on short-term or current intake (i.e., food records or recalls) are generally of limited usefulness for chronic disease research.

FFQs are designed to capture standardized, semiquantitative data on current or past, long-term diet. Although these questionnaires vary, they usually include three sections: (1) adjustment questions, (2) the food list, and (3) summary questions. Adjustment questions assess the nutrient content of specific food items. For example, participants are asked what type of milk they usually drink and are given several options (e.g., whole, skim, and soy), which saves space and reduces participant burden compared to asking for the frequency of consumption and usual portion sizes of many different types of milk. Adjustment questions also permit more refined analyses of fat intake by asking about food preparation practices (e.g., removing skin from chicken) and types of added fats (e.g., use of butter vs. margarine on vegetables).

The main section of an FFQ consists of a food or food group list, with questions on usual frequency of intake and portion size. To allow for machine scanning of these forms, frequency responses are typically categorized from "never or less than once per month" to "2+ per day" for foods and "6+ per day" for beverages. Portion sizes are often assessed by asking respondents to mark "small," "medium," or "large" in comparison to a given medium portion size. However, some questionnaires only ask about the frequency of intake of a "usual" portion size (e.g., 3 ounces meat).

The food list in a FFQ is chosen to capture data on: (1) major sources of energy and nutrients in the population of interest, (2) between-person variability in food intake, and (3) specific scientific hypotheses. The choice of a food list is part data-driven and part scientific judgment. One data-based approach uses record/recall data to determine the foods that are the major nutrient sources in the diet (i.e., the contribution of specific foods to the total population intake of nutrients). Information on food sources of nutrients in the American population has been an important part of the NHANES and CSFII surveys and now the integrated "What We Eat in America" survey.[14,15,30] Details about nutrients are limited, though, for foods consumed in specific population groups that may not be included on the food list (e.g., immigrants who retain their food habits) and there are very limited data on bioactive constituents of foods that are not considered nutrients, but nonetheless have biological actions (e.g., isothiocyanates).

However, a food is only informative if intake varies from person to person such that it discriminates between respondents. Therefore, another data-based approach to choosing the food list is to start with an extensive list of foods that is completed by a representative sample of the larger population. Stepwise regression analysis is performed where the dependent variable is the nutrient and the independent variable is frequency of consumption of foods.[28] In this process, the computer algorithm ranks foods by the degree to which they explain the most between-person variance in nutrient intake, which is reflected in change in cumulative R^2. In addition to these two data-driven methods, items are often added to a questionnaire because of specific hypotheses (e.g., does consumption of soy foods reduce breast cancer risk?).

A particularly challenging issue in FFQ food lists has to do with assessing intake of mixed dishes. For example, many FFQs ask about frequency of pizza consumption. However, from a nutrient perspective, there is no accurate way to define "pizza." Depending on whether it is meat or vegetarian, thick or thin crust, tomato or pesto sauce (and so forth), pizza may be either low-fat and high-carbohydrate or extremely high-fat and high-protein. However, it is unreasonable to ask individuals to disaggregate their pizza into servings of: (1) breads, (2) vegetables, (3) meats, (4) cheese, and (5) added fats. Therefore, FFQs typically strike an uneasy compromise between asking about some mixed dishes (e.g., pizza, hamburgers, and tacos) while also asking the respondent to provide information on foods contained in their mixed dishes: "Cheese, including cheese added to foods and in cooking." Unfortunately, asking about both "lasagna" and "Cheese in cooking" presents the peril of double counting. There are little or no data to guide an investigator in making these judgments.

Finally, to save space and reduce respondent burden, similar foods are often grouped into a single line item (e.g., white bread, bagels, and pita bread). When grouping foods, important considerations include whether they are nutritionally similar enough to be grouped and whether the group will make cognitive sense to the respondent. For example, a food group composed of rice, macaroni, and cooked breakfast cereal may be nutritionally sensible. However, this question could be difficult to answer, because it requires summing food consumption events across different meal occasions.

Finally, FFQ summary questions that ask about usual intake of fruits and vegetables are often included in the questionnaire, because the long lists of these foods needed to capture micronutrient intake can lead to over-reporting of intake.[31] Algorithms using the summary question are typically applied to the sum of the line items all fruits and vegetables consumed to give a more conservative estimate of fruit and vegetable consumption.

Assessing the Reliability and Validity of FFQs

Because records and recalls are open-ended, they can (in theory) be applied in a standardized manner across populations with markedly different eating patterns. However, as noted above, FFQs are close-ended forms with limited food lists. Because the food list varies from questionnaire to questionnaire, every FFQ will have different measurement characteristics. In addition, a questionnaire with appropriate foods and portion sizes for one population group (e.g., older non-Hispanic white men) may be wholly inappropriate for another subgroup (e.g., adolescent African American females). Finally, given the changes in the food supply over time, such as the introduction of specially manufactured low-fat or low-carbohydrate foods, questionnaires can become obsolete. Therefore, the measurement characteristics (i.e., reliability and validity) of an FFQ need to be assessed for each new questionnaire and each new population group being assessed.

Reliability generally refers to reproducibility, or whether an instrument will measure an exposure (e.g., nutrient intake) in the same way twice on the same respondents. Validity, which is a higher standard, refers to the accuracy of an instrument. Generally, a validity study compares a practical, epidemiologic instrument (e.g., an FFQ) with a more accurate but more burdensome and expensive method (e.g., dietary recalls).

Reliability and validity of an FFQ are typically investigated using measures of bias and precision. Bias is the degree to which the FFQ accurately assesses mean intakes in a group. Lack of bias is especially important when the goal is to measure absolute intakes for comparison to dietary recommendations or some other objective criteria. For example, when the aim is to estimate how close Americans are to meeting the dietary recommendation to eat five servings of fruits and vegetables per day, it is critical to know whether the assessment instrument being used under- or overestimates fruit and/or vegetable intake. Precision concerns whether an FFQ accurately ranks individuals from low to high nutrient intakes, which is typically the information needed to assess associations of dietary intake with risk of disease. It is important to remember than an instrument can be reliable without being accurate (valid or precise). That is, it can yield the same nutrient estimates two times and be wrong (e.g., biased upward) both times. Alternatively, an instrument can be reliable and consistently yield an accurate group mean (e.g., unbiased), but have poor precision such that it does not accurately rank individuals in the group from low to high in nutrient intake.

A reliability study compares intake estimates from two administrations of the FFQ in the same group of respondents. If an instrument is reliable, the mean intake estimates should not vary substantially between the two administrations. In addition, correlation-coefficients between nutrient intakes estimated from two administrations of the FFQ in the same group of respondents should be high, and are generally in the range of 0.6 to 0.7. Reliability is easy to measure and gives an upper bound as to the accuracy of an instrument. While a high reliability-coefficient does not imply a high validity coefficient, a low reliability-coefficient clearly means poor validity. That is, if an instrument cannot measure a stable phenomenon (such as usual nutrient intake) the same way twice, it clearly cannot be accurate.

In a validity study, bias is assessed by comparing the mean estimates from an FFQ to those from multiple days of records/recalls in the same respondents. This comparison allows us to determine whether nutrient intake estimates from an FFQ appear to be under- or over-reported in comparison to the criterion measure. Precision is measured as the correlation coefficients between nutrient intake estimates from the FFQ in comparison to a criterion measure, and typically range from 0.4 to 0.6. However, lower correlation coefficients (<0.4) are not unusual for nutrients that are poorly estimated with an FFQ, such as energy.[32] In addition, inclusion of dietary supplement use will often markedly improve correlation-coefficients (>0.8), because supplement use may be more accurately assessed and its doses can be extraordinarily high compared to dietary intake, and thereby markedly increase the variability in intake for a nutrient. Some studies also assess precision by ranking nutrient intake estimates, dividing them into categories (e.g., quartiles) and comparing these to similar categories calculated from another instrument. However, classifying a continuous exposure into a small number of categories does not reduce the effects of measurement error, and, therefore, this analysis does not provide additional information above correlation-coefficients.[33]

The theory behind these (so-called) validity studies is that the major sources of error associated with FFQs are independent of those associated with records and recalls, which avoids spuriously high estimates of validity resulting from correlated errors. The errors associated with FFQs are the limitations imposed by a fixed list of foods and the respondents' ability to report usual frequency of food consumption (and usual portion sizes) over a broad time frame. Since recent studies have documented the increase in typical food and meal portion sizes of American meals over the past 30 years, the fixed portion sizes on FFQs may quickly become obsolete.[34,35] For example, most FFQs list a 12-ounce soft drink as a medium portion, when it is more likely a "small" using today's portion standards. In contrast, diet records are open-ended, do not depend on memory, and permit measurement of portion sizes. Errors in food records result from coding errors and changes in eating habits while keeping the records. Errors in recalls results from estimation of portion sizes, participant memory, and coding errors. All dietary assessment methods are limited by the food composition databases used to derive nutrient estimates.

Nonetheless, it is apparent that there are correlated errors between FFQs and records or recalls.[36,37] Social desirability could influence how participants record or recall food intake across all types of dietary assessment instruments.[17,18,38] Participant errors in estimating portion sizes could bias recall and FFQ estimates of intake in similar ways. There are also correlated errors in nutrient databases. Finally, research using doubly labeled water to estimate total energy expenditure and 24-h urine samples to estimate protein consumption have demonstrated significant underreporting of energy and protein intakes from records, recalls, and FFQs.[36,39] This underreporting may vary by participant characteristics such as age, sex, body mass index, and various psychosocial characteristics.[19,20,38] Taken together, current data suggests that it is important to be aware of the limitations of records and recalls as criterion measures of dietary intake and cautiously interpret results using these assessment tools.

A final note is that an FFQ cannot, in and of itself, be validated. Only individual nutrient intake estimates can be validated by comparison of a nutrient estimate from the FFQ to a more accurate measure.

Advantages and Disadvantages of FFQs

The major advantage of FFQs is that they attempt to assess usual long-term diet, either current or in the past. In addition, they have relatively low respondent burden and are simple and inexpensive to analyze, because they can be self-administered and are machine scannable. A disadvantage of these questionnaires is that respondents must estimate usual frequency of consumption of approximately 100 foods and the associated usual portion sizes. These types of questions (i.e., this cognitive task) can be exceedingly difficult for many respondents, as evidenced by the prevalence of energy estimates from FFQs that are well outside of the realm of plausibility.[28,40] For example, it is not unusual for respondents to report usual energy intakes that are less than 500 kcal/day or greater than 5000 kcal/day. In addition, the format of the questionnaire itself is not user-friendly. Because FFQs are machine-scannable, respondents need to indicate their responses by filling in circles in a food-by-frequency matrix, similar to that used in standardized testing. Some population groups may be unfamiliar or uncomfortable with such data collection methods. As might be hypothesized, validity studies of FFQs suggest that these forms may be less valid in less educated respondents.[41] Elderly participants with poor eyesight may have difficulty completing the questionnaire.

Another major disadvantage of these questionnaires is related to the close-ended nature of the form. The limited food list and fixed portion size will not be appropriate for all individuals in a population and different forms have different measurement characteristics across various populations. For example, use of an FFQ with a typical American food list is not likely to be useful in some special populations or in places outside the United States. There is recent work, though, to develop culturally appropriate FFQs. For example, one FFQ is available for use in rural populations in the southern United States[42] and another for use in South Africa.[43] Therefore, data from different FFQs are not directly comparable, nor are data from the same FFQ used in different populations, nor are data from the same FFQ used at different points in time (because of changes in the food supply). Finally, dependent upon the food list chosen by an investigator, the validity of nutrient intake estimates will vary from nutrient to nutrient.

BRIEF DIETARY ASSESSMENT INSTRUMENTS

Comprehensive dietary assessments (records/recalls and FFQs) are not always necessary or practical, which has led to the development of a diverse collection of brief assessment instruments. These brief methods include three general types: (1) ecologic-level measures such as food disappearance data or household food inventories, (2) short instruments that target a limited number of foods and nutrients, and (3) questionnaires that assess dietary behaviors.

Ecologic-Level Measures

One well-known ecologic assessment of dietary intake is per capita food consumption estimated using national data on the total food supply. Publications from the FAO provide data on a country's total food supply from which nonconsumption uses (such as exports, livestock feed, and industrial uses) are subtracted, after which the total remaining food available can be divided by the population to obtain the per capita estimate of intake. These population intakes have been correlated with disease incidence across countries in provocative hypothesis generating studies.[44–47] One caution about the use of these data is that it is not always clear how the nonhuman uses are tallied and subtracted due to fluctuating market demand for the agricultural goods. For example, soybean farmers may sell their crop in 1 year to an oil manufacturer for human use, but in the process of oil purification, some of the by-product may be drawn off and sold for industrial use. Thus, the best use of food supply data is to give an overall snapshot of food availability.

Other ecologic measures, such as supermarket sale receipts, have been developed and evaluated.[48,49] Household food inventories are another example of ecological measures of diet. In one study, the presence (in the house) of 15 high-fat foods was found to correlate with household members dietary fat intake at 0.42 ($p < .001$).[50] Individuals with ≤4 high-fat foods in their house had a mean of 32% energy from fat compared to 37% for those with ≥8 high-fat foods. Poor household food availability has also been shown to be significantly associated with greater individual-level measures of food insecurity.[51] Household inventories may be especially good assessment tools to use with new immigrants where language or cultural barriers may preclude use of records, recalls or FFQs.[52,53]

Targeted Instruments

Dietary assessment instruments that measure a limited number of foods or nutrients are most useful when the target food/nutrient is not distributed throughout the food supply. For example, dietary fat is widely distributed in dairy foods, meats, added fats, desserts, prepared foods, etc. Therefore, short instruments that attempt to estimate fat intake tend to be biased and imprecise.[54,55] Alternatively, intake of the isoflavones genestein and daidzain, which are largely limited to soy foods, can be captured with relatively short instrument (15 foods).[56] Similarly, a focused recall that can be completed in 5 to 7 min has been shown to give carotenoid estimates that are comparable to those obtained from a full 30-min, 24-h recall.[57] In many situations, the lower participant or patient burden, cost, and staff time associated with targeted instruments may be strong motivations for their use.

Food Checklists

Food checklists and food preference lists have been developed primarily for use as screening tools. In format they are similar to a short FFQ but include no portion size information and may be limited to a certain class of foods, such as sweets or fruits and vegetables.[58–61] These checklists may be appropriate to use when monitoring adherence to a dietary intervention or to use as a counseling tool.

Behavioral Instruments

The development of diet behavioral instruments was motivated by problems with assessing dietary intervention effectiveness, particularly low-fat interventions. Traditional comprehensive instruments, such as records and FFQs, yield fairly imprecise estimates of fat intake that may not be sensitive to an intervention focused on changing participants' dietary behavior. One of the best known instruments of this type is the fat-related diet habit questionnaire.[62] This instrument was based on an anthropologic model that described low-fat dietary change as four types: (1) avoiding high-fat foods (exclusion), (2) altering available foods to make them lower in fat (modification), (3) using new, specially formulated or processed, lower-fat foods instead of their higher-fat forms (substitution), and (4) using preparation techniques or food ingredients that replace the common higher-fat alternative (replacement). Although originally developed for intervention assessment, the diet-habits questionnaire has since been used as a short assessment instrument in other research settings.[63,64]

Advantages and Disadvantage of Brief Assessment Instruments

The principal advantage of ecologic measures is that they are simple, inexpensive, nonintrusive, and objective measures of nutritional status. However, these environmental indicators do not provide precise measures of individual intake and it can be difficult to disentangle human consumption from livestock and industrial use.

Targeted questionnaires also tend to yield rather imprecise food or nutrient estimates. For example, short questionnaires for assessing fruit and vegetable intake have been extensively used in surveillance and intervention research. The typical approach uses two summary questions to capture consumption of most fruits and vegetables ("How often did you eat a serving of fruit [not including juices]?" and "How often did you eat a serving of vegetables [not including salad and potatoes]?"), to which are added usual consumption of juice, salad, and potatoes.[65] Comparison of this brief measure with food records, food frequency estimates, and serum carotenoids indicates that this method yields particularly biased (underestimated) and imprecise measures of vegetable intake, likely because vegetables in mixed foods such as casseroles or sandwiches may be forgotten and unreported.[31] However, more detailed, but short, targeted questionnaires are an improvement to the more global questions mentioned above.

The major advantage of the behavioral questionnaires is that they are short and simple (i.e., low respondent burden) and can be easily data-entered and scored. The disadvantage of these tools is that the diet "score" derived from these measures can be difficult to interpret, because it is not comparable to nutrient or food intake measures. In addition, because these questionnaires have typically been "validated" in relation to records or recalls, which have many sources of error and bias, the degree to which these questionnaires accurately reflect dietary intake is unknown.

USE OF DIETARY ASSESSMENT METHODS IN INDIVIDUALS VS. GROUPS

DETERMINATION OF AN INDIVIDUAL'S DIETARY ADEQUACY FOR PURPOSES OF COUNSELING

Records/Recalls

Records and recalls are used in clinical and counseling settings to assess dietary intake and are often used in a qualitative fashion. That is, respondents are asked to describe a usual day's intake and the nutritionist simply "eyeballs" the eating pattern for estimating dietary adequacy or risk, adherence to a prescribed diet, or areas for improving eating habits. The individualized nature of the interview can allow for probing and personalization of the feedback.

Whether these methods are used in a quantitative or qualitative manner, records and recalls can provide useful and understandable information to a respondent. The respondent can observe that the dietary recommendations are based directly on the food intake information provided and can use the advice to alter future food choices, food preparation techniques, or portion sizes. Therefore, on an individual level, records and recalls can serve an important teaching function. In addition, there is a considerable literature indicating the act of keeping records (i.e., self-monitoring) is a significant predictor of success in achieving weight loss or making other dietary changes.[55]

Food Frequency Questionnaires

FFQs tend to produce imprecise dietary intake estimates because of respondent error and inappropriate food lists and fixed portion sizes that may have little relationship to portions actually consumed. In addition, the data input (usual frequency of intake and portion sizes) and nutrient calculation algorithms are a black box to the respondent. Therefore, the respondent cannot easily use this information to make more healthful food choices. For these reasons, FFQs are not generally useful for assessing an individual's nutrient intake for purposes of counseling.

However, data on food consumption from FFQs has been used for individual feedback. For example, Kristal et al. developed computer programs for tailored feedback to participants in a self-help dietary intervention that used FFQ data to provide food-specific recommendations to reach nutritional goals (e.g., "if you use low-fat mayonnaise instead of regular mayonnaise, you will cut your fat by 28 g/week").[66] Because the feedback being provided to the participants is food based and taken directly from their responses (e.g., type of mayonnaise used and frequency consumed), this approach avoids the black box problems associated with using FFQs to estimate nutrient intake.

Brief Assessment Instruments

These instruments are diverse, and, therefore, it is difficult to generalize regarding their use. Ecologic measures are intended to be environmental indicators, and therefore, are generally not appropriate for individuals. However, it is clear that some, simple targeted instruments can be very useful for individual counseling. For example, a rather short set of questions can likely assess usual fruit and vegetable consumption sufficiently well for purposes of advising a respondent whether their intake appears to be adequate or inadequate. These types of questionnaires may also be useful for nutritionists who need to assess an individual or family's food scarcity.

RESEARCH STUDIES OF DIETARY INTAKE AND DISEASE RISK

Records/Recalls

Historically, records and recalls have not generally been used in large-scale studies of diet and disease risk for scientific and practical reasons. Scientifically, records/recalls only assess current, short-term diet and in most etiologic studies of chronic disease risk, usual long-term (and often past) diet is the exposure of biologic significance. Practically, records and recalls are infeasible because of costs and respondent burden. However, records and recalls are often used in subsamples of the parent study for the following purposes:

1. FFQ reliability and validity substudies
2. Evaluating dietary interventions where the goal is to compare mean intakes in the intervention vs. the control group
3. As a check of the main study assessment instrument (such as an FFQ)

Despite the historical tendency for researchers to avoid use of records and recalls in large etiologic studies, recent evidence suggests that this viewpoint deserves reevaluation. Healthy women in England completed an FFQ and a 7-day weighed food diary between 1993 and 1997. As a follow-up in 2000, diets of women who had been subsequently diagnosed with breast cancer were compared with the diets of women who did not develop breast cancer. When data from the food diaries were used in analysis, saturated fat intake was associated with a 20% increase in breast cancer risk per quintile increase in fat intake. However, analyses using the FFQ showed no association of any dietary measures with breast cancer risk.[67] The authors hypothesized that the large amount of measurement error present in the FFQ distorted the analyses to the extent that the FFQ findings were null.[67,68] Obviously, this sort of result has large implications for the field of nutritional epidemiology, because it calls into question the validity of the basic assessment tools used in the field. Other studies are currently underway to determine whether this type of finding will hold up in other research settings using standard food records or recalls.

Food Frequency Questionnaires

As noted above, the major advantage of an FFQ is that it attempts to assess the exposure of interest in most applications: usual dietary intake in an individual. The main use of these instruments is to rank study participants from low to high intake of many foods and nutrients for comparison (on the individual level) with disease risk. However these questionnaires produce food and nutrient estimates containing considerable random error resulting from inadvertently marking the wrong frequency column, skipping questions, and failures in judgment. These errors introduce noise into nutrient estimates such that our ability to find the "signal," such as an association of dietary fat and breast cancer, is masked or attenuated (i.e., biased toward no association).

However, a more important concern in research studies is systematic error. Systematic error refers to under- or over-reporting of intake across the population and person-specific sources of bias. For example, studies indicate that obese people are more likely to underestimate dietary intake than normal-weight people.[19] Systematic error may result in either null associations or spurious associations. Prentice used data from FFQs collected in a low-fat dietary intervention trial to simulate the effects of random and systematic error on an association of dietary fat and breast cancer, where the true relative risk (RR) was assumed to be 4.0.[69] Assuming only random error exists in the estimate of fat intake, the projected (i.e., observed) RR for fat and breast cancer would be 1.4. Assuming both random error and systematic error exists, the projected RR would be 1.1, similar to that reported in a recent meta-analysis on dietary fat and breast cancer.[70] Data on systematic error from biomarker studies, combined with these types of statistical simulations, clearly suggest that measures of self-reported dietary intake may not be adequate to detect many associations of diet with disease, even when a strong relationship exists. It is important to note that records/recalls are not exempt from these biases.

Finally, FFQs cannot provide detailed information on specific foods (e.g., brand names), restaurant type (e.g., fast food), or eating patterns (e.g., meals and snacks per day or consumption of breakfast) that may be important in some research studies.

Brief Assessment Instruments

Most brief instruments were developed for very specific research applications. The biggest concern when using a brief instrument is that it is often impossible to anticipate all the questions regarding diet that may become important by the end of a study.

TABLE 28.1
Summary of the Major Advantages and Disadvantages of Dietary Assessment Methods

Characteristics	Single Record/Recall	Multiple Record/Recalls per Person	Food Frequency Questionnaire	Brief Assessment Instruments
Brief Description	Detailed recording of everything consumed in one day	Multiple days (per person) of recording of everything consumed	Measure of usual intake determined from frequencies of consumption of about 100 foods (or food groups)	Diverse group of short tools developed to target limited number of foods, nutrients, or dietary behavior
Scientific Features				
Advantages	Open-ended format appropriate for all types of eating patterns Provides detailed information on foods consumed Provide data that are comparable across populations and time Recalls cannot affect (past) food choices	(Same as single records/recalls) 3 to 4 days of records/recalls have been used to characterize usual intake in individuals	Captures data on usual, long-term intake Can be used retrospectively	Ideal for studies where comprehensive assessment is not needed Some are nonintrusive and therefore relatively objective Behavioral assessments may be more sensitive to dietary interventions than nutrient estimates
Disadvantages*	Can only capture information on current intake and one day's intake does not characterize usual intake Records can change eating behavior Recalls depend on respondent memory	(Same as single records/recalls) Because of day-to-day variability in intake, even 3 to 4 days of intake only roughly approximates usual intake	Accurate reporting of usual intake of foods is very difficult for some respondents Limited food list will not be appropriate for all respondents Different questionnaires are needed for different populations and therefore do not produce comparable nutrient estimates	Typically provide fairly imprecise estimates of nutrient intakes Because of targeted nature of these instruments, future scientific questions on other foods or nutrients cannot be addressed
Practical Features				
Advantages	Recalls do not require literate respondents Because recalls are interviewer adminis-tered, data can be collected in a standardized way	(Same as single records/recalls)	Fairly low respondent burden Once developed, scannable FFQs are inexpensive and easy to analyze	Low respondent burden Usually simple and inexpensive to code and analyze
Disadvantages	Expensive to collect, code, and analyze	(Same as single records/recalls) Multiple records or recalls are extremely burdensome for participants	FFQ development costs are extremely high	

* All types of dietary self-report are subjective and are subject to underreporting and person-specific biases associated with sex, obesity, social desirability, etc.

Therefore, the choice of a brief instrument limits the future questions that can be addressed. Nonetheless, data collection for research purposes is a compromise between what is ideal and what is practical, and a comprehensive dietary assessment may not always be possible either from the standpoint of study budget or participant burden.

NUTRITION MONITORING OF POPULATIONS

Records/Recalls

Records and recalls have proven very useful for nutrition monitoring. Recalls are the primary assessment tool used in NHANES, CSFII, and the newer integrated survey. These surveys provide the primary data used to make important policy decisions about the nutritional status of Americans. In these large surveys, a single day's recall intake can provide estimates of the average intake of large groups that are comparable to those obtained with more burdensome techniques.[14–16,30] Because these methods are open ended, they are especially useful for assessing mean intake across population groups with markedly different eating patterns.

However, a single day's intake cannot be used to study distributions of dietary intake, because on any one day, an individual's diet can be unusually high (e.g., a celebratory meal) or low (e.g., a sick day). These days are not representative of an individual's intake even though they may be perfectly recorded. This day-to-day variation in intake is random and does not bias the mean intake for a group, although this variability does result in an increased distribution of observed intake (i.e., a wide standard deviation). However, if multiple measures (per person) are collected on a subsample of the population, it is possible to obtain an estimate of the within- vs. between-person variance and calculate the "true" standard deviation around the mean for the population. This procedure allows the investigator to determine the percent of individuals above (or below) a specified cut-point.[28]

Although the use of records/recalls in nutrition monitoring appears straightforward, there is actually considerable subtlety about the data needed to address public health dietary objectives. For example, assume that a public health objective is to reduce total fat intake to less than or equal to 30% energy from fat. A critical clarification of this objective is whether:

1. The population mean intake should be 30% energy from fat, in which case approximately half of the group will have intakes exceeding that level.
   or
2. The entire population should have intakes less than or equal to 30% energy from fat, in which case the group mean will be several percentage points below 30%.

TABLE 28.2
Summary of the Issues Regarding Use of Data from Dietary Intake Assessment Methods

Data	Single record/recall	Multiple record/ recalls per person	Food frequency questionnaire	Brief assessment instruments
Appropriate use of data	To estimate absolute mean values for intakes of foods and nutrients Group means and standard deviations for comparison to other groups	As an approximation of usual intake in an individual if used with caution and recognition that there will be considerable attenuation of associations with other variables	Ranking individuals from low to high intakes for foods or nutrients	Ranking individuals from low to high intakes for the specific food or nutrient being targeted
Inappropriate use of data*	Ranking respondents from low to high intakes For determination of the percent of population above (or below) some cut-point		Estimation of absolute nutrient intakes for comparison to other questionnaires or populations Just because an FFQ has been "validated" does not mean that it assesses all nutrients with good, or equal, accuracy	Estimation of absolute intakes for nutrients
Data not available	These methods cannot be used to assess dietary intake in the past	(Same as single record/ recall)	Eating pattern information (e.g., meals per day). Detailed information on foods consumed, such as brand names	(Same as FFQ)

* Because of considerable random and systematic error, no forms of dietary self-report data should be regarded as "truth."

TABLE 28.3

Summary of Considerations Regarding Use of Dietary Intake Assessment in Individuals vs. Groups

	Single Record/Recall	Multiple Record/ Recalls per Person	Food Frequency Questionnaire	Brief Assessment Instruments
Individual Assessment				
Appropriate Use	Qualitative use in clinical setting Teaching tool regarding food composition For self-monitoring	(Same as single record/recall) 3 to 4 days can be used as an approximation of usual intake	To provide feedback regarding respondent consumption of a food vs. recommended intake	Targeted instrument may be appropriate for individual counseling for the food or nutrient being assessed
Inappropriate Use	As estimate of usual intake		Nutrient intake estimates too imprecise for individual counseling	Reliable estimate of absolute intakes
Research Studies				
Appropriate Use	For comparing mean intakes in control vs. intervention group As a check of FFQ mean intake estimates for a group	(Same as single record/recall) Validity substudies for comparison of nutrient intake estimates to FFQ	For ranking individuals from low to high intakes for determination of associations with disease risk	Where costs or logistic realities prohibit use of a comprehensive assessment instrument
Inappropriate Use	When characterization of usual, long-term diet is the exposure of interest	(Same as single record/recall) In study population where respondent burden will result in poor quality data	For estimation of absolute intakes When comparable data needed across markedly different populations	In cases where there is the potential for important, new research questions to emerge
Nutrition Monitoring of Populations				
Appropriate Use	Nutrition monitoring of group means, including trends analyses Descriptive data on population eating patterns For international comparisons of food and nutrient intake	(Same as single record/recall) 3 to 4 days can approximate usual intake in individuals		
Inappropriate Use	To determine percentage of population meeting a dietary recommendation or at risk		For estimation of absolute intakes For time trends analyses because changing food supply cam make questionnaires obsolete	To estimate absolute intakes

If the public health objective is the first goal listed, then nutrition monitoring can be appropriately performed with a single 24-h record/recall for determination of mean intake in the population. Alternatively, if the public health objective is the second one listed above, then multiple records/recalls (per person) will need to be collected for assessment of the distribution of intakes in the population to determine the proportion of individuals consuming more than 30% energy from fat. These issues have important implications for food labeling and policy decisions.[71]

Food Frequency Questionnaires

FFQs have proven most useful in nutritional epidemiologic studies when the objective is to rank individuals from low to high intake for a food or nutrient. However, as described above, FFQs are close-ended forms with a limited food list and the accuracy of FFQs will vary considerably across groups with different eating patterns. Therefore, when the goal is to assess mean intakes in population subgroups with markedly different dietary patterns, or to track changes in intake over time, the FFQ is not the instrument of choice.

Brief Assessment Instruments

The accuracy of several of these instruments is particularly sensitive to differences in dietary patterns across population groups. For example, the validity of a fat-related behavioral questionnaire depends entirely on knowledge of those dietary behaviors that influence fat intake. In populations with different dietary patterns, the instrument would be useless for assessment of fat intake. Overall it is helpful to remember that brief dietary assessment instruments are developed for very specific objectives and caution needs to be taken when applying them to other populations or using them for other purposes.

SUMMARY

Much of what has been presented here is summarized in Table 28.1 to Table 28.3. Specifically, Table 28.1 summarizes the major scientific and practical advantages and disadvantages of the major dietary assessment methods. Table 28.2 provides an overview of the issues regarding use of data from dietary intake assessment methods. Table 28.3 gives a summary of consideration regarding use of dietary intake assessment in individuals vs. groups.

The use of sophisticated computerized technologies and Internet accessibility has the potential to address many of the practical and logistic limitations of the major dietary intake assessment methods. For example, a computer screen could provide life-size pictures of foods to help respondents more accurately estimate serving sizes. A user-friendly, computer-administered dietary recall could eliminate the costs associated with this method of collecting data. A touch-screen FFQ program, with algorithms for limiting questions to foods eaten with some minimal frequency, could eliminate the unfriendly format of the questionnaire and tailor the food list. Nonetheless, these practical advances will not eliminate the scientific problems inherent in dietary self-report. In particular, the issues of systematic and person-specific biases in self-report can likely only be addressed by use of objective biomarkers for identification, quantification, and correction of random and systematic error.[36,37,72]

It is clear that from this brief overview that choosing the appropriate dietary assessment method is a complex decision based on the specific objective, with an eye toward the competing demands of accuracy and practicality. There is no right or wrong approach, but only the best possible measure given the specific objectives of the assessment. In many cases, multiple measures of dietary assessment may be preferable to a single measure, although this approach certainly has implications for cost and participant or client burden.[14,15] Despite all the challenges and limitations of dietary assessment methods, these data will continue to serve an essential role in efforts to improve the health and longevity of individuals and groups.

REFERENCES

1. Department of Health and Human Services and United States Department of Agriculture. *Dietary Guidelines for Americans*, 2005.
2. Kant AK. *J Am Diet Assoc* 104: 615–635, 2005.
3. World Cancer Research Fund and the American Institute for Cancer Research. *Food, Nutrition and the Prevention of Cancer: a Global Perspective*. Potter J., ed., American Institute for Cancer Research, Washington DC, 1997.
4. Torun B, Chew F. Protein-energy malnutrition, in *Modern Nutrition in Health and Disease*, 9th ed., Shils ME, Olson JA, Shike M, eds., Lea & Febiger, Philadelphia, PA, 1998, 950.
5. Patterson RE. Overview of Nutritional Epidemiology, in *Nutrition in the Prevention and Treatment of Disease*, Coulston M, Rock CL, Monson E, eds., Academic Press, San Diego 2001.
6. Kolar AS, Patterson RE, White E, et al. *Epidemiology* 16: 579–583, 2005.
7. Beasley J, Riley WT, Jean-Mary J. *Nutrition* 21: 672–677, 2005.
8. Wang DH, Kogashiwa M, Ohta S, et al. *J Nutri Sci Vitamin* 48: 498–504, 2002.
9. Tsang MW, Mok M, Kam G, et al. *J Telemedicine and Telecare* 7: 47–50, 2001.
10. Chambers IV E, Godwin SL, Vecchio FA. *J Am Diet Assoc* 100: 891–897, 2000.
11. Godwin SL, Chambers IV E, Cleveland L. *J Am Diet Assoc* 104: 585–594, 2004.
12. Yanek LR, Moy TF, Raqueno JV, et al. *J Am Diet Assoc* 100: 1172–1177, 2000.
13. Shumaker NL, Neils-Strunjas J, Smith R, et al. *J Allied Health* 32: 196–201, 2003.
14. Dwyer J, Picciano MF, Raiten DJ, et al. *J Nutr* 133: 590S–600S, 2003.
15. Dwyer J, Picciano MF, Raiten DJ, et al. *J Nutr* 133: 609S–623S, 2003.
16. Conway JM, Ingwersen LA, Vinyard BT, et al. *Am J Clin Nutr* 77: 1171–1178, 2003.
17. Hebert JR, Clemow L, Pbert L, Ockene IS, Ockene JK. *Int J Epidemiol* 24: 389, 1995.
18. Jansen A. *Br J Clin Psychol* 35: 381, 1996.
19. Johnson RK, Soultanakis RP, Matthews DE. *J Am Diet Assoc* 98: 1136–1140, 1998.
20. Kristal AR, Andrilla CAH, Koepsell TD, et al. *J Am Diet Assoc* 98: 40, 1998.
21. Johnson RK, Friedman AB, Harvey-Berino J, et al. *J Am Diet Assoc* 105: 1948–1951, 2005.
22. Caan BJ, Ballard-Barbash R, Slattery ML, et al. *J Am Diet Assoc* 104: 357–366, 2004.
23. Harnack L, Himes JH, Anliker J, et al. *Am J Epidemiol* 160: 1117–1121, 2004.
24. Buzzard IM, Faucett CL, Jeffery RW, et al. *J Am Diet Assoc* 96: 574, 1996.
25. Kleges LM, Baranowski T, Beech B, et al. *Prev Med* 38: S78–S87, 2004.
26. Baxter SD, Smith AF, Litaker MS. *Ann Epidemiol* 14: 385–390, 2004.
27. Baxter SD, Thompson WO, Davis HC. *J Am Diet Assoc* 100: 911–918, 2000.
28. Willet W. *Nutritional Epidemiology*, 2nd ed, Oxford University Press, New York, 1998.
29. Rebro S, Patterson RE, Kristal AR, et al. *J Am Diet Assoc* 98: 1163, 1998.
30. Cotton PA, Subar AF, Friday JE, et al. *J Am Diet Assoc* 104: 921–930, 2004.
31. Kristal AR, Vizenor NC, Patterson RE, et al. *Cancer Epidemiol Biomarkers Prev* 9: 939–944, 2000.
32. Patterson RE, Kristal AR, Carter RA, et al. *Ann Epidemiol* 9: 178, 1999.

Methods and Tools for Dietary Intake Assessment in Individuals vs. Groups

541

33. Armstrong BK, White E, Saracci R. Principles of Exposure Measurement in Epidemiology, in *Monographs in Epidemiology and Biostatistics*, Oxford University Press, Oxford, 1994.
34. Diliberti N, Bordi PL, Conklin MT, et al. *Obesity Res* 12: 562–568, 2004.
35. Ello-Martin JA, Ledikwe JH, Rolls BJ. *Am J Clin Nutr* 82: 236S-241S, 2005.
36. Subar AF, Kipnis V, Troiano RP, et al. *Am J Epidemiol* 158: 1–13, 2003.
37. Kipnis V, Midthune D, Freedman LS, et al. *Am J Epidemiol* 153: 394–403, 2001.
38. Tooze JA, Subar AF, Thompson FE, et al. *Am J Clin Nutr* 79: 795–804, 2004.
39. Day N, McKeown, Wong M, et al. *Int J Epidemiol* 30: 309–317, 2001.
40. Black AE. *Europ J Clin Nutr* 54: 395, 2000.
41. Kristal AR, Feng Z, Coates RJ, et al. *Am J Epidemiol* 146: 856, 1997.
42. Tucker KL, Maras J, Champagne C, et al. *Pub Health Nutr* 8: 87096, 2005.
43. MacIntyre UE, Venter CS, Vorster HH. *Pub Health Nutr* 4: 63–71, 2001.
44. Armstrong B, Doll R. *Int J Cancer* 15: 617, 1975.
45. Gray GE, Pike MC, Henderson BE. *Br J Cancer* 39: 1, 1979.
46. Prentice RL, Sheppard L. *Cancer Causes Control* 1: 81, 1990.
47. Roberts DC. *Prostaglandins Leukotrienes Essential Fatty Acids* 44: 97, 1991.
48. Ransley JK, Donnelly JK, Botham H, et al. *Appetite* 41: 141–148, 2003.
49. Ransley JK, Donnelly JK, Khara TN, et al. *Publ Health Nutr* 4: 1279–1286, 2001.
50. Patterson RE, Kristal AR, Shannon J, et al. *Am J Publ Health* 87: 272, 1997.
51. Kendall A, Olson CM, Frongillo EA. *J Nutr* 125: 2793, 1995.
52. Satia JA, Patterson RE, Kristal AR, et al. *Publ Health Nutr* 4: 241–247, 2001.
53. Neuhouser ML, Thompson B, Coronado G, et al. *J Am Diet Assoc* 107, 2007.
54. Neuhouser ML, Kristal AR, McLerran D, et al. *Cancer Epidemiol Biomarkers Prev* 8: 649, 1999.
55. Tinker LF, Patterson RE, Kristal AR, et al. *J Am Diet Assoc* 101: 1031–1040, 2001.
56. Kirk P, Patterson RE, Lampe J. *J Am Diet Assoc* 99: 558, 1999.
57. Neuhouser ML, Patterson RE, Kristal AR, et al. *Publ Health Nutr* 4: 73–79, 2000.
58. Yatsuya H, Ohwaki A, Tamakoshi K, et al. *J Epidemiol* 13: 235–245, 2003.
59. Thompson FE, Midthune D, Subar AF, et al. *Publ Health Nutr* 7: 1097–1105, 2004.
60. Smith KW, Hoelscher DM, Lytle LA, et al. *J Am Diet Assoc* 101: 635–647, 2001.
61. Drewnowski A, Hann C, Henderson SA, et al. *J Am Diet Assoc* 100: 1325–1333, 2000.
62. Kristal AR, Shattuck AL, Henry HJ. *J Am Diet Assoc* 90: 214, 1990.
63. Patterson RE, Kristal AR, White E. *Am J Publ Health* 86: 1394, 1996.
64. Neuhouser ML, Kristal AR, Patterson RE. *J Am Diet Assoc* 98: 45, 1998.
65. Thompson FE, Subar AF, Kipnis V, et al. *Europ J Clin Nutr* 52 (suppl): S45, 1998.
66. Kristal AR, Curry SJ, Shattuck AL, et al. *Prev Med* 31: 380, 2000.
67. Bingham SA, Luben R, Weich A, et al. *Lancet* 362 (9379): 212–214, 2003.
68. Prentice RL. *Lancet* 362 (9379): 182–183, 2003.
69. Prentice RL. *J Natl Cancer Inst* 88: 1738, 1996.
70. Hunter DJ, Speigelman D, Adami HO, et al. *N Engl J Med* 334: 356, 1996.
71. Murphy SP, Barr SI. *Nutr Rev* 63: 267–271, 2005.
72. Prentice RL, Sugar E, Wang CY, et al. *Publ Health Nutr* 5: 977–984, 2002.

29 Lessons Learned over 35 Years: Dietary Assessment Methods for School-Age Children

R. Sue McPherson Day, Deanna M. Hoelscher, Carissa A. Eastham, and Erin M. Koers

CONTENTS

INTRODUCTION

During the last three and a half decades unique challenges have plagued researchers' attempts to assess school-age children's dietary intake. Lessons learned during this period from 102 validity and reliability studies of the application of recalls, records, food frequency questionnaires (FFQs), checklists, screeners, and observations among school-age children are summarized in this report. This updated review combines the studies published from 2000 to 2005 with the authors' two previous literature reviews on this topic.[1,2] Major additions include a category of food recall reliability studies and one for diet history validity studies. The category of FFQs was expanded to include checklists and screener type questionnaires. At the close of this review are recommendations for use of the established methods and discussion of the continuing challenges of measuring children's dietary behaviors.

REVIEW METHODOLOGY

This review covers the dietary assessment methods used with children including the 24 h recall (in-person, telephone and computer-assisted; full and partial day), the food record, the FFQ (including food checklist and screener type questionnaires), the diet history, and observation. A total of 74 validity and 28 reliability studies used at least one of these methodologies and met the review criteria: (1) publication in a peer-reviewed English journal between January 1970 and December 2005; (2) inclusion of school children aged 5 – 18 years living in an industrialized country; and (3) reporting of specific reliability and/or validity tests from a minimum sample of 30 children in either the main study sample or a sub-sample (denoted by age, gender, or ethnicity), after the publishing author's exclusions for analyses. Studies were identified by Ovid Medline and PubMed searches using the following key words: diet, nutrition, adolescent, child, adolescent nutrition, child nutrition, nutrition assessment, diet, eating, food, nutrition survey, questionnaires, reproducibility, repeatability, reliability, validity, sensitivity, and specificity. Studies that did not specifically use the word validity, reliability, reproducibility, or repeatability in the results or discussion may not have been identified. Additional articles were identified by cross-referencing from author reference lists. The degree of reliability or validity of the instrument reported was not considered an inclusion factor; however, the referent period for the validity studies reasonably coinciding with that of the stated validation standard for a study was an inclusion factor. Multiple validity or reliability studies that were included in a single article were evaluated and presented separately and are counted as a separate entry with the reference repeated accordingly.

DIETARY ASSESSMENT METHODOLOGIES

Each of the following sections defines a dietary method and refers to the corresponding validity and reliability tables. The format of table entries is described in Table 29.1.

24 H RECALL

The 24 h recall consists of a structured interview in which a trained nutritionist or other professional asks the child and/or adult caregiver to list everything the child ate or drank during a specified time period, typically the previous day (Table 29.2 and Table 29.3). The 24 h recall is an estimate of actual intake that usually incorporates a detailed description of the food, including brand names, ingredients of mixed dishes, food preparation methods, and portion sizes consumed. Prompts for quantification of portion size such as two- or three-dimensional food models or detailed food pictures are typically employed. Nutrient intake can be calculated for the designated day or portion of the day with this level of detail. When conducted with a randomly sampled population, a single 24 h recall is appropriate for estimating group means, but it is not a tool to describe usual individual intake or to predict individual-level health outcomes such as serum cholesterol levels. Because of intra individual variation in intake, multiple recalls are needed to accurately estimate usual food and nutrient intake. Nelson and colleagues have addressed how to calculate the number of days of recalls or records required to estimate intakes of individual nutrients for children aged 2 to 17 years.[3]

Researchers have modified some of these basic techniques to include self-administered recalls using computer-prompted recalls, [4,5] recalls using a structured list of foods as prompts,[23] recalls using food records as a prompt, [12,14,27] recalls using a

---

TABLE 29.1
Table Entry Format

General
- Except for those in Table 29.7, study entries are listed in ascending order by age

Definitions
- *Adults required* — Adults provided all of the intake information or were required to supplement and assist the child's report
- *Quantitative* — Quantity of food consumed was estimated using weights, measures, or food models. Responses were open ended
- *Semiquantitative* — Quantity of food consumed was estimated using a standard portion size, serving, or a predetermined amount, and the respondent was asked about the number of portions consumed
- *Nonquantitative* — Quantity of food consumed was not assessed
- *Self-administered* — Child completed the dietary assessment without assistance
- *Group-administered* — Child completed the dietary assessment with help from a proctor, teacher, or caregiver in a group setting
- *Interviewer-administered* — A trained interviewer elicited the dietary assessment information from the child in a one-on-one setting
- *Phantom foods or intrusions* — Foods reported eaten that were known to have not been eaten
- *Omissions* — Foods not reported eaten that were known to have been eaten
- *Match* — Foods reported eaten that were known to have been eaten
- *Multiple-pass recall* (MPR) — Questioning for a recall than includes a quick list of foods and drinks consumed, a detailed description of each food, and a review for missed foods

Results Section
- Omission of any of the following components indicates it was not provided in the article or was from a sample of less than 30 children. Statistical significance of measures is noted with clarifications as to whether significance testing was shown in the article or only reported via a statement from the publishing authors. The results are ordered as follows:
- Correlations for energy, protein, and total fat between methodologies or administrations
- Range of correlations, Kappa statistic, or Wilcoxin scores between methodologies or administrations for the nutrients or foods assessed
- For validity studies: the absolute values and percent difference in energy intake between the validation standard and the instrument ([instrument−validation standard]/validation standard ×100)
- For reliability studies: the absolute values and percent difference in energy intake between the first and follow-up assessment ([follow-up instrument−first instrument]/follow-up instrument ×100)
- Comparison of mean intake of nutrients assessed
- Comparison of foods or food groups consumed with low to high range of select food items
- Comparison of portion size
- Results by age, gender, or ethnicity

TABLE 29.2
Recall Validity Studies among School-Age Children

Reference[a]	Sample	Age/Grade	Instrument	Validation Standard	Design	Results
Basch et al.[10]	18 m[b] 28 f[b] Latino	4–7 years Adults required[c]	Evening meal recall; quantitative	Observation	Compared mothers' recall of what child ate against observation of the meal. Excerpted evening meal from 24 h recall	Pearson's correlations (energy adjusted) between recalled evening meal and observed evening meal were 0.71 for energy, 0.50 for protein, and 0.52 for total fat. Range of correlations for 18 nutrients assessed was −0.10 for phosphorus to 0.82 for iron. Recalled energy intake was 9% higher than observed intake (507 vs. 465 kcal/meal). Seven nutrients were significantly overestimated by recalled intake of the meal (significance testing not shown). Range of mothers reporting fewer items consumed as compared with the number of items observed consumed was between 4% and 30%. 15.5% of reported portion sizes were smaller and 33.5% of portions were greater than those observed (significance testing not shown)
Eck et al.[11]	33 m&f	4–9.5 years Adults required	Lunch recall; quantitative	Observation	Compared mother's, father's, or both parents' plus child's (consensus) recall of lunch against observation of lunch. Excerpted lunch meal from 24 h recall	Pearson's correlations between consensus recall of lunch and observed lunch were 0.87 for energy, 0.91 for protein (% kcal), and 0.85 for total fat (% kcal). Range of correlations for nine nutrients assessed was 0.75 for carbohydrate (% kcal) to 0.91 for protein (% kcal). Pearson's correlations between observed intake and fathers' recall were 0.83 for energy, 0.79 for protein (% kcal), and 0.72 for total fat (% of kcal). Pearson's correlations between observed intake and mother's recall were 0.64 for energy, 0.56 for protein (% kcal), and 0.65 for total fat (% kcal). Recalled energy intake from the consensus, fathers', and mothers' recalls was 2% (558 kcal/meal), 5% (545 kcal/meal), and 4% (550 kcal/meal) lower than observed intake (572 kcal/meal), respectively. Only mothers' recall of energy from dairy foods/beverages and snacks/desserts was significantly different from observed intake. There were no significant differences in mean nutrient intake between any pairs compared. Qualitative comparison of number of items recalled revealed that only fathers' recalls of nondairy beverages and snacks/desserts differed significantly from observed intake. Consensus approach appeared to reduce the tendency to overreport low intakes and underreport high intakes (flattened slope phenomenon)
Montgomery et al.[12]	32 m 31 f	4.5–6.9 years Adults required	Three 24 h MPR[h]; semiquantitative	TEE[g] by doubly labeled water	Compared mother's recall of child's intake against 10-day TEE	Recalled energy intake was 0.58% higher than TEE (6910 vs. 6870 kJ/day) for males. Recalled intake was 4.67% higher than TEE (6280 vs. 6000 kJ/day) for females
Fisher et al.[13]	76 m 73 f 99 m&f White 50 m&f AA[f]	4.4–11.5 years Adults required	Two to thrree 24 h MPR; semiquantitative	TEE by doubly labeled water	Compared average of child's parent-assisted recalls against 14-day TEE	Correlation between average recalled intake and TEE was 0.27 for energy. Average recalled energy intake was 10% higher than TEE (1881 vs. 1704 kcal/day). No associations were found between reporting accuracy and age, gender, or ethnicity. Underreporting was significantly greater in heavier children

Continued

TABLE 29.2
Continued

Reference[a]	Sample	Age/Grade	Instrument	Validation Standard	Design	Results
Warren et al.[14]	103 m 100 f	5–7 years	Lunch recall; nonquantitative	Observation	Compared child's recall of packed lunch or school lunch 2 h after consumption against observation of lunch with school lunch discards noted and packed lunch checked before and after meal	Correlation between number of recalled and observed lunch foods was 0.22 for children eating packed lunch and 0.16 for children eating school lunch. Percentage of accurate recall of the number of foods was significantly higher for packed lunch (70%) than for school lunch (58%). Percent report of phantom foods was 22% for packed lunch and 11% for school lunch. Main dishes and drinks were items best recalled by packed lunch children while fried accompaniments and main dishes were best recalled by school lunch children. Vegetables were not well recalled by either group
Baxter et al.[15]	12 m AA 12 m White 12 f AAs 12 f White 12 m AA 12 m White 12 f AAs 12 f White	1st grade 1st grade 1st grade 1st grade 4th grade 4th grade 4th grade 4th grade	Lunch recall; semiquantitative	Observation	Compared child's recall of lunch intake using three prompting methods (preferences, food category, or visual) against observation of school lunch	Average recall inaccuracy after specific prompting for all three groups was increased by 0.5 servings for 1st graders and decreased by 0.1 servings for 4th graders
Lindquist et al.[16]	17 m 13 f 17 White 13 AA	6.5–11.6 years Adults required	Three 24 h recalls, one phone, two interview; quantitative	TEE by doubly labeled water	Compared average of three children's parent assisted recalls against 14-day TEE	Pearson's correlation between average recalled intake and TEE was 0.32 for energy. Recalled energy intake was 0.5% higher than TEE from doubly labeled water (7.90 vs. 7.86 mJ/day). Inaccuracy in energy reporting was not predicted by age, gender, ethnicity, social class or adiposity
Reynolds et al.[17]	18 m&f 25 m&f 31 m&f	7–8 years 9–10 years 11–12 years	Three daytime recalls; nonquantitative	Observation	Compared average of three children's recalls of daytime meals against observation of daytime meals. Exchange units of foods were developed from the recalls for analyses	Recalled energy intake was 34% lower for 7–8 year olds (1818 vs. 2751 kcal/daytime meals), 21% lower for 9–10 year olds (2291 vs. 2887 kcal/ daytime meals), and 17% lower for 11–12 year olds (2643 vs. 3185 kcal/daytime meals) than observed intake. Children significantly underestimated their energy, carbohydrate, and fat consumption as compared with observers, with younger children having larger differences. Exact agreement for the nine exchange groups ranged from 94% for lean fat meat to 17% for the fat group. Females were significantly more accurate in reporting medium fat meat exchange units than males, 62% vs. 50%, respectively (significance testing not shown)
Edmunds et al.[18]	204 m&f	7–9 years	24 h recall, Day in the Life Questionnaire (DILQ); group-administered; nonquantitative	Observation	Compared child's recall of fruit and vegetables on school day meals against observation of school morning break and lunch. Excerpted intake of fruits and vegetables from school day meals from 24 h recall	Kappas for the two assessment periods were 68.5 and 74.0 for count of fruit and vegetables. There were no significant gender differences (significance testing not shown)

						Results
Lytle et al.[8]	49 m&f	3rd grade	24 h recall assisted by food record; quantitative	Observation	Compared child's food record assisted recalls against observation of school lunch and breakfast by trained personnel and of other meals at home by parents	Pearson's correlations between recalled and observed intakes were 0.59 for energy, 0.62 for protein (% kcal) and 0.64 for total fat (% kcal). Range of correlations for the eight nutrients assessed was 0.41 for polyunsaturated fat (% kcal) to 0.79 for saturated fat (% kcal). Recalled energy intake was 10% higher than observed intake (1823 vs. 1650 kcal/day). There was an overall 77.9% agreement in the types of food items recalled and observed. Food portions were recalled within 10% of observed portions 35% of the time; overestimation occurred 42% and underestimation occurred 23% of the time
Van Horn et al.[19]	18 m 14 f	8–10 years	24 h recall by phone; quantitative	Observation	Compared child's recall of intake against parent's observation	Pearson's correlations between recalled intake and observation of intake were 0.76 for energy, 0.74 for protein (% kcal), and 0.73 for total fat (% kcal). Range of correlations for the 10 nutrients assessed was 0.64 for saturated fat (% kcal) to 0.93 for iron. Recalled energy intake was 2% lower than recorded intake (1799 vs. 1836 kcal/day). There were no significant differences between child and parent reports of nutrient intake (significance testing not shown)
Weber et al.[9]	54 m&f American Indian	8–10 years	Breakfast and lunch recall assisted by food record; quantitative	Observation	Compared child's food record assisted recalls of school breakfast and lunch against observation of school meals. Excerpted breakfast and lunch meals from 24 h recall	Pearson's correlations between recalled breakfast and lunch combined and observed breakfast and lunch were 0.52 for energy, 0.68 for protein, and 0.57 for total fat. Range of correlations for the seven nutrient measures assessed was 0.52 for energy to 0.86 for both carbohydrate (% kcal) and protein (% kcal). Recalled energy intake was 13% higher than observed intake (862 vs. 761 kcal/daytime meals). There was an overall 75% agreement in the types of food items recalled and observed. Food portions were recalled within 10% of observed portions 57% of the time; overestimation occurred 30% of the time and underestimation occurred 13% of the time
Todd et al.[20]	30 m&f Chinese 31 m&f Hispanic	8–11 years	Breakfast and lunch recall; quantitative	Observation	Compared child's recall of school breakfast and lunch against observation of school meals with plate waste subtracted. Excerpted breakfast and lunch meals from 24 h recall	Pearson's correlations between recalled lunch and observed lunch for Chinese were 0.49 for energy, 0.62 for protein, and 0.25 for total fat and for Hispanics were 0.53 for energy, 0.51 for protein, and 0.46 for total fat. Range of correlations for the 15 nutrients assessed for Chinese was –0.10 for sodium to 0.63 for thiamin and for Hispanics was 0.34 for niacin to 0.81 for vitamin C. Chinese children's recalled energy intake was 10% lower than observed intake (686 vs. 765 kcal/2 meals). Chinese children recalled consistently less food than consumed which was significantly lower for 4 of the 15 nutrients. Hispanic children's recalled energy intake was 6% higher than observed intake (665 vs. 630 kcal/2 meals). Hispanic children recalled intake vs. consumed intake was inconsistent and was significantly higher for 2 nutrients and lower for 1 of the 15 nutrients assessed. For Chinese, food item omissions ranged from 4% for milk to 35% for vegetables. For Hispanics, food item omissions ranged from 0% for juice and milk to 35% for vegetables

Continued

TABLE 29.2
(Continued)

Reference[a]	Sample	Age/Grade	Instrument	Validation Standard	Design	Results
Samuelson[21]	56 m&f 43 m&f	8 years 13 years	Lunch recall; quantitative	Chemical analysis of food	Compared child's recall of lunch against weighed chemical analyses of a double portion of lunch, with plate waste subtracted. Excerpted lunch meal from 24 h recall	Spearman's correlations between recalled lunch and chemical analyses of lunch for 8 and 13 year olds for energy were 0.68 for 8 year olds and 0.71 for 13 year olds. Correlations for protein of 8 and 13 year olds were 0.55 and 0.45 respectively. Correlations for total fat of 8 and 13 year olds were 0.61 and 0.69 respectively. Range of correlations for the 4 nutrients assessed for 8 year olds was 0.55 for protein to 0.68 for energy. Range of correlations for 13 year olds was 0.45 for protein to 0.71 for energy. Among 8 year olds, recalled energy intake was 18% higher than chemical analyses (472 vs. 399 kcal/meal). Among 13 year olds, recalled energy intake was 1% higher than chemical analyses (494 vs. 491 kcal/meal). Median portion size estimated by child compared with weighing was not significantly different for 8 year olds and was 14% lower among 13 year olds (significance testing not shown)
Lytle et al.[22]	238 m 248 f 253 White 146 Asian 73 AA 14 other	4th grade	Lunch recall; quantitative	Observation	Compared child's recall of school lunch against observation of lunch. Excerpted lunch meal from 24 h recall	Pearson's correlation between recalled and observed intake for energy was 0.44. Range of correlations for the five nutrients assessed was 0.39 for β-carotene to 0.61 for vitamin C. Recalled energy intake was 14% higher than observed intake (600 vs. 526 kcal/meal). There were significant differences between recalled and observed nutrient intake for all nutrients except β-carotene (borderline significant). The highest correlation was for servings of fruit, 0.65, and lowest for servings of vegetables, 0.42. No ethnic specific analyses provided
Baxter et al.[23]	120 m 117 f 58 White 179 AA	4th grade	Lunch recall; quantitative	Observation	Compared child's recall of food items from school lunch either the same day or the following day against observation of that lunch	Average matched food rates from recall of lunch and observation of lunch were 84% and 68% for same day and next day intervals, respectively. Rates for omitted or phantom foods were significantly lower for the same day (16% vs. 5%) than next day recalls (32% vs. 13%). Children were least likely to omit beverages and main dishes and most likely to omit condiments and miscellaneous foods. There were no significant gender, ethnic or time interval differences in the accuracy of recalling the amount of food consumed (significance testing not shown)
Baxter et al.[24]	49 m 55 f 53 White 51 AA	4th grade	24 h MPR, semiquantitative	Observation	Compared child's recall of food items from school breakfast and lunch against observation of school meals. Excerpted breakfast and lunch food from 24 h recall	Mean omission rate of foods on the recalls compared with observation was 51% and mean intrusion rate was 39%
Baranowski et al.[5]	91 m&f White, AA, Hispanic, other	4th grade, 9–11 years	24 h MPR by Food Intake Recording Software System (FIRSSt); self-administered; quantitative	Observation	Compared child's recall of school lunch by FIRSSt against observation of lunch. Excerpted lunch foods from 24 h FIRSSt recall	To control for game exploration using FIRSSt by some children, two sets of data were analyzed: restricted (first n foods reported within each meal or snack: n = 5 for breakfast; 3 for morning snack; 6 for lunch; 3 for afternoon snack; 5 for dinner; 3 for evening snack) and unrestricted (all foods reported). For restricted data, there was a mean food match rate of 46%, omission rate of 30%, and intrusion rate of 24%. For unrestricted data, there was a mean food match rate of 40%, omission rate of 36%, and intrusion rate of 23%

Reference	Sample	Age	Method	Comparison	Results
Baranowski et al.[5]	137 m&f White, AA, Hispanic, other	4th grade, 9–11 years	24 h recall by Food Intake Recording Software System (FIRSSt); self-administered; quantitative	24 h MPR	Compared child's recall of food items from school lunch by FIRSSt against child's recall of foods by 24 h MPR. Excerpted lunch foods from FIRSSt recall and 24 h recall	To control for game exploration using FIRSSt by some children, two sets of data were analyzed: restricted (first n foods reported within each meal or snack: $n = 5$ for breakfast; 3 for morning snack; 6 for lunch; 3 for afternoon snack; 5 for dinner; 3 for evening snack) and unrestricted (all foods reported). For restricted data, there was a mean food match rate of 60%, omission rate of 24%, and intrusion rate of 15%. For unrestricted data, there was a mean food match rate of 56%, omission rate of 24%, and intrusion rate of 20%. Hispanic children reported more problems with using FIRSSt than other ethnic groups
Baranowski et al.[5]	91 m&f White, AA, Hispanic, other	4th grade, 9–11 years	24 h MPR; quantitative	Observation	Compared child's recall of lunch foods by 24 h MPR against observation of the lunch. Excerpted lunch meal from 24 h MPR	To control for game exploration using FIRSSt by some children, two sets of data were analyzed: restricted (first n foods reported within each meal or snack: $n = 5$ for breakfast; 3 for morning snack; 6 for lunch; 3 for afternoon snack; 5 for dinner; 3 for evening snack) and unrestricted (all foods reported). For restricted data, there was a mean food match rate of 59%, omission rate of 24%, and intrusion rate of 17%. For unrestricted data, there was a mean food match rate of 26%, omission rate of 20%
Baxter et al.[25]	10 m AA 8 m White 8 f AA 7 f White	4th grade	24 h MPR in person; semiquantitative	Observation	Compared child's recall of school breakfast and lunch from in person interview against observation of school meals. Excerpted breakfast and lunch meals from same-day recall	Mean omission rate of foods on the recalls compared with observation was 34% and mean intrusion rate was 19%. Accuracy of reporting is not significantly different whether obtained in person or by telephone
Baxter et al. 2003[25]	8 m AA 8 m White 11 f AA 9 f White	4th grade	24 h MPR by phone; semiquantitative	Observation	Compared child's recall of school breakfast and lunch from telephone interview against observation of school meals. Excerpted breakfast and lunch meals from same-day recall	Mean omission rate of foods on the recalls compared with observation was 32% and mean intrusion rate was 16%. Accuracy of reporting is not significantly different whether obtained in person or by telephone
Andersen et al.[26]	36 m 49 f	6th grade	24 h recall of fruit, fruit juice and vegetables; group-administered; semiquantitative	7-day food record with precoded list of foods; semi-quantitative	Compared child's recall of fruit, fruit juice, vegetable, and potato intake against child's report of intake on 7-day food records. Excerpted fruit and vegetable intake from 7-day food record with pre-coded list of foods	Reported intake from the 24 h recall was significantly higher than from the 7-day pre-coded food records for fruit, fruit juice, potato, fruit and vegetable without fruit juice and potato, and fruit, fruit juice, vegetable, and potato, but not for vegetable. The same results were found by gender except potato was also nonsignificant (significance testing not shown). Recalled fruit and vegetable (including fruit juice and potato) intake from the 24 h recall was 159% (4.4 mean portions per day) higher than food record intake (1.7 mean portions per day)
Johnson et al.[6]	41 m 55 f	11–13 years	24 h recall of 41 items (10 fatty; 13 sugary; 10 fibrous; 3 low-sugar foods; and 5 alternative fats), FIQ; self-administered; past three months; nonquantitative	3-day food record with interview	Compared child's recall of foods from previous day on FIQ against nutrient intake from child's 3-day food diary 2 weeks later	Pearson's correlation between the 24 h recall scores and 3-day food diary for energy and the fatty group score was 0.20, and for fat (% kcal) and the fatty group was 0.36. Range of correlations for the 4 nutrients and 3 food groups assessed was −0.057 (not significant) for fiber and the fatty group to 0.36 for fat (% kcal) and the fatty group

Continued

TABLE 29.2
(Continued)

Reference[a]	Sample	Age/Grade	Instrument	Validation Standard	Design	Results
Mullenbach et al.[27]	22 m 18 f	6–9th grade Adults required	24 h recall by phone; quantitative	3-day food record	Compared child's parent assisted recall against child's parent assisted 3-day food records completed 2–4 weeks prior to recalls	Pearson's correlations between recall and food records were 0.42 for energy, 0.42 for protein, and 0.33 for total fat. Range of correlations for the 19 nutrients assessed was 0.09 for cholesterol to 0.57 for riboflavin. Recalled energy intake was 12% lower than recorded energy intake (1835 vs. 2097 kcal/day). There were no significant differences between recalled and recorded average nutrient intake, although the 24 h recall estimates were all lower than those from the food record
Vereecken et al.[14]	55 m 46 f	11–14 years	24 h recall computer assisted Young Adolescent's Nutrition Assessment on Computer (YANA-C); self-administered; quantitative	24 h recall	Compared child's recall of intake by the YANA-C against child's 24 h recall	Spearman's correlations between YANA-C and interview were 0.66 for energy, 0.67 for protein, and 0.59 for fat. Range of correlations for the eight nutrients assessed were 0.44 for iron and 0.86 for calcium. Recalled energy intake from the YANA-C recall was 5% higher than recalled intake (8240 vs. 7812 kJ). Spearman's correlations for amount/portion agreement ranged from −0.02 for fish to 0.90 for milk. Percent agreement of food matches ranged from 67% for sauces and butter to 97% for bread
Vereecken et al.[4]	44 m 92 f	12–14 years	24 h recall computer assisted Young Adolescent's Nutrition Assessment on Computer (YANA-C); self-administered; quantitative	1-day food record; quantitative	Compared child's recall of intake by the YANA-C against child's 1-day food record	Spearman's correlations between YANA-C and food record were 0.64 for energy, 0.44 for protein, and 0.58 for fat. Range of correlations for the eight nutrients assessed were 0.44 for protein and 0.79 for vitamin C. Recalled energy intake from the YANA-C recall was 13% higher than food record intake (9336 vs. 8236 kJ). Spearman's correlations for amount/portion agreement ranged from 0.15 for cereals to 0.97 for eggs. Percent agreement of food matches ranged from 76% for pastry and cookies to 97% each for bread, cereals, and fish

[a] Results of all subgroups not reported due to samples below the $N = 30$ criterion.
[b] Males (m), females (f).
[c] Adult assistance required for instrument administration.
[d] N/A — Not applicable.
[e] FFQ — Food frequency questionnaire.
[f] AA — African-American.
[g] TEE — Total energy expenditure.
[h] MPR — Multiple-pass recall.

TABLE 29.3
Recall Reliability Studies among School-Age Children

References[a]	Sample	Age/Grade	Instrument	Design	Results
Edmunds et al.[18]	204 m&f[b]	7–9 years	24 h recall, Day in the Life Questionnaire (DILQ); group-administered; nonquantitative	Compared 2-week test–retest reproducibility of fruit and vegetable intake from DILQ	Wilcoxon test for difference in total number of fruits and vegetables consumed at time 1 vs. 2 were significant for only one school that had documented no servings of vegetable on the lunch menu for the day of the second visit. There were no differences by gender (significance testing not shown)
Andersen et al.[26]	54 m, 60 f	Sixth grade	24 h recall of fruit and vegetables; group-administered; semiquantitative	Compared 2-week test–retest reproducibility of fruit and vegetable intake from 24 h recalls	Reported intakes from the two 24 h recalls were not significantly different for fruit, fruit juice, potato, and vegetable. There were significant differences for the combined groups; fruit and vegetable without fruit juice and potato; and fruit, fruit juice, vegetable, and potato. No differences were seen between the two times for combined genders (significance testing not shown) except for between time 1 and 2 for girls for combined fruits and vegetables without juice and potato, but not for boys
Vereecken et al.[4]	37 m&f	11–14 years	24 h recall computer assisted "Young Adolescent's Nutrition Assessment on Computer (YANA-C)"; self-administered; semiquantitative	Compared 1-week test–retest reproducibility of food and nutrient intake from YANA-C 24 h recall	Wilcoxon p-values were 0.61 for energy, 0.79 for protein, and 0.98 for fat. p-Values ranged from 0.002 for fiber to 0.98 for both fat and iron. Recalled energy intake from the first assessment was 0.25% (8791 kJ) lower than the second assessment (8813 kJ). Wilcoxon p-values for food groups ranged from 0.03 for eggs and 0.98 for potatoes
Johnson et al.[4]	45 m, 53 f	13–14 years	24 h recall of 41 Items (10 fatty; 13 sugary; 10 fibrous; 3 low-sugar foods; and 5 alternative fats), FIQ; self- administered; past 3 months; nonquantitative	Compared 3-month test–retest reproducibility of food intake from child's recall on FIQ	Spearman's correlations between time 1 and 2 were 0.58 for sugary foods, 0.45 for fiber, and 0.59 for fatty foods; correlations between time 1 and 3 were 0.62 for sugary foods, 0.42 for fiber, and 0.55 for fatty foods; correlations between time 2 and 3 were 0.69 for sugary foods, 0.44 for fiber, and 0.59 for fatty foods

[a] Results of all subgroups not reported due to samples below the $N = 30$ criterion.
[b] Males (m), females (f).
[c] Adult assistance required for instrument administration.
[d] N/A — Not applicable.
[e] FFQ — Food frequency questionnaire.
[f] AA — African-American.
[g] TEE — Total energy expenditure.
[h] MPR — Multiple-pass recall.

multiple-pass approach,[5,12,13,24,25] and recalls of foods eaten without obtaining portion size information.[4,14,17,18] The majority of studies reviewed included recalls of only a portion of the day or selected meals and/or foods.

Most of the recall validity studies (63%) used observation of the child as the validation standard, and another 15% used total energy expenditure (TEE) or chemical analyses. The majority (70%) of the studies considered only individual meals or daytime intakes to determine validity. Energy intake was assessed in 16 of the recall validity studies and was overestimated in 11 and underestimated in 5 as compared with the standard. The majority of the studies conducted with children <9 years of age validated only a partial day recall. Multiple-pass recalls (MPRs) have now been tested in some school-age children. Researchers are cautioned not to give too many prompts for young children as it may indeed increase inaccuracy.[8] The MPR review and reinterview on foods may cause phantom foods to appear. Four reproducibility studies of recalls have now been published, three of which are partial day and one a whole day recall period. The heterogeneity of the reliability study designs and populations does not allow for summarization.

FOOD RECORD

Food records are written accounts of actual intake of the food and beverages consumed during a specified time period, usually 3, 5, or 7 days (Table 29.4).[17] A single food record is a measure of actual intake and, as with the 24 h recall, is appropriate for estimating group means and is not a tool to predict individual-level health outcomes. The work of Nelson and colleagues can be used to calculate the number of days of records necessary to determine nutrient intake with precision.[3] Respondents record detailed information about their dietary intake, such as brand names, ingredients of mixed dishes, food preparation methods, and estimates of amounts consumed. By collecting the information at the time of consumption, error due to memory loss is reduced and thus food records often serve as a validation standard. Prompts for quantification of food portions, such as two- or three-dimensional food models, are frequently used to aid respondents. Audio-taping food records have been explored as an alternative to pen and paper records.[19] Two of the validity studies reviewed reported results from partial day records, and seven studies used the entire food record to assess validity. The food records evaluated ranged from 1 to 8 days in length, and 67% required parental assistance for completion. Five of the nine studies used TEE, one used chemical analyses, one used serum, and two used observation as the validation standard.

Accurate completion of food records is greatly dependent on the ability of the child to read and write. Caution is suggested when interpreting studies that used child-completed food records as the validation standard because young children less than 9 years of age have not been shown to accurately complete food records independently. The validity of food records for measuring long-term or usual food intake improves with increased number of days of recording,[5] which indicates that multiple records may be needed. Multiple food records/recalls can introduce compliance issues for children because of the high respondent burden. As a high degree of cooperation is required from children for food records, it is essential that children be motivated to participate and be cognitively able to complete the records or be provided assistance.

FFQs AND CHECKLISTS

FFQs are used to determine usual food intake and are often used in epidemiologic studies because they are relatively easy to administer, less expensive than other assessment methods, and easily adapted for population studies (Table 29.5 and Table 29.6). A measure of usual intake can be used to rank respondents by intake levels and is useful for predicting health outcomes at both the group and individual level. Respondents report their usual intake over a defined period of time in the past year, month, or week, although frequency of intake on the previous day has also been assessed. The FFQ can be self-administered, interviewer-administered, or group-administered. The burden of work for the researcher is on the front-end developing the food list for the FFQ. The appropriateness of the FFQ food list for the population is the key to the accuracy of usual intake estimates. Respondents are asked to report frequency of consumption and sometimes portion size for a defined list of foods. FFQs can be classified as quantitative, semiquantitative, or nonquantitative. Data from nonquantitative FFQs are generally used to assess frequency of consumption of food; however, these frequencies may also be associated with standard portions to estimate nutrient amounts. Semiquantitative FFQs have generally not used portion sizes adjusted for children's level of intake. This may enhance the lack of agreement between the FFQ and the validation standard if the latter defined standard portions differently than the FFQ.

Researchers developed short food-frequency-type questionnaires, called checklists or screeners, to assess intake of a specific list of foods or food groups. These short FFQs typically did not assess portion size and ranged between 4 and 40 items. Twenty-four of the FFQ validity studies included an instrument with less than 97 items, and the range of FFQ items from all studies was from 4 to 190 items. Multiple food records and/or recalls were used 78% of the time as the validation standard for the FFQs. Sixty percent of the FFQs were semiquantitative and 38% nonquantitative. Adults were needed to assist children under <9 years of age with completion of the FFQs. FFQs consistently overestimated children's intake using nutrients or food measures with few exceptions. The mean percentage of energy overestimation was 27%, with a range of 1 to 87%. FFQs were frequently

TABLE 29.4
Food Record Validity Studies among School-Age Children

Reference[a]	Sample	Age/Grade	Instrument	Validation Standard	Design	Results
O'Connor et al.[28]	22 m[b] 25 f[b]	6–9 years Adults required[c]	3-day food record; quantitative	TEE[g] by doubly labeled water	Compared average of child's parent-assisted food record against 10-day TEE	Mean recorded energy intake was 4% greater than TEE from doubly labeled water (7.51 vs. 7.4 mJ/day). Dietary fat intake was the most significant predictor of misreporting with higher fat intake being associated with overreporting. Misreporting was not associated with sex or body composition.
Lindquist et al.[16]	17 m 13 f 17 White 13 AA[f]	6.5–11.6 years Adults required	3-day audio-taped food record; quantitative	TEE by doubly labeled water	Compared average of child's parent-assisted reports of intake from audio-taped food records against 14-day TEE	Mean recorded energy intake from records was 14% lower than TEE from doubly labeled water (6.73 vs. 7.86 mJ/day). Age was significantly related to reporting accuracy with underestimation of energy intake from audio-taped food records increasing with age
Knuiman et al.[29]	30 m	8–9 years Adults required	3-day lunch food record; quantitative	Observation	Compared average of child's parent-assisted record of lunch intake against observation of lunch with weighed duplicate portions. Excerpted lunch meal from 7-day nonconsecutive food records collected over 15-days	Correlations between mean values from recorded lunch intake and observed lunch intake were 0.71 for energy, 0.66 for protein, and 0.63 for total fat. Range of correlations for 14 nutrients (i.e., both absolute and density values) assessed was 0.62 for saturated fatty acids (% kcal) to 0.92 for polyunsaturated fat (% kcal). Recorded energy intake was 25% higher than observed intake (456 vs. 365 kcal/meal). Ten nutrients were significantly overestimated by recorded intake of lunch as compared with observation
Knuiman et al.[29]	68 m	8–9 years Adults required	7-day dinner food record; quantitative	Chemical analysis of food	Compared average of mothers' record of dinner intake against chemical analyses of duplicate portions of dinner. Excerpted dinner from 7-day nonconsecutive food records collected over 15-days	Correlations between mean values from recorded dinner intake and chemical analyses of dinner were 0.52 for energy, 0.56 for protein, and 0.58 for total fat. Range of correlations for the 14 nutrients (i.e. both absolute and density values) assessed was 0.45 for polyunsaturated fat (% kcal) to 0.85 for cholesterol. Recorded energy intake was 31% higher than chemical analysis of food (647 vs. 495 kcal/meal). Nine nutrients were significantly overestimated by mother's record of dinner as compared with chemical analysis of dinner
Van Horn et al.[13]	33 m&f	8–10 years	1-day food record audio taped; quantitative	Observation	Compared child's report of intake from audio-taped food record against parent's observation recorded as a food record	Pearson's correlations between child's record and parent's record were 0.68 for energy, 0.82 for protein (% kcal) and 0.82 for total fat (% kcal). Range of correlations for the 10 nutrients assessed was 0.68 for energy to 0.96 for iron. Child's recorded energy intake was 2% lower than parents' recorded energy intake (1882 vs. 1913 kcal/day). There were no significant differences between child and parent reports of nutrient intake (significance testing not shown)
Bandini et al.[19]	109 f White, AA, Hispanic, other	8–12 years Adults required	7-day food record; quantitative	TEE by doubly labeled water	Compared average of child's adult assisted food record against 14-day TEE	Mean recorded energy intake was 13% lower than TEE from doubly labeled water (7.00 vs. 8.03 mJ/day). Age was significantly related to reporting accuracy with underestimation of energy intake from food records increasing with age. There were no significant differences by ethnicity
Champagne et al.[31]	60 m 58 f 56 AA 62 White	9–12 years Adults required	8-day food record; quantitative	TEE by doubly labeled water	Compared average of child's parent-assisted food record against 8-day TEE	Mean recorded energy intake was 24% lower than TEE from doubly labeled water for males (1953 vs. 2555 kcal/day) and 27% lower for females (1633 vs. 2232 kcal/day). Mean recorded energy intake was 28% lower than TEE from doubly labeled water for AAs (1678 vs. 2346 kcal/day) and 22% lower for whites (1909 vs. 2441 kcal/day)

Continued

TABLE 29.4 (Continued)

Reference[a]	Sample	Age/Grade	Instrument	Validation Standard	Design	Results
Livingstone et al.[32]	6 m	12 years	7-day weighed food record; quantitative	TEE by doubly labeled water	Compared average of child's parent-assisted food record against 10–14 day TEE	Energy intake from weighed food records was less than TEE in 29 of 34 children
	6 m	15 years				
	5 m	18 years				
	6 f	12 years				
	6 f	15 years				
	5 f	18 years				
	Adults required					
Green et al.[33]	14 f	16 years	3-day food record; quantitative	Serum folate, red blood cell (RBC) folate, and serum vitamin B_{12}	Compared average of child's food record against serum micronutrient levels collected 1 week before food records	Pearson's correlations between recorded folate intake and serum folate were 0.65, between recorded folate intake and RBC folate were 0.50, and between recorded vitamin B_{12} intake and serum B_{12} were 0.32
	19 f	17 years				
	29 f	18 years				
	43 f	19 years				

[a] Results of all subgroups not reported due to samples below the $N = 30$ criterion.

[b] Males (m), females (f).

[c] Adult assistance required for instrument administration.

[d] N/A — Not applicable.

[e] FFQ — Food frequency questionnaire.

[f] AA — African-American.

[g] TEE — Total energy expenditure.

[h] MPR — Multiple-pass recall.

TABLE 29.5
Food Frequency Questionnaire (FFQ) and Checklist Validity Studies among School-Age Children

Reference[a]	Sample	Age/Grade	Instrument	# Response Categories (Range)	Validation Standard	Design	Results
Blom et al.[34]	13 m[b] 17 f[b]	2–16 years Adults[c]	36-items (sucrose, protein, fat, fiber, nitrite, vitamin C); self-administered; referent period not specified; nonquantitative	Unknown (<1/week to ≥4 times/day)	7-day food record	Compared child's parent assisted report of intake on FFQ[e] of foods with high content of sucrose, protein, fat, fiber, nitrite, and vitamin C against child's parent- and other adult-assisted report of intake on 7-day consecutive food record completed 6–8 weeks before the FFQ	Spearman's correlations between FFQ and food records for frequency of food groups with high content of protein and fat were 0.69 and 0.69, respectively. Range of correlations for 6 food groups assessed was 0.52 for sucrose to 0.76 for vitamin C. Compared with the food record, 2 food groups were significantly overestimated and 3 were significantly underestimated by the FFQ. Of the 34 food items, 5 were significantly overestimated and 8 were significantly underestimated by the FFQ
Taylor et al.[35]	26 m 41 f	3–6 years Adults[c]	35-items (calcium); self-administered; past year; semiquantitative	Open-ended (never to number of times/month)	4-day food record	Compared parent's report of child's frequency of intake of calcium foods on FFQ against parent's report of child's 4-day food record	FFQ significantly overestimated mean calcium intake by 18% compared with the food record (942 vs. 798 mg/day)
Kaskoun et al.[36]	22 m 23 f White & Native American	4–6 years Adults[c]	<111-items; self-administered; past year; semiquantitative; adult portions	9 (<1/month to ≥6 times/day)	TEE[g] by doubly labeled water	Compared parent's report of child's frequency of intake of foods on FFQ against 14-day TEE completed after or at the same time as the FFQ	FFQ significantly overestimated total energy intake by 59% compared with TEE (9.12 vs. 5.74 mJ/day)
Persson et al.[37]	477 m&f	4 & 8 years Adults[c]	27-items; interviewer administered; referent period not specified; nonquantitative	8 (none to ≥4 times/day)	7-day food record	Compared parent's report of child's frequency of intake of foods on FFQ against parent's report of child's intake on 7-day food records. Foods from the records were translated into food categories of the FFQ	FFQ significantly overestimated intake of 15 food items and underestimated intake of 9 food items as compared with the food record
Wilson et al.[38]	61 f 50 White 10 AA[f] 1 Asian	4–9 years Adults[c]	109 Items; (Block98 FFQ) interviewer-administered; past year; quantitative	9 (none or <1/month to 2+ times/day); 3 portion sizes	3-day food record	Compared parent's child assisted report of frequency of intake of foods on FFQ against parent's report of child's intake from 3-day food record	Correlations between Block98 FFQ and food records ranged from 0.40 to 0.55 for energy and 3 macronutrients. Block98 FFQ energy intake was 25% higher than the diet record (2180 vs. 1749 kcal/day)

Continued

TABLE 29.5
Continued

Reference[a]	Sample	Age/Grade	Instrument	# Response Categories (Range)	Validation Standard	Design	Results
Hammond et al.[39]	150 m&f	5–11 years Adult[c]	35-items (fat, energy, fiber); self-administered; past month; nonquantitative	10 (none to 7 days/week)	14-day food checklists	Compared child's parent assisted report of frequency of intake of foods on FFQ against child's parent assisted report of intake on 14-day food checklists. Food checklists consisted of two sets of 7-day consecutive food records 1 & 2 months after the FFQ and contained the same food categories as the FFQ	Median difference in days/week consumption between the FFQs and food checklists was: equal to 0 for 17 foods, >0 for 5 foods, and <0 for 13 foods (significance testing not shown). Differences ranged from −1 (cakes, chips) to 1 (green vegetables). Percentage of responders classified by FFQ to within ±1 day per week of frequencies reported on checklists ranged from 46.8% for low-fiber cereal to 99.3% for lamb, other fish and liver
Byers et al.[40]	43 m 54 f White & AA	6–10 years Adults[c]	35-items (15 fruits, 20 vegetables); self-administered; past 3 months; semiquantitative; adult portions	9 (none or <1 time/month to ≥6 times/day)	Serum carotenoids vitamins A, C, and E	Compared parent's report of child's frequency of intake on FFQ of fruit and vegetables against child's serum micronutrient levels	Spearman's correlations between dietary and serum nutrients were 0.16 for carotene, 0.39 for vitamin C, 0.14 for vitamin A, and 0.32 for vitamin E. Correlations between serum levels of carotene, vitamin C, vitamin A, and vitamin E and frequencies of intake of total fruits and vegetables were 0.24, 0.29, 0.14, and 0.17, respectively. There were no differences by gender or ethnicity (significance testing not shown)
Arnold et al.[41]	77 f	7–12 years Adults[c]	160-items; self-administered; past year (inferred); semiquantitative; adult portions	Open-ended (none to number of months/year)	14-day food record	Compared child's parent assisted report of frequency of intake of foods from two FFQ administrations against child's parent assisted report of intake on 14-day food records. Records consisting of two sets of 7-day consecutive food records were completed 1 month after the first FFQ and 6 months later	Pearson's correlations (log-transformed, energy-adjusted) between the first FFQ and the first food record and the second FFQ and second food record were 0.13 to 0.22 for energy, 0.20 to 0.30 for protein, and 0.28 to 0.46 for fat, respectively. Range of correlations for 16 nutrients assessed was 0.06 for starch to 0.61 for vitamin B_2. For the first FFQ, energy intake was 24% higher than the first food record (2319 vs. 1861 kcal/day). For the second FFQ, energy intake was 16% higher than the second food record (2205 vs. 1902 kcal/day). Both administrations of the FFQ overestimated intake for all 16 nutrients compared with the food records (significance testing not shown)
Baranowski et al.[42]	1530–1570 m&f White & AA	3rd grade	7-items (3 fruit 4 vegetables); group-administered; past month; semiquantitative; "serving" portions	10 (none to ≥5 times/day)	7-day food record	Compared child's report of servings of fruits and vegetables against child's report of intake on 7-day food records. Foods from the records were abstracted into the FFQ categories by a dietitian	Pearson's correlations between FFQ and food records for fruits and vegetables, fruits and juices, and vegetables were 0.20, 0.24, and 0.15, respectively. Total servings of fruits and vegetables/week as measured by the FFQ were 50.9 and by food record was 15.9. The FFQ significantly overestimated intake of food items in all seven food categories, both aggregate and individual items (significance testing not shown)

Reference	Sample	Age	Instrument		Reference method	Comparison	Results
Bellu et al.[43]	165 m 158 f	8–10 years Adults[c]	116-items; self-administered; past 6 months; semiquantitative; "average" portions	Unknown	24 h recall	Compared parent's report of child's frequency of intake on FFQ of foods against mother's report of child's intake on 24 h recall	Mean energy estimates from the FFQ were 27% higher than the 24 h recall for females (2156 vs.1703 kcal/day) and 25% higher for males (2281 vs. 1821 kcal/day). Among females, of the 10 nutrients, the FFQ significantly overestimated 1 nutrient and significantly underestimated 2. Among males, 3 nutrients were significantly overestimated and 1 was significantly underestimated by the FFQ
Perks et al.[44]	23 m 27 f	8–16 years	131-items Youth/Adolescent Questionnaire (YAQ); self-administered; past year; semiquantitative; child portions	Dependent on type of food	TEE by doubly labeled water	Compared child's report of frequency of intake of foods on YAQ against TEE. Child completed YAQ within one year of TEE measurement	Mean recorded energy intake from YAQ was 1.93% higher, yet not significant, than TEE from doubly labeled water (10.03 vs.9.84 mJ/day). Body weight and percentage body fat were found to be significantly correlated to the discrepancy in energy intake (YAQ-TEE)
Bellu et al.[45]	39 m 49 f	9–12 years Adult[c]	116-items; self-administered; past 6 months; semiquantitative; "average" portions	Unknown	14-day food record	Compared parent's report of child's frequency of intake of foods on FFQ against parent's report of child's intake on 14-day weighed food records. Records consisted of two sets of 7-day consecutive food records at the beginning of the study and 6 months later, before and after the FFQ	Pearson's correlations between FFQ and food records were 0.46 for energy, 0.34 for protein, and 0.39 for fat. Range of correlations for 18 nutrients assessed was 0.07 for vitamin A to 0.52 for carbohydrates. FFQ energy intake was 40% higher than the diet record (2620 vs. 1865 kcal/day). The FFQ significantly overestimated six nutrients and significantly underestimated five nutrients compared with the food records
Rockett et al.[46]	122 m 139 f 96% White	9–18 years	131-items Youth/Adolescent Questionnaire (YAQ); self-administered; past year; semiquantitative; child portions	Dependent on type of food	Three, 24 h recall	Compared child's report of frequency of intake of foods (mean of two administrations 1 year apart) on YAQ against child's report of intake on three 24 h recalls. Recalls were collected by telephone using research dietitians in the year between YAQ administrations	Pearson's correlation (unadjusted log-transformed values) between YAQ and recalls were 0.35 for energy, 0.30 for protein, and 0.41 for fat. Range of correlations for 28 nutrients assessed was 0.09 for copper to 0.46 for vitamin C. YAQ energy intake was 1% higher than the recalls (2196 vs. 2169 kcal/day). Of 31 nutrients assessed, 16 were overestimated by the YAQ and 8 were underestimated (significance testing not shown). Correlations did not show a consistent pattern by gender or age (significance testing not shown)

Continued

TABLE 29.5
(Continued)

Reference[a]	Sample	Age/Grade	Instrument	# Response Categories (Range)	Validation Standard	Design	Results
Domel et al.[47]	160–165 m&f White & AA	4–5th grade	45-items (15 fruit, 30 vegetables); group-administered; past month; semiquantitative; "serving" portions	7 (none or <1/month to several per day)	22-day food record	Compared child's report of frequency of fruit and vegetable intake (mean of two administrations) against child's report of intake on 22 consecutive days of food records. Records were collected between FFQ administrations; foods from the records were abstracted by a dietitian into servings of fruit and vegetables	Spearman's correlations between month 1 FFQ and food records and month 2 FFQ and food records were 0.12 and 0.17 for total fruit, −0.04 and 0.02 for total vegetables, and −0.05 and 0.01 for total fruit and vegetable. Range of correlations for 8 fruit/vegetable groupings assessed was −0.05 for total fruit and vegetables to 0.32 for fruit and vegetable juice. Mean daily servings of total fruit and vegetables were 409% higher for the month 1 FFQ compared with the corresponding food records (11.7 vs. 2.3), and 135% higher for the month 2 FFQ compared with the food records (5.4 vs. 2.3). Both administrations of the monthly FFQ significantly overestimated mean daily servings for all 8 fruit/vegetable groupings compared with the corresponding food records
Domel et al.[47]	154–156 m&f White & AA	4–5th grade	45-items (15 fruit, 30 vegetables); group-administered; past week; semiquantitative; "serving" portions	5 (none or <1/week to several per day)	7-day food record	Compared child's report of frequency of fruit and vegetable intake (mean of two administrations) against child's report of intake on 7-day food records. Records were collected between FFQ administrations; foods from the records were abstracted by a dietitian into servings of fruit and vegetables	Spearman's correlations between week 1 FFQ and food records and week 2 FFQ and food records were 0.18 and 0.18 for total fruit, −0.01 and 0.11 for total vegetable, and 0.00 and 0.05 for total fruit and vegetable. Range of correlations for 8 fruit/vegetable groupings assessed was −0.01 for total vegetable to 0.25 for total legumes and fruit. Mean daily servings of total fruits and vegetables were 295% higher for week 1 FFQs compared with the corresponding food record (8.3 vs. 2.1), and 306% higher for week 2 FFQ (7.3 vs. 1.8). Both administrations of the weekly FFQ significantly overestimated mean daily servings for all 8 fruit and vegetable groupings compared with the corresponding food records

Study	Sample	Grade	Instrument	Response options	Reference method	Comparison	Results
Field et al.[48]	51 m&f 58 m&f 84% AA	4–5th grade 6–7th grade	97-items (11 fruit & fruit juice, 14 vegetable); group-administered to 4–5th grades; self-administered to 6–7th grades; past year; semiquantitative; child portions	Dependent on type of food	Four 24 h recalls	Compared child's report of frequency of intake of foods on FFQ against child's report of intake from four, nonconsecutive 24 h recalls administered 3 months apart and within 1 year of FFQ. Recalls were not conducted during the summer or on Saturdays	Pearson's correlations (unadjusted log transformed values) between FFQ and mean of recalls among 4–5th graders were 0.26 for energy, 0.20 for protein, and 0.26 for fat. Correlations among 6–7th graders were 0.34 for energy, 0.23 for protein, and 0.24 for fat. Range of correlations among 4–5th graders for the 10 nutrients assessed was 0.01 for fat (% kcal) to 0.31 for saturated fat. Range among 6–7th graders was from 0.04 for fat (% kcal) to 0.50 for vitamin C. Spearman's correlations (unadjusted) between FFQ and recalls among 4–5th graders ranged from −0.01 for servings of fruits and juice to 0.16 for vegetables. Among 6–7th graders the range was from 0.13 for vegetables to 0.30 for fruit juice. Median FFQ energy intake was 87% higher than recalls (3136 vs.1677 kcal/day) among 4–5th graders. Median FFQ energy intake was 15% higher than recalls (2297 vs. 1992 kcal/day) among 6–7th graders
Vereecken et al.[49]	101 m&f 52% m 48% f	5–6th grade	15-items (fiber, calcium foods, and foods relevant to youth food culture) Health Behavior in School-Aged Children (HBSC) FFQ; group-administered; yesterday; nonquantified	7 (Never to more than once a day)	7-day food record structured on meal segments	Compared child's report of frequency of intake of foods on HBSC against child's report of frequency of food items abstracted from food record. To identify misclassification and percent agreement, the HBSC and records were translated into 3 comparable categories of frequency of consumption	Spearman's correlations between the HBSC and food record ranged from 0.10 for crisps to 0.65 for semiskimmed milk. The Wilcoxon test used to compare mean consumption indicates the HBSC significantly overestimated intake for all items except two: cheese and soft drinks. Percentage agreement ranged from 34% for vegetables (excluding composite dishes) to 66% for crisps. Percentage gross misclassification ranged from 1% for chips to 21% for diet soft drinks
Koehler et al.[50]	66 m 54 f American Indian, non-Hispanic-White, Hispanic	5–8th grade	33-items Yesterday's Food Choices-(YFC); self-administered; past day; non quantitative	3 Yes, not sure, and no	24 h recall	Compared child's report of frequency of intake of particular foods on YFC against child's 24 h recall, both completed on same day	Spearman's correlations between scores on the YFC and 24 h recall were 0.71 for low fat foods, 0.35 for high fiber foods, 0.29 for fruits and vegetables, and 0.40 for high fat foods.
Andersen et al.[26]	36 m 49 f	6th grade	16-items (7 fruit & vegetable); self-administered; past 3 months; nonquantitative	10 (never to several times a day)	7-day food record with pre-coded list of 277 foods	Compared child's report of fruit and vegetable intake on FFQ against child's report of intake on 7-day food records. Excerpted fruit and vegetable intake from 7-day food record with pre-coded list of foods	Spearman's correlations between FFQ and food record were 0.21 for fruit, 0.21 for potato, 0.23 for fruit, fruit juice, vegetable and potato, 0.28 for vegetable, 0.28 for fruit juice, and 0.32 for fruit and vegetable without fruit juice and potato. Percent correctly classified by tertiles for six food groups ranged from 35% for fruit to 47% for fruit, fruit juice, vegetable and potato. Spearman's correlation coefficients were generally higher among females than males (significance testing not shown)

Continued

TABLE 29.5
(Continued)

Reference[a]	Sample	Age/Grade	Instrument	# Response Categories (Range)	Validation Standard	Design	Results
Jenner et al.[51]	61 m 57 f	~11–12 years	175-items; group-administered; past week; nonquantitative	6 (none to every day)	14-day food record	Compared child's report of frequency of food intake on FFQ against child's report of intake on 14-day diet records. Seven sets of two consecutive day records were collected in the 3 months following administration of the FFQ. Nutrient estimates from FFQ completed by parents were also compared with the 14-day diet records	Pearson's correlations (log-transformed) between the child's FFQ and diet records were 0.25 for energy, 0.18 for protein and 0.19 for total fat. Range of correlations for 13 nutrients assessed was 0.11 for monounsaturated fat to 0.42 for complex carbohydrates. Correlations between the parents' FFQs and diet records were 0.38 for energy, 0.26 for protein and 0.30 for total fat. Range of correlations was 0.26 for protein to 0.47 for complex carbohydrates. Children's FFQ energy intakes were 36% higher than diet records (10.9 vs. 8.0 mJ/day). Parents' FFQ estimates of children's energy intake were 21% higher than children's diet records (9.7 vs. 8.0 mJ/day). All 13 nutrients were overestimated by both the child and the parent FFQ (significance testing not shown)
Lietz et al.[52]	37 m&f	11–13 years	unknown number of items, European Prospective Investigation of Cancer (EPIC) FFQ; Interviewer-administered; past year; semiquantitative	9 (<1 time/mo to >6 times/day)	7-day weighed food record	Compared child's report of intake from frequency of intake of foods on EPIC against child's 7-day weighed food record completed 1 day after the EPIC interview	Spearman's correlations (unadjusted) between EPIC and food records were 0.33 for energy, 0.30 for protein, and 0.52 for total fat. Range of correlations for 13 nutrients assessed was 0.27 for potassium and 0.61 for total fat (% kcal). Energy-adjusted correlations were 0.31 for protein, 0.66 for fat and ranged from 0.26 for sodium to 0.66 for total fat. FFQ energy intake was 30% higher than the diet record (10.4 vs. 8.0 MJ/day). Percent correctly classified into tertiles by the two methods ranged from 29.7% for total fat (% kcal) to 48.6% for potassium and total carbohydrate. Percent misclassified in opposite thirds ranged from 8.1% each for calcium, potassium, carbohydrate (% kcal), and sugar (% kcal) to 16.2% for Englyst fiber (median 10.8%)
Yaroch et al.[53]	57 f AA	11–17 years	18-items; (13 related to low-fat or high-fat eating behaviors) Qualitative Dietary Fat Index Questionnaire (QFQ): usual; interviewer-administered; nonquantitative	4 (never to always)	Three 24 h recalls	Compared child's report of food intake on QFQ against the mean of three 24 h recalls administered within 2 weeks after QFQ. The 18 low-fat and high-fat items were summed to create a total QFQ score with a higher score indicating lower-fat intake behaviors	Pearson's correlations (log transformed) between QFQ score and mean of recalls were −0.23 for energy, −0.31 for total fat, and −0.23 for fat (% kcal)

Reference	Sample	Age/Grade	Instrument	Response Options	Comparison Method	Results
Smith et al.[54]	243 m&f	7th grade	40-items; (foods high in total fat, saturated fat and sodium) Child and Adolescent Trial for Cardiovascular Health (CATCH) Food Checklist (CFC); group-administered; yesterday; nonquantitative	Yes/No	24 h recall	Compared child's reported frequency of intake of foods on CFC against child's 24 h recall. Children were in two groups, the first group completed the recall at least 2 h after the CFC and the second group completed the recall at least 2 h before the CFC. For each of the 40 foods a score of 0 (low intake) to 5 (high intake) was assigned and a total score summed for each nutrient — total fat, saturated fat and sodium	Pearson's correlations between CFC nutrient scores and the 24 h recall using equal weights were 0.22 for percent total fat, 0.23 for percent saturated fat and 0.24 for sodium. Kappa statistics between the CFC food items and foods on recall ranged from 0.21 for butter to 0.84 for pizza and lasagna. The mean kappa value was higher for students who completed the CFC after the recall (kappa = 0.45) than for those who completed the CFC first (kappa = 0.60); suggesting that recognition memory enhanced validity measures. Male students reported greater intake of all three nutrients on the CFC than females; however, CFC scores were only significantly different for sodium
Cullen et al.[55]	89 m&f, 41% m, 59% f, 54% AA, 46% Hispanic	7–8th grade	152-items Youth/Adolescent Questionnaire (YAQ); group-administered; past year; semiquantitative; child portions	Dependent on type of food	6-day food record	Compared nutrient intake from child's report of frequency of food intake on YAQ against child's report of intake from food records	Spearman's correlations between YAQ and mean of food records were 0.19 for energy and 0.09 for fat (% kcal). Spearman's correlations for the 4 fruit and vegetable groupings ranged from 0.02 for high-fat vegetables to 0.23 of regular vegetables. Among AA's the Spearman's correlations ranged from 0.002 for fruit to 0.25 for juice and among Hispanics ranged from −0.06 for high-fat vegetables to 0.38 for regular vegetables.
Prochaska et al.[56]	59 m&f, 37% m, 63% f, 37% White, 25% Asian, 12% Hispanic, 3% AA	7–12th grade	21-items (21 high-fat foods) PACE+; self-administered; past 7 days; nonquantitative	6 (Did not eat it this week to more than twice each day)	3-day food record	Compared child's scores from report of frequency of food intake on PACE+ and fat measure against child's report of intake on 3-day food records	Pearson's correlation between PACE+ and fat score and food records was 0.36 for total fat (% kcal), $p < .01$
Prochaska et al.[56]	59 m&f, 37% m, 63% f, 37% White, 25% Asian, 12% Hispanic, 3% AA	7–12th grade	4-categories (4 high-fat food groups); self-administered; past 7 days; nonquantitative	6 (Did not eat it this week to more than twice each day)	3-day food record	Compared fat measure scores from child's report of frequency of food intake against child's report of intake on 3-day food records	Pearson's correlation between 4-category fat measure and food records was 0.12 for total fat (% kcal), $p < .31$
van Assema et al.[57]	50 m&f	12–18 years	35-items (19 foods high in total fat and saturated fat) Fat List; self-administered; past 6 months; semiquantitative	Open-ended	7-day food record	Compared child's total fat score from Fat List against child's report of intake on 7-day food records kept consecutively after the Fat List was completed. For each of the 19 foods a fat score of 0 (low fat intake) to 5 (high fat intake) was assigned and a total score summed for all foods	Pearson's correlations between Fat List score and food records were 0.56 for energy and 0.61 for fat. Range of correlations for five nutrients assessed was 0.14 for saturated fat (% kcal) to 0.61 for fat

Continued

TABLE 29.5
(Continued)

Reference[a]	Sample	Age/Grade	Instrument	# Response Categories (Range)	Validation Standard	Design	Results
Hoelscher et al.[58]	103 m 106 f 79 White 36 AA 85 Hispanic 9 other	8th grade	63-items (17 items tested for validity) School-Based Nutrition Monitoring Questionnaire (SBNM); group-administered; yesterday; nonquantitative	4 (0 times/day to 3+ times/day)	24 h recall	Compared child's report of frequency of intake of foods on SBNM against child's report of intake of 24 h recall. Using two groups, the first group completed the recall at least 2 hours after the SBNM and the second group completed the recall at least 2 hours before the SBMN. Excerpted foods from recall to match the 17 SBNM food items	Spearman's correlations between SBNM items and recall ranged from 0.32 for any type of bread, bun, bagel, tortilla, roll to 0.68 for milk and for beans. Kappa statistics ranged from 0.12 for any type of bread, bun, bagel, tortilla, roll to 0.59 for beans. Percentage agreement ranged from 38% for any type of bread, bun, bagel, tortilla, or roll to 89% for gravy
Johnson et al.[59]	1822 m&f 32% m 68% f 1666 White 144 non-White 36 unknown	13–16 years	23-items; Adolescent Food Habits Checklist (AFHC); self-administered; usual intake; nonquantified	True/False (10 items also have a nonapplicable option)	Number of portions of fruits and vegetables; Dietary Instrument for Nutrition Education (DINE) FFQ	Compared child's score from AFHC against child's report of fruit and vegetables portions and frequency of intake using DINE FFQ. AFHC score was number of "healthy" responses * (23/number of items completed)	Pearson's correlations between AFHC score and Dine FFQ were −0.46 for dietary fat, 0.16 for dietary fiber and 0.45 for portions of fruit and vegetable intake. Among females the correlations were 0.44 for fruit and vegetable intake and −0.41 for dietary fat and 0.18 for dietary fiber. Among males the correlations were 0.45 for fruit and vegetable intake and −0.46 for dietary fat, and 0.24 for dietary fiber
Kinlay et al.[60]	57 m 48 f	13–17 years Adults required	12-items (fat, saturated fat); self-administered; past week; semiquantitative	Dependent on type of food	FFQ[e]	Compared child's parent-assisted report of frequency of specific fatty food intake against child's parent assisted report of food intake on a FFQ	Spearman's correlations between the brief FFQ and the FFQ were 0.40 for total fat as % of kcal and 0.54 for saturated fat as % of kcal
Field et al.[61]	102 m&f 50% m 50% f 35% White 24% AA 15% Hispanic	9–12th grade	27-items (12 fruit, 15 vegetables) Youth/Adolescent Questionnaire (YAQ): self-administered; past year; semiquantitative	Unknown (<1/month to ≥2 times/day)	Three 24 h recalls	Compared child's report of frequency of fruit and vegetable intake on YAQ against child's report of intake on three nonconsecutive 24 h recalls completed 2 weeks apart. YAQ was administered 2–4 weeks after the third recall	Spearman's correlations between the YAQ and mean of three 24 h recalls were 0.33 for fruit only, 0.29 for fruit juice, 0.33 for fruit and juice, 0.32 for vegetables, and 0.41 for fruit (including juice) and vegetables

Study	Sample	Age	Instrument	Frequency	Reference	Results
Field et al.[61]	102 m&f 50% m 50% f 35% White 24% AA 15% Hispanic	9–12th grade	4-items (2 fruit, 2 vegetable) Youth Risk Behavior Surveillance System Questionnaire (YRBSS); self-administered; past day; semiquantitative	Unknown (none to ≥3 times/day)	Three 24 h recalls	Compared child's report of fruit and vegetable intake on YRBSS against child's mean intake of fruits and vegetables calculated with an algorithm using three nonconsecutive 24 h recalls completed 2 weeks apart. YRBSS was administered 2–4 weeks after third recall	Spearman's correlations between YRBSS items and mean of 24 h recalls were 0.17 for fruit only, 0.07 for fruit juice, 0.21 for fruit and juice, 0.24 for vegetables, and 0.28 for fruit (including juice) and vegetables
Field et al.[61]	102 m&f 50% m 50% f 35% White 24% AA 15% Hispanic	9–12th grade	6-items (2 fruit, 4 vegetable) Behavioral Risk Factor Surveillance System Questionnaire (BRFSS); self-administered; past day; semiquantitative	Unknown none to ≥3 times/day	Three 24 h recalls	Compared child's report of frequency of fruit and vegetable intake against child's reported mean intake of fruits and vegetables calculated with an algorithm using two nonconsecutive 24 h recalls completed 4 weeks apart. BRFSS was administered halfway between the two recalls	Spearman's correlations between past day BRFSS and mean of 24 h recalls were 0.33 for fruit only, 0.30 for fruit juice, 0.34 for fruit and juice, 0.14 for vegetables, and 0.30 for fruit (including juice) and vegetables
Field et al.[61]	100 m&f 50% m 50% f 35% White 24% AA 15% Hispanic	9–12th grade	6-items (2 fruit, 4 vegetable) Behavioral Risk Factor Surveillance System Questionnaire (BRFSS); self-administered; past year; semiquantitative	Unknown (none to ≥5 times/day)	Three 24 h recalls	Compared child's report of frequency of fruit and vegetable intake on BRFSS against child's reported mean intake of fruits and vegetables calculated with an algorithm using three nonconsecutive 24 h recalls completed 4 weeks apart. BRFSS was administered preceding the third recall	Spearman's correlations between past year BRFSS and mean of 24 h recalls were 0.36 for fruit only, 0.36 for fruit and juice, 0.35 for vegetables, and 0.43 for fruit (including juice) and vegetables
Green et al.[33]	14 f 19 f 29 f 43 f	16 years 17 years 18 years 19 years	116-items; self-administered; past year; semiquantitative	Unknown	Serum folate, red blood cell (RBC) folate, and serum vitamin B_{12}	Compared child's report of frequency of intake of foods on FFQ against serum micronutrient levels	Pearson's correlations were 0.48 between folate intake from the FFQ and serum folate, 0.42 between folate intake from the FFQ and RBC folate, and 0.25 between vitamin B_{12} intake from the FFQ and serum B_{12}

Continued

TABLE 29.5 (Continued)

Reference[a]	Sample	Age/Grade	Instrument	# Response Categories (Range)	Validation Standard	Design	Results
Andersen et al.[62]	13 m 36 f	11th grade Adults required	190-items; group administered; past year; semi quantitative	Dependent on type of food	7-day weighed food record	Compared child's parent assisted report of frequency of food intake on FFQ against child's report of intake on 7-day weighed food records completed 2–3 months after FFQ administration. Records consisted of four consecutive days, a 1 week interval, and 3 consecutive days	Spearman's correlations between FFQ and food records were 0.51 for energy, 0.48 for protein, and 0.57 for total fat. Range of correlations for 18 nutrients assessed was 0.14 for vitamin D to 0.66 for monounsaturated fat. FFQ energy intake was 24% higher than diet records (10.7 vs. 8.6 mJ/day). The FFQ significantly overestimated 16 of the 18 nutrients. The FFQ significantly overestimated intake of 8 of 13 food items as compared with diet records
Vereecken et al.[49]	7072 m&f 47.4% m 52.6% f	11–18 years	15-items (fiber, calcium foods, and foods relevant to youth food culture) Health Behavior in School-Aged Children (HBSC) FFQ; group-administered; yesterday; nonquantitative	7 (Never to more than once a day)	24 h Food Behavior Checklist (FBC)	Compared child's report of frequency of intake of foods on HBSC against child's report of intake of foods on FBC adjusted for weekly time period	Percent agreement of foods with responses 'never' or 'once a day, every day' and 'everyday, more than once' on HBSC with the FBC foods ranged from 89% for other milk products to 99.3% for alcohol, with a mean agreement for all food items of 95.3% (data not shown). No differences were found between genders or between students aged 11–12, 13–14, 15–16, and 17–18 (significance testing not shown)

[a] Results of all subgroups not reported due to samples below the $N = 30$ criterion.

[b] Males (m), females (f).

[c] Adult assistance required for instrument administration.

[d] N/A — Not applicable.

[e] FFQ — Food frequency questionnaire.

[f] AA — African-American.

[g] TEE — Total energy expenditure.

[h] MPR — Multiple-pass recall.

TABLE 29.6
Food Frequency Questionnaire (FFQ) and Checklist Reliability Studies among School-Age Children

References[a]	Sample	Age/Grade	Instrument	Response Categories (Range)	Design	Results
Basch et al.[63]	166 m&f[b] Latino	4–7 years Adults required[c]	~116-items; interviewer administered; past 6 months; semiquantitative; child portions	9 (none or <1/month to ≥6/day)	Compared both 3-month and 1-year test–retest reproducibility of nutrient estimates from FFQs[e] completed by the parent	Pearson's correlations (log-transformed) between the two FFQs at 3 months were 0.53 for energy, 0.49 for protein, and 0.56 for total fat. Range of correlations for 12 nutrients assessed at 3 months was −0.06 for sucrose to 0.61 for crude fiber. At 1 year, correlations were 0.46 for energy, 0.40 for protein, and 0.47 for total fat. Range of correlations for 12 nutrients assessed at 1 year was 0.06 for sucrose to 0.57 for polyunsaturated fat
Metcalf et al.[64]	90 m&f	5–14 years Adults required	117-items Children's Nutrition Survey FFQ; past 4 weeks; self-administered; past 4 weeks; semiquantitative	7 (never or less than once per month to two or more times per day)	Compared a 2-week test–retest repeatability of FFQs completed by parent/caregiver or parent/caregiver and child	Pearson's correlations (log-transformed) between the two FFQs for the 17 food groups ranged from 0.35 for bread (slices) to 0.86 for rice among 5–9 year olds and from 0.49 for spreads to 0.91 for red meats among 10–14 year olds. Spearman's correlations (log-transformed) between the two FFQs for the 17 food groups ranged from 0.38 for bread (slices) to 0.85 for rice among 5–9 year olds and from 0.54 for mixed meat dishes to 0.89 for convenience meals among 10–14 year olds. Standardized Cronbach's alpha between the two FFQs ranged from 0.52 for bread (slices) to 0.92 for rice among 5–9 year olds and from 0.64 for spreads to 0.95 for red meats among 10–14 year olds. Pearson's and Spearman's correlations and Cronbach's alpha were generally lower among 5–9 year olds compared with 10–14 year olds
Arnold et al.[41]	77 f	7–12 years Adults required	160-items; self-administered; past year; semiquantitative; adult portions	5 (open-ended, none to number of months/year)	Compared 6-month test–retest reproducibility of nutrient estimates from FFQs completed by the parent and child	Pearson's correlations (log-transformed, energy adjusted) between the two FFQs were 0.60 for energy, 0.51 for protein, and 0.14 for total fat. Range of correlations for 16 nutrients assessed was 0.14 for total fat to 0.71 for fiber. Mean energy intake was 5% higher in the first FFQ compared with the second (2319 vs. 2205 kcal/day). Mean intake of 15 nutrients was higher in the first FFQ compared with the second; 1 nutrient was lower (significance testing not shown)
Domel et al.[47]	146 m&f AA[f] & White	4–5th grade	45-items (15 fruit, 30 vegetable); group administered; past week; semiquantitative; "serving" portions	5 (none or <1/week to several per day)	Compared 1-week test–retest reproducibility of fruit and vegetable intake from FFQs completed by the child. Order of fruit (15 items) and vegetables (30 items) was reversed between first and second administrations	Spearman's correlations between the 2 FFQs were 0.50 for total fruit, 0.48 for total vegetable, and 0.54 for total fruit and vegetable intake. Range of correlations for 8 fruit and vegetable groupings assessed was 0.39 for fruit and vegetable juice to 0.54 for total fruit and vegetables. Mean daily servings of total fruits and vegetables was 12% higher for Week 1 FFQ compared with Week 2 FFQ (8.3 vs. 7.3). Mean daily servings of 6 fruit and vegetable groupings of eight assessed were higher for Week 1 FFQ compared with Week 2 FFQ (significance testing not shown)

Continued

TABLE 29.6
Continued

References[a]	Sample	Age/Grade	Instrument	Response Categories (Range)	Design	Results
Domel et al.[47]	156 m&f AA & White	4–5th grade	45-items (15 fruit, 30 vegetable); group administered; past month; semiquantitative; "serving" portions	7 (none or <1/month to several per day)	Compared 1-month (3.5-week) test–retest reproducibility of fruit and vegetable intake from FFQs completed by the child. Order of fruit (15 items) and vegetables (30 items) was reversed between first and second administrations	Spearman's correlations between the 2 FFQs were 0.43 for total fruit, 0.37 for total vegetable, and 0.47 for total fruit and vegetable intake. Range of correlations for 8 fruit and vegetable groupings assessed was 0.28 for fruit and vegetable juice to 0.47 for both legumes and total fruit and vegetable intake. Mean daily servings of total fruits and vegetables was 54% higher for Month 1 FFQ compared with Month 2 FFQ (11.7 vs. 5.4). Mean daily servings of 8 fruit and vegetable groupings were higher for Month 1 FFQ compared with Month 2 FFQ (significance testing not shown)
Field et al.[48]	35 m&f 34 m&f	4–5th grade 6–7th grade	97-items (11 fruit and fruit juice, 14 vegetable); group-administered to 4–5th grades; self-administered to 6–7th grades; past year; semiquantitative; child portions	Dependent on type of food	Compared a 1-year test–retest reproducibility of FFQs completed by child	Spearman's correlations between the 2 FFQs among 4–5th graders were 0.24 for energy, 0.25 for protein, and 0.15 for total fat. Correlations between the 2 FFQs among 6–7th graders were 0.21 for energy, 0.23 for protein, and 0.18 for total fat. The range of correlations for the 11 nutrients assessed was from 0.03 for phosphorous to 0.30 for carbohydrates among 4–5th graders. Among 6–7th graders correlations ranged from 0.18 for total fat to 0.47 for iron. Spearman's correlations between the two FFQs among 4–5th graders were −0.26 for vegetables, 0.07 for fruit and vegetables, 0.36 for fruit, and 0.40 for fruit juice. Among 6–7th graders correlations were 0.18 for fruit juice, 0.28 for vegetables, 0.29 for fruit and vegetables, and 0.33 for fruit
Buzzard et al.[65]	415 m&f 46% m 54% f 56% White 32% AA 12% Asian, Latino, or Indian	6th grade 11–14 years	35-items (25 food frequency questions measuring fat, fiber, and fruit and vegetable intake, Goals for Health); self-administered; usual intake; nonquantitative	7 (never to 3 or more times a day)	Compared a 4-month test–retest reliability of nutrient scores from FFQs completed by child	Pearson's correlations (log-transformed) between nutrient scores from the two FFQs were 0.58 for total fat, 0.49 for fiber, and 0.51 for fruit and vegetables. Correlations of the 25 frequency items ranged from 0.24 for donuts, sweet rolls, muffins to 0.59 for mayonnaise on sandwiches. The mean correlation was 0.41. In comparing excluded and included students, males were somewhat more likely to be excluded (59% of exclusions, $p < .05$)
Andersen et al.[22]	54 m 60 f	6th grade	16-items (7 fruit and vegetable); self-administered; past 3 months; nonquantitative	10 (never to several times a day)	Compared a 2-week test–retest of fruit and vegetable intake from FFQs completed by the child	Spearman's correlations between the 2 FFQs were 0.62 for fruit, 0.70 for vegetable, 0.75 for fruit and vegetable without fruit juice and potato, 0.77 for fruit juice, 0.78 for fruit, fruit juice, vegetable, and potato, and 0.83 for potato
Speck et al.[66]	31 m&f 42% m 58% f 56% White 44% AA	6–8th grade	140-items (14 food habit questions, 83 food frequency questions past week, and 43 quantity of foods eaten/day questions) Eating Habits Questionnaire (EHQ); group-administered; past week; quantitative	5 for food items (never to almost every day); 6 for beverage items (never to 3 or more times a day); 4 for quantity items (0 to 5 or more servings)	Compared a 48 h test–retest reliability of FFQs completed by the child	Pearson's correlations between the 2 FFQs for the 10 food groupings ranged from 0.46 for dairy to 0.85 for meats/fish/casseroles

Speck et al.[66]	31 m&f 55% m 45% f 57% White 43% AA	6–8th grade	140-items (14 food habit questions, 83 food frequency questions past week, and 43 quantity of foods eaten/day questions) Eating Habits Questionnaire (EHQ); group-administered; past week; quantitative	5 for food items (never to almost every day); 6 for beverage items (never to 3 or more times a day); 4 for quantity items (0 to 5 or more servings)	Compared a 2-week test–retest reliability of FFQs completed by the child	Correlations between the initial and 2-week FFQ ranged from 0.08 for dairy to 0.76 for sweet snacks
Smith et al.[54]	122 m&f	7th grade	40-items; (foods high in total fat, saturated fat and sodium) Child and Adolescent Trial for Cardiovascular Health (CATCH) Food Checklist (CFC); group administered; yesterday; nonquantitative	Yes/No	Compared a morning and afternoon test–retest reliability of CFCs completed by child. The second administration of the CFC occurred at least 2 h after the first administration	Pearson's correlations between scores from the two CFCs were 0.89 for total fat, 0.85 for saturated fat and 0.86 for sodium. Kappa statistics for individual items between the 2 CFC food items ranged from 0.66 for pork to 0.94 for pickles/olives and for pretzels (median = 0.85)
Cullen et al.[55]	89 m&f 41% m 59% f 54% AA 46% Hispanic	7–8th grade	152-items Youth/Adolescent Questionnaire (YAQ); group-administered; past year; semiquantitative; child portions	Dependent on type of food	Compared a 3-week test–retest reliability of YAQs completed by child	Spearman's correlations between the two YAQ were 0.72 for energy and 0.19 for total fat (% kcal). Correlations for the five fruit and vegetable groupings ranged from 0.37 for fruit juice to 0.67 for total fruit, juice and vegetables. Mean daily consumption values were higher in the first YAQ than the second YAQ for all items assessed except total fat (% kcal). Correlations between the two YAQ among Hispanics were 0.61 for energy and 0.11 for total fat (% kcal) and for the five fruit and vegetable groupings ranged from 0.30 for high-fat vegetables to 0.68 for total fruit, juice and vegetables. Among AA children correlations between the two YAQ were 0.80 for energy and 0.31 for total fat (% kcal) and for the five fruit and vegetable groupings ranged from 0.44 for juice to 0.66 for total fruit, juice and vegetables. The reliability coefficients were generally lower for the Hispanic children compared with the AA children
Hoelscher et al.[58]	254 m&f 48% m 52% f 74% White 6% AA 16% Hispanic 5% Other/missing	8th grade	63-items (19 food items tested for reproducibility) School-Based Nutrition Monitoring Questionnaire (SBNM); group-administered; yesterday; nonquantitative	4 (0 times/day to 3+ times/day)	Compared a morning and afternoon test–retest reproducibility of SBNM completed by child. Second administration of SBNM occurred after lunch and at least 2 h after first administration from Tuesdays through Fridays	Spearman's correlations between the two SBNM for the 19 food groupings ranged from 0.66 for French fries or chips to 0.97 for gravy. Kappa statistics ranged from 0.54 for French fries or chips to 0.93 (adjusted) for gravy. Percentage agreement ranged from 70% for any type of bread, bun, bagel, tortilla, or roll and 70% for French fries or chips to 98% for gravy. No significant gender differences were detected

Continued

**TABLE 29.6
(Continued)**

References[a]	Sample	Age/Grade	Instrument	Response Categories (Range)	Design	Results
Hoelscher et al.[58]	259 m&f 49% m 51% f 75% White 6% AA 14% Hispanic 5% Other/missing	8th grade	63-items (11 food habit items tested for reproducibility) School-Based Nutrition Monitoring Questionnaire (SBNM); group-administered; usual intake; nonquantitative	4 (0 times/day to 3+ times/day)	Compared a 9- to 14-day test–retest reproducibility of SBNM completed by child. The SBNM was administered Tuesdays through Fridays, and was not administered after a holiday	Spearman's correlations between the 2 SBNM for 11 food and meal choice behaviors ranged from 0.43 for eating dinner to 0.87 for type of milk (fat content). Kappa statistics ranged from 0.41 for eating dinner to 0.79 for type of milk (fat content). Percentage agreement ranged from 62% for type of sweet roll, doughnuts, cookies, brownies, pies cakes (fat content) to 96% for vegetarian status. No significant gender differences were detected
Rockett et al.[67]	75 m 101 f 3 N/A[d] multi-ethnic	9–18 years	151-items Youth/Adolescent Questionnaire (YAQ); self-administered; past year; semiquantitative; adult portions	9 (none or <1/month to ≥6/day)	Compared 1-year test-retest reproducibility of nutrient estimates from YAQs completed by the child	Pearson's correlations (log-transformed, energy-adjusted) between the two YAQs were 0.49 for energy, 0.26 for protein, and 0.41 for total fat. Range of correlations for 7 nutrients assessed was 0.26 for protein and iron to 0.58 for calcium. Mean energy intake was 10% higher in the first YAQ compared with the second (2477 vs. 2222 kcal/day). Mean intake of six nutrients assessed was significantly higher in the first YAQ compared with the second. Range of correlations for eight food groups assessed was 0.39 for meats to 0.57 for soda. Pearson's correlations (log-transformed) for fruits servings/day were 0.49 for fruits, 0.48 for vegetables, and 0.48 for fruits and vegetables. Of the eight food groups, mean serving frequencies of 5 were significantly higher in the first YAQ compared with the second. Reproducibility of nutrient intake was significantly higher for females than males (mean correlation for all nutrients was 0.44 and 0.34, respectively). There were no significant differences by age or ethnicity
Vereecken et al.[49]	207 m&f 43% m 57% f	11–12 years	15-items (fiber, calcium foods, and foods relevant to youth food culture) Health Behavior in School-Aged Children (HBSC) FFQ; group-administered; yesterday; nonquantitative	7 (never to more than once a day)	Compared a 7- to15-day test-retest reliability of HBSC completed by child	Spearman's correlations between the 2 HBSCs for the 15 foods ranged from 0.52 for chips to 0.82 for semiskimmed milk. Mean weighted kappa value between the 2 HBSCs was 0.58. The range of kappa values for the 15 foods was 0.44 for other milk products to 0.70 for semiskimmed milk. Percentage perfect agreement between the 2 HBSCs ranged from 39% for other milk products to 87% for alcoholic beverage with an overall mean perfect agreement of 55%
Prochaska et al.[56]	40 m 26 f 57 m 104 f 41% White 26% AA 16% Asian 4% Hispanic	7–8th 7–8th 9–12th 9–12th grades	21-items (21 high-fat foods) PACE+; self-administered; past 7 days; nonquantitative	6 (did not eat it this week to more than twice each day)	Compared a 1- to 2-week test-retest reproducibility of high-fat food intake from FFQs completed by the child	Intraclass correlation of the fat intake measures between the 2 FFQs was 0.64 for the full sample of males and females grade 7–12, 0.62 for males grade 7–8, 0.55 for males grade 9–12, and 0.68 for females grade 9–12. Internal consistency, as calculated by coefficient α, was 0.88 at time 1 and 0.87 at time 2

Source	Sample	Grade/age	Instrument	Response categories	Comparison	Results
Prochaska et al. [56]	40 m 26 f 57 m 104 f 41% White 26% AA 16% Asian 4% Hispanic	7–8th 7–8th 9–12th 9–12th grades	4-categories (4 high-fat food groups); self-administered; past 7 days; nonquantitative	6 (did not eat it this week to more than twice each day)	Compared a 1- to 2-week test–retest reproducibility of high-fat food intake from FFQs completed by the child	Intraclass correlations of the fat intake measures between the 2 FFQs were 0.65 for the full sample of males and females grade 7–12, 0.50 for males grade 7–8, 0.71 for males grade 9–12, and 0.65 for females grade 9–12. Internal consistency, as calculated by coefficient α, was 0.74 at Time 1 and 0.76 at Time 2
Frank et al. [68]	189 m&f AA & White	12–17 years	64-items; group administered; past week; semi quantitative; adult portions	6 (none to >3 times/day)	Compared 2-week test–retest reproducibility of food intake from FFQs completed by the child	Two-thirds of the children reported similar responses for the frequency of consumption of low-fat milk, diet carbonated soft drinks and shellfish. Twelve food groups had percent agreement of 50% or better (significance testing not shown)
Vereecken et al. [49]	560 m&f 60% m 40% f	13–14 years	15-items (fiber, calcium foods, and foods relevant to youth food culture) Health Behavior in School-Aged Children (HBSC) FFQ; group-administered; yesterday; nonquantified	7 (Never to more than once a day)	Compared a 6- to 10-day test–retest reliability of traditional paper FFQ and a computerized version of FFQ completed by child	Spearman's correlations between the 2 FFQs for the 15 foods ranged from 0.57 for chips and for other milk products to 0.78 for brown bread. Mean weighted kappa value between the 2 FFQ was 0.55. The range of kappa values for the 15 foods was 0.43 for other milk products to 0.66 for white bread and for brown bread. Percentage perfect agreement between the 2 FFQs ranged from 37% for other milk products to 68% for chips with an overall mean perfect agreement of 52%
Turconi et al. [69]	68 m&f	14–17 years	106-items (28 food frequency and 14 food habit/portion questions); self-administered; usual day or weekly intake; semiquantitative	Dependent on question	Compared a 1-week test–retest reliability of FFQs completed by the child	Pearson's correlations for 28 items in the food frequency section ranged from 0.45 for pasta/rice/bread/potatoes and sweets to 0.90 for milk/milk and coffee/cappuccino/yogurt and beer. Pearson's correlation for food habit scores between FFQs was 0.88, with a Cronbach's of 0.75
Andersen et al. [62]	53 m 50 f	11th grade Adults required	190-items; group administered; past year; semiquantitative	Dependent on type of food	Compared 6-week test–retest reproducibility of nutrient estimates from FFQs completed by the child and parent	Spearman's correlations (energy-adjusted) between the 2 FFQs were 0.87 for energy, 0.86 for protein, and 0.86 for total fat. Range of correlations for 18 nutrients assessed was 0.72 for vitamin C to 0.91 for alcohol. Median energy intake was 11% higher in the first FFQ compared with the second (12.3 vs. 10.9 mJ/day). Median intake of 15 nutrients was significantly higher in the first FFQ compared with the second FFQ. Differences in median correlations for nutrient intake were not significant between females and males (0.78 vs. 0.74, respectively)

a Results of all subgroups not reported due to samples below the $N = 30$ criterion.

b Males (m), females (f).

c Adult assistance required for instrument administration.

d N/A — Not applicable.

e FFQ — Food frequency questionnaire.

f AA — African-American.

g TEE — Total energy expenditure.

h MPR — Multiple-pass recall.

used to classify children into groups of low and high intakes of nutrients and foods. The number of FFQ reliability studies published since 2000 has tripled. Results from these studies indicate that the FFQ has an acceptable reproducibility for select nutrients and foods. The studies indicated that girls and older youth had more reliable FFQ reports than younger youth. Shorter intervals between administrations of the FFQ typically resulted in higher agreement between foods or nutrients. The intervals between administrations of FFQs ranged from a few hours up to 1 year.

DIET HISTORY

Diet histories assess the past diet of an individual in the form of usual meal patterns, food intake, and food preparation practices through an extensive interview or questionnaire (Table 29.7).[7] The diet history provides a measure of usual intake that is appropriate for ranking individuals and predicting health outcomes. In contrast to other methods of dietary assessment, a diet history is usually more qualitative than quantitative, allowing detailed information about food preparation, eating habits, and food consumption to be collected by a highly trained interviewer. This method requires children or parents to recall dietary intake from the past, understand spatial relationships, be able to apply math skills, and have the stamina to complete the typically 1 to 2 h long interview. Because of the respondent burden, diet histories are not often used to assess children's diets. One diet history validity study and one reliability study has been reported.

OBSERVATION

Observation is useful for assessing children who are preliterate (third grade or younger), either in a lunchroom setting with school meals or in controlled school or group activities (Table 29.7). Intensively trained observers unobtrusively watch the children, sometimes many at a time, to ascertain foods, brand names, and portion sizes consumed. A single observation provides a measure of actual intake that is appropriate for estimating group means and cannot be used to predict health outcomes. Multiple observations can provide a measure of usual intake. The recordings are interpreted after the collection process and coded to a nutrient database to calculate nutrient intake for each child. Adult observations of children were used in 63% of the recall validity studies in the last three and half decades, and yet there have been no validity studies reported for this technique. Only one reliability study of adult observations of children eating has been published.

CHALLENGES

In the 5 years since our previous review there has been a doubling in the number of studies on this topic. This heightened attention to dietary assessment methods resulted in the appearance of several recall reliability studies and one diet history validity study. Also, the number of recall validity studies doubled and the number of FFQ reliability studies tripled. There was also an increase in new styles of food-frequency-type questionnaires called checklists and screeners.

This review allows comparison of dietary methods to determine the most effective dietary data collection instruments to use with particular study designs and research questions.[70,71] The reader may, for example, scan each table for instruments with higher or lower nutrient correlations with a particular validity standard — instruments that children can complete without adult assistance, those with no portion size estimation, or instruments specific to assessing intake of food groups, all by age or grade. Applications of the dietary assessment methods are summarized in Table 29.8, which provides advantages and disadvantages for using the dietary assessment methods, applicable study designs, and brief highlights of their validity.

It is evident that many of the validation standards used in the reviewed articles are imperfect, especially for children. In this review, food records or recalls were the most common choices for validation standards, and information on the validity of these methods for children noted in the review are mixed. Observations were the most common validity standard for recall validity studies, and there are no studies regarding the validity of this measure for assessing children's intake. Thus, the validation standards used may have inconsistent validity, or use a referent period that differs from that used for the instrument. Heterogeneity of the studies also makes it difficult to draw conclusions; the differences in study administrations and study populations often make comparisons uncertain both within a type of assessment method and between methods.

In evaluating validation studies, the effect of correlated errors between the method being evaluated and the validation standard should be considered. All dietary assessment methods have inherent errors; for validation studies, it is important that these errors be as independent as possible.[72] For example, if errors between the methods are similar (e.g., both methods such as FFQ and recalls rely on dietary information from a respondent), correlations between the two methods will be artificially inflated. In contrast, errors inherent in physiologic measures (e.g., doubly labeled water measurements or serum micronutrients) or observational data do not rely on information provided by respondents, and would be a more independent comparison to a respondent-based measure.[73] Comparisons of physiologic end points, such as blood nutrient levels, with dietary assessment methods have not been widely used with school-age children and offer other problems as food intake may not be directly correlated with physiologic end points.

Selecting a validation standard can be a difficult task because often there is no dietary assessment tool available with the same referent period as the assessment tool. Thus, a compromise may need to be made in the study design. For example, a FFQ

TABLE 29.7
Diet History and Observation Validity and Reliability Studies among School-Age Children

Validity	Sample	Age/Grade	Instrument	Response Categories (Range)	Validation Standard	Design	Results
Reference[a]							
Sjöberg et al.[74]	51 f	15–16 years	Diet history; habitual intake; interviewer assisted group administration and interview; quantitative	Fixed categories of frequency and amount of foods	7-day diet record	Compared child's report of diet history of foods, nutrients and meals against child's 7-day food record	Spearman's correlations between diet history and records were 0.63 for energy, 0.67 for protein, and 0.63 for total fat. Range of correlations for 11 nutrients assessed were 0.25 for alcohol to 0.71 for fiber. Mean daily energy intake was 8% higher in the diet history as compared with the 7-day records (8.1 MJ vs. 7.5 MJ). Spearman's correlations for 20 food groups ranged from 0.30 for buns, pastry, and biscuits and ice cream to 0.71 for sweets
Reliability Reference[a]				**Design**			
Rasanen[75]	47 m&f[b] 50 m&f 37 m&f Adults required[c]	5 years 9 years 13 years	Diet history; past year; interviewer-administered; quantitative			Compared 7-month test–retest reproducibility of nutrient intake from diet histories completed by child and parent	Pearson's correlations between the first and second interviews were 0.59 for energy, 0.60 for protein, and 0.57 for total fat. Range of correlations for 11 nutrients assessed was 0.41 for ascorbic acid to 0.60 for protein. Mean daily energy intake was 27% higher in the first diet history interview as compared with the second interview (3256 vs. 2573 kcal/day)
Simons-Morton et al.[76]	45 m&f Adults required	3–5th grade	Observation; lunch only; quantitative			Compared two simultaneously collected adult observers' estimates of nutrient intake and food items from observations of lunch	Intraclass correlations between paired observers ranged from 0.81–0.90 for energy and from 0.74–0.88 for fat. Of the 6 nutrients assessed, intraclass correlations were lowest for total fat (0.74–0.88) and highest for vitamin A (0.96–0.98). Interobserver percent differences in mean energy intake ranged from 0.1–6.8%. Overall agreement on food items between observers was 84%; percent agreement was highest for chips and condiments, and lowest for desserts. Differences in portion size estimates accounted for most of the energy and nutrient differences between observers

[a] Results of subgroups not reported due to samples below the $N = 30$ criterion.
[b] Males (m), Females (f).
[c] Adult assistance required for instrument administration.
[d] N/A — Not applicable.
[e] FFQ — Food frequency questionnaire.
[f] AA — African-American.
[g] TEE — Total energy expenditure.
[h] MPR — Multiple-pass recall.

TABLE 29.8
Summary of Dietary Assessment Methods for School-Age Children

Method and Number of Studies Reviewed	Ages Evaluated	Energy Validity[a]	Protein Validity[a]	Total fat Validity[a]	Energy Intake Compared with Standard[b]	Study Design Applications	Advantages	Disadvantages
Food recall Validity — 27 Reliability — 4	4–14 years adult assistance needed for <8 years	0.27–0.87	0.42–0.91	0.25–0.85	–34%–18%	Cross-Sectional Intervention Monitoring Clinical Epidemiologic	Short administration time Defined recall time Intake can be quantified Procedure does not alter habitual dietary patterns Low respondent burden Can be telephone-administered Procedure can be automated	Recall depends on memory Portion size difficult to estimate Trained interviewer required Expensive to collect and code
Food record Validity — 9 Reliability — 0	6–19 years adult assistance needed for <8 years	0.52–0.71	0.56–0.82	0.58–0.82	–28%–31%	Cross-Sectional Intervention Monitoring Clinical Epidemiologic	Record not rely on memory Defined record time Intake can be quantified Training can be group-administered Procedure can be automated	Recorder must be literate High respondent burden Food eaten away from home less accurately recalled Procedure alters habitual dietary patterns Validity may decrease as recording days increase Expensive to collect and code
Food frequency Validity — 37 Reliability — 22	2–19 years adult assistance needed for <8 years	0.13–0.56	0.18–0.48	0.12–0.61	1%–87%	Cross-Sectional Intervention Monitoring Epidemiologic	Trained interviewers not needed Interviewer or self-administered Relatively inexpensive to collect Procedure does not alter habitual dietary habits Low respondent burden Total diet or selected foods or nutrients can be assessed Can be used to rank according to nutrient intake Procedure can be automated	Recall depends on memory Period of recall imprecise Quantification of intake imprecise because of poor recall or use of standard portion sizes Specific food descriptions not obtained
Diet history Validity — 1 Reliability — 1	5–16 years adult assistance needed for all ages	n/a				Monitoring Clinical Epidemiologic	Literacy not required Procedure does not alter habitual dietary habits Can obtain highly detailed descriptions of foods and preparation methods	Recall depends on memory Highly trained interviewers required Period of recall imprecise Very high respondent burden Requires long interview time Quantification of intake imprecise because of poor recall or use of standard portion sizes Expensive to administer
Observation Validity — 0 Reliability — 1	8–10 years					Intervention Monitoring Epidemiologic	Literacy not required Procedure does not alter habitual dietary habits Procedure does not rely on memory Defined observation time Intake can be quantified Multiple days give measure of individual or group intake	Highly trained observers required Requires long observation period Expensive to administer

[a] Pearson's and Spearman's correlations of nutrients both unadjusted and adjusted for percentage of kilocalories.

[b] Calculation of percentage = ([instrument–validation standard]/validation standard).

measures usual food consumption over a period of 6 months to a year, whereas a food record generally is used to measure food consumption on a day-to-day basis. In order to validate a FFQ, it would be necessary to complete several sets of food records over the referent period for the FFQ. Clearly, validation studies that use a week of continuous consecutive food records may not capture seasonal variation in diet. Similarly, a food recall, which is generally used to measure one complete day of consumption, should be validated by a method that assesses an entire day and not just a portion of the day.

The problem of referent periods also influences the experimental design for reliability studies. Because there is much day-to-day variation in diet, readministration should be close enough in time to reflect the same referent period. As some methods reflect diet over a short span of time (e.g., 1 day records and 24 h recalls), theoretically the reliability testing should be completed on the same day as the assessment tool, which may allow memory effects from the first assessment to bias the readministration. Studies that examine reliability should alternate administrations in order to eliminate bias as much as possible. Because FFQs usually include a longer referent period, it is easier to develop reproducibility studies for this method.

The studies reviewed adapted adult dietary assessment methods for administration to a pediatric population. Specific adaptations included incorporating parental or adult assistance, adjusting portion size information, using shorter referent times, using food pictures, using computer programs designed for children, and administering the instrument in the school setting. Children younger than 8 to 9 years of age need adult assistance to provide accurate dietary information for all the methods because they usually have limited reading skills and adults control most of the food offered, including the timing and frequency of eating occasions.[77,78] This review found that almost all of the validity and reliability studies among children less then 8 to 9 years of age, with the exception of a few of the recall and FFQ studies, included adult participation. This participation varied from completion of the entire form to obtaining only supplemental information from parents or surrogates, such as child-care providers, or secondary sources such as school food service observations.

Children generally have difficulty estimating portion sizes.[36,79,80] A recent review of portion size aids was unable to make guidelines for portion size estimation for children or even adults.[81] Both two- and three-dimensional models have been used to enhance children's portion size estimation.[8,10,11,19,27,29,63,75,76,82–84] Pictures of food and portions have been incorporated in assessments to enhance children's understanding; however, the addition of pictures did not increase accuracy among third graders.[85] Among the newer tools for dietary assessment are reference books with life-size photographs of portion sizes, which have been credited as being both easy and accurate.[86–89] Training to improve portion size estimation among children has been attempted with significant improvements in estimation; however, even with training some errors were reported to be as high as 100%.[90] Until portion size issues are adequately addressed children's intakes will continue to be biased.

RECOMMENDATIONS

Many of the same challenges noted in the earlier review still exist and have not been overcome. Despite the extensive dietary intake data available to nutritionists, epidemiologists, and pediatricians, this review identifies methodological concerns associated with the assessment tools currently used to determine dietary intake of school-age children. Generally, comparisons across studies were limited by differences in instruments, research design, validation standards, and populations. The paucity of data in many areas also made it difficult to draw generalized conclusions.

Although it is not possible to make solid recommendations regarding the use of each dietary assessment technique with children, it is possible now with the data available from the last 35 years of work to provide recommendations regarding some assessment methods. Overall results indicate that food records tend to underestimate children's energy intake less and overestimate intake more than recalls. FFQs consistently overestimate usual energy and macronutrient intake at a higher percentage than other methods. FFQs are best used for ranking children's intake. Younger children underestimate intakes more frequently than older children, and as age increases overestimation increases.

The most extensive body of validation work has occurred with food recalls and FFQs, with a limited number of validation studies and even fewer reliability studies of the other methods among school-age children. In the future, evaluations of dietary assessment techniques for children need to be conducted that give particular attention to experimental design, careful use of validation standards, and inclusion of different age, gender, ethnic, and body-size subgroups. As with adults, there is no perfect method of assessing dietary intake in children. Special consideration must be given to the age and cognitive ability of the child as well as methodological issues associated with nutrient analyses, food coding, and portion sizes. Both age and cognitive ability relate to the child's understanding of the method used and the thought processes that contribute to self-reporting of food choices.

Selection of the measure of truth for validation studies will be challenging, as there is not always a good choice when the referent periods differ so markedly between instruments and the potential effect of correlated errors is considered. Physiologically based measures, such as doubly labeled water, chemical analyses of food, or serum micronutrient concentrations, represent a type of standard with considerable appeal and merit further study, as these measures are not affected by respondent error. In addition, studies that compare multiple validation standards for a particular assessment method would allow comparisons of the validation standards best suited for particular situations. Future studies need to address the timing of the referent period that best suits the assessment instrument in the design phase.

New approaches and modifications to existing dietary assessment approaches for use among school-age children are being explored and need refinement. Computer-prompted recalls, lists to prompt recalls, and short FFQ checklists and screeners are examples of such techniques. The dietary habits of children, especially young children who are preliterate, are inherently difficult to study. Unfortunately, assessment techniques that work reasonably well among adult men and women may not be useful for youth, especially those less than 8 to 9 years of age, who may need assistance from a proxy or special prompting techniques to estimate portion size. Because parents/adults are often the respondents for young children, the methods used to interview them may resemble those used best with adults, whereas methods for the child need to be age-appropriate. Creative portion-size tools must be developed to estimate children's portion sizes to enhance the quality of nutrient estimates. Systematic evaluations of children's ability to estimate portion size utilizing various approaches by age, gender, ethnicity, and body size are needed.

This review found little research on the effects of age, gender, or ethnicity. Given the multiplicity of minority groups in the United States, and the rising obesity epidemic among children, it is essential to determine the accuracy of these dietary assessment tools within major subgroups. Other areas, such as the effect of body size on reporting of dietary intake, need further study. For example, a recent study suggested that children with central fat distribution had higher rates of underreporting of energy intake than lean or obese children, or those with peripheral fat distribution.[29] Another study reported that energy intake was significantly lower in obese children than nonobese children when compared with doubly labeled water as a percentage of energy expenditure.[91] Underreporting of dietary intake by obese adolescents is consistent with recent findings that obese adults underreport their dietary intake.[91] With the increasing prevalence of obesity among children and adolescents, it is essential to determine whether body size differences significantly affect accuracy of dietary assessment instruments.[92]

In summary, we have made progress in understanding the accuracy of dietary assessment methods for youth; however, the work is not complete. This 35-year review serves as a guide to the status of dietary assessment methods for school-age children. Recalls and records generally agreed more with the validation standards than did FFQs. Administration protocols differed greatly, the recalls and records often represented only meals or portions of the day, and the FFQ food lists varied from a few items to the total diet. Some researchers compared very specific foods and food groups for the validation study using analytic approaches that widely differed, hindering the ability to compare the instrument's validity in this review. The key to advancing the field is to build on our current base of methods, refine those techniques that are useful, and develop new approaches to overcome obstacles that have been identified in study designs and data collection and analysis procedures. We must be able to accurately assess the dietary intake of school-age children so that we can monitor dietary intake trends, make accurate research and policy decisions, and develop and effectively evaluate nutrition interventions.

ACKNOWLEDGMENTS

The authors would like to thank Stephanie Carter for assisting with manuscript preparation.

REFERENCES

1. McPherson, RS, Hoelscher, DM, Alexander, M et al., *Prev Med* 31: S11; 2000.
2. McPherson, RS, Hoelscher, DM, Alexander, M, Scanlon, KS, Serdula, MK, *Handbook of Nutrition and Food*, Berdanier, CD, Ed., CRC Press, Boca Raton, 2002, Chapter 22.
3. Nelson, M, Black, AE, Morris, JA et al., *Am J Clin Nutr* 50: 155; 1989.
4. Vereecken, CA, Covents, M, Matthys, C et al., *Eur J Clin Nutr* 59: 658; 2005.
5. Baranowski, T, Islam, N, Baranowski, J et al., *J Am Diet Assoc* 102: 380; 2002.
6. Johnson, B, Hackett, A, Roundfield, M et al., *J Hum Nutr Diet* 14: 457; 2001.
7. Thompson, FE, Byers, T, *J Nutr* 124: 2245S; 1994.
8. Lytle, LA, Nichaman, MZ, Obarzanek, E et al., *J Am Diet Assoc* 93: 1431; 1993.
9. Weber, JL, Lytle, L, Gittelsohn, J et al., *J Am Diet Assoc* 104: 746; 2004.
10. Basch, CE, Shea, S, Arliss, R et al., *Am J Public Health* 80: 1314; 1990.
11. Eck, LH, Hanson, CL, Klesges, RC, *J Am Diet Assoc* 89: 784; 1989.
12. Montgomery, C, Reilly, JJ, Jackson, DM et al., *Am J Clin Nutr* 80: 591; 2004.
13. Fisher, JO, Johnson, RK, Lindquist, C et al., *Obes Res* 8: 597; 2000.
14. Warren, JM, Henry, CJ, Livingstone, MB et al., *Public Health Nutr* 6: 41; 2003.
15. Baxter, SD, Thompson, WO, Davis, HC, *J Am Diet Assoc* 100: 911; 2000.
16. Lindquist, CH, Cummings, T, Goran, MI, *Obes Res* 8: 2; 2000.
17. Reynolds, LA, Johnson, SB, Silverstein, J, *J Pediatr Psychol* 15: 493; 1990.
18. Edmunds, LD, Ziebland, S, *Health Educ Res* 17: 211; 2002.
19. Van Horn, LV, Gernhofer, N, Moag-Stahlberg, A et al., *J Am Diet Assoc* 90: 412; 1990.
20. Todd, KS, Kretsch, MJ, *Nutr Res* 6: 1031; 1986.
21. Samuelson, G, *Nutr Metab* 12: 321; 1970.

22. Lytle, LA, Murray, DM, Perry, CL et al., *J Am Diet Assoc* 98: 570; 1998.
23. Baxter, SD, Thompson, WO, Davis, HC et al., *J Am Diet Assoc* 97: 1293; 1997.
24. Baxter, SD, Thompson, WO, Litaker, MS et al., *J Am Diet Assoc* 102: 386; 2002.
25. Baxter, SD, *J Nutr Educ Behav* 35: 124; 2003.
26. Andersen, LF, Bere, E, Kolbjornsen, N et al., *Eur J Clin Nutr* 58: 771; 2004.
27. Mullenbach, V, Kushi, LH, Jacobson, C et al., *J Am Diet Assoc* 92: 743; 1992.
28. O'Connor, J, Ball, EJ, Steinbeck, KS et al., *Am J Clin Nutr* 74: 643; 2001.
29. Knuiman, JT, Rasanen, L, Ahola, M et al., *J Am Diet Assoc* 87: 303; 1987.
30. Bandini, LG, Cyr, H, Must, A et al., *Am J Clin Nutr* 65: 1138S; 1997.
31. Champagne, CM, Baker, NB, DeLany, JP et al., *J Am Diet Assoc* 98: 426; 1998.
32. Livingstone, MB, Prentice, AM, Coward, WA et al., *Am J Clin Nutr* 56: 29; 1992.
33. Green, TJ, Allen, OB, O'Connor, DL, *J Nutr* 128: 1665; 1998.
34. Blom, L, Lundmark, K, Dahlquist, G et al., *Acta Paediatr Scand* 78: 858; 1989.
35. Taylor, RW, Goulding, A, *Eur J Clin Nutr* 52: 464; 1998.
36. Kaskoun, MC, Johnson, RK, Goran, MI, *Am J Clin Nutr* 60: 43; 1994.
37. Persson, LA, Carlgren, G, *Int J Epidemiol* 13: 506; 1984.
38. Wilson, AM, Lewis, RD, *J Am Diet Assoc* 104: 373; 2004.
39. Hammond, J, Nelson, M, Chinn, S et al., *Eur J Clin Nutr* 47: 242; 1993.
40. Byers, T, Trieber, F, Gunter, E et al., *Epidemiology* 4: 350; 1993.
41. Arnold, JE, Rohan, T, Howe, G et al., *Ann Epidemiol* 5: 369; 1995.
42. Baranowski, T, Smith, M, Baranowski, J et al., *J Am Diet Assoc* 97: 66; 1997.
43. Bellu, R, Riva, E, Ortisi, MT et al., *Nutr Res* 16: 197; 1996.
44. Perks, SM, Roemmich, JN, Sandow-Pajewski, M et al., *Am J Clin Nutr* 72: 1455; 2000.
45. Bellu, R, Ortisi, MT, Riva, E et al., *Nutr Res* 15: 1121; 1995.
46. Rockett, HR, Breitenbach, M, Frazier, AL et al., *Prev Med* 26: 808; 1997.
47. Domel, SB, Baranowski, T, Davis, H et al., *J Am Coll Nutr* 13: 33; 1994.
48. Field, AE, Peterson, KE, Gortmaker, SL et al., *Public Health Nutr* 2: 293; 1999.
49. Vereecken, CA, Maes, L, *Public Health Nutr* 6: 581; 2003.
50. Koehler, KM, Cunningham-Sabo, L, Lambert, LC et al., *J Am Diet Assoc* 100: 205; 2000.
51. Jenner, DA, Neylon, K, Croft, S et al., *Eur J Clin Nutr* 43: 663; 1989.
52. Lietz, G, Barton, KL, Longbottom, PJ et al., *Public Health Nutr* 5: 783; 2002.
53. Yaroch, AL, Resnicow, K, Petty, AD et al., *J Am Diet Assoc* 100: 1525; 2000.
54. Smith, KW, Hoelscher, DM, Lytle, LA et al., *J Am Diet Assoc* 101: 635; 2001.
55. Cullen, KW, Zakeri, I, *J Am Diet Assoc* 104: 1415; 2004.
56. Prochaska, JJ, Sallis, JF, Rupp, J, *Prev Med* 33: 699; 2001.
57. van Assema, P, Brug, J, Ronda, G et al., *J Hum Nutr Diet* 14: 377; 2001.
58. Hoelscher, DM, Day, RS, Kelder, SH et al., *J Am Diet Assoc* 103: 186; 2003.
59. Johnson, F, Wardle, J, Griffith, J, *Eur J Clin Nutr* 56: 644; 2002.
60. Kinlay, S, Heller, RF, Halliday, JA, *Prev Med* 20: 378; 1991.
61. Field, AE, Colditz, GA, Fox, MK et al., *Am J Public Health* 88: 1216; 1998.
62. Andersen, LF, Nes, M, Lillegaard, IT et al., *Eur J Clin Nutr* 49: 543; 1995.
63. Basch, CE, Shea, S, Zybert, P, *Am J Public Health* 84: 861; 1994.
64. Metcalf, PA, Scragg, RK, Sharpe, S et al., *Eur J Clin Nutr* 57: 1498; 2003.
65. Buzzard, IM, Stanton, CA, Figueiredo, M et al., *J Am Diet Assoc* 101: 1438; 2001.
66. Speck, BJ, Bradley, CB, Harrell, JS et al., *J Adolesc Health* 28: 16; 2001.
67. Rockett, HR, Wolf, AM, Colditz, GA, *J Am Diet Assoc* 95: 336; 1995.
68. Frank, GC, Nicklas, TA, Webber, LS et al., *J Am Diet Assoc* 92: 313; 1992.
69. Turconi, G, Celsa, M, Rezzani, C et al., *Eur J Clin Nutr* 57: 753; 2003.
70. Cullen, KW, Baranowski, T, Baranowski, J et al., *J Am Diet Assoc* 99: 849; 1999.
71. Eldridge, AL, Smith-Warner, SA, Lytle, LA et al., *J Am Diet Assoc* 98: 777; 1998.
72. Willett, W., *Nutritional Epidemiology*, 2nd ed., Oxford University Press, New York, 1998.
73. Bingham, SA, *Am J Clin Nutr* 59: 227S; 1994.
74. Sjöberg, A, Hulthen, L, *Eur J Clin Nutr* 58: 1181; 2004.
75. Rasanen, L, *Am J Clin Nutr* 32: 2560; 1979.
76. Simons-Morton, BG, Forthofer, R, Huang, IW et al., *J Am Diet Assoc* 92: 219; 1992.
77. Frank, GC, *Am J Clin Nutr* 59: 207S; 1994.
78. Baranowski, T., *Handbook of Health Behavior Research I: Personal and Social Determinants*, Gochman, D S, Ed., Plenum Press, New York, 1997, Chapter 9.
79. Buzzard, IM, Sievert, YA, *Am J Clin Nutr* 59: 275S; 1994.
80. Contento, I, Balch, GI, Bronner, Y et al., *J Nutr Educ* 27: 284; 1995.
81. Cypel, YS, Guenther, PM, Petot, GJ, *J Am Diet Assoc* 97: 289; 1997.

82. Crawford, PB, Obarzanek, E, Morrison, J et al., *J Am Diet Assoc* 94: 626; 1994.
83. Frank, GC, Berenson, GS, Schilling, PE et al., *J Am Diet Assoc* 71: 26; 1977.
84. McPherson, RS, Nichaman, MZ, Kohl, HW et al., *Pediatrics* 86: 520; 1990.
85. Baranowski, T, Dworkin, R, Henske, JC et al., *J Am Diet Assoc* 86: 1381; 1986.
86. Nelson, M, Atkinson, M, Darbyshire, S, *Br J Nutr* 72: 649; 1994.
87. Nelson, M, Atkinson, M, Darbyshire, S, *Br J Nutr* 76: 31; 1996.
88. Faggiano, F, Vineis, P, Cravanzola, D et al., *Epidemiology* 3: 379; 1992.
89. Hess, M. A. Portion Photos of Popular Foods. 1997.
90. Weber, JL, Cunningham-Sabo, L, Skipper, B et al., *Am J Clin Nutr* 69: 782S; 1999.
91. Bandini, LG, Schoeller, DA, Cyr, HN et al., *Am J Clin Nutr* 52: 421; 1990.
92. Goran, MI, *Pediatrics* 101: 505; 1998.

30 Anthropometric Assessment: Historical Perspectives

George A. Bray

CONTENTS

QUETELET

Lambert-Adolf-Jacques Quetelet is credited with the concept of the body mass index (BMI). The proposal was made in a monograph in 1835 on the development of the human body. As Frudenthal says, "With Quetelet's work in 1835 a new era in statistics began … . The work gave a description of the average man as both a static and dynamic phenomenon." [1] It was Quetelet who introduced the concept of quantitative measurement of the human being and thus provided a framework for epidemiology and statistics. Quetelet, with his mathematical background, took statistical methods into new arenas. He was a pioneer in the application of statistics to human biology, anthropology, and criminology.

Quetelet was interested in the underlying factors that were responsible for the distribution of such events as births, marriages, deaths, and the prevalence of various types of crime. In his work, he noted the seasonal distribution of births, deaths, and marriages. He also noted a seasonal distribution of crime, and that crimes against property appeared more frequently in cold months, while crimes against the person were more common in the summer. In commenting on the constancy of crimes from year to year, he said, "Thus we pass from one year to another with the sad perspective of seeing the same crimes reproduced in the same order and calling down the same punishments in the same proportions. Sad condition of humanity … ." [2] Fortunately, the human being has been able to change this apparent constancy by education, laws, and better government. Much of the work in his 1835 book *On the Development of Man and His Faculties* (commonly referred to as *Sur l'homme*) was translated in 1842. In his publications, Quetelet spent a significant amount of space dealing with height and weight. The concept of the "average man" originated with Quetelet and is one of his seminal contributions. To quote from Chapter 2 of the English translation of his work, Quetelet says:

> If man increased equally in all his dimensions, his weight at different ages would be as the cube of his height. Now, this is not what we really observe. The increase in weight is slower, except during the first year after birth; then the proportion which we have just pointed out is pretty regularly observed. But after this period, and until near the age of puberty, the weight increases nearly as the square of the height. The development of the weight again becomes very rapid at the time of puberty, and almost stops at the 25th year. In general, we do not err much when we assume that, *during development, the square of weight at different ages are as the fifth powers of the height*; which naturally leads to this conclusion, in supposing the specific gravity constant, that the transverse growth of man is less than the vertical.
>
> However, if we compare two individuals who are fully developed and well-formed with each other, to ascertain the relations existing between the weight and stature, we shall find that *the weight of developed persons, of different heights, is nearly as the square of the stature*. Whence it naturally follows, that a *transverse section, giving both the breadth and thickness, is just proportioned to the height of the individual*. We furthermore conclude that, proportion still being attended, width predominates in individuals of small stature.

These two paragraphs succinctly summarize the concept of the BMI according to Quetelet and the rationale on which he developed his concept. [2]

LIFE INSURANCE TABLES

Nearly 80 years after Quetelet, the life insurance industry in the United States began to weigh in on the importance of excess weight as a risk for early death. They also noted that a central distribution of weight was important. The 1922 *Statistical Bulletin* of the Metropolitan Life Insurance Company says.[3]

> It is generally recognized that weight of the human body in relation to its height plays a part in determining the health and longevity of the individual. It is only recently, however, that the long experience of the insurance companies has made possible the crystallization of this impression into a series of definite propositions. We know now, for example, that overweight is a serious impairment among insured lives, the gravity increasing with the excess in weight over the average for the height and age. But, even this statement has its exceptions because, at younger ages, a limited amount of overweight is apparently an advantage. Such persons have uniformly lower death rates from tuberculosis. It is after the age of 35 that overweight, even in relatively small amounts, begins to be dangerous. The seriousness increases with advancing age and with the amount of overweight.[3]

From the 1920s to the 1980s, "weight tables" of appropriate, desirable, or ideal weight were developed by the life insurance industry.[3] The Framingham Study, the first American effort at a long-term community population-based evaluation of health risks, used the Metropolitan Life Insurance Table of 1959 as the standard for comparing the weights of people living in Framingham. They termed this the "Metropolitan Relative Weight," which was the weight-for-height of an individual to the expected weight-for-height from the Metropolitan Life Insurance Table median frame group. The final Metropolitan Life Insurance Table of Desirable Weights was published in 1983.

VARIOUS INDICES PROPOSED

Several indices relating height to weight have been proposed. The BMI, or what might more appropriately be called the Quetelet Index (QI), is described above. A comparison of the BMI to using skinfolds as the "standard" was published in 1972 by Keys et al.[4] They evaluated the Wt/Ht, the $Wt/(Ht)^2$ (QI), and the $Ht/(Wt)^{1/3}$ (Ponderal Index). Of these three, the BMI (QI) had a slightly better correlation with fatness than Wt/Ht. The Ponderal Index was clearly the worst.

GRADUAL ADOPTION OF THE BMI

In 1971, Benn showed that a simple index of $Wt/(Ht)^p$ could be derived for each population in which p was a power for the formula where weight had the lowest relation to height for that population.[5] For most populations this number was between 1 and 2. The ratio that Quetelet proposed in 1835 had a power of 2 $(Wt(Ht)^2)$. Lee, Kolonel, and Hinds, in an effort to apply a Wt/Ht index to a variety of populations living in Hawaii, found different indices useful for ranking the different populations.[6] However, these authors did not measure fatness, and since all of these weight-to-height indices are strongly related to weight,[7] their data are unhelpful in resolving the value of the QI vs. the Benn Index as estimates of fat. Keys et al. examined the relationship of weight-to-height indices.[4] In a study of 12 different populations, they found that $Wt(Ht)^2$ had the best correlations with body fat, as estimated from skinfolds. The correlations of the BMI with fat ranged from $R = .611$ and $R = .850$. In a detailed evaluation of four large study populations, Garn and Pesick[7] showed a strong correlation between any index and weight which approximated $R = .90$. In this study, the population-specific indices, as proposed by Benn $(Wt(Ht)^2)$, ranged between 1.18 and 1.83. These population-specific indices provided no advantage over $Wt/(Ht)^2$ when related to skinfolds.

Garrow and Webster have examined the BMI as a measure of fatness in a group of obese subjects.[8] Fat was measured by three separate techniques including densitometry, measurement of total body water, and measurement of total body potassium (K) using γ emission from naturally occurring ^{40}K. As Garrow and Webster[8] point out, there is considerable variation in estimating fat between the methods that they selected for this study. The accuracy for measuring fat was greater for men than for women by all methods. The standard deviations for estimating fat by the BMI, however, were only slightly larger than those for density, body water, and body potassium. The relationship of $Fat/(Ht)^2$ plotted against $Wt(Ht)^2$, yielded very similar slopes for men (0.715) and for women (0.713). This indicates that men and women of similar height differ in weight by tissue, which is approximately 75% fat and 25% nonfat. In their analysis, there was an important difference in the fatness between men and women, such that a woman with 0 (zero) body fat would have a QI of 13.7 kg/m², whereas a man with zero body fat would have a QI of 16.9 kg/m². Garrow and Webster thus conclude that "Quetelet's Index has been underrated as a measure of obesity in adults. It provides a measure of fatness not much less accurate than specialized laboratory methods."[8] As they point out, this index can be applied over the entire weight range, while such measurements as skinfold thickness are severely limited in obese individuals and nearly useless in very obese individuals.

Gallagher et al.[9] have used a four-compartment model to compare body fat and BMI in a large group of men and women. Their findings support Garrow and Webster, and show that as BMI rises, body fat rises in parallel for men and women, with women having 10 to 12% more body fat at any given BMI. Table 30.1 shows BMI values for weights and heights.

TABLE 30.1
A Table of BMI Values

Height	Good Weights							Over Weight					Obese									
	19	20	21	22	23	24	25	26	27	28	29	30	31	32	33	34	35	36	37	38	39	40
4'10"	91	96	100	105	110	115	119	124	129	134	138	143	148	153	158	162	167	172	177	181	186	191
4'11"	94	99	104	109	114	119	124	128	133	138	143	148	153	158	163	168	173	178	183	188	193	198
5"	97	102	107	112	118	123	128	133	138	143	148	153	158	163	168	174	179	184	189	194	199	204
5'1"	100	106	111	116	122	127	132	137	143	148	153	158	164	169	174	180	185	190	195	201	206	211
5'2"	104	109	115	120	126	131	136	142	147	153	158	164	169	175	180	186	191	196	202	207	213	218
5'3"	107	113	118	124	130	135	141	146	152	158	163	169	175	180	186	191	197	203	208	214	220	225
5'4"	110	116	122	128	134	140	145	151	157	163	169	174	180	186	192	197	204	209	215	221	227	232
5'5"	114	120	126	132	138	144	150	156	162	168	174	180	186	192	198	204	210	216	222	228	234	240
5'6"	118	124	130	136	142	148	155	161	167	173	179	186	192	198	204	210	216	223	229	235	241	247
5'7"	121	127	134	140	146	153	159	166	172	178	185	191	198	204	211	217	223	230	236	242	249	255
5'8"	125	131	138	144	151	158	164	171	177	184	190	197	203	210	216	223	230	236	243	249	256	262
5'9"	128	135	142	149	155	162	169	176	182	189	196	203	209	216	223	230	236	243	250	257	263	270
5'10"	132	139	146	153	160	167	174	181	188	195	202	209	216	222	229	236	243	250	257	264	271	278
5'11"	136	143	150	157	165	172	179	186	193	200	208	215	222	229	236	243	250	257	265	272	279	286
6"	140	147	154	162	169	177	184	191	199	206	213	221	228	235	242	250	258	265	272	279	287	294
6'1"	144	151	159	166	174	182	189	197	204	212	219	227	235	242	250	257	265	272	280	288	295	302
6'2"	148	155	163	171	179	186	194	202	210	218	225	233	241	249	256	264	272	280	287	295	303	311
6'3"	152	160	168	176	184	192	200	208	216	224	232	240	248	256	264	272	279	287	295	303	311	319
6'4"	156	164	172	180	189	197	205	213	221	230	238	246	254	263	271	279	287	295	304	312	320	328

Source: Copyright 1997 George A. Bray.

An additional feature of the BMI is the similarity of the mortality and morbidity curves plotted against BMI for men and women. Whether related to excessive deaths or to morbidity from various diseases, the minimum BMI is similar for both sexes at comparable ages. Yet, at all ages, the quantity of body fat in women is higher than men for any given height/weight combination. This implies that the extra fat in women (the zero fat BMI values noted above of 3.2) is not associated with increased risk of mortality.

SUMMARY

In summary, the relationship between height and weight $(Wt(Ht)^2)$ proposed by Quetelet in 1835 and termed the BMI has stood the test of time. In tribute to his contribution and its validation from a number of sources, it would be appropriate to refer to it as the QI and replace the frequently used BMI with this new nomenclature.

REFERENCES

1. Freudenthal, H., *Lambert-Adolph-Jacques Quetelet. Dictionary of Scientific Biography*. C. C. Gillespie. New York, Charles and Sons. 1975; 236–8.
2. Bray, G. A., *Obes Res* **2**(1): 68–71, 1994.
3. Bray, G. A., *Obes Res* **3**(1): 97–9, 1995.
4. Keys, A. et al., *J Chronic Dis* **25**(6): 329–43, 1972.
5. Benn, R. T., *Br J Prev Soc Med* **25**(1): 42–50, 1971.
6. Lee, J. et al., *Int J Obes* **6**(3): 233–9, 1982.
7. Garn, S. M. and Pesick, S. D., *Am J Clin Nutr* **36**(4): 573–5, 1982.
8. Garrow, J. S. and Webster, J., *Int J Obes* **9**(2): 147–53, 1985.
9. Gallagher, D. et al., *Am J Epidemiol* **143**(3): 228–39, 1996.

31 Anthropometric Assessment: Stature, Weight, and the Body Mass Index in Adults

William Cameron Chumlea, Michael J. LaMonte, and George A. Bray

CONTENTS

INTRODUCTION

Anthropometric measurements and indices describe body size, shape, and composition. They infer information about the body at the tissue level, and they are affected by and reflect changes due to aging and disease. Weight is a limited indicator because it is related to stature, for example, on average, tall people are heavier than short people. This limitation is reduced in weight-divided-by-stature indices, such as the body mass index (BMI). Stature and weight are covariates in statistical models of body composition,[1] and BMI values are associated with morbidity and mortality.[2] Standardized anthropometric techniques are required to compare clinical and research data, and text and video media describing these techniques are available.[3,4] Those needing to use anthropometric methods and equipment should also consult these several resources for additional information.

KEY MEASUREMENTS

STATURE

Stature describes general body size and length, and variation in stature from the normal range can be associated with disease. Measuring stature is useful in screening for osteoporosis and in interpreting body weight. Stature is easily measured with a variety of fixed or portable commercially available stadiometers. There are also methods of predicting stature when it can not be measured, such as in disabled persons or in those with mobility impairments.[5,6] In some instances, recumbent length can be substituted but an adjustment of 1.5 cm is subtracted to account for the systematic differences between recumbent length and stature. Reference data for stature are available from the Centers for Disease Control, National Center for Health Statistics (CDC/NCHS; http://www.cdc.gov/nchs) and from the World Health Organization (WHO; http://www.who.int/en).

Measurement Technique

Measurement of stature requires a vertical surface with an attached metric rule and a horizontal headboard attached to the vertical surface that is brought into contact with the most superior point on the head. The subject is barefoot or wears thin socks and little clothing so that the position of the body is clear. The subject stands upright without assistance, with heels close together, legs straight, arms at the sides, and shoulders relaxed. The subject stands erect facing away from the vertical portion of the sta-diometer. The buttocks, shoulders, and head are positioned to be in contact with the vertical portion of the stadiometer, and the heels are placed together so that the subject stands straight when viewed from the side. It may not be possible for some subjects to place their buttocks, shoulders, and head against the stadiometer because of adipose tissue on the buttocks. These subjects are positioned with only the buttocks in contact with the vertical portion of the stadiometer, and the body is positioned vertically above and below the waist so that the subject stands straight when viewed from the side. The head is positioned vertically from left to right with the subject looking straight ahead, and the head is positioned horizontally so that a line from the lower margin of the bony socket containing the eye and the opening of the external ear is parallel to the floor. The subject inhales deeply and stands fully erect, and the horizontal measuring piece is lowered to make contact with the top of the head. Hair ornaments, buns, braids, etc., are removed as necessary to obtain an accurate measurement. The measurer's eyes should be level with the headpiece to avoid reading errors due to parallax. The subject's stature is recorded to the nearest 0.1 cm. Mean intermeasurer differences range from 1.4 mm (SD = 1.5 mm) to 2.1 mm (SD = 2.1 mm) for adults between 20 and 85 years of age.[3]

WEIGHT

Weight is an overall composite measure of total body size and composition, and changes in weight reflect corresponding changes in body water, fat, and lean tissues. A weight change with or without the presence of chronic disease is a possible indicator of potential health problems. Weight tends to increase through middle age because of increased fatness; thus, it is the obvious mea-sure of overweight and obesity as most adults with high body weights tend to have high amounts of body fat. However, this is not always true, as in the case of athletes who can have high body weights due to increased bone and skeletal muscle mass rather than high amounts of fat, or in elderly persons with sarcopenic obesity, in which stable or even low body weights occur with increased percentage of body fatness.[7] Reference data for weight are available from CDC/NCHS: http://www.cdc.gov/nchs, and from the WHO: http://www.who.int/en.

Measurement Technique

Weight is the most commonly recorded anthropometric variable, and generally it is measured accurately. Weight is measured using a beam scale or a calibrated digital scale that must be level and resting on a hard or firm surface. The subject stands in the middle of the scale platform with head held straight and eyes looking straight ahead. Light indoor clothing can be worn, excluding shoes, dresses, long trousers, and sweaters, but it is best to standardize the clothing, for example, a disposable paper gown. It is not necessary to subtract the weight of the paper gown from the observed weight. In studies to assess short-term changes, weights must be recorded at standardized times, but this is not necessary for a single measurement. Weight is recorded to the nearest 100 g, and mean intermeasurer differences are 1.5 g (SD = 3.6 g) and intermeasurer and intrameasurer technical errors are about 1.2 kg for pairs of measurements made 2 weeks apart.[3]

Handicapped subjects, those with amputations and mobility impairments, can be weighed using a chair scale or bed scale. Scales that can be moved from one location to another are useful, but they must be calibrated each time they are moved.

BODY MASS INDEX

Weight is related to stature in that a weight of 100 kg has a completely different meaning if it is associated with a stature of 150 cm compared with 190 cm as are the corresponding associations with body fatness. An index of weight, independent of stature, should be a better descriptor of body fatness than weight alone. The BMI is weight divided by stature squared, and Lambert-Adolf-Jacques Quetelet developed this concept in 1835.[8] In the middle of the twentieth century, several indices incorporating weight divided by stature raised to a power of one-third and greater were proposed, which reduced the association of weight with stature. The BMI has been compared against several of these indices by Keys et al., Benn, and many others.[9–13] The current consensus is that there is little, if any, significant improvement or utility of these other weight-for-stature indices over that of the BMI in describing associations with body fatness. Another advantage of BMI over other indices is the availability of extensive national reference data worldwide, its established relationships with levels of body composition, and its strong association with the risk of developing chronic diseases and with premature mortality.[14] Reference data for BMI are available from the CDC/NCHS: http://www.cdc.gov/nchs, and from the WHO: http://www.who.int/en.

Measurement Technique

BMI includes measures of stature and weight that are recorded accurately in metric units or converted from English values to kilograms and centimeters. BMI is calculated easily with a calculator or from one of many Web sites that perform this task using either English or metric measurement values.

BMI, Race, and Ethnicity

Race and ethnic variations in BMI and body composition are associated with differences in socioeconomic status, diet, health care utilization, and degrees of genetic admixture within and between countries.[12,15] For example, African-American and Hispanic women tend to have higher mean levels of BMI and body fatness than non-Hispanic White women. Compared with African-American and non-Hispanic White men, Hispanic men tend to have higher mean levels of body fat, but not BMI.[16] Race- and age-specific reference data for BMI in the United States population are available from the CDC/NCHS: http://www.cdc.gov/nchs.

BMI, Weight, and Obesity

Weight and BMI are used to screen for and monitor the effectiveness of treatment of overweight and obesity, but both measurements are imperfect tools for evaluating fatness. A weight change of 3.5 kg is necessary to produce a one unit change in BMI. Body builders, wrestlers, and athletes can have high weight and BMI values due to high levels of muscularity rather than high body fatness. Conversely, in the elderly BMI and weight may be normal or even low, in spite of a high level of relative body fatness, because of declines in stature, bone mass, and fat-free mass with age.[17] Correlations between BMI values and standardized measures of body fat range from <0.1 to >0.8 depending on the initial percentage of body fatness, levels of physical activity and fitness, gender, race, and age, that is, a BMI of 28 does not have the same meaning in relation to body fatness in all adults but must be used in context with other related factors.[18] On an individual basis, weight and BMI can be of limited value, but for the "average" adult, they are both useful and important screening tools.

The WHO categorizes grades of BMI values in relation to health risk associated primarily with obesity (Table 31.1). Adults with BMI levels below 18 and above 25 have higher risks for health problems than adults with BMI levels from 18 to 25. A BMI of 30 or greater defines obesity (Table 31.1), and based on this criteria, the prevalence of obesity is 20% to 30% for non-Hispanic White, non-Hispanic Black, and Mexican-American men, 25% to 40% for non-Hispanic White and Mexican-American women, and is as high as 46% to 53% for non-Hispanic Black women, and the prevalence of BMI-defined overweight in each of these groups is higher.[2] Similar health associations and prevalence of overweight and obesity exists for adult populations in Europe and among urban areas of Mexico, the Middle East, India, and China.[19–22]

BMI and Central Obesity

Obese adults typically have increased amounts of intraabdominal fat, which is not assessed by BMI. A measure of abdominal circumference is a valuable addition in assessing weight-related health risk. The ratio of abdominal circumference (sometime incorrectly referred to as "waist" circumference) to the hip circumference has also been used to describe adipose tissue distribution or fat patterning,[23,24] but this ratio poorly describes levels of intraabdominal adipose tissue, and the abdominal circumference is now the reference measure to screen for and assess health risks due to intraabdominal fatness.[25–29] Abdominal circumference thresholds define components of the metabolic syndrome, a cluster of interrelated risk factors that, when coexisting, significantly increase the risk of cardiovascular disease (CVD) events and type 2 diabetes.[30,31] Its relationship with total body fatness and mortality risk are affected by age, sex, and fitness levels,[32–34] and cut-points for abdominal circumference associated with BMI have been established according to risk for developing chronic disease, particularly type 2 diabetes and mortality.[19,35] Abdominal circumference cut-points are reported to be independent of BMI,[36–38] and thus their recommended clinical application is to refine BMI-defined assessment of health risk.[39,40] Abdominal circumference is potentially of greater clinical utility than BMI in describing obesity,[41] but this utility is not universally recommended.[42] Abdominal thickness reflects levels of abdominal obesity because a large abdomen can be a thick abdomen, but standardizing this measurement is inconsistent and little reference data is available.[25]

TABLE 31.1

BMI Value Ranges, Health Classifications and Comorbidity Risk

BMI Ranges	Health Classification	Risk of Comorbidity
≤18.5	Possible wasting	Increased
18.5–24.9	Normal	Average
25–29.9	Overweight	Increased
30.0–34.9	Obese class I	Moderate
35–39.9	Obese class II	Severe
≥40	Obese class III	Very severe

BMI, Morbidity, and Mortality

As a result of the WHO classification of BMI values and their relation to increasing risk of developing chronic diseases and premature mortality, BMI is commonly used in epidemiologic studies of adults.[22,43] BMI values of 18 and less are potential indicators of possible wasting conditions, such as malnutrition, tuberculosis, depression, chronic obstructive pulmonary disease, and lung and stomach cancers. The morbidities associated with BMI values of 30 and higher include impaired mobility, compromised cardiovascular and pulmonary function, sleep apnea, increased prevalence and incidence of cerebrovascular and CVD, diabetes, a number of specific cancers, and a high prevalence of chronic disease risk factors, including impaired glucose intolerance, dyslipidemia, and *Hypertension*, and a high risk for continued obesity, chronic disease, and hospitalization.[19,39,44] This descriptive utility of BMI depends, in part, on its positive association with overall levels of body fatness,[9,45,46] but this association and that with risk of disease deteriorates with age, sex, and ethnicity.[18,36,47–49]

The relationship between BMI and total and cause-specific mortality in adults is characterized as linear in some studies but curvilinear in others.[2,22,39,50,51] The patterns of association between BMI and mortality also vary by age, sex, race/ethnicity, smoking status, and cause of death.[18,36,39,47–49] The association between BMI and mortality further varies within population subgroups in the United States.[52] When adjusted for poverty, smoking, and elevated blood pressure, a high BMI is associated with a slightly increased mortality risk in White men but not in White women, while in the Framingham Heart Study, the relationship of BMI with mortality was positive in nonsmoking men and women over 65 years of age.[53] However, adults with BMI levels above the 70th percentile (28.5 for men; 28.7 for women) had lower survival than those with moderate BMI levels. Underlying these population differences in the BMI–mortality relationship is, in part, the previously mentioned differences in the relationship between BMI and levels of body fat among population subgroups.[9,45,46,54] There are major challenges to disentangling the complex multifactorial etiology of obesity and health outcomes, and limited epidemiologic information is available regarding the concurrent linkage of BMI with body fatness, central fat distribution, and subsequent mortality.[32,55,56]

In many, but not all, studies, the strength of association between mortality and BMI and body composition is reduced when physical activity or cardiovascular fitness is a covariate.[32,57–61] These relationships are illustrated in Figure 31.1 and Figure 31.2 in data on 21,925 men aged 30 to 83 years whose percentage of body fat and cardiovascular fitness were measured at baseline,

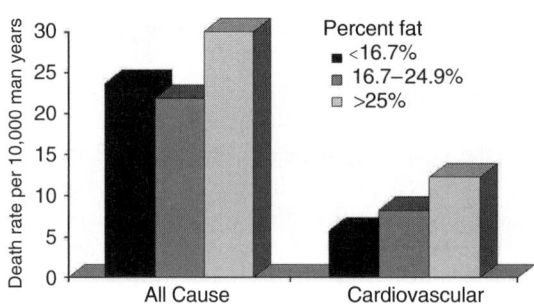

FIGURE 31.1 All-cause and CVD death rates by levels of percentage of body fat in 21,925 men in the Aerobics Center Longitudinal Study, 1971–1989. The numbers of deaths in each incremental level of body fat were 82, 187, and 159 for all-cause mortality, and were 18, 65, and 61 for CVD mortality.

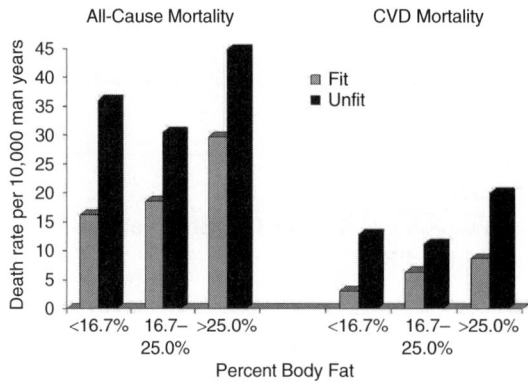

FIGURE 31.2 Rates of all-cause and CVD mortality according to levels of cardiorespiratory fitness and percentage of body fat in 21,925 men in the Aerobics Center Longitudinal Study, 1971–1989. The number of deaths for each bar from left to right were 68, 14, 127, 60, 65, and 94 for all-cause mortality, and 13, 5, 43, 22, 19, and 42 for CVD mortality.

and who were followed up for an average of 8 years for total and CVD mortality.[32] In Figure 31.1, a curvilinear J-shaped association is seen between incremental levels of body fat and all-cause mortality, much as that noted with BMI, but a linear relationship occurred between body fat and CVD mortality. Next, the men were grouped into categories of fit (upper 80% of exercise duration) and unfit, and mortality rates were cross-tabulated on body fat and fitness levels. In each incremental category, fit men had a lower rate of total and CVD mortality than unfit men (Figure 31.2). In fact, men in the highest category of fatness who were fit had lower death rates than their unfit lean counterparts.

Physical inactivity potentially is an antecedent or a consequence of obesity,[62,63] but it is difficult to know how much of the increased morbidity and mortality associated with high BMI results from excessive body fat, from physical inactivity, or both. Data from exercise intervention studies have shown that increases in physical activity result in weight loss and changes in body composition and fat distribution.[64–66] Higher levels of physical activity and fitness are also associated with favorable chronic disease risk factor profiles in men and women,[67–70] and several studies report an inverse association between physical activity or fitness exposures and the occurrence of nonfatal diseases such as *Hypertension*,[71–76] diabetes,[76–84] metabolic syndrome,[76,85] myocardial infarction,[86,87] stroke,[87,88] and certain cancers.[89–91] Several studies have also demonstrated a strong, graded, and inverse association between physical activity or fitness exposures and mortality.[88,92–94] This pattern of association is generally consistent in all adults and is independent of conventional risk factors including body weight and BMI.[93,95] Recently, three expert panels concluded that low levels of physical activity and fitness are likely to be causal factors in the development of overweight and obesity, and that improvements in physical activity and fitness levels will result in favorable changes in chronic disease risk factors and lower risk of morbidity and mortality in the normal weight and overweight alike.[96–98]

BMI Paradox

Several studies have shown a U-shaped relationship of BMI with all-cause mortality characterized by increased risk among adults with a BMI < 18.5, little or no risk observed across BMI levels between 18.5 and 30, and increasingly pronounced mortality risk beyond a BMI of 30.[19,22,39] This U-shaped relationship is associated with an age-related paradox. Between about 40 and 60 years of age, both a low and a high BMI are associated with increased mortality risk. However, after about 70 years of age, only a low BMI is associated with a higher mortality, whereas little if any excess mortality is seen at high BMI levels,[99] although high levels of BMI are reported by others to be related to increased risk of hospitalization and all-cause mortality.[44] This has been interpreted to indicate that a moderate weight gain in later years might be beneficial to health.[2,100] However, there is no clear description of a favorable association between changes in weight or BMI status and the occurrence or severity of disease across the middle and later years of life. A key to clarifying this paradox may require a more thorough evaluation of the purported link between changes in weight from middle to old age and subsequent health status. Age-related weight loss associated with worsening health conditions typically occurs in those persons who have the greatest weight between 40 and 60 years of age, but if health is maintained during aging, then a low body weight often is not an important risk factor.[99] Some important issues must be considered in regard to existing information on this paradox. Most analyses associated with the BMI–mortality paradox are limited to individuals less than 70 years of age, and little is known about this issue among persons of more advanced ages.[99] Data on body weight are often self-reported, which can lead to misclassification of initial weight status as well as erroneous tracking of weight changes. Thus, the underlying changes in body composition (e.g., fat and lean mass) that are associated with the patterns of change in weight from middle to old age cannot be quantified. Therefore, the interaction of changes in weight and body composition with health conditions remains unknown. However, in a recent follow-up study of women and men in the National Health and Nutrition Examination Survey (NHANES) I and II cohorts that found a U-shaped relationship between baseline BMI and all-cause mortality, fat free mass (FFM) had a monotonically inverse relationship with mortality and fat mass had a monotonically positive relationship with mortality.[101] This study shows that, because BMI is not able to discriminate fat from lean tissue, it might mask important underlying mechanisms linking body composition with disease that could be detected with measures of fat distribution such as waist circumference. Leanness might have beneficial effects on longevity that to some degree counters the negative effects of excessive adiposity. Most studies do not have longitudinal data with serial measures of body weight and composition and fat distribution in women and men over a large age range to track relationships with health status during the middle to later years of life. In addition, the effects of smoking, diet, levels of physical activity, and genetic susceptibility confound many of these associations.

SUMMARY

Stature, weight, and BMI are useful measures of body size and indices of body composition in adults, and there are extensive reference data available in many countries that describe the current status of the distributions of these descriptors in their populations. With the increased prevalence of overweight and obesity worldwide among adults, weight, and weight-for-stature indices such as BMI have significant health importance in describing health risk relationships in screening for chronic disease and the risk of early mortality.

ACKNOWLEDGMENTS

This work was supported by grants HD12252, HL072838, HL069995, and DK071485 from the National Institute of Health, Bethesda, MD (Dr. Chumlea), and by grants AG06945, HL62508, and the Communities Foundation of Texas on recommendation of Nancy Ann and Ray L. Hunt (Dr. LaMonte).

REFERENCES

1. Sun SS, Chumlea WC, *Human Body Composition*, Heymsfield SSB, Lohman TTG, Wang Z, et al., eds., Human Kinetics Publishers, Champaign, IL, 2005. 151.
2. Flegal KM, Graubard BI, Williamson DF, et al., *JAMA* 293: 1861; 2005.
3. Lohman TG, Roche AF, Martorell R, et al., *Anthropometric Standardization Reference Manual*, Human Kinetics Publishers, Champaign, IL, 1988, vi, 177.
4. Kuczmarski RJ, Chumlea WC, *J Gerontology* 37: 246; 1997.
5. Chumlea WC, Guo SS, Steinbaugh ML, *JADA* 94: 1385; 1994.
6. Chumlea WC, Guo SS, Wholihan K, et al., *JADA* 98: 137; 1998.
7. Gallagher D, Ruts E, Visser M, et al., *Am J Physiol Endocrinol Metab* 279: E366; 2000.
8. Quetelet LA, *Sur l'homme et le developpement de ses facultes, ou essai de physique sociale*, Bachelier, Paris, 1835.
9. Keys A, Fidanza F, Karvonen MJ, et al., *J Chronic Dis* 25: 329; 1972.
10. Garn SM, Pesick SD, *Am J Clin Nutr* 36: 573; 1982.
11. Benn RT, *Br J Prev Soc Med* 25: 42; 1971.
12. Gallagher D, Visser M, Sepulveda D, et al., *Am J Epidemiol* 143: 228; 1996.
13. Abdel-Malek AK, Mukherjee D, Roche AF, *Hum Biol* 57: 415; 1985.
14. French SA, Folsom AR, Jeffery RW, et al., *Am J Epidemiol* 149: 504; 1999.
15. Wildman RP, Gu D, Reynolds K, et al., *Am J Clin Nutr* 80: 1129; 2004.
16. Chumlea WC, Guo SS, Kuczmarski RJ, et al., *Int J Obes Relat Metab Disord* 26: 1596; 2002.
17. Donini LM, Chumlea WC, Vellas B, et al., *J Nutr Health Aging* 10: 52; 2006.
18. Gallagher D, Heymsfield SB, Heo M, et al., *Am J Clin Nutr* 72: 694; 2000.
19. WHO, *Obesity: Preventing and Managing the Global Epidemic*, Geneva, Switzerland, 1998, 1.
20. James PT, Leach R, Kalamara E, et al., *Obes Res* 9 (Suppl 4): 228S; 2001.
21. Deitel M, *Obes Surg* 13: 329; 2003.
22. Gu D, He J, Duan X, et al., *JAMA* 295: 776; 2006.
23. Seidell JC, Oosterlee A, Thijssen MA, et al., *Am J Clin Nutr* 45: 7; 1987.
24. Fujimoto WY, Newell-Morris LL, Grote M, et al., *Int J Obes* 15 (Suppl 2): 41; 1991.
25. Pouliot MC, Despres JP, Lemieux S, et al., *Am J Cardiol* 73: 460; 1994.
26. Despres JP, Prud'homme D, Pouliot MC, et al., *Am J Clin Nutr* 54: 471; 1991.
27. Bray GA, *Present Knowledge in Nutrition*, International Life Sciences Institute, Washington DC, 1994, 19.
28. Nicklas BJ, Penninx BW, Cesari M, et al., *Am J Epidemiol* 160: 741; 2004.
29. Okosun IS, Chandra KM, Boev A, et al., *Prev Med* 39: 197; 2004.
30. Grundy SM, *Endocrinol Metab Clin North Am* 33: 267; 2004.
31. Katzmarzyk PT, Janssen I, Ross R, et al., *Diabetes Care* 29: 404; 2006.
32. Lee CD, Blair SN, Jackson AS, *Am J Clin Nutr* 69: 373; 1999.
33. Kuk JL, Lee S, Heymsfield SB, et al., *Am J Clin Nutr* 81: 1330; 2005.
34. Janssen I, Katzmarzyk PT, Ross R, et al., *Obes Res* 12: 525; 2004.
35. Yarnell JW, Patterson CC, Thomas HF, et al., *J Epidemiol Commun H* 54: 344; 2000.
36. Van Pelt RE, Evans EM, Schechtman KB, et al., *Int J Obes Relat Metab Disord* 25: 1183; 2001.
37. Iwao S, Iwao N, Muller DC, et al., *Obes Res* 9: 685; 2001.
38. Bigaard J, Frederiksen K, Tjonneland A, et al., *Int J Obes* (Lond) 29: 778; 2005.
39. NHLBI, *Clinical Guidelines on the Identification, Evaluation, and Treatment of Overweight and Obesity in Adults: The Evidence Report*, Rockville, MD, 1998, 1.
40. Zhu S, Heymsfield SB, Toyoshima H, et al., *Am J Clin Nutr* 81: 409; 2005.
41. Wang Y, Rimm EB, Stampfer MJ, et al., *Am J Clin Nutr* 81: 555; 2005.
42. Rexrode KM, Buring JE, Manson JE, *Int J Obes Relat Metab Disord* 25: 1047; 2001.
43. Lamon-Fava S, Wilson PW, Schaefer EJ, *Arterioscler Thromb Vasc Biol* 16: 1509; 1996.
44. Yan LL, Daviglus ML, Liu K, et al., *JAMA* 295: 190; 2006.
45. Garrow JS, Webster J, *Int J Obes* 9: 147; 1985.
46. Kuczmarski RJ, Flegal KM, *Am J Clin Nutr* 72: 1074; 2000.
47. Rimm EB, Stampfer MJ, Giovannucci E, et al., *Am J Epidemiol* 141: 1117; 1995.
48. Stevens J, Plankey MW, Williamson DF, et al., *Obes Res* 6: 268; 1998.
49. Fernandez JR, Heo M, Heymsfield SB, et al., *Am J Clin Nutr* 77: 71; 2003.
50. Van Itallie TB, *Ann Intern Med* 103: 983; 1985.

51. McGee DL, *Ann Epidemiol* 15: 87; 2005.
52. Tayback M, Kumanyika S, Chee E, *Arch Intern Med* 150: 1065; 1990.
53. Harris T, Cook EF, Garrison R, et al., *JAMA* 259: 1520; 1988.
54. Jackson AS, Stanforth PR, Gagnon J, et al., *Int J Obes Relat Metab Disord* 26: 789; 2002.
55. Hubbard VS, *Am J Clin Nutr* 72: 1067; 2000.
56. Katzmarzyk PT, Craig CL, Bouchard C, *Int J Obes Relat Metab Disord* 26: 1054; 2002.
57. Church TS, LaMonte MJ, Barlow CE, et al., *Arch Intern Med* 165: 2114; 2005.
58. Wei M, Kampert JB, Barlow CE, et al., *JAMA* 282: 1547; 1999.
59. Katzmarzyk PT, Church TS, Janssen I, et al., *Diabetes Care* 28: 391; 2005.
60. Wei M, Gibbons LW, Kampert JB, et al., *Ann Intern Med* 132: 605; 2000.
61. Barlow CE, Kohl III HW, Gibbons LW, et al., *Int J Obes Relat Metab Disord* 19 (Suppl 4): S41; 1995.
62. Di Pietro L, Dziura J, Blair SN, *Int J Obes Relat Metab Disord* 28: 1541; 2004.
63. Petersen L, Schnohr P, Sorensen TI, *Int J Obes Relat Metab Disord* 28: 105; 2004.
64. Stefanick ML, *Exerc Sport Sci Rev* 21: 363; 1993.
65. Ross R, Katzmarzyk PT, *Int J Obes Relat Metab Disord* 27: 204; 2003.
66. Ross R, *Sports Med* 24: 55; 1997.
67. Cooper KH, Pollock ML, Martin RP, et al., *JAMA* 236: 166; 1976.
68. Gibbons LW, Blair SN, Cooper KH, et al., *Circulation* 67: 977; 1983.
69. LaMonte MJ, Eisenman PA, Adams TD, et al., *Circulation* 102: 1623; 2000.
70. Dannenberg AL, Keller JB, Wilson PW, et al., *Am J Epidemiol* 129: 76; 1989.
71. Paffenbarger Jr. RS, Wing AL, Hyde RT, et al., *Am J Epidemiol* 117: 245; 1983.
72. Hayashi T, Tsumura K, Suematsu C, et al., *Ann Intern Med* 131: 21; 1999.
73. Hu G, Barengo NC, Tuomilehto J, et al., *Hypertension* 43: 25; 2004.
74. Blair SN, Goodyear NN, Gibbons LW, et al., *JAMA* 252: 487; 1984.
75. Sawada S, Tanaka H, Funakoshi M, et al., *Clin Exp Pharmacol Physiol* 20: 483; 1993.
76. Carnethon MR, Gidding SS, Nehgme R, et al., *JAMA* 290: 3092; 2003.
77. Helmrich SP, Ragland DR, Leung RW, et al., *N Engl J Med* 325: 147; 1991.
78. Hu FB, Sigal RJ, Rich-Edwards JW, et al., *JAMA* 282: 1433; 1999.
79. Wannamethee SG, Shaper AG, Alberti KG, *Arch Intern Med* 160: 2108; 2000.
80. Wei M, Gibbons LW, Mitchell TL, et al., *Ann Intern Med* 130: 89; 1999.
81. Sawada SS, Lee IM, Muto T, et al., *Diabetes Care* 26: 2918; 2003.
82. Manson JE, Nathan DM, Krolewski AS, et al., *JAMA* 268: 63; 1992.
83. Manson JE, Rimm EB, Stampfer MJ, et al., *Lancet* 338: 774; 1991.
84. Hu G, Lindstrom J, Valle TT, et al., *Arch Intern Med* 164: 892; 2004.
85. Laaksonen DE, Lakka HM, Salonen JT, et al., *Diabetes Care* 25: 1612; 2002.
86. O'Connor GT, Hennekens CH, Willett WC, et al., *Am J Epidemiol* 142: 1147; 1995.
87. Salonen JT, Slater JS, Tuomilehto J, et al., *Am J Epidemiol* 127: 87; 1988.
88. Lee IM, Skerrett PJ, *Med Sci Sports Exerc* 33: S459; 2001.
89. Slattery ML, Edwards S, Curtin K, et al., *Am J Epidemiol* 158: 214; 2003.
90. Oliveria SA, Kohl III HW, Trichopoulos D, et al., *Med Sci Sports Exerc* 28: 97; 1996.
91. McTiernan A, Kooperberg C, White E, et al., *JAMA* 290: 1331; 2003.
92. DHHS CDC, *Physical Activity and Health: A report of the Surgeon General*, NCCDPHP, Atlanta, GA, 1996.
93. Blair SN, Cheng Y, Holder JS, *Med Sci Sports Exerc* 33: S379; 2001.
94. Kohl III HW, *Med Sci Sports Exerc* 33: S472; 2001.
95. Blair SN, Brodney S, *Med Sci Sports Exerc* 31: S646; 1999.
96. Grundy SM, Blackburn G, Higgins M, et al., *Med Sci Sports Exerc* 31: S502; 1999.
97. Jakicic JM, Clark K, Coleman E, et al., *Med Sci Sports Exerc* 33: 2145; 2001.
98. Saris WH, Blair SN, van Baak MA, et al., *Obes Rev* 4: 101; 2003.
99. Losonczy KG, Harris TB, Cornoni-Huntley J, et al., *Am J Epidemiol* 141: 312; 1995.
100. Andres R, Muller DC, Sorkin JD, *Ann Intern Med* 119: 737; 1993.
101. Allison DB, Zhu SK, Plankey M, et al., *Int J Obes Relat Metab Disord* 26: 410; 2002.

32 The How and Why of Body Composition Assessment in Adults

William Cameron Chumlea, Karen E. Remsberg, and Marta D. Van Loan

CONTENTS

INTRODUCTION

A variety of direct and indirect methods are available to quantify human body composition at the following levels: (1) the atomic level for the elements of carbon, calcium, potassium, and hydrogen, (2) the molecular level for amounts of water, protein, and fat, (3) the cellular level for extracellular fluid and the body cell mass, and (4) the tissue level for amounts and distributions of adipose, skeletal, and muscle tissues. This methodology is based on assumptions regarding the concentrations of elements, water, and electrolytes, the density of body tissues, biological interrelationships between body components and body tissues, and their distributions among groups of normal-weight adults. Detailed aspects of body composition methodology, its theories, general applications, equipment, and analytical techniques are found in several excellent texts, [1-3] and readers interested in a specific method and its details should consult these references.

In most instances, body composition assessments quantify amounts of lean or fat-free mass (FFM) and fat mass (FM). Other reasons for a body composition assessment may include, but are not limited to, the determination of: (1) bone mineral content (BMC) and bone mineral density (BMD) to screen for and diagnosis osteoporosis, (2) total body water (TBW) and extracellular water (ECW) in adults with end-stage renal disease or other disorders affecting body fluids, or (3) monitoring changes in body composition during clinical treatment. Direct assessments like neutron activation and total body counting quantify chemical elements in the body from the atomic level up to the tissue level. Indirect methods estimate body composition from the molecular level through the tissue level using data collected from and validated against another method and a reference sample. Indirect methods view the body as a compartmental system consisting of TBW, ECW, BMC, FFM, and FM. These compartments are quantified from models using the hydration level, density, chemical composition, and BMC of FFM; the density of FM; and the reference samples used to validate them; they are not "gold standards" for *in vivo* body composition assessment.

Indirect methods quantify body components by measuring a body property such as its volume (total and molecular), density, and conductivity or describe amounts and distributions of muscle and adipose tissues via x-ray or magnetic imaging techniques. Some indirect methods can quantify only total body composition, while others quantify both total and regional body composition. All indirect methods depend on biological interrelationships between directly measured body components and tissues and their distributions among normal adults. Indirect methods include hydrometry (isotope dilution), densitometry, bioelectrical impedance analysis (BIA), dual energy x-ray absorptiometry (DXA), computed x-ray tomography (CT), and magnetic resonance imaging (MRI). Large errors can occur when using indirect methods, and the results are affected by individual and sample specificity and the presence of disease. Some indirect methods rely on prediction equations to estimate body composition that are developed from direct and other indirect methods and their reference samples. Prediction equations using anthropometry are also available to estimate body composition values. However, prediction equations lose accuracy when applied to individuals or groups differing from the validation group, and the predicted results will vary and can require interpretation. In this chapter, current indirect body composition assessments are reviewed and evaluated regarding their methodologies, applications, and limitations in adults.

INDIRECT BODY COMPOSITION METHODS

HYDROMETRY

TBW is quantified by isotope dilution using deuterium or tritium in urine, saliva, or plasma with mass spectrometry, infrared spectrometry, or nuclear magnetic resonance spectroscopy.[4,5] There are good levels of agreement in TBW estimates among subjects, isotopes, specimens, and laboratory methods, but some differences for individuals are as much as 2 to 3 L. These differences are within the range expected in comparisons between body composition methods. The accepted equilibration time for isotope dilution is about 2 to 3 h, but this time is not well documented, and the variations in equilibration times with body size are poorly documented. TBW measures need to be corrected for natural abundance and isotope exchange,[1] especially for deuterium, which is a naturally occurring isotope. ECW is also quantified by dilution using bromide as $NaBr^{96}$ or other chemical elements similar to chloride,[6,7] that estimate the volume of chloride space, which is all extracellular. Bromide concentration in plasma can be measured by either high-pressure liquid chromatography or by colorimetric assay using gold chloride. It is not necessary to measure the natural abundance of bromide in the body, but this increases accuracy.

Body water is easy to measure in an adult, because it does not require undressing or any real physical participation, but this methodology is limited in the obese. Hydrometry presupposes FFM can be calculated from TBW based on an assumed average proportion of TBW in FFM of 73%, but this proportion ranges from 67 to 80%.[8,9] In addition, about 15 to 30% of TBW is present in adipose tissue as ECW, and this proportion increases with the degree of adiposity, but available reference values are out-of-date. These proportions are higher in women than men, higher in the obese, and can produce underestimates of FFM and overestimates of FM. Variation in the distribution of TBW due to diseases associated with obesity, such as diabetes and renal failure, further affects estimates of FFM and FM.

DENSIOMETRY

Densiometry estimates body composition using measures of body weight and body volume corrected for residual lung volume. Densiometry uses an adult's body weight to displace a volume of either air or water as in Archimedes' principle of underwater weighing. Underwater weighing requires a large tank of water sufficient for an adult to completely submerge and have his or her weight recorded at full expiration. Air displacement measures the change in the volume of air created by the presence of the body within a closed container of known volume, but it is hampered by potentially faulty assumptions.[10] Accurate and reliable measures by both water and air displacement are compromised for overweight or obese adults. It is difficult for an overweight or obese adult to submerge underwater, and weight belts can help correct the difficulty with submersion but not all other aspects of performance. Air displacement devices[10–12] are limited to adults who are "moderately" obese at best. Regardless, most overweight and obese adults are reluctant to put on a bathing suit and participate in body density measurements.

Historically, body density has been converted to the percentage of body weight as fat using the two-compartment models of Siri[9] or Brozek and coworkers,[13] but more recently, a multicompartment model has been used.[14] Two-compartment models divide the body into FM and FFM based on densities of 0.9 and 1.10 g/ml, respectively. The density of FM has little interindividual variation across age, but the density of FFM varies depending upon the relative proportions of water, protein, and osseous and nonosseous mineral, as well as the sex, race, and age.[15] Two-compartment models are not sex and race specific, and thus, a variation of only 0.02 g/ml in the density of FFM can produce an error of 5% body fat. Multicompartment models combine body density with measures of bone density from DXA and TBW volume to calculate body fatness.[16] Multicompartment models estimate body composition more accurately than two-compartment models, because they include measures of bone mineral and water that better reflect between-individual variance in body composition estimates across age, race, and sex.

BIOELECTRIC IMPEDANCE ANALYSIS

Bioelectric impedance at a frequency of 50 kHz is used to estimate TBW or FFM and, subsequently, FM by measuring the resistance of the body as a conductor to a very small amperage alternating electric current,[17,18] and bioelectric impedance at multiple frequencies from 1 to 1000 kHz can also differentiate the proportions of intra- and extracellular fluid volumes.[19] Body composition estimates from single- and multifrequency bioelectrical impedance in healthy individuals are well established, but all bioelectrical impedance methods employ some form of predictive modeling to estimate outcomes.[19] Bioelectrical impedance is useful in describing body composition for groups, but large errors for an individual limit its clinical use, especially in the presence of disease or with repeated assessments. The predictive errors for an individual are large so that repeated estimates are insensitive to small responses to treatment.

The tetrapolar method was the common way to measure single- and multifrequency BIA. Early measures of impedance were taken with the subject supine and the electrodes were connected to the right hand-wrist and right ankle-foot, but BIA measurements now depend on the model and manufacturer of the BIA analyzer. For several available BIA instruments, an adult stands barefoot on a metal platform similar to the common bathroom scale, in which the electrodes are imbedded in the platform.

The conductor of the body is its water content, and all BIA machines measure the impedance of this fluid conductor. Impedance is the vector relationship between resistance and reactance measured at a current frequency. Resistance is the opposition of the conductor to the alternating current as in nonbiological conductors, and reactance is from the capacitant effect of cell membranes, tissue interfaces, and nonionic tissues.[19] From Ohm's Law, a conductor's volume is proportional to its length squared divided by its resistance, and BIA utilizes this same relationship in the body where stature (S) is squared and divided by resistance (R) as an index of body volume; thus, S^2/R, is directly related to the volume of TBW. The impedance index (S^2/R) is used to estimate FFM and FM, but this is based upon the fraction of 73% of TBW in FFM. Since the hydration fraction of FFM is not constant, S^2/R is combined with anthropometric data to predict body composition based on results from other methods.

The theory behind multifrequency BIA is the same as that of single-frequency BIA, except that multifrequency BIA uses at least two different frequencies. At low frequency, the current cannot pass through the cell membrane due to its capacitance, so that low-frequency currents are conducted only through ECW of the body. High-frequency currents penetrate cell membranes and are thus used to estimate TBW.

When predicting body fluid volumes with multifrequency BIA, the analysis is adjusted for the effects of the fluid containing materials of differing conductive capacity. This is done using mixture theory,[20,21] which adjusts for the nonlinear relationship between R and water volume in a mixed medium system. The mixture effects are greatest at low frequency, because the conductive volume, presumably ECW, is a smaller proportion of the total volume. Hanai[20] developed an equation to describe the effect on the conductivity of a conducting material having nonconductivity entities in suspension, and hypothesized that the theory could be applied to tissues with nonconductivity materials ranging from 10 to 90%. This approach has been used successfully by a number of investigators to monitor changes in ECW, TBW, and FFM under a variety of conditions.[22–25]

Numerous BIA prediction equations for estimating body composition have been published that describe statistical associations based on biological relationships for a specific population. As such, the equations are useful only for adults who closely match the reference population in body size and shape. BIA has been applied to overweight or obese samples[26,27] in a few studies, but the majority of BIA prediction equations are not applicable to overweight or obese adults. The ability of BIA to predict fatness in obese adults is further limited, because there is a large proportion of body mass and body water accounted for by the trunk, the hydration of FFM is lower, and the ratio of ECW to TBW is increased. There are also prediction equations resident in commercial single frequency impedance analyzers, and these equations are not recommended unless sufficient information is provided by the manufacturer regarding the predictive accuracy, errors, and the samples used to develop them. While BIA is used most often to determine whole-body composition, it can be used for segmental assessments also.

DUAL ENERGY X-RAY ABSORPTIOMETRY

DXA is the most popular method for quantifying amounts of total body and regional fat, and lean and skeletal tissues. The primary use of DXA is measuring BMC and BMD of the hip and spine for diagnosing osteoporosis. The two low-radiation energy levels used in DXA and their differential attenuation through the body and subsequent computer calculations allow discrimination and quantification of total body adipose and soft tissues. DXA is an easy and convenient method for measuring body composition in the majority of the population, and it is currently included in the ongoing National Health and Nutrition Examination Survey (NHANES).[28] DXA software has inherent assumptions regarding levels of hydration, potassium content, and density in estimating fat and lean tissue, and these assumptions vary by manufacturer.[29,30] DXA estimates of body composition are also affected by differences among manufacturers in the technology, models, and software employed, methodological problems and intra- and intermachine differences.[31,32]

A computer printout provides the DXA body composition analysis for body segments and the whole body. Adipose or fat tissue weight is given on the printout, and total body FFM is calculated as the sum of the weights of soft tissue and BMC. The sum of the total body weights of FFM, BMC, and FM should approximate measured body weight within 2.0 kg; otherwise, concern should be raised for measurement and machine accuracy. Intermachine and intermethod comparisons of DXA body composition estimates should be made cautiously. DXA accurately measures BMC compared to neutron activation, and several studies have shown that DXA soft tissue estimates of FFM and FM are equivalent to results obtained from other methods in weight-stable individuals. Regular maintenance and calibration are needed to preserve the accuracy of DXA machines.

The DXA methodology is limited by restrictions on body weight, length, thickness, and width as a function of the available table scan area with each manufacturer and type of DXA machine, that is, pencil or fan beam. Although some innovative adaptations have been proposed, many overweight and obese adults are too wide and too thick for a whole body DXA scan that requires lying supine with current machines.[33] Jebb and colleagues[34,35] reported that estimates of BMD were affected by tissue depth or thickness, with an increasing error when measuring BMD in tissue greater than 20 cm in depth. In weight-stable adults, measurement of soft tissue composition is similar to reference techniques, but concern about BMD in large adults is warranted.[31]

IMAGING METHODS

Imaging systems, such as computed tomography (CT) and MRI are frequently limited to clinical situations and are not practical for obese adults. CT accommodates large body sizes but has high radiation exposures and is inappropriate for whole body assessments, though it has been used to measure intra-abdominal fat. MRI is not able to accommodate large body sizes in many instances but can be used for whole-body assessments and poses no known health risks. Both these methods require time and software to provide whole body and regional quantities of FM and FFM.

COMPUTED TOMOGRAPHY

Computed tomography (CT) is an x-ray device for specific medical diagnoses with an unacceptable radiation dose except for clinical examinations and studies. Rossner et al.[36] compared adipose tissue depths measured directly from cadavers to CT images from 21 cross-sectional abdominal images and found a significant relationship between the two methods for total adipose tissue ($R = .94$) and intra-abdominal adipose tissue ($R = .83$). Work by Ross and colleagues on rats demonstrated a relationship between CT images and chemical analysis of lipids ($R = .98$).[37] Validation and checking the accuracy of this technique are constrained by the need for human cadaver analysis or chemical analysis of animals.

MAGNETIC RESONANCE IMAGING

MRI involves an interaction between a very strong magnet field and the nucleus of the hydrogen atom. Hydrogen is the most abundant element in the body, and the proton in the hydrogen nucleus acts like a tiny magnet. The very strong magnetic field of the MRI instruments aligns the hydrogen protons in a known direction, at which time a pulsed radio frequency is applied to the body part within the magnetic field. The hydrogen protons absorb the radio energy and change alignment or directional orientation like a spinning gyroscope falling out of position. When the radio frequency is turned off, the protons release the absorbed energy and return to their normal position or orientation within the magnetic field. The released energy is detected and converted into images by the computer software.

Foster and coworkers[38] first reported MRI measures of adipose tissue and adjacent muscle tissue, and this work continued with carcass and cadaver. Work by Abate et al.[39] demonstrated that MRI measurements of adipose tissue in humans were similar to direct measurement of visceral and subcutaneous adipose tissue on cadavers. Supporting documentation for the accuracy of MRI has compared MRI to CT scan results,[40] and in general, the relationship between CT and MRI for the assessment of adipose tissue is good, with correlations ranging from 0.79 for subcutaneous, to 0.98 for visceral, and 0.99 for total adipose tissue. MRI is now used regularly to measure intra-abdominal amounts of visceral adipose tissue in epidemiological studies related to risk of cardiovascular disease and the metabolic syndrome.

MRI images involve no radiation, making them a low-risk method for body composition assessment. MRI, like CT imaging, requires multiple scans in order to obtain adipose tissue distribution information. Two different research teams used multiple MRI images over the entire body. Fowler and colleagues[41] acquired 28 images from head to foot, while Ross and coworkers[37] obtained 40+ images from head to foot to determine adipose tissue and lean tissue distribution in both males and females. Fowler demonstrated that as few as four MRI images could be used, while Ross showed that one image at the level of the L4 to L5 lumbar vertebrae could be used to predict total adipose tissue volume.

STATISTICAL MODELS OF BODY COMPOSITION

Statistical modeling can predict body composition for groups or individuals[42] using regression equations. For example, one such model might use age and sex to predict the amount of central adiposity as measured by MRI. The selection of predictor variables depends on their biological and statistical relationships to the outcome variable of interest, because the strength of these relationships affects the accuracy or precision of the prediction equation. Several regression methods are available such as forward selection, stepwise, and backward elimination regression. These are used if the predictor variables are not very interrelated. Predictor variables such as stature and weight are interrelated, and if used together in the same equation can reduce the precision and accuracy of the predictions. In such cases, a maximum R^2 or an all-possible subsets of regression procedure are appropriate analytical choices.

Regression analysis assumes bivariate relationships between an outcome and its predictor variables are linear; otherwise, the prediction equations have large errors and poor performance. It is assumed that the dependent variable is normally distributed in order to allow statistical inferences about the significance of the regression parameters. A large sample results in more precise and accurate prediction equations than a small sample, but the necessary sample size is a function of the correlations between the outcome and predictor variables. The sample size required to achieve accuracy on cross-validation depends on the number of predictor variables, the bivariate relationships among the dependent variable and the predictor variables, and the variance of the dependent variable in the cross-validation sample.

Numerous prediction equations for TBW, FFM, FM, and %FM from anthropometry and for TBW and FFM from bioelectrical impedance for non-Hispanic white, non-Hispanic black, and Mexican-American adults have been published.[16] Unless specified, these equations are not recommended for obese adults or groups. Many of these equations are for whites only, but there are a limited number for Native-American, Hispanic-American, and non-Hispanic black American samples.[43,44] Using a multicomponent body composition validation model, BIA prediction equations for TBW and FFM are available for non-Hispanic white, non-Hispanic black, and Mexican-American adults.[16] These anthropometrical and BIA equations provide reasonable prediction for individuals except at the extremes of the body composition distribution.

AVAILABLE REFERENCE DATA

Body composition references are available from national survey data collected by the National Center for Health Statistics, Centers for Disease Control and Prevention. These surveys use multiple methods of data collection, including interviews, physical examinations, physiological testing, and biochemical assessments from large representative samples of the U.S. population to monitor the nation's health and nutritional status. Plots of estimated means from single-frequency BIA for TBW, FFM, FM, and %FM of non-Hispanic white, non-Hispanic black, and Mexican-American adults from the third NHANES are presented in Figure 32.1 to Figure 32.4.[45] The data in these figures represent estimates for these groups of American adults between 1988 and 1994. More recent data based on the body mass index (BMI) have been published for data collected since 1998, and these body composition estimates will be replaced shortly by body composition values measured by DXA in the current NHANESs.[28]

SPECIAL POPULATIONS AND METHODOLOGICAL ISSUES

Direct and indirect assessment methods and their reference data are applicable to adults, but exclude most of the obese and many of the elderly. Obese (and wasted) adults have metabolic and hormonal profiles accompanied by comorbid conditions that alter assumptions underlying the validity of body composition methods applicable to normal-weight individuals.[46] Body composition assessments are of limited use among most obese adults, because their bodies are too large for the available equipment.

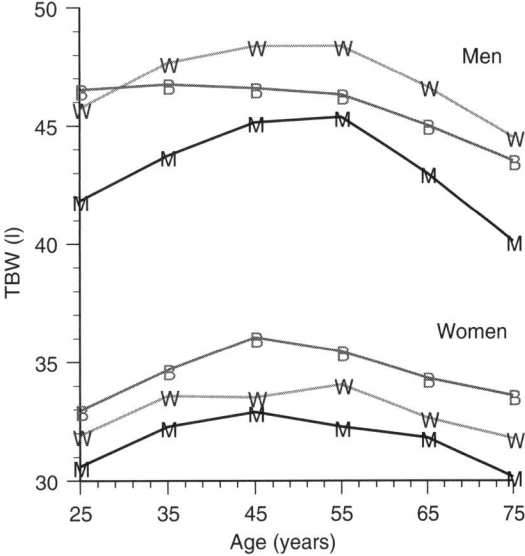

FIGURE 32.1 Estimated means for TBW from NHANES III by 10-year age groups from 20 to 80 years for non-Hispanic white (W), non-Hispanic black (B), and Mexican-American (M) men and women.

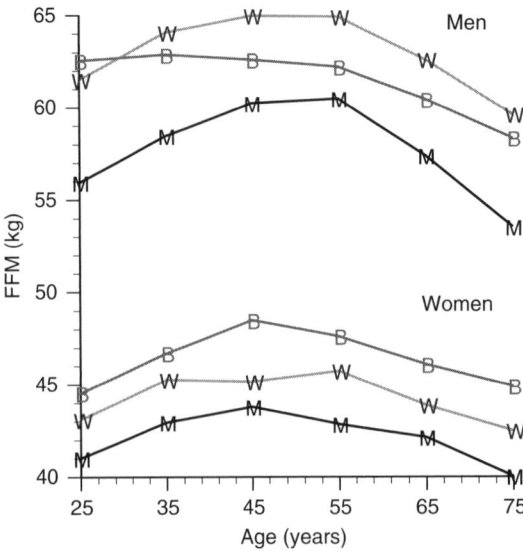

FIGURE 32.2 Estimated means for FFM by 10-year age groups from 20 to 80 years for non-Hispanic white (W), non-Hispanic black (B), and Mexican-American (M) men and women.

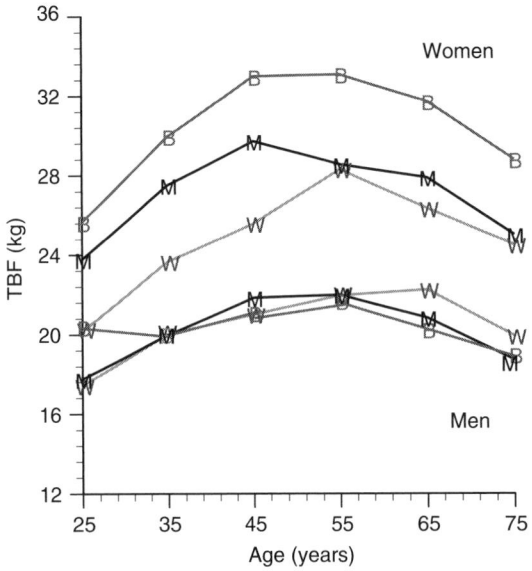

FIGURE 32.3 Estimated means for total body fat (TBF) by 10-year age groups from 20 to 80 years for non-Hispanic white (W), non-Hispanic black (B), and Mexican-American (M) men and women.

Because of the challenges of collecting such data from sufficient numbers of obese individuals, epidemiological and national obesity prevalence data are not based completely on actual measures of body fatness. It is also difficult to monitor and treat obesity without a commonly accepted assessment method or index and a reference population. There is no universally accepted method of clearly measuring body fatness or quantifying overweight and obesity. Current body composition analysis is hampered by problems of nonuniversal assumptions, limited by the application of methodology, or affected by chronic disease or subject size and performance, and these are special problems for the obese patient.

It is important in interpreting results from any body composition assessment to recognize its limitations. Direct assessments have an error of about 2 to 3% body fat at best when compared with corresponding results from other direct methods. With indirect methods, an error of about 5% body fat is expected, and an error of 5 to 10% is more realistic for predicted body composition. In addition, many assessments use technology and software that are proprietary to a manufacturer. Basic understanding of this technology is important, as is understanding the accuracy and reliability of the equipment; these equipment details are frequently available only from the manufacturer and should be evaluated critically.

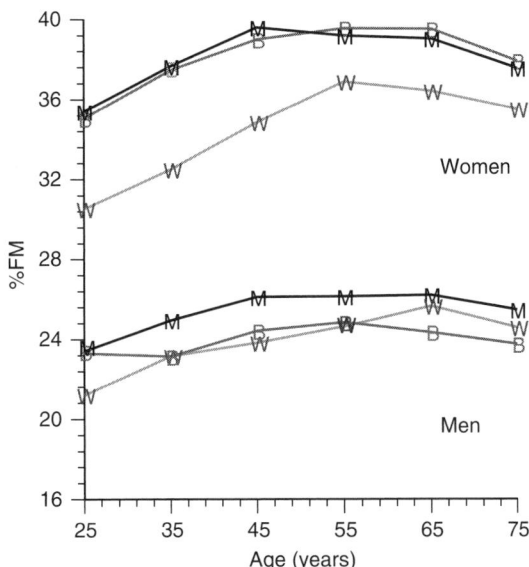

FIGURE 32.4 Estimated means for %FM by 10-year age groups from 20 to 80 years for non-Hispanic white (W), non-Hispanic black (B), and Mexican-American (M) men and women.

CONCLUSION

Researchers and clinicians currently have the ability to assess body composition in a variety of ways. Direct and some indirect methods are impractical for most clinical examinations or community studies because of the scarcity of equipment and testing centers. CT and MRI are used to image the total body or specific body parts for the presence of pathology, disease, or injury. These methods can be used to quantify body fat and lean tissue amounts with multiple exposures and specific software. However, this use is frequently limited due to other clinical needs for these instruments. DXA machines are commonly utilized for both clinical diagnosis and in large community-based studies. Although DXA examinations are conducted clinically, the methodology is practical for both the patient and the testing center. Estimating body composition through prediction equations is the easiest for the patient or study participant and works fairly well for population trends, but is not always the best estimate for an individual. When choosing the most appropriate body composition assessment method for a particular study, the characteristics of the patient population should be balanced with equipment needs and availability, and appropriate interpretations of the results.

ACKNOWLEDGMENTS

This work was supported by the following National Institutes of Health (Bethesda, MD) grants: HD12252, HL072838, HL069995, DK071485 (Dr. Chumlea), HD12252, and DK064482 (Dr. Remsberg).

REFERENCES

1. Roche AF, Heymsfield SB, Lohman TG, *Human Body Composition*, Human Kinetics Books, Champaign, IL, 1996, 366.
2. Lohman TG, *Advances in Body Composition Assessment*, Human Kinetics Publishers, Champaign, IL, 523, 1992.
3. Heymsfield SB, Lohman TG, Wang Z, *Human Body Composition*, 2nd, Human Kinetics Press, Champaign, IL, 160, 2005.
4. Khaled MA, Lukaski HC, Watkins CL, *Am J Clin Nutr* 45: 1; 1987.
5. Rebouche CJ, Pearson GA, Serfass RE, et al., *Am J Clin Nutr* 45: 373; 1987.
6. Cheek D, *J Ped* 58: 103; 1961.
7. Vaisman N, Pencharz P, Koren G, et al., *Am J Clin Nutr* 46: 1; 1987.
8. Chumlea WC, Guo SS, Zeller CM, et al., *Kidn Intl* 59: 2250; 2001.
9. Siri W, *Techniques for Measuring Body Composition*, Henschel A ed., National Academy Press, Washington DC, 1961, 223.
10. Demerath EW, Guo SS, Chumlea WC, et al., *Int J Obes & Relat Disor* 26: 389; 2002.
11. McCrory MA, Gomez TD, Bernauer EM, et al., *Med Sci Sports Exerc* 27: 1686; 1995.
12. Dempster P, Aitkens S, *Med Sci Sports Exerc* 27: 1692; 1995.
13. Brozek J, Grande F, Anderson J, et al., *Ann NY Acad Sci* 110: 113; 1963.
14. Guo SS, Chumlea WC, Roche AF, et al., *Int J Obes & Relat Disor* 21: 1167; 1997.
15. Lohman TG, *Exerc Sport Sci Rev* 14: 325; 1986.

16. Sun SS, Chumlea WC, Heymsfield SB, et al., *Am J Clin Nutr* 77: 331; 2003.
17. Lukaski HC, Johnson PE, Bolonchuk WW, et al., *Am J Clin Nutr* 41: 810; 1985.
18. Chumlea WC, Guo SS, *Nutr Rev* 52: 123; 1994.
19. Chumlea WC, Sun SS, *Human Body Composition*, Heymsfield SB, Lohman TG, Wang Z, et al. eds., Human Kinetics Publishers Champaign IL, 2005, 79.
20. Hanai T, *Emulsion Science*, Sherman P ed., Academic Press, London, 354, 1968.
21. MacDonald J, *Impedance Spectroscopy*, John Wiley & Sons, New York, 616, 1987.
22. Van Loan M, Withers P, Mattie J, et al., *Human Body Composition: In Vivo Methods, Models, and Assessment*, Ellis K, Eastman J eds., Plenum Publishers, New York, 1993, 67.
23. De Lorenzo A, Andreoli A, Matthie J, et al., *J Appl Physiol* 82: 1542; 1997.
24. Van Loan MD, Strawford A, Jacob M, et al., *Aids* 13: 241; 1999.
25. Van Loan M, Koop L, King J, et al., *J Appl Physiol* 78: 1037; 1995.
26. Gray DS, Bray GA, Gemayel N, et al., *Am J Clin Nutr* 50: 255; 1989.
27. Kushner RF, Kunigk A, Alspaugh M, et al., *Am J Clin Nutr* 52: 219; 1990.
28. Binkley N, Kiebzak GM, Lewiecki EM, et al., *J Bone Miner Res* 20: 195; 2005.
29. Kohrt WM, *Med Sci Sports Exerc* 27: 1349; 1995.
30. Roubenoff R, Kehayias JJ, Dawson-Hughes B, et al., *Am J Clin Nutr* 58: 589; 1993.
31. Schoeller DA, Tylavsky FA, Baer DJ, et al., *Am J Clin Nutr* 81: 1018; 2005.
32. Guo SS, Wisemandle WA, Tyleshevski F, et al., *J Health Nutr Aging* 1: 29; 1997.
33. Tataranni PA, Ravussin E, *Am J Clin Nutr* 62: 730; 1995.
34. Jebb SA, Goldberg GR, Jennings G, et al., *Human Body Composition: In Vivo Methods, Models and Assessment*, Ellis K, Eastman J eds., Plenum Press, New York, 1993, 129.
35. Jebb SA, Goldberg GR, Jennings G, et al., *Clin Sci (Lond)* 88: 319; 1995.
36. Rossner S, Bo WJ, Hiltbrandt E, et al., *Int J Obes* 14: 893; 1990.
37. Ross R, Leger L, Morris D, et al., *J Appl Physiol* 72: 787; 1992.
38. Foster MA, Hutchison JM, Mallard JR, et al., *Magn Reson Imaging* 2: 187; 1984.
39. Abate N, Burns D, Peshock RM, et al., *J Lipid Res* 35: 1490; 1994.
40. Seidell JC, Bakker CJ, van der Kooy K, *Am J Clin Nutr* 51: 953; 1990.
41. Fowler PA, Fuller MF, Glasbey CA, et al., *Am J Clin Nutr* 54: 18; 1991.
42. Sun SS, Chumlea WC, The body cell mass and its supporting environment in: *Human Body Composition*, Heymsfield SSB, Lohman TTG, Wang Z, et al. eds., Human Kinetics Publishers Champaign IL, 2005, 151.
43. Lohman TG, Caballero B, Himes JH, et al., *Int J Obes Relat Metab Disord* 24: 982; 2000.
44. Wagner DR, Heyward VH, Kocina PS, et al., *Med Sci Sports Exerc* 29: 969; 1997.
45. Chumlea WC, Guo SS, Kuczmarski RJ, et al., *Int J Obes & Relat Disor* 1596; 2002.
46. Moore FD, W B Saunders Company, Philadelphia–London, 1963.

33 Height, Weight, and Body Mass Index in Childhood

Christine L. Williams and Mary Horlick

CONTENTS

INTRODUCTION

In childhood, height (stature) and weight are the two most frequently used measures of growth and nutritional status. In addition, indices of weight for height, especially BMI, are used as a proxy for body fatness or obesity. As growth is the most sensitive indicator of overall health in childhood, it is essential that accurate measurements be made on a regular basis during routine health supervision of children and adolescents to identify and address significant deviations in a timely manner.

Pediatric health professionals take two basic anthropometric measurements on each child: *recumbent length* (for children *under* 2 years of age) or *standing height* (for children *over* 2 years of age), and *weight*. From these two measurements, *body mass index (BMI)* can be derived from a reference chart or calculated by formula. This chapter will focus on these measures: height (or length), weight, and BMI. For each measurement the following aspects will be discussed: definition, normal patterns of change, measurement techniques, and interpretation of values using reference growth charts. As most practicing pediatricians in the United States, as well as other health professionals who care for children, record their measurements in inches and pounds, these units will be used in the discussion.

HEIGHT

DESCRIPTION

Height, or stature, is a linear measure from the base on which the child is standing to the firm top of the child's head. Height is measured in children over 2 years of age. It is measured with the child standing with erect posture and without shoes. From birth to 2 years of age, the infant or toddler's stature is measured as recumbent length. This is the total length of the child-from the bottom of the feet (positioned at a 90° angle) to the top of the head. Recumbent length is slightly greater than standing height measured in the same individual.

NORMAL PATTERNS OF LINEAR GROWTH IN CHILDHOOD

Normal changes in height (or length): During the first year of life, babies increase in recumbent length about 10 in. on average, from about 20 in. at birth to 30 in. by their first birthday. During the second year of life their length increases by 4 to 5 in., or about ⅓ in./month. After age 2 years, height is measured in the standing position. Growth continues at a slower but steady rate of about 2½ in./year until about the age of 11 in girls and 13 in boys, when the growth spurt associated with puberty usually begins. Puberty is characterized by a greater rate of growth, culminating in a peak height velocity (inches grown per year) comparable to the rate of growth during the second year of life. The peak height velocity for girls is about 2 ½ to 4 ½ in./year, and for boys is about 3 to 5 in./year. For both boys and girls, however, puberty and the pubertal "growth spurt" may occur several years earlier or later than average and still be within a normal range. Normal growth stops when the growing ends of the bones fuse, which usually occurs between 14 and 16 years of age for girls and between 16 and 18 years of age for boys.

Normal Growth Rates during Childhood and Adolescence

	Growth Rate (per Year)	
Age	Inches (in.)	Centimeters (cm)
0–1 year	7–10	18–25
1–2 years	4–5	10–13
2 years to puberty	2–2 ½	5–6
Girls: Pubertal growth spurt	2 ½–4 ½	6–11
Boys: Pubertal growth spurt	3–5	7–13

MEASURING LENGTH

The stature of subjects less than 2 years of age is measured as recumbent length. This is done most accurately with a measuring "box" or "board" that has an inflexible headpiece against which the top of the head is positioned, and a moveable footboard against which the feet are placed at a 90° angle. If possible, the child should be relaxed, the legs should be fully extended, and the head should be positioned so that a line connecting the outer margin of the eyes with the ears is at a 90° angle with the bottom of the measuring box. Recumbent length is measured from the top of the head to the bottom of the feet. It should be measured to the nearest quarter inch and recorded in the child's chart. Measurement of recumbent length on an examining table without a "box" should also be from the top of the head to the bottom of the feet, which are positioned at a 90° angle. It is recommended that the same examiner measure the child at each visit to minimize interexaminer variability.

Because recumbent length is slightly greater than standing height, it is recommended that measurements of both length and height be obtained for two visits between 2 and 3 years of age. With these simultaneous recumbent length and standing height values, measurement discrepancy can be distinguished from actual change in growth rate.

MEASURING HEIGHT

The height of subjects older than 2 years of age is measured, without shoes, with a stadiometer. A stadiometer consists of a measuring tape affixed to a vertical surface, such as a wall or a rigid free-standing measuring device, and a movable block, attached to the vertical surface at a right angle, which can be brought down to the crown of the head. In the absence of a stadiometer, height can be measured on a platform scale, but this is less accurate than the stadiometer. In either case, the subject should stand with heels together and back as straight as possible; the heels, buttocks, shoulders, and head should touch the wall or the vertical surface of the measuring device. The weight of the subject is distributed evenly on both feet and the head is positioned in the horizontal plane. The arms hang freely by the sides with the palms facing the thighs. The subject should be asked to inhale deeply and maintain a fully erect position. The examiner positions the movable block until it touches the head, applying sufficient pressure to compress the hair. The height marker is read while pressing firmly on the headpiece. The number on the height bar immediately behind the indicator line of the height marker is read. The examiner's eyes should look directly at the indicator line at about the same height in order to avoid parallax in reading the measurement. The height is measured to the nearest quarter inch, and then recorded on the child's chart. It is recommended that a second reading be taken to check accuracy.

Height has diurnal variation. Children are tallest in the morning, and shrink as much as a centimeter during the course of a day as the fibrous intervertebral cartilaginous disks are compressed. Diurnal variation in height is completely due to changes in the height of the vertebral column, and full height is regained when the child lies down flat for about 30 min.

Interpretation of Height Measurements

Depending on the statural genes that a child inherits from their parents, children tend to gravitate toward a specific percentile or channel of the reference length (or height) charts during the first 2 to 3 years of life. Thereafter, most children track close to that percentile or channel, maintaining a stable position relative to their peers.

Children who track consistently along the lowest height percentiles may have *familial short stature,* in which the parents are short and the child has inherited the same statural genes. Other short children may have *constitutionally delayed growth* characterized by a slower rate of growth in the first 2 to 3 years of life, followed by normal growth velocity that tracks along a height percentile or channel lower than expected for the family. These children often have later onset of puberty and its accompanying growth spurt, as well as a parent who followed a similar pattern of growth as a child. Final adult height is generally appropriate for parental height expectations.

Children who decelerate in linear growth and shift gradually downward to a lower percentile deserve medical evaluation. Poor linear growth may reflect inadequate nutrition, an underlying disease affecting a major organ system, or a genetic abnormality. Children whose linear growth accelerates and shifts upward to a higher percentile also deserve medical evaluation. Increased rate of linear growth may reflect overnutrition, early or precocious onset of puberty, or another endocrine or genetic abnormality.

Reference Charts for Height (and Length)

Growth charts are simple grids that are used to plot out a child's height according to age and sex. Pediatric health professionals should measure and plot height on a growth chart at every visit, at least every 6 months before school age and annually thereafter. Growth charts are derived from the heights of large numbers of healthy children of all ages, separating the wide ranges of normal heights into percentiles by statistical techniques. The spaces between the percentile lines are called channels. Age in years is plotted along the horizontal axis at the bottom of the chart and height in inches (or centimeters) is plotted along the vertical axis on the left of the chart. The 50th percentile, representing the average height for a given age, is drawn as a heavy line. Growth charts are commonly drawn for values between the 5th and 95th or 3rd and 97th percentiles of the population distribution values.

In 2000 the Center for Disease Control (CDC) published 16 growth charts for boys and girls from birth to 20 years, a revision of the 1977 National Center for Health Statistics (NCHS) growth charts for ages from birth to 17 years, using new national survey data and improved statistical smoothing procedures. The CDC revision includes charts for plotting linear growth including length-for-age (birth to 36 months) and stature-for-age (2 to 20 years) (Figure 33.1 to Figure 33.4). The World Health Organization is developing new international growth standards for birth to 5 years using data from a large sample of breast-fed infants; however, the current and available CDC 2000 infant charts represent the ethnically and geographically diverse population of the United States with both breast- and formula-fed infants included. These charts may be downloaded from the CDC Web site: http://ww.cdc.gov/growthcharts.

WEIGHT

Description

Body *weight* is a measure of body mass, which is a composite of each contributing tissue (e.g., fat, muscle, bone, etc.). Although weight should ideally be measured without clothing, this is often impractical. Most commonly, weight is measured with the child in underwear only or in light indoor clothing, without shoes.

Normal Patterns of Weight Gain in Childhood

Newborn infants commonly double their birth weight by 6 months of age, and triple it by their first birthday. Boys on average increase from 8 lb at birth to 23 lb at 1 year; while girls on average increase from slightly less than 8 lb at birth to 21 lb at age 1 year. From 1 to 2 years of age, toddlers who are tracking along the 50th percentile for weight gain about 5 to 6 lb, or about ½ lb/month, and during the third year of life weight gain averages about 4 lb. Children tracking along higher percentiles gain more, and those tracking on the lower percentiles gain proportionately less.

Measurement Techniques

Weight should be measured in the clinical setting using a standard balance beam scale with moveable weights or with an instrument of equivalent accuracy. It is recommended that the scale be calibrated at least monthly using standard weights. It is preferable to

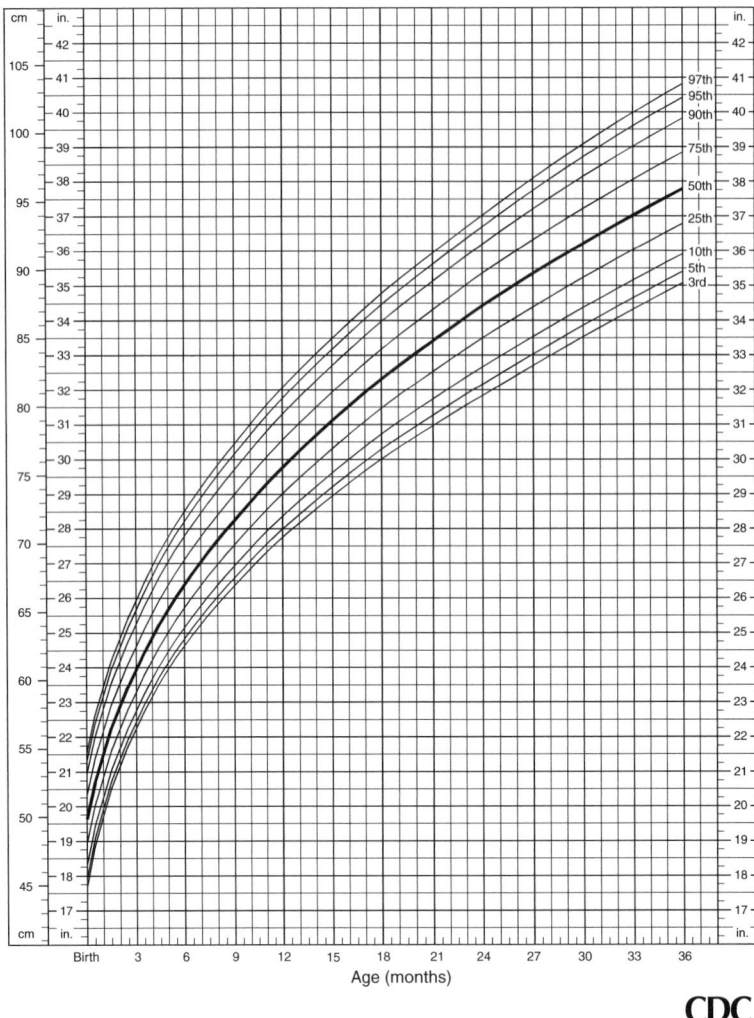

FIGURE 33.1 Length-for-age percentiles: boys, birth to 36 months.

weigh the child without clothing, or in light indoor clothing, but the child's shoes and heavy outer clothing should be removed. With older children, heavy belts and other items carried in their pockets should be removed. The beam of the platform scale must be graduated so that it can be read from both sides. The subject stands still over the center of the platform with body weight evenly distributed between both feet. Weight is recorded to the nearest quarter pound.

Weight, like height, has diurnal variation. In contrast to height, however, weight is lowest in the morning after emptying the bladder, and increases gradually through the day, depending on diet and physical activity.

INTERPRETATION OF WEIGHT MEASUREMENTS

Body weight and patterns of weight gain and adiposity in childhood are the result of gene–environment interactions. A child's genotype reflects the genes inherited from his or her parents. The phenotype expressed, however, with respect to body weight and fatness, is also heavily influenced by environmental factors such as diet and physical activity. Most children gravitate toward a specific percentile curve of the standard weight charts during the first few years of life. However, in the present situation of increasing prevalence of childhood obesity in the United States, it is not uncommon for children's weights to gradually cross upward across percentiles, rather than maintaining a consistent percentile position relative to their peers. It is recommended that body weight, height, and calculated BMI values all be monitored carefully during routine health supervision so that children and adolescents who begin to deviate from normal growth patterns may receive further evaluation and treatment.

Children's weight percentile may be similar to their height percentile, or may be somewhat above or below and still be "normal" or healthy if their BMI is below the 85th percentile for age.

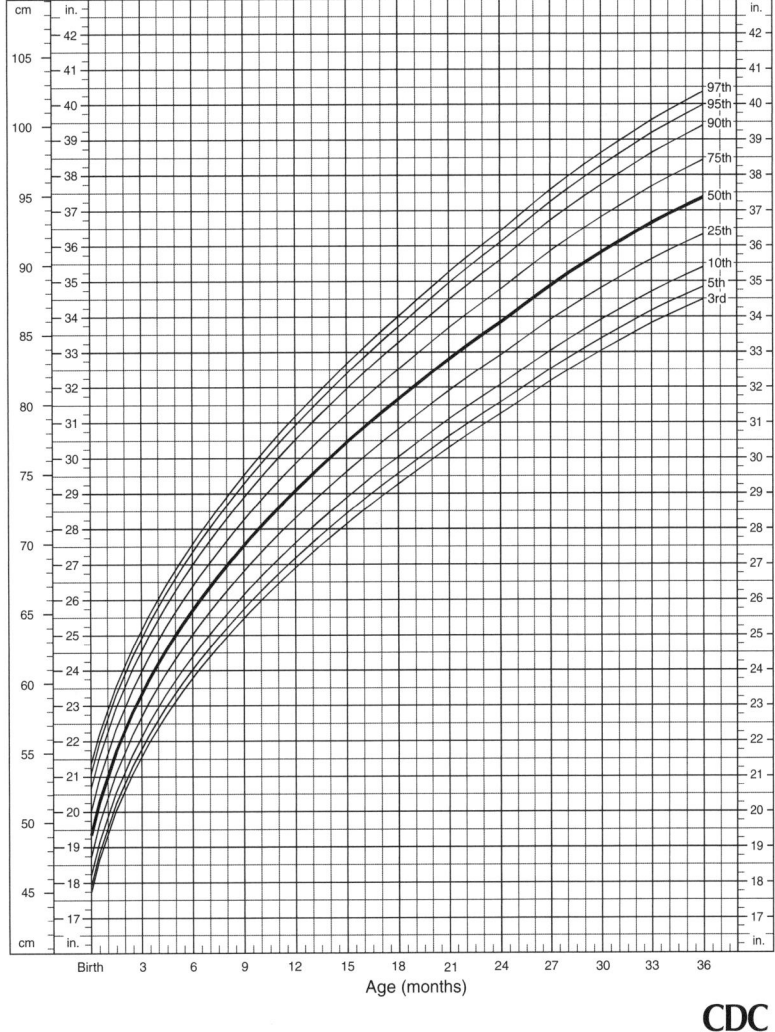

FIGURE 33.2   Length-for-age percentiles: girls, birth to 36 months.

Healthy children who consistently track along the lower weight percentiles throughout childhood are considered normal if their weight is proportionate to their height (close to the same percentile) and consistent with parental heights and weights

Children whose weight gains decelerate and shift downward to a lower percentile, or who actually lose weight (with the exception of overweight children on medically supervised treatment), should be medically evaluated to determine the cause. Poor weight gain or unexplained weight loss may reflect inadequate nutrition, an eating disorder, an underlying disease affecting a major organ system, depression, or other psychological problems.

Overweight children who are placed on medically supervised treatment to either slow the rate of weight gain or lose weight should be carefully monitored to ensure adequate intake of (a) essential nutrients through a balanced calorie-controlled diet and (b) calories to maintain linear growth throughout treatment.

REFERENCE CHARTS FOR WEIGHT

Weight charts, similar to height charts, are available to plot a child's weight according to age and sex. Weight charts are also constructed from the weights of large numbers of healthy children of all ages, separating the wide range of weights into percentiles by statistical techniques. As for the height charts, the spaces between percentile lines are called channels. Age in years is plotted along the horizontal axis at the bottom of the chart and weight in pounds (or kilograms) is plotted along the vertical axis on the left of the chart. The 50th percentile, representing the average weight for a given age, is drawn as a heavy line. Weight charts most commonly provide percentile channels between the 5th and 95th percentile, but are also available now for a distribution between the 3rd and 97th percentiles.

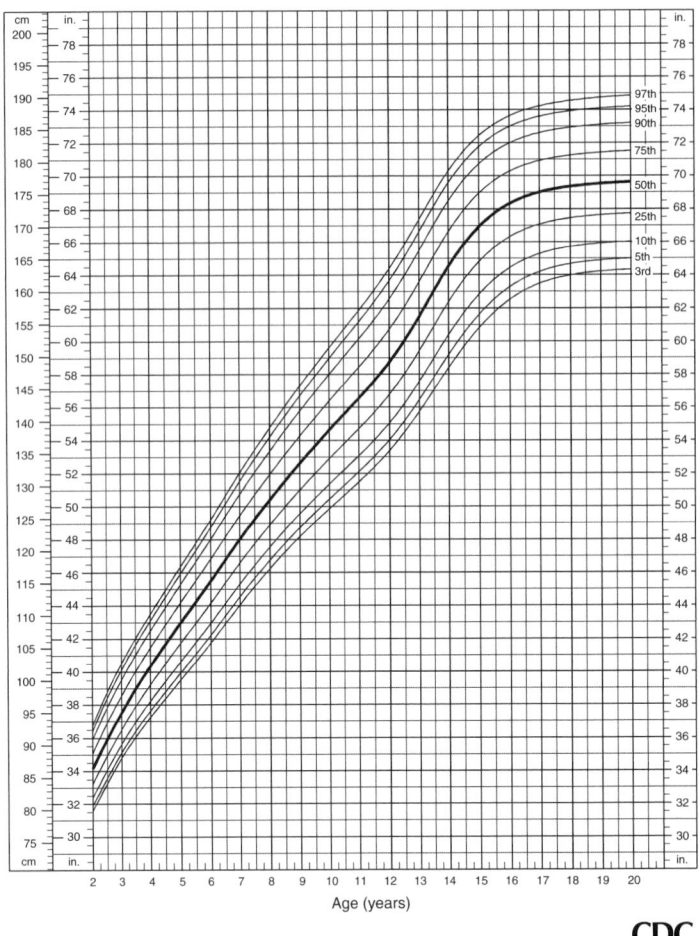

FIGURE 33.3 Stature-for-age percentiles: boys, 2 to 20 years.

The CDC 2000 Growth Charts for boys and girls from birth to 20 years include charts for weight. The process of revision of the 1977 National Center for Health Statistics (NCHS) growth charts included opinions from experts on how to resolve the issue of the increase in overweight observed in the new national survey data. The Growth Charts for weight-for-age (birth to 36 months and 2 to 20 years), weight-for-length (birth to 36 months), and weight-for-stature (77 to 121 cm) for boys and girls may be downloaded from the CDC Web site (see Figure 33.5 to Figure 33.12): http://ww.cdc.gov/growthcharts.

BODY MASS INDEX

BODY MASS INDEX

Body Mass Index, or BMI (weight/height^2), provides a guideline based on weight and height to determine underweight or overweight status. BMI is not an exact measure of fatness because levels of fatness vary among children at a given BMI. This is so because BMI reflects (1) frame size, (2) leg length, and (3) the amount of lean and fat tissue. Although BMI correlates less well with the percent of body weight that is fat than more direct measures of fat such as triceps skin-fold thickness or other body composition techniques, the readily available weight and height data make BMI a more useful tool for clinical assessment of overweight or underweight.

BMI in children and adolescents compares well with laboratory measurements of body fat. Children and adolescents with a BMI-for-age above the 95th percentile are classified as overweight. BMI values above the 95th percentile applied as a definition of overweight in children and adolescents (1) reflects adiposity, (2) is consistent across age groups, and (3) is predictive of morbidity.

The percentage of children and adolescents who are overweight in the United States has more than tripled since the 1960s, and the sharpest increase has occurred in the last 15 to 20 years, since the late 1980s. Currently, among 6- to 17-year-old youth, about 16% are overweight (BMI >95th percentile reference value), and an additional 16% are "at-risk" of overweight (BMI 85th to <95th percentile).

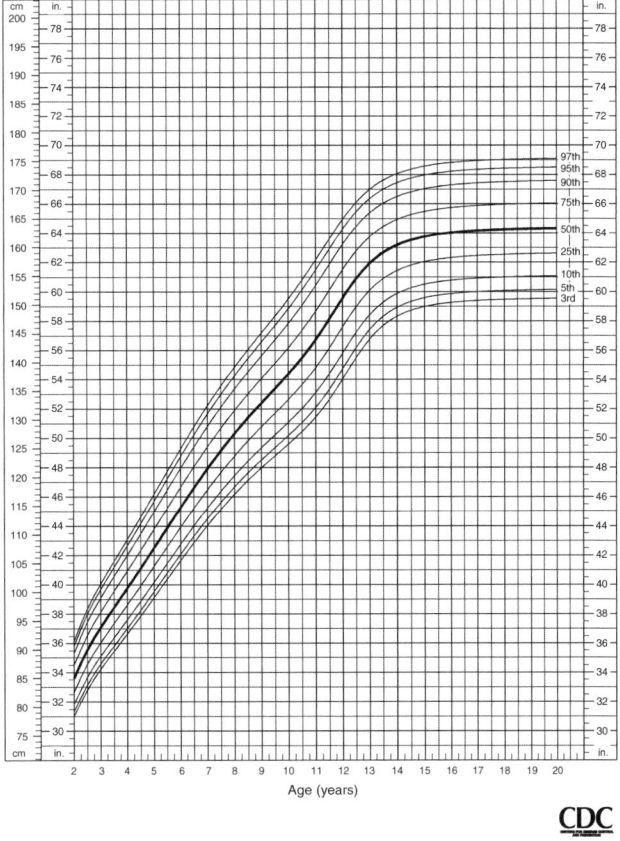

FIGURE 33.4 Stature-for-age percentiles: girls, 2 to 20 years.

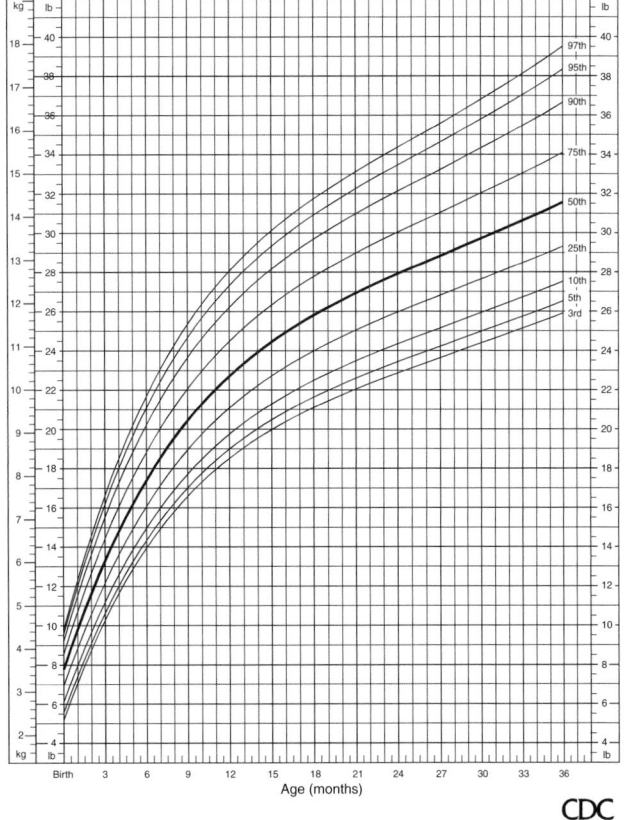

FIGURE 33.5 Weight-for-age percentiles: boys, birth to 36 months.

The rationale for proposing a pediatric BMI classification is based on studies indicating that BMI is related to health risks. Overweight children are likely to become overweight adults, with risk increasing with severity and duration of the problem. Sixty percent of youth with a BMI-for-age above the 95th percentile have at least one risk factor for cardiovascular disease, while 20% have two or more risk factors. High blood pressure, abnormal blood lipid levels (elevated total cholesterol, low-density lipoprotein [LDL] cholesterol, and/or triglycerides; and low levels high-density lipoprotein [HDL] cholesterol), insulin resistance, and type II diabetes mellitus are some of the risk factors observed in overweight children and adolescents. Overweight children are also at increased risk of a wide range of other medical and psychological problems.

NORMAL PATTERNS OF BMI DURING CHILDHOOD AND ADOLESCENCE

For U.S. children, BMI increases rapidly during the first year of life, and then decreases to its lowest value on average between 4 and 6 years of age. After reaching this nadir, BMI again begins a slow increase throughout the rest of childhood and adolescence. The upward shift of the BMI curve, after reaching the lowest point, has been termed "adiposity rebound." Studies suggest that children who begin their adiposity rebound earlier than average are at greater risk for being overweight as older adolescents and young adults.

MEASUREMENT OF BMI

BMI, also known as the weight–height index or Quetelet index, is calculated as the quotient of weight divided by height squared:
The *English formula* (in inches and pounds) is as follows:

$$\text{Weight in pounds} \div \text{Height in inches} \div \text{Height in inches} \times 703 = \text{BMI}$$

The *metric formula* (in meters and kilograms) is as follows:

$$\text{Weight in kilograms} \div \text{Height in meters} \div \text{Height in meters} = \text{BMI}$$

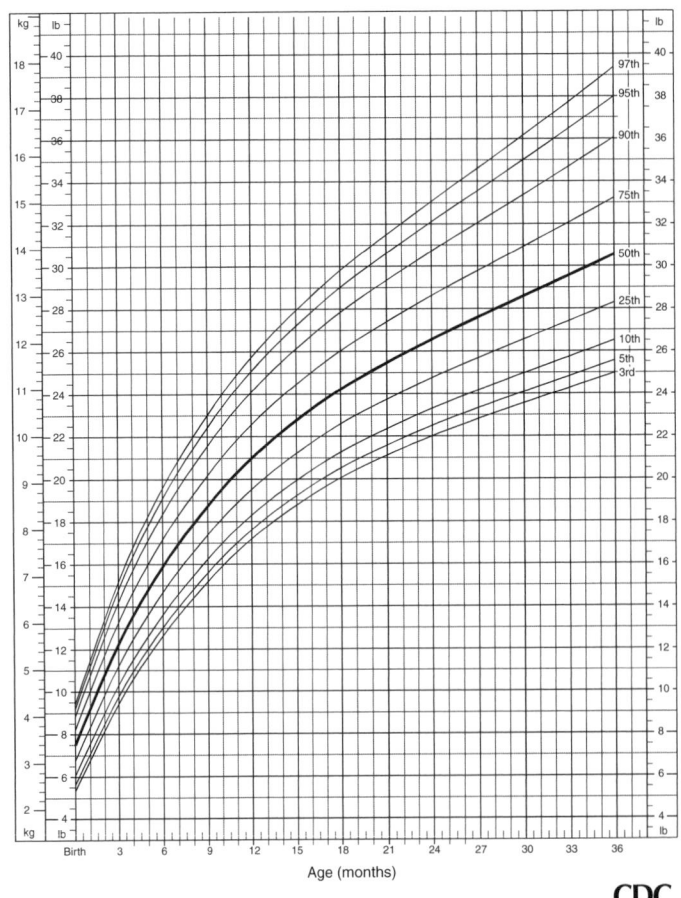

FIGURE 33.6   Weight-for-age percentiles: girls, birth to 36 months.

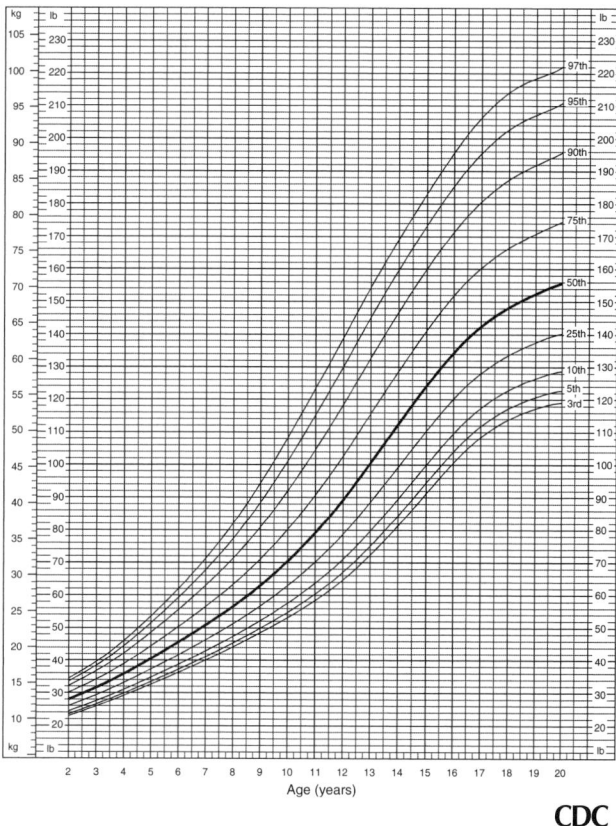

FIGURE 33.7 Weight-for-age percentiles: boys, 2 to 20 years.

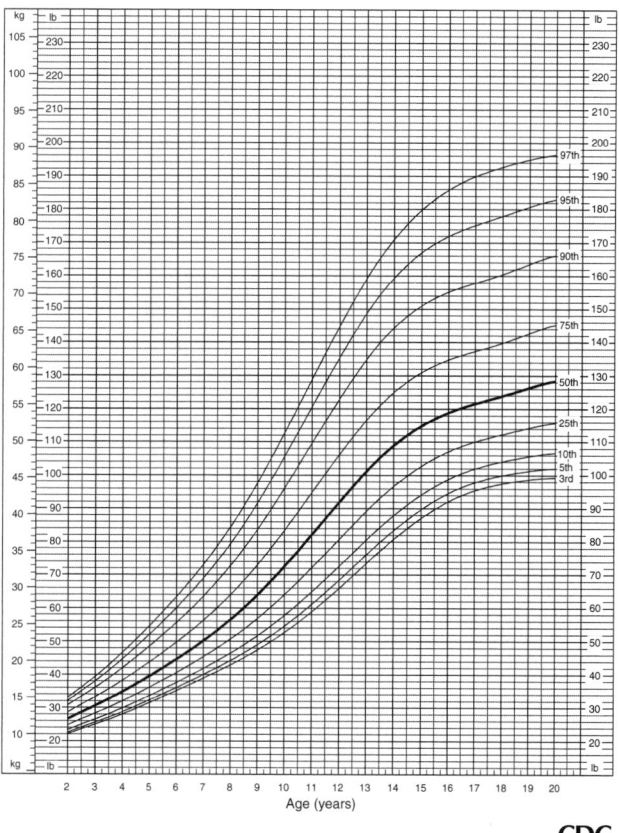

FIGURE 33.8 Weight-for-age percentiles: girls, 2 to 20 years.

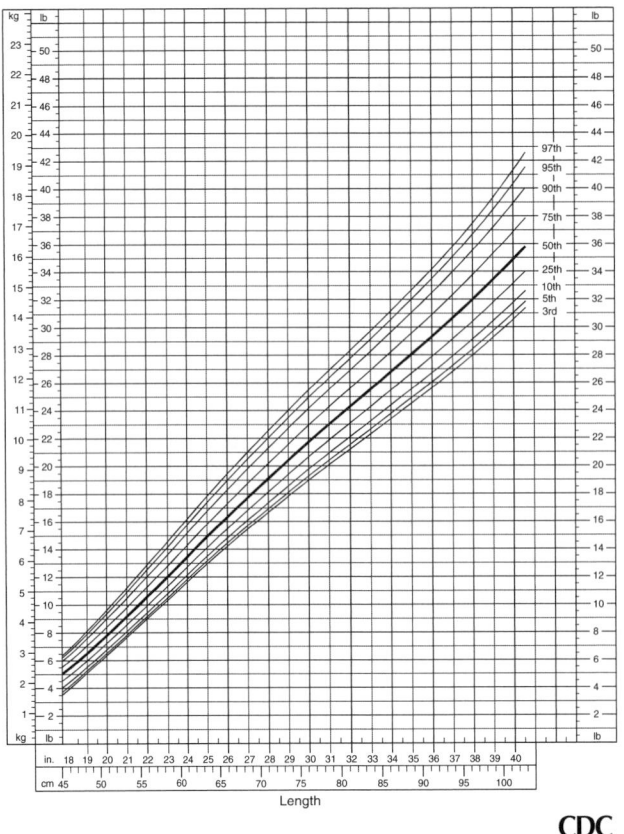

FIGURE 33.9   Weight-for-length percentiles: boys, birth to 36 months.

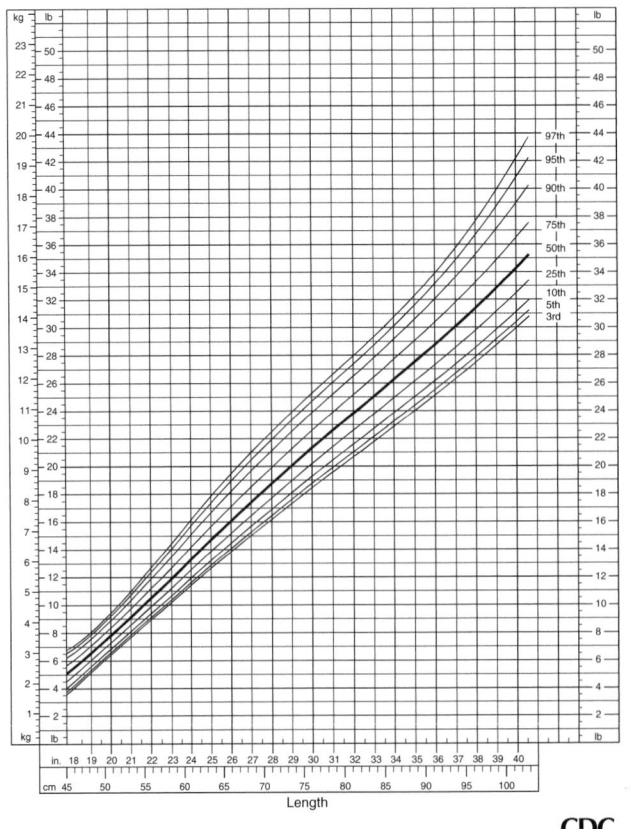

FIGURE 33.10   Weight-for-length percentiles: girls, birth to 36 months.

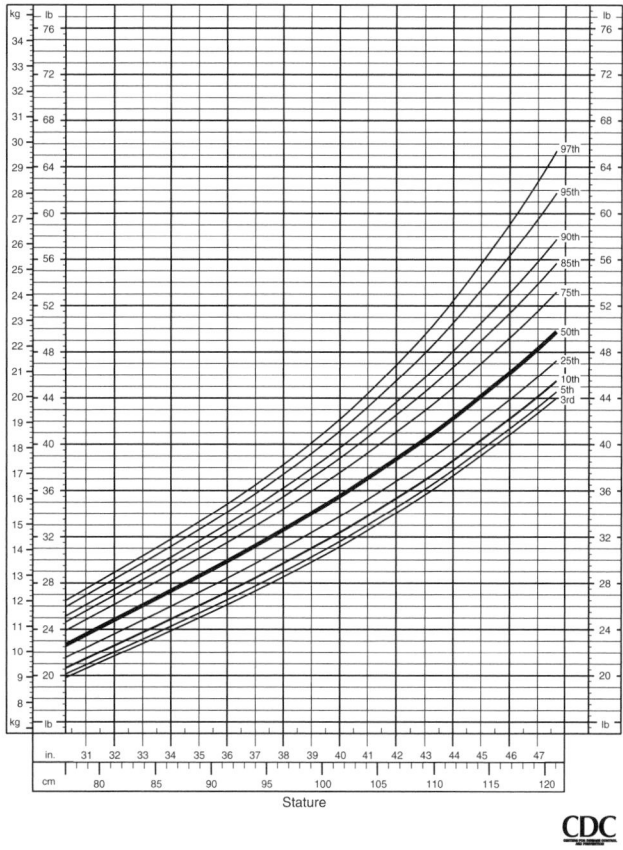

FIGURE 33.11   Weight-for-stature percentiles: boys.

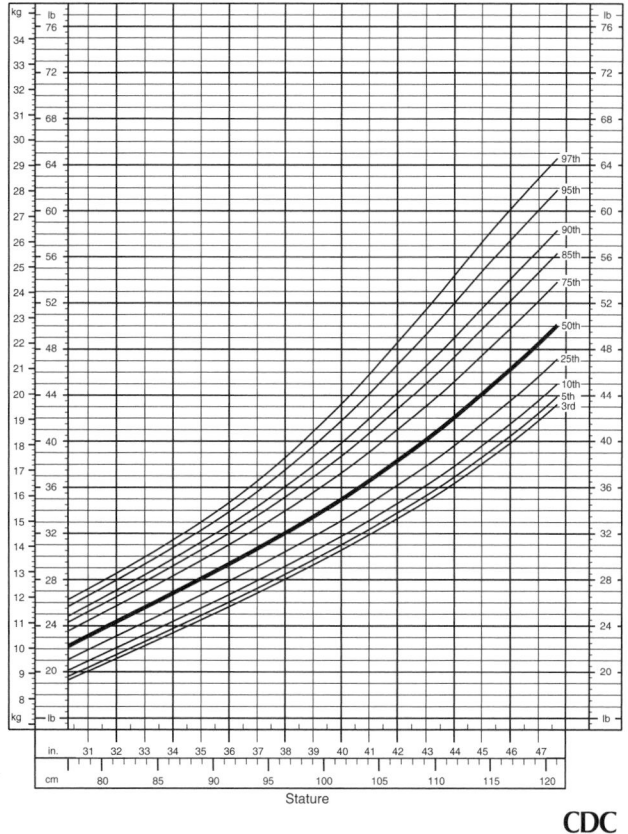

FIGURE 33.12   Weight-for-stature percentiles: girls.

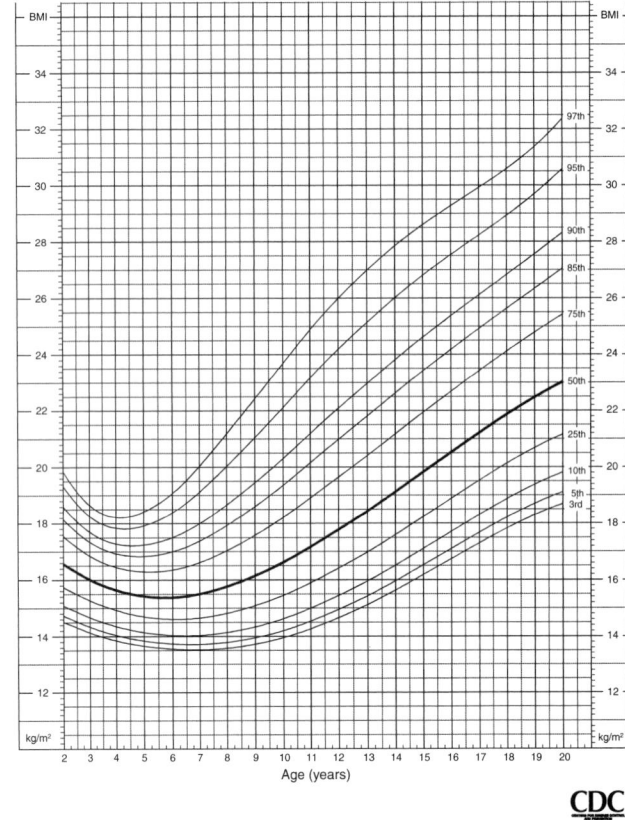

FIGURE 33.13   Body mass index-for-age percentiles: boys, 2 to 20 years.

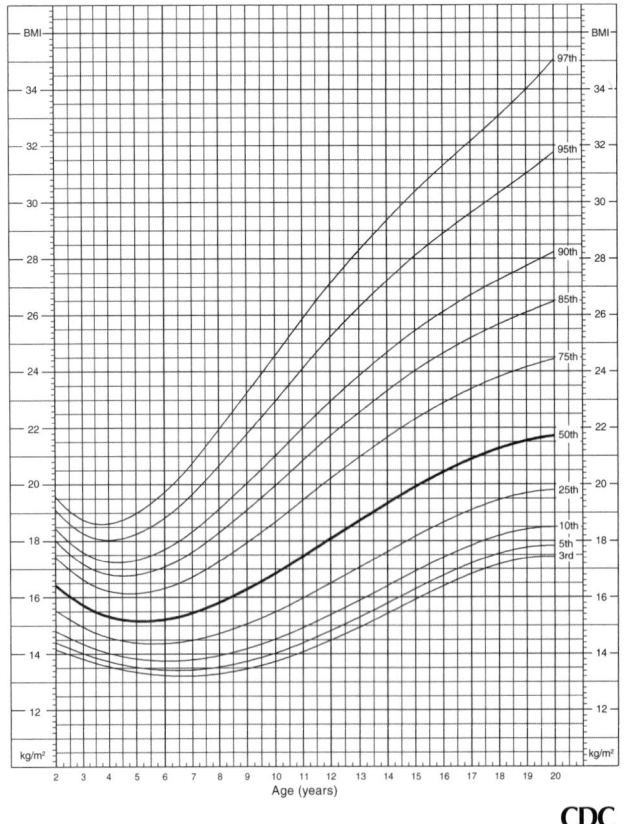

FIGURE 33.14   Body mass index-for-age percentiles: girls, 2 to 20 years.

INTERPRETATION OF BMI VALUES

Interpretation of BMI depends on the sex and age of the child, as boys and girls differ in their body fatness as they mature. Therefore, BMI is plotted on age- and sex-specific charts. Established cutoff points are used to identify children and adolescents who are underweight or overweight. BMI values that should raise clinical concern are the following:

Underweight	BMI-for-age <5th percentile
"At-Risk" of Overweight	BMI-for-age 85th to <95th percentile
Overweight	BMI-for-age ≥95th percentile

REFERENCE CHARTS FOR BMI

The Center for Disease Control (CDC) has published BMI-for-age charts; one for boys, ages 2 to 20 years, and another for girls, 2 to 20 years of age (Figure 33.13 and Figure 33.14). These charts may be downloaded from the CDC Web site: http://www. cdc.gov/nccdphp/dnpa/bmi-for-age.htm. In addition, from the same site, a CDC Table for Calculated Body Mass Index Values for Selected Heights and Weights for Ages 2 to 20 Years may also be downloaded. Clinicians can avoid having to calculate BMI values by using this extensive set of tables covering heights from 29 to 78 in. and weights from 18 to 250 lb.

FURTHER READING

Barlow SE, Dietz WH. Obesity evaluation and treatment: Expert committee recommendations. *J Ped* 1998;102(3):e29.

Deschamps l, Desleuz JF, Machinot S et al. Effects of diet and weight loss on plasma glucose, Insulin, and free fatty acids in obese children. *Ped Res* 1978;12:757–760.

Dietz WH, Bellizzi MC. Introduction: The use of BMI to assess obesity in children. *Am J Clin Nutr* 1999;70(suppl):123s–125s.

Dietz WH. Health consequences of obesity in youth: Childhood predictors of adult disease. *Pediatrics* 1998;101:518–525.

Freedman DS et al. The relation of overweight to cardiovascular risk factors among children and adolescents: The Bogalusa Heart Study. *Pediatrics* 1999;103:1175–1182.

Gam SM. Continuities and changes In fatness from infancy through adulthood. *Curr Prob Ped* 1985;15:1–47.

Guo SS, Chumlea WC. Tracking of BMI In children in relation to overweight in adulthood. *Am J Clin Nutr* 1999;70(suppl): 145s–148s.

Guo SS et al. The predictive value of childhood BMI values for overweight at age 35 years. *Am J Clin Nutr* 1994:59:810–819.

Guo SS, Khoury PR, Sprecker B. Prediction of fat-free mass in black and white preadolescent girls from anthropometry and impedance. *Am J Human Biol* 1993;5:735–745.

Gutin B, Basch C, Shea S et al. Blood pressure, fitness, and fatness in 5- and 6-year-old children. *JAMA* 1990;264:1123–1127.

Himes JH, Deitz WH. Guidelines for overweight in adolescent preventive services: recommendations form an expert committee. *Am J Clin Nutr* 1994;59:307–316.

Kelsey JL, Acheson RM, Keggi KJ. The body build of patients with slipped capital femoral epiphysis. *Am J Dis Child* 1972;124:276–281.

Kuczmarski RJ, Ogden CL, Grummer-Strawn LM et al. CDC growth charts: United States. Advance data from vital statistics; no. 314. National Center for Health Statistics, 2000.

Lazarus R et al. BMI in screening for adiposity in children and adolescents: Systematic evaluation using receiver operator curves. *Am J Clin Nutr* 1996;63:500–506.

Morrison JA, Payne G, Barton BA, Khoury PR, Crawford P. Mother-daughter correlations of obesity and cardiovascular disease risk factors in black and white households: the NHLBI Growth anf Health Study. *AJPH* 1994;84:1761–1767.

Ogden CL, Kuczmarski RJ, Flegal KM et al. Centers for Disease Control and Prevention 2000 Growth Charts for the United States: Improvements to the 1977 National Center for Health Statistics Version. Pediatrics 2002;109:45–60

Parra A, Schultz RS, Graystone JE et al. Correlative studies in obese children and adolescents concerning body composition and plasma Insulin and growth hormone levels. *Ped Res* 1971;5:606–613.

Pietrobelli A, Faith M, Allison DB, Gallagher D, Chiumello G, Heymsfeld SB. Body Mass Index as a measure of adiposity among children and adolescents: A validation study. *J Ped* 1998;132:204–210.

Rames LK, Clark WR, Connor WE et al. Normal blood pressures and the evaluation of sustained blood pressure elevation in childhood: The Muscatine study. *Pediatrics* 1978;61:245–251.

Shear CL, Freedman DS, Burke GL et al. Body fat patterning and blood pressure in children and young adult — The Bogalusa Heart Study. *Hypertension* 1987;9:236–244.

Tracy W, De NC, Harper JR. Obesity and respiratory infection in infants and young children. *BMJ* 1971;1:16–18.

Whitaker RC, Pepe MS, Wright JA, Seidel KD, Dietz WH. Early adiposity rebound and the risk of adult obesity. Ped 998;101(5):URL: http://www.pediatrics.org/cgi/content,/full/101-3/e5.

34 Frame Size, Circumferences, and Skinfolds

Barbara J. Scott

CONTENTS

INTRODUCTION

Numerous studies conducted over the past 80 years provide a large body of knowledge and evidence that simple methods of quantifying body size and proportions can be used with different populations to estimate body composition and regional fat distribution. This chapter will discuss the strengths and weaknesses and potential best applications of three field anthropometric methods: frame size, skinfolds, and circumferences. These methods have been widely studied and are commonly used, because they yield valid and reliable results when applied correctly, they are noninvasive, inexpensive, portable, and relatively simple to perform.

APPLICATIONS TO PRACTICE

Important applications for the measurement and analysis of body composition and body dimensions using these methods include:

- Evaluating how individuals or groups are faring in general or in response to changing economic or political situations (new leadership, prolonged drought or famine, war, decreased expenditures for health services, increase in number of individuals or families living in poverty, increased cost of food, etc.)
- Monitoring individual response to specific therapeutic interventions (surgery, medication, chemotherapy etc.)
- Making comparisons of actual with "ideal" (weight for height (BMI), waist-to-hip circumference ratio, and level of body fatness etc.)
- Formulating exercise or dietary programs/regimens
- Providing prognostic indicators in certain disease states linked to body composition (diabetes, certain types of cancer, osteoporosis, cystic fibrosis, HIV/AIDS, etc.)
- Providing periodic feedback regarding achievement of goals resulting from lifestyle modifications (diet, exercise, smoking cessation, etc.)
- Assessing level of potential risk for (cardiovascular, cancer, diabetes, and osteoporosis) and monitoring relative risk over time

While more precise methods for measuring body composition, such as computed tomography (CT), magnetic resonance imaging (MRI), and dual-energy x-ray absorptiometry (DEXA), are becoming more available, indirect field methods will likely continue to be widely used as their selection is often dependent on practical considerations of cost, availability of equipment, staff (number of personnel and expertise), and portability. The degree of precision needed is also a factor in selection of the method to be used, and may be based on study sample size and purpose for which the information is being collected. For example, methods yielding less precision may be acceptable if the focus is on generalized risk assessment or documenting change in a diet or exercise program than if the information is needed for establishing health policy or making clinical decisions about disease treatment or prognosis. Ongoing research using more accurate reference methods to validate or refine equations for skinfold, frame size, and circumference measurements with different populations will provide clinicians with the necessary information and tools to continue using these practical methods with confidence.

There appears to be greater standardization of methodology in many of the body composition validation studies done over the past decade with greater adherence to and more detailed documentation of use of commonly accepted measurement protocols, inclusion of both a test and a validation sample in the study design, and use of similar statistical methods to examine results. With regards to the analysis of results, more studies are using what has become known as the Bland-Altman method whereby agreement between measurements is examined using a plot of the difference between methods against their mean.[1] This standardization should be helpful to clinicians and field researchers as they make decisions as to selection of the best methods to use in practice.

APPLICATION TO DIFFERENT POPULATIONS

Many variables have been found to affect the validity of measurements of body composition including age, gender, ethnicity, measurement site selection, weight status, and health status.[2] Therefore, it is imperative that methods selected are those that are best suited to the persons or population being measured or studied. Depending on the setting and application, it may be necessary to use different methods, different anatomical sites, or to apply different equations to the same methods. This is particularly critical, because the population in the United States and other countries has become more overweight and more ethnically diverse, and more people are living to be very old. Indeed, because so many of the longstanding prediction equations were developed on very homogenous samples, the preponderance of recent studies have been done to examine the validity of these existing prediction equations on specific population groups of interest (children, elderly, pregnant, overweight or obese persons, dialysis patients, Hispanic adults, etc.). Studies have been selected for summarization in this chapter to represent these diverse populations.

REFERENCE METHODS: "GOLD STANDARDS"

Many different methods have been employed over the past eight decades to measure the composition of the human body,[3] and new technological developments and findings from validation studies both inform and complicate decisions about which methods to select for a given purpose. A primary consideration in the selection of a method is whether it can provide valid information for the specific application and population being studied. Many different statistical tests have been employed to compare body composition derived from experimental or indirect methods (predictor variables) with those from a direct method or a reference standard method (dependent or outcome variables). These include: analysis of variance (examining differences), correlation coefficients (examining similarities), standard error, coefficient of variation (examining the size of the standard deviation relative to the mean; focusing on variability), level of bias (difference between the "gold standard" and experimental measure), regression analyses (examining the unique and additive contributions of different measures in improving the predictive power of body composition equations), and intra- and interobserver variance. Development of greater consensus and understanding by researchers regarding statistical methods for comparing clinical measurement methods and reporting results is adding clarity to this body of knowledge.

From the practical standpoint, there is no one perfect method to use to measure and find the true value for body composition in living humans. However, the more body compartments that can be directly measured, the greater is the accuracy. Conversely, the fewer compartments that are measured and the more assumptions that have to be made, the less is the accuracy, because the assumptions are often violated due to wide difficulty in assessing variations, particularly in hydration and bone mineral content between people who differ by age, gender, ethnicity, or health status.

There appears to be consensus that a four compartment (body cell mass, extracellular water fat free extracellular solids and body fat) model for body composition is an excellent standard against which to compare and validate other methods. However, because the four-compartment model uses a variety of methods to independently estimate body fat (hydrostatic weighing, deuterium oxide dilution, and DEXA), it is not practical to perform on a large number of subjects. Therefore, use of the DEXA (that employs a three-compartment body composition model, which directly measures fat mass, lean mass, and bone[4]) is gaining acceptance as a practical reference model. It has essentially replaced hydrostatic weighing (employing a two-compartment model that divides body composition into fat and fat-free components and assumes constant densities for these tissues that in reality are not universally applicable[4]) as the measurement against which the majority of field measures of frame size, circumferences, and skinfolds are now being evaluated and is currently included in the periodic National Health and Nutrition Examination Survey (NHANES) studies. However, while the DEXA technology is easier and more convenient for the operator and subject, it has a number of limitations.[5] The software used to interpret results relies on and uses assumptions about levels of hydration, potassium content, and tissue density, and these assumptions may vary by manufacturer. The machines must be routinely calibrated, they utilize different scan types (pencil or fan), and they impose physical limitations on the size (weight, length, thickness, etc.) of individuals to be scanned. Therefore, ideally it is wise not to rely on a single method, but rather use multiple methods whenever possible to simultaneously measure the different body compartments to establish and validate field methods on diverse populations.[6]

Direct methods used in recent studies to examine amount and location (subcutaneous vs. intra-abdominal) of central body fat as a risk factor for cardiovascular disease (CVD) include computed tomography (CAT scan) and Magnetic Resonance Imaging (MRI). Additional methods of body composition analysis that have been used in recent studies to validate or compare results from field methods include bioelectrical impedance analysis (BIA) and air displacement plethysmography (the "BOD POD").

MEASUREMENT ERROR

Once a field method has been selected as appropriate to the application at hand, adherence to guidelines for achieving acceptable levels of measurement error[7,8] are needed to ensure the quality of data collected (see Table 34.1).

Guidelines for training and certification of measurers direct a repeated-measures protocol where the trainee and trainer measure the same subjects until the difference between them is very small. However, the definition or description of "small difference" is constrained to some extent by the technique (how precise it can be), the equipment (how exactly it can be calibrated, how fine the scale is), and by the magnitude of the potential size of the measurement itself (measured in many centimeters such as height vs. in few millimeters such as some skinfolds).

Some targets for difference to be achieved that are acceptably small to certify competency have been proposed (Table 34.2).[11] Given the limits of what level of accuracy is possible, investigators must also be aware of the proportion of the total measurement that is represented by the acceptable difference.[12]

METHODS

Even though literally hundreds of anthropometric studies have been done comparing methods and developing predictive equations,[13] there is neither clear evidence nor scientific consensus as to which methods, sites, or equations should be used. Thus, best practice is to select a method with a preponderance of supporting evidence for the specific setting, population, and application, to use good equipment, train staff well, understand the limitations, and be able to interpret the results within these limitations. Specific instructions for taking measurements or locating anatomical sites will not be covered in this chapter because excellent detailed anthropometric manuals are available.[14,15]

Once a method and site of measurement has been selected as appropriate to the purpose for which the information is needed, the next steps include the "logistics" of selecting, calibrating, and using equipment and training and certifying staff in the actual measurement procedures.

TABLE 34.1
Data Quality and Anthropometric Measurement Error[9,10]

Goal of Quality Measurement	Terminology, Definitions, and Causes or Contributing Factors
Repeated measures give the same value	**Reliability:** Differences between measures on a single subject (within-subject variability) are not caused by errors in measurement (site or technique) or physiologic variation
	Imprecision: Different results are obtained for a single subject when measurements are done either by one person (intra-observer differences) or two or more persons (inter-observer differences) and reflect measurement errors
	Undependability: Different results are due to physiologic factors (such as differences over the course of a day in weight due to weight of food eaten or fullness of the bladder) or height (due to compression of the spine)
	Unreliability: The sum of errors due to imprecision and undependability

TABLE 34.2
Recommendations for Evaluating Differences between Trainer and Trainee

Measurement	Difference Between Trainer and Trainee			
	Good	**Fair**	**Poor**	**Gross error**
Height (length) (cm)	0–0.5	0.6–0.9	1.0–1.9	2.0 or >
Weight (kg)	0–0.1	0.2	0.3–0.4	0.5 or >
Arm circumference (cm)	0–0.5	0.6–0.9	1.0–1.9	2.0 or >
Skinfolds (any) (mm)	0–0.9	1.0–1.9	2.0–4.9	5.0 or >

FRAME SIZE

It seems intuitive that it is fat weight that is unhealthy and that persons with larger frames can weigh more and still be healthy. While there is general agreement that frame is a valid consideration in the assessment of weight for height, identifying an exact method for classifying frame size has been problematic.[16] The literature includes a variety of different concepts of frame size: body type and body proportions (length of trunk relative to total height), bone and skeletal size and thickness, and muscularity. There are two general "schools of thought" about frame; one that frame is primarily a skeletal concept, and the other that it also encompasses the fat-free mass (everything that is not fat including bone and muscle). Most researchers agree that a valid measure of frame must be independent of body fatness, while others believe that it must also be somewhat independent of height to be of value in the assessment of weight. However, studies have shown varying degrees of correlation of different measures of skeletal size and dimension with height (the linear dimension of the skeleton) and correlation of measures of both bone and muscle with body weight and fatness. Therefore, additional criteria for validity of frame size measures have been proposed: (1) the correlation of the measure with fat free mass (FFM) should be greater than the correlation of height alone with FFM; and (2) the measure should have little or no association with body fat beyond that accounted for by the association of FFM with fat.[17]

Others have proposed more generalized methods or observations for classifying frame according to body type or morphology. The categories of leptomorph, metromorph, or pyenomorph[18] follow the idea that the human body is like a cylinder, and its mass is determined by height, breadth, and depth.

The main purpose for assessing frame size is to evaluate weight and recommend an optimal weight that would be associated with the best present state of health and longest life expectancy. One of the first proposed common uses of frame size was with weight tables published by the Metropolitan Life Insurance Company in 1954 that were based on mortality rates of insured adults in the United States and Canada.[19] These early tables suggested "ideal" weights by gender and by ranges of height and frame size (small, medium, and large), but provided no method or instructions for assessing frame.[20] The tables were updated in 1983 and provided instructions for measuring elbow breadth and applying cut-offs for classifying frame size using data from the U.S. National Health and Nutrition Examination Survey (HANES, 1971–1975) that were to result in approximately 50% of persons falling in medium frame and 25% in small- and large-frame categories, respectively (see Table 34.3).[21] When these cutoffs were subsequently tested on a large Canadian sample ($n = 12,348$ males and 6,957 females), they were found to classify only a small percentage of the sample as having large frames, thereby increasing the probability of misclassification into incorrect frame size categories and consequent unrealistic weight recommendations.[22]

Practical evaluation of measures of frame size is complicated by several factors, including a lack of national reference standards for any measure except elbow breadth (see Table 34.4). Because frame size cannot be directly measured by any single

TABLE 34.3
Approximation of Frame Size by 1983 Metropolitan Height and Weight Tables

Women		Men	
Height (in.) in 1″ Heels	Elbow Breadth (in.)	Height (in.) in 1″ Heels	Elbow Breadth (in.)
58–59″ (4′10″–4′11″)	2 1/4–2 1/2″	62–63″ (5′2″–5′3″)	2 1/2–2 7/8″
60–63″ (5′0″–5′3″)	2 1/4–2 1/2″	64–67″ (5′4″–5′7″)	2 5/8–2 7/8″
64–67″ (5′4″–5′7″)	2 3/8–2 5/8″	68–71″ (5′8″–5′11″)	2 3/4–3″
68–71″ (5′8″–5′11″)	2 3/8–2 5/8″	72–75″ (6′–6′3″)	2 3/4–3 1/8″
72″ (6′0″)	2 1/2–2 3/4″	76″ (6′4″)	2 7/8–3 1/4″

TABLE 34.4
Frame Size by Elbow Breadth by Gender and Age[23]

Age (Years)	Males			Females		
	Small Frame	Medium Frame	Large Frame	Small Frame	Medium Frame	Large Frame
18–24	≤6.6	>6.6 and <7.7	≥7.7	≤5.6	> 5.6 and <6.5	≥6.5
25–34	≤6.7	>6.7 and <7.9	≥7.9	≤5.7	>5.7 and <6.8	≥6.8
35–44	≤6.7	>6.7 and <8.0	≥8.0	≤5.7	> 5.7 and <7.1	≥7.1
45–54	≤6.7	>6.7 and <8.1	≥8.1	≤5.7	>5.7 and <7.2	≥7.2
55–64	≤6.7	>6.7 and <8.1	≥8.1	≤5.8	>5.8 and <7.2	≥7.2
65–74	≤6.7	>6.7 and <8.1	≥8.1	≤5.8	>5.8 and <7.2	≥7.2

parameter, there is no "gold standard" by which to judge proposed surrogate measures. Neither is there consensus on how to assign cut points for categorizing small, medium, or large frames, or a standard upon which to base expectations of how frame size is (or should be) distributed in a normal population. Different conceptualizations include:

- Distribution by percentiles
- Terciles (equal numbers in each of three frame categories)
- Distribution by quartiles where the lowest and highest quartiles constitute the small and large frame categories, respectively, with the middle two quartiles combined to indicate medium frame
- Distribution by varying "border values" defined at the 15th, 20th, or 25th and 75th, 80th, or 85th percentiles for small and large frames
- Defining cut-points by standard deviations with medium frame falling within plus or minus one standard deviation of the mean and those with small and large frames falling below or above these values

Many different skeletal measurements, including segmental lengths, breadths, circumferences, and radiographs have been examined for assessing frame size (see Table 34.5). These include:

- Wrist and arm circumference
- Elbow, knee, shoulder, chest, hip, wrist, and ankle breadths
- Combination measurements
- Ratio of wrist circumference to height
- Frame index ([elbow breadth (mm)/height (cm)] ×100)
- Regression of the sum of bitochanteric and biacromial breadths (large calipers) on height
- Ratio of sitting to standing height

TABLE 34.5
Selected Validation Studies of Determinants of Frame Size (FS)

Frame Size Measure	Subjects[a]	Methods and Criterion[b,c]	Results
Bony chest breadth[24]	$n = 2201$, ♂, Scotland	a. Bony chest breadth measured by x-ray b. Criterion tested: 1, 3 and sig > in wt with > in FS	a. Correlation of bony chest breadth to wt > correlation of Ht to Wt b. Wt > about 3.7 kg/cm>in bony chest breadth c. Wt > about 12 kg/FS (S → M → L) d. Wt to bony chest breadth ratio correlated with FFM
Ratio of height (cm) to wrist circumference (cm)[25]	100% and ♀ adult patients at a university medical center, United States	a. Wrist measured distal to styloid process at wrist crease on right arm b. Frame size (S, M, L) assigned using this ratio by gender	a. Method for assigning frame size not stated. It appears that some sort or "normal" distribution was applied, but no other criteria of validity were tested b. FS assigned by Ht to wrist ratio:
Elbow and bitrochanteric breadths[26]	$n = 16,494$; age range: 18–74; ♂ and ♀; black and white; United States NHANES 1971–1974	a. Criterion tested: 1, 3 and 4 b. Body fat determined by sum of triceps and subscapular skinfolds	a. Correlation coefficients of weight, elbow, bitrochanteric breadth to log-transformed sum of skinfold values done by gender by three age groups by race demonstrate lowest correlation with elbow breadth b. Categories of SML FS established for elbow breadths with cut points at the 15th and 85th percentiles (values given by gender, race, and age group) demonstrate significant gender differences and some racial differences c. Greater differences were observed for mean weights of subjects when they were categorized by FS (S, M, L) vs. height (short, medium, and tall) demonstrating that FS is more effective in weight discrimination
Elbow breadth[24]	$n = 21,752$; "adults" age range: 25–54; "elderly" age 55–74; ♂ and; multiracial; United States NHANES I and II	Based on this large data set, percentiles of weight, skinfolds (triceps, and subscapular), and bone-free upper arm muscle were developed by height, gender, and FS (using elbow breadth) for two age groups	a. Values of elbow breadth for S, M, and L FS are given for males and females by age. (See Table 34.4) b. These standards can be used to identify persons who are at risk of being undernourished or overfat

Continued

TABLE 34.5
(Continued)

Frame Size Measure	Subjects[a]	Methods and Criterion[b,c]	Results
Height (H) and sum of biacromial (A) & bitochanteric (T) (HAT method) Body fatness estimated by hydro-static weighing[27]	mean age = 22; n = 113 ♂, 182 ♀; ♈; university students; Ht & Wt representative of U.S. population for this age group; Caucasian, United States	a. Criterion: 3,5 b. Bivariate model developed based on height (H) and sum of biacromial (A) and bitochanteric (T) breadths c. Boundaries for FS (S,L) set by gender using mean ht + 1 sd	a. Criterion satisfied b. For ♂ differences in Wt between FS primarily due to differences in FFM c. For & there was small but sig. increase in FM per FS but no increase in FFM per FS d. FS equations: ♂ ht (8.239) + (A + T); & ht (10.357) + (A + T) e. HAT FS boundaries: ♂ S < 1459.3; M 1459.4–1591.9; L > 1592.0; ♀ S < 1661.9; M 1662.0–1850.7; L > 1850.8
Wrist, biacromial, elbow, hip, knee, and ankle breadths Body fatness estimated by hydro-static weighing[17]	n = 225 ♂ and 215 ♀; age range = 18–59; Canada, Quebec City, French descent. Tended to be leaner than either Canadian or U.S. reference populations	a. Criterion: 5–6 b. differences in lean weight between FS categories (assigned by terciles) > differences in % body fat	a. All bone breadth measures were shown to be associated with FFM b. Biacromial, elbow, hip, and knee did not meet criterion 6 c. Both criterion satisfied for wrist and ankle breadths. (Data not shown for FS cut points)
Actual FS (AFS)[d] Body composition determined by JP, Br[28]	n = 17; 0 age = 20.9 ± 1.4; ♈; ♂; Caucasian; United Kingdom	Criterion: 1–5 and correlation with proposed measure AFS	a. Lack of agreement in assigning FS between methods 2–5 b. Criterion satisfied: ankle breadth & elbow breadth 1–5; AFS and hand length 1–3 & 5; HAT 1–3; chest breadth 1–4; wrist breadth 2,3; height:wrist 3 c. Additional correlations: ht → wt r = 0.68 (s); ht → ffm r = 0.70 (s); ffm → fm r = 0.20 (ns)
Frame index 5[29]	n = 21,648 ♂; 21,391 and (sample size planned for 96 ♂ statistical confidence); age range = 18–70; Germany	a. Developed: b. Percentile curves for weight, height, BMI by gender, and age c. Three categories of frame index using 20th and 80th percentiles as border values d. Median values for BMI and %BF by gender and age for each FS	a. Graph of median curves for frame-specific BMI by age (18–64) demonstrate important differences with age and gender and consistently higher BMI with for larger frame b. Graph of median curves for frame-specific %BD by age (18–64) also demonstrate age and gender differences and consistently higher body fat with larger FS c. Values used for cut points for frame index (at the 20th and 80th percentiles by gender and age) are not given for this sample. However, those published by Frisancho (derived from U.S. NHANES data) could be used for other studies
Biacromial, bi-iliocristal, wrist, and knee diameters and sitting height Body composition: DW[30]	n = 2512♂ age range = 45–59 South Wales	Criterion of effectiveness, improvement in correlation of BMI with body fatness when BMI is adjusted for FS	a. All four breadth frame measures were positively associated with BF (range of r = .16 [wrist]–.45) and with height (range of r = .32–.43). (Correlation of sitting height with BF or total Ht not reported.) b. Adjusting BMI for FS did not improve the association of BMI with BF c. Correlations of the BMI adjusted for FS by wrist and sitting height (both r = .74) were essentially the same as for BMI alone (r = .76) d. Correlations of the BMI adjusted for FS by biacromial, bi-iliocristal and knee diameters (range of r = .60–.66) were lower than for BMI alone (r = .76), indicating a possible inflating effect of subcutaneous fat on these diameter measures
Elbow breadth and height-to-wrist ratio Body composition: BIA-Lu[31]	n = 42 ♀ and 38♂ age range = 18–55; United States	Criterion tested: 3, measures result in normal distribution of FS, and produce the same FS in an individual	a. Criterion 3 met for ♂ but not ♀ b. Both measures resulted in a FS distribution highly skewed to small frame (53–73% of subjects) with 0–3% in large frame c. These two FS measures produced the same FS in 69% of the subjects
Arm and wrist circumferences; ankle, elbow, and wrist breadths; subscapular skinfolds; frame index 2; Ht and Ht; visual assessment[32]	n = 300 (71♂ and 229 ♀); mean age = 72.6 ± 5.1; ♈; Caucasian; Midwest, United States	Criterion tested: #3 and agreement across methods in classifying FS	a. Distribution of FS designation varied by determinant but was not influenced by age b. Visual assessment and elbow breadth[19] classified about 75% of subjects as medium frame. Elbow breadth[21] and Frame Index 2 5 resulted in more even distribution of FS c. Association with "fatness" (subscapular skinfold) was noted for women with elbow breadth and for men with height:wrist d. Ankle and wrist breadth had lowest correlations with subscapular skinfold, but lack of population based standards limits their application

Continued

TABLE 34.5
(Continued)

Frame Size Measure	Subjects[a]	Methods and Criterion[b,c]	Results
Wrist and knee width used as FS measures; Ht and Wt; sitting Ht Slenderness index (Ht/wrist + knee width) %BF measured by UWW and BIA.[33]	$n = 120$, matched for age, gender, and BMI. China (Singapore and Beijing Chinese) and Netherlands (Caucasian)	a. Measured ♂BF compared by matched BMI between ethnic groups b. ♂BF calculated from BMI compared to measured c. Skeletal mass calculated from ht, wrist and knee width	a. ♂BF differences observed between groups for the same BMI, with %BF > with > FS b. ♂BF calculated vs. measured not different for Beijing Chinese and Dutch c. ♂BF calculated underpredicted true value by 4% in Singapore Chinese d. Differences in FS are at least partially responsible for differences in relationship of BMI → %BF among different ethnic groups
Wrist circumference (WC) and elbow breadth (EB)[34]	$n = 224$; (127♂; 117 ♀); adults; Υ; Venezuela	Distribution of FS (S, M, L) determined by two methods: WC (Grant, 1980) and EB (Frisancho, 1989) and used to compare weight for height classification	Distribution of FS: a. WC: S = 57♂; M = 38♂; L = 6♂ b. EB: S = 16♂; M = 60♂; L = 25♂ Significant differences are observed in weight for height classification within the same group of persons depending on frame size method used. EB achieved more "normal" distribution

Abbreviations: FS = frame size; S, M, L= small, medium, large; ht = height; wt = weight; ffm = fat free mass; fm = fat mass; ♂BF = percent body fat; r = correlation coefficient; sig = statistically significant; ns = not statistically significant; sd = standard deviation.

[a] Subjects (all information provided in the original reference is given): n = number of subjects; age in years; health status: Υ = healthy; gender: ♂ = male; ♀ = female.

[b] Criterion applied: 1 = highly correlated with weight; 2 = highly correlated with fat free mass (FFM); 3 = minimally correlated with body fatness; 4. minimally correlated with height; 5. correlation with FFM is greater than the correlation of height alone with FFM; 6. little or no association with body fat beyond that accounted for by the association of FFM with fat.

[c] Methods for determining body composition: UWW = underwater weighing; BIA = bioelectrical impedance analysis; JP = regression equations of Jackson and Pollock[35,36]; Br = formula of Brozek et al.[37]; DW = regression equation of Durnin and Wormersley[38]; BIA-Lu = bioelectrical impedance analysis using the equations of Lukaski et al.[39]

[d] In this study, the authors propose a reference measure "actual FS" comprised of the sum of a battery of 22 different skeletal measures (11 breadths, 9 lengths, and 2 depths) as described in text of Lohman et al.[14]

CIRCUMFERENCES

Circumference measurements have been widely examined because of advantages of being relatively easy to perform, inexpensive, noninvasive, and requiring only a tape measure and minimal training of personnel. Primary applications include:

- Monitoring brain growth in children
- Monitoring effectiveness of treatments (including physical exercise) to measure reduction or increase in selected body areas
- As a marker of protein-energy malnutrition
- Estimation of the relative proportion of body weight from fat vs. lean both as an independent measure and as a measure of frame size
- Describing body shape or the relative distribution of body weight using single measures or ratios of two circumference measures such as waist and hip

Techniques for taking circumference measures are relatively simple. However, significant errors can result from improper positioning or placement of the tape and from differences in tension applied. In general, the tape is placed perpendicular to the long axis of the body, but exceptions include head and neck where the measurement is made at the widest and narrowest point, respectively. In almost all cases except the head, the tension on the tape is just enough to place it snug against the skin without causing an indentation. However, if the purpose of the circumference is to estimate frame size (or skeletal size), it is not entirely clear whether the tape should be pulled more tightly to get as close to the bone as possible. "Equipment" includes a flexible but nonstretchable tape measure that is relatively narrow (0.7 cm) that has metric measures on one side and English measures on the other. Special anthropometric tapes are available such as those that are already interlocked to slip over the arm or head with arrows to make reading the measurement or finding the midpoint of the back of the arm easier. Detailed instructions for technique for measurement of the head, neck, chest, waist, abdomen, hops or buttocks, thigh, calf, ankle, forearm, and wrist are described by Callaway et al, who recommend intra- and intermeasurer limits of agreement of 0.2 cm for relatively small sites (calf, ankle, wrist, head, arm, and forearm) and 1.0 for the large sites (waist. abdomen, buttocks, and chest).[40]

TABLE 34.6
Circumferences Used to Estimate Percent Body Fat

Young Women (Ages 17–26)	Older Women (Ages 27–50)	Young Men (Ages 17–26)	Older Men (Ages 27–50)
Abdomen	Abdomen	Right upper arm	Buttocks
Right thigh	Right thigh	Abdomen	Abdomen
Right forearm	Right calf	Right forearm	Right forearm

One of the most commonly measured and clinically practical anthropometric indices is the arm muscle area that was originally developed for use in the field for the evaluation of undernourished children.[41] Arm circumference and tricep skinfold measurement can be used to compare an individual to a reference population[42] and to estimate the relative proportion of fat and muscle[43] or to estimate the severity of undernutrition in seriously ill hospitalized patients.[44] The use of arm circumference has importance when either undernutrition or overnutrition is of concern, and it can be easily used in the field, hospital, or community setting. Similarly, head circumference is a common measurement for infants in the first 2 to 3 years of life that can be plotted on standard growth charts to be compared with population norms.

Because of some of the difficulties of applying traditional height–weight tables to individuals who are either very lean or very fat and because of the practicality of doing circumference measurements, various researchers have evaluated the validity of using circumferences to estimate body composition and physical fitness. Using underwater weighing as the "gold standard," tables such as Table 34. 6 have been developed to estimate percent body fat within 2.5 to 4% for women and men.[45]

The U.S. Navy requires personnel to pass certain physical fitness screening tests including having an appropriate weight for height. In this setting, it is quite important to use a method that provides more specific information than traditional height–weight indices in differentiating individuals who have excess lean weight from those individuals with excess fat. Because of the large numbers of potential recruits and enlisted personnel being measured, practicality is also very important. Equations using circumference measures have been used to estimate percent body fat and body density since the early 1980s. (See Table 34.7 for selected studies of circumference measures.)

SKINFOLD MEASUREMENTS

The skinfold (sometimes referred to as *fat fold*) technique is performed by pinching the skin and underlying fat at a given location between the thumb and forefinger, pulling the fold slightly away from the body, placing the calipers on the fold, and measuring its thickness. Some skinfold sites are relatively easy to locate and measure while others are not. There are many individual factors that affect the accuracy of skinfold measurements:

- Degree of leanness or fatness
- Muscle tone (including presence of muscle wasting)
- Changes with growth
- Younger or older age (as this affect accuracy of assumptions about tissue composition, muscle tone, skinfold compressibility, and elasticity)
- Subject cooperation (small children may be frightened or uncooperative)
- Ethnicity
- Health status (bedridden vs. ambulatory)
- Hydration status

Use of this method relies on two main assumptions: (1) skinfolds provide good measures of subcutaneous fat; and (2) there is a good relationship between subcutaneous fat and total body fat. The ability to predict total body fat varies by site, with some sites highly correlated with total fat and others relatively independent of total fat. Studies show that the relationship between subcutaneous and total body fat (ranging from 20 to 70%) is affected by age, gender, degree of fatness, and race.[54–56] Thus, as has been mentioned previously, it is important to review the literature carefully and select sites and predictive equations that have been validated for the population being measured and provide sufficient precision for the desired application.

Guidelines for skinfold measurement technique, location of measurement sites, and information on reliability of measurement at the various sites have been published.[57] Considerable supervised practice is required before an individual can take accurate skinfold measurements. Training by an experienced person should be conducted, and measures practiced until consistency is achieved between the expert and trainee and by the trainee on within-subject repeated measures. Experts agree on the importance of using standardized techniques in both locating the site and using calipers to take the measurement, yet some argue

TABLE 34.7
Selected Studies of Circumference Measures

Circumference Sites	Subjects[a]	Methods	Results
Neck, abdomen, thigh[46]	$n = 5710$ ♂ and 477 ♀, Navy personnel, United States	%BF estimated from standardized Navy equations for men {♂ Body Fat = $(0.740 \times$ abdomen$)$ − $(1.249 \times$ neck$) + 0.528$[47] Body Density = $-[.19077 \times$ Log10 (abdomen − neck)] + $[.15456 \times$ Log10 (height)] + 1.0324; Percent body fat = $[(4.95/\text{body density}) - 4.5] \times 100$}[48] and women {♂ Body Fat = $(1.051 \times$ Biceps$)$ − $(1.522 \times$ forearm$)$ − $(0.879 \times$ neck$)$ + $(0.326 \times$ abdomen$)$ + $(0.597 \times$ thigh$) + 0.707$}[49] ♂ BF estimates correlated with 3 measures of physical fitness	[a]Estimates of percent body fat derived from these circumference measurements and equations correlated better with performance on the Navy's physical fitness tests than did commonly used weight-height indices
Waist, hip[50]	$n = 32{,}978$; age range = 25–64; participants in 19 ♂ and 18 ♀ populations participating in a WHO MONICA project	Identification of obesity compared by cut points for waist circumference at 2 levels (1. ♂ ≥ 94 cm; ♀ ≥ 80 cm; 2. ♂ ≥ 102 cm; ♀ ≥ 88 cm) vs. cut points for BMI (≥ 25 kg/m^2) and WHR (♂ ≥ 0.95; ♀ ≥ 0.80)	[a]Sensitivity was lowest in populations with fewer overweight individuals and highest in populations with more overweight. Use of waist cut points vs. BMI or WHR cut points would correctly identify most people without obesity but miss some with obesity. Optimal screening cut-off points for waist circumference may be population specific
Waist, hip umbilical[51]	$n = 91$, ♀; age range 20–54; BMI:18–34 kg/m^2	♂ BF by DEXA compared with ♂ BF from predictive equations	Comparability and precision of %BF estimates from predictive equations can be improved by adjusting for umbilical circumference and BMI
Waist, hip[52]	$n = 385$ (140 ♂ and 245 ♀); mean age = 80 (range = 65–96); United States	♂ BF by DEXA and BIA. BF distribution by skinfolds	♂ BF < ♂ vs. ♀, upper body obesity > ♂ vs. ♀ even in older age Strong age adjusted correlations among obesity measures (BMI, ♂ BF [DEXA ♀ BIA], skinfolds) were observed for both ♂ and ♀ Weak associations among measures of upper body obesity differed by gender
Neck[53]	$n = 979$ (460 ♂ and 519 ♀); mean age = 51 + 17 years); visiting Family Medicine clinic for any reason; Israel	Examined correlation between neck circumference (NC) and measures of obesity (BMI, weight, waist and hip circumference and ratio	NC simple and time saving measure can be used to identify potentially overweight patients. Men with NC < 37 cm and women with NC < 34 cm not considered overweight. Men with NC > 37 and women with NC > 34 require additional evaluation of overweight or obesity status
Waist, hip, waist to hip ratio[52]	$n = 385$ (140 ♂; 245 ♀); age range = 65–96. United States	♂ body fat by DEXA	For both ♂ and ♀ waist circumference is more strongly correlated with BMI and ♂ BF by DEXA that W:H For subjects >80 years a. W:H not correlated with any measure of obesity or fat distribution for ♂ and only with subscapular sf in ♀ b. Waist correlated significantly with almost all measures of central obesity

Abbreviations: IAF= intraabdominal fat; WHR = waist to hip ratio; ht = height; wt = weight; BMI = body mass index; ffm = fat free mass; fm = fat mass; %BF = percent body fat; r = correlation coefficient; sig = statistically significant; ns = not statistically significant; sd = standard deviation.

[a] Subjects (all information provided in the original reference is given): n = number of subjects; health status: ϒ = healthy; gender: ♂ = male; ♀ = female

[b] Methods for determining intra-abdominal fat: MRI = magnetic resonance imaging.

[c] Methods for determining body composition: UWW = underwater weighing; DEXA = dual energy x-ray absorptiometry; DD = deuterium dilution; TBK = total body potassium; BIA = bioelectrical impedance analysis; SKF = JP = regression equation of Jackson and Pollock;[35,36] Br = formula of Brozek et al;[37] DW = regression equation of Durnin and Wormersley;[38] BIA-Lu = bioelectrical impedance analysis using the equations of Lukaski et al.[39]

that in light of the many biologic variables affecting body composition, technical errors in skinfold measurement are of comparatively little importance.[58] Nonetheless, given a standard level of training and care in measurement, high levels of reliability can be achieved (see Table 34.8).

Many different models of skinfold calipers are available, but only those that are designed to maintain a constant tension (10 g/mm) between the jaws should be used. However, even with the higher-quality calipers, there is a difference in the pressure exerted by the jaws and, therefore, in the degree of compression of the skinfold.[59] Differences in compression have also been attributed to differences in caliper jaw surface area such that calipers with smaller surface area and lighter spring tension (such as the Lange) give larger values than calipers with larger surface area and tighter spring tension (Holtain and Harpenden).[60] Because of these differences attributable to the calipers themselves, it is important to calibrate often[61] and consistently use the same equipment in order to compare data within or across subjects.

The greater availability of DEXA equipment in the past decade and recognition of the four compartment model as the best reference standard have allowed for the reexamination of some of the most widely used equations using skinfold measures to predict percent body in different populations. The results of some of these studies are summarized in Table 34.9.

TABLE 34.8
Reliability of Selected Skinfold Measurement Sites

Site	Intermeasurer Error	Intrameasurer Error
Subscapular	SEM: 0.88–1.53 mm	SEM: 0.88 to 1.16 mm
Midaxillary	SEM: ± 0.36; 1.47 mm (children); ± 0.64 mm (adults)	SEM: Children: ± 0.95 mm Adults: ± 1.0,1.22, 2.08 mm
Pectoral (chest)	R: .9, .93, .97; SEM: 2.1 mm	R: .91 to .97 mm; SEM: ± 1–2 mm
Abdominal		R: .979; SEM: 0.89 mm
Suprailiac	SEM: 1.53 mm (children); 1.7 mm (adults)	R: .97; SEM: 0.3–1.0 mm
Thigh	R: > .9, .97, .975; SEM: ± 2.1, ± 2.4, 3–4 mm	R: .91, .98, .985; SEM: 0.5–0.7 mm, 1–2 mm
Medial calf		R: .94, .98, .99; SEM: 1.0–1.5 mm
Tricep	SEM: 0.8–1.89 mm	SEM: 0.4–0.8 mm
Bicep	SEM: ± 1.9 mm	SEM: 0.2–0.6, ± 1.9 mm

Abbreviations used: SEM: Standard error of measurement; R: reliability coefficient.
Multiple error estimates represent differing results from different studies.

Source: Information in this table has been summarized from Harrison GG, Buskirk ER, Carter JEL, et al. Skinfold Thickness and Measurement Technique. In: Lohman TG, Roche AF, Martorell R. Anthropometric standardization reference manual. (1988) Champaign, IL: Human Kinetics. pp 55–80. This chapter includes the specific citations for the reliability studies.

TABLE 34.9

Selected Update and Validation Studies Examining the Utility of Field Methods in Predicting or Estimating Body Composition in Different Populations

Subjects	Methods	Results
Healthy young to middle-age adults: $n = 681$ (360 ♂; 321 ♀); mean age ~35. Primarily Caucasian (FELS study), United States[2]	♂ body fat (♂BF) measured by four compartment model (4CM) compared with ♂BF estimated using common sf equations (Durnin ♀ Womersley, Jackson and Pollack)	♂BF from skinfold (sf) thickness equations < ♂BF from 4CM Results from new predictive equations developed from sf yielded results close to 4CM ♂: 22.7♂ (sf) vs. 22.8♂ (4CM) ♀: 32.6♂ (sf) vs. 32.8♂ (4CM)
Fit and healthy young adults: $n = 52$ (21 ♂; 31 ♀); mean age ~22. United Kingdom[63]	♂BF measured by DEXA and 4CM model (♀ only) compared with ♂BF estimated from upper body skinfolds (UBSf) vs. lower body (LBSf)	Thigh skinfold had highest correlation with ♂BF by DEXA ♂ and ♀; and also with ♂BF by four compartment model for ♀ Sum of the LBSf explained more of variance in ♂BF by DEXA than did sum of the UBSf Authors conclude: important to include lower body sf when assessing ♂BF in young adults

Continued

TABLE 34.9
(Continued)

Subjects	Methods	Results
Healthy young to middle-age men: $n = 160$; age range = 18–62; primarily Caucasian; United States[64]	%BF measured by DEXA compared with %BF estimated using 3 of the most common and professionally recommended equations (Jackson and Pollack: 7 site and 2 different 3 site equations)	%BF from sf equations underestimated by ~3% compared to DEXA New predictive equation developed using sum of 7 sf (chest, midaxillary, triceps, subscapular, abdomen, and thigh) and age
Healthy adults: $n = 117$ (46 ♂; 71 ♀); Normal weight and obese (BMI:19–39); mean age validation group ~48 years; cross-validation group ~58 years.; age range = 26–67 years; Caucasian; Germany[65]	%BF by DEXA compared with %BF by Sf (equations by Durnin and Wormersley and Peterson). Additional measures collected (Sf: chin, biceps, triceps, subscapular, chest, abdomen, hip, thigh, knee, calf; circumferences: waist, hip, thigh, calf; breadths: chest, elbow, knee, wrist, ankle, and chest depth)	New predictive equations developed combining sf, circumferences and breadths: a. Men: waist circumference and Sf (log triceps, subscapular, abdomen) b. Women: hip circumference, Sf (log chin, triceps, subscapular) and knee breadth %BF estimates from new equations showed excellent correspondence to DEXA and had negligible tendency to underestimate %BF in subjects with higher BMI
Asian ($n = 242$) and White ($n = 445$) Adults: age 18–94; United States[66]	Correlations examined between BMI and %BF by DEXA and 6 circumferences and 8 sf compared for Asians vs. whites	Asians had lower BMI but higher %BF. Sf revealed greater subcutaneous fat in Asians and different fat distribution (> upper body) than whites. Magnitude of difference between races > in women vs. men New predictive equations developed for each race and gender based on BMI, age, and sf
African-American Women: $n = 134$; age range = 18–40, premenopausal, United States[67]	%BF estimated from five different sf equations: Jackson and Pollack (three and seven sites), Durnin and Womersley (generalized and age-specific equations), and Wang compared with DEXA	Comparison of predictive accuracy of the five equations found Jackson-Pollack seven sites to be most valid, explaining 75% of variance in reference body density and no significant difference from %BF by DEXA
Pregnant women: $n = 200$. United States[68]	%BF measured by four compartment model (DEXA done 2–4 weeks postpartum)	Estimates of %BF measured at gestation weeks 14 and 37 (early and late pregnancy) using four widely used predictive equations yielded significantly higher values than the four-compartment model New predictive equations developed that were found to be valid for pregnant women with different prepregnancy BMI, different pregnancy weight gains, and different ethnicity and SES Field methods used in these equations include: a. Change in fat mass: thigh sf b. Fat at term: biceps sf, thigh sf, wrist circ
Young children: $n = 98$ (49 ♂; 49 ♀); mean age = 6.6; Caucasian, United States[69]	%BF by sf (using Slaughter equation based on triceps and calf sf) and BIA with DEXA	%BF by DEXA significantly < than %BF by sf or BIA New predictive equations developed for this age and ethnic group
Children: $n = 86$ (34♂; 52♀); mean age = 11; range = 7–18; African American (~30% of sample) and Caucasian, United States[70]	%BF estimated from triceps sf (Dezenberg equation[71]) compared with %BF from DXA and air-displacement plethysmography (ADP)[72]	Triceps sf accounted for only 13% of the variance in %BF change Authors conclude: a. There appears to be no noninvasive, simple method to measure changes in children's %BF change accurately and precisely b. ADP could prove useful for measuring change %BF in children
Children in adiposity rebound period: $n = 75$ (34 ♂; 41♀); mean age ~6; range = 3–8); Hispanic (~16% of sample) and Caucasian, United States[73]	%BF estimated from sf (using equations of Slaughter [method 1 and 2],[74] Duerenberg,[75] and Dezenberg) compared with BIA and DEXA	All methods except Duerenberg significantly underestimated %BF as determined by DEXA BMI underestimated more than Sf or BMI Correlations with %BF by DEXA: a. Slaughter method 2: high ($r = .82$) b. BMI: moderate ($r = .61–.75$) BIA: low ($r = .30$)
Latino children: $n = 96$; mean age ~11; range = 7–13; Hispanic, United States[76]	%BF estimated using equations of Dezenberg (weight, triceps, gender) compared with DEXA	%BF by method of Dezenberg et al significantly different (-3.43 ± 4.32 kg) than DEXA New predictive equations developed Authors conclude: weight (as single most significant predictor) can be used alone to estimate %BF. Adding age and gender increases precision

Continued

TABLE 34.9
(Continued)

Subjects	Methods	Results
African American (AA) and White (W) Adolescent Girls: n = 112 (40 AA; 72 W), mean age = 13; United States[77]	♂ BF from 4CM compared with ♂ BF estimated from sf using eight equations (three logarithmic, two quadratic, three linear) Bland-Altman plot method used to determine bias and limits of agreement	[2]♂ BF estimated using quadratic equations agreed most closely with 4CM [b]The quadratic equation of Slaughter et al recommended for population studies in adolescent females because of accuracy and simplicity (uses triceps and calf sites vs. "invasive" subscapular, suprailiac, or thigh skinfolds, or buttocks circumference) ♂ BF can be over- or underestimated in an individual by ~ 10♂ when this equation is used (Hence recommendation for use in population studies) ♂ BF significantly underestimated by Slaughter and Dezenberg equations compared with DEXA New predictive equations developed: Boys: triceps, biceps, subscapular, suprailiac, and thigh Girls: biceps, subscapular, suprailiac, and thigh calf
Black African children: n = 214 (118 ♂; 96♀); prepubescent; mean age = 9.5 years; Tanner Stage 1; South Africa[78]	♂ BF estimated using equations of Slaughter and Dezenberg compared with DEXA. Validation and cross-validation samples. Bland-Altman plot method used to determine bias and limits of agreement	
Adolescent girls: n = 59; age 14–17 years; eumenorrheic; ballet dancers; Israel[79]	♂ BF estimated from sum of four sf (triceps, biceps, subscapular, and suprailiac) and compared to DEXA and bioelectrical impedance (BIA)	Correlation of sf with DEXA (r=.8) > BIA with DEXA Authors conclude: skinfold measures can be successfully used to estimate ♂ BF in homogeneous group of female ballet dances and by used to determine minimal healthy body weight
Elderly (>80 years): n = 67; ♂; age=20–95; Italy[80]	♂ BF estimated from age-specific equations using sf and BMI compared with BIA and DEXA. Results for subjects >80 years examined separately	Equations based on BMI and BIA systematically overestimated ♂ BF as compared to DEXA in all ages ♂ BF difference sf vs. DEXA < differences BMI or BIA vs. DEXA, but in subjects > 80 years, ♂ BF by sf significantly underestimated Authors conclude: Age related differences in total body bone mineral mass and fat-free mass mineralization in elderly > 80 require further research to develop and validate practical field methods for estimating ♂ BF
Elderly: n = 204 (76 ♂; 128♀); age range = 60–87; healthy; Netherlands[81]	♂ BF by sf (triceps, biceps, subscapular, suprailiac [all subjects], and umbilicus, quadriceps, fibula [subset of subjects]) compared with ♂ BF by hydrostatic weight (UW)	♂ BF predicted from sf using existing published equations generally underestimated ♂ BF from UW Three new predictive equations developed found to be valid for elderly based on gender and: a. Sum of two sf (biceps, triceps) (SEE ♂ BF = 5.6♂) b. Sum of four sf (biceps, triceps, suprailiac, and subscapular (SEE ♂ BF = 5.4♂) c. BMI (SEE ♂ BF = 4.8♂)
Elderly: n = 286 (125 ♂; 161♀); age = 75; Sweden[82]	♂ BF by 4CM compared with ♂ BF estimated from sf using three equations: Durnin and Wormersley (DW), Deurenberg (D), and Visser (V) Bland-Altman plot method used to assess limits of agreement	Difference ♂ BF by 4CM vs. sf equation: a. DW: overestimate in ♂ by 3.12♂ and underestimate in ♀ by 1.06♂ b. D: overestimate ♂ by 3.26♂ and ♀ by 9.56♂ c. V: overestimate ♂ by 3.63♂ and ♀ by 9.23♂ New predictive equation developed using $\log_{10}$ sum of biceps, triceps, subscapular, suprailiac sf, gender, weight, and height (r = .86; mean difference ♂ BF 4CM — ♂ BF new equation = 0) Authors conclude: population-based prediction equations preferable in the elderly
Obese women: n = 16 nonobese (BMI~22; mean age = 28.6) and 21 obese (BMI~34.5; mean age 39.3); Turkey[83]	♂ BF by DEXA compared with BIA and Sf (biceps, triceps, subscapular, and suprailiac) using equation of Durnin and Wormersly	Preliminary analysis using correlation coefficients: Non-obese: DEXA-BIA r^2 = .93; DEXA-Sf r^2 = .89 Obese: DEXA-BIA r^2 = .84; DEXA-Sf r^2 = .75 Re-analysis of data by Bland-Altman method: a. lack of agreement between DEXA-BIA and DEXA-Sf methods in obese subjects b. ♂ BF underestimated by BIA and SF as compared to DEXA in both groups Authors conclude: DEXA should be considered method of choice in obese patients
Dialysis patients: n = 30 (15 ♂; 15♀); mean age = 47; clinically stable; Brazil[84]	♂ BF by DEXA compared with BIA and Sf (biceps, triceps, subscapular, and suprailiac) using equation of Durnin and Wormersly	For all patients, ♂ BF estimates not significantly different between methods. Bland-Altman plot revealed agreement between DEXA and Sf (0.47 ± 2.8 kg) and DEXA and BIA (−0.39 ± 3.3 kg) When results examined by gender, BIA had greater variability and mean prediction error after variability and mean

[a] Subjects (all information provided in the original reference is given): n = number of subjects; health status; Υ = healthy; gender: ♂ = male; ♀ = female

IMPORTANCE OF FRAME SIZE, SKINFOLDS, AND CIRCUMFERENCES TO DISEASE RISK

A variety of approaches have been employed to better understand the validity of using these field measurements for the assessment of risk for the most prevalent and serious diseases: heart disease, diabetes, cancer, and osteoporosis. Major interest has been in evaluating these measures for their ability to measure, estimate, or predict:

- Total fat or percent body fat
- Fat or weight patterning or distribution
- Skeletal size or density
- Biochemical markers such as lipids, insulin sensitivity/resistance
- Health outcomes such as elevated blood pressure, morbidity, or mortality (cancer, diabetes, coronary artery disease, and myocardial infarction)

The preponderance of studies relating anthropometric measures to disease have been in the area of cardio vascular desease (CVD) in an attempt to identify potentially modifiable body factors and to understand potential markers for and predictors of disease. An extensive summary of studies done in men illustrates the methodological and statistical difficulties that are encountered when assessing the relationship between CVD and various body measurements.[85] In general, studies have not shown a consistent relationship between obesity using a variety of measures (weight for height, relative weight, total body fat, etc.) and CVD. The strength of association between central fat distribution and CVD is stronger than that of body fat alone, yet a large percent (30 to 50%) of the variation remains unexplained. Potential sources of difficulty in conducting these studies include inability to identify adequate surrogates for obesity, confounding effects of cigarette smoking or subclinical disease, short follow-up periods, and inadequate methodology for identifying subgroups of obese persons who are at risk.

There is general agreement that persons who have a greater central distribution of body fat have higher risk for cardiovascular disease, diabetes, hypertension, and possibly some cancers, and several studies suggest that those who develop this pattern early in life may have even greater disease risk.[86,87] While one study of three distinct populations found a consistent direct association between abdominal obesity as measured by waist circumference and waist-to-hip ratio and dyslipidemia;[88] others have found the sagittal abdominal diameter to be a better predictor of risk than BMI, waist circumference, or waist to hip ratio.[89,90] Recent studies have been conducted using MRI or CT scans and DEXA as reference standards against which to compare the utility of more practical field methods in estimating total central fat and partitioning it into intra-abdominal vs. subcutaneous fat. Results of selected studies conducted with samples of varying age and ethnicity are summarized in Table 34.10.

Several studies evaluating the ability of simple anthropometric measures to identify those at risk for low bone mass and fractures, have found a strong association between weight and bone mineral density (BMD) while others have not (see Table 34.11.)

TABLE 34.10
Selected Studies Examining the Utility of Field Methods in Predicting or Estimating Central Body Fat

Anthropometric Measures	Subjects	Methods	Results
Weight, BMI, waist circumference, waist to hip ratio, subscapular skinfold[91]	n = 157 (97 ♂; 60 ♀); age range = 48–68; predominantly Caucasian; United States	Field methods compared to results from reference standard: MRI Intra-abdominal fat (IAF) and subcutaneous abdominal fat area (SAF) measured	Gender differences identified: a. ♀ had more > SAF and = IAF than ♂ and tend to deposit IAF at a constant rate as weight > b. ♂ have more IAF at relatively lower weight than ♀ and fat is more uniformly deposited at higher body weights After correction for age, IAF associated with BMI, waist, weight, and subscapular sf ♂: quadratically ♀: linear relationship Anthropometric measures tended to predict less of total variance in IAF for ♂ than for ♀ Anthropometric indices linearly associated with SAF and predicted more of variance in SAF than IAF
Waist circumference, saggital diameter[92]	n = 150 (75 ♂; 75 ♀); age range = 70–79; African American and Caucasian; Netherlands	Visceral fat (VF) and total abdominal fat (TAF) by reference standard CT compared to TAF by DEXA with and without field methods	TAF: good correlation between DEXA and CT but DEXA underestimated TAF by ~ 10♂ VF: Association of VF by CT with DEXA comparable to association of CT with saggital diameter. Combination of information from DEXA + anthropometrics gave only limited improvement in predicting VF

Continued

TABLE 34.10
(Continued)

Anthropometric Measures	Subjects	Methods	Results
Abdominal skinfold and waist circumference[93]	$n = 113$; prepubertal children age range = 4–10 years; African-American and Caucasian; United States	IAF and SAF measured by CT. Total fat and trunk fat measured by DEXA	IAF by CT most strongly and similarly correlated with abdominal sf and trunk fat by DEXA SAT most strongly correlated with trunk fat and total fat by DEXA and waist circumference Authors' conclusion: IAF and SAF can be accurately estimated in this population from anthropometry with or without DEXA data
Waist (WC) and hip circumference, waist-to-hip ratio (W:H); abdominal saggital diameter (ASD)[94]	$n = 76$; age range = 20–80; Caucasian; United States	TAF and VF measured by CT	For both and WC and ASD but not W:H strongly associated with TAF ($r = .87–.93$) and VF ($r = .84–.93$) from CT
Waist, waist:hip[95]	$n = 40$ (18 ♂ and 22 ♀); age range = 26–57; BMI: ≥ 30 Scotland	Observational, cross sectional study Reference methods: IAF measured by MRI and central abdominal fat (CAF) measured by DEXA	Obese ♀: waist, waist:hip and CAF by DEXA equally well correlated with IAF by MRI Obese ♂: waist, waist:hip not sig. correlated with IAF; CAF by DEXA moderately correlated with IAF by MRI
Waist, hip, wrist, and arm circumferences; waist:hip; saggital diameter[96]	$n = 692$ (Black: 91 ♂; 137 ♀; White: 227 ♂; 237 ♀); age range = 17–65; United States	VF and SAF measured by CT. ♂ Body Fat (♂BF) determined by hydrostatic weighing	VF of White ♂ and ♀ > than Black ♂ and ♀ (independent of BMI, W:H, wrist circumference, and age.) VF of ♂ > ♀ Using VF from CT as reference: combination of saggital diameter, SAF, age, and race accounted for 84♂ of variance in ♂ and 75♂ in ♀ Two valid generalized field equations for predicting VF using: (1). BMI, W:H, age, race ($r^2 = .78$ ♂; 73 ♀); (2). BMI (♀ only), wrist, age, race ($r^2 = .78$ ♂; .72 ♀). Accuracy of predictive ability decreases as VF increases
Sf (bicep, tricep, subscapular, suprailiac, midaxillary, and abdominal) and circumferences (midarm, abdomen, hip, midthigh, and calf)[97]	$n = 129$ (54 ♂; 75 ♀); mean age 60.4 at baseline (followed 9.4 years); United States	VF and TAF measured by CT. ♂ Body Fat (♂BF) determined by hydrostatic weighing	Subcutaneous fat = while total fat > Waist and hip circumference changes were best anthropometric predictors of total fat change Thigh circumference change more strongly associated with fat-free mass change than with fat mass change in women Authors conclude: Sf cannot be used to assess changes in BF because of age-related fat redistribution. Waist and thigh girths should be considered for use in longitudinal studies in the elderly to capture information about increased abdominal adiposity and sarcopenia

[a] Subjects (all information provided in the original reference is given): n = number of subjects; health status; ϒ = healthy; gender: ♂ = male; ♀ = female

Possible factors affecting the relationship between body weight and size and bone mineral density include simple mechanical loading (because a larger and heavier body will need a stronger skeletal support), the influence of endogenous sex steroids, and possibly muscularity (either directly by its contribution to total body weight or indirectly by its association with increased activity). For these reasons, anthropometric measures related to gender-related weight distribution (central vs. lower body), frame size, and measures of muscularity/adiposity have been investigated for their value in estimating BMD.

CONCLUSION

Findings from recent studies using more precise reference methods have added important information to the already extensive body of literature in this area, thus improving our ability to use field methods of frame size, circumferences, or skinfolds to estimate body composition, predict disease risk, or evaluate treatment outcomes. In particular, data from well-designed studies on specific sub-groups (age, gender, ethnicity, condition, etc.) provide a more solid evidence base from which clinicians and researchers can select and apply these practical, inexpensive, and portable techniques when evaluating individuals and populations.

TABLE 34.11

Selected Studies Examining the Relationships between Anthropometric Measures and Bone Mass or Bone Mineral Density

Anthropometric Measures	Subjects	Methods	Results
Frame: biacromial, biiliac, bicofemoral, bicohumeral, and wrist breadths Skinfold: triceps, biceps, forearm, subscapula, suprailium, calf, abdomen, and thigh Circumferences: calf, waist, upper arm, abdomen Height and Weight[98]	$n = 342$; mean age = 44.1 (range = 25–79); ♀; United States	Correlation of anthropometric measures to: a. Measured (photon absorptiometry) bone mineral density (g/cm^2) at the radius, femoral neck, Ward's triangle, trochanter, lumbar spine b. Constructed summary bone density score (radius, spine, and femoral neck) Muscle mass (termed "muscularity") estimated from circumferences and skinfolds[99] Multiple regression models constructed to test the usefulness of measures in predicting bone mass	a. For all skeletal sites one frame measure (biacromial width [BW]), one skinfold (subscapular [SSF]) and one circumference (calf [CC]) provided the strongest correlations b. The greater trochanter was more strongly correlated with all anthropometric measures than any other skeletal site c. After inclusion of age, BW, SSF, and muscularity in multiple regression model, BW was a significant predictor for all sites except the radius and SSF and muscularity were significant for all sites d. Neither height nor weight contributed significantly to the model after BW, SSF, and CC or muscularity were included e. Despite the strength of the associations, none of the models accounted for more than 40–45♂ of the variability in bone mass at any site and therefore are not adequate to predict bone mass for individuals f. No measures of distribution of body fat were significantly associated with bone mass g. Cross-sectional data not adequate to address questions of rates of bone loss
Elbow breadth Height, Weight and BMI Waist:hip ratio[100]	$n = 6705$; ♀ mean age = 71.2 ± 5, Non-black, United States	Bone mineral density (BMD) measured by single-photon (proximal and distal radius and calcaneus) and dual-energy x-ray absorptiometry (lumbar spine and proximal femur) Adiposity measured by bioelectrical impedance	a. Weight was the major determinant of BMD at all sites, explaining 6–20♂ of the variability. (Weight explained more of the variability at direct weight bearing sites — proximal femur and os calcis.) Effect of weight on BMD did not seem to vary with age. (Age had independent significant effect on BMD decline.) b. Although the measures of BMI, elbow breadth, height, and waist-to-hip ratio resulted in statistically significant ($p < 0.001$) improvements in fit of the model, they added very little explanatory power over weight alone c. A modest proportion of the weight effect was explained by adiposity (36–63♂ at weight bearing sites and 8–12♂ at forearm sites) d. These data suggest that both mechanical loading and metabolic mechanisms affect BMD
Waist to hip ratio, wt, BMI, arm muscle, and fat area[101]	$n = 1873$ ♀ (97♀ postmenopausal), Italy	Bone mineral content (BMC) and density (BMD) evaluated by DEXA as normal (N), osteopenic (OPN) or osteoporotic (OPR)	[a]Body wt., BMI, arm muscle, and fat sig > in N than either OPN or OPR groups [b]WHR not different between groups [c]Wt and age sig predictors of BMC and BMD but high levels of variation in BMC for the same level of wt (under, normal, over) negate its usefulness as a predictive indicator
Skinfolds at 4 sites, waist, hip, waist:hip, BMI[102]	$n = 100$; postmenopausal ♀, mean age = 55; Turkey	BMC, BMD and whole body composition (lean and fat) determined by DEXA	[d]Lean mass (but not fat mass) correlated with BMD at all sites measured (range $r = .312$–.636$; all $p < .01$)

[a] Subjects (all information provided in the original reference is given): n = number of subjects; health status; ϒ = healthy; gender: ♂ = male; ♀ = female

REFERENCES

1. Bland, JM, Altman, DG. *Lancet* 1:307; 1986.
2. Wang, J, Thornton, JC, Kolesnik, S, Pierson, RN, Jr. *Ann N Y Acad Sci* 904:317; 2000.
3. Sutcliffe, JF. *Phys Med Biol* 41:791; 1996.
4. Wagner, DR, Heyward, VH. *Res Q Exer Sport* 70:135; 1999.
5. Chumlea, WC, Guo, SS. *Endocrine* 13:135; 2000.
6. Heyward, VH, *Sports Med* 22:146; 1996.
7. Frisancho, AR. *Anthropometric Standards for the Assessment of Growth and Nutritional Status.* Ann Arbor, MI: University of Michigan Press, 1990.
8. Ulijaszek, SJ, Mascie-Taylor, CGN (eds). *Anthropometry: The Individual and the Population,* Cambridge: Cambridge University Press, 1994.
9. Ulijaszek, SJ, Kerr, DA. *Br J Nutr* 82:165; 1999.
10. Nordhamm, K, S dergren, E, Olsson, E et al. *Int J Obes* 24:652; 2000.
11. Zerfas, AJ. *Checking Continuous Measures: Manual for Anthropometry.* Division of Epidemiology, School of Public Health, University of California, Los Angeles, 1985.
12. Ulijaszek, SJ, Lourie, JA. *Coll Antropol* 21:429; 1997.
13. Fuller, NJ, Sawyer, MB, Elia, M. *Int J Obesity* 18:503; 1994.
14. Lohman, TG, Roche, AF, Martorell, R. *Anthropometric Standardization Reference Manual.* Human Kinetics, Publisher, Champaign, IL, 1988.
15. Heyward VH, Stolarczyk LM. *Applied Body Composition Assessment.* Champaign, IL: Human Kinetics, 1996.
16. Van Itallie, TB. *Am J Public Health* 75:1054; 1985.
17. Himes, JH and Bouchard, C. *Am J Public Health* 75:1076; 1985.
18. Kretschmer E. K̄rperbautypus und Charakter. Berlin, Gottingen: Springer, 1921.
19. Metropolitan Life Insurance Co. New weight standards for men and women. *Stat Bull* 40:1; 1959.
20. Weigley, ES. *J Am Diet Assoc* 1984; 84:417; 1984.
21. Metropolitan Life Insurance Co. Metropolitan height and weight tables. *Stat Bull* 64:2; 1983.
22. Faulkner, RA, Dailey, DA. *Can J Public Health* 80:369; 1989.
23. Frisancho, AR. *Am J Clin Nutr* 40:808; 1984.
24. Garn, SM, Pesick, SD, Hawthorne, VM. *Am J Clin Nutr* 37:315; 1983.
25. Grant, JP. *Handbook of Total Parenteral Nutrition.* Philadelphia: WB Saunders, 1980.
26. Frisancho, AR, Flegel, PN. *Am J Clin Nutr.* 11:418; 1983.
27. Katch, VL, Freedson, PS. *Am J Clin Nutr* 36:669; 1982.
28. Peters, DM, Eston, R. *J Sports Sci* 11:9; 1993.
29. Greil, H, Trippo, U. *Coll Antropol* 2:345; 1998.
30. Fehily, AM, Butland, BK, Yarnell, JWG. *Eur J Clin Nutr* 44:107; 1990.
31. Nowak, RK, Olmstead, SL. *J Am Diet Assoc* 87:339; 1987.
32. Mitchell, MC. *J Am Diet Assoc* 1993; 93:53; 1993.
33. Deurenberg, P, Deurenberg, YM, Wang, J et al. *Int J Obes Relat Metab Disord* 23:537; 1999.
34. Hernandez, RA, Hernandez deValera, Y. *Arch Lat Nutr* 48:13; 1998.
35. Jackson, AS, Pollock, ML. *Br J Nutr* 40:497; 1978.
36. Jackson, AS, Pollock, Ward, A. *Med Sci Sports Exerc* 12:175; 1980.
37. Brozek, J, Grande, F, Anderson, JT et al. *Ann NY Acad Sci* 110:113; 1963.
38. Durnin, JVGA, Womersley, J. *Br J Nutr* 32:77; 1974.
39. Lukaski, HC, Johnson, PE, Bolonchuk, WW, Lykken, GI. *Am J Clin Nutr* 41:1985; 1984.
40. Callaway, CW, Chumlea, WC, Bouchard, C et al. In: Lohman, TG, Roche, AF, Martorell, R. (ed.), *Anthropometric Standardization Reference Manual.* Champaign, IL: Human Kinetics Books, 1988, pp. 39–54.
41. Jelliffe, EFP, Jelliffe, DB. *J Trop Pediatr* 15:179; 1969.
42. Frisancho, AR. *Am J Clin Nutr* 34:2540; 1981.
43. Gurney, JM, Delliffe, DB *Am J Clin Nutr* 26:912; 1973.
44. Heymsfield, SB, McManus, C, Smith, J et al. *Am J Clin Nutr* 36:680; 1982.
45. Katch, FI, McArdle, WD. *Nutrition, Weight Control, and Exercise.* Philadelphia: Lea & Febiger, 1988.
46. Conway, TL, Cronan, TA, Peterson, KA. *Aviat Space Environ Med* 60:433; 1989.
47. Wright, HF, Dotson, CO, Davis, PO. *U.S. Navy Med* 72:23; 1981.
48. Hodgdon, JA, Beckett, MB. *Prediction of percent body fat for US Navy men from body circumferences and height.* Technical Report No. 84–29, Naval Health Research Center, San Diego, CA, 1984.
49. Wright, HF, Dotson, CO, Davis, PO. *U.S. Navy Med* 71:15; 1980.
50. Molarius, A, Seidell, JC, Sans, S et al. *J Clin Epidemiol* 52:1213; 1999.
51. Rutishauser, IHE, Pasco, JA, Wheeler, CE. *Eur J Clin Nutr* 49:248; 1995.
52. Goodman-Gruen, D, Barrett-Connor, E. *Am J Epidemiol* 143:898; 1996.
53. Ben-Noun, L, Sohar, E, Laor, A. *Obes Res* 9:470; 2001.

54. Vickery, SR, Cureton, KJ, Collins, MA. *Hum Biol* 60:135; 1988.
55. Behnke, AR. In: Wilson, NL (ed.), *Obesity.* Philadelphia: FA Davis, 1969.
56. Lohman, TG. *Hum Biol* 53:181; 1981.
57. Harrison, GG, Buskirk, ER, Carter, JEL et al. In: Lohman, TG, Roche, AF, Martorell, R., (eds.), *Anthropometric Standardization Reference Manual.* Champaign, IL: Human Kinetics, 1988, pp 55–80.
58. Durnin, JVGA, DeBruin, H, Feunekes, GIJ. *J Nutr* 77:3; 1997.
59. Schmidt, PK, Carter, JEL. *Hum Biol* 62:369; 1990.
60. Gruber, JJ, Pollack, ML et al. *Res Q* 61:184; 1990.
61. Gore, CJ, Woolford, SM, Carlyon, RG. *J Sports Sci* 13:355; 1995.
62. Peterson, MJ, Czerwinski, SA, Siervogel, RM. *Am J Clin Nutr* 7:1186; 2003.
63. Eston, RG, Rowlands, AV, Charlesworth, S et al. *Eur J Clin Nutr* 59:695; 2005.
64. Ball, SD, Altena, TS, Swan, PD. Comparison of anthropometry to DXA: A new prediction equation for men. *Eur J Clin Nutr* 58:1525; 2004.
65. Garcia, AL, Wagner, K, Hothorn, T et al. *Obes Res* 13:626; 2005.
66. Wang, J, Thornton, JC, Russell, M et al. *Am J Clin Nutr* 60:23; 1994.
67. Irwin, ML, Ainsworth, BE, Stolarczyk, LM, Heyward, VH. *Med Sci Sports Exerc* 30:1654; 1998.
68. Paxton, A, Lederman, SA, Heymsfield, SB et al. *Am J Clin Nutr* 67:104; 1998.
69. Goran, MI, Driscoll, P, Johnson, R et al. *Am J Clin Nutr* 63:299; 1996.
70. Elberg, J, McDuffie, JR, Sebring, NG et al. *Am J Clin Nutr* 80:64; 2004.
71. Dezenberg, CV, Nagy, TR, Gower, BA et al. *Int J Obes Relat Metab Disord* 23:253; 1999.
72. Dempster, P, Aitkens, S. *Med Sci Sports Exerc* 27:1692; 1995.
73. Eisenmann, JC, Heelan, KA, Welk, GJ. *Obes Res* 12:1633; 2004.
74. Slaughter, MH, Lohman, TG, Boileau, RA et al. *Hum Biol* 60:709; 1988.
75. Deurenberg, P, Pieters, JJ, Hautvast, JG. *Br J Nutr* 63:293; 1990.
76. Huang, TTK, Watkins, MP, Goran, MI. *Obes Res* 11:1192; 2003.
77. Wong, WW, Stuff, JE, Butte, NF et al. *Am J Clin Nutr* 72:348; 2000.
78. Cameron, N, Griffiths, PL, Wright, MM et al. *Am J Clin Nutr* 80:70; 2004.
79. Eliakim, A, Ish-Shalom, S, Giladi, A et al. *Int J Sports Med* 21:598; 2000.
80. Ravaglia, G, Forti, P, Mailoi, F et al. *J Gerontol A Biol Sci Med Sci* 54:M70; 1999.
81. Visser, M, Van Den Heuvel, E, Deurenberg, P. *Br J Nutr* 71:823; 1994.
82. Gause-Nilsson, I, Deay, DK. *J Nutr* 9:19; 2005.
83. Erselcan, T, Candan, F, Saruhan, S, Ayca, T. *Ann Nutr Metab* 44:243; 2000.
84. Kamimura, MA, Avesani, CM, Cendoroglo, M et al. *Nephrol Dial Transplant* 18:101; 2003.
85. Williams, SRP, Jones, E, Bell, W, Cavies, B, Bourne, MW. *Eur Heart J* 18:376; 1997.
86. Freedman, DS. *Am J Med Sci* 310:S72; 1995.
87. Van Lenthe, FJ, Kemper, HCG, Van Mechelen, W, Twist, JWR. *Int J Epidemiol* 25:1162; 1996.
88. Paccaud, F, Schluter-Fasmeyer, V, Wietlisbach, V, Bovet, P. *J Clin Epidemiol* 53:393; 2000.
89. Hrval, M, Berglund, L, Vessby, B. *Int J Obes* 24:497; 2000.
90. Gustat, J, Elkasabany, A, Srinivasan, S, Berenson, GS. *Am J Epidemiol* 151:885; 2000.
91. Schreiner, PJ, Terry, JG, Evans, GW et al. *Am J Epidemiol* 15:335; 1996.
92. Snijder, MB, Visser, M, Dekker, JM et al. *Int J Obes Relat Metab Disord* 26:984; 2002.
93. Goran, MI, Gower, BA, Treuth, M, Nagy, TR. *Int J Obes Relat Metab Disord* 22:549; 1998.
94. Clasey, JL, Bouchard, C. Teates, CD et al. *Obes Res* 7:256; 1999.
95. Kamel, EG, McNeill, G, Van Wijk, MC. *Obes Res* 8:36; 2000.
96. Stanforth, PR, Jackson, AS, Green, JS et al. *Int J Obes Relat Megab Disord* 28:925; 2004.
97. Hughes, VA, Roubenoof, R, Wood, M et al. *Am J Clin Nutr* 80:475; 2004.
98. Slemenda, CW, Hui, SL, Williams, CJ et al. *Bone Miner* 11:101; 1990.
99. Ross, WD, Crawford, SM, Kerr, DS et al. *Am J Phys Anthropol* 77:169; 1988.
100. Glauber, HS, Vollmer, WM, Nevitt, MC et al. *J Clin Endocrinol Metab* 80:1118; 1995.
101. Bedogni, G, Simonini, G, Viaggi, S et al. *Ann Hum Biol* 26:561; 1999.
102. Sahin, G, Polat, G, Baethis, S et al. *Rheumatol Int* 23:87; 2003.

35 Psychological Assessment for Adults and Children

Craig A. Johnston, Chermaine Tyler, and John P. Foreyt

CONTENTS

PSYCHOLOGICAL TESTS

Psychological factors play a significant role in many nutritional abnormalities. These factors include mood (e.g., depression, anger, and anxiety), emotional eating, distorted body image, low self-esteem, poor self-efficacy and quality of life, dietary restraint, stress, susceptibility to external cues to eat, and locus of control. They contribute to a number of nutritional abnormalities including obesity, anorexia nervosa (AN), bulimia nervosa (BN), and binge eating disorder (BED). In this chapter we discuss instruments that assess psychological factors relevant to nutritional goals and concerns.

OBESITY

Obesity is epidemic in our modern society.[1–3] In the United States from 1994 to 2000, the prevalence of obesity has increased from 21 to 28% in men, and from 26 to 34% in women.[1] The prevalence of childhood overweight has also increased during this time period from 11 to 15% in 6 to 11 year olds and from 11 to 16% in 12 to 19 year olds.[3] The abundance of good tasting, energy-dense food is a significant factor fueling this increasing prevalence of obesity. Aromas, advertisements, and social gatherings are some of the environmental cues that trigger eating behavior. An individual's susceptibility to external cues to eat, perceptions of ability to control behavior, and feelings of self-efficacy and self-esteem are factors that interact with the environment to determine behavioral responses.

Despite awareness of the seriousness of obesity in the United States and the chronic and debilitating conditions related to it, many people do not attempt to change behaviors that contribute to the problem. Though a number of reasons for this failure to act have been given (e.g. lack of self-confidence, perception of change as too difficult, and lack of knowledge), to date research has not definitively shown why people maintain unhealthy habits. Of those who do attempt change, the majority fail to maintain their weight-loss goals.

The ability to measure psychological states and traits may facilitate the planning of the treatment for disordered eating. We have identified instruments that measure these characteristics in adults and children (Table 35.1 and Table 35.2) and described them in this chapter. Each description explains what the instrument measures, how it measures it, why it is important, administration and scoring procedures, norms, psychometrics, and availability. Many of the instruments do not provide norms for obese populations; however, in light of the evidence indicating no significant differences in levels of psychopathology between obese and nonobese individuals, the lack of obesity-specific norms may not be a major problem.[4,5]

TABLE 35.1
Adult Psychological Instruments and What They Measure

	Mood	Body Image	Quality of Life	Self-Efficacy	Eating Disorders	Restrained Eating	Locus of Control	Stage of Change
SCL90-R	X							
BDI	X							
FRS		X						
EDI2		X			X			
SF-36			X					
GWD			X					
ESES				X			X	
BES				X	X			
EDE					X			
EI						X		
DEBQ						X	X	
DBS							X	
SOCA								X
URICA								X

TABLE 35.2
Child Psychological Instruments and What They Measure

	Mood	Body Image	Quality of Life	Eating Disorders	Restrained Eating	Locus of Control
SCL90-R	X					
BASC	X					
CDI	X					
EDI2		X		X		
PedsQL			X			
KEDS		X		X		
DEBQ					X	X

EATING DISORDERS

AN, BN, and BED are eating disorders described in the *Diagnostic and Statistical Manual*, fourth edition, Text Revised (DSM-IV-TR), published by the American Psychiatric Association.[6] AN is marked by a failure to maintain a minimal healthy body weight and a fear of gaining weight. BN is characterized by the uncontrollable eating of unusually large amounts of food (binge eating) followed by compensatory behavior such as vomiting. BED was proposed as an eating disorder for inclusion in the DSM-IV-TR. Although it was not accepted as a formal disorder, DSM-IV-TR included research criteria to encourage further investigation of the condition.[6] BED is characterized by recurrent episodes of eating unusually large amounts of food within discrete periods of time associated with feelings of being out of control. Three of the following features must also be present to meet the DSM-IV-TR criteria for BED: rapid eating; eating until uncomfortably full; eating when not physically hungry; and feelings of embarrassment, disgust, depression, and guilt. Additionally, the behavior must occur at least 2 days per week for a period of 6 months.[6]

These eating disorders are often comorbid with other psychological abnormalities. For example, the cardinal features of AN include fear of being out of control and distorted body image.[7] Comorbid major depression or dysthymia has been reported in 50 to 75% of AN patients.[8] According to Maxmen and Ward,[7] 75% of BN patients develop major depression. Increased rates of anxiety were reported in 43% of individuals with AN.[8] Restrained eating and emotional eating due to stress are believed to be related to BED.[9] Large and unplanned changes in body weight are often symptoms of depression.[6] Instruments assessing these eating disorders are also described in this section.

MOOD

SYMPTOM CHECKLIST 90-R

The Symptom Checklist 90-R (SCL90-R)[10] is a 90-item self-report instrument designed to assess current pathology along nine dimensions: somatization, obsessive–compulsive, interpersonal sensitivity, depression, anxiety, hostility, phobic anxiety, paranoid ideation, and psychosis. The scales of particular interest to clinicians are anxiety, hostility, and depression because they measure characteristics that may be related to abnormal eating behaviors.[7] The items describe physical and psychological conditions, and subjects are asked to assess the degree to which the conditions have affected them over the past 7 days. Responses are selected from a 5-point Likert scale that ranges from "not at all" (0) to "extremely" (4). The subscale scores are determined by averaging the scores of the items in each subscale.

SCL90-R has extensive normative data for psychiatric and nonpsychiatric populations, White and non-White subjects, men, women, and adolescents.[10] The subscales have good internal consistency with alpha coefficients ranging from 0.77 to 0.90.[11] Investigations yielded Pearson Product Moment Coefficients ranging from 0.78 to 0.90, which indicates good test–retest reliability.[11]

A weakness of SCL90-R is a lack of evidence supporting the discriminant validity of the subscales. The test appears to have the ability to measure general distress; however, its ability to discriminate between types of distress is not supported. SCL90-R is available from Pearson Assessments. The Web address for this instrument is http://www.pearsonassessments.com/tests/scl90r.htm.

BEHAVIOR ASSESSMENT SYSTEM FOR CHILDREN

An instrument similar to SCL90-R that can be used with children as young as 2 years of age is the Behavior Assessment System for Children (BASC).[12] BASC provides a multidimensional approach to evaluating behavior and personality in children. It includes Teacher Rating Scales (TRS), Parent Rating Scales (PRS), and a Self-Report of Personality (SRP). The clinical scales provided include Hyperactivity, Aggression, Conduct Problems, Anxiety, Depression, Somatization, Atypicality, Withdrawal, Attention Problems, and three adaptive scales (i.e., Adaptability, Social Skills, and Leadership). This instrument produces four composite scores including Externalizing Problems, Internalizing Problems, Behavioral Symptom Index, and Adaptive Skills. The TRS includes the aforementioned scales with an additional Learning Problems clinical scale, Study Skills adaptive scale, and a School Problems composite score.

Adequate reliability and validity have been shown for this measure.[12] Specifically, internal consistency for all scales averages above 0.80, with the internal consistency for the composite scores ranging from the middle 0.80s to the 0.90s. The most current version of BASC is the second edition (BASC-2), which is available from Pearson Assessments. The Web address for this instrument is http://www.pearsonassessments.com/tests/basc.htm.

BECK DEPRESSION INVENTORY

The comorbidity of depression and eating disorders is well documented.[13,14] Depressive symptoms are more severe among obese subjects who also binge eat than among nonbingers.[15] Its assessment in people receiving treatment for these conditions is important because the depression may have a negative impact on program adherence.[16] Intervention outcome for depressed patients receiving treatment for eating-related disorders may be improved by treating the depression first.[17,18]

The Beck Depression Inventory (BDI)[19] is a 21-item instrument commonly used to measure depression. The items explore changes in mood, activity level, self-concept, and feelings of self-worth. BDI has been used with a broad array of subjects ranging from young adolescents to adults. It is easy to understand and takes only about 10 min to complete.

Each item offers a choice of four self-descriptive statements that range in severity from 0 to 3. The instrument is scored by summing the values of the individual items. The range of possible scores is 0 to 63. Cutoff scores for interpretation of the instrument are 0 to 9, normal; 10 to 18, mild to moderate depression; 19 to 29, moderate to severe depression; and 30 to 63, severe depression.[20] Individuals scoring above 16 should receive further screening.

The reliability of BDI is good. Test–retest reliability has been consistently reported in the range of 0.60 to 0.84 in non-psychiatric populations.[20] Internal consistency ranges from 0.73 to 0.92.[20] The most current edition is the second edition (BDI-II) and is available from The Psychological Corporation, San Antonio, Texas. The Web address for this instrument is http://harcourtassessment.com/.

CHILDREN'S DEPRESSION INVENTORY

Similar to BDI, the Children's Depression Inventory (CDI)[21] is a 27-item self-report questionnaire that is scored on six domains including total score, negative mood, interpersonal problems, ineffectiveness, anhedonia, and negative self-esteem. The CDI has been used with children as young as 6 years. For quick screening purposes, a short form of 10 items is also available. The reading level of CDI is at the first grade, which is the lowest reading level for any measure of depression in children.[21]

Each item offers a choice of three possible answers that range in severity from 0 to 2. The range of possible scores is 0 to 54. Separate norms were developed for children aged 6 to 12 years and 13 to 17 years. Reliability has been found to be good with internal consistency ranging from 0.71 to 0.89.[21] The CDI is available from Pearson Assessments. The Web address for this instrument is http://www.pearsonassessments.com/tests/cdi.htm.

BODY IMAGE

FIGURE RATING SCALE

The Figure Rative Scale (FRS)[22] is a popular instrument used to assess an individual's level of dissatisfaction with physical appearance. Dissatisfaction with aspects of physical appearance is very common among people with weight and eating problems. Indeed, it is part of the DSM-IV criteria for diagnosing anorexia and bulimia.[6]

The instrument consists of a set of nine figures of increasingly larger size. Administration is done in two parts. First, respondents are asked to select the figure that most closely resembles their current size. They are then asked to select the figure that most closely resembles their ideal size. The difference (discrepancy score) between selections represents their level of body dissatisfaction.

Despite its popularity, little reliability and validity data exist for this instrument. Measurement of internal consistency is not applicable with this type of scale. A two-week test–retest reliability was 0.82 for ideal size and 0.92 for current size in a sample of 34 men, and 0.71 for ideal size and 0.89 for current size in a sample of 58 women.[23] In a sample of 146 women, correlations between discrepancy scores and other measures of self-image were moderate to strong.[23] These results suggest that the FRS has adequate validity and good test–retest reliability. The scale appears in chapter by Stunkard, Sorenson, and Schlusinger.[22]

The use of figure scales for children has been discouraged for several reasons. First, most of the instruments are age specific. This is problematic because the shape of children's bodies change so rapidly, and images from one age group to another do not generalize. Second, reliability coefficients for most of the scales fall well below 0.70.[24] Finally, most of the stimuli were made using obvious Caucasian characteristics.[25] For a measure of body dissatisfaction in children, the reader is directed to the description of the Eating Disorders Inventory-2 (EDI2) and the Kids Eating Disorder Survey (KEDS) provided in the following sections.

EATING DISORDER INVENTORY-2

EDI2[26] is a popular 91-item self-report instrument used to assess eating attitudes and behaviors along three subscales: drive for thinness, bulimia, and body dissatisfaction. Measurement of these factors is important because of their relation to serious nutrition-related conditions such as anorexia and bulimia.

The drive for thinness and the bulimia subscales assess attitudes and behaviors toward weight and eating, respectively. The body dissatisfaction scale is closely related to body image. It assesses attitudes and behaviors toward the shapes of nine different body parts. Subjects indicate the degree to which they relate to statements by choosing from six possible answers ranging from "never" to "always." The three most pathological responses are scored 3, 2, and 1 in order of descending severity. The three least pathological responses are not scored. Scores are computed by summing all responses for each subscale. Normative data are available for male and female college-age eating-disordered and non-eating-disordered subjects,[27] as well as for adolescents.[28] The body dissatisfaction subscale has been found reliable with children as young as 8 years.[28]

In reports on internal consistency, reliability estimates of the eight scales ranged from 0.82 to 0.93. One-year test–retest reliability in a sample of nondisordered subjects ranged from 0.41 to 0.75.[27] Test–retest reliability after a 3-week span was above 0.80 on all scales in a similar sample.[29] The most current version is the EDI-3, which is available from Psychological Assessment Resources, Odessa, Florida. The Web address for this instrument is http://www3.parinc.com./products/product. aspx?Productid=EDI-3.

QUALITY OF LIFE

MEDICAL OUTCOMES STUDY SHORT-FORM 36 HEALTH STATUS SURVEY

Quality of life is a global construct that incorporates emotional, social, and physical functioning. It provides a comprehensive assessment of both physical and psychosocial factors that may impact a patient. Quality of life may be used as an outcome to determine if an intervention has improved multiple areas of a patient's life. Health-related quality of life has been shown to be significantly impaired in people who are overweight, and as weight increases, quality of life decreases.[30] The quality of life of obese children has also been shown to be lower than that of healthy children and similar to that of children with cancer.[31]

The Short-Form 36 (SF-36)[32] was developed to provide a general assessment of health status. The measure has 36 items, representing eight domains: physical functioning, pain, social functioning, vitality, general health, emotional well-being, role limitations caused by physical problems, as well as those caused by emotional problems. Participants self-report their responses, and domains are scored separately with scores ranging from 0 (low) to 100 (high). Thus, SF-36 is useful as an indicator of the extent to which weight presents problems in various aspects of health. The use of SF-36 has been supported in diverse groups of participants, and the measure is available in numerous languages. This instrument is widely accepted as a valid measure of health-related quality of life with reliability coefficients for the domains ranging from 0.65 to 0.94.[33] There is an updated second version of the SF-36, which is SF-36v2. The Web address for this instrument is www.sf-36.org.

GENERAL WELL-BEING SCHEDULE

The General Well-Being (GWB) Schecule [34] comprises 18 items indicating subjective feelings of psychological well-being and distress. GWB total scores are computed by summing across all 18 items and subtracting 14, as the items are on both 6- and 11-point Likert scales. Scores range from 0 to 110, with low scores representing greater distress.[34] Proposed cutoffs representing three levels of distress are 0 to 60 (severe distress), 61 to 72 (moderate distress), and 73 to 110 (positive well-being). In addition, this measure assesses six hypothesized dimensions including anxiety, depression, general health, positive well-being, self-control, and vitality.[35]

Adequate test–retest reliability has been reported for the GWB total, with reliability coefficients ranging from 0.68 to 0.85.[36,37] High internal consistency has been demonstrated for GWB, with all correlations reported to be over 0.90.[37] Previous studies have also consistently demonstrated correlational validity between the GWB and depression scales[38] and with use of psychiatric services.[36] The GWB is available in a book by McDowell and Newell.[39]

PEDIATRIC QUALITY OF LIFE SCALE

The Pediatric Quality of Life Scale (PedsQL) 4.0[40] is a 23-item self-report measure that assesses health-related quality of life in children and adolescents. Each item is answered using a 5-point scale that ranges from "Never" to "Almost Always." The measure yields four generic core scales of functioning (physical, 8 items; emotional, 5 items; social, 5 items; and school, 5 items) and three summary scales (total scale, 23 items; physical health, 8 items; and psychosocial health, 15 items).

The scale has demonstrated reliability with a Cronbach's alpha reliability coefficient of 0.90 for the total scale score and with all subscale scores exceeding Cronbach's alpha of 0.70.[41] Validity of the scale is supported based on its ability to distinguish between healthy and physically ill children. In addition, the scale has been shown to respond to clinical change over time and has been normed and used in a variety of ethnic minority groups.[41] The Web address for this instrument is www.pedsql.org/conditions.html.

SELF-EFFICACY

EATING SELF-EFFICACY SCALE

For many people, today's environment is filled with opportunities and encouragement to consume large quantities of food. This is especially challenging for those who eat in response to stress. Understanding a person's behavioral response in the presence of gastronomical opportunities and stress is important in the design of programs to normalize eating.

The Eating Self-Efficacy Scale (ESES)[42] is a self-report instrument designed to measure perceived ability to control eating behavior in 25 challenging situations. Perceived ability to control eating is evaluated along two subscales: control in socially acceptable situations and control when experiencing negative affect.

The ESES is a 25-item Likert scale that presents answers in a 7-point format. Ten of the items make up the social acceptability subscale and the other 15 make up the negative affect subscale. Subscale scores are computed by summing the scores of the associated items.

The instrument appears to have good internal consistency across subscales. Alpha coefficients for a sample of 484 female undergraduates were 0.85 on the negative affect subscale and 0.85 on the social acceptability subscale.[42] Seven-week test–retest reliability using a sample of 85 female undergraduates was 0.70.[42] The ESES appears in an article by Glynn and Ruderman.[42]

EATING DISORDERS

EATING DISORDERS EXAMINATION

The Eating Disorders Examination (EDE)[43] is a 62-item semistructured interview that measures the presence of disorders along four subscales: shape concern, weight concern, eating concern, and dietary restraint. Shape concern is related to general feelings of dissatisfaction and preoccupation with issues related to body image. Weight concern relates to the desire to lose weight and the importance given to it. The eating concern subscale measures fear and guilt about eating as well as any preoccupation with food. The dietary restraint scale attempts to quantify the degree to which the subject is guided by strict rules concerning type and quantity of food.

In addition to subscale items, the examination also has items used in making a clinical diagnosis of eating disorders. EDE was originally developed with individuals suffering from BN and AN. Hence, the examination is useful in determining specific areas of concern, as well as in making formal clinical diagnoses of eating disorders. It is a mature instrument that underwent many revisions before publication.

The items used in calculating the four subscales are scored using a severity indicator expressed by a Likert scale that ranges from 0 to 7. These items are organized within a set of 23 higher-order categories such as pattern of eating, restraint, and fear of losing control. The four subscales comprise the 23 higher order items, with the restraint scale consisting of 5 items, the eating concern scale 5, the weight concern scale 5, and the shape concern scale 8. Subscale values are computed by summing the severity indicators of the related items and then dividing by the number of valid items. A global score, defined as the sum of the individual subscale scores divided by the number of valid subscales, may also be computed. The diagnostic items are scored in terms of frequency (e.g., frequency of binge days over the preceding 2 months).

EDE has become the preferred method for the assessment of binge eating. It is designed to be administered and scored by trained interviewers familiar with eating disorders. It measures eating behavior using a 28-day recall method, although some questions extend to the previous 3 and 6 months. Even when administered by trained interviewers, requiring subjects to recall what they ate more than 14 days previously is problematic.

Administration may take 1 h or more when properly given. The authors of the instrument recommend that the interviewer first seek to develop a rapport with the subject. The belief is that good rapport and a feeling of trust facilitates disclosure and contributes in a positive way to the validity of the process.

EDE appears to have satisfactory internal consistency. With a sample of 100 eating disordered patients and 42 controls, Cooper et al.[44] reported alpha coefficients ranging from 0.68 to 0.82 for the four subscales. Another study measuring internal consistency in a sample of 116 eating-disordered people reported alpha coefficients ranging from 0.68 to 0.78.[45] In studies of interrater reliability, very good correlations were reported across all items.[46,47] EDE appears in an article by Fairburn and Cooper.[43]

KIDS EATING DISORDER SURVEY

The KEDS[48] is a 12-item questionnaire used to assess symptoms of eating disorders in children.[49] It is completed by the child. There are two subscales, purging/restriction and weight dissatisfaction, which have been shown to discriminate children with and without eating disorders.[49] Scores of 16 or more are considered to be elevated on either scale. A KEDS total score is also provided. Two administered items are not accounted for on either of the subscales but are included in the total score.[49]

The questionnaire has been found reliable and valid in children between 10 and 13 years of age.[48] However, an interview format has been used to assist younger children interpret questions.[50] Results have indicated that KEDS has adequate internal consistency (alpha = 0.73) and good test–retest reliability ($R = .83$).[48] Overall, KEDS was found to be useful in identifying children with eating disorders as determined by a clinical interview.[49] KEDS appears in an article by Childress et al.[49]

RESTRAINED EATING

EATING INVENTORY

The Eating Inventory (EI),[51] also known as the Three-Factor Eating Questionnaire (EFEQ-R), is a 51-item self-report instrument that was developed as a measure of behavioral restraint in eating. Measuring restraint is important in the nutritional context of obesity because severe caloric restriction may lead to binge eating and increased metabolic efficiency, promoting weight gain.[52,53] Restriction also has nutritional sequelae such as vitamin deficiency and related morbidity.

The instrument is divided into two parts. The first part consists of 36 true/false questions. The second part has 14 questions presented in a four-level Likert format with choices ranging from "rarely" to "always," plus an additional question, which is a 6-point rating of perceived self-restraint. Questions ask about cues to eat, ability to control eating, and willingness to diet. Respondents are asked to indicate how often each statement applies to their personal behavior patterns.

The questionnaire has three subscales:

1. Cognitive control of eating
2. Disinhibition
3. Susceptibility to hunger

The first subscale is related to one's awareness of, and ability to cognitively control or restrain, eating behavior. The second subscale refers to one's tendency to periodically lose control of eating, and the third relates to one's ability to resist cues to eat.

Scoring is described in the EI Manual.[54] The control subscale has 21 questions, the disinhibition subscale has 16, and the hunger subscale has 14. Each question has a value of 0 or 1. Individual subscale scores are calculated by summing the scores of the related questions. Scores above 13, 11, and 10 are considered to be in the clinical range for the control, disinhibition, and hunger subscales, respectively.

The EI appears to have good construct validity. Food diaries and doubly labeled water techniques have been used to assess the construct validity of the subscales. These studies have shown that high scores on the restraint scale are correlated in the hypothesized direction with low levels of caloric intake.[55,56]

The test has good internal consistency (>0.80)[51] and test–retest reliability of 0.91 over 2 weeks.[57] The inventory appears in an article by Stunkard and Messick.[51] The inventory and related scoring materials are available from the Psychological Corporation, San Antonio, Texas. The Web address for this instrument is http://harcourtassessment.com/.

DUTCH EATING BEHAVIOR QUESTIONNAIRE

The Dutch Eating Behavior Questionnaire (DEBQ)[58] is a 33-item self-report instrument that measures eating behavior along three subscales: restrained eating, emotional eating, and eating in response to external cues. The diagnostic capabilities of this instrument are useful for identifying overeating triggers when designing effective behavioral interventions, as well as for the identification of individuals with restrained eating patterns. The reading level of this instrument is between the fifth and eighth grade.[59] In research, it has been used with children as a measure of dieting behavior.[60,61]

The instrument consists of questions related to eating behavior. Each item is presented in a 5-point Likert response format with possible answers being: never, seldom, sometimes, often, and very often. Some of the items have an additional "not relevant" category. Subscale scores are computed by summing the scores of the related items and dividing by the number of items. Items scored as not relevant are omitted from the subscale score.

The restraint scale has received most of the research attention. Some norms are available for the restraint scale.[62] In general, they indicate that women have higher restraint scores than men, and that obese people have higher restraint scores than the nonobese. Internal consistency of the scales was reported in the range from 0.80 to 0.95.[62] A two-week test–retest reliability of the restraint scale was 0.92.[57] DEBQ is published in an article by Van Strien et al.[58]

BINGE EATING SCALE

The Binge Eating Scale (BES)[63] is a 16-item scale designed to assess binge eating in obese subjects. It has also been used with nonobese populations. Eight items of BES measure binge eating behavior and the other eight measure associated feelings and thoughts. Each item consists of a cluster of self-statements. Respondents are asked to select the statement that most closely resembles their feelings. Responses are given different weights. The scale score is computed by summing weighted scores of the 16 items. BES does not assess all of the information necessary to make a clinical diagnosis, but it does measure behavioral features and cognitions associated with binge eating. The scale score has been interpreted as an indication of severity of binge eating.[64] The range of potential scores is 0 to 46. The higher the score, the more severe the binge eating. A score above 27 suggests severe binge eating.

The original work by Gormally et al.[63] suggests that BES has adequate internal consistency. The scale discriminates well between individuals with BN (nonpurging) and normal controls.[64] BES has good test–retest reliability.[65] BES, along with norms and instructions for scoring, appears in an article by Gormally et al.[63]

LOCUS OF CONTROL

DIETING BELIEFS SCALE

The Dieting Beliefs Scale (DBS)[66] is a 16-item scale that measures weight-specific loci of control. Weight locus of control is a method for categorizing beliefs about factors influencing weight. Individuals with an internal locus of control have the expectancy that they can control, to some extent, their own weight. An external locus of control implies a more fatalistic orientation marked by beliefs that weight is determined by factors outside of personal control, for example, genetics, environment, and social context.

The utility of this instrument is in the planning of treatment of obese and overweight individuals. Theoretically, individuals who believe that they have control over factors determining their weight would be expected to have greater success in weight management programs. Identifying individuals with an external locus of control might be valuable in the process of treatment planning because it would cue the counselor to be particularly mindful to avoid interventions that might inadvertently reinforce preexisting negative expectations. For example, very modest and frequently measured short-term goals may be set for individuals with external loci of control in an effort to encourage them toward more positive expectations.

The 16 items are statements expressing either internal or external locus of control viewpoints: eight are internal and eight are external. The items are presented in a 6-point Likert format ranging from "not at all descriptive of my beliefs" (1) to very "descriptive of my beliefs" (6). Eight of the items are reverse scored. The instrument is scored in the internal direction so that high scores indicate more of an internal locus of control.

DBS has three subscales: internal control, uncontrolled factors, and environmental factors. The internal control subscale is related to the belief that individuals can control their weights through internal means such as willpower and effort. The uncontrolled factors subscale is associated with belief in the importance of factors such as genetics and fate. The environmental factors subscale is related to beliefs in the importance of context and social setting. The subscales are scored by summing the individual items that make up the scale.

The scale demonstrates moderate internal consistency (Chronbach's alpha = 0.69) and good stability in a sample of undergraduate students.[66] The DBS is published in an article by Stotland and Zuroff.[66]

STAGE OF CHANGE

STAGES OF CHANGE ALGORITHM

The Stages of Change Algorithm (SOCA)[67] is a self-report instrument that assesses weight-loss activities and intentions. The instrument is based on the transtheoretical model,[68] which conceptualizes change as a six-stage process. The stages are precontemplation, contemplation, preparation, action, maintenance, and termination. The purpose of the model is to maximize successful behavior change. The model posits that optimal intervention strategies vary according to a person's position in the change process. The purpose of the SOCA is to facilitate treatment planning by identifying the individual's position in the process. Persons in the precontemplation stage may not be at all concerned with their condition. These individuals might benefit from efforts to raise their awareness and to personalize their risk factors. People in the contemplation stage may be concerned but not yet decided on taking action. Such people might benefit from information regarding possible treatment alternatives. The preparation stage is characterized by having decided to do something about the condition and have taken some steps aimed at changing. Encouragement to take action and to make a commitment to their health may help people move to the action stage. Individuals in the action stage shown recent behavior change and may benefit most from behavioral interventions such as goal setting and self-monitoring. Moral support and recognition might be best for people in the maintenance stage as they have implemented changes over a period of time. SOCA uses only four of the stages: precontemplation, contemplation, action, and maintenance. The model is of particular interest in the context of nutrition because of the refractory nature of dysfunctional eating behavior.

The SOCA consists of four yes/no items. The scoring is simple and the determination of the person's stage of change is quickly determined.[67] Data describing the reliability of the SOCA for weight loss is not available. SOCA was found to be reliable when applied to similar problems. For example, in their investigation of the processes of change in smoking-related behavior, Prochaska et al.[69] observed alpha coefficients ranging from 0.69 to 0.92, with the majority being above 0.80. SOCA is published in an article by Rossi et al.[67]

UNIVERSITY OF RHODE ISLAND CHANGE ASSESSMENT SCALE

The University of Rhode Island Change Assessment Scale (URICA)[70,71] is a 32-item Likert scale designed to measure a person's position in the four-stage change process: precontemplation, contemplation, action, and maintenance. It is similar in concept to SOCA. It is different in that it has 28 more items, and each stage of change is implemented as a scale. The URICA produces a score for each scale. When viewed together, the scale scores can be interpreted as a profile. This approach is richer than SOCA because it provides a framework that allows attitudes and behaviors characteristic of different stages of change to coexist in a single individual. Thus, URICA may be able to detect gradual shifts from one stage to another. URICA is general in format and not specific to any particular problem area. It has been widely used across an array of problem areas.

Items are presented in a 5-point format. Scale scores are computed by summing the responses to the scale items. Good internal consistency is indicated by numerous studies reporting alpha coefficients ranging from 0.69 to 0.89 across all scales.[70–72]

The general version of URICA is published in an article by McConnaughy et al.[70] A version designed for use in a weight-control context is available in an article by Rossi et al.[67]

STAGE OF CHANGE FOR CHILDREN

Although no specific algorithm for stages of change is readily available for children, several researchers have provided direction in this area. Kristal[73] and colleagues were the first to specifically propose using parental stage of change to determine the appropriateness of intervening with a child. Based on this suggestion, Rhee et al.[74] examined this with parents of overweight children between the ages of 2 and 12 years. More specifically, questions regarding increasing fruit and vegetable intake, decreasing juice consumption, and changing to lower-fat food items were included. A flow chart of questions to be asked is included in an article by Rhee et al.[74]

SUMMARY

Having a better understanding of a person's psychological state should facilitate planning of nutritional interventions for both adults and children. The instruments presented in this chapter are used for such purposes. Brief explanations of the psychological factor to be measured as well as the importance of the factor have been presented. Additionally, instrument-specific information has been included to assist the health care professional in determining the usefulness of the measure for a particular patient. Although not exhaustive, these measures represent factors relevant to nutrition-related treatment.

ACKNOWLEDGMENTS

Thanks to Victor Pendleton for his contributions to an earlier version of this chapter. Preparation of this paper was supported, in part, by USDA ARS 2533759358.

REFERENCES

1. Flegal KM, Carroll MD, Ogden CL, Johnson CL. 1999–2000. *JAMA*. 288:1723–1727; 2002.
2. Mokdad AH, Serdula MK, Dietz WH, et al. *JAMA*. 282:1519; 1999.
3. Ogden CL, Flegal KM, Carroll MD, Johnson CL. *JAMA*. 288:1728; 2002.
4. Perri MG, Nezu AM, Viegener BJ. *Improving the Longterm Management of Obesity: Theory, Research, and Clinical Guidelines.* New York, NY: John Wiley and Sons; 1992.
5. Zeller MH, Saelens BE, Roehrig H, et al. *Obes Res.* 12:1576; 2004.
6. *Diagnostic and Statistical Manual of Mental Disorders*, 4th Edition, Text Revision. Washington, DC: American Psychiatric Association; 2000.
7. Maxmen JS, Ward NG. *Essential Psychopathology and Its Treatment*, 2nd Edition. New York, NY: W. W. Norton & Company; 1995.
8. Halmi KA, Eckert E, Marchi P, et al. *Arch Gen Psychiatr.* 48:712; 1991.
9. Polivy J, Herman CP. In: Fairburn CG, Wilson G, eds. *Binge Eating: Nature, Assessment, and Treatment*. New York, NY: Guilford Press; 1993:173–205.
10. Derogatis LR. *Symptom Checklist-90-R (SCL-90-R) Administration, Scoring and Procedures Manual*, 3rd Edition. Minneapolis, MN: National Computer Systems; 1994.
11. Derogatis LR, Cleary PA. *J Clin Psychol.* 33:981; 1977.
12. Reynolds CR, Kamphaus RW. *The Clinician's Guide to the Behavior Assessment System for Children*. New York, NY: Guilford; 2002.
13. Garner DM, Olmsted MP, Davis R, Rockert W. *Internat J Eating Disord.* 9:1; 1990.
14. Strober M, Katz JL. *Internat J Eating Disord.* 7:171; 1987.
15. Marcus MD. In: Fairburn CG, Wilson G, eds. *Binge Eating: Nature, Assessment and Treatment*. New York, NY: Guilford Press; 1993:77–96.
16. Webber EM. *J Psychol.* 128:339; 1994.
17. Clark MM, Niaura R, King TK, Pera V. *Addict Behav.* 21:509; 1996.
18. Tanco S, Wolfgang L. *Intl J Eating Disorders*. 23:325; 1998.
19. Beck A, Ward C, Mendelson M, et al. *Arch Gen Psychiatry*. 4:561; 1961.
20. Beck AT, Steer RA, Garbin MG. *Clin Psychol Rev.* 8:77; 1988.
21. Kovacs M. *Manual for the Children's Depression Inventory*. North Tonawanda, NJ: Multi-Health Systems; 1992.
22. Stunkard A, Sorenson T, Schlusinger F. In: Kety S, et al. eds. *The Genetics of Neurological and Psychiatric Disorders*. New York, NY: Raven Press; 1983:115.
23. Thompson J, Altabe MN. *Intl J Eating Disorders*. 10:615; 1990.

24. Thompson JK. In: Thompson JK, ed. *Body Image, Eating Disorders, and Obesity*. Washington, DC: American Psychological Association; 1996:49–81.

25. Altabe M. In: Thompson JK, ed. *Body Image, Eating Disorders, and Obesity*. Washington, DC: American Psychological Association; 1996:129–148.

26. Garner DM, Olmstead MP, Polivy J. *Intl J Eating Disorders*. 2:15; 1982.

27. Espelage DL, Mazzeo SE, Aggen SH, et al. *Psychol Assess*. 15:71; 2003.

28. Garner D. *Manual for the Eating Disorder Inventory-2 (EDI-2)*. Odessa, FL: Psychological Assessment Resources; 1991.

29. Wear RW, Pratz O. *Intl J Eating Disorders*. 6:767; 1987.

30. Hassan MK, Joshi AV, Madhavan SS, Amonkar MM. *Intl J Obes Related Metab Disorders*. 27:1227; 2003.

31. Schwimmer JB, Burwinkle TM, Varni JW. *JAMA*. 289:1813; 2003.

32. Ware JE, Sherbourne CD. *Med Care*. 30:473; 1992.

33. McHorney C, Ware JE, Lu J, Sherbourne CD. *Med Care*. 32:40; 1994.

34. Dupay HJ. Paper presented at: American Public Health Association Meeting; October 17, 1978; Los Angeles, CA.

35. Brook RH, Ware JE, Davies-Avery A, et al. *Med Care*. 17:1; 1979.

36. Edwards DW, Yarvis RM, Mueller DP, et al. *Eval Quart*. 2:275; 1978.

37. Monk M. *Clin Invest Med*. 4:183; 1981.

38. Simpkins C, Burke FF. *Comparative Analyses of the NCHS General Well-Being Schedule: Response Distributions, Community vs. Patient Status Discriminations, and Content Relationships (Contract No. HRA 106-74-13)*. Nashville, TN: Center for Community Studies, George Peabody College; 1974.

39. McDowell I, Newell C. *Measuring Health: A Guide to Rating Scales and Questionnaires*. New York, NY: Oxford University Press; 1987.

40. Varni JW, Seid M, Rode CA. *Med Care*. 37:126; 1999.

41. Varni JW, Seid M, Kurtin PS. *Med Care*. 39:800; 2001.

42. Glynn SM, Ruderman AJ. *Cogn Ther Res*. 10:403; 1986.

43. Fairburn CG, Cooper Z. In: Fairburn CG, Wilson GT, eds. *Binge Eating: Nature, Assessment, and Treatment*. New York, NY: Guilford Press; 1993:317–360.

44. Cooper Z, Cooper PJ, Fairburn CG. *Brit J Psychiatry*. 154:807; 1989.

45. Beumont P, Kopec-Schrader E, Touyz S. *Aus and N Zealand J Psychiatr*. 27:506; 1993.

46. Cooper Z, Fairburn C. *Intl J Eating Disorders*. 6:1; 1986.

47. Wilson G, Smith D. *Intl J Eating Disorders*. 8:173; 1989.

48. Childress AC, Jarrell MP, Brewerton TD. *Eating Disorders: J Treat Prev*. 1:123; 1993.

49. Childress AC, Brewerton TD, Hodges EL, Jarrell MP. *J Am Acad Child and Adoles Psychiatry*. 32:843; 1993.

50. Epstein LH, Paluch RA, Saelens BE, et al. *J Pediat*. 139:58; 2001.

51. Stunkard AJ, Messick S. *J Psychosomatic Res*. 29:71; 1985.

52. Klesges RC, Isbell TR, Klesges LM. *J Ab Psychol*. 101:668; 1992.

53. Polivy J, Herman C. *Am Psychol*. 40:193; 1985.

54. Stunkard AJ, Messick S. *Eating Inventory Manual*. San Antonio, TX: Harcourt Brace Jovanovich; 1988.

55. Laessle RG, Tuschl RJ, Kotthaus BC, Prike KM. *J Ab Psychol*. 98:504; 1989.

56. Tuschl RJ, Laessle RG, Platte P, Pirke KM. *Appetite*. 14:9; 1990.

57. Allison DB, Kalinsky LB, Gorman BS. *Psychol Assess*. 4:391; 1992.

58. Van Strien T, Frijters JE, Van Staveren WA, et al. *Intl J Eating Disorders*. 5:747; 1986.

59. Allison DB, Franklin RD. *Psychother Priv Pract*. 12:53; 1993.

60. Hill AJ, Oliver S, Rogers PJ. *Brit J Clin Psychol*. 31:95; 1992.

61. Wardle J, Marsland L. *J Psychosomatic Res*. 34:377; 1990.

62. Gorman BS, Allison DB. In: Allison DB, ed. *Handbook of Assessment Methods for Eating Behaviors and Weight-Related Problems: Measures, Theory, and Research*. Thousand Oaks, CA: Sage Publications, Inc.; 1995:149–184.

63. Gormally J, Black S, Daston S, Rardin D. *Addict Behav*. 7:47; 1982.

64. Marcus MD, Wing RR, Hopkins J. *J Consult Clin Psychol*. 56:433; 1988.

65. Wilson G. In: Fairburn CG, Wilson GT, eds. *Binge Eating: Nature, Assessment, and Treatment*. New York, NY: Guilford Press; 1993:227–249.

66. Stotland S, Zuroff DC. *J Personality Assess*. 54:191; 1990.

67. Rossi JS, Rossi SR, Velicer WF, Prochaska JO. In: Allison DB, ed. *Handbook of Assessment Methods for Eating Behaviors and Weight-Related Problems: Measures, Theory, and Research*. Thousand Oaks, CA: Sage Publications, Inc.; 1995:387–430.

68. Prochaska JO, DiClemente CC, Norcross JC. *Am Psycholog*. 47:1102; 1992.

69. Prochaska JO, Velicer WF, DiClemente CC, Fava J. *J Consul Clin Psychol*. 56:520; 1988.

70. McConnaughy EA, DiClemente CC, Prochaska JO, Velicer WF. *Psychotherapy: Theory, Research, Practice, Training*. 26:494; 1989.

71. McConnaughy EA, Prochaska JO, Velicer WF. *Psychotherapy: Theory, Research & Practice*. 20:368; 1983.

72. DiClemente CC, Hughes SO. *J Substance Ab*. 2:217; 1990.

73. Kristal AR, Glanz K, Curry SJ, Patterson RE. *JADA*. 99:679; 1999.

74. Rhee KE, De Lago CW, Arscott-Mills T, et al. *Pediatrics*. 116:94; 2005.

36 Energy Assessment: Physical Activity

Nancy L. Keim and Cynthia A. Blanton

CONTENTS

INTRODUCTION

Physical activity is an important element in the total energy expenditure (TEE). Physical activity can vary greatly within an individual from day-to-day, or between individuals because preferred physical activities, practices, and routines differ from one person to the other. These variations affect total daily energy expenditure (EE) and could potentially change the energy balance. Accurately measuring the physical activity levels (PALs) of individuals is challenging due to the multifaceted nature of movement, the limitations of measurement devices and self-report, and the potentially high respondent burden it imposes on those who are being measured.

The purpose of this chapter is to provide an overview of physical activity assessment, describe important assessment issues, and discuss relevant aspects to be considered when selecting a method for assessing physical activity, and review the different methods available and present some advantages and disadvantages of each. There is no single measure able to accurately assess physical activity in all individuals or groups of the population, in all settings, and for all aspects and types of physical activity.[1] Some methods that are more accurate and valid in individuals are not feasible for use in large population studies because the costs may be prohibitive. Careful consideration of the accuracy, validity, and feasibility of the available methods to assess physical activity is necessary to best meet each study's objectives.

CONCEPTS AND DEFINITIONS

Physical activity is defined as bodily movement resulting in increased EE over resting levels; exercise is a more vigorous form of physical activity that is structured and repetitive and can result in improved physical fitness.[2] TEE has three components: resting energy expenditure (REE), thermic effect of food (TEF), and physical activity energy expenditure (PAEE). REE represents the amount of energy expended under restful conditions and typically accounts for about 60 to 70% of TEE; within-subject variability is small and can be predicted from body size and age with reasonable accuracy for the majority of individuals.[3] TEF, or diet-induced thermogenesis, represents the energy needed for eating, digesting, absorbing, transporting, metabolizing, and storing useable forms of energy derived from food. Generally, this represents about 10% of TEE. PAEE represents the energy used for bodily movement, and because persons choose to be inactive, moderately active, or very active, the contribution of this component to TEE can be small to large and highly significant.

Physical activity includes all types of bodily movement, including structured exercise, complex sports, recreational activities, occupational and household tasks, hard physical labor, and nonexercise activity thermogenesis (such as fidgeting).[4] Quantitative dimensions of physical activity include frequency, intensity, and duration. Efficiency of performing activity may alter its EE.[5] Depending on the type of activity, its associated EE may vary with body size, so individuals of different body sizes may expend different amounts of energy while performing the same activity.

The unit of measurement for activity-related EE is total kilocalories (or kilojoules), and it can be expressed per unit of time (min) or per unit of body mass (kg), or both. The intensity of activity can be defined in qualitative terms (light, moderate, or vigorous) or in quantitative terms related to actual EE. The energy expended in physical activity or exercise is often expressed in metabolic equivalents (METs). A MET is a numerical value that represents a multiple of REE for a given activity. The Compendium of Physical Activities provides MET values for a large selection of physical activities.[6,7] MET values between 1.0 and 1.5 are considered *sedentary*, and values ranging between 2.0 and 12.0 represent the typical physical activity spectrum from light to intense. In general, activities with MET values ranging from 3.0 to 4.5 are of moderate intensity and are associated with health benefits. For aerobic-type exercises, it is also common to see intensity described in terms of oxygen uptake values relative to maximal oxygen uptake (VO_2max). When performing exercise against resistance, such as weight lifting, pedaling against a load, or running up a flight of stairs, power output can be measured. These power tests measure work accomplished per unit time, and the results are expressed in watts, joules, Newton-meters, or kilogram-meters.

An individual's PAL is a quantitative summary of the different types of physical activity engaged in for various amounts of time during a specified time period, usually 24 h. PAL is defined as the ratio of TEE to REE and can be determined directly by measuring TEE using the doubly labeled water (DLW) method and REE using indirect calorimetry. In the absence of these measures, PAL can be estimated as a weighted average of MET values assigned to all activities constituting the 24-h period, including sleep and rest. The current Dietary Reference Intakes for Macronutrients[2] define PAL values for *sedentary* ≥1.0 to <1.4; *low active* ≥1.4 to <1.6; *active* ≥1.6 to <1.9; and *very active* ≥1.9 to <2.5.

WHY IT IS IMPORTANT TO ASSESS PHYSICAL ACTIVITY

Evidence obtained from epidemiological studies suggests a causal association between low levels of physical activity and increased risk of several chronic diseases such as cardiovascular disease, type 2 diabetes mellitus, obesity, and some forms of cancer.[8] These relationships have largely been established using self-reported physical activity. Some investigators have reported associations between disease risk and aerobic fitness levels.[9,10] Nevertheless, there is some inconsistency in the evidence supporting the association between physical activity and breast cancer[11] and in studies examining the effects of physical activity interventions[12] that may be related to lack of precision of some physical activity measures. These authors and others[13] emphasized the need to develop and utilize standardized methods that are valid, reliable, nonreactive, and precise. Such instruments will facilitate determination of the specific type and amount of habitual physical activity necessary to gain protective effects against degenerative diseases, to maintain a healthy body weight, and to improve metabolic fitness. Further evaluation of existing methods and the development of new or alternative methods of activity assessment are required if we are to improve our understanding of critical activity–disease relationships.

It also is important to assess physical activity for surveillance purposes. We need to determine whether individuals of all ages are meeting public health physical activity recommendations and whether or not patterns are changing over time. Assessing physical activity will provide valuable information to public health professionals, teachers, researchers, policymakers, and others responsible for physical activity interventions.

IMPORTANT ASPECTS TO CONSIDER IN CHOOSING THE MOST APPROPRIATE MEASURE

Whether evaluating a physical activity intervention program, determining the prevalence of activity in a population, establishing the associations between physical activity and health outcomes, or determining whether activity guidelines are being met, it is necessary to choose an appropriate physical activity assessment method. A perfect method for assessing physical activity would be accurate, valid, simple, not time consuming, inexpensive, and suitable for use in a wide range of individuals under a wide range of conditions. However, such a method has not yet been developed. Many of the available methods have acceptable validity and reliability, but all have limitations. Choosing the most appropriate method or methods depends on various factors.

PURPOSE OF THE ASSESSMENT

The purpose and objectives of a research study or an intervention program are the primary factors to consider when selecting the physical activity assessment method. If the purpose is population surveillance of physical activity, it may be sufficient to classify individuals into broad activity categories such as sedentary, moderately active, or highly active. This can be accomplished by relatively simple and inexpensive methods, such as completion of a short questionnaire on general activity patterns. Physical inactivity has been identified as an important public health concern for adults and children; therefore, assessing sedentary activities may be equally as important as measuring physical activity in observational or intervention studies.

To investigate the relationship between activity and health outcomes, additional issues must be considered. The specific health outcome(s) of interest should guide the choice of activity assessment method. For example, if the health outcome is osteoporosis, specific attention should be given to weight-bearing and strength-building activities. For cardiovascular disease or diabetes outcomes, an aerobic activity such as walking might be emphasized.

Intervention studies typically involve tens or hundreds of participants, whereas population surveillance and epidemiological studies of physical activity and health require thousands or tens of thousands of participants. The small number of participants in intervention studies requires detailed information on physical activity to have sufficient statistical power to detect differences between groups. Another factor to consider in selecting a physical activity assessment method in an intervention study is the content of the intervention. If the study will emphasize fitting more walking into daily routines, a detailed questionnaire on walking times, amounts, intensity, frequency, and duration would be appropriate, and the use of a pedometer as an assessment tool would provide an objective measure. In clinical counseling situations, it is often important to assess an individual's activity level for the purposes of self-monitoring, goal setting, and evaluating progress. In this case, it is necessary to have data that accurately reflect the person's activity. Thus, a combination of self-assessment and objective monitoring would be ideal.

WHAT TO ASSESS (CHARACTERISTICS OF PHYSICAL ACTIVITY)

Specific dimensions of physical activity may have different effects on various health outcomes. Often, it is important to characterize physical activity using both quantitative and qualitative methods.[5] Particular dimensions of physical activity related to health include EE, aerobic intensity, weight bearing, flexibility, and strength.[14] The overall amount or volume of physical activity is generally measured in terms of the energy expended, and is often expressed in kilocalories. Indirect calorimetry and a stable isotope dilution method using DLW are valid methods of measuring activity-related EE. However, it is not feasible to use indirect calorimetry for assessing physical activity outside of the laboratory setting. The use of DLW is appropriately applied to free-living individuals, but it can only provide an estimate of PAEE averaged over a number of days and one must assume that REE and TEF remain constant over that time. Also, there are qualitative and quantitative aspects of physical activity that cannot be measured by DLW (i.e., type, duration, and frequency of physical activity) that may also be important in the regulation of energy balance and health.

PHYSICAL ACTIVITY PATTERNS (DAY, WEEK, SEASON, AND YEAR)

It is important to know how regularly an individual engages in physical activity and also how the patterns of activity vary at different times. The majority of health benefits are acquired as chronic adaptations to exercise, and this requires that habitual patterns of physical activity be assessed. Generally, adults have relatively regular daily patterns that may only change for different seasons or during holidays, whereas children have more erratic patterns of activity. Climate may influence greatly the type and frequency of activities undertaken. Significant differences have been found between weekdays and weekends in type and amount of activity.[15]

NATURE OF THE STUDY POPULATION (AGE, GENDER, AND CULTURE)

The nature of the population to be examined is an important consideration for choosing an assessment method. Methods developed for adults may not be appropriate for children. Since children appear to have more variation than adults in patterns of activity, and they perform activities over shorter time periods, their intermittent and frequently changing pattern of activity requires a different strategy than that used for adults.[16] Physical activity has been assessed in children and adolescents by various methods, including self-report by questionnaire or interview, which is probably of limited value in younger children, and report by proxies such as parents or teachers. Objective measures such as heart rate monitors, motion sensors, DLW, and indirect calorimetry have been used frequently in small-scale studies. A comprehensive approach to measurement issues in assessing children's physical activity has been presented by Welk et al.[16] Points to be considered when selecting a physical activity measurement for children and adolescents are that 7 days of monitoring are required to obtain stable estimates of overall activity patterns,[17] both weekend and weekdays need to be included in the assessment,[18] and motion sensors need to be worn for the entire day or at least for multiple times over the course of the day.[17]

In adults, other considerations include age, gender, and socioeconomic factors also may possibly often be important. For example, activity patterns between female and male executives may be similar, whereas women who are homemakers with child care responsibilities may have very different activity patterns than men of the same household who work outside the home. Newer information is available on specific activity assessment methods for specific racial or ethnic groups.[19] It is important to consider the various types of activity that are likely to be present in a population when planning what assessment method to use.

If the study group is a general population sample, it will probably be necessary to include a wide range of activities, including occupational, household, caretaking, leisure time, walking or cycling for transportation to work or on errands, and sports. If the project is to be conducted in a group of business executives, it is probably reasonable to evaluate leisure-time physical activity in detail, since these are the activities that provide most of the EE beyond Reating Energy Expenditure (REE) and TEF in this group. For these executives, it is reasonable to give only limited attention to occupations and household activities.

Physical activity varies with age, with general population data showing a gradual decline and the highest prevalence of sedentary behavior observed in elderly persons, especially women.[8] However, there may be substantial differences in activity patterns in retired individuals. For some, most of the activity might be housework and yard work, for others it might be walking, and perhaps for those living in retirement centers the major activities might be recreational activities such as golf or dancing. It is not possible to select a single activity assessment method for use with older individuals, but it is important to consider the type of older population that will be included in the project.

In summary, the nature of the population to be monitored is important to consider when selecting a physical activity assessment method. In general, younger persons are more active than older individuals, men are more active than women, and members of minority groups tend to be less active than non-Hispanic whites. Nonetheless, it is not possible to simply select a method based on age, gender, or racial/ethnic group status. Many other factors such as educational level, health status, geography, climate, and occupational group must be considered. Ideally, it would be useful to collect some pilot data, perhaps by open-ended questionnaires and conducting focus groups, to obtain information on types of activity most often reported by the target population.

SAMPLE/POPULATION SIZE

The characteristics or the size of a sample must be taken into account before selecting the activity measure. A national survey or a large population study is not likely to use labor-intensive or high-cost techniques. A validation study or clinical trial with a relatively small sample means that the cost, time, logistical complexity, and other resources per person can be increased, allowing the use of more sophisticated, time-consuming, and accurate techniques.

PERIOD OF MEASUREMENT

For instruments that measure activity over periods of time, an important question is the appropriate length of the monitoring period. This may differ for adults as compared with children and adolescents. According to Janz et al.,[20] 4 or more days of activity monitoring are needed to achieve satisfactory reliability, although Gretebeck and Montoye[21] suggested that at least 5 or 6 days of monitoring are needed to minimize intraindividual variance. More recently, Trost et al.[17] concluded that a 7-day monitoring period was required for accelerometers to assess usual activity in children and adolescents and account for apparent differences between weekday and weekend activity behaviors in the same way as within daily differences. Similarly, Matthews et al.[22] found that reliable accelerometer measures of activity in adults require at least 7 days of monitoring.

In addition to considering the length of the monitoring period, it is also necessary to consider whether multiple periods need to be monitored over the course of a year. It is obvious that seasonal or climatic effects could have an influence on physical activity, but this has not been studied adequately. Most epidemiological studies on physical activity and health have obtained activity measurements at one time point. However, some of these approaches have asked about activity over periods of various lengths — past week, past month, past 3 months, past year, or usual activity. There is insufficient evidence to determine whether any single approach is better than any other, so at this time investigators should simply select the recall period that seems logical for their specific population.

COST AND FEASIBILITY

Although objective measures are probably more accurate than self-reports for assessing physical activity, the high cost of these methods does not allow them to be used in some studies. For example, the use of methods such as DLW is not feasible in epidemiological studies because of cost and participant burden. Motion sensors (reviewed in more detail later) are objective and show promise, and the cost of such instruments has been decreasing. However, they still may be too expensive for use in some large studies, and technical support may be required, which further increases the cost. Some of the objective methods also impart a greater participant burden than questionnaire approaches. Use of DLW or motion sensors requires multiple visits to the study laboratory and requires participant cooperation and involvement over longer periods.

SUMMARY

It is not possible to give a few simple guidelines for selecting a physical activity assessment method, and we have presented several factors that need to be considered when making a decision. The purpose of the study, type of physical activity that is of interest, nature of the study group, size, and complexity of the study, and the available resources are all essential elements to be evaluated in order to select the most appropriate method for measuring physical activity. It is important to spend sufficient time in planning and selecting an assessment method to avoid later problems.

PHYSICAL ACTIVITY ASSESSMENT METHODS

Physical activity assessment methodology is a growing field, stimulated by a recent surge in obesity-prevention research and public interest in personal health. Extensive varieties of methods exist for obtaining qualitative and quantitative measures of physical activity. Matching one's study objectives, participant population, and resources with the appropriate physical activity measurement tools requires knowledge of the uses, strengths, and limitations of different approaches. A summary of methods, divided into subjective and objective categories, is provided below and in Table 36.1.

SUBJECTIVE METHODS

Subjective measures of physical activity rely on study participant or proxy self-report. Information is obtained by questionnaire or diary/log through manual or computer-assisted means. Time and materials costs vary across methods, as does the degree of detail in data collected. The benefits of flexibility in mode of administration (e.g., telephone, Internet, or in-person; self-administered or interviewer assisted) and relatively simple scoring for subjective assessment methods must be weighed against their susceptibility to participant misreporting. Also important to consider is the influence of mode of questionnaire administration on response bias.[23,24] Self-report methods are not recommended for use in children younger than 10 years of age due to the diverse range and sporadic nature of children's activities and their inability to accurately recall and record multiple aspects of physical activity.[25,26]

Questionnaires: Questionnaires are self-completed by the subject or proxy, or administered by research staff. Large-scale epidemiological studies frequently use questionnaires to evaluate the relationship between physical activity and health outcomes. Three general types of physical activity questionnaires, listed in increasing length and degree of detail, are global self-report, recall, and quantitative history. Questionnaires commonly measure occupational, household, and leisure activity separately and assign scores to answers, which are then converted to general activity levels or specific EE values. Guidelines have been published for using information derived from questionnaires to select an appropriate PAL factor in calculating TEE.[27] The accuracy, repeatability, and utility of self-report physical activity measures have been reviewed.[1,28–31] A compilation of physical activity questionnaires can be found in related literature.[32]

Records/diaries and logs: The terms *physical activity records*, *diaries*, and *logs* are used variously in the literature but generally refer to a detailed, ongoing account of physical activity performed over a defined period of time.[33] At regular time intervals, subjects record the duration of time spent performing specified types of physical activity. The listing of physical activity categories can be customized for evaluating a particular population (e.g., the elderly) or outcome measure (e.g., exercise intensity). EE scores are calculated by multiplying the summed time spent in each physical activity category by the rate of EE (or MET) for that category. Important to note, methods using average MET values listed in the Compendium of Physical Activity[6,7] to estimate PAEE may not produce accurate results for individuals. This limitation has been discussed by the Compendium authors[6,7] and was investigated by Bryne et al.[34] Another factor to consider is the substantial effort required of subjects and staff to keep and score, respectively, physical activity records. Handheld computerized versions of PA logs are gaining popularity as simple-to-use, accurate tools.[35] Ecologic Momentary Assessment (EMA), which captures information on the context of a behavior in real time, has been applied successfully to physical activity assessment by means of electronic diary.[36]

OBJECTIVE METHODS

Objective approaches to physical activity assessment utilize an external measure of activity, such as electronic activity monitors or direct observation. Objective methods carry generally higher costs for purchase, maintenance, and operation than do subjective methods, yet they avoid inaccuracies associated with subject misreport and are appropriate for use across most populations, including children. Common objective tools are described below and in Table 36.1.

Direct observation: In direct observation, the subject's physical activity is coded according to type, intensity, duration, etc., by a trained observer. Direct observation is used as a criterion measure and is frequently employed to assess physical activity in children.[37–39] Coding can be performed in real time or during review of a camera recording. Direct observation allows multiple dimensions of physical activity, such as social and physical context, to be reliably and objectively assessed, but the number of subjects observed and the time period and location of observation are limited.

Indirect calorimeters: Indirect calorimetry determines EE from VO_2 consumption and VCO_2 production, and is frequently used to measure PAEE. As an established method, it is often used as a criterion measure to validate other physical activity assessment methods. Respiratory gas exchange is measured within a whole-room calorimeter[40,41] or, more commonly, by means of

TABLE 36.1
Methods of Physical Activity Assessment

Instrument	Unit of Measurement	Period of Measurement	Field Measure	Activity parameters assessed					Cost	Subject Burden	Sample Size
				Total Volume	Duration	Intensity	Type	Frequency			
Subjective Measures											
I. Questionnaires[32,53]	Activity index; METs; kcal/day; kcal/kg day	Day to year	x	x	x	x	x	x	$	Light	Large
Retrospective quantitative history[70,71] Global[72,73] Recall[31,74]											
II. PA Records/Diary[35,55,75]	kcal/day	Days	x	x	x	x	x	x	$-$$	Heavy	Small
Objective Measures											
I. Direct Observation[38,39]	Min activity	Hours	x		x	x	x	x	$$	None	Small
II. Indirect Calorimetry[40]											
Whole-Room Calorimetry[41]	TEE, PAEE	1–3 days	x	x	x	x	x	x	$$$	Very heavy	Small
Metabolic Cart[42]	PAEE, REE	<1 h		x	x	x	x	x	$$$	Heavy	Small
Portable Gas Analyzer[44]	PAEE	Hours	x	x	x	x			$$	Heavy	Small
III. DLW[46]	TEE (PAEE-derived)	7–14 days	x	x	x				$$$	Light	Small–Medium
IV. Pedometers[76,77]	Steps; EE*	Days, weeks	x	x	x			x	$	Light	Medium–Large
V. Accelerometers[51,78] MTI (www.mtiactigraph.com) Actical (www.minimitter.com) Tritrac (www.stayhealthy.com)	Counts, PAEE; TEE*	1–2 weeks	x	x	x	x		x	$$	Light	Medium–Large
VI Heart Rate (HR) Monitors[56] Polar (www.polarheartratemonitor.com)	HR, PAEE; TEE*	Days	x	x	x	x		x	$$	Light–Moderate	Medium
VII. Recent Developments											
IDEEA (www.minisun.com)[57,58]	PAEE, TEE, qualitative measures	Days	x	x	x	x	x	x	$$$	Heavy	Small
Actiheart (www.minimitter.com)[59,60]	HR, PAEE, TEE	Days	x	x	x	x		x	$$	Light	Small–Medium
SenseWear Armband (www.bodymedia.com)[61–64]	HR, PAEE, TEE	Days	x	x	x	x		x	$$	Light–Moderate	Small–Medium

* Estimated by some models.

Cost: $ = Low, $$ = Moderate, $$$ = High.

an automated metabolic gas analyzer.[42] Recent advances in instrumentation have produced small, portable gas analyzers that can be used in field settings otherwise inaccessible to stationary metabolic carts.[43,44] While these newer compact devices enable measurement of free-living PAEE, they are cumbersome to wear and expensive at this stage of development.

DLW: This is considered the gold standard for measuring TEE.[45,46] In this method, stable isotopes of water (deuterium and oxygen-18) are orally administered to the subject and CO_2 production is estimated from analysis of the isotopes remaining in urine samples collected over time (usually 7 to 14 days). From this, average 24-h TEE is calculated using regression analysis.[47] PAEE is derived by subtracting measured or calculated[48] resting metabolic rate and TEF from TEE. The DLW method imposes minimal burden on free-living subjects; however, it is a technically complex and expensive technique that provides no descriptive physical activity information (e.g., type, duration, and frequency).

Activity monitors: Activity monitors comprise a variety of electronic and mechanical devices that include pedometers (step counters) and accelerometers (acceleration detectors). Pedometers record the number of steps accumulated over a period of time. Their low weight, low cost (for most models), and ability to provide feedback to the wearer are ideal for use in large-scale walking intervention studies. More detailed physical activity assessment requires the sophistication of an accelerometer. Most accelerometers contain a piezoelectric sensor that generates a voltage in response to movement in one or more planes of motion. The voltage is translated by a microprocessor to create a digital count value that can be further processed to yield EE. Typical accelerometer output displays the duration and energy cost of physical activity by intensity category for each recording hour. Accelerometers are easy to wear on the waist, wrist, or ankle, yet their operation and data management are significantly more complicated than that of pedometers. Reviews of accelerometry, including validation and reliability studies, are available.[49–52]

Heart rate monitors: Heart rate monitoring is a common method used to describe the intensity and duration of physical activity. The premise of this method is the linear relationship between heart rate and oxygen uptake across a range of aerobic activities. Most monitors have software for converting heart rate data into an estimate of EE. However, when a higher level of data accuracy is desired, a graded exercise test is required in order to calibrate the individual's heart rate to simultaneous oxygen consumption. From this, a calibration curve can be constructed for estimating EE at moderate to strenuous levels of exercise. A limitation of employing heart rate as a surrogate for EE is that the relationship between heart rate and VO_2 is weak at low activity levels, which are the levels characteristic of most sedentary individuals. For example, in a seated subject, heart rate can rise or fall solely in response to emotions, caffeine intake, ambient temperature, smoking, or illness.[53] Another important consideration in utilizing heart rate monitors for physical activity assessment is usability. Depending on model design, heart rate monitor chest transmitters are uncomfortable for some subjects to wear, resulting in poor compliance.[54,55] Suggested reviews of heart rate monitoring as a marker for physical activity are available.[30,50,56]

Recent developments: Devices that render novel applications to or combine traditional physical activity assessment methods have been introduced in recent years. One is a sophisticated system for recording posture and movement, called the Intelligent Device for Energy Expenditure and Activity (IDEEA). It is composed of a microcomputer worn on the hip with flexible wire extensions that attach to the feet, legs, and chest. Data output describes physical activity by type, intensity, duration, and energy cost. Validity and reliability studies have been conducted with encouraging results.[57,58]

Two examples of combination methods are Actiheart (heart rate monitor and accelerometer) and SenseWear Armband (accelerometer and multiple temperature sensors). Actiheart has shown reliability and validity (against indirect calorimetry) in estimating PAEE[59] and has demonstrated superior accuracy compared to accelerometry alone.[60] SenseWear Armband is a portable device worn on the upper arm that contains an accelerometer, temperature sensors, and a receiver capable of recording transmissions from a heart rate monitor. Studies evaluating SenseWear offer mixed results[61,62] and suggest that exercise-specific algorithms are necessary to accurately estimate PAEE.[63,64]

Global positioning system (GPS) technology has been applied to physical activity assessment methodology, particularly as a complement to accelerometry.[65] GPS contributes spatial data on locomotion, such as position, speed, incline, and stride length and frequency, all which influence the energy cost of movement.[66,67]

SUMMARY

The scope of physical activity assessment methodology has expanded in response to the need for comprehensive, accurate approaches to quantifying and qualifying physical activity. Exciting advances in electronic and computer technologies have resulted in increasingly small, portable devices capable of measuring multiple aspects of free-living physical activity. Changing demographics, including increased cultural diversity and a growing elderly population in the United States and other nations, has led to the development of population-specific physical activity questionnaires (e.g., for Spanish-speaking[68] and older individuals[69]). Such methodological advancements have not only improved the accuracy and descriptiveness of physical activity assessment but have also increased the accessibility of physical activity measurement tools to a wide range of health care and research professionals. The unique perspectives contributed by these investigators in the context of a global effort to promote physical activity will continue to spur the progress of physical activity assessment methodology.

REFERENCES

1. Sallis JF, Saelens BE. *Res Q Exerc Sport* 71:S1; 2000.
2. Institute of Medicine, Food and Nutrition Board. Dietary Reference Intakes for Energy, Carbohydrate, Fiber, Fat, Fatty Acids, Cholesterol, Protein, and Amino Acids (Macronutrients), 2004.
3. Frankenfield D, Roth-Yousey L, Compher C. *J Am Diet Assoc* 105:775; 2005.
4. Levine JA. *Nutr Rev* 62:S82; 2004.
5. Goran MI, Sun M. *Am J Clin Nutr* 68:944S; 1998.
6. Ainsworth BE, Haskell WL, Leon AS, et al. *Med Sci Sports Exerc* 25:71; 1993.
7. Ainsworth BE, Haskell WL, Whitt MC, et al. *Med Sci Sports Exerc* 32:S498; 2000.
8. Physical Activity and Health: A Report of the Surgeon General. Mental Health. US Department of Health and Human Services, 1996:135.
9. Blair SN, Kohl III HW, Paffenbarger Jr. RS, Clark DG, Cooper KH, Gibbons LW. *JAMA* 262:2395; 1989.
10. Blair SN, Kohl III HW, Barlow CE, Paffenbarger Jr. RS, Gibbons LW, Macera CA. *JAMA* 273:1093; 1995.
11. Ainsworth BE, Sternfeld B, Slattery ML, et al. *Cancer* 83:611; 1998.
12. Stone EJ, McKenzie TL, Welk GJ, Booth ML. *Am J Prev Med* 15:298; 1998.
13. Melanson Jr. EL, Freedson PS. *Crit Rev Food Sci Nutr* 36:385; 1996.
14. Paffenbarger Jr. RS, Lee IM, Kampert JB. *World Rev Nutr Diet* 82:210; 1997.
15. Tudor-Locke C, Bassett DR, Swartz AM, et al. *Ann Behav Med* 28:158; 2004.
16. Welk GJ, Corbin CB, Dale D. *Res Q Exerc Sport* 71:S59; 2000.
17. Trost SG, Pate RR, Freedson PS, et al. *Med Sci Sports Exerc* 32:426; 2000.
18. Sallis JF. *J Sch Health* 61:215; 1991.
19. Masse LC, Fulton JE, Watson KL, et al. *Res Q Exerc Sport* 70:212; 1999.
20. Janz KF, Witt J, Mahoney LT. *Med Sci Sports Exerc* 27:1326; 1995.
21. Gretebeck RJ, Montoye HJ. *Med Sci Sports Exerc* 24:1167; 1992.
22. Matthews CE, Ainsworth BE, Thompson RW, Bassett Jr. DR. *Med Sci Sports Exerc* 34:1376; 2002.
23. Pridemore WA, Damphousse KR, Moore RK. *Soc Sci Med* 61:976; 2005.
24. Perlis TE, Des Jarlais DC, Friedman SR, et al. *Addiction* 99:885; 2004.
25. Sallis JF, Buono MJ, Roby JJ, et al. *Med Sci Sports Exerc* 22:698; 1990.
26. Sallis JF, Buono MJ, Roby JJ, et al. *Med Sci Sports Exerc* 25:99; 1993.
27. Black AE. *Int J Obes Relat Metab Disord* 24:1119; 2000.
28. Shephard RJ. *Br J Sports Med* 37:197; 2003.
29. Lamonte MJ, Ainsworth BE. *Med Sci Sports Exerc* 33:S370; 2001.
30. Haskell WL, Kiernan M. *Am J Clin Nutr* 72:541S; 2000.
31. Matthews CE. Use of Self-Report Instruments to Assess Physical Activity. In: Welk GJ, ed. *Physical Activity Assessments for Health-Related Research*. Champaign, IL: Human Kinetics, 2002.
32. Pereira MA, FitzerGerald SJ, Gregg EW, et al. *Med Sci Sports Exerc* 29:S1; 1997.
33. Conway JM, Seale JL, Jacobs Jr. DR, Irwin ML, Ainsworth BE. *Am J Clin Nutr* 75:519; 2002.
34. Byrne NM, Hills AP, Hunter GR, et al. *J Appl Physiol* 99:1112; 2005.
35. Kretsch M, Blanton C, Baer D, Staples R, Horn W, Keim N. *JADA* 104 (Suppl 2):Abstracts; 2004.
36. Dunton GF, Whalen CK, Jamner LD, et al. *Am J Prev Med* 29:281; 2005.
37. Reilly JJ, Coyle J, Kelly L, et al. *Obes Res* 11:1155; 2003.
38. Robertson RJ, Goss FL, Aaron DJ, et al. *Med Sci Sports Exerc* 38:158; 2006.
39. Trost SG, Sirard JR, Dowda M, et al. *Int J Obes Relat Metab Disord* 27:834; 2003.
40. Levine JA. *Public Health Nutr* 8:1123; 2005.
41. Chen KY, Sun M. *J Appl Physiol* 83:2112; 1997.
42. Macfarlane DJ. *Sports Med* 31:841; 2001.
43. Duffield R, Dawson B, Pinnington HC, Wong P. *J Sci Med Sport* 7:11; 2004.
44. McNaughton LR, Sherman R, Roberts S, Bentley DJ. *J Sports Med Phys Fitness* 45:315; 2005.
45. Schoeller DA, Ravussin E, Schutz Y, et al. *Am J Physiol* 250:R823; 1986.
46. Schoeller DA. *J Nutr* 118:1278; 1988.
47. Racette SB, Schoeller DA, Luke AH, et al. *Am J Physiol* 267:E585; 1994.
48. Frankenfield DC, Rowe WA, Smith JS, Cooney RN. *JADA* 103:1152; 2003.
49. Chen KY, Bassett Jr. DR. *Med Sci Sports Exerc* 37:S490; 2005.
50. Ainslie P, Reilly T, Westerterp K. *Sports Med* 33:683; 2003.
51. Welk GJ, Blair SN, Wood K, Jones S, Thompson RW. *Med Sci Sports Exerc* 32:S489; 2000.
52. Welk GJ. Physical Activity Assessments for Health-Related Research. Champaign, IL: Human Kinetics, 2002.

53. Montoye HJ. *Measuring Physical Activity and Energy Expenditure*. Champaign, IL: Human Kinetics, 1996.
54. Lof M, Hannestad U, Forsum E. *Br J Nutr* 90:961; 2003.
55. Forrest A, Gustafson-Storms M, Gale B, et al. *FASEB J* 18:A112; 2004.
56. Janz KF. Use of Heart Rate Monitors to Assess Physical Activity. In: Welk GJ, ed. *Physical Activity Assessments for Health-Related Research*. Champaign, IL: Human Kinetics, 2002.
57. Zhang K, Pi-Sunyer FX, Boozer CN. *Med Sci Sports Exerc* 36:883; 2004.
58. Zhang K, Werner P, Sun M, et al. *Obes Res* 11:33; 2003.
59. Brage S, Brage N, Franks PW, et al. *Eur J Clin Nutr* 59:561; 2005.
60. Corder K, Brage S, Wareham NJ, Ekelund U. *Med Sci Sports Exerc* 37:1761; 2005.
61. Fruin ML, Rankin JW. *Med Sci Sports Exerc* 36:1063; 2004.
62. King GA, Torres N, Potter C, et al. *Med Sci Sports Exerc* 36:1244; 2004.
63. Cole PJ, LeMura LM, Klinger TA, et al. *J Sports Med Phys Fitness* 44:262; 2004.
64. Jakicic JM, Marcus M, Gallagher KI, et al. *Med Sci Sports Exerc* 36:897; 2004.
65. Rodriguez DA, Brown AL, Troped PJ. *Med Sci Sports Exerc* 37:S572; 2005.
66. Schutz Y, Herren R. *Med Sci Sports Exerc* 32:642; 2000.
67. Terrier P, Ladetto Q, Merminod B, Schutz Y. *Med Sci Sports Exerc* 33:1912; 2001.
68. Elosua R, Garcia M, Aguilar A, et al. *Med Sci Sports Exerc* 32:1431; 2000.
69. Stewart AL, Mills KM, King AC, et al.. *Med Sci Sports Exerc* 33:1126; 2001.
70. Reiff GG, Montoye HJ, Remington RD, et al. *J Sports Med Phys Fitness* 7:135; 1967.
71. Taylor HL, Jacobs Jr. DR, Schucker B, et al. *J Chronic Dis* 31:741; 1978.
72. Schechtman KB, Barzilai B, Rost K, Fisher Jr. EB. *Am J Public Health* 81:771; 1991.
73. Weiss TW, Slater CH, Green LW, et al. *J Clin Epidemiol* 43:1123; 1990.
74. Sallis JF, Haskell WL, Wood PD, et al. *Am J Epidemiol* 121:91; 1985.
75. Irwin ML, Ainsworth BE, Conway JM. *Obes Res* 9:517; 2001.
76. Schneider PL, Crouter SE, Bassett DR. *Med Sci Sports Exerc* 36:331; 2004.
77. Tudor-Locke C, Ainsworth BE, Thompson RW, Matthews CE. *Med Sci Sports Exerc* 34:2045; 2002.
78. Bassett Jr. DR, Ainsworth BE, Swartz AM, et al. *Med Sci Sports Exerc* 32:S471; 2000.

37 Environmental Challenges and Assessment

Suzanne Phelan and Gary D. Foster

CONTENTS

INTRODUCTION

The prevalence of obesity in the United States has increased dramatically over the last 20 years. Data from the 1999–2002 National Health and Nutrition Examination Survey (NHANES) show that 65% of the adult population in the United States is overweight, which is defined as having a body mass index (BMI) greater than 25 kg/m^2, compared with 46% seen in NHANES I, conducted between 1971–1974 (Figure 37.1).[5,10] The prevalence of obesity, defined as BMI greater than 30 kg/m^2, has increased dramatically from 14 to 30% over the same time frame (Figure 37.1).[10] Children are also affected, with the prevalence of obesity in children and adolescents up by 10% (from 6 to 16%) during this period (Figure 37.2). Based on prevalence data over the past 30 years, Foreyt and Goodrick[11] predicted that the entire U.S. population will be obese by the twenty-third century. The World Health Organization (WHO) has declared overweight as one of the top ten risk conditions in the world and one of the top five in developed nations.[12]

In this chapter, the major environmental factors that have contributed to the rise in obesity will be examined. In addition, methods of assessing environmental influences at the population and clinical levels will be reviewed.

ETIOLOGY OF OBESITY

Obesity is the result of an energy imbalance in which intake exceeds expenditure. Both biological and behavioral factors play a role in the development of obesity.[13] Research over the past 15 years has underscored the importance of genetic factors in the etiology of obesity.[5,6] However, genetic composition has not changed dramatically in the last few decades to explain the accelerating trend in obesity. Therefore, attention has shifted toward environmental factors as the driving force behind the obesity epidemic.[14,15] The environment of industrialized countries has been viewed as so severely promoting of obesity that it has been labeled "toxic."[16,17] In order to combat the "toxic environment," extreme measures have been proposed, including

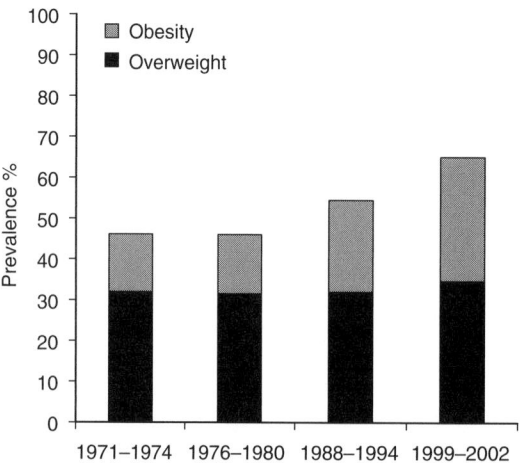

FIGURE 37.1 Prevalence of overweight (BMI ≥25 to 29.9 kg/m^2) and obesity (BMI ≥30 kg/m^2) in the United States from 1960 to 2002. (*Source:* Based of data from the NHANES.[5,8])

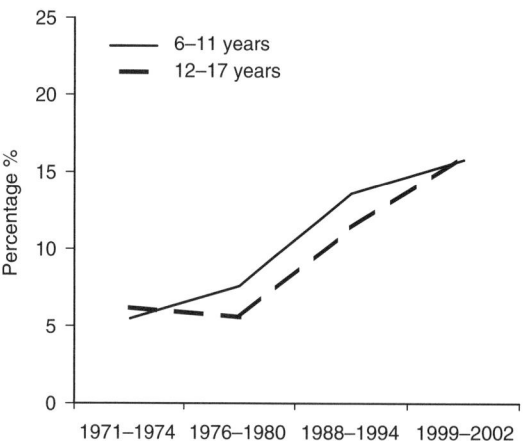

FIGURE 37.2 Prevalence of overweight and obesity (BMI ≥95th percentile) in children and adolescents in the United States, 1963–2002. (*Source:* National Center for Health Statistics[7]; Froiano, Flegal, et al., 1995[9]; Hedley, Ogden, Johnson et al., *JAMA.* 291:2847; 2004. With permission et al.[5])

a tax on high-fat, low-nutrition foods.[18–20] In order to better understand the environmental influences on obesity, both energy intake and expenditure must be examined.

ENVIRONMENTAL FACTORS

ENERGY INTAKE

Food consumption in industrialized and Western nations has increased significantly over the past few decades. U.S. data from NHANES indicate that between 1971 and 2000 the average energy intake for men increased from 2450 to 2618 kcals/day and, for women, from 1542 to 1877 kcals/day.[21]

Similarly, data from the United States Department of Agriculture (USDA) indicate that the food supply has also increased, most significantly over the past few decades (Figure 37.3). Specifically, the amount of food available for consumption per capita per day has increased from 3500 kcal per capita/day in 1909 to an average of 3900 kcal per capita/day in 2000, representing a 10% increase.[4] Other indicators, including increases in portion sizes and the widespread availability of high-fat and energy-dense foods further suggest that increases in energy intake account, in part, for the rising prevalence of obesity.[22]

Larger Portions and Decreased Costs

Although little empirical data examining secular trends in portion sizes exist, the "supersizing" of America is ubiquitous. Whereas once only 8 oz servings of soft drinks were available, today 16, 32, 20, and 64 oz drinks can be purchased at convenience stores

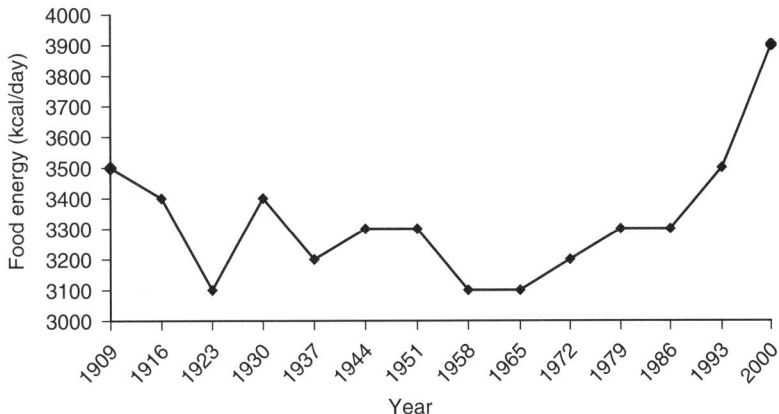

FIGURE 37.3 Food energy per capita per day in the United States. (*Source:* USDA Center for Nutrition Policy and Promotion, 2004.[4])

TABLE 37.1
Typical vs. Recommended Serving Sizes

	Typical	USDA
Medium baked potato	7 oz	4 oz
Medium bagel	4 oz	2 oz
Medium muffin	6 oz	2 oz

USDA = United States Department of Agriculture.

Source: Young and Nestle, *JADA*. 98:458; 1998.

and restaurants nationwide.[16] A "king size" McDonald's soft drink in the 1950s is equivalent to the "child size" of today.[14] Similarly, a McDonald's "medium" serving of French fries was reclassified as a "small" in order to make room for a new supersized serving of French fries. Candy bars and potato chips sizes have also increased dramatically from their "traditional" sizes.[23] In addition, recommended serving sizes are often much smaller than people's perceptions. For example, research participants selected as a single serving a "medium" bagel that was twice the size of the recommended USDA serving, and chose a "medium" muffin that was three times the recommended serving size (Table 37.1).[24] These trends are concerning, as studies have demonstrated that increased portion sizes encourage increased consumption.[25]

Consumption of larger portions is further enhanced by attractive size/quantity discounts. "Value meals" offering larger burgers, fries, and soft drinks for only a small increase in cost have continued to gain in popularity. Similarly, a 22 oz soft drink at a movie theatre costs $2.50 while a drink twice the size (i.e., 44 oz) costs only 50 cents more. In addition, marketing data suggest that supersizing and multiple unit-pricing (i.e., "two for $1.00" instead of "50 cents each") translate into greater food consumption.[16] In one study,[25] subjects poured themselves 20% more bottled water when it came in a 2 l container than when it came in a 1 l container. Interestingly, when the containers were labeled "tap water," participants poured the same amount from each container, suggesting that consumption is influenced by perceived cost/value. Other research has shown that reducing the price of health foods increases sales of these items.[26,27]

High-Fat, Energy-Dense, and Convenience Foods

Of all the nutrients, fat is the most energy dense, providing 9 kcal/g compared with 7 kcal/g for alcohol and 4 kcal/g for protein and carbohydrate. As fat is the most calorically dense macronutrient, its consumption is likely to increase the risk of subsequent weight gain.[28–31]

Surprisingly, based on surveys of individual intake, there has been a decrease in percentage of energy intake from fat over the past few decades. NHANES data indicate that between 1971 and 2000 the percentage of kilocalories from total fat decreased from 36.9 to 32.8% ($p < .01$) for men and from 36.1 to 32.8% ($p < .01$) for women.[21] In addition, the percentage of kilocalories from saturated fat decreased from 13.5 to 10.9% ($p < .01$) for men and from 13.0 to 11.0% ($p < .01$) for women. The decrease in fat intake may reflect, in part, the increase in total calories consumed over this time frame. However, since 1909, the amount of fats and oils in the U.S. food supply has nearly doubled, and consumption of sweets has increased by 7% (Figure 37.4).[3]

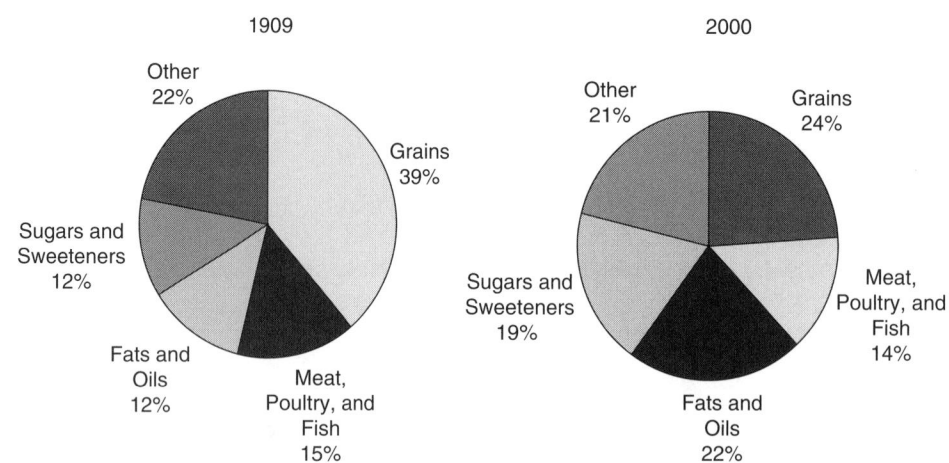

FIGURE 37.4 Sources of food energy in the U.S. food supply. (*Source:* USDA Center for Nutrition Policy and Promotion, 2004.[4])

In addition, the increased availability of high-fat, energy-dense food is observable in the proliferation of food courts, service station minimarts, fast food restaurants, and drive-through windows. Increasingly, fast food restaurants are found at schools and hospital cafeterias. McDonald's stated goal is to have no American more than 4 min from a McDonald's restaurant. Furthermore, an estimated three new McDonald's restaurants are opened each day.[12] Estimates suggest that 37% of adults and 42% of children eat in a fast food restaurant on any given day.[32] Continued fast food consumption has been shown to predict increased BMI in both children and adults.[23,33–35] Moreover, adults and children who report eating fast food have higher intakes of total energy, fat, saturated fat, sodium, and carbonated soft drinks, and lower intake of vitamins A and C, milk, fruits, and vegetables.[32,35]

Correspondingly, consumer purchases of high-fat foods are on the rise. The proportion of money spent at fast food and other restaurants has risen from 26.9% in 1974 to 38.2% in 1994.[36] In addition, home purchases of high-fat, energy-dense foods have risen. Specifically, the proportion of home food purchases of fats, oils, prepackaged foods, and frozen meals has increased more than any other category of food since the 1980s, even after controlling for changes in food prices.[37] The second largest increase was in cereal and bakery products, including cookies, cakes, and doughnuts. Interestingly, the percentage of Americans consuming low-fat products has also increased from 19% in 1978 to 76% in 1991.[38] The added sugars in low-fat foods, and the belief that larger portions are more acceptable, may offset any caloric benefit of consuming low-fat products.[39]

Soft drink consumption has increased by 131% since 1977.[40] This huge increase has contributed to the added sugars that comprised 16% of total energy intake in the American diet; intake of sugars is even higher among adolescents, comprising 20% of total energy intake.[41] As soft drink consumption has increased, milk consumption has decreased (Figure 37.5), and there are data to suggest that soft drinks are displacing milk consumption among children and adolescents.[3,14,41] The increasing availability of soft drink vending machines could be contributing to the increase in soft drink consumption. In 1999, 2.8 million soft drink vending machines dispensed 25.9 billion drinks.[42]

Summary

The available research, based principally on self-reports, reveals significant increases in dietary intake over the past few decades. The principal factors that appear to be responsible are increasing portion sizes and accessibility to high-fat, energy-dense foods at an affordable price.

ENERGY EXPENDITURE

Although nearly one-third of U.S. adults do not engage in any physical activity during their leisure time, there is little evidence that physical activity levels have changed significantly over the past decade (Figure 37.6).[43] Nonetheless, it is generally accepted that, with the modernization of society, energy expenditure has decreased and is at least partly responsible for the increasing prevalence of obesity.[13,44,45] The decrease in energy expenditure is most likely due to changes in activities of daily living.[45]

Table 37.2 lists some of the ways time (and energy) is saved each day. In particular, computers have clearly changed the American workplace, as their numbers have increased exponentially in the last two decades. It has been suggested that sending an e-mail rather than walking to the office next door to communicate information may decrease energy expenditure by half.[14] Computer use in the home has also increased dramatically, from 8% in 1984 to 61.8% in 2003.[46] Parallel increases have been observed in purchases of cable television (Figure 37.7).[1,47] Estimates suggest that adults spend an average of 28 h/week watch-

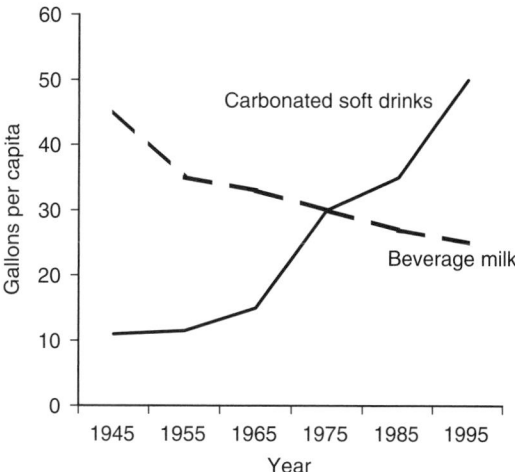

FIGURE 37.5 Per capita consumption of milk and carbonated soft drinks, 1945–1995. (*Source:* Putnam and Gerrior. Trends in the US Food Supply, 1970–1997. *America's Eating Habits: Changes and Consequences.* Washington DC: USDA Economic Research Service; 1999.)

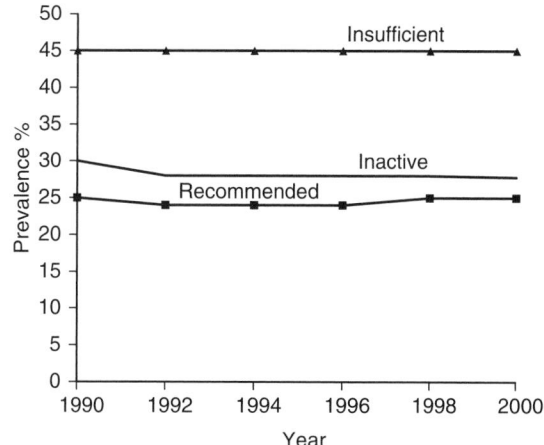

FIGURE 37.6 Trends in leisure time physical activity of adults aged 18+ years, Behavioral Risk Factor Surveillance System, United States, 1990–2000. (*Source:* US Department of Health and Human Services.[6,79]) (Recommended level=moderate intensity activity ≥5 times/week for ≥30 min each time per day or vigorous intensity ≥3 times/week for ≥200 min each time, or both; insufficient= some activity but not enough to be classified as moderate or vigorous; inactive=no leisure time physical activity during the preceding month.)

ing television, and children and adolescents watch an average of 25 h/week.[48] Children spend more time watching television than any other activity, with the exception of sleeping, and by the age of 18 the average teenager has spent more time watching television than learning in the classroom.[22,49] Television viewing is strongly related to the increasing prevalence of obesity among children[50–52] and to the level of obesity in adults.[53,54]

Automobiles are clearly the preferred mode of travel over walking in both the United States (Figure 37.8)[7] and United Kingdom,[55] and people are less likely than in previous years to walk or bike. The environmental barriers to bicycling and walking include lack of bike trail access, safety concerns (e.g., crime), lighting, and traffic, lack of changing facilities at work, lack of employer support, and inconvenience.[56] More research is needed on trends in other laborsaving devices or on their potential impact on physical activity levels, such as escalators and leaf blowers.

CULTURAL AND SOCIAL FACTORS

The increasing prevalence of overweight is also associated with cultural and social factors. The prevalence of obesity in the United States is greatest among non-Hispanic Blacks and Mexican-American women (Figure 37.9).[5] This may reflect cultural values and beliefs that limit the motivation for weight control and effectiveness of weight-control programs or specific behav-

TABLE 37.2
Energy Savers

Personal computers
Telecommuting
Cellular phones
Email/Internet
Shopping by phone
Food delivery services
Phone extensions
Dishwashers
Escalators/Elevators
Cable movies
Drive-through windows
Computer games
Intercoms
Moving sidewalks
Remote controls
Garage-door openers
Snowblowers
Riding lawn mowers

Source: Based on data from the NHANES.[5,8]

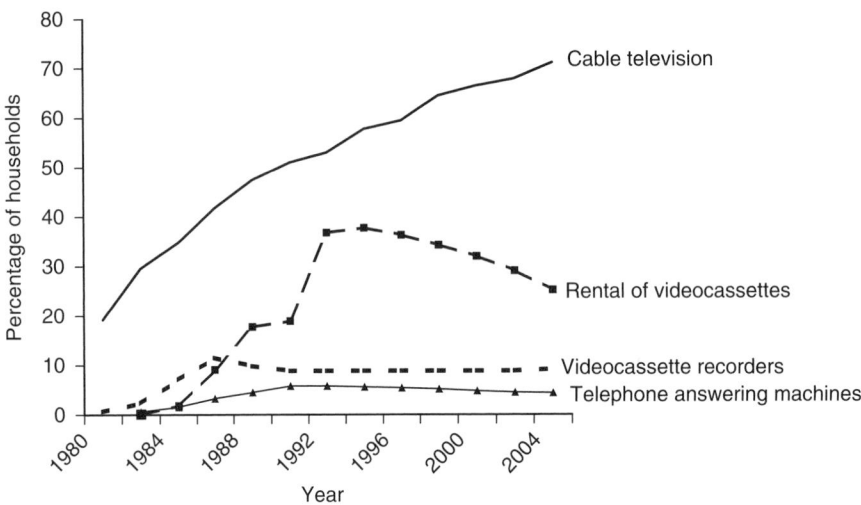

FIGURE 37.7   Percentage of households reporting expenditures, 1980–2004. (*Source:* US Bureau of Labor Statistics, 1992.[1])

iors such as lower levels of physical activity.[57,58] Metabolic factors may also play a role, including decreased energy expenditure among obese African-American women relative to Caucasian women.[59]

Obesity is also more common among low-income populations.[60] Low-income populations often experience differential access to health care services[61,62] due to cost barriers, unavailability of health insurance, and discrimination in health care.[63,64] Economic status may also impact families' nutritional patterns, level of concern about nutrition, and knowledge of foods to purchase and consume.[65,66]

ASSESSMENT OF ENVIRONMENTAL CHALLENGES

A detailed review of measures of food intake and physical activity can be found in Chapters 26 to 29, 36, 49, and 51 of this book and other comprehensive texts (e.g., References 67 and 68) Therefore, only a brief review of assessment tools will be provided here.

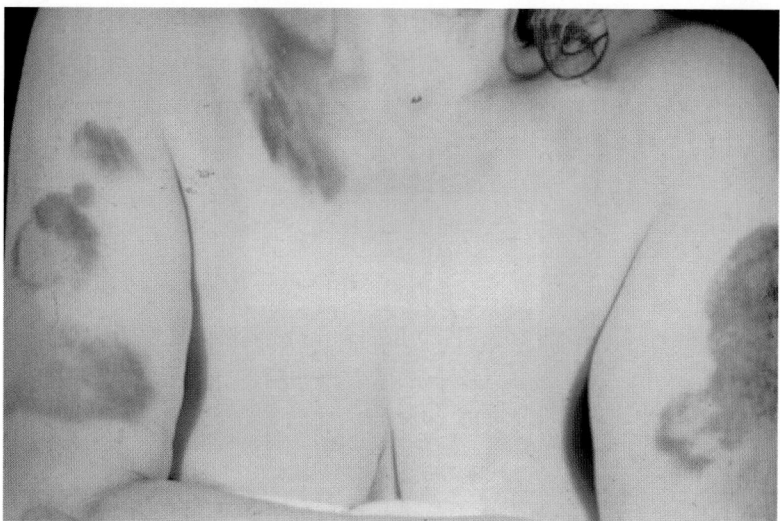

COLOR FIGURE 9.1   Adult female patient with severe vitamin K deficiency illustrating multiple purpuric areas accuring spoentaneously. (Photo courtesy of Elaine B. Feldman.)

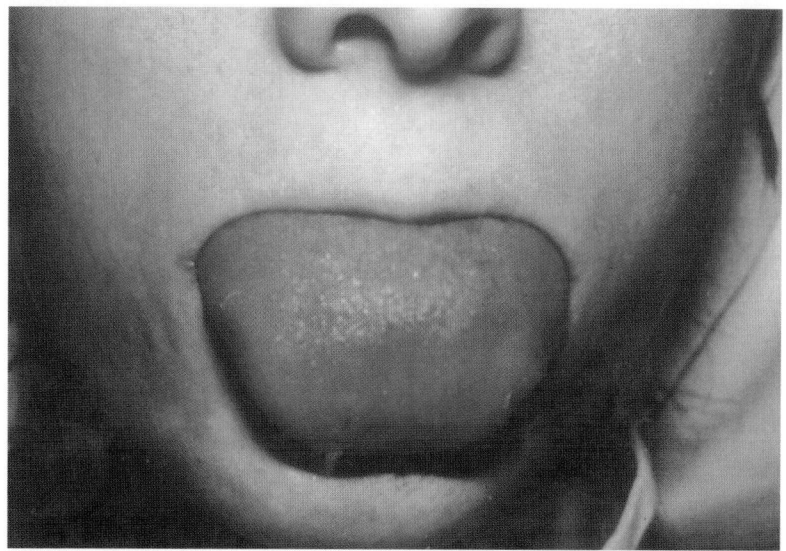

COLOR FIGURE 9.2   Adult female patient with advanced deficiency of riboflavin (vitamin B_2) illustrating large, red, smooth tongue, Paller and Cheelosis. (Photo courtesy of Elaine B. Feldman, MD.)

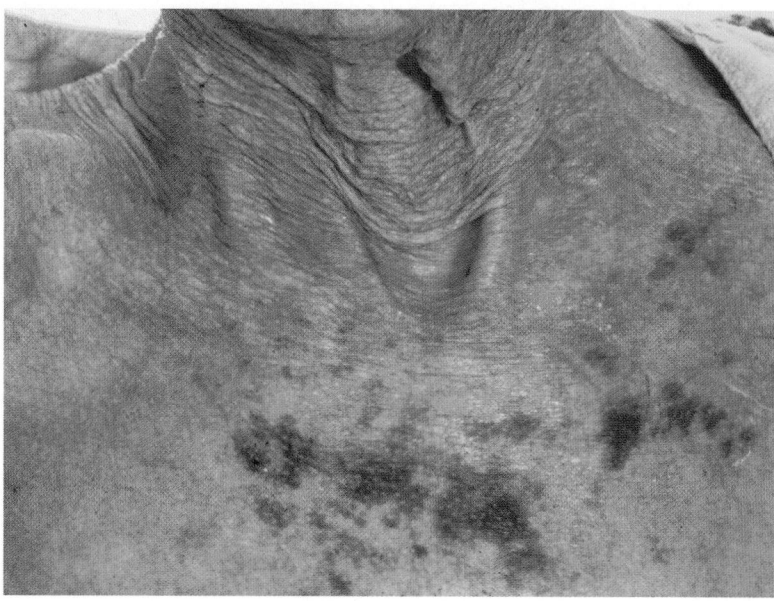

COLOR FIGURE 9.3   Adult male patient with advanced lesions of pellagra resulting from severe, prolonged main deficiency illustrating a dark scaly, eruptier over the skin particularly the seen exposed areas. (Photo courtesy of Elaine B Feldman MD.)

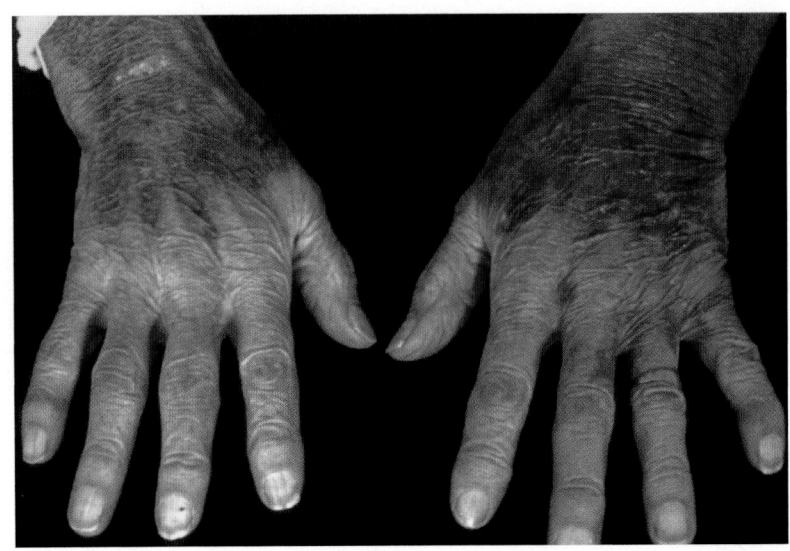

COLOR FIGURE 9.4   Same patient as in Figure 9.3 showing hands with dark, scaly thickened skin lesions. (Photo courtesy of Elaine B. Feldman MD.)

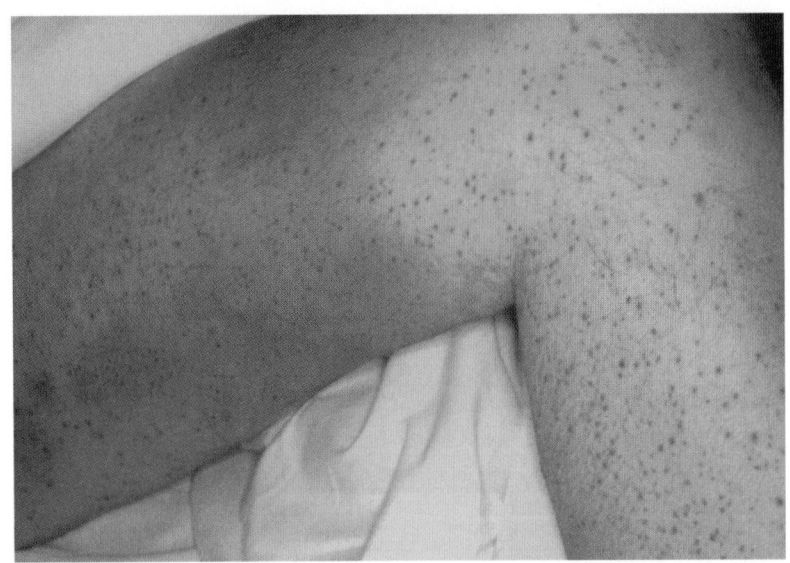

COLOR FIGURE 9.5   Adult female patient with advanced scurvy resulting from severe deficiency of vitamin C illustrating multiple perifollicular hemorrhages and sore corkscrew hairs. (Photo courtesy of Elaine B Feldman MD.)

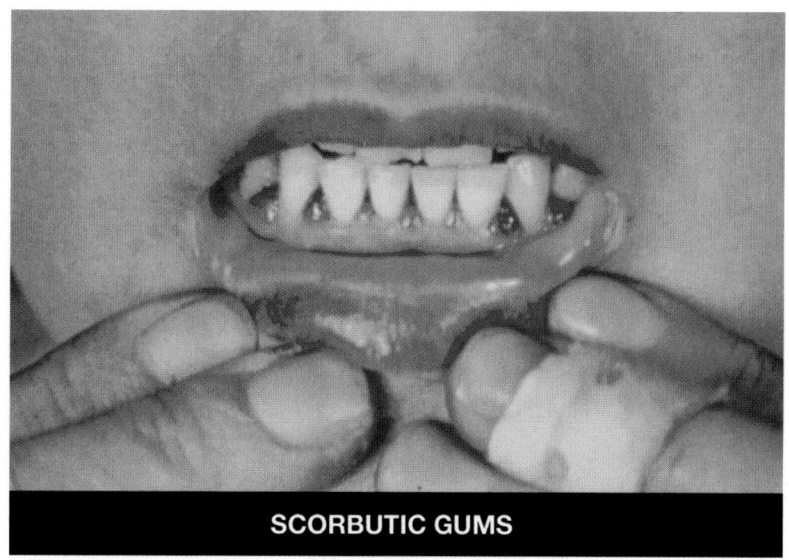

SCORBUTIC GUMS

COLOR FIGURE 9.6   Same patient as in Figure 9.5 showing bleeding, swollen gingeval tissues. (Photo courtesy of Elaine B Feldman MD.)

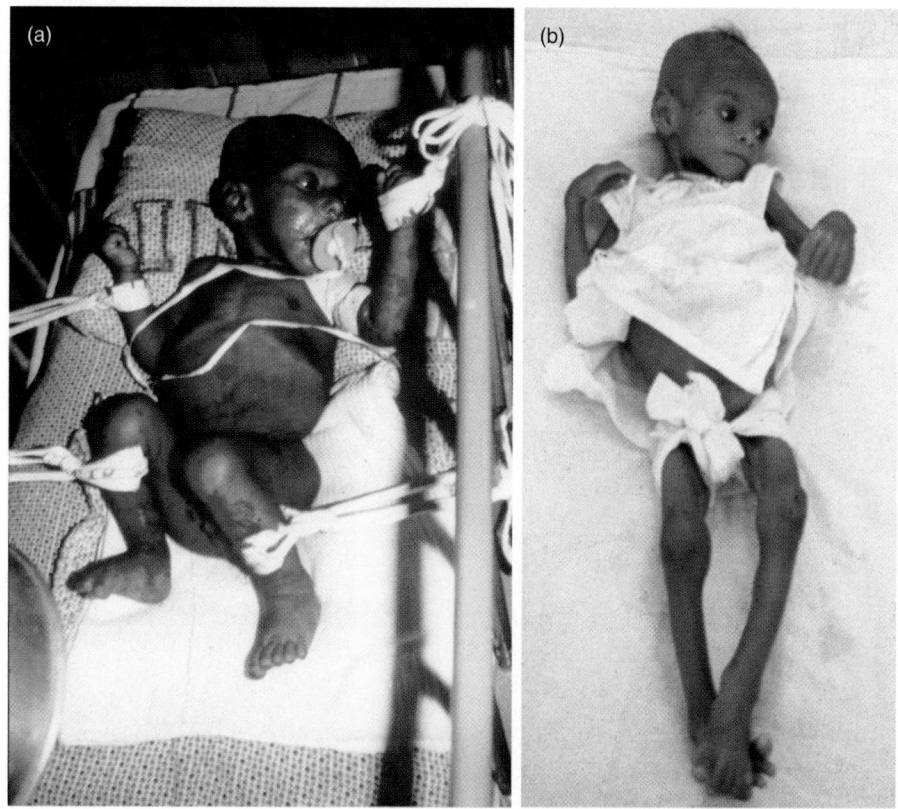

COLOR FIGURE 39.1   (a) Marasmic infant. (b) Kwashiorkor in a child. (Photographs are from Brazil and were provided by Dr. T. Kuske. They are reproduced from Feldman, EB, *Essentials of Clinical Nutrition*, Philadelphia, PA, F.A. Davis, 1988, pp. 321–325. With permission.)

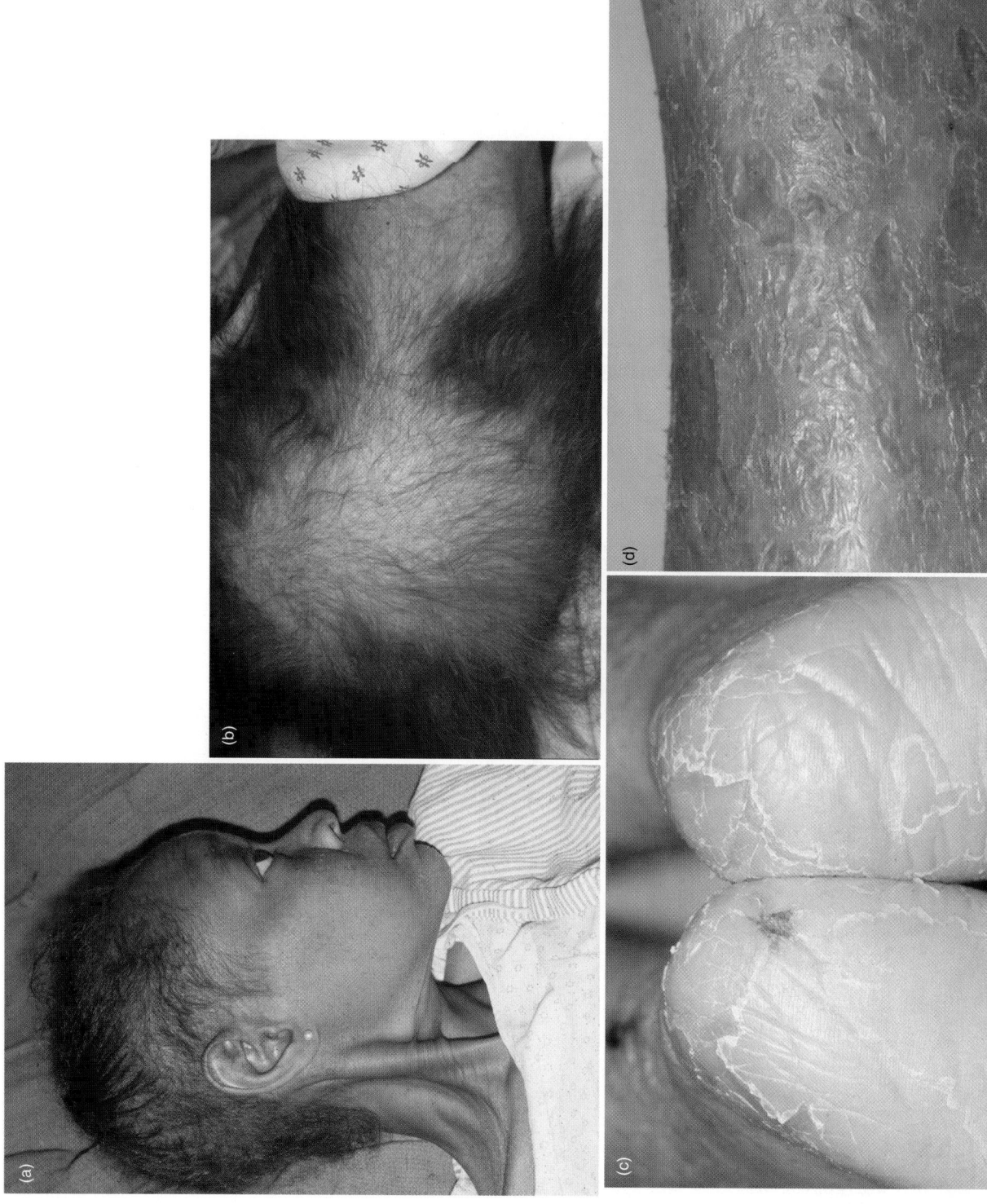

COLOR FIGURE 39.2 EExamples of some of the physical findings associated with PEM. (a) reddish hair (b) hair loss (c) flaking skin of the heels (d) 'flaking paint' dermatosis-darkly pigmented patches that may peal like old, sun-baked and blistered paint. (Photographs are provided by Dr. E.B. Feldman of patients at the Medical College of Georgia, Augusta.)

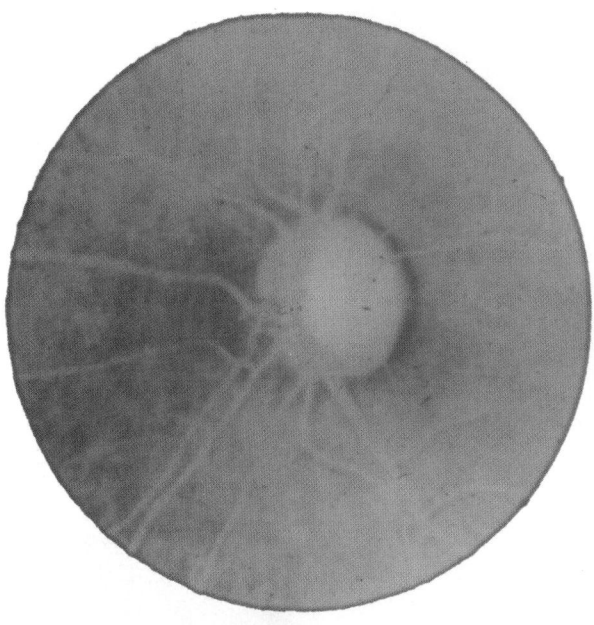

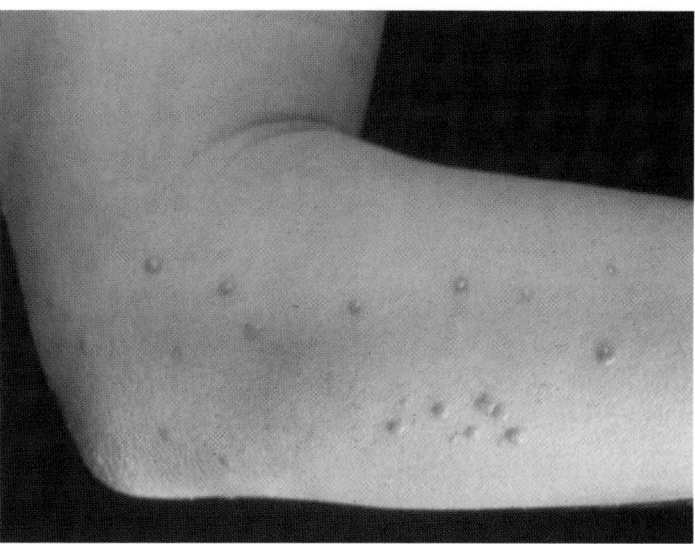

COLOR FIGURE 42.2 Eruptive xanthomas observed in a patient with chylomicronemia.

COLOR FIGURE 42.1 Lipemia retinalis visualized in the optical fundus of a patient with chylomicronemia with TAG levels exceeding 3000 mg/dl.

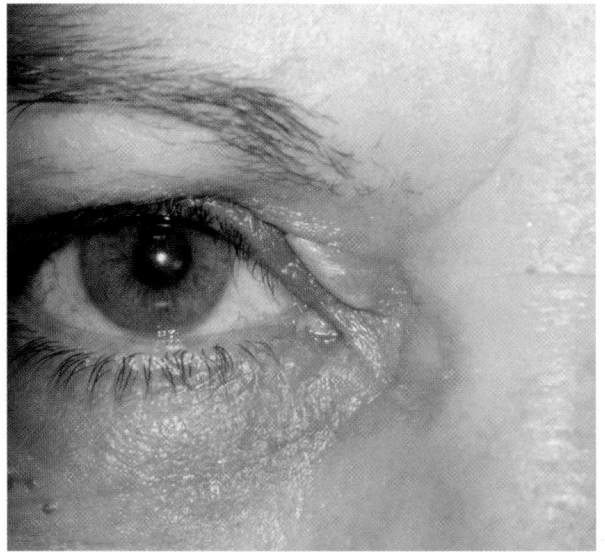

COLOR FIGURE 42.3 Eyelid xanthelasma from a woman with familial hypercholesterolemia.

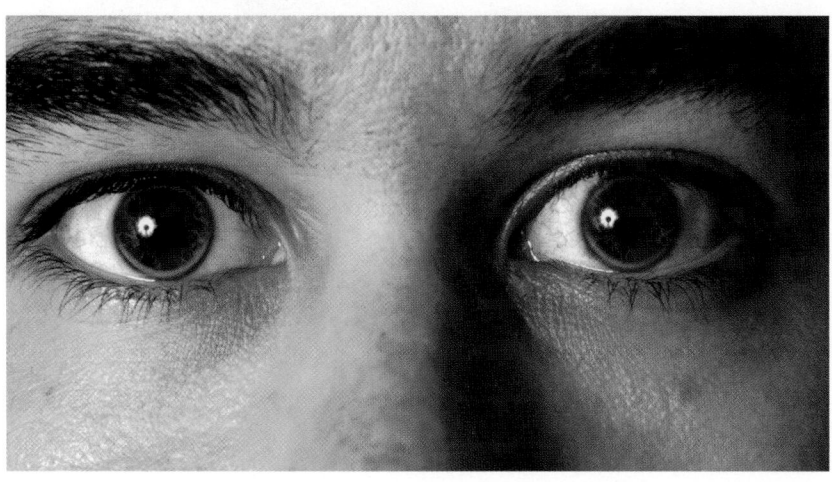

COLOR FIGURE 42.4 Corneal arcus observed in a 31-year-old man with familial hypercholesterolemia.

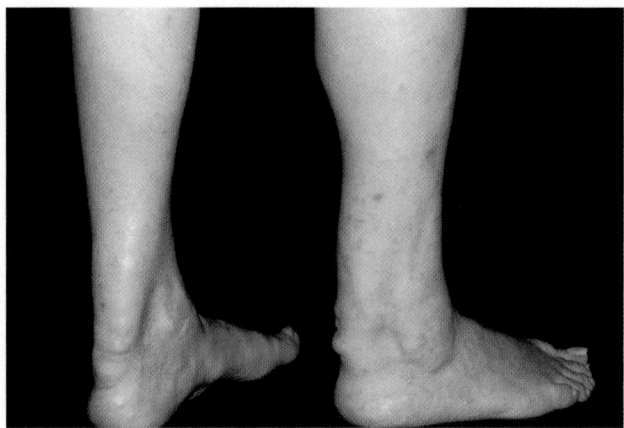

COLOR FIGURE 42.5 Xanthomas of the Achilles tendon of a patient with familial hypercholesterolemia.

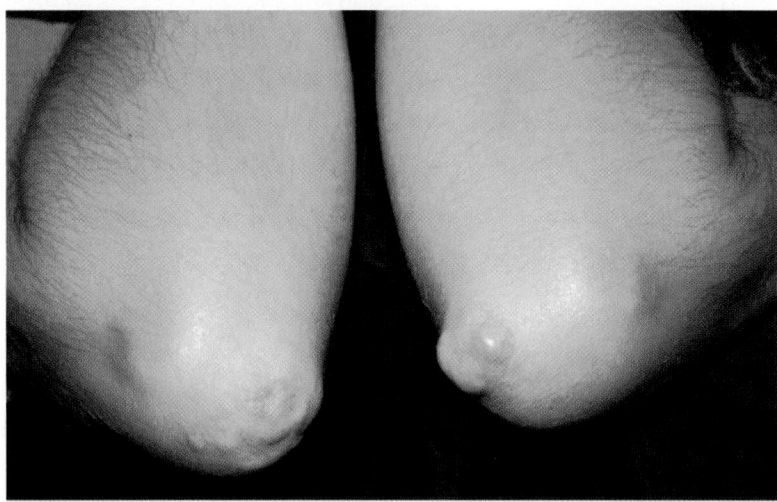

COLOR FIGURE 42.6 Tuberous xanthomas in the skin of the elbows of a teenage girl with familial hypercholesterolemia.

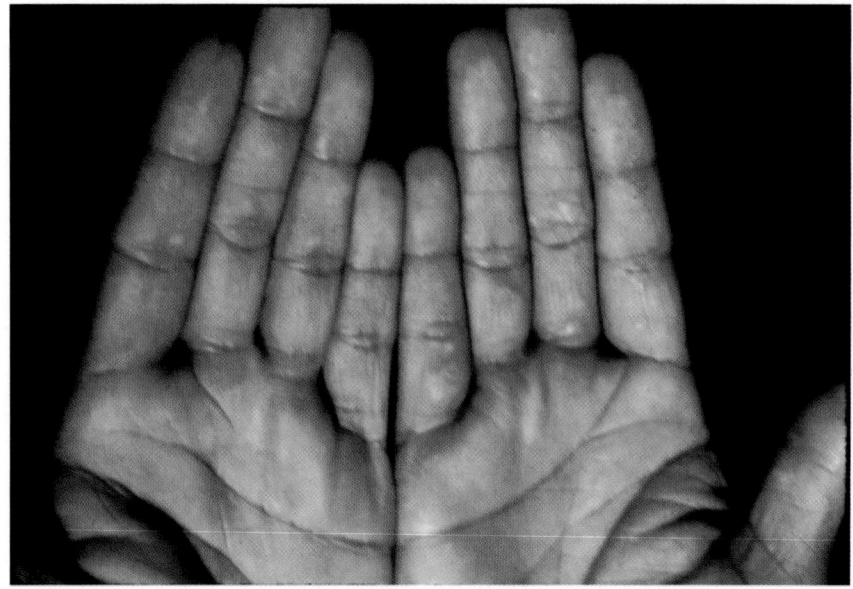

COLOR FIGURE 42.7 Yellow linear deposits in the creases of the fingers and palms of the hands of a 33-year-old man with Type III hyperlipoproteinemia.

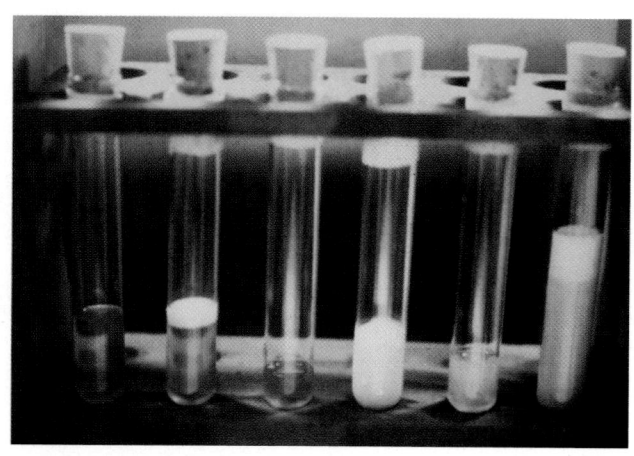

COLOR FIGURE 42.8 The appearance of plasma, refrigerated overnight, from fasting patients. The tubes with plasma samples are taken from (left to right): a subject with normal lipid levels and clear plasma (similar to a patient with Type IIa); a patient with chylomicronemia (Type I) with a creamy top layer above a clear infranatant; a patient with hypercholesterolemia (Type IIa) with clear plasma; a patient with Type III hyperlipoproteinemia with diffusely turbid plasma; a patient with Type IV hyperlipoproteinemia also showing diffuse turbidity; and a patient with Type V hyperlipoproteinemia with plasma exhibiting a creamy top layer over a turbid infranatant.

Red blood cell development

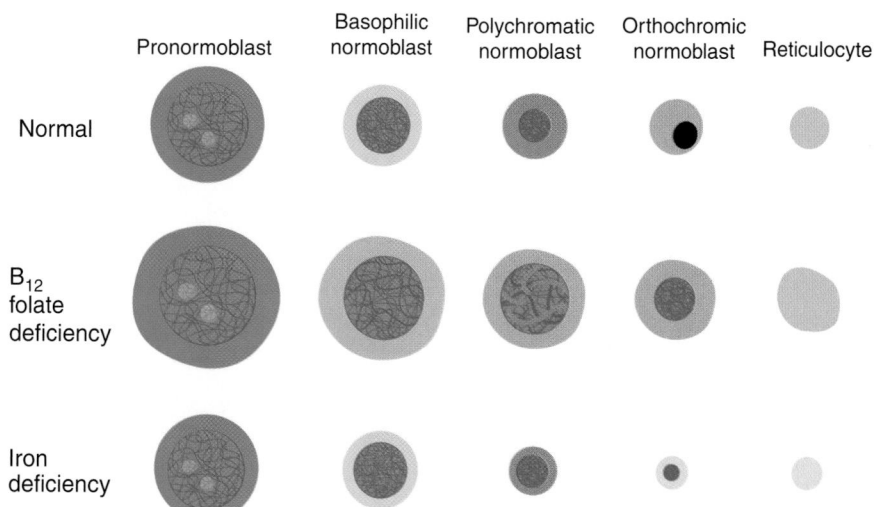

COLOR FIGURE 65.1 Erythropoiesis as it is affected by states of iron deficiency and vitamin B_{12} or folate deficiency.

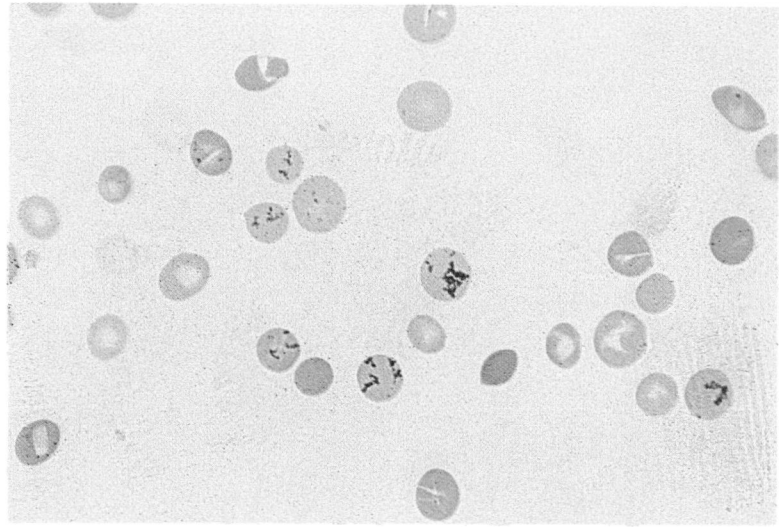

COLOR FIGURE 65.2 Reticulocytes. The appearance of young, newly produced RBCs, reticulocytes, as seen in the peripheral blood smear that has been stained with new methylene blue.

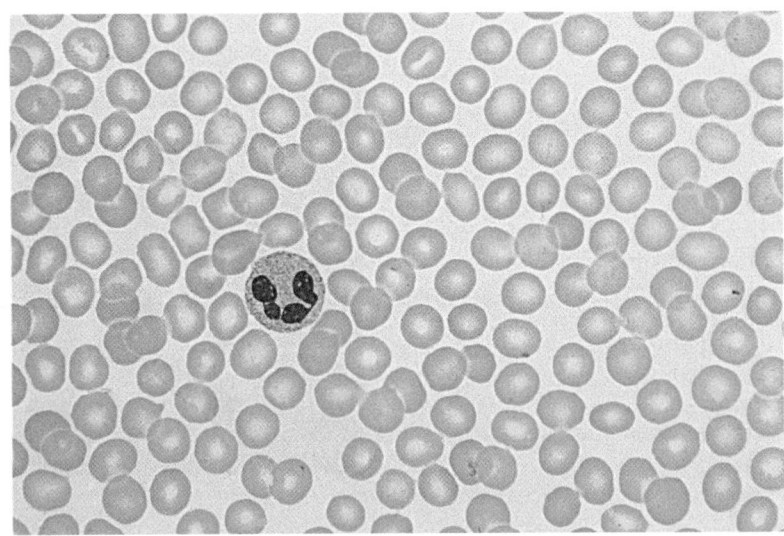

COLOR FIGURE 65.4 A normal peripheral blood smear.

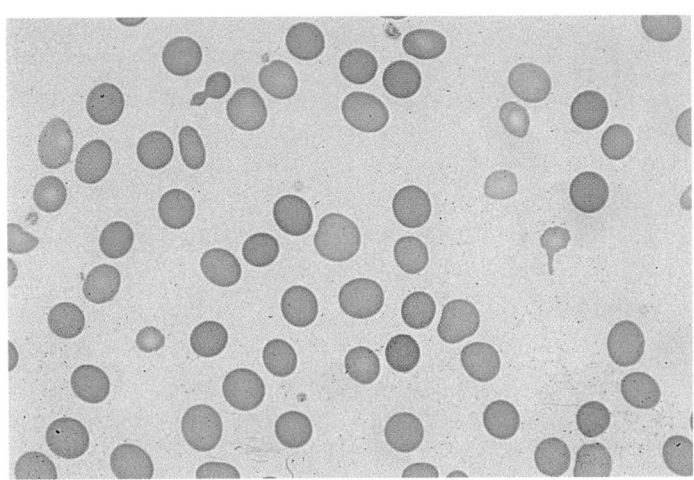

COLOR FIGURE 65.5 Macrocytic RBCs. RBCs that are larger than normal (macrocytic) and white blood cells that have nuclei with multiple segments (hypersegmented neutrophils) are characteristic of a vitamin B_{12} deficiency anemia.

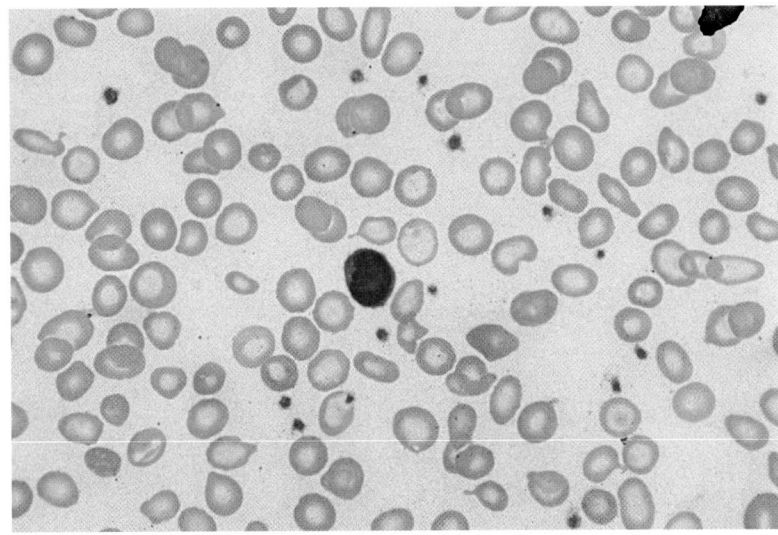

COLOR FIGURE 65.6 Microcytic RBCs. RBCs that are smaller than normal and have pale features (microcytic and hypochromic) are characteristic of Fe deficiency anemia.

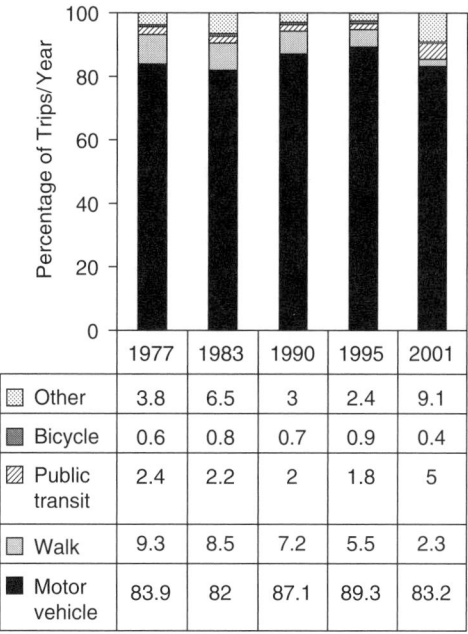

FIGURE 37.8 Mode of travel in the United States from 1997 to 2001. (*Source:* Nationwide Personal Transportation Surveys, 1998, 2001.[2])

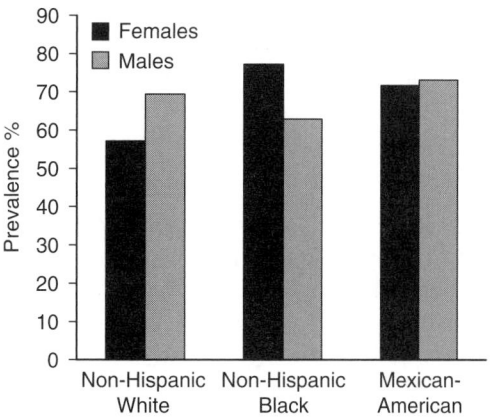

FIGURE 37.9 Prevalence of overweight (BMI ≥ 25 kg/m^2) in the United States by race/ethnic group for men and women aged 20 to 74 years, 1999–2002. (*Source:* Hedley, Ogden, Johnson et al., *JAMA.* 291:2847; 2004.)

EPIDEMIOLOGIC ASSESSMENT

Physical Activity

Although physical activity tends to be overreported,[43,69] questionnaires are frequently used in epidemiologic studies to classify levels of physical activity.[70,71] Although several physical activity measures exist (e.g., diaries and retrospective histories), recall surveys appear to be the least likely to influence behavior and generally require the least amount of effort by respondents.[43,70] Among the most frequently used measures are the Physical Activity Recall (PAR)[72] and the Paffenbarger.[73] The PAR is available in interviewer- and self-administered versions[72] and categorizes activities by their intensity; the Paffenbarger is a one-page questionnaire that evaluates habitual daily and weekly activity. Measures of sedentary promoting behaviors, such as television viewing and computer use, are only beginning to be utilized and validated. However, sedentary behavior can be simply assessed by the number of reported minutes per day spent in sedentary behaviors (e.g., watching television, using the computer playing, videogames, and driving).

Food Intake

As noted earlier, food intake tends to be underreported, particularly in obese individuals.[74] Nonetheless, several methods of assessment exist to measure nutrient intake. The 24 h recall has been used in many large-scale studies (e.g., the NHANES) to assess nutrient intake. The 24 h recall is typically administered by trained interviewers. It takes about 20 min to complete, requires no record keeping on the part of respondents, and, unlike other measures (e.g., food diaries), does not cause subjects to alter their intake.[75] Alternatively, if assessment of subjects' average, long-term intake is needed (rather than a more precise measurement of short-term consumption), food frequency questionnaires (FFQ) are an appropriate alternative. FFQ (e.g., the Block[76]) assess the frequency and quantity of habitual consumption of food items listed on a questionnaire in reference to the past week or month. These are easy to administer and do not require trained interviewers.

CLINICAL ASSESSMENT

Physical Activity

The questionnaires reviewed above (i.e., the PAR[72] and the Paffenbarger[73]) may also be useful in assessing physical activity in the clinical setting. Alternatively, a few simple questions may provide a practical and efficient means of assessing physical activity. These include, "How many minutes do you spend each week in planned physical activity?" "Approximately how many city blocks to you walk each day?" and "How many flights of stairs do you climb each day?" Television viewing, computer and videogame use, and driving time may also be evaluated in the clinical setting by weekly number of minutes for each activity. Finally, pedometers, which provide a count of the total number of steps taken each day, can be very useful in monitoring changes in physical activity.

Food Intake

The most commonly used means to assess energy and nutrient intake in the clinical setting is the food record. Food records are patients' daily notations of the type, quantity, and calories of food and liquid consumed. Patients are instructed to record all meals, drinks, and snacks immediately after eating. Patients may also record the number of fat grams consumed, place of consumption, and minutes of television viewing per day. It should also be noted that food records are also commonly used as an intervention tool.[77] If a less reactive and more immediate assessment of intake is required, FFQ or 24 h recalls may be used. Restaurant eating can be assessed at the time of the clinic assessment with the question, "How many times per week, on average, do you eat at restaurants?"

ASSESSMENT MODEL

The ultimate challenge of environmental assessment is to integrate the multiple factors that influence obesity. As Figure 37.10 illustrates that food intake and physical activity may result from a combination of influences (e.g., large portion sizes and use of laborsaving devices) that interact with cultural and social factors to promote obesity. In this model, excess food intake may be due to larger portion sizes at restaurants, but other factors must also be considered. For example, cultural taste preferences and economic status may also influence restaurant selection. Although distinguishing among the several overlapping environmental influences can be difficult, an awareness of such interrelationships is critical for designing public health and clinical interventions aimed to decrease the rising prevalence of obesity.

SUMMARY AND CONCLUSION

In summary, obesity is due to an imbalance of energy intake and expenditure. Both biological and behavioral factors are implicated. Several environmental changes have occurred over the past few decades that appear to contribute to the increase in obesity in industrialized nations. In particular, portion sizes have increased and high-fat, energy-dense foods are heavily marketed and readily available at a low cost. In addition, the amount of energy expended in activities of daily living appears to have declined.

The problem of obesity may be instructive to understanding other nutrition-related disorders affected by environmental factors, including high cholesterol, hypertension, and osteoporosis. As in the case of obesity, it is likely that a combination of cultural, societal, and other environmental forces leads to the development of nutritional problems in the world today. Clearly, promoting healthy nutrition will require targeting multiple environmental components and a partnership among various sectors of society, including the government, food industry, and the media.[78]

REFERENCES

1. US Bureau of Labor Statistics. *Consumer Expenditures: 1990–2004.* In: US Department of Labor, ed: Data provided by the US Bureau of Labor Statistics; 2005.
2. Center for Urban Transportation Research. *Public Transit in America: Results from the 2001 National Household Travel Survey.* Tampa: National Center for Transit Research; 2005.

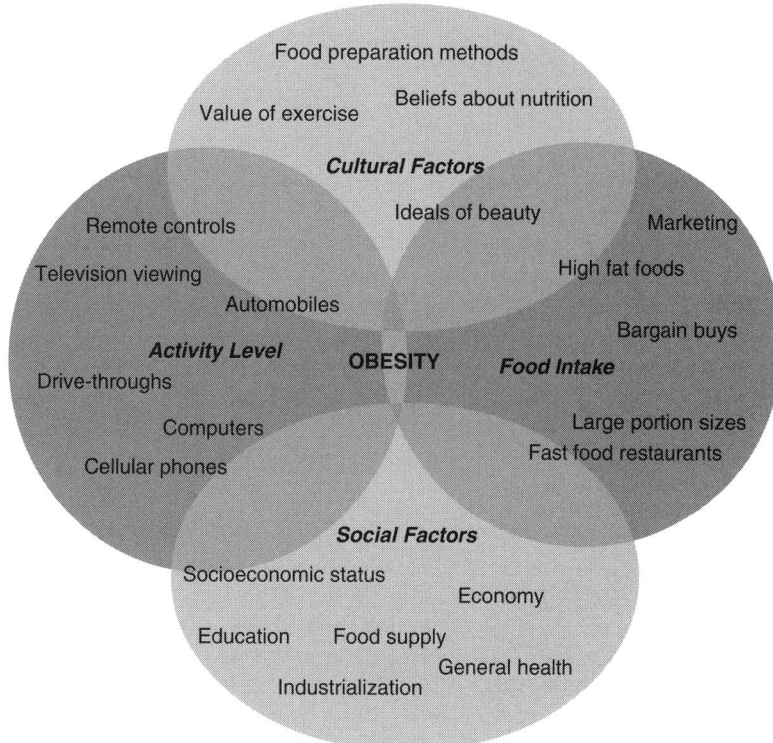

FIGURE 37.10 Environmental influences on obesity.

3. Putnam JJ, Gerrior S. Trends in the US Food Supply, 1970–1997. *America's Eating Habits: Changes and Consequences.* Washington DC: USDA Economic Research Service; 1999.

4. Gerrior S, Bente L, Hiza H. *Nutrient Content of the U.S. Food Supply, 1909–2000: A Summary Report:* US Department of Agriculture, Center for Nutrition Policy and Promotion; 2004.

5. Hedley AA, Ogden CL, Johnson CL, et al. *JAMA.* 291:2847; 2004.

6. Centers for Disease Control and Prevention (CDC). Physical activity trends — United States, 1990–1998. *MMWR Morbidity and Mortality Weekly Report.* 50(9):166–169; 2001.

7. Pickrell D, Schimek P. Trends in Personal Motor Vehicle Ownership and Use: Evidence From the Nationwide Personal Transportation Survey. In: Transportation USDo, ed: 1998.

8. Flegal KM, Carroll MD, Kuczmarski RJ, Johnson CL. *Int J Obes.* 22:39; 1998.

9. Centers For Disease Control and Prevention (CDC). Prevalence of physical activity, including lifestyle activities among adults — United States, 2000–2001. *MMWR Morbidity and Mortality Weekly Report.* 52:764; 2003.

10. National Center for Health Statistics/Division of Data Services. www.cdc.gov/nchs/data/hus/hus05.pdf#chartbookontrends; 2005.

11. Foreyt JP, Goodrick GK. *Lancet.* 346:134; 1995.

12. World Health Organization. www.who.int/nut/obs.htm; 2005.

13. Weinsier RL, Hunter GR, Heine AF, et al. *Am J Med.* 105:145; 1998.

14. French SA, Story M, Jeffery RW. *Ann Rev Pub Health.* 22:309; 2001.

15. Hill JO, Wyatt HR, Reed GW, Peters JC. *Science* 299:853; 2003.

16. Center for Science in the Public Interest. *Nutrition Action Health Letter.* 25:3; 1998.

17. Battle DE, Brownell KD. *Addict Behav.* 21:755; 1996.

18. Brownell KD. *New York Times.* A29; 1994

19. Horgan KB, Brownell KD. In: Miller, Heather, eds. *Treating Addictive Behaviors.* New York: Plenum; 1998: 105.

20. Ahmad S. *U.S. News and World Report.* 1997:62–63.

21. Centers for Disease Control and Prevention: Morbidity and Mortality Weekly Report. *Trends in Intake of Energy and Macronutrients — United States,* 1971–2000; 2004.

22. Brantley PJ, Myers VH, Roy HJ. *J Louis St Med Soc.* 156:S19; 2005.

23. French S, Story M, Neumark-Sztainer D. *Int J Ob Relat Metab Disord.* 25:1823; 2001.

24. Young LR, Nestle M. *JADA.* 98:458; 1998.

25. Wansink B. *J Marketing.* 60:1; 1996.

26. French S, Jeffery R, Story M, Hannan P, Snyder M. *Am J Public Health.* 87:849; 1997.

27. Jeffery RW, French SA, Raether C, Baxter JE. *Prev Med.* 23:788; 1994.

28. Golay A, Bobbioni E. *Int J Obes.* 21:S2; 1997.

29. Lissner L, Levitsky DA, Strupp BJ, et al. *Am J Clin Nutr.* 46:886; 1987.
30. Stubbs RJ, Harbron CG, Murgatroyd PR. *Am J Clin Nutr.* 62:316; 1995.
31. Thomas CD, Peters JC, Reed GW. *Am J Clin Nutr.* 55:934; 1992.
32. Paeratakul S, Ferdinand DP, Champagne CM, et al. *JADA.* 103:1332; 2003.
33. Jeffery RW, French S. *Am J Public Health.* 88:277; 1998.
34. Pereira MA, Kartashov AI, Ebbeling CB, et al. *Lancet.* 367:36; 2005.
35. Bowman SA, Vinyard BT. *J Amer Coll Nutr.* 23:163; 2004.
36. Kinsey JD. *J Nutr.* 124:1878S; 1994.
37. Bureau of Labor Statistics. *Monthly Labor Review.* Vol December; 3; 1998.
38. Heini AF, Weinsier RL. *Am J Med.* 102:259; 1997.
39. Rolls BJ, Miller DL. *J Amer Coll Nutr.* 16:535; 1997.
40. Subar AF, Heimendinger J, Patterson BH, et al. *Health Promotion.* 9:352; 1995.
41. Guthrie JF, Morton JF. *JADA.* 100:43; 2000.
42. Sanford T. *Vending Times.* 39:15; 1999.
43. US Dept of Health and Human Services. The Surgeon General's Report on Nutrition and Health. In: Department of Health and Human Services, ed: Government Printing Office; 1996:88-50210.
44. Prentice AM, Jebb SA. *Br Med J.* 311:437; 1995.
45. Hill JO, Wyatt HR, Melanson EL. *Med Clin N Am.* 84:333; 2000.
46. US Bureau Census. Web-Site Database; 2005.
47. Bureau of Labor Statistics. Consumer spending on durables and services in the 1980's. *Monthly Labor Review.* Vol May; 1992:18–26.
48. Nielsen Media Research. *2000 Report on Television: The First 50 Years.* New York: AC Nielsen Co.; 2000.
49. Kotz K, Story M. *JADA.* 94:1296; 1994.
50. Dietz WH, Gortmaker SL. *Pediatrics.* 75:807; 1985.
51. Gortmaker SL, Must A, Sobol AM, et al. *Arch Pediatr Adolesc Med.* 150:356; 1996.
52. Andersen RE, Crespo CJ, Bartlett SJ, et al. *JAMA.* 279:938; 1998.
53. Tucker LA, Friedman GM. *Am J Public Health.* 79:516; 1989.
54. Tucker LA, Bagwell M. *Am J Public Health.* 81:908; 1991.
55. DiGuiseppi C, Roberts I, Li L. *Br Med J.* 314:710; 1997.
56. US Department of Transportation. *Final Report: The National Bicycling and Walking Study: Transportation Choices for a Changing America.* Washington, DC; 1994. FHWA-PD-023.
57. Kumanyika S, Wilson JF, Guilford-Davenport M. *JADA.* 93:416; 1993.
58. Kumanyika S, Morssink C, Agurs T. *Ethnicity Disease.* 2:166; 1992.
59. Foster GD, Wadden TA, Swain RM, et al. *Am J Clin Nutr.* 69:13; 1999.
60. Sobal J, Stunkard AJ. *Psych Bull.* 105:260; 1989.
61. Ginzberg E. *JAMA.* 262:238; 1991.
62. Finucane TE, Carrese JA. *J Gen Int Med.* 5:120; 1990.
63. Wenneker MB, Epstein AM. *JAMA.* 261:253; 1987.
64. Carlisle DM, Leake BD, Shapiro MF. *Am J Public Health.* 85:352; 1995.
65. US Department of Health Education and Welfare. Ten-State Nutrition Survey, 1968–1970. In: Health Education and Welfare, ed: Center for Disease Control; 1972.
66. Hulshof KF, Lowik MR, Kik FJ. *Eur J Clin Nutr.* 45:441; 1991.
67. Allison DB. *Handbook of Assessment Methods for Eating Behaviors and Weight-Related Problems: Measures, Theory, and Research.* Thousand Oaks: Sage; 1995.
68. St. Jeor ST. *Obesity Assessment: Tools, Methods, Interpretations.* New York: Chapman & Hall; 1997.
69. Lichtman SW, Pisarska K, Berman ER. *N Engl J Med.* 327:1893; 1992.
70. LaPorte RE, Montoye HJ, Caspersen CJ. *Pub Health Report.* 100:131; 1985.
71. Caspersen CJ. *Exerc Sport Science Rev.* 17:423; 1989.
72. Blair SN. In: Matarazzo JD, Weiss SM, Herd JA, Miller NE, eds. *Behavioral Health: A Handbook of Health Enhancement and Disease Prevention.* New York: Wiley; 1984:424–427.
73. Blair SN, Haskell PH, Paffenbarger RS, *Am J Epidemiol.* 122:794; 1985.
74. Schoeller DA. *Metabolism.* 44:18; 1995.
75. Wolper C, Heshka S, Heymsfield SB. In: Allison DB, ed. *Handbook of Assessment Methods for Eating Behaviors and Weight Related Problems. Measures, Theory and Research.* Sage: Thousand Oaks; 1995:215–240.
76. Block G, Woods M, Potosky A, Clifford C. *J Clin Epidemiol.* 43:1327; 1990.
77. Foster, GD, Makris, AP, Bailer, BA. *Am J Clin Nutr.* 82:230S; 2005.
78. WHO. *Obesity: Preventing and Managing the Global Epidemic.* Geneva; 1998.

Part V

Clinical Nutrition

38 Medical Nutritional Evaluation

Elaine B. Feldman and Carolyn D. Berdanier

CONTENTS

INTRODUCTION

Family physicians, pediatricians, and internists are the usual providers of primary medical care for adults, with gynecologists/ obstetricians increasingly performing this task for women. The assessment of nutritional status should be carried out in their offices and in hospital settings.[1] The most common reasons for office visits that may require nutritional intervention are problems related to hypertension, diabetes mellitus, degenerative joint disease, heart disease, asthma, abdominal pain, pregnancy care, and obesity. Nutritional status assessment may also be a part of a general medical examination.[2]

Nutritional science should be applied to many aspects of primary care delivery.[1,3,4] The patient's medical and family history, the physical examination, and appropriate laboratory assessments can then be used to assess nutritional status. NHANES methodology is available should the examination warrant such use.[5] As a result of medical nutrition evaluation, patients may be categorized as normal, malnourished, or at risk of malnourishment. Dietary history, anthropometric measurements, and specific physiological and biochemical laboratory tests should be appropriately elaborated in patients with malnutrition or in those at risk for malnutrition. These usually require referrals. In order to communicate effectively with patients, physicians should know the components of a healthy diet in terms of foods and the nutrients that these foods contain, as well as the patterns of consuming food in meals. Details of food composition, however, are more likely in the knowledge base of dietitians and nutritionists.

The physician should obtain specific information about the patient's body weight and height, its change over time, the patient's recent meal intake (quantitative as well as qualitative), and his or her appetite. The physician will also want to know about the patient's physical activity, special diets, and diet supplements.

Height and weight are vital signs and should be measured directly under standardized conditions. Weight should be measured each time the patient visits. A complete blood count (CBC) and serum albumin provide clues to nutritional anemia and protein nutritional status. The patient who is starved or who has a malabsorption problem or who has hepatic, pancreatic or renal disease, trauma, sepsis, cancer, or who requires critical care should be given special attention with regard to nutritional status assessment and subsequent nutritional therapy. A registered dietitian is an invaluable resource in assessing dietary intake by dietary recall, prospective food records, or food frequency questionnaires.

The physician needs to ask about the use of dietary supplements (vitamins, minerals, and others). Vitamin/mineral supplements are often used to optimize nutritional health and forestall disease development. Over-the-counter remedies are also often used and are marketed with little restriction with respect to their efficacy or active ingredient content. Often, patients do not report the use of such supplements and over-the-counter remedies. This can set the stage for deleterious interactions with respect to prescribed drugs or further problems in the management of a particular disease state. Toxic adverse interactions between herbals and medications or foods can occur (see Chapters 74 & 75), and patients need to be counseled to avoid unorthodox remedies.

The health professional should be aware of good food sources of essential nutrients (see Chapter 1), appropriate serving sizes, and the foods that are nutrient fortified. Encouraging patients to read food labels will improve their nutrition knowledge and health (see Chapter 2). Appropriate food choice can reduce the risk of cardiovascular and cerebrovascular diseases, hypertension, and cancer. Chapter 42 – 45, and Chapters 70 to 72 address these issues in more detail.

In a primary care practice a miscellany of special circumstances, when suspected, may warrant nutritional interventions. While serious nutritional deficiencies have largely disappeared in affluent countries they still exist especially in patients who have other predisposing conditions. One such condition is alcoholism (see Chapter 57). If possible, that condition should be addressed and nutritional support provided. The special needs of menstruating women are another of these special circumstances. The regular loss of menstrual fluids means that women are at risk of anemia (see Chapter 65), and nutritional supplements may be needed to address their potential deficiencies of iron, copper, and some of the B vitamins (see Chapter 10 on the use of such supplements). The postmenopausal woman is at risk of calcium loss from her bones (see Chapter 64), and this too can be addressed from the nutritional point of view as well as pharmacologically. Vegetarianism could be a concern if the patient is unaware of the need to ingest sufficient vitamin B_{12} and balanced protein (see Chapter 20). The special nutrient needs of pregnant and lactating women should also be a special consideration (see Chapter 13). Meeting the periconceptual need for folic acid is a related special circumstance (see Chapter 55). Gender differences need to be recognized with respect to body size, body composition, and metabolic/hormonal differences. All of these can impact nutritional status. Lastly, with increasing age and the effects of age on nutrient need, there should be concern about the nutritional status of the elderly. A number of instances of diseases common in the elder population have nutrition components. Conditions such as vascular disease, dementia, and osteoporosis all have nutrition components (see Chapter 17 and Chapter 18). Intervention strategies instituted in middle life could be instrumental in delaying the development and onset of these degenerative diseases. Patients who cannot or will not eat should be evaluated for possible enteral or parental nutrition support (see Chapter 67 and Chapter 68). Finally, all physicians should be educated in the principles of a health-promoting diet.[6]

PATIENT EVALUATION

The medical history will provide 80 to 90% of the information leading to a diagnosis.[7–9] The evaluation of nutritional status will emphasize certain elements of the medical history and social background that will differ depending on the patient's gender, age, and the presenting problem. The usual level of physical activity and the degree of stress should be noted. It is imperative to distinguish whether any impairment is caused by a patient's disease or is directly related to an abnormal intake of nutrients or to an unbalanced diet. Malnutrition resulting from disease can be managed effectively only if the underlying disease is controlled or cured. For example, is there a physiological or anatomical loss of gastrointestinal function, or is the degree of weight change out of proportion to the food consumed indicating hyper or hypometabolism? Does the patient have diabetes mellitus? Is there excessive blood loss from menstruation?

FAMILY HISTORY

Many nutritional disorders are familial or inherited. Thus, a history of cancer, cardiovascular disease, metabolic diseases, gastrointestinal disease, liver disease, diabetes mellitus, or obesity, etc., should alert the examiner in the patient evaluation. Table 38.1 outlines the questions that should be asked when taking a patient's medical history. Table 38.2 outlines questions that should be asked about the patient's socioeconomic history.

DIET HISTORY AND EVALUATION

An extensive assessment is best done by the professionally trained dietitian and is required in patients who have nutritional problems or appear at risk of malnutrition. Nevertheless, the physician should acquire basic knowledge of the patient's food intake, meal pattern, and dietary habits, including the use of supplements. This will allow for the assessment of general nutritional status and help identify potential problems that may need to be addressed. The physician has the opportunity to practice preventive medicine (through nutrition) by evaluating the patients energy balance (intake, activity, and body weight) and the consumption of dietary components predisposing to vascular disease, cancer and other chronic diseases. In the inpatient setting, it is important to note the diet prescribed and whether the time constraints of diagnostic tests or interventional therapies preclude the patient's eating the meals that were ordered.

GENERAL PHYSICAL EXAMINATION

Height and weight should be considered vital signs and should be measured and recorded with careful attention to accuracy and precision. Height should be measured annually and weight at most office visits. Weight measurements should also be taken at regular intervals in the hospitalized patient. The body mass index or BMI (see Chapter 30 for table) is a useful parameter for monitoring body size. A body weight that is decreased profoundly alerts the physician to increasing morbidity or mortality. A weight loss of ~20% of ideal body weight increases the chances of infection; a weight loss of 40% of ideal body weight predicts dying. Few individuals survive at a loss of 50% of their ideal body weight.[10]

Observation, inspection, and measurement are the primary tools of the examination. The physical signs of malnutrition are listed and categorized according to anatomic site and organ system in Table 38.3.

TABLE 38.1
Medical History

The elements of a medical history include the present illness, past medical and surgical history, family history, a medication list, and a review of systems

Pertinent questions to ask are:
- What is the patient's usual weight?
- Has there been any recent change in weight?
- If so, how much and over what period of time?
- What were the maximum and minimum weights?
- What were the weights one year ago and five years ago?

A rapid and profound weight loss is probably the single most important clue to malnutrition. This leads the history taker into evaluation of normal and abnormal food and nutrient intake. Are there:
- Changes in smell or taste
- Depression, alcoholism
- Dental problems, poor dentition, sore tongue, swallowing difficulties, loss of appetite, loss of enjoyment of eating
- Poverty, low socioeconomic status, limited access to food, limited transportation options to purchase food, and limited food preparation facilities
- Special diet prescriptions
- Food idiosyncrasies (e.g., pica), food fads, excessive use of dietary supplements
- Mechanical problems in eating due to muscle weakness, joint deformities, tremors, and fracture of jaw and associated structures due to injury
- Altered memory or dementia interfering with food and water intake
- Digestion and absorption problems: medications such as antacids, laxatives, oral contraceptives, anticonvulsants; parasites, surgical resection of the gastrointestinal tract, and malabsorption syndromes (e.g., lactose intolerance, gluten-induced enteropathy, etc.)
- Utilization: Anticonvulsants, oral contraceptives, antimetabolites, isoniazid, and inborn errors of metabolism
- Losses: Blood loss, diarrhea (change in bowel habits), vomiting, draining wounds, fistulas, ostomies, burns, proteinuria, and dialysis
- Destruction: fevers, sepsis, hypermetabolism, multiple trauma, burns, constipation, and obstipation
- Special requirements: chronic disease, recent major surgery, alcohol abuse, hormone replacement therapy, chemotherapy, immunosuppressive therapy, behavior, excessive use of caffeine, alcohol abuse, fad diets, and excessive use of dietary supplements
- Miscellaneous: Neurologic symptoms, for example, numbness, dizziness, weakness, skin rash, dryness, flaking, and hair loss

TABLE 38.2
Socioeconomic History

The psychosocial evaluation should generate information concerning the patient's living conditions. This is especially important in the elderly
- Does the patient live alone?
- Does he or she have access to shopping?
- Are the facilities for storing and cooking food adequate?
- Does the patient have a history of smoking?
- Are financial resources adequate?
- Are there assistance programs available?

LABORATORY TESTS

Some routine laboratory tests can assist in the nutritional assessment and diagnosis. These include the CBC, and blood chemistry panels (glucose, electrolytes, minerals, lipids, and indices of renal and hepatic function). Tests of blood coagulation can also be informative.

Hemoglobin levels will show the presence of anemia (see Chapter 65 for more details) that may be vitamin specific or mineral related and can indicate chronic disease. The red cell size and hemoglobin content and concentration can provide clues to liver disease, alcoholism, and specific nutritional deficiencies. While serum albumin is not a sensitive indicator of protein status, it does provide a clue. Low levels may indicate a limiting amount of substrate for hepatic protein synthesis. On the other hand, nonnutritional factors may be responsible for hypoalbuminemia such as expanded extracellular fluid, accelerated protein breakdown, and impaired renal and hepatic function. Albumin levels may also be unreliable indicators of protein status in the postoperative or acutely injured patient. Some enzyme tests are indicators of nutritional cofactor status, for example, alkaline phosphatase for zinc or aminotransferase for vitamin B_6. Laboratory tests useful in Clinical Nutritional Assessment are provided in Table 38.4. Table 38.5 and Table 38.6 provide normal values for blood and urine with respect to micronutrients.

TABLE 38.3
Physical Signs of Malnutrition

Area of Body Examined	Common Signs of Malnutrition	Deficiency/Abnormality
Appearance in general	Significant overweight or underweight. Apathetic or hyperirritable	Energy imbalance
	Loss or slowness of ankle or knee reflexes. Pitting edema	Protein
Eyes	Paleness, dryness, redness, or pigmentation of membranes (conjunctiva)	Vitamin A, riboflavin
	Foamy patches or conjunctiva (Bitot's spots)	Iron B_{12}, folate, and copper
	Dullness, softness, or vascularization of the cornea	Excess, Wilson's disease
	Redness or fissures on eyelids	hypercholesterolemia
Face	Rash, seborrhea, and pallor	Riboflavin, iron, and folate B_{12}
Gums	Receded. "Spongy" and bleeding. Swelling of the gingiva	Vitamin C
Hair	Dullness. May be brittle and easily plucked without pain. Sometimes lighter in color than normal (depigmentation may be bandlike when hair is held up to a source of light).	Protein
Lips	Swollen, red, corners, and cracked (cheilosis)	Riboflavin
Muscles	Wasting and flabbiness of muscle. Bleeding into muscle	Protein, iron, folate, and B_{12}
Nails	Brittle and ridged nails	Spooning protein, iron
Heart	Racing heartbeat (over 100 beats per minute)	
	Enlargement	Selenium
	Failure	Thiamin
	Abnormal rhythm of heart	Magnesium, potassium, calcium
Organs	Palpable enlargement of liver or spleen	Alcohol abuse
	Ascites	Protein
Skeleton	Softening, swelling, or distorted shapes of bones and joints	Vitamins C and D
Skin	Roughness (follicular hyperkeratosis), dryness, or flakiness	Protein
	Irregular pigmentation, black and blue marks, lesions	Niacin
	Symmetrical, reddened lesions, rash, and edema	Protein
	Looseness of skin (lack of subcutaneous fat)	Energy
	Flakiness, peeling, and dry	Protein, and zinc
Teeth	Caries. Mottled or darkened areas of enamel	Fluoride excess
Tongue	Atrophy of papillae (the tongue is smooth) or hypertrophy of papillae	B_{12}, folate, and riboflavin
	Swollen, scarlet, magenta (purple colored), or raw tongue	
	Irregularly shaped and distributed white patches	Iron

TABLE 38.4
Laboratory Tests Useful in Clinical Nutritional Assessment

Test	Index for
Hemoglobin, hematocrit, red and white cell counts, and differential (calculate total lymphocyte count)	Anemia, protein status
Urea, creatinine, glucose, sodium, potassium chloride, and CO_2	Renal function, diabetes, acid–base balance
Cholesterol, triglycerides, and lipoproteins	Lipid disorders
Total protein, albumin, and uric acid	Renal/hepatic function
Calcium, phosphate, magnesium, bilirubin, alkaline phosphatatse	Skeletal disorders
Aminotransferases, iron, and ferritin	Anemia, iron status
Transferrin, transthyretin, retinol-binding protein	Iron status
Prothrombin time, partial prothrombin time	Vitamin K status

EDUCATING PHYSICIANS IN NUTRITION

Nutrition plays an important role in the etiology, prevention, or treatment of many chronic diseases. Thus, an appropriate knowledge of nutrition principles should be part of the education and training of physicians, especially those in primary care.[5,11] Family medicine specialists have developed guidelines for incorporating nutrition into their medical education and residency training programs.[12–14] The current guidelines are presented in Table 38.7 and can be accessed on the web site of the American Academy of Family Physicians, www.aafp.org.

TABLE 38.5
Normal Values for Micronutrients in Blood

Nutrient	Range of Normal Values
Ascorbic acid, plasma	0.6–1.6 mg/dl
Calcium, serum	4.5–5.3 meq/l
β-carotene, serum	40–200 μg/dl
Chloride, serum	95–103 meq/l
Lead, whole blood	0–50 μg/dl
Magnesium, serum	1.5–2.5 meq/l
Sodium, plasma	136–142 meq/l
Vitamin A, serum	15–60 μg/dl
Retinol, plasma	>20 μg/dl
Phosphorus	3.4–4.5 mg/dl
Potassium	3.5–5.0 meq/l
Riboflavin, red cell	>14.9 μg/dl cells
Folate, plasma	>6 ng/ml
Pantothenic acid, plasma	$\geq$6 μg/dl
Pantothenic acid, whole blood	$\geq$80 μg/dl
Biotin, whole blood	>25 ng/ml
B_{12}, plasma	>150 pg/ml
Vitamin D 25(OH)-D_3, plasma	>10 ng/ml
α-Tocopherol, plasma	>0.80 mg/dl

For more information on blood analyses see: *NHANES Manual for Nutrition Assessment*, CDC, Atlanta, GA; ICNND *Manual for Nutrition Surveys*, 2nd ed, 1963, US Government Printing Office, Washington, DC; Sauberlich et al. 1974 *Laboratory Tests for the Assessment of Nutritional Status*, CRC Press, Boca Raton, FL.

TABLE 38.6
Normal Values for Micronutrients in Urine

Nutrient	Range of Normal Values
Calcium, mg/24 h	100–250
Chloride, meq/24 h	110–250
Copper, μg/24 h	0–100
Lead, μg/24 h	<100
Phosphorus, g/24 h	0.9–1.3
Potassium, meq/24 h	25–100
Sodium, meq/24 h	130–260
Zinc, mg/24 h	0.15–11.2
Creatinine, mg/kg body weight	15–25
Riboflavin, μg/g creatinine	>80
Niacin metabolite[a], μg/g creatinine	>1.6
Pyridoxine, μg/g creatinine	$\geq$20
Biotin, μg/24 h	>25
Pantothenic acid, mg/24 h	$\geq$1
Folate, FIGLU[b] after histidine load	<5 mg/8 h
B_{12}, methylmalonic acid after valine load	<2 mg/24 h

For more information on urine analysis see: ICNNO, 1963, *Manual for Nutrition Surveys*, 2nd ed. US Government Printing Office Washington, DC; *NHANES Manual for Nutrition Assessment*, CDC Atlanta, GA; Gibson, RS, 1990 *Principles of Nutrition Assessment* Oxford University Press, NY.

[a] N1-methylnicotinamide.

[b] Formiminoglutamic acid.

TABLE 38.7
Recommended Nutrition Guidelines for Family Practice

Develop attitudes that recognize:

Nutrition is a major part of wellness, disease prevention, and treatment of disease

Poor nutrition can cause disease

Family, ethnic, and religious attitudes affect nutrition behavior

Socioeconomic factors are important in nutrition excess and deficiency

Different nutritional considerations at different times are required in the life cycle

Nutritionists and dietitians are important in the area of the patient's nutritional status, education, and disease prevention

Develop knowledge of:

Basic nutritional requirements/recommended allowances and intakes

Nutritional content of food and the food pyramid

Nutritional information from public and private sources

The role of qualified nutritional professionals as consultants

The changing nutritional requirements of infancy, childhood, adolescence, pregnancy, lactation, menopause, and aging

Nutritional requirements of disease processes and exercise

Clinical effects of dietary fat, carbohydrate, proteins, and fiber

Basic concepts of vegetarianism

The role of nutrition in the treatment and prevention of disease: hypertension, heart, dental, gastrointestinal, hepatic and renal disease, diabetes, alcoholism, anemia, and cancer

Signs and symptoms of nutrient deficiencies

Breast feeding and formula feeding

Use of vitamin and mineral supplements

Weight reduction and dieting

Food and drug interactions

Allergies and food intolerances

Eating disorders

Refeeding syndromes

Nutrition Quackery

Develop skills in:

Assessing nutritional status during the history and physical examinations

Assessing nutritional status and needs of hospitalized patients

Ordering laboratory and metabolic studies to detect nutritional deficiencies and assess adequacy of the nutrition provided

Counseling patients and family about specific nutritional needs related to their life cycle and disease process, the role of diet in preventing disease, safe weight reduction, and dieting, including health benefits

Educating patients about food marketing and nutritional quackery

Prescribing and managing oral supplementation, tube feeding, peripheral nutrition, and total parenteral nutrition

Preventing and managing refeeding syndromes

Recognizing and appropriately referring patients with disordered eating habits

Adapted from: *Physician's Curriculum in Clinical Nutrition.* STFM, Kansas City 1995. Web sites providing clinical tools for assessment are: http://bms.brown.edu/nutrition/ and http://www.medicine.wisc.edu/mainweb/DOMPages. php?section=naa&page=metabolic

These websites not only provide tools for nutrition assessment, they also provide tools for metabolic syndrome assessment.

REFERENCES

1. Feldman, EB. In *Laboratory Medicine; The Selection and Interpretation of Clinical Laboratory Studies.* Roe, DA, Rock, RC, eds. Williams & Wilkins, Baltimore, 1993, ch 10.
2. Kolasa, KM. *Eur. J. Clin. Nutr.* 53: S89; 1999.
3. Feldman, EB. *Southern Med. J.* 88: 204; 1995.
4. Feldman, EB. *Nutrition* 16: 649; 2000.
5. http://www.CDC.NHANES
6. Feldman, FB. *Nutrition Screening Initiative. Incorporating Nutrition Screening and Interventions into Medical Practice.* A Monograph for Physicians. 1010 Wisconsin Ave, NW Suite 800, Washington DC, 2007. The nutrition Screening Initiative. 1994.
7. Feldman, EB. *Essentials of Clinical Nutrition.* FA Davis, Philadelphia, 1988, ch 3.
8. Newton, JM, Halsted, CH. In *Modern Nutrition in Health and Disease*, Shils, ME, Olson, JA, Shike, M, Ross, AC, eds., 9th ed., Williams and Wilkins, Baltimore, 1999, ch 55.

 9. Owen, GM. In *Nutrition Assessment, A Comprehensive Guide for Planning Intervention*, Simko MD, Cowell C, Gilbride JA, eds., 2nd ed., Aspen Publishers, Inc., Gaithersberg, MD, 1995, ch 6.
10. Feldman, EB. *Essentials of Clinical Nutrition*. FA Davis, Philadelphia, 1988, ch 13.
11. Feldman, EB. *Am. J. Clin. Nutr.* 54: 618; 1991.
12. Feldman, EB. *Society for Teachers of Family Medicine Working Group on Nutrition Education, Physician's Curriculum in Clinical Nutrition*. STFM Kansas City, 1995.
13. Feldman, EB. American Academy of Family Physicians (AAFP) *Recommended Core Educational Guidelines on Nutrition for Family Practice Residents*. American Academy of Family Physicians, Kansas City, 1989, revised 1995.
14. Feldman, EB. *Society for Teachers of Family medicine. Physicians Guide to Outpatient Nutrition.* www.fmdrl.org

39 Protein-Energy Malnutrition

Naomi K. Fukagawa

CONTENTS

INTRODUCTION

Protein-energy malnutrition (PEM) is not limited to the severe cases seen in developing countries. Individuals with varying degrees of malnutrition are seen in both inpatient and outpatient settings in the United States, and all ages may be affected. By definition, PEM results from inadequate intakes of protein, energy fuels, or both. Deficiencies of protein and energy usually occur together, but when one predominates and the deficit is severe, kwashiorkor (primarily protein deficiency) or marasmus (predominantly energy deficiency) ensues (Figure 39.1). However, in many cases, it is difficult to recognize which deficit predominates.

Marasmus means "wasting." Marasmus results from an overall deficiency of both protein and calories and is characterized by emaciation. "Kwashiorkor," a West African word that means "the disease that occurs when the next baby is born" and first used by Williams in 1933,[1] refers to an inadequate protein intake with a fair or normal intake of energy. The classic finding in kwashiorkor is edema, which often masks the degree of wasting. However, because individuals often present with a mixed picture of marasmus and kwashiorkor, the term protein-calorie malnutrition was suggested by Jelliffe to include the entire spectrum of undernutrition.[2] In 1973, the World Health Organization (WHO) renamed it PEM.[3] Table 39.1 summarizes the classification of PEM based on standard measures. The best anthropometric measure in children is based on measurements of weight and height, or length, and records of age to calculate the two indices: weight-for-height as an index of current nutritional status and height-for-age as an index of past nutritional history. The body mass index (BMI, or Quetelet's index) defined as weight in kilograms divided by the square of height in meters is often used for adolescents and adults. Women have more body fat than men at all three cutoff points, but this is an intrinsic biological phenomenon, and so the same BMI cutoffs may be used for both sexes. Recently, because of potential difficulties in obtaining accurate weight and height measures, the use of the mid-upper arm circumference (MUAC) was compared with the weight-for-height ratio and shown to perform at least as well for predicting subsequent mortality among severely malnourished children in rural Kenya.[5] Further evaluation is needed in other settings, but the data suggest that alternatives to classic anthropometrics are feasible.

Weight loss is the main feature of mild and moderate PEM with a decrease in subcutaneous fat. Physical activity and energy expenditure also decline.[6,7] Other functional indicators such as immunocompetence and gastrointestinal function or behavior may be altered.[8,9] In adults, capacity for prolonged physical work is reduced, but this is usually apparent only in those engaged in intense, energy-demanding jobs. Malnourished women have a higher probability of giving birth to low-birth-weight infants.[10] The diagnosis of severe PEM is principally based on dietary history and clinical features, described later and in the section on nutritional assessment.

ETIOLOGY AND EPIDEMIOLOGY

Causes of PEM may be primary, that is, as a result of inadequate food intake, or secondary, when it is the result of other diseases that lead to limited food intake, poor nutrient absorption or utilization, or increased nutrient requirements or losses. Factors that may modify the expression of PEM include the age of the patient, the cause of the deficiency, and the association with other

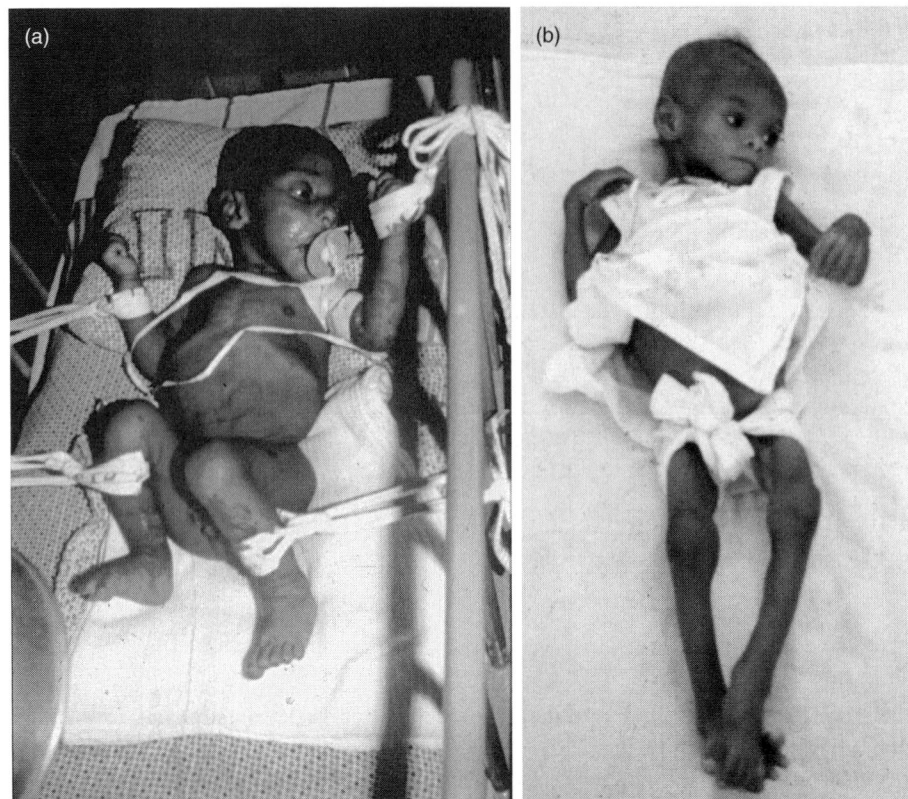

FIGURE 39.1 **(See color insert following page 654.)** (a) Marasmic infant. (b) Kwashiorkor in a child. (Photographs are from Brazil and were provided by Dr. T. Kuske. They are reproduced from Feldman, EB, *Essentials of Clinical Nutrition*, Philadelphia, PA, F.A. Davis, 1988, pp. 321–325. With permission.)

TABLE 39.1
Classification of Protein-Energy Malnutrition

	Mild	Moderate	Severe
Children			
Weight-for-height[a] (deficit = wasting)	80–89	70–79	<70 or with edema
Height-for-age[a] (deficit = stunting)	90–94	85–89	<85
Adults			
Weight:height[b], percentage of standard	90–95	80–90	<80
Triceps skin fold[c], percentage of standard	60–90	40–60	<40
Body Mass Index[d] (wt/ht^2, kg/m^2)	17.0–18.4	16.0–16.9	<16.0

[a] Percentage relative to modern NCHS standards.[4]

[b] Midrange of medium-frame values of the 1959 Metropolitan Life Insurance Tables.

[c] Men 12.5 mm, Women 16.5 mm.

[d] James WP, Ferro-Luzzi A, Waterlow JC. *Eur J Clin Nutr* 42: 969; 1988.

nutritional defects or infectious disease. PEM is the most important nutritional disease in developing countries, especially because of its impact on childhood mortality and growth and development. In more developed countries, PEM is often seen in chronically ill patients, the elderly and hospitalized individuals. PEM often develops gradually and is characterized by a series of metabolic and behavioral responses due to an attempt to adapt to the reduced food intake. Some of the causes of PEM are listed in Table 39.2.

The global magnitude of PEM is difficult to estimate because mild cases are often not recorded, and many of those afflicted do not receive medical attention. It is estimated that there are about 852 million undernourished people in the world. Most malnourished persons live in developing countries (Africa, Southern and Eastern Asia, Latin America, and the Caribbean). PEM primarily affects infants and preschool children, making it the main cause of growth retardation. About 31% of the children less than 5 years of age in developing countries are moderately to severely underweight, 39% are stunted, and 11% are wasted, based on a deficit of more than two standard deviations below the WHO/National Center for Health Statistics (NCHS) reference

---

TABLE 39.2
Causes of Protein-Energy Malnutrition

Primary
- Insufficient food intake (protein, energy, or micronutrients)
- Ingestion of proteins of poor nutritional quality
- Poverty, ignorance, low food supply, or insufficient household food security

Biologic Factors
- Maternal malnutrition prior to and/or during pregnancy
- Infectious diseases

Environmental
- Overcrowded and/or unsanitary life conditions
- Agricultural, climatic, or man-made catastrophe (war, civil disorder or forced migration)
- Poor food storage

TABLE 39.3
Characteristics of Patients at High Risk for Developing PEM

- Gross underweight (<80% weight-for-height)
- Gross overweight (because requirements often overlooked)
- Recent weight loss of >10% body weight
- Alcoholism
- NPO orders >10 days on 5% dextrose in water solution intravenously
- Protracted nutrient losses (gut, fistulas, dialysis, extensive exudative or exfoliative cutaneous lesions, or deep decubitus ulcerations)
- Increased metabolic needs
- Catabolic, anorexogenic or antinutrient therapies (steroids, chemotherapy, or immunosuppression)
- Aged with polypharmacy and concurrent illness
- Infections, especially in those with marginal nutritional status

---

values.[11] There has been a gradual improvement in the prevalence of childhood malnutrition, if countries are not ravaged by natural or man-made disasters such as war, drought, economic crisis, etc., or by increased prevalence of infectious diseases such as HIV/AIDS. Nevertheless, the total number of malnourished children worldwide has not really decreased overall because of the rise in populations in countries where malnutrition is prevalent.

In industrialized countries, primary PEM is seen among young children of the lower socioeconomic groups, the elderly living alone, adults addicted to alcohol and drugs, or individuals with chronic diseases who have limited food intake. Of interest is the fact that, in the United States, 1% of the children under five are considered moderately to severely underweight, 1% is wasted, and 2% are stunted.[11] Kwashiorkor has been reported in the United States owing to peculiar dietary habits imposed upon children by their parents (e.g., unbalanced vegetarian diets), almost total removal of protein in diets of children considered (often incorrectly) to have cow's milk sensitivity, and replacement of milk by low-protein nondairy creamers. The prevalence of PEM in adults in developed countries is high when considering those who are hospitalized, suffer from chronic diseases, or are disabled. In a recently published study on 369 patients older than 70 years admitted to a general medical service, 24% were moderately malnourished and 16% severely malnourished.[12] Malnutrition in these patients was associated with greater mortality, delayed functional recovery, and higher rates of nursing home use. These findings emphasize the importance of recognizing and treating PEM if we are to have any impact on the health and well-being of the world population. Some of the characteristics that place patients in the hospital at high risk for PEM are listed in Table 39.3.

DIAGNOSIS

The classical feature of mild to moderate PEM is weight loss ($\geq$5% in 1 month or $\geq$10% in 6 months in adults; weight-for-height <80% of the standard in children). A reduction in subcutaneous adipose tissue is apparent as well as in lean tissue, particularly skeletal muscle, resulting in a marked reduction in upper arm circumference, temporal muscle, and generalized muscle wasting.

TABLE 39.4
Physical Findings Associated with PEM

General
- Poor growth
- Decreased subcutaneous tissue
- Muscle wasting
- Edema

Skin
- Dry, scaling, flaking dermatitis
- Altered skin pigmentation

Hair
- Dull, altered texture, depigmented, or reddish
- Alopecia

Nails
- Transverse ridging, fissuring

Lips
- Cheilosis

Tongue
- Atrophic lingual papillae

Abdomen
- Distention, hepatomegaly

In infancy and early childhood, poor weight gain is the earliest and most consistent finding with PEM, followed by slowing of linear growth. Some of the physical findings suggestive of PEM are listed in Table 39.4 and illustrated in Figure 39.2.

Biochemical information is often not consistent in mild and moderate PEM. Laboratory data related to low protein intake may include low urinary excretion of urea nitrogen and creatinine, altered plasma amino acid patterns (decreased branched-chain amino acids), decreased serum concentrations of albumin and transferrin, and reduced total lymphocyte counts. Severe PEM may be characterized by biochemical changes such as a decline in transport proteins (e.g., transferrin, ceruloplasmin, retinol, binding protein, cortisol-, and thyroxine-binding proteins, and α- and β-lipoproteins) and decreased enzyme concentrations (e.g., amylase, pseudocholinesterase, and alkaline phosphatase). In addition, serum or plasma transaminase concentrations may be increased while the urea cycle or other enzymes associated with degradation (e.g., xanthine oxidase, glycolic acid oxidase, and cholinesterase) may be lower. Enzymes utilized in amino acid synthesis may be increased in both forms of PEM. Recently, leptin, the adipocyte-derived hormone, has been deemed more important as a starvation hormone than as a satiety signal.[13] Stein et al.[14] concluded that the ratio of soluble leptin receptor to leptin levels may be a better marker of nutritional status than IGF-1 in PEM during recovery.

PEM develops over weeks or months, allowing for a series of metabolic and behavioral adjustments that decrease nutrient demands and result in a nutritional equilibrium compatible with a lower level of nutrient availability for the cells. Some of the adaptive responses are shown in Table 39.5.[15,16] Many are directed at preserving body protein and essential protein-dependent functions. Energy deficits are initially responded to by a decrease in energy expenditure.[17,18] When compensation fails, fat is mobilized to produce fuel for energy production.[19] This may be followed by protein catabolism with visceral protein preserved longer.[20] The adaptive response is also characterized by endocrine changes aimed at regulating fuel availability and utilization.[21] As in acute fasting, weight loss early in semistarvation is rapid but gradually slows even if there is no change in the starvation diet. The reduction in total energy expenditure helps to bring the starving individual back to energy equilibrium, which is further maintained by a reduction in lean tissue mass.

Successful adaptation involves the process of controlled protein loss, which should stop when just enough has been sacrificed to permit energy balance. Because the rate of lean tissue loss is roughly proportional to the amount of lean mass, it automatically slows as the mass of lean tissue decreases.[22] Simultaneously, there is increased efficiency of dietary protein retention until a new state of protein equilibrium is reached.[15] An inverse relationship exists between the amount of lean tissue and the efficiency of retention of protein in the diet. This relationship is affected by the concentration of protein in the diet. As starvation progresses and the lean tissue store diminish, the rate of protein depletion slows as the amount of protein retained from each meal increases. A new equilibrium is established and lean tissue loss ceases when the line depicting the relationship between amount of lean tissue and rate at which it is depleted crosses over the line describing the relationship between the amount of lean tissue and the efficiency of retention of protein in the diet. The "price" paid to achieve this physiologic adaptation is the reduction in lean tissue stores. This analytical approach illustrates that a high-protein diet may permit protein equilibrium only

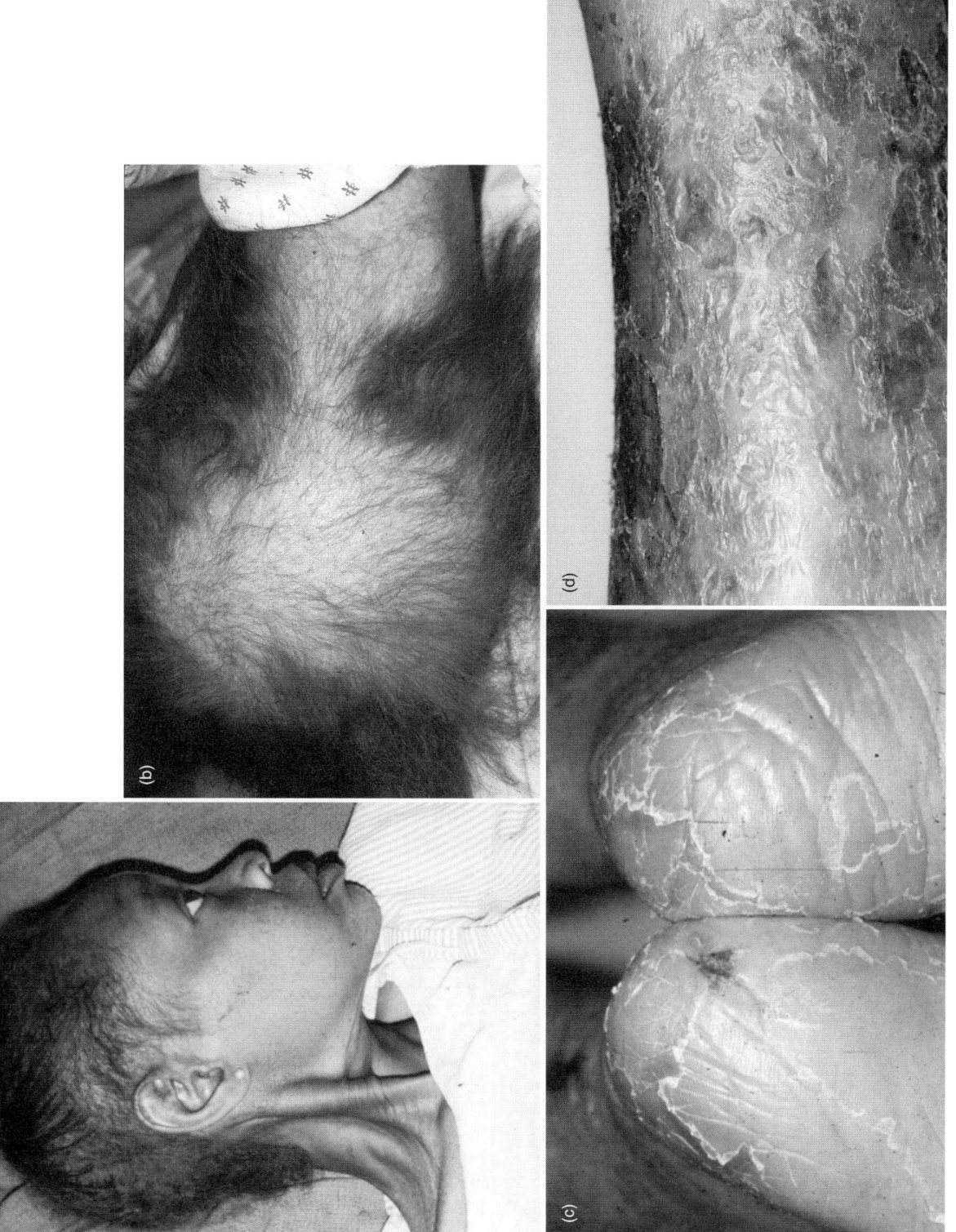

FIGURE 39.2 (See color insert following page 654.) Examples of some of the physical findings associated with PEM. (a) reddish hair (b) hair loss (c) flaking skin of the heels (d) 'flaking paint' dermatosis–darkly pigmented patches that may peal like old, sun-baked and blistered paint. (Photographs are provided by Dr. E.B. Feldman of patients at the Medical College of Georgia, Augusta.)

TABLE 39.5

Adaptive Responses to Protein-Energy Starvation

- Hypometabolism ($\downarrow$ energy expenditure, $\downarrow$ physical activity, $\downarrow$ protein turnover)
- Endocrine changes ($\downarrow$ serum T_3, $\downarrow$ insulin, $\uparrow\downarrow$ catecholamines, $\downarrow$ IGF-1)
- Cardiovascular and renal function ($\downarrow$ cardiac output, $\downarrow$ heart rate, $\downarrow$ blood pressure, $\downarrow$ renal plasma flow, $\downarrow$ glomerular filtration)
- Immune system (lymphocyte depletion, $\downarrow$ complement components, alterations in monokines or cytokines)

TABLE 39.6

Approach to Treatment of Mild and Moderate PEM

Setting
- Ambulatory setting preferred

Foods
- Home diet supplemented with easily digested foods containing proteins of high-biologic-value, high-energy-density, and adequate micronutrients

Intake Goals
- At least twice the protein and 1.5 times the energy requirement (e.g., preschool child: 2–2.5 g protein and 500–625 kJ (120–150 kcal)/kg body weight)

Food Facts
- Appetizing, ready-made, or easy to prepare, little commercial value outside the home to avoid sale of items for cash

Special Attention
- Avoid a decrease in breastfeeding for infants, ensure adequate vitamins and minerals, perhaps with the use of fortified foods

after moderate lean tissue wasting and that a low-protein diet may also be compatible with protein equilibrium, but the cost, in terms of protein wasting, will be greater.[15]

The intimate relationship between dietary energy and the maintenance of body protein should be underscored. Many studies have shown that energy intake influences nitrogen (N) balance at a constant protein intake.[23] The effect of energy is most potent in the modest submaintenance range of protein and energy intake.[15,24] The amount of dietary energy in surplus or in deficit after energy expenditure is accounted for will influence N balance, making the assessment of energy balance important in managing therapy.[15,24]

MANAGEMENT

MILD TO MODERATE PEM

If semistarvation is the principal cause for the development of PEM, the patient's response to complete nutrition support is excellent. The response is characterized by marked efficiency of protein utilization when protein intakes increase from the Recommended Daily Allowances (RDA) of 0.8 g/kg to a high of 1.5 g/kg and when energy intakes are increased from main-tenance to surfeit. In the case of mild to moderate PEM, treating the precipitating event and increasing protein and energy on the basis of the actual height in children and ideal weight in adults may be sufficient. Specific supplementation of individual nutrients is indicated by the presence of signs of specific nutrient deficiency. Table 39.6 outlines the general approach to the treatment of mild to moderate PEM. In children, treatment of mild and moderate PEM corrects the acute signs of the disease but catch-up growth in height takes a long time or might never be achieved. Weight-for-height can be restored early, but the child may remain stunted. Many severely malnourished children appear to have residual behavioral and mental problems, but the causal role of PEM and poor living conditions are difficult to dissociate.

SEVERE PEM

Mortality rates in severe PEM can be as high as 40% with the immediate cause of death being infection. Treatment strategies of severe PEM can be divided into three stages: (1) resolving the life-threatening conditions, (2) restoring nutritional status with-out disrupting homeostasis, and (3) ensuring nutrition rehabilitation. The most frequent life-threatening conditions associated with severe PEM are described in Table 39.7, and particular attention must be paid to children with HIV infection or AIDS.

Assessing dehydration in severe PEM is not easy because the classic signs (sunken eyeballs and decreased skin turgor) may also be found in well-hydrated malnourished patients. Furthermore, hypovolemia may coexist with subcutaneous edema. Because of the peculiarities of water and electrolyte disturbances in severe PEM (Table 39.7), the therapeutic approach differs from that used in well-nourished individuals (Table 39.8). Fluid repletion should allow a diuresis of at least 200 ml per 24 h in children and 500 ml in adults.[25] Whenever possible, oral or nasogastric rehydration should be used. The need to reduce the high sodium content of common ORS has led to a new formulation.[26] The WHO ORS packet for 1 L contains 3.5 g sodium chloride, 2.9 g trisodium citrate dihydrate, 1.5 g potassium chloride, and 20 g glucose. The recipe for ReSoMal (Rehydration Solution for the Malnourished) is 2 l water, one 1 L WHO-ORS packet, 50 g sucrose, and 40 ml of the electrolyte/mineral solution (Table 39.9). Table 39.9 shows the composition of an electrolyte/mineral mix that can complement the diet or be combined with WHO's regular ORS and sucrose to prepare the new formulation. ReSoMal contains ~ 45 mmol Na, ~40 mmol K, and ~3 mmol Mg/l , and its osmolarity is 245 mOsm/l. The solution has the magnesium necessary to replenish the body stores and will help potassium retention as well as replace other minerals deficient in severe PEM. An approach for rehydration is outlined in Table 39.10.

Nasogastric tubes may be used in children who vomit constantly or cannot be fed orally. Small portions are the key, but if hydration is not improved after 4 h, intravenous, rehydration may be used. Hypoosmolar solutions (200 to 280 mOsm/l) must be used and sodium should not be >3 mmol/kg/day. Potassium (not >6 mmol/kg/day) may be added when urination is established. Glucose should provide approximately 63 to 126 kJ (15 to 30 kcal)/kg/day. The approach to intravenous rehydration is described in Table 39.11.[16]

TABLE 39.7
Life-Threatening Conditions Associated with Severe PEM

Fluid and Electrolyte Disturbances
- Hypoosmolarity with moderate hyponatremia (but intracellular Na excess)
- Intracellular K^+ depletion without hypokalemia
- Mild to moderate metabolic acidosis
- Hypocalcemia
- Decreased body magnesium with or without hypomagnesemia

Severe Vitamin A Deficiency

Infections

Hemodynamic Alterations
- Cardiac failure secondary to intravenous fluids or after introduction of high-protein and high-energy feeding or a diet with high Na^+ content
- Pulmonary edema

Severe Anemia
- Treat only if hemoglobin <4 g/dl

Hypothermia

Hypoglycemia

TABLE 39.8
General Approaches to Therapy

Fluid Repletion
- Allow diuresis of at least 200 ml/24 h in children; 500 ml in adults
- Oral or nasogastric rehydration preferred

Electrolytes (if urinating)
- ~6 mEq K
- 2–3 mEq Na
- 2–3 mEq Ca^{+2}

Antibiotics
- Not used prophylactically
- Choice depends on suspected etiology

Anemia
- Treat only in severe cases (hemoglobin <4 g/dl)

Vitamin A Deficiency
- 50,000–100,000 IU for infants and children on day 1
- 100,000–200,000 IU for older children and adults on day 1
- Followed by 5,000 IU orally each day for the duration of treatment

TABLE 39.9
Concentrated Electrolyte/Mineral Solution for ReSoMal and to Complement Liquid Foods

Salt	Amount (g)	Molar Content of 20 ml
Potassium chloride: KCL	224	24 mmol
Tripotassium citrate: $C_6H_5K_3O_7.H_2O$	81	2 mmol
Magnesium chloride: $MgCl_2.6H_2O$	76	3 mmol
Zinc acetate: $Zn(H_3COO)_2.H_2O$	8.2	300 μmol
Copper sulfate: $CuSO_4.5H_2O$	1.4	45 μmol
Water: make up to	2500 ml	

1 mmol K = 39.1 mg; 1 mmol Mg = 24.3 mg; 1 mmol Zn = 65.4 mg; 1 mmol Cu = 63.5 mg

Notes:

Add selenium if available (sodium selenate 0.028 g, NaSeO4 10H2O) and iodine (potassium iodide 0.012 g, KI) per 2500 ml.

Add 20 ml of electrolyte/mineral solution to 1000 ml of milk feed or 40 ml to 21 preparation of ReSoMal.

Taken from WHO Web site http://www.who.int/child-adolescent-health/New_Publications/.

TABLE 39.10
Approach to Oral Rehydration for Severe PEM

Initiation
- Small sips to provide 70–100 ml/kg body weight over 12 h (10 ml/kg/h during first 2 h for mild to moderate dehydration; up to 30 ml/kg/h for severe dehydration)

Compensation for Ongoing Losses
- 50–100 ml after each loose stool or vomiting for those under 2 years of age; 100–200 ml for older children
- Continue breast-feeding

Evaluation
- Monitor every hour; as soon as improvement is seen (usually 4–6 h after initiation), small amounts of liquid dietary formula with potassium, calcium, magnesium, and other electrolytes may be offered every 2 to 3 h.

Persistent Dehydration
- Continue ORS for another 12 h
- If signs of overhydration (puffy eyelids, ↑ edema, distended jugular veins, ↑ respiratory rate), use breast milk or liquid diet instead of ORS

TABLE 39.11
Suggested Intravenous Rehydration Regimen

Solutions
- 1:1 mixture of 10% dextrose with isotonic saline or Ringer's lactated solution (δ5% glucose in 0.5 N saline)

Rate
- 10–30 ml/kg for the first hour followed by 5% dextrose in 0.2 N saline at 5–10 ml/kg/h
- Add K^+ when patient is urinating
- Patients with severe hypoproteinemia (<30 g/l), anemia, and signs of impending circulatory collapse should be given 10 ml plasma per kg in 1 to 2 h followed by 20 ml/kg/h of a mixture of 2 parts 5% dextrose and one part isotomic saline for 1–2 h. If diuresis does not improve, the dose of plasma may be repeated 2 h later

Hypocalcemia may occur secondary to magnesium deficiency. If magnesium levels cannot be determined, it is necessary to give both calcium and magnesium. Intramuscular or oral magnesium should follow initial parenteral magnesium until repletion with magnesium is complete. A general guideline is intravenous magnesium as a 50% solution of magnesium sulfate in doses of 0.5, 1, and 1.5 ml for patients who weigh less than 7, between 7 and 10, and more than 10 kg, respectively. This may be repeated every 12 h until there is no recurrence of hypocalcemic symptoms. Calcium replacement may be discontinued when the symptoms disappear or serum Ca^{+2} levels rise to normal. Oral magnesium supplementation of 0.25 to 0.5 mmol magnesium (0.5 to 1 mEq)/kg/day can be given later as described for maintenance therapy.

Infections are frequently the immediate cause of death in severe PEM, and when suspected, appropriate antibiotic therapy should be started immediately. The choice depends on the suspected etiology, patterns of drug resistance, and severity of the disease. Prophylactic antibiotics are not recommended but may be used if close monitoring for signs of infection by experienced personnel is not available. Clinicians should be aware that PEM may alter drug metabolism and that detoxification mechanisms may be compromised.[25] Delayed absorption, abnormal intestinal permeability, reduced protein binding, changes in volume of distribution, decreased hepatic conjugation or oxidation, and decreased renal clearance may all occur. Treatment for intestinal parasites should be deferred until nutritional rehabilitation is underway as this is rarely urgent. Vaccination against measles for every child over 6 months should be carried out with a second dose after discharge because seroconversion may be impaired.

Hemodynamic alterations may occur in severe PEM, especially in the presence of severe anemia, during or after administration of intravenous fluids or shortly after the introduction of high-protein and high-energy feeding or of a diet with high sodium content. Diuretics such as furosemide (10 mg intravenously or intramuscularly, repeated as necessary) may be given, and other supportive measures taken. The use of diuretics merely to accelerate the disappearance of edema in kwashiorkor, however, is contraindicated. Routine use of blood transfusions for anemia endangers the patients; therefore, it should be given only to those with severe anemia with hemoglobin of <4 g/dl, <12% packed cell volume (hematocrit), clinical signs of hypoxia, or impending cardiac failure. In countries with a high prevalence of infection with HIV and few or no resources for screening the blood supply, the risk of transmission of HIV is significant. Therefore, use of blood transfusions should be restricted except in life-threatening situations. Whole blood (10 ml/kg) can be used in marasmic patients, but it is better to use packed red blood cells (6 ml/kg) in edematous PEM. Transfusions must be given slowly, over 2 to 3 h, and may be repeated as necessary after 12 to 24 h. At signs of heart failure, 2.5 ml blood/kg should be withdrawn before the transfusion is started and at hourly intervals until the total volume of blood transfusion equals volume of anemic blood removed.

Hypothermia, defined as body temperature below 35.5°C, and hypoglycemia, defined as plasma glucose concentrations below 3.3 mmol/l (or 60 mg/dl), may be due to impaired thermoregulation, reduced fuel substrate availability, or severe infection. Asymptomatic hypoglycemia is usually treated by feeding with the small volumes of glucose- or sucrose-containing diets described earlier, whereas severe symptomatic hypoglycemia must be treated with intravenous 50% glucose solution followed by oral or nasogastric administration of 10% glucose solutions at 2 h intervals. Low body temperature will usually rise with frequent feedings of glucose-containing diets or solutions, but patients must be closely monitored when external heat sources are used to reduce the loss of body heat because they may become rapidly hypothermic when the heat source is removed.

Vitamin A deficiency is usually associated with severe PEM, and therefore a large dose of vitamin A should be given on admission. Water-miscible vitamin A as retinol should be given orally or intramuscularly on the first day at a dose of 52 to 105 μmol (15,000–30,000 μg or 50,000–100,000 IU) for infants and preschool children or 105 to 210 μmol (30,000–60,000 μg or 100,000–200,000 IU) for older children and adults followed by 5.2 μmol (1,500 μg or 5,000 IU) orally each day for the duration of treatment. Corneal ulceration should be treated with ophthalmic drops of 1% atropine solution and antibiotic ointments or drops until the ulcerations heal.[16]

The refeeding syndrome may develop in severely wasted patients during the first week of nutritional repletion.[27–29] Hyperinsulinemia stimulated by increased carbohydrate consumption results in an antinatriuretic effect.[30] Increased body sodium also results from increased sodium intake. In addition, hypophosphatemia and hypocalemia, as well as hypomagnesemia, can occur as a result of a stimulation of glycogen synthesis with the refeeding of carbohydrate. Close monitoring is therefore necessary to avoid acute deficiencies especially of phosphorous and potassium.

Following the attention to life-threatening conditions as described in the preceding text, the next objective of therapy is to restore nutritional status as rapidly and as safely as possible. This may be done with liquid formula diets fed orally or by a nasogastric tube, and for older children and adults with a good appetite, the liquid formula can be substituted with solid foods that have a high density of high-quality and easily digested nutrients. The marasmic patient may require larger amounts of dietary energy after 1 or 2 weeks of dietary treatment, which can be provided by adding vegetable oil to increase the energy density of the diet. Intravenous alimentation is not justified in primary PEM and can actually increase mortality.[31] The protein source in all foods must be of high biologic value and easily digested. Cow's milk protein is frequently available, and although there is concern about lactose malabsorption, cow's milk is usually well tolerated. Eggs, meat, fish, soy isolates, and some vegetable protein mixtures are also good sources of good protein. Vitamin and mineral supplements should be included at doses slightly higher than the RDA, which can be accomplished by adding the appropriate amounts of the mineral mix outlined in Table 39.9. Older children and adults should have their diets tailored to their age and general food availability. Initial maintenance treatment should provide average energy and protein requirements followed by a gradual increase to about 1.5 times the energy and 3 to 4 times the protein requirements by the end of the first week. Marasmic patients may need to have further increase in dietary energy intake. Initially, responses to the diet may be no change in weight or a decrease because of the loss of edema and a large diuresis. After 5 to 15 days, there is usually a period of rapid weight gain or "catch-up," but this is usually slower in marasmic patients than kwashiorkor patients.

The final step is ensuring nutritional rehabilitation in patients treated for PEM and usually begins 2 to 3 weeks after admission. Traditional foods should be introduced into the dietary regimen, and for the malnourished child, emotional, and physical stimulation are important. Adult patients should exercise regularly with gradual increases in their cardiorespiratory workload. Although the major emphasis of this chapter appears to be for infants and children, the same physiologic changes and principles apply to adolescents and adults with severe PEM. A brief summary of the approach is provided in Table 39.12. Because adults and adolescents often do not want to eat anything other than habitual foods and resist the intake of formula diets, added sugar and oil may be used to increase the energy density of the traditional diet. Liquid diets with vitamins and minerals can be given between meals and at night.

MONITORING

Monitoring the individual's response to initial therapy encompasses the same principles used to monitor the treatment of life-threatening conditions. Table 39.13 lists the characteristics associated with poor prognosis in patients with PEM. Treatment until full recovery from PEM should not be in the hospital. Ideally, the patient should be followed up in a nutrition clinic or rehabilitation center to continue treatment until after all life-threatening conditions have been controlled and the appetite is good, edema and skin lesions have resolved, and the patient appears content and interacts with the staff and other patients. The caretaker of the individual must understand the importance of continuing a high-energy, high-protein diet until full recovery has taken place. An increase in plasma protein or albumin concentration indicates a good response but not full recovery. The most practical criterion for recovery is weight gain, and almost all fully recovered patients should reach the weight expected for their height. Weight-for-height measures do not necessarily indicate protein repletion, and therefore it is good to use it in conjunction with other body composition indices such as creatinine–height index (CHI).[32–35] Table 39.14 summarizes guidelines for CHI and N balance.[35] Premature termination of treatment increases the recurrence of malnutrition. If body composition cannot be assessed, dietary therapy must continue for a month after the patient admitted with edematous PEM reaches an adequate weight-for-height without edema and clinical and overall performances are adequate, or for 15 days after the marasmic patient reaches that weight.[16] The minimum normal limits should be 92% for weight expected for height or one standard deviation below the reference mean. For children, assuring continual growth at a normal rate with no functional impairments is important.

TABLE 39.12
Dietary Treatment of Adolescents and Adults with Severe PEM

Initial
- Energy and protein appropriate for age (45 kcal and 0.75 g protein/kg/day for adolescents; 40 kcal and 0.6 g protein/kg/day for adults)
Rehabilitation
- Gradual increase to 1.5 times the energy and 3–4 times the protein requirements
- RDA for minerals and vitamins
- Vitamin A — single dose of 210 μmol (60 mg or 200,000 IU) retinol should be given to all except pregnant women
Monitoring
- Supplementary feeding should continue until BMI exceeds 15, 16.5, and 18.5 kg/m^2 for adolescents 11 to 13 years old, 14 to 17 years old, and adults, respectively

TABLE 39.13
Characteristics Associated with Poor Prognosis in Patients with PEM

- Age ≤6 months or ≥65 years
- Significant deficits in weight for age >40% or weight-for-height >30%
- Infections, especially bronchopneumonia or measles, or septicemia
- Total serum proteins ≤3 g/dl
- Severe anemia with signs of hypoxia
- Hypoglycemia
- Hypothermia
- Circulatory collapse or signs of heart failure, or respiratory distress
- Coma, stupor, or other changes in awareness
- Severe dehydration or electrolyte disturbance

TABLE 39.14

Guidelines for Creatinine–Height Index and Nitrogen Balance

Creatinine–Height Index (CHI)(34)

CHI = observed creatinine excretion/expected creatinine excretion × patient ideal weight for height,

Where expected = 18 mg/kg (women) or 23 mg/kg (men)

60–80% = moderate muscle mass depletion

<60% = severe muscle mass depletion

Nitrogen Balance

Dietary nitrogen (g protein/6.25) – (urinary urea N + 4 g)

Catabolic Index (CI)

Urinary urea N – (0.5 dietary N intake + 3 g)

CI = 0, no significant stress

CI = 1 to 5, mild stress

CI = >5, moderate to severe stress

TABLE 39.15

Factors Contributing to PEM in End-Stage Liver Disease

- Reduced energy intake
- Vomiting
- Fat malabsorption
- Abnormal carbohydrate and protein metabolism
- Increased energy requirements
- Vitamin and mineral deficiencies

Nitrogen balance (Table 39.14) is useful for estimating the degree of catabolism and monitoring the response to treatment. N balance is the difference between the quantity of dietary N ingested and the amount of N lost. Because dietary protein is assumed to have an average N content of 16%, protein intake is multiplied by 0.16 or divided by 6.25 to convert protein to N. As most of the N is lost in urine as urea, total N excretion may be estimated by adding a correction factor of 4 g to measured urea N: 2 g N for fecal and cutaneous losses and 2 g for nonurea nitrogenous compounds. One gram of N represents approximately 30 g of lean tissue. The catabolic index (CI) (Table 39.14) may be used as an estimate of the degree of stress in an individual. In this case, the amount by which the measured value exceeds the estimated amount is an indicator of the level of stress.[36]

The goal is complete nutritional recovery within 3 to 4 months. In children, clearly measurable laboratory changes may be seen within 2 to 3 weeks and anthropomorphic changes from 3 weeks onwards. Changes in adults are slower unless the PEM was acute and of short duration. Comprehensive programs of nutrition education, psychosocial stimulation, and progressive increments in physical activity must be undertaken.

IMPACT ON PROGNOSIS, MORBIDITY, AND MORTALITY FOR OTHER ILLNESSES, ESPECIALLY IN THE ELDERLY

PEM is also common in hospitalized patients and individuals with chronic diseases. This has been known since the early 1970s.[37] PEM is an inevitable consequence of chronic liver disease, and reversal of malnutrition is one of the key aims of liver transplantation.[38] Some of the factors contributing to PEM in end-stage liver disease are listed in Table 39.15. Patients with renal disease requiring dialysis are also at significant risk for PEM.[39,40] One of the challenges is to provide adequate nutrition to dialysis patients. Approaches often include dietary supplements, enteral tube feeding, intradialytic parenteral nutrition, and total parenteral nutrition. Appetite stimulants (e.g., megestrol acetate) and growth factors (e.g., anabolic steroids, recombinant growth hormone, or insulin-like growth factor-1) have been used.[41] Another prevalent disease with high incidence of PEM is HIV/ AIDS. PEM is one of the more common findings in AIDS. Chronic inflammatory bowel disease (e.g., Crohn's disease), anorexia nervosa, or other eating disorders are also commonly associated with PEM.

An important complication of PEM is its impact on wound healing and the development of pressure sores or decubitus ulcers. The majority of studies have looked at the relationship between nutritional factors and the development of pressure ulcers in hospitalized and nursing home patients, most of whom were elderly. Nutritional factors associated with the development of decubitus ulcers include inadequate energy and protein intake, making it one of the many risk factors that are potentially reversible.[42] Providing a diet that is complete in nutrient requirements results in the optimum environment for recovery and healing. A reasonable provision of protein is 1.0 to 1.5 g/kg/day and caloric intake ranging from 30 to 35 kcal/kg/day. Two other nutrients important for wound healing are vitamin C and zinc. Studies have shown that supplements of specific nutrients in patients who are not clinically deficient have little effect on the healing of pressure ulcers.[42] However, as the diagnosis of a subclinical deficiency status is difficult to make, physiologic replacement of dietary deficiencies is prudent when the diet is obviously lacking in sources of vitamins and minerals.

The group at greatest risk for PEM comprises the elderly, either with or without underlying diseases. Severe PEM occurs in 10 to 38% of older outpatients,[43–45] 5 to 12% of homebound patients,[46] and 5 to 85% of institutionalized older individuals.[47–49] As discussed earlier, a significant number of older hospitalized patients are also at risk for PEM.[12] Unfortunately, the presence of PEM is rarely recognized by physicians and, even when recognized, rarely treated.[45] A number of screening tests for malnutrition risk have been developed, but SCALES (Table 39.16) was developed to be used as a screening tool in the clinic. It has been cross-validated with the Mini-Nutritional Assessment (MNA), developed for older subjects.[50] SCALES appears to have superior ability to MNA in identifying subsequent nutritionally associated problems but has the disadvantage of requiring blood tests. Weight loss remains one of the most sensitive indicators of malnutrition. A useful mnemonic for causes of weight loss, especially in the elderly, is shown in Table 39.17. These tables and statistics, however, cannot replace the astute physician or health care provider who remains sensitive to the needs of the elderly and cognizant of this commonly overlooked problem — PEM. Table 39.18 provides a simple checklist that may be useful in the prevention and treatment of PEM in any hospitalized patient.

TABLE 39.16
Scales: Rapid Screen for Risk of PEM

S: Sadness
C: Cholesterol <4.14 mmol/l (160 mg/dl)
A: Albumin <40 g/l (4 g/dl)
L: Loss of weight
E: Eating problems (cognitive or physical)
S: Shopping problems or inability to prepare a meal

Source: From Morley, JE, *Proc Nutr Soc* 57: 587; 1998. With permission.

TABLE 39.17
"Meals on Wheels" Mnemonic for the Causes of Weight Loss

M: Medications
E: Emotional (depression)
A: Alcoholism, anorexia tardive[a], or abuse of elders
L: Late-life paranoia
S: Swallowing problems (dysphagia)
O: Oral problems
N: No money (poverty)
W: Wandering and other dementia-related problems
H: Hyperthyroidism, pheochromocytoma
E: Enteric problems (malabsorption)
E: Eating problems
L: Low-salt, low-cholesterol diet
S: Stones

[a] New onset of food refusal related to a desire to maintain a thin body habitus [51]

Source: From Morley, JE, *Proc Nutr Soc* 57: 587; 1998. With permission.

TABLE 39.18
Checklist of Procedures to Prevent and Treat PEM

Accurate record of admission height and weight and weekly follow-up weights

Write specific diet orders; monitor ability to eat and maintain weight

Consult dietician to assess follow-up. Collaborate on oral- and tube-feeding regimens

Regularly check to be sure nutrition composition is sufficient to cover basal and stress-related needs

Know your standard nutrition diets and supplements available

Do not wait >3–5 days before adding protein, calories and other nutrients. Avoid prolonged use of 5% dextrose in water and saline solutions

Use anthropometric measures and available laboratory data to assess and monitor nutritional status

Be cognizant that "hospital food", withholding meals for tests and anorexia from medications and illness can contribute to malnutrition

Consult Nutrition Support Service when in doubt

Be especially cognizant of patients at high risk (see Table 39.3 and Table 39.15)

Source: Adapted from Marliss, EB, *Protein Calorie Malnutrition, Cecil Textbook of Medicine*, 17th ed., Wyngaarden, JB, Smith, Jr, LH, WB Saunders Co., 1985.

REFERENCES

1. Williams, CD, *Arch Dis Childhood* 8: 423; 1933.
2. Jelliffe, DB, *J Pediatr* 54: 227; 1959.
3. Waterlow, JC, *Br Med J* 3: 566; 1972.
4. Waterlow, JC, in: *Nutrition in Preventive Medicine*, World Health Organization, Geneva, 1976.
5. Berkley, J, Mwangi, I, Griffiths, K et al., *JAMA* 294: 591; 2005.
6. Shetty, PS and Kurpad, AV, *Eur J Clin Nutr* 44: 47; 1990.
7. Minghelli, G, Schutz, Y, Charbonnier, A, et al., *Am J Clin Nutr* 51: 563; 1990.
8. Chandra, RK, *Am J Clin Nutr* 53: 1087; 1991.
9. Suskind, RM and Lewinter-Suskind, L, in: *The Malnourished Child*, Raven Press, New York, 1990.
10. Habricht, JP, Lechtig, A, and Yarborough, C, in: *Size at Birth,* Elsevier, New York, 1974. (Elliott, K & Knight, I, eds)
11. Habricht, JP, Lechtig, A, and Yarborough, C, UNICEF, *The State of the World's Children 2000*, United Nations Publications, New York, 2000.
12. Covinsky, KE, Martin, GE, Beyth, R et al., *J Am Geriatr Soc* 47: 532; 1999.
13. Prentice, AM, Moore, SE, Collinson, AC, and O'Connell, MA, *Nutr Rev* 60: S56; 2002.
14. Stein, K, Vasquez-Garibay, E, Kratzsch, J et al., *J Clin Endocrinol Metab* 91: 1021; 2006.
15. Hoffer, LJ, in: *Modern Nutrition in Health and Disease,* 9th ed., Williams and Wilkins, Baltimore, 1999. Shills, M ed.
16. Torun, B and Chew, F, in: *Modern Nutrition in Health and Disease*, 9th ed., Williams and Wilkins, Baltimore, 1999. Skills, M ed.
17. Torun, B, International Dietary Energy Consultancy Group 335; 1990.
18. Viteri, FE and Torun, B, *Bol Saint Panam* 78: 54; 1975.
19. Torun, B. and Viteri, F. E., *United Nations Univ Food Nutr Bull* 229; 1981.
20. Bistrian, BR, in: *Nutritional Assessment*, Blackwell Science Publications, Boston, 1984. Wright RA & Hemofield, S eds. Heymofield.
21. Becker, DJ, *Ann Rev Nutr* 3: 187; 1983.
22. Grande, F, in: *Handbook of Physiology: Adaptation to the Environment*, APS, Washington, DC, 1964. Dill DB ed
23. Elwyn, DH, Gump, FE, Munro, HN, et al. *Am J Clin Nutr* 32: 1597; 1979.
24. Calloway, DH, in: *Protein Quality in Humans: Assessment and In Vitro Estimation*, AVI Pub Co, Westport, CT, 1981.
25. Mehta, S, in: *The Malnourished Child*, Raven Press, New York, 1990. Suskind, RM & Le Winter-Suskind, L, Eds.
26. Muller, O and Krawinkel, M, *CMAJ* 173: 279; 2005.
27. McMahon, MM, Farnell, MB, and Murray, MJ, *Mayo Clin Proc* 68: 911; 1993.
28. Graham, GG, *N Eng J Med* 328: 1058; 1993.
29. Solomon, SM and Kirby, DF, *J Parenteral Enteral Nutr* 14: 90; 1990.
30. Barac-Nieto, M, Spurr, GG, Lotero, H et al., *Am J Clin Nutr* 32: 981; 1979.
31. Janssen, F, Bouton, JM, Vuye, A, and Vis, HL, *J Parenteral Enteral Nutr* 7: 26; 1983.
32. McMahon, MM and Bistrian, BR, *Disease-A-Month* 36: 373; 1990.
33. Walser, M, *J Parenteral Enteral Nutr* 11: 73S; 1987.
34. Viteri, FE and Alvarado, J, *Pediatrics* 46: 696; 1970.
35. Bistrian, BR, Blackburn, GL, Sherman, M, and Scrimshaw, NS, *Surg Gynecol Obstet* 141: 512; 1975.
36. Bistrian, BR, *Surg Gynecol Obstet* 148: 675; 1979.
37. Bistrian, BR, Blackburn, GL, Vitale, J, et al., *JAMA* 235: 1567; 1976.
38. Protheroe, SM and Kelly, DA, *Baillieres Clin Gastroenterol* 12: 823; 1998.

39. Kopple, JD, *J Nutr* 129: 247S; 1999.
40. Bistrian, BR, McCowen, KC, and Chan, S, *Am J Kidney Dis* 33: 172; 1999.
41. Kopple, JD, *Am J Kidney Dis* 33: 180; 1999.
42. Thomas, DR, *Clin Geriatr Med* 13: 497; 1997.
43. Miller, DK, Morley, JE, Rubenstein, LZ et al., *J Am Geriatr Soc* 38: 645; 1990.
44. Wallace, JI, Schwartz, RS, LaCroix, AZ et al., *J Am Geriatr Soc* 43: 329; 1995.
45. Wilson, MM, Vaswani, S, Liu, D et al., *Am J Med* 104: 56; 1998.
46. Morley, JE, *Proc Nutr Soc* 57: 587; 1998.
47. Sandman, PO, Adolfsson, R, Nygren, C et al., *J Am Geriatr Soc* 35: 31; 1987.
48. Silver, AJ, Morley, JE, Strome, LS et al., *J Am Geriatr Soc* 36: 487; 1988.
49. Morley, JE and Silver, AJ, *Ann Intern Med* 123: 850; 1995.
50. Guigoz, Y, Vellas, RJ, and Garry, PJ, *Facts Res Gerontol* 4: 15; 1994.
51. Miller, DK, Morley, JE, Rubenstein, LZ, and Pietreszka, FM, *J Am Geriatr Soc* 39: 462; 1991.

40 Assessment of Lipids and Lipoproteins

Elaine B. Feldman and Gerald R. Cooper

CONTENTS

INTRODUCTION

The circulating lipids include free cholesterol, cholesterol esterified with long-chain fatty acids, triacylglycerols (triglycerides [TG]), phospholipids, and unesterified or free fatty acids. Lipids are transported in the blood plasma in the form of lipoproteins. The lipoproteins include:

- Chylomicrons
- Very-low-density lipoproteins (VLDL)
- Intermediate-density lipoproteins (IDL, beta-VLDL)
- Low-density lipoproteins (LDL)
- High-density lipoproteins (HDL)

The chemical and physical properties of the lipoproteins are shown in Table 40.1. As the size of the lipoprotein decreases, from chylomicrons to HDL, the concentration of total cholesterol (TC), phospholipids (PL), and proteins increase gradually while the concentration of TG decreases.[1] This chapter summarizes preanalytical (biological and environmental) factors influencing lipid and lipoprotein levels, describes methodology for assays in common clinical use and provides data on the range of normal values.

CHOLESTEROL

Cholesterol is synthesized by all animal cells, but in mammals, this synthesis is greatest in hepatic cells. De novo synthesis is referred to as endogenous synthesis. Plants synthesize very little. Until recently it was thought that plants synthesize none, but improved analytical techniques have shown that some is synthesized (~50 mg/kg) and is present in plant cell membranes and surface lipids.[2] In a study of genes encoding sterol biosynthetic enzymes in plants, cholesterol, campesterol, and sitosterol were found essential for optimal vegetative growth including plant embryonic development, cell growth, plant growth, and fertility.[3] It has been confirmed that methyltransferase-1 controls the levels of cholesterol in plants.[4]

Circulating cholesterol in animals comes not only from endogenous synthesis, but from food sources as well. This cholesterol is called exogenous cholesterol. Food sources are listed in Chapter 43. Endogenous synthesis provides the majority of the cholesterol in circulation, and cholesterol is needed to support the synthesis of several hormones as well as vitamin D. It is also an important component of the cellular membranes. Circulating cholesterol levels vary with age, beginning to increase in both males and females from puberty and continuing to increase in males until the fifth decade of life and in women until the sixth decade of life (Table 40.2).[5,6] Levels in women are lower than in men from age 30 to 50 and higher than men above age 50. In men from age 30 to age 70, TC levels increase from an average 190 to 214 mg/dl (4.94 to 5.59 mmol/l) and women from an

TABLE 40.1
Plasma Lipoproteins in Humans[a]

					Chemical Composition, %				
					Surface			Core	
Class	Particle Diameter(nm)	Flotation Density	Electrophoretic Mobility	Major Apoproteins	Proteins	Phospholipids	Cholesterol	Cholesterol Esters	TG
Chylomicrons	80–500	<0.95	a2	B, E, A-1,A-4,C	2	7	2	3	86
VLDL	30–80	0.95–1.006	pre-β	B, E, C	8	18	7	12	55
IDL	25–35	1.006–1.019	slow pre-β	B, E	19	19	9	29	23
LDL	18–28	1.019–1.063	β	B	22	22	8	42	6
HDL$_2$	9–12	1.063–1.125	αl	A-I, A-II	40	33	5	17	5
HDL$_3$	5–9	1.125–1.210	αl	A-I, A-II	55	25	4	13	3

[a] Modified from Feldman, EB. *Essentials of Clinical Nutrition*, FA Davis, Philadelphia, PA, 1988, p. 433.

Note: Abbreviation: VLDL, Very-low-density lipoprotein; IDL, intermediate-density lipoprotein; LDL, low-density lipoprotein; HDL, high-density lipoprotein.

TABLE 40.2
Average Levels of Circulating Lipids[a,b]

Age (Years)	TC mmol/l	TC mg/dl	LDL-C mmol/l	LDL-C mg/dl	HDL-C mmol/l	HDL-C mg/dl	TG mmol/l	TG mg/dl
White men								
15–19	3.95	152	2.42	93	1.20	46	0.77	68
20–24	4.13	159	2.63	101	1.17	45	0.88	78
25–29	4.58	176	3.02	116	1.14	44	0.99	88
30–34	4.94	190	3.22	124	1.17	45	1.15	102
35–39	5.04	194	3.41	131	1.12	43	1.23	109
40–44	5.30	204	3.51	135	1.12	43	1.39	123
45–49	5.46	210	3.67	141	1.17	45	1.34	119
50–54	5.49	211	3.72	143	1.14	44	1.45	128
55–59	5.56	214	3.77	145	1.20	46	1.32	117
60–64	5.59	215	3.72	143	1.27	49	1.25	111
65–69	5.54	213	3.80	146	1.27	49	1.22	108
70+	5.56	214	3.69	142	1.25	48	1.30	115
White women								
15–19	4.08	157	2.42	93	1.33	51	0.72	64
20–24	4.29	165	2.65	102	1.33	51	0.90	80
25–29	4.6	178	2.81	108	1.43	55	0.86	76
30–34	4.63	178	2.83	109	1.43	55	0.82	73
35–39	4.84	186	3.02	116	1.38	53	0.94	83
40–44	5.02	193	3.17	122	1.46	56	0.77	68
45–49	5.30	204	3.30	127	1.51	58	1.06	94
50–54	5.56	214	3.48	134	1.61	62	1.16	103
55–59	5.95	229	3.77	145	1.56	60	1.25	111
60–64	5.88	226	3.87	149	1.59	61	1.18	105
65–69	6.06	233	3.93	151	1.61	62	1.33	118
70+	5.88	226	3.82	147	1.56	60	1.24	110

[a] See Table 40.1 for abbreviations of lipoproteins; Total C: cholesterol; TG: triglycerides.
[b] Adapted from Cohn, JN, Hoke, L, Whitwam, W, et al. Lipid Res Clin Program, *JAMA* 251: 351; 1984.

average 178 to 233 mg/dl (4.63 to 6.06 mmol/l). About two-thirds of the plasma cholesterol is transported as LDL, and levels of LDL-cholesterol (LDL-C) parallel those of TC (Table 40.2). HDL transports about one-quarter of the plasma cholesterol, with levels averaging about 1.17 mmol in men, and are 0.23 to 0.44 mmol higher in women (Table 40.2). Table 40.3 provides data on the upper limits of normal for LDL- and HDL-cholesterol (HDL-C). Table 40.4 provides data on mean values for lipids and lipoproteins in men and women from National Health and Nutrition Examination Survey (NHANES) III data.[7]

Mean serum TC levels in U.S. adults aged 20 to 74 have consistently declined over the time period 1976 to 1991, documented by four different time period national surveys.[7] The reference values in Table 40.2 were collected during a time period before the development of the powerful cholesterol-lowering drugs (statins) and thus represent cholesterol and lipoprotein reference values associated only with the variation in diet of the U.S. population before 1980. The average serum TC decreased from 220 mg/dl (5.69 mmol/l) in 1960 to 205 mg/dl (5.30 mmol/l) in 1991. All 5-year age groups for men and women showed similar reductions in serum TC.[7] The trends in serum lipids and lipoproteins of adults have been summarized from 1960 to 2002.[8]

Representative lipid, lipoprotein, and apolipoprotein clinical laboratory assays and available reference methods are listed in Table 40.5. Clinical laboratories are automated for the lipid analyses. Specific methods are provided as kits by the manufacturer of the analytical instrument in use. Desktop methodologies also are available for outpatient facilities (physicians' offices and clinics) but are not as accurate or precise as the commercial or hospital laboratory procedures. The Clinical Laboratory Improvement Amendments (CLIA) passed by Congress in 1988 established standards for clinical laboratory testing on human specimens in U.S. clinical laboratories for health assessment.[9]

The ATP111 suggested cutoffs for classification of TC values are as follows:

- Optimal (with other cardiovascular disease risk factors: 170 mg/dl(4.40 mmol/l)
- Desirable: <200 mg/dl (5.17 mmol/l)
- Borderline, High: 200–239 mg/dl (5.17–6.18 mmol/l)
- High: <240 mg/dl (6.21 mmol/l)

TABLE 40.3
Levels of Circulating Lipids Warranting Attention[a,b]

Age (Years)	LDL-C 75th Percentile		HDL-C 25th Percentile		TG 90th Percentile	
	mmol/l	mg/dl	mmol/l	mg/dl	mmol/l	mg/dl
White men						
15–19	2.83	109	1.01	39	1.41	125
20–24	3.07	118	0.99	38	1.64	146
25–29	3.59	138	0.96	37	1.92	171
30–34	3.74	144	0.99	38	2.41	214
35–39	4.00	154	0.94	36	2.81	250
40–44	4.08	157	0.94	36	2.84	252
45–49	4.24	163	0.99	38	2.84	252
50–54	4.21	162	0.94	36	2.74	244
55–59	4.37	168	0.99	38	2.36	210
60–64	4.29	165	1.07	41	2.17	193
70+	4.26	164	1.04	40	2.27	202
White women						
15–19	2.89	111	1.12	43	1.26	112
20–24	2.07	118	1.14	44	1.52	135
25–29	3.28	126	1.22	47	1.54	137
30–34	3.33	128	1.20	46	1.58	140
35–39	3.61	139	1.14	44	1.91	170
40–44	3.80	146	1.25	58	1.81	161
45–49	3.90	150	1.22	47	2.02	180
50–54	4.16	160	1.30	50	2.14	190
55–59	4.37	168	1.30	50	2.6	229
60–64	4.37	168	1.33	51	2.36	210
65–69	4.78	184	1.27	49	2.49	221
70+	4.42	170	1.25	48	2.13	189

[a] See Table 40.1 for abbreviations.

[b] Adapted from Cohn, JN, Hoke, L, Whitwam, W, et al. Lipid Res Clin Program, *JAMA* 251: 351; 1984.

TABLE 40.4
Lipid Levels U.S. NHANES III Population[a,b]

Lipid Level (mg/dl)	Mean ± SD (mg/dl)
Mean TC	225 ± 45
Men	218 ± 42
Women	237 ± 47
Mean LDL-C	142 ± 37
Men	139 ± 35
Women	147 ± 40
Mean HDL-C	50 ± 16
Men	47 ± 14
Women	56 ± 17
Median TG	140 ± 120
Men	137 ± 129
Women	144 ± 108
Mean total-C/HDL-C	4.9 ± 2.1
Men	5.1 ± 1.7
Women	4.7 ± 2.6
Mean LDL-C/HDL-C	3.1 ± 1.5
Men	3.2 ± 1.2
Women	2.9 ± 1.9
Apolipoprotein A_1	147 ± 27
Men	139 ± 23
Women	158 ± 29
Apolipoprotein B	116 ± 26
Men	115 ± 24
Women	119 ± 27

[a] See Table 40.1 for abbreviations.
[b] With permission from DHHS NCHS. Third National Health and Nutrition Examinations Survey, 1988–1994, NHANES III, Hyattsville, MD, 1996.

TRIACYLGLYCEROLS (TGS)

Circulating TG levels average about 1.13 mmol/l in young adults after overnight fasting. Levels increase from 50 to 75% with age, and are lower in women compared to men (Tables 40.2 and 40.3). Median TG values range from 0.90 to 1.47 mmol/l. TG levels are labile, varying by up to 50% daily, depending on the recent diet. In the fasting state, TGs are transported in the VLDL, whereas chylomicrons transport newly absorbed fat. Upper limits of normal for TG are given in Table 40.3.

TG assays and reference methods[22–28] are listed in Table 40.5.

The National Cholesterol Education Program (NCEP) Working Group on lipoprotein measurement recommends that clinical laboratories measure serum TG concentrations with an accuracy and confidence value of ±5%.[10] The NCEP Expert Panel on Detection, Evaluation, and Treatment of serum TG analytical results[11] are as follows:

- *Normal*: <150 mg/dl (<1.70 mmol/l)
- *Borderline high*: 150–199 mg/dl (1.70–2.25 mmol/l)
- *High*: 200–499 mg/dl (2.26–5.64 mmol/l)
- *Very high*: 500 mg/dl (5.65 mmol/l)

The TG cutoff for risk to coronary heart disease was decreased based on findings that TG values above 150 mg/dl combined with HDL-C below 40 mg/dl (1.03 mmol/l). This was associated with an increase in small dense highly pathogenic LDL. When high TG concentrations in the serum is found with the metabolic syndrome, (low HDL-C, abdominal obesity, elevated blood pressure, insulin resistance, hyperhomocysteinemia, and elevated chronic inflammatory hsCRP measurements) the clinician recognizes this metabolic syndrome as a secondary target of LDL-C. TG are then measured in the clinical laboratory for three major purposes:

- To establish TG status
- To assess risk of coronary heart disease
- To calculate LDL-C concentration when LDL-C cannot be determined directly[12]

TABLE 40.5

Tests for Plasma Lipids, Lipoproteins, and Lipolytic Enzymes

Assay	Principle of Method	Reference or Usual Clinical Method	Performance Criteria
TC	Chemical	Abell et al[22]	CV ≤3%
	Spectrophotometric		Bias <3%
	Modified Liebermann-Burchard		
	Automated enzymatic	Allain[23]	
	Colorimetric	Rautela[24]	
TG	Glycerol assay	Van Handel-Zilversmit[25]	
	Spectrophotometric		CV <5%
	Automated enzymatic		Bias <5%
	Spectrophotometric	Sampson[26]	
		Hagen[27]	
		Rautela[28]	
VLDL			
VLDL remnant	Ultracentrifugation	Nakajima[29]	
LDL-calculate	TC-{HDL-C + TG/5}	Friedewald[30]	CV <4%
			Bias <4%
LDL ultracentrifuge	C in d <1.006–HDL-C	Havel-Eder-Bragdon[31]	
		Krauss[32]	
LDL direct	Precipitation of chylomicrons, VLDL, IDL, HDL by antibodies to apo-E and apo A-I	McNamara[33]	
Lp(a), ELISA		Marcovina[34]	
HDL	Heparin-Mn or dextran-Mg precipitation of VLDL, LDL; analyze C in supernatant	Burstein[36] Warnick[37]	CV <4% Bias <5%
Apo A-I	Immunoassay	Albers[40]	CV 6%
Apo B	Immunoassay	Warnick[41]	
PL	Lipid phosphorus (lipid extract)	Bartlett[42]	
FFA	Titration of extracted plasma	Dole-Meinertz[43]	
Fatty acid composition	Gas-liquid chromatography of fatty acid methyl esters	Nelson[44]	
Lipoprotein lipase (LPL)	Hydrolysis of radioactive lipid emulsion by post-heparin plasma	Olivecrona[46]	3–5% accuracy
Plasma pool			
Hepatic lipase (HL)	Antiserum to HL		
NaCl inhibition of LPL		Huttunen[47]	Values lower in women
Lecithin–cholesterol acyl transferase (LCAT)	Double antibody radioimmunoassay	Albers[48]	

Note: CV = coefficient of variation, abbreviations used: PL, phospholipical; TC, Total cholestrol; TG, Total Triglyceride FFA, free faty acids, see Table 40.1 for Lipoprotein abbreviations.

LIPOPROTEINS

Lipoprotein assays[29–41] are given in Table 40.5.

CHYLOMICRONS

These particles originate in the small intestine when fat is absorbed, and are absent in plasma from fasting normal subjects. They are visibly highly turbid in freshly collected blood when TG levels exceed 700 mg/dl (7.90 mmol/l) (Figure 43.8, Chapter 43). When the blood or plasma is allowed to sit overnight in the refrigerator, the chylomicrons form a creamy top layer. At higher TG levels, the standing plasma will show a creamy top layer. Chylomicrons are transported into the lymphatic system, delivered into the blood, and removed by the action of the enzyme LPL to produce remnant particles that are taken up by specific receptors in the liver (Figure 40.1). The composition of chylomicrons is listed in Table 40.1.

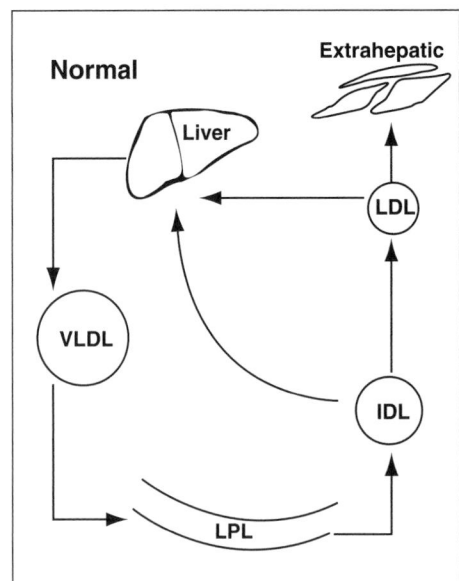

FIGURE 40.1 Production of lipoproteins, delivery into blood, and removal by tissues. See Table 40.1 for abbreviations. LPL = lipoprotein lipase.

VERY-LOW-DENSITY LIPOPROTEIN

These particles are produced in the liver and result from *in vivo* synthesis from carbohydrate precursors or from free fatty acids mobilized from adipose tissue and delivered to the liver. VLDL composition is given in Table 40.1. The standing plasma begins to appear diffusely turbid when TG levels exceed 250 mg/dl or 2.83 mmol/l. The source of this diffuse turbidity is the VLDL. LPL action produces VLDL remnants, or IDL, that are rapidly removed from the blood by receptors in the liver (Figure 40.1). An assay for VLDL remnants that has been developed for research studies[29] is under consideration by laboratory manufacturers for clinical applications. The cholesterol in the VLDL is usually calculated from the value of TG/5.[30]

INTERMEDIATE-DENSITY LIPOPROTEIN

This TG-rich particle is relatively enriched in the proportion of cholesterol esters compared to its precursor VLDL (Table 40.1). The atherogenic beta-VLDL is a related cholesterol-rich particle with interactions with the LDL and remnant receptors (Figure 40.1). This particle is evanescent in the plasma of healthy normolipidemic subjects. Elevated concentration of serum IDL is associated with the diagnosis of hyperlipoproteinemia type III. This lipoproteinemia is also associated with xanthomas on the hands.

LOW-DENSITY LIPOPROTEIN

This particle is the main transporter of cholesterol in the blood and is considered the most atherogenic lipoprotein. The LDL cholesterol level reflects changes in lipoprotein composition. LDL delivers cholesterol to cells and is taken up by specific cell surface receptors (Figure 40.2). LDL assays are listed in Table 40.5. LDL cholesterol may be calculated as:

$$LDL = [TC] - [HDL\text{-}C] - [TG/5]^{13}$$

Optimal cutoff values have been decreased over time but there has not been a significant decline in coronary heart disease (CHD) in relation to these values in recent years.[8-11]

The cutoff values are as follows:

- *Optimal*: <100 (2.59)
- *Near optimal*: Between 100 and 129 (2.59–3.34)
- *Borderline high*: Between 130 and 159 (3.36–4.11)
- *High*: 160–189 (4.14–4.89)
- *Very high*: <190 (<4.91)

The NCEP Laboratory Standardization Panel specifies criteria for acceptable LDL-C analytical performance in clinical laboratories as accuracy within 4% of reference values and precision consistent with CV of <4% (10A).

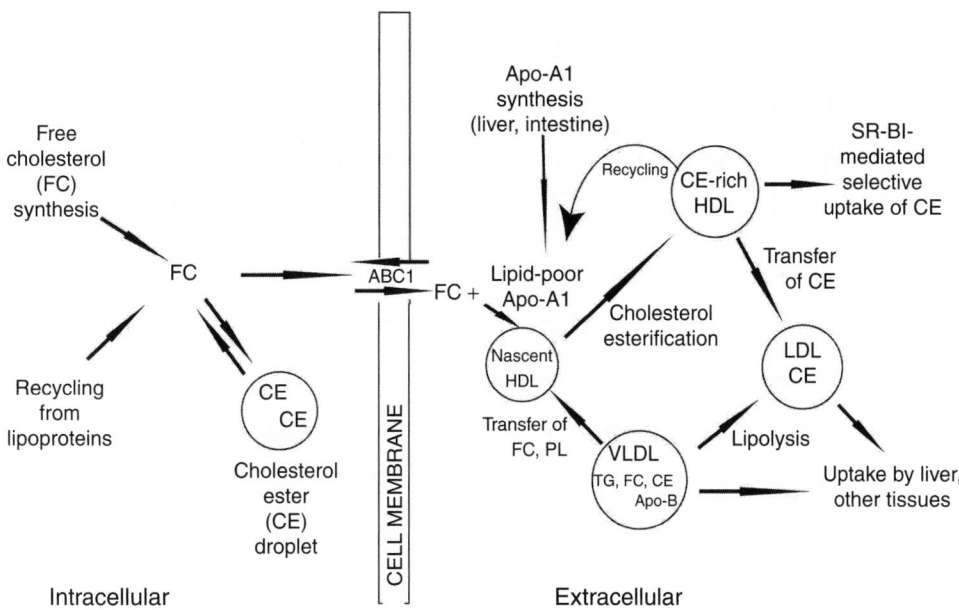

FIGURE 40.2 The generation of HDL and the interrelations of the lipoproteins, their production, and removal. ABC 1 = ATP-binding-cassette transporter. SRB 1 = Scavenger receptor binder. (With permission from Young, SG, Fielding, CJ. *Nat Genet* 22: 316; 1999.)

TABLE 40.6
Lipoprotein Subclasses[a]

Particle	Diameter	nm	Association with Risk of CVD
VLDL 1	Large	80	Higher
VLDL 12	Medium	70	Intermediate
VLDL 13	Small	60	Lower
IDL 1	Large	40	Higher
IDL 12	Small		
LDL I	Large	30	Lower
LDL II a			
LDL II b			
LDL III a	Medium		Intermediate
LDL III b			
LDL IV a	Small		Higher
LDL IV b		20	
HDL 2 b	Large	10	Negative risk
HDL 2 a		9	
HDL 3 a	Small	8	Positive risk
HDL 3 b		7	
HDL 3 c		6	

[a] See Table 40.1 for abbreviations.

Alternatively, LDL can be measured by ultracentrifugation (beta-quantification, or beta-quant)[31] or directly, using an immunologic procedure[32] (Table 40.5).

LDL particle size is variable, ranging from large and buoyant to small and dense (Table 40.6). The small dense particle, oxidative changes in LDL, and the presence of a variant of LDL, Lp(a), raise the atherogenicity of LDL. Lp(a) levels range from undetectable to 1000 mg/l. The risk of atherosclerosis increases as values exceed 300 mg/l. The Lp(a) assay[34] is listed in Table 40.5.

HIGH-DENSITY LIPOPROTEIN (HDL)

The HDL particle is generated by the transfer of surface lipids from TG-rich lipoproteins during lipolysis[35] (Figure 40.2). The HDL 2 and HDL 3 particles differ in size and composition, and particles vary in their content of the specific apolipoproteins, apo A-I and A-II (Tables 40.1 and 40.6). HDL is protective against atherosclerosis, enhancing removal mechanisms by reverse cholesterol transport. Methods of assay[36,37] are described in Table 40.5.

New cutoff HDL-C values were recommended for CHD risk from HDL-C and are as follows:

- *High risk*: <40 mg/dl (1.03 mmol/l) for men and <50 mg/dl (1.29mmol/l) for women
- *Low risk*: <60 mg/dl (1.55 mmol/l)
- *Negative risk*: a HDL-C value above 60 mg/dl (1.55 mmol/l) is a negative risk factor that removes one risk factor from the total count of risk factors.

The NCEP Laboratory Panel recommended that the analytical performance of HDL-C measurements in the clinical laboratory meet CV of 4% and bias of <5% (10B).

NON-HDL (OR APO B) LIPOPROTEINS

This equals TC minus HDL-C or cholesterol in VLDL, IDL and LDL-C. It is equivalent to apo B measurement. It is attractive to laboratory workers, because it measures the risk contributed by apo B in all lipoproteins. The average value attributed to apo B lipoproteins is LDL-C average value plus 30 mg/dl (0.78 mmol/l).

STANDARDIZATION OF ASSAYS

Blood samples for assays of serum or plasma lipids and lipoproteins should be obtained under standardized conditions of a stable diet, avoiding alcohol, and in the morning after an overnight fast. Serum and plasma values differ, as do values of cholesterol when the subject is supine, sitting, or standing. A recent meal has minor effects on cholesterol and predominantly-cholesterol-containing lipoproteins (LDL and HDL), but has a major influence on the levels of TG and TG-containing lipoproteins (VLDL). Optimally, determinations should be carried out on plasma samples obtained by using EDTA as anticoagulant and prepared and stored carefully. The biological variation of cholesterol, within the normal range, approximates 16%.[38] Laboratory accuracy and precision should be standardized with reference materials or reference laboratories.[15] Because of variability, more than one sample of plasma or serum lipids should be drawn, with an interval of several weeks of unchanged lifestyle, and analyzed in order to evaluate lipid status or therapy.[39]

A simple clue to lipid/lipoprotein values is provided by the standing plasma test (Figure 43.8, Chapter 43). Plasma is refrigerated overnight and examined for turbidity. Hypercholesterolemia does not cause the plasma to become cloudy, whereas elevated TG, either as VLDL, remnants, or chylomicrons will produce diffuse turbidity with or without a creamy supernatant layer (see Chapter 43).

The Center for Desease Controle (CDC) conducts a CDC-NHLBI Lipid Standardization Program to assist standardization of epidemiologic studies, clinical investigations, public health CVD prevention programs and lipid methodology research laboratories.[13]

Since many thousands of clinical laboratories operate in the United States, it is impossible to offer a standardization program directly to them. A cholesterol Reference Method Laboratory Network (CRMTN) was, therefore, established to offer standardization services to manufacturers and distributors of lipid and lipoprotein analytical systems and reagents for the manufacturer to standardize their particular diagnostic products before distribution to clinical laboratories. [14]

APOPROTEINS

Apolipoproteins (or apoproteins) determine the metabolic fate of lipoprotein particles and the solubility of lipoprotein lipids in plasma. They include:

Apo A-I
Apo A-II
Apo A-IV
Apo B-100
Apo B-48
Apo C-I
Apo C-II
Apo C-III
Apo-D
Apo E-2
Apo E-3 {E-phenotype: E2/2, 2/3, 2/4, 3/3, 3/4, 4/4}
Apo E-4

Apo-F
Apo-G
Apo-H
Apo-J
Apo (a)

Their distribution among the lipoproteins is shown in Table 40.1.

The assay methods available in some clinical laboratories[29–41] are provided in Table 40.5. The mean values in plasma are provided in Table 40.7. The apoprotein level indicates the number of lipoprotein particles in plasma (i.e., concentration). The apoprotein composition and levels are determined in some genetic and lipid laboratories using electrophoretic and immuno-logic methods. The ATPIII recommends clinical acceptance of an initial evaluation profile of TC < LDL-C <TG and HDL-C labo-ratory measurements of the patients serum. It is strongly advised that all persons know their TC number. A large panel of lipid and other metabolic laboratory tests combined with clinical tests were found effective in uncovering unsuspected early CVD.[15,40,44,46]

OTHER LIPID ASSAYS

Phospholipids are determined by measuring lipid phosphorus after lipid extraction.[42]

Free fatty acids in plasma can be analyzed, usually in relation to metabolic abnormalities, such as diabetes mellitus, and related to values of glucose and insulin. The assay is listed in Table 40.5.[43]

The fatty acid composition of plasma lipids, and separated and isolated free fatty acids, cholesterol esters, phospholipids, or TG, can be quantified.[28] This may be useful in the diagnosis of essential fatty acid deficiency and some inborn errors of metabolism.

Fecal fat can be measured as free fatty acids or TG fatty acids in order to test for malabsorption syndromes.[29]

REGULATORS OF LIPID METABOLISM

Enzymes, receptors, and transporters involved in the regulation of lipid and lipoprotein metabolism are listed in Chapter 42 and Table 42.1. Their values are determined primarily in lipid research laboratories rather than as part of the usual clinical lipid profile for patient assessment. Methods for the determination of postheparin lipolytic activity, LPL,[46] HL,[47] and LCAT[48] are listed in Table 40.5.

ACKNOWLEDGMENT

The authors would like to acknowledge the assistance of Virgil W Brown and Carolyn D. Berdanier in the preparation of this chapter for publication.

TABLE 40.7
Average Levels of Apoproteins in Plasma (mg/l)[a,b]

Apoprotein	Mean ± SD
A-I	1200 ± 200 (men)
	1350 ± 250 (women)
A-II	330 ± 50 (men)
	360 ± 60 (women)
B	1000 ± 200
C-I	70 ± 20
C-II	40 ± 20
C-III	130 ± 50
D	60 ± 10
E	50 ± 20

[a] SD = standard deviations.

[b] Adapted from Albers, in Eleventh Internatio-nal Congress of Clinical Chemistry (Keuser, E, Giabal, F, Muller, MM, et al., eds.) Walter de Greyter, Berlin, 1982.

REFERENCES

1. Feldman, EB. *Essentials of Clinical Nutrition*, FA Davis, Philadelphia, PA, 1988.
2. Behrman, EJ, Gopolan,V. *J Chem Edu* 82: 1791; 2005.
3. Schaller, H. *Prog in Lipid Res* 42: 162; 2003.
4. Diener, AC, Li, H, Zhou, W, et al. *Plant Cell* 12: 853; 2000.
5. The Lipid Research Clinics Program Epidemiology Committee. *Circulation* 60: 427; 1979.
6. Heiss, G, Tamir, I, Davis, CE, et al. *Circulation* 61: 302; 1980.
7. Johnson, CL, Rifkind, BM, Sempos, CT, et al. *JAMA* 269: 3002; 1993.
8. Carroll, MD, Lacher, DA, Sorlie, PD, et al. *JAMA* 294: 1773; 2005.
9. Benson, CC, Chenault, VM. In: *Handbook of Lipoprotein Testing* (Rifai, N, Warnick, GR, Dominiczak, MH, eds.) 2nd edition, AACC Press, Washington, DC, pg 767, 2000.
10. Stein, EA, Myers, GL. *Clin Chem* 41: 1414; 1995.
11. Bachorik, PS, Ross JW. *Clin Chem* 41: 1414; 1995.
12. Warnick, GR, Wood, PD. *Clin Chem* 41: 1427; 1995.
13. Warnick, GR, Wood, PD. *JAMA* 285: 2486; 2001.
14. Cole, TG, Klotzsch, SG, McNamara, JR. In: *Handbook of Lipoprotein Testing* (Rifai, N, Warnick, GR, Dominiczak, MH, eds.) 2nd edition, AACC Press, Washington, DC, pg 207; 2000.
15. Myers, GI, Cooper, GR, Greenberg, N, et al. In: *Handbook of Lipoprotein Testing* (Rifai, N, Warnick, GR, Dominiczak, MH, eds.) 2nd edition, AACC Press, Washington, DC, pg 717; 2000.
16. Myers, GI, Kimberly, MM, Waymack, PP, et al. *Clin Chem* 46: 1762; 2000.
17. Cohn, JN, Hoke, L, Whitwam, W, et al. *Am Heart J* 146: 679; 2003.
18. Cohn, JN, Hoke, L, Whitwam, W, et al. Lipid Res Clin Program *JAMA* 251: 351; 1984.
19. Cohn, JN, Hoke, L, Whitwam, W, et al. NHANES III *JAMA* 269: 3000; 1993.
20. Liebermann, C. *Ber Deut Chem Ges* 18: 1803; 1885.
21. Burchard, H. *Chem Zentraalbl* 610: 25; 1890.
22. Abell, LL, Levy, BB, Brodie, BB, Kendall, FE. *J Biol Chem* 195: 357; 1952.
23. Allain, CC, Pool, NS, Chan, CSG, et al. *Clin Chem* 20: 470; 1974.
24. Rautela, SS, Liedtke, RJ. *Clin Chem* 24: 108; 1978.
25. Van Handel, E, Zilversmit, DB. *J Lab Clin Med* 50P: 152; 1957.
26. Sampson, EG, Demers, LM, Kreig, AF. *Clin Chem* 21: 1983; 1975.
27. Hagen, JR, Hagen, PB. *Can J Biochem Physiol* 40: 1129; 1962.
28. Rautela, SS. *Clin Chem* 20: 857; 1974.
29. Nakajima, K, Sato, T, Tamura, A, et al. *Clin Chim Acta* 223: 53; 1993.
30. Friedewald, WT, Levy, RI, Fredrickson, DS. *Clin Chem* 18: 499; 1972.
31. Havel, RJ, Eder, HA, Bragdon, JH. *J Clin Invest* 34: 1345; 1955.
32. McNamara, JR, Cole, TG, Contols, JH, et al. *Clin Chem* 46: 232; 1995.
33. Krauss, RM, Burke, DJ. *J Lipid Res* 12: 97; 1983.
34. Marcovina, SM, Albers, JJ, Gabel, B, et al. *Clin Chem* 41: 246; 1995.
35. Young, SG, Fielding, CJ. *Nat Genet* 22: 316: 1999.
36. Burstein, M, Scholnick, HR, Mortin, R. *J Lipid Res* 11: 283; 1970.
37. Warnick, GR. *Clin Chem* 28: 1379; 1982.
38. Cooper, GR, Myers, GL, Smith, SJ, Schlant, RC. *JAMA* 267: 1652; 1992.
39. Smith, SJ, Cooper, GR, Myers, GL, Sampson, EJ. *Clin Chem* 39: 1012; 1993.
40. Albers, JJ. In: *The Determination of Apoproteins and Their Diagnostic Value in Clinical Chemistry* (Kaiser E, Gabal F, Muller MM, et al., eds.) Eleventh International Congress of Clinical Chemistry, Walter de Gruyter, Berlin; 1982.
41. Warnick, GR, Cheung, MC, Albers, JJ. *Clin Chem* 25: 596; 1979.
42. Bartlett, GR. *J Biol Chem* 223: 466; 1959.
43. Dole, VP, Meinertz, H. *J Biol Chem* 231: 2959; 1960.
44. Dole, VP, Meinertz, H. In: *Blood Lipids and Lipoproteins Quantitation, Composition and Metabolism* (Nelson, GH, ed.) Wiley Interscience, New York; 1972.
45. Van de Kamer, JH, Huinink, HTB, Weijers, HA. *J Biol Chem* 177: 347; 1949.
46. Bengtsson-Olivecrona, O, Olivecrona, T. In: *Lipoprotein Analysis: A Practical Approach* (Skinner, RE, Converse, CA, eds.) Oxford University Press, Oxford, pg 169; 1992.
47. Huttunen, Y, Enholm, C, Kinnunen, PKJ, Nikkila, EA. *Clin Chim Acta* 63: 335; 1975.
48. Albers, JJ, Chen, C-H, Lacco, AG. *Methods Enzymol* 129: 763; 1986.

41 Clinical Nutrition Studies: Maximizing Opportunities and Managing the Challenges

Colin D. Kay, Penny M. Kris-Etherton, Tricia L. Psota,
Deborah Maddox Bagshaw, and Sheila G. West

CONTENTS

INTRODUCTION

Clinical nutrition research continues to be the hallmark for establishing nutrient requirements throughout life. Over the years, it also has provided the basis for the evolution of dietary guidelines for the prevention and treatment of chronic disease. More recently, nutrition research has focused on overconsumption and associated chronic degenerative diseases. Moreover, the current trend is the evaluation of dietary patterns that have beneficial effects on multiple risk factors for several chronic diseases. This chapter addresses practical issues for designing studies and conceptual developments that aim to guide future clinical nutrition research.

Clinical nutrition research has yielded an impressive database showing the importance of diet in potently modulating multiple risk factors for chronic disease. In part, this progress has resulted from the use of more complex and powerful study designs. Much has been learned from sequential designs in which hypotheses are tested in a stepwise manner where the first experiment frames the hypothesis to be evaluated in subsequent work. In addition, a growing list of risk factors is being evaluated, thereby extending our understanding of the many "targets" that diet affects. Contemporary clinical nutrition tests hypotheses in many different populations, establishing the efficacy of diet in high-risk populations and diverse ethnic groups. Because of these important developments, this chapter will review the design and results of a selection of landmark clinical nutrition studies conducted since the 1990s. The goal is to illustrate the best practices in the design of high-impact studies and to provide guidance to researchers about how to incorporate these practices into smaller-scale studies. The primary focus is on interventions that target cardiovascular disease (CVD) risk factors because of the great progress that has been made in understanding the role of nutrition in modulating CVD risk (see Chapter 42 and Chapter 43 for more information on CVD). Importantly, many of these practices can be used in studies designed to assess nutrient requirements as well as effects of diet and dietary factors on risk of other chronic diseases.

This chapter provides practical advice for scientists conducting clinical nutrition research. We recognize that, while many investigators do not have the resources to conduct large-scale, multicenter studies, there is great merit in smaller studies for many reasons that include gathering essential pilot data to justify larger studies and conducting experiments that can require intensive subject participation or gaining a better understanding about mechanisms of action. For example, well-designed clinical studies can advance the field by identifying subgroups of patients with the largest response to a given intervention by testing implementation of a specific diet intervention in free living subjects and by suggesting potential mechanisms that explain the diet response. In Table 41.1, we have included a number of important resources that describe the key aspects of designing and conducting clinical studies. These books and journal articles provide detailed and comprehensive information regarding all aspects of conducting nutrition research with human participants. However, there are many novel study designs with inherent challenges in defining participant populations, food or supplement distribution, and diet design. For the most part, these issues have not been discussed in detail in the references listed in Table 41.1. In Table 41.2 are listed online resources for information needed for the Institutional Review and Protection of Human subjects. In Table 41.3 to Table 41.10 and Figure 41.1, we provide a variety of forms developed at the Metabolic Diet Study Center at Penn State University that we have used for our human studies research. Other investigators may find these useful and will want to adapt them for their own purposes. Finally, we discuss emerging trends in biological science with important implications for clinical nutrition.

NEW DESIGN APPROACHES

Dietary intervention studies have shifted from focusing on a single nutrient, such as saturated fat or cholesterol, to testing effects of a complete dietary pattern, such as the Mediterranean diet. Furthermore, nutrition intervention studies vary in what they emphasize — specific food components (i.e. the Portfolio studies),[1–4] a structured nutrient profile (i.e. the Dietary Effects on Lipoproteins and Thrombogenic Activity, the DELTA study),[5] or a dietary pattern (i.e. the Dietary Approaches to Stop Hypertension [DASH] diet studies).[6–8] During some interventions, all foods are provided to participants, whereas in others only certain foods or supplements are provided. In supplement studies, participants may be instructed to consume their habitual diet or a modified diet. The study population also is an important component of nutrition intervention studies. Large-scale studies may assess dietary interventions that target disease prevention in the general population; whereas smaller-scale studies are useful for determining the effects of diet for secondary prevention of chronic diseases.

Often, clinical nutrition research uses "sequential" designs, in which a series of related studies are conducted that evaluate responses to a single nutrient, a single food, a food group, or a dietary pattern across a range of conditions varying in the degree of experimental control. The DASH study series is an example of a sequential design that targeted a dietary pattern and then focused on the effect of a single nutrient e.g. sodium within that pattern. In the Portfolio diet series, a sequential design

---

TABLE 41.1
Resources for Information on the Conduct of Clinical Nutrition Studies[5,25,44–48,57,58]

Allison, DB, Gadde, K, Ryan, D, Pi-Sunger, F.X., Design, analysis and interpretation of Randomized Clinical Trials in Obesity, 2006

Dennis BH, Ershow AG, Obarzanek E, Clevidence BA. *Well-Controlled Diet Studies in Humans.* Chicago, IL: The American Dietetic Association, 1999

Dennis BH, Stewart P, Hua-Wang C, Champagne C, Windhauser M, Ershow A, Karmally W, Phillips K, Stewart K, Van Heel N, Farhat-Wood A,
  Kris-Etherton PM. Diet design for a multicenter controlled feeding trial: The DELTA Program. *JADA* 98:766, 1998

Dennis BH, Kris-Etherton PM. *Designing, Managing, and conducting a Clinical Nutrition Trial. In: Research, Successful Approaches.* 2nd Edition Edited by
  E. Monsen. Chicago, IL: The American Dietetic Association, 2003

Greenberg RS, Daniels SR, Flanders WD, Eley JW, Boring JR. *Medical Epidemiology,* 4th ed. The McGraw-Hill Companies, Inc., 2004

Griel, AE, Psota, TL, Knis-Etherton, PM. Guidelines for Implementing Clinical Nutrition Studies, chapter 9 2007

Monsen, E.R. (ed) *Research: Successful Approaches,* 2nd ed., Chicago, IL: The American Dietetic Association, 2003

Obarzanek E, Moore TJ. The dietary approaches to stop hypertension (DASH) trial. *J Am Diet Assoc* 1999;8: S1–S104

Windhauser M, Ershow A, Obarzanek E, Dennis B, Swain J, Kris-Etherton P, Karmally W, Blackwell S. The multicenter approach to human feeding studies.
  In: *Well-Controlled Diet Studies in Humans.* Edited by Dennis B, Ershow A, Obarzanek E, Clevidence, B. Chicago, IL: The American Dietetic Association,
  1999:390–403

Refer to Table 41.2 for references for Institutional Review and Protection of Human Subjects.

TABLE 41.2
Resources on Institutional Review and Protection of Human Subjects

(a) Internet References for Institutional Review and Protection of Human Subjects

Resource	Source	Web Address
Regulatory Compliance	The United States Department of Health and Human Services	www.hhs.gov/ohrp
Ethical Issues in Research Involving Human Participants	National Institutes of Health	www.nlm.nih.gov/pubs/cbm/hum_exp.html
Bioethics Resources	National Institutes of Health	www.nih.gov/sigs/bioethics/IRB.html
Research on Human Specimens	National Institutes of Health	www.cdp.ims.nci.nih.gov/brochure
Guidance for Institutional Review Boards, Clinical Investigators, and Sponsors	U.S. Food and Drug Administration	www.fda.gov/oc/ohrt/irbs/default
Biomedical Ethics in U.S. Public Policy	Office of Technology Assessment; Congress of the United States	www.wws.princeton.edu/ota/disk1/1993/9312_n.html
Medical Research Involving Human Subjects	World Medical Association	www.wma.net/e/policy/b3.htm
Ethics in Human Research	National Council on Ethics in Human Research	www.ncehr-cnerh.org
Tri-Council Policy on Ethical Conduct for Research Involving Humans	Government of Canada	www.pre.ethics.gc.ca

(b) Published References for Institutional Review and Protection of Human Subjects[49-56]

Title	Authors	Source
Challenges in human subjects protection	Nightingale SL	Food Drug Law J, 1995; 50:493–501
Local institutional review boards (IRBs), multicenter trials, and the ethics of internal amendments	Jansen LA	IRB, 2005; 27(4):7–11
Looking into the institutional review board: observations from both sides of the table	Burke GS	J Nutrition, 2005; 135(4):921–924
What must research subjects be told regarding the results of completed randomized trials?	Markman M	IRB, 2004; 26(3):8–10
Variation in Institutional Review processes for a multisite observational study	Vick CC, Finan KR, Kiefe C, Neumayer L, Hawn MT	Am J Surg, 2005; 190(5):805–809
Searching for an efficient institutional review board review model: Interrelationship of trainee-investigators, funding, and initial approval	Dominguez RA, Feaster DJ, Twiggs LB, Altman NH	J Laborat Clin Med, 2005; 145(2):65–71
Variations among Institutional Review Board reviews in a multisite health services research study	Dziak K, Anderson R, Sevick MA, Weisman CS, Levine DW, Scholle SH	Health Serv Res, 2005; 40(1):279–290
Ethical and institutional review board issues	Skolnick BE	Adv Neurol, 1998; 76:253–262

There are numerous resources outlining guidelines for obtaining IRB and ethical approval. Such resources include your University Office of Regulatory Compliance, the United States Department of Health & Human Services (www.hhs.gov/ohrp), and various Bioethics resources as presented by the NIH (www.nih.gov/sigs/bioethics/IRB.html). Most of these sites list necessary resources for the implementation of clinical research, including biosafety, as well as animal subject (IACUC) and human subject (IRB) regulations. Most of this material also applies to other human ethics review boards as found outside of the United States such as the Canadian Tri-Council Policy on Ethical Conduct for Research Involving Humans (www.pre.ethics.gc.ca) and international guidelines on ethics principles for medical research involving human subjects as endorsed by the world medical association (www.wma.net/e/policy/b3.htm). Specific resources, both internet and print, outlining guidelines and tips for obtaining Institutional Review Board (IRB) approval and for the protection of human subjects are listed in the following tables.

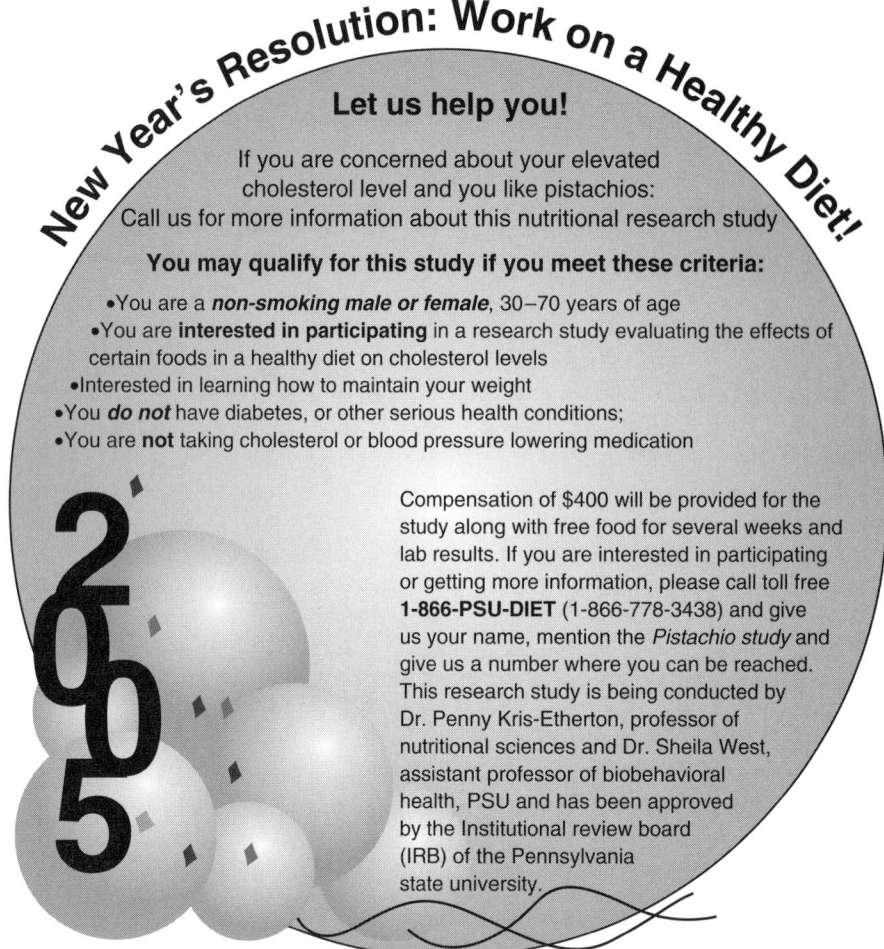

New Year's Resolution: Work on a Healthy Diet!

Let us help you!

If you are concerned about your elevated
cholesterol level and you like pistachios:
Call us for more information about this nutritional research study

You may qualify for this study if you meet these criteria:

- You are a *non-smoking male or female*, 30–70 years of age
- You are **interested in participating** in a research study evaluating the effects of certain foods in a healthy diet on cholesterol levels
- Interested in learning how to maintain your weight
- You *do not* have diabetes, or other serious health conditions;
- You are **not** taking cholesterol or blood pressure lowering medication

Compensation of $400 will be provided for the study along with free food for several weeks and lab results. If you are interested in participating or getting more information, please call toll free **1-866-PSU-DIET** (1-866-778-3438) and give us your name, mention the *Pistachio study* and give us a number where you can be reached. This research study is being conducted by Dr. Penny Kris-Etherton, professor of nutritional sciences and Dr. Sheila West, assistant professor of biobehavioral health, PSU and has been approved by the Institutional review board (IRB) of the Pennsylvania state university.

FIGURE 41.1 Sample recruitment advertisement for recruiting.

was used to test a dietary pattern, components of which were selected from numerous studies focusing on individual foods and supplements. In both examples, initial studies determined efficacy (the maximum effect of the interventions in a controlled feeding setting), while later studies determined effectiveness (the magnitude of intervention effects attainable in the free-living environment) (see Chapter 44 and Chapter 45 for further information on hypertension).

The first example of a sequential progression in research is the DASH trial,[9] which was followed by the DASH-Sodium trial,[10] and then the PREMIER trial.[11] A unique feature of the DASH trial was that it tested a dietary pattern rather than a single nutrient.[6] In the DASH trial, the DASH combination diet (high in fruits, vegetables, whole cereal products, low-fat dairy products, fish, chicken, and lean meats; low in saturated fat and cholesterol; moderate in protein; and high in minerals and fiber) was compared with a control diet relatively low in potassium, magnesium, calcium, and fiber and with a diet rich in fruits and vegetables that matched the DASH diet for potassium, magnesium, and dietary fiber (F&V diet). The DASH trial was a parallel arm, controlled-feeding study in 456 healthy men and women, aged ≥22 years, with systolic blood pressure (SBP) <160 mmHg and diastolic blood pressure (DBP) between 80 and 95 mmHg. After 8 weeks, both treatment diets significantly decreased blood pressure compared with the control diet (DASH diet: SBP −5.5/DBP −3.0 mmHg; F&V diet: SBP −2.8/DBP −1.1 mmHg). Declines in blood pressure were significantly greater in the DASH diet group; and patients with stage 1 hypertension showed the largest responses.[9]

The findings of this trial raised the question of whether the DASH diet would augment the demonstrated blood pressure reductions that are typically observed with sodium restriction.[9] The DASH Diet, Sodium Intake and Blood Pressure trial (DASH-Sodium), was conducted to evaluate this question. The study population consisted of individuals with above-optimal blood pressure (120–139/80–90 mmHg) and stage 1 hypertension (140–159/90–95 mmHg). In this controlled-feeding trial, there were two parallel arms in which an average American diet (AAD) and a DASH diet were compared. Within these two arms, a three-way crossover was implemented to compare the effects of three levels of sodium intake (50, 100, and 150 mmol/day), which represented average U.S. consumption (high intake), the upper limit of the U.S. recommendation at the time (intermediate intake), and a targeted lower sodium level (low intake).[10] After 30 days of reduced sodium intake, SBP decreased significantly in both diet groups (high to intermediate: –2.1 mmHg during control diet [p <.001] and –1.3 mmHg during DASH diet [p = .03]; intermediate to low: –4.6 mmHg during control diet [p <.001] and –1.7 mmHg during DASH diet [p <.01]).[7] Thus, this study suggests that sodium restriction has independent blood-pressure-lowering effects, and these effects also are expected in patients who are already consuming a diet high in fruits, vegetables, and low-fat dairy foods. This trial illustrates a complex design that targets the effect of one specific nutrient within the context of two dietary patterns.

The PREMIER trial extended the findings of the DASH and DASH-Sodium trials by testing behavioral lifestyle interventions (weight loss if overweight, reduced sodium intake, increased physical activity, and limited alcohol intake) in addition to dietary modifications.[11] To test the effectiveness of the intervention, participants with higher than optimal blood pressure or stage 1 hypertension were randomly assigned to an advice only (standard care) group, a behavioral lifestyle modification group, or a behavioral lifestyle modification plus DASH diet group in the free-living environment. After subtracting the change in the advice only group, SBP decreased significantly in both lifestyle intervention groups after 6 months (behavior modification only: –3.7 mmHg [p <.001]; Behavior plus DASH: –4.3 mmHg [p <.001]), indicating that multiple lifestyle changes can lower blood pressure.[8] However, these results were no longer significant at the 18 month follow-up, thereby illustrating the need for a sustained intervention to achieve long-term adherence for implementation of a DASH dietary pattern.

The progression of the DASH, DASH-Sodium, and PREMIER trials determined the effect of the DASH diet alone, in conjunction with reductions in sodium intake, and in combination with lifestyle modifications. Furthermore, the large sample sizes in these studies allowed for multiple subgroup analyses by age,[12] race,[7,13] blood pressure values,[7-9,14,15] and inflammatory state.[16] Taken together, this integrated series of state-of-the-art multicenter trials showed that sequential design is an effective research approach for determining the specific effects of food groups and a target nutrient (sodium) on markers of health.

The Portfolio diet studies[1-4] are examples of a series of related nutrition interventions in a specific subpopulation of hyper-cholesterolemic men and postmenopausal women. These studies incorporated food components that have Food and Drug Administration (FDA)-permitted health claims for coronary heart disease risk reduction[17-20] and were designed to determine if the combination of these dietary components results in additive effects, synergistic effects, or lessening of their individual cholesterol-lowering properties.[1] The efficacy of the Portfolio diet, a vegetarian diet rich in soy protein, almonds, plant sterols, and viscous fibers, on risk factors of CVD was tested first.[1] This diet significantly improved CVD risk factors[1] and was more effective than a Step II diet in a subsequent parallel arm study.[2] The next step in this series of studies was to compare the Portfolio diet to low-dose statin therapy and a Step II diet in a three-way crossover study.[3] This study demonstrated that the Portfolio diet, which utilizes a unique combination of foods, was equally as effective at improving CVD risk factor status as drug therapy. All study foods were provided, except fruits and vegetables, for which participants were reimbursed. In this controlled clinical setting, the dietary Portfolio was able to decrease total cholesterol levels by 22 to 37% and low-density lipoprotein (LDL) cholesterol levels by 22 to 35% after 4 weeks of treatment,[1-3] which was comparable to statin therapy.[3]

The subsequent study tested implementation of the Portfolio diet in free-living subjects on self-selected diets, and allowed consumption of red meat if desired.[4] This free-living study tested the effectiveness of dietary advice, encouraging the consumption of the same four dietary components as were tested in the previous metabolic studies (soy protein, almonds, plant sterols, and viscous fibers). Although meat was not encouraged, if it was consumed, advice was given to limit the amount eaten and to select lower-fat options. Although CVD risk factors significantly improved after 1 year (total cholesterol –10% and LDL cholesterol –13%), these benefits were not as great as those achieved in the controlled-feeding studies.[4] Reductions in total and LDL cholesterol were one-half to one-third of those attainable in the metabolic studies. Furthermore, only one-third of the participants achieved LDL reductions ≥20%, while one-third attained 10 to 20% and the remaining third <10%. The majority of the subjects found it difficult to follow the strict advice of the Portfolio diet, with only 7 of the 55 subjects consuming a vegan or vegetarian diet and ~50% following the advice for viscous fiber and soy protein. Compliance was 79% for almonds and 67% for the sterol-enriched margarine. Thus, this study quantified the effectiveness of the Portfolio dietary pattern under real-world conditions. This provides important information for clinical dieticians for individual diet counseling, as well as for policymakers who are developing population-based dietary recommendations.

In summary, utilization of more complex research designs that build on previous studies is critical to advance the field of clinical nutrition. Studying the effects of single bioactive agents in a way that minimizes potentially confounding variables can be very challenging in clinical nutrition studies because it often is not possible to change one variable without altering others. Often, the only way to approach this challenge is with a series of carefully nested studies, each of which must be adequately powered to focus on a small number of testable hypotheses. The DASH and Portfolio studies are excellent examples of sequential designs in which the initial experiments establish efficacy and frames the questions for subsequent studies.

SUCCESSFUL EXECUTION OF CONTROLLED-FEEDING STUDIES

In this section, we provide practical advice for obtaining approval from the institutional review board (IRB) and suggestions for kitchen management, subject enrollment, and assessment of adherence in dietary studies. This information is provided for investigators and their staff who are new to the conduct of highly controlled clinical nutrition studies. More experienced investigators are referred to the discussion of new concepts and state-of-the-art techniques that follow this section. One reason that a discussion of basic management issues is so important is the increasing complexity of clinical nutrition studies. Consequently, many aspects of the study become more complicated, including logistics, staffing issues, costs, and the increased expectations placed on the subjects. These are all very important considerations when scaling up a study.

TIPS FOR SUCCESSFUL APPLICATIONS TO THE IRB

There are numerous current resources that provide detailed descriptions of the guidelines for obtaining IRB approval for protocols involving human subjects (see Table 41.2). For university researchers, the best resource is often the Office of Regulatory Compliance or Office of Research Protections on campus. Most hospitals, contract research organizations, and industry groups have similar regulatory branches, which are responsible for ensuring safety and ethical treatment of human subjects. Our recent work suggests three primary issues that should be considered prior to submission of an application to the IRB: (1) issues of safety when control diets are prescribed, (2) inclusion of new, more sophisticated end points/outcomes, and (3) archiving of blood and other samples for as yet undefined secondary analyses, which may be proposed years in the future.

With regard to the safety of control diets, this issue is potentially of greater importance when clinical intervention studies enroll individuals with a clinical diagnosis, such as hypercholesterolemia, hypertension, or symptomatic CVD. It is common in nutrition studies for patients to be randomized to a control diet that is typical of U.S. consumption patterns (and is therefore not optimal for managing the patient's medical condition). This raises both ethical and safety questions. We recently completed a randomized crossover study examining the effects of the DASH diet on blood pressure in individuals with stage 1 hypertension. The IRB was concerned that, although the control diet was quite consistent with current dietary patterns of many adults consuming a Western diet, patients with hypertension may have been consuming a more restrictive diet before they entered the study and would therefore be potentially at risk for blood pressure increases when they began the study. This concern was addressed by including "safety checks," daily blood pressure measurements collected during the first week of each new diet period, with weekly follow-up thereafter. This approach was cost-effective and highly appropriate to protect subject safety. Fortunately, none of the subjects exhibited worsening of their hypertension during the study, which would have required them to seek treatment and exit the study. In addition to the use of safety monitoring procedures, the use of a crossover study design (or wait-list control) improves the risk/benefit ratio for individual subjects because they are entitled to receive the active treatment as part of their participation in the study. Obviously, it is important to ensure that control or placebo diets are as brief as possible to ensure subject safety.

There is great interest in defining conditions under which consent can be requested for archiving blood and other samples for later analysis, particularly when the assay targets are not defined when the study is underway. This is critical for preliminary studies or studies with minimal funding because the availability of additional funding, new assay techniques, or new hypotheses could substantially improve the study's contribution to the literature. For example, we designed a study to assess the lipid-lowering effects of adding soy protein to a Step-I diet.[21] Moderately hypercholesterolemic adults consumed a low-fat, high-fiber Step-I diet with the addition of either 25 g/day of milk protein or soy protein isolate in a crossover design. We found that the low-fat, high-fiber diet significantly lowered LDL cholesterol, regardless of soy or milk protein content, and concluded that changes in the lipid profile may not be the primary mechanism for lowered CVD risk in people who consume high amounts of soy protein. In order to explore whether individual differences in responsiveness to soy could be explained by differences in metabolism of soy isoflavones, archived urine samples were analyzed for newly identified metabolites of isoflavones. Additional assays of this type, added to an approved study protocol, may require additional review and approval from the IRB unless the consent form specifies in advance that such post hoc analyses are permitted.

In the same study, the availability of carefully preserved serum archives allowed us to reprocess samples at a later date to measure C-reactive protein (CRP) and various inflammatory cytokines.[22] Results from this secondary analysis indicated that the inflammatory status of the individuals was not influenced by either protein source. However, individuals without evidence of inflammation at study entry (as indicated by low baseline CRP concentrations) exhibited a significant decrease in LDL cholesterol and LDL/HDL ratio in response to the Step-I diet, whereas those with high baseline CRP exhibited worsening of the LDL/HDL ratio, apolipoprotein B, and lipoprotein(a) during treatment. By planning ahead and archiving samples, we were able to derive important additional information that enhanced the impact and value of the final reports from the study. Local IRBs should be consulted for ways to obtain consent to store and later analyze blood and other samples, even if the analyses have not yet been determined. Implicit to subsequent analyses at a later time is that the sample is stored in a way that maximizes long-term stability. In addition, it is important to note that post hoc analysis of genetic material may require that subjects be reconsented because of unique ethical issues associated with genotyping.

RECRUITING PARTICIPANTS

Recruitment tactics should be specifically tailored to the inclusion and exclusion criteria for the study. Additionally, the IRB or equivalent ethics review board must approve all recruiting materials to assure that the information is neither misleading nor coercive and that critical information is provided. Depending on the available budget and the specific characteristics of the

TABLE 41.3
Recruiting Strategies

Advertisement strategy	Tips	Advantages	Disadvantages
Local newspapers	Careful attention should be given to wording and exclusion criteria should be mentioned in order to limit the number of calls from ineligible participants	Reaches a large audience	Often expensive
Local radio and television advertisement	• In many areas, broadcast public service announcements can be used as a low-cost method of recruiting • Invest in a memorable toll-free number for subject contact (e.g., 1-888-PSU-DIET)	Reaches a large audience	May be cost-prohibitive and advertisements are limited in the amount of information that can be disseminated
Speaking at local community organizations, church groups, or health fairs	• Offering free health screening (i.e., glucose monitoring, blood pressure measurement, etc.) can be a productive method of recruiting	Targets a very specific audience, relatively cheap	Time-consuming
Posting flyers	• Post flyers on bulletin boards in supermarkets, drug stores, or doctors' offices	Targets a specific audience and is inexpensive	Labor-intensive, may require permission, some chain stores do not allow it
Developing relationships with physicians	• Develop relationships with physicians who provide patient referrals • Develop an easy to administer screening checklist that can be completed rapidly by busy clinicians	Very useful in recruiting subjects with defined baseline characteristics	Requires highly motivated physician, and a simple and easy to complete screening tool
Mass mailings (brochure, postcard or letter)	• Yields for direct mail campaigns are typically quite low (~0.5 to 1.0%), but they can be effective within a larger recruiting strategy	Effectively targets a specific population	Somewhat labor-intensive and costly for materials, mailing lists, and postage
Internet postings	• Must implement an effective procedure for managing the list, particularly for people who "opt out"	May allow you to target a specific population	Sometimes requires the purchase of a mailing list
Patient specific databases maintained by a clinical center or hospital	• Requires considerable up-front investment and careful attention to HIPAA regulations	Easily allows targeted recruitment	Not practical for individual investigators unless database exists

target population, we have developed a range of recruiting methods which vary in their expense, yield rates, and time required to return results. Advantages and disadvantages of several approaches are presented in Table 41.3. Our recent recruiting efforts have typically included: advertisements in local newspapers, radio, and television; speaking at local community organizations, church groups, or health fairs; posting flyers on bulletin boards in supermarkets, drug stores, or doctors' offices; developing relationships with physicians who provide patient referrals; mass mailings of brochures and postcards; and Internet postings and e-mail. An example of a newspaper recruitment ad is shown in Figure 41.1.

Regardless of the recruitment method used, careful records are required to track recruiting progress (and to note the success of various methods), and, more importantly, to document that eligibility criteria are being met. If recruitment is advancing too slowly, summary data on reasons for exclusion can be the basis for deciding whether eligibility criteria can be loosened. Therefore, recruitment methods should be flexible enough that volunteers can be recontacted if the decision is made to alter enrollment criteria. The IRB typically requires that investigators obtain consent to recontact participants or refer them to other studies for which they are eligible, and this should be anticipated in the IRB application. The practice of referring interested volunteers to other active protocols is a productive method for building community interest in research participation.

SCREENING POTENTIAL PARTICIPANTS

Initial contact by phone is often used to exclude those who do not meet the most easily identifiable criteria, and this strategy avoids including participants in expensive clinic visits. Inexperienced telephone interviewers faced with dozens of phone calls to return may wish to focus only on whether a prospective volunteer meets the eligibility criteria. However, callers are uncomfortable answering detailed personal questions without a basic understanding of the study's purpose and requirements. We find it valuable to structure the screening questions within a scripted phone conversation to standardize the information provided across interviewers (see Telephone Interview Form, Table 41.4). Our interview typically inquires about health conditions and medication usage early in the conversation because these are the most common reasons for ineligibility. In addition, some subjects will refuse to participate in a study if weight maintenance is a strict requirement, and we recommend that this issue be discussed early in the screening process.

Next, a face-to-face meeting is often required to assess whether a volunteer is willing and able to adequately follow the protocol, and this is of particular importance in nutrition studies. During such a visit, general dietary information may be gathered

TABLE 41.4
Telephone Interview Form

Date _____   Interviewer: _____

Before asking any questions, please read the following paragraph to obtain verbal consent to conduct the telephone interview:

"We received your message that you are interested in participating in our Study. I will first read a brief description of the study. In this study we will give you all food and beverages for 14 weeks. There will be one, 2-week feeding period and three, 4-week feeding periods. There will be a 2-week break in-between each diet period for a total time commitment of 18 weeks. During each of these three 4-week feeding periods we will provide you with three meals and a snack every day and beverages. You will come to the Metabolic Diet Study Center on the Penn State campus Monday through Friday for breakfast or dinner, where meals will be prepared and provided for you. On Friday evenings, you will be given a cooler that contains your Friday dinner and Saturday and Sunday meals and snacks. All the foods provided will be typical foods available in local grocery stores. We will ask that you not consume any other foods or beverages other than those provided during each 4-week interval. We will draw blood from you nine times during the study, once at screening and on two consecutive days at the end of the 2 week run-in period and at week 4 of each feeding period to determine your blood fat levels. At the end of each diet period we will measure your blood vessel function which will take about 1 h and your stress reactivity which will take about 2 h. Please note that this is not a weight-loss study, so we will weigh you daily to ensure you are not gaining or losing weight. You should be aware that the compensation for this study ($400) is considered income. If you are a Penn State employee, it will be taxed; if you are not, it is reportable income. Are you still interested in the study?"

        YES _____ (continue with interview)

        NO _____ (thank them for their time and interest)

"I will now ask you a series of questions about your past medical history and your current lifestyle. If you agree to answer these questions, and it is then determined that you meet the criteria for this study, we will schedule you for a screening visit. Are you willing to answer these questions, which will take about 15 min?"

        YES _____ (continue with interview)

        NO _____ (thank them for their time and interest)

1. Please give us your:

Name _____ Date of Birth _____

Home address _____

        _____

Daytime Phone Number _____ Evening Phone Number _____

2. What is your age? _____   **Interviewer:**

   Your height (ft and in.) _____   Age between 30 and 70 years   Yes   No

   Your weight (lb) _____   BMI 21–35   Yes   No

3. For women only:

   (a) Are you currently pregnant or wishing to become pregnant during the next 6 months?   Yes   No

   (b) Are you currently lactating or been lactating any time during the last 6 weeks?   Yes   No

   (c) Are you currently taking an oral contraceptive?   Yes   No

If yes, please specify the type of medication used and duration of use:

_____

_____

4. Have you donated blood in the past 2 months?   Yes   No

   If yes, how long has it been since you donated? _____

   If not, would you abstain from donating blood during the study?   Yes   No

5. Have you lost any weight during the past 6 months?   Yes   No

   If yes, how much: _____   **Interviewer:**
   Weight loss >10% body weight   Yes   No

6. Are you currently on a weight-loss diet or program?   Yes   No

   If yes, please specify: _____

   How long have you been on this weight loss diet? _____

   How much weight have you lost? _____

Continued

TABLE 41.4
(Continued)

7. Will you be in the area for the entire 20 weeks of the study?	Yes	No
8. Do you have access to the following appliance at home:		
Refrigerator	Yes	No
Freezer	Yes	No
Microwave, oven or toaster oven	Yes	No
9. Do you have any of the following medical conditions:		
a. Heart disease	Yes	No
b. Stroke	Yes	No
c. TIA (mini stroke)	Yes	No
d. Diabetes	Yes	No
e. High blood pressure	Yes	No
f. Renal or kidney disease	Yes	No
g. Rheumatoid arthritis, lupus or other autoimmune diseases	Yes	No
h. Gastrointestinal disease (such as Crohn's disease, irritable bowel syndrome, ulcer or history of bowel surgery, lactose intolerance)	Yes	No
i. Blood clotting disorder	Yes	No
j. Liver disease or cirrhosis	Yes	No
k. Any condition that requires the use of steroids	Yes	No
l. Gout (requiring treatment)	Yes	No
m. Anemia (or sickle cell anemia)	Yes	No
n. Lung disease (such as bronchitis, emphysema, asthma)	Yes	No
o. Cancer within the last 10 years	Yes	No
p. Thyroid disease	Yes	No
q. Problems with immune system (such as chronic fatigue syndrome, hepatitis, AIDS)	Yes	No
r. Peripheral vascular disease or circulation problems such as Reynaud's	Yes	No
s. Any other medical conditionNot specified in this list	Yes	No

Specify_____

Explain any "yes" answers: _____

_____

_____

10. Do you take any medication prescribed by a doctor? (This includes medications for any diseases, any type of pain medicine, and any drugs for treatment of depression or other mental health problems.)	Yes	No

If yes, please specify the type of medication used, duration of use and reason:

_____

11. Do you take any blood pressure or cholesterol-lowering medication?	Yes	No

Example: Captopril, Hydrochlorothiazide, Atenol or Zocor, Ezetimibe, Questran, Colestid, Orlistat

12. Are you taking any OTC cholesterol-lowering substances?	Yes	No

Example: psyllium, fish capsules, soy lecithin, phytoestrogen; if so, what? _____

13. Do you take any medication **not** prescribed by a doctor? Or any type of nutritional supplement, herb or vitamin?	Yes	No

If yes, please specify the type of medication used, duration of use and reason: _____

_____

_____

If yes, are you willing to discontinue use during the study?	Yes	No

Continued

TABLE 41.4
(Continued)

14. Do you have any food or nut allergies?	Yes	No

If yes, please specify foods:

_____

15. Are you allergic to latex?	Yes	No
16. Are you lactose intolerant or allergic to dairy products?	Yes	No
17. Do you have any food restrictions related to religious practices? Or are there any foods you refuse to eat?	Yes	No

If yes, please specify: _____

18. Are you on a special diet prescribed by a doctor or self-prescribed?	Yes	No

If yes, please specify (specifically ask about vegetarian) _____

Interviewer: Vegetarian	Yes	No
19. Do you exercise intensely more than 10 h a week or play sports regularly?	Yes	No

If yes, please specify: _____

20. Do you have any problems with your speech or when speaking to other people?	Yes	No

If yes, please explain: _____

21. Do you currently smoke?	Yes	No
If no, have you ever smoked before?	Yes	No

Explain: _____

22. Do you consume alcohol?	Yes	No

If yes, how much/how often?_____

23. Do the investigators have permission to recontact you for future studies?	Yes	No
24. Would you like to have your name referred for research projects in other labs?	Yes	No

SUBJECT MAY BE CONSIDERED ELIGIBLE FOR THE STUDY IF NO BOLDED RESPONSES ARE CHECKED ON THE TELEPHONE INTERVIEW FORM

If subject is eligible, schedule visit to General Clinical Research Center for Clinic Visit 1.

Yes, subject eligible   Date of screening: _____

No, subject is not eligible — Reason: _____

Give the subject directions to the General Clinical Research Center in Noll Lab on the PSU campus. Please have them meet the study staff at the second floor nurse's station. Enter the GCRC through the door that faces Atherton street. Instruct them to put on their flashers, go to the nurse's station to get a parking permit and then return to their car and put the permit on their mirror and turn off their flashers. The first visit will take approximately 1 h to complete all of the paperwork and testing.

to identify participants who cannot or will not eat specific foods because of religious reasons, allergies, intolerance, food aversions, or physical discomfort. In addition, it is important to assure that potential subjects are willing to give up foods that they consider "essential" in their habitual diets but which are not included in the test diets. It is also valuable to identify family or work situations or extensive travel plans that may make adherence to the protocol difficult. Questions that probe these issues are included in our telephone screening form; however, if adhering to a specific dietary pattern is important to the study's objectives, we find it valuable to ask these questions more than once. Participants meeting the telephone screening criteria are generally required to come to the study site for clinical laboratory tests or other measurements to assure that they are otherwise healthy and meet all the study eligibility criteria, as well as to give informed consent. If the study requires control for menstrual cycle phase or information about menopausal status, the questions listed in Table 41.5 will be of great help in establishing eligibility and scheduling appointments.

Be prepared to spend a significant amount of time recruiting and screening potential participants. Depending on the complexity of eligibility criteria, many more subjects will generally be screened than those enrolled in the study. Our efforts to

---

TABLE 41.5
Women's History Form

Date: _____   Subject: _____

1. Have you had a baby within the last 6 months?	Yes	No
2. Are you breast-feeding?	Yes	No
3. Are you pregnant or planning to become pregnant?	Yes	No
4. Are you currently taking oral contraceptives?	Yes	No

    If yes, specify: _____

    How long have you been taking this oral contraceptive? _____

5. Is your menstrual status:

a. Regular	Yes	No
Does it occur at least once/month?	Yes	No

    How many days between the first day of one period and the first day of the next period? _____

    How many days do you typically experience menstrual flow each cycle:

      1 2 3 4 5 >5 days

    In the past 3 months, how many cycles have you had? _____

    In the past 6 months, how many cycles have you had? _____

    How would you characterize your menstrual flow in the first two days of menses?

    Heavy   Moderate   Light

b. Irregular	Yes	No

    If yes, explain: _____

c. Not menstruating	Yes	No

    If you are not menstruating, what is the reason?

i. Natural menopause (no period w/in last year)	Yes	No
date of last period? _____		
ii. Hysterectomy	Yes	No
If yes, did you have your ovaries removed?	Yes	No
iii. Other _____	Yes	No
6. Are you taking HRT for "hot flashes" or other symptoms of menopause?	Yes	No

    If yes, specify: _____

    How long have you been taking this HRT? _____

Do you take the same dose every day or are your pills taken on a "cycle"?	Same dose	Cycle
Does it cause bleeding?	Yes	No

Subject is considered eligible for the study if no bolded responses are checked.

---

identify healthy adults with hypercholesterolemia who are willing to enroll in a controlled feeding protocol for 26 weeks typically yield one eligible subject from every 10 to 15 contacts. Willingness to participate obviously decreases with increasing subject burden. In a recent investigation by our group, over 600 individuals responded to an advertisement and inquired about the investigation by phone. Of those, only 74 were eligible after the phone interview for clinical screening and only 28 met the clinical inclusion criteria and were admitted into the study.

ORIENTATION SESSION

For studies that require significant changes in participant behavior, an orientation session is required to ensure that they understand the protocol and any measurement tools that they must master in order to provide accurate data. A manual or handout that lists guidelines for successful participation in the study should be reviewed during an orientation session immediately prior to the study start date. An example of helpful information for the subjects enrolled in a complex controlled-feeding study is shown in Table 41.6. Typically, our reminder lists include:

- Complete lists of all foods and beverages to be administered or allowed so that allergies or refusal to eat specific foods can be determined early in the process
- A statement of the requirement for complete consumption of all foods and beverages and the need for timely completion of daily record forms
- A request that subjects check the completeness of meals packed for them by research staff before they leave the site
- Instructions for typical problems (e.g., what to do if they feel too full or too hungry to follow the protocol)
- Heating directions for take-out foods
- A list of contact persons with telephone numbers should problems arise
- Instructions for safe handling of foods that are to be consumed off site

Assuring Diet Adherence

Although several biomarkers of dietary intake have been proposed (particularly for consumption of sodium, potassium, and dietary fats and fatty acids), most nutrition studies rely on participant self-report of adherence to the protocol. We find that compliance to even complex study protocols is enhanced when subjects are aware of the benefits of study participation and when they are provided their lipid and lipoprotein profile results at the completion of the study. A participant who views enrollment in a dietary intervention study as a preferred alternative to pharmacological treatment has great motivation to adhere to the protocol in order to validate the effects of diet on their own cardiac/chronic disease risk profile.

Adherence is usually assessed on a daily basis (see Daily Monitoring Form, Table 41.7). These records should be reviewed frequently by study staff, and the results should be discussed with participants to determine if new strategies can be devised to enhance compliance. Participants must be encouraged to record their behaviors honestly and must not feel that their participation is threatened by their candid responses. Nonetheless, they must understand that compliance is an expectation of study subjects. However, on occasion, small deviations from study protocol are to be expected. Data from these daily checklists may be used to calculate a compliance score. A daily diary, daily log, or food and beverage intake form may also be used to gather information for the following broad categories:

- The type and amount of study foods not eaten
- The type and amount of nonstudy foods eaten
- The type and amount of discretionary or "allowed" food items consumed
- The type and amount of beverages consumed, including coffee, tea, soft drinks, water, and alcoholic beverages
- The number of unit foods or calorie adjusters eaten
- Dietary supplements or over-the-counter medications taken
- Feedback regarding concerns or questions related to participation in the study

These forms may also be used to track other important study variables, such as phase of menstrual cycle and fluctuations in body weight. On a weekly basis, the participant may complete another form that asks about general-health-related items that might influence food intake or study outcomes (see Weekly Monitoring Form, Table 41.8). It is also important for the staff to document deviations from the protocol observed during on-site meals and those reported to staff during off-site meals. The data may then be adjusted for compliance measures and energy or nutrient calculations.

Supplement studies (in which the intervention consists of a prepared nutritional supplement) have unique challenges. Researchers need to consider whether it will be administered in tablet or pill form, incorporated in different ways into whole foods, or if it will be consumed through supplementation of specific foods such as flaxseed, almonds, walnuts, tomatoes, etc. If the pharmacokinetics of the active compound are known, or if there are problems with acceptability or side effects, researchers may choose to administer the supplement in multiple doses throughout the day.

Exit Interviews

At the end of the study, an exit interview may be planned for individuals or for a group of participants. Information offered to the participants could include clinical laboratory data gathered during the study, such as health risk assessments and appropriate educational materials. The IRB must approve which data can be released to patients and what interpretation, if any, the researchers may offer to explain the results provided. In addition, anonymous input from participants about their experiences and views is helpful for planning future studies. Typically, we ask about favorite foods and disliked foods served in the test diets, factors that made it easy or difficult to follow the study protocol, an evaluation of how they were treated by study staff, and whether they would recommend participating in this study to their friends. This information can be invaluable for improving future studies by increasing menu acceptability, identifying omissions in data collection, and making participation in a study a more enjoyable experience.

TABLE 41.6
Study Reminders

Here are some dos, don'ts and hints for you. We recognize that participating in a controlled feeding study is a significant commitment — if you have any problems, concerns or questions please ask any of the staff — we will try to help you as best we can

Study Contact Info: Diet Center: XXX-XXXX (Contact Name)
Research Study Office: XXX-XXXX (Contact Name)

Please let us know if you are not coming at your "regular" time or are having any problems; fill out a "pack out request" if you need meals packed out for a trip or meeting

<u>Allowed Beverages</u>

1. Caffeine free diet or unsweetened beverages may be consumed in any amount desired
   Water
   Calorie-free mineral water
   Diet caffeine-free soda
   Crystal Light or sugar-free KoolAid (the Crystal Light cannot be calcium fortified)
   Decaf Coffee and Tea

2. Caffeinated no-calorie diet soda beverages and caffeinated coffee and tea are limited to 5 servings/day. For soda: 1 serving is one 12 oz can. Coffee and tea: 1 serving is 8 oz

Beverages those are limited or not allowed:
1. Alcoholic beverages are limited to 2/week for this study. (1 alcoholic drink is considered to be a 12 oz beer, 5 oz of wine or 1.5 oz of hard liquor and if you drink hard liquor the mixer must be noncaloric, that is, diet soda, water, etc.)
2. Regular soda or beverages with calories are not allowed, this includes all fruit juices, vegetable juices, etc.

Allowed Seasonings: Lemon Pepper Seasoned Salt Mixes (Mrs. Dash); Pepper, Tabasco, or hot pepper sauce; Lemon Juice; and **any seasoning in the dining room at Diet Center (in glass case)**

Limited Seasonings: The following condiments are allowed in limited amounts (you may have up to 5 units/day). One unit is listed for each

Catsup	1 packet
Mustard	2 packets
Horseradish	1 TBSP

Allowed sweeteners: Equal, Sweet-n-Low, Splenda, or any other noncaloric sweetner

Caloric sweeteners are **not** allowed: including sugar of any kind, honey or syrup

<u>Allowed Medications</u>
During the study, you will be asked on a daily basis if you have been ill and if so, did you take any medication. If necessary, and on an occasional basis, it is OK to take over-the-counter and prescription medication as listed below. For any medication not listed below, please ask

Headache/Pain Medications	Tylenol — check before taking any other pain medication (such as Advil, Ibuprofen, etc.)
Sleep/Sedative Medications	OTC Preparations — check with study staff
Cold/Allergy Medications	check with study staff
Laxatives	Senna-only for occasional use; please notify staff if you are experiencing a problem for more than a day or two
Antidiarrheal	Lomotil, Kaopectate-only for occasional use; please notify staff if you are experiencing a problem for more than a day
Cough	check with study staff

Do not take Aspirin, or Vitamin/herb supplements. If you need to take an antibiotic please check with the study staff before taking it

Other: Sugar-free chewing gum is allowed

<u>Fasting Blood Draws:</u> Please be sure to fast for 12 h prior to each blood draw. You may only drink water during these fasting periods. Also, please do not drink alcohol for 48 h prior to each blood draw. We will remind you when the blood draws are approaching so that you will remember about the fasting and alcohol restriction

<u>Exercise:</u> Please do not alter your level of physical activity during this study. Ideally, we would like you to maintain a consistent level of activity, with very few changes to your normal routine. Also, it is important not to engage in very strenuous activity (i.e., aerobics class, jogging, etc.) on the day before a blood draw

Other hints:
1. If you are a coffee or tea drinker, you may use some of the milk from your breakfast in your beverage. You may **NOT** use additional milk
2. If you feel there is too much butter with breakfast, you may eat it with that day's dinner entrée, vegetable, or roll

Thank you for your participation!!!! Questions?? Please ask study staff.

TABLE 41.7
Daily Monitoring Form

To be completed by study staff:

Week: DP1 — 1   2   3   4   DP2 — 1   2   3   4

  1. Past 24-h caloric intake: 1800   2100   2400   2700   3000

  2. Past 24-h unit food intake: _____

Participants, please complete the remainder of this form at the end of each day, based on the past 24 h
(or based on the past weekend if today is Monday)

  3. **Did you consume any caffeine containing beverages**?   Yes   No

      If yes, specify: Description (e.g., coffee)   Amount (oz)

                                    _____   _____

                                    _____   _____

                                    _____   _____

                                    _____   _____

                                    _____   _____

  4. **Did you drink any alcoholic beverages?**   Yes   No

      If yes, specify type and amount: _____   _____oz

                                       _____   _____oz

  5. **Did you fail to eat/drink any study foods/drinks?**   Yes   No

      if yes, specify: Description   Amount (oz or part of portion)

                                    _____   _____

                                    _____   _____

  6. **Did you eat/drink any nonstudy foods/drinks?**   Yes   No

      If yes, specify: Description   Amount (oz or part of portion)

                                    _____   _____

                                    _____   _____

  7. How many ounces of caffeine-free beverages (water, diet/caffeine free soda, etc.) did you drink? _____ _____ oz

  8. Did you consume any sodium-containing foods, beverages, or condiments? Please list below

      Description: amount (oz or portion size)

      _____   _____

      _____   _____

      _____   _____

      _____   _____

      _____   _____

      _____   _____

                                                                       Total mg sodium

  9. **Did you take any medications?**   Yes   No

      a. If yes, specify:

      Description (e.g., Aspirin)   Amount   Reason

      _____   _____   _____

      _____   _____   _____

      _____   _____   _____

  10. Comments?

TABLE 41.8
Weekly Monitoring Form

To be completed by study staff:

Week   DP1 – 1   2   3   4   DP2 – 1   2   3   4

1. In the past week has your exercise level changed?		Yes	No
If yes, was it:		More Active	
		Less Active	
		No Exercise	

Please remember to keep your exercise level constant throughout the study

2. Have you taken any prescription or nonprescription drugs in the past week?   Yes   No

If yes, specify: Description   Amount

     _____   _____

     _____   _____

3. Have you taken any vitamins, minerals or other supplements   Yes   No
   in the past week?

If yes, specify: Description   Amount

     _____   _____

     _____   _____

4. Have you been ill in the past week?   Yes   No

     If yes, describe illness: _____

     _____

5. If you were ill in the past week, did your eating change as a result?   Yes   No

     If yes, describe: _____

FOOD PRODUCTION AND MEAL ASSEMBLY

Used in conjunction with standardized recipes, a food production form is followed for the preparation and portioning of all menu items (see Food Production form, Table 41.9). An established menu sequence will determine which menu is to be served on each day of the study. For each menu, portion sizes for the various calorie levels are listed. The food is prepared according to tested, reproducible recipes and portioned according to the list, and then the staff responsible initials the item in the space provided. A tray assembly check sheet is also valuable for assuring that all participants receive each menu item. Similar procedures may be followed for packed meals, checking off each item as it is placed in the take-out container (see Packed Meal Check Sheet, Table 41.10). Another practical form for packed meals or snacks is a checklist of the menu items that participants use to verify that all items have been packed in their take-out container. The form is attached to or placed inside the container, and the participant is instructed to contact a kitchen staff member if any item on the form is missing from the container.

It is imperative that all staff involved in the preparation and delivery of research diets understand the strict procedures necessitated by the protocol. For example, they must know the acceptable ranges for weights when portioning various food items, how to read the food production forms, and cooking procedures. The development of a training manual is useful so that staff can periodically review the standard procedures and have a reference available to answer any questions that may arise during the course of a study. During the regular production of the menus, duplicate meals should be prepared and collected at random points throughout the study for monitoring quality assurance of the diets and for chemical analysis of target nutrients if necessary. For each test diet, a menu cycle (in duplicate) is homogenized for subsequent chemical analysis of nutrients of interest. Details of menu validation and quality control nutrient monitoring have been described in References 5, 23, and 24.

OTHER ISSUES IN THE MANAGEMENT OF RESEARCH KITCHENS

The use of food service sanitary inspection checklists for personnel, food handling, equipment, storage practices, dishwashing, and other kitchen areas are standard practice. Inspection of refrigerator and freezer temperatures also should be conducted on a regular basis. In a research kitchen, regular accuracy checks of the electronic balances should be documented. If foods are donated to the study, their expected delivery, date received, and accuracy may be tracked on a form that also includes a description of the food items, company, address, contact person, and telephone number.

TABLE 41.9
Food Production Form for Use by Kitchen Staff

PARTICIPANT Name:

Calorie Level:

BREAKFAST	g
Orange juice, prepared from concentrate	235
Thomas Honey Wheat English muffin	52
Jelly (**1 = 14 g**)	14
Margarine	4
General Mills Wheaties cereal	25
Kellogg's All Bran cereal	20
Skim milk	250
LUNCH	
Healthy Choice deli cooked ham, sliced	70
Swiss cheese, sliced	30
Rye bread	60
Dijon mustard sauce (**see recipe**)	15
Pineapple, canned in juice	85
Unit Foods	
DINNER	
Lentil Pasta Sauce (**see recipe**)	140
Couscous, cooked	150
Romaine lettuce, torn pieces	60
Tomato, sliced	55
Carrots, grated	50
Kraft Free fat free French dressing	38
Pepperidge Farm-dinner roll	30
Butter	5.5
Egg yolk, cooked	16.5
SNACK	
Chocolate Truffle Brownie (**recipe**)	52
Sliced strawberries, frozen	80

TABLE 41.10
Packed Meal Form. One Copy is Kept in the Kitchen and One Copy is Provided to Research Participants

Name _____ I.D. _____Telephone Contact (___)____-_____

Day M T W T F Sat Sun   Date ___ ___ ___   Packed by _____   Meal   A   B   C   D

   (Circle One)   mm dd yy

Instructions to study participants: Before leaving the diet center, please review this packing list and make sure that everything listed on this form is actually in your cooler. Please alert the staff if anything is missing and return this form

BREAKFAST	LUNCH	DINNER	UNIT FOODS		SNACK
Packed	**Packed**	**Packed**	**# of Units Packed**		**Packed**
Orange Juice	Deli Cooked Ham	Lentil and Couscous	_____	Step I Honey Muffin	Chocolate Truffle Brownie
Honey Wheat English Muffin	Swiss Cheese	Salad			Sliced Strawberries, Frozen
Jelly	Rye Bread	Fat Free French			
Margarine	Dijon Mustard	Dinner Roll			
Wheaties	Pineapple, Canned	Butter			
All Bran					
Skim Milk					

UNIQUE STUDY CHALLENGES AND STRATEGIES FOR ADDRESSING THEM

Clinical nutrition studies may present challenges at every stage, for example, with experimental design, menu development, recruitment of participants, the preparation and delivery of the experimental diets, and, finally, data analysis. Obstacles must be overcome for a successful outcome. As an illustration, we describe several of our previous studies that have dealt with unique and challenging situations with regards to the population studied, experimental design employed, and experimental diets fed to participants. The conduct of multicenter clinical nutrition trials present their own challenges, which are discussed elsewhere.

Recruitment and Retention

We designed a study to evaluate the effects of diets high in both n-6 and n-3 polyunsaturated fatty acids (n-6 PUFA accounted for 13 and 11% of energy for the linoleic acid [LA]-rich and α-linolenic acid [ALA]-rich diets; ALA accounted for 4 and 7% of energy for the LA and ALA diets, respectively), derived from walnuts and walnut oil with different levels of n-6/n-3 FA ratios (9:1 vs. 4:1), on multiple risk factors for CVD.[26] We targeted healthy adults ages 45 to 65 years so that the results could be generalized to a typical middle-aged population in the United States. The participants were to be overweight or mildly obese, with moderate hypercholesterolemia (LDL between the 40th to 90th percentile for age and gender according to NHANES III data) and taking no medications. Several of the study end points, including vascular reactivity, serum cytokines, and the release of tumor necrosis factor-α (TNFα) and interleukin (IL) 6 by polymorphonuclear cells, are known to be affected by the menstrual cycle. This dictated that premenopausal women be excluded because it is very challenging to synchronize menstrual cycle phase with the end of a dietary treatment. In addition, another of our studies had shown that postmenopausal females taking hormone replacement therapy (HRT) exhibited smaller lipid reductions during a low-fat diet, and this suggested that women taking HRT should be excluded or enrolled in sufficient numbers to test for unique subgroup effects of diet.

These criteria made recruiting very challenging. Many people within this age group were taking nutrient supplements, cholesterol-lowering drugs, or medications for hypertension, diabetes, or rheumatoid arthritis, and so were not eligible for the study. Although it is possible for subjects to discontinue use of prescription drugs in order to enroll in a study, this must be approved by the IRB and their personal physician. Secondly, family commitments make it difficult for one or both parents (if both are involved in the study) to come to the clinical site for breakfast and dinner each weekday for three 6-week dietary periods. Third, at the time the study began, postmenopausal women who were not taking HRT accounted for only a small proportion of women with cholesterol elevations.

Various recruitment strategies were used, such as advertising by posters, in newspapers, and on television, and sending advertising fliers to churches, senior or retired communities, and to individuals who were between the ages of 45 to 65. We even agreed to feed both members of a married couple in order to recruit one of them who qualified to be a study participant. Other clinical centers provide guest meal passes so that family members or friends may regularly join the study participants for meals. Creative retention strategies are needed when the time commitment exceeds 3 months and frequent visits to the study site are required. Additional suggestions for retention and recruiting are provided in subsequent sections of this chapter.

Other challenges arose in two studies of young females. We sought participants with low iron status in order to observe the overloading effect of an iron supplement.[27] We targeted females, ages 19 to 47, because as a group they have lower iron levels than males. They were required to have regular menstrual periods, because menstruation reduces iron levels. Difficulties in recruiting occurred for several reasons. During the summer months, the overall student population at the university diminishes greatly and this reduces the potential participant pool. Also, the prospect of strictly adhering to a controlled diet during the relaxing summer months provided another hurdle. To enhance adherence, the 2-week break between diet periods was planned around the July 4th holiday and the summer arts festival to avoid further recruiting obstacles.

For this study, and another one that required females 18 to 22 years of age,[28] weight concerns proved to be a barrier for recruiting. Many young women were trying to lose weight and did not want to maintain their current weight as was required by the study protocols. In addition, women in this age group tend to be "fat phobic" and very cautious about their fat consumption. They were hesitant to consume diets that contained more fat than their usual diets. Therefore, it was important that the fats and oils were discreetly added to the study diets. This was accomplished by choosing meals, such as turkey with dressing and mashed potatoes, or stuffed flounder, which would readily accept the oils and fats without drawing attention.

Providing specialized, prepackaged meals or foods to participants for daily consumption may make recruiting easier (i.e., more participants are willing to eat prepackaged foods at home, rather than having all meals served through a metabolic kitchen), and yet challenges still abound as in other clinical nutrition studies. At one site of a year-long, multicenter study testing the effect of a prepackaged meal plan on multiple CVD risk factors, 70 men and women with hyperlipidemia, hypertension, and type 2 diabetes mellitus were recruited.[29] Finding enough participants who met the entry criteria proved to be challenging in a small college town. Thus, the study was conducted simultaneously in a more urban location 90 mi away. Once all the participants were recruited, the greatest challenge was the weekly home delivery of the prepackaged, frozen meals. The food could not be left without a signature, which sometimes proved to be a significant obstacle. Occasionally, participants received meals that were different from those they ordered. They also became bored with their limited food selection during the year-long study.

Thus, although a prepackaged meal appears to be a simple solution to conducting a controlled-feeding study off-site, care is needed to anticipate these potential problems.

FOOD PRODUCTS AND MENU PLANNING

Cocoa powder is a rich source of antioxidants in the form of flavonoids; however, its distinctive flavor and aroma made it difficult to integrate into many foods. The Cocoa Study was designed to evaluate the effects of a diet high in cocoa powder (22 g/day) and dark chocolate (16 g/day) on LDL oxidative susceptibility and total antioxidant capacity of plasma.[30] The study employed a two-period, crossover design. Using a randomized diet assignment, participants were fed the cocoa powder/dark chocolate diet (cocoa products) and an AAD (control) for 4 weeks each. The cocoa powder and dark chocolate were incorporated into only one experimental diet, making it impossible to employ a blinded experimental diet design. Planning a study of chocolate would appear to be easy, but controlling for dietary factors in cocoa powder and associated menu development were difficult.

In addition to issues of taste and blinding, it was necessary to match the control diet for other components present in the cocoa products in order to "isolate" the contribution of cocoa-derived flavonoids to the observed antioxidant effects. To do this, an identical amount of cocoa butter was included in the control diet. Diets also had to be matched for caffeine, theobromine, and fiber as cocoa powder and dark chocolate contain these compounds in addition to the flavonoids. The caffeine was supplemented in the control diet with diet cola and 431 mg/day of pure theobromine in a gel capsule. The fiber was held constant across diets with bran cereal. In addition, the diets were designed to be low in flavonoids from other dietary sources. Thus, foods that were limited or excluded included: tea, coffee, wine, onions, apples, beans, soybeans, orange juice, and grape juice. This example is provided to guide thoughtful design of studies incorporating foods with distinctive flavors and which contain multiple bioactive agents.

BAKED GOODS AS A VEHICLE FOR INGREDIENT DELIVERY

We conducted a study to evaluate the effects of 31 g/day of an isoflavone-rich soy powder (equivalent to 25 g soy protein) on plasma lipids and lipoproteins, and vascular reactivity in hypercholesterolemic, but otherwise healthy, male and female participants.[21,22] Participants were first fed a Step-I (run-in) diet followed by either a Step-I diet plus soy protein or a Step-I diet with milk protein. Because isoflavones are cleared rapidly from the plasma after ingestion, soy-containing menu items were incorporated throughout the day to maintain plasma levels. The barrier to overcome was incorporating the protein isolates into baked products at an acceptable level without sacrificing the quality and palatability of the product. Acknowledging the importance of this, we worked with a colleague with expertise in food product design who prepared several great tasting products for the study. Thus, with considerable product development effort it was possible to employ a blinded study design.

FORTIFICATION OF COMMONLY AVAILABLE FOODS

Folate fortification of foods in the United States created obstacles for menu development in a study examining effects of a low-folate diet with milk (8 oz milk, 3 times/day) or with no milk (8 oz apple juice, 3 times/day) on folate absorption and blood homocysteine levels.[28] For the low-folate diet, it was necessary to purchase foods from countries that did not fortify their food products. Pasta imported from Italy became a staple in these menus and was used for lunch salads and dinner items. Foods manufactured for individuals with celiac sprue are naturally low in folate because they are made with rice flour and cornstarch rather than wheat flour. Some of these items included crackers, pretzels, and a delicious chocolate truffle brownie. Sources for these low-folate foods were identified by searching specialty food shops and Internet research. Given the limited number of foods that could be included in a low-folate diet, this study only included a 4-day cycle of unique daily menus. A short menu rotation may contribute to monotony and boredom, and so encouraging adherence may require extra effort.

ADHERENCE AND ACCEPTABILITY

High monounsaturated fatty acid (MUFA) diets have been studied extensively in order to evaluate their effects on plasma lipids and lipoproteins. Previous studies have generally used olive oil as the MUFA source, whereas other MUFA-rich food sources have not been evaluated. The peanut study was conducted to evaluate the effects of experimental diets high in peanuts and peanut products (e.g., peanut butter and peanut oil) that are rich MUFA sources on lipid and lipoprotein risk factors for CVD.[31] The greatest challenge with this study was the demand on participants (6 months of controlled feeding) and the number of crossover treatments (five diets, lasting 6 weeks each). In a long-term study such as this, it is imperative that special efforts be made to sustain the commitment of the participants. Participants were allowed time off during one of the scheduled diet periods to allow time for a vacation, family activities, or food-based celebrations. Thus, we scheduled six diet periods from which each subject chose any five that were convenient for their schedule. Despite participants' initial enthusiasm, some found it difficult to complete the study. Nonetheless, providing some scheduling flexibility did help with adherence. Incentives for the participants, such as T-shirts, coffee mugs, and movie tickets, also were advantageous in maintaining long-term adherence. Interestingly, as the study progressed, it was increasingly challenging for the staff to maintain their enthusiasm as well. Theme parties without food (i.e., Halloween night and Thanksgiving celebration) helped participants and staff members maintain a positive attitude throughout the study.

A study designed to achieve weight maintenance after a weight-loss phase presented interesting situations with participant adherence to the controlled-feeding study.[32] Moderately overweight adults were assigned to one of two energy-restricted diets designed to achieve a weight loss of 2 lb/week. Following a 6-week weight-loss period, they were fed the same diets, but with calories sufficient to maintain their weight. Despite using a metabolic cart to calculate energy needs, about 20% of the participants continued to lose weight during the weight maintenance phase. Because of this, treatment periods longer than 4 weeks were necessary to establish a stable body weight.

In general, people enjoy participating in controlled weight-loss studies, and consequently adherence is ideal. For this study, the weight-loss aspect was tremendously motivating, as well as the weekly incentives that also were provided. The greatest challenge was getting the participants to eat all of their food during the weight maintenance phase. Most wanted to continue to lose weight and had to be encouraged into adhering to the study protocol. In addition, two people enrolled in the weight-loss study had eating disorders that were not recognized at enrollment. Of course, this made it difficult for them to comply with a protocol in which calories were restricted for several weeks and then increased for the remainder of the study. This problem suggested the need for a screening questionnaire that would help identify people with eating disorders at study entry. However, given the complexity of this problem, staff should be alerted to monitor participant behaviors and offer referrals when appropriate.

In summary, these examples are provided to illustrate the challenges that could develop for which contingency plans must be in place for conducting rigorously-controlled-feeding studies. These situations can arise even with a dedicated metabolic kitchen, motivated staff and students, and participants who work hard to adhere to the protocol. New investigators should seek the advice of experienced investigators when designing new controlled-feeding studies so that appropriate controls are included in the menu design.

NEW CONCEPTS AND STATE-OF-THE-ART TECHNIQUES

Clinical nutrition studies have become increasingly more complex as a result of advances in technologies including food processing, biochemical analysis, and biomedical and genetic screening. As we have gained faster, cheaper, and more sensitive analytical techniques, there is an associated need to carefully integrate these methodologies into different aspects of a controlled clinical nutrition study. The following text will introduce important concepts associated with nutraceuticals and functional foods, nutrigenomics, risk factor profiling, and other modern assays and techniques. This is by no means a comprehensive list, and we direct the reader to more complete references.

NUTRACEUTICALS AND FUNCTIONAL FOODS

The growing interest in identifying physiologically active components in foods from both plants and animals has led to the concept of "functional foods" and "nutraceuticals." A "functional food" is similar in appearance to, or may be, a conventional food. Functional foods are consumed as part of a usual diet and are demonstrated to have physiological benefits and to reduce the risk of chronic disease beyond basic nutritional functions. A "nutraceutical" is a product isolated or purified from foods that is generally sold in medicinal forms not usually associated with food. A nutraceutical is demonstrated to have a physiological benefit or provide protection against chronic disease (as defined by Health Canada).[33] Although there is evidence that certain functional foods or food ingredients can play a role in disease prevention and health promotion, safety considerations should be of principal concern. The safety issues related to herbs, and nutraceuticals specifically have received increasing attention. With the potency of phytochemicals, such as phytoestrogens and phytosterols, great caution must be taken in designing trials involving novel foods containing these compounds. Adequate toxicological and ethical considerations must be ensured before human feeding can be implemented. Evaluation of safe dosage, bioaccumulation, and long-term safety must be considered. For in-depth discussions on the implications of nutraceuticals and functional foods refer to References 34 to 37.

NUTRIGENOMICS

Nutritional genomics, also known as nutrigenomics, is the scientific study of how specific genes and bioactive food components interact.[38] Specifically, this field of study identifies specific (and multiple) genes that are regulated by nutrients/bioactive compounds, as well as gene expression profiles that seem to be associated with phenotypic responses to various diet constituents. Nutrigenomics provides a powerful means for increasing our understanding of how nutrients and bioactive compounds modulate gene expression and how changes in expression of many genes affect cell function and metabolism.[39] Findings from nutrigenomics research will increase our knowledge of how environment and behavioral factors influence phenotype and its relationship to health. An important aspect of contemporary nutrigenomics is that we have tools available to assess how different nutrients and bioactive compounds affect gene expression of a large array of genes and even the genome. Nutrigenomics is an important "tool" to use for understanding mechanisms of action that are due to changes in gene expression, either an increase or decrease in transcription of genes. Consequently, nutrigenomics will be useful in understanding the biological mechanisms involved in nutrient–disease interactions.[40] In addition, assessing changes in global gene expression (via array analyses) will be used to identify different "profiles" of gene expression that may be used to predict diet response, and, thus, be used for prescribing the optimal diet (referred to as personalized nutrition).

A challenge in conducting this research is that many nonnutrient bioactive compounds, as well as nutrients, are ligands for transcription factors, either directly altering gene expression or indirectly affecting gene expression by affecting signal transduction and chromatin structure.[40] Although not all chemicals in our diets alter gene expression, many diet constituents can alter gene expression in various ways (both directly and indirectly). For example, the phytoestrogen genistein directly alters gene expression by regulating estrogen-responsive genes. This occurs because genistein binds to the active site where the endogenous ligand estradiol normally binds. Although genistein binds with less affinity than the native ligand, it still promotes transcription.[41]

Preparing for sample collection to be used in a nutrigenomic study, as with all end point samples, should be done early in the study planning process. The types of samples that may prove useful for this kind of assay are cheek cells taken with a swab, lymphocytes or monocytes isolated from whole blood or other cells from which DNA and RNA can be isolated. There are numerous commercially available "kits" for collecting cheek cells and whole blood for cell isolation. The samples need to be processed as quickly as possible and carefully stored in a monitored –70°C freezer. Freeze–thaw cycles will cause sample deterioration. Of note, is that additional IRB approval will be necessary with special consideration given to how the results of genetic testing will be handled and kept confidential.

Modern Assays/Techniques (Oxidation, Inflammation, and Cell Adhesion)

With the vast number of risk factors for CVD known today, emerging techniques allow for the identification of complex associations, such as those between diet, circulating metabolites, cells, and vascular function. For example, interventions may aim to determine how altering the fatty acid profile of the diet affects fatty acid substrates and metabolites associated with inflammatory and oxidative response, which may, in turn, affect how the vascular system, responds to these occurrences (vascular reactivity). For instance, a recent study involving feeding the n-3 fatty acid ALA to hypercholesterolemic subjects was conducted to determine its effects on vascular inflammation and endothelial dysfunction. In this study, we measured serum fatty acids and a combination of biomarkers such as CRP, intracellular and vascular adhesion molecules, (markers of endothelial activation) and lipoproteins in subjects undergoing the controlled-feeding protocol. We found that including ALA in the diet potentially reduces the CVD risk profile above and beyond its known lipid and lipoprotein-lowering effects by inhibiting vascular inflammation and endothelial activation.[26] This study showed a link between consumption of an n-3 fatty acid (ALA) and vascular function, and also provided insight into the potential mechanism for the vascular response.

Risk Profiling/Multiple Risk Factor Analysis

Although the main concept in medicine is the treatment of illness and disease, there is an increasing emphasis in nutritional health research on disease prevention. In the case of chronic degenerative diseases such as CVD and diabetes, there are multiple risk factors, many of which cluster and even interact synergistically. Additionally, many individuals who develop disease may not display traditionally recognizable risk facts risk such as high blood pressure, triglycerides, or LDL cholesterol. Risk profiling is a way of identifying total risk by measuring multiple risk factors of a specific disease.[42] With the advent of technologies including autoanalyzers, and economical and efficient commercial assays, the average laboratory can now analyze multiple end points in a relatively short period of time, utilizing a small portion of resources and very little sample. For instance, CVD risk factor profiling may include clotting factors, adhesion molecules, vascular reactors, inflammatory cytokines, blood pressure, various cholesterol and lipoprotein fractions, glucose and insulin, triglycerides, coronary artery calcification scoring, genetic phenotyping, biomarkers of oxidation, and stress proteins. Although researchers may produce a significant amount of data from a single investigation, statistical considerations must be taken into account during the design and interpretation of a study. For example, risk factors for the same disease are often intercorrelated, and this requires care in analysis. In addition, markedly increasing the number of outcome variables may also increase the risk of a type I error (a false-positive finding). For a more complete review of risk profiling refer to Reference 42.

Defining Mechanisms of Action

An important aspect of clinical nutrition research is identifying the underlying biological mechanisms that explain the responses observed. There are a multitude of approaches for studying biological mechanisms that typically range from evaluating how blood-based bioactives are linked to physiological responses, to assessing how a nutrient or phytochemical affects transcriptional regulation. An example of this comes from clinical and basic research that we have conducted to evaluate dietary effects on lipids, lipoproteins, and inflammatory markers. In this study, a diet high in ALA significantly decreased CRP as well as vascular cell adhesion molecule-1 (VCAM-1), suggesting an anti-inflammatory response of ALA.[26] This clinical study was designed in tandem with two cell culture studies to elucidate mechanism of action. At the end of each diet period, monocytes were isolated from blood samples of the subjects exposed to the controlled-feeding protocols. We used these cells to test whether exposure to the diets changed cellular release of cytokines. In a second study, human monocyte THP-1 cells (from an established cell line) were incubated with the same fatty acids that had been identified as having an anti-inflammatory response in the clinical study. The THP-1 cell line is widely used to study monocyte biology and responsiveness to nutrients and other stimuli We found that cells that were pretreated with ALA exhibited decreased gene expression of IL-6, IL-1B, and TNFα, as well as secretion of these proteins. Additionally, nuclear factor (NF)-κB DNA-binding activity was decreased and peroxisome proliferator-activated receptor-gamma (PPAR-γ) was increased.[43] These three studies illustrate how clinical and basic research may complement one another to infer the potential mechanisms of action of dietary treatments.

CONCLUSIONS

Well-controlled clinical nutrition studies have been invaluable in advancing our understanding of diet–disease relationships and for informing evidence-based recommendations for dietary patterns and nutrient intakes. There have been many recent publications that describe quality control procedures for controlled-feeding studies (see Table 41.1). However, additional practical advice is needed, particularly for new investigators, because clinical nutrition studies are not easily modeled on the reductionistic designs of pharmacology. One goal of this chapter is to provide detailed examples of how we, and others, have resolved logistical challenges in preparing and delivering food, enhancing adherence, and designing carefully matched control diets. Although many of these issues have not been discussed in-depth in the literature, resolving them is absolutely essential to the conduct of successful work in this area.

In addition to these practical issues, we also have addressed larger questions of study design in order to illustrate best practices in cutting-edge nutrition research. We highlight emerging themes in the field of nutrition, including the design of clinical studies that integrate hypotheses about mechanisms of action with the study of nutrigenomics, functional foods and nutraceuticals, and multiple risk factor profiling. Advances in this area will require continued interdisciplinary collaboration with experts in cellular and molecular biology, lipid chemistry and metabolism, genomics, behavioral science, physiology, etc. The National Institutes of Health has defined clinical and translational research as a primary goal for federally funded research programs. To meet this challenge, nutrition studies must be designed with a multilevel, biobehavioral approach that tests both the *efficacy* and *effectiveness* of new interventions while simultaneously examining underlying biological mechanisms. We believe that clinical nutrition is perfectly poised to play a major role in this effort.

REFERENCES

1. Jenkins DJ, Kendall CW, Faulkner D, et al. *Metab* 51:1596, 2002.
2. Jenkins DJ, Kendall CW, Marchie A, et al. *Metab* 52:1478, 2003.
3. Jenkins DJ, Kendall CW, Marchie A, et al. *JAMA* 290:502, 2003.
4. Jenkins DJ, Kendall CW, Faulkner DA, et al. *Am J Clin Nutr* 83:582, 2006.
5. Dennis BH, Stewart P, Wang CH, et al. *JADA* 98:766, 1998.
6. Sacks FM, Obarzanek E, Windhauser MM, et al. *Ann Epidemiol* 5:108, 1995.
7. Sacks FM, Svetkey LP, Vollmer WM, et al. *N Eng J Med* 344:3, 2001.
8. Appel LJ, Champagne CM, Harsha DW, et al. *JAMA* 289:2083, 2003.
9. Harsha DW, Lin PH, Obarzanek E, et al. *JADA* 99:S35, 1999.
10. Svetkey LP, Sacks FM, Obarzanek E, et al. *JADA* 99:S96, 1999.
11. Svetkey LP, Harsha DW, Vollmer WM, et al. *Ann Epidemiol* 13:462, 2003.
12. Bray GA, Vollmer WM, Sacks FM, et al. *Am J Cardiol* 94:222, 2004.
13. Svetkey LP, Simons-Morton D, Vollmer WM, et al. *Arch Intern Med* 159:285, 1999.
14. Vollmer WM, Sacks FM, Ard J, et al. *Ann Intern Med* 135:1019, 2001.
15. Appel LJ, Moore TJ, Obarzanek E, et al. *N Eng J Med* 336:1117, 1997.
16. Erlinger TP, Miller III ER, Charleston J, Appel LJ. *Circulation* 108:150, 2003.
17. FDA. United States Food and Drug Administration: Food Labeling: Health Claims; Docket No. 96P-0338. Washington DC, 1998.
18. FDA. United States Food and Drug Administration: Federal Register 64:57699-57733. Washington DC, 1999.
19. FDA. United States Food and Drug Administration: FDA Authorizes New Coronary Heart Disease Health Claim for Plant Sterol and Plant Stanol Esters. Washington DC, 2000.
20. FDA. United States Food and Drug Administration: Food Labeling: Health Claims; Docket No. 95P-0197, 15343-15344. Washington DC, 2001.
21. West SG, Hilpert KF, Juturu V, et al. *J Womens Health (Larchmt)* 14:253, 2005.

22. Hilpert KF, Kris-Etherton PM, West SG. *J Nutr* 135:1075–1079, 2005.
23. Swain JF, Windhauser MM, Hoben KP, et al. *JADA* 99:S54, 1999.
24. Phillips KM, Stewart KK, Karanja NM, et al. *JADA* 99:S60, 1999.
25. Windhauser M. In: Dennis B, ed. *Well-Controlled Diet Studies in Humans: The American Dietetic Association ADA*, Chicago, IL 1999:390–403.
26. Zhao G, Etherton TD, Martin KR, et al. *J Nutr* 134:2991, 2004.
27. Binkoski AE, Kris-Etherton PM, Beard JL: *J Nutr* 134:99, 2004.
28. Picciano MF, West SG, Ruch AL, et al. *Am J Clin Nutr* 80:1565, 2004.
29. McCarron DA, Oparil S, Chait A, et al. *Arch Intern Med* 157:169, 1997.
30. Wan Y, Vinson JA, Etherton TD, et al. *Am J Clin Nutr* 74:596, 2001.
31. Kris-Etherton PM, Pearson TA, Wan Y, et al. *Am J Clin Nutr* 70:1009, 1999.
32. Pelkman CL, Fishell VK, Maddox DH, et al. *Am J Clin Nutr* 79:204, 2004.
33. Health. Canada: Coordination of Natural Health Product Research in Canada: CCAB-3-0285 Final Report submitted to the Natural Health Products Directorate, 2004.
34. Arvanitoyannis IS, Van Houwelingen-Koukaliaroglou M. *Crit Rev Food Sci Nutr* 45:385, 2005.
35. Ferrari CK. *Biogerontology* 5:275, 2004.
36. Halsted CH. *Am J Clin Nutr* 77:1001S, 2003.
37. Hasler CM. *J Nutr* 132:3772, 2002.
38. Trujillo E, Davis C, Milner J. *JADA* 106:403, 2006.
39. Afman L, Muller M. *JADA* 106:569, 2006.
40. Kaput J, Rodriguez RL. *Physiol Genomics* 16:166, 2004.
41. Kaput J. *Ann NY Acad Sci* 1055:64, 2005.
42. Sigurdsson EL, Thorgeirsson G. *Scand J Prim Health Care* 21:68, 2003.
43. Zhao G, Etherton TD, Martin KR, et al. *Biochem Biophys Res Commun* 336:909, 2005.
44. Dennis B, Ershow A, Obarzanek E, Clevidence B. Chicago, IL: Well Controlled Diet Studies in Human The American Dietetic Association, 1999.
45. Dennis BH, and Kris-Etherton, PM. *Designing, Managing and Conducting a Clinical Nutrition Study*. In: Research: Successful approaches 2nd Edition; Monsen, E. Editor ADA, Chicogo, IL. 2003.
46. Greenberg RS, Daniels SR, Flanders WD, Eley JW, Boring JR. *Medical Epidemiology*, 4th ed. The McGraw-Hill Companies, Inc., NY, NY. 2004.
47. Monsen ER. *Research: Successful Approaches*, 2nd ed. Chicago, IL: The American Dietetic Association, 2003.
48. Obarzanek E, Moore TJ. *JADA* 99:S9, 1999.
49. Nightingale SL. *Food Drug Law J* 50:493, 1995.
50. Jansen LA. *Local IRBs, Multicenter. IRB* 27:7, 2005.
51. Burke GS. *J Nutr* 135:921, 2005.
52. Markman M. *IRB* 26:8, 2004.
53. Vick CC, Finan KR, Kiefe C, et al. *Am J Surg* 190:805, 2005.
54. Dominguez RA, Feaster DJ, Twiggs LB, Altman NH. *J Lab and Clin Med* 145:65, 2005.
55. Dziak K, Anderson R, Sevick MA, et al. *Health Services Res* 40:279, 2005.
56. Skolnick BE. *Adv in Neurol* 76:253, 1998.
57. Allison DB, et al. *Design, Analysis and Interpretation of Randomized Clinical Trials in Obesity*. Vidio prodeedings of NIH-funded conference. 2006. available at http://main.nab.edu/shrp/default.aspx?pid=97738
58. Griel AE, Psota, TL, Kris-Etheton, PM. *Guidelines for Implementing Clinical Nutrition Studies*, Chapter 9. Research: Successful Approaches, 3rd Ed. Monsen, E, and Van Horn, L, Editors. ADA, 2007.

42 Hyperlipidemias: Major Gene and Diet Effects

Elaine B. Feldman, Patty Siri-Tarino, and Ronald M. Krauss

CONTENTS

The production and metabolism of serum lipids and lipoproteins can be influenced by genetic variation, as well as by nutrients in the diet.[1,2] A number of factors are involved in the regulation of lipid metabolism (Table 42.1), and their abnormal expression or activity can result in changes in lipid or lipoprotein levels that may predispose an individual to atherosclerosis. Diet may be an important component in the modulation of the lipid and lipoprotein phenotype, and while these effects depend in part on an individual's genetic background, general trends for nutrient effects have been observed. These are outlined in Table 42.2.

HYPERLIPIDEMIAS

These lipid disorders reflect abnormal increases in one or another serum lipid component and lipoprotein carrier (Table 42.3 and Table 42.4). The abnormalities are often inherited and can be influenced by diet. Their management requires accurate diagnosis and evaluation with consideration for the possibility that other diseases may induce secondary hyperlipidemia.[3] The dietary intervention, if unsuccessful, should be followed by appropriate medication that normalizes the lipids and lipoproteins in order to prevent complications of atherosclerotic disease (myocardial infarction and peripheral vascular disease) or pancreatitis.[4]

Persons with hyperlipidemia have lipid levels generally above the 90th percentile for their age and sex (Table 42.3). Blood samples should be obtained after a 12- to 14-h fast in individuals consuming their usual diet. At least three blood samples should be evaluated, 2 or 3 weeks apart. The lipid studies may need to be more elaborate than the usual lipid screen or profile (see Chapter 40). Ultracentrifugation of the plasma is often necessary, usually performed in a specialized lipid laboratory. These lipid disorders can be suspected from the patient's history, family history, and physical examination. First-degree relatives should also be investigated in order to detect others with the disorder and to characterize the genetics.

TYPES OF HYPERLIPIDEMIAS

CHYLOMICRONEMIA (TYPE I HYPERLIPOPROTEINEMIA)

Dietary TAGs that are transported as chylomicrons are increased in Type I.[3–7] This rare disorder results from a defect in removal of chylomicrons from the blood due to the presence of a recessive gene that results in deficiency of lipoprotein lipase

TABLE 42.1

Factors Involved in the Formation and Metabolism of Lipoproteins

Type	Action
Apoproteins	
Apo A-I	Antiatherogenic: facilitates reverse cholesterol transport
Apo A-II	Apo A-II-containing lipoproteins are not effectively metabolized by lipoprotein lipase (defective lipolysis)
Apo A-IV	Antiatherogenic
Apo A-V	Reduces plasma triglyceride by lowering VLDL production and enhancing lipolysis
Apo B100	Ligand for the LDL receptor
Apo B48	Primary protein of chylomicrons
Apo C-I	Blocks apo E binding to receptors
Apo C-II	Activates lipoprotein lipase (LPL)
Apo C-III	Impairs TAG hydrolysis by inhibiting LPL, thereby delaying clearance of remnant particles; decreases LDL binding to receptors; displaces apo E from lipoprotein particles
Apo E	Ligand for the LDL receptor; interacts with the LDL-receptor-related protein (LRP); enhances lipolysis
Apo H	Antiatherogenic protein component of lipoprotein particles
Enzymes	
Lipoprotein lipase (LPL)	Hydrolyzes TAGs to free fatty acids in chylomicrons and VLDL to form chylomicron remnants and IDL
Hepatic lipase (HL)	Functions as a phospholipase and TAG hydrolase. Converts IDL to LDL as well as larger HDL (HDL2) to smaller HDL (HDL3)
Diacylglycerol acyl transferase (DGAT)-1 and DGAT-2	Acyl transferases required for synthesis of TAG molecule
Lecithin:cholesterol acyltransferase (LCAT)	Catalyzes the esterification of free cholesterol to cholesterol ester on plasma lipoproteins
Acyl CoA:cholesterol acyltransferase (ACAT)	Catalyzes cholesterol esterification
HMG CoA reductase	Rate-limiting enzyme of cholesterol biosynthesis
Receptors	
LDL receptor	Binds apo B-containing lipoproteins, such as LDL
LDL-receptor-related protein (LRP)	Takes up chylomicron remnants
Scavenger receptor A (SR-A)	Binds LDL modified by oxidation
CD-36, a scavenger receptor on macrophages	Binds modified LDL
Scavenger receptor B1 (SR-B1)	Selectively removes cholesterol esters from HDL and apo B-containing lipoproteins
VLDL receptor	
Transfer Proteins	
Cholesterol ester transfer protein (CETP)	Transfers cholesterol esters synthesized in HDL to the apo B-containing lipoproteins in exchange for TAG
Phospholipid Transfer Protein (PLTP)	Associated with increased apo B-containing lipoprotein concentrations
ATP-binding-cassette transporter-A1 (ABC-A1) and ABC G-1	Actively transports free cholesterol out of cells and into HDL particles
ABC-G5 and ABC-G7	Transport plant sterols from intestinal cells to intestinal lumen, preventing absorption into the bloodstream
Microsomal triglyceride transfer protein (MTP)	Necessary to generate apo B-containing lipoprotein particles
Transcription Factors	
Sterol Response Element Binding Protein (SREBP)-1a and SREBP-1c	Regulate fatty acid biosynthesis and metabolism
SREBP2	Regulates cholesterol biosynthesis and metabolism
Insig1 + Insig2	Regulate SREBP activation
Peroxisome-proliferator-activated receptor-∝ (PPAR-∝)	Promotes free fatty acid oxidation by decreasing apo C-III and increasing LPL activity
PPAR-γ	Promotes adipocyte differentiation and fatty acid uptake

(LPL, Table 42.4).[6] A similar disorder results from the absence or abnormal function of the apo C-II activator of LPL,[7] or from the presence of a circulating inhibitor of LPL. Type I may present in infants and children. It does not usually predispose to vascular disease, but patients are at risk of recurrent severe pancreatitis. Signs of lipemia retinalis (Figure 42.1), eruptive xanthomas (Figure 42.2), and hepatosplenomegaly may be present. The plasma shows a chylomicron creamy layer over a clear infranatant. Plasma TAG levels usually exceed 17 mmol/l.

TABLE 42.2
Effects of Diet and Lifestyle on Lipid and Lipoprotein Profiles

Factor	Effect
Saturated fat	Increases total, LDL and HDL cholesterol; downregulates LDL receptor activity
Omega-6 fatty acids	Decrease triglyceride, lower LDL and HDL cholesterol
Omega-3 fatty acids	Lower triglyceride and increase HDL cholesterol
Trans fatty acids	Increase total and LDL cholesterol and reduce HDL cholesterol
Carbohydrate	Increases the secretion of triglyceride enriched apo B-containing lipoproteins
Calories	Excessive intake results in oversecretion of triglyceride rich, apo B-containing lipoproteins that can drive atherogenic dyslipidemia, that is, high triglyceride, low HDL cholesterol, and small, dense LDL
Exercise	Increases energy utilization and insulin sensitivity; improves atherogenic dyslipidemia

TABLE 42.3
Classification (Type) of Hyperlipidemia and the Underlying Lipoprotein Abnormality

Type	Lipoprotein Abnormality
I	Increased exogenous triacylglycerols (TAG) in the form of chylomicrons
IIa	Hypercholesterolemia with increase in LDL and normal TAG levels
IIb	Hypercholesterolemia combined with mild hypertriglyceridemia (increase in LDL and VLDL particle number, overproduction of apo B)
III	Remnant hyperlipemia; hypercholesterolemia with hypertriglyceridemia and increase in IDL
IV	Mild to moderate endogenous hyperlipemia; increased VLDL with TAG 2.8-7.9 mmol/l or 250–700 mg/dl
V	Mixed hyperlipemia; moderate to severe hypertriglyceridemia (>11.3 mmol/l or 1000 mg/dl) with mixed VLDL and chylomicrons

TABLE 42.4
Genetic Basis of Familial Hyperlipidemias

Type	Abnormality	Mutation
I	Familial lipoprotein lipase deficiency	40 known missense and nonsense mutations of gene encoding
	Familial lipoprotein lipase inhibitor	enzyme
	Familial apo C-II deficiency	14 defects identified
	Familial hepatic lipase deficiency	
IIa	Familial hypercholesterolemia	400 deletions/point mutations in five classes of the LDL gene
	Familial defective apo B_{100}	Apo B 3500 mutation impairs binding to the LDL receptor
	Polygenic hypercholesterolemia	Apo A-I/C-III/A-IV gene clusters
IIb	Familial combined hyperlipidemia	Apo A-I/C-III/A-IV
		LCAT
		Mn superoxide dismutase linkage
		Partial LPL deficiency
III	Familial dysbetalipoproteinemia	Apo E gene polymorphism affects amino acid coding
		E2/E2 phenotype
IV	Familial hypertriglyceridemia (mild)	Apo A-I/C-III/A-IV/A-V
		Hepatic lipase deficiency
V	Familial hypertriglyceridemia (severe)	Apo A-I/C-III/A-IV
	Familial lipoprotein lipase deficiency	Apo A-II
	Apo C-II deficiency	

Numerous mutations have been associated with the various types of familial hyperlipoproteinemias (Table 42.4).[5] More than half the variability in serum cholesterol (low-density lipoprotein, LDL cholesterol) among individuals is attributable to genetic variation, presumably polygenic. Polymorphisms in apo E or apo B are examples. The remaining variability in cholesterol levels may be attributable to the diet, diet–gene interactions, or postulated genes that control variability of response to the environment. The prevalence of hyperlipidemias is increased in patients with premature coronary heart disease (CHD), that is, <55 years of age.

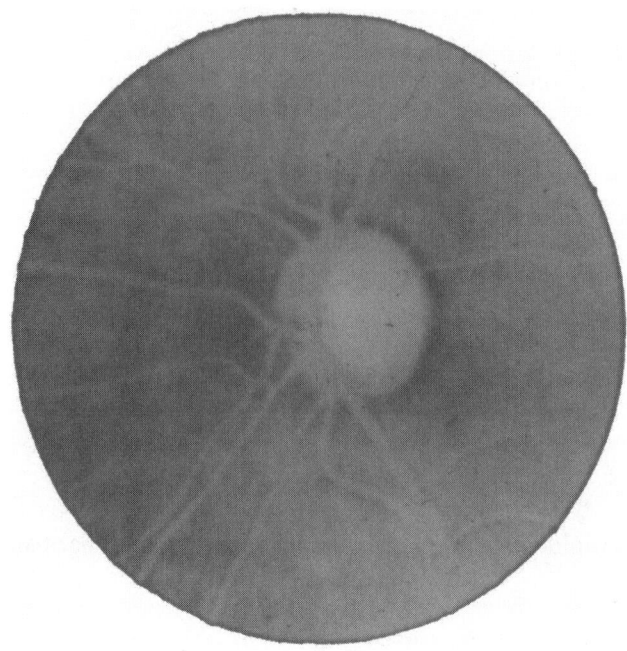

FIGURE 42.1   (See color insert following page 654.) Lipemia retinalis visualized in the optical fundus of a patient with chylomicronemia with TAG levels exceeding 3000 mg/dl.

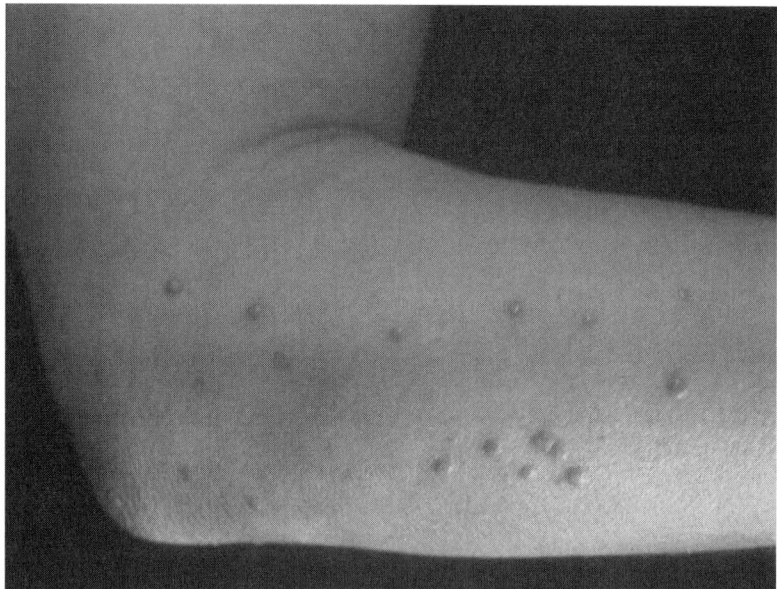

FIGURE 42.2   (See color insert following page 654.) Eruptive xanthomas observed in a patient with chylomicronemia.

HYPERCHOLESTEROLEMIA (TYPE IIA AND TYPE IIB HYPERLIPOPROTEINEMIAS)

In Type IIa hypercholesterolemia, increased LDL is present with normal levels of TAGs.[3,4,8] Familial hypercholesterolemia (FH) is a single-gene defect of the cell surface receptor that binds circulating LDL and delivers cholesterol to cells.[9] To date, more than 400 mutations have been characterized in five classes.[5,8] In the heterozygote, receptor number or activity is about half normal. LDL cholesterol does not enter the cell and does not suppress the activity of hydroxymethylglutaryl coenzyme A (HMG CoA) reductase, the rate-limiting step in cholesterol synthesis. Cholesterol synthesis continues and esterified cholesterol accumulates in the cell, suppressing LDL receptor synthesis. The LDL cholesterol level in blood doubles (to about 9 mmol/l) and the fractional catabolic rate of LDL is halved. In the FH homozygote with no receptors, LDL production is greatly enhanced and removal severely decreased. LDL cholesterol levels average 19 mmol/l.

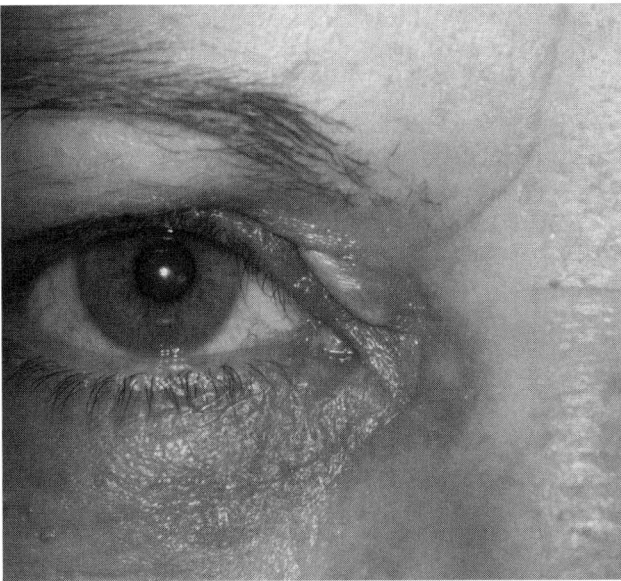

FIGURE 42.3   (See color insert following page 654.) Eyelid xanthelasma from a woman with familial hypercholesterolemia.

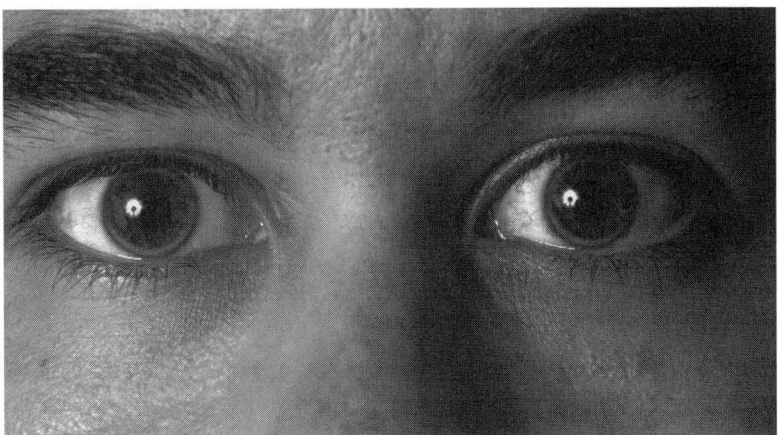

FIGURE 42.4   (See color insert following page 654.) Corneal arcus observed in a 31-year-old man with familial hypercholesterolemia.

Signs of FH include lipid deposits such as eyelid xanthelasma (Figure 42.3), corneal arcus (Figure 42.4), and tendon and tuberous xanthomas of the skin (Figure 42.5 and Figure 42.6) that appear in the second or third decade of life. Hypercholesterolemia is present from birth.[10] FH homozygotes may have xanthomas in infancy or early childhood. The incidence of CHD is increased 25-fold in FH patients and occurs prematurely (before age 50). In FH homozygotes, CHD may be present in infancy and early childhood, with death occurring by age 21.

Patients with familial defective apo B (Table 42.4) may exhibit a phenotype identical to FH[5] In Type IIb, hypercholesterolemia is combined with hypertriglyceridemia, with LDL and very-low-density lipoprotein (VLDL) increased, and overproduction of apo B. Familial combined hyperlipidemia (FCH) is the most common hyperlipidemic syndrome in patients with premature CHD. In this condition, Apo B is overproduced, with increased levels of atherogenic remnants and small, dense LDL.[11-13]

TYPE III HYPERLIPOPROTEINEMIA (DYSBETALIPOPROTEINEMIA, BROAD-BETA OR FLOATING-BETA DISEASE)

In this syndrome, hypercholesterolemia is combined with hypertriglyceridemia.[14] Intermediate density lipoprotein (IDL) remnants are increased, at times mixed with chylomicrons. The disorder is due to homozygosity for the apo E2 variant. Apo E2 protein has defective LDL receptor binding, resulting in a lesser rate of removal and increase in the circulating level of IDL.[15] Preparative ultracentrifugation demonstrates increased cholesterol relative to TAG in the VLDL fraction, with more rapid

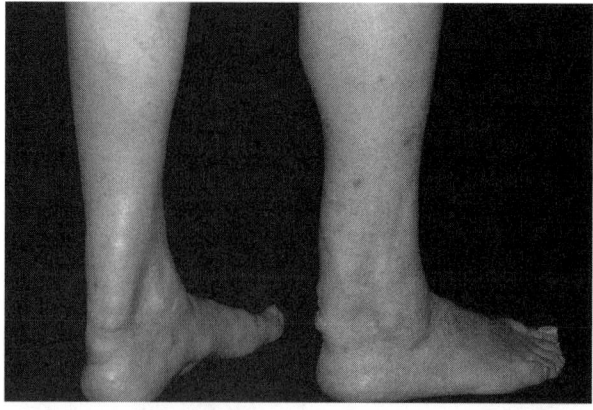

FIGURE 42.5   (See color insert following page 654.) Xanthomas of the Achilles tendon of a patient with familial hyper-cholesterolemia.

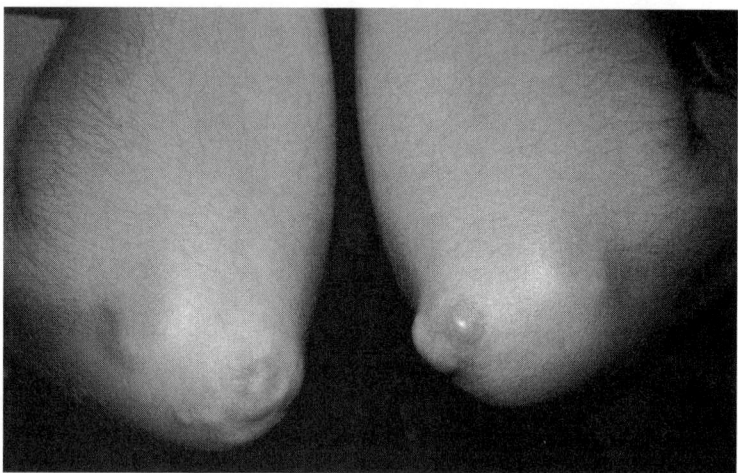

FIGURE 42.6   (See color insert following page 654.) Tuberous xanthomas in the skin of the elbows of a teenage girl with familial hypercholesterolemia.

migration of the lipoprotein on electrophoresis. Apo E isoforms should be determined by phenotype analysis. Alternatively, apo E2 may be determined by genotype analysis. Patients show planar xanthomas of the palms (Figure 42.7) and tuberous xanthomas as early as the third decade of life. Patients have premature peripheral vascular disease and CHD.[16]

TYPE IV HYPERLIPOPROTEINEMIA

Endogenous hypertriglyceridemia is characterized by mild to moderate increase in TAG levels (3 to 8 mmol/l, 250 to 700 mg/dl), with increase in VLDL.[5,17,18] Both overproduction and decreased removal of VLDL TAG may be responsible. LDL cholesterol levels are within the normal range. Usually HDL cholesterol is decreased. These subjects may be at increased risk of atherosclerosis, and hypertriglyceridemia per se may be an independent risk factor for cardiovascular disease (CVD).[17,18] Patients often have no signs or symptoms other than the abnormal lipid and lipoprotein values, and may present initially with cardiovascular events. Underlying mechanisms and genetic defects are multiple.[5] See also "atherogenic dyslipidemia" below.

TYPE V HYPERLIPOPROTEINEMIA

Moderate to severe increases in TAG levels exceeding 11.3 mmol/l or 1000 mg/dl characterize this disorder, often termed the chylomicronemia syndrome.[3,4,6,16] Chylomicrons appear along with increased levels of VLDL. Patients exhibit eruptive xanthomas and lipemia retinalis (TAG levels >34 mmol/l, 3000 mg/dl) (Figure 42.1 and Figure 42.2). They are at high risk for recurrent episodes of acute pancreatitis, at times resulting in pancreatic insufficiency. Fifty percent or more of these patients have diabetes mellitus that must be controlled to effectively lower TAG levels. Alcohol intake or estrogen treatment may convert a Type IV patient to Type V, or worsen Type V and precipitate pancreatitis.[3] Underlying mechanisms and genetic defects are a mixture of those of Type I and Type IV (Table 42.4).

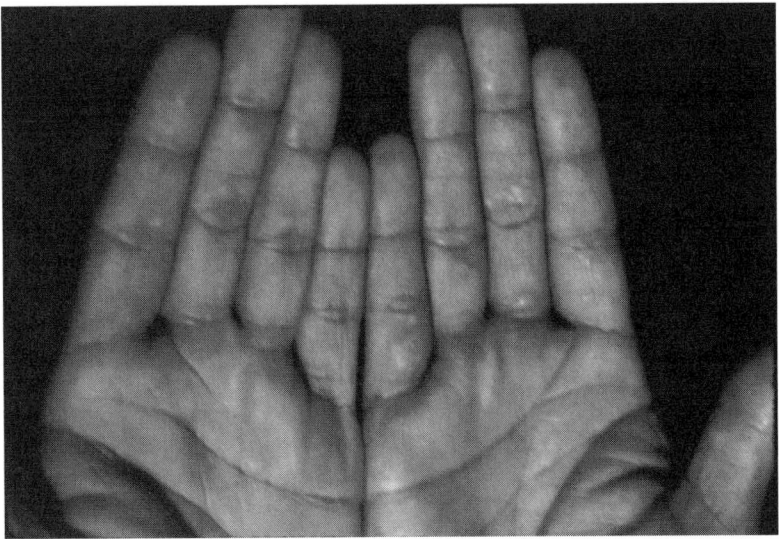

FIGURE 42.7 **(See color insert following page 654.)** Yellow linear deposits in the creases of the fingers and palms of the hands of a 33-year-old man with Type III hyperlipoproteinemia.

TABLE 42.5
Metabolic Syndrome Risk Factors

Insulin resistance
Elevated triacylglycerides
Decreased size and buoyancy of LDL
Low HDL cholesterol
Hyperinsulinemia
Glucose intolerance
Hypertension
Prothrombotic state
Truncal obesity
Premature CVD

DYSLIPOPROTEINEMIA (ATHEROGENIC DYSLIPIDEMIA)

Of increasing prevalence in the United States and most of the world is the phenotype of atherogenic dyslipidemia, which is defined by elevations in triglyceride levels, smaller and denser LDL, and low HDL cholesterol. There are other CVD risk factors that often cluster together with atherogenic dyslipidemia in what has come to be known as the metabolic syndrome or Syndrome X, and these include insulin resistance, abdominal obesity, and hypertension (Table 42.5). Persons with the metabolic syndrome are at an increased risk of atherosclerosis.[1,7]

In most cases, atherogenic dyslipidemia can be ameliorated with weight loss through reductions in caloric intake and increases in physical activity. Pharmacological management may also be required.[19] Furthermore, several gene associations have been identified in the determination of metabolic syndrome risk, including polymorphisms in PPAR gamma[20] and LPL.[21]

EVALUATION OF PATIENTS WITH HYPERLIPIDEMIA

Table 42.6 enumerates the details of the history, physical examination, and laboratory tests used for the evaluation of subjects who may have one of the hyperlipidemic syndromes (Figure 42.8).

DIETARY MANAGEMENT OF HYPERLIPIDEMIAS

Appropriate diet tailored to the lipid abnormality is the initial intervention. Results of recent randomized clinical trials have shown significant benefits within 1 to 2 years of dietary intervention in reducing fatal and nonfatal events as well as coronary disease mortality.[22] In particular, dietary interventions that include omega-3 fatty acids have been shown to have a particular

TABLE 42.6
Evaluation of Patient for Hyperlipidemia

History of:
Vascular disease, angina, MI, angioplasty, bypass surgery, and claudication
Abdominal pain
Diabetes
Thyroid, hepatic, renal, disease, and gout
Smoking habits, exercise, and medications
Body weight
Family history of vascular disease, diabetes, and gout
Diet history: alcohol, supplement use, amount and type of fat and cholesterol, energy,
    protein, carbohydrate, and sucrose intakes (best done by a dietitian)

Physical examination:
Blood pressure, height, and weight
Corneal arcus, xanthelasma, retinopathy, lipemia retinalis
Xanthomas of skin and tendons
Dry skin and hair loss
Bruits, murmurs, absent pulses, and arrhythmias
Liver and spleen size

Laboratory:
Blood, after 12–14-h overnight fast, cholesterol, TAG, HDL cholesterol, and glucose
Plasma turbidity
Apoproteins, ultracentrifugation, and electrophoresis
Post-heparin lipolytic activity
Tests of renal, hepatic, and thyroid function
Electrocardiogram

FIGURE 42.8   (See color insert following page 654.) The appearance of plasma, refrigerated overnight, from fasting patients. The tubes with plasma samples are taken from (left to right): a subject with normal lipid levels and clear plasma (similar to a patient with Type IIa); a patient with chylomicronemia (Type I) with a creamy top layer above a clear infranatant; a patient with hypercholesterolemia (Type IIa) with clear plasma; a patient with Type III hyperlipoproteinemia with diffusely turbid plasma; a patient with Type IV hyperlipoproteinemia also showing diffuse turbidity; and a patient with Type V hyperlipoproteinemia with plasma exhibiting a creamy top layer over a turbid infranatant.

rapid time to benefit (within 3 to 6 months). Treatment goals are to normalize lipids, or in patients with vascular disease, to lower these to optimal levels, which promote regression of atherosclerotic disease and stabilize plaque. According to the most recent Adult Treatment Panel guidelines, the optimal goal for LDL cholesterol in very high-risk patients, such as those with or without Type 2 diabetes, is less than 70 mg/dl.[23] HDL cholesterol and triglyceride concentrations are classified as low and high respectively, when they are less than 60 mg/dl and greater than 200 mg/dl, respectively. Lipid levels should be monitored at 6- to 8-week intervals. After a 3- to 6-month trial of diet, depending on the response and the severity of the disease, appropriate cholesterol- and triglyceride-lowering medication should be added. The diet is continued (unless the response is adverse) so that medication dose can be lower, thereby minimizing side effects and cost. Treatment is lifelong.

Diets to Lower Serum Cholesterol and LDL Cholesterol

Cholesterol lowering is achieved by a diet that regulates calories to achieve desirable weight, and includes an exercise regimen.[3,4] Depending on the severity of hypercholesterolemia, saturated fat should be reduced to <10% or <7% of calories with the remainder of total fats derived from polyunsaturated and monounsaturated fatty acids.[24] Dietary cholesterol intake should be limited to less than 200 mg/day. Consumption of fruits, vegetables, nuts, legumes, whole grains, fatty fish, poultry and lean meats as well as low fat and fat free dairy products and liquid vegetable oils and dietary fiber should be emphasized. Of significant interest is the recent demonstration that consumption of such a portfolio of cholesterol-lowering foods is as effective in reducing cholesterol as low dose statin treatment.[25]

See Table 42.7 for food choices and menu plans for patients with Type II hyperlipidemia or FH.[26,27] Compliance with and response to these changes may lower total and LDL cholesterol by 10 to 20%.

TABLE 42.7

Guidelines of Food Choices and Menu Plans for Patients with Severe Hypercholesterolemia (FH)[a]

Very Low-Fat Diet-Meal Plan			Goal 10-15% Fat Kcals	
Food	Total Kcal	Fat (g)	Sat Fat (g)	Cholesterol (mg)
Breakfast				
Orange juice, fresh, 6 fl. oz	84	0	0	0
Banana slices, 1/2 med	52	0.5	0	0
Shredded wheat, spoon size, 1 c	170	0.5	0	0
Milk, fat-free, 8 fl. oz	86	0.4	0.3	4
Breakfast subtotal	392	1.4	0.3	4
Lunch				
Turkey sandwich:				
Turkey breast, fat-free luncheon meat, 2 oz	52	0.4	0.2	23
Mayonnaise, light, 1 Tbsp	50	5	1	0
Whole wheat bread, two slices	130	2	0.4	0
Sliced tomato, 1/2 med	13	0.2	0	0
Apple, 1 med	81	0.5	0.1	0
Lunch subtotal	326	8.1	0.7	23
Dinner				
Pork tenderloin, marinated, 4 oz	140	4	1.5	65
Baked potato, w/skin, 8 oz	220	0.2	0.1	0
Fat-free sour cream, 2 Tbsp	35	0	0	5
Margarine, Promise Ultra fat free, 1 Tb	5	0	0	0
Broccoli, steamed, 1 c	44	0.6	0	0
Angel food cake, 1/12	130	0	0	0
Strawberries, fresh, 1/2 c	23	0.6	0	0
Whipped topping, fat-free, 2 Tbsp	15	0	0	0
Dinner subtotal	612	5.4	1.6	70
Snacks				
Non-fat vanilla yogurt, 8 fl oz	200	0	0	5
Honeydew melon, cubed pieces, 1c	60	0.2	0	0
Snacks subtotal	298	0.7	0	5
Daily Total	1628	15.6	2.6	102
		8.6%	1.4%	

19% Protein

72% Carbohydrate

[a] Prepared by Sandra Leonard, M.S., R.D.

DIETS TO LOWER SERUM TAG

TAG in VLDL are decreased when calories are restricted, especially the intake from refined carbohydrates and alcohol. N-3 fatty acids in fish and fish oils lower TAG by increasing free fatty acid oxidation. [3,4,28,29] In addition, reduction of total dietary carbohydrate, particularly carbohydrates that elicit a high postprandial glucose response (i.e., high-glycemic carbohydrates), can lower plasma triglyceride concentrations and raise HDL cholesterol. [30,31] Chylomicron TAG are lowered by limiting fat intake severely to 50 g or less daily, or to less than 20% of calories. Patients with Type V who become pregnant may require placement on diets with the fat content lowered to 20 g/day. Alcohol should be eliminated from the diet, which also controls calories and increases exercise to optimize weight. Table 42.8 indicates some food choices and menu plans for TAG lowering in patients with more severe forms of hypertriglyceridemia (Type V). [27] Patients may respond rapidly to withdrawal of dietary fat, with TAG levels falling by 50%/day.

TABLE 42.8
Guidelines of Food Choices and Menu Plans for Patients with Severe Hypertriglyceridemia (Type V)[a]

Triglyceride-Lowering Meal Plan			Goals:	<30% Fat <10% Sat Fat Low Refined Sugar Low Cholesterol	
Food	Total Kcal	Fat (g)	Sat Fat (g)	Sugar (g)	Cholesterol (g)
Breakfast					
Cheerios, 1 1/2 c	165	3	0	1.5	0
Milk, 1%, 8 fl. oz	102	2.6	1.6	*N/A	10
Blackberries, fresh, 1/2 c	37	0.3	0	*N/A	0
Orange juice, 1/2 c	56	0.2	0	8	0
Breakfast subtotal	360	6.1	1.6	9.5	10
Lunch					
Ham and cheese sandwich					
Lean ham, 2 oz	69	2.2	0.8	1.8	29
Cheese, cheddar, low-fat, 1 oz	49	2	1.2	0	6
Mustard, 1 Tbsp	0	0	0	0	0
Whole wheat bread, 2 slice	130	2	0.4	4	0
Peach, fresh, 1 med	37	0.1	0	*N/A	0
Tea, with sugar substitute	0	0	0	0	0
Lunch subtotal	285	6.3	2.4	5.8	35
Dinner					
Pink salmon, broiled, 6 oz	254	7.6	1.2	0	114
Salad:					
Romaine, 1 c	8	0.2	0	1.2	0
Tomato, 1/2 med	13	0.2	0	1.7	0
Ranch dressing, light, 2 Tbsp	100	8.0	1.0	1.0	5
Pasta, cooked, 1/2 c	100	0.5	0	0	0
Marinara sauce, 1/4 c	55	2.5	0.8	4.0	0
Asparagus, 6 spears	22	0.3	0.1	1.4	0
Lemon juice	0	0	0	0	0
Cherries, sweet and fresh, 10	49	0.7	0.1	*N/A	0
Dinner subtotal	601	20	3.2	9.3	119
Snacks					
Pear, raw, 1 med	98	0.7	0	*N/A	0
Triscuits, reduced fat, 8 wafers	130	3	0.5	0	0
Snacks subtotal	228	3.7	0.5	0	0
Daily Total	1474	36.1	7.7	24.6	164
		22%	4.7%		

19% Protein
56% Carbohydrate

* N/A = Not Available.

[a] Provided by Sandra Leonard, M.S., R.D.

Diet and Lp(a)

Saturated fat lowers Lp(a) levels whereas trans fats have no effects on Lp(a) concentrations when compared to a diet of cis-fatty acids, or oleic acid. [32] Niacin has been shown to effectively lower Lp(a). [33] The general advice to individuals with elevated Lp(a) is to aggressively treat any known risk factors for CHD, especially elevated levels of LDL cholesterol.

DRUG MANAGEMENT OF HYPERLIPIDEMIAS

Patients with severe hypercholesterolemia (FH) are unlikely to reach desirable levels in terms of CHD prevention with diet alone. [4,34–38] Therefore the trial of diet should be shortened and medication added. The diet trial is worthwhile in order to ascertain whether the subject is diet responsive. Patients with CHD and hypercholesterolemia who are at higher risk also may be placed on medication after a shortened diet trial period. Drug treatment should be monitored for efficacy and safety, and medication needs to be taken throughout life.

Drugs to Lower Cholesterol

The first line therapy for hypercholesterolemia is statin treatment.[34,35] A number of statins exist (lovastatin, pravastatin, simvastatin, atorvastatin, fluvastatin, cerivastatin, etc.) with differing potencies, biochemical properties, and routes of metabolism.[19] Statins inhibit the rate-limiting step in cholesterol biosynthesis, leading to decreased intracellular cholesterol levels which upregulate LDL receptors and thereby clear plasma LDL cholesterol. Other drugs that lower total and LDL cholesterol include bile acid-binding resins, cholestyramine and colestipol, and niacin. More recently, ezetimibe has been identified as a cholesterol-lowering agent that reduces total and LDL cholesterol by ~25% by inhibiting its absorption at the intestinal level. The relative efficacy of some of these classes of drugs is depicted in Figure 42.9. Niacin and statins also increase HDL cholesterol. Side effects with resins (constipation) and niacin (flushing and hepatotoxicity) are more common and serious than those encountered with statins (hepatotoxicity and myositis). Drugs may need to be used in combination in the management of severe hypercholesterolemia. Timing of medication and efficacy in combination with food vary among these drugs, so that the patient must be advised appropriately by health caregiver or pharmacist.

Plasmapheresis has been used successfully for treating severe forms of FH that are poorly controlled with diet and multiple medications. Liver transplant may improve patients with homozygous FH.

Drugs Affecting TAG and HDL Concentrations

Fibric acid derivatives (clofibrate, gemfibrozil, and fenofibrate) and niacin are potent TAG-lowering medications that also increase HDL cholesterol. [36,37] Effects of fibrate may be mediated by their stimulatory effects on PPAR-α. Niacin is most effective at increasing HDL cholesterol at lower doses and can be used when low HDL cholesterol is the only clinical abnormality. These medications should be added to the diet early in patients with Type V with severe elevations of TAG in order to prevent attacks of acute pancreatitis. At times, the LDL levels will increase with fibric acid derivatives as VLDL and chylomicrons decrease, so that a statin may need to be combined with the initial agent. Side effects of fibric acid derivatives include lithogenic bile and gallstones, gastrointestinal distress, and myositis. Oral contraceptives, estrogens, or corticosteroids may worsen hypertriglyceridemia. TAG levels should be monitored carefully in patients with Type V using these drugs.

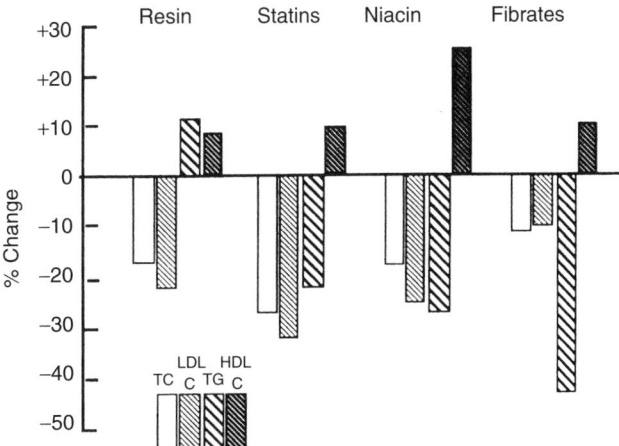

FIGURE 42.9 The efficacy of various lipid-lowering drugs in treating patients with hypercholesterolemia. Data represent the percent change in lipoprotein lipid levels from levels obtained from patients ingesting a baseline lipid-lowering diet.

Additional relevant information may be found in Chapter 40, that addresses the laboratory assessment of lipids and lipoproteins and Chapter 43, which discusses the role of nutrition in preventing and modifying cardiovascular risk factors.

REFERENCES

1. Semenkovich, CF. In *Modern Nutrition in Health and Disease*, 9th ed., Shils, ME, Olson, JA, Shike, M, Ross, AC, Eds, Williams & Wilkins, Baltimore, 1999, ch. 74.
2. Havel, RJ, Kane, JP. In *The Metabolic and Molecular Bases of Inherited Disease*, 7th ed., Scriver, CL, Beaudet, AL, Sly, WS, Valle, D, Eds, McGraw Hill, NY, 1995, ch. 56.
3. Feldman, EB. In *Modern Nutrition in Health and Disease*, 8th ed., Shils, ME, Olson, JA, Shike, M, Eds, Lea & Febiger, Philadelphia, 1993, ch. 72.
4. Grundy, SM. In *Modern Nutrition in Health and Disease*, 9th ed., Shils, ME, Olson, JA, Shike, M, Ross, AC, Eds., Williams & Wilkins, Baltimore, 1999, ch. 75.
5. Humphries, SE, Peacock, R, Gudnason, V. In *Lipoproteins in Health and Disease*, Betteridge DJ, Illingworth DR, Shepherd J, Eds., Oxford University Press, NY, 1999.
6. Brunzell, JD. In *The Metabolic and Molecular Bases of Inherited Disease*, 7th ed., Scriver CL, Beaudet AL, Sly WS, Valle D, Eds, McGraw Hill, NY, 1995, ch. 59.
7. Santmarina-Fojo, S. *Curr Opin Lipidol* 3: 186; 1992.
8. Goldstein, JL, Hobbs, HH, Brown, MS. In *The Metabolic and Molecular Bases of Inherited Disease*, 7th ed., Scriver CL, Beaudet AL, Sly WS, Valle D, Eds, McGraw Hill, NY, 1995, ch. 62.
9. Brown, MS, Goldstein, JL. *Science* 232: 34; 1986.
10. Sohar, E, Bossak, ET, Wang, CI, Adlersberg, D. *Science* 123: 461; 1957.
11. Aouizerat BE, Allayee H, Cantor RM et al. *Arterioscler Thromb Vasc Biol* 19: 2730; 19XX.
12. Kwiterovich PO, Jr. *Curr Opin Lipidol* 4: 133; 1993.
13. Campos H, Dreon DM, Krauss RM. *J Lipid Res* 34: 397; 1993.
14. Mahley RW, Rall SC, Jr. In *The Metabolic and Molecular Bases of Inherited Disease*, 7th ed, Scriver CL, Beaudet AL, Sly WS, Valle D, Eds, McGraw Hill, NY, 1995, ch. 61.
15. Eichner, JE, Dunn, ST, Perveen, G et al. *Am J Epidemiol* 155: 487; 2002.
16. Feldman EB. In *Essentials of Clinical Nutrition*. FA Davis, Philadelphia, 1988, ch.
17. Brewer HB, Jr. *Am J Cardiol* 83: 3F; 1999.
18. Austin MA, Hokanson HE, Edwards KL. *Am J Cardiol* 82: 7B; 1999.
19. Kreisberg, RA, Oberman, A. *J Clin Endocrinol Metab* 88: 2445; 2003.
20. Altshuler, D, Hirschhorn, JN, Klannemark M et al. *Nat Genet* 26: 76; 2000.
21. Goodarzi, MO, Guo, X, Taylor, KD et al. *Diabetes* 53: 214; 2004.
22. Denke, MA. *Am J Cardiol* 96: 3F; 2005.
23. Grundy, SM, Cleeman, JI, Merz, CN et al. *Circulation* 110: 227; 2004.
24. Grundy, SM, Cleeman, JI, Merz, CN et al. *JAMA* 285: 2486; 2001.
25. Jenkins, DJ, Kendall, CW, Faulkner, DA et al. *Am J Clin Nutr* 83: 582; 2006.
26. Greene, JM, Feldman, EB. *J Am Coll Nutr* 10: 443; 1991.
27. Bloch, AS, Shils, ME. In *Modern Nutrition in Health and Disease*, 9th ed., Shils, ME, Olson, JA, Shike, M, Ross, AC, Eds, Williams & Wilkins, Baltimore, 1999, pp. A167, 170.
28. Kris-Etherton, PM, Harris, WS, Appel, LJ. *Arterioscler Thromb Vasc Biol* 23: 151; 2003.
29. Harris, WS. *Curr Opin Lipidol* 7: 3; 1996.
30. Mensink, RP, Katan, MB. *Arterioscler Thromb* 12: 911; 1992.
31. Parks, EJ, Hellerstein, MK. *Am J Clin Nutr* 71: 412; 2000.
32. Clevidence, BA, Judd, JT, Schaefer, EJ et al. *Arterioscler Thromb Vasc Biol* 17: 1657; 1997.
33. Carlson, LA. *J Intern Med* 258: 94; 2005.
34. Lipid Research Clinics Program. *JAMA* 251: 351; 1984.
35. Jones P, Kalonek S, Laurora I, Hunninghake D. For the CURVES Investigators, *Am J Cardiol* 81: 582; 1998.
36. Knopp RH, Waldaen CE, Rezlaff BM et al. *JAMA* 278: 1509; 1997.
37. Goldberg, AC, Schonfeld, G, Feldman, EB et al. *Clin Ther* 11: 69; 1989.
38. Lockman, AR, Tribastone, AD, Knight, KV, Franko, JP. *Am Fam Physician* 71: 1137; 2005.

43 Effects of Diet on Cardiovascular Disease Risk

Patty Siri-Tarino, Elaine B. Feldman, and Ronald M. Krauss

CONTENTS

INTRODUCTION

Coronary heart disease (CHD) is the leading cause of death in both men and women in the United States and throughout most of the world. In the United States, 49% of men and 32% of women will develop CHD.[1] Evidence suggesting that nutritional practices can influence cardiovascular health is derived from numerous epidemiologic studies as well as some rigorously controlled dietary interventions. In part, the effects of diet on CHD risk may be mediated by effects on prevalent metabolic disorders such as obesity, hypertension, and abnormal lipid profiles, all of which have been independently associated with increased CHD risk.

General dietary guidelines for cardiovascular health have been issued in recent years by the American Heart Association, the Adult Treatment Panel III of the National Cholesterol Education Program, the National Heart, Lung, and Blood Institute (NHLBI) Joint National Committee for the Prevention, Detection, Evaluation and Treatment of High Blood Pressure, and the NHLBI Clinical Guidelines on the Identification, Evaluation, and Treatment of Overweight and Obesity in Adults. Overall, these expert panels recommend diets that emphasize intake of fruits and vegetables, whole grains, nuts and legumes, fatty fish, poultry and lean meats, low-fat and fat-free dairy products, and liquid vegetable oils. Such foods tend to contain high concentrations of micronutrients and fiber, moderate amounts of unsaturated fatty acids, particularly omega-3 fatty acids, and lower amounts of saturated and *trans*-fatty acids. They also tend to contain less sugar and starches with a high glycemic effect.

This chapter will focus on the effects of overall dietary patterns — in terms of relative carbohydrate, fat, and protein composition — on morbidity and mortality from cardiovascular disease (CVD). The nutritional modulation of major CVD risk factors, such as obesity, dyslipidemia, and hypertension, will also be examined. Finally, the role of nutrition in the determination of homocysteine, C-reactive protein (CRP), and oxidant stress levels will be examined in the context of CVD risk.

EFFECTS OF NUTRIENT COMPOSITION ON CVD RISK

TOTAL DIETARY FAT

Studies documenting effects of diet composition on morbidity and mortality from CVD have been mostly epidemiologic in nature, although, more recently, larger-scale clinical studies have been carried out. Observational studies from the 1950s first suggested a relationship between fat intakes — in particular, saturated fat intake — and CVD risk. These studies showed a positive

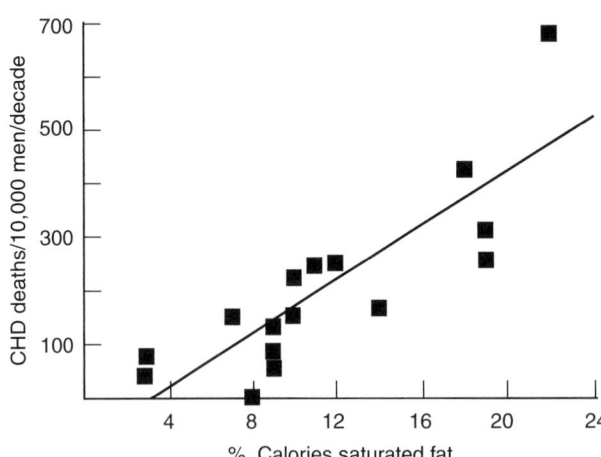

FIGURE 43.1 Death rates from CHD and the intake of saturated fat in the Seven Countries Study. The ordinate represents deaths from coronary heart disease that occurred over a 10-year period per 10,000 men enrolled in the study. The cohorts are from sites in seven countries: the United States, Japan, Greece, Italy, Yugoslavia, the Netherlands, Finland. The regression equation is $y = -83 + 25.1x$, $r + 0.84$. (Adapted from Keys, A. *Seven Countries Study — A Multivariate Study of Death and Coronary Heart Disease*, Harvard University Press, Cambridge, 1980.)

and dose-dependent correlation between saturated fat consumption and death due to CVD. Furthermore, the impact of dietary fat on disease appeared to be modulated by effects on serum cholesterol. Ecologic studies demonstrating an increased prevalence of CHD in countries with higher fat consumption provided corroborating evidence for an association of diet pattern and risk of disease. More recently, however, a large epidemiologic study in which 78,778 American women free of CVD were evaluated over 20 years showed contrasting results.[2] In this cohort of healthy women, total fat intake had no effect on risk of CHD. Instead, intake of *trans*-fats was positively associated with death from CHD, while polyunsaturated fat intake was inversely associated with CHD mortality (Figure 43.1).

Early secondary prevention trials also failed to show an association between reductions in total fat and reductions in cholesterol or CHD events.[3] More recently, the Lifestyle Heart Trial showed significant decreases in diameter stenosis and cardiac events in an intervention group consuming a very-low-fat diet relative to controls. However, the intervention included other features including aerobic exercise training, stress management, smoking cessation, and psychosocial support. The effectiveness of the intervention could therefore not be specifically attributed to the low-fat component of the intervention.

In the largest long-term randomized dietary intervention trial to date, the Women's Health Initiative (WHI) Randomized Controlled Dietary Modification Trial[4] was designed to test the hypothesis that a diet low in fat and high in fruit, vegetable, and grain would lead to a reduction of CVD events. Nearly 50,000 postmenopausal women were randomized to an intervention group receiving regularly scheduled individualized dietary consultations or to a comparison group receiving diet-related education materials only. Despite achieving a reduction in total fat intake between the intervention and control groups (28.8% vs. 37% of calories [$p < 0.001$], respectively), no effects of the intervention on CHD, stroke, or CVD were observed during the 8-year follow-up. The authors suggested that the lack of benefit on CVD end points might have been related to the minimal changes in low-density lipoprotein (LDL) cholesterol observed owing to the counterbalancing effects of saturated fat and polyunsaturated fats. Nevertheless, the results of WHI support the increasingly accepted concept that modulation of total dietary fat does not alter CVD risk.

Dietary guidelines recommending limitation of total fat to less than 30% of total energy have since been revised.[5] Originally, limitation guidelines were set in an effort to reduce the energy intake as fat is the most energy-dense nutrient (9 kcal/g compared with 4 kcal/g for carbohydrate and protein). This guideline was also set in an effort to decrease saturated fat intake, because the consumption of saturated fat has been positively associated with total fat consumption. However, the lack of evidence for a beneficial effect of low-fat diets as well as some evidence that such diets may induce adverse effects have called such recommendations into question.[6] Furthermore, the benefit of diets rich in polyunsaturated fat have been supported by a number of clinical investigations.

TYPE OF FAT

In contrast to the ambiguous data available for the effects of total fat on CHD risk, there is more evidence from prospective epidemiologic studies,[7] controlled feeding studies,[8] and randomized clinical trials[6] that types of fat may be relevant in the determination of CHD risk. The Finnish Mental Hospital Study,[9] the Veterans Administration Study, and the Oslo Diet Heart Study[10]

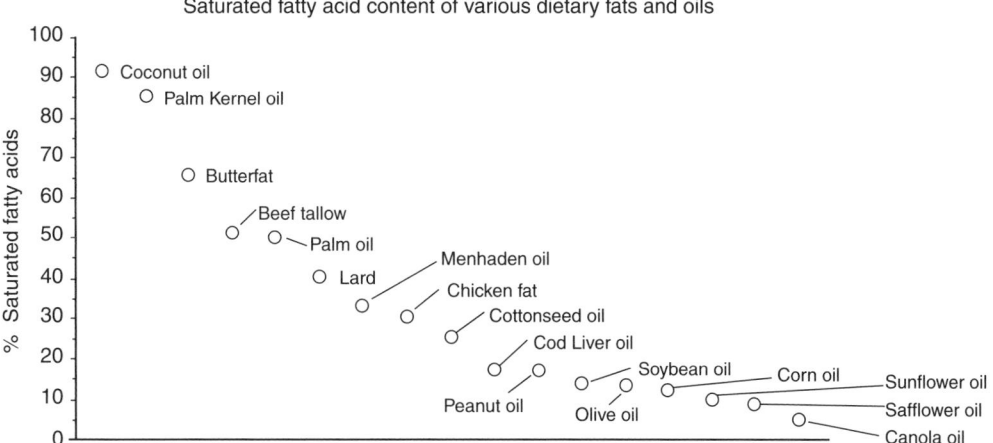

FIGURE 43.2 The saturated fatty acid content of various fats and oils.

were among early randomized clinical trials that showed that diets high in polyunsaturated fatty acids (PUFA) were associated with decreased CHD incidence. In particular, PUFA-enriched diets may most benefit cardiovascular health when they replace saturated fatty acids and *trans*-fatty acids (Figure 43.2).[11]

Long-chain omega-3 polyunsaturated fatty acids, in particular, have been shown to contribute to cardiovascular health. In the Diet and Reinfarction Trial (DART), consumption of fatty fish twice a week or fish oil capsules (1.5 g/day) led to decreased total and coronary mortality in a group of over 2000 postmyocardial infarction Welsh men relative to controls.[3] Singh et al.[12] showed decreased cardiac events in persons supplemented with fish oil (containing 1.8 g/day of eicosapentanoic acid [EPA] +decosahexanoic acid [DHA] or mustard oil (2.9 g/day of α-linolenic acid) relative to controls taking placebo. The Gruppo Italiano per lo Studio della Sopravvivenza nell'Infarto Miocardico (GISSI) trial, a study of 11,000 Italian postinfarct patients, found that the consumption of omega-3 fatty acids (1 g/day) was associated with decreased rates of coronary death relative to controls not consuming the fatty acid supplement.[13] The Lyon Diet Heart Study also showed that a diet rich in omega-3 fatty acids, that is a Mediterranean diet, reduced the incidence of CHD events in postinfarct patients.[14,15] Of particular note, no differences were observed in lipid parameters between the intervention and the control groups in this study, suggesting that the improvement in CVD risk was mediated through mechanisms independent of lipid pathways. Omega-3 fatty acids may prevent death after acute myocardial infarction through their antiarrhythmic properties,[16,17] which effectively increases the threshold for ventricular fibrillation;[18] they may also decrease the tendency for thrombosis and improve endothelial dysfunction.[19]

There is some, albeit weaker, evidence linking omega-6 fatty acid concentrations with risk of CVD. In an epidemiologic study comparing heart disease mortality rates in four European regions, linoleic acid concentrations in adipose tissue were inversely correlated with CVD mortality even after adjustment for other major risk factors.[20] The balance of omega-6 (linoleic acid) and omega-3 fatty acids (linolenic acid and its products, EPA and DHA) has also been suggested to be relevant in the determination of CVD risk,[21] with a ratio of 6:1 for omega-6 and omega-3 fatty acids, respectively, considered optimal.

Increased monounsaturated fat (MUFA) intake has also been associated with decreased CVD risk,[7] particularly when it replaces saturated fats and *trans*-fats. Generally, the effects of MUFA are less potent than those of PUFA.

DIETARY CARBOHYDRATE

Dietary carbohydrate may alter CVD risk through its effects on lipid profiles, insulin sensitivity, and inflammatory processes. As with dietary fat, the type of carbohydrate may be the salient factor in the determination of CVD risk. The glycemic index primarily reflects the rate of starch digestion and absorption from the small intestine. Dietary carbohydrates with high glycemic indices elicit a relatively high postprandial glucose and insulin response compared to those with low glycemic indices. High-glycemic-index diets have been associated with chronic hyperinsulinemia and insulin resistance in some epidemiologic studies.[22] Several studies have documented reduced CVD risk with increased consumption of low-glycemic-index foods such as whole grains.[23,24] Of particular note, a protective effect of fiber, particularly water-soluble fiber, on risk of myocardial infarction, CVD death, and other CVD outcomes has been documented in a number of prospective epidemiologic studies.[25–27]

DIETARY PROTEIN

A positive relationship between diets high in animal protein and CVD risk has been suggested by ecologic and animal studies.[28] In the Nurses' Health Study, high protein intake was associated with lower risk of ischemic heart disease such that persons in the highest quintile of protein consumption had a relative risk of CHD that was 0.76 times the risk of persons in the lowest quintile of total protein intake.[29] More recently, in the Iowa Women's Health Study, a reduced risk of coronary death was observed when vegetable protein was substituted for animal protein or carbohydrate.[30] Inverse associations have been observed for animal protein and risk of intraparenchymal hemorrhage in women.[31] In this study, lower consumption of saturated fat was also associated with increased risk of hemorrhagic stroke, particularly in women with hypertension.[31] Although these epidemiologic studies point to a possible role for protein in the determination of CVD risk as defined by CVD events or mortality, long-term clinical trials testing this relationship are lacking.

MODULATION OF RISK FACTORS FOR CVD BY DIET

The effects of diet on CVD risk may be mediated by risk factors for CVD, in particular, obesity, plasma lipids and lipoproteins, and blood pressure. Also relevant are effects of diet on homocysteine, inflammation, and oxidative stress.

OBESITY

At least in part, CHD risk over the last several decades may be attributable to the significant increase in the prevalence of obesity.[32] Certainly, excess caloric intake can lead to metabolic imbalances such that insulin resistance underlies a cascade of events leading to increases in plasma triglyceride, decreases in high-density lipoprotein (HDL) cholesterol, and increases in small, dense LDL cholesterol. Each of these lipid abnormalities has been associated with increased CHD risk. Overweight and obesity are also commonly associated with numerous other comorbidities, including hypertension, diabetes, and metabolic syndrome.[33,34] Weight loss has been shown to be an effective modulator of CVD risk and can lead to the amelioration of the metabolic abnormalities commonly associated with weight excess.

Guidelines to managing weight emphasize matching caloric intake to caloric needs and maintaining a level of physical activity that achieves fitness and balances or exceeds (if the goal is weight reduction) energy intake. Importantly, weight loss can be achieved with caloric restriction irrespective of the macronutrient composition of the diet. Nonetheless, considerable debate has taken place among nutrition experts as to the most effective means of weight loss. There have been some reports that diets high in protein or monounsaturated fats may not only facilitate weight loss[35] but also lead to greater weight loss in the short-term, that is, periods less than 6 months, compared with diets with more conventional amounts of carbohydrate. A meta-analysis of the five most rigorously conducted clinical trials in this regard confirmed evidence of improved triglyceride and HDL cholesterol concentrations in the low-carbohydrate, high-protein, high-fat group compared with conventional diet.[36] However, these were also associated with increases in LDL and total cholesterol. In a population of obese women, weight loss induced by a high-protein diet led to improvements in metabolic parameters without an increase in LDL cholesterol.[37] Another recent clinical study by Luscombe-Marsh et al.[38] compared high-protein to high-fat diets in the setting of carbohydrate restriction. The study suggested that the most important determinant of improved metabolic profiles was restriction of carbohydrate, a finding in agreement with the findings of a recently published study by Krauss et al., which showed significant weight-loss-independent benefits of low-carbohydrate diets relative to conventional diets.[39]

High-protein diets may facilitate weight loss by increasing satiety, decreasing postprandial insulin responses, and increasing thermogenesis.[28] Nonetheless, the long-term effects of high-protein diets on CVD risk await the results of long-term clinical trials. Of concern are the high concentrations of saturated fats and *trans*-fats generally associated with such diets, the lack of fruits and vegetables, the questionable ability to adhere to the program over a longer period of time, and other potential adverse effects in the setting of renal or hepatic impairment.

ABNORMAL LIPIDS AND LIPOPROTEINS

As previously described, lipid and lipoprotein concentrations are important determinants of CVD risk. Dietary carbohydrate can promote atherogenic dyslipidemia through its effects on triglyceride-rich lipoprotein metabolism.[40] Specifically, exogenous carbohydrate can stimulate lipogenesis and impair clearance of lipoprotein particles. Increased triglyceride availability drives the secretion of hepatically derived particles whose triglyceride enrichment leads to more rapid lipolysis and the production of LDL particles that are smaller and denser. In addition, the excess triglyceride on these particles can be exchanged for HDL cholesterol, thereby leading to the reduction of plasma concentrations of HDL.

The replacement of dietary carbohydrate with dietary fat, irrespective of type, has been shown to effectively decrease plasma triglyceride concentrations[41] and improve the atherogenic dyslipidemia thereby associated. Replacement of dietary carbohydrate with protein has also been shown to be effective in decreasing LDL cholesterol and triglyceride while raising HDL cholesterol in persons with normolipidemia,[42] mild hypercholesterolemia,[43] and familial hypercholesterolemia.[44]

Polyunsaturated fats, in particular, have been shown to decrease LDL and HDL cholesterol most effectively. Linoleic acid, an omega-6 fatty acid, has been shown to decrease plasma total and LDL cholesterol via enhanced receptor-dependent clearance of LDL and decreased LDL production. Its availability also modulates the cholesterolemic potential of other fatty acids such that saturated fats and *trans*-fats exert a more exaggerated effect on LDL cholesterol when linoleic acid concentrations are below a certain threshold value (<3% of energy).[21]

The omega-3 fatty acids have been shown to be particularly effective in decreasing triglyceride concentrations. Two to four grams of EPA + DHA per day can lower triglyceride levels by 20 to 40%.[45] Omega-3 fatty acids have been shown to be effective in cases of marked hypertriglyceridemia as well as in type 2 diabetes.[46] Moreover, the effect of omega-3 fatty acids is dose-dependent and extends to postprandial lipemia.[47] Slight increases in LDL cholesterol may be observed (5 to 10%) with minimal changes in HDL cholesterol.

Saturated fat increases LDL cholesterol, at least in part through its downregulation of LDL receptors. The increase in LDL cholesterol may be specific to larger- and medium-sized LDL particles, and effects of saturated fat may be genetically modulated.[39] Lauric acid is associated with the greatest increase in LDL cholesterol followed by myristic and palmitic acids. Saturated fat, and lauric acid in particular, is also associated with significant increases in HDL cholesterol. Whereas lauric acid is found in tropical oils, such as coconut and palm oil, palmitic acid is found in meats, dairy fats, and palm oil. Using predictive equations based on a meta-analysis of dietary trials, Mensink and Katan have shown that LDL cholesterol lowering is most effectively achieved when saturated fat is replaced with polyunsaturated fat followed by monounsaturated fat. Replacement of saturated fat with carbohydrate also lowers LDL cholesterol, but it concomitantly decreases HDL cholesterol; therefore, no change in the LDL-to-HDL ratio, or total-cholesterol-to-HDL ratio, for that matter, is observed in this dietary replacement scenario.

trans-Fats have been shown to be particularly detrimental to lipid and lipoprotein profiles as they increase LDL cholesterol and decrease HDL cholesterol concentrations. Increased intake of *trans*-fats has been associated with a rise in the total-cholesterol-to-HDL-cholesterol ratio. Of note, replacement of *trans*-fats with a mix of carbohydrates and unsaturated fats leads to improvements in the total-cholesterol-to-HDL-cholesterol ratio that are twice as large as those when replacing saturated fat.[8]

Plant stanols and sterols at a dose of 2 g/day have been shown to decrease LDL cholesterol by as much as 15% and can therefore be considered as part of dietary therapy.[48] In postmenopausal women, plant stanol esters have been shown to effectively lower LDL cholesterol by approximately half the reduction that was observed with statin therapy, making this dietary modulation an attractive alternative to pharmacological intervention.[49]

The effectiveness of a comprehensive dietary program in modulating lipid profiles was confirmed in a study examining multiple dietary components known to reduce blood cholesterol concentrations. A dietary portfolio high in plant sterols, soy protein, viscous fibers, and almonds was shown to be as effective as 20 mg/day of lovastatin in lowering LDL cholesterol and, presumably, cardiovascular risk.[50] That dietary modulation could yield results comparable to pharmacological intervention was a striking observation and provides even more evidence to support lifestyle and dietary intervention as the first line of therapy in persons who present with hypercholesterolemia.

HYPERTENSION

Dietary sodium plays an important role in the determination of blood pressure, and reductions in sodium intake by 1.8 g/day have been associated with reductions in systolic and diastolic blood pressure of approximately 4 and 2 mmHg, respectively (see Chapter 44 and Chapter 45).[51] The Dietary Approaches to Stop Hypertension (DASH) diet, a carbohydrate-rich diet that emphasized fruits, vegetables, and low-fat dairy products and reduced saturated fat, total fat, and dietary cholesterol, showed significant effects on reducing hypertension at all levels of salt intake.[52] More recently, in the follow-up study entitled the OMNI-HEART study, replacement of carbohydrate with protein or unsaturated fat led to even greater decreases in blood pressure in prehypertensive and stage 1 hypertensive participants.[53] A reduction in LDL and HDL cholesterol was seen when carbohydrate was replaced with protein but not with unsaturated fat.

In the CARDIA study, 4304 young adults were followed for over 15 years in a multicenter, population-based, prospective study of CVD risk evolution. Diets rich in whole grains, refined grains, fruits, vegetables, nuts, or legumes were found to be inversely related to blood pressure, while positive effects of red and processed meat intake on blood pressure were observed.[54] In an epidemiologic study of approximately 1700 persons, those consuming 14 or more servings of fruit or vegetables per day were likely to have less of an increase in blood pressure than persons consuming less than 14 servings per day of fruits and vegetables after a 7-year follow-up.

OTHER CVD RISK FACTORS AND THEIR NUTRITIONAL MODULATORS

HOMOCYSTEINE

Elevated levels of homocysteine have been associated with increased risk for atherosclerosis. *In vitro* and *in vivo* data have suggested that homocysteine promotes oxidant stress, inflammation, thrombosis, endothelial dysfunction, and cell proliferation.

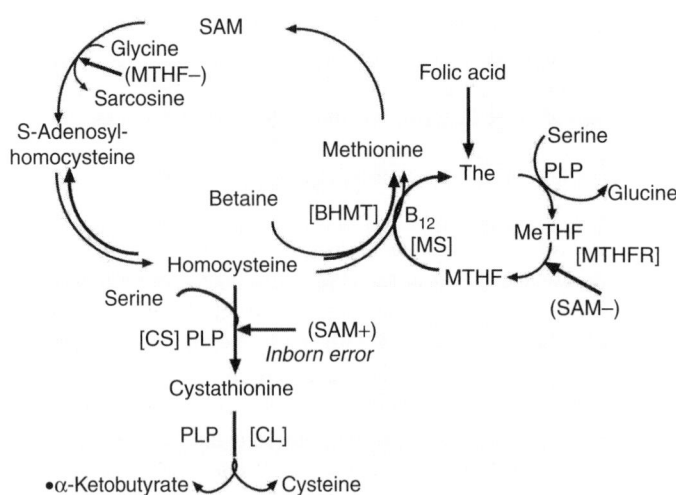

FIGURE 43.3 Homocysteine metabolism is regulated by enzymes dependent on folate and vitamins B₆ and B₁₂. + = activation, – = inhibition. Abbreviations: THF = tetrahydrofolate; MeTHF = methylene tetrahydrofolate; MTHF = methyltetrahydrofolate; SAM = *S*-adenosylmethionine; PLP = pyridoxalphosphate (biological active form of vitamin B₆); CS + cystathionine synthase; CL = cystathionine lyase; MS = methionine synthase; MTHFR = methylene tetrahydrofolate reductase; BHMT = betaine homocysteine methyl transferase.

An examination of data available from prospective observational studies led the Homocysteine Studies Collaboration to conclude that a 25% reduction in homocysteine is associated with a risk reduction of ischemic heart disease and stroke (11% and 19%, respectively).[55] A reduction of recurrent events has also been shown to be associated with a reduction in serum levels of homocysteine.[56]

The metabolism of homocysteine occurs through pathways dependent on vitamins B₆ and B₁₂ and folate (Figure 43.3). In the transsulfuration pathway, vitamin B₆ acts as an enzymatic cofactor to convert homocysteine to cystathione and subsequently to cysteine. Folate and vitamin B₁₂ are necessary components of the remethylation pathway that leads to the production of methionine. In animal studies and clinical trial,[15,57] supplementation with B-vitamins led to reductions in serum homocysteine levels as well as improvements in CVD risk profiles, providing the basis for the design and conduct of larger-scale randomized clinical trials.

Three secondary prevention trials aimed at reducing homocysteine concentrations, and thereby coronary events in patients with established CVD, have recently been completed. The Vitamin Intervention for Stroke Prevention (VISP),[58] the Norwegian Vitamin (NORVIT),[59] and the Heart Outcomes Prevention Evaluation (HOPE) 2 trials [60] provided patients (*n* = 3680, 3749, and 5522, respectively) with a daily dose of folic acid, vitamin B₆, and vitamin B₁₂. In all three studies, homocysteine levels were successfully lowered. However, no differences were observed in CVD end points after 2 to 5 years of follow-up. Though marginal trends towards fewer strokes in the vitamin supplementation group were observed in the NORVIT and HOPE 2 trials, there was a near significant trend toward more myocardial infarction in the vitamin group in the HOPE 2 study.

The lack of efficacy of B-vitamin supplementation in reducing coronary risk through reduction of homocysteine levels speaks of the complexity of the metabolic pathways involved. B-vitamin supplementation may affect CVD risk adversely through other pathways. Alternatively, homocysteine concentrations may only be a marker for another factor that is the "true" atherogenic determinant. In light of these recent clinical trials, recommendations regarding use of B-vitamins in the prevention of CVD are unwarranted.

C-REACTIVE PROTEIN

C-reactive protein (CRP) as a biomarker of inflammation is a well-established risk factor for CVD that may be modulated by diet.[61] Elevated CRP concentrations have been associated with obesity,[62] and weight loss has been linearly correlated with percentage reduction in CRP levels in a comparison of multiple dietary interventions.[63] There is some evidence that α-linolenic acid and oleic acid may reduce CRP levels, whereas fish oil and conjugated linoleic acid generally have been shown to have no effect. The data regarding saturated fats and *trans*-fats are equivocal, with a limited number of studies showing positive associations with increased consumption of these fats.

Diets high in glycemic load have been positively associated with elevations in CRP.[64] Dietary protein as arginine has been associated with decreased CRP concentrations,[65] as has alcohol intake in healthy[66] and diabetic men.[67] Importantly, a dietary portfolio known to reduce serum cholesterol levels as well as statin therapy also reduced CRP levels to a comparable extent.[50]

OXIDATIVE STRESS

Although oxidative stress is recognized as an important contributor to atherogenesis, data to support the concept of using anti-oxidants — in particular, vitamins A, C, and E and β-carotene — to reduce risk of CVD are controversial and inconclusive.[68] Although a number of observational studies have provided support for a relationship between antioxidant intake and risk of CVD, the results of randomized clinical trials testing the efficacy of antioxidant supplementation have generally shown no benefit and have in some cases shown potentially hazardous effects of supplementation. A meta-analysis of 15 randomized clinical trials of vitamin E or β-carotene supplementation ($n = 81,788$ and $138,113$ persons, respectively) showed no effects of vitamin E supplementation on CVD end points and a small but significant increase in total mortality as well as mortality from CVD in patients receiving β-carotene supplements.[69] Recently, in the Women's Health Study, supplementation with 600 IU of vitamin E on alternate days also showed no effect on major CVD events or total mortality, although CVD mortality was decreased significantly.[70] Antioxidant supplementation may even interfere with cardioprotective effects of statin and niacin treatment as was shown when the lipid-lowering effects of the drugs were attenuated.[71] More recently, treatment with vitamins C and E in conjunction with intense atorvastatin treatment showed no additional benefit on CVD health.[72] Finally, in a study of the effects of hormone and antioxidant therapy in postmenopausal women, antioxidant therapy did not improve endothelial vaso-dilator function.[73] These findings were in line with earlier study findings that showed no benefit but possible harm of vitamin supplementation on cardiovascular health.[74] Based on the available evidence to date, recommendations for use of antioxidant therapies cannot be made.

REFERENCES

1. Lloyd-Jones, DM, Larson, MG, Beiser, A, Levy, D. *Lancet* 353: 89; 1999.
2. Oh, K, Hu, FB, Manson, JE, et al. *Am J Epidemiol* 161: 672; 2005.
3. Burr, ML, Fehily, AM, Gilbert, JF, et al. *Lancet* 2: 757; 1989.
4. Howard, BV, Van Horn, L, Hsia, J, et al. *JAMA* 295: 655; 2006.
5. Krauss, RM, Eckel, RH, Howard, B, et al. *Circulation* 102: 2284; 2000.
6. Sacks, FM, Katan, M. *Am J Med* 113: 13S; 2002.
7. Hu, FB, Stampfer, MJ, Manson, JE, et al. *N Engl J Med* 337: 1491; 1997.
8. Mensink, RP, Zock, PL, Kester, AD, Katan, MB. *Am J Clin Nutr* 77: 1146; 2003.
9. Turpeinen, O, Karvonen, MJ, Pekkarinen, M, et al. *Int J Epidemiol* 8: 99; 1979.
10. Leren, P. *Circulation* 42: 935; 1970.
11. Sacks, F. *J Cardiovasc Risk* 1: 3; 1994.
12. Singh, RB, Niaz, MA, Sharma, JP, et al. *Cardiovasc Drugs Ther* 11: 485; 1997.
13. Gruppo Prevenzione Investigators. *Lancet* 354: 447; 1999.
14. de Lorgeril, M., Renaud, S., Mamelle, N., et al. *Lancet* 343: 1454; 1994.
15. de Lorgeril, M, Salen, P, Martin, JL, et al. *Circulation* 99: 779; 1999.
16. Billman, GE, Hallaq, H, Leaf, A. *Proc Natl Acad Sci USA* 91: 4427; 1994.
17. Leaf, A. *Circulation* 99: 733; 1999.
18. Sellmayer, A, Witzgall, H, Lorenz, RL, Weber, PC. *Am J Cardiol* 76: 974; 1995
19. Hu, FB, Willett, WC. *JAMA* 288: 2569; 2002.
20. Riemersma, RA, Wood, DA, Butler, S, et al. *Br Med J (Clin Res Ed)* 292: 1423; 1986.
21. Wijendran, V, Hayes, KC. *Ann Rev Nutr* 24: 597; 2004.
22. Liu, S, Willett, WC, Stampfer, M J, et al. *Am J Clin Nutr* 71: 1455; 2000.
23. Jacobs, DR, Jr., Meyer, KA, Kushi, LH, Folsom, AR. *Am J Clin Nutr* 68: 248; 1998.
24. Liu, S, Stampfer, MJ, Hu, FB, et al. *Am J Clin Nutr* 70: 412; 1999.
25. Bazzano, LA, He, J, Ogden, LG, Loria, CM, Whelton, PK. *Arch Intern Med* 163(16), 1897; 2003.
26. Wolk, A, Manson, JE, Stampfer, MJ, et al. *JAMA* 281: 1998; 1999.
27. Liu, S, Buring, JE, Sesso, HD, et al. *J Am Coll Cardiol* 39: 49; 2002.
28. Hu, FB. *Am J Clin Nutr* 82: 242S; 2005.
29. Hu, FB, Stampfer, MJ, Manson, JE, et al. *Am J Clin Nutr* 70: 221; 1999.
30. Kelemen, LE, Kushi, LH, Jacobs, DR, Jr., Cerhan, JR. *Am J Epidemiol* 161: 239; 2005.
31. Iso, H, Stampfer, MJ, Manson, JE, et al. *Circulation* 103: 856; 2001.
32. Hedley, AA, Ogden, CL, Johnson, CL, et al. *JAMA* 291: 2847; 2004.
33. Eckel, RH. *Circulation* 96: 3248; 1997.
34. Mokdad, AH, Ford, ES, Bowman, BA, et al. *JAMA* 289: 76; 2003.
35. Foster, GD, Wyatt, HR, Hill, JO, et al. *N Engl J Med* 348: 2082; 2003.
36. Nordmann, AJ, Nordmann, A, Briel, M, et al. *Arch Intern Med* 166: 285; 2006.
37. Noakes, M, Keogh, JB, Foster, PR, Clifton, PM. *Am J Clin Nutr* 81: 1298; 2005.

38. Luscombe-Marsh, ND, Noakes, M, Wittert, GA, et al. *Am J Clin Nutr* 81: 762; 2005.
39. Krauss, RM, Blanche, PJ, Rawlings, RS, et al. *Am J Clin Nutr* 83: 1025; 2006.
40. Parks, EJ, Hellerstein, MK. *Am J Clin Nutr* 71: 412; 2000.
41. Mensink, RP, Katan, MB. *Arterioscler Thromb* 12: 911; 1992.
42. Wolfe, BM, Piche, LA. *Clin Invest Med* 22: 140; 1999.
43. Wolfe, BM, Giovannetti, PM. *Metabolism* 40: 338; 1991.
44. Wolfe, BM, Giovannetti, PM. *Clin Invest Med* 15: 349; 1992.
45. Kris-Etherton, PM, Harris, WS, Appel, LJ. *Arterioscler Thromb Vasc Biol* 23: 151; 2003.
46. Montori, VM, Farmer, A, Wollan, PC, Dinneen, SF. *Diabetes Care* 23: 1407; 2000.
47. Kris-Etherton, PM, Harris, WS, Appel, LJ. *Arterioscler Thromb Vasc Biol* 23: e20; 2003.
48. Grundy, SM. *Am J Cardiol* 96: 47D; 2005.
49. Cater, NB, Garcia-Garcia, AB, Vega, GL, Grundy, SM. *Am J Cardiol* 96: 23D; 2005.
50. Jenkins, DJ, Kendall, CW, Marchie, A, et al. *JAMA* 290: 502; 2003.
51. Graudal, NA, Galloe, AM, Garred, P. *JAMA* 279: 1383; 1998.
52. Sacks, FM, Svetkey, LP, Vollmer, WM, et al. *N Engl J Med* 344: 3; 2001.
53. Appel, LJ, Sacks, FM, Carey, VJ, et al. *JAMA* 294: 2455; 2005.
54. Steffen, LM, Kroenke, CH, Yu, X, et al. *Am J Clin Nutr* 82: 1169 and quiz 1363; 2005.
55. Homocysteine Studies Collabration. *JAMA* 288: 2015; 2002.
56. Wald, DS, Law, M, Morris, JK. *Brit Med J* 325: 1202; 2002.
57. Zhou, J, Moller, J, Ritskes-Hoitinga, M, et al. *Atherosclerosis* 168: 255: 2003.
58. Toole, JF, Malinow, MR, Chambless, LE, et al. *JAMA* 291: 565; 2004.
59. Bonaa, KH, Njolstad, I, Ueland, PM, et al. *N Engl J Med* 354: 1578; 2006.
60. Lonn, E, Yusuf, S, Arnold, MJ, et al. *N Engl J Med* 354: 1567; 2006.
61. Basu, A, Devaraj, S, Jialal, I. *Arterioscler Thromb Vasc Biol* 26: 995; 2006.
62. Visser, M, Bouter, LM, McQuillan, GM, et al. *JAMA* 282: 2131; 1999.
63. Dietrich, M, Jialal, I. *Nutr Rev* 63: 22; 2005.
64. Liu, S, Manson, JE, Buring, JE, et al. *Am J Clin Nutr* 75: 492; 2002.
65. Wells, BJ, Mainous, AG, 3rd, Everett, CJ. *Nutrition* 21: 125; 2005.
66. Estruch, R, Sacanella, E, Badia, E, et al. *Atherosclerosis* 175: 117; 2004.
67. Shai, I, Rimm, EB, Schulze, MB, et al. *Diabetologia* 47: 1760; 2004.
68. Hasnain, BI, Mooradian, AD. *Cleve Clin J Med* 71: 327; 2004.
69. Vivekananthan, DP, Penn, MS, Sapp, SK, et al. *Lancet* 361: 2017; 2003.
70. Lee, IM, Cook, NR, Gaziano, JM, et al. *JAMA* 294: 56; 2005.
71. Brown, BG, Zhao, XQ, Chait, A, et al. *N Engl J Med* 345: 1583; 2001.
72. Stone, PH, Lloyd-Jones, DM, Kinlay, S, et al. *Circulation* 111: 1747; 2005.
73. Waters, DD, Alderman, EL, Hsia, J, et al. *JAMA* 288: 2432; 2002.
74. Kelemen, M, Vaidya, D, Waters, DD, et al. *Atherosclerosis* 179: 193; 2005.

Nutritional Treatment of Blood Pressure: Nonpharmacologic Therapy

L. Michael Prisant

CONTENTS

Blood pressure is a continuous variable like temperature and heart rate.[1] The level of blood pressure gradually increases from birth to age 18 years. The dividing line between normal and abnormal blood pressure is arbitrary. However, there is a continuous relationship between the level of blood pressure and various cardiovascular events, including myocardial infarction, strokes, chronic heart failure, renal failure, and mortality.[2] An optimal blood pressure is a systolic blood pressure less than 120 mmHg and diastolic blood pressure less than 80 mmHg. Hypertension is defined by the average of multiple measurements with either a systolic blood pressure ≥140 mmHg or a diastolic blood pressure ≥90 mmHg.

The hallmark of hypertension is an elevated systemic vascular resistance. Hypertension may be caused by various adrenal tumors producing cortisol, aldosterone and norepinephrine, hyperthyroidism, hypothyroidism, hyperparathyroidism with increased parathormone and calcium, acromegaly with increased growth hormone, renal failure, renal artery stenosis resulting in renal ischemia and increased renin, obstructive sleep apnea, and various drugs that cause salt and water retention, increase renin, or activate the sympathetic nervous system. The majority of patients with essential hypertension do not have a known cause.

Why does the prevalence of essential hypertension increase with aging, and what causes it to remain an enigma?[3] It is likely that what is called essential hypertension may be the result of diverse causes, including loss of distensibility of the aorta with ageing. Multiple factors alter the level of blood pressure. The sympathetic nervous system is important for modifying the tone of blood vessels. Circulating renin, angiotensin, aldosterone, norepinephrine, and endothelin are vasoconstrictors. The kidney is necessary to regulate sodium excretion and volume. Endothelial damage due to abnormal lipids, glucose intolerance, tobacco use, hyperinsulinemia, and circulating vasoconstrictors cause blood vessels to be less responsive to local endogenous vasodilators such as nitric oxide. Essential hypertension is not a homogenous disease state; it is likely a polygenic trait.

Hypertension affects 41.4% of blacks and 28.1% of whites in the U.S. adult population.[4] Since essential hypertension accounts for 90 to 95% of all causes and the prevalence increases with each decade of life, there is an interest in the role of nutrients and foods for both the etiology and treatment of hypertension. Epidemiologists and researchers advocate a primary prevention approach.

NUTRIENTS/FOODS AND BLOOD PRESSURE

SODIUM

A large body of data relates salt intake to the level of blood pressure. In a study using a colony of 26 chimpanzees that normally eat a fruit and vegetable diet (low sodium and high potassium intake), half had salt (up to 15 g/day) added gradually to their diet over 20 months.[5] Sodium chloride resulted in a blood pressure increase of 33/10 mmHg, which could be reversed within 6 months of removing sodium chloride from the diet. Similar studies have convinced the medical community that salt may be responsible for the higher prevalence of hypertension in modern society compared to more primitive communities. However, sodium may not be the sole culprit. Studies suggest that the chloride anion with sodium is necessary for an increase in blood pressure since giving sodium with other anions does not increase blood pressure.[6,7]

The INTERSALT (International Study of Salt and Blood Pressure) Cooperative group examined 10,079 men and women (20 to 59 years) by measuring urine sodium excretion and blood pressure at 52 centers throughout the world.[8] The average intake of sodium was between 100 and 200 mmol (6 to 12 g NaCl or 2.5 to 5 g sodium). The relationship of sodium excretion and systolic blood pressure correlated positively in 33 of 52 centers after correcting for age, gender, body mass index, alcohol consumption, and urine potassium excretion, but was significant in only eight centers. Negative correlations were observed in 19 centers. For the entire cohort, the adjusted effect of sodium for systolic blood pressure was +2.17 mmHg/100 mmol of 24-h sodium excretion ($p < .001$). There was not a significant adjusted effect for diastolic blood pressure. Among the centers with a low body mass index (21.8 kg/m^2) and a low sodium intake (26.7 mmol), the mean prevalence of hypertension was 1.7%. For the sites with a low body mass index (22.2 kg/m^2), but with a high sodium intake (187.7 mmol), the prevalence of hypertension was 11.9%.[9] Alternatively, the Scottish Heart Health Study of 7354 men and women aged 40 to 59 years reported a weak positive correlation of urinary sodium excretion and either systolic or diastolic blood pressure.[10] The correlation was not significant after adjustment for age, body mass index, alcohol consumption, and urinary-potassium excretion.

The implication of INTERSALT is that if the population reduces daily sodium intake by 100 mmol or 1 teaspoon of salt/day, the systolic blood pressure would decrease 2 to 3 mmHg.[9] This could have the potential to reduce coronary deaths by 4 to 5%, stroke deaths by 6 to 8%, and total mortality by 3 to 4%. The impact would be greater over a lifetime for a whole population, reducing total, coronary, and stroke mortality by 13, 16, and 23%, respectively. Processed foods contain excess sodium. The public policy sodium intake goal is 6 g/day.[11]

However, not every person's blood pressure increases with salt. Salt-sensitivity refers to those individuals whose blood pressure rises with increased salt intake and decreases with reduced salt intake. Perhaps, up to 50% of hypertensives are salt sensitive. The blood pressure response to sodium chloride is determined by genetic and environmental factors. African Americans, obese patients, low-renin hypertensives, chronic renal insufficiency patients, and the elderly may benefit more than other groups by reducing sodium intake.

To assess the impact of sodium chloride on blood pressure, trials have been conducted by either restricting or supplementing dietary sodium. Sodium supplementation trials are conducted less commonly (see Table 44.1).[12] In the Study of Sodium

TABLE 44.1
Randomized Double-Blind Trials of Sodium Supplementation

Author, Year	Study Group	Design	n	Group Differences in Na$^+$ Excretion, mEq/24 h	Sodium Effect on Blood Pressure (Δ Systolic/Δ Diastolic) mmHg
Australian National Council, 1989	Hypertensive	Parallel	103	43	+4.8/+2.8
Dodson, 1989	Hypertensive Type 2 Diabetes	Parallel	9	+76	+9.7/+5.1
McCarron, 1997	Hypertensive	Crossover	99	55	+4.9/+2.9
MacGregor, 1982	Hypertensive	Crossover	19	146	+10/+5
MacGregor, 1989	Hypertensive	Crossover	20		
High intake				141	+16/+9
Moderate intake				59	+8/+4
Mascioli, 1991	Normotensive	Crossover	48	60	+3.6/+2.3
Palmer, 1989	Elderly	Crossover	7	—	+11.0/+8.6
Watt, 1983	Hypertensive	Crossover	18	56	+0.5/+0.4

Source: Updated and modified from Mascioli.[12]

and Blood Pressure, 48 normotensive subjects participated in a randomized, double-blind crossover trial, using a placebo or 96 mEq sodium capsules in 4-week treatment periods, that was separated by a 2-week washout period.[12] Overnight urinary sodium excretion decreased 51-mEq/8 h from baseline to 9-mEq/8 h after the low-sodium-diet run-in period, before treatment periods were initiated. Differences in systolic and diastolic blood pressure between sodium and placebo treatment periods were significant: + 3.6 mmHg ($p < .001$) for systolic blood pressure and +2.3 mmHg ($p = .005$) for diastolic blood pressure. Sodium excretion increased + 20.4 meq/8 h ($p < .001$). Of the study participants, 65% and 69% experienced an increase of systolic and diastolic blood pressure, respectively, with the salt capsules.

A number of meta-analyses have sought to summarize the impact of sodium restriction on blood pressure.[13–23] One meta-analysis of 2635 subjects with 32 randomized trials on sodium reduction required random allocation, no confounding variables, an objective measure of a change in sodium intake (i.e., urine sodium excretion), and no adolescents,[17] updating an earlier analysis by the same authors.[14] The individual studies are listed in Table 44.2 and Table 44.3. The largest meta-analysis of 4294 subjects included 58 trials of hypertensive and 56 trials of normotensive persons.[18] The mean reduction of blood pressure by sodium restriction in hypertensive individuals was –3.9/–1.9 mmHg ($p < .001$ for both systolic and diastolic blood pressure) and in normotensives was –1.2/–0.26 mmHg ($p < .001$ for systolic only). Table 44.4 and Table 44.5 provide a comprehensive list of the trials used in that meta-analysis. The authors concluded that the cumulative blood-pressure-lowering effect has been stable since 1985 in individual sodium restriction trials of both normotensive and hypertensive populations. No future trials are likely to change the average treatment effect noted above.

The reduction of sodium intake for primary prevention as well as nonpharmacologic treatment of hypertension has become somewhat controversial in recent years.[24–27] In one study, 2937 hypertensive men on no medication for 3 to 4 weeks provided 24-h urine collections for sodium determination.[27] After 3.8 years of average follow-up, 117 cardiovascular events, including 55 myocardial infarctions, occurred. There was an inverse relationship between baseline urinary sodium excretion and myocardial infarction rate. A recent meta-analysis indicated that renin, aldosterone, norepinephrine, total cholesterol, and low-density

TABLE 44.2
Descriptive Summary of Sodium-Reduction Trials in Normotensive Subjects*

Author, Year	n	Duration, mo	Blinding	Δ Urinary Na, mmol/24 h	Changes in Confounders	Δ Systolic BP, mmHg	Δ Diastolic BP, mmHg
Crossover Trials							
Skrabal, 1981	20	0.5	NR	–170	Wt, (K)§	–2.7	–3.0
Cooper, 1984	113	2	BP obs	–68	Wt, (K)	–0.6	–1.4
Watt, 1985 (H)	35	1	DB	–74	(Wt), K	–1.4	1.2
Watt, 1985 (L)	31	1	DB	–60	(Wt), K	–0.5	1.4
Teow, 1985	9	0.5	BP obs	–210	(Wt), K	–0.6	–2.7
Myers, 1989	172	1	BP obs	–130	(Wt), (K)	–3.5†	–1.9†
Hargreaves, 1989	8	0.5	DB	–106	(Wt), (K)	–6.0†	–3.0†
Mascioli, 1991	48	1	DB	–20.2/8 h	NR	–3.6†	–2.3†
Parallel Trials‡							
Puska , 1983	19, 19‡	0.5	BP obs	–117	Wt, K, Alc, (P:S)	–1.5	–1.1
HPT, 1990	174, 177	36	BP obs (RZ)	–16	(Wt), K	0.1	0.2
Cobiac, 1992	26, 28	1	DB	–71	(Wt), (K)	–1.7	0.8
TOHP, 1992	327, 417	18	BP obs (RZ)	–44	(Wt), (K), (Ca), (Mg), (Alc), (fat)	–1.7†	–0.9†
Nestel, 1993 (Females)	15, 15	6	DB	–94	(Wt), (K)	–6.0†	–2.0†
Nestel, 1993 (Males)	17, 19	6	DB	–76	(Wt), (K)	–2.0†	–1.0†

* NR, not reported; Wt, body weight; K, potassium excretion; BP obs, observers blinded; H, high blood pressure; L, low blood pressure; DB, double blind; Alc, alcohol intake; P:S, ratio of polyunsaturated to saturated fat; HPT, Hypertension Prevention Trial; RZ, random zero manometer; TOHP, Trials of Hypertension Prevention; Ca, calcium intake; Mg, magnesium intake; fat, fat intake.

† $p < .05$.

‡ Values are the number of subjects in the sodium-reduction treatment and control groups, respectively.

§ Parentheses denote controlled factors; no parentheses denote possible confounders.

Source: Modified from Cutler.[17] Reproduced with permission from *Am J Clin Nutr.*, 65(2 Suppl): 643S–651S, 1997. Copyright *Am. J. Clin. Nutr.* American Society for Clinical Nutrition.

TABLE 44.3

Descriptive Summary of Sodium-Reduction Trials in Hypertensive Subjects*

Author, Year	n	Duration, mo	Blinding	Δ Urinary Na, mmol/24 h	Changes in Confounders	Δ Systolic BP, mmHg	Δ Diastolic BP, mmHg
Crossover Trials							
Parijs,1973	15	1	NR	−98	(Wt)[¶]	−6.7	3.2
MacGregor, 1982	19	1	DB	−76	Wt, (K)	−10.0[†]	−5.0[†]
Watt,1983	18	1	DB	−56	(Wt), (K)	0.5	−0.3
Richards, 1984	12	1–1.5	NR	−105	(Wt), K	−5.2	−1.8
Grobbee, 1987	40	1.5	DB	−72	(Wt), (K)	−0.8	−0.8
MacGregor, 1989	20	1	DB	−82	(Wt), (K)	−8.0[†]	−5.0[†]
Dodson,1989	9	1	DB	−76	(Wt), (K)	9.7[†]	−5.1
ANHMRC,1989	88	2	DB	−67	(K)	−2.6[†]	−2.1[†]
Benetos, 1992	20	1	DB	−78	(Wt), (K), (Ca)	−6.5[†]	−3.7[†]
Parallel Trials[‡]							
Morgan, 1978	31, 31[‡]	24	BP obs	−27	NR	−1.5[†]	−6.9[†]
Morgan,1981	6, 6	2	BP obs	−98	K	NR	−6.02
Morgan, 1981	6, 6	2	BP obs	−78	K	NR	−4.0
Costa, 1981	20, 21	12	NR	NR[§]	NR	−18.3[†]	−5.9[†]
Silman, 1983	10, 15	12	BP obs (RZ)	−53	(Wt), (K)	−8.7	−6.3
Puska, 1983	15, 19	1.5	BP obs	−117	Wt, K, Alc, (P:S)	1.8	0.5
Fagerberg, 1984	15, 15	2.3	NR	−89	(Wt), (K), (Alc)	−13.3[†]	−6.7[†]
Maxwell,1984	18, 12	3	NR	−171	Wt	−2.0	2.0
Erwteman,1984	44, 50	6	BP obs (RZ)	−58	NR	−2.7	−3.4[†]
Chalmers,1986	48, 52	3	NR	−54	(K)	−5.1[†]	−4.2[†]
Logan,1986	37, 38	6	BP obs	−32	Wt, (K)	−1.1	−0.2
Dodson, 1989	17, 17	3	BP obs	−59	(Wt), (K)	−13.0[†]	−1.8
ANHMRC, 1989	50, 53	2	DB	−71	(Alc)	−5.5[†]	−2.8[†]
Sciarrone, 1992	46, 45	2	DB	−84	(Wt), (K)	−6.0[†]	−1.0
Parker,1990, low ethanol	16, 15	1	DB	−80	(Wt), (Alc), (K), (Ca), (Mg)	2.2	0.5
Parker,1990, normal ethanol	15, 13	1	DB	−52	(Wt), (Alc), (K), (Ca), (Mg)	−0.1	0.8

* NR, not reported; Wt, body weight; DB, double blind; K, potassium intake/excretion: ANHMRC, Australian National Health and Medical Research Council; Ca, calcium intake/excretion; BP obs, observers blinded: RZ, random zero manometer; Alc, alcohol intake; P:S, ratio of polyunsaturated to saturated fatty acid; Mg, magnesium excretion.

[†] $p < .05$.

[‡] *n* values given for each study are the number of subjects in the sodium-reduction treatment and control groups, respectively.

[§] −23% intracellular sodium.

[¶] Parentheses denote controlled factors; no parentheses denote possible confounders.

Source: Modified from Cutler.[17] Reproduced with permission from *Am J Clin Nutr.,* 65(2 Suppl): 643S–651S, 1997. Copyright *Am. J. Clin. Nutr.* American Society for Clinical Nutrition.

lipoprotein cholesterol increased with sodium restriction.[18] Other hazards of moderate sodium restriction include a potential rise in blood pressure in 15% of patients, increased sympathetic activity and sleep disturbances, the potential of simultaneous restriction of grain products, meat, poultry, and fish, and dairy products (which provide ~50% of sodium intake), decreased iodine intake, decreased susceptibility of the elderly to respond to blood loss or heat stress, and the potential for fetal growth retardation during pregnancy.[26]

POTASSIUM

Intracellular potassium is the major cation that is responsible for establishing the membrane potential. The blood pressure of normotensives increases with potassium depletion.[28] Observational studies suggest an inverse relationship between potassium intake and blood pressure.[29] Often, there is an inverse relationship with dietary potassium and sodium or a positive relationship between urinary Na^+/K^+ ratio and blood pressure.[8,29] In the Scottish Heart Health Study, the relationship between blood

TABLE 44.4

Characteristics of Trials of Sodium Restriction and Blood Pressure in Normotensive Populations*

Author, Year	Design	Duration, Days	n	Age, year	NU	SR	CI	Cum SR	CI	Effect SBP	CI	Effect DBP	CI	Cum SBP	CI	Cum DBP	CI	Z SBP	Z DBP
Bruun, 1990	Op, CO	4	10	46	1	341	41	131	5	5.0	11.1	1.0	8.7	1.1	0.8	0.3	0.7	3.6	1.1
Burnier, 1993	Op, CO	6	16	29	1	186	19	136	4	1.0	8.6	-0.5	6.3	1.4	0.6	0.4	0.5	4.7	1.9
Burnier, 1993	Op, CO	6	7	29	1	218	27	137	4	1.0	7.9	-1.2	10.3	1.4	0.6	0.4	0.5	4.7	1.8
Cobiac, 1992	DB, P	28	52	66	2	75	30	194	4	3.1	4.6	2.8	2.4	1.3	0.7	0.4	0.6	4.3	1.8
Cobiac, 1992	DB, P	28	54	67	2	73	30	192	4	2.7	4.6	-0.6	2.4	1.3	0.7	0.4	0.6	4.4	1.7
Cooper, 1984	SB, CO	24	54	16	1	72	24	107	9	-0.3	2.0	-0.7	3.0	1.3	1.2	2.7	1.2	1.3	2.6
Cooper, 1984	SB, CO	24	59	16	1	55	20	111	9	1.4	2.0	3.4	2.8	2.0	1.4	3.5	1.3	1.6	3.0
Dimsdale, 1990	Op, CO	5	19	34	2	183	14	129	6	-1.4	2.3	-4.1	2.1	1.2	0.8	0.5	0.8	3.7	1.6
Dimsdale, 1990	Op, CO	5	23	34	2	178	20	132	6	-1.0	3.9	-4.4	2.5	1.2	0.8	0.3	0.8	3.6	1.0
Donovan, 1993	SB, CO	5	8	36	1	152	17	164	3	2.0	10.0	-1.0	6.7	1.4	0.6	0.4	0.5	5.1	1.6
El Ashry, 1987	SB, CO	14	13	24	1	222	87	111	7	0.0	11.4	4.0	10.7	1.3	0.8	0.8	0.8	3.4	1.9
El Ashry, 1987	SB, CO	14	13	27	1	232	34	115	6	0.0	8.5	1.0	11.9	1.3	0.8	0.8	0.8	3.3	1.9
Feldmann, 1996	DB, CO	7	5	27	1	176	56	164	3	-5.0	3.9	-5.0	3.9	1.2	0.6	0.2	0.5	4.5	1.1
Fliser, 1993	SB, CO	8	8	25	2	190	13	167	3	1.3	8.8	1.3	8.8	1.4	0.6	0.3	0.5	4.9	1.5
Fliser, 1993	SB, CO	8	8	26	2	181	18	167	3	0.6	9.4	0.6	9.4	1.4	0.6	0.3	0.5	4.8	1.5
Friberg, 1990	Op, CO	13	10	33	3	117	32	120	6	0.0	0.0	1.0	4.5	1.4	0.8	1.0	0.8	4.0	2.4
Fuchs, 1987	Op, CO	9	11	20	3	93	19	111	6	1.1	10.0	-1.0	6.9	1.3	0.8	0.8	0.8	3.5	1.8
Fuchs, 1987	Op, CO	9	6	20	3	99	45	113	7	5.8	9.7	-3.0	9.8	1.3	0.8	0.8	0.8	3.6	1.9
Grey, 1996	DB, CO	7	34	23	1	133	18	164	3	-1.0	5.0	-1.0	3.0	1.4	0.6	0.3	0.5	5.0	1.5
Hargreaves, 1989	DB, CO	14	8	23	2	106	46	119	6	6.0	13.3	3.0	10.6	1.3	0.8	0.8	0.8	3.4	1.7
HPT, 1990	SB, P	1100	228	40	1	23	18	125	6	-0.3	2.6	-0.1	2.2	1.1	0.7	0.3	0.7	3.5	0.9
Lawton, 1988	Op, CO	6	13	24	1	313	44	119	6	2.0	7.8	-2.0	5.7	1.3	0.8	0.8	0.8	3.3	1.7
Mascioli, 1991	DB, CO	28	48	52	5	70	32	197	5	3.6	1.8	2.3	1.6	1.3	0.7	0.4	0.7	4.3	1.5
Miller, 1997	Op, CO	7	10	—	2	194	19	163	3	-1.0	9.3	-1.0	9.3	1.2	0.6	0.2	0.5	4.4	1.1
Miller, 1997	Op, CO	7	12	23	2	182	23	163	3	1.0	4.8	1.0	4.8	1.2	0.6	0.2	0.5	4.5	1.1
Mtabaji, 1990	Op, P	7	30	—	1	272	62	121	6	9.0	5.9	9.0	5.9	1.4	0.8	1.0	0.8	4.0	2.3
Myers, 1982	Op, CO	14	136	39	1	130	11	133	11	3.3	1.8	2.7	1.6	2.4	1.7	2.4	1.5	1.1	2.2
Nestel, 1993	DB, P	42	60	65	4	73	22	165	3	6.0	5.6	2.0	4.7	1.4	0.6	0.4	0.5	5.1	1.7
Nestel, 1993	DB, P	42	72	66	4	56	21	166	3	2.0	5.0	1.0	3.2	1.4	0.6	0.3	0.5	4.9	1.6
Puska, 1983	SB, P	72	38	40	3	90	21	123	10	1.5	8.6	2.1	5.0	2.4	1.7	2.2	1.5	1.1	2.2
Richards, 1986	SB, CO	4	8	36	4	181	50	114	7	2.0	10.6	-7.0	8.5	1.3	0.8	0.9	0.8	3.5	2.2
Ruppert, 1991	SB, CO	7	24	36	3	275	11	190	5	-6.0	3.3	-6.0	3.3	0.9	0.7	0.1	0.7	2.9	0.4
Ruppert, 1991	SB, CO	7	25	46	3	262	11	198	4	7.5	4.7	7.5	4.7	1.0	0.7	0.2	0.7	3.3	0.9
Ruppert, 1991	SB, CO	7	98	35	3	275	6	179	5	-0.3	3.0	-0.3	3.0	1.1	0.8	0.3	0.7	3.5	1.0
Ruppert, 1993	SB, CO	7	108	36	3	275	7	160	3	1.4	2.5	-1.2	1.7	1.4	0.6	0.4	0.5	5.2	2.1
Ruppert, 1993	SB, CO	7	25	35	3	280	11	165	3	-5.9	6.3	-8.0	3.8	1.4	0.6	0.3	0.5	4.9	1.5
Ruppert, 1993	SB, CO	7	30	46	3	270	9	146	4	12.6	6.6	5.6	3.3	1.4	0.6	0.4	0.5	5.1	2.3

Continued

TABLE 44.4
(Continued)

Author, year	Design	Duration, days	n	Age, year	NU	SR	CI	Cum SR	CI	Effect SBP	CI	Effect DBP	CI	Cum SBP	CI	Cum DBP	CI	Z SBP	Z DBP
Schmid, 1990	SB, CO	7	9	32	1	190	37	128	5	3.0	10.8	0.0	8.2	1.1	0.8	0.3	0.7	3.5	1.0
Schorr, 1996	DB, CO	28	16	64	2	61	17	162	3	1.0	13.6	0.0	7.5	1.2	0.6	0.2	0.5	4.4	1.0
Schorr, 1997	SB, CO	7	27	25	7	208	21	163	3	5.6	4.9	5.6	4.9	1.3	0.6	0.3	0.5	4.6	1.3
Schorr, 1997	SB, CO	7	76	25	7	208	12	165	3	-2.8	7.6	-2.8	7.6	1.2	0.6	0.3	0.6	4.5	1.2
Sharma, 1990	SB, CO	7	15	24	2	192	32	127	5	0.9	9.7	3.7	8.0	1.1	0.8	0.3	0.7	3.4	1.1
Sharma, 1991	SB, CO	6	10	24	3	247	40	198	4	6.4	9.1	5.9	6.7	1.1	0.7	0.2	0.7	3.7	1.1
Sharma, 1991	SB, CO	6	13	25	3	246	37	198	4	3.0	3.2	-0.5	3.6	1.1	0.7	0.2	0.7	3.6	0.9
Sharma, 1993	SB, CO	7	16	24	3	224	26	166	3	0.8	3.6	0.5	5.0	1.4	0.6	0.3	0.5	4.9	1.5
Skrabal, 1981	Op, CO	14	20	23	1	150	52	147	27	2.7	6.9	3.0	6.0	-2.7	4.3	0.7	3.8	-1.0	0.4
Skrabal, 1984	Op, CO	14	22	23	1	167	28	113	8	7.7	5.2	4.6	4.8	1.5	1.1	2.4	1.1	1.9	2.7
Skrabal, 1984	Op, CO	14	30	23	1	137	34	109	8	-1.4	4.5	-0.8	3.4	1.2	1.1	2.3	1.1	1.0	2.2
Skrabal, 1985	SB, CO	14	28	23	1	163	28	118	7	5.8	2.3	3.3	1.6	1.4	1.0	2.0	0.9	3.3	3.9
Skrabal, 1985	SB, CO	14	34	23	1	144	30	115	8	0.1	1.2	0.6	1.4	0.9	1.0	1.9	1.0	1.9	2.8
Steegers, 1991	SB, P	140	36	27	5	63	31	195	4	-2.0	9.6	-2.0	7.9	1.3	0.7	0.4	0.7	4.1	1.4
Sullivan, 1980	Op, CO	4	27	29	1	146	32	146	31	-7.1	6.1	-1.1	5.4	-7.1	5.8	-1.1	5.1	-2.2	-0.4
Teow, 1986	Op, CO	14	9	25	1	200	58	112	7	0.6	6.2	2.7	6.9	1.3	0.8	0.9	0.8	3.6	2.9
TOHP, 1992	SB, P	550	744	43	3	47	4	135	4	1.7	1.2	0.9	0.8	1.4	0.6	0.4	0.5	4.7	2.0
Watt, 1985	DB, CO	28	31	23	4	60	27	114	7	0.5	1.6	-1.4	1.8	1.3	0.9	1.4	0.9	3.4	3.3
Watt, 1985	DB, CO	28	35	22	4	75	22	111	7	1.4	1.4	-1.2	1.8	1.3	0.8	0.9	0.8	3.7	2.8

* Op: open label; SB: single blind; DB: double blind; P: parallel; CO: crossover; n: number of persons in trial; Age: mean age of persons in trial; NU: number of urine collections per person per treatment period; SR: sodium reduction, mmol/24 h; Cum: cumulative; CI: 95% confidence interval of previous column. SBP: systolic blood pressure; DBP: diastolic blood pressure; Z: summary statistic.

Source: Personal Communication from NA Graudal of unpublished data from his manuscript.[1]

TABLE 44.5
Characteristics of Trials of Sodium Restriction and Blood Pressure in Hypertensive Populations*

Author, Year	Design	Duration, Days	n	Age, Year	NU	SR	Cum CI	SR	CI	Effect SBP	CI	Effect DBP	CI	Cum SBP	CI	Cum DBP	CI	Z SBP	Z DBP
Ambrosioni, 1982	SB, CO	42	25	23	6	60	19	91	12.4	2.2	5.6	0.4	3.9	3.9	2.77	2.6	2.32	1.3	1.7
ANHMRC, 1989	Op, P	48	103	58	4	63	18	89	5.2	5.5	3.1	2.9	1.6	4.6	1.30	2.7	0.94	5.2	4.8
Beard, 1982	Op, P	84	90	48	3	124	20	95	9.8	5.2	7.0	3.4	4.2	5.4	2.32	3.0	1.78	2.2	2.5
Benetos, 1992	DB, CO	28	20	42	1	78	34	103	4.5	6.5	7.3	3.7	4.1	4.1	1.08	2.3	0.77	6.5	5.1
Bruun, 1990	Op, CO	4	12	47	1	331	32	103	4.6	8.0	9.0	4.0	9.0	4.2	1.18	2.4	0.86	5.8	4.8
Buckley, 1994	SB, CO	5	12	49	1	296	46	106	3.8	8.7	6.2	8.7	6.2	3.7	0.96	1.6	0.66	6.8	5.0
Cappuccio, 1997	DB, CO	30	47	67	2	83	21	118	3.7	7.3	3.9	3.2	2.1	3.9	0.85	1.9	0.57	7.7	6.0
Carney, 1991	DB, CO	42	11	54	4	102	74	106	4.6	1.0	17.4	-1.0	11.1	3.9	1.15	2.3	0.83	5.8	4.8
Chalmers, 1986	SB, P	84	100	53	6	70	23	91	6.4	4.8	4.7	4.2	1.9	3.3	1.56	2.3	1.04	3.0	3.5
Del Rio, 1993	DB, CO	14	30	49	1	151	17	106	4.3	1.4	6.5	0.5	3.9	4.0	1.07	2.2	0.76	6.5	5.1
Dimsdale, 1990	Op, CO	5	16	34	2	178	24	93	4.9	6.4	4.8	-2.0	5.3	4.9	1.26	2.7	0.90	6.0	5.0
Dimsdale, 1990	Op, CO	5	17	34	2	198	23	98	4.8	0.1	4.2	-0.8	4.5	4.6	1.22	2.6	0.88	6.0	4.9
Dodson, 1989	SB, P	90	34	62	3	44	41	90	5	13.0	16.6	1.8	6.8	4.8	1.29	2.8	0.92	5.8	5.2
Egan, 1991	DB, CO	7	27	39	1	194	26	106	4.6	1.1	2.9	1.1	2.9	3.9	1.13	2.3	0.83	5.9	4.8
Erwteman, 1984	SB, P	28	94	46	4	58	18	91	7.4	2.7	4.6	2.5	3.5	3.3	1.88	2.0	1.26	2.5	2.9
Fagerberg, 1984	Op, P	63	30	51	4	99	37	92	7.2	3.7	12	3.1	7.2	3.3	1.81	2.0	1.21	2.6	2.9
Feldmann, 1996	DB, CO	7	8	27	1	178	64	120	3.7	-2.0	5.2	-2.0	5.2	3.8	0.89	1.8	0.60	7.4	5.7
Ferri, 1996	DB, CO	14	61	47	2	264	17	120	3.7	7.4	3.2	3.5	2.1	3.9	0.89	1.8	0.61	7.6	5.9
Fotherby, 1993	DB, CO	35	17	73	2	79	28	105	3.8	8.0	7.0	0.0	4.0	3.6	0.97	1.5	0.66	6.5	4.7
Grobbee, 1987	DB, CO	42	40	24	4	72	13	88	5.8	0.8	5.4	0.8	4.5	3.1	1.51	2.3	1.06	3.0	3.5
Jula, 1994	Op, P	365	76	44	3	57	32	105	3.8	6.7	6.5	3.8	2.8	3.7	0.95	1.7	0.64	6.9	5.2
Koolen, 1984	Op, CO	14	20	41	2	213	34	97	8.4	6.5	10.7	4.9	5.5	3.4	2.16	1.9	1.42	2.2	2.5
Kurtz, 1987	DB, CO	7	5	58	2	217	46	91	5.7	16.0	5.5	8.4	5.5	4.7	1.45	2.6	1.03	4.6	4.3
Lawton, 1988	Op, CO	6	9	25	1	328	54	91	5.5	1.0	12.4	-4.0	11.5	4.4	1.38	2.6	0.99	4.7	4.4
Logan, 1986	Op, P	180	86	47	1	43	24	92	6.7	1.1	5.6	0.2	4.4	3.1	1.66	1.9	1.12	2.8	2.9
MacGregor, 1982	DB, CO	28	19	49	2	76	27	89	11.1	10.0	5.2	5.0	3.6	5.4	2.44	3.0	1.99	2.0	2.2
MacGregor, 1987	DB, CO	30	15	52	2	100	32	88	5.7	13.0	6.6	9.0	6.4	3.6	1.47	2.4	1.04	3.6	3.9
MacGregor, 1989	DB, CO	30	20	57	2	150	28	91	5.1	16.0	8.4	9.0	5.9	4.8	1.29	2.8	0.93	5.6	5.2
Mark, 1975	Op, CO	10	6	28	1	305	41	216	27.4	13.1	9.1	7.7	8.9	9.8	5.33	-0.1	3.64	2.7	0.4
Maxwell, 1984	Op, P	84	30	46	4	161	74	92	7.4	2.0	11.4	-2.0	7.6	3.3	1.84	1.9	1.23	2.5	2.8
McCarron, 1997	DB, CO	28	99	52	1	56	19	119	3.8	4.9	3.6	2.9	2.3	3.8	0.87	1.8	0.59	7.4	5.7
Morgan, 1978	SB, P	90	62	60	2	23	24	114	18.3	1.0	6.4	2.0	3.2	6.2	3.93	1.2	2.42	2.6	0.9
Morgan, 1981	SB, P	56	12	38	2	67	52	106	16.6	—	—	4.0	8.7	—	—	1.9	3.03	—	1.1
Morgan, 1981	SB, P	56	12	40	2	92	74	104	15.9	—	—	8.0	8.7	—	—	3.0	2.90	—	1.7
Morgan, 1987	SB, P	60	20	58	5	57	36	90	5.6	6.0	19.6	4.0	7.8	4.7	1.44	2.6	1.02	4.5	4.4
Morgan, 1988	SB, CO	14	16	63	1	50	31	89	5.5	3.0	3.2	4.0	4.3	4.5	1.39	2.7	0.99	4.7	4.6
Mühlhauser, 1996	DB, P	28	16	36	4	107	69	120	3.7	2.0	13.5	0.0	6.4	3.8	0.88	1.8	0.60	7.2	5.5
Overlack, 1995	DB, CO	7	11	61	3	240	23	109	3.9	9.9	7.8	9.9	7.8	3.9	0.95	1.8	0.63	7.4	5.8

Continued

TABLE 44.5 (Continued)

Author, year	Design	Duration, Days	n	Age, Year	NU	SR	Cum CI	SR	CI	Effect SBP	CI	Effect DBP	CI	Cum SBP	CI	Cum DBP	CI	Z SBP	Z DBP
Overlack, 1995	DB, CO	7	27	40	3	249	17	114	3.8	0.8	5.6	0.8	5.6	3.8	0.94	1.8	0.63	7.3	5.8
Overlack, 1995	DB, CO	7	8	43	3	234	36	115	3.7	-6.0	11.1	-6.0	11.1	3.7	0.93	1.7	0.63	7.1	5.6
Parijs, 1973	Op, CO	28	15	41	1	98	39	98	35.9	6.7	7.5	-3.2	4.7	6.7	6.86	-3.2	4.31	1.6	-1.2
Parker, 1990	DB, P	28	28	54	4	49	56	97	4.7	-1.9	6.1	-1.8	6.3	4.1	1.19	2.4	0.86	5.6	4.7
Parker, 1990	DB, P	28	31	50	4	73	33	97	4.8	-1.9	5.2	0.1	2.8	4.3	1.20	2.4	0.87	5.8	4.9
Puska, 1983	SB, P	72	34	40	3	90	23	91	8.6	-1.8	10.5	-0.5	5.8	3.3	2.07	1.8	1.46	2.0	2.3
Redon–Mas, 1993	Op, P	28	418	55	1	104	6	105	3.8	-1.0	2.5	-1.9	1.2	3.5	0.98	1.6	0.67	6.3	4.7
Resnick, 1985	Op, CO	5	12	—	1	190	36	96	7	3.0	5.9	1.0	5.0	3.3	1.74	1.9	1.17	2.7	2.9
Richards, 1984	SB, CO	28	12	36	2	100	29	97	8.1	4.0	5.6	3.0	4.2	3.4	2.05	2.0	1.35	2.4	2.7
Ruilope, 1993	DB, P	21	19	—	1	69	108	106	4.3	4.0	17.5	4.0	6.2	4.0	1.07	2.3	0.75	6.4	5.1
Schmid, 1990	SB, CO	7	9	36	1	181	31	99	4.7	6.0	16.3	1.9	9.9	4.1	1.19	2.4	0.86	5.7	4.7
Sciarrone, 1992	DB, P	56	91	54	1	82	14	104	4.5	5.8	4.1	0.4	2.9	4.0	1.09	2.2	0.79	6.4	4.9
Shore, 1988	SB, CO	5	6	—	5	97	52	91	5.4	9.0	16.3	5.6	14.5	4.5	1.37	2.6	0.99	4.8	4.4
Silman, 1983	Op, P	90	28	55	4	63	51	91	9	-3.5	23.2	-0.5	5.9	3.5	2.14	1.9	1.52	2.1	2.4
Singer, 1991	DB, CO	30	21	54	2	91	37	106	4.7	9.0	6.3	3.0	4.2	4.0	1.13	2.3	0.81	6.1	4.9
Sullivan, 1980	Op, CO	4	19	27	1	153	39	121	17.3	-1.2	7.6	1.2	8.5	4.6	3.55	1.2	3.16	2.2	0.9
Watt, 1983	DB, CO	28	18	52	4	56	30	92	9.2	0.5	3.2	0.3	1.9	3.6	2.07	2.0	1.58	2.3	2.5
Weir, 1995	SB, CO	14	11	60	5	127	94	106	3.9	-4.0	15.8	-5.0	8.0	3.8	0.96	1.7	0.63	7.1	5.5
Weir, 1995	SB, CO	14	11	60	5	146	68	106	3.8	9.0	17.4	7.0	8.0	3.8	0.96	1.8	0.64	7.2	5.7
Zoccali, 1994	SB, CO	7	15	45	1	163	43	106	3.8	14.0	10.7	8.0	4.8	3.8	0.95	1.7	0.64	7.2	5.6

* Op: open; SB: single blind; DB: double blind; P: parallel; CO: crossover; n: number of persons in trial; Age: mean age of persons in trial; n: number of urine collections per person per treatment period; SR: sodium reduction, mmol/24 h; Cum: cumulative; CI: 95% confidence interval of previous column. SBP: systolic blood pressure; DBP: diastolic blood pressure; Z: summary statistic.

Source: Personal Communication from NA Graudal of unpublished data from his manuscript.[18]

pressure and the urinary Na^+/K^+ ratio was stronger than the relationship between blood pressure and the excretion of sodium or potassium individually.[10] After adjusting for age, gender, body mass index, ethanol intake, and urinary sodium intake, the INTERSALT study reported that the systolic blood pressure was 2.7 mmHg lower for each 60 mmol/day higher excretion of potassium.[8] Since African Americans have a lower intake of potassium due to decreased consumption of fresh fruits and vegetables, this observation has been offered as an explanation of the higher prevalence of hypertension among blacks compared to whites.[29–32] Potassium supplementation (80 mmol/day), compared to placebo, reduced systolic and diastolic blood pressure (–6.9/–2.5 mmHg) significantly in African Americans consuming a diet low in potassium for 21 days.[33]

Whether anions other than chloride with potassium supplementation lower blood pressure have been studied and found to lower blood pressure in many studies.[34–36] Explanations for the hypotensive effects of potassium include direct vasodilatation, a direct natriuretic effect, altered baroreceptor function, increased urinary kallikrein, or suppression of the renin–angiotensin–aldosterone axis or sympathetic nervous system.[11]

Studies using the Dahl salt-sensitive rat show a protective effect of potassium supplementation, reducing mortality by 93% in the hypertensive rats.[37] In a 12-year prospective population study of 859 older persons, the relative risk of stroke-associated mortality in the lowest tertile of potassium intake, as compared with that in the top two tertiles combined, was 2.6 times higher in men ($p = .16$) and 4.8 times higher in women ($p = .01$).[38] A 10-mmol increase in daily potassium decreased stroke-associated mortality by 40% ($p < .001$) in a multivariate analyses. In the Health Professionals Follow-up Study, a multivariate analysis demonstrated that the greater the potassium intake, the lower the relative risk of stroke ($p = .007$) (Figure 44.1).[39] Furthermore, the use of potassium supplements, especially among men taking diuretics, was inversely related to the risk of stroke. However, after further adjustment for fiber and magnesium intake, the relative risk of stroke was similar, but no longer statistically significant.

There have been several meta-analyses examining potassium supplementation.[40–42] The largest meta-analysis (see Table 44.6 and Table 44.7) observed a significant reduction in both systolic and diastolic blood pressure (–4.44/–2.45 mmHg, $p < .01$ for both) for oral potassium supplementation.[41] There was a greater decrease in blood pressure (–4.91/–2.71 mmHg, $p < .01$ for both systolic and diastolic) when trials were examined that achieved a net change in urinary potassium 20 mmol/day or greater. If trials excluded concomitant antihypertensive drugs, the change in blood pressure was –4.85/–2.71 mmHg ($p < .01$ for both). The change in blood pressure was lower for normotensives (–1.8/–1.0 mmHg) compared with hypertensives (–4.4/–2.5 mmHg) patients. The change for systolic blood pressure among black subjects was greater than white subjects (–5.6 vs. –2.0 mmHg, $p = .03$); however, the change for diastolic blood pressure was not significant (–3.0 vs. –1.1 mmHg, $p = .19$).

Interestingly, there was no overall association between 24-h urinary potassium excretion and change in systolic or diastolic blood pressure; however, the higher the urinary sodium excretion at follow-up (see Figure 44.2), the greater the decline in both systolic ($p < .001$) and diastolic blood pressure ($p < .001$).[41] This explains the lack of benefit seen in a study that combined sodium restriction and potassium supplementation in patients.[43] This randomized, placebo-controlled, double-blind trial of 287 men assessed the effect of 96 mmol of microcrystalline potassium chloride or placebo on a sodium-restricted diet. After the withdrawal of their antihypertensive medication at 12 weeks, there was no significant difference in either systolic or diastolic blood pressure between the two groups at any point in time up to an average of 2.2 years.[43]

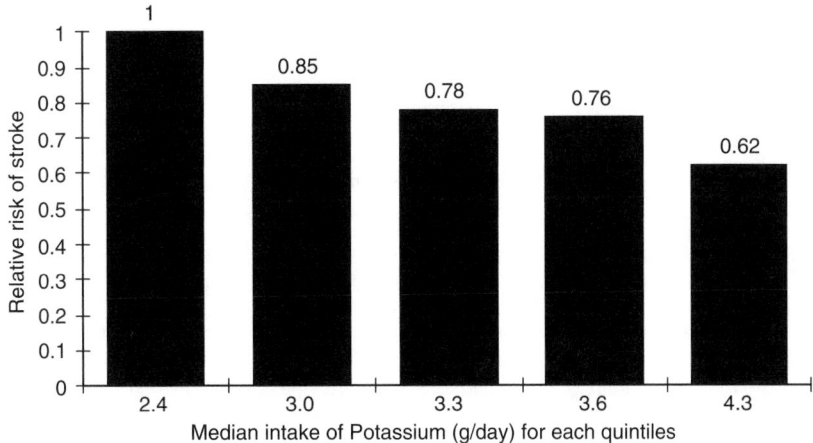

FIGURE 44.1 Multivariate-adjusted relative risk of stroke of 43,738 U.S. men, 40 to 75 years by quintile of potassium intake: Adjusted for age, total energy intake, smoking, alcohol consumption, history of hypertension and hypercholesterolemia, family history of premature myocardial infarction, profession, body mass index, and physical activity ($p = .007$ for trend). With permission from Ascherio.[39]

TABLE 44.6

Participant and Study Design Characteristics in 33 Potassium Supplementation Trials

Left Panel

Author, Year	Number of Subjects	Mean Age, Years	Age Range, Years	% Male	% White	% HTN[†]	Anti-HTN Medication	Study Design*	Study Duration, Weeks
Skrabal, 1981									
(a)	20	—	21–25	100	—	0	No	XO	2
(b)	20	—	21–25	100	—	0	No	XO	2
MacGregor, 1982	23	45	26–66	52	78	100	No	XD	4
Khaw and Thom, 1982	20	—	22–35	100	—	0	No	XD	2
Richards, 1984	12	—	19–52	67	—	100	No	XO	4–6
Smith, 1985	20	53	30–66	55	90	100	No	XD	4
Kaplan, 1985	16	49	35–66	38	19	100	Yes[‡]	XD	6
Zoccali, 1985	19	38	26–53	53	100	100	No	XD	2
Bulpitt, 1985	33	55	—	45	—	100	Yes[‡]	PO	12
Matlou, 1986	32	51	34–62	0	0	100	No	XS	6
Barden, 1986	44	32	18–55	0	—	0	No	XD	4
Poulter and Sever, 1986	19	—	18–47	100	0	0	No	XD	2
Chalmers, 1986									
(a)	107	52	—	85	—	100	No	PO	12
(b)	105	52	—	86	—	100	No	PO	12
Grobbee, 1987	40	24	18–28	85	—	100	No	XD	6
Siani, 1987	37	45	21–61	62	—	100	No	PD	15
Svetkey, 1987	101	51	—	74	88	100	No	PD	8
Medical Research Council, 1987	484	—	35–64	56	—	100	Yes[‡]	PS	24
Grimm, 1988	312	58	45–68	100	—	100	Yes[‡]	PD	12
Cushman and Langford, 1988	58	54	26–69	100	47	100	No	PD	10
Obell, 1989	48	41	23–56	44	0	100	No	PD	16
Krishna, 1989	10	—	20–40	100	100	0	No	XD	10 day
Hypertension Prevention Trial, 1990	391	39	25–49	64	83	0	No	PO	3 year
Mullen and O'Connor, 1990									
(a)	24	25	22–31	100	9	0	No	XD	2
(b)	24	25	22–31	100	92	0	No	XD	2
Patki, 1990	37	50	—	22	—	100	No	XD	8
Valdes, 1991	24	50	—	54		100	No	XD	4
Barden, 1991	37	32	—	0		0	No	XD	4 day
Overlack, 1991	12	37	25–59	67	—	100	No	XS	8
Smith, 1992	22	67	≥60	57	71	100	No	XD	4 day
Fotherby and Potter, 1992	18	75	66–79	28	—	100	No	XD	4
Whelton, 1995	353	43	30–54	72	86	0	No	PD	24
Brancati, 1996	87	48	27–65	36	0	0	No	PD	3

* XO indicates crossover open; XS, crossover single blind; XD, crossover double blind; PO, parallel open; PS, parallel single blind; PD, parallel double blind; No data indicated by—

[†] HTN indicates hypertensive; BP indicates blood pressure; SBP, systolic BP; and DBP, diastolic BP. Sitting BP was used in the studies by Khaw and Thom, Matlou, Poulter and Sever, Chalmers, Svetkey, Grimm, Hypertension Prevention Trial, Barden, and Overlack.

[‡] Study participants were treated with thiazide or thiazide-like diuretics, hydrochlorothiazide 25–75 mg/day or chlorthalidone 50 mg/day, and in addition, clonidine 0.1 mg twice daily in one subject (Kaplan); bendrofluazide 2.5–10 mg/day, cyclopenthiazide 25–50 mg/day, hydrochlorothiazide 25 mg/day, furosemide 40–80 mg/day, and chlorthalidone 50–100 mg/day (Bulpitt); bendrofluazide 5–10 mg/day (Medical Research Council); chlorthalidone or hydrochlorothiazide (84%), β-blockers (43%) other medications, for example, reserpine (6%), hydralazine (6%), and methyldopa (5%): doses not specified (Grimm).

Source: Table Modified from Whelton PK.[41] Reproduced with permission from May 28, *JAMA*, 277(20): 1624–1632, 1997. Copyright 1997, American Medical Association.

Continued

TABLE 44.6
(Continued)

Right Panel

Intervention	Control	Baseline Supine BP, mmHg[†]	Baseline Urinary Electrolytes, mmol/Day K^+/Na^+	Baseline K^+ mmol/L
200 mmol K from diet, 200 mmol NaCl	80 mmol KCl, 200 mmol NaCl	—	—/—	4.7
200 mmol K from diet, 50 mmol NaCl	80 mmol KCl, 50 mmol NaCl	—	—/—	4.6
64 mmol KCl	Placebo	154/99	68/152	4.0
64 mmol KCl	Placebo	118/74	73/138	—
200 mmol K from diet, 180 mmol NaCl	60 mmol KCl,180 mmol NaCl	140–180/90–105	—/—	3.8
64 mmol KCI, 70 mmol NaCl	Placebo,70 mmol NaCl	163/103	72/68	3.9
60 mmol KCI	Placebo	131/96	46/166	3.0
100 mmol KCI	Placebo	154/96	—/—	3.8
64 mmol KCl	Usual care	150/95	66/...	3.7
65 mmol KCl	Placebo	154/105	62/172	3.8
80 mmol KCl	Placebo	118/71	50/131	—
64 mmol KCl	Placebo	113/69	39/123	—
100 mmol K from diet	Normal diet	150/95	71/155	—
100 mmol K from diet, low Na	Low Na	152/95	68/148	—
72 mmol KCI, low Na	Placebo, low Na	143/78	71/141	3.8
48 mmol KCI	Placebo	145/92	60/190	4.4
120 mmol KCI	Placebo	145/95	—/—	4.4
17–34 mmol KCl	Usual care	161/98	—/—	4.2
96 mmol KCI, low Na	Placebo, low Na	124/80	79/166	4.2
80 mmol KCl	Placebo	150/95	52/176	—
64 mmol KCl	Placebo	174/100	59/171	4.0
90 mmol KCI	10 mmol KCl	120/77	70/164	3.2
100 mmol K from diet, low Na	Low Na	124/82	64/161	—
75 mmol KCI	Placebo	117/69	77/153	4.2
75 mmol K citrate	Placebo	117/69	77/153	4.2
60 mmol KCl	Placebo	155/100	62/196	3.6
64 mmol KCl	Placebo	147/96	57/155	3.8
80 mmol KCl	Placebo	105/63	53/105	—
120 mmol K citrate and bicarbonate	Placebo	150/100	62/169	4.4
120 mmol KCI	Placebo	152/87	70/192	3.9
60 mmol KCl	Placebo	187/96	63/115	4.2
60 mmol KCl	Placebo	122/81	59/153	—
80 mmol KCl	Placebo	125/78	47/147	—

Source: Reproduced with permission from May 28, *JAMA*, 277(20):1624–1632, 1997.[41] Copyright 1997, American Medical Association.

CALCIUM

Most body calcium is found in the skeleton. Calcium is important for its role in smooth muscle relaxation and contraction, especially the vascular smooth muscle that alters peripheral vascular resistance directly. An inverse relationship between water hardness and blood pressure has stimulated an interest in the role of calcium supplementation on blood pressure.[44] Paradoxically, data from the first Health and Nutrition Examination Survey found that daily calcium intake was lower in 1012 hypertensive vs. 8541 normotensive persons (608 vs. 722 mg, $p < .01$).[45] However, it was not associated with blood pressure when age and body mass index were controlled. For 58,218 women nurses with a calcium intake of at least 800 mg/day, the reduction in the risk of hypertension was 22% when compared with an intake of less than 400 mg/day.[46] For men, calcium was inversely associated with baseline blood pressure but not with a change in blood pressure; furthermore, intake of calcium in men was not inversely associated with an increase risk of stroke.[39,47] Other observational studies have reported both positive and negative correlations with blood pressure, but many studies did not adjust for weight and alcohol, vitamin D, sodium, and other nutrient intake and are based on dietary recall.[48] Also, it has been suggested that calcium supplementation is important in African Americans since intake of dairy products is especially low and the prevalence of hypertension much higher than Caucasians. In addition, sodium

TABLE 44.7
Urinary Electrolyte Excretion, Body Weight, and Blood Pressure during Follow-up in 33 Potassium Supplementation Trials*

Author, Year	Mean Net Change in Urinary Electrolytes, K⁺/Na⁺, mmol/Day	Urinary Sodium Excretion During Follow-up, mmol/Day	Mean Net Change in Body Weight, kg	Mean Net Change in Blood Pressure, Systolic/Diastolic, mmHg
Skrabal, 1981				
(a)	44/–55	155	–0.9	–1.7/–4.5
(b)	107/–12	28	–0.2	0.4/–0.5
MacGregor, 1982	56/29	169	–0.2	–7.0/–4.0
Khaw and Thom, 1982	52/9	164	—	–1.1/–2.4
Richards, 1984	129/5	200	0.8	–1.9/–1.0
Smith, 1985	50/7	80	0.1	–2.0/0
Kaplan, 1985	46/1	168	0.8	–5.6/–5.8
Zoccali, 1985	81/13	195	—	–1.0/–3.0
Bulpitt et al, 1985	40/10	149	1.2	2.3/4.8
Matlou et al, 1986	62/35	165	–0.4	–7.0/–3.0
Barden et al, 1986	68/5	130	—	–1.4/–1.4
Poulter and Sever, 1986	38/1	114	–0.1	–1.2/2.0
Chalmers et al, 1986				
(a)	22/7	150	—	–3.9/–3.1
(b)	12/25	79	—	–1.0/1.6
Grobbee, 1987	57/12	69	0.4	–2.5/–0.6
Siani, 1987	30/6	189	—	–14.0/–10.5
Svetkey, 1987	—/—	—	—	6.3/–2.5
Medical Research Council, 1987	—/—	—	—	0.8/–0.7
Grimm, 1988	80/–9	114	—	0.7/1.4
Cushman and Langford, 1988	36/177	177	—	—/–0.1
Obel, 1989	39/—	172	—	–41.0/–17.0
Krishna, 1989	47/44	144	–0.6	5.5/–7.4
Hypertension Prevention Trial, 1990	0/–6	155	0.2	–1.3/–0.9
Mullen and O'Connor, 1990				
(a)	23/–12	141	–0.1	0/3.0
(b)	34/–15	138	–0.2	–2.0/2.0
Patki, 1990	22/–14	184	—	–12.1/–13.1
Valdes, 1991	68/19	166	–1	–6.3/–3.0
Barden, 1991	72/15	120	—	–1.7/–0.6
Overlack, 1991	105/–13	156	0	2.8/3.0
Smith et al, 1992	109/29	221	0.2	–4.3/–1.7
Fotherby and Potter, 1992	39/13	136	–0.7	–10.0/–6.0
Whelton, 1995	42/6	144	—	–0.3/0.1
Brancati, 1996	70/20	141	–0.1	–6.9/–2.5

No data indicated by—

Source: Table Modified from Whelton PK et al.[41] Reproduced with permission from May 28, *JAMA*, 277(20): 1624–1632, 1997. Copyright 1997, American Medical Association.

excretion and calcium intake interact in salt-sensitive individuals: increased ingested calcium facilitates sodium excretion.[49] Calcium supplementation is associated with controversy because of the association of hyperparathyroidism and hypertension, the pressor effect of hypercalcemia in normotensives, and the direct relationship of calcium and blood pressure.[50] However, responders to calcium supplementation may be a subset of hypertensives with a low renin level, high parathormone level, and low ionized calcium.[49]

In a randomized, double-blind study of 48 hypertensive persons and 32 normotensive persons, 1000 mg/day of calcium or placebo was given for 8 weeks.[51] Supine blood pressure decreased significantly –3.8/–2.3 mmHg in the hypertensive subjects; 25%, 23%, and 13% of subjects achieved a blood pressure goal of systolic less than 140 mmHg, diastolic less than 90 mmHg and

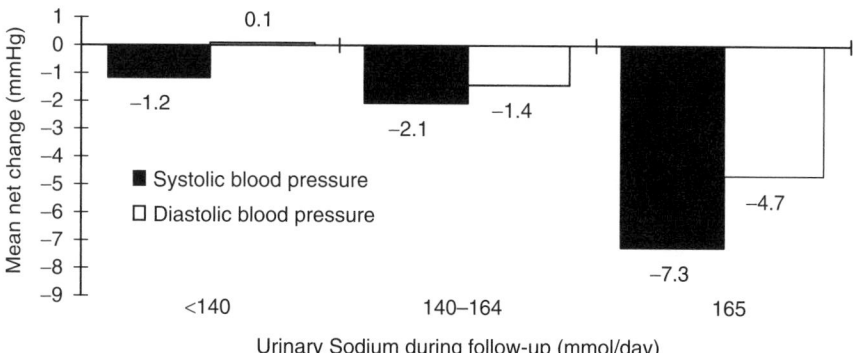

FIGURE 44.2   Effect of potassium supplementation on net blood pressure reduction according urinary sodium excretion during follow up: The greater the sodium excretion, the greater the blood pressure reduction with potassium supplementation ($p <.001$ for both systolic and diastolic blood pressure). With permission from Whelton.[41]

both systolic and diastolic less than 140/90 mmHg, respectively. Calcium did not lower blood pressure in the normotensives. Forty-four percent of hypertensive and 19% of normotensive subjects lowered their standing systolic blood pressure greater than 10 mmHg.

There have been at least 67 randomized trials of calcium supplements in nonpregnant study populations. There have been several meta-analyses to assess the effect of dietary and nondietary interventions on blood pressure.[48,52–57] A larger effect of calcium supplementation on systolic blood pressure was observed with increasing age and among women.[54] The subgroup of hypertensive subjects had a greater reduction in blood pressure than the normotensives (–4.30/–1.50 vs. –0.27/–0.33 mmHg).[55] The change in systolic and diastolic blood pressure was significant for the hypertensives, but not the normotensives.[55] The largest meta-analysis (see Table 44.8 and Table 44.9) reported a reduction of blood pressure of –1.44/–0.84 mmHg ($p < .001$ for each).[56] There was no difference in the change in blood pressure comparing 33 nondietary trials (–1.09/–0.87 mmHg) and the nine dietary trials (–2.01/–1.09 mmHg). The authors concluded that the small reduction in blood pressure of calcium supplements did not merit its use in mild hypertension, and further suggested that the use of calcium must weigh the benefits of reducing cardiovascular disease and increasing bone density vs. the risk of nephrolithiasis.

Despite this modest benefit in nonpregnant subjects, a meta-analysis (see Table 44.10 and Table 44.11) of calcium supplementation in pregnancy observed a blood pressure reduction of –5.40/–3.44 mmHg and a decrease in the rate of preeclampsia (odds ratio = 0.38, 95% CI: 0.22 to 0.65).[57] Since the publication of the meta-analysis, the National Institutes of Health sponsored trial, Calcium for Preeclampsia Prevention, has been completed.[58] This placebo-controlled, randomized, multicenter trial assigned 4589 nulliparous women 13 to 21 weeks pregnant to 2 g of calcium carbonate or placebo. There was no benefit on the rate of preeclampsia (6.9 vs. 7.3%), the prevalence of gestational hypertension (15.3 vs. 17.3%) or pregnancy-associated proteinuria (3.4 vs. 3.3%) in the calcium ($n = 2295$) and placebo ($n = 2294$) groups.

MAGNESIUM

Magnesium is a divalent intracellular cation. The adult body contains about 25 g distributed between the skeleton (60%) and soft tissues (40%).[59] It serves as a cofactor for many enzyme systems. Intracellular calcium increases and blood pressure rises as magnesium depletion occurs in rats. The hypotensive effect of magnesium is observed best when given in preeclampsia and toxemia. Magnesium supplementation in 400 normotensive primigravida women given 13 to 24 weeks gestation did not lower blood pressure or the incidence of preeclampsia.[60] However, among 2138 hypertensive women admitted in labor, intramuscular magnesium sulfate was superior to phenytoin in preventing eclamptic seizures (0 vs. 0.92%, $p = .004$).[61]

Magnesium and calcium contributes to water hardness. There is an inverse relationship between water hardness[62] and blood pressure.[63,64] However, epidemiologic studies assessing the role of magnesium and blood pressure often do not control for potential confounders, including caloric, ethanol, sodium, potassium, and calcium intake and use of antihypertensive medication.[64] Thus, observational studies using 24-h dietary recall, food records, and food frequency questionnaires have not always shown a consistent correlation, but they generally show a negative correlation with both systolic and diastolic blood pressure after adjustment.[64] In the Health Professionals Follow-up Study, the relative risk of a stroke among 43,738 men between the lowest quintile of magnesium intake and highest quintile, after adjustment for age, body mass index, various risk factors, family history, profession, and physical activity, was 0.62 ($p < .002$).[39] In the Atherosclerosis Risk in Communities Study of four U.S. communities ($n = 15,248$ participants), an early report suggested a low serum and dietary magnesium may be related to the etiology of hypertension; however, a subsequent report found no association between dietary magnesium intake and incident hypertension.[65,66]

TABLE 44.8
Randomized Controlled Trials Examining the Relationship of Calcium on Blood Pressure

Study Design, Author, Year	No. of Subjects (Active/Control)	Quality Score*	Calcium Formulation	Elemental Calcium, mg/Day	Study Duration, Weeks
Nondietary Interventions					
Belizan, 1983	30/27	4	Calcium gluconate	1000	22
Sunderrajan, 1984[cx]	17/17	0	Calcium carbonate	1000	4
Johnson, 1985	59/56	2	Calcium carbonate	1500	208
McCarron, 1985[cx]	80/80	3	Calcium carbonate	1000	8
Grobbee, 1986	46/44	4	Calcium citrate	1000	12
Nowson, 1986	31/33	3	Calcium carbonate	1600	8
Resnick, 1986[cx, ci]	8/8	0	Calcium carbonate	2000	8
Strazzullo, 1986[cx, ci]	17/17	3	Calcium gluconate	1000	15
Van Berestyn, 1986	29/29	3	Calcium carbonate	1500	6
Cappuccio, 1987[cx]	18/18	4	Calcium gluconate	1600	4
Lyle, 1987	37/38	4	Calcium carbonate	1500	12
Meese, 1987[cx]	19/17	3	Calcium carbonate	800	8
Siani, 1987[cx]	8/8	4	Calcium gluconate	1000	3
Thomsen, 1987	14/14	3	Calcium gluconate	2000	52
Vinson, 1987	4/5	4	Calcium carbonate	500	7
Zoccali, 1987[cx, ci]	11/11	3	Calcium gluconate	1000	2
Siani, 1988[cx]	14/14	5	Calcium gluconate	1000	4
Zoccali, 1988[cx]	21/21	3	Calcium gluconate	1000	8
Orwoll, 1990[ci]	34/28	3	Calcium carbonate	1000	156
Tanji, 1991[cx]	28/28	3	Calcium carbonate	1200	12
Cutler, 1992	237/234	6	Calcium carbonate	1000	26
Lyle, 1992	21/21	3	Calcium carbonate	1500	8
Galloe, 1993[cx]	20/20	4	Calcium gluconate	2000	12
Jespersen, 1993[cx]	7/7	5	Calcium carbonate	1000	8
Pan, 1993[cx]	14/15	1	Calcium citrate and placebo Vitamin D	800	11
Weinberger, 1993[cx]	46/46	4	Calcium carbonate	1500	8
Petersen, 1994[ci]	10/10	1	Calcium gluconate	2000	26
Zhou, 1994	30/27	3	Calcium carbonate	1000	14
Gillman, 1995	51/50	4	Calcium citrate malate	600	12
Sacks, 1995[ci]	34/31	5	Calcium carbonate	1000	26
Lijnen, 1996[ci]	16/16	5	Calcium gluconate	2000	16
Davis, 1997	17/17	3	Calcium gluconate	1500	4
Sanchez, 1997	10/10	4	Calcium gluconate	1500	8
Dietary Interventions					
Margetts, 1986[cx, ci]	39/39	3	Other dietary manipulation	1076	6
Rouse, 1986	18/18	3	Other dietary manipulation	1177	6
Bierenbaum, 1988[cx]	50/50	1	Milk/dairy product supplement	1150	26
Morris, 1988	142/139	4	Other dietary manipulation	1500	12
Hakala, 1989	31/37	3	Other dietary manipulation	1163	52
Van Beresteijn, 1990	28/25	3	Milk/dairy product supplement	1180	6
Kynast-Gales, 1992[cx]	7/7	1	Milk/dairy product supplement	1515	4
McCarron, 1997	274/274	4	Milk/dairy product supplement	1886	10
Appel, 1997	151/154	4	Milk/dairy product suppl	1265	8

[cx] crossover study; [ci] cointervention.

* A quality score of six corresponds to the highest quality level.

Source: Modified with permission from Griffith LE, et al., *Am J Hypertens.*[56]

TABLE 44.9
Randomized Controlled Trial Studying the Effect of Calcium Supplementation on Blood Pressure

Author, Year	Position of Blood Pressure Measurement	Mean BP at Study End*	Systolic Mean Baseline, mmHg	Systolic Mean Difference, mmHg (SD)[†]	Mean Diastolic Baseline, mmHg	Diastolic Mean Difference, mmHg (SD)[†]
Nondietary Interventions						
Belizan, 1983						
Women	Lateral	1	102	−2.40 (1.03)	68	−4.50 (1.46)
Men	Lateral	1	113	−0.80 (1.05)	71	−6.00 (1.94)
Sunderrajan, 1984						
Normotensive	Sitting	2	NA	1.89 (2.78)	NA	1.89 (2.50)
Hypertensive	Sitting	2	NA	−1.63 (5.93)	NA	−4.13 (2.50)
Johnson, 1985						
Normotensive	Sitting	2	120	0.00 (3.01)	74	0.00 (1.67)
Hypertensive	Sitting	2	141	−13.0 (6.52)	86	0.00 (2.79)
McCarron, 1985						
Normotensive	Standing	2	113	1.30 (2.00)	75	1.00 (2.62)
Hypertensive	Standing	2	144	−5.60 (2.10)	92	−2.30 (1.40)
Grobbee, 1986	Sitting	1	143	−0.40 (2.27)	83	−2.40 (1.90)
Nowson, 1986						
Normotensive	Sitting	1		0.00 (2.97)		0.30 (2.33)
Hypertensive	Sitting	1	157	1.60 (3.83)	92	1.30 (2.90)
Resnick, 1986						
Salt-sensitive	Sitting	1	NA	NA	NA	−8.0 (6.0)
Salt-insensitive	Sitting	1	NA	NA	NA	7.0 (6.0)
Strazzullo, 1986	Standing	2	145	−8.60 (4.98)	98	−1.70 (2.56)
Van Berestevn, 1986	Supine	1	115	−1.36 (1.88)	65	0.79 (1.66)
Cappuccio, 1987	Standing	2	156	2.00 (4.17)	112	0.40 (2.64)
Lyle, 1987						
White	Sitting	1	115	−2.44 (2.00)	75	−1.89 (2.31)
Black	Sitting	1	114	−3.63 (3.85)	71	4.02 (5.67)
Meese, 1987	Sitting	2	143	−5.00 (4.21)	95	−2.00 (2.83)
Siani, 1987	Supine	2	154	5.10 (8.01)	96	1.30 (4.10)
Thomsen, 1987	Supine	2	124	−0.50 (6.10)	76	−1.30 (3.78)
Vinson, 1987	Supine	2	114	7.90 (4.93)	74	2.40 (2.05)
Zoccali, 1987	Sitting	1	141	6.45 (3.35)	88	4.64 (2.21)
Siani, 1988	Supine	2	139	2.20 (4.94)	91	0.70 (3.68)
Zoccali, 1988	Sitting	1	142	−2.80 (2.97)	88	−2.80 (2.47)
Orwoll, 1990	Sitting	1	131	2.60 (3.54)	84	3.08 (2.63)
Tanji, 1991	Sitting	1	146	3.00 (4.20)	95	2.00 (2.40)
Cutler, 1992	Sitting	1	126	−0.46 (0.67)	84	0.20 (0.46)
Lyle, 1992	Sitting	1	133	−5.90 (1.99)	87	−7.20 (1.71)
Galloe, 1993	Sitting	1	168	2.20 (4.49)	97	3.30 (2.75)
Jespersen, 1993	Supine	1	148	−0.57 (7.20)	93	−0.86 (3.88)
Pan, 1993	Sitting	1	136	−7.09 (7.89)	72	−0.87 (3.29)
Weinberger, 1993						
Normotensive	Sitting	2	116	1.00 (3.00)	72	−1.00 (2.64)
Hypertensive	Sitting	2	131	−2.00 (5.68)	87	−1.00 (2.92)
Petersen, 1994	Sitting	2	145	4.50 (13.2)	81	−8.20 (5.10)
Zhou, 1994	Sitting	1	158	−14.6 (4.48)	103	−7.11 (2.43)
Gillman, 1995	Sitting	1	102	−2.20 (11.0)	58	−0.80 (7.16)
Sacks, 1995	Sitting	1	NA	3.70 (2.45)	NA	3.60 (2.32)
Lijnen, 1996	Supine	1	114	−5.70 (2.18)	73	−3.50 (1.79)
Davis, 1997	Mean 24-h ambulatory blood pressure	1	125	−1.72 (1.20)	91	−0.49 (0.35)
Sanchez, 1997	Sitting	1	166	1.60 (1.60)	99	0.40 (1.21)

Continued

TABLE 44.9
(Continued)

Author, Year	Position of Blood Pressure Measurement	Mean BP at Study End*	Systolic Mean Baseline, mmHg	Systolic Mean Difference, mmHg (SD)†	Mean Diastolic Baseline, mmHg	Diastolic Mean Difference, mmHg (SD)†
Dietary Interventions						
Margetts, 1986	Sitting	1	NA	–3.50 (1.75)	NA	–1.20 (1.00)
Rouse, 1986	Sitting	2	NA	1.90 (2.30)	NA	2.30 (1.40)
Bierenbaum, 1988	Sitting	2	119	–2.00 (2.19)	79	–1.00 (1.33)
Morris, 1988						
Normotensive	Standing	1	113	–1.00 (1.04)	77	–0.90 (0.80)
Hypertensive	Standing	1	145	–3.60 (1.50)	94	–1.20 (0.86)
Hakala, 1989	Sitting	1	129	3.80 (11.9)	84	3.20 (4.53)
Van Beresteijn, 1990	Supine	1	114	–2.82 (1.83)	63	0.43 (1.89)
Kynast-Gales, 1992	Supine	1	136	–8.29 (8.12)	83	–0.14 (6.15)
McCarron, 1997	Sitting	1	134	–1.80 (0.78)	85	–1.20 (0.46)
Appel, 1997	Sitting	1	131	–2.70 (0.83)	84	–1.90 (0.60)

* For mean blood pressure at study end, 1 indicates change and 2 indicates mean.

† SD, standard deviation

Source: Modified with permission from Griffith LE, et al., *Am J Hypertens.*[56]

The mechanism most often cited for the apparent antihypertensive effect of magnesium is a calcium antagonist property. Other mechanisms include stimulation of vascular prostacyclin release, renal vasodilation, acceleration of the cell membrane sodium pump, and alterations in vascular responsiveness to vasoactive agents.[67] One 1988 analysis concluded that there were inadequate data from the four randomized, controlled trials to suggest a hypotensive effect.[63] Since that report, there have been a number of trials reported with mixed results (see Table 44.12). A meta-analysis reported –0.6/–0.8 mmHg decline in blood pressure, which was not significant.[68] When single-blind studies were excluded, the decrease in systolic blood pressure was significant for the 16 double-blind studies and the 14 trials of hypertensive patients. There was a dose-dependent decline in blood pressure for each 10-mmol/day increment in magnesium on both systolic and diastolic blood pressure (–4.3/–2.3 mmHg, $p < .001$ for systolic only).

It has been suggested that combinations of cations may act in concert; however, in a randomized, double-blind, multicenter trial of 125 participants, there was no hypotensive effect of magnesium in combination with either calcium or potassium.[67] In normotensive women, whose reported intake of magnesium was between the 10th to 15th percentiles, 16 weeks of a daily supplement of magnesium 14 mmol had no significant treatment effect on blood pressure (–0.9/–0.7 mmHg). The administration magnesium with potassium did not enhance the effect of potassium alone.[69]

ω-3 POLYUNSATURATED FATTY ACIDS

ω-3 Polyunsaturated fatty acids refer to fish oil, the very long chain fatty acids, eicosapentaenoic (EPA) and docosahexaenoic (DHA) acids. ω-3 polyunsaturated fatty acids are thought to lower blood pressure by altering the balance of the vasoconstrictor thromboxane A_2 and the vasodilator prostacyclin prostaglandin I_3, by modulating the vasoconstrictor response to pressors, or by decreasing blood viscosity.[11] In addition, the membrane physical-chemical properties and red blood cell fluidity may be altered by the incorporation of ω-3 polyunsaturated fatty acids in phospholipids. Furthermore, arterial elasticity may be improved.[70]

A meta-analysis by Appel identified 40 studies testing the impact of ω-3 polyunsaturated fatty acids on blood pressure; however, 23 were eliminated because of design, including concurrent antihypertensive medications, no control group, an unhealthy study population, concurrent use of ω-3 polyunsaturated fatty acids in the control group, or insufficient data.[71] Most trials used a combined dose of 3 g daily of EPA and DHA, which is equal to 6 to 10 capsules of commercial fish oil supplements or two 100-g servings of the fish that are high in ω-3 polyunsaturated fatty acids. The overall change in blood pressure, –1.5/–1.0 mmHg, was significant. For normotensives, the change in blood pressure, –1.0/–0.5 mmHg, was significant for the systolic blood pressure only. However, the decline in blood pressure, –5.5/–3.5 mmHg, for hypertensives was significant by both systolic and diastolic blood pressure ($p < .001$). Interestingly, the higher the blood pressure, the greater was the reduction ($p < .05$); however, the change in blood pressure was not a function of the dose of the ω-3 polyunsaturated fatty acids, duration of treatment, type of intervention (food vs. oil capsules), or the age of the participants. Side effects summarized include the unpleasant or fishy taste, gastrointestinal symptoms, eructation, loose stool or diarrhea, and obstipation occurring in 28% of experimental subjects and 13% of the control group ($p < .001$).[71]

TABLE 44.10
Randomized Controlled Trials of Calcium Supplementation in Pregnancy

Author, Year	No. of Participants, Calcium Supplementation/ Placebo	Calcium Formulation	Elemental Calcium Equivalent, mg/Day	Type of Control	Weeks of Gestation	Treatment Duration, Week	Compliance Cointervention	Quality Assessed	Score[†]
Trials Providing Data on Treatment Effects of Systolic and Diastolic Blood Pressure									
Belizan, 1983	11/14	Calcium Sandoz	2000	Placebo	15	22	NA*	NA	3
Marya, 1987	188/182	Unknown calcium supplement	375	Placebo	22	18	No	Yes	5
Villar,1987	25/27	Os-Cal tablets	1500	Placebo	26	14	Yes	Yes	0
Lopez-Jaramillo, 1989	49/43	Calcium gluconate	2000	Placebo	23	17	No	Yes	1
Repke, 1989	16/18	Os-Cal tablets	1500	Placebo	25	10	No	Yes	4
Lopez-Jaramillo,1990	22/34	Elemental calcium	2000	Placebo	30	10	No	No	4
Belizan, 1991	579/588	Calcium carbonate	2000	Placebo	20	20	No	Yes	2
Felix, 1991	14/11	Elemental calcium	2000	Placebo	20	20	No	Yes	3
Knight, 1992	10/10	Os-Cal tablets	1000	Normal diet	12	20	Yes	Yes	5
Sanchez-Ramos, 1993	36/39	Unknown calcium supplement	NA	Unknown	22	18	No	No	6
Sanchez-Ramos,1994	29/34	Calcium carbonate	2000	Placebo	25	15	No	Yes	4
Levine, 1997‡	2294/2295	Calcium carbonate	2000	Placebo	17	21	No	Yes	6
Trials Providing Data on Binary Outcomes Exclusively									
Montanaro, 1990	84/86	Calcium carbonate	2000	Placebo	24	16	No	No	1
Villar and Repke, 1990	95/95	Os-Cal tablets	2000	Placebo	23	20	Yes	Yes	2
Cong, 1993	50/50	Shen gu capsules	Unknown	Placebo	22	18	No	No	0

* NA indicates not applicable.

[†] Quality scores range from 0 to 6 with 6 indicating the highest quality score.

‡ Calcium for the Preeclampsia Prevention Trial (Not in the original meta-analysis).

Source: Modified from Bucher HC.[57] Reproduced with permission from April 10, *JAMA*, 275(14): 1113–1117, 1996. Copyright 1996, American Medical Association.

TABLE 44.11

Change in Blood Pressure in Randomized Controlled Trials of Calcium Supplementation in Pregnancy

Author, Year	Mean Difference in Systolic Blood Pressure, mmHg	Mean Difference in Diastolic Blood Pressure, mmHg
Belizan, 1983	–5.10	–5.70
Marya, 1987	–6.90	–3.40
Villar, 1987	–4.10	–4.90
Lopez-Jaramillo, 1989	–8.70	–6.60
Repke, 1989	–2.50	–2.77
Lopez-Jaramillo, 1990	–13.10	–11.80
Belizan 1991	–1.70	–0.90
Felix, 1991	–6.30	–5.80
Knight and Keith, 1992		
Normotensive	–2.70	0.50
Hypertensive	+4.8	0
Sanchez-Ramos, 1993	+4.6	–0.82
Sanchez-Ramos, 1994	–4.08	–3.00
Levine, 1997*	–0.3	+0.3

* Calcium for the Preeclampsia Prevention Trial (Not in the original meta-analysis).

Source: Modified from Bucher HC.[57] Reproduced with permission from April 10, *JAMA*, 275(14): 1113–1117, 1996. Copyright 1996, American Medical Association.

Another meta-analysis included 31 of 52 studies with a placebo group and a report of pre- and post-treatment blood pressures (see Table 44.13).[72] Like the previous meta-analysis, hypertensives (–3.4/–2.0 mmHg) had a greater blood pressure decline than normotensives (–0.4/–0.7 mmHg), but the dose of the fish oil was higher in the hypertensive group (5.6 g/day) than in the normotensive group (4.2 g/day). There also was a statistically significant dose-dependent decline in blood pressure: ≤3g/day, –1.3/–0.7 mmHg; >3 to 7g/day, –2.9/–1.6 mmHg; and 15g/day, –8.1/–5.8 mmHg. The effect of fish oil on blood pressure was maximally manifested by 3 to 4 weeks.

In the most current meta-analysis, fish oil reduced blood pressure more in older vs. younger subjects (>45 years) and hypertensive vs. normotensive patients.[73] However, this observation was no longer statistically significant after multivariate analysis. There was no relationship between the dose of fish oil and the change in blood pressure.

Whether EPA or DHA reduces blood pressure was addressed in a double-blind, parallel, placebo-controlled trial.[74] A group of 59 overweight, mildly hyperlipidemic men were randomized to 4 g/day of purified EPA, DHA, or olive oil (placebo) capsules and continued their usual diet for 6 weeks. Of these, 56 subjects completed the study. Only DHA significantly reduced 24-h and daytime ambulatory blood pressure ($p < .05$). In 63 overweight hypertensives, combining a daily meal of fish with a weight-reduction regimen led to additive reduction on ambulatory blood pressure and decreased heart rate.[75]

Olive oil, a monounsaturated fatty acid, is often used as placebo in studies testing the benefit of fish oils on blood pressure. However, some small studies suggest an antihypertensive effect of olive oil. A group of 31 treated elderly hypertensives were compared to 31 elderly normotensives that were randomized sequentially to receive virgin olive oil or sunflower oil for 4 weeks followed by a 4-week washout period.[76] Systolic blood pressure was significantly reduced among the hypertensive participants. Another study assigned 23 treated hypertensive patients to a diet high in monounsaturated or polyunsaturated fats for 6 months.[77] Blood pressure decreased significantly more with the monounsaturated diet (–7/–6 mmHg), compared to the polyunsaturated diet (+1/0 mmHg). The daily dosage of antihypertensive medication was also significantly reduced (48 vs. 4%, $p = .005$). Thus, olive oil does not appear to be an appropriate control for studies of fish oil supplementation to evaluate blood pressure.

Dietary Protein

Protein intake was thought to increase blood pressure due to adverse effects on renal function in partially nephrectomized rats. Cross-sectional studies show that dietary protein intake is inversely related to blood pressure, although a direct relationship was considered to exist.[78] The mechanism of action of high dietary protein intake is not clear, because there is a possibility that multiple nutrients may correlate with each another and complicate the analysis. Certain amino acids (e.g., tryptophan, tyrosine, arginine) may affect hormones or neurotransmitters that ultimately alter blood pressure.[79] For instance, in a double-blind, placebo-controlled trial, the sulfonic amino acid taurine given 6 g for 7 days in 19 young hypertensive subjects decreased blood

TABLE 44.12
Randomized Trials of Magnesium Supplementation

Author, Year	n	Mean Age, Year	Men, %	Cohort	BP Meds	Mg salt, mmol mg/Day	Study Design*	Duration, Weeks	Control ΔSBP/ΔDBP, mmHg	Magnesium ΔSBP/ΔDBP, mmHg
Cappuccio, 1985	17	52	53	Hypertensive	No	Aspartate, 15	DB, CO	4	-3/-3	0/-2
Doyle, 1999	26	23	0	Normotensive	No	Oxide, 10.3	DB, CO	8		-1.8/-1.5
Dyckner, 1983	20	65	33	90% Hypertensive	Yes	Aspartate, 15	O,PC	24	-0/-4	-12/-8
Ferrara, 1992	14	47.5	57	Hypertensive	No	Pidolate, 15	DB, PC	24	-17/-4	-7/-7
Henderson, 1986	41	62	?	Hypertensive	Yes	Oxide, 12.5	DB, PC	24	-3/-1	-4/-3
Itoh, 1997	33	65	33	Mixed	?	Hydroxide, 17–23	DB, PC	4	+1/-1	-5/-2
Kawano, 1998	60	58	57	Hypertensive	Some	Oxide, 20	CO	8		-3.7/-1.7
Lind, 1991	71	61	52	Hypertensive	No	Mixed†, 15	DB, PC	24	-2/-4.2	+1/-2
Motoyama, 1989	21	44	100	Hypertensive	No	Oxide, 24.7	O, PC	8		6§
Nowson, 1989	25	63	68	Hypertensive	No	Aspartate, 10	DB, PC	8	-2/-3	+2/+1
Patki, 1990	37	50	22	Hypertensive	No	Chloride, 20	DB, CO	8		+3.6/+3.5¶
Plum-Wirell, 1994	39	39	62	Hypertensive	No	Aspartate, 15	DB, CO	8	-0.8/-0.4	-2.4/-0.4
Purvis, 1994	28	53.8	86	Diabetes (no insulin)	?	Chloride, 15.7	DB, CO	6		-7.4/-2.3
Reyes, 1984	21	57	19	Hypertensive	Yes	Chloride, 15.8	DB, PC	3	-13/-4	-11/-7
Sacks, 1998	153	39	0	Normotensive	No	Lactate, 14	DB, PC	16	+0.4/+0.2	-0.5/-0.5
Saito, 1998	20	57	75	Hypertensive	Yes	Oxide, 24.7	O, PC	8		-7.5/3.0
Sanjuliani, 1996	15	36–65	47	Hypertensive	No	Oxide, 25	DB, CO	3	+1.7/-1.0	-7.6/-3.8
Sibai, 1989	374	18	0	Pregnancy	No	Aspartate, 15	DB, PC	21	+16/+18	+15/+16
TOHP, 1992‡	461	43	70	Normotensive	No	Diglycine, 15	DB, PC	24	-2.9/-2.7	-3.0/-2.9
de Valk, 1998	50	62.5	56	Diabetes (insulin)	?	Aspartate, 15	DB, PC	12	-10.4/-0.8	-7.7/-0.3
Widman, 1993	17	50	88	Hypertensive	No	Hydroxide, 15–40	DB, CO	9	-1/0.0	-7.9/-8.2
Wirell, 1994	39	26–69	77	Hypertensive	Yes	Aspartate, 15	DB, CO	8	+3.2/+2.3	-3.8/-1.7
Witteman, 1994	91	57	0	Hypertensive	No	Aspartate, 20	DB, PC	24	+0.2/+0.1	-3.3/-2.4
Zemel, 1990	13	~49	86	Hypertensive	No	Aspartate, 40	DB, PC	12	-1/+1	+3/+2

* DB = double blind, PC = Placebo controlled, CO = crossover, O = open label.

† 4.58 mmol Mg lactate + 0.42 Mg citrate.

‡ TOHP, Trials of Hypertension Prevention (phase I).

§ Only mean arterial pressure reported: difference between placebo period and active treatment.

¶ Magnesium added to potassium 30 mmol/15ml.

TABLE 44.13
Characteristics of the 31 Trials of Meta-analysis of Fish Oil and Blood Pressure

Study, Year	Study Design*	Blinding Subject	Blinding Observer§	Duration, Weeks	n, Treatment*	ω-3 dose, g/Day‡	ω-3 dose, Gender (Age, Range)	Baseline BP, mmHg	Δ SBP/DBP, mmHg¶
Healthy Subjects									
Mortensen, 1983	XO	+	+	4	20 Fish oil 20 Mixed oil	3.3	Men (25–40 year)	120/76	−4.0/−4.0
Bruckner, 1987	PG	+	−	3	10 Fish oil 11 Olive oil	3.9	Men (19–40 years)	119/80	+5.0/+1.0
v Houwelingen, 1987									
Maastricht	PG	−	+	6	19 Fish 20 Meat	4.7	Men (20–45 years)	121/77	+1.1/−0.9
Tromso	PG	−	+	6	11 Fish 12 Meat	4.7	Men (20–45 years)	118/77	+0.1/−0.9
Zeist	PG	−	+	6	10 Fish 10 Meat	4.7	Men (20–45 years)	115/73	−3.7/−3.0
Flaten, 1990	PG	+	+	6	27 Fish oil 29 Olive oil	6.5	Men (35–45 years)	119/80	+1.5/+0.8
Ryu, 1990	PG	NS†	NS	4	10 Fish oil 10 Wheat germ	3	Men (20–39 years)	124/73	−4.3/−2.0
TOHP, 1992	PG	+	+	24	175 Fish oil 175 Olive oil	2.4	Both (30–54 years)	123/81	−0.2/−0.6
Hypertensive Subjects									
Norris, 1986	XO	+	+	6	16 Fish oil 16 Placebo	NS	Both (45–74 years)	161/95	−10.0/−2.0
Knapp, 1989	PG	−	−	4	8 Fish oil 8 Saturated mix	3	Men (age NS)	137/94	−2.6/−0.1
Meland, 1989	PG	+	+	6	20 Fish oil 20 Mixed oil	6	Men (26–66 years)	149/101	+1.0/−1.0
Bonaa, 1990	PG	NS	NS	10	78 Fish oil 78 Corn oil	5.1	Both (34–60 years)	144/95	−6.4/−2.8
Levinson, 1990	PG	+	+	6	8 Fish oil 8 Saturated mix	15	Both (18–75 years)	147/94	−8.0/−9.0
Wing, 1990	XO	+	+	8	20 Fish oil 20 Olive oil	4.5	Both (32–75 years)	139/81	+0.6/−0.3
Radack, 1991	PG	+	+	12	16 Fish oil 17 Safflower	2	Both (mean, 46 year)	136/95	−7.2/−6.7
Margolin, 1991	PG	+	+	8	22 Fish oil 24 Corn oil	4.7	Both (60–80 years)	164/94	+1.1/+0.1
Morris, 1992	XO	+	+	6	18 Fish oil 18 Olive oil	4.8	Both (32–64 years)	130/87	−2.4/−1.8
Hypercholesterolemic Subjects									
Demke, 1988	PG	+	+	4	13 Fish oil 18 Safflower	1.7	Both (18–60 years)	119/74	−3/+1.0
Bach, 1989	PG	+	+	5	30 Total saturated	2.5	Both (mean, 31 year)	130/85	−9.0/−4.0
Dart, 1989	XO	NS	NS	8	21 Fish oil 21 Olive oil	6	Both (mean, 46 year)	125/77	−5.3/−2.0
Wilt, 1989	XO	NS	NS	12	38 Fish oil 38 Safflower	6	Men (mean, 42 year)	124/84	−2.7/−1.8
Kestin, 1990	PG	+	+	6	11 Fish oil 11 Linoleic	3.4	Men (mean, 46 year)	124/75	−5.1/0.0
Cobiac, 1991	PG	−	−	5	12 Fish 13 Fish oil 6 Saturated mix	4.5	Men (30–60 years)	128/79	−0.6/+1.3
Davidson, 1986	PG	+	+	4	30 Total olive oil	6	Age, sex: NS†	142/88	−9.8/−3.2

Continued

TABLE 44.13
(Continued)

Study, Year	Study Design*	Blinding Subject	Blinding Observer§	Duration, Weeks	n, Treatment*	ω-3 dose, g/Day‡	ω-3 dose, Gender (Age, Range)	Baseline BP, mmHg	Δ SBP/DBP, mmHg¶
Cardiovascular Disease Subjects									
Mehta, 1988	XO	+	+	4	8 Fish oil	5.4	Men (52–73 years)	138/80	−10.0/−4.0
					8 Placebo				
Solomon, 1990	PG	+	+	12	5 Fish oil	4.6	Both (42–64 years)	142/87	−16.8/−9.6
					5 Olive oil				
Gans, 1990	PG	+	+	16	16 Fish oil	3	Both (mean, 66 year)	148/80	+9.0/+1.0
					16 Corn oil				
Diabetic Subjects									
Haines, 1986	PG	−	−	6	19 Fish oil	4.6	Both (30–59 years)	136/82	+1.0/+1.7
					22 Olive oil				
Jensen, 1989	XO	+	+	8	18 Fish oil	4.6	Both (22–47 years)	148/89	−9.0/−4.0
					18 Olive oil				
Hendra, 1990	PG	+	+	6	40 Fish oil	3	Both (mean, 56 year)	143/83	+0.4/−0.6
					40 Olive oil				
Mixed Sample†									
Rogers, 1987	PG	+	+	4	30 Fish oil	3.3	Men (22–65 years)	130/76	−3.1/−5.0
					30 Olive oil				

* The number of subjects in each treatment period is listed for crossover studies. XO, crossover, PG, parallel group. The number of subjects in each treatment group was not reported for Davidson, 1986 and Bach, 1989. Saturated mix is a mixture of saturated and other oils; mixed oil is a mixture of corn and olive oils.

† NS, not specified. Mixed sample indicates that there were no inclusion criteria for health of the sample.

‡ ω-3 Dose represents EPA acid plus DHA acid. The ω-3 dose for Bruckner, 1987, reported as 1.5g/10 kg body weight, is estimated based on a mean weight of 85 kg.

§ Blinded to treatment status.

¶ Average blood pressure at baseline for active and control groups for parallel group studies and blood pressure during the placebo period for crossover studies. SBP, systolic blood pressure; DBP, diastolic blood pressure; NS, not specified. Change in BP attributed to fish oil treatment.

Source: Tabulated from Tables 2 and 3 from Morris.[72]

pressure −9.0/−4.1 mmHg compared with to −2.7/−1.2 mmHg in the placebo-treated subjects.[80] L-Arginine supplementation with natural foods or supplements lowered blood pressure in healthy volunteers.[81] Perhaps, other protein metabolites have natriuretic or diuretic activity.

Human observational studies on protein and blood pressure show in aggregate that increased protein intake, determined by food records or recall or by urine studies of sulfate and urea nitrogen, is associated with decreased blood pressure.[78] The relationship of blood pressure and vegetable protein vs. animal protein is unclear. After adjustment for age, body mass index, alcohol consumption, urinary sodium excretion, dietary intake, and resident area, He and Whelton observed that one standard deviation of a higher level of dietary protein intake (39 g) resulted in a 3.55 mmHg lower systolic blood pressure.[82] In a cross-sectional epidemiologic study (*n* = 4680), there was an inverse relationship between a higher vegetable protein intake of 2.8% kilocalories and lower blood pressure (−1.11/−0.71 mmHg), after adjusting for confounders, height and weight.[83] The amino acid content among individuals eating a high vegetable and low animal protein diet contained more glutamic acid, cystine, proline, phenylalanine, and serine. However, there was no direct relationship between animal protein intake and blood pressure. Most intervention trials have been conducted in normotensive subjects, were not designed to assess the relationship between protein and blood pressure or determine a dose relationship, and were not powered adequately or randomized.[78,82]

Soy is a legume. Soybean and soy foods (tofu, tempeh, soy flours, etc.) are rich in soy protein and isoflavones. The isoflavones, phenolic compounds, are produced by soy.[84] The most prominent isoflavones in soy are daidzein, genistein, glycitein, and their glucosides (the biologically inactive daidzein, genistein, and glycitein). The effectiveness of soy protein on blood pressure has been frequently tested (see Table 44.14). A meta-analysis calculated an insignificant reduction in blood pressure (−1/−1 mmHg) in examining 22 studies.[84] When women taking antihypertensive medications were excluded from the analyses, they had insignificant increases in systolic blood pressure. A recent scientific advisory from the American Heart Association stated that there was no blood pressure reduction with soy protein.[85]

TABLE 44.14
Controlled Clinical Trials of Soy Protein Supplementation

Author, Year	n	Study Design*	Duration, Week	Mean Age, Year	Men, %	Cohort*	BP* Meds	Control Group	Soy Protein Intake/Day	Control ΔSBP/ΔDBP, mmHg	Soy Protein ΔSBP/ΔDBP, mmHg
Atkinson, 2004	177	R, DB, PC	52	55	0	Perimenopausal	?	Placebo	43.5 mg red-clover isoflavone/day	+2.0/–3.0	–2.0/–2.0
Burke, 2001	36	R, PL	8	55	50	Hypertensive	Yes	Maltodextrin	66 g soy protein / 66 g soy protein and psyllium	+2.3/+1.4† / +2.3/+1.4†	–0.1/–1.0† / –8.4‡/–2.3†
Chiechi, 2002	113	R, PL	26	53	0	Postmenopausal	?	Usual diet	40–60 mg isoflavones to diet	–3.1/+2.8	–3.4/+0.2
Cuervas, 2003	18	R, DB, CO	4	59	0	Postmenopausal Hypercholesterolemia	?	Caseinate	40 g soy protein powder (80 mg isoflavones)	–5/–4	–5/–3
Han, 2002	80	R, DB, PC	13	49	0	Postmenopausal	?	Placebo	100 mg isoflavones	0/0	0/+1
Harrison, 2004	112	R, BB, PC	5	52	53	SBP >130 mmHg or Hypercholesterolemia	No	White bread rolls, cereal bars, cracker biscuits	25 g soya protein (50 mg isoflavones)	–9.0/–4.0	–9.0/–5.0
He, 2005	276	R, DB, PC	12	51	46	Hypertensive & Normotensive	No	Complex carbohydrate	40 g soybean protein supplement	–8.7/–2.6	–13.0/–5.4‡
Hermansen, 2001	20	R, DB, CO	6	63	70	Type 2 Diabetes	?	Casein 50 g/day	50 g soy protein (isoflavone 165 mg/day, cotyledon fiber 20 g/day)	–1.0/–1.0	0/–1.0
Hodgson, 1999	59	DB, PC	8	56	78	Normotensive	No	Placebo	55 mg isoflavones		–1.4/–0.8†¶
Hutchins, 2005	8	R, DB, CO	2	56	0	Postmenopausal	No	Placebo	isoflavones 5 mg/kg	?	+8‡/+2∥
Jayagopal, 2002	32	R, DB, CO	12	62	0	Postmenopausal & Type 2 Diabetes	?	Placebo	30 g isolated protein (132 mg isoflavones)	+2.3/–0.4	–2.2/–0.8
Jenkins, 2002	41	R, CO	4	62	56	Hyperlipidemic men or postmenopausal women	Some	Low fat diet	52 g soy protein (isoflavones 10 mg) / 50 g soy protein (isoflavones 73 mg)	–2/0 / –2/0	–4‡/–2 / –1/–1

Study	n	Design				Population	Some	Milk protein	Intervention		
Kreijkamp-Kaspers, 2005	175	R, DB, PC	52	67	0	Postmenopausal	?	Milk protein	26.5 g soy protein powder	-3.5/-1.7	+0.8†/+0.3
Kurowska, 1997	34	R, CO	4	55	50	Hypercholesterolemia	?	Milk, 2% fat	31 g soy milk	-8‡/-4‡	-3‡/0
Meyer, 2004	23	R, PC, CO	5	54	57	Hypercholesterolemia or hypertensive	No	Low fat milk/yoghurt	30 g soy milk/yoghurt (80 mg isoflavones)	+1/+2	0/0
Nestel, 1997	21	R, CO	5	54	0	Postmenopausal	?	Placebo	80 mg isoflavones	-6	-6
Puska, 2004	143	R, DB, PC	8	58	?	Hypercholesterolemia	?	Placebo yoghurt	Yoghurt 41.4 g soy protein	-1.1/0.2	-0.4/0.1
Rivas, 2002	40	R, DB, PC	12	48	63	Hypertensive	No	Cow's milk	18 g soy milk 1000 ml/day	-1.4/-3.7	-18.4‡/-15.9‡
Sagara, 2003	61	R, DB, PC	5	52	100	SBP >130 mmHg or TC>220 mg/dL	No	Placebo	20 g soy powder baked goods (80 mg isoflavones)	-3.6/-1.7	-10.8‡/-5.1‡
Simons, 2000	20	R, DB, CO	8	59	0	Postmenopausal	No	Placebo	80 mg isoflavones	-9/-5	-10/-5
Squadrito, 2002	60	R, DB, PC	26	56	0	Postmenopausal	?	Placebo	54 mg genistein	+1/+1	-3/-1
Teede, 2001	179	R, DB, PC	13	61	55	Normotensive	No	Casein	40 g soy protein (118 mg isoflavones)	-3.6/-1.9	-7.5‡/-4.3‡
Vigna, 2000	73	R, DB, PL	12	53	0	Postmenopausal	No	Caseinate	60 g soy protein (76 mg isoflavones)	-8.6/-3.1	-3.2/-0.1
Washburn, 1999	42	R, DB, CO	6	51	0	Perimenopausal	?	20 g complex carbohydrate supplement	20 g soy protein supplement (34 mg phytoestrogen)	-5.4/-3.6	-8.0/-5.9
									40 g soy protein supplement (68 mg phytoestrogen)	-5.4/-3.6	-6.7/-8.5‡

* R, randomized; DB, double-blind; PC, placebo-controlled; PL, parallel; CO, crossover; BP, blood pressure; SBP, systolic BP; TC, total cholesterol; ?, data not given.

† Ambulatory blood pressure measurements.

‡ Significant change in blood pressure.

§ Mean arterial pressure.

¶ Difference between placebo groups.

DIETARY FIBER

Dietary fiber, a nonstarch polysaccharide, describes plant substances that resist enzyme digestion in the gastrointestinal tract. Cellulose, hemicelluloses, and lignin are insoluble sources of fiber derived from whole-grain products; whereas pectins, gums, and mucilages are natural gel-forming soluble fiber, derived from fruits, vegetables, pulses (edible seeds of pod-bearing plants: peas, beans, lentils, etc.), and oats. Vegetarians and other persons with high fiber intakes have lower average blood pressures than persons with low fiber intakes. The explanation for lower blood pressure with fiber is unclear. Suggested mechanisms include reduced insulin resistance, increased intake in dietary potassium, magnesium, and vitamin C, reduced weight, and decreased sodium intake.[86]

In the Coronary Artery Risk Development in Young Adults (CARDIA) Study, fiber intake predicted insulin levels, weight gain, and other cardiovascular risk factors more potently than did fat consumption.[87] High intake of fiber was associated with lower systolic and diastolic blood pressure in whites but not African Americans. Among 30,681 white male health professionals, only dietary fiber had an independent inverse association with hypertension after four years of follow-up.[47] The relative risk of hypertension was 1.57 times greater for men with a fiber intake of less than 12 vs. greater than 24 g/day. In the Health Professionals Follow-up Study (43,738 men), high intakes of cereal fiber and magnesium were inversely associated with the risk of all strokes after 8 years.[39] Among 827 Chinese men, a 10 g higher intake of dietary fiber was significantly associated with a reduced systolic and diastolic blood pressure (–2.2/–2.1 mmHg).[88]

Among controlled studies, the average intake of fiber (primarily cereal) was increased by 14 g, resulting in an average reduction of blood pressure of –1.6/–2.0 mmHg.[89] One meta-analysis examined 25 randomized trials of dietary fiber.[90] Only hypertensive subjects had a significant decline in blood pressure (–5.9/–4.2 mmHg). Trials that were 8 weeks or longer had a greater reduction in blood pressure than shorter-duration studies (–3.1/–2.6 vs. +0.3/–0.6 mmHg). An intermediate fiber intake (7.2 to 18.9 g/day) was associated with a greater blood pressure reduction (–3.4/–2.0 mmHg) than a lower (–1.3/–1.8 mmHg) or high fiber intake (+2.6/–1.0 mmHg). Thus, there was no dose effect of fiber supplementation demonstrated. Another meta-analysis examined 24 trials (see Table 44.15) and calculated a blood pressure reduction of –1.1/–1.3 mmHg (significant only for diastolic).[91] In a multivariate model, systolic blood pressure was reduced more in subjects older than 40 years compared to younger subjects (–3.0 vs. –0.19 mmHg, $p = .04$). The fiber source (soluble, insoluble, or mixed), dose, and duration were not significant factors for the blood pressure response. Clearly more trials need to be conducted.

ASCORBIC ACID (VITAMIN C) AND ANTIOXIDANT COMBINATIONS

Ascorbic acid is an antioxidant and a free-radical scavenger. Low vitamin C levels might decrease the production of nitric oxide and increase blood pressure by increasing free-radical formation.[92] In hypertensive patients, intraarterial infusion of vitamin C improves the impaired vasodilatation of acetylcholine, but not nitroprusside.[93] Other mechanisms include decreased vasodilating prostaglandin formation, modified leukotriene metabolism, altered vascular sodium content, or nutrient multicollinearity.[94] Several studies have suggested an inverse relationship between blood pressure or stroke and vitamin C levels. The difference in nutrient intakes between hypertensives and normotensives are shown in Figure 44.3.[95]

It has been observed that the association of vitamin C and blood pressure could also be explained by a low potassium.[96] In 722 Eastern Finnish men in the Kuopio Ischemic Heart Disease Risk Factor Study, both plasma ascorbic acid and serum selenium concentrations had independent inverse associations with the blood pressure.[92] However, neither vitamin E or vitamin C supplements reduced the risk of stroke in the Health Professionals Follow-up Study of 43,738 men.[97] In 168 healthy subjects, plasma concentrations of ascorbic acid (but not α-tocopherol, selenium, or taurine) were significantly inversely related to systolic and diastolic blood pressure.[94] Intravenous vitamin C, thioproline, and glutathione (all antioxidants) individually demonstrated an acute decrease in blood pressure in 20 unmedicated hypertensive and 20 diabetic subjects.[98] In a 17-week dietary depletion and repletion study, higher plasma ascorbic acid levels were associated with lower systolic and diastolic blood pressure.[99]

Few studies assessed the impact of ascorbic acid supplementation alone. Ascorbic acid, 500 mg twice daily in 21 subjects, lowered blood pressure –4.2/–2.9 mmHg in a pilot study.[100] In double-blind, randomized, crossover study, ascorbic acid 200 mg twice daily or placebo for 4 weeks was given to 27 elderly hypertensives.[101] No significant treatment effect was observed. Following a 2-week run-in phase, 48 untreated elderly hypertensive subjects in a randomized, double-blind, placebo-controlled 6-week study received ascorbic acid 250 mg twice daily or placebo.[102] The change in blood pressure in the vitamin C group was –10.3/–5.9 mmHg and in the placebo group was –7.7/–4.7 mmHg (not significant). In a controlled trial, 20 subjects received placebo and 19 subjects received a 2 g bolus of ascorbic acid followed by 500 mg daily for 30 days.[103] Systolic blood pressure decreased –13 mmHg ($p < .05$); the change in diastolic blood pressure was not significant. Table 44.16 summarizes several trials of vitamin C supplementation on blood pressure. The effect on systolic blood pressure is consistently greater than diastolic blood pressure.

Several studies have combined several antioxidants to assess an effect on blood pressure. In a randomized, placebo-controlled, clinical trial, 297 retired teachers were randomly assigned to 2 to 4 months of an antioxidant capsule (vitamin E 400 IU/day, vitamin C 500 mg/day, and β-carotene 6 mg/day) or placebo. The antioxidant combination capsule had no significant

TABLE 44.15

Randomized Trials of Dietary Fiber

Author, Year	Design*	n	Duration, Weeks	Age, Years	Men, %	Blood Pressure Δ, mmHg	Fiber Dose, g/Day	Fiber Type	Fiber Source
Arvil, 1995	CO, DB	63	4	47	100	−3.43/−0.27	3.9	Supplement	Soluble
Birketved, 2000	PL, DB	53	24	40	0	0.60/−2.30	4.7	Supplement	Insoluble
Brussaard, 1981	PL, O	31	5	23	65	3.50/3.90	10.0	Supplement	Soluble
Brussaard, 1981	PL, O	32	5	23	65	3.60/1.00	19.0	Supplement	Insoluble
Burke, 2001	PL, O	36	8	57	50	−6.50/−1.90	12.0	Supplement	Soluble
Eliasson, 1992	PL, DB	63	12	48	62	−0.34/−4.30	6.0	Supplement	Insoluble
Fehily, 1986	CO, SB	201	4	37	73	−0.40/0.20	12.0	Diet	Soluble
Hagander, 1989	CO, O	12	8	62	58	−3.00/2.00	25.6	Supplement	Soluble
He, 2004	PL, DB	102	12	48	40	−1.79/−1.24	10.0	Supplement	Soluble
Jenkins, 2002	CO	82	8	60	83	−0.7/−0.3	8.0	Diet	Soluble
Keenan, 2002	PL, SB	18	6	44	50	−8.80/−6.00	5.5	Diet	Soluble
Little, 1990	PL, SB	78	8	58	51	−0.30/−0.40	36.4	Diet	Mixed
Margetts, 1987	CO, SB	88	6	39	58	−1.20/−1.10	42.6	Diet	Mixed
Nami, 1995	PL, DB	16	2	46	38	−14.3/−5.40	3.5	Supplement	Mixed
Önning, 1999	CO, DB	52	5	63	100	−1.60/−1.50	6.8	Supplement	Soluble
Pins, 2002	PL, DB	88	12	48	51	−6.0/−5.0	11.67	Diet	Soluble
Rigaud, 1990	PL, DB	52	24	37	21	−1.30/2.50	6.0	Supplement	Insoluble
Rössner, 1987	PL, DB	54	8	39	0	3.00/0.00	5.0	Supplement	Mixed
Rössner, 1987	PL, DB	41	12	39	0	0.00/−5.00	7.0	Supplement	Mixed
Rössner, 1988	PL, DB	62	12	40	0	1.00/−3.00	6.5	Supplement	Mixed
Ryttig, 1989	PL, DB	97	11	39	0	0.10/−2.90	7.0	Supplement	Insoluble
Ryttig, 1990	CO, DB	19	2	25	53	3.0/?	7.0	Supplement	Soluble
Schlamowitz, 1987	PL, DB	46	12	?	?	−11.0/−3.00	7.0	Supplement	Mixed
Solum, 1987	PL, DB	60	12	35	0	−9.0/−5.00	5.0	Supplement	Insoluble
Swain, 1990	CO, DB	20	6	30	20	3.00/2.00	20.5	Supplement	Soluble
Törrönen, 1992	PL, DB	28	8	41	100	6.00/1.00	15.1	Supplement	Soluble
Van Horn, 1991	PL, O	80	8	42	50	0.50/−1.40	4.2	Supplement	Soluble

* CO = crossover; DB = double blind; O = open; PL = parallel; SB = single blind; ?, data not provided.

Source: Table updated and modified from Streppel MT.[91]

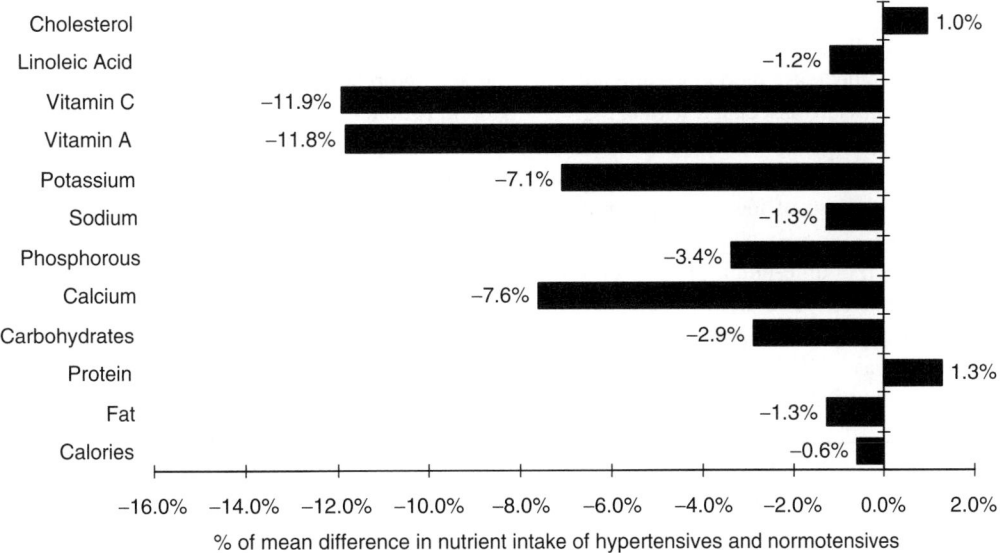

FIGURE 44.3 Health and Nutrition Examination Survey I: % mean difference in average nutritional consumption between hypertensives and normotensive persons, adjusted for age. With permission from McCarron.[95]

TABLE 44.16
Trials of Ascorbic Acid and Blood Pressure

Study	n	Design*	Cohort	Age or Range, Year	Duration, Week	Ascorbate Dose (mg/Day)	Blood Pressure Treatment Effect, mmHg
Darko, 2002	35	R, DB, PC	Type 2 Diabetes	56	3	1500	NS/NS
Duffy, 1999	39	R, DB, PC	Hypertension	48	4	2000 PO then 500	$-11^{\dagger}/-6$
Eskurza, 2004	10	SB	Young	18–30	4	500	$-1/0$
	10		Older	60–79	4	500	$-1/-1$
Feldman, 1992	21	SB	Healthy	43	4	1000	$-4.2/-2.9$
Fotherby, 2000	40	R, DB, CO	Older	60–80	24	500	$-2^{\dagger}/0^{\ddagger}$
Hypertensive	17						$-3.7^{\dagger}/-1.2$
Ghosh, 1994	48	R, DB, PC	Untreated hypertension	49	6	500	$-2.5/-1.2$
Hajjar, 2002	31	R, SB	Treated hypertension	62	24	500–2000	$-4.5^{\dagger}/-2.8^{\dagger}$
Hutchins, 2005	8	R, DB, CO	Postmenopause	56	2	500	$+2/-1$
Kim, 2002	378	R, DB, PC	Atrophic gastritis	40–69	260	50 or 500	$+1.3^{\dagger}/+0.9$
Lovatt, 1993	27	R, DB, CO	Hypertension	60–83	4	400	-2 to $-5.3^{\dagger}/-0.2$ to $-1.9^{\dagger}$
Magen, 2004	31	R, SB, PC	Hypertension, dyslipidemia	53	8	500	NS/NS‡
Mullan, 2002	30	R, DB, PC	Type 2 diabetes	45–70	4	500	$-9.9^{\dagger}/-4.4^{\dagger}$
Osilesi, 1991	20	R, CO, PC	Mixed population	58	6	1000	$-6.3^{\dagger}/0.6$
Pellegrini, 2004	8	R, DB, CO	Healthy smokers	43	5	1000	NS/NS
Ward, 2005	36	R, DB, PC	Treated Hypertension	62	6	500	$-1.8^{\dagger}/+1.5^{\ddagger}$

* R, Randomized; SB, single-blind; DB, double-blind; PC, placebo-controlled; CO = crossover; NS, not significant.

† Significant.

‡ Ambulatory blood pressure.

hypotensive effect.[104] In a randomized, double-blind, crossover, placebo-controlled study, 21 hypertensives and 17 normotensives were assigned to receive either 8 weeks of placebo followed by 2 weeks washout, then 8 weeks of combined antioxidants (zinc sulfate 200 mg, ascorbic acid 500 mg, α-tocopherol 600 mg and β-carotene 30 mg) daily, or the opposite sequence. Only systolic blood pressure (−5.3 mmHg) decreased significantly at the end of the antioxidant phase compared with the placebo phase (+3.7 mmHg) in hypertensive subjects ($p < .01$).[105]

GARLIC (*ALLIUM SATIVUM*)

Garlic has been reported to decrease blood pressure and attenuate the age-related increase in aortic stiffness, which could alter the rise in systolic blood pressure associated with aging.[106–110] Allicin is believed to be the component that is responsible for the medicinal effects of garlic. In rabbits and dogs, garlic elicits a dose-dependent diuretic-natriuretic response.[111,112] In a randomized, placebo-controlled, double-blind trial, 47 subjects with mild hypertension (diastolic blood pressure from 95 to 104 mmHg) took garlic powder or a placebo of identical appearance for 12 weeks.[106] The supine diastolic blood pressure in the garlic treatment group decreased 13 mmHg after 12 weeks ($p < .01$); however, there was no significant change in the placebo group. A randomized, multicenter, double-blind, placebo-controlled, 12-week parallel treatment study using garlic powder (Kwai®) 300 mg 3 times/day in hypercholesterolemic subjects found no benefits in lowering lipids or blood pressure.[113] The authors of this paper emphasized that negative studies tend not to be submitted or published, suggesting that the current literature on garlic represents a publication bias.[113,114]

A meta-analysis of eight trials (415 subjects), using dried garlic powder 600 to 900 mg, observed a decrease in blood pressure of −7.7/−5.0 mmHg.[114] In hypertensive subjects, a decline in blood pressure (−11.1/−6.5 mmHg) was reported. The authors observed that blinding might have been difficult due to the odor of garlic. Furthermore, they emphasized that their quality assessment of the trials was poor, because the authors did not state their technique to achieve effective randomization.

In an analysis of 27 small, randomized trials, there were mixed, but never a large treatment effect of garlic on blood pressure reduction (see Table 44.17).[115] Most studies did not observe a significant decline in subjects randomized to garlic compared to placebo. Uncertain randomization procedures, lack of intention-to-treat analyses, missing data, and variability in blood pressure measurement techniques does not support the use of garlic to lower blood pressure.

TABLE 44.17
Randomized-Controlled Trials of Garlic on Blood Pressure*

Study	n	Design	Age, Year	Male, %	Cohort	Intervention	Baseline BP, mmHg	Duration, Week	Garlic (% SBP/DBP Δ)	Control (% SBP/DBP Δ)
Auer, 1990	47	DB, PC	46	45	Hypertensive	Kwai ® vs. placebo	Sp 171/102	4	–4/–8 Sp	–4/–5 Sp
							Sd 171/101	12	–11/–13 Sp	–5/–4 Sp
									–12/–11 Sd	–6/–4 Sd
Barrie, 1987	20	DB, PC, CO	46	?	None	Cold pressed garlic oil vs. placebo	St M 94	4	–5.4 St M	–2.3 St M
Czerny, 1996	30	DB, PC	55	?	Hyperlipidemic/PVD	Garlic oil macerate vs. placebo	Uc 162/100	4	–7/–2	–2/–4
								12	–13/–12	–5/–7
								13	–11/0	–4/0
								26	–17/–11	–1/0
de Santos, 1993	60	DB, PC	52	53	Hyperlipidemic	Kwai ® vs. placebo	Uc 145/91	4	–8/–7	–4/0
de Santos, 1995	80	SB	56	35	Hyperlipidemic	Kwai ® vs. Hoefels Original Garlic Oil ®	Kwai ® St 151/96 Garlic Oil St 138/88	16	Kwai®: –17/–18 St	Garlic oil: NC/–2 St
Gardner, 1999	53	DB, PC	52	51	Hyperlipidemic	Dehydrated tablet vs. placebo	Not stated	12	NS	NC
Holzgartner, 1992	98	DB, PC	57	39	Hyperlipidemic	Kwai ® vs. antilipidemic	Uc 143/83	12	–5/–5 Uc	NS
Isaacsohn, 1998	50	DB, PC	58	54	Hyperlipidemic	Kwai ® vs. placebo	St 121/72	12	+2/+1 St	0/+4 St
Jain, 1993	42	DB, PC	52	45	Hyperlipidemic	Kwai ® vs. placebo	St 128/83	12	+1/–1 St	–1/–1 St
Kandziora, 1988	40	DB	43–65	?	Hypertensive	Kwai ® and antihypertensive vs. antihypertensive	Sp 178/100	4	–6/–12 Sp	–2/–7 Sp
							Sd 174/99		–6/–12 Sd	–3/–7 Sd
									–9/–15 Sp	–3/–9 Sp
								12	–9/–16 Sd	–3/–8 Sd
Kandziora, 1988	40	SB	56	83	Hypertensive	Kwai ® vs. antihypertensive	Sp 176/99	4	–6/–11 Sp	–6/–11 Sp
							Sd 178/100		–5/–12 Sd	–6/–11 Sd
								12	–7/–14 Sp	–7/–14 Sp
									–6/–15 Sd	–7/–14 Sd
Kannar, 1998	90	DB, PC	54	54	Hyperlipidemic	Cotter Foods® vs. placebo	St 126/76	12	–1/+1.4 St	–2.8/+0.3 St
Kiesewetter, 1991	60	DB, PC	24	30	SWISA	Kwai® vs. placebo	Uc 116/74	4	–9.5/? Uc	NS
Kiesewetter, 1993	80	DB, PC	60	54	PVD	Kwai® vs. placebo	Uc D 85	12	NC/–3.5 Uc	NC/–2 Uc
Luley, 1996	34	DB, PC, CO	?	?	Hyperlipidemic	Dehydrated tablet vs. placebo	Not given	6	NC	NC
Luley, 1996	51	DB, PC, CO	?	?	Hyperlipidemic	Dehydrated tablet vs. placebo	Not given	6	NC	NC
Mansell, 1996	60	PC	63	76	Diabetics	Dehydrated tablet vs. placebo	Not given	?	NS	NS
McCrindle, 1998	31	DB, PC	14	52	Hyperlipidemic/CAD	Kwai® vs. placebo	Uc 102/62	8	+2/0 Uc	NS
Saradeth, 1994	72	DB, PC	39	29	Age 18 to 50	Kwai® vs. placebo	Uc 125/81	5	–1/0 Uc	–3/0 Uc
								15	+2/+2 Uc	–1/–1 Uc
Simons, 1995	31	DB, PC, CO	54	52	Hyperlipidemic	Kwai® vs. placebo	Uc 127/80	12	NS	NS
Steiner, 1996	52	DB, PC, CO	32–68	100	Hyperlipidemic	"Aged garlic extract™," vs. placebo	Uc 134/84	13	–7/–2 Uc	–4/–7 Uc
								26	–7/–2 Uc	–3/–4 Uc

Continued

TABLE 44.17 (Continued)

Study	n	Design	Age, Year	Male, %	Cohort	Intervention	Baseline BP, mmHg	Duration, Week	Garlic (% SBP/DBP Δ)	Control (% SBP/DBP Δ)
Superko, 2000	50	DB, PC	53		Hyperlipidemic	Kwai® vs. placebo	Not given	12	NS	NS
Turner, 2004	62	DB, PC	50	39	40–60 years	Garlic powder vs. placebo	Su 115/75	12	+2/0 Su	+3/+0.5
Ventura, 1990	40	DB, PC	59	38	Hyperlipidemic	Dehydrated tablet /hawthorn vs. placebo	Uc 164/84	8	–8/–2 Uc	–2/–2 Uc
Vorberg, 1990	40	DB, PC	50	53	Hyperlipidemic	Kwai® vs. placebo	Sp 146/92	4 / 12 / 16	–1/–3 Sp / –1/–4 Sp / –3/–4 Sp	0/0 Sp / +1/+3 Sp / +2/+3 Sp
Yeh, 1997	34	DB, PC	48	100	Hyperlipidemic	"Aged garlic extract™" vs. placebo	Uc 121/82	8 / 16 / 20	+2/–5 Uc / +5/+2 Uc / +2/+1 Uc	–5/–4 Uc / +1/–1 Uc / +1/0 Uc

* DB, double blind; SB, single blind; CO, crossover; BP, blood pressure; CAD, Coronary artery disease; PVD, peripheral vascular disease; SWISA, Elevated spontaneous platelet aggregation; M, mean BP; SBP, systolic BP; DBP, diastolic BP; Sd = standing; Sp = supine BP; St = sitting BP; Uc = BP position unclear; Cr, crossover study; NS, not significant; NC, no change; ?, data not provided.

Source: Modified and derived from Mulrow C et al.[115]

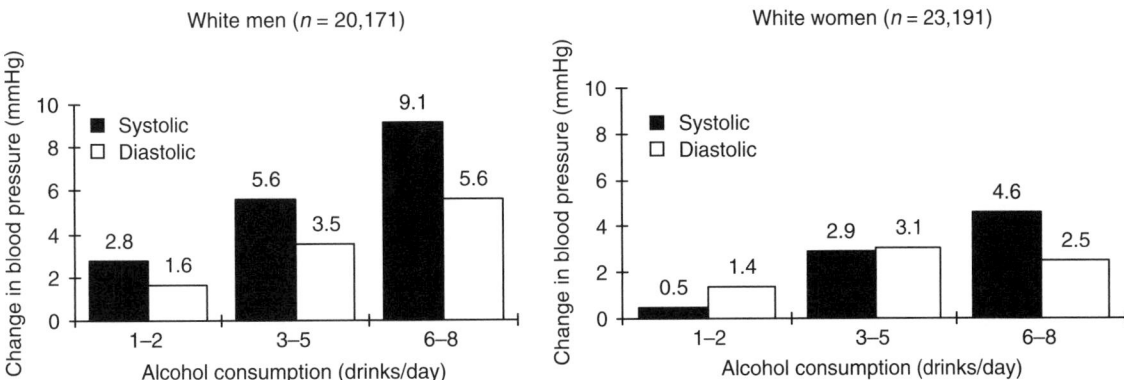

FIGURE 44.4 The effect of ethanol consumption on the change in blood pressure independent of other factors. With permission from Klatsky.[121]

ETHANOL

Alcohol consumption increases the risk of development of hypertension.[116,117] The risk increases above 28 g of ethanol/day (which is equivalent to 24 oz of beer, 10 oz wine, and 3 oz of distilled spirits).[118] The maximum addition to the prevalence of hypertension of alcohol usage greater than two drinks daily is estimated to be 5 to 7%; however, the 11% risk in men is greater than in women because of greater alcohol intake.[119] In another study, alcohol consumption greater than 20 g/day increased the risk of hypertension among women.[120] The relationship of alcohol intake to blood pressure is graded and continuous with the effect clearer in men than in women (see Figure 44.4) and more consistent in whites than in blacks.[121] The effect of alcohol consumption on systolic blood pressure is independent of the effects of age, obesity, cigarette smoking, and physical activity.[122] In the INTERSALT Study ($n = 10,079$), both body mass index and heavy alcohol consumption were significantly and independently correlated with both systolic and diastolic blood pressure ($p < .001$).[123] The effect of alcohol consumption on blood pressure was independent of and additive to body mass index and urinary excretion of sodium and potassium.[124] The effect of alcohol on change in blood pressure, independent of other risk factors, is displayed in Figure 44.4.[121] Resting plasma concentrations of norepinephrine, epinephrine, renin activity, angiotensin II, aldosterone, and cortisol are similar in drinkers and nondrinkers.[125] In the Scottish Health Heart Study, alcohol consumption showed a weak positive correlation with blood pressure among 7354 men, but the correlation was greater than for sodium.[10] In a prospective study of 7735 middle-aged British men, the prevalence of measured hypertension and level of blood pressure were significantly higher on Mondays and lower on Fridays than on other weekdays.[126] This suggests a withdrawal effect of weekend ethanol consumption.

Modest alcohol intake has been associated with a protective effect on ischemic heart disease events. Heavy alcohol intake has been associated with an increased rate of hemorrhagic strokes.[127,128] However, mild-to-moderate consumption in men reduced the risk of ischemic stroke without increasing the risk of hemorrhagic stroke.[129]

Several trials have been conducted to assess the impact of alcohol intake reduction on blood pressure using either cognitive and behavioral techniques or low-alcohol beer substitution (see Table 44.18).[130] The meta-analysis of these trials reported a significant reduction in blood pressure in both normotensives and hypertensive subjects. The studies with the highest baseline blood pressure had the greatest decline in blood pressure. Furthermore, there was a dose-response relationship between the amount of alcohol reduction and the degree of blood pressure reduction.

The Prevention and Treatment of Hypertension Study (PATHS) was designed to assess alcohol intake reduction in nondependent moderate to heavy drinkers.[118,131] Six-hundred and forty-one outpatient hypertensive and nonhypertensive veterans with a diastolic blood pressure of 80 to 99 mmHg were randomized to observation or a behavioral cognitive intervention. To qualify for enrollment, self-reported alcohol intake had to be ≥294 g/week or ≥21 drinks/week for the preceding 6 months. The goal of behavioral cognitive intervention was to reduce alcohol intake to the lesser of either 50% of baseline intake or 14 drinks/week. For the entire cohort, the average reduction of alcohol intake at 6 and 24 months between groups was 131 and 124 g/week ($p < .001$ for each). Among the hypertensive subjects ($n = 265$), the average reduction at 6 and 24 months was 157 and 135 g/week (each $p < .001$). At 6 and 12 months, this translated to an insignificant reduction in blood pressure (i.e., treatment effect) for the entire cohort of –1.0/–0.6 and –0.9/0.6 mmHg. For the hypertensive participants, the insignificant treatment effect at 6 and 12 months was –1.9/–0.6 and –1.6/–0.4 mmHg. There was no significant difference in the incidence of hypertension at 24 months: 16.6% intervention group and 21.8% in the control group. Weight declined more in the intervention group by –0.5 and –1.0 kg at 6 and 24 months.

PATHS was designed to achieve a two-drink reduction in alcohol between treatments, but only achieved a reduction of 1.3 drinks/day. Furthermore, it was anticipated that 60% of the intervention group and 20% of the control group could reduce

TABLE 44.18
Randomized Controlled Trials of Alcohol Reduction on Blood Pressure*

Author, Year	n	Mean Age, Year	Male, %	HTN, %	Rx, %	Study Design	Duration, Week	Intervention	Alcohol Reduction, %	Δ Blood Pressure, mmHg	Mean Weight Δ, kg
Cox, 1993	72	36.6	100	0	0	PO	4	Substitute	85	-4.71/-1.92	-0.43
Cushman, 1998	641	57.3	99	42	0	PO	104	Counseling	29	-2.00/-1.91	-0.50
Howes, 1986	10	26.5	100	0	0	XO	1	Substitute	100	-3.04/-3.12	?
Kawano, 1998	34	?	100	100	82.5	XO	8	Counseling	84	-3.00/-2.00	-1.00
Lang, 1995	129	42.5	95	100	19.5	PO	104	Counseling	16	-6.32/-1.73	?
Mahaswaran, 1992	41	44.6	100	100	51.2	PO	8	Counseling	50	-2.22/-6.00	-0.50
Parker, 1990	63	52.0	100	100	100	PO	4	Substitute	85	-5.40/-3.20	-1.00
Puddey, 1985	46	35.0	100	0	0	XO	12	Substitute	80	-3.83/-1.43	-0.70
Puddey, 1986	44	?	100	100	100	XO	12	Substitute	86	-5.02/-3.01	-0.90
Puddey, 1992	86	44.3	100	0	0	PO	18	Substitute	85	-4.82/-3.37	?
Rakic, 1998	14	45.5	100	0	0	XO	8	Substitute	76	-1.00/0.00	-0.42
Rakic, 1998	41	45.5	100	0	0	XO	8	Substitute	76	-2.00/-2.00	-0.42
Ueshima, 1987	50	44.5	100	100	22.0	XO	4	Counseling	51	-1.35/-0.63	-0.62
Ueshima, 1993	54	44.5	100	100	0	XO	6	Counseling	54	-3.67/-1.91	?
Wallace, 1988	909	42.7	58	?	0	PO	52	Counseling	46	-2.12/?	?

* HTN, hypertensive; Rx, antihypertensive medication; XO, crossover, open design; PO, parallel open design; ?, data not specified; Substitute intervention uses a low-alcohol beer.

Note: Counseling intervention reduces alcohol intake by cognitive and behavioral methods.

Source: Derived and modified from Xin X et al.[130]

baseline alcohol intake to less than 50%; however, at 6 months, the level for the control group was 23% and the intervention group was 44%.

CAFFEINE

Caffeine has an acute effect on blood pressure. Caffeine may increase peripheral vascular resistance by blocking the adenosine receptors and increasing epinephrine, norepinephrine, and cortisol. Whether chronic caffeine use increases the incidence of hypertension is controversial. Two recent large cohort studies examining men ($n = 1017$) and women ($n = 155,594$) did not establish a relationship between caffeine consumption and the incidence of hypertension.[132,133]

There are several randomized, controlled trials assessing the impact of coffee consumption on blood pressure.[132,133] A study, using ambulatory blood pressure to examine nonsmoking men and women older than 50 years, reported a +4.8/+3.0 mmHg higher 24-h blood pressure for 14 hypertensive coffee drinkers of 5 cups/day for 2 weeks compared to 13 hypertensive abstainers after a mandatory period of abstention of caffeine-containing foods for 2 weeks.[134] A early meta-analysis reviewed 36 studies and identified 11 controlled trials with 522 subjects.[62] The median duration of the trials was 56 days. They estimated the overall pooled treatment effect attributable for a median coffee intake of 5 cups/day was +2.4/+1.2 mmHg. Only one of the 11 trials included a hypertensive cohort. This meta-analysis did not observe a treatment effect on blood pressure based on treatment duration, the type of coffee (instant or not), whether coffee was filtered, or the type of coffee control (decaffeinated or no coffee). Age, coffee consumption, and sample size were independently associated with both systolic and diastolic blood pressure. Blood pressure increased +0.8/+0.5 mmHg per cup of coffee consumed. A more recent meta-analysis (see Table 44.19),

TABLE 44.19
Randomized Controlled Studies of Coffee or Caffeine

Author, Year	Study Design*	n	Duration, Days	Age, Year	Males, %	Intervention Group	Dose‡	Control Group	Δ Blood Pressure, mmHg
Arciero, 1998	CO, DB	10	28	71	100	Caffeine tablet	295	Placebo	+12.0/+2.0
Bak, 1990	OL, PL†	62	63	26	54	Boiled coffee	700 (441)	No coffee	+6.0/+2.8
Bak, 1990	OL, PL†	66	63	26	53	Filtered coffee	700 (469)	No coffee	+6.1/+3.0
Bak, 1991	PL, DB	62	63	25	55	Caffeine Tablet	375	Placebo	−0.6/+0.6
Burr, 1989	OL, CO†	54	28	35	65	Instant coffee	1235 (741)	Decaffeinated coffee	+1.7/−1.1
Burr, 1989	OL, CO†	54	28	35	65	Instant coffee	1235 (741)	No coffee	+2.9/−0.9
Dusseldorp, 1989	CO, DB	45	42	38	49	Filtered coffee	750 (435)	Decaffeinated coffee	+1.5/+1.0
Dusseldorp, 1991	OL, PL†	42	79	39	52	Boiled, filtered coffee	900 (798)	No coffee	+0.4/+0.4
Dusseldorp, 1991	OL, PL†	43	79	39	51	Boiled coffee	900 (774)	No coffee	+3.5/+0.9
Eggertsen, 1993	CO, DB	23	14	56	57	Instant coffee	525 (263)	Decaffeinated coffee	+0.3/−0.1
Höfer, 1994	OL, PL	120	9	32	50	Instant coffee	998 (335)	Decaffeinated coffee	−0.7/−1.0
James, 1994	CO, DB	18	7	23	0	Caffeine Tablet	336	Placebo	+1.5/+1.3
James, 1994	CO, DB	18	7	23	100	Caffeine Tablet	410	Placebo	+2.1/+1.6
MacDonald, 1991	OL, CO†	50	14	47	46	Instant coffee	450 (225)	Decaffeinated coffee	−0.8/−0.3
MacDonald, 1991	OL, CO†	50	14	47	46	Instant coffee	450 (225)	No coffee	−0.7/+0.1
Rakic, 1999	OL, PL	21	14	72	29	Instant coffee	750 (300)	No coffee	−1.6/−0.2
Rakic, 1999	OL, PL	27	14	77	15	Instant coffee	750 (300)	No coffee	+3.6/+4.7
Robertson, 1984	PL, DB	17	7	30	41	Caffeine Tablet	750	Placebo	+8.5/+5.0
Rosmarin, 1990	OL, CO	21	56	36	100	Filtered coffee	540 (270)	No coffee	+2.1/−2.4
Superko, 1991	OL, PL†	120	56	46	100	Filtered coffee	1067 (615)	No coffee	+1.3/+0.2
Superko, 1991	OL, PL†	123	56	47	100	Filtered coffee	1090 (629)	Decaffeinated coffee	+2.7/−0.7
Superko, 1994	OL, PL†	103	56	47	100	Filtered coffee	1067 (615)	Decaffeinated coffee	+1.6/+1.1
Superko, 1994	OL, PL†	99	56	44	100	Filtered coffee	1067 (615)	No coffee	+1.4/+0.7
Watson, 2000	CO, DB	12	84	38	0	Caffeine Tablet	400	Placebo	+5.0/−1.0
Watson, 2000	CO, DB	22	84	38	100	Caffeine Tablet	400	Placebo	+2.0/+1.0

* OL, Open-label; PL, parallel; CO, crossover; DB, double-blind.

† Various interventions were compared to the same control group or placebo.

‡ In coffee trials, the coffee dose (ml/day) is reported. For caffeine tablet trials, the mg/day given is reported.

Source: Derived and modified from Noordzij M, et al.[135]

which included 1010 subjects, calculated a significant increase in systolic blood pressure (+2.04/+0.73 mmHg) after combining coffee and caffeine tablet trials; however, caffeine tablets produced a larger increase in blood pressure (+4.16/+2.41 mmHg).[135]

SUMMARY

Table 44.20 is a summary of all the meta-analyses that have been reported on the nonpharmacologic intervention of blood pressure. The importance of the amount of change in blood pressure depends on whether you are a clinician or an epidemiologist.

TABLE 44.20
Meta-Analyses of Nonpharmacologic Intervention on Blood Pressure

Intervention	Author, Year	Number of Trials	Δ Systolic BP (95% CI), mmHg	Δ Diastolic BP (95% CI), mmHg
Aerobic exercise*	Ebrahim, 1998[23]	7		
Normotensive		4	−0.7 (−2.8 to +1.5)	+0.3 (−1.6 to +1,1)
Hypertensive		3	−0.8 (−5.9 to +4.2)	− 3.7 (−7.4 to 0)
Aerobic exercise	Whelton, 2002[139]	54	−3.84 (−4.97 to −2.72)	− 2.58 (−3.35 to −1.81)
Normotensive		27	−4.04 (−5.32 to −2.75)	− 2.33 (−3.14 to −1.51)
Hypertensive		15	−4.94 (−7.17 to −2.70)	− 3.73 (−5.69 to −1.77)
Caffeine supplementation	Jee, 1999[62]	11	+2.4 (+1.0 to +3.7)	+1.2 (+0.4 to +2.1)
Normotensive		10	+2.4 (+1.0 to +3.8)	+1.2 (+0.4 to +2.1)
Caffeine supplementation	Noordzij, 2005[135]	16	+2.0 (+1.1 to +3.0)	0.7 (+0.14 to 1.31)
Calcium supplementation	Cappuccio, 1989[53]	15	−0.13 (−0.46 to +0.19)	+0.03 (−0.17 to +0.22)
Hypertensive		10	+0.06 (−0.59 to +0.72)	+0.03 (−0.21 to +0.27)
Calcium supplementation	Cutler, 1990[48]	19	−1.8 (−3.0 to −0.6)	−0.7 (−1.5 to +0.2)
Normotensive		9	−1.3 (−3.2 to +0.8)	−1.3 (−2.6 to −0.1)
Hypertensive		12	−2.1 (−3.6 to −0.6)	−0.1 (−1.3 to +1.0)
Calcium supplementation	Allender, 1996[54]	22	−0.89 (−1.74 to −0.05)	−0.18 (−0.75 to +0.40)
Normotensive		13	−0.53 (−1.56 to +0.49)	−0.28 (−0.99 to +0.42)
Hypertensive		16	−1.68 (−3.18 to −0.18)	+0.02 (−0.96 to +1.00)
Calcium supplementation	Buchner, 1996[55]	33	−1.27 (−2.25 to −0.29)	−0.24 (−0.92 to +0.44)
Normotensive		33	−0.27 (−1.80 to +1.27)	−0.33 (−1.56 to +0.90)
Hypertensive		6	−4.30 (−6.47 to −2.13)	−1.50 (−2.77 to −0.23)
Calcium supplementation	Griffith, 1999[56]	42	−1.44 (−2.20 to −0.68)	−0.84 (−1.44 to −0.24)
Ethanol Reduction	Xin, 2001[130]	15	−3.31 (−2.52 to −4.10)	−2.04 (−2.58 to −1.49)
Normotensive		6	−3.56 (−4.61 to −2.51)	−1.80 (−3.03 to −0.58)
Hypertensive		7	−3.90 (−5.04 to −2.76)	−2.41 (−3.25 to −1.57)
Fiber supplementation	He, 1996[89]	20	−1.6 (−2.7 to −0.4)	−2.0 (−2.9 to −1.1)
Fiber supplementation	Whelton, 2005[90]	25	−1.15 (+0.39 to −2.68)	−1.65 (−2.70 to −0.61)
Normotensive		20	+0.14 (−1.10 to +0.82)	−0.78 (−1.70 to +0.13)
Hypertensive		5	−5.95 (−9.50 to −2.40)	−4.20 (−6.55 to −1.85)
Fiber supplementation	Streppel, 2005[91]	24	−1.13 (−2.49 to +0.23)	−1.26 (−2.04 to −0.48)
Normotensive		17	−1.00 (−1.94 to −0.06)	−0.81 (−1.60 to −0.02)
Hypertensive		8	−2.42 (−5.28 to +0.45)	−1.83 (−3.52 to −0.14)
Garlic supplementation	Silagy, 1994[114]	8	−7.7 (−11.0 to −4.3)	−5.0 (−7.1 to −2.9)
Hypertensive		2	−11.1 (−17.2 to −5.0)	−6.5 (−9.6 to −3.4)
Magnesium supplementation	Jee, 2002[68]	20	−0.6 (−2.2 to +1.0)	−0.8 (−1.9 to +0.4)
Hypertensive		14	−3.3 (−0.1 to +6.8)	−2.0 (−1.0 to +5.6)
ω-3 fatty acids supplementation	Appel, 1993[71]	17	−1.5 (−2.4 to −0.6)	−1.0 (−1.6 to −0.4)
Normotensive		11	−1.0 (−2.0 to 0.0)	−0.5 (−1.2 to +0.20)
Hypertensive		6	−5.5 (−8.1 to −2.9)	−3.5 (−5.0 to −2.1)
ω-3 fatty acids supplementation	Morris, 1993[72]	31	−3.0 (−4.5 to −1.5)	−1.5 (−2.2 to −0.8)
Normotensive		8	−0.4 (−1.6 to +0.8)	−0.7 (−1.5 to +0.1)
Hypertensive		9	−3.4 (−5.9 to −0.9)	−2.0 (−3.3 to −0.7)

Continued

TABLE 44.20
(Continued)

Intervention	Author, Year	Number of Trials	Δ Systolic BP (95% CI), mmHg	Δ Diastolic BP (95% CI), mmHg
ω-3 fatty acids supplementation	Geleijnse, 2002[73]	36	–2.1 (–1.1 to –3.1)	–1.6 (–1.0 to –2.2)
Normotensive		27	–1.2 (–2.7 to +0.2)	–1.1 (–0.3 to –2.0)
Hypertensive		23	–3.7 (–1.6 to –5.7)	–2.5 (–1.3 to –3.7)
Potassium supplementation	Cappuccio, 1991[40]	18	–4.0 (–4.7 to –3.2)	–2.4 (–3.0 to –1.8)
Hypertensive		12	–5.3 (–6.2 to –4.4)	–3.0 (–3.7 to –2.3)
Potassium supplementation	Whelton, 1997[41]	32	–3.11 (–4.31 to –1.91)	–1.97 (–3.42 to –0.52)
Normotensive		12	–1.8 (–2.9 to –0.6)	–1.0 (–2.1 to 0.0)
Hypertensive		20	–4.4 (–6.6 to –2.2)	–2.5 (–4.9 to –0.1)
Potassium supplementation	Geleijnse, 2003[42]	30	–2.42 (–3.75 to –1.08)	–1.57 (–2.65 to –0.50)
Normotensive		11	–0.97 (–3.07 to +1.14)	–0.34 (–2.04 to +1.36)
Hypertensive		19	–3.51 (–5.31 to –1.72)	–2.51 (–3.96 to –1.06)
Sodium reduction	Cutler, 1991[14]	23	–2.91 (–3.67 to –2.15)	–1.60 (–2.09 to –1.11)
Normotensive		6	–1.70 (–2.68 to –0.72)	–0.97 (–1.62 to –0.32)
Hypertensive		18	–4.92 (–6.19 to –3.65)	–2.64 (–3.46 to –1.82)
Sodium reduction	Midgley, 1996[16]	56	–0.5 (–1.17 to –0.07)	–1.6 (–2.10 to –1.02)
Normotensive		28	–0.1 (–0.76 to +0.63)	–0.5 (–1.16 to +0.14)
Hypertensive		28	–2.0 (–3.57 to –0.49)	–2.7 (–3.77 to –1.58)
Sodium reduction	Cutler, 1997[17]	32	–2.81 (–3.39 to –2.23)	–1.52 (–1.90 to –1.14)
Normotensive		12	–1.90 (–2.62 to –1.18)	–1.09 (–1.57 to –0.61)
Hypertensive		22	–4.83 (–5.87 to –3.79)	–2.45 (–3.13 to –1.77)
Sodium reduction	Graudal, 1998[18]	114		
Normotensive		56	–1.2 (–1.8 to –0.6)	–0.26 (–0.3 to +0.9)
Hypertensive		58	–3.9 (–4.8 to –3.0)	–1.9 (–2.5 to –1.3)
Sodium reduction*	Ebrahim, 1998[23]	8		
Normotensive		2	–1.3 (–2.7 to +0.1)	–0.8 (–1.8 to +0.2)
Hypertensive		6	–2.9 (–5.8 to 0)	–2.1 (–4.0 to –0.1)
Sodium supplementation†	Alam, 1999[22]	11	+5.58 (+4.31 to +6.95)	+3.50 (+2.61 to +4.38)
Sodium reduction‡	Hooper, 2002[21]	11		
6 to 12 months		7	–2.5 (–3.8 to –1.2)	–1.2 (–1.8 to –0.7)
13 to 60 months		4	–1.1 (–1.83 to –0.41)	–0.61 (–1.54 to +0.31)
>60 months		1	–3.8 (–7.9 to +0.3)	–2.2 (–4.8 to +0.4)
Sodium reduction§	He, 2002[20]	28		
Normotensive		11	–2.03 (–2.56 to –1.50)	–0.97 (–1.39 to –0.55)
Hypertensive		17	–4.96 (–5.75 to –4.17)	–2.73 (–3.21 to –2.25)
Sodium reduction	Geleijnse, 2003[42]	47	–2.54 (–3.16 to –1.92)	–1.96 (–2.41 to –1.51)
Normotensive		19	–1.26 (–2.08 to –0.43)	–1.14 (–1.76 to –0.51)
Hypertensive		28	–5.24 (–6.56 to –3.93)	–3.69 (–4.69 to –2.69)
Sodium reduction	Jurgens, 2004[19]	115		
Normotensives		57	–1.27 (–1.76 to –0.77)	–0.54 (–0.94 to –0.14)
Hypertensives		58	–4.18 (–5.08 to –3.27)	–1.98 (–2.46 to –1.32)
Soy protein supplementation	Balk, 2005[84]	22	–1.0 (–3.0 to +1.0)	–1.0 (–2.0 to 0)
Weight reduction*	Ebrahim, 1998[23]	8		
Normotensive		4	–2.8 (–3.9 to –1.8)	–2.3 (–3.2 to –1.4)
Hypertensive		4	–5.2 (–8.3 to –2.0)	–5.2 (–6.9 to –3.4)
Weight reduction	Neter, 2003[137]	25	–4.78 (–5.76 to –3.80)	–3.56 (–4.31 to –2.81)
Normotensive		17	–4.46 (–5.71 to –3.21)	–2.62 (–3.83 to –1.42)
Hypertensive		17	–4.73 (–6.40 to –3.06)	–4.36 (–5.72 to –3.00)

* Included trials of follow-up duration ≥6 months and age ≥45 years.

† Older patients ~60 years.

‡ Included trials of follow-up duration ≥6 months.

§ Included trials of modest salt intake reduction to ~5 g and duration >4 weeks.

REFERENCES

1. Prisant, L. M., in Current Diagnosis 9, 9th ed., Conn, R. B., Borer, W. Z. and Synder, J. W., eds., W. B. Saunders Company, Philadelphia, PA, 1997, 349.
2. Chobanian, A. V., et al., *Hypertension*, 42: 1206, 2003.
3. Gifford, R. W. and Prisant, L. M., in Hypertension in the Elderly, 1st ed., Prisant, L. M., ed., Humana Press, Totowa, NJ, 2005, 3.
4. Hertz, R. P., et al., *Arch Intern Med.*, 165: 2098, 2005.
5. Denton, D., et al., *Nat Med.*, 1: 1009, 1995.
6. Kurtz, T. W., Al-Bander, H. A. and Morris, R. C., *N Engl J Med.*, 317: 1043, 1987.
7. Boegehold, M. A. and Kotchen, T. A., *Hypertension*, 17: I158, 1991.
8. INTERSALT Cooperative Research Group. *BMJ.*, 297: 319, 1988.
9. Stamler, R., *Hypertension*, 17: I16, 1991.
10. Smith, W. C., et al., *BMJ.*, 297: 329, 1988.
11. National High Blood Pressure Education Program Working Group. *Arch Intern Med.*, 153: 186, 1993.
12. Mascioli, S., et al., *Hypertension*, 17: I21, 1991.
13. Grobbee, D. E. and Hofman, A., *BMJ.*, 293: 27, 1986.
14. Cutler, J. A., et al., *Hypertension*, 17: I27, 1991.
15. Law, M. R., Frost, C. D. and Wald, N. J., *BMJ.*, 302: 819, 1991.
16. Midgley, J. P., et al., *JAMA.*, 275: 1590, 1996.
17. Cutler, J. A., Follmann, D. and Allender, P. S., *Am J Clin Nutr.*, 65: 643S, 1997.
18. Graudal, N. A., Galloe, A. M. and Garred, P., *JAMA.*, 279: 1383, 1998.
19. Jurgens, G. and Graudal, N. A., Effects of low sodium diet versus high sodium diet on blood pressure, renin, aldosterone, catecholamines, cholesterols, and triglyceride. Cochrane Database Syst Rev [Electronic]. March 1, 2004; CD004022. Available at: http://www.ncbi.nlm.nih.gov/entrez/query.fcgi?cmd=Retrieve&db=PubMed&dopt=Citation&list_uids=14974053. Accessed January 23, 2006.
20. He, F. J. and MacGregor, G. A., *J Hum Hypertens.*, 16: 761, 2002.
21. Hooper, L., et al., *BMJ.*, 325: 628, 2002.
22. Alam, S. and Johnson, A. G., *J Hum Hypertens.*, 13: 367, 1999.
23. Ebrahim, S. and Smith, G. D., *J Public Health Med.*, 20: 441, 1998.
24. Alderman, M. H., *Am J Hypertens.*, 10: 584, 1997.
25. Alderman, M. H., Cohen, H. and Madhavan, S., *Lancet*, 351: 781, 1998.
26. Alderman, M. H. and Lamport, B., *Am J Hypertens.*, 3: 499, 1990.
27. Alderman, M. H., et al., *Hypertension*, 25: 1144, 1995.
28. Krishna, G. G., Miller, E. and Kapoor, S., *N Engl J Med.*, 320: 1177, 1989.
29. Langford, H. G., *Ann Intern Med.*, 98: 770, 1983.
30. Grim, C. E., et al., *J Chronic Dis.*, 33: 87, 1980.
31. Veterans Administration Cooperative Study Group on Antihypertensive Agaents. *J Chronic Dis.*, 40: 839, 1987.
32. Adrogue, H. J. and Wesson, D. E., *Semin Nephrol.*, 16: 94, 1996.
33. Brancati, F. L., et al., *Arch Intern Med.*, 156: 61, 1996.
34. Morris Jr., R. C., et al., *Semin Nephrol.*, 19: 487, 1999.
35. Franzoni, F., et al., *Biomed Pharmacother.*, 59: 25, 2005.
36. He, F. J., et al., *Hypertension*, 45: 571, 2005.
37. Tobian, L., et al., *Hypertension*, 7: I110, 1985.
38. Khaw, K. T. and Barrett-Connor, E., *N Engl J Med.*, 316: 235, 1987.
39. Ascherio, A., et al., *Circulation*, 98: 1198, 1998.
40. Cappuccio, F. P. and MacGregor, G. A., *J Hypertens.*, 9: 465, 1991.
41. Whelton, P. K., et al., *JAMA.*, 277: 1624, 1997.
42. Geleijnse, J. M., Kok, F. J. and Grobbee, D. E., *J Hum Hypertens.*, 17: 471, 2003.
43. Grimm Jr., R., et al., *N Engl J Med.*, 322: 569, 1990.
44. Stitt, F. W., et al., *Lancet*, 1: 122, 1973.
45. Gruchow, H. W., Sobocinski, K. A. and Barboriak, J. J., *JAMA.*, 253: 1567, 1985.
46. Witteman, J. C., et al., *Circulation*, 80: 1320, 1989.
47. Ascherio, A., et al., *Circulation*, 86: 1475, 1992.
48. Cutler, J. A. and Brittain, E., *Am J Hypertens.*, 3: 137S, 1990.
49. Resnick, L. M., *Am J Hypertens.*, 12: 99, 1999.
50. Subcommittee on Nonpharmacological Therapy of the 1984 Joint National Committee on Detection, Evaluation, and Treatment of High Blood Pressure. *Hypertension*, 8: 444, 1986.
51. McCarron, D. A. and Morris, C. D., *Ann Intern Med.*, 103: 825, 1985.
52. Cappuccio, F. P., Siani, A. and Strazzullo, P., *J Hypertens.*, 7: 941, 1989.
53. Cappuccio, F. P., et al., *Am J Epidemiol.*, 142: 935, 1995.
54. Allender, P. S., et al., *Ann Intern Med.*, 124: 825, 1996.
55. Bucher, H. C., et al., *JAMA.*, 275: 1016, 1996.

56. Griffith, L. E., et al., *Am J Hypertens.*, 12: 84, 1999.

57. Bucher, H. C., et al., *JAMA.*, 275: 1113, 1996.

58. Levine, R. J., et al., *N Engl J Med.*, 337: 69, 1997.

59. Appel, L. J., in *Hypertension* Primer. The Essentials of High Blood Pressure, 2nd ed., Izzo, J. H. and Black, H. R., eds., Lippincott Williams & Wilkins, Dallas, 1999, 253.

60. Sibai, B. M., Villar, M. A. and Bray, E., *Am J Obstet Gynecol.*, 161: 115, 1989.

61. Lucas, M. J., Leveno, K. J. and Cunningham, F. G., *N Engl J Med.*, 333: 201, 1995.

62. Jee, S. H., et al., *Hypertension*, 33: 647, 1999.

63. Whelton, P. K. and Klag, M. J., *Am J Cardiol.*, 63: 26G, 1989.

64. Mizushima, S., et al., *J Hum Hypertens.*, 12: 447, 1998.

65. Ma, J., et al., *J Clin Epidemiol.*, 48: 927, 1995.

66. Peacock, J. M., et al., *Ann Epidemiol.*, 9: 159, 1999.

67. Sacks, F. M., et al., *Hypertension*, 26: 950, 1995.

68. Jee, S. H., et al., *Am J Hypertens.*, 15: 691, 2002.

69. Sacks, F. M., et al., *Hypertension*, 31: 131, 1998.

70. McVeigh, G. E., et al., *Arterioscler Thromb.*, 14: 1425, 1994.

71. Appel, L. J., et al., *Arch Intern Med.*, 153: 1429, 1993.

72. Morris, M. C., Sacks, F. and Rosner, B., *Circulation*, 88: 523, 1993.

73. Geleijnse, J. M., et al., *J Hypertens.*, 20: 1493, 2002.

74. Mori, T. A., et al., *Hypertension*, 34: 253, 1999.

75. Bao, D. Q., et al., *Hypertension*, 32: 710, 1998.

76. Perona, J. S., et al., *Clin Nutr.*, 23: 1113, 2004.

77. Ferrara, L. A., et al., *Arch Intern Med.*, 160: 837, 2000.

78. Obarzanek, E., Velletri, P. A. and Cutler, J. A., *JAMA.*, 275: 1598, 1996.

79. Elliott, P., *Proc Nutr Soc.*, 62: 495, 2003.

80. Fujita, T., et al., *Circulation*, 75: 525, 1987.

81. Siani, A., et al., *Am J Hypertens.*, 13: 547, 2000.

82. He, J. and Whelton, P. K., *Clin Exp Hypertens.*, 21: 785, 1999.

83. Elliott, P., et al., *Arch Intern Med.*, 166: 79, 2006.

84. Balk, E., et al., Effects of Soy on Health Outcomes. Evidence Report/Technology Assessment No. 126, AHRQ Publication No. 05-E024-2., Agency for Healthcare Research and Quality, Rockville, MD, 2005.

85. Sacks, F. M., et al., *Circulation*, 113: 112, 2006.

86. Singh, R. B., et al., *Am J Cardiol.*, 70: 1287, 1992.

87. Ludwig, D. S., et al., *JAMA.*, 282: 1539, 1999.

88. He, J., et al., *J Hypertens.*, 13: 1267, 1995.

89. He, J., Whelton, P. K. and Klag, M. J., *Am J Hypertens.*, 9: 74A, 1996.

90. Whelton, S. P., et al., *J Hypertens.*, 23: 475, 2005.

91. Streppel, M. T., et al., *Arch Intern Med.*, 165: 150, 2005.

92. Salonen, J. T., *Ann Med.*, 23: 295, 1991.

93. Taddei, S., et al., *Circulation*, 97: 2222, 1998.

94. Moran, J. P., et al., *Am J Clin Nutr.*, 57: 213, 1993.

95. McCarron, D. A., et al., *Science*, 224: 1392, 1984.

96. Bulpitt, C. J., *J Hypertens.*, 8: 1071, 1990.

97. Ascherio, A., et al., *Ann Intern Med.*, 130: 963, 1999.

98. Ceriello, A., et al., *Clin Sci.*, 81: 739, 1991.

99. Block, G., et al., *Hypertension*, 37: 261, 2001.

100. Feldman, E. B., et al., *Ann NY Acad Sci.*, 669: 342, 1992.

101. Lovat, L. B., et al., *J Hum Hypertens.*, 7: 403, 1993.

102. Ghosh, S. K., et al., *Gerontology*, 40: 268, 1994.

103. Duffy, S. J., et al., *Lancet*, 354: 2048, 1999.

104. Miller, E. R., et al., *J Cardiovasc Risk*, 4: 19, 1997.

105. Galley, H. F., et al., *Clin Sci.*, 92: 361, 1997.

106. Auer, W., et al., *Br J Clin Pract Suppl.*, 69: 3, 1990.

107. Vorberg, G. and Schneider, B., *Br J Clin Pract Suppl.*, 69: 7, 1990.

108. Steiner, M., et al., *Am J Clin Nutr.*, 64: 866, 1996.

109. Breithaupt-Grogler, K., et al., *Circulation*, 96: 2649, 1997.

110. Ernst, E., *Pharmatherapeutica*, 5: 83, 1987.

111. Pantoja, C. V., et al., *J Ethnopharmacol.*, 31: 325, 1991.

112. Pantoja, C. V., Norris, B. C. and Contreras, C. M., *J Ethnopharmacol.*, 52: 101, 1996.

113. Isaacsohn, J. L., et al., *Arch Intern Med.*, 158: 1189, 1998.

114. Silagy, C. A. and Neil, H. A., *J Hypertens.*, 12: 463, 1994.

115. Mulrow, C., et al., Garlic: Effects on Cardiovascular Risks and Disease, Protective Effects Against Cancer, and Clinical Adverse Effects. Evidence Report/Technology Assessment No. 20., AHRQ Publication No. 01-E023, Agency for Healthcare Research and Quality, Rockville, MD, 2000.
116. Klatsky, A. L., et al., *N Engl J Med.*, 296: 1194, 1977.
117. Beilin, L. J., *Ann NY Acad Sci.*, 676: 83, 1993.
118. Cushman, W. C., et al., *Am J Hypertens.*, 7: 814, 1994.
119. MacMahon, S., *Hypertension*, 9: 111, 1987.
120. Witteman, J. C., et al., *Am J Cardiol.*, 65: 633, 1990.
121. Klatsky, A. L., Friedman, G. D. and Armstrong, M. A., *Circulation*, 73: 628, 1986.
122. Arkwright, P. D., et al., *Circulation*, 66: 60, 1982.
123. The INTERSALT Co-operative Research Group. *J Hypertens Suppl.*, 6: S584, 1988.
124. Marmot, M. G., et al., *BMJ.*, 308: 1263, 1994.
125. Arkwright, P. D., et al., *Circulation*, 66: 515, 1982.
126. Wannamethee, G. and Shaper, A. G., *J Hum Hypertens.*, 5: 59, 1991.
127. Iso, H., et al., *Stroke*, 26: 767, 1995.
128. Camargo, C. A., *Stroke*, 20: 1611, 1989.
129. Berger, K., et al., *N Engl J Med.*, 341: 1557, 1999.
130. Xin, X., et al., *Hypertension*, 38: 1112, 2001.
131. Cushman, W. C., et al., *Arch Intern Med.*, 158: 1197, 1998.
132. Klag, M. J., et al., *Arch Intern Med.*, 162: 657, 2002.
133. Winkelmayer, W. C., et al., *JAMA.*, 294: 2330, 2005.
134. Rakic, V., Burke, V. and Beilin, L. J., *Hypertension*, 33: 869, 1999.
135. Noordzij, M., et al., *J Hypertens.*, 23: 921, 2005.
136. Expert Panel on the Identification, Evaluation, and Treatment of Overweight and Obesity in adults. *Arch Intern Med.*, 158: 1855, 1998.
137. Neter, J. E., et al., *Hypertension*, 42: 878, 2003.
138. Blair, S. N., et al., *JAMA.*, 276: 205, 1996.
139. Whelton, S. P., et al., *Ann Intern Med.*, 136: 493, 2002.

45 Nutritional Treatment of Blood Pressure: Major Nonpharmacologic Trials of Prevention or Treatment of Hypertension

L. Michael Prisant

CONTENTS

PRIMARY PREVENTION TRIALS

PRIMARY PREVENTION OF HYPERTENSION (PPH) TRIAL

The purpose of PPH was to determine whether intense lifestyle modifications would reduce the incidence of hypertension and lower blood pressure in the intervention vs. the monitored (control) group.[1] Hypertension-prone individuals between the ages of 30 and 44 years were screened. Diastolic blood pressure <90 mmHg was required for enrollment. Greater than 50% above desirable weight, excess alcohol use, diabetes mellitus, and major cardiovascular diseases precluded participation in the trial. Diastolic blood pressure ≥90 mmHg or initiation of antihypertensive drug therapy was the primary end point. Interventions by nutrition counselors and physicians included (1) the greater of a 4.5 kg decrease or a 5% weight loss in overweight subjects, (2) decreased sodium intake to ≤1800 mg (4.5 g NaCl), (3) reduced alcohol intake (≤26 g), and (4) increased physical activity (30 min for 3 days/week).

The group that did not receive the intervention was monitored. Baseline characteristics are shown in Table 45.1. The incidence of hypertension was 8.8% of 102 intervention subjects and 19.2% of monitored subjects (*p* = .027) over 5 years. The odds ratio for hypertension development in the control group was 2.4 (90% confidence interval [CI] 1.2–4.8, *p* < .027).

HYPERTENSION PREVENTION TRIAL (HPT)

Men and women between the ages of 25 and 49 years with a diastolic blood pressure ≤89 mmHg were randomized.[2] Group counseling and individual dietary counseling were performed. This primary prevention trial allocated subjects

TABLE 45.1

Nonpharmacologic Interventions in High Normal Blood Pressure

Trial	n	Mean Age (Years)	% Male	% White	Study Duration	Intervention	Initial Blood Pressure (mmHg)	Systolic/Diastolic Change (mmHg)	Relative Risk of Hypertension[a]
Primary Prevention of Hypertension[1]	201	38	87	82	5 years	↓ calories and NaCl ↓ ethanol ↑ physical activity	123/83	−1.3/−1.2	0.46[b]
Hypertension Prevention Trial[2]	252	38	68	80	3 years	↓ calories	125/83	−2.4/−1.8	0.77
	392	39	62	84	3 years	↓ NaCl	124/83	+0.2/+0.1	0.79
	255	39	62	82	3 years	↓ calories and NaCl	125/83	−1.0/−1.3	0.95
	391	38	63	85	3 years	↓ NaCl and KCl	124/83	−1.2/−0.7	0.77
Trials of Hypertension Prevention[3] (Phase I)	564	43	72	79	18 months	↓ Calories and ↑ physical activity	124/84	−2.9/−2.3	0.49[b]
	744	43	72	797	18 months	↓ NaCl	125/84	−1.7/−0.9	0.76
	562	43	71	84	18 months	Manage Stress	125/84	−0.5/−0.8	1.07
	471	43	68	85	6 months	↑ Calcium	126/84	−0.5/+0.2	0.91
	461	43	68	85	6 months	↑ Magnesium	125/84	−0.2/−0.1	0.63
	351	43	72	87	6 months	↑ Potassium	122/81	+0.1/−0.4	0.87
	350	43	70	86	6 months	↑ Fish Oil	123/81	−0.2/−0.6	1.11
Trials of Hypertension Prevention[4] (Phase II)	1191	43	66	79	36 months	↓ calories	127/86	−1.3/−0.9	0.81[b]
	1190	43	67	80	36 months	↓ NaCl	128/86	−1.2/−0.7	0.88
	1193	43	69	79	36 months	↓ Calories and NaCl	127/86	−1.1/−0.6	0.84[b]

[a] Defined as diastolic blood pressure of ≥90 mmHg or antihypertensive drug therapy during follow-up.

[b] $p < .05$.

Source: Modified from *Arch Intern Med* 153: 186, 1993; Used with permission and Copyright 1993, American Medical Association.

(see Table 45.1) on the basis of body mass index (BMI) into several interventions. Low-BMI subjects (men <25 kg/m^2 and women <23 kg/m^2) were randomized to: (1) a control group, (2) sodium restriction ≤70 mmol/day (≤1610 mg/day), or (3) sodium restriction and potassium augmentation ≥100 mmol/day (3900 mg/day). High-BMI individuals were randomized to: (1) control, (2) caloric restriction, (3) sodium restriction, (4) sodium and caloric restriction, or (5) sodium restriction and potassium augmentation.

The mean change in blood pressure for the interventions is displayed for both systolic and diastolic blood pressure at 6 months in Table 45.2. Caloric restriction reduced blood pressure significantly. Caloric and sodium restriction was a less effective strategy in this cohort. Sodium restriction with or without caloric restriction or potassium supplementation had no effect on blood pressure reduction. After 3 years, weight reduction was still significant (3.5 kg, $p < .001$) and was associated with a significant blood pressure reduction of −2.4/−1.8 mmHg. After 3 years, the incidence of hypertension was significantly reduced in the low-BMI group only ($p < .01$), and only marginally so in the high-BMI group ($p = .066$) as shown in Figure 45.1.

TRIALS OF HYPERTENSION PREVENTION (TOHP), PHASE I

The Trials of Hypertension Prevention (Phase 1) was designed to assess the effect of various nonpharmacologic interventions in nonhypertensive subjects to lower blood pressure and to determine the long-term impact on preventing the development of hypertension (see Table 45.1).[3] The trial was a multicenter, randomized study that examined three lifestyle interventions — weight reduction ($n = 308$), sodium restriction ($n = 327$), stress management ($n = 242$), compared with usual care ($n = 589$) — and various nutritional supplements in two stages with an intervening washout period: (1) 25 mmol or 1 g q.d. of calcium carbonate ($n = 237$), 15 mmol or 360 mg q.d. of magnesium diglycine ($n = 227$), and placebo ($n = 234$) and (2) 6 g of fish oil containing 3 g of omega-3 fatty acids ($n = 175$), 60 mmol or 4.5 g of potassium chloride ($n = 178$), and placebo ($n = 175$). Weight reduction was attempted with a combination of caloric reduction, exercise increase, and behavioral self-management. Stress management involved teaching slow breathing, progressive muscular relaxation, mental imagery, stretching, and managing stress perceptions, reactions, and situations. The lifestyle modifications lasted 18 months and used blinded measurement of blood pressure as an end point. The nutritional supplements were placebo-controlled, doubled-blinded, and lasted 6 months.

TABLE 45.2
Hypertension Prevention Trial (HPT): 6-Month Change in Interventions

	High Body Mass Index				Low Body Mass Index		
	Control	Calories	Sodium	Sodium/Calories	Control	Sodium	Sodium/Potassium
Number of Subjects	121	112	109	113	191	173	180
Δ SBP/DBP (mmHg)	−1.8/−2.5	−6.9[†]/−5.3[‡]	−3.6/−3.4	−5.8/−4.0	−2.1/−3.0	−3.8/−3.4	−3.4/−3.7
Δ Weight (kg)	+0.18	−5.58[†]	−0.04	−3.90	+0.27	+0.00*	+0.27
Δ Na[+] Excretion (mmol/8h)	−4.5	−4.2	−7.8	−8.4	−3.9	−9.4**	−11.4
Δ K[+] Excretion (mmol/8h)	0.3	−1.1	0.9	−0.1	−0.1	0.2	1.2

* $p = .025$; [†] $p < .001$; [‡] $p < .01$; ** $p = .002$ for intervention vs. control group.

Source: Derived from Hypertension Prevention Trial Research Group. *Arch Intern Med*, 150: 153, 1990.

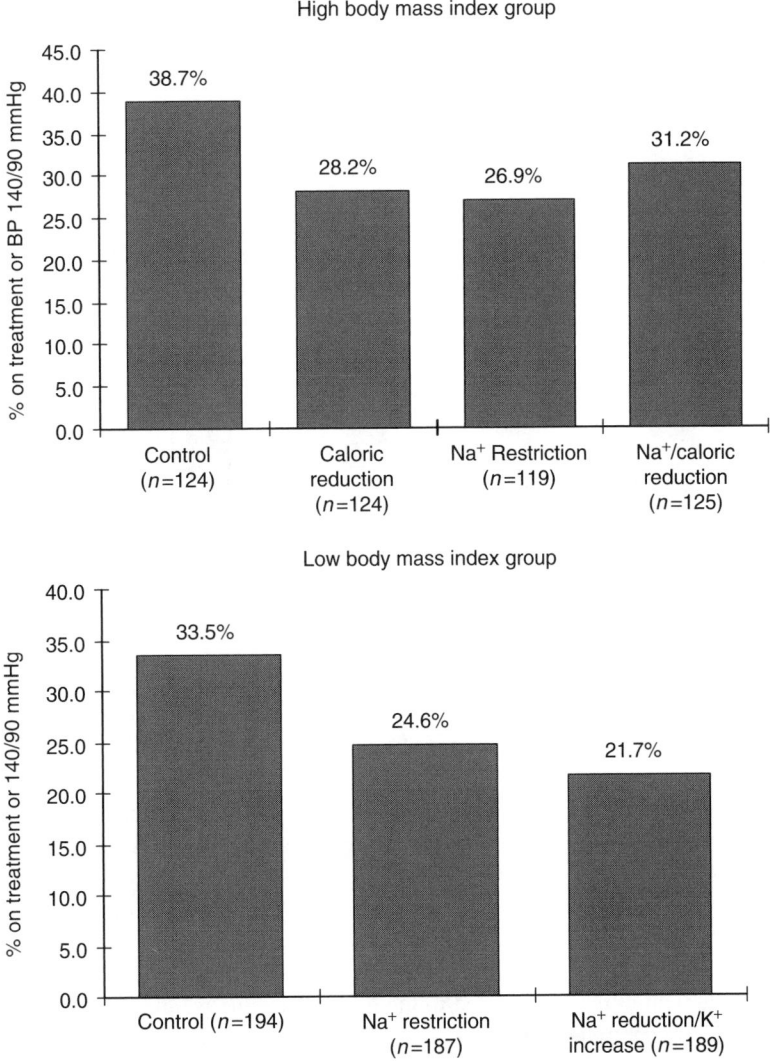

FIGURE 45.1 Hypertension Prevention Trial: 3-year rate of elevated blood pressure or treatment for hypertension, according to BMI and intervention.

TABLE 45.3

Intervention Outcome Treatment Effect and Blood Pressure Effect (Active–Control) in Trial of Hypertension Prevention (Phase I)

Intervention	Outcome treatment effect	Blood pressure effect (mmHg)
18-Months Maximum Follow-up		
Sodium Excretion (mmol/24 h)	$-43.86^{\dagger}$	$-1.69^{\dagger}/-0.85^{*}$
Weight Change (kg)	$-3.90^{\dagger}$	$-2.90^{\dagger}/-2.28^{\dagger}$
Stress Score Frequency/Intensity	$+2.35^{\dagger}/-0.01$	$-0.47/-0.82$
6-Months Maximum Follow-up		
Magnesium Excretion (mmol/24 h)/Serum (mmol/l)	$1.31^{\dagger}/+0.04^{\dagger}$	$-0.20/-0.05$
Calcium Excretion (mmol/24 h)	$0.91^{\dagger}$	$-0.46/+0.20$
Potassium Excretion (mmol/24 h)	$42.29^{\dagger}$	$+0.06/-0.42$
Percentage of Eicosapentaenoic/Docosahexaenoic Fatty Acid	$2.90^{\dagger}/2.04^{\dagger}$	$-0.22/-0.62$

$^{*} p < .05;\ ^{\dagger}p < .01$ for active treatment vs. control (usual care).

Source: Derived from the Trials of Hypertension Prevention Collaborative Research Group. *JAMA*, 267: 1213, 1992.

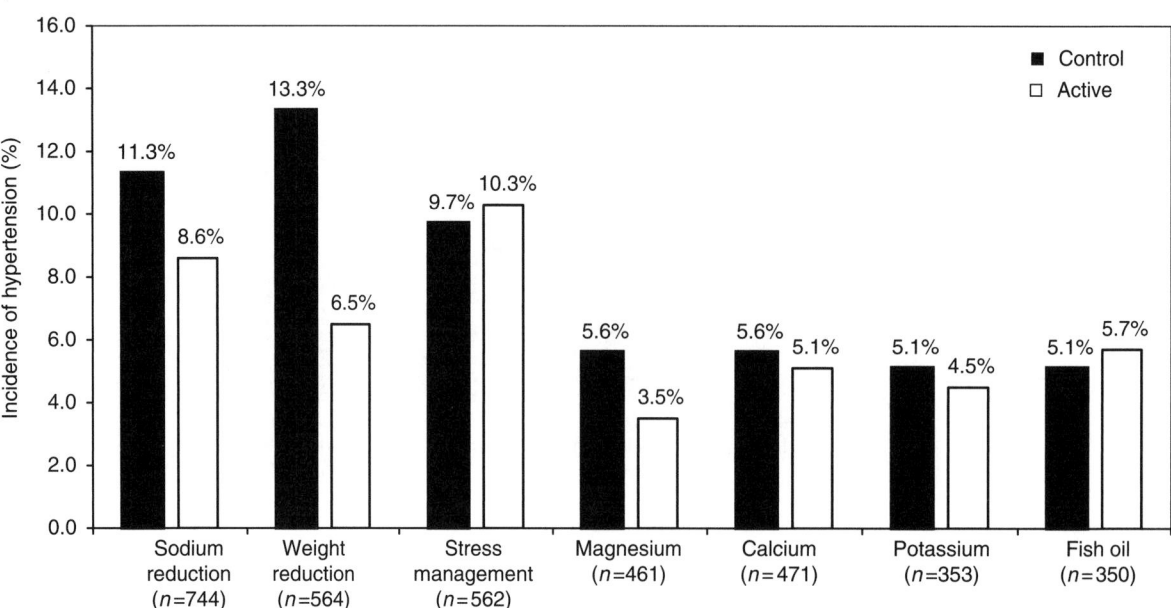

FIGURE 45.2 Trials of Hypertension Prevention (Phase I): incidence of hypertension in each lifestyle change and nutritional supplement group. Only weight reduction significantly reduced incidence of hypertension, relative risk = 0.49 (95% CI, 0.29 to 0.83). (Derived from Corrected Table The Trials of Hypertension Prevention Collaborative Research Group. *JAMA*, 267: 2330, 1992.)

The primary outcomes are displayed in Table 45.3 and Figure 45.2. Only weight reduction significantly lowered blood pressure and reduced the development of hypertension at maximal follow-up at 18 months. Sodium restriction significantly lowered systolic and diastolic blood pressure, −1.7/−0.09 mmHg, but did not significantly reduce the incidence of hypertension.

The weight-loss goal was 4.5 kg for the enrolled participants with 115 to 165% of desirable body weight. In the intervention group, 45% of men and 26% of women, compared with 12% of men and 18% of women in the control group, met the weight-loss goal at 18 months. The net change in weight at 18 months was 4.7 kg for men and 1.8 kg for women ($p < .01$). Rather than being related to gender, the treatment effect was related to the higher baseline weight in males. In fact, the amount of blood pressure change by gender related more to the quintile of weight change, as shown in Table 45.4.

TRIALS OF HYPERTENSION PREVENTION (TOHP II), PHASE II

The randomized Trials of Hypertension Prevention (Phase II) was conducted as a 2 × 2 factorial design study to assess the effect of weight reduction, sodium restriction, or both compared with usual care in lowering blood pressure and preventing the development of hypertension after 3 to 4 years of follow-up.[4] Eligible patients were 30 to 54 years old. Patients with treated

TABLE 45.4

Trials of Hypertension Prevention (Phase I) Effect of Weight Change on Blood Pressure Reduction at 18 Months by Gender

	Quintile of Weight Change (kg)				
	<−9.5	−9.5 to <−4.5	−4.5 to <−2.0	−2.0 to <1.0	≥1.0
Δ Systolic Blood Pressure (mmHg)					
Men	−9.0	−6.6	−4.8	−3.3	−1.6
Women	−5.7	−7.5	−5.0	−0.8	−1.2
Δ Diastolic Blood Pressure (mmHg)					
Men	−9.4	−6.8	−5.5	−4.2	−2.6
Women	−9.1	−7.1	−4.3	−4.9	−4.1

Source: Derived from The Trials of Hypertension Prevention Collaborative Research Group. *JAMA*, 267: 1213, 1992.

TABLE 45.5

Baseline Characteristics and Outcome of the Trials of Hypertension Prevention (Phase II)

	Weight Loss	Sodium Restriction	Combined	Usual Care
Number	595	594	597	596
Age (year)	43.4	44.2	43.6	43.2
Male (%)	63.0	64.8	68.8	68.3
White (%)	78.0	81.1	78.4	79.5
Weight (kg)	93.4	94.0	93.6	93.6
Baseline sodium excretion (mmol/day)	180.9	186.1	179.3	188.0
Baseline blood pressure (mmHg)	127.6/86.0	127.7/86.1	127.4/86.0	127.3/85.8
Six-Month Follow-up				
Weight Change (kg)	−4.4	−1.1	−4.1	0.1
	$p < 0.001$[a]	$p < 0.001$[a]	$p < 0.006$[a]	
Sodium Excretion Change (mmol/d)	−18.2	−78.0	−64.3	−27.6
	$p = 0.48$[a]	$p < 0.001$[a]	$p = 0.006$[a]	
Change in Blood Pressure (mmHg)	−6.0/−5.5	−5.1/−4.4	−6.2/−5.6	−2.2/−2.8
	$p < 0.001/<0.001$[b]	$p < 0.001/<0.001$[b]	$p < 0.001/<0.001$[b]	
Incidence of Hypertension (%)	4.2	4.5	2.7	7.3
	$p = 0.02$[a]	$p = 0.04$[a]	$p < 0.001$[a]	
36-Month Follow-up				
Weight Change (kg)	−0.2	+1.7	−0.3	+1.8
	$p < 0.001$[a]	$p = 0.92$[a]	$p < 0.001$[a]	
Sodium Excretion Change (mmol/d)	−9.0	−50.9	−34.1	−10.5
	$p = 0.79$[a]	$p < 0.001$[a]	$p < 0.001$[a]	
Change in Blood Pressure (mmHg)	−0.8/−3.2	−0.7/−3.0	−0.5/−3.0	+0.6/−2.4
	$p = 0.01/0.04$[†]	$p = 0.02/0.10$[b]	$p = 0.05/0.19$[b]	
Incidence of Hypertension (%)	31.9	34.4	32.8	39.2

[a] Significance vs. usual-care group.

[b] Significance of systolic and diastolic blood pressure vs. usual group.

Source: Derived from Trials of Hypertension Prevention Collaborative Research Group *Arch Intern Med*, 157: 657, 1997.

hypertension, cardiovascular disease, diabetes mellitus, and renal insufficiency were excluded. Diastolic blood pressure was required to be 83 to 89 mmHg at the third screening visit and weight 110% to 165% of desirable body weight. Intervention goals for the weight reduction group were weight loss ≥4.5 kg and for the sodium reduction group a decrease in sodium intake ≤80 mmol/day. Blinded observers measured blood pressure, and 2382 subjects were recruited.

Baseline and treatment outcomes are displayed in Table 45.5. By 6 months, neither the weight loss nor sodium restriction goals were met by the groups; however, the net blood pressure reduction compared with the usual-care group was significant ($p<.001$ for each intervention): weight loss, −3.7/−2.7 mmHg; sodium restriction, −2.9/−1.6 mmHg; and the combination,

−4.0/−2.8 mmHg. At 36 months, many of the treatment effects were lost. The 38% incidence of hypertension was similar in all treatment groups, compared with 44% in the usual-care group, and did not appear additive at 36 months. The relative risk of hypertension (compared with the usual-care group) was 0.87 for the weight-loss group (p = .06), 0.86 for the sodium reduction group (p = .04), and 0.85 for the combined intervention group (p = .02).[4]

Subsequent analyses compared the sodium restriction and the usual-care groups, which included 1159 Black (17%) and White participants[5,6] After 36 months, urine sodium excretion decreased from baseline by a greater amount in men (−60.1 mmol/24 h) than in women (−34.4 mmol/24 h) assigned to the sodium reduction group; however, the baseline was higher in men (203.8 mmol/24 h) than women (153.4 mmol/24 h).[5] Compared with the usual-care group; there was a greater difference in urinary sodium excretion in men (−51.3 mmol/24 h) than women (−19.8 mmol/24 h) among sodium-restricted patients. Comparing the change in urine sodium excretion between the usual-care and sodium reduction groups after 36 months, the greatest difference was seen among Black men (−74.6 mmol/24 h) and the least among White women (−18.4 mmol/24 h). Overall only 21% of study participants achieved a urinary sodium level <80 mmol/24 h. More attendance at intervention sessions predicted a greater reduction in sodium excretion. After 36 months, the treatment effect of sodium restriction (subtracted from the usual-care group) on blood pressure was −1.1/−0.3, +0.5/+1.4, −1.5/−1.4 and −3.0/−2.4 mmHg for White men, Black men, White women, and Black women, respectively. Overall, the incidence of hypertension was 6% lower in sodium-restricted group compared with the usual-care group, and 7%, 4%, 2%, and 12% lower among White men, Black men, White women, and Black women, respectively. The effect of the degree of urinary sodium excretion on blood pressure was studied.[6] At 36 months for both groups, there was a −3.0/−0.5 mmHg (p = .005 for systolic only) greater reduction in blood pressure for the quintile that had greatest change in urinary sodium excretion from baseline compared with the group that had the least.

SECONDARY PREVENTION TRIALS

DIETARY INTERVENTION STUDY IN HYPERTENSION (DISH)

Participants in DISH were former medicated participants of the Hypertension Detection and Follow-up Program.[7] The cohort (n = 496) was grouped into obese (≥120% of ideal body weight) or nonobese. The obese group was randomized into one of four groups: (1) continue drug therapy or (2) discontinue drug therapy, and (a) receive no dietary intervention, the control group, (b) decrease sodium intake, or (c) lose weight. The nonobese group was randomized to (1) continue drug therapy or (2) discontinue drug therapy and (a) receive no dietary intervention, the control group, or (b) decrease sodium intake.

Demographics and outcomes are shown in Table 45.6. Among overweight persons, 46.3% lost an average of 5% of weight or >4.5 kg after 56 weeks. The average weight loss in this group was 4.0 kg (p < .05 vs. the no-medication control group). Among obese and nonobese persons who were sodium restricted, the mean decrease in urine sodium output was −59 mEq/24 h and −44 mEq/24 h (each p < .05 vs. the no-medication control group) after 56 weeks. The percentage not taking antihypertensive medication among obese individuals was 35.3% in the control group, 44.9% in the sodium-restricted group, and 59.5% in weight-loss group (p = .0015 vs. control). In the lean group, the percentage not taking antihypertensive medication was 45% in the control group and 53.4% in the sodium-restricted group (not significantly different).

TABLE 45.6
Dietary Intervention Study in Hypertension: Demographics and Outcome

	Obese				Lean		
	Drug Therapy Control	No Drug Control	Sodium Restriction	Weight Reduction	Drug Therapy Control	No Drug Control	Sodium Restriction
Number	48	89	101	87	33	70	68
Age (years)	59	57	57	56	58	57	56
Percentage of Blacks	75	70	64	62	58	73	56
Percentage of Women	69	64	59	68	52	50	47
BP[a] (mmHg)	131/80	128/80	128/81	128/81	126/80	124/80	127/81
Δ Weight (kg)	−0.46	−0.46	0	−4.0	+0.46	0	+0.46
Δ Urine Na$^+$ (mEq/day)	−13	−10	−59	0	+2	−5	−44
No BP[a] Drugs (%)	0	35.3	44.9	59.5	0	45.0	53.4

[a] BP = blood pressure.

Source: Derived from Langford, H. G. et al., *JAMA*, 253: 657, 1985.

THE HYPERTENSION CONTROL PROGRAM (HCP)

Participants in HCP were former drug-treated participants of the Hypertension Detection and Follow-up Program.[8] Subjects ($n = 189$) were randomized to three groups: (1) discontinue antihypertensive therapy and reduce weight, excess salt, and alcohol; (2) stop medication without nutritional intervention (the control group); or (3) continue drug treatment with no nutritional program. The primary end point was the percentage of subjects remaining hypertensive in the intervention vs. the control group.

As shown in Table 45.7, in the nutritional intervention group, weight decreased ($p < .001$) and sodium excretion increased ($p < .001$) significantly after 4 years. Of the nutritional therapy group, 39% were maintained on no drug therapy compared with only 5% of the control group ($p < .001$).

TRIAL OF ANTIHYPERTENSIVE INTERVENTION AND MANAGEMENT (TAIM)

This multicenter, placebo-controlled, 3×3 designed trial randomized 787 overweight (110 to 160% ideal body weight) hypertensive (baseline diastolic pressure 90 to 100 mmHg) men and women to one of three drugs (placebo, chlorthalidone 25 mg q.d., or atenolol 50 mg q.d.) and three dietary interventions (usual diet, weight loss, or sodium decrease/potassium increase).[9] The weight-loss goal was the greater of 10% of baseline weight or 4.54 kg decrease. Sodium reduction was 52 to 100 mmol/day and potassium augmentation 62 to 115 mmol/day, depending on weight. Both weight reduction and electrolyte changes required group nutritional counseling weekly for 10 weeks and individually thereafter every 6 to 12 weeks. There was no change in the drugs or their dosages during the first 6 months of the trial, unless critical diastolic blood pressures were reached (treatment crossovers). Change in diastolic blood pressure, treatment failure (as assessed by the need to increase drug treatment), quality of life, and calculated cardiovascular risk were measured.

Table 45.8 shows the change in systolic and diastolic blood pressure from baseline to 6 months in the treatment groups. In the weight-loss group, the average decrease in weight was 4.5 kg after 6 months. Weight loss was more effective than the usual

TABLE 45.7
Hypertension Control Program: Demographics and Outcome

	No BP[a] Drugs		BP Drugs
	Nutritional Therapy	No Nutritional Therapy	No Nutritional Therapy
Number	97	44	48
Age (years)	57	55	55
Percentage of Females	35	39	38
Percentage of Blacks	11	21	15
BP (mmHg)	122/78	118/77	119/79
Δ Weight (kg)[b]	−1.8*	+2.0	+2.0
Δ Urinary Na$^+$ (mEq/day)	−60*	+20	−5
Δ Ethanol (g/day)[c]	−12.5	−7.1	−10.2
Percentage without BP Drugs	39*	5	0

* $p < .001$.

[a] Blood Pressure.

[b] Among obese subjects only.

[c] Among drinkers only.

Source: Derived from Stamler, R. et al., *JAMA*, 257: 1484, 1987.

TABLE 45.8
Trial of Antihypertensive Intervention and Management: Change in Blood Pressure (mmHg) from Baseline by Treatment Group at Six Months

	Usual Diet	Weight Loss	Low Na$^+$/High K$^+$
Placebo	−10.34/−7.96 ($n = 90$)	−11.49/−8.78 ($n = 90$)	−8.66/−7.91 ($n = 79$)
Chlorthalidone	−17.41/−10.78 ($n = 87$)	−21.72/−15.06 ($n = 87$)	−19.51/−12.18 ($n = 89$)
Atenolol	−15.06/−12.43 ($n = 87$)	−18.11/−14.81 ($n = 88$)	−18.29/−12.76 ($n = 90$)

Source: Derived from Langford, H. G. et al., *Hypertension*, 17: 210, 1991.

TABLE 45.9

Trial of Antihypertensive Intervention and Management: Change in Diastolic Blood Pressure (mmHg) for >4.5 kg Weight Change-Comparable to Low-dose Drug Therapy

	Usual Diet	>4.5 kg Weight Loss
Placebo	−7.0 (n = 71)	−11.6 (n = 33)*
Chlorthalidone	−11.1 (n = 80)	−15.3 (n = 53)†
Atenolol	−12.4 (n = 79)	−18.4 (n = 26)‡

* $p < .01$; † $p = .002$, ‡ $p = .0005$ compared to usual diet.

Source: Derived from Wassertheil-Smoller, S. et al., Arch Intern Med, 152: 131, 1992.

diet ($p = .001$) or low sodium/high potassium diet ($p = .019$) in lowering diastolic blood pressure. Weight loss in combination with a diuretic added significantly to blood pressure reduction compared with the usual diet with a diuretic (−15.1 mmHg vs. −10.8 mmHg, $p = .002$). The combination of weight loss with a β-blocker did not add to the effect of the drug alone on a usual diet (−14.8 mmHg vs. −12.4 mmHg, $p = .07$).

Of the weight-loss cohort, 45% lost ≥4.5 kg. For patients who were not treatment crossovers, placebo and usual diet ($n = 71$) was associated with a 7 mmHg decrease in diastolic blood pressure and a 0.63 kg weight loss and was less effective than placebo diet, which was associated with >4.5 kg weight loss and diastolic blood pressure decrease of 11.6 mmHg ($p < .01$). There was a graded relationship with the amount of weight reduction and diastolic blood pressure reduction: <2.25 kg, −6.9 mmHg; −2.25 to 4.5 kg, −8.9 mmHg; and >4.5 kg, −11.6 mmHg. The change in diastolic blood pressure inversely correlated with the baseline plasma renin indexed to the 24 h urinary sodium in the weight-loss diet group.[10] Also, the change in diastolic blood pressure with >4.5 kg weight change is comparable with that in low-dose drug therapy as seen in Table 45.9. After 24 months, there was gradual return of weight toward the baseline.[11] Among the weight-loss diet patients, the least mean change in weight occurred among atenolol-treated subjects. Furthermore, among atenolol-treated subjects assigned to usual diet or electrolyte modification, there was a mean weight gain. The 5-year incidence of treatment failure was lower in the weight-loss group (49.8 per 100 subjects) than in the usual diet group (56.7 per 100 subjects).[12]

In the low-sodium/high-potassium group, the average decrease in urinary sodium was 27.4 mmol/day and the average increase in urinary potassium 10.9 mmol/day. The effect of the low-sodium/high-potassium diet on blood pressure was not different when compared with the usual diet ($p = .347$). The low-sodium/high-potassium diet did not further lower diastolic blood pressure, but the baseline urinary sodium excretion was already relatively low (133 mmol/day). However, in the placebo group, when urinary sodium excretion ≤70 mEq/day was achieved, systolic and diastolic blood pressure reduction was greater than in the usual diet group (−23.7/−13.9 mmHg vs. −9.6/−7.0 mmHg, each $p < .005$).[13]

After 3 years, compared with the usual diet, the net difference of urinary sodium excretion reduction was 30 mmol/day and urinary potassium excretion augmentation was 11 mmol/day.[14] There was a 41% decrease ($p = .01$) in the risk of treatment failure for women and a 34% decrease ($p = .03$) among less obese patients. After 3.5 years, among patients assigned to low-sodium/high-potassium diet, treatment failures occurred in 68% of placebo-, 47% of diuretic-, and 35% of β-blocker-assigned subjects.

Quality of life was improved with weight reduction.[15] Weight reduction significantly reduced symptoms of physical problems, especially sexual problems, and improved satisfaction with physical health. Weight reduction reduced symptoms of sexual problems in both men and women significantly. Weight loss improved reported erectile dysfunction with chlorthalidone and usual diet (12.1% vs. 26.2%).[16] The low-sodium/high-potassium diet with placebo was associated with greater fatigue (34.3%) than was either with usual diet (18.1%, $p = .04$) or weight reduction (14.6%, $p = .009$). The electrolyte intervention group in combination with chlorthalidone (32.0%, $p = .04$) was associated with more sleep disturbances than with chlorthalidone and a usual diet (16%). A nonsignificant ($p = .07$) similar trend was observed with atenolol.

Overall calculated cardiovascular risk worsened with chlorthalidone therapy in the usual diet group at 6 months because of the changes in cholesterol and glucose.[17] Those persons treated with atenolol or weight reduction showed the lowest relative risk.

Trial of Nonpharmacologic Interventions in the Elderly (TONE)

This was a randomized, multicenter, controlled trial of 975 men and women aged 60 to 80 years with a blood pressure <145/<85 mmHg on a single hypertensive drug.[18] Patients were randomized to treatment based on their body habitus. 585 obese patients received: (1) usual care, (2) sodium restriction (a dietary intake <80 mmol/d as measured by 24-hour urine sodium collection), (3) a weight-loss program to achieve a loss of ≥4.5 kg, or (4) a combination of sodium restriction and weight loss. 390 nonobese patients were randomized to usual care or sodium restriction.

The mean change in blood pressure prior to attempted medication withdrawal for each group was: (1) sodium reduction, −3.4/−1.9 mmHg; (2) weight reduction, −4.0/−1.1 mmHg; (3) combination intervention, −5.3/−3.4 mmHg; and (4) usual care, −0.8/−0.8 mmHg. Sodium reduction, weight loss and the combination intervention lowered blood pressure significantly more than usual care. After 3 months of nonpharmacological therapy, antihypertensive medication withdrawal was attempted. After 30 months, 44% of patients in the combined sodium and weight reduction group were free of a primary endpoint (sustained blood pressure of 150/90 mmHg or higher, pharmacologic treatment of hypertension, or occurrence of a clinical cardiovascular event). Compared to 16% in the usual-care group, 34% of the sodium restriction group and 37% of the weight reduction group did not have a primary endpoint at 30 months. The sodium restricted group reduced average sodium intake about 40 mmol/d. In the weight-loss group, average body weight decreased by 3.5 kg. Sodium restriction was equally effective in the obese and lean subjects; however, the combined intervention was not more effective than either single intervention. Predictors of successful long-term withdrawal of pharmacologic treatment include lower baseline systolic blood pressure, shorter duration of hypertension or drug treatment, and the absence of a history of cardiovascular disease.[19]

Diet, Exercise, and Weight Loss Intervention Trial (DEW-IT)

This trial assessed the effect of a DASH diet (see the following section), weight loss, reduced sodium intake (100 mmol/day), and regular aerobic exercise on 24 h ambulatory blood pressure.[20] The study was conducted over a period of 9 weeks. Overweight (BMI > 25 kg/m^2), hypertensive patients receiving monotherapy or a fixed combination antihypertensive medication were selected. Using a random-zero sphygmomanometer, the entry blood pressure was 130 to 170 mmHg for systolic and 80 to 100 mmHg for diastolic blood pressure, based on the average two measurements per visit at each of the three visits. All meals were provided at the clinic site or home. Alcohol was limited to 2 drinks/day and caffeinated beverages to 3 drinks/day. The weight-loss goal was 4.5 kg (10 lb), and the exercise goal was 30 to 45 min of moderate aerobic exercise (brisk walking or a cycle ergometer) 3 days each week. The control group was provided nutritional and lifestyle counseling.

Forty-five patients were randomized to this carefully conducted trial. The baseline characteristics included a mean age of 54 years, BMI 33.5 kg/m^2, 62% African-Americans, and 62% women. The mean reduction in 24 h ambulatory blood pressure after 9 weeks was greater in the intervention group than the control group (−10.5/−5.9 vs. −1.1/−0.6 mmHg, $p \leq .002$ for systolic and diastolic). The rate of blood pressure control (<135/85 mmHg) using 24 hour ambulatory blood pressure was greater in the intervention group than the control group (75% vs. 35%, $p = .012$). The change from baseline after 9 weeks was significantly improved in the lifestyle group compared with the control group for 24 h urine potassium (+13 vs. −4 mmol/l, $p = .009$), BMI (−1.9 vs. −0.2 kg/m^2, $p < .001$), weight (−5.5 vs. −0.6 kg, $p < .001$), heart rate (−14.8 vs. −6 beats/min, $p = .011$), and low-density lipoprotein (LDL) cholesterol (−5 vs. +12 mg/dl, $p = .005$). The change from baseline in 24 h urine sodium excretion and triglycerides was not different between groups; however, the change in high-density lipoprotein (HDL) cholesterol was significantly lower in the lifestyle group compared with the control group (−9 vs. −3 mg/dl, $p < .001$).

MIXED-POPULATION PREVENTION TRIALS

Dietary Approaches to Stop Hypertension (DASH)

The DASH trial was a multicenter, randomized feeding study that sought to assess the impact of nutrients naturally occurring in food in contrast to nutritional supplements.[21] Subjects were required to have a systolic blood pressure less than 160 mmHg and a diastolic blood pressure 80 to 95 mmHg. Persons consuming greater than 14 alcoholic beverages per week were excluded from the study. After screening, all subjects completed a 3-week control diet. The control diet included magnesium, potassium, and calcium at the 25th percentile of consumption and fiber at the average level of consumption. After the control period, 459 study participants were randomized to a control diet, a fruit and vegetable diet, or a combination diet for 8 weeks. The fruit and vegetable diet provided magnesium and potassium at the 75th percentile of consumption and was also high in fiber. The composition of the combination diet was: (1) high in protein and fiber, (2) high in calcium, magnesium and potassium to the 75th percentile of consumption, and (3) low in total fat, total cholesterol, and saturated fat. The sodium content (~3000 mg/day) was similar for all three diets. Caloric intake was adjusted so that weight gain did not occur in the study.

The average age of the subjects was 44 years, 60% were African-American, and 49% were women. About 14% of study participants had a diastolic blood pressure ≥90 mmHg, and 23.5% had a systolic blood pressure ≥140 mmHg. The change in the diastolic blood pressure was the primary outcome. The change in blood pressure in the combination group (corrected for the change in the control group) was −5.5/−3.0 mmHg ($p < .001$ for systolic and diastolic blood pressure). The change in blood pressure among hypertensive subjects was larger than nonhypertensive subjects (−11.4/−5.5 mmHg vs. −3.5/−2.1 mmHg), and among minority subjects was larger than in nonminority subjects (−6.8/−3.5 mmHg vs. −3.0/−2.0 mmHg). The change in blood pressure in the fruits and vegetables group minus the change in the control group was −2.8/−1.1 mmHg ($p < .001$ for systolic and diastolic blood pressure). Hypertensive subjects had a greater blood pressure reduction (−7.2/−2.8 mmHg) on the fruits and vegetables diet.

The combination diet demonstrated superiority over the fruits and vegetables in reducing blood pressure significantly by an average of −2.5/−1.9 mmHg more. The combination diet lowered systolic blood pressure significantly more in African-Americans

(6.8 mmHg) than in Whites (3.0 mmHg), and in hypertensive subjects (11.4 mmHg) than in nonhypertensive subjects (3.4 mmHg) ($p < .05$ for both).[22]

DIETARY APPROACHES TO STOP HYPERTENSION-SODIUM (DASH-SODIUM)

To assess the effect of the level of sodium intake on blood pressure, a multicenter trial randomized 412 participants to a control diet or the DASH diet.[23] Sodium intake targets were low (50 mmol/day), intermediate (100 mmol/day), or high (150 mmol/day), corresponding to the hypothesized optimal antihypertensive effect, the national guideline recommendation, and the typical consumption. Food was provided to all subjects, and the caloric content was adjusted to ensure that weight did not change during the trial. A high-sodium control diet was given for 2 weeks. Then, using a parallel-group design, subjects were assigned to one of two diets and, in a random sequence, each of the three sodium levels for 30 days. Blood pressure, using a random-zero sphygmomanometer, and 24 h urinary electrolytes were measured.

The population included patients with a blood pressure of 120–159/80–95 mmHg. Screened patients with heart disease, renal insufficiency, diabetes that was poorly controlled or requiring insulin, hypertensive individuals on antihypertensive medications, or alcohol intake exceeding 14 drinks/week were excluded. Average age was 48 years, 57% were women, 57% were Black, and 41% were hypertensive. The BMI was 30 kg/m^2, blood pressure 135/86 mmHg, and urinary sodium excretion 155 mmol/day.

Weight was stable in each sodium level group although the weight in the control diet group was 2.8 to 3 kg higher than the DASH group. Urinary sodium excretion was 65, 107, and 1440 mmol/day in the low-, intermediate-, and high-sodium-intake groups, respectively. Urinary potassium excretion was 35 to 40 mmol/day higher among DASH diet participants. Compared with control diet, the DASH diet lowered blood pressure in the high-sodium ($-5.9/-2.9$ mmHg, $p < .001$ for systolic and diastolic), intermediate-sodium ($-5.0/-2.5$, $p < .001$ for systolic and $p < .01$ for diastolic blood pressure), and low-sodium groups ($-2.2/-1.0$ mmHg, $p < .05$ for systolic blood pressure only). For control diet, the change in blood pressure from high sodium to low sodium intake was $-6.7/-3.5$ mmHg and for the DASH diet $-7.2/-3.5$ mmHg.

Subgroup analyses comparing the lower-sodium-intake DASH diet with the higher-sodium-intake control diet observed a blood pressure reduction of $-11.5/-5.7$ mmHg for hypertensives (vs. $-7.1/-3.7$ mmHg for nonhypertensives, $p < .01$ systolic only), $-9.6/-5.0$ mmHg for Blacks, $-7.8/-3.7$ mmHg for non-Blacks, $-10.5/-4.7$ mmHg for females (vs. $-6.8/-4.2$ mmHg for males, $p < .05$ for systolic only), and $-11.6/-5.5$ mmHg for subjects >45 years (vs. $-5.6/-3.3$ mmHg for younger subjects, $p < .01$ for systolic and $p < .05$ for diastolic).[24] There were no systolic blood pressure differences among participants according to BMI (-7.8 mmHg for ≥30 kg/m^2 vs. -9.5 mmHg for <30 kg/m^2). Compared with the high-sodium diet, there was a powerful graded reduction of blood pressure with low-sodium diet according to age among control diet ($-4.8/-2.4$ mmHg for 23 to 41 years, $-5.9/-3.4$ mmHg for 42 to 47 years, $-7.5/-4.2$ mmHg for 48 to 54 years, and $-8.1/-3.7$ mmHg for 55 to 76 years) and DASH diet patients ($-1.0/-0.9$ mmHg for 23 to 41 years, $-1.8/-1.4$ mmHg for 42 to 47 years, $-4.3/-1.8$ mmHg for 48 to 54 years, and $-6.0/-2.8$ mmHg for 55 to 76 years).[25] Dietary sodium intake did not influence LDL cholesterol, HDL cholesterol, or triglyceride levels on either diet.[26] Total, LDL, and HDL cholesterol was lower on the DASH diet at each level of sodium intake.

PREMIER TRIAL

The purpose of PREMIER was to determine the effectiveness of two multicomponent interventions on blood pressure and hypertension status at 6 months.[27,28] 810 participants were randomized to one of three groups: (1) advice only, (2) behavioral, or (3) behavioral with the DASH diet. The advice group received a single, individual counseling session by a registered dietician, who discussed weight, sodium intake, physical activity, and the DASH diet. The behavioral group received four individual counseling sessions and 14 group meetings to achieve a weight-loss goal of 15 lb (if the body mass index was 25 kg/m^2 or more), moderate-intensity physical exercise of 180 min/week, dietary sodium restriction to 100 mEq, and alcohol restriction of 1 oz/day for men and ½ oz/day for women. The behavioral with DASH diet group was additionally educated on the details of the DASH diet. However, unlike the DASH trial, this was not a feeding study. Blood pressure measurements were taken with a random-zero sphygmomanometer by staff masked to treatment group assignment.

The study population included individuals 25 years or older with a BMI of 18.5 to 45 kg/m^2. Individuals not on antihypertensive medications were eligible if their blood pressure was 120–159/80–95 mmHg based on duplicate measurements at three screening visits. Cardiovascular disease, target organ damage, diabetes mellitus, cancer, and heavy ethanol consumption (21 drinks/week) were the main exclusion factors. Dietary recall of nutrients and food groups was assessed twice both at baseline and 6 months. Physical activity recall for a 1-week period and a submaximal stress test were also performed. In addition, an alcohol intake questionnaire and 24 h urinary electrolytes were collected.

The study population was 50 years, 62% women, 34% African-American, and 95% overweight. Of the study participants, 37 to 38% were hypertensive. Weight loss occurred in each group; however, weight loss in the advice group (-1.1 kg) was less than the behavioral group (-4.9 kg, $p < .001$) or the behavioral and DASH group (-5.8 kg, $p < .001$). There was no difference in physical activity and alcohol intake among the three groups, but fitness assessed by submaximal exercise heart rate improved more in both behavioral intervention groups. The percentage of individuals attaining intervention goals is displayed in Table 45.10.

TABLE 45.10
Attained Intervention Goals in PREMIER Trial: Percent Change from Baseline

	Advice Only	Behavioral Only	Behavioral and DASH
Weight loss >15 lb (%)	6.2	28.6*	34.3[†]
Urine sodium ≤100 mmol/d (%)	7.9	19.8*	12.8[†‡]
Alcohol Intake Goal (%)	−0.9	1.3	1.3
≥9 servings/day of fruits and vegetables (%)	3.5	1.3	26.9[†‡]
≥2 servings/day of dairy products (%)	2.6	−3.5	23.0[†‡]
≤25% kcal/day of total fat (%)	3.5	14.6*	42.2[†‡]
≤7% kcal/day of saturated fat (%)	3.9	13.6*	36.9[†‡]

* $p < .05$: Behavioral only vs. advice only.

[†] $p < .05$: Behavioral and DASH vs. advice only.

[‡] $p < .05$: Behavioral and DASH vs. behavioral only.

Source: Derived from data of Appel L. J. et al., *JAMA*, 289: 2083, 2003.

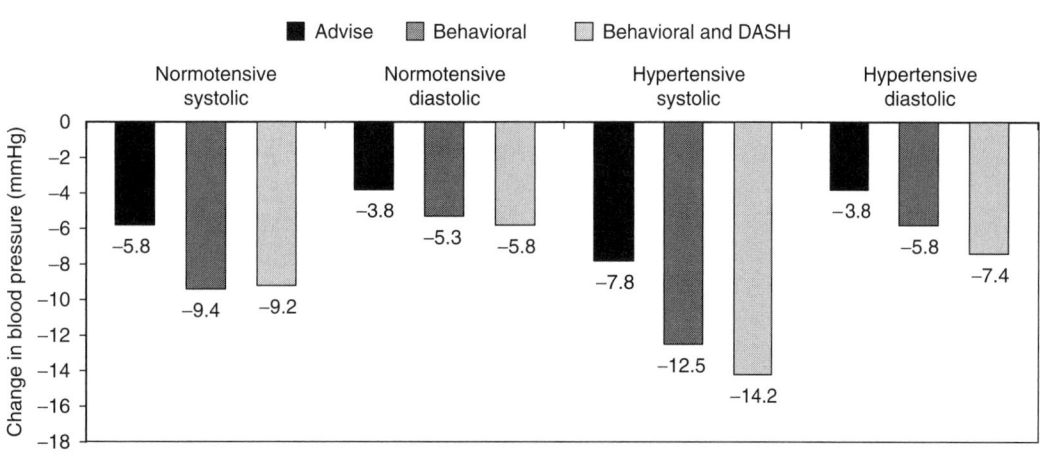

FIGURE 45.3 PREMIER Trial: change in blood pressure (mmHg) from baseline to 6 months according to hypertensive status and treatment category. (Derived from data of Appel, L. J. et al., *JAMA*, 289: 2083, 2003.)

The mean change in blood pressure from baseline to 6 months was −6.6/−3.8 mmHg in the advice group, −10.5/−5.5 mmHg in behavioral group, and −11.1/−6.4 mmHg in the behavioral and DASH group. The change in blood pressure in both behavioral intervention groups was greater than the advice group ($p < .001$); however, the change in blood pressure between the behavioral groups was not significant. Figure 45.3 displays the mean change in blood pressure in hypertensive and normotensive subjects according the treatment assignment. Among the normotensive patients at baseline, the percentages that were hypertensive at 6 months were 11%, 8%, and 6% in the advice, behavioral, and behavioral and DASH groups (no significant difference among the groups); among the hypertensive patients, the corresponding percentages were 52%, 34% ($p = .01$ vs. advice group), and 23% ($p < .001$ vs. advice group). An optimum blood pressure (<120/80 mmHg) was attained less commonly in the advice group (19%) compared with the behavioral (30%, $p = .005$ vs. advice group) and behavioral and DASH (35%, $p < .001$ vs. advice group) interventions. Table 45.11 shows the change in systolic blood pressure from baseline to 6 months according treatment, race, gender, and age.[29] African-American women did not achieve a significant reduction in systolic blood pressure from both behavioral interventions compared with the advice group. Of the 52 subjects tested with an intravenous glucose tolerance test at baseline and 6 months, insulin sensitivity improved only in the behavioral and DASH group.[30]

OPTIMAL MACRONUTRIENT INTAKE TRIAL TO PREVENT HEART DISEASE (OMNIHEART)

Although the carbohydrate-rich DASH trial reported benefits in lowering blood pressure and LDL cholesterol, HDL cholesterol also decreased.[31] The purpose of OmniHeart was to compare which macronutrient (protein, carbohydrate, or unsaturated fat) should replace saturated fats to optimally lower blood pressure and lipids.[32] This was a randomized, three-period crossover design comparing three diets that were low in saturated fats after a 6-day run-in period. The order of diets was randomized

TABLE 45.11
PREMIER Trial: Change in Systolic Blood Pressure (mmHg) in Demographic Groups According to Treatment Group

	Advice Only	Behavioral Only	Behavioral and DASH
Black women	−6.2	−7.7	−8.6
Black men	−6.4	−11.8*	−10.2*
Non-Black women	−7.6	−11.9*	−11.6*
Non-Black men	−6.2	−10.7*	−12.2*
Age ≥50	−7.1	−10.6*	−13.5*
Age <50	−6.4	−10.3*	−8.3*

* $p < .05$ compare to advice group.

Source: Derived from data of Svetkey, L. P. et al., *J Hum Hypertens*, 19: 21, 2005.

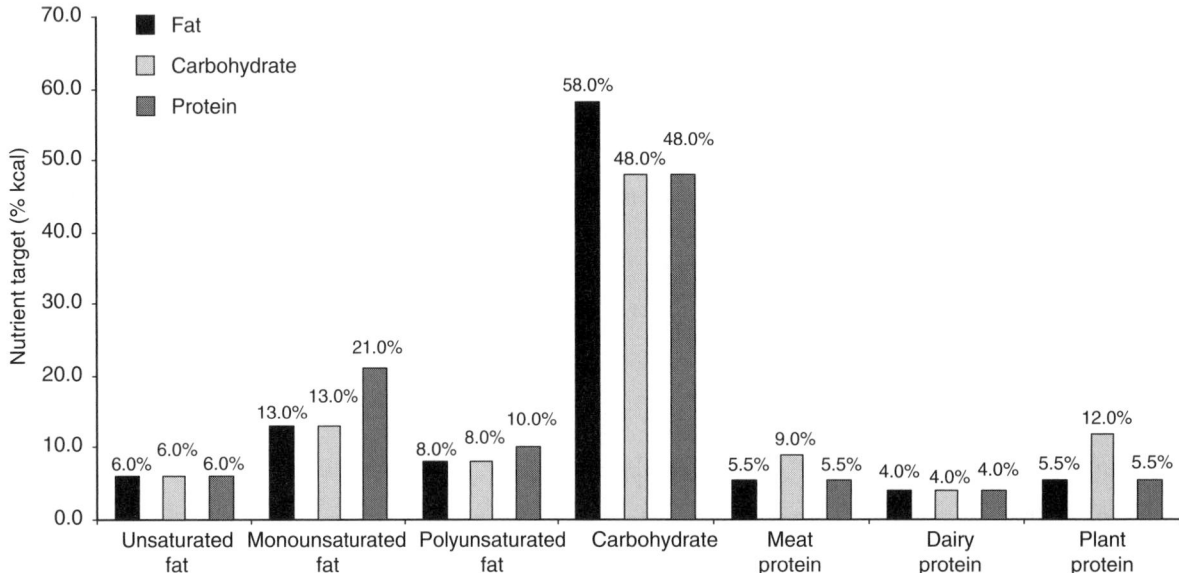

FIGURE 45.4 Optimal Macronutrient Intake Trial to prevent heart disease: nutrient targets of foods by diet at 2100 kcal. (Derived from Appel, L. J. et al., *JAMA*, 294: 2455, 2005.)

to one of six sequences of 6 weeks duration with a washout period of 2 to 4 weeks between feeding periods. Weight was maintained by adjusting the caloric content at the meal site. The nutritional targets for the carbohydrate, protein, and unsaturated fat diets are displayed in Figure 45.4. The carbohydrate diet was similar to the DASH, except that carbohydrate content was increased by 3% of kilocalories and the protein content reduced by 3% of kilocalories. 191 participants were enrolled, and 160 to 161 subjects were used in analysis.

Patients 30 years or older were included with a blood pressure of 120–159/80–99 mmHg. African-Americans were recruited to a target of about 50%. Patients who were excluded had cardiovascular disease, diabetes, medications affecting blood pressure or lipids, LDL cholesterol >220 mg/dl, fasting triglycerides >750 mg/dl, weight >350 lb, and >14 alcoholic beverages per week.

Adherence to the diet was high, 95 to 96%. Compared with baseline, each diet was associated with a decline in blood pressure, LDL and HDL cholesterol, and triglycerides (except the carbohydrate diet). The blood pressure decline (between-diet difference compared with the carbohydrate diet) was −1.4/−1.2 mmHg ($p \leq .002$ for systolic and diastolic) for the protein diet and −1.3/−0.8 mmHg ($p \leq .02$ for systolic and diastolic) for the unsaturated fat diet. Of the 32 hypertensive subjects, more remained hypertensive on the carbohydrate diet (38%) than on the protein (22%) or the unsaturated fat diet (19%). There was no blood pressure difference between the protein and unsaturated fat diet. Compared with the carbohydrate diet, the protein (1.5 mmHg, $p = .009$) and the unsaturated fat diet (1.2 mmHg, $p = .05$) lowered systolic blood pressure by a greater amount in Blacks.

LDL cholesterol was lowered by 3 mg/dl more on the protein diet compared with the carbohydrate diet. HDL cholesterol decreased more on the protein diet compared with carbohydrate (−1.3 mg/dl, $p = .02$) and unsaturated fat diet (−2.3 mg/dl, $p < .001$); however, HDL increased more on the unsaturated fat diet compared with the carbohydrate diet (+1.1 mg/dl, $p = .03$).

The protein (−15.7 mg/dl, $p < .001$) and saturated fat (−9.6 mg/dl, $p = .02$) diets lowered triglycerides more than the carbohydrate diet, and the protein diet lowered triglycerides more than the unsaturated fat diet (−7.1 mg/dl, $p = .03$).

SUMMARY

The primary prevention trials prove that sodium restriction and weight reduction are effective in reducing the rate of development of hypertension. However, the behavioral changes are difficult to sustain over a 36-month period, and the treatment effects are modest. Individual strategies of potassium, calcium, magnesium, or fish oil supplementation are not effective in nonhypertensive subjects in lowering blood pressure or preventing the development of hypertension.

The secondary prevention trials document a clear benefit for sodium restriction and weight reduction in controlling blood pressure. However, the combination of weight reduction and sodium restriction was not additive. Weight loss was additive to diuretic therapy and improved quality of life, including sexual dysfunction. Whereas, individual dietary components of potassium, calcium, magnesium, and fish oil supplementation have not been successful strategies for primary prevention, the DASH feeding study, which reduced intake of total fat, total cholesterol, and saturated fat and increased protein, fiber, fruit, and vegetable intake, demonstrates the potential that can be achieved with nonpharmacological interventions. The PREMIER Trial shows that patients can implement the DASH diet with multicomponent lifestyle changes, especially with intense behavioral counseling.

REFERENCES

1. Stamler, R. et al., *JAMA*, 262: 1801, 1989.
2. Hypertension Prevention Trial Research Group. *Arch Intern Med*, 150: 153, 1990.
3. The Trials of Hypertension Prevention Collaboration Research Group. *JAMA*, 267: 1213, 1992.
4. The Trials of Hypertension Prevention Collaboration Research Group. *Arch Intern Med*, 157: 657, 1997.
5. Kumanyika, S. K. et al., *J Hum Hypertens*, 19, 33, 2005.
6. Cook, N. R. et al., *J Hum Hypertens*, 19: 47, 2005.
7. Langford, H. G. et al., *JAMA*, 253: 657, 1985.
8. Stamler, R. et al., *JAMA*, 257: 1484, 1987.
9. Langford, H. G. et al., *Hypertension*, 17: 210, 1991.
10. Blaufox, M. D. et al., *JAMA*, 267: 1221, 1992.
11. Davis, B. R. et al., *Hypertension*, 19: 393, 1992.
12. Davis, B. R. et al., *Arch Intern Med*, 153: 1773, 1993.
13. Wassertheil-Smoller, S. et al., *Arch Intern Med*, 152: 131, 1992.
14. Davis, B. R. et al., *Am J Hypertens*, 7: 926, 1994.
15. Wassertheil-Smoller, S. et al., *Ann Intern Med*, 114: 613, 1991.
16. Wassertheil-Smoller, S. et al., *Am J Hypertens*, 5, 37, 1992.
17. Oberman, A. et al., *Ann Intern Med*, 112: 89, 1990.
18. Whelton, P. K. et al., *JAMA*, 279: 839, 1998.
19. Espeland, M. A. et al., *Arch Fam Med*, 8: 228, 1999.
20. Miller, E. R. 3rd et al., *Hypertension*, 40: 612, 2002.
21. Appel, L. J. et al., *N Engl J Med*, 336: 1117, 1997.
22. Svetkey, L. P. et al., *Arch Intern Med*, 159: 285, 1999.
23. Sacks, F. M. et al., *N Engl J Med*, 344: 3, 2001.
24. Vollmer, W. M. et al., *Ann Intern Med*, 135: 1019, 2001.
25. Bray, G. A. et al., *Am J Cardiol*, 94: 222, 2004.
26. Harsha, D. W. et al., *Hypertension*, 43: 393, 2004.
27. Svetkey, L. P. et al., *Ann Epidemiol*, 13: 462, 2003.
28. Appel, L. J. et al., *JAMA*, 289: 2083, 2003.
29. Svetkey, L. P. et al., *J Hum Hypertens*, 19: 21, 2005.
30. Ard, J. D. et al., *Diabetes Care*, 27: 340, 2004.
31. Obarzanek, E. et al., *Am J Clin Nutr*, 74: 80, 2001.
32. Appel, L. J. et al., *JAMA*, 294: 2455, 2005.

46 Nutrition in Diabetes Mellitus

Maria F. Lopes-Virella and Carolyn H. Jenkins

CONTENTS

INTRODUCTION

Diabetes mellitus is a common metabolic disorder.[1,2] The hallmark of diabetes is fasting and postprandial hyperglycemia. Hyperglycemia results from insulin deficiency or interference with its action (insulin resistance), or both. Uncontrolled diabetes leads to widespread metabolic derangement. An estimated 16 million people in the United States have diabetes mellitus. The prevalence of diabetes is increasing at an alarming rate in all age groups, from children to the elderly. Diabetes is progressively more common with advancing age. It is estimated that 50% or more of the population after 80 to 90 years of age has glucose intolerance or diabetes. Diabetes is the sixth leading cause of death due to disease in the United States and decreases the average life expectancy up to 15 years when compared to the population without diabetes. Diabetes has an enormous social impact, mostly due to its chronic microvascular (retinopathy, nephropathy, and neuropathy) and macrovascular complications. Diabetic retinopathy is the leading cause of blindness in the United States. In people with diabetes, aged 20 to 74 years, there are 12,000 to 24,000 new cases of blindness each year. Diabetic nephropathy occurs in 20 to 40% of patients with diabetes and is the leading cause of end-stage renal disease. In 1996, more than 130,000 people with diabetes underwent either dialysis or kidney transplantation.

Diabetic neuropathy is present in 60 to 70% of all patients with diabetes. Besides increasing the risk for sudden death and silent myocardial infarction, diabetic neuropathy leads to impotence, and 50% of men with diabetes experience it. Diabetic neuropathy, together with peripheral vascular disease, is responsible for more than 200,000 cases of foot ulcers and 80,000 limb amputations each year. Finally, diabetes is also responsible for macrovascular complications, including peripheral vascular disease, stroke, and cardiovascular disease. Cardiovascular disease is the leading cause of death in diabetes (80% of all patients with diabetes die of cardiovascular disease). An estimated 75% of cardiovascular mortality in diabetes is from coronary heart disease, and 25% from cerebral or peripheral vascular disease. Coronary heart disease, peripheral vascular disease, and stroke account for nearly 1 million hospital admissions each year among patients with diabetes. In women, diabetes carries yet another burden since it may lead to problems during pregnancy mainly congenital malformations in babies born from diabetic mothers. The rate of major congenital malformations is 10%, compared to 2% in nondiabetic women, and fetal mortality occurs in 3 to 5% of pregnancies.

CLASSIFICATION AND DIAGNOSTIC CRITERIA OF THE SEVERAL SUBTYPES OF DIABETES AND INTERMEDIATE SYNDROMES

CLASSIFICATION OF DIABETES MELLITUS

Type 1 Diabetes

Type 1 diabetes is characterized by pancreatic β cell destruction usually leading to absolute insulin deficiency.[3,4] Its etiology is likely due to a combination of genetic and environment factors. Most type 1 diabetes is an organ-specific auto-immune disease characterized by T-cell-mediated autoimmune destruction of the pancreatic β cells. In a few cases, there is no evidence of an auto-immune process, and these cases are classified as idiopathic.

Type 2 Diabetes

Type 2 diabetes is characterized by insulin resistance and an insulin secretory defect.[3,4] Type 2 diabetes is the most prevalent type of diabetes and comprises 90% of the population with diabetes. As with type 1 diabetes, type 2 diabetes has both a genetic and an environment component. Type 2 diabetes may range from cases with predominantly insulin resistance and relative insulin deficiency to cases with a predominantly secretory defect and some degree of insulin resistance.

Other Specific Types of Diabetes

Genetic defects in β cell function or in insulin action, as well as in several diseases of the exocrine pancreas, endocrinopathies, infections, drugs or chemicals, uncommon forms of immune-mediated diabetes, and other genetic syndromes that may lead to hyperglycemia, are included under the definition of other specific types of diabetes. A comprehensive list is included in Table 46.1.

TABLE 46.1
Etiologic Classification of Diabetes Mellitus

I. Type 1 diabetes[a] (β-cell destruction, usually leading to absolute insulin deficiency)
  A. Immune mediated
  B. Idiopathic
II. Type 1I diabetes[a] (may range from predominantly insulin resistance with relative insulin deficiency to a predominantly secretory defect with insulin resistance)
III. Other specific types
  A. Genetic defects of β-cell function
    1. Chromosome 12, HNF-1a (MODY3)
    2. Chromosome 7, glucokinase (MODY2)
    3. Chromosome 20, HNF-4a (MODY1)
    4. Mitochondrial DNA
    5. Others
  B. Genetic defects in insulin action
    1. Type A insulin resistance
    2. Leprechaunism
    3. Rabson-Mendenhall syndrome
    4. Lipoatrophic diabetes
    5. Others
  C. Diseases of the exocrine pancreas
    1. Pancreatitis
    2. Trauma/pancreatectomy
    3. Neoplasia
    4. Cystic fibrosis
    5. Hemochromatosis
    6. Fibrocalculous pancreatopathy
    7. Others
  D. Endocrinopathies
    1. Acromegaly
    2. Cushing's syndrome
    3. Glucagonoma
    4. Pheochromocytoma
    5. Hyperthyroidism
    6. Somatostatinoma
    7. Aldosteronoma
    8. Others
  E. Drug-or chemical-induced
    1. Vacor
    2. Pentamidine
    3. Nicotinic acid
    4. Glucocorticoids
    5. Thyroid hormone
    6. Diazoxide
    7. β-adrenergic agonists
    8. Thiazides
    9. Dilantin
    10. α-interferon
    11. Others
  F. Infections
    1. Congenital rubella
    2. Cytomegalovirus
    3. Others
  G. Uncommon forms of immune-mediated diabetes
    1. "Stiff-man" syndrome
    2. Antiinsulin receptor antibodies
    3. Others
  H. Other genetic syndromes sometimes associated with diabetes
    1. Down's syndrome
    2. Klinefelter's syndrome
    3. Turner's syndrome
    4. Wolfram's syndrome
    5. Friedreich's ataxia
    6. Huntington's chorea
    7. Laurence-Moon-Biedl syndrome
    8. Myotonic dystrophy
    9. Porphyria
    10. Prader-Willi syndrome
    11. Others
IV. Gestational diabetes mellitus (GDM)

[a] Patients with any form of diabetes may require insulin treatment at some stage of their disease. Such use of insulin does not, of itself, classify the patient.

Source: Reprinted with authorization from American Diabetes Association. *Diabetes Care*, 23 (Suppl 1): 6, 2000.

Gestational Diabetes

Gestational diabetes is defined as any degree of glucose intolerance that is initially recognized during pregnancy. The type of treatment required managing glucose intolerance in pregnancy and whether or not the glucose intolerance continues after pregnancy does not affect the diagnosis. After 6 or more weeks of pregnancy, it is necessary to reclassify the patient and to determine whether diabetes, impaired glucose tolerance, impaired fasting glucose, or normoglycemia is present. About 4% of all pregnancies are complicated by gestational diabetes, and the diagnosis is commonly made during the third trimester. The prevalence may range from 1 to 14% of all pregnancies, depending on the population studied.[5]

At present, it is not recommended that all women be screened for gestational diabetes. Screening in patients considered at lower risk for the development of glucose intolerance is not considered cost-effective.[5] Low-risk group includes women who (1) are less than 25 years of age, (2) have normal body weight, (3) have no family history of diabetes (4) have no history of abnormal glucose metabolism, (5) have no history of poor obstetric outcome, and (6) are not members of an ethnic/racial group with a high prevalence of diabetes (Hispanic American, Native American, Asian American, African American, or Pacific Islander). Risk assessment should be undertaken at the first prenatal visit, and patients at risk should undergo glucose testing as soon as possible. If the screening is negative, it should be repeated between 24 to 28 weeks of gestation. A fasting plasma glucose level above 126 mg/dl or a casual level of glucose above 200 mg/dl meets the criteria to diagnose diabetes. If the levels are not conclusive, a glucose challenge test using a 50-g load of glucose should be performed. If the screening test is positive, a 100-g diagnostic loading test needs to be performed.

Impaired Glucose Tolerance and Impaired Fasting Glucose

These two syndromes are usually associated with a metabolic stage intermediate between normal glucose metabolism and diabetes. Impaired glucose tolerance is associated with levels of plasma glucose ≥ 100 mg/dl but <126 mg/dl or 2 h values in the oral glucose tolerance test (OGTT) of >140 mg/dl, but less than 200 mg/dl. Patients with glucose intolerance are often hyperglycemic if challenged with an oral glucose load but in normal conditions, they may have normal or near-normal plasma glucose levels and hemoglobin A1c. Impaired fasting glucose corresponds to fasting levels of plasma glucose ≥ 100 mg/dl but <126 mg/dl. *Per se*, neither of these two syndromes is a disease, but they are considered risk factors for the development of macrovascular disease and diabetes since they are associated with the metabolic syndrome that includes abdominal or visceral obesity, dyslipidemia including hypertriglyceridemia and low-HDL cholesterol, as well as hypertension. The two syndromes can also be observed in the disease processes listed in Table 46.1. Interestingly, however, a recent study by Tominaga, et al.,[6] examining the cumulative survival rates from cardiovascular disease in a Japanese population of 2534 individuals with either normal glucose tolerance, impaired glucose tolerance, impaired fasting glucose, or diabetes showed no significant difference between the survival rates from cardiovascular disease in subjects with normal glucose tolerance and subjects with impaired fasting glucose. Nevertheless, it showed a significant decrease in survival in subjects with impaired glucose tolerance and diabetes. Therefore, they concluded that impaired glucose tolerance was a risk factor for cardiovascular disease, but impaired fasting glucose was not.

DIAGNOSTIC CRITERIA

In the past, the diagnostic criterion for diabetes conventionally used was that recommended by the National Diabetes Data Group[3] or WHO;[1] the revised criteria are shown in Table 46.2. For epidemiological studies determining prevalence and incidence of diabetes, the first criterion (fasting plasma glucose >126 mg/dl) can be used, but it will lead to slightly lower estimates

---

TABLE 46.2
Criteria to Diagnosis Diabetes Mellitus[a]

1. Symptoms of diabetes plus casual plasma glucose concentration ≥ 200 mg/dl (11.1 mmol/l). *Casual* is defined as any time of day without regard to time since last meal. The classic symptoms of diabetes include polyuria, polydipsia, and unexpected weight loss

   or

2. FPG ≥ 126 mg/dl (7.0 mmol/l). Fasting is defined as no caloric intake for at least 8 h

   or

3. 2-h PG ≥ 200 mg/dl (11.1 mmol/l) during an OGTT. The test should be performed as described by WHO (2), using a glucose load containing the equivalent of 75-g anhydrous glucose dissolved in water

[a] In the absence of unequivocal hyperglycemia with acute metabolic decompensation, these criteria should be confirmed by repeat testing on a different day. The third measure (OGTT) is not recommended for routine clinical use.

Source: Reprinted with authorization from American Diabetes Association. *Diabetes Care*, 28(Suppl 1): S41, 2005.

TABLE 46.3

Estimated Prevalence of Diabetes in the United States in Individuals 40 to 74 Years of Age Using Data from the NHANES III

Diabetes Diagnostic Criteria	Prevalence (%) of Diabetes by Glucose Criteria Without a Medical History of Diabetes[a]	Total Diabetes Prevalence (%)[b]
Medical history of diabetes	—	7.92
WHO (2) criteria for diabetes:		
FPG ≥140 mg/dl (7.8 mmol/l) or 2-h PG ≥200 mg/dl (11.1 mmol/l)	6.34	14.26
FPG ≥126 mg/dl (7.0 mmol/l)	4.35	12.27

a Diabetes prevalence (by glucose criteria) in those without a medical history of diabetes x (100 %- prevalence of diabetes by medical history).

b First column of data plus 7.92.

Source: Data are from K. Flegal, National Center for Health Statistics, personal communication. Reprinted with authorization from American Diabetes Association. *Diabetes Care*, 23(Suppl 1): 11, 2000.

of prevalence/incidence than the combined use of the fasting plasma glucose and oral glucose tolerance test. That is clearly demonstrated by the data obtained in NHANES III[2] (National Health and Nutrition Examination Survey), as summarized in Table 46.3. WHO criteria were based on the fact that the prevalence of retinopathy and nephropathy would rise markedly when the level of glucose 2 h after a standardized glucose load was >200 mg/dl. The revised criteria are based on results of several studies showing that fasting plasma level >126 mg/dl, like a 2–h, post-glucose load of >200 mg/dl, is associated with a marked rise in the prevalence of vascular complications.[4] In other words, levels of glucose ≥126 mg/dl reflect a serious metabolic disorder associated with the development of serious chronic diabetic complications.

Impaired fasting glucose is defined by glucose levels ≥100 mg/dl and <126 mg/dl after an 8-h fast. Impaired glucose tolerance is defined by a level of glucose ≥140 mg/dl but <200 mg/dl 2 h after a 75-g oral glucose load. The impaired glucose tolerance criteria will identify more people with impaired glucose homeostasis than the criteria of impaired fasting glucose.

CRITERIA FOR SCREENING FOR DIABETES

Generally, patients with type 1 diabetes have an acute presentation with marked hyperglycemia and acute symptoms of diabetes, and they are diagnosed soon after the symptoms develop. Type 1 diabetes is commonly an auto-immune process, characterized by a variety of auto-antibodies against intracellular or surface protein epitopes in the β cell. The markers that may identify patients at risk before development of the disease are many. However, the levels of the markers that would permit the diagnosis of high-risk patients are not well established. Furthermore, the methodology is not easily accessible, and there is no consensus about what to do if high levels of auto-antibodies are observed. Thus, screening for auto-antibodies related to type 1 diabetes as a means to screen for type 1 diabetes is not recommended now. Nowadays, there is no effective and safe treatment to prevent the development of type 1 diabetes. A number of clinical studies are being conducted to test various methods of preventing type 1 diabetes in high-risk individuals, such as siblings of patients with type 1 diabetes. If these studies uncover effective means to prevent type 1 diabetes, targeted screening may be appropriate in the future for patients at high risk for developing type 1 diabetes.

Screening for type 2 diabetes is, however, highly recommended. Undiagnosed type 2 diabetes is very common in the United States. Approximately one-third of patients with type 2 diabetes are undiagnosed. Individuals at high risk to develop type 2 diabetes should be screened for diabetes and prediabetes. Some epidemiological studies have shown that retinopathy will start developing 7 years prior to making the diagnosis of diabetes.[8] Even more worrisome is the fact that patients with undiagnosed diabetes are at significantly higher risk of developing premature macrovascular disease. [9] The risk of developing type 2 diabetes increases with age, obesity, and lack of physical activity. Furthermore, diabetes is more common in certain racial/ethnic groups (Hispanic, Asian, Afro-Americans, Native Americans, and Pacific Islander), in women with gestational diabetes, and in individuals with a family history of diabetes, hypertension, or dyslipidemia. The major risk factors for developing diabetes are listed in Table 46.4.

The ADA recommends screening at 3-year intervals for individuals of age above or equal to 45 and BMI ≥25 kg/m^2 and a more frequent testing in individuals with additional risk factors, such as those listed in Table 46.4. The incidence of type 2 diabetes in children and adolescents has markedly increased in the last years; thus, children and youth at increased risk to develop diabetes should also be screened.[10] The criteria for screening type 2 diabetes in children are depicted in Table 46.5. Either fasting plasma glucose measurement or an oral glucose tolerance test is adequate to perform screening for diabetes. Fasting, as mentioned before, represents a period of at least 8 h without food or beverage other than water. When an oral glucose tolerance test is performed, a load of 75 g of anhydrous glucose is considered as the standard load for adult testing. Interpretation of the results is crucial, and it should be made according to the criteria shown in Table 46.6. Fasting plasma glucose is the preferred

---

TABLE 46.4
Major Risk Factors for Diabetes Mellitus

Age ≥45 years, particularly those with BMI ≥25 kg/m^2
Age <45 years in those with BMI ≥25 kg/m^2 and additional risk factors such as:
Physical inactivity
Family history of diabetes (first degree relative with diabetes)
Race/ethnicity (i.e., African-Americans, Hispanic-Americans, Native Americans, Asian-Americans, and Pacific
  Islanders)
Previously identified IFG or IGT
Hypertension (≥140/90 mm Hg)
HDL cholesterol level ≤35 mg/dl (0.90 mmol/l) and/or a triglyceride level ≥250 mg/dl (2.82 /l)
    Polycystic ovary syndrome
    Clinical conditions associated with insulin resistance such as acanthosis nigricans
History of GDM or delivery of babies over 9 lb
Established Vascular Disease

Source: Reprinted with authorization from American Diabetes Association. *Diabetes Care*, 28(Suppl 1): S6, 2005.

TABLE 46.5
Criteria for Testing for Type 2 Diabetes in Children

Overweight (BMI over 85th percentile for age and sex, weight for height above 85th percentile or weight above 120% of
  ideal for height) and two or more of the following risk factors
Family history of diabetes (first or second degree relative with diabetes)
Race/ethnicity (i.e., African-Americans, Hispanic-Americans, Native Americans, Asian-Americans, and Pacific Islanders);
Signs of insulin resistance or conditions associated with insulin resistance (acanthosis nigricans, polycystic ovary
  syndrome, hypertension, or dyslipidemia)
Age of initiation: age 10 years or at onset of puberty if puberty occurs at an earlier age
Frequency: every 2 years
Test preferred: Fasting Plasma-Glucose

Source: Reprinted with authorization from American Diabetes Association. *Diabetes Care*, 28(Suppl 1): S6, 2005.

TABLE 46.6
Criteria to Diagnose Impaired Glucose Metabolism and Diabetes Mellitus (in mg/dl)

Normoglycemia	Impaired Glucose Metabolism	DM[a]
FPG <100	FPG ≥100 and <126	FPG ≥126
2-h PG[b] <140	2-h PG[b] ≥140 and <200	2-h PG[b] ≥200
		Symptoms of DM and random plasma glucose concentration ≥200

a A diagnosis of diabetes must be confirmed, on a subsequent day, by measurement of FPG, 2-h PG or random plasma glucose (if symptoms are present.) The FPG test is greatly preferred because of ease of administration, acceptability to patients, and lower cost. Fasting is defined as no caloric intake for at least 8 h. DM, diabetes mellitus; 2-h PG, 2-h postload glucose.

b This test requires the use of a glucose load containing of 75 g anhydrous glucose dissolved in water.

TABLE 46.7
Screening and Diagnosis Scheme for GDM^a

Plasma Glucose	75-g Oral Glucose Load (mg/dl)	100-g Oral Glucose Load (mg/dl)
Fasting	95	95
1-h	180	180
2-h	155	155
3-h	not done	140

[a] The diagnosis of GDM requires any two or more plasma glucose values obtained during the test to meet or exceed the values shown above.

Source: Reprinted with authorization from American Diabetes Association. *Diabetes Care*, 28(Suppl 1): S6, 2005.

---

test to screen for prediabetes and diabetes. However, oral glucose tolerance test can also be used in high-risk adults. It is important to remember that certain drugs, including furosemide, gluco-corticosteroids, thiazides, estrogen-containing preparations, β-blockers, and nicotinic acid, may induce hyperglycemia. In community screening tests, it is sometimes impossible to use a fasting plasma glucose assay and, therefore, a fasting capillary whole-blood glucose test is performed due to its convenience and simplicity of measurement. The levels are not, however, as accurate as those measured in plasma and they are lower. If the measurement is made in capillary whole blood, individuals with blood glucose ≥110 mg/dl should be referred to a physician for further evaluation and testing. Criteria for diagnosis of GDM (Gestational Diabetes Mellitus) are summarized in Table 46.7.

DIABETIC COMPLICATIONS: MICROVASCULAR

RETINOPATHY

Diabetic retinopathy is a specific microvascular complication present in both type 1 and type 2 diabetes, strongly correlated with the duration of diabetes. After 20 years of diabetes, nearly all patients with type 1 diabetes and more than 60% of the patients with type 2 diabetes will have some degree of retinopathy.[11]

Retinopathy can be defined as damage to the retina, a cell layer in the posterior part of the eye, which contains the photoreceptors necessary for vision. Retinopathy can be classified as mild, nonproliferative (also called background retinopathy), or moderate-to-severe nonproliferative retinopathy, characterized by hard exudates and retinal blot hemorrhages. This type of retinopathy advances to a preproliferative phase when retinal ischemia becomes more severe. Proliferative retinopathy is the most advanced stage of retinopathy, and it is characterized by the growth of new blood vessels on the retina and posterior surface of the vitreous. Proliferative retinopathy usually leads to loss of vision due to retinal detachment, and it is the leading cause of blindness in persons of 30 to 65 years of age. Vision loss may also occur in patients without proliferative retinopathy when vascular leakage (macular edema) and occlusion occurs in the area of the macula. Maculopathy is more common in type 2 compared to type 1 diabetes and it is an important cause for decreased visual acuity in this group of patients.

Screening

Screening for the presence of retinopathy depends on the rates of progression of diabetic retinopathy and on the risk factors that may alter these rates. Most of the available data is based on studies on Caucasian populations, and it is not certain whether or not these data can be applied to the ethnic groups with the highest incidence of diabetes and complications. The guidelines for screening and follow-up of patients for diabetic retinopathy are summarized in Table 46.8.

Influence of Glycemic Control and Treatment of Hypertension and Dyslipidemia

Data from the Diabetes Control and Complications Trial (DCCT) clearly show a definitive and direct relationship between glycemic control and diabetic microvascular complications, including retinopathy.[12,13] The DCCT shows that intensive-insulin therapy of type 1 diabetes reduced or prevented the progression of diabetic retinopathy by 27% when compared with conventional therapy. Similar results were observed in type 2 diabetes, as shown by the United Kingdom Prospective Diabetes Study (UKPDS).[14,15] The earlier intensive control is started in the course of diabetes, the more effective it is in preventing the development of retinopathy.[13] Besides poor glycemic control, proteinuria is also associated with retinopathy. Hypertension is a known

TABLE 46.8
Screening and Follow-up of Patients with Diabetes for Retinopathy

	Recommended Ophthalmologic Examination[a]	Recommended Minimum Follow-Up
Type 1 diabetes >10 years of age	Within 5 years after onset of disease	Yearly or more often if retinopathy is progressing
Type 2 diabetes	At the time of diagnosis of diabetes	Yearly or more often if retinopathy is progressing
Diabetic patients during pregnancy	Prior to conception if programmed and during the first trimester	As often as necessary, according to physician
Patients with macular edema, severe proliferative retinopathy	Immediately after diagnosis of the condition	As often as necessary, according to physician

[a] The ophthalmologic exam recommended is a dilated and comprehensive exam by an ophthalmologist or optometrist.

TABLE 46.9
Classification of Diabetic Neuropathy

Diabetic polyneuropathies	Diabetic mononeuropathies
Distal symmetrical	Peripheral
Chronic sensorimotor	Cranial
Autonomic	Radiculopathy
Proximal motor	Isolated nerve lesions
Acute sensory	

risk factor for the development of macular edema (see below) and is associated with the presence of proliferative diabetic retinopathy. Lowering blood pressure as shown in the UKPDS study decreases progression of retinopathy. Finally, maculopathy consists of edema and lipid exudates; since the lipid exudates observed in cases of maculopathy originate from circulating blood lipids, aggressive treatment of lipid abnormalities is also important in the prevention of retinopathy/maculopathy. It has also been shown that pregnancy and the post-partum period in type 1 diabetes may aggravate retinopathy transiently, but laser photocoagulation surgery can minimize the risk.[16,17]

The main reason screening, for diabetic retinopathy, is essential because of the well-known efficacy of laser photocoagulation therapy in patients with proliferative retinopathy and macular edema. The surgery, as demonstrated well in the Early Treatment Diabetic Retinopathy Study and the Diabetic Retinopathy Study, is extremely efficient in preventing loss of vision, but has not much impact in reversing visual acuity, if already diminished. Since proliferative retinopathy and macular edema are quite often asymptomatic, screening is crucial.

NEUROPATHY

Symptomatic and potentially disabling neuropathy affects nearly 50% of diabetic patients. Neuropathy can be symmetrical or focal and often involves the autonomic nervous system. The prevalence of symmetrical neuropathy is similar in type 1 and type 2 diabetes, but the focal forms of neuropathy are more common in the older type 2 diabetic patient. The classification of neuropathy is made according to the areas affected due to the relative poor understanding of the pathogenic mechanisms of this diabetic complication. Table 46.9 includes the most commonly accepted classification of diabetic neuropathic syndromes.

The cause for mononeuropathies is unknown, but they usually have a sudden onset and that suggests a vascular component in their pathogenesis. They usually tend to resolve with time, and despite occurring in diabetes, they are not the typical neuropathic lesions of diabetes. Diabetic polyneuropathies are the main problems for diabetic patients, and they will be discussed in some detail. To assess diabetic neuropathy, history of clinical symptoms and physical exam, electrodiagnostic studies, quantitative sensory testing, and autonomic function testing should be performed. Table 46.10 summarizes the clinical signs and symptoms of diabetic polyneuropathy and Table 46.11 summarizes the functional changes associated with autonomic failure. In Table 46.12, adequate diagnostic testing to assess diabetic neuropathy is summarized.

Influence of Glycemic Control

Data from the DCCT and UKPDS clearly show a definitive and direct relationship between glycemic control and diabetic microvascular complications, including neuropathy.[12-15] The DCCT data showed that intensive insulin therapy, when compared with

TABLE 46.10

Symptoms and Signs of Diabetic Polyneuropathy

	Symptoms	Signs
Polyneuropathy	Pain and paresthesias most common at night	Diminished sensation to touch, temperature, pain, and vibration. Loss of reflexes Atrophy of intrinsic hand muscles, sensory impairment

TABLE 46.11

Functional Changes Associated with Autonomic Failure

Systems Involved	Manifestations
Cardiovascular	Resting tachycardia, impaired exercise-induced cardiovascular responses, cardiac denervation, orthostatic hypotension, heat intolerance, impaired vasodilatation, and impaired venoarteriolar reflex (dependent edema)
Eye	Decreased diameter of dark-adapted pupil (dark-adapted meiosis)
Gastrointestinal	Esophageal enteropathy, gallbladder atony, impaired colonic motility (diarrhea, constipation), and anorectal sphincter dysfunction (incontinence)
Genitourinary	Neurogenic vesical dysfunction (decreased bladder sensitivity/incontinence/retention), sexual dysfunction, (male: penile Erectile failure and retrograde ejaculation; female: defective lubrication)
Sudomotor	Anhidrosis/hyperhidrosis (heat intolerance), gustatory sweating
Endocrine	Hypoglycemia-associated autonomic failure

Source: Reprinted with authorization from American Diabetes Association. *Diabetes Care*, 19(Suppl 1): 82, 1996.

TABLE 46.12

Electrodiagnostic Studies, Sensory Testing, and Autonomic Function Testing for the Diagnosis of Diabetic Neuropathy

Sensory Testing	Electrodiagnosis	Autonomic Function Testing
Vibration/touch thresholds	Motor and sensory nerve conduction studies	R–R variations, orthostasis, Valsalva
Thermal thresholds		Resting heart rate
Pain thresholds	Needle electromyography of extremity and paraspinal muscles	QTc, DAPS, NPT, CMG + BST
		REPs, QSART, TST
		Solid Phase Gastric Motility
		Clamped Hypoglycemia
		Clamped insulin infusion test

Abbreviations: QTc-corrected QT interval on EKG; DAPS-dark-adapted pupil size; NPT-nocturnal penile tumescence, CMG + BST-cystometrogram + Bethanechol supersensivity test; REPs-reflex-evoked potentials; QSART-quantitative sudomotor axon reflex test; TST-thermoregulated sweat test.

conventional therapy, reduced or prevented the progression of diabetic neuropathy in patients with type 1 diabetes. The UKPDS showed the same results in patients with type 2 diabetes.

NEPHROPATHY

Diabetic nephropathy is characterized by persistent albumin excretion (≥300 mg/24 h), a progressive decline in the glomerular filtration rate (GFR), and increased blood pressure.[18] The earliest clinical evidence of nephropathy is the increased excretion of albumin in the urine. This phase of incipient nephropathy is designated as microalbuminuria. The levels of albumin excretion in the microalbuminuria stage of nephropathy range from 30 to 299 mg/24 h. Table 46.13 summarizes the cut-off levels for diagnostic purposes, as well as the correspondent values in spot urine collections. Measurement of creatinine and albumin

TABLE 46.13
Definition of Abnormalities in Albumin Excretion

	24-h Collection	Spot Collection (mg/g Creatinine)
Normal	<30 mg/24 h	<30
Microalbuminuria[a] (incipient nephropathy)	30–299 mg/24 h	30–299
Nephropathy[a]	≥300 mg/24 h	≥300

[a] Two out of three urine specimens collected within a 3–6 month period should be abnormal before diagnosing a patient as having incipient nephropathy or nephropathy. Exercise within 24 h, infection, fever, CHF, marked hyperglycemia, and marked hypertension may elevate urinary albumin excretion over baseline levels.

excretion simultaneously in the same urine specimen is necessary when a spot urine sample is collected and it is also recommended in timed specimens to ensure that a proper urine collection was obtained. Interpretation of microalbuminuria needs to take into consideration factors such as hyperglycemia, level of exercise preceding the urine collection, uncontrolled hypertension, urinary tract infections, acute febrile illnesses, and heart failure since all of these conditions may lead to increased albuminuria. Diagnosis of nephropathy needs to be based on data from three urine specimens collected within a 3-to-6-month period. At least two of the specimens may be concordant to allow establishment of a valid diagnosis.

About 20 to 40% of patients with type 1 or type 2 diabetes develop nephropathy. A high percentage of subjects with type 2 diabetes are found to have microalbuminuria shortly after their initial diagnosis for two different reasons: either diabetes has been present for many years and not diagnosed, or microalbuminuria in type 2 diabetes is less specific of diabetic nephropathy, as shown by renal biopsy studies.

Persistent albuminuria in the range of 30 to 299 mg/24 h has been shown to be the earliest stage of diabetic nephropathy in type 1 diabetes and a marker for development of nephropathy in type 2 diabetes. Microalbuminuria is also a well-established marker of increased CVD risk.[19] Approximately 80% of individuals with type 1 diabetes who develop sustained microalbuminuria will progress to overt nephropathy over a period of 10 to 15 years. Once overt nephropathy occurs and if there is no therapeutic intervention, 50% of these patients will progress to end-stage renal disease in 10 years and 75% in 20 years. The progression to overt nephropathy in type 2 diabetes, without therapeutic intervention, is less than in type 1 diabetes (approximately in 20 to 40% of the cases), and only approximately 20% will progress to end-stage renal disease. Marked racial/ethnic variability exists, however, as far as progression to end-stage renal disease in type 2 diabetes. Native Americans, Mexican-Americans, and African-Americans have a much higher risk of developing end-stage renal disease than the other populations with type 2 diabetes. In the United States, diabetic nephropathy is responsible for one-third of all cases of end-stage renal disease and that is a terrible burden in the country's economy. Regardless of the fact that subjects with type 1 diabetes are more prone to progress to end-stage renal disease, due to the higher prevalence of type 2 diabetes in the population, half of the patients with diabetes on dialysis have type 2 diabetes.

Two major risk factors that can be easily intervened upon are involved in the progression of nephropathy: hypertension and hyperglycemia. The standards of care for hypertension and hyperglycemia in diabetes will be discussed later in this chapter.

Influence of Hypertension and Glycemic Control

In type 1 diabetes, hypertension is usually caused by the underlying diabetic nephropathy and is typically detected at the time microalbuminuria becomes apparent. In type 2 diabetes, hypertension is present at the time diabetes is diagnosed in one-third of the patients. The hypertension may be related to the underlying diabetic nephropathy or be secondary to other diseases or is a coexisting disease "essential hypertension." Commonly, subjects with type 2 diabetes before being diagnosed as having diabetes have been found to have an insulin resistance syndrome, which basically comprises a cluster of problems including hypertension, obesity, dyslipidemia, and glucose intolerance. The UKPDS provided strong evidence that control of blood pressure reduces the development of nephropathy in type 2 diabetes.[20] In addition, large prospective randomized studies in patients with type 1 diabetes have shown that lowering of systolic blood pressure with angiotensin-converting enzyme (ACE) inhibitors is more efficient in delaying the progression of nephropathy and can slow the decline in glomerular filtration rate in patients with macroalbuminuria.[20–22] In addition, ACE inhibitors have been shown to reduce severe cardiovascular disease (CVD), further supporting the use of these agents in microalbuminuria.[23] ACE receptor blockers (ARBs) have also been shown to reduce the rate of progression of microalbuminuria to macroalbuminuria in patients with type 2 diabetes. Thus, in the setting of albuminuria or nephropathy, patients should be treated with ACE inhibitors or ARBs, but if they are unable to tolerate either of these drugs, the use of nondihydropyridine calcium channel blockers (non-DCCBs), β-blockers, or diuretics for the management of hypertension should be considered.[24]

Hyperglycemia has been shown to have a major impact in the development of microvascular complications including nephropathy. Intensive treatment of diabetes to obtain near-normal glucose and hemoglobin A1c levels has significantly reduced the risk of development of microalbuminuria and overt nephropathy.[14–15,25]

Influence of Protein Restriction and Treatment of Lipid Disorders

It is well known that microalbuminuria is a marker for increased cardiovascular mortality and morbidity in patients with either type 1 or type 2 diabetes. In reality, microalbuminuria is considered as an indicator to screen patients for macrovascular complications (see macrovascular complications). Interestingly, there is also some preliminary evidence showing that lowering cholesterol leads to a reduction in the level of proteinuria. More work is needed to adequately validate this observation. Protein restriction has been shown to be of great benefit in animal studies to reduce progression of renal disease, including diabetic nephropathy. However, studies in humans are less clear. Several small studies seem to indicate that patients with overt nephropathy treated with a diet containing protein at 0.7 g/kg of body weight had mild retardation in the fall of the glomerular filtration rate. A recent study of patients with renal disease in which 3% had type 2 diabetes failed to show any benefit of protein restriction. In reality, marked decrease of protein intake in patients with end-stage renal disease on dialysis showed that the main predictive factor of mortality was low albumin due to protein-energy malnutrition.

Follow-up for Diabetic Nephropathy

The role of annual microalbuminuria assessment is less clear when the patient has been diagnosed as having microalbuminuria, and therapy has been instituted with ACE inhibitors or ARBs and blood pressure control. However, continued surveillance to assess both response to therapy and progression of disease is recommended and should be performed. In addition, calculation of GFR should be made by accessing www.kidney.org/professionals/dogi/gfr_calculator.cfm, and when the GFR drops to values below 60 ml/min^{-1}.1.73 m^{-2} or difficulties in managing hypertension or hyperkalemia are present, referral to a specialist in the treatment of diabetic nephropathy should be considered. If GFR drops below 30 ml/min^{-1}.1.73 m^{-2}, a nephrologist should be consulted. Recommendations concerning follow-up of diabetic nephropathy are summarized in Table 46.14.

DIABETIC COMPLICATIONS: MACROVASCULAR DISEASE

GENERAL CONSIDERATIONS

Macrovascular disease, which includes CAD, cerebrovascular disease, and peripheral vascular disease, is the leading cause of mortality in people with diabetes. Individuals with diabetes have at least a twofold to fourfold increased risk of having cardiovascular events and stroke and an eightfold increased likelihood of peripheral vascular disease compared with age-matched subjects without diabetes. The atherosclerotic process in diabetic patients is indistinguishable from that affecting the nondiabetic population, but it begins earlier and is more severe. Most deaths in the diabetic population are due to complications of CAD. Although diabetic patients have a higher prevalence of traditional CAD risk factors (i.e., hypertension, dyslipidemia, and obesity) compared with people without diabetes, these risk factors account for less than half the excess mortality associated with diabetes. Thus, the diagnosis of diabetes is a major independent risk factor for the development of CAD and adverse outcomes following a myocardial event. Other abnormalities induced by diabetes such as increased levels of small dense atherogenic LDL,

---

TABLE 46.14
Recommendations for Treatment of Nephropathy

General Recommendations: To reduce the risk or slow the progression of nephropathy optimize glucose control and blood pressure control
Specific Recommendations:
Use either ACE inhibitors or ARBs in the treatment of micro and macroalbuminuria except during pregnancy (In patients with type 1 diabetes, ACE inhibitors have been shown to delay progression of nephropathy. In type 2 diabetes, both ACE inhibitors and ARBs have been shown to delay progression of nephropathy.)
If ACE inhibitors are not tolerated they should be substituted by ARBs and vice versa
If ACEs or ARBs are not tolerated consider using non-DCCBs, β-blockers, or diuretics for the management of hypertension. Use of non-DCCBs may reduce albuminuria, even during pregnancy
If ACEs, ARBs, or diuretics are used monitor serum potassium levels
Consider referral to a physician with experience in diabetic nephropathy if GFR falls below 60 ml.min^{-1}.1.73m^{-2} or if difficulties occur in the management of hyperkalemia or hypertension

Source: Adapted from American Diabetes Association. *Diabetes Care*, 28(Suppl 1): S6, 2005.

oxidized or glycated LDL, increased platelet aggregation, hyperviscosity, endothelial cell dysfunction, decreased fibrinolysis, and increased clotting factors and fibrinogen are likely responsible for accelerated atherosclerosis in diabetic patients.

CURRENT TREATMENT AND PREVENTION STRATEGIES

Current treatment of macrovascular complications includes reduction of cardiovascular risk factors (obesity, smoking, and sedentary lifestyle) with special emphasis on the treatment of hypertension and dyslipidemia. Diabetic patients with existing or incipient macrovascular disease in general require multiple modifications of lifestyle and diet, as well as a poly-pharmaceutical approach to address the optimization of lipids level, blood pressure, and other disease risk factors. Glycemic control seems also to contribute to a reduction in macrovascular events both in type 1 and type 2 diabetes, but its impact is much less marked than impact of treatment of cardiovascular risk factors such as dyslipidemia and hypertension.

Treatment of Hypertension

Hypertension accelerates not only atherosclerosis but also nephropathy and retinopathy. Thus, in diabetes, it is important to treat even minimal elevations of blood pressure that in nondiabetic patients might be dismissed. The normal nocturnal fall in blood pressure may be lost in diabetic patients, leading to a more sustained hypertension throughout the day. In type 1 diabetes, hypertension is often the result of diabetic nephropathy. In type 2 diabetes, hypertension may be part of the "metabolic syndrome" (i.e., obesity, hyperglycemia, and dyslipidemia), which is associated with high rates of CVD. Randomized clinical trials have shown the importance of lowering blood pressure to levels below 130/80 mmHg in order to reduce CVD event rates, stroke, and nephropathy progression.[20,26] During pregnancy in diabetic women with hypertension, target blood pressure goals of systolic blood pressure are 110 to 129 mmHg and of diastolic blood pressure are 65 to 79 mmHg. Lower blood pressure can, however, be associated with impaired fetal growth, and it needs to be avoided. Although there are no well-controlled trials of diet and exercise in patients with diabetes, weight loss, exercise training, sodium restriction, and avoiding excessive consumption of alcohol are good hygienic measures that are affective in lowering blood pressure as well as lipids and blood glucose levels. Drug therapy is indicated in addition to the above lifestyle changes. Among the various therapeutic options, ACE inhibitors, ARBs, β-blockers, diuretics, and calcium channel blockers have been shown to be effective in reducing CVD events. Several studies suggest that ACE inhibitors may be superior to dihydropyridine calcium channel blockers (DCBBs) in reducing CVD events.[27] In contrast, the non-DCCB, verapamil, demonstrated a similar reduction in CVD mortality as β-blockers and that hold true in diabetes.[24] In pregnancy ACEs and ARBs are contraindicated since they may lead to fetal damage, but methyldopa, labetolol, diltiazem, clonidine, and prazosin are safe for use in pregnancy.

Treatment of Dyslipidemia

Dyslipidemia is common in subjects with diabetes. The more common lipid abnormalities in diabetes are increased triglycerides and low HDL cholesterol levels. Small (cholesterol-poor) dense LDL particles are also common in patients with hypertriglyceridemia and the insulin resistance syndrome. Dense LDL is more readily oxidized and more atherogenic. Aggressive treatment of dyslipoproteinemia is crucial to prevent the development and progression of macrovascular complications in diabetes.[28] Recommendations by the ADA concerning goals for therapy of hyperlipidemia as well as guidelines for lifestyle modifications, physical activity, smoking cessation, and drug treatment have been widely promulgated. Glucose control, together with weight loss and adequate physical activity, is also essential for the treatment of dyslipidemia, particularly in patients with high triglycerides and low-HDL cholesterol. Optimal triglyceride levels in diabetes are below 150 mg/dl, as in nondiabetic patients. HDL cholesterol levels above 40 mg/dl in men and 50 mg/dl in women are the targeted levels. In the past decade, however, it became apparent that lowering LDL cholesterol levels in diabetes led to a significant reduction in the risk of a major CHD event and therapy to lower LDL to a target level of less than 100 mg/dl or at least a reduction of 40 to 50% became first priority in the treatment of dyslipidemia in diabetes. The reduction of CVD events in diabetes after treatment with statins was shown in several clinical trials, including two major secondary prevention trials: Scandinavian Simvastatin Survival Study[29] and CARE trial.[30] More recently, the Heart Protection Study[31] demonstrated that, in people with diabetes with total cholesterol greater than 135 mg/dl and over the age of 40, lowering of LDL by approximately 30%, after simvastatin therapy, led to a decrease of 25% in first events for major CAD, independently of baseline LDL, preexistent CAD, glycemic control, and duration of diabetes. The Collaborative Atorvastatin Diabetes Study (CARDS) also show that patients with type 2 diabetes treated with atorvastatin had a significant reduction in CVD events, including stroke.[32] More recently, studies in high-risk patients (established CVD disease or acute coronary syndromes) show that further reduction of LDL to a goal of less than 70 mg/dl led to a significant reduction in further CAD events.[33,34] Most of the data obtained has been in type 2 diabetes. The Heart Protection Study included approximately 600 individuals with type 1 diabetes and the results were similar, but due to the relatively small number did not reach statistical significance. However, it is felt that similar consideration should be given to treatment of dyslipidemia in type 1 and type 2 diabetes. Although the large majority of the trials show the effect of treatment with statins, there is also evidence that treatment with fibric acid derivatives, which lower triglycerides and increase HDL, also lead to reduction of CVD events.[35,36] The same is true for Niacin. Thus, besides lowering LDL cholesterol, raising HDL and lowering triglycerides is also recommended. When HDL is less than 40 mg/dl, addition of a fibrate or niacin to the therapy is highly recommended. Niacin dosage needs to be kept at modest levels (750 mg to 2 g/day) to avoid serious disturbances in glucose homeostasis. Combination therapy is nowadays the recommended approach for patients who need treatment for LDL cholesterol, triglycerides, and HDL cholesterol. The possible side effects need to be taken into consideration and watched for, but they should not preclude the use of combination in these patients. Trials to assess the efficacy of combination therapy are needed, but are unfortunately not yet available.

Anti-Platelet Therapy

Aspirin has been recommended as primary and secondary therapy to prevent CVD events, both in diabetic and nondiabetic patients. Many trials have shown a 30% decrease in myocardial infarction and a 20% decrease in stroke in a wide range of patients (males, females, young, and middle age, with and without history of CVD). Dosages in most trials ranged from 75 to 325 mg. Clopidogel has been shown to reduce CVD rates in diabetic individuals.[37] It may be useful as additional therapy in patients at high risk for CVD or in those who are aspirin-intolerant.

Smoking Cessation

Multiple studies have shown a relationship between cigarette smoking and health risks. Smoking contributes to one of every five deaths in the United States, and it is a modifiable cause of premature death. Most of the studies do not separate the effect of smoking in health by subsets, suggesting that patients with diabetes have at least an equivalent risk to that of nondiabetics. Studies performed in patients with diabetes consistently show an increased risk of morbidity and premature death due to macrovascular disease in smokers. Smoking is also associated with the development of microvascular complications. Thus, it is important to enroll the patients in smoking cessation counseling and to assess the degree of nicotine dependence to address the difficulty in treating and the likelihood of a relapse.

INDICATIONS FOR CHD SCREENING

Annual screening for CVD risk factors is necessary. Risk factors include dyslipidemia, hypertension, smoking, family history for premature CVD, and the presence of micro- or macroalbuminuria. Asymptomatic CAD and silent MI are quite frequent subjects with diabetes. Thus, early diagnosis of CAD in patients with diabetes is very important and allows earlier implementation of preventive programs aimed at the reducing risk of future coronary morbidity and mortality, initiation of treatment with antiischemic medications in silent ischemia, and earlier identification of patients in whom revascularization is appropriate. Indications for cardiac testing are summarized in Table 46.15.

DIABETIC COMPLICATIONS: HYPOGLYCEMIA

It is well established that glycemic control will prevent specific long-term complications of diabetes. However, in order to prevent complications, intensive treatment of diabetes is necessary and unfortunately, it may lead to hypoglycemia. It is obvious that even in optimal conditions hypoglycemia is the limiting factor in the management of patients with type 1 diabetes.

TABLE 46.15
Indications for Cardiac Testing in Diabetic Patients

Testing for CAD is warranted in patients with the following:
1. Typical or atypical cardiac symptoms
2. Resting EKG suggestive of ischemia or infarction
3. Peripheral or carotid occlusive arterial disease
4. Sedentary lifestyle, age ≥35 years, and plans to begin a vigorous exercise program
5. Two or more of the risk factors listed below (a-e) in addition to diabetes
   (a) Total cholesterol ≥240 mg/dl, LDL cholesterol ≥160 mg/dl, or HD cholesterol <35 mg/dl
   (b) Blood pressure >140/90 mm Hg
   (c) Smoking
   (d) Family history of premature CAD
   (e) Positive micro/macroalbuminuria test

Source: Adapted from American Diabetes Association. *Diabetes Care*, 28(Suppl 1): S6, 2005.

Hypoglycemia is defined as a blood glucose of ≤60 mg/dl that may occur with or without symptoms.[38] During the course of the DCCT trial and even under optimal conditions the incidence of severe hypoglycemia was more than three times higher in patients on intensive therapy when compared with patients treated with conventional therapy. The effects of hypoglycemia cannot be ignored since they can be devastating particularly on the brain. The first signs of hypoglycemia are shakiness, sweating, tachycardia, hunger, irritability, and dizziness. These symptoms are followed by inability to concentrate, confusion, slurred speech, irrational behavior, blurred vision, and extreme fatigue. Finally, the symptoms of severe hypoglycemia are seizures, unresponsiveness, and loss of consciousness. Symptoms of hypoglycemia may occur at any time and therefore patients with diabetes should always be prepared to address them.

The level of glucose that leads to symptoms of hypoglycemia varies from person to person and also varies in the same individual under different circumstances. Hypoglycemia is a much less frequent problem for people with type 2 diabetes except in the elderly, mainly when they have associated diseases that require the use of beta blockers. Hypoglycemia usually occurs gradually and in general is associated with warning signs, including rapid heart beat, perspiration, shakiness, anxiety, and hunger. However, warning symptoms of hypoglycemia may be absent, causing the clinical syndrome of hypoglycemia unawareness. This syndrome results from excessive insulin in the setting of absent glucagon secretory responses to falling glucose levels. These episodes in turn cause reduced autonomic responses and lead to further decrease of the warning symptoms of hypoglycemia. That creates a vicious cycle that can only be broken by avoiding inducing iatrogenic hypoglycemia. The most common causes of hypoglycemia include: (1) skipping, delaying, or reducing the size of the meals and snacks; (2) increased physical activity without adequately adjusting therapy; (3) alcohol intake mainly on an empty stomach; and (4) treatment with excessively high levels of insulin or other antidiabetic medications. Hypoglycemia occurs mainly when the patient is being treated with insulin or sulfonylureas. In theory, biguanidines, thiazolidinediones, and α-glucosidase inhibitors would not be expected to induce hypoglycemia, since by themselves they will not increase the level of plasma insulin. However, it is conceivable that any intervention that limits hepatic glucose production, favors glucose utilization or both may lead to hypoglycemia, since increased hepatic glucose production and limited glucose utilization are mechanisms of defense against a drop in plasma glucose levels. In the elderly, it is not uncommon to have hypoglycemia episodes, and they may be dangerous since, not infrequently, these subjects live alone. A recent study examining the risk of sulfonylurea induced hypoglycemia in elderly type 2 diabetic patients concluded that therapy with sulfonylureas is well tolerated by the elderly and that the primary mechanisms of protection against hypoglycemia is an increase in epinephrine secretion. [39] That suggests that glucagon secretion in elderly patients is diminished and supports the concept that treatment of these patients with sulfonylureas or insulin when they are also being treated with β-blockers may be dangerous, and a close follow-up is needed. Oral antidiabetic agents other than sulfonylureas are probably better candidates for the treatment of these patients if their hyperglycemia is relatively modest. Although hypoglycemia during treatment with these agents may also occur, it is likely to be less frequently observed and less severe.

STANDARDS OF MEDICAL CARE FOR DIABETIC PATIENTS

Standards of medical care for diabetic patients have been markedly influenced by the results of recent major clinical trials. Some of the trials were specifically designed to address the importance of intensive glycemic control in subjects with type 1 or type 2 diabetes (DCCT and UKPDS). Some of the clinical trials although not designed to specifically address questions related with diabetic patients had a sufficiently large number of patients with type 2 diabetes and glucose intolerance to allow drawing conclusions on the effect of lipid-lowering therapy in the development of macrovascular complications (CARE, 4S, AF-CAPS/TEX-CAPS). Recently, CARDS[32] (Collaborative Atorvastatin Diabetes Study) confirmed the effect of lipid-lowering therapy in reducing CVD events in type 2 diabetes. Data published concerning these trials as well as the technical reviews of the ADA[40] will provide evidence for the standard of care measures proposed by the ADA for the treatment of patients with diabetes.

Standards of diabetes care are expected to provide health care providers taking care of patients with diabetes the means to establish treatment goals, assess the quality of the diabetes treatment provided, to identify areas where more self-management is needed, and to define situations when referral to specialists is necessary. Also, the same standards of diabetes care should allow patients with diabetes to assess the quality of medical care that they receive, understand their role in the treatment of their disease, and compare their treatment outcomes with standard goals.

GENERAL PRINCIPLES

It is accepted that lowering blood glucose levels to normal or near-normal levels will reduce: (1) the danger of acute decompensation due to diabetic ketoacidosis or hyperosmolar hyperglycemic nonketotic syndrome; (2) the symptoms of blurred vision and symptoms/signs usually accompanying diabetes (polyuria, polydipsia, weight loss with polyphagia, and fatigue) as well as vaginitis or balanitis; (3) the development or progression of diabetic retinopathy, nephropathy, and neuropathy; and (4) triglycerides leading to a less atherogenic lipid profile. It is also well accepted that lowering lipid levels will result in a decrease in diabetic macrovascular complications.

Thus, proper standards of diabetes care should include: (1) appropriate frequency of self monitoring of blood glucose; (2) adequate medical nutrition therapy (3) regular exercise; (4) adequate regimens with insulin and or oral glucose-lowering agents; (5) instructions in the prevention and treatment of hypoglycemia; (6) instructions in the prevention and treatment of acute and chronic diabetes complications (7) adequate regimens of lipid lowering therapy; (8) continuing education and reinforcement programs; and (9) periodic assessment of treatment goals.

SPECIFIC GOALS FOR MANAGEMENT OF DIABETES

An overview of the steps, goals, and treatment needed to obtain optimal care of patients with diabetes is summarized in Table 46.16.

TABLE 46.16
Recommended Diabetes Management Guidelines

Parameters to Assess	Frequency of Evaluation	Goal	Action Indicated if:	Recommended Treatment
Assessment of Metabolic Control				
HbA1c	Quarterly	<7%	>7%	Diet, exercise, oral agents, and/or insulin
Self-monitoring of blood glucose				
Preprandial	As necessary for	90–130 mg/dl	>130 mg/dl	Stepped adjustment of
Peak Postprandial	glycemic control	<180 mg/dl	>180 mg/dl	medication/diet to obtain adequate glycemic control
Technique check	Annually	Proficient	Not proficient	Referral for teaching
Hypoglycemic episodes	Each visit	No episodes	Episodes occur	Change in lifestyle, diet, and drug treatment
Hyperglycemic episodes/ketonuria	Each visit	No episodes	Episodes occur	Change in lifestyle, diet, and drug treatment
Assessment Macrovascular Complications				
Blood Pressure	Each visit	<130/80 mm Hg	>130/80 mm Hg	ACE Inhibitors, ARBs and other antihypertensive medications
Lipid Profile:				
LDL Cholesterol	At least yearly.	<100 mg/dl**	>100 mg/dl	Stepped approach to lipid control with lipid
HDL Cholesterol	Quarterly or	>40 mg/dl (men)	<40 mg/dl	lowering medications, diet, and exercise
Triglycerides	more frequently	>50 mg/dl (women)	<50 mg/dl	Low dosage aspirin for patients with established
	if levels are	<150 mg/dl	>150 mg/dl	macrovascular disease or patients with several
	abnormal			risk factors for macrovascular disease
EKG	Annually	Normal	Abnormal	Stress test and referral to cardiology
Ankle/brachial ratio	Annually	Normal	Abnormal	Peripheral vascular assessment and referral to vascular surgery
Peripheral pulses	Each visit	Normal	Abnormal	see above
Assessment of Microvascular Complications				
Retinopathy:				
				Referral to Ophthalmology
Dilated Eye Exam by Eye Care Specialist	Annually	Normal	Abnormal	Adequate glycemic control
Nephropathy:				
Microalbumin	Annually or	<30 mg/24 h		Adequate Glycemic Control
	quarterly	or	≥30 mg/24 h or	Adequate treatment with ACE inhibitors/ARBs and
	if abnormal	<30 mg/g of	≥30 mg/g of	other anti-hypertensives
		creatinine	creatinine (spot	Adequate treatment of hyperlipidemia
		(spot urine)	urine)	Referral to nephrology if necessary
Neuropathy:				Protective and preventive education
Peripheral Sensory	Annually	Intact sensation	Abnormal	Adequate glycemic control
				Drug treatment for symptomatic disease
Feet Exam	Each Visit	No complications	Corns, Calluses, ulcers, wounds, infections	Referral to podiatry and/or vascular surgery specialist
				Adequate control of lipid abnormalities and blood glucose
				Treatment of infections if present

Continued

TABLE 46.16
(Continued)

Parameters to Assess	Frequency of Evaluation	Goal	Action Indicated if:	Recommended Treatment
Assessment of Other Complications				
Oral/Periodontal	Each Visit Dental visit and hygiene every 6 months	Healthy gums/teeth	If no routine dental visits and hygiene are being performed	Referral for dental hygiene and care Adequate glycemic control*
Other infection	Each Visit	Absence of infection	If infection is present	Adequate glycemic control* Appropriate treatment of infection and referral to ID if necessary
Lifestyle Assessment				
Exercise	Each Visit	20–45 min on most days	<3 times weekly	Exercise counseling related to type, frequency, duration, and intensity.
Smoking, Tobacco Use	Each Visit	No use	Any use	Smoking cessation counseling.
Weight	Each Visit	Ideal body weight	Patient is over- or underweight	For overweight: diet adjustment for short-term weight loss of 0.2–0.5 kg/week; for long-term weight loss as much as needed to attain IBW For underweight: Consult NST, if severe If mild-assess the reasons for weight loss and treat accordingly
Nutrition	Each visit, annual in-depth assessment by RD	Healthy eating daily Weight control Metabolic control	Poor glucose or lipid control or increased weight	Referral for nutrition counseling In-depth nutrition assessment, plan, and follow-up by RD
Overall Diabetes Self-Management Practices	Each visit, annual in-depth assessment and self-management update	Healthy diabetes management with metabolic control and at least annual diabetes assessment and self-management education update	Early signs of complications and early signs of poor self-management of diabetes	Referral to diabetes educator or formal diabetes education classes for assessment, plan, evaluation, and follow-up by CDE

Severe gum disease or any local or systemic infection is associated with higher glucose levels. Treatment of infection improves glycemic control.

Special Considerations

Pregnancy

To reduce the risk of fetal malformations and maternal and fetal complications, pregnant diabetic women require excellent glycemic control. Follow-up by a multidisciplinary team including a diabetologist, internist or family physician, obstetrician, and diabetes educator is essential. Other specialists need to be called upon if necessary. Self-management skills essential for glycemic control and preparation for pregnancy include: (1) designing an appropriate meal plan, with timing of meals and snacks and an appropriate physical activity plan; (2) self-monitoring blood glucose levels, choosing the time and site for insulin injections, using therapy with glucagon or carbohydrate intake for treatment of hypoglycemia and self-adjusting insulin dosages; and (3) reducing stress and coping with denial. Before conception, it is essential to have a good laboratory evaluation including HbA1c, baseline assessment of renal function, thyroid function tests, and lipid profile. Other tests may need to be added according to medical history and physical exam. Conception should be deferred until the initial evaluation is completed and specific goals of therapy including glucose control and dietary and physical activity adherence are attained. Since the safety of oral antidiabetic agents is not well established for the fetus, the patients need to be switched to insulin therapy. The goals for blood glucose are between 70 and 100 mg/dl preprandial and <140 or <120 mg/dl, respectively, 1 or 2 h postprandial. HbA1c should be less than 6%. Hypertension, retinopathy, nephropathy, gastroparesis, and other neuropathies as well as elevated lipid levels need to be stabilized prior to conception. Pregnancy will exacerbate and accelerate acute and long-term complications of diabetes. Continuing care by a team of professionals is essential in the management of pregnant diabetic patients.

TABLE 46.17

Treatment Decisions Based on LDL Cholesterol Levels in Adults

	Medical Nutrition Therapy		Drug Therapy	
	Initiation Level	LDL Goal	Initiation Level	LDL Goal
Initiation level LDL goal				
With CAD, PVD, or CVD	>100	<70[a]	>100	<70[a]
Without CAD, PVD, or CVD	>100	<100	>100	<100

Data are given in mg/dl.

[a] Optional

Source: Adapted from American Diabetes Association. *Diabetes Care,* 23(Suppl 1): 58, 2000 and *Diabetes Care,* (Suppl 1): 28, S16, 2005.

Macrovascular Disease

Recommendations listed in Table 46.16 for LDL and HDL cholesterol levels as well as for triglycerides have as a goal to reduce the risk for development of coronary heart disease and to stop progression or cause regression in patients with already established macrovascular disease. The goal for LDL cholesterol levels is of 100 mg/dl for all diabetics and less than 70 mg/dl in high-risk patients with overt CVD. Lipid-lowering drug therapy should be initiated in patients with established vascular disease (coronary heart disease, peripheral vascular, or cerebrovascular disease) if the levels of LDL cholesterol are above 100 mg/dl. In diabetic patients without established macrovascular disease, lipid-lowering drug therapy is recommended for LDL cholesterol of 130 mg/dl or above. The recommendations for treatment of elevated LDL cholesterol are summarized in Table 46.17. Pharmacological therapy should be initiated after behavioral interventions are used. However, in patients with clinical CAD or very high LDL cholesterol levels (i.e., ≥200 mg/dl), pharmacological therapy should be initiated at the same time that behavioral therapy is started. The ADA guidelines recommend that diabetic subjects with clinical CAD and an LDL cholesterol level of >100 mg/dl be treated with pharmacological agents. For diabetics without preexisting CAD, the current ADA recommendations for starting pharmacological therapy are LDL cholesterol levels ≥130 mg/dl.

A point to consider in diabetic patients is the method used to measure LDL cholesterol. Due to the prevalence of dense LDL in these patients, the conventional method to calculate LDL cholesterol is inappropriate, and the levels determined are in general falsely low.

Increased triglyceride levels are also recognized as a target for intervention. The levels of triglycerides considered acceptable are <150 mg/dl, and the acceptable HDL cholesterol levels are >40 mg/dl in men and more than 50 mg/dl in women. The initial therapy for hypertriglyceridemia is behavioral modification with weight loss, increase physical activity, and no alcohol consumption. In the case of severe hypertriglyceridemia (≥1000 mg/dl), severe dietary fat restriction (15 to 20% of calories as fat) in addition to pharmacological therapy is necessary to reduce the risk of pancreatitis. These patients are hard to manage and improving glycemic control rather tightly is a very effective measure for reducing triglyceride levels and should be aggressively used before the introduction of fibric acid derivatives.

NUTRITIONAL RECOMMENDATIONS AND PRINCIPLES FOR THE DIETARY, TREATMENT OF DIABETICS

GOALS OF NUTRITION THERAPY

The goals of medical nutrition therapy for people with diabetes are to optimize health, and to prevent and treat the chronic complications of diabetes by attaining and maintaining optimal metabolic outcomes including blood glucose and A1c level, LDL and HDL cholesterol and triglyceride levels, blood pressure and body weight control, and prevent or delay its complications.[41] The goals are summarized in Table 46.18. MNT is individualized for the person with diabetes so as to integrate the therapy into the daily routine of living. A registered dietitian completes a nutritional assessment and diagnosis, establishes behavioral goals, develops the individualized meal plan, and behavioral interventions with the person with diabetes and the family, and then provides nutrition monitoring and evaluation.[42] The effectiveness of the dietary interventions in helping the person with diabetes achieve the identified goals should be evaluated routinely until goals are achieved. If goals are not met, changes in the overall management plan are needed. When goals are achieved, reassessment, continuing education, and evaluation should occur at least annually, and more often with changes in lifestyle, to ensure optimal control of diabetes and maintenance of health.

TABLE 46.18
Goals of Medical Nutrition Therapy for Diabetes

- Achieve and maintain metabolic outcomes, including
  - A1c levels and blood glucose concentrations as close to normal as is safely possible to prevent or reduce the risk for complications of diabetes
  - Lipid and lipoprotein profiles that reduce the risk for macrovascular disease
  - Blood pressure levels that reduce the risk for vascular disease
- Modify nutrient intake and lifestyle for the prevention and treatment of long-term complications of diabetes, such as obesity, hypertension, nephropathy, retinopathy, and cardiovascular diseases
- Improve overall health and wellness through healthy food choices and physical activity.
- Provide optimal nutrition for individual nutrition needs, while taking into consideration personal and cultural preferences and lifestyle, within the context of respecting the individual's wishes and willingness to change

Source: Based on the 2004 American Diabetes Association Position Statement "Nutrition Principles and Recommendations in Diabetes" *Diabetes Care*, 27(Suppl 1): S36, 2004.

TABLE 46.19
Survival Skills for Managing Diabetes

- To acquire an adequate knowledge of:
  - Basic food and meal guidelines (including when eating out)
  - Effect of carbohydrates on blood glucose
  - Amount of carbohydrates taken daily
  - Carbohydrate food groups, portion sizes, and label information
- To coordinate insulin administration with food intake
- To be able to perform self-monitoring of blood glucose
- To schedule exercise according to food intake and glucose control
- To acquire knowledge of how to treat hypoglycemia:
  (in general, 15 g of carbohydrates should raise blood glucose 50–100 mg/dl in 15 min).
- To know that alcohol intake may cause hypoglycemia (by inhibiting gluconeogenesis in liver).
- To know why, when, and how to call the health care provider and dietitian.
- To have an established plan for recording self-management and returning for continuing care

---

NUTRITION THERAPY FOR DIFFERENT TYPES OF DIABETES

Type 1 Diabetes

The person with type 1 diabetes is typically thin or within recommended weight range. Prior to diagnosis, the patient may have experienced weight loss, frequent urination (polyuria), thirst and increased fluid intake (polydipsia), and hunger (polyphagia). The initial goals of medical nutrition therapy (MNT) are to replace fluids, normalize blood glucose and lipids, and provide appropriate calories for healthy living. Food, insulin administration, and physical activity need to be well balanced to obtain optimal control. It is essential that the person with diabetes coordinates the eating and exercise patterns with the onset of action and the duration of the insulin. The person with newly diagnosed type 1 diabetes may be overwhelmed with changes in daily routine; thus, the focus is initially on survival skills for managing diabetes (Table 46.19), followed by teaching self-management knowledge and skills, and behavior changes that are needed to optimally control diabetes and its complications.[43,44] Dietary changes to optimize health can be made more slowly over time. Figure 46.1 outlines the two approaches to nutrition therapy currently recommended by the ADA.[45] Blood glucose levels need to be monitored, and insulin doses and food intake to control blood glucose should be adjusted to achieve recommended levels of blood glucose control (Table 46.16).

Type 2 Diabetes

The person with newly diagnosed type 2 diabetes may have had asymptomatic type 2 diabetes for a number of years prior to diagnosis, and may present with one or more complications. Most are obese or have increased percentage of body fat distributed predominately in the abdominal region. The goals of therapy for persons with type 2 are summarized in Table 46.18 and

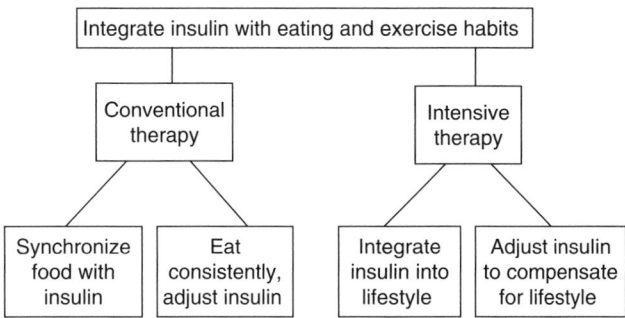

FIGURE 46.1 Nutrition therapy for type 1 diabetes. (Reprinted with permission from *Maximizing the Role of Nutrition in Diabetes Management*, American Diabetes Association, Alexandria, 1994.)

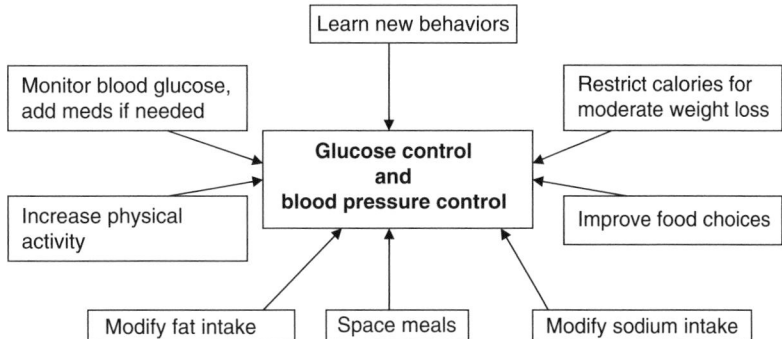

FIGURE 46.2 Nutrition therapy for type 2 diabetes. (Adapted with permission from *Maximizing the Role of Nutrition in Diabetes Management*, American Diabetes Association, Alexandria, 1994.)

focus on achieving and maintaining glucose, lipid, blood pressure, and body weight within recommended ranges. Weight loss is recommended for all overweight or obese adults with type 2, and the primary approach is therapeutic lifestyle change with at least 1000 to 1200 kcal/day for women and 1200 to 1600 kcal/day for men. [41] Methods for attaining these goals are outlined in Figure 46.2. There is no clear indication as to which goal should have first priority; however, the UKPDS researchers found that blood pressure control produced the most improved outcomes. [46] The desired outcomes of medical nutrition therapy for persons with type 2 diabetes are outlined in Tables 46.16.

Diabetes in Pregnancy

The goal of nutrition therapy for diabetes in pregnancy is to produce a healthy baby at term and maintain optimal health for the mother. If type 1 or type 2 diabetes is diagnosed prior to pregnancy, counseling is recommended to attain optimal control of diabetes prior to conception and throughout pregnancy. The pregnant woman is defined as having gestational diabetes if first diagnosed during the present pregnancy. GDM does not exclude the possibility that diabetes may have been unrecognized prior to pregnancy; thus, risk assessment for GDM should be undertaken at the first prenatal visit. [47] However, GDM typically occurs around the twenty-fourth week of pregnancy and screening is recommended for all high-risk and average-risk women between the 24th and 28th weeks of pregnancy, which includes about 90% of all pregnant women. [47, 48] Women diagnosed with GDM in a prior pregnancy have a 30 to 65% probability of developing GDM in a subsequent pregnancy. Studies also show that women with GDM have a 22 to 30% probability of developing type 2 diabetes in 7 to 10 years and a 50 to 60% risk of developing diabetes in their lifetime. Additionally, the offspring have an increased risk of obesity and GDM. [49]

The overall goals for MNT for diabetes in pregnancy are shown in Table 46.20, [47,50] and blood glucose goals are shown in Table 46.21. [47] To accomplish these goals, meal patterns, nutrient composition, and caloric needs are reviewed in Table 46.22, [42,50] and meal/snack patterns need to be individualized to meet the needs of the person with diabetes.

NUTRITIONAL RECOMMENDATIONS

Guidelines for nutrient consumption and other nutrition components such as sweeteners and cholesterol, along with technical reviews of the evidence for the guidelines, have been published by the ADA[43,51–53] and are summarized in Table 46.23.

TABLE 46.20
Goals for Medical Nutrition Therapy in GDM

- To consume food-providing nutrients necessary for maternal and fetal health
- To achieve and maintain maternal normoglycemia
- To teach good nutrition patterns to the family "gatekeeper"
- To develop nutritional patterns that prevent or forestall recurrence of GDM and onset of type 2 diabetes mellitus

Source: Based on American Diabetes Association: Thomas-Dobersen,D, et al: Clinical Diabetes 1, 172, 1999, and Thomas, AM and Gutierrez, YM. American Dietetic Association Guide to Gestational Diabetes Mellitus, 2005.

TABLE 46.21
Target Plasma Blood Glucose in Pregnancy

	mg/dl	mmol/l
Fasting	60–95	5.3
Postprandial 1 h	<140	7.2
Postprandial 2 h	<120	6.7

Source: Reprinted with permission from American Diabetes Association. Gestational Diabetes Mellitus. *Diabetes Care*, 27(Suppl 1): S88–90, 2004.

TABLE 46.22
Summary of Nutritional Therapy for GDM

Meal pattern

Three meals plus 2–4 small snacks (2–3 h intervals)

(Breakfast carbohydrate load may need to be as low as 15–30 g)

Carbohydrate intake individualized

Composition

40–45% carbohydrate >175 g. minimum

20–25% protein ($\geq$1.1 g/kg desirable body weight)

30–40% fat (mono or polyunsaturated emphasized, and saturated and trans fat minimized)

Nonnutritive sweeteners are generally safe, but use in moderation

Caffeine should be limited to <300 mg/day

Alcohol should be avoided

Estimated Energy Requirements (EER)

First trimester = Adult EER = 0

Second trimester = Adult EER + 160 kcal (8 kcal/week × 20 weeks) + 180 kcal

Third trimester = Adult EER + 272 kcal (8 cal/week × 34 weeks) + 180 kcal.

EER = 354 – (6.91 x age in years) + PA x (9.36 × weight in kg + 726 x height in meters

PA = Physical activity coefficients ranging from 1.0 (sedentary), 1.12 (low active), 1.27 (active),and 1.45 (very active)

Weight gain

Adjust kilocalorie level to achieve appropriate weight gain for prepregnancy BMI category

	Prepregnancy BMI	Recommended Total Weight Gain
Underweight	<18.5	28–40 lb (12.5–18 kg)
Normal weight	18.5–24.9	25–35 lb (11.5–16 kg)
Overweight	25–29.9	15–25 lb (7–11.5 kg)
Obesity	30–34.9	minimum 15 lb (7.1 kg)
Twins gestation		35–45 lb (15.9–20.5 kg.)

Source: Adapted from Thomas, AM, Gutierrez, YM. American Dietetic Association Guide to Gestational Diabetes Mellitus, 2005 and Ross, TA, Boucher, JL, and O'Connel, BS. American Dietetic Association Guide to Diabetes Medical Nutrition Therapy and Education, 2005.

TABLE 46.23
Medical Nutrition Therapy Nutrient and Other Nutrition Component Recommendation

Nutrient	Recommendation	Comments
Protein Sources: chicken, fish, meat, eggs, milk, tofu, nuts, and peanut butter	10–35% of total calories should come from protein sources	Research indicates needs are similar for people with or without diabetes With onset of nephropathy, limit protein to adult RDA (0.8 g/kg/day) Some research studies suggest vegetable protein may not be as harmful to the kidneys as animal protein
Carbohydrate Sources: starch (grains, bread, pasta, rice, potato, and beans), milk, fruit, vegetables, sugar, honey, jam, molasses, etc	65–90% of calories are divided between carbohydrate and fats based on individual risk factors and needs. Depending on nutritional assessment and medical nutritional therapy goals, this generally equates to 45–65% of total calories from carbohydrate Not <130 g/day	Total carbohydrate intake has greater impact on blood glucose control than source of carbohydrate, that is, whether complex carbohydrate or sucrose Sucrose and sucrose-containing foods should be consumed within the context of a healthful diet. These foods are often high in total carbohydrate and fat and low in vitamins and minerals
Sugars and Other Sweeteners **Source:** Sucrose, Fructose, Corn sweeteners such as corn syrup, fruit juice, or fruit juice concentrate honey, molasses, dextrose, and maltose. Sorbitol, mannitol, xylitol (sugar alcohols)	% of calories will vary and is individualized based on usual eating habits, glucose, and lipid goals. Sucrose and other sugars/sweeteners can be integrated into a healthy eating pattern for persons with diabetes	Sucrose and sucrose-containing foods should be consumed within the context of a healthful diet. These foods are often high in total carbohydrate and fat and low in vitamins and minerals Individuals can be taught to substitute sucrose-containing foods for other carbohydrate foods in their meal plan
Nonnutritive sweeteners such as saccharin, aspartame, acesulfame K, and sucralose	All are approved by the FDA, and the FDA determines an acceptable daily intake (ADI) which includes a 100-fold safety factor. Actual intake by persons with diabetes is well below the ADI	
Fat Sources: Monounsaturated: olive and canola oils, avocado, and nuts	65–90% of calories are divided between fats and carbohydrates. Most of fat calories (>90%) are divided between monounsaturated fats and carbohydrates	Individuals with diabetes, normal lipid levels, and reasonable body weight should limit total fat to <30% of total calories and <300 mg of dietary cholesterol per day
Polyunsaturated: safflower, sunflower, corn, and soy oils	At least 10% of calories should be from polyunsaturated fats	If obesity and weight management are the primary issues, reducing total fat to reduce total calories and increasing exercise should be recommended If low-density lipoprotein cholesterol is the primary concern, progression to National Cholesterol Education Program step II dietary guidelines (<7% of total calories from saturated fat and <200 mg cholesterol per day) should be implemented
Saturated: butter, lard, shortening, animal fats, coconut, and palm oils	No more than 7–10% of total calories should be from saturated fats	Guidelines for reducing cardiovascular risk are emphasized — nobody should exceed 10% of total calories from saturated fats
	Depending on nutritional assessment, total fat intake equates to 25–35% of total calories	If elevated triglyceride and very low density lipoprotein cholesterol are the primary concerns, a moderate increase in monounsaturated fat intake, with <10% of total calories from saturated fat, and a more moderate (slight decrease) in carbohydrate can be tried. Some studies have shown that a diet with increased total fat from monounsaturated fats can lower plasma triglycerides, glucose, and insulin levels more than a high-carbohydrate diet in some individuals. In individuals with triglycerides >1000, reduction of all types of dietary fats to reduce levels of plasma dietary fat in the form of chylomicrons should be implemented

Continued

TABLE 46.23
(Continued)

Nutrient	Recommendation	Comments
Fat		
Sources: (*Continued*)		
Trans fats:	Minimized	Effective in 2006, trans fats are listed on the nutrition
Some stick margarine and shortening, some processed and fast foods		labels and intake should be minimized to reduce the risks of CVD
		Trans fatty acids appear to be particularly deleterious because, in addition to increasing LDL cholesterol, they reduce HDL cholesterol
Fat Replacers	Foods with fat replacers can be substituted	Food products that contain <20 calories or 5 g of
Typically fall into three categories based on their nutrient content:	in an individual's meal plan based on the nutrient profile of the food product	carbohydrate per serving have a negligible effect on metabolic control
Carbohydrate based includes carrageenan, cellulose gum, corn syrup solids, dextrin, guar gum, hydrolyzed corn starch, maltodextrin, modified food starch, pectin, polydextrose, sugar beet fiber, tapioca dextrin, and xanthan gum		Foods containing 20 calories per serving should be limited to 3 servings spread throughout the day
Protein based includes microparticulated egg white and milk protein (Simplesse, K-Blazer), whey protein concentrate		
Fat based includes		
caprenin, olestra (Olean), salatrin (Benefat) and others		
Dietary cholesterol	<300 mg/day	MNT typically reduces LDL Cholesterol 15–25 mg/dl (0.40–40.65 mmol/l)
Fiber	20–35 g/day-same recommendation as for individuals without diabetes[a]	Research suggests that in the amounts typically consumed fiber intake has very little impact on blood glucose levels
Sodium	Same as for general population: <3000 mg/day	There is an association between hypertension and both IDDM and NIDDM, with an increased level for obese people with NIDDM. There is also evidence that individuals with NIDDM are more salt-sensitive
	If hypertensive, individuals should reduce sodium intake to <2400 mg/day	
	Food selection guidelines: <400 mg sodium per single serving of food; <800 mg sodium per entree or convenience meal	
Alcohol	Insulin users: Limit to 2 drinks per day and do not cut back on food	Abstinence is recommended for those with history of alcohol abuse or alcohol-induced hypertriglyceridemia and during
1 drink = 12 oz. beer, 5 oz. wine, 1 oz. 80 proof liquor	Noninsulin users: Substitute alcohol for fat	pregnancy
		Drink only with food. Alcohol can lead to hypoglycemia via inhibition of gluconeogenesis
		Limit for weight loss and elevated triglycerides
Micronutrients	The vitamin and mineral needs of people who are healthy appear to be adequately met by the RDAs, which include a generous safety factor	Individuals who are at greatest risk for vitamin/mineral deficiency include those on weight loss diets, strict vegetarians, the elderly, pregnant, or lactating women, those taking medications known to alter micronutrient metabolism, people with poor glycemic control (i.e., glycosuria), people with malabsorption disorders, and people with congestive heart failure or myocardial infarction

[a] Exception in patients with autonomic neuropathy who should not have increased fiber in their diet.

Source: Adapted, expanded, and updated from Karlsen, M., Khakpour, D., and Thomson, L.L. *Clinical Diabetes*, 14: 54, 1996.

The energy nutrients can be converted into blood glucose and glucose can be produced by the body from stored energy nutrients. Table 46.24 summarizes the estimated absorption time and the potential energy from each of the nutrients. Protein and fats have minimal or no effect on blood glucose except in patients whose diabetes is poorly controlled, since these nutrients may lead to a rapid increase in gluconeogenesis and deteriorated glycemic control.[53] Many persons with diabetes initially think that only sugar can increase blood glucose; thus, diabetes education about the effect of all carbohydrates, as well as "sugar-free" and "fat-free" foods containing calories, is essential to good control.

FOOD GUIDES AND PLANNING FOOD INTAKE FOR PERSONS WITH DIABETES

Historically, the approaches to planning food intake for persons with diabetes have ranged from starvation diets (during the preinsulin era) to high-fat, low-carbohydrate diet plans to our present system of more liberalized food intake. Various food guides and methods for planning food intake have been used. An overview of the meal planning approaches for providing MNT to persons with diabetes is reviewed in Table 46.25. A meal planning approach that provides the desired outcomes (decrease of complications and optimal health and satisfaction) is desirable. Carbohydrate counting is one method that allows maximum flexibility as well as excellent glycemic control. The different ways to count carbohydrates are reviewed in Table 46.26.

FOOD LABELING

Teaching patients with diabetes how to read a food label is especially important to those persons who count carbohydrate, fat, or protein in their meal plan. For persons using exchange lists for meal planning, information about how to use the nutrition

---

TABLE 46.24
Energy Nutrients, Their Calories, and Absorption

Nutrient	Calories/ Gram	% Nutrient Converted to Glucose Through Gluconeogenesis	Estimated time for absorption[a]
Carbohydrate	4	100	
Simple			5–30 min
Complex			1–3 h
Protein[b]	4	50–60	3–6 h
Fat[b]	9	10	3–8 h

[a] The absorption time is affected by the nutrient mix. For example, the sugar from a candy bar with high fat content is more slowly absorbed that a piece of candy that contains no fat.

[b] The effect of these nutrients on blood glucose is considered minimal or none with normal intake; however, determine the potential effect if carbohydrate intake is restricted and protein and fat are needed as major sources of energy.

TABLE 46.25
Meal Planning Approaches

Approach	Benefits	Drawbacks
Plate method	Easy to follow and remember	Little emphasis on sizes of portions
Food guide pyramid	Well known by the general public	Little focus on meal spacing
Health food choices	Mixes guidelines with meal plan	Often perceived as diet
Exchange lists for meal planning	Places emphasis on all nutrient groups	Concept difficult to understand by the lay person
Counting plans	Good approach for specific nutrient intervention	Requires committed learner
Carbohydrate indications:	Useful for adequate glucose control	Ignores other nutrients
Protein indications:	Addresses diabetic nephropathy	Ignores other nutrients
Fat indications:	Addresses weight or hyperlipidemia	Ignores other nutrients

Source: Reprinted with permission from American Diabetes Association: Karlsen, M., Khakpour, D., and Thomson, L.L., *Clincal Diabetes*, May/June, 54, 1996, and updated with addition of plate method.

TABLE 46.26
Ways to Count Carbohydrates

Method	Description	Ease vs. Accuracy	Calculation[a]
Premeal or bolus dose			
1. Counting carbohydrates exchanges (interchanges)	Count each serving of starch, fruit, and milk as one carbohydrate exchange and consider them equal in carbohydrate value	Easiest method but also the least accurate Requires the least math skill	Calculate premeal dose units/exchange
2. Counting food exchanges	Add the carbohydrates values of all exchanges that contain carbohydrates (including vegetables) to obtain the carbohydrate total for a meal	Easy and fairly accurate	Calculate premeal dose as units/exchange, counting vegetables as carbohydrates or calculate the bolus by dividing the total grams of carbohydrate in the meal by the insulin-to-carbohydrate ratio
3. Carbohydrate gram counting	Add carbohydrate gram values for all foods eaten to obtain the intake per meal	More time consuming than methods 1 and 2 but also quite accurate Requires more math skill to add and divide 2- and 3-digit numbers	Calculate premeal dose by dividing the total grams of carbohydrate in the carbohydrate total meal by the insulin-to-carbohydrate ratios
4. Calculating available glucose	Count grams of carbohydrate for all foods eaten. Then calculate the glucose available from protein and add this value to the carbohydrate grams to obtain the meal total	Most difficult. Requires the most math skill of all methods	Multiply grams of protein in meal by 0.6 to obtain available glucose, add to grams of carbohydrate Calculate the dose by dividing this total by the insulin-to-carbohydrate ratio
5. Evaluating glycemic index of carbohydrates	Glycemic index (GI) is a measure of the change in blood glucose after ingestion of carbohydrate-containing foods	May provide additional benefit for evaluating post meal glucose values as compared to total carbohydrate in some Individuals	Use table for GI values of carbohydrate foods High-GI foods are ≥ 70 while low GI is <55

[a] Short-acting insulin administered before meals to control the meal-related glucose rise. The calibration of insulin to food intake is recommended for individuals with type 1 diabetes, especially those following intensive therapy.

information to fit foods into the exchange lists is helpful (and essential for combination foods). The key question for the provider is to ask "how can I help my client or patient with diabetes use the food label to better control diabetes," and for the patient to ask is "how does this food, based on the nutritional information, fit into my food plan for controlling diabetes."[54]

DIABETES AND PHYSICAL ACTIVITY

Exercise can be used as a therapeutic tool for controlling diabetes, and the person with diabetes needs to incorporate exercise into the lifestyle for healthy living with diabetes.

PATIENT EVALUATION BEFORE EXERCISE

The person with diabetes should undergo a medical evaluation with appropriate diagnostic studies and should be screened for complications that may be worsened by the exercise program.[36,56] If complications are present, the patient should have an individualized exercise program prescription that specifies the frequency, intensity, and duration of exercise, along with specific precautions for minimizing risks. The benefits of physical activity are many, including cardiovascular fitness and psychological well-being. However, the risks of exercise for the person with diabetes are many, including fluctuations in blood glucose control, ketosis, lower-extremity injury, and exacerbation of preexisting conditions.

EXERCISE RECOMMENDATIONS

For Persons with Cardiovascular Disease

People with diabetes at risk of or with diagnosed cardiovascular disease should undergo a medical evaluation of cardiac status and special evaluation for exercise tolerance before participating in increased physical activities. Supervised cardiovascular risk reduction or rehabilitation programs often provide the patient and his family with increased support for increasing physical activities. Positive effects of regular exercise on reducing blood pressure have been consistently demonstrated in hyperinsulinemic persons.

For Persons with Peripheral Arterial Disease

Following an evaluation of peripheral arterial disease, the basic treatment is a supervised exercise program and cessation of smoking, carried out under the supervision of a physician. A walking program may improve muscle metabolism and collateral circulation for a person with intermittent claudication. If pain is severe and does not improve, further evaluation and possible limitation of exercises involving the lower extremities may be considered.

For Persons with Retinopathy

Following a dilated eye exam, if proliferative diabetic retinopathy is present, the person with diabetes may need to avoid anaerobic exercise and exercise that involves straining, jarring, or Valsalva maneuvers and any other activities that increase systolic blood pressure. Medical status dictates the level of risks associated with exercise; however, low-impact cardiovascular conditioning such as swimming, walking, low-impact aerobics, stationary cycling, and endurance exercises are considered low risk.

For Persons with Nephropathy

Specific exercise recommendations have not been developed for persons with nephropathy, but some patients may self-limit exercise, based on a reduced capacity for activity. High-intensity or strenuous exercises should probably be discouraged for persons with overt nephropathy, but other low-intensity physical activities may increase sense of well-being and socialization.

For Persons with Neuropathy

a. *Peripheral*: For the person who has loss of protective sensation in the feet on testing, weight-bearing exercises are contraindicated. These include use of treadmill, prolonged walking, jogging, and step exercises. Recommended exercises include swimming, bicycling, rowing, chair and arm exercises, along with other non-weight-bearing exercises.
b. *Autonomic*: Autonomic neuropathy increases the risks of exercise-related problems, and certain precautions need to be taken to tailor the exercise prescription to each individual patient following an in-depth evaluation. Thermoregulation may be difficult, so avoiding exercise in hot or cold environments and special attention to adequate hydration are most important.

EXERCISE AND GLYCEMIC CONTROL

Regular exercise activities (30 or more minutes on most days) have demonstrated consistent beneficial effects on carbohydrate metabolism and insulin sensitivity, as well as enhanced weight loss. Current recommendations for exercise suggest that those who need to reduce or maintain a reduction in body weight may need up to 90 min of physical activity on most days.

Exercise for Persons with Type 1 Diabetes

Persons with type 1 diabetes, who do not exhibit some of the limiting complications previously discussed or poor glycemic control, can enjoy all types of exercise.[56,37] The key is regulating the glycemic response to exercise. The person should avoid exercise if fasting glucose levels are >250 mg/dl with ketosis present or if glucose levels are >300 mg/dl. If glucose levels are <100 mg/dl prior to exercise, additional carbohydrates are recommended. Food adjustments for exercise for persons with type 1 diabetes are shown in Table 46.27. Food and fluids should be readily available for persons with type 1 diabetes during exercise. If the duration of exercise is 30 min or more during peak action time of insulin and blood glucose is in good control, reduction of insulin is recommended. The reduction of insulin is based on duration and intensity of exercise and usually ranges from 5 to 60% of daily requirements. After exercise, an extra carbohydrate snack may be necessary. Frequent monitoring of blood glucose and adequate food/fluid intake to prevent hypoglycemia are essential for self-management and maintaining a healthy lifestyle.

Exercise for Persons with Type 2 Diabetes

Many persons with type 2 diabetes may have some of the previously mentioned complications at diagnosis, and also may have been sedentary for many years. Thus, before beginning an exercise program, an in-depth physical examination and recommendations for exercise frequency, intensity, and duration is recommended.[57,38] Beginning with 5-to-10-min sessions with gradual increase is usually successful and safe. Unless treated with insulin or glucose-lowering medications, the person with type 2

TABLE 46.27
Food Adjustments for Exercise for Persons with Type 1 Diabetes

Types of Exercise and Examples	If Blood Glucose is:	Increase Food Intake by:	Suggestion of Food Exchanges to Use:
General guidelines			
Short-duration, low-to-moderate intensity (walking a half mile or leisurely bicycling for <30 min)	<100 mg/dl	10 to 15 g of carbohydrates (CHO)	1 fruit or 1 starch
	≥100 mg/dl	None	
Moderate intensity (1 h of tennis, swimming, jogging, leisurely bicycling, golfing, etc.)	<100 mg/dl	25 to 50 g CHO before exercise, then 10 to 15 g/h of exercise	1 meat sandwich with a milk or fruit
	100–180 mg/dl	10 to 15 g CHO	1 fruit or 1 starch
	180–300 mg/dl	None	
	≥300 mg/dl	Do not begin exercise until blood glucose is under control	
Strenuous (about 1–2 h of football, hockey, racquetball, or basketball; strenuous bicycling or swimming; shoveling heavy snow)	<100 mg/dl	50 g CHO, monitor blood glucose carefully	1 meat sandwich (2 slices of bread) with a milk and fruit
	100–180 mg/dl	25 to 50 g CHO depending on intensity and duration	meat sandwich with a milk and fruit
	180–300 mg/dl	10 to 15 g CHO	1 fruit or 1 starch
	≥300 mg/dl	Do not begin exercise until blood glucose is under better control	

* Self-blood glucose monitoring is essential for all persons to determine their carbohydrate needs. Persons with type 2 diabetes usually do not need an exercise snack. During periods of exercise, all individuals need to increase fluid intake.

Source: Adapted with permission from Franz, MJ, Barry, B, *Diabetes and Exercise: Guidelines for Safe and Enjoyable Activity,* American Diabetes Association, Alexandria, p.16, 1996.

diabetes does not usually need additional food before, during, or following exercise, except for exercise that is intense or of long duration. Recent attention has focused on the useful role of exercise in preventing or delaying the onset of type 2 diabetes.

Exercise for the Older Adults with Diabetes

Exercise in older adults with diabetes is recommended and may lead to an improved quality of life and fewer chronic diseases. The same precautions should be taken with the older adults with and without diabetes.

HOSPITAL ADMISSION GUIDELINES FOR PERSONS WITH DIABETES

If the standard of care of a diabetic patient is adequate, seldom will a diabetic patient require hospitalization. According to the guidelines of the ADA, inpatient care may be required in:

- Life-threatening acute metabolic complications of diabetes
- Newly diagnosed diabetes in children and adolescents
- Patients with chronic poor metabolic control that necessitates close monitoring to determine the problem behind the poor control and changes in therapy
- Patients with severe chronic complications that require intensive treatment either of diabetes or of conditions that significantly affect diabetes control and further development of complications
- Uncontrolled or newly discovered insulin-requiring diabetes during pregnancy
- Patients in whom institution of insulin-pump therapy or other intensive insulin regimens are being contemplated

TRANSLATION OF MEDICAL NUTRITION THERAPY FOR DIABETES TO HEALTH CARE INSTITUTIONS

Today's recommendations for MNT in health care facilities are based on individualized needs of the patients with diabetes. One of the approaches that is more frequently used is the "consistent carbohydrate diabetes meal plan"; a plan for developing a menu is shown in Table 46.28.

TABLE 46.28

Developing a Consistent Carbohydrate Diabetes Meal Plan Menu for Health Care Facilities

1. Establish the desired calorie range

Determine the desired percentages of macronutrients (carbohydrate, protein, saturated fat, and total fat)

Determine the numbers of CHO choices to be given at each meal, and if included, at bedtime snack

Determine how often to include sucrose-containing desserts and the maximum number of CHO choices to be allotted to each dessert

Analyze current fat-modified menus for distribution of macronutrients (% carbohydrate, protein, saturated fat, and total fat) to determine if they meet goal ranges of new diabetic menus

Determine how many grams of carbohydrate or CHO choices are in each item in the fat-modified menu (i.e., fruits, salads, starches, casseroles, desserts, milk, and juices)

For nonselective menus, adjust the fat-modified menus to provide the established number of CHO choices, and include a bedtime snack if desired

For facilities with menu selections, identify the CHO choices for each carbohydrate item, and include instructions on the menu regarding the number of carbohydrate choices to make at each meal

For long-term care facilities that wish to base their diabetic diet (consistent carbohydrate diet) on regular menus, use the same process as for fat-modified menus

Source: Reprinted with permission from Schafer, R.G. *Pract Diabetol*, 16: 3, 48, 1997.

ACUTE HEALTH CARE FACILITIES

Approximately one out of seven hospital beds is occupied by a person with diabetes. In the acute care facility, many of the patients have complex health problems, in addition to diabetes. Thus, the challenge is to maximize health potential and provide foods that are culturally acceptable to the patient, while lowering the risks of complications. Each acute care facility has different meal planning systems that best meet their needs. The consistent carbohydrate menu plan can be used to improve metabolic control. The ideal meal plan reflects the diabetes nutrition recommendations and does not unnecessarily restrict sucrose.[58]

LONG-TERM HEALTH CARE FACILITIES

Since the risk of diabetes increased with age, the patient population in long-term care includes many individuals with diabetes. Additionally, malnutrition is a recognized challenge in the older adult population. Food intake should be adequate and not overly restricted. Regular menus, with consistent amounts of carbohydrate at meals and snacks are the recommended approach. Monitoring of blood glucose and hemoglobin A1C should be used to evaluate glycemic control, with individualized approaches to achieve goals of MNT.

SELF-MANAGEMENT EDUCATION FOR PERSONS WITH DIABETES

Diabetes self-management education and continuing nutrition care is essential for meeting the goals of MNT and diabetes control. The outpatient and home setting is the ideal environment. If the patient is hospitalized with multiple other priorities, usually the concern of the patient and the family is not focused on diabetes self-management education. Learning readiness is the cornerstone for self-management education. At discharge from the inpatient facility, plans are made for continuing education and follow-up by the health care team.

EDUCATION FOR HEALTH CARE PROFESSIONALS AND ADMINISTRATORS

The role of MNT in helping the teams (including the person with diabetes) to attain the desired treatment goals is cost-effective and leads to quality health services.[59,60] One of the roles of the registered dietitian is to translate nutrition recommendations for the diabetes care team and to integrate these recommendations into the overall care of the person with diabetes. Team members should have access to simplified guidelines for patient nutrition care until a registered dietitian is available.

THIRD PARTY REIMBURSEMENT FOR DIABETES CARE, SUPPLIES, AND SELF-MANAGEMENT EDUCATION

Currently, 46 states and the District of Columbia require state regulated health insurance plans to cover basic diabetes care; states currently not providing coverage include Alabama, Idaho, North Dakota, and Ohio.[62] The coverage is at risk in a growing number of states as almost half-considered provisions to roll back or eliminate laws requiring state regulated health insurance plans to cover diabetes supplies and services during recent legislative sessions.[61] The website of the American Diabetes Association (http://www.diabetes.org) usually has the latest information related to diabetes reform laws in the states; however, examination of each state's reform laws is necessary to determine the extent of coverage. Current Medicare regulations Part B provide for both diabetes self management training (DSMT) and MNT.[62] Currently, at a minimum, the qualified beneficiary with diabetes obtains a referral from the treating physician for MNT, and either a physician or qualified nonphysician practitioner may order DSMT. The person with diabetes may receive an initial 10 h of DSMT and 3 h of MNT if not provided on the same day and 2 h of follow-up DSMT annually and up to 2 h of MNT annually. Additional hours may be ordered if there is a significant change in medical condition, diagnosis, or treatment regime that requires a change in MNT.[62] Medicaid, a federal–state partnership program for persons unable to afford health care and private third-party insurance, offers coverage for MNT in some states. To determine if your state offers coverage, contact your state's Medicaid program.

The frequency of dietitian contact with the patient and the essential care processes for MNT have not been clearly delineated; yet quality health care today requires consistently applied, evidence-based care that leads to positive outcomes for most patients. The Diabetes Care and Education Practice Group of the American Dietetic Association reports that the use of guidelines resulted in changes in dietitian practices and produced greater improvement in patient blood glucose outcomes at 3 months, as compared to usual care. Self-management education is critical to successful diabetes management, and medical treatment without self-management education is regarded as substandard and unethical. Numerous studies have demonstrated that self-management education and MNT improve outcomes for persons with diabetes.[42]

LIST OF ABBREVIATIONS

ADA — American Diabetes Association
CAD — Coronary Artery Disease
CHO — Carbohydrates
DCCT — Diabetes Control and Complications Trial
GDM — Gestational Diabetes Mellitus
GI — Glycemic index
HDL — High density lipoproteins
LDL — Low density lipoproteins
MI — Myocardial Infarction
MNT — Medical Nutrition Therapy
NCPR0 — National Cholesterol Education Program
NHANES III — The Third National Health and Nutritional Examination Survey
UKPDS — UK Prospective Diabetes Study
WHO — World Health Organization

REFERENCES

1. World Health Organization: *Diabetes Mellitus: Report of a WHO Study Group*. Geneva, World Health Org., 1985 (Tech. Rep. Ser. no. 727).
2. Harris, MI, Flegal, KM, Cowie, CC, et al., *Diabetes Care*, 21: 518, 1998.
3. National Diabetes Data Group: Classification and diagnosis of diabetes mellitus and other categories of glucose intolerance. *Diabetes* 28: 1039, 1979.
4. Expert Committee on the Diagnosis and Classification of Diabetes Mellitus, *Diabetes Care*, 21(Suppl. 1), 5, 1998.
5. American Diabetes Association, *Diabetes Care*, 28(Suppl 1): S7, 2005.
6. Tominaga, M, Eguchi, H, Manaka, H, et al., *Diabetes Care*, 22: 920, 1999.
7. Harris, MI, Hadden, WC, Knowler, WC, Bennett, PH, *Diabetes*, 36: 523, 1987.
8. Harris, MI, *Diabetes Care*, 16: 642, 1993.
9. Klein, R, *Diabetes Care*, 18: 258, 1995.
10. Engelgau, MM, Narayan, KM, Herman, WH, *Diabetes Care*, 23: 1563, 2000.
11. Aiello, LP, Gardner TW, King, GL, et al., *Diabetes Care*, 21: 143, 1998.
12. The Diabetes Control and Complications Trial Research Group, *N Engl J Med*, 329: 997, 1993.
13. The Diabetes Control and Complications Trial Research Group, *N Engl J Med*, 342: 381, 2000.
14. UK Prospective Diabetes Study Group, *Lancet*, 352: 837, 1998.
15. UK Prospective Diabetes Study Group, *Lancet*, 352: 854, 1998.
16. Fong, DS, Aiello, LP, Ferris, FL, Klein, R, *Diabetes Care*, 27: 2540, 2004.
17. The Diabetes Control and Complications Trial Research Group, *Diabetes Care*, 23: 1084, 2000.
18. DeFronzo, RA, *Diabetes Reviews*, 3: 510, 1995.
19. Klausen, K, Borch-Johnsen, K, Feldt-Rasmussen, B, et al., *Circulation*, 110: 32, 2004.

20. UK Prospective Diabetes Study Group, *Br Med J*, 317: 703, 1998.
21. Laffell, LM, McGill, JB, Gans, DJ., *Am J Med*, 99: 497, 1995.
22. Bakris, GL,Williams, M, Dworkin, L, et al., *Am J Kidney Dis*, 36: 646, 2000.
23. Heart Outcomes Prevention Evaluation Study Investigators. *Lancet*, 355: 253, 2000.
24. Pepine, CJ, Handberg, EM, Cooper-De-Hoff, RM, et al., *JAMA*, 290: 2805, 2003.
25. The Diabetes Control and Complications Trial Research Group. *Kidney Int*, 47: 1703, 1995.
26. Chobanian, AV, Bakris GL, Black, HR, et al., *JAMA*, 289: 2560, 2003.
27. Estacio, RO, Jeffers, BW, Hiatt, WR, et al., *N Engl J Med*, 338: 645, 1998.
28. Haffner, SM, *Diabetes Care*, 21: 160, 1998.
29. Pyorala, K, Pederson, TR, Kjekshus, J, et al., *Diabetes Care*, 20: 614, 1997.
30. Sacks, FM, Pfeffer, MA, Moye, LA, et al., *N Engl J Med*, 335: 1001, 1996.
31. Heart Protection Study Collaborative Group, *Lancet*, 361: 2005, 2003.
32. Colhoun, HM, Betteridge, DJ, Durrington, PN, et al., *Lancet*, 364: 685, 2004.
33. Cannon, CP, Braunwald, E, McCabe, CH, et al., *N Engl J Med*, 350: 1495, 2004.
34. Nissen, SE, Tuzcu, EM, Scoenhagen, P, et al., *JAMA*, 291: 1071, 2004.
35. Frick, HM, Elo, O, Haapa, K, et al., *N Engl J Med*, 317: 1237, 1987.
36. Rubins, HB, Robins, SJ, Collins, D, et al., *N Engl J Med*, 341: 410, 1999.
37. Bhatt, DL, Marso, SP, Hirsch, AT, et al., *Am J Cardiol*, 90: 625, 2002.
38. Cryer, PE, Fisher, JN, Shamoon, H, *Diabetes Care*, 17: 734, 1994.
39. Burge, MR, Schmitz-Firentino, K, Fischett, C, et al., *JAMA*, 279: 137, 1998.
40. Weir, GC, Nathan, DM, Singer, DE, *Diabetes Care*, 17: 1514, 1994.
41. American Diabetes Association. Standards of Medical Care. *Diabetes Care*, 29(Suppl 1): S12, 2006.
42. Poss, TA, Boucher, JL, O'Connell, BS, *American Dietetic Association Guide to Diabetes Medical Nutrition Therapy and Education.* American Dietetic Association, Chicago, 6–8, 2005.
43. Franz, MJ, Bantle, JP, Beebe, CA, et al., *Diabetes Care*, 25: 148, 2002.
44. Warsi, A, Wang, PS, Lavalley, MP, et al., Self-management education programs in chronic disease: A systematic review and methodological critique of the literature. *Arch Intern Med*, 164: 1641, 2004.
45. American Diabetes Association, *Maximizing the role of nutrition in diabetes management*, American Diabetes Association, Alexandria, 1994, Chap. 5, 6.
46. UKPDS — Blood pressure.
47. American Diabetes Association, *Clinical Practice Recommendations 2006, Diabetes Care*, 29(Suppl 1): S7, 2006.
48. Agency for Healthcare Research and Quality. *The Guide to Clinical Preventive Services 2005*, AHRQ Pub. No. 05-0570, 2005, 147–148.
49. Thomas-Dobersen, D. *Clin Diabetes*, 17, 179, 1999.
50. Thomas, AM, Gutierrez, YM, *American Dietetic Association Guide to Gestational Diabetes Mellitus.* Chicago, American Dietetic Association, 2005.
51. American Diabetes Association. *Diabetes Care*, 27(Suppl 1): S36, 2004.
52. American Diabetes Association. *Diabetes Care*, 27(Suppl 1): S88, 2004.
53. Lewis, G, Thomson, LL, *Optimizing Glycemic Control with Diabetes Technology and Diabetes Medical Nutrition Therapy with Advanced Insulin Management.* Chicago: American Diabetes Association, 2005.4e
54. Wheeler, ML, Franz, M, Heins, J, *Diabetes Care*, 17: 489, 1994.
55. Wasserman, DH, Zinman, B, *Diabetes Care*, 17: 924, 1994.
56. Schneuider, SH, Ruderman, NB, *Diabetes Care*, 13, 785, 1990.
57. American Diabetes Association, *Diabetes Care*, 22(Suppl 1): S47, 2000.
58. Schafer, RG, Bohannon, B, Franz, M, et al., *Diabetes Care*, 20: 96, 1997.
59. Steed, L. Cooke, D, Newman, S, *Patient Education Counseling*, 51: 5, 2003.
60. Pastors, JG, Franz, M, Warshaw, H, et al., *J Am Diet Assoc*, 103: 827, 2003.
61. American Diabetes Association. Available at http://www.diabetes.org/advocacy-and-legalresources/state-legislation/healthinsurance.jsp Accessed on February 1, 2006.
62. CMS. Medical Nutrition Therapy Available at http://www.cms.hhs.gov/MedicalNutritionTherapy/ Accessed February 9, 2006.

47 Renal Nutrition

Lynn Thomas and Roxanne Poole

CONTENTS

INTRODUCTION

The kidneys play a vital role in the maintenance of normal blood volume/pressure and the regulation of acid–base balance. Approximately one-fourth of the cardiac output is filtered through the kidneys each minute. Urinary excretion is the pathway for removal of the waste products of absorption and metabolism. These include ammonia, urea, creatinine, phosphorus, water, sodium, and potassium. Normal bone health is facilitated by activation of vitamin D and regulation of calcium and phosphorus. The kidney produces the hormone erythropoietin. Deficiency of this hormone results in profound anemia.

A decrease in kidney function greatly affects metabolism and nutritional status. These patients are at risk for protein-energy malnutrition. Common manifestations include edema, uremia, hypertension, anemia, and metabolic acidosis. The medical nutrition therapy for kidney failure becomes increasingly complex as the renal disease advances. The diet prescription is matched to the stage of renal failure in order to keep the diet as liberal as possible. Table 47.1[1] defines the terms used in this chapter.

NUTRITIONAL ASSESSMENT IN THE RENAL PATIENT

It is a recommended standard of practice that all renal patients be considered at risk for nutritional compromise. Protein-energy malnutrition is a common finding among these patients. Acute and chronic renal failure patients should receive baseline assessments as soon as they are identified or admitted to the hospital. The National Kidney Foundation's Dialysis Outcomes Quality Initiative (NKF-DOQI) provides clinical practice guidelines. Under these guidelines new dialysis patients are expected to receive a nutritional assessment within 30 days of the initial treatment. Reassessments are completed annually. Monthly follow-up

TABLE 47.1
Explanation of Terms Used in This Chapter

Term	Explanation
Acute renal failure	Sudden onset secondary to shock, trauma, hypertension, exposure to nephrotoxic substances of bacteria. Reversible in many cases
Azotemia	Elevated concentrations of nitrogenous wastes in blood serum.
Chronic renal failure (CRF) or insufficiency (CRI)	Gradual progression terminating with end-stage renal disease requiring dialysis or transplant. Causes include obstructive disease of the urinary tract such as congenital birth defects, systemic diseases such as diabetes mellitus or systemic lupus erythematosis, glomerular disease, and overdosing on analgesic medications. Patients follow an increasingly restricted diet as renal failure progresses.
Hemodialysis	Removal from blood of the waste products of metabolism by use of a semipermeable membrane and a dialysis treatment machine. This process takes 3 to 6 h three times a week in an outpatient clinic or hospital. Some patients, with appropriate training and assistance, can dialyze at home. Hemodialysis patients follow a diet restricted in sodium, potassium, phosphorus, and fluids.
Nephrotic syndrome	Failure of the glomerular basement membrane to filter waste products appropriately. Large amounts of protein are found in the urine. Patients frequently have edema secondary to hypoalbumenemia.
Peritoneal dialysis	Removal of the waste products of metabolism by perfusion of a sterile dialysate solution throughout the peritoneal cavity. This method of dialysis is done at home. Dialysate exchanges are performed several times a day or continuously at night with the aid of a peritoneal dialysis machine. Peritoneal dialysis patients follow a liberalized diet as dialysis is daily. The diet is normally a low-sodium diet with diabetes mellitus restrictions as necessary.
Uremia	A toxic systemic syndrome caused by retention of high levels of urea.

TABLE 47.2
Components of the Nutrition Assessment

Component	Approach
Medical history and physical exam	One way to organize findings is to use a "review of systems" approach. Note any medical problems or surgical procedures that could impact on nutritional status. Look for recent changes in weight and potential drug–nutrient interactions. Measure the patient's height, weight, and other anthropometric measurements. Check for edema and signs of muscle wasting. Activity levels and urine output are helpful in determining energy needs and fluid restriction
	Another useful tool for assessment is the Subjective Global Assessment (SGA). It is a five-component screen that uses weight change, dietary intake, gastrointestinal symptoms, functional capacity, and comorbidities, plus three components of a brief physical examination (muscle wasting, fat stores, and malnutrition related changes in fluid status). A form is used to give an overall SGA rating with ranges from well nourished to severely malnourished
Laboratory values	Look for laboratory values within expected ranges according to the patient's stage of disease. Consider causes for abnormal findings and corrective actions to take
Food intake assessment	A diet history should be taken using a 24 h recall or food frequency questionnaire. It is important to determine if the recall is typical and if there have been any changes in appetite. Also ask about use of dietary or nutritional supplements. Determine if the patient practices pica (ingestion of nonfood substances such as ice, cornstarch, or clay). Consider if the current intake is adequate and, if not, how the problem can be corrected
Environmental factors	Determine if the patient has an understanding about the necessity for changes in the diet. Investigate psychological and socioeconomic status. Is there someone who helps the patient follow the diet at home? Who does the grocery shopping and cooking? What is the educational level of the patient?

notes and 6-month nutritional updates are also required. Any significant changes in weight, laboratory values, or medical status generate an in-depth investigation. One of the primary goals of the baseline assessment is to develop a diet prescription tailored to a patient's individual needs. The diet should be as liberal as possible and include favorite foods. Every patient should be provided with written or otherwise appropriate educational materials covering the major points. The diet should be modified on a regular basis as indicated. Table 47.2[2–8] and Table 47.3[6,9–12] provide guidelines for various components of the nutrition assessment.

STAGES OF RENAL FAILURE

The treatment methods and nutrition recommendations vary as the patient progresses through the various stages of renal failure. The normal kidney removes excess fluid and waste products from the body and maintains acid–base balance. The kidney also regulates blood pressure, stimulates red blood cell production, and regulates the metabolism of calcium and phosphorus. Nephrotic syndrome is a dysfunction of the glomerular capillaries. Symptoms include urine losses of plasma proteins, low serum albumin,

TABLE 47.3

Interpretation of Laboratory Results for Hemodialysis and Peritoneal Dialysis Patients

Test	Range in Renal Disease	Reference Range	Comments
Albumin g/l (depends on method of analysis)	35–50	35–55 Infant: 44–55 <3 years: 40–59	Higher values are more desirable — mortality is 50% higher when albumin is <39
Alkaline phosphatase UL	42–128	42–128	High in bone disease
BUN (mmol/l)	14.4–28.6	3.6–7.1 Infant and child: 1.8–6.4	Varies with protein intake and dialysis adequacy
Calcium (mmol/l)	2.3–2.8	2.3–2.8	Low with insufficient vitamin D; high with excess
Cholesterol (mmol/l)	<5.2	<5.2	High with nephrotic syndrome, or hereditary disorders of lipid metabolism
High-density lipoprotein cholesterol (mmol/l)	>1.5	>1.5	
Low-density lipoprotein cholesterol (mmol/l)	<2.6	<2.6	
Triglycerides (mmol/l)	<1.7	<1.7	
Creatinine (μmol/l)	177–1326	44.2–97.2 Infant: 17.7–35.4 Child: 26.5–62 Teen: 44.2–88.4	Low in extreme muscle wasting
C-reactive protein (mg/dl)	<0.8	<0.8	High in infection and inflammation
Ferritin (pmol/l)	>225–1798	27–674 male 23–337 female Infant >2 months: 112–449 Child:15–319	High in inflammatory states
Glucose (mmol/l)	3.9–6.1	3.9–6.1	Monthly clinic labs usually are nonfasting
Hematocrit (%)	33–36	42–52 male 37–47 female Infant: 30–49 Child: 30–42 Teen: 34–44	Target for EPO therapy: 33
Hemogloblin (mmol/l)	6.8–7.4	8.7–11.2 male 7.4–9.9 female Child to teen: 6.2–10.57	
Intact Parathyroid Hormone (iPTH) (pg/ml)	150–300	10–65	
Iron (μmol/l)	13–31	13–31 Child: 50–120	Day-to-day variations common
Phosphorus (mmol/l)	1.1–1.9	0.97–1.45 Child:1.45–2.1	High serum levels common — binders and low PO_4 diet are used for control
Potassium (mmol/l)	3.5–5.0	3.5–5.0	High serum levels common — low K diet used for control
Prealbumin/Transthyretin (mg/l)	150–360	>300	Low in malnutrition and inflammation
Sodium (mmol/l)	136–145	136–145	Varies with fluid status

edema, and elevated blood lipids. In acute renal failure, the nephrons lose function or the glomerular filtration rate (GFR) drops suddenly. Symptoms include increased blood urea nitrogen, catabolism, negative nitrogen balance, elevated electrolytes, acidosis, increased blood pressure, and fluid overload. Nephrotic syndrome and acute renal failure are usually reversible conditions. The GFR declines gradually. In chronic renal failure in early stages compensation occurs by enlarging the remaining nephrons. Symptoms similar to those in acute renal failure appear when the kidney is at 75% of normal function. When the GFR is 10% or less of the normal rate, the patient is considered to be in end-stage renal disease. Dialysis is started to replace diminished kidney function. Electrolytes, fluids, anemia, and diet are monitored monthly by a registered dietician. Some patients in end-stage renal failure receive a kidney transplant. This restores kidney function and the patient is able to return to a more liberal diet.

ACUTE RENAL FAILURE: DAILY NUTRIENT AND FLUID NEEDS

Table 47.4[13–16] outlines basic nutritional requirements for children who have acute renal failure. Table 47.5[6,16–20] outlines basic nutritional requirements for adults who have acute renal failure. Guidelines are adjusted for individuals depending on the stress level, phase of disease, and dialysis treatments.

TABLE 47.4
Daily Nutrient and Fluid Needs for Pediatric Patients with
Acute Renal Failure

Age (Years)	Energy (Kcal/kg)	Protein (g/kg)
Birth to 1 year	>100	1.0–2.0
1–3	>100	1.5–1.8
4–10	70–90	1.0–1.5
11–18	55	0.8–1.5

Nutrient	Recommendations
Sodium	Monitor and adjust as needed
Potassium	Monitor and adjust as needed
Fluids	Maintain envolemic state
Calcium	Maintain normal serum levels
Phosphorus	Maintain normal serum levels. Use binders as needed
Vitamins and minerals	Follow daily RDA/DRI or therapeutic levels depending on needs

Note: Fluids and electrolytes and micronutrients either are unrestricted or individualized by patient rather than age. The Holliday–Segar method is frequently used to estimate maintenance. Energy and fluid needs for pediatric patients older than 14 days. The method uses actual body weight.

TABLE 47.5
Daily Nutrient and Fluid Needs for Adults with
Acute Renal Failure

Nutrient	Recommendations
Energy	25–35 kcal/kg
Protein[a]	0.6–0.8 g/kg
Sodium[b]	1–2 g/day
Potassium[b]	2 g/day
Fluids	Output plus 500 cc
Calcium	Keep serum values within normal limits
Phosphorus	Keep serum values within normal limits
Vitamins and minerals	Follow daily RDA/DRI or therapeutic levels (depending on needs)

[a] Increase as renal function improves or if dialysis is started.
[b] Replace in diuretic phase of disease.

CHRONIC RENAL FAILURE: DAILY NUTRIENT AND FLUID NEEDS

Table 47.6[13–16] outlines basic nutritional requirements for children who have chronic renal failure. Children have an increased incidence of renal osteodystrophy due to higher rate of bone turnover. Radiographic studies of the wrist should be performed annually. Table 47.7[6,16–21] outlines basic nutritional requirements for adults who have renal insufficiency but have not yet started dialysis. Guidelines are adjusted depending on GFR (ml/min 1.72 m^2) as contained in the NKF K-DOQI Clinical Practice Guidelines. Guidelines also can be adjusted for comorbidites and age.

POST KIDNEY TRANSPLANT: DAILY NUTRIENT AND FLUID NEEDS

Table 47.8[6,14–16,24] outlines basic nutritional requirements for children who have received renal transplants. Guidelines can be adjusted for comorbidity. Table 47.9[6,16–24] outlines basic nutritional requirements for adults who have received a kidney transplant. Guidelines can be adjusted for comorbidites and advanced age. As posttransplant patients are at increased risk for

TABLE 47.6
Daily Nutrient and Fluid Needs for Pediatric Patients with Chronic Renal Failure

Age (Years)	Energy (Kcal/kg)	Protein (g/kg)
Birth to 6 months	>100	2.2
6 months to 1 year	~100	1.6
1–3	~100	1.2
4–10	70–90	1.0–1.2
11–18	>40–50	0.9–1.0

Nutrient	Recommendations
Sodium	Monitor and adjust with level of renal function
Potassium	Monitor and adjust with level of renal function
Fluids	Maintain envolemic state
Calcium	Maintain normal serum levels
Phosphorus	Maintain normal serum levels. Use binders as needed
Vitamins and minerals	Follow daily RDA/DRI or therapeutic levels depending on needs

Note: Fluids, electrolytes, and micronutrients are either unrestricted or individualized by patient rather than age. The Holliday–Segar method is frequently used to estimate maintenance Calorie and fluid needs for pediatric patients older than 14 days. The method uses actual body weight.

TABLE 47.7
Daily Nutrient and Fluid Needs for Adults with Chronic Renal Failure

Nutrient	Recommendations
Energy	30–35 kcal/kg
Protein[a]	0.6–0.8 g/kg
Sodium[b]	1–2 g
Potassium[b]	Unrestricted
Fluids[c]	Unrestricted
Calcium[d]	1.0–1.5 g
Phosphorus	10–12 mg/g protein
Vitamins and minerals	Follow daily RDA/DRI or therapeutic levels depending on needs

[a] 0.8–1.0 g/kg in nephrotic syndrome, do not adjust for urine protein losses.

[b] Possible restriction when gomerular filtration rate <10 ml/min or when serum values become elevated.

[c] Start restriction when urine output diminishes.

[d] Include amounts from calcium containing binders.

hyperlipidemia, the diet should incorporate the principles from the Dietary Guidelines for Healthy Americans: American Heart Association.

PERITONEAL DIALYSIS: DAILY NUTRIENT AND FLUID NEEDS

Table 47.10[14,15] outlines basic nutritional requirements for children undergoing daily peritoneal dialysis. Guidelines can be adjusted for any comorbidity. Supplemental tube feedings may be required for those unable to meet nutritional requirements for growth with oral intake. Table 47.11[16,17,21,25] outlines basic nutritional requirements for adults undergoing daily peritoneal dialysis. Guidelines can be adjusted for comorbidites and advanced age.

TABLE 47.8
Daily Nutrient and Fluid Needs for Pediatric Patients Post Kidney Transplant

Age (Years)	Energy (Kcal/kg)	Protein <3 Months Post-Transplant (g/kg)	Protein >3 Months Post-Transplant (g/kg)
Birth to 5 months	≥108	3.0	2.2
5 months to 1 year	≥98	3.0	1.6
1–3	102	2.0–3.0	1.3
4–6	90	2.0–3.0	1.2
7–10	70	2.0–3.0	1.0
11–14 (girls)	47	1.5–2.0	1.0
15–18 (girls)	40	1.5–2.0	0.9
11–14 (boys)	55	1.5–2.0	1.0
15–18 (boys)	45	1.5–2.0	0.9

Nutrient	Recommendations
Sodium	1–3 g postoperative, then as tolerated
Potassium	As tolerated
Fluids	Unrestricted
Calcium	Supplement as needed
Phosphorus	Unrestricted
Vitamins and minerals	Follow daily RDA/DRI or therapeutic levels depending on needs

TABLE 47.9
Daily Nutrient and Fluid Needs for Adults Post Kidney Transplant

Nutrient	Recommendations
Energy	30–35 kcal/kg
Protein[a]	0.8–1.0 g/kg
Sodium	2–4 g/day
Potassium	Unrestricted
Fluids	Unrestricted
Calcium	0.8–1.5 g
Phosphorus	Unrestricted
Vitamins and minerals	Follow daily RDA/DRI or therapeutic levels depending on needs

[a] Higher end for postoperative recovery.

HEMODIALYSIS: DAILY NUTRIENT AND FLUID NEEDS

Table 47.12[14,15,16,26] outlines basic nutritional assessment parameters for children undergoing hemodialysis at least three times a week. Guidelines can be adjusted for any comorbidity. Table 47.13[17,18,21,27] outlines basic nutritional requirements for adults undergoing hemodialysis three times a week. Guidelines can be adjusted for comorbidites and advanced age.

SPECIAL NUTRITION FOCUS

According to the 2004 United States Renal Data Systems (USRDS) Renal Data Report,[28] the number of dialysis patients has reached ~300,000. Practitioners often encounter dialysis patients who have medical nutrition therapy needs beyond the average patient. These patients require intense nutritional management to improve, and then maintain, good nutritional status, either for the short term as in pregnancy or for the long term as in patients with diabetes or acquired immunodeficiency disease (AIDS).

TABLE 47.10
Daily Nutrient and Fluid Needs for Pediatric Patients Undergoing Peritoneal Dialysis

Age (Years)	Energy[a] (Kcal/kg)	Protein (g/kg)	Calcium (mg)
Birth to 5 months	≥108	2.5–4.0	400
5 months to 1 year	≥98	2.0–2.5	600
1–3	102	2.0–2.5	800
4–6	90	2.0–2.5	800
7–10	70	2.0–2.5	800
11–14 (girls)	47	1.5	1200
15–18 (girls)	40	1.5	1200
11–14 (boys)	55	1.5	1200
15–18 (boys)	45	1.5	1200

Nutrient	Recommendations
Sodium	As tolerated, 1–4 g
Potassium	As tolerated
Fluids	Usually unrestricted
Phosphorus	As tolerated
Vitamins and minerals	Follow daily RDA/DRI or therapeutic levels depending on needs

[a] Includes kcal from dialysate (3.4 kcal/g).

TABLE 47.11
Daily Nutrient and Fluid Needs for Adults Undergoing Peritoneal Dialysis

Nutrient	Recommendations
Energy[a]	30–35 kcal/kg
Protein	1.2–1.3 g/kg
Sodium	2–4 g
Potassium	3–4 g
Fluids	As tolerated
Calcium[b]	2.0–2.5 g
Phosphorus	12–15 mg/g protein
Ascorbic acid	60–100 mg
Pyridoxine	5–10 mg
B_{12}	3 μg
Folic acid	400 μg
No A or K	
Zinc	15 mg
Riboflavin	1.8–2.0 mg
Niacin	20 mg
Thiamin	1.5–2.0 mg
Biotin	20–30 μg
Vitamin E	10–15 IU
Pantothenic acid	10 mg
Iron and active vitamin D	Individualized

[a] Includes kcal from dialysate (3.4 kcal/g).
[b] Include amounts from any calcium containing binders.

TABLE 47.12
Daily Nutrient and Fluid Needs for Pediatric Patients Undergoing Hemodialysis

Age (Years)	Energy (kcal/kg)	Protein (g/kg)	Calcium (mg)
Birth to 5 months	≥108	2.6	400
5 months to 1 year	≥98	2.0	600
1–3	102	≥1.6	800
4–6	90	≥1.6	800
7–10	70	≥1.4	800
11–14 (girls)	47	1.3–1.5	1200
15–18 (girls)	40	1.3–1.5	1200
11–14 (boys)	55	1.3–1.5	1200
15–18 (boys)	45	1.3–1.5	1200

Nutrient	Recommendations
Sodium	As tolerated, 4 g/day maximum
Potassium	1–3 mEq/kg
Fluids	Replace urine output and insensible losses
Phosphorus	Unrestricted, 600–800 mg/day if serum levels elevated
Vitamins and minerals	Follow daily RDA/DRI or therapeutic levels depending on needs

TABLE 47.13
Daily Nutrient and Fluid Needs for Adults Undergoing Hemodialysis

Nutrient	Recommendations
Energy	30–35 kcal/kg
Protein	≥1.2 g/kg
Sodium	2–3 g
Potassium	2–3 g
Fluids	Urine output plus 1000 cc
Calcium[a]	2.0–2.5 g
Phosphorus	10–12 mg/g protein
Ascorbic acid	60–100 mg
Pyridoxine	5–10 mg
B_{12}	3 μg
Folic acid	400 μg
No A or K	
Zinc	15 mg
Riboflavin	1.8–2.0 mg
Niacin	20 mg
Thiamin	1.5–2.0 mg
Biotin	20–30 μg
Vitamin E	10–15 IU
Pantothenic acid	10 mg
Iron and active vitamin D	Individualized

[a] Include amounts in calcium containing binders.

Pregnant Hemodialysis Patients

The frequency of pregnancy in female dialysis patients is approximately ~10 per 1000. Fifty-two percent of these women will carry to term. Dialysis time usually is increased to an average of 24 h/week. Predialysis Blood Urea Nitrogen (BUN) is best kept below 60 mg/dl. Table 47.14[16,29–34] lists the recommendations for nutrients for pregnant women undergoing hemodialysis or peritoneal dialysis. Adequate nutrition and an individualized dialysis regimen are the hallmarks of a successful pregnancy.

TABLE 47.14
Pregnant Hemodialysis Patients

Nutrient	Recommended Amount
Energy	35 kcal/kg + 300 kcal[a]
Protein	1.0–1.5 g/kg + 10 g[b]
Sodium	Individualize[c]
Potassium	Individualize[c]
Fluids	Individualize[c]
Calcium	1300–2000 mg/day including binders
Phosphorus	Balance between diet and binders
Vitamins and minerals	Consider increased dose of renal vitamins B & C plus zinc (15 mg/day)and folic acid (600 μg/day), 1,25(OH)$_2$D$_3$ PRN, fat soluble vitamins A, E, and K are not usually supplemented

[a] Adjust for adequate weight gain.
[b] Second and third trimesters.
[c] Liberalize with increased dialysis treatments.

TABLE 47.15
Special Nutrition Focus: Adult Patients with Diabetes Mellitus

	Recommended Amount		
Nutrient	Predialysis	Hemodialysis	Peritoneal Dialysis
Energy[a,b] (kcal/kg)	25–35	30–35	25–35[b]
Protein (g/kg)	0.8–1	1.2–1.4	1.5–2.0
Sodium (g)	2–4	2	2–4
Potassium	Not restricted	2–3 g	Individualize
Fluids	Not restricted	Urine output plus 1000 cc	Urine output plus 2000 cc
Calcium[c] (g)	2.0–2.5	2.0–2.5	2.0–2.5
Phosphorus (mg/g protein)	10–12	12–15	12–15
Vitamins and other minerals	Daily RDA/DRI for most vitamins and minerals (fat soluble vitamins and magnesium are not supplemented)		

[a] <10% of Energy from saturated fats (<7% in individuals with high LDL cholesterol), remaining Energy from fats should be divided between monounsaturated and polyunsaturated fats. Limit dietary cholesterol to 300 mg daily (<200 mg in patients with high LDL cholesterol).
[b] Includes kcal from dialysate (3.4 kcal/g). Many patients will require adjustment of insulin regimens.
[c] Includes calcium from binders.

ADULT DIALYSIS PATIENTS WITH DIABETES MELLITUS

Carbohydrate and fat are individualized for diabetic patients with renal disease. Total fat is generally limited to less than 30%. Serum lipid levels are monitored. Goals of therapy are the same as for nondialysis diabetic patients, that is, fasting plasma glucoses of <120 mg/dl for Chronic Kidney Disease (CKD), <140 mg/dl for hemodialysis, and <160 mg/dl for peritoneal dialysis. HbA1c should be <7%, independent of treatment modality. Table 47.15[16,35–42] lists recommendations for nutrients for diabetic patients who are pre-ESRD or are End-stage Renal Disease (ESRD) and undergoing hemodialysis or peritoneal dialysis.

DIALYSIS PATIENTS WITH AIDS NEPHROPATHY

Intestinal malabsorption and diarrhea occur in most AIDS patients. It is therefore not uncommon for the patient to be very malnourished when AIDS nephropathy leads to dialysis. Improving and maintaining nutrition status is a special challenge in this population. Table 47.16[16, 43–45] lists the nutrient recommendations for dialysis patients with AIDS.

TABLE 47.16

Special Nutrition Focus: Dialysis Patients with AIDS Nephropathy

	Recommended Amount	
Nutrient	Hemodialysis	Peritoneal Dialysis
Energy (kcal/kg)	45–50	45–50[a]
Protein (g/kg)	1.4–2.0	1.5–2.0
Sodium (g)	2–3	2–4
Potassium	1 mEq/kg	Individualize supplement as needed
Fluids	Urine output plus 1000–1200 cc	Urine output plus 2000 cc
Calcium (g)	1.0–1.5	1.0–1.5
Phosphorus[b] (mg/g protein)	12–15	12–15
Vitamins and minerals	Same as non-AIDS patients	

[a] Includes kcal from dialysate (3.4 kcal/g).

[b] Lift restriction if PO intake poor.

OSTEODYSTROPHY MANAGEMENT IN CHRONIC KIDNEY DISEASE

The management of the osteodystrophy that is associated with chronic kidney disease revolves around a therapy triad: an adequate source of calcium, a binder for dietary phosphate, and a source of activated vitamin D.

PHOSPHATE BINDERS

With the decrease in kidney function, phosphorus excretion decreases and serum phosphorus increases. Treatment for elevated phosphorus includes dietary restriction of high-phosphorus foods and the use of a phosphate binder. Products used for phosphate binding are taken with or immediately after eating meals and snacks.

Phosphate Binders/Calcium-Based Supplements

Calcium supplements are used to supplement therapeutic diets that are low in calcium due to the restriction of dairy products and many other foods high in calcium. Calcium products used for supplementation are taken between meals. Calcium products are also used to bind dietary phosphorus in order to change the route of elimination from urine to stool. The recommendation for the amount of elemental calcium per day provided by calcium based binders is 1500 mg. Iron supplements should not be taken with calcium supplements. End-stage renal patients do not need to take calcium products with added vitamin D. When vitamin D supplementation is needed, it will be prescribed as an activated form or as a vitamin D analog. Table 47.17[46,47] lists sources for calcium supplementation/binders.

Phosphate Binders/Non-Calcium-Based Supplements

In the past, aluminum-containing products were used to bind dietary phosphorus when calcium supplements were not effective or not medically appropriate. A consequence of the use of aluminium-containing products was elevated serum aluminum. With the introductions of non-calcium-, non-aluminium-containing supplements, aluminum products are not routinely used. If phosphorus is elevated >7.0, and the medical team chooses to use aluminium-based binders, the recommendation is only to use for short-term (4 weeks) therapy and then to replace with another phosphate binder. Renagel® is a polymetric phosphate binder that contains no calcium. Fosrenol™, a phosphate binder containing lanthanum carbonate, does not contain calcium or aluminum. Magnesium binders in combination with calcium carbonate are also an alternative in certain situations. The information in Table 47.18[46,47] is a list of current products. There may be other products as well.

VITAMIN AND MINERAL SUPPLEMENTS

Vitamin and Mineral supplements for renal patients are generally limited to water-soluble vitamins and essential amounts of minerals. Table 47.19(a)[16,21,27,48] gives general vitamin and mineral renal formulations. Table 47.19(b) gives a sampling of vitamin and mineral supplements suitable for the population with chronic kidney disease. Supplements for children need to be individualized depending on requirements for growth. Oral iron supplements are routinely used in conjunction with intravenous Epoetin

TABLE 47.17
List of Products to Provide Suitable Source of Calcium for Patients with Renal Disease[a]

Generic Name	Name Brand	Elemental Ca^{++} (mg)	Source
Calcium acetate	PhosLo® Tablet or Gelcap	169	Nabi Bio-pharmaceuticals
	Calphron®	169	NephroTech
Calcium carbonate[b]	Calci-chew®	500	R&D Laboratories
	Calci-mix®	500	
	Caltrate® 600	600	Wyeth Consumer Healthcare
	Maalox® Quick Dissolve (regular strength)	222	Novartis Consumer Health, Inc.
	Nephro-Calci®	600	R&D Laboratories
	Oscal® 500	500	GlaxoSmithKline
	Rolaids® Soft chews EX	471	Pfizer Consumer
	TUMS® regular	200	GlaxoSmithKline
	TUMS® EX	300	
	TUMS® Ultra	400	
Calcium citrate[c]	Citracal®	200	Mission Pharmacal

[a] Manufacturer's information.

[b] Efficacy of different brands of calcium carbonate varies due to ability to dissolve. A tablet of calcium carbonate placed in 6 oz of vinegar at room temperature and stirred frequently should disintegrate within 30 min.

[c] Not generally recommended for renal patients secondary to enhanced aluminum absorption.

TABLE 47.18
Phosphate Binders (Non-Calcium-Based)[a]

Active Ingredient	Unit	Amount	Brand Name	Manufacturer
Aluminum hydroxide	5 ml	208 mg Al	AlternaGEL® suspension	Johnson & Johnson
Lanthanum carbonate	1 tablet	250/500 mg	Fosrenol™	Shire US, Inc.
Magnesium carbonate/ calcium	1 tablet	200/450 mg 57 mg elemental MG/160 mg elemental Ca^{++}	MagneBind® 200	Nephro-Tech, Inc.
Magnesium carbonate/ calcium	1 tablet	300/300 mg 85 mg elemental MG/100 mg elemental Ca^{++}	MagneBind® 300	Nephro-Tech, Inc.
Sevelamer hydrochloride	1 capsule	403 mg	Renagel®	Genzyme Pharmaceuticals
Sevelamer hydrochloride	1 tablet	400 mg	Renagel®	Genzyme Pharmaceuticals
Sevelamer hydrochloride	1 tablet	800 mg	Renagel®	Genzyme Pharmaceuticals

[a] Manufacturer's information.

alfa (EPO) therapy to control anemia in dialysis patients. EPO is an amino acid glycoprotein manufactured by recombinant DNA technology. It has the same biological effects as endogenous erythropoietin in stimulating red blood cell production. Aranesp® and Procrit® are also products used in stimulating erythropoiesis and are used in the predialysis population. Some intravenous supplements need to be given as a test dose before actual therapy to assess the potential for allergic reaction. Oral supplements can have gastrointestinal side effects such as nausea, vomiting, and constipation. Table 47.20[49] lists some of the available iron supplements for use with renal patients.

ENTERAL NUTRITION SUPPLEMENTS FOR THE RENAL PATIENT

Nutritional supplements are frequently used to provide nutrients for persons who, even after liberalization of the diet, cannot consume adequate oral nutrition or to supply a complete source of nutrition for patients who are nourished through an enteral

TABLE 47.19(a)
General Vitamin and Mineral Renal Formulations

Vitamin	Recommended Amount/Day	Vitamin	Recommended Amount/Day
Vitamin C	60–100 mg	Thiamin(B_1)	1.4 mg
Riboflavin (B_2)	1.1–1.3 mg	Niacin	14–35 mg
Pyroxdine (B_6)	1.3–2 mg	Cobalamin (B_{12})	2.4 μg
Folic acid	400–800 μg[a]	Pantothenic acid	5 mg
Biotin	30 μg	Zinc	12.5 mg

[a] As dietary folate equivalents. 1 DFE = 1 μg food folate = 0.6 μg of folic acid from fortified food/supplement.

TABLE 47.19(b)
Sample Vitamin/Mineral Supplement Product List[a]

Product	Manufacturer
Vitamins	
Dialyvite® Tablets, Dialyvite® with Zinc Tablets, Dialyvite® 3000 tablets	Hillestad Pharmaceuticals, Inc.
Diatx® Tablets, Diatx® Zn Tablets	Pamlab, L.L.C.
Foltx® Tablets	Pamlab, L.L.C.
NephPlex® RX Tablets, RenaPlex® Tablets	NephroTech, Inc.
Nephrocaps® Softgels	Fleming & Company
Nephronex Caplets®, Nephronex Liquid®	Llorens Pharmaceutical Corporation
Nephro-Vite® B&C Complex Tablets	R&D Laboratories
Nephro-Vite® RX	R&D Laboratories
Renax® Caplets	Everett Laboratories
Vitamins with iron	
Neprhon FA®	Nephro-Tech
Nephro-Vite® + FE	R&D Laboratories
Active vitamin D	
Calcijex® (Calcitriol Injection)	Abbott Laboratories
Hectoral® (doxercalciferol), Hectoral® capsules (doxercalciferol)	Genzyme Corporation
Rocaltrol® (oral)	Roche Laboratories
Zemplar® (Paracalcitol Injection), Zemplar® capsules (Paracalcitol)	Abbott Laboratories

[a] Manufacturer's information.

feeding tube. There are many products from which to choose that will meet the nutrition requirements for most types of medical nutrition therapy. In addition to a variety of normal nutrition products, there are specialty products available for persons with acute or chronic renal failure including end-stage disease. Selecting the appropriate product can be a challenge as there is such a wide variety from which to choose. Many renal patients are successfully managed with normal supplements, which tend to be less expensive than the specialty formulas. In selecting a formula, the following points should be considered:

1. Goal of therapy: more protein, more calories or both
2. How much of the patient's needs are being met by the diet
3. How much of the patient's fluid restriction can be spared for the supplement
4. Which products are affordable and available in the patient's area

The location of the tube must be considered in making the formula selection. The feedings must be timed in order to allow time for dialysis without compromising the nutrition therapy. Table 47.21(a) is a partial listing of complete ready-to-feed nutrition products suitable for use with the renal population. Table 47.21(b) lists modular products also suited for use with this clientele.

TABLE 47.20
Sampling of Iron Supplements[a]

Source of Iron	Elemental Iron	Brand Name	Form
Ferrous bis-glycinate	70 mg	Chromagen® (Ther-Rx)	PO
Ferrous fumarate	150 mg	Ferrimin 150 (Hillestad)	PO
	106 mg	Hemocyte™ (US Pharmaceuticals)	
	115 mg	Nephro-Fer® (R&D Labs)	
Ferrous gluconate	27 mg	Fergon® (Bayer Pharmaceuticals)	PO
Ferrous sulfate	65 mg	Feosol® (GlaxoSmithKline)	PO
	50 mg	Slow Fe® (Novartis)	
Heme iron polypeptide	12 mg	Proferrin®-ES (Proctor & Gamble)	PO
Polysaccharide iron	150 mg	Niferex 150®	PO
	60 mg	Niferex® caps (Ther-Rx)	
	150 mg	Nu-Iron® Merz Pharmaceuticals	
Iron dextran	50 mg/ml	InFeD® (Watson Pharmaceuticals)	IV
Iron sucrose	20 mg/ml	Venofer® (American Regent)	IV
Sodium ferric gluconate	62.5 mg/5 ml	Ferrlecit® (Watson Pharmaceuticals)	IV

[a] Manufacturer's information.

TABLE 47.21a
Sampling of Ready-to-Feed Enteral Nutrition Products for Renal Patients[a]

Product	Kcal/ml	CHO (g/l)	PRO (g/l)	FAT (g/l)	K (mg/l)	PO$_4$ (mg/l)	%H$_2$O/l
Boost® (Novartis)	1.0	173	42	17.8	1690	1310	85
Boost Plus® (Novartis)	1.5	200	59	58	1610	1310	78
Ensure Plus®(Ross)	1.5	200	54.9	53.3	2114	840	77
Magnacal® Renal (Novartis)	2	200	75	101	1270	800	71
Nepro® (Ross)	2	222	70	95.6	1060	685	70
Novasource® Renal (Novartis)	2	200	74	100	810	650	70
NutriRenal® (Nestlé)	2	204	70	104	1256	700	70
Re/Gen HP/HC® (Nutra/balance)	2	240	80	80	200	340	n/a
Suplena®(Ross)	2	255	30	95.6	1120	730	71

[a] Manufacturer's information.

TABLE 47.21(b)
Modular Enteral Nutrition Supplements for Renal Patients[a]

Product	Unit	Kcal	CHO/g	PRO/g	FAT/g	K/mg	PO$_4$/mg
Casec® (Novartis)	1 Table spoon (T)	17	0	4	0.1	0	35
Egg Pro Powder® (Nutra/Balance)	1 T	15	0.6	4	0	50	8
MCT Oil (Novartis)	1 ml	8	0	0	1	0	0
Microlipid® (Novartis)	1 ml	4.5	0	0	0.5	0	0
Polycose® (Ross)	1 T	23	6	0	0	<1	<1
Procel® (Global Health Products)	1 scoop	28	0	5	0.5	35	27
ProMod® (Ross)	1 scoop	28	0.7	5	0.6	45	33
Pro-Stat™ 101 (Medical Nutrition USA)	30 ml	101	15	10	0	12	12
Pro-Stat™ 64 (Medical Nutrition USA)	30 ml	64	15	1	0	12	12
Protein Fortified Cookies (Nutra/Balance)	2 oz Cookie	250	28	6	14	140	57
Proteinex® (Llorens Pharmaceuticals)	30 ml	60	0	15	0	11	0
Resource® Beneprotein® Instant Protein Powder (Novartis)	1 scoop	25	0	6	0	35	20

[a] Manufacturer's information.

PRACTICAL APPLICATION OF THE DIET

The renal diet is complicated by various and often changing restrictions. The diet is adjusted for every stage of chronic kidney disease and every dialysis modality.

FOOD CHOICES TO CONTROL POTASSIUM AND PHOSPHORUS

Potassium is widely distributed in foods. As the kidneys primarily excrete this nutrient, dietary intake of potassium is an important aspect of the diet of patients with end-stage renal disease. The diet should initially be individualized for each patient based on food likes and dislikes and modified if indicated. Although the potassium content of foods varies greatly, most foods can be incorporated into the diet of the hemodialysis patient by limiting quantities or by altering method of preparation. Dietary potassium is usually not a problem with peritoneal dialysis as the patients are dialyzed daily. Some foods very high in potassium are listed in Table 47.22.[51] Serum phosphate level is almost impossible to control in end-stage renal disease by diet alone. Phosphate binders are necessary to maintain acceptable blood levels. It is also important that the patient limit the intake of dietary phosphorus. Dietary restrictions should be individualized for each patient depending on food preferences and compliance with binders. Table 47.23[51] lists some foods very high in phosphorus.

SUGGESTED MEAL PLANS AND SAMPLE MENUS

Listed in Table 47.24[52–54] are suggested meal plans for four different calorie levels of the diet for patients with end-stage renal disease. Additional modifications may be indicated when other disease states are also present. In clients with diabetes, emphasis should be placed on complex carbohydrates. It is difficult to achieve energy and protein goals using complex carbohydrate sources exclusively from foods that must be limited because of their potassium, phosphorus, and sodium content. Carbohydrates should be

TABLE 47.22
Some Foods Very High in Potassium

Food	Portion	Amount of Potassium (mg)
Orange Juice, fresh	1 cup	496
Banana	Medium sized	451
Cantaloupe	1 c pieces	494
Honeydew Melon	1 c pieces	461
Prunes, dried, cooked	1/2 cup	354
Peanuts, oil roasted	1/2 cup	573
Potato with skin, baked	1 large (202 g)	844
Black-eyed peas, fresh-cooked	1/2 cup	347
Sweet Potato, baked	1 medium (114 g)	397
Spinach, cooked from raw	1/2 cup	419

TABLE 47.23
Some Foods Very High in Phosphorus

Food	Portion	Amount of Phosphorus (mg)
Bran Cereal, 100%	1/2 cup	344
Milk, 2%	1 cup	232
Whole Wheat Bread	1 slice	65
Cheese, cheddar	1 oz	145
Black-eyed peas, frozen, boiled	1 cup	208
Peanuts, oil roasted	1 oz	145
Peanut Butter, creamy smooth	2 tbsp	103
Lima Beans, boiled	1 cup	208
Yogurt, low-fat-fruit flavor	8 oz	247
Cocoa, dry unsweetened	2 T	74

TABLE 47.24
Sample Menus

1800 kcal[a]	2000 kcal[b]	2200 kcal[c]	2400 kcal[d]
Breakfast			
1/2 cup grits	1/2 cup grits	1 cup grits	1 cup grits
1 piece toast	1 piece toast	1 piece toast	1 piece toast
1/2 c grape juice	1/2 c apple juice	1/2 c apple juice	1/2 c apple juice
1/2 c 2% milk	1/2 c 2% milk	1/2 c 2% milk	1/2 c 2% milk
1 t margarine	1 t margarine	1 t margarine	1 t margarine
Lunch			
1 c rice	1 c rice	1 c rice	1 c rice
1 slice bread	1 slice bread	1 slice bread	1 slice bread
1 c garden salad	1 c garden salad	1 c garden salad	1 c garden salad
3 oz skinless chicken breast	1/2 c pears	1/2 c corn	1/2 c pears
1 t margarine	3 oz skinless chicken breast	3 oz skinless chicken breast	1/2 c corn
1 T salad dressing	1 t margarine	1 t margarine	3 oz skinless chicken breast
	1 T salad dressing	1 T salad dressing	1 t margarine
			1 T salad dressing
Afternoon snack			
10 thin pretzels	2 slices bread	6 2 1/2 in. graham crackers	6 2 1/2 in. graham crackers
	1 oz lean ham	1/2 c pears	1/2 c pears
1/2 c cottage cheese	1 t mayonnaise	1/2 c cottage cheese	1/2 c cottage cheese
Dinner			
1/2 c mashed potatoes	1/2 c mashed potatoes	1/2 c mashed potatoes	1/2 c mashed potatoes
1 roll	1 roll	1 roll	2 rolls
1 c greens	1 c greens	1 c greens	1 c greens
1/2 c fruit cocktail	1/2 c fruit cocktail	1/2 c fruit cocktail	1/2 c fruit cocktail
3 oz lean beef	3 oz lean beef	3 oz lean beef	3 oz lean beef
1 t margarine	2 t margarine	1 t margarine	1 t margarine
2 sugar cookies	2 sugar cookies	2 sugar cookies	2 sugar cookies
Bedtime snack			
3–2 1/2 in. square graham crackers	5 vanilla wafers	1 slice bread	2 slices bread
		1 t mayonnaise	1 t mayonnaise
1/2 cup pears	1/2 c pineapple	1 c strawberries	1/2 c peaches
		1 oz turkey breast	1 oz turkey breast

[a] 80 g protein, <2000 mg sodium, <2000 mg potassium, <1200 mg phosphorus.
[b] 80 g protein, <2000 mg sodium, <3000 mg potassium, <1200 mg phosphorus.
[c] 90 g protein, <3000 mg sodium, <3000 mg potassium, <1200 mg phosphorus.
[d] 100 g protein, <3000 mg sodium, <3000 mg potassium, <1300 mg phosphorus.

included with meals rather than as snacks to help slow absorption. Emphasis should also be placed on consistent meal content, especially of carbohydrate, and timing of meals and snacks to facilitate glycemic control. Fat should be from unsaturated sources, preferably monounsaturated. The percentage of calories provided by fat will most likely need to be higher than the recommended 30% in order to provide adequate kilocalories. Hyperlipidemia, especially elevated triglycerides, is often present in renal disease. Because of the high risk for cardiovascular disease in renal patients, a diet high in complex carbohydrates and containing less that 30% of calories from fat may be more appropriate, but in view of other restrictions this may not be top priority. Providing fat calories from monounsaturated and polyunsaturated sources can reduce saturated fat and cholesterol from dietary intake.

EMERGENCY SHOPPING LIST

End-stage renal disease patients are dependent on dialysis to sustain life. Emergencies such as earthquakes, hurricanes, tornadoes, or floods may limit access to dialysis in a specific area. The patient must then use a diet that is restricted in fluids, protein, and electrolytes to survive until dialysis is once again available. Table 47.25[55,56] lists some guidelines for use in the event of a disaster or emergency.

TABLE 47.25
Emergency Shopping List for the Dialysis Patient

(Food for 2–3 days)

Food stored in the refrigerator or freezer should be used first. Limit fluid intake as much as possible

Bottled water: allow 2–3 quarts (~2–3 l) for hygiene purposes plus usual fluid restriction

Loaf of white bread

Dry cereal: corn flakes, rice Krispies, Cheerios, puffed wheat and rice, or shredded wheat

Box of vanilla wafers of other plain cookies

Box of graham crackers

Box of unsalted crackers

Small jars of mayonnaise (open one each day)

Small cans of chicken or tuna (open, eat, and then throw away leftovers. Do not try to save without refrigeration)

Can of lemonade or Kool-Aid mix

Granulated sugar

Peanut butter

Lemon candy

Hard candy in different flavors

Powdered milk or boxed milk

Small cans of evaporated milk

Canned fruit: peaches, fruit cocktail, pears, and applesauce

Fresh apples, lemons, carrots, if available

Jelly: apple, grape, strawberry, blueberry, blackberry

Marshmallows

Boxed juices

Plastic dinnerware and utensils

Paper towels and napkins

TABLE 47.26
Renal and Manufacturer Web Sites

Abbott Laboratories www.abbott.com

American Association of Kidney Patients
   www.aakp.org

American Regent www.americanregent.com

Bayer Corporation www.bayerpharma.com

Everett Laboratories www.everettlabs.com

Fleming & Company www.flemingcompany.com

Genzyme Pharmaceuticals www.genzyme.com

GlaxoSmithKline www.gsk.com

Global Health Products www.globalhp.com

Hillestad Pharmaceuticals www.hillestadlabs.com

Johnson and Johnson www.jnj.com

Llorens Pharmaceutical Corp. www.llorenspharm.com

Merz Pharmaceuticals www.nuiron.com

Mission Pharmaceuticals www.missionpharm.com

Medical Nutrition USA www.pro-statinfo.com

Nabi Pharmaceuticals www.nabi.com

National Kidney Foundation www.kidney.org

National Kidney and Urologic Diseases Information Clearinghouse
   http://kidney.niddk.nih.gov/

National Renal Diet www.eatright.org

NephroTech www.nephrotech.com

Nestlé Nutrition www.nestle-nutrition.com

Novartis Nutrition www.novartisnutrition.com

Nutra/Balance Products www.nutra-balance-products.com

Pamlab, L.L.C. www.pamlab.com

Pfizer Consumer www.pfizer.com

Proctor and Gamble www.pg.com

R&D Laboratories www.snclavalin.com

Roche Laboratories www.rocheusa.com

Ross Products, Division of Abbott Laboratories www.ross.com

Shire US, Inc. www.shire.com

Ther-Rx Products www.Ther-Rx.com

US Pharmaceuticals www.uspharm.com

Watson Pharmaceuticals www.watsonpharm.com

Wyeth Consumer Healthcare www.wyeth.com

SUMMARY

Patients with acute or chronic renal disease are susceptible to the development of profound malnutrition. Protein-energy imbalances worsen prognosis regardless of disease stage. A complete nutrition assessment plus frequent monitoring can help identify malnutrition before there is significant depletion in visceral protein stores and weight loss. Important treatment objectives are to communicate with the patient, to monitor appropriate laboratory indices, and to plan the appropriate continuum of nutritional therapy. Table 47.26 houses a list of useful renal Web sites plus the Web site addresses of manufacturers referenced in this chapter.

REFERENCES

1. Miller, B., Klahr, S. Effects of Renal Insufficiency on Endocrine Function and Nutrient Metabolism. *Handbook of Nutrition and the Kidney*, 5th Edition. Mitch, W., Klahr, S., Editors. Lippincott, Williams, & Wilkins, Philadelphia, PA, 29–46, 2005.

2. Blackburn, G., Bistrian, B., Mainai, B., et al. *JPEN*, 11:1 1977.

3. Druml, W. Nutrition Support in Acute Renal Failure. *Handbook of Nutrition and the Kidney*, 5th Edition. Mitch, W., Klahr, S., Editors. Lippincott, Williams, & Wilkins, Philadelphia, PA, 95–114, 2005.

4. Kopple, J., Massry, S., Editors. *Nutritional Management of Renal Disease*. Williams & Wilkins, Baltimore, MD, 1997.

5. McCann, L., Editor. *Pocket Guide to Nutrition Assessment of the Renal Patient*, 3rd Edition. National Kidney Foundation, New York, NY, Chapter 1, 2002.

6. National Kidney Foundation. Dialysis Outcomes Quality Initiative. Online document: August 2005. Available at: www.kidney.org/professionals/KDOQI

7. Norwood, K., Collins-Thayer, P. Nutrition Assessment in Chronic Renal Failure. *A Clinical Guide to Nutrition Care in End Stage Renal Disease*, Stover, J., Editor. American Dietetics Association, Chicago, IL, 5–16, 1994.

8. Steiber, A., et al. *JRN*, 14(4): 191–200, 2004.

9. American Diabetes Association Standards of Medical Care in Diabetes. *Diabetes Care*, 28: S1–79, 2005.

10. McCann, L., Editor. *Pocket Guide to Nutrition Assessment of the Renal Patient*, 3rd Edition. National Kidney Foundation, New York, NY, Chapter 2, 2002.

11. National Cholesterol Education Program. ATP III guidelines. Online document: September 2005. Available at www.nhlbi.nih.gov/guidelines/cholesterol/ataglance.pdf

12. Systéme International (SI) Conversion Table in author instructions. Online document: September 2005. Available at www.jama-assn.org

13. Holliday, M., Segar, W. *Pediatrics*, 19: 823–852, 1957.

14. Nelson, P., Stover, J. Nutrition Recommendations for Infants, Children, and Adolescents with End-Stage Renal Disease. *A Clinical Guide to Nutrition Care in End-Stage Renal Disease*, Stover, J., Editor. The American Dietetic Association, Chicago, IL, 79–98, 1994.

15. Rock, J., Secker, D. Nutrition Management of Chronic Kidney Disease in the Pediatric Patient. *Nutrition Care in Kidney Disease*, Byham-Gray, L., Wiesen, K., Editors. American Dietetic Association, Chicago, IL, 127–149, 2004.

16. Food and Nutrition Board, Institute of Medicine, National Academies of Science. *Dietary Reference Intakes 1997–2001*. Available at www.nap.edu

17. Beto, J. *JADA*, 95: 898, 1995.

18. Boxall, M., Goodship, T. Nutritional Requirements in Hemodialysis. *Handbook of Nutrition and the Kidney*, 5th Edition. Mitch, W., Klahr, S., Editors. Lippincott, Williams, & Wilkins, Philadelphia, PA, 218–227, 2005.

19. Klahr, S., Levey, A., Beck, G., et al. *NEJM*, 330: 877, 1994.

20. Kopple, J., Greene, T., Chumlea, W., et al. *Kidney International*, 57: 1688, 2000.

21. McCann, L., Editor. *Pocket Guide to Nutrition Assessment of the Renal Patient*, 3rd Edition. National Kidney Foundation, New York, NY, Chapter 3, 2002.

22. Fouque, D., Laville, M., Boissel, J. P., et al. *Br Med J*, 304: 216, 1992.

23. Guichard, S. Nutrition in the Kidney Transplant Patient. *Handbook of Kidney Transplantation*. Danovitch, G., Editor. Lippincott, Williams, & Wilkins, Philadelphia, PA, 475–494, 2005.

24. Dietary Guidelines for Healthy Americans. September 2005. Available at: www.americanheart.org

25. Ikizler, T. *Nutrition and Peritoneal Dialysis. Handbook of Nutrition and the Kidney*, 5th Edition. Mitch, W., Klahr, S., Editors. Lippincott, Williams, & Wilkins, 228–244, 2005.

26. McCann, L., Editor. *Pocket Guide to Nutrition Assessment of the Renal Patient*, 3rd Edition. National Kidney Foundation, New York, NY, Chapter 11, 2002.

27. Masud, T. Trace Elements and Vitamins in Renal Disease. *Handbook of Nutrition and the Kidney*, 5th Edition. Mitch, W., Klahr, S., Editors. Lippincott, Williams, & Wilkins, Philadelphia, 196–217, 2005.

28. US Renal Data System. September 2005. Available at: www.usrds.org

29. Stover, J. Nutrition Management of Chronic Kidney Disease in the Pediatric Patient. *Nutrition Care in Kidney Disease*. Byham-Gray, L., Wiesen, K., Editors. American Dietetic Association, Chicago, 121–126, 2004.

30. Grossman, S., Hou S. Obstetrics and gynecology. *Handbook of Dialysis*, 3rd Edition. Daugirdas, J., Blake, P., Ing. I., Editors. Lippincott, Williams, & Wilkins, Baltimore, MD, 624–636, 2000.

31. Stover, J., Editor. *A Clinical Guide to Nutrition Care in End Stage Renal Disease*, American Dietetics Association, Chicago, IL, 199–206, 1994.

32. Grossman, S. D., Hou, S., Moretti, M., Saran, M. *Journal of Renal Nutrition*, 3(2): 5, 1993.

33. Henderson, N. *J Renal Nutr*, 6(4): 222, 1996.

34. Hou, S. H. *Am J Kidney Dis*, 23: 60, 1994.

35. Diabetes Standards of Care. *Diabetes Care*, 28(1): 4–36, 2005.

36. Davis, M. Nutrition Management of the Patient with Diabetes and Renal Disease. *A Clinical Guide to Nutrition Care in End-Stage Renal Disease*, Stover, J., Editor. The American Dietetic Association, Chicago, IL, 69–78, 1994.

37. Pagenkemper, J. Nutrition Management of Diabetes in Chronic Kidney Disease. *Nutrition Care in Kidney Disease*, Byham-Gray, L., Wiesen, K., Editors. American Dietetic Association, Chicago, IL, 93–105, 2004.

38. Pagenkemper, J. J., Foulks, C. J. *J Renal Nutr*, 1: 119, 1991.

39. Dikow, R., Ritz, E. Nutritional Requirements of Diabetes with Nephropathy. *Handbook of Nutrition and the Kidney*, 5th Edition. Mitch, W., Klahr, S., Editors. Lippincott, Williams, & Wilkins, Philadelphia, PA, 138–159, 2005.

40. American Diabetes Association website. November 21, 2004. Available at: www.diabetes.org

41. McCann, L., Editor. *Pocket Guide to Nutrition Assessment of the Renal Patient*, 3rd Edition, National Kidney Foundation, New York, NY, Chapter 4, 2002.

42. Renal Dietitians Dietetic Practice Group. *National Renal Diet: Professional Guide*, American Dietetics Association, chicago IL, 1993.

43. Goldstein-Fuchs, J. Nutrition Management of HIV/AIDS in Chronic Kidney Disease. *Nutrition Care in Kidney Disease*, Byham-Gray, L., Wiesen, K., Editors. American Dietetic Association, Chicago, IL, 87–92, 2004.

44. Plourd, D. *J Renal Nutr*, 5(4): 182, 1995.

45. McCann, L., Editor. *Pocket Guide to Nutrition Assessment of the Renal Patient*, 3rd Edition, National Kidney Foundation, New York, NY, Chapter 9, 2002.

46. Clinical Practice Guidelines of Bone Metabolism and Disease in Chronic Kidney Disease. National Kidney Foundation. Dialysis Outcomes Quality Initiative online document. November 2005. Available at: www.kidney.org/professionals/KDOQI

47. Bone Metabolism and Disease. National Kidney Foundation. Dialysis Outcomes Quality Initiative. Online document. November 2005. Available at: www.kidney.org/professionals/KDOQI

48. Rocco, M., Makoff, R. *Semin Dialysis*, 10: 272–277, 1997.

49. Treatment of Anemia of Chronic Renal Failure update. National Kidney Foundation. Dialysis Outcomes Quality Initiative. Online document. November 2005. Available at: www.kidney.org/professionals/KDOQI

50. Stover, J., Editor. *A Clinical Guide to Nutrition Care in End Stage Renal Disease*, American Dietetics Association, Chicago, IL, 187–189, 1994.

51. Pennington, J. *Bowes and Church's Food Values of Portions Commonly Used*, 18th Edition. Lippincott, Williams, & Wilkins, Philadelphia, PA, 2004.

52. Dudek, S. *Nutrition Essentials for Nursing Practice*, 5th Edition. Lippincott, Williams, & Wilkins, Philadelphia, PA, 604–605, 2005.

53. A Healthy Food Guide for People on Dialysis. The American Dietetic Association, Chicago, IL, 2002.

54. A Healthy Food Guide for People with Kidney Disease. The

55. Appendix G: Disaster Diet Information for Hemodialysis Patients. *A Clinical Guide to Nutrition Care in End Stage Renal Disease*, Stover, J., Editor. American Dietetics Association, Chicago, 227–229, 1994.

56. Appendix E: Emergency Meal Planning. *Nutrition Care in Kidney Disease*. Byham-Gray, L., Wiesen, K., Editors. American Dietetic Association, Chicago, 237–242, 2004.

48 Genetics of Human Obesity

Chenxi Wang, Richard N. Baumgartner, and David B. Allison

CONTENTS

INTRODUCTION

Obesity has substantially increased in prevalence[1] to the point where many believe the label "epidemic" is appropriate today.[2] It is also among the leading causes of disability[3] and a source of premature death.[4] It is an established risk factor for cardiovascular disease, hypertension, diabetes, and certain types of cancer.[5] Although the increase in the prevalence of obesity during the past two decades strongly suggests that environmental causes are involved,[6] considerable variation exists both within and between populations in susceptibility to obesity that is likely to be genetic in origin. Populations also differ on the associations of obesity with disease risk, indicating genetic susceptibility to the effects of obesity. Thus, research on genetic susceptibility to obesity is important for a better understanding of the etiology and pathophysiology of obesity and associated diseases, for developing more effective means as well as for preventing and treating obesity.

In this chapter, we review the success, merits, and limitations of past and current research approaches and future prospects of research on the genetics of human obesity, with the emphasis on common obesity rather than on single gene defects. Because human obesity is a heterogeneous condition, with a variety of pathophysiological pathways and potential clinical manifestations, we include all of the obesity-related phenotypes such as body mass index (BMI), body fat distribution, serum leptin, etc.

RATIONALE AND SCOPE OF HUMAN GENETIC STUDIES OF OBESITY

EVIDENCE OF GENETIC CONTRIBUTIONS IN HUMAN OBESITY

The genetic contribution to obesity has been confirmed by numerous family, twin, and adoption studies. Family studies detect the familial aggregation of obesity and provide the first line of evidence. They generally report significant correlations of BMI among relatives[7] and higher relative risks for first-degree relatives of obese patients than for the general population.[8] Twin studies are most frequently used to estimate the heritability of obesity, which is defined as the proportion of total variance in a trait that is attributable to genes. In twin studies, heritability is estimated by comparing the difference in concordance between monozygotic (MZ) and dizygotic (DZ) twin pairs for a specific characteristic or trait. MZ twins are genetically identical, and DZ twins share half of the genome.[9] Theoretically, any variances within MZ pairs are due to environmental factors. Higher concordance among MZ than DZ pairs indicates a stronger genetic than environmental contribution to a trait. Twin studies can still be confounded by shared environment, if the equal environments assumption is violated,[10] yet evidence suggests this is not a major problem in obesity research.[11,12] Adoption studies can separate genetic and environmental factors by comparing concordance between the adoptee and the biological and adoptive parents but are poor at estimating complex and nonadditive genetic influences.

Maes et al.[13] comprehensively reviewed the genetic contribution to BMI and adiposity. The estimated heritability of BMI depended on study design. Twin studies usually reported the highest heritability estimates, in the range of 0.5 to 0.9, whereas adoption studies usually reported the lowest estimates, in the range of 0.2 to 0.6. Estimates from family studies are intermediate between twin and adoption studies. Reasons for these differences have been reviewed elsewhere.[13,14] The twin studies are regarded as more accurate with a realistic estimate of heritability.[11,12] The reason for the discrepancy between twin and nontwin studies is that the former capture the substantial nonadditive genetic effects on obesity better. Genetic components are also known for other obesity-related traits, such as metabolic syndrome,[15] serum leptin and leptin receptor (LEPR),[16] and eating behavior.[17] Overfeeding studies in twins also provide suggestive evidence of gene-by-environment interaction.[18,19]

GENETIC ARCHITECTURE OF OBESITY

Obesity can be classified into three categories: (1) monogenic obesity, (2) Mendelian obesity syndromes, and (3) common obesity. Monogenic obesity results from high-risk single-gene mutations. At least 20 Mendelian syndromes have been identified with obesity as an important clinical feature.[20] Both types of obesity may exhibit a simple Mendelian inheritance pattern.

However, most obesity may be the result of multiple environmental factors, genetic susceptibilities, and, perhaps most importantly, the interaction of environmental and genetic factors that has no simple pattern of inheritance. Two hypotheses regarding the genetic architecture of complex diseases are applicable to the scenario of common obesity. The common disease–common variants hypothesis[21–24] proposes that common diseases result from the overall effects of many common genetic variants. In contrast, the rare variants hypothesis[25,26] proposes that common diseases result from many rare mutations, each of which accounts for a very small population risk. To date, evidence is insufficient to prove or disprove either of these hypotheses; that is, common obesity may result either from the effects of multiple common gene variants (and their interaction with other genetic and environmental factors), each with a small individual effect, or from multiple rare gene mutations, each of which accounts for a very small proportion of obesity cases. Of course, things are unlikely to be as simple as either hypothesis and there are likely to be cases of obesity due to rare alleles with massive effects and many common alleles with small effects.

SEARCHING FOR NOVEL GENES OF SMALL EFFECT

In any case, it is reasonable to postulate that common obesity is the result of many genes with small individual effects because of the complexity of pathophysiological pathways involved in energy metabolism, the lack of evidence of major gene effects, and the high likelihood of interaction between genes.[27] It was estimated that more than 80% of genetic variance of BMI can be attributed to the interactive effects of susceptibility genes,[11] which only imply small marginal effects of individual genes.

However, genes with small individual effects are not necessarily less important than those with large effects, and their discovery may greatly aid in identifying epistatic effects among genes that may have an effect that is larger than the individual effects. Furthermore, the discovery of such genes may reveal new pathways, furthering our understanding of obesity etiology and helping to guide new treatments. The discovery of the OB gene[28] is one example that significantly advanced our knowledge of the regulation of energy metabolism and provided new targets for potential therapies.

In addition, the candidate gene approach, which tests the effects of already identified genes on obesity, has had limited success. Therefore, searching for novel genes with small effects on obesity should be one of the major aims of human genetic research in this context.

CURRENT FINDINGS OF HUMAN GENETIC STUDIES

MONOGENIC OBESITY AND OBESITY SYNDROMES

There has been some success in the identification of susceptibility genes for monogenic obesity and obesity syndromes. Mutations on a total of 10 genes of 173 monogenic obese cases have been reported.[29] Homologues of mouse obesity genes have been found in humans including leptin (LEP), LEPR, proopiomelanocortin (POMC), and melanocortin 4 receptor (MC4R). These genes regulate energy intake, and rare mutations may account for most human monogenic obesity. More than 50 mutants have been found in MC4R gene, representing an extreme example of allelic heterogeneity.

There are more than 20 Mendelian syndromes manifesting obesity. The genetic defects in these syndromes have been mapped and most causal genes have been identified.[29] Among these Mendelian syndromes, Prader–Willi syndrome is the most common. Eight chromosomal regions have been mapped for the Bardet–Biedl syndrome (BBS), and all susceptibility genes in these regions have been cloned, which is a good example of locus heterogeneity.

A complete list of these Mendelian diseases can be found at the Online Mendelian Inheritance in Man database (OMIM).[30]

COMMON OBESITY

Linkage Studies

Linkage analysis tests the cosegregation of genetic variants (markers) with phenotypes in related subjects. When the pattern of inheritance of a phenotypic trait agrees with the cosegregation of the genetic variants, one can infer that the locus identified includes a gene that determines the trait. The use of a genome scan in linkage analysis requires no prior knowledge about gene functions and can be based on as few as 400 markers to screen the whole genome for susceptible genes. The first two genome scans for obesity-related phenotypes, published in early 1997,[31,32] reported three quantitative trait loci (QTLs). With the development of high-throughput genotyping techniques and reduction in cost, genome-wide scanning is being used increasingly and may become the standard approach for linkage studies. The new technology also allows for high-density genome scans (i.e., thousands rather than hundreds of markers) and may include variants with and without known functions.

More than 50 genome scans and more than a dozen follow-up scans for previously identified candidate chromosomal regions have been published.[29] More than 200 QTLs have been reported of which several show significant evidence of linkage according to the criteria suggested by Lander and Kruglyak.[33] At least 10 QTLs located on chromosomes 2p, 3q, 4p, 5p, 6p, 7q,10p, 11q, 17p, and 20q were independently replicated three times.[29] Emerging, although still limited, evidence suggests that these regions harbor causal candidate genes[34,35] that need to be further investigated.[36,37] In summary, this "shot-gun" approach to identifying obesity susceptibility genes has been moderately successful.

QTLS SUPPORTED BY INDEPENDENT REPLICATIONS

Interestingly, the QTL with the strongest evidence of linkage for obesity comes from one of the very first genome scans,[32] which was a general pedigree-based multipoint linkage analysis with more than 5000 relative pairs of Mexican Americans (San Antonio Family Heart Study, SAFHS). A log of odds (LOD) score of 4.9 found at chromosome location 2p.22.3 accounted for 47% of the variation in serum leptin in this population sample. The LOD score was 2.8 for fat mass on the same locus. In a follow-up study with additional markers, the LOD increased to 7.5 in a subset of the original sample.[38] Linkage between this locus and BMI in whites was further replicated in the Cleveland Family Study ($p = .006$)[39] and the Framingham Heart Study[40] (LOD = 3). Other studies produced evidence of linkage for markers close to this region with LEP,[41,42] serum adiponectin,[43] and diabetes,[44,45] which has been reviewed by Loos and Bouchard.[45] Recently, another genome scan in a cohort of Mexican American from SAFHS found a linkage signal in this region for saturated fat intake.[46]

The highest reported LOD score for an obesity-related QTL is 9.2 on 4p15.1.[47] Initially, Perusse et al.[48] reported a QTL on 4p15.2 (marker D4S2937; LOD = 2.3) in the Quebec Family Study of 156 families with 521 subjects. One year later, Stone et al.[47] (2002) reported a genome scan using 37 large multigeneration pedigrees with at least three extreme (BMI $\geq$ 40) obese members. The multipoint LOD score was 6.2, with a nonparametric linkage score of 5.3,[49] for female obesity. Genotyping 73 additional genetic markers in a 60-cM interval centered on D4S2632 on 4p15.1 and including more pedigrees increased the LOD score to 9.2 and the non parametric linkage (NPL) to 11.3.[47] Arya et al.[50] replicated this finding in an independent genome scan among 27 largest pedigrees in the SAFHS with 430 individuals and reported a LOD score of 4.5 for marker D4S2912 on 4p15.1.

The chromosome 7q31-33 region, which harbors the OB gene coding LEP, has been frequently replicated for linkage with obesity-related traits. Three studies reported weak evidence for linkage of the marker D7S1875 on 7q32.2 with BMI ($p = .04$),[51] waist-to-hip ratio ($p = .009$),[52] and abdominal subcutaneous fat (LOD = 2).[48] Marker D7S504 on the same region was reported by two earlier, small candidate gene studies.[53,54] A genome scan with 243 markers reported a LOD score of 4.9 for marker D7S1804 on 7q32.3 among 401 white families of 3027 subjects in the National Heart, Lung, and Blood Institute (NHLBI) Family Heart Study.[55]

The Family Heart Study is a population-based, multicentered study that includes the Framingham Heart Study, the Utah Health Family Tree Study, and the Atherosclerosis Risk in Communities Study. This finding was replicated in a candidate gene study with a small number of extreme[14] obese (BMI >35) pairs.[56] Another large-scale genome scan for BMI, which combined eight samples from multiple ethnic populations from the NHLBI Family Blood Pressure Program for a total of 1055 sib pairs, reported suggestive linkage of marker D7S2847 on 7q31.31 with BMI.[57] Taken together with other evidence,[58,59] there is now a full line of supportive evidence for an obesity-related QTL within 7q31-33.

Initially, Hager et al.[41] reported linkage of marker D10S204 on 10p12 with a LOD score of 4.9 among French families. An independent replication[60] reported suggestive linkage (LOD = 2.24) of the same marker with obesity among German children and adolescents. Four more studies found linkage of markers on 10p12 with obesity,[61,62] LEP,[59] and adiponectin.[43] Dong et al.[61] also found interactions between these markers and markers on chromosome 20 in extreme obesity.

Other chromosomal regions were also reported to show linkage with obesity-related traits with at least three independent replications. The 6p21-23 region was reported in multiple studies to have suggestive[63–70] (LOD ≥ 2) or significant linkage (LOD ≥3).[71–73] The 11q22-23 region was reported to show linkage with obesity-related traits in multiple ethnic groups, including Pima Indians,[31,74–76] Mexican Americans,[47,50] African,[75] Old Order Amish (a relatively isolated and homogenous population),[77] as well as whites.[40] The last region to highlight is the 20q12-13 region. There is suggestive-to-borderline significant linkage of the 20q12 region with BMI,[47,78,79] and the adjunct region 20q13 is also linked to both anthropometric measurements[47,79,80] and macronutrient intake.[81] Motivated readers are referred to other excellent resources for near-complete listings of obesity-related QTLs.[29,45,82]

FROM QTLs TO GENES

Follow-up and Fine Mapping Studies

More than a dozen follow-up and fine-mapping studies have tried to confirm previously reported QTLs. The follow-up studies usually use denser markers, which help to map the QTLs in finer scale and independent samples. Some studies have simultaneously published the original genome scan result with the fine mapping with additional markers at the locus with the peak linkage signal.[47] Most follow-up fine-mapping studies focus on previously reported QTLs with suggestive-to-significant linkages. Some of these follow-up studies report even stronger linkage[50,78,83] than the initial studies. Most, however, report weaker but still suggestive linkage compared with the initial findings.[35,42,61,62,84,85] There are also negative follow-up studies[86]. Exclusion mapping[87] is a linkage analysis based on LOD scores that is designed to exclude QTLs that are not likely to contribute to phenotypes. Thus, the null hypothesis in this approach is that the QTL does not account for the phenotype or will be accepted (contrary to rejected) if the LOD score is lower than –2. A recent exclusion mapping study purported to exclude chromosomal regions 7q and 11q for both BMI and percent of body fat.[88] However, given that this finding contradicts findings listed above, the complexity of BMI and adiposity as phenotypes, and the plausibility of differential effects across populations, we urge caution before definitively excluding any these or any regions from consideration.

Candidate Gene Studies

The next logical step is to identify candidate genes by an association study (positional candidate genes) for the QTLs confirmed and narrowed by fine-mapping studies.

Only a handful of studies have identified promising putative genes.[34,35] Boutin et al.[35] fine-mapped chromosome 10p, initially mapped by Hager et al.,[41] with 16 additional markers between D10S191 and D10S220 in 188 French nuclear families. Two linkage peaks at markers D10S197 (maximum LOD score MLS = 3.2) and D10S600 (MLS = 3.4) were identified, one of which is on the GAD2 gene that codes the glutamic acid decarboxylase enzyme catalyzing γ-aminobutyric acid production. Novel mutations were screened in 24 obese patients from families showing linkage at the candidate locus. Common single-nucleotide polymorphisms (SNPs) on GAD2 were genotyped, and association studies were conducted in two sets of unrelated morbidly obese patients and nonobese controls both separately and combined. As reviewed by Tiwari et al.,[36,37] Boutin et al.[35] found significant and seemingly impressive associations of GAD2 SNPs and haplotypes with obesity. Yet, a recent, large independent association study failed to confirm the association of GAD2 SNPs with obesity.[89] Similarly, Groves et al.[90] performed a genome-wide linkage scan for BMI in 573 U.K. pedigrees. They identified a statistically significant linkage peak in the region of GAD2. They subsequently examined eight SNPs in GAD2 and observed marginally significant (.01 < p < .05) associations between four common SNPs and BMI, but these SNPs did not account for their linkage evidence and did not replicate previous GAD2 associations. They concluded that GAD2 is not likely an important contributor to obesity.

Another promising positional candidate gene is SLC6A14 on chromosome Xq24. Suviolahti et al.[34] fine mapped a 15-Mb region on Xq24 that was initially reported by the same group of investigators to show linkage.[91] Haplotype analysis reduced the 15-cM region to 4 Mb with three functional candidate genes. Of these three genes, SLC6A14 showed significant association with obesity in a group of 117 cases and 182 controls (p = .0007). Suviolahti et al.[34] further confirmed this association in a combined group of Finnish and Swedish with 837 cases and 968 controls. A recent independent replication in a French population also found a significant association between SLC6A14 with obesity.[92]

Although both GAD2 and SLC6A14 need to be further confirmed by functional analysis as causal candidate genes for obesity,[36,37] these two findings provide evidence of the potential success of the positional cloning strategy. We may conservatively expect more positional candidate gene searching activities with the further harvest of QTLs.[93]

Association Studies

Association studies test association between genetic variants with phenotypes in unrelated subjects. The association study is relatively simple in design and sampling and more powerful in mapping genes with small effects than linkage analysis.[94] However, association studies may be confounded by population stratification, which can result in false-positive findings. Methods, such as genomic control[95] and structured analysis[96] were developed to help control the potential false-positive rate in association studies but have not been extensively used in association studies of genes for obesity.

By the end of October 2004, 358 studies reported significant associations between obesity-related traits and 113 candidate genes.[29] Both the number of significant reports and the list of associated candidate genes are growing rapidly. In 2004 alone, 81 new studies and 21 new candidate genes were published.[29] Hundreds of published studies, however, failed to find significant associations. Among the list of reported candidate genes, only a few have been replicated by three or more independent studies (Table 48.1).[38,97–132] The candidate genes in Table 48.1 can be divided into five groups according to the putative functions of

TABLE 48.1
Candidate Genes for Human Obesity Reported By Multiple Independent Replications

Putative Function	Gene (Abbreviation)	Location	Reference*
Food intake	Agouti-related protein (AGRP)	16q22	Argyropoulos et al.[97]
	Dopamine-R D2 (D2DRD2)	11q23.2	Comings et al.[98]
	Melanocortin 4-R (MC4R)	18q22	Chagnon et al.[99]
	Proopiomelanocortin (POMC)	2p23.3	Hixson et al.[38]
	Leptin (LEP)	7q31.3	Shintani et al.[100]
	Leptin Receptor (LEPR)	1p31	Thompson et al.[101]
Energy expenditure	Adrenergic-R 2A (ADR2A)	10q24-26	Oppert et al.[102]
	Adrenergic-R 2B (ADRB2)	5q31-32	Large et al.[103]
	Adrenergic-R 3B (ADRB3)	8p12-p11.2	Clement et al.[104]
	ATPase 1A2 (ATP1A2)	1q23.1	Deriaz et al.[105]
	Cytochrome P450 (CYP19A1)	15q21.1	Baghaei et al.[106]
	Peroxisome proliferator-activated-R G (PPARG)	3p25	Deeb et al.[107]; Meirhaeghe et al.[108]; Ristow et al.[109]
	Uncoupling protein 1 (UCP1)	4q28-31	Fumeron et al.[110]
	Uncoupling protein 2 (UCP2)	11q13.3	Walder et al.[111]
	Uncoupling protein 3 (UCP3)	11q13	Argyropoulos et al.[112]
Adiopocyte metabolism	Adiponectin (ACDC)	3q27	Stumvoll et al.[113]
	Interleukin 6 (IL6)	7p21	Berthier et al.[114]; Kubaszek et al.[115]
	Insulin (INS)	11p15.5	Weaver et al.[116]
	Lipase-E (LIPE)	19q13.2	Magre et al.[117]
	Lipoprotein Lipase (LPL)	8p21.3	Jemaa et al.[118]
	Tumor necrosis factor alpha (TNFA)	6p21.3	Fernandez-Real et al.[119]
Lipid metabolism	Apolipoprotein A-IV (APOA4)	11q23.3	Fisher et al.[120]
	Apolipoprotein B (APOB)	2p24.2	Rajput-Williams et al.[121]
	Apolipoprotein E (APOE)	19q13.32	Oh et al.[122]
Other hormones/receptors	Angiotensin (AGT)	1a42.2	Hegele et al.[123]
	Androgen-R (AR)	Xq11.2-12	Gustafson et al.[124]; Zitzmann et al.[125]
	Estrogen-R1 (ESR1)	6q25.1	Deng et al.[126]
	G-protein beta(3) (GNB3)	12p13.31	Hegele et al.[127]; Siffert et al.[128,129]
	5-hydroxytryptamine-R 2C (HTR2C)	Xq24	Yuan et al.,[130] 2000
	Glucocorticoid-R 3C1 (NR3C1)	5q31	Buemann et al.,[131] 1997
	Vitamin D-R (VDR)	12q13.11	Ye et al.[132]

* Only the first report is shown here. Please see text, Perusse et al. (2005), and OGMD (2005) for more complete references.

gene products: genes regulating food intake, energy expenditure, adipose metabolism, lipid metabolism, and other hormones or receptors. These groups are not mutually exclusive. For example, the adrenergic receptor regulates energy expenditure through adipose metabolism and, therefore, can be classified in either group. There are several excellent reviews of association studies covering most of the frequently replicated candidate genes.[45,133,134] and the very recent update of human obesity gene map.[99] Hence, we will highlight just a few candidate genes with emphasis on energy intake and expenditure pathways and methodology issues.

Genes Regulating Energy Intake

Genes on the food intake pathway, especially human homologues of animal obesity genes, are under intensive investigation. Mutations on the LEP and LEPR genes result in early onset extreme obesity. Both LEP (7q31) and LEPR (1p31) are on or close to previously identified QTLs (see "Linkage studies"). The effects of LEP and LEPR genes on common obesity, however, are weak. Both LEP and LEPR gene polymorphisms have been reported to be associated with BMI, body weight change, and LEP levels,[29] but there are more positive reports for LEPR than LEP. LEPR is associated with 24-h energy expenditure,[135] hyperlipidemia,[136] and diabetes.[137] A meta-analysis[138] with a total 3263 subjects found no significant association between LEPR genes and BMI or waist circumstance but found that certain LEPR alleles might have population-specific effects.

Melanocortin 4 Receptor

MC4R knockout causes obesity in mice, and polymorphisms were detected that seem to induce obesity in other animals.[139] Antagonists of MC4R are known to induce feeding.[140] MacKenzie[141] opines that MC4R agonist drugs will probably be successfully developed in the near future, providing effective antiobesity treatment alone or with other approaches. MC4R has been touted as the gene with the most common obesity-promoting alleles in humans.

MC4R polymorphisms, presumed to cause severe obesity, have been found with a higher frequency in MC4R than in other genes.[142–144] As Kublaoui and Zinn[144] describe, this receptor is involved in food intake regulations. In 1998 the first reports appeared of heterozygous MC4R mutations being associated with severe early onset obesity. Subsequently, over 70 polymorphisms were reported, many purportedly associated with severe obesity. Hyperphagia, rapid height growth in childhood, and increased bone mineral density have been reported as associated characteristics. Even here, the results have been inconsistent. One of the largest single studies conducted found no association.[143] Other recent studies were not especially supportive of an important role for spontaneously occurring MC4R mutations in contributing to variations in adiposity among humans. In an editorial commenting on two of the largest and most recent studies, Kublaoui and Zinn[144] wrote:

> These studies demonstrate several difficulties in this field. Mutations that clearly impair MC4R function are found with significant frequency in only the most severely obese cohorts. ... The fact that four large studies with more than 3000 obese patients shared only one pathogenic MC4R mutation underscores the rarity of individual mutations and the need for very large multicenter studies of highly selected populations and extremely large prospective, population-based cohort studies (on the order of 200,000 subjects... to understand the spectrum of human MC4R mutations and associated phenotypes. The present studies also suggest that the yield of MC4R testing in clinical diagnosis of obesity is likely to be low except in highly selected patients.

Genes Regulating Energy Expenditure

Currently genes putatively associated with the energy expenditure pathway draw the most attention in association studies, because more known factors are involved in this pathway than in food intake pathways. At least nine genes in this pathway (Table 48.1) have been frequently replicated.[29]

All three beta adrenergic receptor subtypes promote lipolysis, a key component of energy expenditure and adipose metabolism in human adipose tissue.[145] The β_2-adrenergic receptor (ADRB2) was reported to be associated with a variety of obesity-related traits, including BMI,[103,146,147] body fat,[103,146] body weight change,[146–148] LEP,[149] and lipolysis[150] in Caucasians,[147,148,151] African Americans,[151] and Asians.[152]

The β_3-adrenergic receptor (ADRB3) has a very low level of expression in adults. Nonetheless, the Trp64Arg polymorphism in ADRB3 was reported to be associated with obesity-related traits in multiple populations.[104,153,154] Four meta-analyses were done on the data for this polymorphism.[155–158] Allison et al.[155] combined 23 studies including 36 subgroups and a total of 7399 subjects and found marginally significant evidence (mean difference .19, $p = .07$) of association for Trp64Arg and BMI. Fujisawa et al.[156] analyzed a moderately large sample size (31 studies, 48 subgroups with 9236 subjects) and reported moderate evidence of association (mean difference 0.30, CI: 0.13–0.47). Both meta-analyses concluded that the effects of the Trp64Arg polymorphism are homogeneous across different ethnic groups. Kurokawa et al.'s meta-analysis[157] with only Japanese subjects also found a significant but similar mean difference. Zhan and Ho[158] confirmed the moderate effects of the Trp64Arg polymorphism on insulin resistance in obese and diabetic Asians. In summary, evidence is consistent with small effects of the beta-adrenergic receptors, especially ADRB3, on obesity-related traits.[159]

Proteins in the mitochondrial respiration chain, such as uncoupling proteins (UCPs), ATPase, and cytochrome P450, are important for thermogenesis. Therefore, genes coding these proteins are good candidates for association studies and have been reported most frequently. UCPs uncouple substrate oxidation from ATP synthesis.[160,161] Several studies reported significant associations of UCP1, UCP2, and UCP3 and obesity-related traits, although UCP1 is expressed primarily in infant brown adipose tissue and only to a limited extent in adults.[29] In addition to commonly tested phenotypes, certain sophisticated energy metabolic traits may be associated with UCP1 (resting metabolic rate),[162] UCP2 (respiratory quotient[163], resting energy expenditure and resting glucose oxidation rate[164], and 24-h metabolic rate[111]), and UCP3 (resting metabolic rate[162] and resting energy expenditure[165]). Several reports showed an association of SNPs in the ATPase (ATP1A2) and cytochrome P450 (CYP19A1) genes, but more data are needed to fully evaluate these associations.[29]

The peroxisome-proliferator-activated receptor gamma (PPARG) is a subtype of PPAR, a group of nuclear hormone receptor transcription factors. PPARG regulates the transcription of various genes involved in adipocyte differentiation and lipid and glucose metabolism.[166] Two common polymorphisms of PPARG gene, Pro12Ala and C161T, were found. Most association studies have focused on the Pro12Ala polymorphism.[45] Masud and Ye[167] pooled 30 studies with a total of 19,136 subjects in a meta-analysis and reported that the Ala12 allele was associated with higher BMI, but the effect was very small (0.07, CI: 0.01–0.12) and was not observed in the nonobese group (BMI ≤ 27). There was significant heterogeneity among studies in the meta-analysis.

Evidence for interactions among genes in the energy expenditure pathway is increasing. Three studies reported that the -3826 A-to-G polymorphism of UCP1 gene has a significant synergistic effect with the Trp64Arg polymorphism in ADRB3 on BMI,[168] basal metabolic rate,[169] and autonomic nervous system activity.[170] This synergistic effect was also observed on weight change.[171–173] Interactions were reported between ADRB3 and PPARG[174,175] and between UCP2 and PPARG[176] for obesity-related traits. Interactions of the LEP gene with the UCP3[177] and ADRB3[178] genes were reported, which indicates possible coordination of food intake and energy expenditure pathways.

Other Candidate Genes

A growing body of evidence indicates that genes regulating adipose tissue and lipid metabolism, and receptors for hormones, are also associated with common obesity (Table 48.1). For example, a recent meta-analysis that pooled 31 studies found an association between the G-308A polymorphism in tumor necrosis factor-α and obesity and insulin resistance.[179] However, more data are needed to confirm these associations.

NONREPLICATION IN GENETIC STUDIES OF OBESITY

Independent replication is the mainstay for confirmation of scientific findings. Both linkage and association studies of complex traits in general and in obesity in particular suffer from nonreplication.

POTENTIAL FACTORS ACCOUNTING FOR NONREPLICATION

This is a difficult field of study: Flaws in study design, population sampling, statistical modeling, and measurement errors in genotyping and phenotyping make reproducibility across studies difficult. Most human studies are limited to observational designs that are subject to a combination of well-recognized but difficult-to-control selection and information (measurement) biases. For example, selection bias in association studies that compare samples of affected cases with nonaffected controls can produce either false-positive results or obscure true ones, regardless of the issue of covert population stratification. Linkage studies in samples of related subjects are also not immune to selection bias.

Small sample size and statistical power are often cited as problems in nonreplication across studies. Association studies are generally considered to be more powerful (as well as easier to conduct) than linkage studies of similar sample size. However, modern studies using genomic scans involving hundreds if not thousands of markers and functional polymorphisms present a complex multiple-testing, signal-to-noise problem requiring either very large samples or unconventional approaches for determining significance. This sample size problem is further exacerbated when interactions among multiple genes or between multiple genes and environmental factors are to be investigated. The pervasive problem of sample size has led to efforts to pool findings from several studies in meta-analyses, but this may not be an optimal solution for the issue of nonreplication.

As for many complex traits, the genetic makeup of obese patients is not homogeneous because of incomplete penetrance and phenocopy, genetic (locus) heterogeneity, allelic heterogeneity, and polygenic inheritance.[21] Moreover, obesity is not a homogeneous phenotype. People with the same BMIs may have quite different body composition in terms of percent body fat, fat distribution, and muscle mass. Obese people may also differ considerably for obesity-related metabolic characteristics, such as resting energy expenditure, and disease risk factors, such as lipid profile, glucose tolerance, and blood pressure.

Association studies are vulnerable for population stratification and genetic admixture. Population stratification occurs when subpopulations with different allelic frequencies and phenotype distributions are present within a sample, but not accounted for, which may cause a false positive result in a test for association. Admixed populations have two or more ancestral populations with distinct genetic backgrounds. Population stratification and admixture are ubiquitous and may exist in apparently homogeneous populations.[180] Without proper control, such population structures can result in spurious associations.[181,182] Although it is not clear whether population stratification accounts for a large share of nonreplication in association studies, it needs to be carefully evaluated when association studies are designed and conducted. A number of statistical methods have been developed to control the confounding due to population structure, including the family based transmission disequilibrium test,[183–186] the genomic control test,[95] and the structured association test.[96,187,188]

Nonrandom mating is another important confounding factor. A small degree of assortative mating can result in a significant inflation of false-positive rates.[189] Structured association tests addressing the population structure issue may be used, at least partially, to detect and control the spurious association due to the nonrandom mating.

Inadequate control of significance levels,[190] inadequate power in replication studies,[191,192] together with publication bias seem to account for most of the nonreplication in association studies. A stringent significance level, large sample size, and postanalysis power calculation indicating the probability of observing the reported effect are reasonable ways to address the low power issue.[193]

CONSTRUCTIVE REPLICATION

Nonreplication is not unusual in scientific research. For example, Siefe[165] summarized some studies in which the initial 5-sigma findings (at least five standard deviations above the threshold with corresponding p-value at the 10^{-7} magnitude) vanished upon attempted replication. As already mentioned, follow-up studies of obesity candidate genes and QTLs generally tend to be either less significant or nonsignificant compared with the initial findings. A recent example is the association of a polymorphism of the INSIG2 gene and obesity.[194] To our knowledge, it is the first genome-wide association study screening for obesity-associated genes. The initial finding came by use of a self-replication method and was confirmed by four of five separate samples but not in a sample of 2726 subjects from the Nurses' Health Study. Froguel[195] also failed to observe the result in a separate sample of 10,000 subjects. This seems like a 5-sigma anomaly. It underscores the need for truly independent replications, or what Lykken[196] would have referred to as constructive replication. Lykken[196] described different types of replication and suggested that perhaps we should be most confident in a finding when we can replicate it using the most disparate methods relative to those that produced the original finding. Perhaps there is a need for the scientific community to begin more formal investigations of how to conduct and evaluate replication studies.

FUTURE DIRECTIONS

Here, we highlight a few important future directions.

NONMAMMALIAN ANIMAL MODELS

Many basic metabolic pathways that are involved in the regulation of energy balance and that may lead to obesity may be highly conserved across species.[197] Thus, experimental genetic studies in nonhuman species may be informative. For a long time, mammalian, especially murine, models have been the models of choice for obesity research. However, some nonmammalian organisms, such as fruit flies and soil nematodes, are valuable alternatives. Major advantages of such organisms include a small yet highly sophisticated genome, low cost, markedly shorter lifespan, large number of offspring, mutant stock supplies, and well-characterized inbred lines. These make identifying trait-conferring genetic variants in such species a markedly more tractable problem than it is in mammalian species. Genes identified as playing a role in adiposity in these species are not guaranteed to have human homologues. Nevertheless, these species are outstanding tools for identifying physiological pathways and novel targets for future drug development.

POOLING DATA

A major concern of obesity genetic studies is the inadequate power of many if not all studies. As these many studies accumulate, there is great potential to seek greater power, precision, and clarity via pooling data analysis. We use the term "pooling data analysis" to refer to any activity that uses the data (whether raw data or published summary statistics) from two or more studies in a formal and quantitative manner to estimate quantities or test hypotheses. Meta-analysis has long been used to analyze data from studies with similar designs, statistical analyses, and study populations. An emerging trend is to integrate data within and across several domains, such as genomic, transcriptomic, and proteomic data, or even to integrate data from a variety of species.

META-ANALYSIS

Meta-analysis is very useful when narrative review is inadequate to draw meaningful conclusion. It can be used to integrate the latest results in the context of existing research and to refine estimates of an effect or association. Meta-analytic techniques for association studies are well established. For example, as mentioned, four different meta-analyses examined the association between the TRP64ARG polymorphism of ADRB3 and obesity-related traits.[155–158] Although they differed with respect to their conclusions about statistical significance depending on the amount of data available and the populations studied, all of them suggested that ADRB3 has a small association with BMI. In other words, the magnitudes of point estimates of the association were very consistent. In contrast, methods of meta-analysis for linkage studies[170–185,198–213] still need further development.

INTEGRATION OF DATA WITHIN AND ACROSS DOMAINS

A growing body of investigators have expressed the belief that we will learn more about genotype-phenotype relations by integrating "omic" data across data types (e.g., mRNA expression, protein, linkage, disequilibrium, sequence, and ontology data) as well as across species. Systematic, quantitative methods for integrating information across "omic" domains are still in their infancy. The few methods that have been articulated to date are typically ad hoc in nature and often somewhat subjective and informal. Moreover, the operating characteristics or properties of these methods have rarely been demonstrated via thorough analyses of biological data in which the correct answers are known, through mathematical proofs or computational simulations. Nevertheless, this approach, termed "integromics," [214] represents a promising direction.

There is much enthusiasm about the benefits of integromic research. Obesity is a somewhat unique trait in that its most commonly used anthropometric indicators — BMI in humans and body fat mass in both humans and model organisms — are relatively easily and commonly measured by most biomedical researchers even if they are not primarily obesity researchers. Perhaps for that reason, there have been many genetic studies of obesity or obesity-related traits. As these studies accumulate, the opportunity to seek greater power, precision, and clarity via integrative analysis comes to the fore. Most integrative omic analyses have been meta-analyses within a single domain and species.[57,89,138,155–158,167,179,215–225] Most used challenging but semiconventional meta-analytic methods. An informal but creative approach was published by Meyre et al.,[221] who combined eight genome scans to identify a locus on chromosome 6 (6q16.3-q24.2). By looking for regions of overlap in multiple different genome scans, they identified a risk haplotype in the gene ENPP1 for severe obesity.

A few integromic obesity studies integrated data across domains or species.[188,189] For example, Hult et al.[188] analyzed lipin transcript levels in both human and mouse adipose tissues and also polymorphisms in the lipin gene in relation to BMI. By using this cross-species and multiple-data-type approach, they were able to identify associated allelic haplotypes that seem to influence both adiposity and metabolic phenotypes. These early studies have begun to yield promising results suggesting the power of integrative analysis. We believe that by adding more formal, rigorous, and powerful omic approaches to these integrative efforts, we can help the field move forward further still.

REFERENCES

1. Ogden, C. L. et al. *JAMA 295*: 1549; 2006.
2. Flegal, K. M. *Int J Epidemiol 35*: 72; discussion 81; 2006.
3. Liou, T. H., Pi-Sunyer, F. X., and Laferrere, B. *Nutr Rev 63*: 321; 2005.
4. Fontaine, K. R. et al. *JAMA 289*: 187; 2003.
5. Klein, S. et al. *Circulation 110*: 2952; 2004.
6. Keith, S., Redden, D. T., Katzmarzyk, P. et al. *Internat J Obes.* 30: 1585; 2006.
7. Bouchard, C., and Perusse, L. In *The Genetics of Obesity*; Bouchard, C., Ed.; CRC Press: Boca Raton, FL, 1994, p 79–92.
8. Allison, D. B., Faith, M. S., and Nathan, J. S. *Int J Obes Relat Metab Disord 20*: 990–999; 1996.
9. Neale, M. C., and Cardon, L. R. *Methodology for Genetic Studies of Twins and Families*; Kluwer Academic Publishers: Dorchrect, The Netherlands, 1992.
10. Eaves, L., Foley, D., and Silberg, J. *Twin Res 6*: 486; 2003.
11. Segal, N. L., and Allison, D. B. *Int J Obes Relat Metab Disord 26*: 437; 2002.
12. Allison, D. B. et al. *Int J Obes Relat Metab Disord 20*: 501; 1996.
13. Maes, H. H., Neale, M. C., and Eaves, L. J. *Behav Genet 27*: 325; 1997.
14. Allison, D. B., Matz, P., Pietrobelli, A., Zannolli, R., and Faith, M.S. In *Primary and Secondary Preventive Nutrition*; Bendich, A., and Deckelbaum, R. J., Eds.; Humana Press: Totowa, NJ, 2001, p 147–164.
15. Lin, H. F. et al. *Diabetologia 48*: 2006; 2005.
16. Li, H. J. et al. *J Clin Endocrinol Metab 90*: 3659; 2005.
17. Tholin, S. et al. *Am J Clin Nutr 81*: 564; 2005.
18. Bouchard, C. et al. *Prog Food Nutr Sci 12*: 45; 1988.
19. Bouchard, C. et al. *Int J Obes 14*: 57; 1990.
20. Bray, M. S., and Allison, D. B. In *Animal Models — Disorders of Eating Behavior and Body Composition Disorders*; Owen, J. B., Treasure, J. L., and Collier, D. A., Eds.; Kluwer Academic Publishers: Dordrecht, The Netherlands, 2001, p 1–18.
21. Lander, E. S., and Schork, N. J. *Science 265*: 2037; 1994.
22. Cargill, M. et al. *Nat Genet 22*: 231; 1999.

23. Chakravarti, A. *Nat Genet 21*: 56; 1999.
24. Reich, D. E., and Lander, E. S. *Trends Genet 17*: 502; 2001.
25. Pritchard, J. K. *Am J Hum Genet 69*: 124; 2001.
26. Pritchard, J. K., and Cox, N. J. *Hum Mol Genet 11*: 2417; 2002.
27. Allison, D. B., and Schork, N. J. *Behav Genet 27*: 401; 1997.
28. Zhang, Y. et al. *Nature 372*: 425; 1994.
29. Perusse, L. et al. *Obes Res 13*: 381; 2005.
30. OMIM. Online Mendelian Inheritance in Man. Accessed throught www.ncbi.nlm.nih.gov/omim.
31. Norman, R. A. et al. *Am J Hum Genet 60*: 166; 1997.
32. Comuzzie, A. G. et al. *Nat Genet 15*: 273; 1997.
33. Lander, E., and Kruglyak, L. *Nat Genet 11*: 241; 1995.
34. Suviolahti, E. et al. *J Clin Invest 112*: 1762; 2003.
35. Boutin, P. et al. *PLoS Biol 1*: E68; 2003.
36. Tiwari, H. K. et al. *Nutr Rev 63*: 315; 2005.
37. Tiwari, H. K., and Allison, D. B. *J Clin Invest 112*: 1633; 2003.
38. Hixson, J. E. et al. *J Clin Endocrinol Metab 84*: 3187; 1999.
39. Palmer, L. J. et al. *Am J Hum Genet 72*: 340; 2003.
40. Moslehi, R. et al. *BMC Genet 4 (Suppl 1)*: S97; 2003.
41. Hager, J. et al. *Nat Genet 20*: 304; 1998.
42. Rotimi, C. N. et al. *Diabetes 48*: 643; 1999.
43. Comuzzie, A. G. et al. *J Clin Endocrinol Metab 86*: 4321; 2001.
44. Vionnet, N. et al. *Am J Hum Genet 67*: 1470; 2000.
45. Loos, R. J., and Bouchard, C. *J Intern Med 254*: 401; 2003.
46. Cai, G. et al. *Am J Clin Nutr 80*: 1410; 2004.
47. Stone, S. et al. *Am J Hum Genet 70*: 1459; 2002.
48. Perusse, L. et al. *Diabetes 50*: 614; 2001.
49. Camp, N. J. et al. *Genet Epidemiol 21 (Suppl 1)*: S461; 2001.
50. Arya, R. et al. *Am J Hum Genet 74*: 272; 2004.
51. Roth, H. et al. *Exp Clin Endocrinol Diabetes 105*: 341; 1997.
52. Bray, M. S., Boerwinkle, E., and Hanis, C. L. *Genet Epidemiol 16*: 397; 1999.
53. Reed, D. R. et al. *Diabetes 45*: 691; 1996.
54. Rutkowski, M. P. et al. *Hypertension 31*: 1230; 1998.
55. Feitosa, M. F. et al. *Am J Hum Genet 70*: 72; 2002.
56. Clement, K. et al. *Diabetes 45*: 687; 1996.
57. Wu, X. et al. *Am J Hum Genet 70*: 1247; 2002.
58. Duggirala, R. et al. *Am J Hum Genet 59*: 694; 1996.
59. Hsueh, W. C. et al. *J Clin Endocrinol Metab 86*: 1199; 2001.
60. Saar, K. et al. *Pediatrics 111*: 321; 2003.
61. Dong, C. et al. *Am J Hum Genet 72*: 115; 2003.
62. Price, R. A. et al. *Diabetologia 44*: 363; 2001.
63. Zhu, X. et al. *Diabetes 51*: 541; 2002.
64. Steinle, N. I. et al. *Am J Clin Nutr 75*: 1098; 2002.
65. Cassell, P. G. et al. *Diabetologia 43*: 1558; 2000.
66. Geller, F., Dempfle, A., and Gorg, T. *BMC Genet 4 (Suppl 1)*: S91; 2003.
67. Heijmans, B. T. et al. *Twin Res 7*: 192; 2004.
68. Bell, C. G. et al. *Diabetes 53*: 1857; 2004.
69. Chagnon, Y. C. et al. *Metabolism 49*: 203; 2000.
70. Chen, W. et al. *Int J Obes Relat Metab Disord 28*: 462; 2004.
71. Arya, R. et al. *Diabetes 51*: 841; 2002.
72. Fox, C. S. et al. *Diabetes 53*: 1399; 2004.
73. Meyre, D. et al. *Diabetes 53*: 803; 2004.
74. Hanson, R. L. et al. *Am J Hum Genet 63*: 1130; 1998.
75. Adeyemo, A. et al. *Obes Res 11*: 266; 2003.
76. Lindsay, R. S. et al. *Diabetes 50*: 2850; 2001.
77. Platte, P. et al. *Am J Med Genet C Semin Med Genet 121*: 71; 2003.
78. Hunt, S. C. et al. *Hum Genet 109*: 279; 2001.
79. Lee, J. H. et al. *Am J Hum Genet 64*: 196; 1999.
80. Borecki, I. B. et al. *Obes Res 2*: 213; 1994.
81. Collaku, A. et al. *Am J Clin Nutr 79*: 881; 2004.
82. OGMDB; Obesity Gene Map Database. 2005. Internet: http://obesitygene.pbrc.edu/ (accessed 18 June 2006).
83. Luke, A. et al. *Diabetes 52*: 1284; 2003.

84. Hinney, A. et al. *J Clin Endocrinol Metab 85*: 2962; 2000.
85. Li, W. D. et al. *Diabetes 52*: 1557; 2003.
86. Iliadou, A. et al. *Twin Res 6*: 162; 2003.
87. Ott, J. *Analysis of Human Genetic Linkage*; Revised Edition; Johns Hopkins University Press: Baltimore, MD, 1991.
88. Guo, J. J. et al. *Biochem Biophys Res Commun 332*: 602; 2005.
89. Swarbrick, M. M. et al. *PLoS Biol 3*: e315; 2005.
90. Groves, C. J. et al. *Diabetes 55*: 1884; 2006.
91. Ohman, M. et al. *J Clin Endocrinol Metab 85*: 3183; 2000.
92. Durand, E. et al. *Diabetes 53*: 2483; 2004.
93. Blangero, J. *Curr Opin Genet Dev 14*: 233; 2004.
94. Risch, N., and Merikangas, K. *Science 273*: 1516; 1996.
95. Devlin, B., Roeder, K., and Wasserman, L. *Theor Popul Biol 60*: 155; 2001.
96. Pritchard, J. K. et al. *Am J Hum Genet 67*: 170; 2000.
97. Argyropoulos, G. et al. *J Clin Endocrinol Metab 87*: 4198; 2002.
98. Comings, D. E. et al. *Biochem Med Metab Biol 50*: 176; 1993.
99. Chagnon, Y. C. et al. *Mol Med 3*: 663; 1997.
100. Shintani, M. et al. *Diabetologia 39*: 1398; 1996.
101. Thompson, D. B. et al. *Hum Mol Genet 6*: 675; 1997.
102. Oppert, J. M. et al. *Obes Res 3*: 249; 1995.
103. Large, V. et al. *J Clin Invest 100*: 3005; 1997.
104. Clement, K. et al. *N Engl J Med 333*: 352; 1995.
105. Deriaz, O. et al. *J Clin Invest 93*: 838; 1994.
106. Baghaei, F. et al. *Obes Res 11*: 578; 2003.
107. Deeb, S. S. et al. *Nat Genet 20*: 284; 1998.
108. Meirhaeghe, A. et al. *Hum Mol Genet 7*: 435; 1998.
109. Ristow, M. et al. *N Engl J Med 339*: 953; 1998.
110. Fumeron, F. et al. *Int J Obes Relat Metab Disord 20*: 1051; 1996.
111. Walder, K. et al. *Hum Mol Genet 7*: 1431; 1998.
112. Argyropoulos, G. et al. *J Clin Invest 102*: 1345; 1998.
113. Stumvoll, M. et al. *Diabetes 51*: 37; 2002.
114. Berthier, M. T. et al. *J Hum Genet 48*: 14; 2003.
115. Kubaszek, A. et al. *Diabetes 52*: 558; 2003.
116. Weaver, J. U., Kopelman, P. G., and Hitman, G. A. *Eur J Clin Invest 22*: 265; 1992.
117. Magre, J. et al. *Diabetes 47*: 284; 1998.
118. Jemaa, R. et al. *Int J Obes Relat Metab Disord 19*: 270; 1995.
119. Fernandez-Real, J. M. et al. *Diabetes 46*: 1468; 1997.
120. Fisher, R. M. et al. *J Lipid Res 40*: 287; 1999.
121. Rajput-Williams, J. et al. *Lancet 2*: 1442; 1988.
122. Oh, J. Y., and Barrett-Connor, E. *Clin Genet 60*: 132; 2001.
123. Hegele, R. A., Brunt, J. H., and Connelly, P. W. *Circulation 92*: 1089; 1995.
124. Gustafson, D. R., Wen, M. J., and Koppanati, B. M. *Int J Obes Relat Metab Disord 27*: 75; 2003.
125. Zitzmann, M. et al. *Diabetologia 46*: 31; 2003.
126. Deng, H. W. et al. *J Clin Endocrinol Metab 85*: 2748; 2000.
127. Hegele, R. A. et al. *Genome Res 9*: 972; 1999.
128. Siffert, W. et al. *J Am Soc Nephrol 10*: 1921; 1999.
129. Siffert, W. et al. *J Hypertens 17*: 1095; 1999.
130. Yuan, X. et al. *Diabetologia 43*: 373; 2000.
131. Buemann, B. et al. *Obes Res 5*: 186; 1997.
132. Ye, W. Z. et al. *Eur J Endocrinol 145*: 181; 2001.
133. Clement, K. *proc. nutr. Soc 64*: 133; 2005.
134. Bell, C. G., Walley, A. J., and Froguel, P. *Nat Rev Genet 6*: 221; 2005.
135. Stefan, N. et al. *Int J Obes Relat Metab Disord 26*: 1629; 2002.
136. van der Vleuten, G. M. et al. *Int J Obes (Lond) 30*: 892; 2006.
137. Park, K. S. et al. *J Hum Genet 51*: 85; 2006.
138. Heo, M. et al. *Int J Obes Relat Metab Disord 26*: 640; 2002.
139. Meidtner, K. et al. *Anim Genet 37*: 245; 2006.
140. Pontillo, J. et al. *Bioorg Med Chem Lett 15*: 2541; 2005.
141. MacKenzie, R. G. *Peptides 27*: 395; 2006.
142. Clement, K. *Horm Res 66*: 70; 2006.
143. Hirschhorn, J. N., and Altshuler, D. *J Clin Endocrinol Metab 87*: 4438; 2002.
144. Kublaoui, B. M., and Zinn, A. R. *J Clin Endocrinol Metab 91*: 1671; 2006.

145. Barbe, P. et al. *Br J Pharmacol 117*: 907; 1996.
146. Garenc, C. et al. *Obes Res 11*: 612; 2003.
147. van Rossum, C. T. et al. *Int J Obes Relat Metab Disord 26*: 517; 2002.
148. Meirhaeghe, A. et al. *Lancet 353*: 896; 1999.
149. Rosmond, R. et al. *J Intern Med 248*: 239; 2000.
150. Hoffstedt, J. et al. *Br J Pharmacol 133*: 708; 2001.
151. Ellsworth, D. L. et al. *Int J Obes Relat Metab Disord 26*: 928; 2002.
152. Yamada, K. et al. *J Clin Endocrinol Metab 84*: 1754; 1999.
153. Kadowaki, H. et al. *Biochem Biophys Res Commun 215*: 555; 1995.
154. Walston, J. et al. *N Engl J Med 333*: 343; 1995.
155. Allison, D. B. et al. *Int J Obes Relat Metab Disord 22*: 559; 1998.
156. Fujisawa, T. et al. *J Clin Endocrinol Metab 83*: 2441; 1998.
157. Kurokawa, N. et al. *Obes Res 9*: 741; 2001.
158. Zhan, S., and Ho, S. C. *Obes Res 13*: 1709; 2005.
159. Shuldiner, A. R., and Sabra, M. *Obes Res 9*: 806; 2001.
160. Ledesma, A., de Lacoba, M. G., and Rial, E. *Genome Biol 3*: 3015; 2002.
161. Ricquier, D. *Proc Nutr Soc 64*: 47; 2005.
162. Ukkola, O. et al. *Eur J Clin Nutr 55*: 1008; 2001.
163. Cassell, P. G. et al. *Diabetologia 42*: 688; 1999.
164. Le Fur, S. et al. *Diabetes 53*: 235; 2004.
165. Kimm, S. Y. et al. *Am J Clin Nutr 75*: 714; 2002.
166. Kersten, S., Desvergne, B., and Wahli, W. *Nature 405*: 421; 2000.
167. Masud, S., and Ye, S. *J Med Genet 40*: 773; 2003.
168. Evans, D. et al. *Int J Obes Relat Metab Disord 24*: 1239; 2000.
169. Valve, R. et al. *Diabetologia 41*: 357; 1998.
170. Shihara, N. et al. *Int J Obes Relat Metab Disord 25*: 761; 2001.
171. Clement, K. et al. *Int J Obes Relat Metab Disord 20*: 1062; 1996.
172. Fogelholm, M. et al. *J Clin Endocrinol Metab 83*: 4246; 1998.
173. Sivenius, K. et al. *Int J Obes Relat Metab Disord 25*: 1609; 2001.
174. Ochoa, M. C. et al. *Int J Obes Relat Metab Disord 28 (Suppl 3)*: S37; 2004.
175. Hsueh, W. C. et al. *Diabetes Care 24*: 672; 2001.
176. Cho, Y. M. et al. *Diabetologia 47*: 549; 2004.
177. Gomez-Ambrosi, J., Fruhbeck, G., and Martinez, J. A. *Cell Mol Life Sci 55*: 992; 1999.
178. Ramis, J. M. et al. *Metabolism 53*: 1411; 2004.
179. Sookoian, S. C., Gonzalez, C., and Pirola, C. J. *Obes Res 13*: 2122; 2005.
180. Campbell, C. D. et al. *Nat Genet 37*: 868; 2005.
181. Cardon, L. R., and Palmer, L. J. *Lancet 361*: 598; 2003.
182. Wacholder, S., Rothman, N., and Caporaso, N. *J Natl Cancer Inst 92*: 1151; 2000.
183. Spielman, R. S., McGinnis, R. E., and Ewens, W. J. *Am J Hum Genet 52*: 506; 1993.
184. Allison, D. B., and Neale, M. C. *Theor Popul Biol 60*: 239; 2001.
185. Zhao, H. *Stat Methods Med Res 9*: 563; 2000.
186. Whittaker, J. C., and Morris, A. P. *Ann Hum Genet 65*: 407; 2001.
187. Satten, G. A., Flanders, W. D., and Yang, Q. *Am J Hum Genet 68*: 466; 2001.
188. Hoggart, C. J. et al. *Am J Hum Genet 72*: 1492; 2003.
189. Redden, D. T., and Allison, D. B. *Behav Genet 36*: 678; 2006.
190. Colhoun, H. M., McKeigue, P. M., and Davey Smith, G. *Lancet 361*: 865; 2003.
191. Risch, N. J. *Nature 405*: 847; 2000.
192. Lohmueller, K. E. et al. *Nat Genet 33*: 177; 2003.
193. Redden, D. T., and Allison, D. B. *J Nutr 133*: 3323; 2003.
194. Herbert, A. et al. *Science 312*: 279; 2006.
195. Couzin, J. In *ScienceNOW Daily News*; 2006.
196. Lykken, D. T. *Psychological Bulletin 70*: 151; 1968.
197. Ruden, D. M. et al. *Annu Rev Nutr 25*: 499; 2005.
198. Dempfle, A., and Loesgen, S. *Ann Hum Genet 68*: 69; 2004.
199. Etzel, C. J., and Guerra, R. *Am J Hum Genet 71*: 56; 2002.
200. Goffinet, B., and Gerber, S. *Genetics 155*: 463; 2000.
201. Gu, C. et al. *Genet Epidemiol 15*: 609; 1998.
202. Gu, C., Province, M., and Rao, D. C. *Genet Epidemiol 17 (Suppl 1)*: S599; 1999.
203. Gu, C., Province, M. A., and Rao, D. C. *Adv Genet 42*: 255; 2001.
204. Guerra, R. et al. *Genet Epidemiol 17 (Suppl 1)*: S605; 1999.
205. Koziol, J. A., and Feng, A. C. *Ann Hum Genet 68*: 376; 2004.

206. Koziol, J. A., and Feng, A. C. *BMC Bioinformatics 6*: 32; 2005.
207. Li, Z., and Rao, D. C. *Genet Epidemiol 13*: 377; 1996.
208. Pardi, F., Levinson, D. F., and Lewis, C. M. *Bioinformatics 21*: 4430; 2005.
209. Wise, L. H., Lanchbury, J. S., and Lewis, C. M. *Ann Hum Genet 63*: 263; 1999.
210. Wise, L. H., and Lewis, C. M. *Genet Epidemiol 17 (Suppl 1)*: S767; 1999.
211. Zintzaras, E., and Ioannidis, J. P. *Genet Epidemiol 28*: 123; 2005.
212. Zintzaras, E., and Ioannidis, J. P. *Bioinformatics 21*: 3672; 2005.
213. Cooper, M. E. et al. *BMC Genet 6 (Suppl 1)*: S42; 2005.
214. Weinstein, J. N. *Breast Dis 19*: 11; 2004.
215. Keightley, P. D., and Knott, S. A. *Genet Res 74*: 323; 1999.
216. Hult, M. et al. *Mol Cell Endocrinol 248*: 26; 2006.
217. Suviolahti, E. et al. *Hum Mol Genet 15*: 377; 2006.
218. Hubner, N. et al. *Nat Genet 37*: 243; 2005.
219. Yagil, C. et al. *Circ Res 96*: 617; 2005.
220. Mehrabian, M. et al. *Nat Genet 37*: 1224; 2005.
221. Meyre, D. et al. *Nat Genet 37*: 863; 2005.

49 Metabolic Assessment of Overweight Patients

Shawn C. Franckowiak and Ross E. Andersen

CONTENTS

INTRODUCTION

Often, patients seeking to lose weight implore nutrition specialists and dieticians for advice on how many calories they should consume each day. This chapter introduces the clinician to the various components of metabolism and provides methods to calculate the energy needs of a patient trying to lose weight. Included in this chapter is an overview of the actual measurement of metabolic rate and prediction methods for determining the individual energy needs of the patient. It concludes with a brief review of the effects of exercise, activity, and caloric restriction on metabolic rate.

PRODUCING WEIGHT LOSS

To produce weight loss, a negative energy balance needs to exist whereby the patient consumes less energy than he or she expends in a day. The total energy needs of a person are expressed as:

Total energy needs = BMR + TEF + TEA + energy needed for growth, reproduction, lactation, or healing from injury.

BMR: Basal metabolic rate
TEF: Thermic effect of feeding
TEA: Thermic effect of activity

The total amount of energy a person expends in a 24 h period is termed total energy expenditure (TEE) and is composed of three different components: the resting metabolic rate (RMR), the thermic effect of feeding (TEF), and the thermic effect of activity (TEA) (Figure 49.1). RMR is the energy expenditure needed to sustain the basic biochemical reactions of the body in a resting state. A resting state is when a person is fasting (not starving), awake in a thermoneutral environment (not sweating, shivering, or fidgeting), and lying still without any skeletal muscle movement. This component of metabolism is also referred to as basal metabolic rate (BMR); the differences between BMR and RMR will be covered later in this chapter. The TEF is the energy expenditure attributed to the digestion, absorption, and excretion of food. TEF can be thought of as the difference in energy use between the fed and fasting state. The TEA is the energy expenditure associated with skeletal muscle movement. We have maximum control of this component of TEE because a person can choose to do variable amounts of physical activity that ultimately involve skeletal muscle movement. TEA consists of both purposeful exercise and a subcomponent called non-exercise activity thermogenesis (NEAT) that comprises daily activities such as sitting, standing, walking, and talking.[1,2] The RMR accounts for approximately 60 to 75% of TEE, the TEF approximately 7 to 10%, and the TEA 15 to 30% of daily energy expenditure.

DEFINITIONS OF ENERGY UNITS AND COMPONENTS OF METABOLISM

Before introducing the definition of RMR and other components of metabolism, it is important to define the energy unit. This is the "kilocalorie" or "kilojoule." The kilocalorie is the amount of heat content or energy required to raise the temperature of 1 kg of water by 1°C at 15°C; it is used in measurements of the heat production of chemical reactions including those of

24-hour energy expenditure

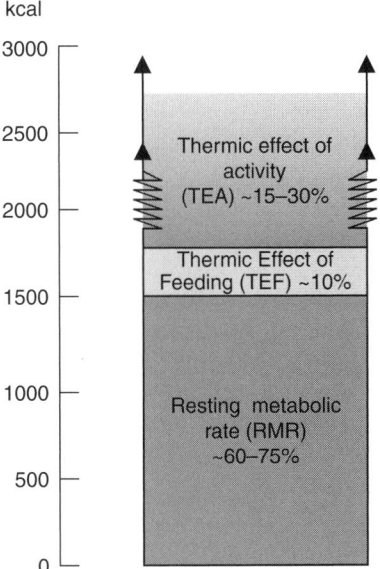

FIGURE 49.1 The components of the total daily energy expenditure (TEE): An approximate percentage of contribution towards TEE and a brief description of each component. RMR: resting metabolic rate, TEF: thermic effect of feeding, NEAT: nonexercise activity thermogenesis, TEA: thermic effect of activity.

biological systems.[3] At any given time in the human body, there are continuous biochemical reactions consisting of the breakdown of adenosine triphosphate (ATP) to a smaller molecule of adenosine diphosphate (ADP) and energy to serve the functional element of cells.[4] This reaction produces energy measurable in kilocalories. The word kilocalorie (or Calorie) may be used to define the amount of energy in the food a person consumes; it can also quantify the amount of energy a person expends.

RMR is typically presented as a measure of energy expressed as the amount of kilocalories expended in a day, represented as kcal/d. However, the kilocalorie may also be expressed as the kilojoule to achieve uniformity of SI unit measuring system.[3] One kilocalorie equals 4.184 kilojoules. Although the joule may be a uniform standard unit that scientists use in the research setting, the layperson will be better served when measurement of energy intake and expenditure is presented as kilocalories as this term is more relevant to food labels and packaging used in everyday life. Those seeking to lose weight pursue a negative energy balance whereby they expend more kilocalories than those consumed. A negative energy balance can be achieved by increasing TEE or decreasing overall caloric intake. Calorie is a word that many people associate with food labels to define the energy richness of a food item; it is often seen on exercise machinery stating the quantity of calories expended for a person of a given body weight for each minute of exercise. When investigating energy balance, it is important to understand the concept that a calorie is a measure of energy, and energy that is expended is measurable using different techniques. Most of this chapter will be devoted to defining RMR and several components that make up TEE, and it provides an overview of the methodology, implementation, and interpretation of the RMR.

TEE

TEE in free-living populations can be measured using doubly labeled water ($^{2}H_{2}{}^{18}O$). Measurement of TEE by doubly labeled water involves using stable isotopes of hydrogen and oxygen. A urine specimen is collected from the subject at baseline; the administered dosage of doubly labeled water is determined by body weight. Although this is the "gold standard" for the measurement of TEE, doubly labeled water is very costly and is almost exclusively used by scientists involved in measuring TEE and various components of the metabolism for clinical research studies.

Usually, clinicians do not have the option of estimating TEE by doubly labeled water. Therefore, TEE is typically estimated by measuring the RMR and estimating energy expenditure of physical activity. Physical activity patterns may be assessed using accelerometers or by administering a valid questionnaire.

RMR

RMR can be defined as the energy required to sustain bodily functions and maintain body temperature at rest. It is quantitatively the largest component of energy expenditure in humans. Typically it can account for 60% to 75% of the total daily expenditure.[5] RMR is often used to estimate the daily energy needs of the individuals for population-based studies and it is a useful tool in the clinical management of obesity.[5] Researchers have defined RMR as being different from that of BMR; BMR is the energy expenditure of a person at rest (not asleep) in a fasting state and at sexual repose in a thermoneutral environment (neither shivering, sweating, or fidgeting). To obtain a BMR measurement, patients should sleep in the lab and measurements should be taken upon awakening. The RMR is defined as a the energy expenditure measured on an outpatient basis.[6] For clinical purposes, the RMR can be assumed to be similar to the BMR.[6] Furthermore, RMR measurements can be both less expensive and less of a burden for the participant.

The RMR is the component of daily metabolism that is difficult to influence. Clinicians working with overweight patients will be quick to point out that their overweight clients often believe that they have low or sluggish RMR, and consequently feel that this is the reason for their inability to lose or maintain weight. Often, RMR values are not as low as the patient believes. RMR measurements are frequently within the normal range for the patient's age, gender, height, and weight.

TEF

Although thermogenesis via dietary means will be covered in more detail in its own section of this chapter, we will briefly describe TEF here. TEF is occasionally called dietary-induced thermogenesis (DIT) and accounts for approximately 7 to 10% of the TEE of a person.[7] TEF represents the energy expenditure associated with the ingestion, digestion, absorption, and excretion of food. There is an increase in the metabolic rate when a person has eaten food. This is why the assessment of RMR typically requires individuals to be fasted for a minimum of 12 h prior to the assessment of that component of the metabolism. TEF can be quantified by taking the measurements of a valid RMR assessment and comparing these measurements to values attained using the same testing procedures after the ingestion of a meal of known energy value and composition. The difference between the RMR and the energy used for digestion and absorption is the TEF (TEF + RMR = Energy expended after a meal is consumed).

TEA

The TEA is the only component of the TEE that we can directly influence. TEA is the amount of energy that is expended as a direct result of the voluntary skeletal muscle movement. TEA is made up of both programmed exercise and nonexercise physical activity involvement. Overall, TEE differs between active and sedentary persons. Sedentary persons expend less energy than active persons, and thus their TEA as a percentage of their total energy expenditure is less than that of active persons.

THERMOGENESIS

Additional caloric expenditure can also occur via a condition called thermogenesis. This is defined as energy expenditure above RMR that is not associated with physical activity. TEF is the dietary aspect of thermogenesis and makes up approximately 7% to 10% of the calories expended daily. However, thermogenesis can also be produced from medications and cold exposure. Many of the recent research studies involving the study of thermogenesis are also investigating the influence of fidgeting or changes in posture on TEE.[1,8–10] The term explaining the nonvolitional muscle activity, muscle tone, and fidgeting in a person is nonexercise activity thermogenesis (NEAT).[11] Researchers of NEAT have speculated that inadequate modulation of NEAT along with being sedentary may be important in understanding obesity.[2] These topics will be covered later in this chapter. To avoid overlap with authors covering prescribed weight-loss medications in other chapters of this book, only a review of the influence of over-the-counter weight-loss medications on thermogenesis will be provided in this chapter.

TECHNIQUES FOR MEASURING RMR

RMR can be measured using two different methods: direct calorimetry and indirect calorimetry. Direct calorimetry is the measurement of overall heat liberated by a body mass. Heat production is proportional to the body surface area available (kcal/m^2) for the release of heat by radiation or transvection.

Indirect calorimetry involves measuring oxygen (O_2) consumption and carbon dioxide (CO_2) production to determine RMR by calculation using the Weir equation.[12] To produce values for indirect calorimetry in kilocalories per day, the measurement of 1 L of oxygen consumed generates 3.9 kcal, and 1 L of carbon dioxide produced generates 1.1 kcal.[13] The original Weir equation involves measurement of gases that are consumed and produced at rest plus the collection of total 24 h urine nitrogen during the same day of measurement. However, a second abbreviated Weir equation has been developed that has less than 2% measurement error when compared with the longer equation.[12] This abbreviated Weir formula is as follows:

$$RMR = [3.9(VO_2) + 1.1\,(VCO_2)]1.44$$

Variables: VO_2 = oxygen consumption in ml/min

VCO_2 = carbon dioxide production in ml/min

Note: This equation is to determine resting energy expenditure (REE), so for determining RMR the patient must be in a 12 h fasted and rested state.

DIRECT CALORIMETRY

The measurement of energy needs of an adult who is neither gaining nor losing weight can be made using a whole-body calorimeter. This instrument measures the heat released by the body as a result of its metabolism.[13-15] It is a composite value in that it is not only the result of baseline metabolic reactions that produce heat but also the heat that results from the ingestion, digestion, and absorption of foods, in addition to that from muscular activity. Subjects must remain in the whole-body calorimeter for hours at a time so that sufficient data can be accumulated. This technique is extremely expensive and has limited clinical potential.[13]

INDIRECT CALORIMETRY

For most applications, a viable alternative is the indirect calorimeter or metabolic cart. Indirect calorimetry measures the gas exchange of an individual.[14,16] The gases detected by the metabolic cart are compared with the environmental conditions of the surrounding room's gases at standard temperature, pressure, and humidity (STPD). STPD is a symbol indicating that a gas volume has been expressed as if it were at standard temperature (0°C) and standard pressure (760 mmHg absolute) and were dry (no water vapor); under these conditions, 1 mol of a gas occupies 22.4 l. The testing environment should be controlled for temperature, barometric pressure, and humidity. Depending on the instrumentation, the measurement conditions are entered prior to beginning the assessment and correction factors applied to standardize the results. The room temperatures should also be kept between 68°F and 74°F. Furthermore, the room should be dimly lit, and spare blankets should be offered to individuals who may experience coldness when sitting for prolonged periods of time.

The measurement of gas exchange allows for the calculation of the respiratory quotient (RQ). ($RQ = CO_2/O_2$). The RQ specifies cellular metabolism and is a reflection of heat production (direct calorimetry). This value is an indication of the fuel mixture being oxidized.[14] Different fuels such as fats, carbohydrates, and proteins require different amounts of oxygen for oxidation to CO_2 and water. Thus, the RQ varies depending on the ratio of fat to carbohydrate in the fuel mixture.[17] In starvation, the major fuel is fat, and the RQ is 0.70. Usually a mixture of fuels (carbohydrate and fat) is oxidized. The various substrates and their RQ values are shown in Table 49.1.

INSTRUMENTATION AVAILABLE

There are two indirect calorimetry systems: open-circuit and closed-circuit systems. Both techniques require devices to measure the concentration of O_2, CO_2, gas volume or flow rate, temperature, and time. In the closed-circuit system, the patient breathes from a reservoir (mixture of gases resembling ambient air), and the decrease in oxygen over time is used to calculate VO_2. Closed-circuit systems are usually simpler in design and less costly than open systems. Open-circuit systems are more versatile and can be more easily used in the clinical setting.[13] The patient breathes from a reservoir of air of known composition in the closed-circuit system; the depletion of oxygen, VCO_2, and VO_2 are calculated.[13] In the open-circuit technique (see Figure 49.2), the patient breathes room air and expires into a gas-sampling system, which eventually vents the expired air back into the room. Open-circuit systems are more commonly used to measure RMR in the clinical setting as they are more versatile and can be used in a variety of clinical conditions. The techniques described in this chapter will therefore focus on the open-circuit indirect calorimetry system.

TYPES OF COLLECTION SYSTEMS

There are many types of accessories that allow for the collection of consumed and expired gases of the person being tested, including face masks, mouthpieces, chambers, and ventilated hoods.

TABLE 49.1

Respiratory Quotient and Energy Content of Various Substrates

Fuel (Substrate)	Energy Content (Kcal μg^{-1})	Respiratory Quotient (RQ)
Carbohydrate	4.1	1.00
Fat	9.3	0.70
Protein	4.3	0.80

Source: Adapted from American College of Sports Medicine. *Guidelines for Exercise Testing and Prescription.* Malvern, PA: Lea and Febiger, 1991, p. 14.

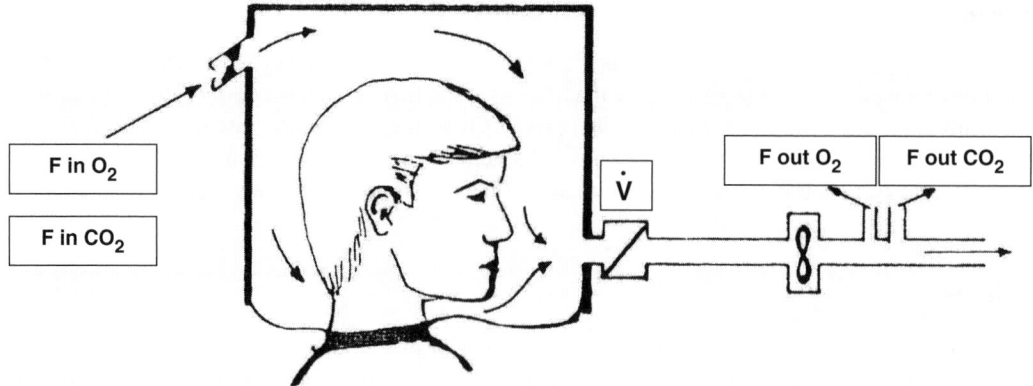

FIGURE 49.2 Open-circuit technique of indirect calorimetry using a canopy hood. Labels: FinO$_2$: forced inspiratory oxygen; FinCO$_2$: forced inspiratory carbon dioxide; gas flow; FoutO$_2$: forced expiratory oxygen; FoutCO$_2$: forced expiratory carbon dioxide. (Reprinted from Ferrannini E, *Metabolism* 37: 296: 1988. ©1988, with permission from Elsevier.)

FACE MASKS

Similar to face masks that are used by firefighters and military personnel, the face mask collection system provides a sealed environment around the nose and mouth of the person in order to collect all gases. The face mask has an elastic head harness that encompasses the back of the head. This device works well for collection of gases; however, these devices do have some drawbacks. The first drawback is that some patients may find a face mask to be invasive and may have difficulty tolerating a face mask being strapped to the head and face. Secondly, if using the face mask collection system, it is important to have several sizes of masks on hand to optimize fit. Although not as comfortable as some of the other collection devices, the face mask is very easily used with portable gas analyzers and is useful for the field settings or where exercise-induced energy expenditure is measured.[18]

MOUTHPIECES

The mouthpiece collection system is similar to a snorkel that is used to allow breathing underwater. The mouthpieces used for RMR measurement are usually identical to those mouthpieces used for maximal VO$_2$ testing in an exercise laboratory. In order for the mouthpiece to be able to work correctly, the subject being tested needs to maintain a tight seal around the mouthpiece and have a nose clip sealing of the nasal passageway. There is a certain amount of discomfort that may be experienced from a static contraction of the jaw muscles to keep a tight seal around the mouthpiece. Therefore, this collection system is not often used to assess RMR.

VENTILATED (CANOPY) HOOD

The ventilated hood is the most widely used collection system. This collection system is advantageous for a number of reasons: it allows for easy spontaneous breathing in apparently healthy individuals, there is no error associated with the facial features such as beard or facial hair of the test subject, it has been found to accurate in long-term measurement of RMR, and it is a relatively noninvasive gas collection system. When using this collection system, a plastic, transparent hood is placed directly over the entire head of the person in a semirecumbent position.

COMPARISON OF COLLECTION DEVICES

There are both advantages and disadvantages for each collection device. In the clinical setting, the ventilated hood may offer a more relaxed and unobtrusive measurement environment. However, for claustrophobic patients, the lights of the laboratory may need to be dimmed to reduce feelings of being confined. The face masks work well for collection of gases; however, structural differences in the size of the face may make it necessary to use different sized masks. Furthermore, facemasks are expensive, and a variety of masks are necessary to achieve valid measurements. Finally, although mouthpieces may seem to have no limitations, patients may find it difficult to achieve a tight seal around the mouthpiece for long periods of time. Moreover, a nose clip must be placed on the patient's nose during measurement to prevent any escape of nonmeasured gas, and this can be unpleasant for the patient as well.

CLINICAL APPLICATIONS AND USEFULNESS OF RMR

Understanding the energy requirement of an individual can be useful in prescribing a personal dietary intake. The interpretation of values produced from RMR measurements should be done by an experienced clinician. Typically, university hospitals and established university weight-loss centers will have access to metabolic carts to perform RMR assessments. An accurate measure of RMR will allow the clinician to tailor the energy intake of the individual (and increase overall energy expenditure via the thermic effect of activity) in order to produce a negative energy balance. This information may also be important in the estimation of TEE. The values of RMR may be multiplied by an activity factor to produce best estimates of TEE, as outlined in the Table 49.2. It may be helpful to get detailed recent exercise histories from patients to help assess the appropriate level of general activity. Bear in mind that most people overestimate their activity levels.

HELPING PATIENTS GAIN WEIGHT

RMR values attained from indirect calorimetry can also be used for certain anabolic circumstances. Often, hospital clinicians will measure RMR in patients suffering from severe burns or frail, elderly patients as a result of the onset of disease. For these instances, the values attained at bedside are important in tailoring meal plans to facilitate weight gain in life-threatening medical situations.

Those individuals seeking to gain weight for performance purposes can also benefit from accurate measures of RMR. Individuals who seek to increase their overall lean body mass (or fat-free mass) may wish to understand how much energy is required above maintenance to produce a safe rate of weight gain. The values attained from RMR in conjunction with counseling on an appropriate activity and exercise program may be helpful to individuals training for body-building or sports performance-related events. Two case studies depicting the usefulness of values attained from assessment or prediction of RMR are contained in the following section.

CASE STUDIES

Person Seeking Weight Loss

A 40-year-old woman with a height of 5′6″ and weight of 185 lb (BMI of 30 kg/m²) seeks to lose 20 lb. This person seeks treatment from a dietician in a hospital that does not have a metabolic cart. Therefore, an equation to predict RMR will be used.

TABLE 49.2
Factors for Estimating Total Daily Energy Needs of Activities for Men and Women (Aged 19 to 50 Years)

Level of General Activity	Activity Factor (Multiplied by REE[a])	Energy Expenditure (Kcal/kg/Day)
Very light		
Men	1.3	31
Women	1.3	30
Light		
Men	1.6	38
Women	1.5	35
Moderate		
Men	1.7	41
Women	1.6	37
Heavy		
Men	2.1	50
Women	1.9	44
Exceptional		
Men	2.4	58
Women	2.2	51

[a] REE = Resting energy expenditure.

Source: Reprinted with permission from Recommended Dietary Allowances, 10th ed., ©1989 by the National Academy of Sciences, courtesy of the National Academies Press, Washington, DC, p. 29. See Heshka S, Feld K, Yang M-U, Allison DB, Heymsfield SB. *J Am Diet Assoc* 93: 1031; 1993 for a comparison of various prediction equations.

Using a prediction equation that has a table with value of kilocalories based on age and gender multiplied by body surface area,[19] the RMR is predicted to be 1498 kcal/day. Furthermore, the woman participates in 30 min of vigorous aerobic exercise on 4 days of the week. Therefore, to determine her predicted TEE, we multiply her RMR by an activity factor that is equal to that of a moderately active person. This activity factor is 1.5. Multiplying 1498 by 1.5 yields a TEE of 2247 kcal/day. To predict a safe rate of weight loss of 1.5 lb/week, the energy intake needs to be restricted by 750 kcal/day, equaling a consumption of approximately 1447 kcal/day (if 3500 kcal equals 1 lb of weight loss).

Person Seeking Weight Gain

A 20-year-old man who is participating in strength and agility training over a 15-week period seeks to gain 15 lb for the start of fall football season. He is 6′5″, weighs 270 lb, and has 18% body fat. Fortunately, he lives near a university hospital that has dieticians who specialize in sports nutrition and also have access to a metabolic cart. When assessed for RMR, the man has a baseline RMR of 2653 kcal/day. The man's training habits, which involve 2 h of strength and agility training each day, warrant that his RMR be multiplied by an activity factor of 1.7. His determined TEE is therefore 4510 kcal/day. However, he seeks to gain weight and not to remain weight stable. Therefore, in order to predict an average of 1 lb of weight gain per week, the man needs to ingest 500 kcal/day more than his predicted TEE. This value is equal to 5010 kcal/day.

PREDICTING RMR

As direct measurement of RMR is often not available to those outside a hospital setting, clinicians can use prediction equations to estimate RMR as an alternative. These prediction equations have mostly been developed using regression analysis to fit functions according to gender, age, height, weight, and other available clinical variables.[20] A majority of these equations were developed using normal-weight persons who were relatively sedentary. Unfortunately, this poses a problem when predicting RMR in the obese population, considering that RMR is correlated with the fat-free mass (FFM) of the individual[21–25] and that the obese person has a larger distribution of adipose tissue and a decreased proportion of FFM when compared with their normal-weight counterparts.[26] Furthermore, although some prediction equations have worked well when comparing the estimated RMR with actual values in large samples, there may be large individual errors when using these equations.[27] Some of these equations used for the prediction of RMR for the normal-weight and overweight populations are contained in Table 49.3.

HARRIS–BENNEDICT EQUATION

For normal-weight individuals (determined by BMI or body composition analysis), the prediction equation of Harris and Bennedict[30] is appropriate:

$$\text{For Men: kcal/day} = 66.4730 + 13.751W + 5.0033L - 6.750A$$

$$\text{For Women: kcal/day} = 655.0955 + 9.563W + 1.8496L - 4.6756A$$

where W = weight (kg); L = height (cm); and A = age (years).

These equations were developed in 1919 and are currently widely used by clinicians. However, as these equations rely so heavily on body weight as a function of predicting RMR, they may overestimate RMR in obese individuals.[27] Furthermore, given the increased prevalence of overweight in industrialized countries such as the United States,[36] it is important for the clinician to use prediction equations that have been validated using overweight persons.[37]

ROBERTSON–REID AND FLEISCH EQUATIONS

Three prediction equations may potentially offer reasonable predictions of RMR for the overweight patient. The prediction equations of Robertson and Reid[19] and Fleisch[31] have been recommended for obese populations.[20] The Robertson–Reid and Fleisch equations will be presented in this section as viable prediction equations for the obese patient. For the Robertson–Reid equation, predicted RMR was derived from the actual measurement of RMR of 987 men and 1323 women aged 3 to 80 years. The equation requires that the clinician find a value for heat output (in table form) based on the patient's age and gender. Subsequently, this value is multiplied by the body surface area of the person (in m^2) to determine kcal/h; this number is then multiplied by 24 to yield daily RMR. The basis of this prediction equation is that there is constant heat output that corresponds to surface area within people that are the same gender and age:

$$\text{RMR in kcal/day} = \text{Heat output in kcal} \times \text{Body surface area in m}^2 \times 24 \text{ h}$$

$$\text{Heat output} = \text{Value derived for men and women from a table developed by Robertson and Reid}[19]$$

$$\text{Body surface area (BSA)} = [0.007184 \times (\text{weight in kg})]^{0.425} \times (\text{height in cm})^{0.725}$$

$$\text{Time} = 24 \text{ h}$$

TABLE 49.3
Equations for Estimating Resting Metabolic Rate (RMR) in kcal/24 h[a]

Reference	Equations	Reference
Bernstein, et al.	W: 7.48(kg) − 0.42(cm) − 3.0(year) + 844	120
	M: 11.0(kg) + 10.2(cm) − 5.8(year) − 1,032	
Cunningham	501.6 + 21.6 (LBM); where	121
	for W: LBM = [69.8 − 0.26(kg) − 0.12(year)] × kg/73.2	
	for M: LBM = [79.5 − 0.24(kg) − 0.15(year)] × kg/73.2	
Harris and Benedict	W: 655 + 9.5(kg) + 1.9(cm) − 4.7(year)	28
	M: 66 + 13.8(kg) + 5.0(cm) − 6.8(year)	
Fleisch[a]	W/M: kcal/m^2 of BSA from Fleisch table × [[0.007184 × (kg)]$^{0.425}$ × (cm)$^{0.725}$] × 24	31
James	W: 18–30 year: 487 + 14.8(kg)	122
	30–60 year: 845 + 8.17(kg)	
	>60 year: 658 + 9.01(kg)	
	M: 18–30 year: 692 + 15.1(kg)	
	30–60 year: 873 + 11.6(kg)	
	>60 year: 588 + 11.7(kg)	
Mifflin, et al.	W: 9.99(kg) + 6.25(cm) − 4.92(year) − 161	32
	M: 9.99(kg) + 6.25(cm) − 4.92(year) + 5	
Owen, et al.	W: 795 + 7.18(kg)	123
	M: 879 + 10.2(kg)	
Pavlou, et al.	M: −169.1 + 1.02(pRMR)	124
Robertson and Reid[a]	W/M: kcals/m^2 of BSA from Robertson and Reid table × [[0.007184 × (kg)]$^{0.425}$ × (cm)$^{0.725}$] × 24	19

W = Women, M = Men, pRMR = predicted RMR from the Harris and Benedict equation.

[a] This equation uses tabled values for kcal/m^2.

Source: Reprinted from Heshka S, Feld K, Yang M-U, Allison DB, Heymsfield SB. *J Am Diet Assoc* 93: 1033; 1993. ©1993, with permission from American Dietetic Association.

The equation of Fleisch uses the same concept as the Robertson and Reid equation. However, the values of heat output differ, and Fleisch provides a separate table to calculate the predicted RMR.[31] The Fleisch equation is as follows:

$$\text{RMR in kcal/day} = \text{kcal/m}^2 \text{ of BSA from Fleisch table}^{31} \times [[0.007184 \times (kg)]^{0.425} \times (cm)^{0.725}] \times 24$$

MIFFLIN, ET AL. EQUATION

A third prediction equation for the obese population comes from Mifflin, et al.[33] This equation was derived using linear regression analysis on a subset of patients (247 females, 251 males) who had their RMRs measured using indirect calorimetry. In an unpublished research study at the Johns Hopkins University School of Medicine, the equation has provided predicted RMR values in obese patients at a university weight-loss center that are not different than those produced by actual measurement. Furthermore, a systematic review of the accuracy of some of the more popular RMR prediction equations revealed that the Mifflin, et al. equation was the most reliable equation to predict RMR within 10% of measured values in obese individuals.[38] The equation is as follows:

$$\text{RMR in kcal/day (men)} = 9.99(kg) + 6.25(cm) − 4.92(\text{years of age}) + 5$$

$$\text{RMR in kcal/d (women)} = 9.99(kg) + 6.25(cm) − 4.92(\text{years of age}) − 161$$

PRETESTING PROCEDURES FOR MEASUREMENT OF RMR

The testing procedures for determining RMR necessitate that a strict protocol be followed to ensure that the measurement of RMR is accurate. Individuals should be provided with pretesting requirements prior to RMR measurement. The subject should be questioned about his/her adherence to the pretest procedures prior to performing the assessment. If one or more of these procedures are not followed, the individual should be rescheduled at a later date to reduce measurement error.

WEIGHT STABLE

If the subject has experienced recent weight loss, the measurement of RMR may not be valid. The measurement of RMR should be avoided if the person being tested has lost weight from weight-loss efforts or prolonged sickness, or if he or she has gained more than 1 lb in the past week. To reduce error associated with physiological responses to weight loss, a period of weight stabilization of 2 weeks is necessary prior to an RMR assessment.

WELL RESTED

RMR measurement should be administered as close to the time a person awakes as possible. Additionally, the individual being tested should get a restful night's sleep prior to coming to the clinic or hospital for testing. If an individual sleeps poorly on the night prior to the assessment of RMR, confounding environmental influences may unduly increase the metabolic expenditure of the individual. Measurement should occur before 10:00 a.m.; measurements taken in the late morning may be suspect to increased metabolic activity.

FASTED

Measurements should be taken first thing in the morning after a 12 h overnight fast.[39] A light meal the night before measurement should be encouraged; RMR is the energy expended at rest in a fasted state, and therefore any lasting effects of food or drink would add additional energy expenditure from diet-induced thermogenesis. Early morning coffee or tea should be avoided, and only minimal amounts of water can be ingested prior to measurement. Clinicians can determine if the patient is fasting by examining the RQ values during testing.

MEASUREMENT IN RELATION TO LAST EXERCISE BOUT

Testing performed at least 24 h after rest from exercise has been shown to eliminate any residual effects from the most recent training session.[40] Hence, the person being testing should be instructed to abstain from programmed exercise for at least a day prior to measurement of RMR.

LOCATION AND ACCLIMATION TO THE TESTING ENVIRONMENT

Studies have shown that there are no differences in measurements of RMR performed with or without an inpatient overnight stay.[6] Therefore, to avoid excessive costs associated with inpatient stays, an outpatient procedure is usually recommended. Upon arrival at the lab where the RMR assessment will occur, the individual should be instructed to rest in a sedentary supine or semirecumbent position for at least 30 min prior to the assessment. During this time, the person should remain still. The subject should be asked if they have to void, as it is necessary that they are comfortable during the entire test. Some laboratories will further acclimatize the individual by placing the collection system (canopy hood) over of the subject to ensure that he or she is comfortable with the measurement setting.

ANALYSIS

The metabolic cart will often express resting metabolic rate as the mean of multiple minute measurements. However, the cart will also provide continuous measurements of VO_2 and VCO_2 each minute. Many researchers suggest that the calculation of RMR be the average of five of these continuous minute measurements of steady state.[24,41] Steady state is 5 min of measurement of VO_2 and VCO_2 that possess an intravariability of 5% or less.[41]

Table 49.4 is a simple checklist to ensure that the assessment of RMR is valid.

FACTORS AFFECTING RMR

A variety of factors have been shown to influence RMR, including genetics, age, gender, total body weight, fat-free weight, aerobic fitness level, total energy flux through the body, body and/or environmental temperature, hormonal factors, drugs, and stress.[42] Of these factors, the strongest correlation exists between an individual's FFM and RMR,[42] and collectively, FFM, age, sex and physical activity account for 80 to 90% of the variance in RMR.[43]

EXERCISE

As exercise training has been associated with increases in FFM, this is one factor that can be manipulated to potentiate resting metabolism. Some cross-sectional studies have demonstrated that aerobically trained individuals have higher RMRs for their metabolic size than their untrained counterparts.[44–47] More recently, a study investigating men and women aged 20 to 75 years

TABLE 49.4
Checklist for RMR Testing

Pretesting Subject Requirements

- 12 h Fast. Water is allowed ad libitum
- Refrain from strenuous physical activity/exercise for 48 h prior to testing
- Well Rested. Make sure subject has at least 8 h of sleep
- Minimize activity the morning of test. Light grooming allowed. Shower the night prior
- Keep food diaries for 48 h prior to testing. Dinner meal should be <1000 kcal night prior

Laboratory Requirements

- Room should be isolated to reduce any external noise
- Room should be dimly lit, but not dark
- Temperature should be controlled and ideally at 22°C to 24°C. Blankets should be used if subject is cold
- The bed or comfortable chair should be semi-recumbent and not flat; having a slight incline of approximately 10°

Testing Procedures

- Monitor subject during testing. Direct subject to avoid any: talking, fidgeting, and sleeping
- Acclimate patient to test. Possibly perform practice test prior to actual procedure
- Rest subject in semi-recumbent position for at least 30 min prior to testing
- If able to, use HR monitor to track HR the day before, morning of and during test

Authors would like to thank Dr. Jack Wilmore for the helpful suggestions for the RMR checklist.

involved in 24 weeks of strength training showed an absolute increase in RMR of 7% after 24 weeks of training.[48] This increase in RMR remained statistically significant even after adjusting for FFM. However, when analyzing men and women separately, women showed no overall increase in RMR after the strength-training program, while the men increased RMR by 9%.[48]

AGE

Age is another variable that has been found to have a significant impact on an individual's resting metabolism. In fact, the decline in RMR is one of the most consistent physiological changes that occur with age.[49] Recent studies have suggested a curvilinear reduction in RMR with advancing age that is accelerated beyond middle age and postmenopausal years.[49] Several studies attribute the age-related decline in RMR primarily to the loss of FFM that often accompanies aging; however, there remains uncertainty whether other physiological factors may also contribute to the reduction of RMR.[49] The term sarcopenia describes the condition in which profound changes in body composition (increased fat mass, decreased FFM, and decreased strength) occur.[50] The hormonal changes associated with sarcopenia are not well understood, but researchers suggest that the effects of sarcopenia can occur as early as the fourth decade of life in humans.[51] The effects of sarcopenia may be a function of decreased RMR, secondary to decreased activity levels and onset of various diseases.[51]

GENDER

Gender differences in resting metabolism have also been reported, with males having a higher RMR by approximately 50 kcal/day than females.[43] This difference is independent of the gender difference in FFM, and is consistent across the life span.[43] Menopausal status has also been pinpointed as an influence on RMR in women. Studies have found lower RMR in postmenopausal women relative to premenopausal women, which was again primarily attributable to reductions in lean mass and a decline in aerobic fitness.[49,52]

RACE

Information on the effect of race on RMR has been mixed. In a cross-sectional study by Jakacic and Wing,[53] obese (BMI = 32.6 kg/m^2) African-American women had significantly lower RMRs than their Caucasian counterparts, even after adjusting for body weight and FFM. A more recent cross-sectional study by Jones and colleagues in 2004 found that RMR was lower in African-American women compared with Caucasian women in a group of 521 moderately overweight individuals (BMI = 25.5 kg/m^2).[54] In this particular study,[54] although the African-American women had RMRs that were approximately 38 kcal/day less than the Caucasian women, RMRs of the two groups were not statistically different. One explanation for ethnic differences between African-American and Caucasian women may be a discrepancy in heat-producing tissues and organs between races, and these differences actually may increase as a function of age.[54] In one particular study, researchers have discovered that African-American women actually have greater amounts of low-metabolic-rate skeletal muscle and bone than their Caucasian counterparts.[54] Interestingly, when Glass and colleagues examined physiological changes in a small cohort of African-American and Caucasian women after a 13-week diet and exercise behavior modification program, they observed no differences between the races for the changes in RMR accompanying weight loss.[55]

ENVIRONMENT

Environmental factors may also influence RMR, with people in tropical climates typically experiencing RMRs of 5 to 20% higher than that of their counterparts living in more temperate areas.[56] Cold climates also have a significant impact on RMR that is dependent on an individual's body fat content and the amount and type of clothing worn.[56] During extreme cold stress at rest, metabolic rate can double or triple with shivering as the body attempts to maintain a stable core temperature.[56]

CIGARETTE SMOKING

Some studies have also documented the influence of substances such as cigarettes, caffeine, alcohol, and certain medications on RMR. Many laypersons believe that cigarette smoking may be helpful in maintaining body weight,[57] and many smokers are unwilling to quit because of their fear of weight gain. Over time, studies have demonstrated that the increase in metabolic rate resulting from cigarette smoking is transient.[57] In a recent cross-sectional study of 374 women by Clemens, et al., the women who smoked cigarettes had significantly higher RMRs compared with their nonsmoking counterparts.[58] Furthermore, another study found no effect in habitual smokers when assessment of RMR did not begin until 25 to 30 min after smoking. Thus, it is thought that the acute metabolic effects of cigarettes are not significant beyond 30 min after smoking. Yet, given the typical ~30 min between cigarettes for most smokers, RMR may remain slightly elevated throughout the day as a result of these "acute" effects.[57]

CAFFEINE

Caffeine has been identified as a substance that elevates metabolic rate, and caffeine ingestion has also been shown to increase work performance and promote lipid oxidation during prolonged exercise.[59–61] In a study investigating the influence of caffeine on the RMR of exercise-trained and inactive subjects found that metabolic rate was increased in response to a stimulus of approximately two cups of coffee (300 mg).[59] This study also compared regular and nonregular caffeine consumers to investigate the effects of consumption levels on metabolic response. This investigation confirmed previous findings that, with regular consumption, the physiological and stimulatory effects of caffeine were not diminished.[59]

ALCOHOL

Alcohol is another substance that has been found to influence RMR. Alcohol is decidedly the most commonly consumed psychoactive drug in the United States, and because of its energy density, it is widely believed to be a causal factor in the development and maintenance of obesity.[62] However, in a study utilizing data gathered in two national cross-sectional surveys — the Second National Health and Nutrition Examination Survey (NHANES II; $n = 10929$) and the Behavioral Risk Factor Surveys (BRFS; $n = 18388$) — it was found that alcohol consumption had a slight negative effect on the body weights of men and a profound negative effect on the body weights of women.[62,63] This negative effect was not a result of lowered dietary intake among drinkers. In fact, in controlled isoenergetic dietary studies, subjects tended to lose weight on alcohol-containing regimens.[64,65] This has lead to the hypothesis that alcohol intake may increase REE.[62] Early studies found inconsistent evidence regarding the effects of alcohol on REE.[62,66] However, recent studies have found evidence in support of the hypothesis that alcohol may increase REE,[62,67] although further investigations are needed to explain the mechanism by which alcohol suppresses body weight.[62]

MEDICATIONS

Medications are also known to have an impact on resting metabolism. Beta-blocking medications, for example, are prescribed to several million Americans with cardiovascular disease to treat conditions such as hypertension and angina.[68] Unfortunately, despite their widespread use in medical practice, beta-blocking medications have many side effects. One such side effect is the influence on RMR. Research indicates that RMR and, perhaps, the energy needs of individuals treated with beta-blockers are reduced.[68] The magnitude of this reduction in RMR has been found to vary between 8% and 17%.[68] One study reported a reduction in RMR of approximately 17% or 4 kcal/kg/day in a group of healthy subjects taking 80 mg twice daily of propranolol for 5 days.[68] This could result in significant weight gain in a patient receiving beta-blockers long term if no changes were made to both dietary and exercise habits.[68]

RMR AND WEIGHT LOSS

America currently has a preoccupation with weight loss, and as a result, for many years scientists have been interested in identifying interventions that might attenuate the drop in RMR that accompanies weight reduction in overweight and obese patient populations.[42] Factors causing a decrease in RMR would make weight maintenance or weight loss difficult, or possibly result in weight gain. Conversely, anything that increases RMR would potentially facilitate weight loss and maintenance of the weight that is lost.[69]

Energy restriction and RMR

Over the past decade, there has been a dramatic increase in the prevalence of overweight and obesity in adults as well as children and adolescents. Using data from the most recent National Health and Nutrition Examination Survey (NHANES Continuous; 1999–2000),[70] it has been reported that 64.5% of U.S. adults are overweight (BMI ≥ 25 kg/m^2) and 30.5% of U.S. adults are obese (BMI ≥ 30 kg/m^2). These data represent an increase in the prevalence of obesity of approximately 8% since the Third National Health and Nutrition Survey (NHANES III; 1988 to 1994)[71] was conducted less than 10 years previously.[70] Paradoxically, dieting has become a way of life for many Americans. In a study utilizing data from the 1996 state-based Behavioral Risk Factor Surveillance System, it was reported that 28.8% and 43.6% of men and women, respectively, trying to lose weight at any given time.[72] Researchers have been exploring the consequences of dieting — particularly those related to changes in the RMR.[41] Several investigators have found that a restrictive diet depresses RMR,[26,41,73] which may contribute to the regaining of weight that is often observed after treatment. One such study found that the RMR among obese individuals decreased during a protein-sparing modified fast, and remained depressed for 2 months after treatment despite increased energy consumption to a level that allowed body weight stabilization.[73] Similar findings were reported by Heshka, et al.[26] in participants of a conservative weight-loss program. It was found that RMR declined to a greater degree than would be expected from loss of lean mass alone.[26] Other investigators have found no adverse effects on RMR, and have concluded that any decline in RMR is fully explained by an anticipated reduction in FFM accompanying weight loss.[41] A study examining the short-term and long-term effects of very-low-calorie diets (VLCDs) observed a 17.3% decrease from baseline of resting metabolism after patients consumed 500 kcal/day for just 2 weeks.[74] This reduction in RMR was associated with a weight reduction of only 5.8%. There was, however, an observed rebound in RMR accompanying the patients' return to a 1000 to 1200 kcal/day balanced diet, and the 11% end-of-treatment decline in RMR was paralleled by a 12% reduction in body weight.[74]

It appears that RMR declines rapidly in response to severe energy restriction. Reductions as great as 30% have been reported in some individuals.[42] In a study by Das and colleagues, a group of extremely obese women who underwent gastric bypass surgery, which produces caloric restriction and significant weight reduction, experienced an average decrease in RMR of 573 kcal/day after 14 months of postsurgery weight loss (53 kg).[75] In other weight reduction strategies, very-low-energy diets have been found to be associated with substantial short-term reductions in RMR.[41] This decline, however, appears to be attributable primarily to the caloric restriction, and is largely reversed when dieting is stopped.[41] With weight stability, reductions in RMR have been found to be modest, and are highly related to the changes in FFM.[41] It is thought that physical activity, energy deficit, macronutrient distribution, and rate of weight loss may be key factors in the retention of FFM and, by extension, RMR.

Exercise and RMR

Many effects of exercise are thought to be beneficial to weight loss and weight maintenance. A single bout of exercise produces an increase in energy expenditure, the magnitude of which is dependent on the intensity, duration, and type of exercise.[21] Weight-bearing activities such as walking, jogging, and cross-country skiing lead to energy expenditure that is directly related to body weight, and may be of particular benefit to obese individuals.[21] Muscle-strengthening exercises may give an added advantage by maintaining or increasing muscle mass. Some investigators have proposed a carryover effect of exercise on metabolic rate; however, if any long-term effect exists, it is thought to only occur after very vigorous and sustained physical activity.[21]

Both resistance and endurance training have, therefore, been proposed as interventions that might enhance RMR to facilitate weight loss in overweight and obese patient populations. Findings from several cross-sectional studies have indicated that athletes and active individuals demonstrate a higher RMR than sedentary individuals, and training studies indicate that sedentary individuals who are not restricting energy can increase their RMR by beginning a regular exercise program.[5,76] Despite these findings, the research literature regarding the effects of resistance and endurance training, separately or in combination, on elevating the RMR is mixed, and whether exercise training enhances RMR remains a controversial question.[40]

Resistance Training and RMR

Resistance training is thought to have the potential to increase RMR by increasing FFM.[40] This belief is founded on the significant relation between FFM and RMR. Heavy resistance training promotes skeletal muscle development, which could have a favorable impact on a person's RMR by increasing the total amount of metabolically active tissue (FFM).[42] However, the extent to which resistance training is able to increase RMR has not been well documented, and studies evaluating the impact of high-intensity resistance exercise on body composition and other physiological adaptations during weight loss have reported inconsistent findings. In a study by Lemmer, et al.,[48] RMR increased after 24 weeks of strength training for young and older men, whereas the young and older women in the intervention experienced no increase in RMR. In contrast, in a different longitudinal study by Broeder, et al. comparing the effects of strength training and aerobic exercise on body composition, body weight, and RMR in healthy, nondieting young men, the resistance training was associated with increased strength and FFM, but body weight and RMR did not change significantly.[42] These findings by Broeder, et al. were corroborated by a similar study with untrained female subjects in whom a statistically significant increase in RMR was not observed despite favorable alterations in body composition.[24] Further studies of longer duration are needed to determine whether a significant increase in RMR would be observed with a longer resistance-training program.[24]

Endurance Training and RMR

Physical activity, especially in the form of endurance exercise, significantly affects energy intake and expenditure, and is therefore a key regulatory component in the energy balance equation.

After exercise, oxygen consumption decreases rapidly, but may remain above resting levels for several hours or even days after the bout of activity.[5] The repair of damaged muscle tissue and the resynthesis of substrates such as creatine phosphate (CP), ATP, and glycogen partially account for the excessive postexercise oxygen uptake (EPOC) in the exercised muscles, and may be the cause of the elevated muscle oxygen uptake in recovery. Bullough[77] reported that RMR was greater in trained than in untrained subjects only when trained subjects were in a state of recovery from vigorous exercise. Their data indicate that RMR is influenced by exercise, energy intake, and their interaction. They suggest that higher RMR in trained vs. untrained individuals results from acute effects of high-intensity exercise rather than from a chronic adaptation to exercise training.

Phelain, et al.[77] have examined the effects of low- and high-intensity aerobic exercise of similar energy output on postexercise energy expenditure and substrate oxidation in fit eumenorrheic women. They used continuous indirect calorimetry performed during cycle ergometry exercise and for 3 h after low-intensity exercise (500 kcal at 50% VO_2 max) or high-intensity exercise (500 kcal at 75% VO_2 max). Mean EPOC for the 3 h postexercise period for high-intensity exercise (9.0 ± 1.7 l, 41 kcal) was significantly greater than that for the lower-intensity activity (4.8 ± 1.6 l, 22 kcal). Oxygen consumption (VO_2) following the higher-intensity exercise remained elevated at the end of the 3 h postexercise period, but not so with the low-intensity group. Quinn, et al.[78] reported that exercise duration increases EPOC significantly and that a 60 min bout of aerobic exercise duration yields approximately twice the EPOC than either 20 or 40 min in trained younger women. However, Almuzaini, et al.[79] examined the effects of splitting a 30 min exercise bout of cycling into two equal sessions vs. a single uninterrupted session. They compared the affects of these two exercise trials on EPOC and RMR and concluded that dividing a 30 min exercise session in two parts for these individuals significantly increases magnitude of EPOC but does not affect RMR.

Short and Sedlock[80] also found that fit individuals have faster regulation of postexercise metabolism when exercising at either the same relative or absolute work rate than their untrained counterparts. In another investigation, Gillette and colleagues[81] compared strenuous resistive exercise to steady state endurance exercise of similar estimated energy cost. They found that the resistance training resulted in greater excess postexercise VO_2 compared with the aerobic exercise.

There is minimal information about EPOC affects after engaging in moderate intensity physical activity. However, results from a recently conducted small pilot study (seven younger women) by Imamura and colleagues showed that modest increases in EPOC can accompany 30 to 60 min of moderate-intensity exercise such as stationary cycling.[82] Future studies investigating postexercise energy expenditure may want to further examine the degree of EPOC after moderate-intensity activity, considering that public health guidelines often advocate [83] engaging in moderate-intensity lifestyle activity.

Energy Restriction Combined with Exercise Training: The Effects on RMR

The National Institutes of Health[84] and the American College of Sports Medicine[85] have stressed the importance of including exercise as part of a comprehensive weight management program. Additionally, in clinical practice, exercise when used alone has not been viewed as an optimal method of weight reduction.[86] This may be attributed, in part, to the difficulty many patients have in maintaining an appropriate program of physical activity.

A meta-analysis was conducted to examine how exercise training and gender influence the composition of diet-induced weight loss.[87] The study revealed that diet-plus-exercise (DPE) training groups did not differ from dietary-restriction-only (DO) groups with respect to either the amount of body weight lost (mean = −10 ± 1.4 kg) or fat mass lost (mean = −8 ± 1.1 kg). Exercise training, however, attenuated the amount of body weight lost as FFM compared with DO for the same sex. The percentage of weight lost as FFM for DPE subjects was approximately half ($p < .05$) of that for DO subjects of the same sex. The DO males lost 28 ± 4% of weight as FFM, wheras DPE males lost 13 ± 6%. The DO females lost 24 ± 2% of their weight from lean mass compared with the DPE females, who only lost 11 ± 3% of their weight from the FFM. These data provide evidence that exercise training reduces the amount of FFM lost during diet-induced weight loss. In addition, gender differences do not seem to exist with respect to body composition changes of weight reduction.

The decline of RMR in response to energy restriction has been well documented, and is suspected to decrease the rate of weight loss during periods of energy restriction.[88] Exercise is frequently advocated in the treatment of obesity as a means of increasing energy expenditure and potentially counteracting the negative effects of dietary restriction.[22] Several studies based on the addition of a component of exercise to dietary restriction have been published.[21,22,86,89,90] Some studies have continued to report similar decreases in RMR, whereas others have shown an attenuation of the decrement or an increase in RMR when an element of exercise was added.

Energy Restriction Combined with Resistance Training: The Effects on RMR

In theory, strength training should attenuate the decline of RMR if it preserves FFM by preventing atrophy of skeletal muscle. Skeletal muscle composes more than 50% of the FFM of the body.[90] It is for this reason that resistance training was initially added to weight-loss programs: to reduce or prevent the loss of muscle during energy restriction, which, in theory, should attenuate the drop in RMR typically seen with weight loss.

Few studies have been conducted that combined diet and heavy resistance exercise, and the studies evaluating the impact of high-intensity resistance exercise on body composition and other physiological adaptations during weight loss have reported inconsistent findings.[86] Conflicting results regarding the impact dietary restriction combined with resistance training has on lean body mass have been reported. An additional problem in evaluating the impact of resistance training is the fact that many investigators fail to examine all the physiological variables of interest simultaneously. Two studies incorporating strength training during energy restriction found contradictory results. One study reported an increase in FFM (RMR was not measured),[90,91] whereas the second found no effect of strength training on FFM or RMR, indicating that there are no advantages of a resistance-training program to maintenance of lean body mass and attenuating reductions in RMR.[90,92] The lack of an effect on FFM in this study may have been attributable to the relatively low energy intake of 522 kcal/day overriding the potential benefits of strength training.[90]

In the case of VLCDs, a limited number of studies have combined resistance training with a VLCD.[93] Most studies have found that incorporating resistance training into the very-low-energy diet regimen does not attenuate the loss of FFM or decrease in RMR.[93] It has, however, been reported that significant muscle hypertrophy is possible in an individual undergoing severe energy restriction.[93,94] Hypertrophy was observed only in the exercised muscles, and resistance training was unable to prevent the loss of overall FFM any better than diet alone.[93,94] In a study comparing the benefits of aerobic and resistance training when combined with an 800 kcal liquid diet, it was found that the addition of an intensive, high-volume resistance-training program resulted in preservation of FFM and RMR during weight loss.[93]

The results of studies examining both moderate and severe dietary energy restriction have led to the following hypothesis: there may be a minimum level of dietary intake necessary for significant muscle hypertrophy to occur with resistance training.[93] Researchers have reported that a dietary intake of at least 1000 to 1500 kcal/day is required to attain the positive benefits that exercise training can have on RMR and FFM.[93,95,96] Further studies are therefore necessary to determine whether a diet adequate in protein, fiber, and vitamins and minerals, but low in total energy, can help mediate the expected chronic adaptations to heavy resistance training.[86]

Caloric Restriction Combined with Endurance Training: The Effects on RMR

Aerobic exercise not only increases energy expenditure but may also minimize the reductions in RMR that accompany dieting by potentially increasing sympathetic nervous system activity.[91,95,97] It has also been found to attenuate the loss of FFM.[91,98] In turn, this may prevent reduction in RMR. Several studies examined the effects of incorporating endurance training into weight-loss regimens, with the hypothesis that its addition would attenuate losses of FFM and, by extension, reductions in RMR.[97] Studies have documented favorable effects of aerobic activity on REE in participants who consumed diets providing 1200 to 1500 kcal/day.[97,99–101] In a study designed to examine the effects of diet and exercise training on RMR, participants were placed on a program combining moderate energy restriction and supervised aerobic exercise.[99] It was found that REE, when adjusted for body weight, increased 10% in this group of obese women.[99] In another study examining the effects of exercise on weight, body composition, REE, appetite, and mood in obese women, it was found that participants who consumed diets providing 1200 to 1500 kcal/day and engaged in aerobic activity experienced favorable changes in REE.[97] In addition, the study confirmed the findings of previous investigators regarding the effect of aerobic training in participants consuming VLCDs.[102,103] When participants were prescribed a 925 kcal/day diet, there was no effect of aerobic training on REE. However, when participants terminated their marked dietary energy restriction, a positive effect was observed.[97] In contrast, there have been studies that have found no attenuation of the reduction in RMR in patients consuming a balanced deficit diet consisting of 1200 to 1500 kcal/day. Our laboratory recently examined the physiologic changes after weight reduction with vigorous exercise and moderate-intensity physical activity and found that there were no differences between groups in decreases in RMR.[104] In this study, vigorous aerobic activity did not attenuate reductions in RMR in patients consuming a self-selected diet.[104] The percentage change in RMR for each type of exercise intervention is shown for both men and women in Figure 49.3.

There have also been studies that have failed to find positive effects on RMR of aerobic training in participants consuming VLCDs. In fact, one study found that participants who exercised vigorously while consuming 720 kcal/day had significantly greater reductions in RMR than did nonexercising dieters.[102] Similar findings were reported by Heymsfield, et al.[103] This reduction

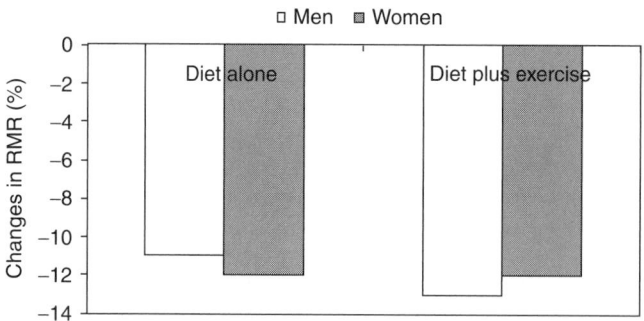

FIGURE 49.3 Changes in resting metabolic rate following a 12-week intervention of diet plus aerobic exercise training or diet plus life-style physical activity. (Data adapted from Andersen RE, et al. *Metabolism* 51: 1528; 2002.)

in RMR appears to be a consequence of compounding the marked caloric deficit introduced by the VLCD with that introduced by exercise.[97] It has therefore been suggested that the most favorable findings for both RMR and FFM are obtained when exercise was combined with diets of 1000 to 1500 kcal/day rather than with VLCDs providing 400 to 800 kcal/day.[97]

THERMOGENESIS

Thermogenesis and Obesity

There is no strong evidence that alterations in thermogenesis contribute to obesity. Thermogenesis, excluding RMR and TEA, only contributes roughly 10% to TEE. Thermic effect of food is the majority of this 10%, which has been reported to be slightly decreased in obese compared with lean subjects in some,[105–111] but not all, studies.[112,113] More importantly, it is not known whether alterations in TEF promoted the obese state, or whether the obese state promotes alterations in TEF. Insight into this question arises from investigations on subjects before and after weight reduction. When subjects are studied after weight loss, TEF is either not different from that of age-matched lean subjects[114] or partially normalized,[115] suggesting that decreased TEF is a result of weight gain and not a causative factor in the development of obesity. Therefore, it is unlikely that alterations in thermogenesis can explain the increased prevalence of obesity today.

Thermogenesis, NEAT, and Alterations in Daily Energy Expenditure

Thermogenesis induced by drugs, food consumption, or cold exposure is of questionable importance in determing TEE because of their transient nature and the relatively small effect on increasing whole-body oxygen consumption. However, fidgeting behavior has recently been described and may contribute significantly to enhance TEE.[116] Levine, et al.[116] quantified energy expenditure during 8 weeks of overfeeding by 1000 kcal/day in 16 nonobese men. The authors of this study coined this energy expenditure nonexercise activity thermogenesis (NEAT) to account for energy expenditure not associated with TEA or TEF. This term was described previously in the section on components of metabolism. Interestingly, the authors reported that changes in NEAT predicted resistance to fat gain during overfeeding (a negative correlation between fat gain and change in activity thermogenesis or NEAT, $r = -.077$; $p < .001$), while no relationship was observed between fat gain and changes in TEF or RMR.[116] The NEAT exhibited marked intravariability and may partially explain why some individuals are more susceptible to obesity than others. An additional study by Levine, et al. investigated the increase in energy expenditure associated with fidgeting in addition to sitting and standing.[9] The increases in energy expenditure above the resting state for fidgeting activities were also quite variable. However, fidgeting while sitting resulted in approximately 37 kcal/h (2.6 kJ/min) more than fidgeting alone in the 24 men and women who were either normal or overweight.[9] Fidgeting while standing resulted in 60 more kcal/h (4.2 kJ/min) beyond that of standing.[9] The increases in energy expenditure above the resting state associated with sitting, standing, and fidgeting for Levine, et al.'s study are presented in Figure 49.4.

Currently, there is no conclusive idea of what determines the magnitude of NEAT, or why such a wide variability may exist from person to person.[116] However, NEAT is an interesting avenue for future research, which may suggest possible lifestyle interventions or drug targets, which could increase the various types of NEAT and promote greater TEE. One should not discount the importance of energy expended by NEAT activities. There has been interesting research on the topic; Levine, et al.[117] have performed a study investigating the energetics of gum chewing, a component of NEAT. The authors reported that gum chewing increased energy expenditure by 11 kcal/h, a 20% increase over RMR. If gum chewing occurred during the waking hours throughout the day with no other lifestyle changes, the authors predicted weight loss of up to 5 kg of body weight in one year. Thus, NEAT activities increase energy expenditure only slightly, but may have important implications for long-term energy balance.

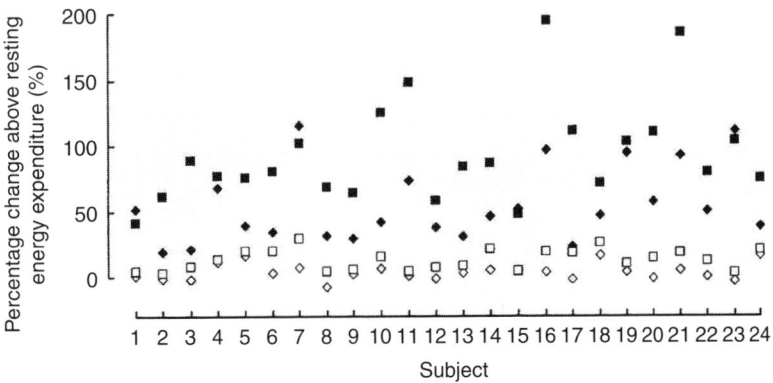

FIGURE 49.4 Percentage change in energy expenditure above resting values while sitting motionless (◇), partaking of fidgeting-like activities while sitting (◆), standing motionless (□), and partaking of fidgeting-like activities while standing (■) in 24 healthy subjects (subjects 1 to 7 were men, subjects 8 to 24 were women). (From Levine JA, Schleusner SJ, Jenson MD. *Am J Clin Nutr* 72: 1451; 2000. Reproduced with permission. © Am *J Clin Nutr.* American Society for Nutrition.)

Furthermore, the latest study by Levine and colleagues examined the individual variation in energy expended via the posture allocation in sitting and standing for both lean and obese persons.[1] Interestingly, during a 10-day baseline period, lean subjects stood for 152 more min/day than their overweight counterparts. After asking the overweight subjects to lose weight for 8 weeks and the lean subjects to gain weight (overfeed) for 8 weeks, the researchers observed no change in postural allocation in the initially lean and obese groups for a follow-up 10-day assessment of NEAT. The authors of the study suggest that this may be an indicator that the postural allocation of NEAT may actually be biologically determined.[1]

Thermic effect of food has the largest influence in dictating changes in TEE excluding physical activity and NEAT. However, diet composition is the most influential moderator of TEF, more so than age, gender, or weight.[113,118–123] Thus, differences between individuals in TEF are mostly due to alterations in macronutrient composition of the diet and have very small effects on changing TEE. It is therefore unlikely that alterations in TEF alone are responsible for changes in TEE in most people. Rather, the amount of planned physical activity far exceeds any small increment in thermogenesis that may be induced by medications, cold, or diet in determining TEE.

SUMMARY

The research literature regarding the effects of dieting plus resistance and/or endurance training, separately or in combination, on RMR is mixed. (Table 49.5 shows a collection of these studies.) Despite the numerous reported benefits of exercise training, many

TABLE 49.5
Collection of Various Studies Investigating Changes in Physiological Variables Associated with Treatment

Study	Intervention	# of Participants	Weight Change (kg)	Fat Change (kg)	FFM Change (kg)	RMR Change (Kcal/Day)
Andersen, et al.[104]	Diet + aerobic	18	−6.27	−5.41	−0.89	−152.2
	Diet + lifestyle	21	−5.21	−4.48	−1.13	−158.9
Belko, et al.[124]	Diet only	5	−7.78	−5.1	−2.68	−109.9
	Diet + aerobic	6	−5.70	−4.7	−0.96	−10.0
Broeder, et al.[125]	Control	19	0.3	0.1	0.2	−17.2
	Strength only	13	0.0	−2.1	2.1	58.5
	Aerobic only	15	−1.1	−1.4	0.3	30.9
Bryner, et al.[93]	Diet + aerobic	10	−18.1	−12.8	−4.1	−210.7
	Diet + strength	10	−14.4	−14.5	−0.8	63.3
Byrne, et al.[126]	Strength	10	2.0	0.1	1.9	44
	Strength + walking	9	1.7	−0.2	1.9	−53
	Control	9	1.0	0.5	0.5	7

Continued

TABLE 49.5
(Continued)

Study	Intervention	# of Participants	Weight Change (kg)	Fat Change (kg)	FFM Change (kg)	RMR Change (Kcal/Day)
Das, et al.[75]	Gastric bypass	30	−53.2	−42.1	−11.3	−573.6
Donelly, et al.[92]	Diet only	26	−20.4	−4.7	−16.1	−138.3
	Diet + aerobic	16	−21.4	−4.8	−16.6	−158.6
	Diet + strength	18	−20.9	−4.7	−16.1	−186.9
	Diet + aerobic + strength	9	−22.9	−4.1	−18.0	−217.0
Doucet, et al.[127]	Diet only (phase 1)	10	−11.9	−10.7	−1.2	−304
(men)	Diet + aerobic (phase 2)	9	−2.0	−3.3	1.3	134
Doucet, et al.[127]	Diet only (phase 1)	7	−7.6	−5.8	−1.8	−148
(women)	Diet + aerobic (phase 2)	7	−1.2	−2.2	1.0	−199
Frey-Hewitt, et al.[128]	Control	41	0.38	−0.27	0.64	27.1
	Diet only	36	−6.68	−5.52	−1.16	−149.0
	Aerobic only	44	−4.10	−4.12	0.01	−22.8
Geliebter, et al.[90]	Diet only	22	−9.5	−6.8	−2.7	−88.2
	Diet + strength	20	−7.8	−6.7	−1.1	−127.2
	Diet + aerobic	23	−9.6	−7.2	−2.3	−148.9
Henson, et al.[129]	Diet + aerobic	7	−9.50	−8.59	−1.1	−247.0
Heymsfield, et al.[103]	Diet only	5	−7.0	−4.4	−2.6	−115.2
	Diet + aerobic	6	−7.5	−5.3	−2.2	−278.4
Hill, et al.[130]	Diet only	3	−7.9	−4.48	−3.44	−211.2
	Diet + aerobic	5	−8.3	−6.13	−2.13	−252.0
Keim, et al.[131]	Diet + aerobic	5	−13.08	−7.3	−4.7	−139.0
	Aerobic only	5	−5.61	−3.9	−1.3	18.0
Kraemer, et al.[132]	Control	6				132
	Diet only	8	−6.2		−0.1	−75
	Diet + aerobic	9	−6.8		1.4	−30
	Diet + aerobic + strength	8	−7.0		−1.7	−143
Kraemer, et al.[86]	Control	6	−0.35	−0.80	−4.84	−93
	Diet only	8	−9.64	−6.68		−80
	Diet + aerobic	11	−8.99	−7.00		−122
	Diet + aerobic + strength	10	−9.90	−9.57		−136
Mathieson, et al.[133]	Diet + Aerobic (high-carbohydrate VLCD)	5	−6.70	NA	NA	−333
	Diet + aerobic (low-carbohydrate VLCD)	7	−8.00	NA	NA	−207
Pavlou, et al.[21]	Diet + aerobic	15	−8.30	−6.91	−1.30	1.0
	Diet only	16	−6.40	−5.47	−0.80	−176.0
Racette, et al.[22]	Diet only	13	−8.30	−6.1	−2.2	−129.0
	Diet + aerobic	10	−10.50	−8.8	−1.7	−129.0
Sum, et al.[134]	Aerobic + strength	42	−16.10	−17.80	1.7	−109.3
Svendson, et al.[135]	Control	20	0.50	0.50	0.60	63.0
	Diet only	50	−9.50	−7.80	−1.20	−86.25
	Diet + aerobic	48	−10.30	−9.60	0.00	−45.95
Van Dale, et al.[136]	Diet only	6	−12.2	−9.4	−2.80	−533.7
	Diet + aerobic	6	−13.2	−10.9	−2.30	−371.5
Van Dale, et al.[137]	Diet only(no yo-yo)	7	−15.2	−11.9	−3.3	−389
	Diet + aerobic(yo-yo)	7	−18.9	−15.2	−3.7	−374
	Diet + aerobic(no yo-yo)	6	−19.4	−15.4	−4.0	−302
Wadden, et al.[41]	Balanced diet + aerobic	9	−18.20	−16.3	−0.70	−203.3
	Very low calorie diet + aerobic	6	−21.60	−15.6	−1.90	−166.5
Wadden, et al.[97]	Diet only	29	−14.40	−11.6	−2.8	−106
	Diet + aerobic	31	−13.70	−10.6	−3.1	−46
	Diet + strength	31	−17.20	−14.0	−3.2	−20
	Diet + aerobic and strength	29	−15.20	−13.4	−1.8	−7
Wilmore, et al.[40]	Aerobic only	77	0.00	−0.60	0.70	16.72

studies have failed to show significant benefits of exercise on changes in weight and body composition or RMR. Consequently, the significance of many of the effects of exercise remains questionable.[22]

The precise cause of the discrepancy among longitudinal studies investigating the effects of exercise training on RMR is unknown. There are, however, several factors that have been suggested as playing a role in the inconsistent findings. The timing of the RMR measurement in regard to the last bout of exercise training, as well as differences in training mode, exercise intensity, duration, frequency, and total training load, have been highlighted as potential factors that may account for some of the discrepancies among studies.[42] Thus, more rigorous, well-controlled longitudinal studies may be needed to elucidate the impact of exercise training, both resistance and endurance, as well as combined strength and endurance, on RMR.

Despite the equivocal findings regarding the impact of exercise training on RMR of dieting individuals, exercise appears to be the single most important behavior for long-term weight control in obese individuals.[138] In addition to the well-known benefits of both resistance and endurance training, it has been found, almost universally, that persons who maintain their weight loss report that they exercise regularly, whereas those regaining weight do not. Exercise should therefore remain a cornerstone in the comprehensive treatment of overweight and obesity.

ACKNOWLEDGMENTS

The authors would like to acknowledge Dr. Bryan C. Bergman and Dr. James O. Hill for their contributions on the sections of this chapter covering thermogenesis. Much of the information on the thermogenesis sections was taken from a book chapter from a previous edition of the *Handbook of Nutrition and Food,* written by Dr. Bergman and Dr. Hill. The authors would also like to acknowledge the support from NIH Grant M400-215-2111 RO1 (Dr. Andersen).

REFERENCES

1. Levine JA, Lanningham-Foster LM, McCrady SK, et al. *Science* 307: 584; 2005.
2. Levine JA. *Am J Physiol Endocrinol Metab* 286: E675; 2004.
3. Stedman's Medical Dictionary. Baltimore, MD: Williams & Wilkins; 1995, p. 262.
4. Moffett DF, Moffett SB, Schauf CL. *Human Physiology: Foundations & Frontiers.* St. Louis, MO: Mosby-Yearbook, 1993, ch 4.
5. Andersen RE. In: *Lifestyle and Weight Management Consultant Manual.* Cotton RT, Ed. San Diego, CA: American Council on Exercise; 1996, p. 95.
6. Bullough RC, Melby CL. *Ann Nutr Metab* 37: 24; 1993.
7. Poehlman ET. *Med Sci Sports Exerc* 21: 515; 1989.
8. Snitker S, Tataranni PA, Ravussin E. *Int J Obes Relat Metab Disord* 25: 1481; 2001.
9. Levine JA, Schleusner SJ, Jensen MD. *Am J Clin Nutr* 72: 1451; 2000.
10. Levine J, Melanson EL, Westerterp KR, et al. *Am J Physiol Endocrinol Metab* 281: E670; 2001.
11. Fruhbeck G. *Lancet* 366: 615; 2005.
12. Weir JBdV. *J Physiol* 109: 1; 1949.
13. Matarese LE. *J Am Diet Assoc* 97: S154; 1997.
14. Webb P. In: *Obesity.* Björntorp P, Brodoff BN, Eds. Philadelphia, PA: J.B. Lippincott Company, 1992, p. 91.
15. Jéquier E. In: *Substrate and Energy Metabolism.* Garrow JS, Halliday D, Eds. London: Libbey 1985, p. 82.
16. Ferrannini E. *Metabolism* 37: 287; 1988.
17. American College of Sports Medicine. *Guidelines for Exercise Testing and Prescription.* Malvern, PA: Lea and Febiger, 1991, p. 14.
18. National Institutes of Health. *Consensus conference on physical activity and cardiovascular health.* 276: 241; 1996.
19. Robertson JD, Reid DD. *Lancet* 1: 940; 1952.
20. Heshka S, Feld K, Yang MU, et al. *J Am Diet Assoc* 93: 1031; 1993.
21. Pavlou KN, Whatley JE, Jannace PW, et al. *Am J Clin Nutr* 49: 1110; 1989.
22. Racette SB, Schoeller DA, Kushner RF, et al. *Am J Clin Nutr* 61: 486; 1995.
23. Seefeldt VD, Harrison GG. In: *Anthropometric Standardization Reference Manual,* Lohman TG, Roche AF, Martorell R, Eds. Champaign, IL, Human Kinetics Books, 1988, p. 111.
24. Cullinen K, Caldwell M. *J Am Diet Assoc* 98: 414; 1998.
25. Haugen HA, Melanson EL, Tran ZV, et al. *Am J Clin Nutr* 78: 1141; 2003.
26. Heshka S, Yang M-U, Wang J, et al. *Am J Clin Nutr* 52: 981; 1990.
27. Foster GD, McGuckin BG. *Obes Res* 9 Suppl 5: 367S; 2001.
28. Bernstein RS, Thornton JC, Yang M-U, et al. *Am J Clin Nutr* 37: 595; 1983.
29. Cunningham JJ. *Am J Clin Nutr* 33: 2372; 1980.
30. Harris JA, Benedict FG. 297: 1919.
31. Fleisch A. *Helv Med Acta* 1: 23; 1951.
32. James WPT. *Postgrad Med J* 60: 50; 1984.
33. Mifflin MD, St. Jeor ST, Hill LA, et al. *Am J Clin Nutr* 51: 241; 1990.

34. Owen OE, Kavle E, Owen RS, et al. *Am J Clin Nutr* 44: 1; 1986.
35. Pavlou KN, Hoeffer MA, Blackburn GL. *Ann Surg* 203: 136; 1986.
36. Kuczmarski RJ, Flegal KM, Campbell SM, et al. *JAMA* 272: 205; 1994.
37. Livingston EH, Kohlstadt I. *Obes Res* 13: 1255; 2005.
38. Frankenfield D, Roth-Yousey L, Compher C. *J Am Diet Assoc* 105: 775; 2005.
39. Berke EM, Gardner AW, Goran MI, et al. *Am J Clin Nutr* 55: 626; 1992.
40. Wilmore JH, Stanforth PR, Hudspeth LA, et al. *Am J Clin Nutr* 68: 66; 1998.
41. Wadden TA, Foster GD, Letizia KA, et al. *JAMA* 264: 707; 1990.
42. Broeder CE, Burrhus KA, Svanevick LS, et al. *Am J Clin Nutr* 55: 795; 1992.
43. Goran MI. *Med Clin North Am* 84: 347; 2000.
44. Poehlman ET, Gardner AW, Ades PA, et al. *Metabolism* 41: 1351; 1992.
45. Poehlman ET, McAuliffe TL, Van Houten DR, et al. *Am J Physiol* 259: E66; 1990.
46. Poehlman ET, Melby CL, Badylak SF. *Am J Clin Nutr* 47: 793; 1988.
47. Poehlman ET, Melby CL, Badylak SF, et al. *Metabolism* 38: 85; 1989.
48. Lemmer JT, Ivey FM, Ryan AS, et al. *Med Sci Sports Exerc* 33: 532; 2001.
49. Poehlman ET, Arciero PJ, Goran MI. *Exerc Sport Sci Rev* 22: 251: 1994.
50. Evans WJ. *J Gerontol A Biol Sci Med Sci* 50 (Spec No): 5; 1995.
51. Karakelides H, Sreekumaran NK. *Curr Top Dev Biol* 68: 123; 2005.
52. Arciero PJ, Goran MI, Poehlman ET. *J Appl Physiol* 75: 2514; 1993.
53. Jakicic JM, Wing RR. *Int J Obes Relat Metab Disord* 22: 236; 1998.
54. Jones A, Jr., Shen W, St Onge MP, et al. *Am J Clin Nutr* 79: 780; 2004.
55. Glass JN, Miller WC, Szymanski LM, et al. *J Sports Med Phys Fitness* 42: 56; 2002.
56. McArdle WD, Katch FI, Katch VL. *Exercise Physiology: Energy, Nutrition, and Human Performance*. Philadelphia: Lea & Febiger; 1991, ch 9.
57. Perkins KA. *J Appl Physiol* 72: 401; 1992.
58. Clemens LH, Klesges RC, Slawson DL, et al. *Int J Obes Relat Metab Disord* 27: 1219; 2003.
59. Poehlman ET, Despres JP, Bessette H, et al. *Med Sci Sports Exerc* 17: 689; 1985.
60. Costill DL, Dalsky GP, Fink WJ. *Med Sci Sports* 10: 155; 1978.
61. Ivy JL, Costill DL, Fink WJ, et al. *Med Sci Sports* 11: 6; 1979.
62. Klesges RC, Mealer CZ, Klesges LM. *Am J Clin Nutr* 59: 805; 1994.
63. Williamson DF, Forman MR, Binkin NJ, et al. *Am J Public Health* 77: 1324; 1987.
64. McDonald JT, Margen S. *Am J Clin Nutr* 29: 1093; 1976.
65. Pirola RC, Lieber CS. *Pharmacology* 7: 185; 1972.
66. Lieber CS. *Nutr Rev* 46: 241; 1988.
67. Suter PM, Schutz Y, Jequier E. *N Engl J Med* 326: 983; 1992.
68. Lamont LS. *J Cardiopulm Rehabil* 15: 183; 1995.
69. Connolly J, Romano T, Patruno M. *Fam Pract* 16: 196; 1999.
70. Flegal KM, Carroll MD, Ogden CL, et al. *JAMA* 288: 1723; 2002.
71. National Center for Health Statistics. Vital Health Stat DHHS Publication No. (PHS)92-1509: 1994.
72. Serdula MK, Mokdad AH, Williamson DF, et al. *JAMA* 282: 1353; 1999.
73. Elliot DL, Goldberg L, Kuehl KS, et al. *Am J Clin Nutr* 49: 93; 1989.
74. Foster GD, Wadden TA, Feurer ID, et al. *Am J Clin Nutr* 51: 167; 1990.
75. Das SK, Roberts SB, McCrory MA, et al. *Am J Clin Nutr* 78: 22; 2003.
76. Gilliat-Wimberly M, Manore MM, Woolf K, et al. *J Am Diet Assoc* 101: 1181; 2001.
77. Phelain JF, Reinke E, Harris MA, et al. *J Am Coll Nutr* 16: 140; 1997.
78. Quinn TJ, Vroman NB, Kertzer R. *Med Sci Sports Exerc* 26: 908; 1994.
79. Almuzaini KS, Potteiger JA, Green SB. *Can J Appl Physiol* 23: 433; 1998.
80. Short KR, Sedlock DA. *J Appl Physiol* 83: 153; 1997.
81. Gillette CA, Bullough RC, Melby CL. *Int J Sport Nutr* 4: 347; 1994.
82. Imamura H, Shibuya S, Uchida K, et al. *J Sports Med Phys Fitness* 44: 23; 2004.
83. U.S. Department of Health and Human Services. *Physical Activity and Health: A Report of the Surgeon General*. Atlanta, GA: U.S. Department of Health and Human Services, Centers for Disease Control and Prevention, National Center for Chronic Disease Prevention and Health Promotion, 1996.
84. National Institutes of Health, National Heart Lung and Blood Institute. *Obesity Education Initiative: Clinical Guidelines on the Identification, Evaluation, and Treatment of Overweight and Obesity in Adults*. U.S. Department of Health and Human Services, 1998.
85. Jakicic JM, Clark K, Coleman E, et al. *Med Sci Sports Exerc* 33: 2145; 2001.
86. Kraemer WJ, Volek JS, Clark KL, et al. *Med Sci Sports Exerc* 31: 1320; 1999.
87. Ballor DL, Poehlman ET. *Int J Obes Relat Metab Disord* 18: 35; 1994.
88. Henson LC, Poole DC, Donahoe CP, et al. *Am J Clin Nutr* 46: 893; 1987.
89. Andersen RE, Wadden TA, Bartlett SJ, et al. *JAMA* 281: 335; 1999.

90. Geliebter A, Maher MM, Gerace L, et al. *Am J Clin Nutr* 66: 557; 1997.
91. Ballor DL, Katch VL, Becque MD, et al. *Am J Clin Nutr* 47: 19; 1988.
92. Donnelly JE, Pronk NP, Jacobsen DJ, et al. *Am J Clin Nutr* 54: 56; 1991.
93. Bryner RW, Ullrich IH, Sauers J, et al. *J Am Coll Nutr* 18: 115; 1999.
94. Donnelly JE, Sharp T, Houmard J, et al. *Am J Clin Nutr* 58: 561; 1993.
95. Poehlman ET, Melby CL, Goran MI. *Sports Med* 11: 78; 1991.
96. Sweeney ME, Hill JO, Heller PA, et al. *Am J Clin Nutr* 57: 127; 1993.
97. Wadden TA, Vogt RA, Andersen RE, et al. *J Consult Clin Psychol* 65: 269; 1997.
98. King AC, Haskell WL, Taylor CB, et al. *JAMA* 266: 1535; 1991.
99. Lennon D, Nagle F, Stratman F, et al. *Int J Obes Relat Metab Disord* 9: 39; 1985.
100. Tremblay A, Fontaine E, Poehlman ET, et al. *Int J Obes Relat Metab Disord* 10: 511; 1986.
101. Nieman DC, Haig JL, de Guia ED, et al. *J Sports Med* 28: 79; 1988.
102. Phinney SD, LaGrange BM, O'Connell M, et al. *Metabolism* 37: 758; 1988.
103. Heymsfield SB, Casper K, Hearn J, et al. *Metabolism* 38: 215; 1989.
104. Andersen RE, Franckowiak SC, Bartlett SJ, et al. *Metabolism* 51: 1528; 2002.
105. Nelson KM, Weinsier RL, James LD, et al. *Am J Clin Nutr* 55: 924; 1992.
106. Segal KR, Blando L, Ginsberg-Fellner F, et al. *Metabolism* 41: 868; 1992.
107. Segal KR, Chun A, Coronel P, et al. *Metabolism* 41: 754; 1992.
108. Segal KR, Edano A, Tomas MB. *Metabolism* 39: 985; 1990.
109. Segal KR, Gutin B, Albu J, et al. *Am J Physiol* 252: E110-E117; 1987.
110. Swaminathan R, King RF, Holmfield J, et al. *Am J Clin Nutr* 42: 177; 1985.
111. Segal KR, Gutin B, Nyman AM, et al. *J Clin Invest* 76: 1107; 1985.
112. D'Alessio DA, Kavle EC, Mozzoli MA, et al. *J Clin Invest* 81: 1781; 1988.
113. Nair KS, Halliday D, Garrow JS. *Clin Sci (Lond)* 65: 307; 1983.
114. Weinsier RL, Nelson KM, Hensrud DD, et al. *J Clin Invest* 95: 980; 1995.
115. Schwartz RS, Halter JB, Bierman EL. *Metabolism* 32: 114; 1983.
116. Levine JA, Eberhardt NL, Jensen MD. *Science* 283: 212; 1999.
117. Levine J, Baukol P, Pavlidis I. *N Engl J Med* 341: 2100; 1999.
118. Karst H, Steiniger J, Noack R, et al. *Ann Nutr Metab* 28: 245; 1984.
119. Tappy L. *Reprod Nutr Dev* 36: 391; 1996.
120. Zed C, James WP. *Int J Obes* 10: 391; 1986.
121. Labayen I, Forga L, Martinez JA. *Eur J Nutr* 38: 158; 1999.
122. Schwartz RS, Ravussin E, Massari M, et al. *Metabolism* 34: 285; 1985.
123. Westerterp KR, Wilson SA, Rolland V. *Int J Obes Relat Metab Disord* 23: 287; 1999.
124. Belko AZ, Van Loan M, Barbieri TF, et al. *Int J Obes Relat Metab Disord* 11: 93; 1987.
125. Broeder CE, Burrhus KA, Svanevick LS, et al. *Am J Clin Nutr* 55: 802; 1992.
126. Byrne HK, Wilmore JH. *Int J Sport Nutr Exerc Metab* 11: 15; 2001.
127. Doucet E, Imbeault P, Almeras N, et al. *Obes Res* 7: 323; 1999.
128. Frey-Hewitt B, Vranizan KM, Dreon DM, et al. *Int J Obes Relat Metab Disord* 14: 327; 1990.
129. Henson LC, Poole DC, Donahoe CP, et al. *Med Sci Sports Exerc* 46: 893; 1987.
130. Hill JO, Sparling PB, Shields TW, et al. *Am J Clin Nutr* 46: 622; 1987.
131. Keim NL, Barbieri TF, Belko AZ. *Int J Obes Relat Metab Disord* 14: 335; 1990.
132. Kraemer WJ, Volek JS, Clark KL, et al. *J Appl Physiol* 83: 270; 1997.
133. Mathieson RA, Walberg JL, Gwazdauskas FC, et al. *Metabolism* 35: 394; 1986.
134. Sum CF, Wang KW, Choo DCA, et al. *Metabolism* 43: 1148; 1994.
135. Svendsen OL, Hassager C, Christiansen C. *Am J Med* 95: 131; 1993.
136. van Dale D, Saris WHM, Schoffelen PFM, et al. *Int J Obes Relat Metab Disord* 11: 367; 1987.
137. van Dale D, Saris WHM. *Am J Clin Nutr* 49: 409; 1989.
138. Kayman S, Bruvold W, Stern JS. *Am J Clin Nutr* 52: 800; 1990.

50 Adult Obesity

Diane K. Smith

CONTENTS

INTRODUCTION

Obesity is a multifactorial disease that is growing in epidemic proportions. It is associated with significant medical risks that may be ameliorated by modest weight loss. Exercise and behavioral modification of diet are the cornerstones of treatment; pharmacotherapy and surgery may be useful adjuncts.

ETIOLOGY

It is estimated that 40 to 70% of the variation in obesity within populations is heritable;[1] however, this predisposition can be overridden by environmental cues and behavior (physical activity and nutrient choices). Less common are secondary causes of obesity (Table 50.1).

GENETIC CAUSES

Genetic background strongly influences the risk of obesity, as demonstrated by adoption studies, where adoptees more closely resembled their biological parents than their adoptive parents,[2] and twin studies that showed a concordance rate in identical twins twice that of fraternal twins.[3] Both positive and negative energy balance studies in twins show greater variations between pairs than within pairs.[4] Although most forms of monogenetic obesity (Table 50.2) are rare to extremely rare, frame shift mutations of the melanocortin-4 (MC4) receptor have been described in 2 to 7% of populations.

More commonly, polygenetic influences are involved. Although extensively studied, candidate genes remain to be identified.[1,5] These genes may influence food intake, metabolism, energy expenditure, and hormones (Table 50.3). Updates of the human obesity gene map are published annually in Obesity Research.[6]

TABLE 50.1
Etiology of Obesity

Primary
Genetic
Nutritional
Environmental

Secondary
Neural
   Hypothalamic lesions
   Amygdala lesions
   Temporal lobe lesions
Endocrine
   Oophorectomy
   Insulinoma, insulin therapy
   Cushing's syndrome, corticoid therapy
Pharmacologic
Viral

TABLE 50.2
Monogenetic Human Obesity

Prader–Willi syndrome
Laurence–Moon–Biedl syndrome
Cohen's syndrome
Kleinfelter's syndrome
Leptin deficiency
Truncated leptin receptor
Proopiomelanocortin deficiency
Melanocortin-4 receptor

TABLE 50.3
Obesity-Related Factors Thought to be
Genetically Modulated

Diet Related
Dietary fat preferences
Appetite regulation
Amount and rate of eating

Metabolism/Nutrient Partitioning
Adipose tissue distribution
Adipose tissue lipolysis
Adipose tissue and muscle lipoprotein lipase (LPL) activity
Muscle composition and oxidative potential
Free fatty acid and β-receptor activities in adipose tissue
Capacities for fat and carbohydrate oxidation

Energy Expenditure
Metabolic rate
Dietary induced thermogenesis
Nutrient partitioning
Propensity for physical activity/inactivity

Hormonal
Insulin sensitivity/resistance
Growth hormone status
Leptin action

ENVIRONMENTAL CAUSES

NUTRITIONAL

The role of nutrient intake in promoting obesity is quantitative, qualitative, and temporal. The increasing availability of food, often in excessive serving sizes, promotes hyperphagia. Hedonic factors such as food texture, temperature, color, appearance, and variety may also lead to overconsumption. Visual cues also influence intake; subjects eating from covertly self-refilling bowls consumed 73% more than subjects eating from normal bowls.[7]

Carbohydrates with a high glycemic response may promote obesity by altering fuel partitioning, that is, promoting postprandial carbohydrate oxidation and sparing fat oxidation.[8] A dramatic increase in high-fructose corn syrup temporally correlates with the development of the obesity epidemic. Compared to glucose, differences in the metabolism of fructose may promote adiposity.[9]

The intake of dietary fat is significantly related to adiposity.[10] Dietary fat is converted to body fat with approximately 25% greater efficiency than carbohydrate. Dietary fat may be less satiating than protein and complex carbohydrates, although foods with a high glycemic index (i.e., rapidly converted to glucose) may stimulate hunger and lead to more frequent eating. The long-chain fatty acid composition of dietary fat influences energy utilization; low ratios of polyunsaturated to saturated fat are associated with lower respiratory quotients (RQ; moles of carbon dioxide produced per mole of oxygen consumed).[11]

The pattern of food intake may play a role in the development of obesity. Widely spaced meals are used less efficiently because of the energy cost of storage. Compared to immediate oxidation, the energy cost of converting glucose into glycogen is 5%, and into fat is 28%.

INACTIVITY

Physical inactivity is increasing as a result of decreased manual labor, the use of labor-saving devices, and a shift in leisure preferences (television, computers, spectator sports, etc.). Based on population studies, increased sedentary behavior may be even more important than dietary excess in contributing to the current obesity epidemic.[12]

PSYCHOSOCIAL FACTORS

A cause-and-effect relationship between low socioeconomic status and obesity has been demonstrated.[13] Societal ideals of desirable weight have various ethnic, cultural, and gender determinants. Emotional distress may promote overeating. The hormonal response to stress has been suggested to promote visceral adiposity.[14]

PHYSIOLOGIC STATES

Environmental factors *in utero* may influence subsequent obesity as well as fat distribution.[15] Both low and high birth weights are associated with obesity. Some women develop excessive adiposity during gestation. Menopause is associated with changes in energy balance and body composition.[16] Similar changes are well documented in aging individuals of either gender.

SECONDARY OBESITY

Endocrine changes secondary to obesity (insulin resistance, decreased growth hormone secretion, blunted prolactin responsiveness, hyperparathyroidism, and decreased serum testosterone in men) may make it difficult to determine whether obesity is primary or secondary. Secondary obesity may result from hypothyroidism, Cushing's syndrome, insulinoma, hypogonadism, Frolich syndrome, hypothalamic tumors, head injury, or drugs (Table 50.4). There are several known animal models of viral-induced obesity. Antibodies to human adenovirus AD-36 (capable of producing obesity in chickens and mice) have been observed more commonly in obese humans than in lean humans.[17] Although a causative relationship in humans has not been demonstrated, recent studies have shown that AD-36 enhanced the differentiation of preadipocytes *in vitro*.[18]

ENERGY BALANCE

Energy balance is the difference between energy intake and energy expenditure. Within groups, there is not a correlation between energy intake and body weight; for the individual, intake does correlate with weight. Therefore, obesity can be viewed as a disorder of energy homeostasis. This variability may be either innate or acquired, and may be the result of hyperphagia, energy partitioning, intermediary metabolism, the efficiency of the coupling of electron transport to ATP generation, the efficiency of

TABLE 50.4
Drugs That May Affect Weight

Weight Promoting	Weight Neutral or Lowering
Neuroleptics	Neuroleptics
Olanzapine	Ziprasidone
Clozapine	Molidone
Haloperidol	Aripiprazole
Respiridone	Quetiapine
Antidepressants	Antidepressants
Mirtazapine	Buproprion
Imipramine	Nafazodone
Amytriptyline	Tranylcypromine
Doxepin	Antiepileptics
Phenelzine	Topiramate
Isocarboxizid	Zonisamide
Lithium	Lamotrigine
Antiepileptics	Antihypertensive agents
Valproate	Calcium channel blockers
Carbamazepine	ACE inhibitors
Gabapentin	Antidiabetic agents
Antihypertensive agents	Metformin
α-Adrenergic blockers	Acarbose
β-Adrenergic blockers	Meglitol
Antidiabetic agents	
Sulfonylureas	
Thiazolidinediones	
Insulin	
Some steroid contraceptives	
Corticosteriods	
Cyproheptadine	
Antihistamines	
Weight variable	
Selective serotonin reuptake inhibitors	

ATPases, degree of physical activity, the magnitude of adaptive thermogenesis, hormonal influences on energy expenditure, and physiological demands (growth, pregnancy, and lactation).

APPETITE REGULATION

The major loci in the central nervous system that regulate feeding behavior are the dorsomedial, paraventricular, arcuate, and lateral nuclei of the hypothalamus, the prefrontal cortex, the amygdala, the nucleus accumbens, and the nucleus of the solitary tract. These sites respond to a variety of stimuli, including deprivation, intracellular glucose concentration, intracellular fat oxidation, food choice, meal timing, desire, mood, stress, metabolic rate, fidgeting, fat stores (via leptin), and ingestive behavior. These areas communicate via complex interactions of neuromodulators that either suppress or stimulate feeding (Table 50.5). Within the central nervous system, appetite is stimulated by neuropeptide Y (directly promotes feeding behavior) and agouti-related protein (blocks the melanocortin type 4 receptor which inhibits appetitie). Appetite suppression is modulated by cocaine- and amphetamine-regulated transcript and proopiomelanocortin (activates the melanocortin type 4 receptor via alpha-melanocyte-stimulating hormone).

Signals from the periphery originate from the gut (ghrelin, peptide YY3-36, cholecystokinin, bombesin, enterostatin, and glucagon-like protein), pancreas (insulin, amylin, glucagon, and pancreatic polypeptide) and adipose tissue (leptin). Other adipose-derived proteins/peptides, such as adiponectin and resistin, may influence appetite via their effects on insulin.

Appetite regulation can also be viewed as several interacting feedback loops. The glucostat theory involves glucose-sensitive neurons that stimulate appetite under conditions of low glucose levels, and glucoreceptors in the liver that provide the afferent signal via the vagus nerve. Leptin, a protein produced by adipocytes, appears to drive the adipostat, which is thought to measure the adequacy of fat stores. Thermogenesis in brown adipose tissue has been proposed as a thermostatic regulator of food intake.[19]

ENERGY PARTITIONING

Genetic, hormonal, nutritional, and physical activity factors influence the partitioning of energy between fat and fat-free mass, as well as preference for carbohydrate versus fat oxidation to meet energy needs. A high RQ has been shown to predict future weight gain.[20,21] Obese subjects have an attenuation of both basal- and epinephrine-stimulated rates of lipolysis[22] that may in part result

---

TABLE 50.5
Neuromodulators of Appetite Regulation

Stimulatory
Norepinephrine (α-2)
Endogenous opioids
Dopamine (physiologic levels)
Neuropeptide Y
Orexins
Galanin
Agouti-related protein
Melanin-concentrating hormone
Ghrelin
Endocannabinoids

Inhibitory
Norepinephrine (β)
Epinephrine (β)
Dopamine (supraphysiologic)
Serotonin
Cholecystokinin
Somatostatin
Glucagon, glucagon-like protein (GLP-1)
Urocortin
Corticotropin-releasing hormone (CRH)
Melanocortin agonists (e.g., proopiomelanocortin,
    melanocyte-stimulating hormone)
Cocaine/amphetamine regulated transcript
Leptin
Peptide YY3-36

from hyperinsulinemia. Dietary fat intake may also influence substrate utilization, with low ratios of polyunsaturated to saturated fats resulting in lower RQs.[23] Substitution of oleic acid for palmitic acid increases fat oxidation and energy expenditure.[24]

A propensity to excessive fat stores may result from increased LPL activity and peroxisome proliferator-activating receptor (PPAR) abnormalities. LPL activity is increased in obesity, although it is unclear if this increase is a cause or result of obesity. Adipose tissue LPL activity increases during caloric restriction and may lead to rapid weight regain when caloric restriction is abandoned. PPARs promote differentiation of preadipocytes. Mutations in gamma-2 PPAR have been described in some severely obese humans.[25]

ENERGY EXPENDITURE

Basal metabolic rate (BMR) is the rate of energy expenditure upon awakening, before any physical activity and 12 to 18 h after the last meal. More commonly assessed is resting energy expenditure (REE), which is obtained in the resting state several hours after the last meal. The difference between BMR and REE is small. This energy component is expended for maintenance of body functions and homeostasis (primarily proton pumping and protein turnover) and accounts for 60 to 75% of total energy expenditure in sedentary individuals. Subjects with low REE gain more weight than persons with normal or elevated REE.[26] The REE is increased in obesity, related to the individual's increase in lean body mass. REE increases with overfeeding. With caloric restriction, REE is decreased by both the caloric deficit and the resultant loss in lean tissue. Exercise may help minimize REE decrease. Physical training, that is, being in the "trained state," can also increase REE independent of body composition or the residual effects of the last bout of exercise.[27]

Energy expenditure on physical activity is the most variable, and is the only component of energy balance that is under volitional control. It includes shivering and fidgeting, as well as physical work. It may range from less than 100 kcal/day in sedentary individuals to greater than 1000 kcal/day with strenuous exercise or labor. Exercise efficiency (energy expenditure/unit work) is not altered by obesity, but because of carrying excess weight, more energy will be expended during weight-bearing activities. In general, the obese are less physically active than the lean. The influence of physical activity on obesity, independent of genotype, has been examined in twins, where discordance for obesity was associated with discordance in activity level.[28]

The thermic effect of food (TEF), also known as diet-induced thermogenesis, is the energy cost of food digestion, absorption, metabolism, and storage, as well as a component resulting from sympathetic nervous system activity. It is lowest for fat and highest for excess carbohydrate stored as fat and protein. It may account for up to 10% of daily energy expenditure and consists of both obiligatory and facultative components. The latter may be decreased in obesity. Weight loss does not normalize TEF and may contribute to weight regain.[29–30] However, longitudinal studies have demonstrated declines in glucose-induced thermogenesis with the evolution of obesity.[31] With caloric restriction, the TEF declines.

Exercise may potentiate TEF, especially in insulin-sensitive subjects. Although study results are inconsistent, at least some obese individuals have lesser magnitudes of energy expenditure than their lean counterparts.

Adaptive thermogenesis is influenced by both genetic and environmental (ambient temperature, food intake, and emotional stress) factors and usually accounts for 10 to 15% of total energy expenditure. Mechanisms include changes in the efficiency of oxidative phosphorylation, rates of protein turnover, NaK pump activity, futile cycles, and activity/inactivity of brown fat (nonshivering thermogenesis). Examples of futile cycles which waste ATP are:

Glucose to pyruvate to glucose
Cyclic lipolysis and reesterification of triglycerides
Glucose to lactate to glucose (Cori cycle)
Glucose to glucose-6-phosphate to glucose
Fructose-6-phosphate to fructose-di-phosphate to fructose-6-phosphate
Pyruvate to phosphoenolpyruvate to pyruvate
Wastage of ATP may also result directly by phosphatases converting ATP to ADP

Nonshivering thermogenesis as a mechanism of heat production is well established in hibernating animals and infants of various species, although its contribution to adult human obesity is controversial. This thermogenesis occurs in mitochondria of brown adipose tissue, where an uncoupling protein (uncoupling protein-1 [UCP-1]) facilitates a proton leak, and thus fat oxidation is dissociated from oxidative phosphorylation. Recently, additional UCPs have been discovered (currently, five are known). Several of the UCPs have genetic linkage to human obesity, but the importance in obesity remains to be delineated. A polymorphism in the UCP-3 gene has been associated with altered REE.[32]

PREVALENCE OF OBESITY

Overweight and obesity are increasing dramatically globally. There has been a greater than 25% increase in the U.S. in the past three decades.[33] The CDC reports an astounding 49% increase in obesity in young adults from 1991 to 1998.[34] For U.S. adults,

33% are overweight (body mass index [BMI] ≥25 to 29.9); and 31% are obese (BMI ≥30).[35] African- and Hispanic-Americans have a higher prevalence of obesity than Anglo-Americans.

ASSESSMENT

Assessment of the patient should include the BMI, waist circumference (measured at the level of the iliac crest), and overall medical risk. Bioimpedance analysis is a simple noninvasive technique that measures total body water and total fat, and calculates lean body mass. Other methods of assessment (underwater weighing, doubly labeled water, calorimetry, dual-energy x-ray absorptiometry [DEXA], computerized tomography [CT] scan, and magnetic resonance imaging [MRI]), are expensive and inaccessible to most practitioners. Although skinfold measurements are inexpensive, they have poor reproducibility, especially with increasing obesity.

BODY MASS INDEX

The BMI is highly correlated with fatness, and minimizes the effect of height. It is calculated as:

$$BMI = wt \text{ (in kg)}/ht^2 \text{ (in meters) or}$$
$$BMI = wt \text{ (in lb)} \times 703/ht^2 \text{ (in inches)}$$

(50.1)

As an index of mass, it does not distinguish between fat and fat-free mass. Consequently, it is possible to be overweight without having excess adiposity (very muscular individuals) as well as obese without being overweight (sarcopenic individuals). Table 50.6 presents classification for BMI.

FAT DISTRIBUTION

In addition to total adiposity, distribution of body fat has medical implications (Table 50.7), with abdominal (visceral) fat presenting a greater health risk than gluteal-femoral fat.[36] A waist circumference >40 in. in men or >35 in. in women reflects

TABLE 50.6
Classification for BMI

BMI	Weight Classification
18.5–24.9	Normal weight
25.0–29.9	Overweight
30.0–34.9	Class 1 obesity
35.0–39.9	Class 2 obesity
≥40	Class 3 obesity

TABLE 50.7
Metabolic Consequences of Upper Body Obesity

Increased insulin secretion
Decreased hepatic clearance of insulin
Insulin resistance
Increased lipolysis
Increased circulating free fatty acids
Increased free fatty acid oxidation
Increased gluconeogenesis and decreased glucose utilization
Effects of hyperinsulinemia (see Table 50.8)
Increased free testosterone and free androstenedione levels associated
  with decreased sex-hormone-binding globulin in women
Decreased progesterone levels in women
Decreased testosterone levels in men
Increased cortisol production

excess abdominal fat. Gluteal-femoral fat, which is thought to be estrogen dependent, serves as an energy store for lactation and increases during each pregnancy. Following menopause, this fat depot decreases, while intraabdominal fat increases.

INSULIN RESISTANCE

Given the key role of hyperinsulinemia on the medical risks of obesity (see below) assessment of insulin resistance is desirable. Most sensitive is the insulin suppression test, although its performance is not practical in the usual care setting. Fasting plasma insulin levels, although less sensitive, are a useful guide.

MEDICAL RISKS OF OBESITY (COMORBIDITIES)

The medical consequences of obesity may result from hyperinsulinemia, mechanical effects of excess weight, and alterations in sex hormones. Especially damaging is hyperinsulinemia (Table 50.8). Increased insulin secretion is related to total body fat; however, decreased hepatic insulin clearance is related specifically to the amount of abdominal fat (may be related to increased androgen effects on the liver). Exhaustion of pancreatic reserves may lead to impaired glucose tolerance. Glucose intolerance relates to increased intra-abdominal visceral fat as opposed to subcutaneous abdominal fat.[37] Other comorbidities associated with hyperinsulinemia include hypertension, hyperlipidemia, atherosclerotic disease, stroke, and polycystic ovarian syndrome.

Mechanical consequences of obesity include congestive heart failure, sleep apnea, restrictive lung disease, surgery risks (pneumonia and wound infection), high risk pregnancy, cellulitis, degenerative arthritis, and steatohepatitis. Alterations in sex hormones contribute to decreased fertility, menorrhagia, oligomenorrhea, and certain cancers (breast and uterus).

Comorbidities are present in approximately two thirds of subjects with a BMI >27. Hypertension is the most common obesity-related health risk and its prevalence increases markedly with increasing levels of obesity, as does the incidence of type 2 diabetes, gallbladder disease, and osteoarthritis. Hypercholesterolemia, while more common in the overweight and obese than

TABLE 50.8
Effects of Hyperinsulinemia

Renal
Uric acid: increased production, decreased clearance
Decreased potassium and sodium excretion

Lipid Metabolism
Increased VLDL
Decreased high-density lipoprotein (HDL)
Decreased clearance of chylomicron remnants and IDL
Increased postprandial lipemia
Increased small, dense LDL
Increased "oxidizabilty" of LDL
Decreased lipolytic activity

Glucose Metabolism
Glucose intolerance

Nervous System
Increased sympathetic activity

Cardiovascular
Increased heart rate

Hypertension
Increased plaque formation
Decreased plaque regression
Smooth muscle and connective tissue proliferation
Enhanced LDL receptor activity

Hemostasis
Increased PAI-1
Increased fibrinogen
Increased von Willibrand factor
Increased factor X
Increased adhesion of mononuclear cells to endothelium

Gonadal
Polycystic ovaries

in normal weight individuals, does not show an increase with increasing levels of obesity. However, the risk of coronary heart disease in women does increase with increasing level of obesity.[33,38] The risk for death from cardiovascular disease, cancer, or other diseases increases with increasing degrees of obesity.[39-40] For more extensive detail, the reader is referred to the NIH Clinical Guidelines,[41] the WHO Consultation on Obesity Report,[42] and recent reviews by Pi-Sunyer[43] and Aronne.[44] A modest (5 to 15% of initial weight) sustained weight loss will improve many of the health complications of obesity.[45-50]

TREATMENT

The most effective weight-loss programs combine diet, exercise, behavior modification, and social support. Pharmacologic agents may be a useful adjunct, but are inappropriate as sole therapy. The patient's motivation can be assessed using the Diet Readiness Questionnaire.[51] For descriptions of popular weight loss programs (see Weighing the Options,[52] pg 66–80.)

GOALS

Practitioners should help patients to set realistic goals to help prevent the patient from being overwhelmed or relapsing. Without guidance, most patients choose goals based on cosmetic criteria that are usually unachievable. A reasonable or healthy weight loss goal needs to take into account health risks, genetic predisposition to obesity, and whether the patient has hyperplastic (excess fat cell number) versus hypertrophic (excess fat cell size) obesity. When fat cells hypertrophy, they develop insulin resistance, resulting in increased medical risk. When adipocytes reach some maximum size (approximately double optimal size), there is a stimulus to proliferate. Hyperplastic obesity is common in patients with childhood/adolescent-onset obesity, morbid obesity, and in some cases of excessive weight gain during pregnancy. When individual fat cells are reduced below a critical size, the body interprets this as under nutrition and compensatory mechanisms are set into play. Because it is impossible to reduce the number of adipocytes, an appropriate goal for the patient with hyperplastic obesity is to reduce excess fat by approximately one half.

For patients with a BMI >30, a 10% weight loss over six months (i.e., 1 to 2 lb or 0.5 to 1.0 kg/week) is a reasonable goal. Slower weight loss is appropriate for those with lesser degrees of obesity. For overweight subjects who are not motivated to lose weight, the goal should be prevention of further weight gain.

CRITERIA FOR CHOOSING A WEIGHT-LOSS PROGRAM

Guidelines for choosing a weight loss program have been developed by the NIH (Table 50.9) and The Institute of Medicine.[52]

DIET

Diets should be individually planned to help create a deficit of 500 to 1000 kcal/day. Successful weight reduction is more likely to occur when consideration is given to a patient's food preferences in tailoring a particular diet. The dietitian should ensure that all of the recommended dietary allowances are met; this may necessitate the use of a dietary or vitamin supplement. The diet should also be realistic, that is, based on dietary modification and practical changes in eating habits. The nutritional recommendations should be based on the patient's current eating habits, lifestyle, ethnicity and culture, other coexisting medical conditions, and potential nutrient–drug interactions.

The diet should be prescribed by the physician and implemented by the dietitian. The active involvement of the physician in such cases is essential, while the role of the dietitian can be invaluable, since caloric intake should be evaluated monthly. Food records should be completed by the patient to assess the relationship of caloric intake to weight loss. However, changes in body weight may not reflect changes in body fat if the patient has edema or has been adding muscle tissue due to an aggressive exercise program. The rate of weight loss can be expected to decline as the patient's energy requirements decline.

TABLE 50.9
NIH Guidelines for Choosing a Weight-Loss Program

The diet should be safe and include all the Recommended Dietary Allowances for vitamins, minerals, and proteins

The program should be directed towards a slow, steady weight loss unless a more rapid weight loss is medically indicated

A doctor should evaluate health status if the client's weight-loss goal is greater than 15 to 20 lb, if the client has any
 health problems, or if the client takes medication on a regular basis

The program should include plans for weight maintenance

The program should give the prospective client a detailed list of fees and costs of additional items

---

Low-Calorie Diets (LCDs)

Caloric restriction is an integral component of weight loss regimens. The restriction can be moderate to severe; however, compliance decreases with unrealistic restrictions. In general, a 500 to 1000 kcal reduction from maintenance caloric requirements is recommended. Maintenance requirements may be determined by the REE recommended by Mifflin et al.[53]:

$$REE = (9.99 \times \text{weight in kg}) + (6.25 \times \text{height in cm}) - (4.92 \times \text{age in years}) +$$
$$(166 \times \text{sex [male} = 1; \text{female} = 0]) - 161 \tag{50.2}$$

Multiply the REE by an activity factor (1.5 for women; 1.6 for men) to determine maintenance requirements.[54]

The Harris–Benedict equation can also be used to calculate REE or BMR; however, this equation overpredicts REE by 5 to 24%.[53] The Harris–Benedict equations are[54]:

$$\text{BMR for males} = 66 + 13.8 \text{ (weight in kg)} + 5 \text{ (height in cm)} - 6.8 \text{ (age in years)} \tag{50.3}$$

$$\text{BMR for females} = 655 + 9.6 \text{ (weight in kg)} + 1.8 \text{ (height in cm)} - 4.7 \text{ (age in years)} \tag{50.4}$$

Subtract 500 to 1000 kcal to determine the caloric intake needed to achieve a weight loss of approximately 1 to 2 lb/week.[52]

Implementation of Diet

The dietitian usually uses the exchange system, or the Food Guide Pyramid, to prescribe a specified number of exchanges (or servings) of foods from each food group, and a defined portion size for each food. Thus, weighing and measuring foods is an important requirement in terms of patient compliance. The subject can choose a variety of foods within each food group, and some higher-calorie foods can be built in, occasionally. Once caloric needs have been determined, Table 50.10 can be used as a guide for various caloric levels. A sample meal plan for a 1500-calorie exchange diet is shown in Table 50.11.

Because overweight individuals need to lose weight over a period of time, it is imperative that the diet be acceptable. The diet must fit the taste preferences and habits of the individual and be flexible enough to allow eating outside the home as well. Dietary education is necessary to assist in the adaptation to an LCD and should address the topics[41] listed in Table 50.12.

Low-Calorie, High-Fiber Diets

Reducing dietary fat, along with an increase in dietary fiber and a decrease in refined sugars, is a sound program for weight loss as well as weight maintenance, especially when consuming the recommended number of servings from the Food Guide Pyramid. Consuming ample fruits, vegetables, and whole grains can aid in weight loss, because increased fiber intake can increase satiety. The National Research Council and the American Heart Association recommend consuming 25 to 35 grams of fiber each day. A fat intake of 20 to 30% of total kilocalories is appropriate, as long as total kilocalories from refined sugars are not excessive. Reducing the percentage of dietary fat alone will not produce weight loss unless total kilocalories are also reduced.[41] Although lower-fat diets without targeted caloric reduction help promote weight loss by producing a reduced kilocalorie intake, lower-fat diets with targeted caloric restriction promote greater weight loss than lower-fat diets alone.[41]

Low calorie, high fiber diets are associated with decreased energy density of foods. Energy density can also be manipulated by incorporation of water or air into food. These techniques have been associated with increased satiety and decreased energy intake.[55,56] Caloric density can also be decreased by food substitutes such as Olestra™ (nonabsorbable fat), Enova™ (diacylglycerol-substituted oil) and "noncaloric" sweeteners including saccharin, acesulfane-K, aspartame and Splenda™, however, consequential weight loss has not been substantiated.

TABLE 50.10
Food Group Exchanges for Various Caloric Levels

	Calorie Level, Kcal		
	1200	**1500**	**1800**
Starch group exchanges	5	6	8
Fruit group exchanges	2	3	4
Vegetable group exchanges	3	4	5
Milk group exchanges	2	2	2
Meat group exchanges	5 oz	6 oz	7 oz
Fat group exchanges	≤3	≤4	≤5
Sweets	Use sparingly	Use sparingly	Use sparingly

TABLE 50.11
Sample Meal Plan for 1500 Calories

Food	Calories (Kcal)
Breakfast	
Whole wheat toast, 2 slices	140
Banana, 1 small	60
Milk, fat-free, 8 fl. oz	90
Margarine, 2 tsp	90
Coffee/tea/water	0
Lunch	
Turkey sandwich	
Turkey breast, 2 oz	70
Bread, 2 slices	140
Mayonnaise, fat-free, 1 Tb	10
Lettuce, 1 leaf	0
Mini carrots, raw, 1 cup	25
Yogurt, fat-free, vanilla, 1 cup	200
Coffee/tea/water	0
Supper	
Fish, baked, 4 oz	140
Potato, baked, 1 med (6 oz)	160
Sour cream, light, 2 Tb	40
Broccoli, steamed, 1 cup	50
Margarine, 1 tsp	45
Strawberries, fresh, 1 1/4 cup	60
Whipped topping, fat-free, 2 Tb	15
Coffee/tea/water	0
Snack	
Popcorn, air-popped, 6 cups	180
Total calories	1515

TABLE 50.12
Educational Topics for Weight Loss Counseling

Energy value of different foods
Food composition — fats, carbohydrates (including dietary fiber), and proteins
Evaluation of nutrition labels to determine caloric content and food composition
New habits of purchasing — give preference to low-calorie foods
Food preparation — avoid adding high-calorie ingredients during cooking (e.g., fats and oils)
Avoid overconsumption of high-calorie foods (both high-fat and high-carbohydrate foods)
Maintain adequate water intake
Reduction of portion sizes
Limiting alcohol consumption

Implementation of Diet

The dietitian should prescribe a caloric level appropriate for a weight loss of one half to 1 lb/week. The dietitian should also recommend the fat intake (20 to 30%) and the fiber goal (25 to 35 g). Advising the patient to gradually increase fiber in the diet will help avoid gastrointestinal side effects such as gas, cramps, and bloating. Increasing fluid intake while increasing fiber intake will prevent constipation. Educating the patient on high-fiber cereals, eating the peels on apples and potatoes, and eating the whole fruit rather than just drinking the juice will help fulfill the requirement for fiber. Beans are also an excellent low-fat source of fiber. Patients should be encouraged to keep food records of total kilocalories, fat, and fiber to monitor compliance. Recommendations of references for counting calories, fat, and fiber should be given to the patient along with sample meal plans. A sample meal plan is shown in Table 50.13.

TABLE 50.13
Sample Meal Plan for Low-Fat, High-Fiber Diet

Food	Calories (Kcal)	Fat (g)	Fiber (g)
Breakfast			
Orange juice, 1/2 cup	56	0	0.5
Fiber One cereal, 1/4 cup	30	0.5	6.5
Fruit 'n Fiber cereal, 1/2 cup	105	1.5	3
Banana, 1/2 med	52	0.2	1.3
Milk, fat-free, 8 fl oz	86	0.4	0
Whole wheat toast, 1 slice	65	2	2
Margarine, light, 1 tsp	17	2.7	0
Coffee/tea/water	0	0	0
Lunch			
Split pea soup, 1 cup	133	1.6	3.7
Triscuit crackers, reduced fat, 8	130	3	4
Chicken breast, grilled, skin removed, 2 oz	95	2.1	0
Hamburger bun, 1	123	2.2	1.2
Honey mustard, 1 Tb	25	0	0
Sliced tomato, 1/2 med	13	0.2	0.7
Lettuce, 1 leaf	2	0	0.3
Pear, 1 med	98	0.7	4
Coffee/tea/water	0	0	0
Supper			
Spinach salad, 1 cup	12	0.2	1.6
Salad dressing, light, 2 Tb	100	8	0
Grouper, baked, 4 oz	133	1.4	0
Brown rice, 1/2 cup	108	0.9	1.8
Asparagus, steamed, 6 spears	22	0.3	1.4
Whole wheat roll, 1	75	1.3	2.1
Margarine, light, 2 tsp	34	5.4	0
Yogurt, fat-free, vanilla, 1 cup	200	0	0
Strawberries, 1 cup	45	0.6	3.4
Coffee/tea/water	0	0	0
Totals	1759	35.2[a]	37.5

[a] Fat calories provide 18% of total kilocalories.

VERY-LOW-CALORIE DIETS

A VLCD is defined as one that provides <800 kcal/day. Such diets may severely restrict carbohydrates and induce ketosis (ketogenic diets) or may simply restrict all macronutrients, and can be either a liquid formulation or a food diet.[57] The following discussion will refer to ketogenic VLCDs. Ketosis produces anorexia and thus improves dietary compliance. This diet is appropriate only when a patient has major health risks and the physician has determined that the diet can be used safely. Indications for patients for VLCDs are a BMI ≥35, or a BMI ≥30, in association with comorbid conditions. The natriuresis associated with ketosis and the rapid reduction in insulin resistance make the diet especially useful in patients with fluid overload and diabetes, respectively. Candidates for VLCDs should have failed prior weight-loss attempts and should demonstrate motivation to adhere to the VLCD. Additionally, the patient should understand that this is a temporary method for weight loss, and that transitioning to a more balanced eating pattern will be necessary for further weight loss and weight maintenance. Patients should not follow this diet for more than 12 to 16 weeks. Contraindications for use of VLCDs are listed in Table 50.14.

VLCDs are not recommended for weight-loss therapy for most patients because they require special monitoring and supplementation.[58] Specialized practitioners experienced in the use of VLCDs are preferable for screening and supervising patients for this diet. Medical monitoring will help the physician detect any patients who may react adversely to the VLCD. Potential complications include excessive loss of lean body mass, orthostatic hypotension, constipation (inadequate fiber in diet), gout (ketones compete with uric acid for excretion), and a likelihood for recidivism. Diuretics should be discontinued to minimize the increased risk of electrolyte imbalance,[59] and diabetic drugs will need to be reduced or discontinued. Clinical trials show that LCDs are as effective as VLCDs in producing sustained weight loss after 1 year.[60] As with any type of weight loss program, including behavioral therapy and physical activity along with the VLCD seems to improve maintenance of weight loss.[58,61]

TABLE 50.14
Contraindications to Very-Low-Calorie Diets (VLCDs)

Recent myocardial infarction
Cerebrovascular disease
Chronic renal failure
Hepatic disease
Type I diabetes mellitus
Severe psychiatric disorders
Alcoholism
Cancer
Infection
Acute substance abuse
Human immunodeficiency virus infection

TABLE 50.15
VLCD Sample Meal Plan

Breakfast
Lean ham, 4 oz
Coffee, 8 fluid oz

Lunch
Lean ground beef, 5 oz
Carrots, raw, 2 whole
Soda, diet, 12 fluid oz

Supper
Baked chicken breast, skinless, boneless, 6 oz
Green beans,1/2 cup cooked
Tea, sugar substitute, 12 fl oz

Implementation of Diet

The VLCD should provide 1.2 to 1.5 g protein/kg of desirable body weight per day. This protein must be of high biologic value in order to maximize preservation of lean body mass. Lean meat, fish, poultry, and egg whites are recommended. The dietitian determines the protein needs of the patient and converts grams of protein to ounces of meat (7 g protein = 1 oz meat). The meat is divided into three meals per day, and the patient is encouraged not to skip meals. The patient is given the following directions:

Choose only lean meats
Prepare meats without adding fats, breading, or sauces
Weigh meat after cooking to comply with prescribed amount
Include two servings of nonstarchy vegetables per day
Drink at least two quarts of noncaloric fluids per day
Take one multiple vitamin–mineral supplement per day
Take a calcium supplement providing 1000 to 1500 mg elemental calcium per day
Test urine for ketones one time per day with KetoStix (available over the counter)
A sample meal plan is shown in Table 50.15 for a VLCD providing 15 oz meat per day

In the case of liquid diets, the protein should be from dairy sources, soy, or albumin. Most liquid formulations provide between 0.8 and 1.5 g protein/kg of desirable body weight, up to 100 g carbohydrate, the minimum of essential fatty acids, and the recommended allowances of vitamins and minerals. Commercial versions of VLCDs include Optifast™, HMR™ (Health Management Resources), and Medifast™.

Refeeding, the process of gradual weaning from the VLCD back to a balanced diet, generally takes 3 to 6 weeks. The dietitian should follow the patient closely at this time and gradually increase the daily caloric intake, because the decline in resting metabolic rate usually continues for about 3 months after the VLCD has been discontinued.[59] Patients should be informed that some water weight will most likely be regained when they return to a balanced diet (reversal of the natriuresis associated with ketosis).

HIGH-PROTEIN, LOW-CARBOHYDRATE DIETS

Diet books such as *Dr. Atkins New Diet Revolution, Protein Power, The Carbohydrate Addict's LifeSpan Program*, *Sugar Busters*, *The Zone* and *The South Beach Diet* all emphasize protein and limit carbohydrates or sugar. These diets are similar in some respects to the VLCDs, but typically are not medically supervised. Some of these diets allow/encourage excessive saturated fat and protein. High intake of protein may promote satiety[62,63] and improve dietary compliance. Studies[64,65] have documented that, compared to more liberal carbohydrate intake, these severely carbohydrate restricted diets are more effective in lowering glucose and triglyceride levels and raising HDL cholesterol levels in subjects who are insulin resistant.

MEAL REPLACEMENT DIETS

As portion control is a primary strategy in weight management, meal replacement diets have been shown to be effective.[66] Meal replacements are foods designed to replace all or part of a meal while providing a known caloric level. Commercial programs based on meal replacement include Jenny Craig™ and NutriSystem™.

CONSEQUENCES OF DIETING

Caloric restriction produces a natriuresis and diuresis that is reversed with resumption of higher kilocalorie levels. This may lead to discouragement and abandonment of dietary efforts. With severe caloric restriction, adaptation to starvation produces hypometabolism. Loss of lean tissue will also reduce the REE. Weight loss also produces a reduced capacity for fat oxidation.[67] However, the evidence thus far does not support adverse effects of weight cycling on REE, body composition, or body fat distribution.[68]

Temporary consequences of weight loss include secondary amenorrhea and hair loss. Gallstones may develop during weight loss; a large percentage of these dissolve spontaneously.

EXERCISE

Adding exercise to a calorie-restricted diet marginally increases weight loss but minimizes the decline in the REE due to the caloric deficit. Exercise promotes preservation of lean tissue and may result in reduction of adipose tissue and decreased insulin resistance in the absence of weight loss.[69] The major benefits of exercise are its effects on health, mood, and maintenance of weight loss (Table 50.16). The slightly greater proportion of fat used with low-intensity aerobic exercise is offset by the greater total energy expended by high-intensity aerobic exercise. Physical training increases oxidation of fatty acids. By increasing muscle mass, resistance exercise is also beneficial.

BEHAVIOR MODIFICATION

Behavior modification refers to tools or skills used to improve compliance with diet and exercise regimens. Table 50.17 outlines several approaches. Behavioral therapy is an essential component of any adequate obesity treatment program. Behavioral treatment may produce weight loss of 8 to 10% during the initial six months of therapy.[70,71]

SURGERY

Surgical options for the treatment of obesity have been reviewed by Kral.[72] The most common are gastroplasty (creation of a small gastric pouch with restricted outlet along the lesser curvature of the stomach) and gastric bypass (construction of a proximal gastric pouch whose outlet is a Roux-en-Y limb of small intestine). Both procedures produce a >50% reduction of excess weight in the majority of patients, with the bypass having superior results. Additional procedures include gastric banding (adjustable band creating a proximal gastric pouch) and biliopancreatic diversion. Jejunoileal bypasses, which have produced severe complications, are not recommended. Candidates for surgical treatment are those with severe obesity (BMI > 35 with comorbidities or >40 without comorbidity) who are well informed and highly motivated, but have failed prior dietary attempts. (See chapters 52 & 53

DRUGS

To be considered for pharmacotherapy, subjects should have a BMI ≥30 without risk factors, or a BMI of ≥27 with obesity-related comorbidities. Centrally acting noradrenergic agents (Table 50.18) are approved for short-term use only. Common side effects of noradrenergic agents are headache, insomnia, nervousness, irritability, and increased blood pressure and pulse.

TABLE 50.16
Proposed Mechanisms Linking Exercise with Successful Weight Maintenance

Increased energy expenditure
Improved body composition
   Fat loss
   Preservation of lean body mass
   Reduction of visceral fat depot
Increased capacity for fat mobilization and oxidation
Control of food intake
   Short-term reduction of appetite
   Reduction of fat intake
Stimulation of thermogenic response
   RMR
   Diet-induced thermogenesis
Change in muscle morphology and biochemical capacity
Increased insulin sensitivity
Improved plasma lipid and lipoprotein profile
Reduced blood pressure
Better aerobic fitness
Positive psychological effects
   Improved mood
   Improved self-esteem
   Increased adherence to diet

TABLE 50.17
Behavior Modification Techniques

Self-monitoring: using food and exercise diaries
Stimulus control: keeping food out of sight
Stress management
Social support
Eating management: eating slower
Behavior substitution: exercising instead of eating
Rewards
Relapse prevention
Cognitive restructuring: positive self-talk
Environmental engineering: eating only at the table
Covert sensitization: imagining unpleasant consequences

TABLE 50.18
Weight Loss Agents

Drug	Usual Dose per Day (mg)
Noradrenergic agents	
Phendimetrazine	105
Phentermine	15–37.5
Mazindol	1–3
Diethylproprion	75
Adrenergic/serotonergic reuptake inhibitors	
Sibutramine	5–15
Gastrointestinal lipase inhibitors	
Orlistat	120 mg tid

Sibutramine (a serotonin and norepinephrine reuptake inhibitor) and orlistat (a lipase inhibitor) have been demonstrated to be effective in promoting weight loss and improving metabolic parameters in long-term, double-blind, randomized, placebo-controlled trials. Both are approved by the FDA for long-term use. Currently, approval for an over-the-counter dose of orlistat is being sought. Sibutramine produces a dose-related weight loss.[73] In addition to the side effects seen with noradrenergic drugs, sibutramine may cause dry mouth. Side effects of lipase inhibitors are a consequence fat malabsorption and may include abdominal pain, diarrhea, oily stools, fecal incontinence, and malabsorption of fat-soluble vitamins. Side effects may be reduced by the concomitant use of fiber such as psyllium.[74]

Rimonabant, a cannabinoid receptor blocker, has been demonstrated to promote significant weight loss. Currently, the Federal Food and Drug Administration (FDA) have issued an "approvable" letter, although final approval has not yet been granted. Medications that are approved for nonobesity indications that have been shown to promote weight loss (considered" off-label usage" when used for weight loss) include buproprion,[75,76] topiramate,[77,78] and zonisamide.[79]

Numerous over-the-counter preparations for weight loss are promoted to the lay public with little scientific data supporting efficacy. A recent review[80] indicates that chitosan, garcinia (active ingredient hydroxycitric acid), guar gum and psyllim are ineffective. Conflicting data exist for pyruvate and yohimbe, whereas slight effectiveness has been demonstrated for chromium picolinate, glucomannan, hydroxy-methylbutyrate and yerba mate (contains caffeine). Ephedra/ephedrine, while effective is associated with significant side effects and has been removed from the market.

The likelihood of long-term effectiveness can be predicted by weight loss during the first month of therapy. Weight loss drugs are not a substitute for a healthy diet and regular exercise, nor are they a cure for obesity. They can, however, promote modest weight loss sufficient to improve health risks.

OUTCOMES

Treatment outcomes have been reviewed by Brownell and Wadden.[81] Predictors of weight loss and weight maintenance are listed in Table 50.19 and Table 50.20, respectively.

TABLE 50.19
Predictors of Weight Loss

Positive Predictors
Personal Factors
    High initial body weight or BMI
    High REE
    High self-management skills

Process Factors
Attendance at program
Weight loss early in program

Treatment Factors
Increased length of treatment
Having social support
Engaging in physical activity

Incorporation of behavior modification techniques
Self-monitoring
Goal setting
Slowing rate of eating

Negative Predictors
Repeated attempts at weight loss
Experiencing perceived stress
(Others include the opposites of the positive
  indicators)

Nonpredictors
Total body fat, fat distribution, and body
  composition
Personality/psychopathology test results
Dietary restraint
Binge eating

TABLE 50.20
Predictors of Maintenance
of Weight Loss

Positive Predictors
Physical activity
Self-monitoring
Positive coping style
Continued contact
Normalization of eating
Reduction of comorbidities

Negative Predictors
Negative life events
Family dysfunction

REFERENCES

1. Comuzzie AG, Allison DB. *Science* 280: 1374, 1998.
2. Stunkard AJ, Sorensen TI, Hanis C, et al. *N Engl J Med* 314: 193, 1986.
3. Stunkard AJ, Foch TT, Hrubec Z. *JAMA* 256: 51, 1986.
4. Poehlman ET, Tremblay A, Depres J, et al. *Am J Clin Nutr* 43: 723, 1986.
5. Lyon AL, Hirschhorn JN. *Am J Clin Nutr* 82: 215S, 2005.
6. Perusse L, Rankinen T, Zuberi A, et al. *Obes Res* 13: 381, 2005.
7. Wansink B, Painter JE, North J. *Obes Res* 13: 93, 2005.
8. Brand-Miller JC, Holt SHA, Pawlak DB, et al. *Am J Clin Nutr* 76: 281S, 2002.
9. Bray GA, Nielsen SJ, Popkin BM. *Am J Clin Nutr* 79: 537, 2004.
10. Bray GA, Popkin BM. *Am J Clin Nutr* 68: 1157, 1998.
11. Jones PJH, Schoeller DA. *Metabolism* 37: 145, 1992.
12. Weinsier RL, Hunter GR, Heini AF, et al. *Am J Med* 105: 145, 1998.
13. Sobal J, Stunkard AJ. *Psychol Bull* 105: 260, 1989.
14. Bjorntorp P. *Obes Res* 1, 206; 1993.
15. Oken E, Gillman MW. *Obes Res* 11: 496, 2003.
16. Poehlman ET, Toth MJ, Gardner AW. *Ann Intern Med* 123: 673, 1995.
17. Dhurandhar NV, Augustus A, Atkinson RL. *FASEB J* 11: A230, 1997.
18. Vangipuram SD, Sheele J, Atkinson RL, et al. *Obes Res* 12: 770, 2004.
19. Himms-Hagen J. *Obes Res* 3: 361, 1995.
20. Zurlo F, Lillioja S, Esposito-Del Puente A, et al. *Am J Physiol* 259: E650, 1990.
21. Eckel RH. *Lancet* 340: 1452, 1992.
22. Wolfe RR, Peters EJ, Klein S, et al. *Am J Physiol* 252: E189, 1987.
23. Jones PJH, Schoeller DA. *Metabolism* 37: 145, 1992.
24. Kien CL, Bunn JY, Ugrasbul F. *Am J Clin Nutr* 82: 320, 2005.
25. Ristow M, Muller-Wieland D, Pfeiffer A, et al. *N Engl J Med* 339: 93, 1990.
26. Ravussin E, Lillioja S, Knowler WC, et al. *N Engl J Med* 318: 462, 1988.
27. Poehlman ET, Horton ES. *Nutr Rev* 47: 129, 1989.
28. Samaras K, Kelly PJ, Chiano MN, et al. *Ann Intern Med* 130: 873, 1999.
29. Golay A, Schutz Y, Felber JP, et al. *Int J Obes* 13: 767, 1989.
30. Astrup A, Andersen T, Christensen NJ, et al. *Am J Clin Nutr* 51: 331, 1990.
31. Golay A, Jallut D, Schutz Y, et al. *Int J Obes* 15: 601, 1990.
32. Argyropoulos G, Brown AM, Willi SM, et al. *J Clin Invest* 102: 1345, 1998.
33. Must A, Spadano J, Coakley EH, et al. *JAMA* 282: 1523, 1999.
34. Mokdad AH, Serdula MK, Dietz WH, et al. *JAMA* 282: 1519, 1999.
35. National Center for Health Statistics. http://www.cdc.gov/nchs/nanes.htm.
36. Bjorntorp P. In: Handbook of Eating Disorders: Physiology, Psychology and Treatment of Obesity, Anorexia, and Bulimia, Brownell KD, Foreyt JP, Eds, Basic Books, New York, 1986, pg 88.
37. Fujioka S, Matsuzawa Y, Tokunaga K, Tarui S. *Metabolism* 36: 54, 1987.
38. Manson JE, Colditz GA, Stampfer MJ, et al. *N Engl J Med* 322: 882, 1990.
39. Calle EE, Thun MJ, Petrelli JM, et al. *N Engl J Med* 341: 1097, 1999.

40. Lee I-M, Manson JE, Hennekens CH, Paffenbarger RS. *JAMA* 270: 2823, 1993.
41. National Institutes of Health, National Heart, Lung and Blood Institute. *Obes Res* 6: 51S, 1998.
42. World Health Organization. Obesity, Preventing and Managing the Global Epidemic, World Health Organization, Geneva, 1998, pg 1.
43. Pi-Sunyer FX. *Obes Res* 10: 97S, 2002.
44. Arrone LJ. *Obes Res* 10: 105S, 2002.
45. Wing RR, Koeske R, Epstein LH, et al. *Arch Intern Med* 147: 1749, 1987.
46. Wood PD, Stefanick MI, Dreon DM, et al. *N Engl J Med* 319: 1173, 1988.
47. Hypertension Prevention Trial Research Group. *Arch Intern Med* 150: 153, 1990.
48. Goldstein D. *Int J Obes* 16: 397, 1992.
49. Van Gaal LF, Wauters MA, De Leeuw IH. *Int J Obes* 21: 5S, 1997.
50. Bosello O, Armellini F, Zamboni M, Fitchet M. *Int J Obes* 21: 10S, 1997.
51. Brownell KD. The LEARN Program for Weight Control, 7th ed, American Health Publishing Company, Dallas, 1998.
52. Thomas PR. Weighing the Options, Criteria for Evaluating Weight-Management Programs, National Academy Press, Washington, DC, 1995, pg 91.
53. Mifflin MD, St Jeor ST, Hill LA, et al. *Am J Clin Nutr* 51: 241, 1990.
54. Frankenfield DC, Muth ER, Rowe WA. *J Am Diet Assoc* 98: 442, 1998.
55. Rolls BJ, Bell EA, Waugh BA. *Am J Clin Nutr* 72: 361, 2000.
56. Rolls BJ, Bell EA, Thorwart ML. *Am J Clin Nutr* 70: 448, 1999.
57. Life Sciences Research Office, Management of Obesity by Severe Caloric Restriction, Federation of American Societies for Experimental Biology, Washington, DC, 1979.
58. National Task Force on the Prevention and Treatment of Obesity, National Institutes of Health. *JAMA* 270: 967, 1993.
59. Prasad N. *Postgrad Med* 13: 39, 1990.
60. Wadden TA, Foster GD, Letizia KA. *J Consult Clin Psychol* 62: 165, 1994.
61. Perri MG, McAdoo WG, McAllister DA, et al. *J Consult Clin Psychol* 55: 615, 1987.
62. Anderson GH, Moore SE. *J Nutr* 134: 974S, 2004.
63. Weigle DS, Breen PA, Matthys CC, et al. *Am J Clin Nutr* 82: 41, 2005.
64. Sharman MJ, Gomez AL, Kraemer WJ, et al. *J Nutr* 134: 880, 2004.
65. Cornier M-A, Donahoo WT, Pereira R, et al. *Obes Res* 13: 703, 2005.
66. Heymsfield SB, van Mierlo CA, van der Knapp HC, et al. *Int J Obes Relat Metab Disord* 27: 537, 2003.
67. Wyatt HR, Grunwald GK, Seagle HM, et al. *Am J Clin Nutr* 69: 1189, 1999.
68. Wing R. *Ann Behav Med* 14: 113, 1992.
69. Ross R, Janssen I, Dawson J, et al. *Obes Res* 12: 789, 2004.
70. Foster GD, Makris, AP, Bailer BA. *Am J Clin Nutr* 82: 230S, 2005.
71. Wadden TA, Butryn ML, Byrne KJ. *Obes Res* 12: 151S, 2004.
72. Kral JG. In: Treatment of the Seriously Obese Patient, Wadden TA, VanItallie TB, Eds, Guilford Press, New York, 1992, pg 496.
73. Bray GA, Blackburn GL, Ferguson JM, et al. *Obes Res* 7: 189, 1999.
74. Cavaliere H, Floriano I, Medeiros-Neto G. *Int J Obes* 25: 1095, 2000.
75. Gadde KM, Parker CB, Maner LG, et al. *Obes Res* 9: 544, 2001.
76. Anderson JW, Greenway FL, Fujioka K, et al. *Obes Res* 10: 633, 2002.
77. Bray GA, Hollander P, Klein S, et al. *Obes Res* 11: 722, 2003.
78. Astrup A, Caterson I, Zelissen R, et al. *Obes Res* 12: 1658, 2004.
79. Gadde KM, Franciscy DM, Wagner II HR, et al. *JAMA* 289: 1820, 2003.
80. Pittler MH, Ernst E. *Amer J Clin Nutr* 79: 529, 2004.
81. Brownell KD, Wadden TA. *J Consulting Clin Psychol* 60: 505, 1992.

ADDITIONAL SOURCES OF INFORMATION ON THE WEB

American Council on Exercise, www.acefitness.org
American Dietetic Association, www.eatright.org
American Heart Association, www.americanheart.org
American Obesity Association, www.obesity.org
American Society for Nutritional Sciences, www.nutrition.org
American Society of Bariatric Physicians, www.asbp.org/bariatrics
Center for Disease Control and Prevention, www.cdc.gov/nccdphp/dnpa/obesity
Center for Nutrition Policy and Promotion, www.usda.gov/cnpp
Centers for Obesity Research and Education, www.uchsc.edu/core
International Association for the Study of Obesity, www.iaso.org
Mayo Clinic, www.mayoclinic.com/health/obesity/DS00314
National Association to Advance Fat Acceptance, www.naafa.org/index.html

National Institutes of Health, www.nhlbi.nih.gov/health/public/heart/obesity
North American Association for the Study of Obesity, www.naaso.org
Shape Up America, www.shapeupamerica.org
Surgeon General's Call to Action on Obesity, www.surgeongeneral.gov/topics/obesity
U.S. Food and Drug Administration, www.fda.gov/loseweight
World Health Organization, www.who.int/topics/obesity/en

51 Childhood Obesity and Exercise

Scott Owens, Bernard Gutin, and Paule Barbeau

CONTENTS

INTRODUCTION

Obesity has become the most common chronic pediatric disease in the modern era.[1] Body mass index (BMI) data from the National Health and Nutrition Examination Survey (NHANES) indicated that, among children aged 6 to 19 years in 1999 to 2002, 16% were overweight (age- and sex-specific BMI ≥95th percentile) with an additional 15% "at risk for overweight" (age- and sex-specific BMI between the 85th and 95th percentiles).[2] Table 51.1 shows the prevalence of overweight and "at risk for over-weight" by age, sex, and racial/ethnic group among 6 to 19 year olds in the United States during 1999 to 2002. As shown in Table 51.2, the prevalence of childhood overweight has increased dramatically over the past three decades among all age groups and in both sexes.[3] Thus, an ever-increasing number of young people are experiencing a host of undesirable social, emotional, and medical complications due to obesity.

DEFINITION AND CLINICAL EVALUATION OF CHILDHOOD OBESITY

As shown in Table 51.3, a variety of criteria have been used to define childhood overweight and obesity.[4–7] Ideally, a definition of obesity should be based on a measurement of body fat.[8] Reference methods for measuring body fat such as dual-energy x-ray absorptiometry (DXA) and hydrodensitometry are important tools in research settings, but because they require use of sophisticated apparatus and techniques, they tend to be impractical for routine clinical use or for large epidemiologic studies.[9] Thus, surrogate measures that calculate excess body weight for height, such as BMI, are more commonly used in assessing childhood overweight and obesity.[9] Widely used references containing BMI cut points for determining obesity or overweight in children and adolescents include those published by the International Obesity Task Force (IOTF)[10] (Table 51.4), and those from the Centers for Disease Control and Prevention (CDC),[11] as shown in Figure 51.1 and Figure 51.2. The IOTF cut points (Table 51.4) are based on international survey data from six large nationally representative cross-sectional growth studies (Brazil, Great Britain, Hong Kong, the Netherlands, Singapore, and the United States) and were derived from centile curves that at age 18 years pass through the widely used adult BMI cut points of 25 kg/m^2 for overweight and 30 kg/m^2 for obesity.[10] The resulting curves were averaged to provide age- and sex-specific BMI cut points for ages 2 to 18 years. The CDC references (Figure 51.1 and Figure 51.2) are based on U.S. NHANES data and define an age- and sex-specific BMI value ≥85th percentile as at risk for overweight and a

TABLE 51.1

Prevalence of At Risk for Overweight and Overweight in Children by Sex, Age, and Racial/Ethnic Group: United States, 1999–2002[a]

		Prevalence, % (SE)							
		At Risk for Overweight and Overweight (BMI for Age ≥85th Percentile)				Overweight (BMI for Age ≥95th Percentile)			
Sex	Age (Years)	All	Non-Hispanic White	Non-Hispanic Black	Mexican American	All	Non-Hispanic White	Non-Hispanic Black	Mexican American
Both	6–19	31.0 (1.1)	28.2 (1.6)[b,c]	35.4 (0.9)[c,d]	39.9 (1.3)[b,d]	16.0 (0.8)	13.6 (1.1)[b,c]	20.5 (0.8)[d]	22.2 (1.1)[d]
	2–5	22.6 (1.5)	20.8 (2.0)	23.2 (2.3)	26.3 (2.7)	10.3 (1.2)	8.6 (1.5)	8.8 (1.5)	13.1 (2.0)
	6–11	31.2 (1.8)	28.6 (2.6)[c]	33.7 (1.6)	38.9 (2.2)[d]	15.8 (1.1)	13.5 (1.5)[b,c]	19.8 (1.4)[d]	21.8 (1.7)[d]
	12–19	30.9 (1.0)	27.9 (1.5)[b,c]	36.8 (1.3)[d]	40.7 (1.6)[d]	16.1 (0.8)	13.7 (1.1)[b,c]	21.1 (1.2)	22.5 (1.3)[d]
Boys	6–19	31.8 (1.4)	29.2 (2.4)[c]	31.0 (1.3)[c]	42.8 (1.6)[b,d]	16.8 (0.8)	14.3 (1.1)[c]	17.9 (1.0)[c]	25.5 (1.3)[b,d]
	2–5	23.0 (2.3)	21.7 (3.2)	20.9 (2.5)	27.6 (3.1)	9.9 (1.6)	8.2 (1.9)	8.0 (1.8)	14.1 (2.1)
	6–11	32.5 (2.3)	29.3 (3.8)[c]	29.7 (2.2)[c]	43.9 (3.0)[b,d]	16.9 (1.3)	14.0 (1.5)[c]	17.0 (1.5)[c]	26.5 (2.2)[b,d]
	12–19	31.2 (1.5)	29.2 (2.3)[c]	32.1 (2.1)[c]	41.9 (1.8)[b,d]	16.7 (0.9)	14.6 (1.3)[c]	18.7 (1.7)	24.7 (1.9)[d]
Girls	6–19	30.3 (1.3)	27.0 (1.7)[b,c]	40.1 (1.4)[d]	36.6 (1.8)[d]	15.1 (1.1)	12.9 (1.6)[b,c]	23.2 (1.1)[d]	18.5 (1.4)[d]
	2–5	22.3 (1.8)	20.0 (2.3)	25.6 (3.0)	25.0 (3.8)	10.7 (1.5)	9.1 (2.0)	9.6 (1.8)	12.2 (3.4)
	6–11	29.9 (2.1)	27.7 (2.8)	37.9 (2.8)	33.8 (2.6)	14.7 (1.6)	13.1 (2.3)[b]	22.8 (2.5)[d]	17.1 (2.0)
	12–19	30.5 (1.3)	26.5 (2.0)[b,c]	41.9 (1.7)[d]	39.3 (2.3)[d]	15.4 (1.2)	12.7 (1.8)[b]	23.6 (1.8)[d]	19.9 (1.9)

Abbreviation: BMI, body mass index, calculated as weight in kilograms divided by square of height in meters.

[a] BMI was rounded to the nearest tenth. Pregnant girls were excluded. All categories included racial/ethnic groups not shown separately.

[b] Significantly different from non-Hispanic blacks at $P < .05$, with Bonferroni adjustment.

[c] Significantly different from Mexican-Americans at $P < .05$, with Bonferroni adjustment.

[d] Significantly different from non-Hispanic whites at $P < .05$, with Bonferroni adjustment.

Source: From Hedley, A.A. et al. *JAMA*, 291: 2847, 2004. With permission.

TABLE 51.2

Trends in Overweight for Children from Birth through 19 Years by Sex and Age Group[a]

	NHES 2 (1963–1965)	NHES 3 (1966–1970)	NHANES I (1971–1974)	NHANES II (1976–1980)	NHANES III (1988–1994)	NHANES (1999–2000)	P-Values for NHANES III vs. NHANES 1999–2000
6–23 months[b]							
Total				7.2 (1.0)	8.9 (0.7)	11.6 (1.9)	.09
Male				8.2 (1.4)	9.9 (0.8)	9.8 (2.2)	.48
Female				6.1 (1.3)	7.9 (1.0)	14.3 (3.5)	.04
2–5 years[c]							
Total			5.0 (0.6)	5.0 (0.6)	7.2 (0.7)	10.4 (1.7)	.04
Boys			5.0 (0.9)	4.7 (0.6)	6.1 (0.8)	9.9 (2.2)	.06
Girls			4.9 (0.8)	5.3 (1.0)	8.2 (1.1)	11.0 (2.5)	.16
6–11 years[c]							
Total	4.2 (0.4)		4.0 (0.5)	6.5 (0.6)	11.3 (1.0)	15.3 (1.7)	.02
Boys	4.0 (0.4)		4.3 (0.8)	6.6 (0.8)	11.6 (1.3)	16.0 (2.3)	.05
Girls	4.5 (0.6)		3.6 (0.6)	6.4 (1.0)	11.0 (1.4)	14.5 (2.5)	.11
12–19 years[c]							
Total		4.6 (0.3)	6.1 (0.6)	5.0 (0.5)	10.5 (0.9)	15.5 (1.2)	<.001
Adolescent boys		4.5 (0.4)	6.1 (0.8)	4.8 (0.5)	11.3 (1.3)	15.5 (1.6)	.02
Adolescent girls		4.7 (0.3)	6.2 (0.8)	5.3 (0.8)	9.7 (1.1)	15.5 (1.6)	.002

[a] Values are expressed as percentage (SE).

[b] A weight-for-length at the 95th percentile or higher is considered overweight.

[c] BMI for age at the 95th percentile or higher is considered overweight.

Source: From Ogden, C.L. et al. *JAMA*, 288: 1728, 2002. With permission.

TABLE 51.3
Anthropometric Definitions of Childhood Overweight/Obesity

Definition	Reference
Body weight >120% of the value predicted from height	4
Body mass index (BMI) >85th percentile	5
Body mass index (BMI) >95th percentile	5
Triceps skin-fold thickness >85th percentile	6
Triceps skin-fold thickness >95th percentile	6
Body fat >25% for boys and 30% for girls as estimated from sum of subscapular and triceps skin folds	7

TABLE 51.4
International Cut Points for BMI for Overweight and Obesity by Sex between 2 and 18 Years[a]

Age (years)	Males	Females	Males	Females
2	18.41	18.02	20.09	19.81
2.5	18.13	17.76	19.80	19.55
3	17.89	17.56	19.57	19.36
3.5	17.69	17.40	19.39	19.23
4	17.55	17.28	19.29	19.15
4.5	17.47	17.19	19.26	19.12
5	17.42	17.15	19.30	19.17
5.5	17.45	17.20	19.47	19.34
6	17.55	17.34	19.78	19.65
6.5	17.71	17.53	20.23	20.08
7	17.92	17.75	20.63	20.51
7.5	18.16	18.03	21.09	21.01
8	18.44	18.35	21.60	21.57
8.5	18.76	18.69	22.17	22.18
9	19.10	19.07	22.77	22.81
9.5	19.46	19.45	23.39	23.46
10	19.84	19.86	24.00	24.11
10.5	20.20	20.29	24.57	24.77
11	20.55	20.74	25.10	25.42
11.5	20.89	21.20	25.58	26.05
12	21.22	21.68	26.02	26.67
12.5	21.56	22.14	26.43	27.24
13	21.91	22.58	26.84	27.76
13.5	22.27	22.98	27.25	28.20
14	22.62	23.34	27.63	28.57
14.5	22.96	23.66	27.98	28.87
15	23.29	23.94	28.30	29.11
15.5	23.60	24.17	28.60	29.29
16	23.90	24.37	28.88	29.43
16.5	24.19	24.54	29.14	29.56
17	24.46	24.70	29.41	29.69
17.5	24.73	24.85	29.70	29.84
18	25	25	30	30

[a] Cut points defined to pass through BMI of 25 and 30 kg/m^2 at age 18, obtained by averaging data from Brazil, Great Britain, Hong Kong, The Netherlands, Singapore, and the United States.

Source: From Cole, T.J. et al. *BMJ*, 320: 1, 2000. With permission from the BMJ Publishing Group.

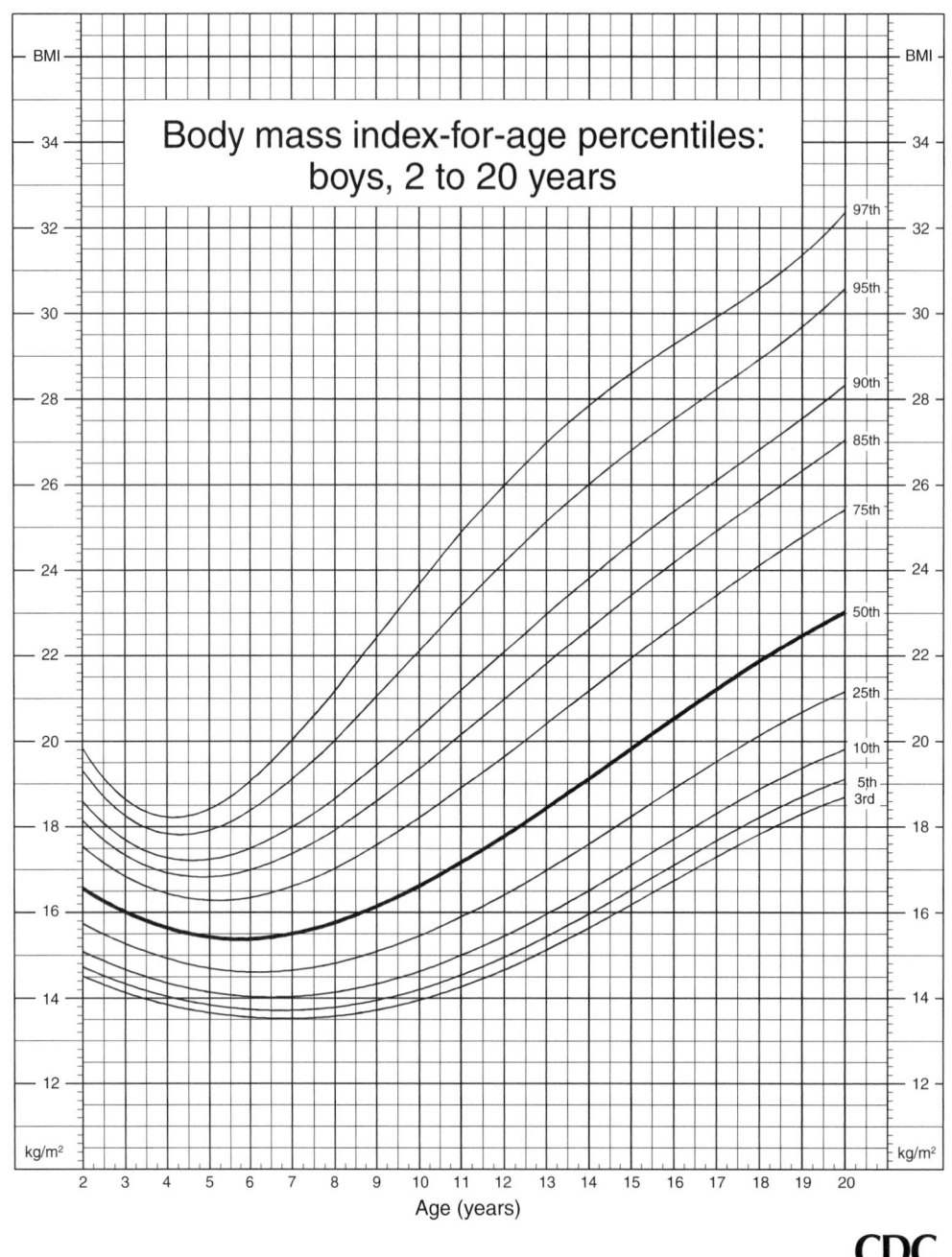

FIGURE 51.1 Growth curves for boys published and distributed by the Centers for Disease Control and Prevention used to estimate an individual's body mass index (BMI) percentile for age and sex.

value ≥95th percentile as overweight.[12] A clinical decision about whether a child with a given BMI is truly overfat may require additional information, such as skin-fold thickness measurements, comorbidity, family history, and recent health history.[13] A careful family history and physical examination can readily diagnose the hormonal and genetic causes of childhood obesity.[14] Table 51.5 lists common hormonal and genetic causes of childhood obesity. Although genetic and hormonal disorders are responsible for less than 10% of childhood obesity, they must be considered, as they require different modes of therapy.[4]

ABDOMINAL OBESITY

In adults and obese children, excess accumulation of abdominal fat, especially in the visceral region, is more highly correlated with risk factors for the development of chronic diseases such as type 2 diabetes, hypertension, and coronary artery disease than is excess peripheral fat or overall obesity as determined by BMI.[15–18] Since accurate measurement of visceral fat requires the

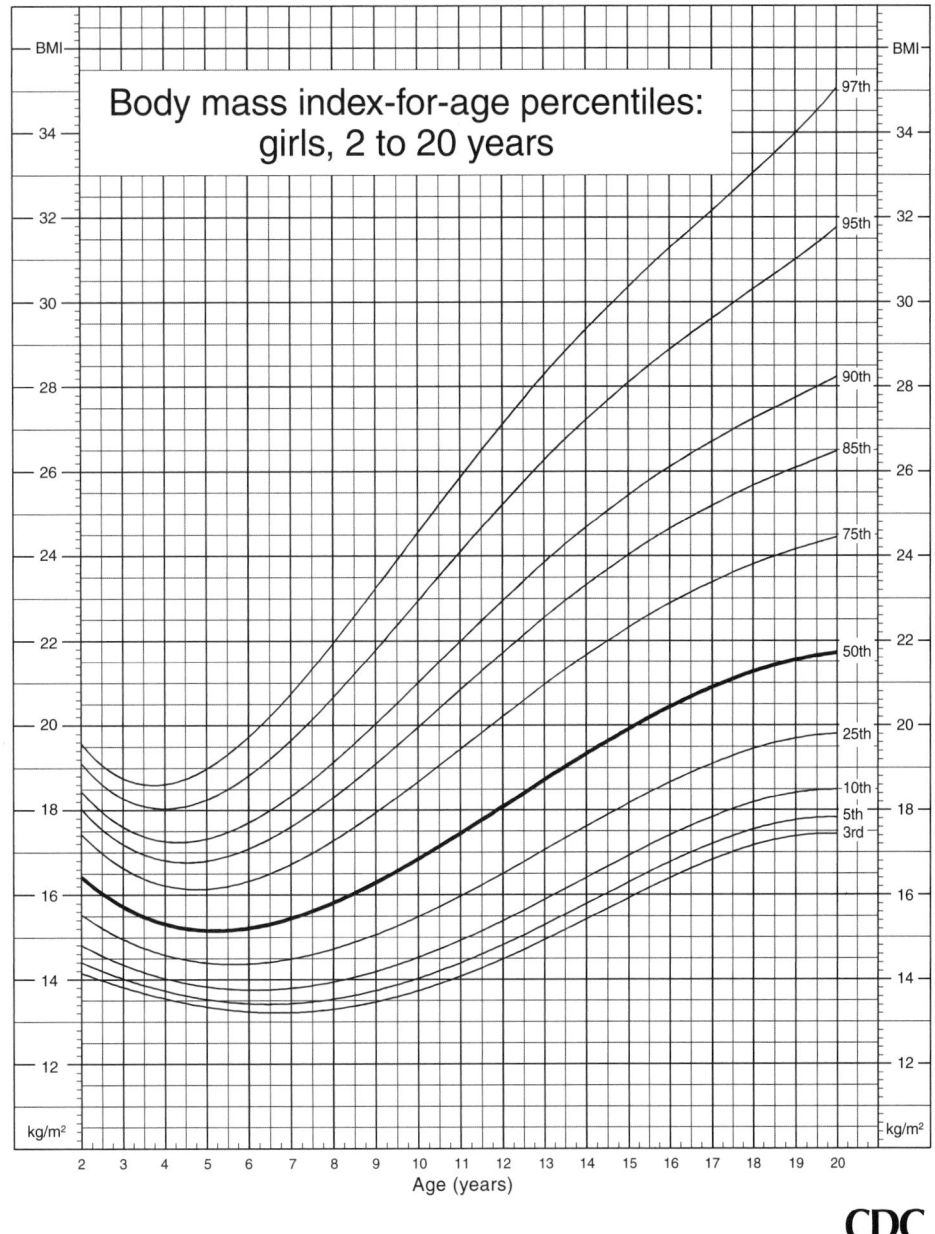

FIGURE 51.2 Growth curves for girls published and distributed by the Centers for Disease Control and Prevention used to estimate an individual's body mass index (BMI) percentile for age and sex.

use of computed tomography or magnetic resonance imaging, both of which are expensive and time consuming, proxy measures of abdominal/visceral fat have been suggested, the most common of which is waist circumference.[19,20] Several authors have recommended that a waist circumference measurement be included in a child's overall obesity assessment.[19–21] Age- and sex-specific waist circumferences ≥90th percentile have been suggested as identifying children and adolescents at increased risk for developing metabolic disorders.[22,23] Table 51.6 to Table 51.9 show age-, sex-, and ethnicity-specific waist circumference percentiles from nationally representative samples of U.S. children and adolescents.

HEALTH RISKS OF CHILDHOOD OBESITY

Childhood obesity is a significant public health problem because of its immediate impact on the physical and psychological health of children and adolescents, and because it is a risk factor for the development of chronic diseases later in life.[24] A variety of additional health problems occur at significantly greater frequencies in obese children (see Table 51.10). There is also some indication that obese children with increased visceral adiposity may be at especially high risk (see Table 51.11).

TABLE 51.5
Hormonal and Genetic Causes of Childhood Obesity

Hormonal Causes	Diagnostic Clues		Genetic Syndromes	Associated Causes
Hypothyroidism	Increased TSH, decreased thyroxine (T_4) levels		Prader–Willi	Obesity, insatiable appetite, mental retardation, hypogonadism
Hypercortisolism	Abnormal dexamethasone test; increased 24 h free urinary cortisol		Laurence–Moon–Biedel	Obesity, mental retardation, spastic paraplegia
Primary hyperinsulinism	Increased plasma insulin, increased C-peptide levels		Alstrom	Obesity, retinitis pigmentosa, deafness, diabetes mellitus
Acquired hypothalamic	Presence of hypothalamic tumor, infection, syndrome trauma, vascular lesion		Cohen	Truncal obesity, mental retardation, hypotonia
			Turner's	Short stature, undifferentiated gonads, cardiac abnormalities, obesity, X genotype
			Weaver	Infant overgrowth syndrome, accelerated maturation

Source: Adapted from Moron R. *Am Fam Phys*, 59: 861, 1999. With permission.

TABLE 51.6
Waist Circumference (cm) by Percentile and Sex for All Children and Adolescents Combined

Age (Years)	Percentile for Boys					Percentile for Girls				
	10th	25th	50th	75th	90th	10th	25th	50th	75th	90th
2	43.2	45.0	47.1	48.8	50.8	43.8	45.0	47.1	49.5	52.2
3	44.9	46.9	49.1	51.3	54.2	45.4	46.7	49.1	51.9	55.3
4	46.6	48.7	51.1	53.9	57.6	46.9	48.4	51.1	54.3	58.3
5	48.4	50.6	53.2	56.4	61.0	48.5	50.1	53.0	56.7	61.4
6	50.1	52.4	55.2	59.0	64.4	50.1	51.8	55.0	59.1	64.4
7	51.8	54.3	57.2	61.5	67.8	51.6	53.5	56.9	61.5	67.5
8	53.5	56.1	59.3	64.1	71.2	53.2	55.2	58.9	63.9	70.5
9	55.3	58.0	61.3	66.6	74.6	54.8	56.9	60.8	66.3	73.6
10	57.0	59.8	63.3	69.2	78.0	56.3	58.6	62.8	68.7	76.6
11	58.7	61.7	65.4	71.7	81.4	57.9	60.3	64.8	71.1	79.7
12	60.5	63.5	67.4	74.3	84.8	59.5	62.0	66.7	73.5	82.7
13	62.2	65.4	69.5	76.8	88.2	61.0	63.7	68.7	75.9	85.8
14	63.9	67.2	71.5	79.4	91.6	62.6	65.4	70.6	78.3	88.8
15	65.6	69.1	73.5	81.9	95.0	64.2	67.1	72.6	80.7	91.9
16	67.4	70.9	75.6	84.5	98.4	65.7	68.8	74.6	83.1	94.9
17	69.1	72.8	77.6	87.0	101.8	67.3	70.5	76.5	85.5	98.0
18	70.8	74.6	79.6	89.6	105.2	68.9	72.2	78.5	87.9	101.0

Source: Adapted from Fernandez, J.R. et al. *J Pediatr*, 145: 439, 2004. With permission.

ETIOLOGY OF CHILDHOOD OBESITY

The rising prevalence of childhood obesity can be explained in part by changes in our environment over the past 30 years, in particular the unlimited supply of convenient, highly palatable, energy-dense foods, coupled with a lifestyle typified by low levels of physical activity.[47] However, obesity is a complex, multifactorial disease that arises as a result of genetic, environmental, and behavioral factors, which may influence individual responses to diet, sedentariness, and physical activity.[47]

GENETICS

Feeding studies with twins have helped to elucidate the role of genetic background in determining obesity. When groups of identical twins are exposed to overfeeding, significantly more variance occurs in the response between pairs of twins

TABLE 51.7

Waist Circumference (cm) by Percentile and Sex for European-American Children and Adolescents

Age (Years)	Percentile for Boys					Percentile for Girls				
	10th	25th	50th	75th	90th	10th	25th	50th	75th	90th
2	52.5	42.9	46.9	47.1	48.6	50.6	43.1	45.1	47.4	49.6
3	55.4	44.7	48.8	49.2	51.2	54.0	44.7	46.8	49.3	51.9
4	58.2	46.5	50.6	51.3	53.8	57.4	46.3	48.5	51.2	54.2
5	61.1	48.3	52.5	53.3	56.5	60.8	47.9	50.2	53.1	56.5
6	64.0	50.1	54.3	55.4	59.1	64.2	49.5	51.8	55.0	58.8
7	66.8	51.9	56.2	57.5	61.7	67.6	51.1	53.5	56.9	61.1
8	69.7	53.7	58.1	59.6	64.3	71.0	52.7	55.2	58.8	63.4
9	72.6	55.5	59.9	61.7	67.0	74.3	54.3	56.9	60.7	65.7
10	75.5	57.3	61.8	63.7	69.6	77.7	55.9	58.6	62.5	68.0
11	78.3	59.1	63.6	65.8	72.2	81.1	57.5	60.2	64.4	70.3
12	81.2	60.9	65.5	67.9	74.9	84.5	59.1	61.9	66.3	72.6
13	84.1	62.7	67.4	70.0	77.5	87.9	60.7	63.6	68.2	74.9
14	86.9	64.5	69.2	72.1	80.1	91.3	62.3	65.3	70.1	77.2
15	89.8	66.3	71.1	74.1	82.8	94.7	63.9	67.0	72.0	79.5
16	92.7	68.1	72.9	76.2	85.4	98.1	65.5	68.6	73.9	81.8
17	95.5	69.9	74.8	78.3	88.0	101.5	67.1	70.3	75.8	84.1
18	98.4	71.7	76.7	80.4	90.6	104.9	68.7	72.0	77.7	86.4

Source: Adapted from Fernandez, J.R. et al. *J Pediatr*, 145: 439, 2004. With permission.

TABLE 51.8

Waist Circumference (cm) by Percentile and Sex for African-American Children and Adolescents

Age (Years)	Percentile for Boys					Percentile for Girls				
	10th	25th	50th	75th	90th	10th	25th	50th	75th	90th
2	43.2	44.6	46.4	48.5	50.0	43.0	44.6	46.0	47.7	50.1
3	44.8	46.3	48.3	50.7	53.2	44.6	46.3	48.1	50.6	53.8
4	46.3	48.0	50.1	52.9	56.4	46.1	48.0	50.2	53.4	57.5
5	47.9	49.7	52.0	55.1	59.6	47.7	49.7	52.3	56.2	61.1
6	49.4	51.4	53.9	57.3	62.8	49.2	51.4	54.5	59.0	64.8
7	51.0	53.1	55.7	59.5	66.1	50.8	53.2	56.6	61.8	68.5
8	52.5	54.8	57.6	61.7	69.3	52.4	54.9	58.7	64.7	72.2
9	54.1	56.4	59.4	63.9	72.5	53.9	56.6	60.9	67.5	75.8
10	55.6	58.1	61.3	66.1	75.7	55.5	58.3	63.0	70.3	79.5
11	57.2	59.8	63.2	68.3	78.9	57.0	60.0	65.1	73.1	83.2
12	58.7	61.5	65.0	70.5	82.1	58.6	61.7	67.3	75.9	86.9
13	60.3	63.2	66.9	72.7	85.3	60.2	63.4	69.4	78.8	90.5
14	61.8	64.9	68.7	74.9	88.5	61.7	65.1	71.5	81.6	94.2
15	63.4	66.6	70.6	77.1	91.7	63.3	66.8	73.6	84.4	97.9
16	64.9	68.3	72.5	79.3	94.9	64.8	68.5	75.8	87.2	101.6
17	66.5	70.0	74.3	81.5	98.2	66.4	70.3	77.9	90.0	105.2
18	68.0	71.7	76.2	83.7	101.4	68.0	72.0	80.0	92.9	108.9

Source: Adapted from Fernandez, J.R. et al. *J Pediatr*, 145: 439, 2004. With permission.

than within pairs for the changes in body weight, suggesting a genetic predisposition for individuals to gain weight.[48] Still, the results from family studies suggest that the maximal heritability for obesity phenotypes ranges from about 30 to 50%, indicating that nongenetic factors play an important role.[49] Quantifying the influence of the nongenetic factors has proven difficult, however.

TABLE 51.9

Waist Circumference (cm) by Percentile and Sex for Mexican-American Children and Adolescents

Age (years)	Percentile for Boys					Percentile for Girls				
	10th	25th	50th	75th	90th	10th	25th	50th	75th	90th
2	44.4	45.6	47.6	49.8	53.2	44.5	45.7	48.0	50.0	53.5
3	46.1	47.5	49.8	52.5	56.7	46.0	47.4	50.1	52.6	56.7
4	47.8	49.4	52.0	55.3	60.2	47.5	49.2	52.2	55.2	59.9
5	49.5	51.3	54.2	58.0	63.6	49.0	51.0	54.2	57.8	63.0
6	51.2	53.2	56.3	60.7	67.1	50.5	52.7	56.3	60.4	66.2
7	52.9	55.1	58.5	63.4	70.6	52.0	54.5	58.4	63.0	69.4
8	54.6	57.0	60.7	66.2	74.1	53.5	56.3	60.4	65.6	72.6
9	56.3	58.9	62.9	68.9	77.6	55.0	58.0	62.5	68.2	75.8
10	58.0	60.8	65.1	71.6	81.0	56.5	59.8	64.6	70.8	78.9
11	59.7	62.7	67.2	74.4	84.5	58.1	61.6	66.6	73.4	82.1
12	61.4	64.6	69.4	77.1	88.0	59.6	63.4	68.7	76.0	85.3
13	63.1	66.5	71.6	79.8	91.5	61.1	65.1	70.8	78.6	88.5
14	64.8	68.4	73.8	82.6	95.0	62.6	66.9	72.9	81.2	91.7
15	66.5	70.3	76.0	85.3	98.4	64.1	68.7	74.9	83.8	94.8
16	68.2	72.2	78.1	88.0	101.9	65.6	70.4	77.0	86.4	98.0
17	69.9	74.1	80.3	90.7	105.4	67.1	72.2	79.1	89.0	101.2
18	71.6	76.0	82.5	93.5	108.9	68.6	74.0	81.1	91.6	104.4

Source: Adapted from Fernandez, J.R. et al. *J Pediatr*, 145: 439, 2004. With permission.

TABLE 51.10

Health Risks Associated with Childhood Obesity

Health Risk	Reference
Elevated triglycerides	25,26
Elevated low-density lipoprotein cholesterol	27
Reduced high-density lipoprotein cholesterol	6,25
Elevated blood pressure	28
Nonalcoholic fatty liver disease (NAFLD)	29,30
Impaired glucose tolerance	31
Elevated insulin	26,27
Insulin resistance	32
Elevated left ventricular mass	33,34
Endothelial dysfunction	35,36
Orthopedic abnormalities (e.g., Blount's disease)	37,38
Gallstone formation	39,40
Asthma	41,42
Sleep disorders	43,44

TABLE 51.11

Visceral Adiposity and Increased Health Risk in Childhood Obesity

Health Risk	Reference
Elevated low-density lipoprotein (LDL) cholesterol and triglycerides associated with visceral fat but not subcutaneous fat in obese children	45
Elevated triglycerides and insulin and lowered high-density lipoprotein (HDL) cholesterol associated with visceral fat in obese but not in nonobese adolescents	46
Visceral fat, but not subcutaneous or total body fat, explained significant proportions of the variance in triglycerides, HDL cholesterol, and LDL particle size in obese children	16
Visceral fat tended to be higher in obese children with impaired glucose tolerance than in obese children with normal glucose tolerance	15

DIET

The extent to which increased energy intake has contributed to the rise in childhood obesity is not entirely clear. On the one hand, a comparison of mean energy intake among youths aged 2 to 19 years using NHANES data collected between 1971 and 1994 showed little evidence of a general increase in daily energy intake.[50] On the other hand, a study of the dietary habits of 2 to 18 year olds based on large representative samples of the U.S. population surveyed between 1977 and 1996 found that daily energy intake increased from 1840 kcal/day in 1977 to 1958 kcal/day in 1996, an increase of 118 kcal/day.[51] Methodological differences between the studies may help explain the divergent findings. In addition to data on mean energy intake, examination of dietary patterns and their relationship to childhood obesity may prove useful. For example, a recent study of 4370 children aged 5 to 6 years found a much lower prevalence of obesity in children who ate four or more meals per day compared with those who ate three meals or fewer per day.[52] Clearly, the relationship between dietary changes and increasing obesity prevalence requires further examination.

RESTING METABOLISM

There is little support for the notion that lowered resting metabolic rate has contributed to the increased prevalence of obesity among young people. Two independent reviews of the isotope dilution (doubly-labeled water) method for measuring energy expenditure concluded that low resting metabolism was probably not responsible for obesity in most children.[53,54]

PHYSICAL INACTIVITY

Several lines of evidence suggest the importance of physical inactivity in the development of childhood obesity. Preschoolers who were classified as inactive were 3.8 times as likely as active children to have increasing triceps skin folds during 2.5 years of follow-up.[55] An analysis of doubly-labeled water studies concluded that low levels of physical activity were associated with higher levels of fatness.[53] Time–motion studies have shown that inactive children are more fat than active children[56,57] even while ingesting less energy.[58] Whether there has been an overall increase in physical inactivity among children in recent decades is anecdotally plausible, but has been difficult to establish empirically.[59,60] If there has been an increase in childhood inactivity, it is not clear whether it has replaced more vigorous activities and thus resulted in a secular decline in daily energy expenditure or simply replaced other sedentary or light-intensity activities such as reading.[59] A reduction in vigorous physical activity might be of particular concern, as a recent study of 421 adolescents reported that the amount of vigorous physical activity was a better predictor of percentage of body fat than was the amount of moderate physical activity.[61]

TREATMENT/MANAGEMENT OF CHILDHOOD OBESITY

Weight management issues are challenging; interventions should involve the family and actively involve the child and parents in adopting healthy eating habits and appropriate levels of physical activity while reducing sedentary behaviors.[62]

DIETARY CONSIDERATIONS

A variety of dietary approaches have been utilized in family-based childhood obesity interventions; some focus on healthy eating habits rather then energy restriction, whereas others prescribe significant caloric reduction. From a behavior change perspective, the specific content of the diet may be less important than how it is presented. The diet should be simple, explicit, and unambiguous so that it is easy to implement and monitor and not subject to confusion or easy rationalization of exceptions.[63] A trained nutritionist can assist the family in evaluating their cooking and eating patterns and by making suggestions relative to the purchasing and preparing of foods. The nutritionist should also help the family understand the concepts of portion size, nutritional contents of foods, and the use of food exchange lists such as the *Exchange Lists for Weight Management*.[64] It is recommended that obese children practice maintaining a food diary. Although in most cases the diary will be inaccurate in figuring total energy intake, it can prove useful for reviewing problem foods and eating patterns.[14,65] Table 51.12 includes summaries of the dietary components from several successful family-based behavioral interventions for childhood obesity.

DECREASING PHYSICAL INACTIVITY

The American Academy of Pediatrics has recommended limiting children's TV and video time to a maximum of 2 h/day.[71] As shown in Table 51.13, several studies have reported improvements in the obesity status of children following decreases in inactivity levels, especially TV watching.

ROLE OF EXERCISE

Exercise should be considered a key component of any obesity management program. Even in the absence of dietary restriction, exercise can result in favorable changes in the obesity status of children and adolescents, as demonstrated by a series of after-school

TABLE 51.12
Selected Family-Based Interventions for Childhood Obesity

Ages	n	Dietary Intervention	Exercise	Outcome	Reference
12–16	36	Nutrition education, emphasis on low sugar, salt, and fat	Increased physical activity encouraged	(1 year) Percentage of overweight declined by 10.7%	66
7–12	4	Hypocaloric diets (600 kcal/day for 10 weeks); 1200 kcal/day next 42 weeks	Gradual increase in physical activity using aerobic points system	(1 year) Percentage of overweight declined by 20%	67
8–12	18	Traffic Light Diet[a], target of 1000–1200 kcal/day	Children reinforced for decreasing sedentary behavior	(1 year) Percentage of body fat (electrical impedance) declined 4.7%	68
7–16	60	Nutrition education, emphasis on healthy eating rather than eating less	Moderate intensity exercise for 30 min/d, lifestyle changes to increase physical activity	(1 year) Percentage of overweight declined by 11%	69
8–16	12	Modified Traffic Light Diet	Moderate intensity exercise for up to 45 min/day, 5–7 day/week	(5 year) Percentage of overweight declined by 23%	70
6–16	64	Nutrition education, hypocaloric diet ~30% below reported intake or 15% below the estimated requirement	Twice/week, supervised 60 min endurance training sessions; one 30–45 min at-home physical activity session	(1 year) Percentage of body fat (skin folds) declined 2.3% in intervention group, increased 3.5% in control group	1

[a] Traffic Light Diet categorizes foods as red (high calorie, low nutrient density), yellow (dietary staples for a balanced diet), green (very low calorie, mostly vegetables).

TABLE 51.13
Studies Examining Relationships between Reduced Physical Inactivity and Changed Obesity Status

Age/Grade	Sample	Inactivity Component	Change in Obesity	Reference
8–12 years	Children from 61 families	Children assigned to groups and reinforced for either (1) decreasing inactivity, (2) increasing physical activity, (3) combination of both	(1 year) Children who decreased inactivity levels had a greater decrease in percentage of body fat (−4.7%) than did children who increased physical activity (−1.3%)	68
Grades 6–8	1295 students in 5 intervention schools and 5 control schools	Intervention schools received curriculum designed to change obesity-related behaviors, including reduced TV watching	(2 year) Among girls (but not boys), reduced TV viewing predicted reduced obesity prevalence	72
Grades 3–4	106 students in the intervention school, 100 in the control school	18-lesson, 6-month classroom curriculum to reduce "screen time" (TV, videotape, video game use)	Screen time reduced 26.3% in the intervention school, 3.6% in the control school. Increases in BMI, skin folds, and waist circumferences were significantly less in the intervention school	73
9–15 years	National sample of 6149 girls and 4620 boys	2 questionnaires, 1 year apart, assessed changes in number of hours of inactive behavior (TV, videos. computer games)	Annual increases in BMI were greater in children who increased the number of hours of inactive behavior	74
8–12 years	10 obese children (7 boys, 3 girls)	Home TV viewing required simultaneous pedaling of a cycle ergometer in the intervention group	By week 12, weekly TV viewing declined from 22.8 to 1.1 h/week in the intervention group. Body fat declined from 44.5 to 43.2% in the intervention group, increased from 37.1 to 38.0% in the control group	75

interventions conducted at the Medical College of Georgia, which are summarized in Table 51.14. Within the context of multicomponent obesity management programs, where diet, exercise, behavior modification, and family involvement are integrated, exercise plays an essential role. Although caloric restriction can result in significant short-term weight loss in obese children, it tends to reduce fat-free mass and resting metabolic rate,[79] thus setting the stage for regain of the lost fat when the dieting stops.[80] Exercise can counter these declines from diet-induced weight loss by attenuating the potentially adverse changes in protein turnover consequent to the hypocaloric diet.[81] Data from a double-labeled water study also suggest that adding exercise to a caloric restriction regimen for obese children can result in total daily energy expenditure above that predicted by the addition of the exercise, perhaps due to the synergistic action of exercise and the sympathetic nervous system on the thermic effect of food.[82]

TABLE 51.14
Medical College of Georgia After-School Exercise Interventions

Subjects	Obesity Status[a]	Exercise Program	Results	Reference
7–11 year girls (n = 25)	Ex = 42.8% fat	Ex = aerobics, 5day/week, 12 weeks	−1.4% fat[b]	76
	C = 43.3% fat	C = lifestyle education only	+ 0.4% fat[c]	
7–11 year boys and girls (n = 74)	Ex = 44.5% fat	Ex = aerobics, 5 day/week, 17 weeks	−2.2% fat[b]	77
	C = 44.1% fat	C = maintain normal activities	no change	
13–16 year boys and girls (n = 41)	All subjects >85th percentile on triceps skinfold	Ex = aerobics, 5day/week, 8 months	−3.6% fat[d]	78
		C = lifestyle education only	+ 0.2% fat	

Significantly different change (p <.001) compared to lifestyle education only group.

[a] Ex is exercise group, C is control group, % fat is percentage of body fat measured with DXA.

[b] Significant change (p <.05) from pre-test.

[c] Non-significant change (p >.05) from baseline.

TABLE 51.15
Behavior Modification Components for Treatment of Childhood Obesity

Component	Comment
Self-monitoring	Utilize food and physical activity log books; monitor body weight changes (usually daily or weekly)
Stimulus control	Limit amount of high calorie foods kept in the house; establish set routines for meals and snacks; model a physically active lifestyle
Reinforcement	Reward targeted behaviors by child with verbal praise by parents; include predetermined (with input from child) tangible rewards that encourage further physical activity (sporting equipment, trips to recreational areas) or healthy eating habits (favorite fruits)
Eating behavior	Avoid second helpings, take smaller bites, put fork down between bites, leave food on plate at meal's end, avoid TV watching while eating
Goal setting and contracting	Parent and child establish realistic goals for physical activity, weight loss, and eating behaviors; use contracts to help maintain focus and provide structure for rewarding desired changes
Managing high-risk situations	Preplan management strategies for holidays, birthdays, parties, and eating in restaurants; practice using role playing

OPTIMAL EXERCISE DOSE

The optimal exercise dose for the treatment of childhood obesity has yet to be established,[59] although examination of Table 51.12 and Table 51.14 suggests that the exercise component of successful obesity treatment programs can vary considerably. Several national bodies have published recommendations regarding daily physical activity goals for children and adolescents. The American Heart Association's Committee on Atherosclerosis, Hypertension, and Obesity in Youth recommended that children older than 2 years of age participate in at least 30 min of moderate physical activity on most days of the week, and preferably every day.[83] A recent CDC-sponsored expert panel recommended that school-aged youth participate daily in 60 min or more of moderate to vigorous physical activity that is developmentally appropriate, enjoyable, and involves a variety of activites.[84] A position statement from The National Association for Sport and Physical Education recommends children aged 5 to 12 years accumulate at least 60 min, and up to several hours, of age-appropriate physical activity on all or most days of the week, adding that this daily accumulation should include moderate and vigorous physical activity with the majority of the time being spent in activity that is intermittent in nature.[85] For the obese child, increasing the level of physical activity gradually is an important consideration so that failure and discouragement do not sabotage both exercise and dietary resolve.[4] Whatever the format, exercise programs should be designed to increase the interaction between parents and children or with other children.[14] Behavioral research also suggests that obese children are more likely to continue being physically active over time if they perceive themselves as having choice and control over being more physically active, rather than attributing control to their parents.[68]

BEHAVIOR MODIFICATION

The work of Epstein et al.[86,87] represents the state of the art in behavioral treatment of childhood obesity.[88] They have systematically studied a progression of behavioral methods and demonstrated long-term effects on weight control.[63] Table 51.15 summarizes components of behavior modification commonly utilized in the treatment of childhood obesity.

TABLE 51.16
Selected Resources on Childhood Obesity

Topic	Resource
Recent review articles on childhood obesity	References 59,88,90–92
Recent books on childhood obesity	1. Keiss, W. (ed), *Obesity in Childhood and Adolescence*, Karger, 2004
	2. Parizkova, J. and Hills, A., *Childhood Obesity: Prevention and Treatment*, CRC Press, 2004
	3. Cameron, N. (ed), *Childhood Obesity: Contemporary Issues*, CRC Press, 2005
	4. Mullen, M. C. and Shield, J. E., *Childhood and Adolescent Overweight: The Health Professional's Guide to Identification, Treatment, and Prevention*, The American Dietetic Association, 2003
Obesity-related professional journals	1. *International Journal of Obesity and Related Metabolic Disorders*
	2. *Obesity Research*
Obesity-related research organizations	1. The NIH Obesity Research Task Force (National Institutes of Health), Bethesda, MD
	2. North American Association for the Study of Obesity (NAASO), The Obesity Society, Silver Spring, MD
	3. Center for Weight and Health (University of California) Berkeley, CA
	4. Center for Health Promotion (International Life Sciences Center) Atlanta, GA
Childhood exercise and fitness	1. *Pediatric Exercise Science*
	2. American College of Sports Medicine (Indianapolis, IN)
	3. American Alliance for Health, Physical Education, Recreation, and Dance (Reston, VA)
	4. President's Council on Physical Fitness and Sports (Washington, DC)
Childhood nutrition	1. Weight Control Information Network (National Institutes of Health), Bethesda, MD
	2. The American Dietetic Association (Chicago, IL)
	3. Division of Nutrition and Physical Activity, National Center for Chronic Disease Prevention and Health Promotion (CDC), Atlanta, GA
	4. Food and Nutrition Information Center, U.S. Department of Agriculture
Pediatric growth charts	Pediatric Growth Charts for the US Population, including BMI http://www.cdc.gov/growthcharts

FAMILY INVOLVEMENT

Studies that have examined successful 5-year[70] and 10-year[86] outcomes for childhood obesity interventions emphasize the importance of family involvement in the weight-loss process and recommend a treatment model that integrates improved dietary habits, increased physical activity, and behavior modification. Active parental participation is a crucial component of the model, given that parenting styles not only influence the development of food preferences but establish the type of family environment that may be conducive to overeating or a sedentary lifestyle. Parents also function as role models and reinforcers for eating and exercise behaviors. Family-based behavioral interventions for childhood obesity typically include an initial, short-term (8 to 16 weeks) treatment phase followed by a longer-term (1 year) maintenance or continued improvement phase.[89] During initial treatment, children typically meet in group settings once a week for 45 to 90 min.[66,70] Follow-up sessions occur once or twice a month for up to 1 year.[66,68] Facilitators for treatment sessions may be pediatricians, child psychologists, or nutritionists.[89]

RESOURCES

Table 51.16 provides a topical list of sources of information on childhood obesity.

REFERENCES

1. Nemet, D. et al. *Pediatrics*, 115: e443, 2005.
2. Hedley, A.A. et al. *JAMA*, 291: 2847, 2004.
3. Ogden, C.L. et al. *JAMA*, 288:1728, 2002.
4. Williams, C.L. et al. *Ann NY Acad Sci*, 817: 225, 1997.
5. Troiano, R.P. et al. *Arch Pediatr Adol Med*, 149: 1085, 1995.
6. Must, A., Dallal, G., and Dietz, W. *Am J Clin Nutr*, 53: 839, 1991.
7. Williams, D. et al. *Am J Pub Health*, 82: 358, 1992.
8. Power, C., Lake, J.K., and Cole, T.J. *Int J Obes Relat Metab Disord*, 21: 507, 1997.
9. Fu, W.P.C. et al. *Int J Obes Relat Metab Disord*, 27: 1121, 2003.
10. Cole, T.J. et al. *BMJ*, 320: 1, 2000.

11. CDC (Centers for Disease Control and Prevention). Growth Charts: United States. Advance data number 314, December 4, 2000 (Revised).
12. Kuczmarski, R.J. et al. *Vital Health Stat*, *11*: 246, 2002.
13. Bellizzi, M.C. and Dietz, W.H. *Am J Clin Nutr*, 70: 173S, 1999.
14. Strauss, R. *Curr Prob Pediatr*, 29: 5, 1999.
15. Weiss, R. et al. *Lancet*, 362: 951, 2003.
16. Owens, S.G. et al. *J Pediatr*, 133: 41, 1998.
17. Bacha, F. et al. *J Clin Endocrinol Metab*, 88: 2534, 2003.
18. Bonora, E. *Int J Obes*, 24: 32S, 2000.
19. Fernandez, J.R. et al. *J Pediatr*, 145: 439, 2004.
20. Hirschler, V. et al. *Arch Pediatr Adolesc Med*, 159: 740, 2005.
21. Steinberger, J. and Daniels, S.R. *Circulation*, 107: 1448, 2003.
22. Cook, S. et al. *Arch Pediatr Adolesc Med*, 157: 821, 2003.
23. Cruz, M.L. et al. *J Clin Endocrinol Metab*, 89: 108, 2004.
24. Eissa, M.A.H. and Gunner, K.B. *J Pediatr Health Care*, 18: 35, 2004.
25. Gidding, S.S. et al. *J Pediatr*, 127: 868, 1995.
26. Gutin, B. et al. *J Pediatr*, 125: 847, 1994.
27. Kikuchi, D.A. et al. *Prev Med*, 21: 177, 1992.
28. Lauer, R.M. et al. *Hypertension*, 18: 174S, 1991.
29. Roberts, E. *Curr Gastroent Rep*, 5: 253, 2003.
30. Lavine, J.E. and Schwimmer, J.B. *Clin Liver Dis*, 8: 549, 2004.
31. Goran, M.I., Ball, G.D.C., and Cruz, M.L. *J Clin Endocrinol Metab*, 88: 1417, 2003.
32. Sinha, R. et al. *N Engl J Med*, 346: 802, 2002.
33. Gutin, B. et al. *J Pediatr*, 132: 1023, 1998.
34. Daniels, S.R. et al. *J Pediatr*, 141: 186, 2002.
35. Treiber, F. et al. *Psychosom Med*, 59: 376, 1997.
36. Watts, K. *J Pediatr*, 144: 620, 2004.
37. Loder, R.T., Aronson, D.D., and Greenfield, M.L. *J Bone Joint Surg*, 75: 1141, 1993.
38. Dietz, W.H., Gross, W.L., and Kirkpatrick, J.A. *J Pediatr*, 101: 725, 1982.
39. Friesen, C.A. and Roberts, C.C. *Clin Pediatr*, 7: 294, 1989.
40. Honore, L.H. *Arch Surg*, 115: 62, 1989.
41. Unger, R., Kreeger, L., and Christoffel, K.K. *Clin Pediatr*, 29: 368, 1990.
42. Kaplan, T.A. and Montana, E. *Clin Pediatr*, 32: 220, 1993.
43. Marcus, C.L. et al. *Pediatr Pulmonol*, 21: 176, 1996.
44. Redline, S. et al. *Am J Resp Crit Care Med*, 159: 1527, 1999.
45. Brambilla, P. et al. *Int J Obes Relat Metab Disord*, 18: 795, 1994.
46. Caprio, S. et al. *Am J Clin Nutr*, 64: 12, 1996.
47. Farooqi, I.S. *Best Prac Res Clin Endocrinol Metab*, 19: 359, 2005.
48. Bouchard, C. et al. *N Engl J Med*, 322: 1477, 1990.
49. Perusse, L. and Bouchard, C. *Ann Med*, 31: 19, 1999.
50. Troiano, R.P. et al. *Am J Clin Nutr*, 72: 1343S, 2000.
51. Nielsen, S.J., Siega-Riz, A.M., and Popkin, B.M. *Obes Res*, 10: 370, 2002.
52. Toschke, A.M. et al. *Obes Res*, 13: 1932, 2005.
53. DeLany, J.P. *Am J Clin Nutr*, 68: 950S, 1998.
54. Goran, M.I. and Sun, M. *Am J Clin Nutr*, 68: 944S, 1998.
55. Moore, L.L. et al. *Am J Epidemiol*, 142: 982, 1995.
56. Goran, M.I. et al. *Int J Obes Res Metab Disord*, 21: 171, 1997.
57. Maffeis, C., Zaffanello, M., and Schutz, Y. *J Pediatr*, 131: 288, 1997.
58. Deheeger, M., Rolland-Cachera, M.F., and Fontvielle, A.M. *Int J Obes Res Metab Disord*, 21: 372, 1997.
59. Rennie, K.L. *Best Prac Res Clin Endocrinol Metab*, 19: 343, 2005.
60. Livingstone, M.B.E. et al. *Proc Nutr Society*, 62: 681, 2003.
61. Gutin, B. et al. *Am J Clin Nutr*, 81: 746, 2005.
62. St. Jeor, S.T. *J Am Dietetic Assn*, 102: 640, 2002.
63. Robinson, T.N. *Int J Obes Res Metab Disord*, 23: 52S, 1999.
64. American Dietetic Association. *Exchange Lists for Weight Management*, Chicago, 2003.
65. Moran, R. *Am Fam Phys*, 59: 861, 1999.
66. Brownell, K.D., Kelman, J.H., and Strunkard, A.J. *Pediatrics*, 71: 515, 1983.
67. Figueroa-Colon, R. et al. *Am J Dis Child*, 147: 160, 1993.
68. Epstein, L.H. et al. *Health Psychol*, 14: 109, 1995.
69. Braet, C., van Winckel, M., and van Leeuwen, K. *Acta Paediatr*, 86: 397, 1997.
70. Johnson, W.G. et al. *Obes Res*, 5: 257, 1997.

71. American Academy of Pediatrics. *Pediatrics*, 112: 424, 2003.
72. Gortmaker, S.L. et al. *Arch Pediatr Adol Med*, 153: 409, 1999.
73. Robinson, T.N. *JAMA*, 282: 1561, 1999.
74. Berkey, C.S. et al. *Pediatrics*, 105: e56, 2000.
75. Faith, M.S. et al. *Pediatrics*, 107: 1043, 2001.
76. Gutin, B. et al. *Obes Res*, 3: 305, 1995.
77. Owens, S. et al. *Med Sci Sports Exer*, 31: 143, 1999.
78. Gutin, B. et al. *Am J Clin Nutr*, 75: 818, 2002.
79. Maffeis, C., Schutz, Y., and Pinelli, L. *Int J Obes Res Metab Disord*, 16: 41, 1992.
80. Schwingshandl, J. and Borkenstein, M. *Int J Obes Res Metab Disord*, 19: 752, 1995.
81. Ebbeling, C.B. and Rodriguez, N.R. *Med Sci Sports Exer*, 31: 378, 1999.
82. Blaak, E.E. et al. *Am J Clin Nutr*, 55: 777, 1992.
83. Williams, C.L. et al. *Circulation*, 106: 143, 2002.
84. Strong, W.B. et al. *J Pediatr*, 146: 732, 2005.
85. National Association for Sport and Physical Activity. *Physical Activity for Children: A Statement of Guidelines*, 2nd edition. Reston, VA: NASPE, 2004.
86. Epstein, L.H. et al. *J Health Psychol*, 13: 373, 1994.
87. Epstein, L.H. et al. *JAMA*, 264: 2519, 1990.
88. Steinbeck, K. *Best Prac Res Clin Endocrinol Metab*, 19: 455, 2005.
89. Owens, S. and Gutin, B. In: *Lifestyle Medicine*, Rippe, J.M. Ed. Malden, MA: Blackwell Science, 1999, ch 50.
90. Ells, L.J. *Best Prac Res Clin Endocrinol Metab*, 19: 441, 2005.
91. Daniels, S.R. et al. *Circulation*, 111: 1999, 2005.
92. Hardy, L.R., Harrell, J.S., and Bell, R.A. *J Pediatr Nurs*, 19: 376, 2004.

52 Bariatric Surgery for Obese Patients: Important Psychological Considerations

Christian R. Lemmon and Paule Barbeau

CONTENTS

INTRODUCTION

The increased prevalence of obesity in people of all ages in the United States has been well documented.[1] About two-thirds of individuals living in the United States are overweight, and of those persons, almost one half are obese. Obesity is associated with a tremendous number of comorbidities that lead to numerous medical and psychological problems. Being 50% above average weight is associated with a twofold increase in mortality rates;[2] in individuals with type 2 diabetes this increases to five and eight times among men and women, respectively. The obesity epidemic, poor responses to more conventional weight loss treatment, improved outcomes of bariatric surgery (BaS) procedures, and the use of the less invasive laparoscopy in BaS have spurned a tremendous growth in BaS. According to the American Society for Bariatric Surgery, 103,000 BaS's were done in 2003. A complete review of the history of BaS, the various procedures currently performed, indications for BaS, and BaS outcomes can be found in this text (see Chapter 53). This chapter will focus primarily on the importance of a comprehensive psychological evaluation of patients being considered for BaS.

Proper nutrition and increased physical activity are paramount in the management of overweight and obese patients. Most multidisciplinary weight-loss programs result in only 5 to 10% loss of excess weight, and the cumulative relapse rate is nearly 100% in 5 years.[3] In the morbidly obese patient it may become increasingly difficult to get any significant change in diet and physical activity habits, even when efforts include state of the art behavior modification programs and antiobesity medications. For severe obesity, very low calorie diets, behavior therapy, and other forms of treatment have, for the most part, proved ineffective.[4] These strategies often prove to be inadequate and may lead to repeated failed weight-loss attempts, feelings of failure, adverse psychological changes and increasing stigmatization from both within the patient and from his or her environment. Simultaneously, the process of attempting to lose weight often leads to significant frustration in those providing these services. Evidence for this can be found in the research performed by Foster, et al.[5] In a survey of more than 600 physicians, physical inactivity was rated as being more important than any other cause of obesity, with overeating and a high-fat diet regarded as the next two greatest causes. Additionally, more than 50% of physicians viewed obese patients as awkward, unattractive, ugly, and noncompliant. Foster, et al.[5] concluded that primary care physicians view obesity largely as a behavioral problem and share our broader society's negative stereotypes about the personal attributes of obese persons. Physicians also regard obesity treatment as less effective than treatment of most other chronic conditions. Almost half of the physicians admit that they do not feel competent prescribing weight loss programs and many others admit spending little time working on weight management issues with their patients.

A recent rigorous meta-analysis of published reports between 1990 and 2003[6] concluded that BaS for morbidly obese patients has proven to be a most effective form of weight loss. Among more than 10,000 patients, the overall percentage of excess weight loss across several types of BaS was 61.2%. Similarly, there was a mean decrease in body mass index (BMI) of 14.2 for more than 8000 patients and a decrease in absolute weight of 39.7 kg in nearly an additional 8000 patients. Furthermore, a significant majority of patients with diabetes (resolved or improved in 77 to 86% of patients), hyperlipidemia (improved in >70% of patients), hypertension (resolved or improved in 62 to 79% of patients), and obstructive sleep apnea (resolved or improved in 84 to 86% of patients) experienced significant improvement, if not complete resolution, post-BaS. In a recent study comparing laparoscopic adjustable gastric banding to an intensive medical program that included very-low calorie diets, pharmacotherapy, and lifestyle change for 24 months in patients with mild to moderate obesity, O'Brien, et al.[7] reported that the banding procedure was significantly more effective than the nonsurgical therapy. More specifically, the surgical group showed greater weight loss, greater resolution of the metabolic syndrome, and improved quality of life (QoL) as compared to the nonsurgical group. For all of these reasons, many researchers and clinicians have suggested that BaS may be the only effective treatment for the severely obese patient.[8]

Despite all of these positive changes that are likely to occur following BaS, one must remember that BaS remains a risky procedure that will require many behavioral changes, with a successful outcome partially dependent upon these behavioral changes.[9–12] Patients should be aware of the mortality rate (<1%) and other complications that may cause morbidity (e.g., infections, dehiscence, hernias, stomal stenosis, thrombophlebitis, gallstones, nutritional deficiencies, and various kinds of leakages).[13] However, it should be noted that the mortality rate in morbidly obese diabetic patients who undergo BaS is significantly lower than in similar patients who do not undergo BaS.[14] Also, 10 to 20% of patients who have had BaS require follow-up procedures to correct complications.[15] It has been suggested that women should avoid pregnancy until their weight is stabilized because of concerns about the possible adverse effects of rapid weight loss and nutritional deficiencies on the developing fetus.[15]

Patient selection, comprehensive preoperative evaluation and education, and comprehensive postoperative follow-up are paramount to BaS.[9,11,12] Several organizations, including the National Institutes of Health[16] and the Veterans Health Administration[17] have recommended that all BaS patients receive comprehensive multidisciplinary evaluation and treatment that includes a preoperative psychological evaluation process. A physician will determine a BaS candidate's medical appropriateness for surgery as indicated by Robert Martindale, M.D. in this text (see Chapter 53). According to Sogg and Mori,[11] the role of the psychologist within this multidisciplinary assessment process is not necessarily to approve or deny the BaS candidate's surgery. Rather, it is the psychologist's responsibility to identify various factors that might affect the success of the surgery. These factors, which will be discussed in greater detail below, include patient knowledge of the surgery, weight and dieting histories, current eating and physical activity habits, psychological and cognitive status, social support, and the patient's plans related to the surgery and his or her postsurgical care.

WHY DO PATIENTS CONSIDER UNDERGOING BaS?

Patients consider BaS for numerous reasons, including health concerns and prompting by their physicians or loved ones. Most individuals consider surgery in an attempt to lose weight after unsuccessfully trying numerous doctor-prescribed, commercial, and self-imposed diets.[18] However, our experiences with patients considering BaS indicate that some have made few, if any, formal attempts to modify their eating or physical activity habits. This anecdotal finding is supported by the research reported by Gibbons, et al.[18] who reported that about 10% of BaS candidates have not participated in any organized weight loss program prior to seeking surgery. It is now widely accepted practice to require BaS candidates to have made at least several attempts to achieve weight loss through dietary, physical activity, and lifestyle modifications, and pharmacological intervention.[16,17]

There is also some variability concerning how much BaS candidates know about the risks and benefits of the surgery, the changes they will need to make postoperatively, and the specifics of postsurgical care. Our experience has shown that the majority of candidates have talked to their primary care physician or surgeon extensively, researched the topic via the Internet, and talked to others who have had both successful and unsuccessful surgeries via friends, acquaintances, and the Internet. However, others indicate that the surgery was simply suggested to them by a family member, friend, or a physician, or they may have seen a program on television that highlighted the surgery. These patients often know very little about the surgery and the lifestyle changes that will be necessary postoperative.

Despite many wanting to believe that the majority of patients seeking BaS are doing so for health reasons, several studies[19,20] and our own clinical experience have shown that social considerations are often a key reason behind patients' desire for BaS. Prospective BaS patients have reported experiencing significant prejudice and discrimination within the workplace, at home and in various social situations.[19] Finally, many BaS candidates report wanting to receive the surgery so that they can lose a significant amount of weight and increase their likelihood of being present and active without pain and ambulatory restraint for their loved ones, and in particular, grandchildren.

PSYCHOSOCIAL STATUS OF THE CANDIDATE FOR BaS

Although some studies have found that the severely obese exhibit no more psychopathology than normal weight persons,[21,22] more studies have revealed strong evidence of psychopathology and other related problems among persons who are considering BaS.[8,21-31] In a comparison of BaS candidates and a matched community sample, Black, et al.[28] used structured interviews and found higher rates of psychopathology among the BaS candidates. More specifically, the BaS patients had a significantly higher prevalence of major depressive disorder, overall mood disorders, agoraphobia, simple phobia, posttraumatic stress disorder, overall anxiety disorders, bulimia, and tobacco dependence. 84% of the BaS candidates met criteria for at least one psychiatric diagnosis, and the BaS patients were also significantly more likely to have more than one psychiatric diagnosis and significantly higher rates of personality disorders as compared to the control group. Recent extensive reviews of this type of research performed by Herpertz, et al.[8] and Greenberg, et al.[30] have revealed similar findings. Herpertz, et al.[8] reported that the prevalence rates of Axis I psychiatric disorders among BaS candidates in studies published between 1980 and 2002 varied between 27.3 and 41.8%. The rates of Axis II disorders varied between 22 and 24%. They also reported that the predominant Axis I diagnoses included mood disorders, anxiety disorders and eating disorders, especially bulimia nervosa and binge eating disorder (BED). The Greenberg, et al.[30] group reviewed the literature on preoperative psychosocial status among BaS candidates between 1980 and 2004 and found higher rates of depression and eating disorders. Finally, Sarwer, et al.[31] concluded that mood and anxiety disorders and BED seem to be the most common comorbid psychiatric conditions found among BaS candidates.

A number of studies have focused more specifically on various forms of eating pathology among BaS candidates. Several studies have found that nearly 50% of female patients considering BaS satisfy DSM[32] criteria for BED[33,34] or engage in binge eating at least once a week,[34,35] and almost 82% reported some sort of eating disturbance, night eating syndrome (NES), or consuming high-calorie drinks.[33,36] Herpertz, et al.[37] reported prevalence rates between 39 and 46% for BED. A review of five other studies revealed a range of 16 to 48% of BED among BaS candidates.[33-36,38] Hsu, et al.[39] reported that over 50% of two different cohorts of female BaS patients had BED or bulimia nervosa prior to their surgery. Associations of body checking with eating restraint, and body avoidance with binge eating also suggest the presence of eating disorder symptoms among BaS candidates.[34] Several researchers have also reported that up to 40% of BaS patients have features of NES,[33,35] an eating mood, and sleep disturbance marked by morning anorexia, evening hyperphagia, nocturnal awakenings, and eating during these periods of wakefulness.[40]

Other psychosocial variables have also been studied among BaS patients with findings in the intuitively expected direction, including marital[41] and sexual[42] dissatisfaction, life stress, low self-esteem, inadequate social support, body image problems,[43] and poor QoL. QoL, and more specifically, health-related QoL (HRQoL) typically refers to the patient's limitations and suffering in physical, emotional, social, and vocational functioning associated with specific disease processes.[44] Many population and clinical studies have shown that severely obese persons report significantly greater bodily pain and physical limitations, as well as social and vocational impairments, as compared to average weight persons.[12] In a study of more than 300 BaS candidates, impairments in HRQoL were found in more than 40% of the patients. The impairments were within physical functioning, physical role limitations, and bodily pain.[45] A review by Greenberg, et al.[30] revealed higher rates of negative body image and low QoL among BaS candidates. Sarwer, et al.[31] indicated that impaired QoL in several areas, including body image, physical health, and functioning within relationships have been found among BaS candidates. Problems in social functioning and low self-esteem have also been shown in BaS patients before surgery.[46]

Given all of these findings and the aforementioned national guidelines, it is quite apparent why a comprehensive psychological evaluation that includes an assessment of psychopathology, eating behaviors, physical activity, problem-solving and coping skills, QoL, and patients' knowledge of BaS and expectations associated with BaS has been determined necessary for BaS candidates. Not only does such an assessment help to identify patients who may encounter special difficulties after their surgeries, but also the evaluation process can help the BaS team to individually tailor follow up programs to meet patients' specific postoperative needs.

PREOPERATIVE PSYCHOLOGICAL EVALUATIONS FOR BaS CANDIDATES

As mentioned previously, The National Institutes of Health Consensus Development Conference in 1991 developed a position statement on BaS for the morbidly obese, declaring that: "Patients judged by experienced clinicians to have a low probability of success with nonsurgical measures, as demonstrated, for example, by failure in established weight control programs or reluctance by the patient to enter such a program, may be considered for surgical treatment."[15] Thus, patients seeking treatment for severe obesity for the first time should be considered first for nonsurgical treatment that includes a dietary intervention, physical activity, behavior modification education and procedures and psychological/psychiatric support. The definition of "failure" in established weight control programs is not currently standardized and may vary widely across insurance companies and other third-party payers who are ultimately approving patients for BaS.[47]

TABLE 52.1

Comprehensive Interdisciplinary Evaluation of BaS Candidates

Medical History	Psychological Evaluation	Eating and Dieting History
Reasons for referral for BaS	Mental status examination	Dieting history
Age	Psychological testing	Baseline food diary
Weight history	Psychiatric history	Nutritional knowledge
BMI	Substance use and abuse/smoking	Food preferences
Medical history and evaluation	Maladaptive eating/dieting behaviors	Food portion size estimation
Medications	Maladaptive drinking	
Sleep patterns	Purging and compensatory behaviors	
Family medical history	Body image	
	Psychodynamic issues and concerns	
	Quality of life	
	Socioeconomic status/financial stress	
Physical activity patterns	**Personal and family history**	**Readiness for BaS**
Physical activity/exercise patterns	Interview with family members	Readiness for change
Barriers to exercise	Family psychiatric history	Knowledge of procedures and risks
Social support system for exercise	Marital/parental marital history	Knowledge of aftercare requirements
	Academic/occupational history	Realistic postoperative expectations
	Interpersonal relations/social support	Ready to allow communication between
		BaS team and primary care physician

Despite the tremendous increase in BaS cited above, few data exist on how best to evaluate BaS candidates and there are no standardized guidelines for the assessment process.[48] Candidates for BaS should receive a thorough biopsychosocial assessment performed by members of an interdisciplinary BaS treatment team that should include the patient's primary care physician, BaS surgeon, psychologist, psychiatrist, dietitian, and exercise physiologist or physical therapist. The team should evaluate the patients across each of the areas outlined in Table 52.1. Which professionals should assess each of these outlined areas varies greatly across BaS centers. In a recent survey of BaS centers designed to determine typical evaluation procedures, it was shown that 86% of the programs require all patients to receive a psychological evaluation and receive approval from a "mental health professional" before surgery, regardless of whether the evaluation process is required for insurance approval.[48] This "mental health professional" varies widely, but programs reported using a psychologist (83%) and a psychiatrist (37%) most of the time for this procedure. Almost half (48%) of the programs utilized formal psychological testing, while 38% performed their evaluations without the aid of formal testing. In addition to psychological testing and a clinical interview, 93% of the programs reported that they routinely include behavioral recommendations as a precursor or adjunct to the BaS as a result of the evaluation process.[48] These researchers also acknowledged that their response rate for programs returning their questionnaires was 43%, thus making it quite possible that screenings are not performed at the rate suggested above. Our own experience with the assessment process has led to our current evaluation protocol, which includes the use of several different professionals (referral source/primary care physician, psychologist, surgeon, dietitian, and physical therapist) who meet with the BaS candidate and assess him or her in their areas of expertise.

Consultation with the patient's primary care physician can prove invaluable as he or she should know more about the patient's medical history and past responses to treatment than anyone else, but a thorough medical history and evaluation should still be conducted. Consensus at this time is that BaS candidates should have a BMI ≥ 40 kg/m^2. Patients with a BMI >35 kg/m^2 but <40 kg/m^2 may also be considered if they have compromising comorbid conditions, including diabetes, obstructive sleep apnea, hypertension or hyperlipidemia, that often accompany morbid obesity. Additionally, there should be no metabolic or endocrine etiology underlying the patient's weight problems.

Wadden & Sarwer,[12] Grothe, et al.[9] and Sogg and Mori[11] recently published helpful guidelines believe should be considered in the psychological evaluation process. Reasons to recommend against BaS will be discussed in a later section of this chapter. Again, the psychological evaluation process should be conducted with careful consideration given to each of the areas outlined in Table 52.1. Most psychological evaluations include a clinical interview along with several standardized self-report measures that take the form of questionnaires or more formal psychological tests. With no consensus about which questionnaires and tests are best, it has typically been the case that BaS programs have developed their own set of instruments that they believe help them to best assess BaS candidates. Wadden & Sarwer[12] presented an outline of the Weight and Lifestyle Inventory (WALI) that they use at the University of Pennsylvania, and Sogg and Mori[11] developed the Boston Interview for Gastric Bypass that they employ during BaS candidate psychological evaluations. Both of these structured interviews cover each of the areas outlined in Table 52.1. Questionnaires specific to depression, anxiety, eating-disordered behavior, and personality functioning are also frequently used during the evaluation process.[9] As indicated by Herpertz, et al.[8] with only one exception, no relationship could be shown between Minnesota Multiphasic Personality Inventory (MMPI-2)[49] scales and the postoperative course of weight change. Specific psychiatric disorders (Axis I) and personality disorders (Axis II) have been shown to influence BaS outcome, and this has lead some clinicians to use psychological tests[9] such as the MMPI-2,[49] the Millon Multiaxial Clinical Inventory (MCMI-III),[50] and the Personality Assessment Inventory (PAI).[51] Other possible reasons for using these tests include their ability to assess the validity of the BaS candidates' self-report.

After assessing the BaS candidates' reading level via questions about their education, literate BaS patients in our practice are sent a preevaluation test packet that includes a questionnaire and several tests designed to gain information about each of these areas in Table 52.1 except for the "readiness for BaS" information. The questionnaire is used to guide the clinical interview so that each of these aforementioned areas is thoroughly assessed. The psychological tests include the Beck Depression Inventory-II,[52,53] the Bulimia Test-Revised,[54] the Eating Disorders Inventory-II,[55] the Binge Scale,[56] the Restraint Scale,[57] The Body Shape Questionnaire,[58] and several other body image, and social anxiety and social functioning tests. Other standardized personality tests may be used only if there is some concern about specific Axis I or Axis II psychiatric disorders.

We have found that many BaS candidates are most often somewhat anxious about this evaluation process, because they regard the psychologist as the "gatekeeper" who will determine whether or not they will get the surgery. We typically try to reduce this concern and assure them that we are part of a multidisciplinary team and that we want to help them decide if the surgery is appropriate for them. We also assure them that the presence of a psychiatric disorder will not necessarily prevent them from getting the surgery. Rather, the information may be used to inform and guide the treatment team in decisions related to preoperative treatment and follow up care. BaS patients' psychological status is determined with the aid of the aforementioned questionnaires and psychological testing results, a mental status examination, and the use of a clinical interview that assesses for psychiatric disorder symptomatology. More specifically, we assess for symptoms of mood and anxiety disorders, substance abuse or dependence, eating disorders, cognitive functioning, intellectual ability, and psychosis. As suggested by Grothe, et al.[9] cognitive functioning is assessed via the mental status examination, and the patients' intellectual ability is estimated indirectly via their vocabulary, educational and occupational histories, their responses to the questionnaires they are asked to complete, and their ability to understand and retain information about their desired surgical procedure and postoperative care. If there are concerns about the patients' cognitive and intellectual abilities, more formal neuropsychological testing may be warranted.[9] We also ask about a history of abuse or trauma, and psychosocial and environmental stressors. If the patient reports a psychiatric history, we routinely ask for permission to talk with their mental health provider, as that person will more than likely know much more about the patient. For those candidates currently in treatment, we provide their health provider with a copy of our evaluation along with pragmatic treatment recommendations designed to help the patient respond best to their surgery. In addition to specific problems, we attend to the patients' appearance, orientation, affect, mood, speech patterns, thought content, attention, concentration, intelligence, judgment, and insight. The presence of possible psychodynamic issues that might contribute to ambivalence and act as barriers to weight loss and adherence to postoperative treatment should also be assessed. These barriers might indirectly prevent or sabotage future weight loss. For example, the patient may think of his or her increased preoperative weight as a protective factor in the avoidance of unwanted sex, or as an excuse for social or occupational failures. One's disability status and the thought of eventually being able to work again might influence weight loss after surgery. Additionally, the severe obesity may have elicited help and concern from others. If present, these issues will need to be addressed at some point. Kral[10] has outlined some of these and other protective factors or subjective benefits of being obese that might influence post-BaS weight loss. Other information obtained during the psychological evaluation is outlined in Table 52.1.

Both the psychologist and a dietitian assess the eating and dieting history of the BaS patient. The psychologist focuses more on current and past evidence of eating disorders (anorexia nervosa, bulimia nervosa, BED, and NES), and other various maladaptive eating patterns that may serve as a barrier to successful adherence to the post BaS diet regimen and weight loss. Although the patient may not have a specific eating disorder, it must be determined if the patient uses food to cope with stress and aversive emotions, and what other coping skills he or she will be able to utilize after the surgery. The dietitian focuses more on nutritional knowledge, food preferences, food portion size estimation, and the specifics of the post-BaS diet regimen. Other important areas to assess include the patients' ability to stick with a structured eating plan, how their new plan will fit into their daily schedule and other family members' schedules, and the need for modification of other behaviors associated with the process of eating. Patients are asked to identify any specific concerns they might have about being able to adhere to the postoperative diet regimen. Physical activity patterns also need to be assessed in order to determine the success of past efforts, barriers encountered, concerns about physical and environmental safety, pain, and social concerns related to exercise, and the likelihood of social support to exercise. We routinely recommend that BaS patients meet with a physical therapist who works with BaS patients and get started with an exercise program before they even receive the surgery. This helps them to become more aware of the importance of physical activity after surgery.

The psychologist also assesses the BaS candidates' personal and family histories as outlined in Table 52.1. Information about their satisfaction with their families and spouses is important to determine, along with information about their living arrangements, social support, and their families' feelings about them getting the surgery need to be determined. There should also be a determination of whether intervention will be necessary within the patient's family given the previously mentioned data pertaining to marital satisfaction among BaS candidates. Consideration should be given to whether the family members have been supportive of the patient's efforts to lose weight in the past, or whether they have contributed to the problem. Will significant weight loss disrupt the family system and contribute to lack of familial support and possible sabotage?

Another important factor is the readiness of the patient seeking BaS. What is motivating the patient to seek BaS? What are their expectations about weight loss after surgery? What is their goal weight after surgery? Is there a specific family member or friend who will be able to assist them in their initial convalescence after surgery? Communication between the patient's primary care provider, surgical provider and those assessing the patient for readiness for surgery is highly recommended. Patients should be well informed, highly motivated, and acutely aware of the procedures, as well as both the risks and benefits of the surgery. The patient and his or her family should have realistic expectations of the postoperative medical care and attention that will be needed (e.g., caring for the wound, dehiscence etc.), and the importance of being able to adhere to the strict diet regimen that will be required of the patient.

EFFECT OF BAS ON PSYCHOSOCIAL OUTCOMES

The literature overall supports improvements in psychosocial outcomes consequent to BaS. Herpertz, et al.[8] reported that prevalence rates of DSM Axis I diagnoses were much lower at follow-up, ranging from no diagnosis present to about one third of the rate present before BaS. As outlined in the review by Sarwer, et al.[31] many other studies reported that patients experience a number of positive psychosocial changes after BaS. Karlsson, et al.[59] reported significant improvements in depression and anxiety in the first year after surgery. Significant improvements in depression were also shown 4 years after surgery.[60]

However, negative findings have also been reported. For example, Karlsson, et al.[59] also found that the improvements in depression and anxiety that were present during the first year began to wane during the following year and a half in the women in the study. However, despite this change, the level of depression and anxiety still remained improved compared to the baseline levels. Another negative finding was reported by Waters, et al.[61] such that they found a higher rate of suicide among postoperative patients 8 years after the surgery.

QoL was improved after surgery in several studies[19,43,46,61–63] and did not seem to be related to the type of surgery nor to postoperative complications.[62] Several studies found significant improvements in depression, self-confidence and mood after BaS.[19,46,61,63] Additionally, significant improvements in patients' self-evaluation of their physical appearance have been reported.[19,43] Short-term follow-up studies showed that these improvements lasted up to 6 months[63] and 1 year.[19,63] One study found that although QoL decreased over time, it was still higher than preoperative levels after 4 years,[62] while another found similar results after 7 years.[46] Conversely, one study found that improvements in psychological well-being had returned to their preoperative states 24 and 36 months after BaS, despite an average weight loss of 103 lbs at 36 months after surgery.[61] Herpertz, et al.[37] reported that obesity-related psychosocial problems decrease dramatically after the weight reductions that accompany BaS. Their review also found that postoperative benefits included improvements in occupational functioning, a more satisfying sexual life, improved self-esteem, and overall satisfaction with the BaS itself.

CAN PREOPERATIVE PSYCHOSOCIAL FACTORS PREDICT OUTCOME AFTER SURGERY?

It is important to note that research on this issue is limited in several ways. First, many studies included only small sample sizes, and the duration of postoperative follow-up was largely limited to less than 2 years. Second, most studies did not include individuals with severe psychiatric problems since most of these patients would be considered ineligible for BaS. Third, the patient drop out rate during follow-up is extremely high. Finally, studies have used inconsistent research designs (e.g., prospective vs. retrospective).[9,31] Therefore, most studies that investigated outcomes after BaS included highly selective samples of patients who were relatively free of significant psychopathology before they ever received the surgery.[8] Despite these limitations, researchers have been encouraged to continue to pursue these types of investigations. The results of such studies will assist clinicians in identifying BaS candidates who may be at risk for poor outcomes and make appropriate pre- and postoperative recommendations related to treatment.

The main outcome predictors related to treatment of the BaS patient are outlined in Table 52.2. The type of BaS (e.g., vertical banded gastroplasty [VGB], adjustable gastric banding, and Roux-en-Y gastric bypass [RGB]) should be chosen to fit the patient's needs, as some forms have proved to be more efficacious than others for certain kinds of patients. For example, a limitation of laparoscopic adjustable gastric banding and VGB is the relative ease with which the patient can resume binge eating and overeating behaviors, which may stretch the pouch, break the band, cause band migration, or create an obstruction. A limitation of the RGB procedure is the possibility of dumping syndrome if too much sugar or large amounts of food are consistently consumed. Hence, RGB appears to be most efficacious for patients who binge eat. There is an association between preexisting eating disorder symptoms and the regaining of lost weight among female VGB patients 2 years after surgery, and although these patients enjoy short-term improvements in their symptoms, they regress back to preoperative levels after about 2 years.[33]

TABLE 52.2

Potential Predictors of Success Postsurgery

- Treatment tailored to the individual's needs and preferences
  - Selecting the appropriate form of BaS
- Preoperative psychological well-being
- Absence of preoperative BED, NES, and bulimia nervosa
- Preoperative QoL
- Postoperative follow-up medical care
- Pre- and postoperative pharmacotherapy
- Pre- and postoperative individual therapy
  - Behavioral/cognitive behavioral treatment
  - Body image treatment
  - Nutritional education and counseling
  - Lifestyles education/physical activity
- Pre- and postoperative group therapy
  - Nutritional education and counseling
  - Lifestyles education/physical activity
- Pre- and postoperative family/marital therapy
- Pre- and postoperative physical therapy

At present, there has been only limited success in identifying preoperative psychosocial predictors of positive postoperative outcomes.[8,9,12,31] The potential predictors most often investigated include the psychosocial variables identified above in our discussion of the psychosocial status of the BaS candidate. Several comprehensive reviews investigated this issue in recent years.[8,30] A history of preoperative psychiatric treatment or a history of counseling for substance abuse was found to be a positive predictor of postoperative weight loss.[64] Clark, et al.[64] suggested that this finding may be due to the counseling these patients received related to skills for lifestyle changes and other coping skills.

Many studies also found that BaS patients' baseline psychiatric status, and their level of depression in particular, did not predict postoperative weight loss.[39,65] One of the more interesting findings concerning postoperative psychological status seen in several studies is that greater baseline depression was associated with greater weight loss.[66,67] More depressed individuals tended to lose greater amounts of weight as compared to less depressed individuals. Dubovsky, et al.[67] suggested that patients who do not express as much distress prior to their surgery might be less dissatisfied with their weight status and body image, and less willing to do the things necessary to promote greater postoperative weight loss.

As mentioned above, a large number of BaS candidates exhibit BED prior to their surgery. One would expect then, that even though it is more difficult to binge eat because of the gastric restrictive procedures, these patients might continue to eat in a manner similar to binge eating and have more difficulties adhering to the strict postoperative diet regimen and exhibit greater medical complications and less weight loss. However, this is not necessarily the case. Some studies reported that preoperative BED predicts less weight loss after surgery,[63,68] while others[35,69] found no relationship between the presence of binge eating preoperatively and subsequent weight loss 2 and 5½ years postoperative. One group of researchers found conflicting results across two of their own studies.[70,71] In the earlier study, Bussetto, et al.[70] found that after surgery, patients with BED had a significantly higher vomiting frequency and a higher frequency of neostoma stenosis than patients without BED. The percentage of excess weight lost was not affected by BED. In the later study,[71] preoperative BED had no significant effect on patient outcome at 3-year follow-up. The authors speculated that the preoperative psychological treatment that they provided to the BaS candidates might have influenced these results. It is important to note that patients with BED may not report postoperative binge eating behavior, because they may find it more difficult to binge eat after surgery due to the gastric restrictive procedures. However, some patients still report feelings of loss of control during the eating process consistent with that found in BED.[33,72] Thus, the inconsistency in the findings of studies related to postoperative binge eating behavior in patients with BED may result from differences in the subjective interpretation of binge eating among both researchers and patients. NES has not been investigated to this point postoperatively.[31]

In our experience, pre- and postoperative treatment, preparation, and education that patients receive are also predictive of BaS success. Treatment strategies may include psychological, psychiatric, dietary, and exercise interventions. Psychological counseling might include efforts to reduce symptoms of psychiatric disorders. Eating behaviors should improve significantly due to anatomical and physiological changes; however, behavioral and cognitive behavioral control procedures can also be introduced to curb excessive snacking, overeating, and binge eating in response to stress, boredom, and aversive emotions. These procedures can also be effective in helping patients to increase physical activity and overcome barriers to increased exercise. Patients should understand the need to alter these behaviors, and that surgery by itself will not improve these behaviors. Preoperative psychiatric intervention using pharmacotherapy may also prove helpful in the presence of mood and anxiety disorders.

Patients and their significant others should also receive appropriate nutritional education and counseling, including basic information about grocery shopping, food choices, food preparation, food groups, dietary reference intakes, and adequate intake of protein, iron, calcium, and various vitamins. Regular nutritional and metabolic evaluations and counseling should be strongly considered.

In summary, few studies have been able to identify specific psychosocial factors that serve as predictors of psychological functioning and weight loss postoperatively. Overall, most studies suggest that psychosocial functioning tends to improve after BaS. However, these changes may be only temporary.[8,9,12,31] In our experience, the extent of pre- and postoperative care given to the patients and their families are also predictive of BaS success.

CONTRAINDICATIONS FOR BaS

There are many contraindications to BaS.[9,17,48] This chapter focuses on the psychosocial and behavioral contraindications; physical contraindications are discussed elsewhere (see Chapter 53). A survey was conducted recently among bariatric programs in the United States to obtain information on what health care professionals involved in BaS consider good practice.[48] As mentioned above, well over 80% of practices require some form of preoperative psychological evaluation of their patients. Most of the evaluations are conducted by psychologists (83%) or psychiatrists (37%). The respondents were also given a list of 37 behavioral, psychiatric, and medical symptoms that may be contraindications for surgery, and asked to rate each one as a definite, possible, or not a contraindication for BaS. The five symptoms identified by over 75% of the respondents as definite contraindications were current illicit drug use (89%), active symptoms of schizophrenia (86%), severe mental retardation (81%), current heavy drinking (78%), and lack of knowledge about BaS (78%).

Only 48% of respondents identified active BED as a definite contraindication, while another 41% identified it as a possible contraindication. A history of BED was considered a possible contraindication by 73% of respondents. The presence of other eating disorders was considered a possible contraindication by 89% of respondents. According to our experience, we would also classify bulimia nervosa as a definite contraindication. Patients who are binge eating and purging several times per week and are unable to implement alternative coping skills in response to aversive emotions and stress will find they are ill-equipped to cope postoperatively. Therefore, we recommend that patients with bulimia nervosa receive treatment targeting both binge eating and purging behaviors prior to surgery. We would classify active BED as a possible contraindication. We recommend that BaS candidates who are binge eating more than once a week in response to stress and aversive emotions receive preoperative counseling targeting this behavior.

Multiple suicide attempts and a recent suicide attempt (within the past year) were identified as definite contraindications by only 62 and 61% of respondents, respectively. We propose that significant suicidal ideation be considered a definite contraindication. These patients may be unable to deal with the increased stress associated with surgery, potential complications, and intensive postoperative regimen. Similar to patients with other psychosocial contraindications, these patients should be referred for psychiatric treatment. The same recommendation applies to any other psychiatric diagnosis that may increase a patient's risk, particularly when the patient is not currently receiving treatment.

PSYCHOLOGICAL FOLLOW-UP AND OTHER TREATMENT RECOMMENDATIONS FOR BaS PATIENTS

Very little is known about postoperative psychosocial factors that may predict long-term outcome of BaS, or on the effects of postoperative psychological treatment. Several of the postoperative determinants of success were discussed in the previous section. As mentioned above, many of the psychosocial benefits seen after BaS seem to fade over time. The large variety of continued health problems, including dumping syndrome, gastric reflux, headaches, and wound infections, may contribute to continued problems in postoperative psychological functioning (feelings of failure, depression, poor HRQoL etc.). Additionally, patients' unrealistic expectations for success may far exceed results. The dramatic weight changes that occur 6 to 12 months after surgery may contribute to initial improvements in psychological functioning.[61] However, the weight loss typically begins to slow down after the first year and this change may contribute to the return to preoperative psychological functioning. It is also a fact that although large amounts of weight may be lost after BaS, most patients will remain obese, albeit at a lesser degree of severity.

It is generally recommended that patients attend group support meetings both before and after BaS.[73] Marcus and Elkins[73] recommended that the group incorporate self-responsibility, aspects of the "relapse prevention" model, and group therapy processes. A survey conducted among patients who attended or did not attend group support meetings found patients who attended meetings tended to lose more weight than those who did not attend.[74] Within attendees, those who came more often lost more weight than those who attended less. Interestingly, patients who reported emotional, psychosocial, dietary, and lifestyle problems were no more likely to attend the meetings. It is unclear why those who could most benefit from the group support meetings are the ones least likely to attend.

It has also been our experience, as it has for others,[75] that the relationship between couples may become strained after BaS. This may be largely due to drastic changes in the patient's self-image and self-confidence. For example, a female patient may become more assertive with her husband, while he becomes less assertive.[75] Men can sometimes become insecure in their relationship with their wife as they see her lose weight and become more attractive. This may even lead to behaviors on the husband's part that may sabotage the patient. Additionally, patients may begin to struggle with other issues related to body image, sexuality, social concerns, or occupational concerns that may have been more easily avoided prior to significant weight loss. The loss of weight may stall or the patient may begin to gain weight again if these concerns are not addressed. Again, many of the postoperative psychosocial factors that may undermine success after BaS can be lessened with appropriate follow-up and counseling, both for the patient and his or her family.

SPECIAL POPULATION CONSIDERATIONS FOR BaS

DIABETIC PATIENTS

The risk for type 2 diabetes is reported to be about two, five, and ten times higher in mildly, moderately and severely obese persons, respectively, in cross-sectional data.[76] A prospective study of nearly 4000 adults found similar results.[77] Estimates of the proportion of BaS patients who are diabetic range from 17 to 56%.[78–80]

BaS has been unequivocally shown to produce significant weight loss (20 to 50%) and improve glycemic control on a long-term basis in the obese diabetic patient.[3] A systematic review[3] of RGB and laparoscopic gastric banding found that RGB resulted in greater improvements in diabetes status compared to gastric banding. RGB was reported to prevent diabetes in 99 to 100% of patients with impaired glucose tolerance, and clinically resolve diabetes in 80 to 90% of the cases. Conversely, gastric banding resulted in clinical resolution of diabetes only 50 to 60% of the time. One meta-analysis found results consistent with the review, namely that improvement or resolution of diabetes ranges from 77 to 86% of patients undergoing various types of BaS,[6] while a more recent meta-analysis found that diabetes improved or was resolved in 64 to 100% of patients.[81] The presence of diabetes in BaS patients has been shown to be associated with poorer postoperative weight loss in patients receiving laparoscopic RGB.[82] Importantly, both types of surgery lead to significantly better improvements in diabetes status than lifestyle changes alone.

BaS is the most effective treatment for type 2 diabetes. In addition to the benefits common to all patients, some benefits are particularly relevant to diabetic people. The mechanisms by which diabetic status is improved are numerous, and still poorly understood. They include weight loss, decreased sympathetic activation, improved pancreatic beta-cell function, and hormonal changes.[83] Interestingly, hormonal changes seem to precede weight changes, as evidenced by a study that showed significant decreases in glucose, insulin, and leptin, three weeks after BaS, despite a very small and nonsignificant decrease in BMI.[84] Importantly, the resolution of glucose levels has been shown to be maintained long term (2 years) after BaS.[85] Furthermore, in the same study, none of the nondiabetic morbidly obese subjects developed diabetes at the same follow up.

PEDIATRIC PATIENTS

The use of surgery to correct obesity in children and adolescents remains somewhat controversial, although BaS within the pediatric population is now being practiced in several countries. However, several factors speak to the necessity of considering BaS in the pediatric population: (1) the current pediatric obesity epidemic, (2) obesity in the pediatric population is associated with the same comorbidities as obesity in adults, and (3) over half of obese children and adolescents will remain obese as adults.[86,87] On the other hand, the pediatric population has special needs that require that it must have specific guidelines.

The International Pediatric Endosurgery Group published guidelines for the surgical treatment of clinically severely obese adolescents in 2003.[88] Several other clinicians have supported these guidelines in literature reviews.[47,89,90] BaS in the pediatric population should be done only in centers that offer a multidisciplinary team approach.[88] The role of the psychologist as a member of the team is particularly important, because it can be difficult to assess the decisional capacity in this population. It is generally understood that children younger than 13 years of age are incapable of understanding the short- and long-term ramifications of such a serious procedure;[89] therefore BaS is generally not recommended in this population. Adolescents are more likely to be able to give informed assent, although parents also have to give informed consent in the case of minors. Another important factor to remember is that the adolescent will be returning to the same environment (i.e., family) that was conducive to the development of obesity in the first place.[91] Thus, it is crucial that both the patient and the family fully understand the procedure, as well as the necessary behavioral changes related to nutrition and physical activity that need to take place postoperatively. The adolescent and parents should be evaluated separately.[89] The psychologist plays an important role in evaluating the adolescent and family's readiness for, and acceptance of the required lifestyle changes.

In addition to psychological maturity, skeletal maturity should be taken into account. It is recommended that adolescents have achieved at least 95% bone maturation before being considered for BaS.[88] This is important because growth requires caloric and nutrient intake that may be difficult to achieve postoperatively, resulting in some stunting of normal growth in adolescents who have not reached physical maturity. It is also very important for the adolescent to have a documented history of failed attempts at weight management for a period of at least 6 months.[88]

Some of the eligibility criteria for BaS in adolescents differ slightly from adults. Adolescents may be considered for surgery if BMI ≥ 40 kg/m^2 in the presence of severe comorbidities, or if BMI ≥ 50 kg/m^2 in the presence of less serious comorbidities.[88] These BMI cutoffs are higher than for adults. It is difficult to predict with 100% accuracy whether an obese adolescent will remain obese during adulthood, although the odds of that happening are high, as noted above. The relative uncertainty associated with the future adult weight status of obese adolescents is one reason to be conservative. Also, the prevalence of comorbidities in adolescents is lower than in adults, although they may still be present. The case of each obese adolescent is unique in that each patient's medical, psychological, social, and environmental factors may differ. Thus each case should be reviewed weighing the pros and cons of BaS for that particular adolescent.

Only a handful of studies have reported on the postoperative effects of BaS on obesity and comorbidities in adolescents,[89,92–95] but the results seem promising. To the best of our knowledge, only three studies have reported on follow-up visits past 30 days postoperative. A study published about 12 years ago reported poor compliance by 34 adolescents to physical activity and dietary regimens at a 6-year follow-up,[96] which is similar to what has been found in adults. Despite this, BMI decreased from 47 to 32 kg/m^2. Another important finding of this study was improvements in psychosocial factors including improved self-esteem, social relationships, and self-image. A more recent study of 58 adolescents found that a significantly lower BMI was maintained (46 kg/m^2 preoperative to 30 kg/m^2) 7 years postoperative.[94] Another recent study reported that BMI decreased from 57 to 36 kg/m^2 at 1-year follow-up in 30 adolescents.[92] This study included a control group of adolescents who underwent a 12-month non-surgical pediatric weight management program. Whereas the surgical group had a decrease in BMI of about 37%, the control group had a decrease of only 3%. There are three main points to note in the previous studies. First, the BMI of adolescents who undergo BaS is generally above the criteria for severe obesity in adults. Second, postoperative BMI will still be within the obese range,[92] which is similar to what has been seen in adults. This speaks again to the importance of ensuring that the adolescent and family members understand the procedure to be performed, have realistic expectations related to postoperative outcomes, and are capable of and agree to follow postoperative regimens. Third, these studies also highlight the importance of regular medical postoperative care. The recommended appointment schedule is weekly during the first month, monthly for the next 6 months, and quarterly for the next 18 months.[91] To date there are no studies that have reported on the preoperative determinants of postoperative success in adolescents.

GERIATRIC PATIENTS

Special consideration also needs to be given to the obese geriatric population.[47] BaS has been performed on this population for a long time, but has been controversial given that elderly people are generally at increased risk when undergoing surgery. The literature comparing morbidity and mortality consequent to BaS in older and younger patients is inconsistent. Some studies reported no significant differences in complication rates between elderly and younger individuals,[97–99] while others reported higher mortality rates.[100–103] Interestingly, a study of Medicare patients found that mortality rates were higher at 90 days and 1-year follow-up in individuals older than 65 years compared to younger individuals.[103] Furthermore, individuals over 75 years of age were five times more likely to die within 90 days postoperative compared to individuals 65 to 74 years of age. There are many confounders in these studies, such as the different procedures used, especially laparoscopic vs. traditional, the specific age range of the "elderly" individuals, and the lack of control conditions. Thus it is unclear whether the geriatric population is at higher risk of morbidity and mortality resulting from BaS.

The obesity epidemic and increasing age of the population will result in an increase in obese elderly individuals. One of the results of obesity in the elderly is an increase in orthopedic problems which can become disabling. BaS and the resultant weight loss in obese elderly individuals also leads to significant improvements in orthopedic problems.[99,104] Some orthopedic surgeons are referring severely obese individuals for BaS before performing orthopedic surgery.[105] The advent of laparoscopic BaS, which has fewer complications than conventional techniques, is likely to increase this practice, thus potentially decreasing the need for more invasive surgery such as hip replacements. It is important to note that despite the risks involved, many clinicians believe that the potential gains outweigh the potential risks for obese elderly individuals. Studies consistently report good outcomes relative to weight and comorbidities,[97–99,102,106,107] although the improvements seen in elderly individuals tend to be smaller than those seen in younger individuals.

SUMMARY

BaS is becoming more common as a treatment alternative for severe obesity in people of all ages. BaS has been shown to be a clearly efficacious treatment of the severely obese, as indicated by significant weight loss and improvement in comorbidities.

However, BaS should be considered only after more conventional and less drastic treatments such as behavioral and pharmacological therapies have failed. There is not much known about the predictors of success for BaS, although preoperative psychological status seems to be a significant risk factor. Psychological evaluation practices for BaS candidates vary widely. The majority of centers implement some form of evaluation. However, many BaS centers fail to implement any psychological evaluation. We recommend that all centers utilize a more formal process that includes a structured clinical interview with the candidate and family members where appropriate, as well as relevant standardized psychological testing. Most importantly, each case should be reviewed on an individual basis, carefully weighing the specific risks and benefits for each candidate.

REFERENCES

1. Ogden CL, Carroll MD, Curtin LR, et al. *JAMA* 295: 1549; 2006.
2. Lew EA, Garfinkel L. *J Chronic Dis* 32: 563; 1979.
3. Leibbrand R, Fichter MM. *Behav Res Ther* 40: 1275; 2002.
4. In *NIH Publication no. 98-4083*. National Heart, Lung, and Blood Institute, Bethesda; 1998.
5. Foster GD, Wadden TA, Makris AP, et al. *Obes Res* 11: 1168; 2003.
6. Buchwald H, Avidor Y, Braunwald E, et al. *JAMA* 292: 1724; 2004.
7. O'Brien PE, Dixon JB, Laurie C, et al. *Ann Intl Med* 144: 625; 2006.
8. Herpertz S, Kielmann R, Wolf AM, Hebebrand J, Senf W. *Obes Res* 12: 1554–69; 2004.
9. Grothe KB, Dubbert PM, O'Jile JR. *Am J Med Sci* 331: 201; 2006.
10. Kral JG. *Intl J Obes Rel Metab Disord* 25 (Suppl 1): S107; 2001.
11. Sogg S, Mori DL. *Obes Surg* 14: 370; 2004.
12. Wadden TA, Sarwer DB, Williams NN. *Obesity* 14 (Suppl 2): 51S; 2006.
13. Mason EE, Cullen JJ. *Curr Surg* 60: 33; 2003.
14. MacDonald Jr. KG, Long SD, Swanson MS, et al. *J Gastrointestinal Sur* 1: 213; 1997.
15. National Institutes of Health. http://win.niddk.nih.gov/publications/gastric.htm
16. National Institutes of Health. *Arch Intern Med* 158: 1855; 1998.
17. Department of Veterans Affairs. http://www.nchpdp.med.va.gov/BariatricSurgery.asp; 2005.
18. Gibbons LM, Sarwer DB, Crerand CE, et al. *Obesity* 14 (Suppl 2): 70S; 2006.
19. Rand CS, Macgregor AM. *South Med J* 83: 1390; 1990.
20. Peace K, Dyne J, Russell G, Stewart R. *N Zealand Med J* 102: 76; 1989.
21. Gertler R, Ramsey-Stewart G. *Aust N Zealand J Surg* 56: 157; 1986.
22. Solow C, Silberfarb PM, Swift K. *N Eng J Med* 290: 300; 1974.
23. Lutfi R, Torquati A, Sekhar N, Richards WO. *Surg Endoscopy* 20: 864; 2006.
24. Wise T, Fernandez F. *Obes Bariatr Med* 8: 83; 1979.
25. Halmi KA, Long M, Stunkard AJ, Mason E. *Am J Psychiatr* 137: 470; 1980.
26. Hutzler JC, Keen J, Molinari V, Carey L. *J Clin Psychiatr* 42: 458; 1981.
27. Gentry K, Halverson JD, Heisler S. *Surgery* 95: 215; 1984.
28. Black DW, Goldstein RB, Mason EE. *Am J Psychiatr* 149: 227; 1992.
29. Sullivan M, Karlsson J, Sjostrom L, et al. *Intl J Obes Rel Metab Disord* 17: 503; 1993.
30. Greenberg I, Perna F, Kaplan M, Sullivan MA. *Obes Res* 13: 244; 2005.
31. Sarwer DB, Wadden TA, Fabricatore AN. *Obes Res* 13: 639; 2005.
32. Sarwer DB, Wadden TA, Fabricatore AN. *American Psychiatric Association, Diagnostic and Statistical Manual of Mental Disorders*. American Psychiatric Association,Washington, DC; 2000.
33. Hsu LK, Sullivan SP, Benotti PN. *Intl J Eating Disord* 21: 385; 1997.
34. Grilo CM, Reas DL, Brody ML, et al. *Beh Res Ther* 43: 629; 2005.
35. Powers PS, Perez A, Boyd F, Rosemurgy A. *Intl J Eating Disord* 25: 293; 1999.
36. Latner JD, Wetzler S, Goodman ER, Glinski J. *Obes Res* 12: 956; 2004.
37. Herpertz S, Kielmann R, Wolf AM, et al. *Intl J Obes Rel Metab Disord* 27: 1300; 2003.
38. De Zwaan M, Mitchell JE, Howell LM, et al. *Obes Res* 10: 1143; 2002.
39. Hsu LK, Benotti PN, Dwyer J, et al. *Psychosomat Med* 60: 338; 1998.
40. Stunkard AJ, Allison KC. *Intl J Obes Rel Metab Disord* 27: 1; 2003.
41. Hafner RJ, Rogers J, Watts JM. *J Psychosomat Res* 34: 295; 1990.
42. Camps MA, Zervos E, Goode S, Rosemurgy AS. *Obes Surg* 6: 356; 1996.
43. Dixon JB, Dixon ME, O'Brien PE. *Obes Surg* 12: 65; 2002.
44. Wadden TA, Phelan S. *Obes Res* 10 (Suppl 1): 50S; 2002.
45. Fabricatore AN, Wadden TA, Sarwer DB, Faith MS. *Obes Surg* 15: 304; 2005.
46. van Gemert WG, Severeijns RM, Greve JW, Groenman N, Soeters PB. *Intl J Obes Rel Metab Disord* 22: 393; 1998.
47. Crookes PF. *Ann Rev Med* 57: 243; 2006.
48. Bauchowitz AU, Gonder-Frederick LA, Olbrisch ME, et al. *Psychosomat Med* 67: 825; 2005.
49. Butcher J, Dahlstrom W, Graham J, et al. *Manual for the Restandardized Minnesota Multiphasic Personality Inventory: MMPI-2*. University of Minnesota Press, Minneapolis, MN; 1989.

50. Millon T. *Manual for the MCMI-III*. National Computer Systems, Minneapolis, MN; 1994.
51. Morey L. *Personality Assessment Inventory: Professional Manual*. Psychological Assessment Resources, Odessa, TX; 1991.
52. Beck AT. *Depression Inventory*. Center for Cognitive Therapy, Philadelphia, PA; 1978.
53. Beck AT, Steer RA, Brown GK. *Beck Depression Inventory II*. Harcourt Assessment, San Antonio, TX; 1996.
54. Thelen M, Farmer J, Wonderlich J, Smith M. *Psychol Assess* 3: 119; 1991.
55. Garner D: *Eating Disorder Inventory-2 Professional Manual*. Psychological Assessment Resources, Odessa, TX; 1991.
56. Hawkins RC, Clement PF. *Addict Behav* 5: 219; 1980.
57. Herman CP, Polivy J. *J Abnor Psychol* 84: 66; 1975.
58. Cooper PJ, Taylor MJ, Cooper Z, Fairburn CG. *Intl J Eating Disord* 6: 485; 1987.
59. Karlsson J, Sjostrom L, Sullivan M. *Intl J Obes Rel Metab Disord* 22: 113; 1998.
60. Dixon JB, Dixon ME, O'Brien PE. *Arch Intern Med* 163: 2058; 2003.
61. Waters GS, Pories WJ, Swanson MS, et al. *Am J Surg* 161: 154 (discussion 57); 1991.
62. van Gemert WG, Adang EM, Greve JW, Soeters PB. *Am J Clin Nutr* 67: 197; 1998.
63. Dymek MP, le Grange D, Neven K, Alverdy J. *Obes Surg* 11: 32; 2001.
64. Clark M, Balsiger B, Sletten C, et al. *Obes Surg* 13: 739; 2003.
65. Dixon JB, Dixon ME, O'Brien PE. *Obes Surg* 11: 200; 2001.
66. Averbukh Y, Heshka S, El-Shoreya H, et al. *Obes Surg* 13: 833; 2003.
67. Dubovsky SL, Haddenhorst A, Murphy J, et al. *Intl J Psychiatr Med* 15: 185; 1985.
68. Kalarchian MA, Marcus MD, Wilson GT, et al. *Obes Surg* 12: 270; 2002.
69. Malone M, Alger-Mayer S. *Obes Res* 12: 473; 2004.
70. Busetto L, Valente P, Pisent C, et al. *Intl J Obes Rel Metab Disord* 20: 539; 1996.
71. Busetto L, Segato G, De Marchi F, et al. *Obes Surg* 12: 83; 2002.
72. Hsu LK, Betancourt S, Sullivan SP. *Intl J Eating Disord* 19: 23; 1996.
73. Marcus JD, Elkins GR. *Obes Surg* 14: 103; 2004.
74. Hildebrandt SE. *Obes Surg* 8: 535; 1998.
75. Hafner RJ, Rogers J. *Intl J Obes* 14: 1069; 1990.
76. Hafner RJ, Rogers J. *Report of the United States National Commission on Diabetes to the Congress of the United States*. 1975. US Gov. Printing Office Washington DC
77. Westlund K, Nicolaysen R. *Scan J Clin Lab Invest* 127S: 1; 1972.
78. Potteiger CE, Paragi PR, Inverso NA, et al. *Obes Surg* 14: 725; 2004.
79. Livingston EH. *Am J Surg* 188: 105; 2004.
80. Residori L, Garcia-Lorda P, Flancbaum L, Pi-Sunyer FX, Laferrere B. *Obes Surg* 13: 333; 2003.
81. Maggard MA, Shugarman LR, Suttorp M, et al. *Ann Intern Med* 142: 547; 2005.
82. Perugini RA, Mason R, Czerniach DR, et al. *Arch Surg* 138: 541 (discussion 45); 2003.
83. Guldstrand M, Ahren B, Wredling R, et al. *Metab* 52: 900; 2003.
84. Rubino F, Gagner M, Gentileschi P, et al. *Ann Surg* 240: 236; 2004.
85. Dixon JB, O'Brien PE. *Diab Care* 25: 358; 2002.
86. Guo SS, Huang C, Maynard LM, et al. *Intl J Obes Rel Metab Disord* 24: 1628; 2000.
87. Freedman DS, Khan LK, Dietz WH, Srinivasan SR, Berenson GS. *Pediatrics* 108: 712; 2001.
88. International Pediatric Endosurgery Group. http://www.ipeg.org/guidelines/morbidobesity.html; 2003.
89. Inge TH, Krebs NF, Garcia VF, et al. *Pediatrics* 114: 217; 2004.
90. Steinbeck K. *Best Practice Res Clin Endocrinol Metab* 19: 455; 2005.
91. Inge T, Zeller M, Kirk S, Daniels S. In *Handbook of Pediatric Obesity: Clinical Management*. Sothern M, Gordon S, von Almen T (eds), CRC Press, Boca Raton, FL, 223; 2006.
92. Lawson ML, Kirk S, Mitchell T, et al. *J Ped Surg* 41: 137 (discussion 37); 2006.
93. Capella JF, Capella RF. *Obes Surg* 13: 826; 2003.
94. Angrisani L, Favretti F, Furbetta F, et al. *Surg* 138: 877; 2005.
95. Dolan K, Creighton L, Hopkins G, Fielding G. *Obes Surg* 13: 101; 2003.
96. Rand CS, Macgregor AM. *South Med J* 87: 1208; 1994.
97. St Peter SD, Craft RO, Tiede JL, Swain JM. *Arch Surg* 140: 165; 2005.
98. Papasavas PK, Gagne DJ, Kelly J, Caushaj PF. *Obes Surg* 14: 1056; 2004.
99. Sugerman HJ, DeMaria EJ, Kellum JM, et al. *Ann Surg* 240: 243; 2004.
100. Livingston EH, Huerta S, Arthur D, et al. *Ann Surg* 236: 576; 2002.
101. Printen KJ, Mason EE. *Surg, Gyne Obstet* 144: 192; 1977.
102. Sosa JL, Pombo H, Pallavicini H, Ruiz-Rodriguez M. *Obes Surg* 14: 1398; 2004.
103. Flum DR, Salem L, Elrod JA, et al. *JAMA* 294: 1903; 2005.
104. Bourdages H, Goldenberg F, Nguyen P, Buchwald H. *Obes Surg* 4: 227; 1994.
105. Parvizi J, Trousdale RT, Sarr MG. *J Arthroplasty* 15: 1003; 2000.
106. Macgregor AM, Rand CS. *Arch Surg* 128: 1153; 1993.
107. Murr MM, Siadati MR, Sarr MG. *Obes Surg* 5: 399; 1995.

53 Bariatric Surgery Overview

Malgorzata Stanczyk, Robert G. Martindale, and Clifford Deveney

CONTENTS

INTRODUCTION

Obesity is a complex disease with psychological, social, and economic ramifications that threatens more than a billion people around the world. It is currently estimated that approximately 65% of U.S. adult population has a body mass index (BMI) ≥ 25 and one in three adults (31%) is considered obese (BMI $\geq$ 30).[1]

Obesity-related deaths are estimated at 400,000 deaths per year, and obesity has become second most common preventable cause of death in the United States, just after smoking (total U.S. deaths in 2000: tobacco 18.1% vs. poor diet and physical inactivity 16.6%).[2] In addition to the obvious physical limitation of obesity, it is widely accepted that obesity adversely affects every major organ system [3–6] (Table 53.1).

The almost uniform failure of nonoperative treatments — exercise and dieting in achieving consistent long-lasting weight loss and weight control — is the main reason surgery has become popular in the management of severe obesity. Following bariatric surgery, the majority of patients not only lose weight but also experience resolution or significant improvement of their comorbidities. Significant reduction of risk for developing cardiovascular, endocrine, infectious, and mental disorders was seen within post-bariatric-surgery patients compared with the nonsurgical control group by Christou et al. in their 2004 study of mortality and morbidity post bariatric surgery.[7] This study also observed a significant reduction in the relative risk of 5-year mortality by 89%.[7]

TABLE 53.1
The Most Common Comorbidities Associated with Obesity[3–6]

System Involved	Comorbidities	Percentage
Cardiovascular	Hypertension	30–69
	Coronary artery disease	3–7
	Peripheral vascular disease/venous stasis	20–25
Pulmonary	Asthma	10–28
	Shortness of breath/dyspnea on exertion	27–97
	Obstructive sleep apnea	20–46
Gastrointestinal	Gallbladder disease	15–27
	Gastroesophageal reflux disease	22–64
Genitourinary	Menstrual irregularity/infertility	4–15
	Urinary stress incontinence	8–48
Musculoskeletal	Abdominal wall hernia	10–15
	Arthritis/degenerative joint disease	27–91
Metabolic	Diabetes mellitus	15–36
	Dyslipidemia	24–71
Neuropsychologic	Depression	7–49
	Pseudotumor cerebri	2–6

TABLE 53.2
NIH Classification of Obesity[8]

Classification	BMI (kg/m^2)
Underweight	<18.5
Normal Weight	18.5–24.9
Overweight	25.0–29.9
Obesity (Class 1)	30.0–34.9
Morbid Obesity (Class 2)	35.0–39.9
Extreme or Superobesity (Class 3)	≥40.0

WHO IS A CANDIDATE FOR BARIATRIC SURGERY?

In 1991 the National Institutes of Health (NIH) Expert Panel gave specific recommendations and guidelines for patient selection for bariatric surgery, using BMI as an indicator. [8] BMI is the ratio of the patient's weight in kilograms (kg) divided by the square of the patient's height in meters (m^2), that is, BMI = Wt /Ht × Ht. All patients were divided into four major classes with three subclasses within the obese group [8] (Table 53.2).

Specific guidelines were developed to assess each potential surgical candidate regarding potential risks and benefits. Good candidates for bariatric surgery should:

1. Have a BMI ≥ 40 kg/m^2 regardless of comorbidities, or BMI ≥ 35 kg/m^2 with a major comorbidity such as DM
2. Have failed serious attempts at nonoperative approaches
3. Be psychologically stable
4. Understand as well as accept the operative risks, be well informed, motivated, and able to participate in and comply with treatment and follow-up

HISTORY OF BARIATRIC SURGERY

The name *bariatric surgery* derives from the Greek word *barys* (heavy) and Latin word *iatria* (relating to treatment), and is one of the newest and fastest growing subspecialties of surgery. Bariatric surgery has evolved considerably since its inception in the early 1950s, when severe obesity was initially being recognized as a serious disease.

In 1954, Kremen and Linner published the first case report of intestinal jejuno–ileal bypass (JIB) as an operation for obesity and weight control. JIB shortened the length of intestine exposed to food from roughly 500 cm to 45 cm and produced dramatic and rapid weight loss by interfering with digestion and absorption secondary to significant shortening of the functional absorptive gut. Unfortunately, JIB was associated with a high morbidity and mortality. The JIB as a bariatric procedure was abandoned in late 1970s, although it continued to be occasionally done in cases of severe hyperlipidemia until the mid-1980s.

In the mid-1960s Mason and Ito introduced two new bariatric procedures — vertical banded gastroplasty (VBG) and loop gastric bypass (loop GBP), which resulted in significant weight loss and had far less long-term morbidity than JIB. VBG was a purely restrictive procedure that limited food intake by surgically creating a small gastric pouch. Loop GBP was also a restrictive procedure, which, in addition, resulted in some malabsorption. In this procedure the small gastric pouch emptied directly into a loop of jejunum brought up to bypass part of the foregut. In the 1970s both these procedures became the new standards in bariatric surgery.

In the early 1980s in Europe (Italy) Scopinaro proposed a different approach. He developed a modified malabsorptive and restrictive procedure — bilio-pancreatic diversion (BPD) (Figure 53.6), which combined the benefits of JIB and GBP. This operation is still performed in its original form as well as with modification, known as duodenal switch (DS) (Figure 53.7). In the 1980s there was increase in the interest in gastroplasties and gastric banding operations (Figure 53.4) — strictly restrictive procedures, less invasive than GBP, BPD, or JIB, and without some of its serious side effects of nutritional deficiencies and the dumping syndrome among others. The popularity of gastric banding is high especially within the European and Australian populations, where it has 15 to 20 years history and good results. Unfortunately all of the bariatric procedures have significant complications related to malabsorption, obstruction, or infections and wound complications.

Bariatric procedures have continued to evolve with the ideal procedure yielding minimum long-term metabolic sequelae and maintaining a weight loss of 60 to 70% of excess body weight (EBW). At present the bariatric procedures most commonly performed are Roux-en-Y gastric bypass (RYGBP), gastric banding, and biliary-pancreatic diversion with or without DS. All of these operations may be performed in a traditional open manner or laparoscopically. Virtually all uncomplicated gastric bands are performed laparoscopically, and an increasing number of RYGBPs and BPD-DSs are being performed laparoscopically.

CURRENT TRENDS IN BARIATRIC SURGERY

The number of bariatric operations has increased considerably over the last two decades and almost exponentially in the past 5 years. The estimated number of bariatric surgical procedures performed increased from 13,000 in 1998 to 72,000 in 2002 and more than 100,000 in 2003.[9,10]

The significant change in type of bariatric procedure performed was noted within this time period — from simple, open gastric restrictive procedures to complex laparoscopic and open procedures with RYGBP being considered the "gold standard." RYGBP currently accounts for more than 80% of all bariatric surgical procedures performed in the United States.[10] In 2003 International Bariatric Surgery Registry (IBSR) study "Trends in Bariatric Surgery," Mason compared information on more than 30,000 patients operated between 1986 and 2001. Over the period studied, it was observed that bariatric procedures were being performed in heavier and older patients (operative BMI increased from 45 to 49 and age at operation increased from 37 to 41 years). As the number of procedures increased, it was recognized that, despite increased complexity of the operation, the length of hospital stay significantly decreased from 5.0 to 3.9 days.[11] This large obesity surgery registry has also reported an increase in percentage of men being operated on (from 12.1 to 14.8 %).[11]

PRINCIPLES OF BARIATRIC SURGERY

Currently, several surgical options are available; these are usually divided by primary mechanism of weight loss:

1. Purely malabsorptive operations
2. Purely restrictive operations
3. Mixed malabsorptive and restrictive operations

PURELY MALABSORPTIVE OPERATIONS

Jejuno–Ileal Bypass (No Longer Recommended and of Historic Value Only)

In the past, the primary malabsorptive procedure was the JIB (Figure 53.1). In general, this procedure consisted of connecting a segment of the proximal small bowel to the distal small bowel or colon and bypassing the main absorptive portion of the gastrointestinal tract. By creation of a long, blind segment of the small intestine, the area of absorption was reduced and included only about 18 in. (45 cm) of the active gastrointestinal tract. Multiple modifications of this procedure were attempted, all with similar poor long-term outcome and high morbidity and mortality.

The advantage of that procedure was rapid and sustained weight loss without a need for change in eating habits. Unfortunately, these procedures had multiple serious side effects, which included severe metabolic abnormalities, oxalate-induced nephropathy and

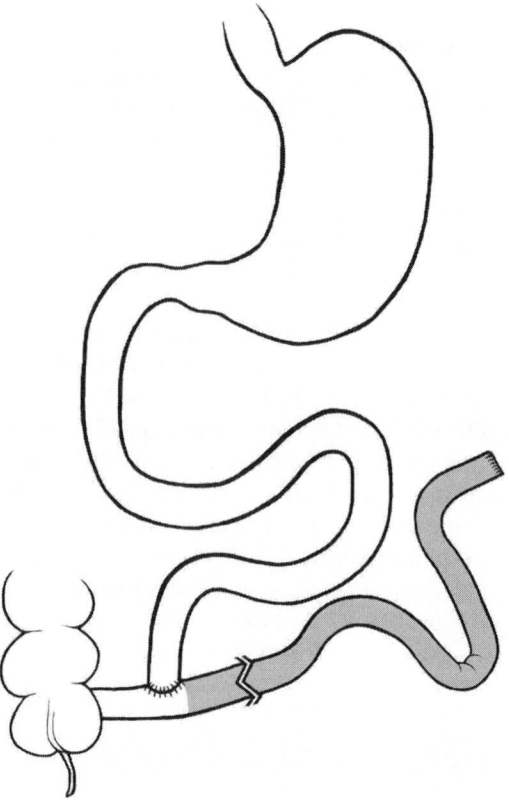

FIGURE 53.1   Jejuno–ileal bypass (JIB), end-to-side anastomosis.

renal calculi, chronic diarrhea and steatorrhea, multiple nutritional deficiencies and a severe electrolyte imbalance, osteomalacia, and high incidence of liver failure.[12] The most lethal long-term complication of JIB was hepatic failure with cirrhosis. This was believed to be secondary to overgrowth of bacteria within bypassed blind intestine loops, resulting in continued absorption of various toxic microbial byproducts into the portal vein, causing progression from hepatic steatosis to cirrhosis to eventual hepatic failure and death. This operation was abandoned in early 1970s and is currently not performed. Many patients who have had this procedure have either it reversed or converted to a safer procedure (e.g., RYGBP).

Purely Restrictive Operations

Purely restrictive procedures work through limitations on intake and, ideally, modifying long-term eating behavior. There are three major types of restrictive operations:

1.   Gastric stapling
2.   VBG
3.   Gastric banding or adjustable gastric banding

Gastric Stapling

A small gastric reservoir called stomach pouch — about 30 ml in size — was created within the stomach by placing a vertical or horizontal staple line (Figure 53.2). Because of frequent stomal widening and staple line dehiscence and availability of better procedures, gastric stapling was essentially abandoned. Gastric stapling frequently failed within 1 to 2 years of operation because of staple line dehiscence.

Vertical Banded Gastroplasty

This modification of gastric stapling was done to avoid the shortcomings of gastric stapling. In VBG the stomach was segmented along its vertical axis and the outlet of stoma was bounded by a plastic mesh or ring to prevent stretching. Some surgeons transected the stomach between several rows of staples to avoid staple line dehiscence and rapid weight gain (Figure 53.3). VBG has the benefit of preserving normal gastrointestinal (GI) transit of the food once it passes the gastric pouch and band. This in effect

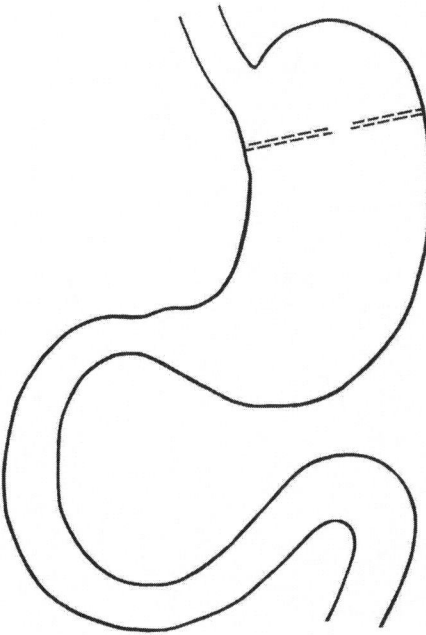

FIGURE 53.2   Gastric stapling (multiple modifications reported).

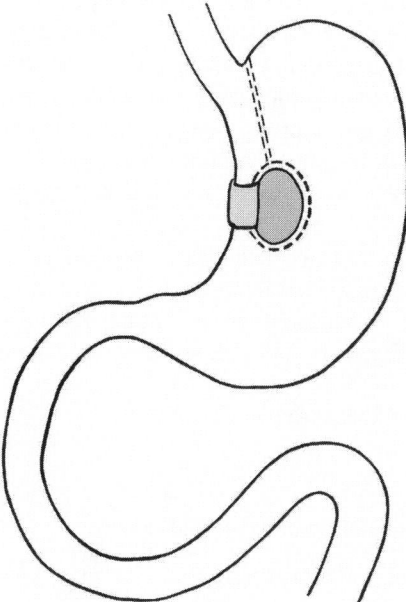

FIGURE 53.3   Vertical banded gastroplasty — (Mason).

prevents the majority of metabolic and nutritional complications. However, the vertical staple line can and often does dehisce in the same manner as with gastric stapling.

Gastric Banding and Adjustable Gastric Banding

Gastric banding provides restriction by placing a band around the stomach near the esophagogastric junction creating a small gastric pouch. The initial gastric banding procedure has been improved by adding an externally adjustable cuff around the stomach, which is attached to the reservoir implanted subcutaneously above the rectus sheath. Injecting the reservoir with saline alters the internal diameter of the gastric band, which provides the ability to change the stoma diameter to induce greater weight loss or alleviate vomiting or excessive weight loss. Currently the most popular restrictive bariatric surgery is the laparoscopic adjustable gastric band, known as the Lap-Band® (Figure 53.4).

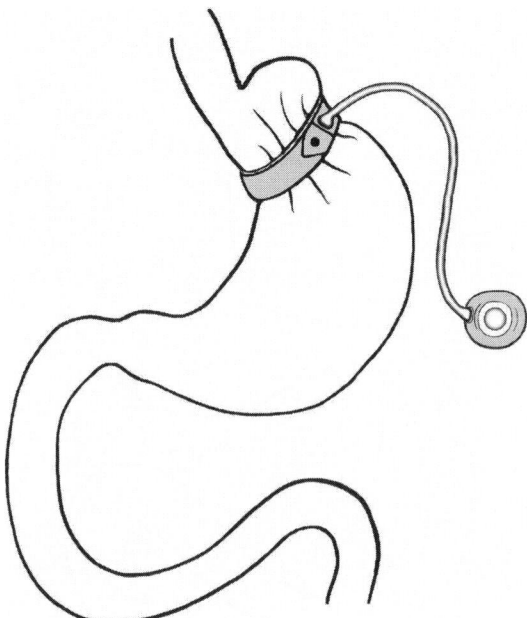

FIGURE 53.4 Adjustable gastric band.

Adjustable gastric banding has been widely used in Australia and Europe, and in 2001, the Lap-Band® was approved by the Food and Drug Administration (FDA) for the use in the United States. The gastric banding surgery is still an evolving procedure. As with any bariatric procedure, disadvantages and a number of complications have now been reported. Slower weight loss, complications with band erosion, and band migration are not uncommon, and occur up to 15 to 20%.[13,14]

In general, the advantage of restrictive only procedures is that they are technically easier in comparison to complex bariatric procedures such as RYGBP. In addition, they preserve GI anatomy and have fewer unwanted GI symptoms such as the dumping syndrome. As no malabsorptive component is involved, fewer mineral and vitamin deficiencies are reported and patients traditionally do not require supplements.

The disadvantage of these procedures is the risk of it being easily overcome by the patient increasing frequency and caloric consumption (high-calorie liquid food, which easily passes through the canal, avoiding the volume limitations).

These procedures are not free from serious complications. Numerous reports of gastroesophageal reflux disease (GERD), stomal stenosis, gastric prolapsed, band erosion or migration, and serious infectious complications are commonly reported.[13–15]

COMBINED RESTRICTIVE AND MALABSORPTIVE OPERATIONS

1. Roux-en-Y Gastric Bypass (RYGBP)
2. Bilio-Pancreatic Diversion (BPD)
3. Bilio-Pancreatic Diversion with Duodenal Switch (BPD-DS)

The combined restrictive and malabsorptive procedures have replaced gastric restrictive procedures in many centers. These procedures traditionally offer more consistent and greater weight loss but significantly alter normal GI physiology.[12,16]

All three of these operations can be performed by laparoscopic or open techniques. The technical disadvantage of the combined malabsorptive and restrictive procedures is the increased technical difficulty compared with restrictive only procedures. Multiple perioperative complications have been reported, most significant being leakage and marginal ulceration of the anastomotic site. Metabolic complications are common following these procedures, including iron deficiency anemia, vitamin B_{12} deficiency, impaired calcium absorption, and numerous other vitamin and mineral deficiencies.[17] Most, if not all, of these deficiencies can be corrected by daily oral supplementation. Rarely, protein-calorie malnutrition can develop if patient dietary compliance is poor and the patient is not monitored regularly and assessed for adequate nutrition parameters.

Roux-en-Y Gastric Bypass

A modification to the original loop gastric bypass was the creation of the Roux-en-Y gastric bypass (RYGBP). This procedure was designed to limit oral intake and create a "physiologic dumping" effect to discourage patient from consuming high concentrations of simple sugars. The Roux-en-Y reconstruction was done to eliminate any bile reflux into the stomach and esophagus, which was commonly experienced following the loop GBP. RYGBP is currently considered the "gold standard" for bariatric surgery and is the most common bariatric procedure being done today in the United States.

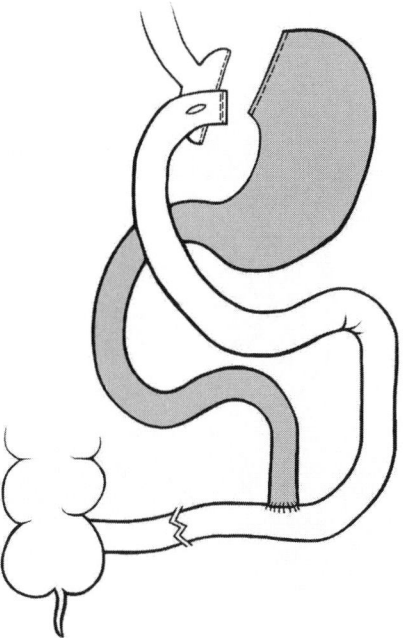

FIGURE 53.5 Roux-en-Y gastric bypass.

In this procedure the upper part of the stomach is divided between the lesser curvature and the angle of His, ideally creating a small gastric pouch (15 to 30 ml in size). The jejunum is divided and it distal portion brought up and anastomosed to the stomach pouch, forming the "Roux limb" and bypassing the remainder of the stomach and the duodenum. The anastomotic opening between the stomach pouch and the jejunum is about 1.2 cm in diameter. The proximal end of the jejunum is attached to the side of the Roux limb at 75 to 150 cm. It is believed that a minimum of 40 cm is required in the Roux limb to limit bile reflux back into the stomach (Figure 53.5). The small size of the pouch restricts food intake and helps to minimize the amount of acid that enters the upper jejunum. The remnant of the native stomach is left in place, and continues to produce gastric secretions, which pass down through the duodenum and mix with hepatic and pancreatic digestive secretions in the duodenum. At the Roux-en-Y anastomosis these secretions mix with food to complete the digestive and absorptive process.

The length of jejunum that is bypassed can be varied to add more malabsorption component if desired. As in all bariatric procedures, complication potentials are numerous and only briefly described here. Additional, more detailed information can be obtained in the references listed.[5,10,18–21]

RYGBP can be associated with the "dumping syndrome," which occurs secondary to a large osmotic load being delivered directly to the jejunum from the stomach pouch. This event produces unpleasant symptoms of flushing, cramping abdominal pain, tachycardia, nausea and/or vomiting, and occasional diarrhea. The dumping syndrome may further reduce intake, especially of simple sugars. RYGBP is a complex, technically difficult procedure, which also has a number of potential problems. There is a risk of anastomotic leak and development of gastric outlet obstruction — a narrowing at the anastomosis between the stomach pouch and the small intestine, which may require dilation. The "Roux stasis syndrome" — a slowing down of the emptying of the "Roux" portion of small bowel — usually results in nausea and vomiting and chronic abdominal pain. Obstructions of the bowel — involving one or both of the Y–limbs — can occur; when these anatomical complications occur, they can lead to development of serious metabolic complications including dehydration, electrolyte disturbances, and vitamin and minerals deficiency.

Cholelithiasis is common following any successful bariatric procedure. This is believed to result from the rapid weight loss precipitating gallbladder stone formation by altering the ratio of bile salts, cholesterol, and lecithin.[22] It is common to remove the gallbladder during these procedures when they are performed in an open manner. When done laparoscopically, the gallbladder is often left in place.

Bilio-Pancreatic Diversion

The multiple serious metabolic complications associated with JIB led to a search for alternative procedures; the BPD procedure, originally described by Scopinaro (Italy) was designed to address some of the shortcomings of the original JIB procedures. Many of the complications were thought to be related to bacterial overgrowth and toxin production and absorption from the blind, defunctionalized segment of the bypassed small bowel. Scopinaro proposed a procedure consisting of two components: a subtotal gastrectomy and a long RYGBP with a diversion for bilio-pancreatic juices into the distal ileum, which in effect prevents creation of defunctionalized segment of small bowel. [23] This procedure creates a 200 to 500 ml gastric pouch, which

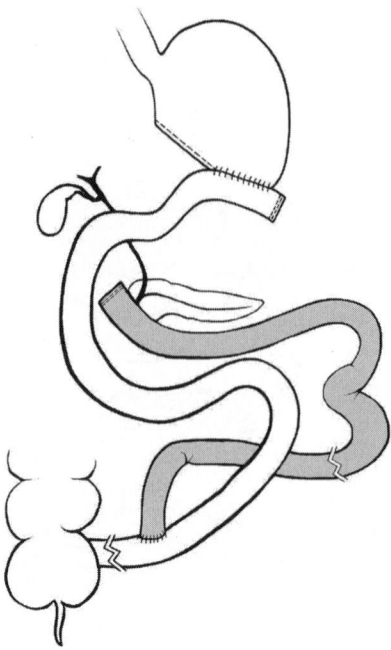

FIGURE 53.6 Bilio-pancreatic diversion.

facilitates reduction of food intake (restrictive component) and a distal Roux-en-Y small bowel bypass resulting in decrease of absorption area (malabsorptive component)[23] (Figure 53.6).

RYGBP is constructed with three separate segments: an "alimentary tract," consisting of 200 cm of ileum connecting the stomach to a common distal segment, and a "biliary tract," a segment between 300 and 400 cm long, which connects the duodenum, jejunum, and remaining ileum to the common distal segment. The third one, called a "common channel" is approximately 50 cm long, where food from the alimentary tract mixes with bilio-pancreatic secretions and digestion and absorption occur. The length of the common segment will influence the degree of malabsorption, particularly of fats and starches.

The disadvantage of this procedure is development of problems including loose stools, excessive and foul odorous flatus, and development of ulceration at the duodeno–ileal anastomosis. Also, many potential nutritional and metabolic complications are reported with this procedure, especially iron deficiency anemia, hypocalcemia, and protein malnutrition.[17,23] Of the current bariatric procedures, BPD has the highest risk of nutritional complications.

As in other bariatric surgeries, development of cholelithiasis is common, and concurrent cholecystectomy is routinely performed when the procedure is performed in an open manner.

Bilio-Pancreatic Diversion with Duodenal Switch or Duodenal Switch

BPD-DS, also called DS, is a modification of the bilio-pancreatic bypass described in the previous section. Instead of performing a distal gastrectomy, a "sleeve" gastrectomy is performed along the vertical axis of the stomach, preserving the pylorus and initial segment of the duodenum, which is then anastomosed to a segment of the ileum, similar to the aforementioned method[24] (Figure 53.7). The basic principle of the procedure is similar to BPD — producing restriction of food intake and selective malabsorption by limiting the food digestion and absorption to a short common distal segment. This modified procedure addressed several of the shortcomings of BPD and is thought to produce fewer and less of the profound metabolic and nutritional complications associated with BPD. Preservation of the pyloric sphincter is designed to be more physiologic and prevent the dumping syndrome. The sleeve gastrectomy decreases the volume of the stomach and also limits the parietal cell mass, which theoretically should decrease the incidence of acid secretion and ulcer formation. However, it is questionable if BPD-DS offers significant advantages over BPD alone.

POTENTIAL FUTURE INVASIVE TREATMENTS OF OBESITY

1. The gastric pacemaker (IGS)
2. Endoscopic vertical gastroplasty (EVG) or endoscopic gastric partitioning
3. Space-occupying devices:
   - Gastric balloons
   - Bezoars (butterfly)

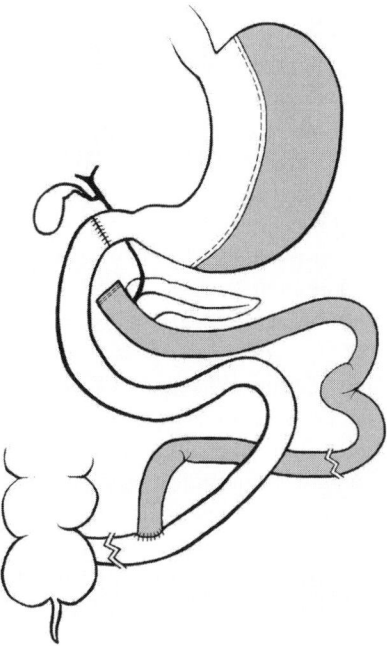

FIGURE 53.7   Bilio-pancreatic diversion with duodenal switch.

The Gastric Pacemaker (IGS)

IGS involves the laparoscopical implantation of bipolar electrode just beneath the seromuscularis of the stomach, along the lesser curvature of the stomach near the esophagogastric junction near the region where the vagus nerves enter the abdominal cavity. These electrodes are attached to a battery-powered stimulator inserted into a subcutaneous pocket in the upper abdomen. The exact mechanism of action is unknown, but it is theorized that the gastric pacemaker alters central nervous system vagal input and induces a feeling of satiety. To have maximum effect, it appears that the pacer should be individually adjusted to provide maximal anorexia with minimum nausea and vomiting. Technically these pacers are relatively easy to place and reported complications are few. To date, it has only been marginally effective.[25]

Endoscopic Vertical Gastroplasty (EVG) or Gastric Partitioning

EVG is currently in the experimental phase of pilot studies and is not routinely available. It is designed as an ambulatory procedure, performed endoscopically, in which the size of the stomach is reduced using an endoscopic stapler or suture to narrow or plicate the gastric inlet.

Patients are able to start eating in 6 h post procedure and are able to resume normal activity the next day. Limited pilot data is available on EVG.[26] Unfortunately, early reports appear to offer minimal long-term results.

Space-Occupying Devices

Several attempts with the use of intragastric-space-occupying devices have been attempted.

Gastric Balloons

The Bioenterics intragastric balloon (BIB) system is made of silicone and designed to partially fill the stomach and mimic an intragastric bezoar. The balloon is placed endoscopically and filled with 400 to 700 ml of sterile saline. It is intended for temporary weight loss, with a maximum placement of about 6 months. The removal of BIB is done endoscopically, usually with general anesthesia. The most frequent complications with gastric balloons include intolerance to the balloon, vomiting, GERD, spontaneous balloon deflation, gastric ulcer or erosions, and abdominal pain.[27]

The Butterfly

This space-occupying device is currently in its experimental phase. It consists of a continuous polyethylene ribbon folded over on it self. The ribbon is approximately 36 m in length. These space-occupying devices are two of several space-filling options, none of which have had much success to date.

COMPLICATIONS POST BARIATRIC SURGERY

All bariatric treatments require a high degree of patient compliance and a through understanding of risks and potential benefits. Outcomes of bariatric operations are difficult to evaluate due in part to the constantly evolving nature of the surgery. Small modifications are commonly made by individual surgeons to decrease the incidence of postoperative and long-term complications.

The overall complication rate of the combined bariatric procedures is approximately 10 to 20% with a mortality rate of about 0.5% (0.1 to 1.5%).[5,10,18–21] Many complications are relatively common and serious, often requiring additional surgical procedures. These include afferent limb obstruction with gaseous distention of the stomach, postoperative leaks, and internal hernias that involve some portion of the intestine, just to highlight a few. Less serious complications include stomal stenosis and marginal ulcers, which often respond to acid suppression therapy.

The recent data from the IBSR 2004 to 2005 Winter Report 19(1), which analyzed data from 38,501 patients who were operated between 1986 and 2005, found that 87.2% had no early postoperative (30-day) complication (3.4% had a major and 9.5% had minor early complication).[28] The most frequently reported major complication was intestinal leak, and the most frequently reported minor complication was wound infection. The mortality rate within 30 days of operation was 0.25%, with pulmonary embolism (PE) being the most frequent cause of death, followed by cardiac events.[28] As the trend to include patients with increasing age and greater comorbidities progress, these rates may increase.

Late complications, which occur more than 90 days post operation, are most often related to weight loss and development of malnutrition or vitamin deficiencies. Most of these complications can be managed nonoperatively or with patients' compliance. Some complications such as incisional hernia, gastric outlet stenosis, or gastric fistula will require additional surgical treatment. Most common early and late complications are listed in Table 53.3 and Table 53.4.

WEIGHT LOSS AFTER BARIATRIC SURGERY

The weight loss and success rate is dynamic and multifactorial and depends on the type of bariatric surgery as well as patient's compliance, initial BMI, and exercise program. Actual postsurgical weight loss will depend on the choice of bariatric procedure

TABLE 53.3
Early Complications Following Bariatric Surgery [5,10,18–21]

	Early Complications	Percentage
1	Gastric or anastomotic leaks	0.7–3
2	Pulmonary embolus	0.4–2
3	Wound complications/dehiscence and infection	1–9
4	Bowel obstruction	1–3
7	GI bleeding	0.6–2
8	Cardiorespiratory failure	0.4–1.3
9	Death	0.25–21

TABLE 53.4
Late Complications Post Bariatric Surgery [5,10,18–21]

	Late Complications	Percentage
1	Inadequate weight loss/weight gain	5–30
2	Gallbladder disease	3–30
3	Incisional ventral hernia	5–20
4	Nutritional deficiencies	5–16
5	Dumping syndrome	2–15
6	Marginal ulceration	3–10
7	Staple line disruption	2–10
8	Band erosion	2–4
9	Gastro-Gastric fistula	1–6
10	Outlet stenosis	1–6
11	Upper GI bleeding	0.2–3
12	Acid reflux/GERD	2–10
13	Nausea and vomiting	4–11

as well as patient's compliance, age, baseline weight, overall health status, motivation, and commitment. Therefore, patient selection becomes a critical process, requiring psychiatric evaluation and a multidisciplinary approach.

Patients with a lower BMI at baseline generally lose a greater percentage of excess weight and come closer to their ideal body weight (IBW) than those with a higher initial BMI. The higher-BMI patient loses more total weight but does not often reach IBW. Older persons and those with type 2 diabetes mellitus tend to achieve a lesser reduction in excess weight loss (EWL) than their younger or nondiabetic counterparts.[29] The outcome of bariatric surgery is measured using different modalities, percentage of EWL or of BMI loss or absolute weight loss. The most popular and widely used is assessment of weight loss according to the patient's percentage of EWL. The definition of successful bariatric surgery is a loss of at least 50% of the patient's EBW and maintaining it for at least 5 years (Reinhold Classification).[30] In 2004 Biron proposed a new set of landmarks for successful outcome of bariatric procedure, with regards to patients initial BMI.[31] The outcome was consider as a successful if the patient with initial BMI $\leq$ 49 reached BMI < 35 or if a superobese patient with initial BMI $\geq$ 50 achieved BMI < 40.[31]

Weight loss after bariatric surgery usually reaches maximum levels at about 18 (12 to 24) months postoperatively and a plateau is commonly reached after that period. A small amount of weight regain can be expected after the weight nadir. Weight loss following placement of the gastric band occur more slowly and may not peak for 36 months.

For gastric restrictive procedures, the weight loss is primarily due to reduced caloric intake, and thus the patient must be committed to eating small meals, reinforced by early satiety. With the exception of the adjustable gastric band, the 5-year percentage of EWL is relatively poor in restrictive-only procedures.

The results for RYGBP shown usually rapid weight loss within the first 6 months and weight stabilization at 18 to 24 months,[28] with a mean EWL of 60 to 85% at 3 years, a 15% weight regain over 14 years, and long-term (5 to 14 years) EWL ranging from 48 to 74%.[20,21,28,30] After BPD-DS, a dramatic early weight loss of as much as 74% EWL has been reported at 1 year, 91% EWL at 5 years, and 78% EWL at 18 years.[32] After BPD without duodenal switch, 18-year results of 78% EWL have been recorded.[23]

In contrast to the dramatic early effects of the complex, restrictive, and malabsorptive procedures (RYGBP and BPD), patients who undergo laparoscopic adjustable gastric banding (LAGB) procedure tend to experience slow and progressive weight loss, with 41 to 53% EWL at 2 years.[33] More recently, O'Brien showed that use of adjustable banding extends the weight loss over 2 to 3 years, with a steady mean weight loss of about 50% of EBW for 6 years.[34] Most other reports are not this optimistic.

DIETARY ISSUES POST BARIATRIC SURGERY

Nutritional deficiencies following bariatric surgery will depend primarily on patient compliance and the type of bariatric procedure performed (Table 53.5). When evaluating for nutritional deficiencies following bariatric surgery, it is critical to obtain as much information as possible on the specifics of the procedure, any radiologic or endoscopic data, patient compliance, and diet history. Generally speaking, most restrictive only procedures (i.e., lap band) will not result in nutritional deficiencies unless they are associated with some anatomic issue limiting intake or dietary compliance is poor. The procedures that result in both restriction of intake and malabsorption (i.e., RYGB, DS, and bilio-pancreatic bypass) commonly develop nutritional deficiencies, with those of vitamin B_{12} and iron being the most common.[35] Suspected etiologies of the B_{12} deficiency are numerous and include inadequate dietary intake, inadequate release of B_{12} from food secondary to low acid and pepsin in pouch, inadequate mixing with R-protein in stomach, decreased availability of intrinsic factor, decrease formation of the B_{12}–IF (intrinsic factor) complex, and possibly bacterial overgrowth of bypassed segment.

The anatomic exclusion of the proximal gut, where iron is primarily absorbed, is the major etiology of iron associated anemia observed in bariatric surgery. The relative achlorhydria induced by the procedure does prevent some cleavage or iron from food and decreases the amount of iron, which remains in the better-absorbed ferrous state. In addition, by following all bariatric

TABLE 53.5
Comparison of Nutritional Deficiencies within Multiple Studies

Study: Author (Year)	Patients Number	Percentage of Patients			
		Iron	Vitamin B_{12}	Folate	Anemia
Halverson (1981)	69	20	26	9	18
Amaral (1985)	150	49	70	18	35
Benotti (1989)	289	28	36		19
Brolin (1990)	124	33	37	16	22
Pories (1995)	20		27		
Provernzale (1992)	608		40		39
Brolin (1998)	348	47	37	35	54
Anthone (2004)	701				16

procedures patients have a tendency to decrease consumption of iron rich foods. Anemia and metabolic bone disease (osteoporosis and secondary hyperparathyroidism) are often seen after malabsorptive procedures.[36] Calcium deficiency, which develops, can be insidious as the serum calcium levels will remain normal until the patient has mobilized a significant percentage of total body calcium. When recommending calcium supplementation, several factors need to be considered. The pharmaceutical preparation (calcium citrate vs. carbonate), age, vitamin D level, timing of intake, gastric acidity, and bioavailability will all influence the calcium available to the patient. The fat-soluble vitamins are commonly deficient in the DS and bilio-pancreatic procedures and are reported in up to 69% of patients.[37] In patients who present with persistent vomiting and marginal oral intake are at risk for acute thiamine deficiency and should be supplemented intravenously if the patient cannot take adequate oral supplementation.

Lifelong daily supplements are required for all malabsorptive procedures. These should include adequate multivitamins and in addition should include additional vitamin B_{12}, iron, and calcium. Vitamin B_{12} supplements are available as oral, sublingual, intranasal, and injections. Other vitamins and minerals may be required depending on the individual patient and presentation.

Women in childbearing years are also advised to take additional folate, iron, and calcium supplements. Numerous other single-nutrient or mixed nutritional deficiencies have been reported following bariatric procedures including night blindness, muscle weakness, dry scaling skin, and the Wernicke–Korsakoff syndrome.

Nutritional deficiency is extremely common following bariatric procedures. Patients should be evaluated for nutritional deficiencies routinely during the first few years post operation and then annually for life. Women who become pregnant following any bariatric procedure require close nutritional monitoring throughout the pregnancy and breast-feeding periods.

LIFE POST BARIATRIC SURGERY

Compliance and lifelong follow-up is necessary for all patients after bariatric surgery. Lifelong monitoring of weight loss, dietary and activity behaviors, comorbidities, and metabolic and nutritional status can provide necessary information to help treat and prevent most of the long-term complications. All patients after bariatric surgery will benefit greatly from physical activity and an active exercise program to improve weight loss and prevent deconditioning.

The importance of vitamin and mineral supplementation cannot be overemphasized, as the signs and symptoms of deficiencies may occur months to years after surgery. Irrespective of the individual bariatric procedure, a vast majority of the patients will not suffer any nutritional deficiency if they are compliant with the postoperative supplement regiment. Nutrition, exercise, and adjustment to the physical and emotional changes associated with significant postoperative weight loss need to be discussed and understood in detail prior to embarking on and any bariatric surgical plan.

REFERENCES

1. Hedley, A.A. et al., *JAMA*, 91, 2847, 2002.
2. Mokdad, A.H. et al., *JAMA*, 291, 1238, 2004.
3. Residori, L. et al., *Obes. Surg.*, 13, 333, 2003.
4. Buchwald, H. et al., *JAMA*, 292, 1724, 2004.
5. Balsiger, B.M. et al., *Mayo Clin. Proc.*, 75, 673, 2000.
6. Livingston, E., *Am. J. Surg.*, 188, 105, 2004.
7. Christou, N.V. et al., *Ann. Surg.*, 240, 416, 2004.
8. *The Practical Guide: Identification, Evaluation, and Treatment of Overweight and Obesity in Adults.* NIH Publication. Number 00-4084, October 2000.
9. Trus, T.L., Pope, G.D., Finlayson, S., *Surg. Endosc.*, 19, 616, 2005.
10. Santry, H.P., Gillen, D.L., Lauderdale, D.S., *JAMA*, 294, 1909, 2005.
11. Mason, E.E. et al., *Obes. Surg.*, 13, 225, 2003 (Abstract) Poster presentation at the ASBS Convention; Boston, MA.
12. Latifi, R., Sugerman, H.J., *Obesity: Mechanisms and Clinical Management*. Philadelphia: Lippincott Williams & Wilkins, 2003.
13. O'Brien, P.E. et al., *Br. J. Surg.*, 86, 113, 1999.
14. Gutschow, C.A. et al., *J. Gastrointest. Surg.*, 9, 941, 2005.
15. Camerini, G. et al., *Obes. Surg.*, 14, 343, 2004.
16. Buchwald, H., Buchwald, J.N., *Obes. Surg.*, 12, 705, 2002.
17. Mason, M.E., Jalagani, H., Vinik, A.I., *Gastroenterol. Clin. N. Am.*, 34, 25, 2005.
18. Livingstone, E.H., *Surg. Clin. N. Am.*, 85, 853, 2005.
19. Maggard, M.A. et al., *Ann. Intern. Med.*, 142, 547, 2005.
20. Fobi. M.A.L. et al., *Obes. Surg.*, 11, 18, 2001.
21. Podnos, Y.D. et al., *Arch. Surg.*, 138, 957, 2003.
22. Shiffman, M.L. et al., *Gastroenterology*, 103, 214, 1992.
23. Scopinaro, N. et al., *World J. Surg.*, 22, 936, 1998.
24. Marceau, P. et al., *World J. Surg.*, 22, 947, 1998.
25. Shikora, S.A., *Obes. Surg.*, 14, 545, 2004.

26. Fogel, R., *Digestive Disease Week*, Abstract 743, May 18th 2005.
27. Evans, J.D., Scott, M.H., *Br. J. Surg.*, 88, 1245, 2001.
28. American Society for Bariatric Surgery. *Rationale for the surgical treatment of morbid obesity.* 2001. Available at: http://ww.asbs. org/html/patients/retionale.html
29. Sugerman, H.J. et al., *Ann. Surg.*, 237, 751, 2003.
30. Reinhold, R.B., *Surg. Gynecol. Obstet.*, 155, 358, 1982.
31. Biron, S. et al., *Obes. Surg.*, 14, 160, 2004.
32. Baltasar, A. et al., *Obes. Surg.*, 11, 54, 2001.
33. Rubenstein, R.B., *Obes. Surg.*, 12, 380, 2002.
34. O'Brien, P.E., Dixon, J.B., *J. Laparoendosc. Adv. Surg. Tech.*, 13, 265, 2003.
35. Brolin, R.E. et al., *Arch. Surg.*, 133, 740, 1998.
36. Goode, L.R. et al., *Obes. Res.*, 12, 40, 2004.
37. Slater, G.H. et al., *J. Gast. Surg.*, 8, 48, 2004.

54 Nutrition-Related Genetic Diseases

Carolyn D. Berdanier

CONTENTS

INTRODUCTION

The genetic material, DNA (deoxyribonucleic acid), in the cell nucleus holds the code that dictates the amino acid sequence of all proteins in the body. A small amount of DNA is also found in the mitochondria (mtDNA). Should there be a change in the sequence of the nucleotides, which comprise DNA and that change in code results in a change in the amino acid used in the synthesis of the gene product, then the sequence of amino acids in the resultant protein could be different. This change in the normal sequence of bases in the DNA is called *mutation*. It can be either a spontaneous mutation or one induced by drugs or a virus or any one of a number of external variants that target the genetic material of the cell. Some changes in the base sequence have no effect on the amino acid used for protein synthesis. This is because many of the amino acids have more than one code in the DNA. When such a base substitution occurs, it is a *polymorphism*, not a mutation. Polymorphisms also occur in the noncoding regions of the DNA and in sections of the DNA that have no relevance when it comes to the function of the gene product.

Whether the substitution of one or more amino acids for another has an adverse effect, on the activity of the protein being synthesized depends wholly on the amino acids in question. If these amino acids have functional groups in their side chains that modify the three-dimensional structure and the function of the protein, then its activity will be abnormal. This chapter describes genetic diseases that have importance in the consideration of nutrient needs and tolerances. The reader is referred to Chapter 7 that describes the various pathways of nutrient metabolism.

GENE EXPRESSION

Before the nutrition-related genetic disorders can be listed and described, a brief overview of gene expression is needed.[1–3] DNA is found in both the nucleus and the mitochondria and is composed of four bases: adenine, guanine, thymine, and cytosine. These bases are condensed to form the DNA chain in a process analogous to the condensation of amino acids in the primary structure of a protein. The chain of nucleotides which comprise DNA is formed by joining adenine, guanine, thymine, and cytosine through phoshodiester bonds. The phosphodiester linkage is between the 5′-phosphate group of one nucleotide and the 3′-OH group of the adjacent nucleotide. This provides a direction (5′ to 3′) to the chain. A typical segment of the chain is illustrated in Figure 54.1. The hydrophobic properties of the bases plus the strong charges of the polar groups within each of the component units, are responsible for the helical conformation of the DNA chain. The bases themselves interact such that in the nucleus, the two chains are intertwined. Hence, the term double helix applies to DNA. In the mitochondria, the DNA, also a double strand, is circular with connections between the light and heavy strands. Hydrogen bonds between the bases stabilize this conformation. Other factors as well serve to stabilize the structure of the DNA. Unwinding a small portion of the DNA, a necessary step in the initiation of nuclear gene transcription, occurs when these stabilizing factors are perturbed and signals are sent to the nucleus that transcription should begin. Unwinding exposes a small (~17 kb) segment of the DNA (the gene), allowing its base sequence to be available for complementary base pairing as happens when messenger RNA is synthesized (transcription). The segment that

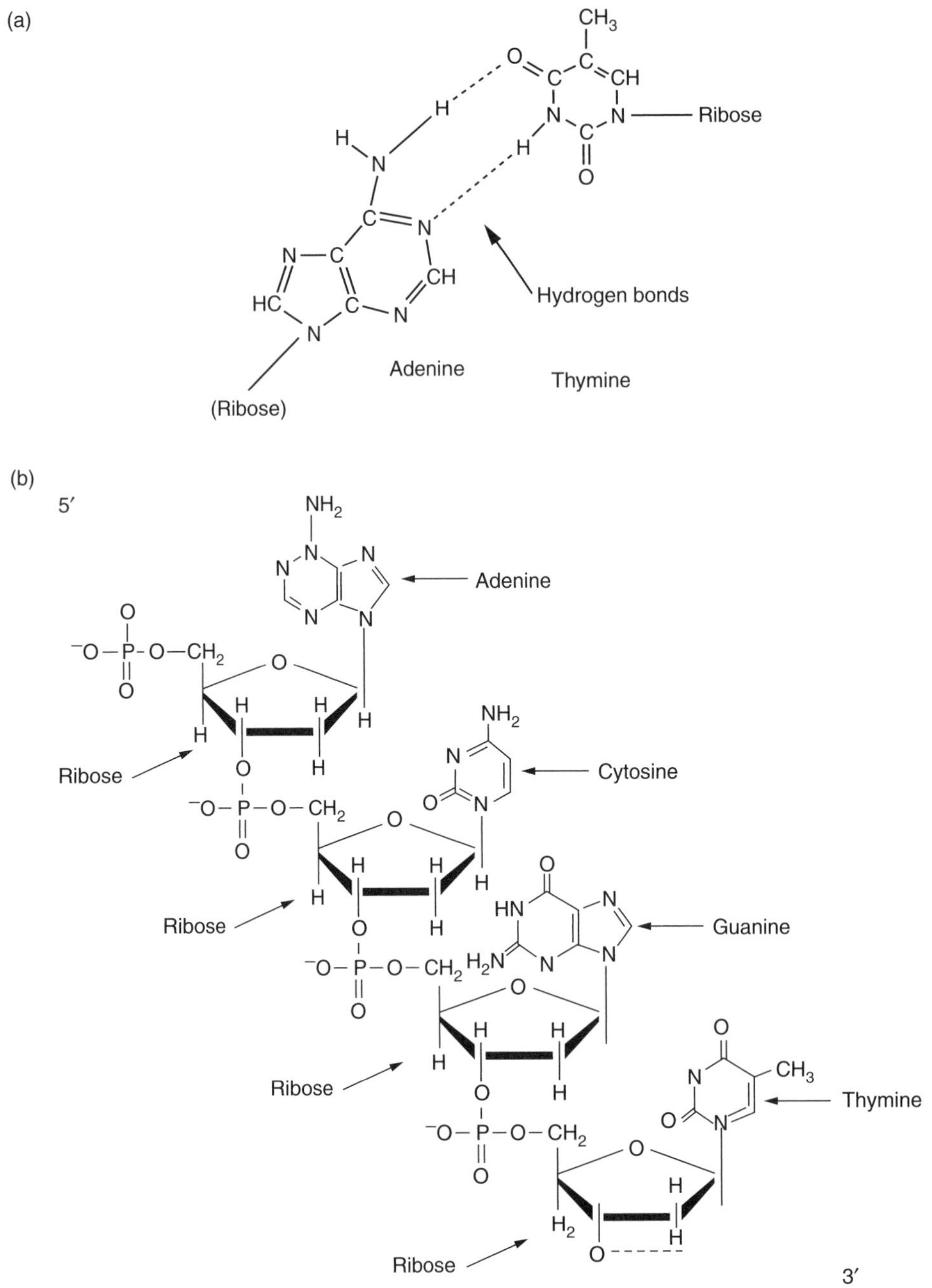

FIGURE 54.1 The bases of DNA are joined together by phosphodiester bonds using ribose as a common link. Hydrogen bonds also form between complementary bases of the strands of DNA or between the bases of the DNA and RNA as it is forming or between the bases of messenger RNA and those of ribosomal RNA and transfer RNA. Adenine complements thymine; guanine complements cytosine. Hydrogen bonding stabilizes the double-helical array of the two strands of DNA.

is exposed contains not only the 600 to 1800 nucleotide-structural genes but also a sequence called the promoter region. The promoter region precedes the start site of the structural gene, and this is said to be upstream of the structural gene. Those bases following the start site are downstream. The nucleotides which code for a specific protein may not be adjacent to each other on the DNA strand but may be located nearby, as the DNA exists in a doubly coiled chain of bases, the double helix.

During cell division, the nuclear DNA, as soon as its replication is completed, becomes highly condensed into distinct chromosomes of characteristic shapes. These chromosomes exist as pairs and are numbered. There are 46 chromosomes in the human. Included in this number are the sex chromosomes, the X and Y chromosomes. If the individual has one X and one Y he is a male; if two X's are present, she is a female. The chromosomes are the result of a mixing of the nuclear DNA of the egg and sperm. Approximately half of each pair comes from each parent. If identical codes for a given protein are inherited from each parent, the resultant progeny will be a homozygote for that protein. If nonidentical codes are inherited, the progeny will be a heterozygote.

Within the heterozygote population, there may be certain codes which are dominant, eye color or hair color, for example. These are dominant traits and are expressed despite the fact that the individual has inherited two different codes for this trait. A mutation in a code that is not expressed is a recessive trait. If, by chance, two identical mutated genes are present that encode a certain protein, the expression of this mutated code will be observed. This is the basis for genetic diseases of the autosomal recessive or dominant type. Autosomal means a mutation in any of the chromosomal DNA except that which is in the X or Y chromosome. A mutation of the DNA in this chromosome is called a sex-linked mutation. If it results in a disease, it is called sex-linked genetic disease. There is another inheritance pattern based on the mitochondrial genome. Because this genome is primarily of maternal origin, certain of the characteristics of the OXPHOS (Oxidative Phosphorylation) system will be inherited via maternal inheritance. A number of mitochondrial mutations result in a number of degenerative diseases.

Having the codes in the nucleus for the synthesis of protein in the cytoplasm implies a communication between the cytoplasm and the nucleus and between the nucleus and the cytoplasm. Signals are sent to the nucleus, which "informs" this organelle of the need to synthesize certain proteins. We do not know what all these signals are. Some are substrates for the needed proteins, some are nutrients, some are hormones, and some are signaling compounds that have yet to be identified. The communication between the nucleus and the cytoplasm is carried out by messenger RNA (mRNA).

TRANSCRIPTION

Messenger RNA is used to carry genetic information from the DNA of the chromosomes to the surface of the ribosomes (Figure 54.2). It is synthesized as a single strand in the nucleus by a process known as transcription. Chemically, RNA is similar to DNA. It is an unbranched linear polymer in which the monomeric subunits are the ribonucleoside $5'$-monophosphates. The bases are the purines, adenine and guanine and the prymidines, uracil and cytosine. Note that thymine is not used in RNA and that uracil is not present in DNA. RNA is single stranded rather than double stranded. It is held together by molecular base pairing and will contract if in a solution of high ionic strength. RNA, particularly the mRNA, is a much smaller molecule than DNA and is far less stable. It has a very short half-life (from minutes to hours) compared to that of nuclear DNA (years). Because it has a short half-life, the bases which comprise it must be continually resynthesized. This synthesis requires a number of micronutrients as well as energy. This explains some of the symptoms of malnutrition. Among these symptoms are skin lesions. This is because the epithelial cells are among the shortest-lived cells and must be constantly renewed. This renewal depends on both an adequate energy and amino acid and on the micronutrients that are involved in mRNA synthesis as well cell renewal.

The synthesis of mRNA from DNA involves three steps: initiation, elongation, and termination. Initiation is the process whereby basal transcription factors recognize and bind the start point for transcription on DNA and form a complex with RNA polymerase II. Most of gene expression can be defined as trans-acting factors or proteins binding cis-acting elements (base sequences). Upstream of the transcription start site on DNA is a region called the promoter (Figure 54.3). Within the promoter, approximately 25 base pairs upstream of the start site, is a consensus sequence called the TATA box, that contains A–T base pairs. One of the basal transcription factors, the TATA binding protein (TBP), recognizes this sequence of DNA and binds there. This begins the process of transcription initiation as the trans-acting TBP binds the cis-acting TATA box and a large complex of basal transcription factors, RNA polymerase II, and DNA is formed. Elongation is the actual process of RNA formation using a DNA template in the $5'$ to $3'$ direction. Shortly after elongation begins, the $5'$ end of mRNA is capped by 7-methylguanosine triphospate. This cap stabilizes the mRNA and is necessary for processing and translation. The third step is the termination of the chain.

The regulation of transcription occurs at the initiation step. The promoter region contains many cis-acting elements, each named for the factor that binds to them. In general, these regions are called enhancers, silencers, or more recently named response elements. Examples include the retinoic acid response element (RARE), heat shock element (HSE), cAMP response element (CRE). The trans-acting factors that bind these elements are in general called transcription factors. They are proteins with at least two domains, DNA binding and transcription activation. Recently, it has been shown that coactivators are needed to bind transcription factors and increase transcription by both interacting with basal transcription factors and altering chromatin structure. Corepressors act to decrease transcription both at the level of basal transcription factors and chromatin structure. Coactivators and corepressors are proteins.

The true regulation of transcription occurs by the regulation of transcription factors. Transcription factors can be regulation by: (1) their rates of synthesis or degradation; (2) phosphorylation or dephosphorylation; (3) ligand binding; (4) cleavage of

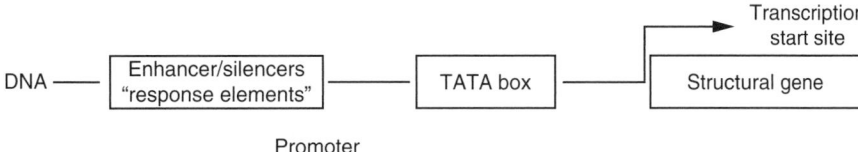

FIGURE 54.2   Detailed structure of the components of a gene.

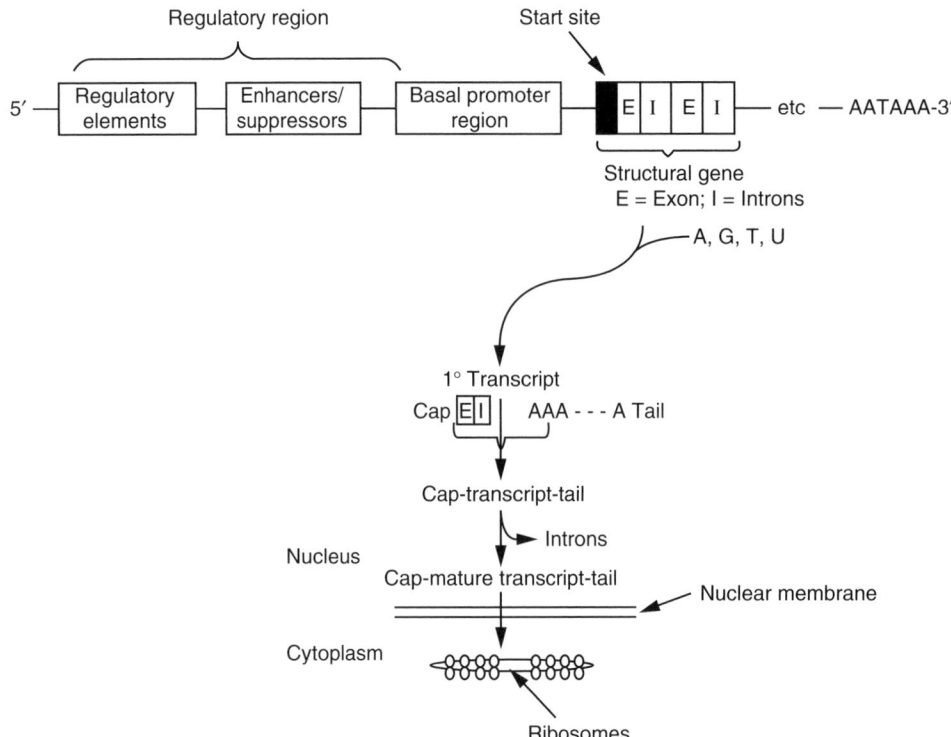

FIGURE 54.3 Transcription: the synthesis of messenger RNA and its editing and migration to the cytosol where it attaches to the ribosomes.

TABLE 54.1
Members of the Nuclear Hormone Receptor Superfamily[1]

Receptor Group[a]	Consensus Half Site	Binding Site	
Group 1			
GR, ER, PR, MR, AR	AGAACA or AGGTCA	→ (3) ←	Homodimers
Group 2			
RXR, RAR, TR, VDR, PPAR, MB67,	AGGTCA	→ (0–5) →	Heterodimerize with RXR
RLD-1, ECR, USP, ARP-1, COUP-TF		→ (0) ←	
Group 3			
NGF1-B, FTZ-F1 (ELP, SF-1) ROR,	(A,T)AAGGTCA	→	Monomers or heterodimerize
Rev-erb, BD73			with RXR
Group 4			
HNF-4	AGGTCA	→ (1) →	Homodimers

[a] It may appear that the names of these receptors are in nonsense code. For ease in identifying specific proteins ligand complexes, letter acronyms have been developed. Some of these codes are readily understood, but others appear more arcane. For example, TR means thyroid hormone binding receptor protein RXR is a protein that binds 9-cis retinoic acid; VDR, a receptor that binds vitamin D ($1,25(OH)_2$ vitamin D), and so forth. Arrows indicate direction of consensus sequence (ex: → (3) ←)is an inverted repeat with three nucleotides spaces in between.

a protranscription factor; or (5) release of an inhibitor. One class of transcription factors important for nutrition is the nuclear hormone receptor superfamily, which is regulated by ligand binding. Ligands for these transcription factors include retinoic acid, fatty acids, vitamin D, thyroid hormone, and steroid hormones. All members of this superfamily contain two zinc fingers in their DNA binding domains. Zinc is bound to histidine and cysteine rich regions of the protein that envelops the DNA in a shape that looks like a finger. The zinc ion plays an enormous role in gene expression because of its central use in the zinc finger. The nuclear hormone receptor superfamily is divided into four groups according to their dimerization potential, their site specificity, and their localization (Table 54.1). Group I receptors bind the steroid hormones and bind DNA as homodimers. Group I response elements are palindromes of either AGAACA or AGGTCA spaced by three nucleotides. The specificity occurs by interactions between the specific nucleotide sequence and the protein sequence of the first zinc finger.

The RXR$\alpha\beta\gamma$ receptor that binds 9-cis retinoic acid binds to either the DR-1 or the IR-O response element. The DR1 response element also binds the PPARα,β, or γ) receptor that in turn binds fatty acids. The PPARγ receptor binds prostaglandin E$_2$. All three of these receptors bind to the same element. If only one were to bind, the process would be called homodimerization. If more than one receptor binds to the same element, we would have heterodimerization.

Group II receptors, also called the Retinoid/Thyroid subfamily, bind nutrients and metabolites such as retinoic acid, vitamin D, and fatty acids. All of these receptors form heterodimers with the retinoid X receptor (RXR). 9-cis retinoic acid binds RXR and has a synergistic effect on transcription when dimerized with most receptors in this group. Generally, these receptors bind to direct repeats of degenerative AGGTCA sequences spaced by (1) (RXR, LXR, PPAR), (2) (alternative RAR, TR), (3) (VDR), (4) (TR, LXR), or (5) (RAR) nucleotides. Specificity occurs due to the spacing between the consensus sequence half sites. In the case of the retinoic acid receptor (RAR) and thyroid receptor (TR) unliganded receptor can bind DNA and repress transcription.

There are numerous proteins aside from those of the steroid receptor superfamily that bind to specific base sequences in the promoter region. Some of these bind minerals, some bind other hormones, and some are by themselves, transcription factors that have control properties.

In addition to the receptor proteins that bind to certain base sequences in the promoter region, we also have smaller molecules that similarly serve to stimulate or suppress transcription. One such is the glucose molecule. It serves to stimulate the transcription of glucokinase that has a glucose sensitive promoter region. Only the β cell and the hepatocyte DNA have this region exposed and only these cell types express the glucokinase gene. Other cells have the gene but do not express it probably because their glucose promoter site is unexposed. Instead, these other cell types express a similar (but different) gene that encodes hexokinase. There are a number of instances in the nutrition science literature where specific nutrients influence the transcription of genes that encode enzymes or receptors or carriers that are important to the use of that nutrient. Shown in Table 54.2 are examples of these influences. All of the above serve to control transcription, a vital step in controlling gene expression.

Once the bases are joined together in the nucleus to form messenger RNA the nucleus must edit and process it. Processing it includes capping, nucleolytic and ligation reactions which shorten it, terminal additions of nucleosides and nucleoside modifications (Figure 54.3). Through this processing less than 25% of the original RNA migrates from the nucleus to the ribosomes where it attaches prior to translation. Editing and processing are needed because immature RNA contains all those bases corresponding to the DNA introns. Introns are those groups of bases that are not part of the structural gene. Introns are intervening sequences that separate the exons or coding sequences of the structural gene. The removal of these segments is a cut and splice process whereby the intron is cut at its 5′ end, pulled out of the way, and cut again at its 3′ end; at the same time, the two exons are joined. This cut and splice routine is continued until all the introns are removed and the exons joined. Some editing of the RNA also occurs with base substitutions made as appropriate. Finally, a 3′ terminal poly A tail is added there.

The editing and processing step is now complete. This mature messenger RNA now leaves the nucleus and moves to the cytoplasm for translation. The nucleotides that have been removed during editing and processing are either reused or totally degraded. Of note is the fact that editing and processing also are mechanisms used to degrade the whole message unit. This serves to control the amount and half-life of messenger RNA. The endonucleases and exonucleases used in the cut and splice processing also come into play in the regulation of mRNA stability. Some mRNAs have very short half-lives (seconds to minutes) while other have longer half-lives (hours). This is important because some gene products are needed for only a short time. Hormones and cell signals must be short lived and, therefore, the body needs to control/counterbalance their synthesis and action. One of the ways

TABLE 54.2
Some Examples of Nutrient Effects on Transcription[2]

Nutrient	Gene	Effect
Retinoic acid	Many genes	Increases transcription through its binding to RXR or RAR, which in turn bind to the AGGTCA sequence in the promoter region
Vitamin B$_6$	Steroid hormone receptor	Suppresses transcription
Vitamin D	Many genes	Increases transcription of genes for calcium-binding proteins
Glucose	Glucokinase	Increases transcription in pancreas and liver
Potassium	Aldosterone synthetase	Increases transcription in adrenal cortex
Fatty acids	Fatty acid synthetase	Suppresses transcription in liver
Selenium	Glutathione peroxidase, 5′ deiodinase	Increases transcription
Sodium	Endothelin 1	Increases transcription
Zinc	Zinc transporters	Increases transcription

to do this is by regulating the amount of mRNA (number of copies of mRNA for each gene product) that leaves the nucleus. Thus, this regulation is a key step in metabolic control.

TRANSLATION

Following transcription is translation (Figure 54.4). Translation is the synthesis of the protein using mRNA to dictate the order with which the amino acids are assembled. This process is also influenced by specific nutrients. The translation of the ferritin gene, for example, is influenced by the amount of iron available in the cell. In iron deficiency, the messenger RNA start site for ferritin translation is covered up by an iron-responsive protein. This protein binds the 3′UTR and inhibits the movement of the 40s ribosome from the cap to the translation start site. When iron status is improved, the start site is uncovered and translation proceeds.

The actual site of translation is on the ribosomes; some ribosomes are located on the membrane of the endoplasmic reticulum, and some are free in the cell matrix. Ribosomes consist almost entirely of ribosomal RNA and ribosomal protein. RNA is synthesized via RNA polymerase I in the cell nucleus as a large molecule; there, it is cleaved and leaves the nucleus as two subunits, a large one and a small one. The ribosome is reformed in the cytoplasm by the reassociation of the two subunits; the subunits, however, are not necessarily derived from the same precursor.

Ribosomal RNA makes up a large fraction of the total cellular RNA. It serves as the "docking" point for the activated amino acids bound to the transfer RNA and the mRNA that dictates the amino acid polymerization sequence. Transfer RNA (tRNA) is used to bring an amino acid to the polysome (ribosome), the site of protein synthesis. Each amino acid has a specific tRNA. Each tRNA molecule is thought to have a cloverleaf arrangement of nucleotides. With this arrangement of nucleotides, there is the opportunity for the maximum number of hydrogen bonds to form between base pairs. A molecule that has many hydrogen bonds is very stable. Transfer RNA also contains a triplet of bases known, in this instance, as the anticodon. The amino acid carried by tRNA is identified by the codon of mRNA through its anticodon; the amino acid itself is not involved in this identification.

A few general statements can be made about the distribution of ribosomes in cells that have different capacities for the synthesis of proteins. (1) Cells which synthesize large numbers of proteins have numerous ribosomes; conversely, cells which synthesize small numbers of proteins contain few. (2) Of the proteins synthesized by a cell to be secreted from that cell for use elsewhere, most of the ribosomes are attached to the endoplasmic reticulum. (3) Those cells, which synthesize protein primarily for intracellular use, have relatively few ribosomes attached to the endoplasmic reticulum membrane. Small groups of ribosomes called *polysomes* are involved in protein synthesis; under physiological conditions, polysomes are bound to the endoplasmic reticulum. The ribosome is bound to the membrane through its large subunit; the small subunit is involved in the binding of mRNA to the ribosome. The ribosomes have two binding sites used in protein synthesis: the amino-acyl site and the peptidyl site. These two sites have specific functions in protein synthesis.

Translation takes place in four stages, as illustrated in Figure 54.4. Each stage requires specific cofactors and enzymes. In the first stage, which occurs in the cytosol, the amino acids are activated by esterifying each one to its specific tRNA. This requires a molecule of ATP. In addition to a specific tRNA, each amino acid requires a specific enzyme for this reaction.

During the second stage, the initiation of the synthesis of the polypeptide chain occurs. Initiation requires that mRNA bind to the ribosome. An initiation complex is formed by the binding of mRNA cap and the first activated amino acid-tRNA complex to

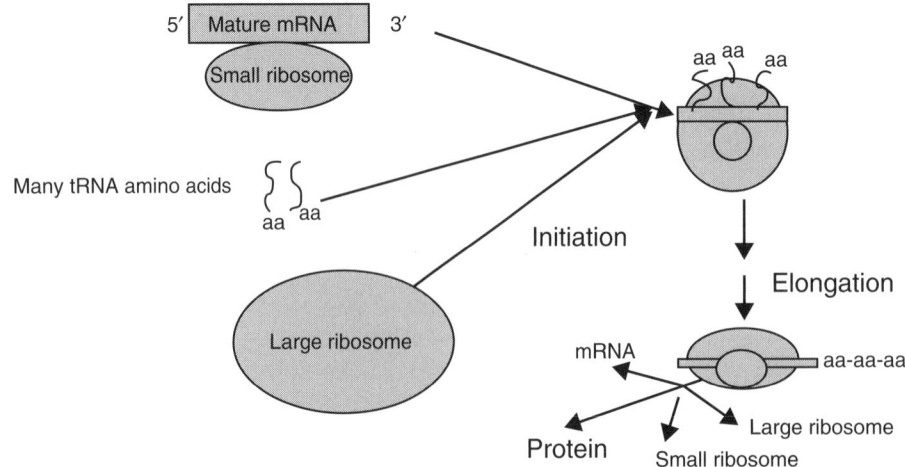

FIGURE 54.4 Translation as a three-step process beginning with initiation, then elongation, and then the release of the ribosomes and the gene product.

the small ribosomal subunit. The ribosome finds the correct reading frame on the mRNA by "scanning" for an AUG codon. The large ribosomal unit then attaches, thus forming a functional ribosome. A number of specific protein initiation factors (eIFs) are involved in this step.

In the third stage of protein synthesis, the peptide chain is elongated by the sequential addition of amino acids from the tRNA complexes. The amino acid is recognized by base pairing of the codon of mRNA to the bases found in the anticodon of tRNA, and a peptide bond is formed between the peptide chain and the newly arrived amino acid. The ribosome then moves along the mRNA; this brings the next codon in the proper position for attachment of the next activated amino acyl-tRNA complex. The mRNA and nascent polypeptide appear to "track" through a groove in the ribosomal subunits. This protects them from attack by enzymes in the surrounding environment.

The final stage of protein synthesis is the termination of the chain. The termination is signaled by one of three special codons (stop codons) in the mRNA. After the carboxy terminal amino acid is attached to the peptide chain, it is still covalently attached to tRNA, which is, in turn, bonded to the ribosome. A protein release factor promotes the hydrolysis of the ester link between the tRNA and the amino acid. Once the polypeptide chain is generated and free of the ribosome, it assumes its characteristic three-dimensional structure.

If there is a mutation in the sequence of bases that comprise the genetic code for a given protein, the amino acid sequence generated in a protein will be incorrect. Whether this substitution of one amino acid for another in the protein being generated affects the functionality of the protein being generated depends entirely on the amino acid in question. In addition, genetic errors in amino acid sequence may pose no threat to the individual if the protein in question is of little importance in the maintenance of health and well-being, or it can have large effects on health if the protein is a critical one. In the synthesis of the important protein, hemoglobin, if the genetic code calls for the use of valine instead of the usual glutamic acid in the synthesis of the β chain in the hemoglobin molecule, the resulting protein is less able to carry oxygen. This amino acid substitution not only affects the oxygen-carrying capacity of the red blood cell, but also affects the solubility of the hemoglobin in the red blood cell cytosol. This, in turn, affects the shape of the red blood cell, changing it from a "dumbbell"-shaped donut to a shape resembling a sickle, hence the name *sickle cell anemia*. The decreased solubility of the hemoglobin can be understood if one remembers the relative polarity of the glutamic acid and valine molecules. The glutamic acid side chain is more ionic and thus contributes more to the solubility of the protein than the nonpolar carbon chain of valine. This change in pH decreases its solubility in water, and, of course, a change in solubility leads to an increased viscosity of the blood as the red cells rupture, spilling their contents into the blood stream.

The amino acid sequence within a given species for a given protein is usually similar. However, some individual variation does occur. An example of an "acceptable" amino acid substitution would be some of the ones that account for the species' differences in the hormone insulin. As a hormone, it serves a variety of important functions in the regulation of carbohydrate, lipid, and protein metabolism. Yet, even though there are species differences in the amino acid sequence of this protein, insulin from one species can be given to another species and be functionally active. Obviously, the species differences in the amino acid sequence of this protein are not at locations in the chains which determine its biological function in promoting glucose use.

After translation is complete, the primary structure is complete. At this point, some post translational modification can occur, and again specific nutrients can influence the process. For example, after the translation of osteocalcin and prothrombin, two proteins that have glutamic-acid-rich regions, these glutamate residues are carboxylated. This posttranslational carboxylation requires vitamin K. Should vitamin K be in short supply, this carboxylation will not occur (or will occur in only a limited way), and these proteins will not be able to bind calcium. Both must bind calcium in order to function; osteocalcin in bone cannot bind calcium, nor can prothrombin. Hence, bone will be more fragile, and blood will not clot as needed.

As the chain of amino acid is produced, the amino acids in that chain begin to interact to form the protein's secondary structure. Then, as the chain twists and turns, more global interactions occur and the tertiary structure becomes apparent. All of these interactions, that is, hydrogen bonding, disulfide bridges, etc., serve to stabilize the protein. Lastly, as these tertiary structures are synthesized, they assemble as subunits of more complex structures (quaternary structures) in the functional protein. Some proteins are very complex and have many subunits; for example, the cytochromes in the mitochondrial respiratory chain, whereas others are not as complex.

MUTATIONS IN THE CODES FOR ENZYMES OF MACRONUTRIENT METABOLISM

There are a number of metabolic diseases affecting nutrient metabolism that are genetically determined.[4] Most of these are quite rare, and most are recessive disorders. Table 54.3 is a list of these disorders, and the mutation responsible for the disorder. This is a partial list, and not all of the genetic diseases are listed. For some of the disorders, there is more than one mutation associated with the disease. For example, there are a number of genetic mutations in the code for red cell glucose-6-phosphate dehydrogenase. The code is carried as a recessive trait on the X chromosome, and thus only males are affected. These mutations are usually silent. That is, the male, having a defective red cell glucose-6-phosphate dehydrogenase, does not know he has the

TABLE 54.3
Genetic Disorders in Nutrient Metabolism [1,4]

Disease	Mutated Gene	Characteristics
Amino acid diseases		
Maple Syrup Urine Disease	Branched chain keto acid dehydrogenase	Elevated levels of a-ketoacids and their metabolites in blood and urine; mental retardation, ketoacidosis, and early death
Homocysteinemia	Cystathionine synthase	Absence of cross-linked collagen, eye malformations, osteoporosis, mental retardation, thromboembolism, and vascular occlusions
Phenylketonuria	Phenylalanine hydroxylase	Mental retardation, decreased neurotransmitter production, shortened lifespan, and six mutations in this gene have been reported
Tyrosinemia	Tyrosine transaminase	Eye and skin lesions, mental retardation
	Fumarylacetoacetate	Normocytic anemia, leukocytosis, and increased serum bilirubin
	Hydroxylase	Increased hepatic enzymes, and prolonged prothrombin time
Albinism	Tyrosinase	Lack of melanin production and sensitivity to sunlight
Alcaptonuria	Homogentisate oxidase	Elevated homogentisate levels in blood, bones, and internal organs; increased susceptibility to viruses and arthritis
Histidinemia	Histidase	Elevated blood and urine levels of histidine and decreased histamine
Hyperprolinemia	Proline oxidase 2 mutations	Mental retardation and seizures
Hyperornithenia	Ornithine-δ-Aminotransferase	Increased levels of ornithine in blood, progression vision loss, and increased urine loss of ornithine
Urea cycle defects	Arginase	Progressive lethargy, mental retardation, and urea cycle failure
	Carbamyl phosphate syntase	Symptoms of ammonia toxicity and early death
	Ornithine transcarbamylase	
	Arginosuccinate syntase	
	Argininosuccinase	
Hyperlysinemia	α-aminoadipic semialdehyde synthase	Elevated levels of lysine in blood and urine; condition is generally benign
Hypermethionemia	Methionine adenyltransferase	Benign
Non-ketotic hyperglycemia	Glycine cleavage system (3 mutations)	Early death, hypoglycemia, mental retardation, and seizures
Gout	?	Excess uric acid production; renal uric acid stones; Uric acid crystals accumulate in joints
Lesch-Nylan	Hypoxanthine phosphoribosyl transferase	Hyperuricemia, choreathetosis, spasticity, mental retardation, self mutilation, and gouty arthritis
Lipid diseases other than those relating to Lipemia		
Tay Sachs	Hexosaminidase A	Early death, CNS degeneration, and ganglioside GM2 accumulation
Gaucher's	Glucocerebrosidase	Hepatomegaly, splenomegaly, erosion of long bones and pelvis, mental retardation, and glucocerebroside accumulation
Fabry's	α galactosidase A	Skin rash, renal failure, pain in legs, and ceramide trihexoside accumulation
Nieman-Pick	Sphinogomyelinase	Enlarged liver and spleen, mental retardation, and sphigomyelin accumulation
Krabbe's	Galactocerebroside	Mental retardation, and absence of myelin
Gangliosidosis	Gandiioside: β galactosidase	Enlarged liver, mental retardation
Sandhoff-Jatzkewitz	Hexaminidase A and B	Same as Tay-Sach's but develops quicker
Fucosidosis	aL-Fucosidase	Cerebral degeneration, spastic muscles, and thick skin
Refsum's	α-hydroxylating enzyme	Neurological problems: deafness, blindness, and cerebellar ataxia
Carbohydrate-related disorders		
Lactose intolerance	Lactase	Chronic or intermittent diarrhea, flatulence, nausea, vomiting, and growth failure in young children
Sucrose intolerance	Sucrase	Diarrhea, flatulence, nausea, and poor growth in infants
Galactose intolerance	Galactose carrier	Diarrhea, growth failure in infants, stools contains large amounts of glucose, galactose, and lactic acid
Galactosemia	Three genes: Galactose-1-P-uridyl transferase	Increased cellular content of galactose-1-phosphate, eye cataracts, mental retardation, and cell galactitol; 3 mutations in this gene
	Galactokinase	Cataracts, cellular accumulation of galactose, and galactitol
	Galactoepimerase	No severe symptoms; 2 mutations in this gene

Continued

TABLE 54.3
(Continued)

Disease	Mutated Gene	Characteristics
Carbohydrate-related disorders		
Fructosemia	Fructokinase	Fructosuria, fructosemia
	Fructose-1-P-aldolase	Hypoglycemia, vomiting after a fructose load, fructosemia, and fructosuria, In children: poor growth, jaundice, hyperbilirubinemia, albuminuria, and amino aciduria
	Fructose 1,6-diphosphatase	Hypoglycemia, hepatomegaly, poor muscle tone, and increased blood lactate
Pentosuria	NADP-linked xylitol Dehydrogenase	Elevated levels of pentose in urine
Hemolytic Anemia	Red cell Glucose-6-phosphate Dehydrogenase	Low red cell NADPH and hemolysis of red cell especially with quinine treatment
	Pyruvate kinase	Nonspherocytic anemia and accumulation of glucose metabolites in red cells Jaundice in the newborn
Type VII glycogen storage disease	Phosphofructokinase	Intolerance to exercise, elevated muscle glycogen levels, and accumulation of hexose monophosphates in muscle
Von Gierke's (Type I glycogen storage)	Glucose-6-phosphatase	Hypoglycemia, hyperlipemia, Brain damage in some pts, excess liver glycogen, shortened lifespan, and increased glycerol utilization
Amylopectinoisis (Type IV glycogenosis)	Branching enzyme, hepatic amylo (1,4→1,6)transglucosidase	Tissue accumulation of long chain glycogen that is poorly branched and intolerance to exercise
Pompe's (Type II glycoenosis)	Lysomal a-1,4-glucosidase (acid maltase)	Generalized glycogen excess in viscera, muscles, nervous system muscle weakness, hepatomegaly, and enlarged heart
	Amylo-1,6-glucosidase (de-branching enzyme)	Generalized glycogen excess in viscera, nervous system, muscles, hepatomegaly, and enlarged heart
Forbes (Type III glycogenosis)	Muscle phosphorylase	Tissue accumulation of highly branched glycogen, hypoglycemia, acidosis muscle weakness, and enlarged heart
McArdle's (Type V glycogenosis)	Liver phosphorylase	Intolerance to exercise
Hers (Type VI glycogenosis)	Phosphorylase kinase	Hepatomegaly, increased liver glycogen content, elevated serum lipids, growth retardation
Micronutrient-related disorders		
Porphyria	Uroporphyrinogen III Cosynthase	Increased red cell porphyrin, excess excretion of δ-aminolevulinic acid (urine), and porphobilinogen (stool); photosensitivity
	Ferrochelatase	Excess Protoporphyrin in stool; photosensitivity
	ALA dehydratase	Neurovisceral symptoms; Excess δ-aminolevulinic acid in urine
	Porphobilinogen deaminase	Neurovisceral symptoms; excess δ-aminolevulenic acid and prophobilinogen in urine
	Coprophyrinogen oxidase	Photosensitivity, neurovisceral symptoms, excess δ-aminolevulenic acid, porphobilinogen, and coproporphyrin in urine
	Protoporphyrinogen oxidase	Photosensitivity, neurovisceral symptoms, excess δ-aminolevulinic acid, porpholbilinogen and coproporphyrin in urine; coproporphyrin, and protophyrin in feces
	Uroporphyrinogen Decarboxylate (2 mutations)	Photosensitivity, uroporphyrin and 7-carboxylate porphyrin in urine, and isocoproporphyrin in feces
Wilson's	?	Reduction in the rate of incorporation of copper into ceruloplasmin
		Reduction in the biliary excretion of copper, increased urinary copper, excess hepatic copper, and liver disease
Menke's	Intestinal copper Carrier	Symptoms of copper deficiency and deficient copper dependent enzymes
Hemochromatosis	?	Excess serum iron, excess liver iron, and excess serum ferritin
Molybdenum Cofactor deficiency	? Neuronal loss and demyelination; early death	Mental retardation, deficient sulfite oxidase, and xanthine dehydrogenase activity
Rickets	25(OH)₂ D hydroxylase	Vitamin D deficient rickets
	D receptor resistance (5 mutations)	Vitamin D deficient rickets

problem unless his cells are tested or unless he is given a drug such as quinine or one of the sulfur antibiotics that increases the oxidation of NADPH⁺H⁺. When this happens, NADPH⁺H⁺ is depleted and is not available to reduce oxidized glutathione. In turn, the red cell ruptures (hemolytic anemia). In almost all cases, the affected male has sufficient enzyme activity to meet the normal demands for NADPH⁺H⁺. It is only when stressed by these drugs that a problem develops.

There are other genomic defects that are silent as well. For example, people unable to metabolize the pentoses found in plums and cherries are unaware of their condition. It may come to light if a non-glucose-specific screening test is used just after the individual has consumed these fruits. There may appear to be an elevated level of sugar in the blood and urine. If a specific assay for glucose (glucokinase) rather than a nonspecific test, the mistake in diabetes diagnosis will not be made. Some individuals may be intolerant of exercise, because they are unable to use the glycogen in their muscles for fuel. Unless forced to exercise, these people might not be aware of their metabolic defect. They may have adopted a very sedentary lifestyle by unconscious realization of their intolerance.

Unconscious food selection has been observed in children with some of the macronutrient intolerances. Children who are lactose intolerant may refuse to consume milk; those who are gluten intolerant may avoid wheat-containing products and so forth. There may be an instinctive avoidance that helps the individual enjoy their food without serious consequences.

Many of the disorders listed in Table 54.3 have no cure and many are characterized by a shortened lifespan. However, for some there are nutrition strategies that may be helpful. Diseases associated with the malabsorption of carbohydrate that is lactose intolerance, galactose intolerance, etc., can be managed by the omission of these carbohydrates from the diet. Some of the amino acid disorders can be managed by the reduction of the dietary intakes of the particular amino acid in question. For example, phenylkentonuria can be managed by a reduction in the phenylalanine content of the diet. This is rather tricky, since enough of this essential amino acid must be provided but not too much, so that there is a surplus that cannot be appropriately metabolized. In addition, since phenylalanine is used to make tyrosine, this amino acid must then be provided in the diet in sufficient amounts to meet the need.

GENETIC DISEASES INVOLVING THE MICRONUTRIENTS

There are two genetic disorders that have assisted scientists in understanding the function and metabolism of copper. In one, Menkes syndrome, copper absorption is faulty. Intestinal cells absorb the copper but cannot release it into the circulation. Parenteral copper corrects most of the condition which resembles copper deficiency but care must be exercised in its administration. Too much can be toxic. In addition, parenterally administered copper does not reach the brain and cannot prevent the cerebral degeneration and premature death characteristic of patients with Menkes disease.

Another genetic disorder in copper status is Wilson's disease. This condition is also associated with premature death and is due to an impaired incorporation of copper into ceruloplasmin and decreased bilary excretion of copper. This results in an accumulation of copper in the liver and brain. Early signs of Wilson's disease include liver dysfunction, neurological disease, and deposits of copper in the cornea manifested as a ring that looks like a halo around the pupil. This lesion is called the Kayser-Fleischer ring. Renal stones, renal aciduria, neurological deficits, and osteoporosis also characterize Wilson's disease. Periodic bleeding, which removes some of the excess copper, can be helpful in managing Wilson's disease, as can treatment with copper-chelating agents such as D-penicillamine and by increasing the intake of zinc, which interferes with copper absorption.

Iron is an essential mineral for hemoglobin formation. However, there are a number of genetic reasons why excess iron and subsequent problems are encountered. These are the porphyrias and hemochromatosis. In the latter, excess iron accumulates and in the former, there are abnormalities in porphyrin metabolism. Some of these disorders are devastating, while others are less so. Vitamin D and the uptake of calcium and phosphate are linked. In the absence of active vitamin D, rickets develops. Some individuals are unable to activate the vitamin. That is, they do not have a normal activity of the renal enzyme, $25(OH)_2D$ hydroylase. As a result, these individuals develop vitamin D rickets. The bones are not appropriately mineralized, because there is a deficiency of the active vitamin. This can be managed by providing the active form of the vitamin. In addition, there is also a resistance to the activity of active vitamin D. The genetic problem here is a deficiency in the receptor for the vitamin. Five different mutations have been reported that accounts for this problem. Patients with these genetic problems also develop rickets and are collectively referred to as having vitamin-D-resistant rickets. Lastly, there are a couple of complex disorders that affect more pathways in addition to those of vitamin D. These include the Franconi syndrome, X-linked hypophosphatemia, and pseudohypoparathyroidism. In each of these, there is a disturbed mineralization of the skeletal system as well as disturbed regulation of calcium status, phosphorus status, and soft tissue mineralization.

GENETIC BASIS FOR LIPOPROTEINEMIA

Hyperlipemia is fairly common in western nations. However, there is no single cause. As with some of the less well-known genetic disorders, more than one mutation has been found that is associated with this characteristic (see Chapters 42, and 43 for further information). Table 54.4 lists the proteins involved in lipid transport as well as mutations (and their estimated frequencies) that result in lipid transport abnormalities. Not all of the genetic diseases of lipid transport are associated with atherosclerosis nor are all associated with elevated serum lipid levels. The genes for the transport proteins, apo A-I, apo A-II, apo A-IV, apo (a), apo B, apo D, apo C-I, apo C-II, apo C-III, apo D, and apo E have been identified. In addition to these transport proteins, we have: the (1) proteins that are the important rate-limiting enzymes, (2) receptors that are involved in lipoprotein

TABLE 54.4

Mutations of Genes Involved in Lipoprotein Metabolism [1,5-7]

Gene	Chromosome Location	Characteristics of Mutation	Frequency of Mutation
apo A-II	1	Transport protein in HDL	?
apo B 48	2 p 23–24	Hypobetalipoproteinemia	1:1,000,000
High-density-lipoprotein-binding protein (HDLBP)	2 q 37		?
apo D	3	Transport protein similar to retinol-binding protein	?
apo (a)	6	Abnormal transport protein for LDL	?
LPL	8 p 22	Defective chylomicron clearance	1:1,000,000
apo A-I	11	Defective HDL production (Tangier's disease)	1:1,000,000
apo C-III	11		?
apo A-IV	11		?
Hepatic LPL (HTGL)	15 q 21	Defective IDL clearance	?
CETP	16 q 22.1		?
LCAT	16 q 22.1	Familial lecithin: cholesterol transferase deficiency. 2 Types	Rare
LDL receptor	19	Familial hypercholesterolemia	1:500
apo B 100	2	Familial defective apo B 100	1:500–501:1000
apo E	19	Type III hyperlipoproteinemia	1:5000
apo C-I	19	Transport protein for VLDL	?
apo C-II	19	Defective chylomicron clearance	1:1,000,000

processing, (3) the peripheral lipoprotein lipase and the hepatic lipoprotein lipase, (4) the lipoprotein receptors on the plasma membrane of the cells which receive and oxidize or store the transported lipids, and (5) the rate-limiting enzymes of lipid synthesis and use. Included in this last category are the fatty acid enzymes of lipid synthesis and use: the fatty acid synthase complex, acetyl CoA carboxylase, HMG CoA reductase, HMG CoA synthase, cholesterol ester transfer protein (CETP), fatty acid binding protein (FABP), lecithin-cholesterol acyltransferase (LCAT), cholesterol 7-hydroxylase, and the high-density-lipoprotein-binding protein (HDLBP). Many of these proteins have been isolated and studied in detail. Several of their cognate genes have been identified and mapped.

Lipoprotein lipase is synthesized by these target cells but is anchored on the outside of the cells by a polysaccharide chain on the endothelial wall of the surrounding capillaries. Should this lipoprotein lipase be missing or genetically aberrant (Type I lipemia or chylomicronemia), so that the chylomicrons cannot be hydrolyzed, these chylomicrons accumulate and the individual would have a lipemia characterized by elevated levels of triacylglyceride and cholesterol containing chylomicrons. Also, characteristic of this condition is the presence of an enlarged liver and spleen, considerable abdominal discomfort and the presence of subcutaneous xanthomas (clusters of hard saturated fatty acid and cholesterol-rich nodules). Like familial hypo-lipoproteinemia, this condition is rare. Of interest is the observation that, despite the very high blood lipid levels of these people, few die of coronary vessel disease. Their shortened lifespan is due to an inappropriate lipid deposition in all of the vital organs that, in turn, has a negative effect on organ function and lifespan.

Failure to appropriately edit the apo B gene in the intestinal cell will result in a disorder called *familial hypobetalipoproteinemia*. In this disorder, there will be a total or partial (depending on the genetic mutation) absence of lipoproteins in the blood. Hypobeta-lipoproteinemia can also develop, should there be base substitutions in the gene for the apo B protein. In addition to very low blood lipids, patients with this disorder also have fat malabsorption (steatorrhea). The feces contain an abnormally large amount of fat and have a characteristic peculiar odor. In this disorder, not only is the triacylglyceride absorption affected, but also are the fat-soluble vitamins. Without the ability to absorb these energy-rich food components and the vital fat-soluble vitamins, the patient does not thrive and survive. Fortunately, this genetic mutation is not very common. It is inherited as an autosomal recessive trait.

Defects in exogenous fat transport are manifested in several ways. As described above, defective chylomicron formation due to mutations in either the apo B gene or its editing leads to and is characterized by fat malabsorption. This includes the malabsorption of fat-soluble vitamins as well. Twenty different mutations have been identified in the gene for the apo B protein. These mutations are inherited via an autosomal recessive mode and are characterized not only by fat malabsorption but also by acanthocytes, retinitis pigmentosa, and muscular neuropathies. To a large extent, these symptoms can be attributed to a relative deficiency of the fat-soluble vitamins due to malabsorption. While a defect in the apo B gene can account for defective fat absorption, there may be another mutation (in the microsomal triglyceride transfer protein) that also might result in fat malabsorption.

This transfer protein is essential for apo B translocation and subsequent synthesis of chylomicrons. Defects in this transfer protein would impair apo B availability and chylomicron formation. In these defects, very low levels of chylomicrons are found in the blood. Persons with this disorder are rare (one in a million). In this circumstance, the severity of the disease is related to the size of the mutated gene product and whether it can associate with the lipids, it must carry. The size of the truncated apo B can vary from apo B-9 (41 residues) to apo B-89 (4487 residues). Except in the case of the apo B-25, the result of a deletion of the entire exon 21, all the truncated forms reported to date are C–T transitions or base deletions. These deletions can involve misaligned pairing-deletion mechanisms. Frameshift mutation can be compensated by a reading frame restoration of the apo B gene.

Familial hyperchylomicronemia is characterized by elevations in chylomicrons having both triglycerides and cholesterol. Hyperchylomicronemia was found to be due to mutations in the genes that encode the enzyme lipoprotein lipase needed for the hydrolysis of chylomicrons. This enzyme is a glycoprotein having an apparent monomeric molecular weight of about 60,000 Da on SDS gel electrophoresis and 48,300 Da by sedimentation-equilibrium ultracentrifugation. The enzyme is linked to the endothelial cells of the capillary system. Lipoprotein lipase is quite similar to hepatic triglyceride lipase, an enzyme found in the hepatic sinusoids. The main difference between the two lipases is that the interstitial lipase has a requirement for the lipid-carrying protein, apo C-II, for full activity, whereas hepatic LPL does not. Mutations in the gene for apo C-II can result in aberrant lipase activity because apo C-II serves as a cofactor in the lipoprotein lipase-catalyzed reaction. Hepatic triglyceride lipase has no such requirement. Aberrations in the hepatic triglyceride lipase results in an accumulation of very-low-density lipoproteins (VLDL), rather than accumulations of chylomicrons. Mutations in the genes for LPL and apo C-II are very rare, occurring at a frequency of one in a million. The gene for LPL has been mapped to chromosome 8 while that for apo C-II has been mapped to chromosome 19 and the hepatic LPL to chromosome 15. Other features of these disorders include an inflammation of the exocrine pancreas and eruptive xanthomas. Chylomicronemia does not appear to be atherogenic. The mutations in the LPL gene appear to be insertions or deletions or due to aberrant splicing, while those in the apo C-II gene seem to be due to splice site mutations or small deletions. Twenty-two mutations in the apo C-II gene have been reported. With respect to the aberrant splicing of the LPL gene in three unrelated humans, Holzl et al. reported a C $\rightarrow$ A mutation in position -3 of the acceptor splice site of intron 6, which caused aberrant splicing. The major transcript showed a deletion of exons 6 through 9 and amounted to about 3% of normal. Trace amounts of both a normally spliced LPL mRNA and a second aberrant transcript devoid of exon 7 were found. In one of these patients, Holzl et al. found a three-splice mutation on one allele, while on the other allele they found a missense mutation resulting in Gly 188 $\rightarrow$ Glu substitution. All three subjects were classed as hyperchylomicronemic due to LPL deficiency.

The absence of LPL activity in certain tissues or in certain individuals can be attributed to mutations in lipoprotein lipase promoter region. Studies of tissue-specific expression of LPL showed that cis acting elements located within -1824-bp of the five flanking regions was required for the expression of LPL. These include nuclear factors recognizing both the CCAAT box and the octamer sequence immediately flanking the transcriptional start site. Those tissues that have no LPL activity lack this promoter region. Since humans and mice have identical CCAAT and octamer sequences, one could suppose that humans having an intact LPL gene of normal sequence but lacking LPL activity might have a deficient or mutated promoter region; proof that this might occur is presently lacking.

Mutations in the gene for hepatic lipoprotein lipase result in elevated blood levels of triglycerides and cholesterol, and these elevations are related to an increased risk for atherosclerosis. Hepatic LPL must be secreted by the hepatocyte into the sinusoids to function as a catalyst for the hydrolysis of core TG and surface phospholipids of chylomicron remnants, HDL, and IDL. Through its activity, it augments the uptake of HDL cholesterol by the liver (reverse cholesterol transport) and is involved in the reduction of HDL size from HDL_2 to HDL_3. Hepatic LPL aids in the clearance of chylomicron remnants by exposing the apo E epitopes for enzymatic action. Missense mutations in the hepatic LPL gene include substitutions of serine for phenylalanine at amino acid position 267, threonine for methionine at position 383, and asparagine for serine at position 291. These mutations result in poorly secreted enzyme, and thus the phenotypic expression of the mutation is low hepatic lipase activity. The frequency of the Asn 291 Ser mutation in a population having premature CVD has been reported as 5.2%.

Defects in chylomicron remnant clearance are much more common than any of the above mutations. Defective clearance due to mutations in the apo E gene results in a lipemia known as Type III hyperlipoproteinemia. It is associated with premature atherosclerosis, and patients with these defects have high serum triglyceride as well as high serum cholesterol levels. Xanthomas are found in nearly three-quarters of the population with these defects. The lipemia is responsive to energy restriction using diets that have 40% of energy from carbohydrate, 40% from fat, and 20% from protein. Weight loss is efficacious for most people with this defect. The apo E gene codes for the protein on the surface of the chylomicron remnant that is the ligand for receptor-mediated clearance of this particle. A number of mutations in the apo E gene have been reported, and the phenotypes of these mutations are grouped into three general groups labeled E_2, E_3, and E_4. Those of the E_2 groups fail to bind the particles to the cell surface receptor for the chylomicron remnant. Those of the E_3 and E_4 groups have generally low remnant clearance rates. The apo E allele and phenotype frequency varies. The E_2 frequency is about 8%, the E_3 about 77%, and the E_4, about 15% of the total population with an apo E mutation. The incidence of apo E gene mutations is about 1% of the population. Since apo E is involved in both endogenous and exogenous lipid transport and clearance, a faulty apo E gene is devastating. Mature human apo E is a 299 amino acid polypeptide. Apo E genes as well as other apolipoproteins contain 11 or 22 amino acid repeated sequences as one of their key features. These appear to encode largely amphipathic helices, which are needed for lipid binding. There is a high degree of conservation among species of nucleotide sequences in the gene fragment that encodes the amino acid repeats. The gene for apo E has been mapped to chromosome 19, as have the genes for apo C-I, apo C-II and LDLR. There appears to be a tight linkage among these genes which coordinates their expression. Among the common mutations are amino acid substitutions at positions 112 and 158, while less-frequent substitutions occur at other positions in the polypeptide chain. Several of these involve the exchange of neutral amino acids for acidic amino acids with the net result of alterations in polypeptide charge and subsequent inadequate binding to the appropriate cell surface receptors. In a rare form of the disorder, the mutation is such that no useful apo E is formed. Transgenic mice have been constructed with an apo E mutation that mimics apo E deficiency. These mice, like humans, develop hypercholesterolemia and increased susceptibility to atherosclerosis. When these mice were fed diets low (5%) or high (16%) in fat, a differential serum cholesterol pattern was observed: those fed the high-fat diet had significantly higher levels of cholesterol and VLDL and LDL than those fed a low-fat or stock diet. The transgenic mice even when fed the stock diet had significantly higher levels of cholesterol and VLDL and LDL than the normal control mice. There was a gender difference as well. Male transgenic mice were less diet responsive in terms of their cholesterol levels than female transgenic mice. As mentioned, there is some sequence homology between humans and mice in the apo E DNA and one could infer that these responses to dietary fat intake in mice could be observed in humans as well. While the above transgenic approach used the gene knockout paradigm (an extreme in the variants of apo E mutants), it nonetheless suggests that variation in the apo E genes could determine the responsiveness of humans with apo E defects to dietary manipulation. Indeed, such nutrient-gene interactions have been reported. The dietary fat clearance in normal subjects appears to be regulated by the genetic variance in apo E sequence and this, in turn, is related to fat intake. Not only is triacylglycerol clearance affected but also is cholesterol clearance. One study reported that the apo E genotype declares the response to cholesterol intake with respect to blood cholesterol levels and that this genotype influences cholesterol synthesis. Those subjects who respond poorly to an oral cholesterol challenge vis-à-vis blood cholesterol clearance had higher rates of cholesterol synthesis than those who could rapidly clear their blood of cholesterol after an oral challenge. One of the more interesting variants of the apo E is called the *Milano variant*. In this variant, blood lipid levels are elevated, but these elevations are not associated with an increased risk of atherosclerosis.

Cholesterol traffic is also controlled by the LDL receptor and the transport protein, apo B-100. Mutations in the gene for the LDL receptor or in the gene for apo B-100, the ligand for the LDL receptor, results in high serum levels of cholesterol. The former results in the disorder called familial hypercholesterolemia and occurs with a frequency of about 1 in 500. Familial hypercholesterolemia is associated with early death from atherosclerosis in man and related primates. Dietary fat saturation affects transcription of LDL receptor mRNA in that feeding a diet containing saturated fat results in decreased LDL receptor mRNA compared to feeding an unsaturated-fat diet. These results suggest that unsaturated fatty acids may interact with proteins that in turn serve as either cis or trans acting elements for this gene in much the same way as polyunsaturated fatty acids affect fatty acid synthetase gene expression.

Familial defective apo B-100 hypercholesterolemia is due to a mutation in the coding sequence of the apo B gene at bp 3500 that changes the base sequence such that glutamine is substituted for arginine. This is in the LDL receptor-binding region of the apo B protein and results in a binding affinity of less than 4% of normal. Polymorphic variation in the genes for both the LDL receptor and the apo B-100 have been reported for mice and this variation has provided the opportunity to identify the genetic and molecular constraints of lipoprotein gene expression. Both apo B and apo E serve as ligands for the LDL receptor. In contrast to apo E, apo B has little homology with the other apolipoproteins. Apo B in mice is quite variable, and this variation imparts or confers a diet responsive characteristic in inbred mouse strains vis-a-vis polypeptide sequence and activity. That is, some mouse strains have reduced levels of plasma apo B when fed a high-fat diet compared to controls fed a stock diet, while other mouse strains are unresponsive to diet vis-à-vis their plasma apo B-100 levels. Such polymorphism also exists in humans. Apo B has been mapped to chromosome 2 and produces two gene products, apo B-100 and B-48. In the intestine, the apo B primary transcript is co- or post-transcriptionally modified. This modification converts codon 2153 from a glutamine (CAA) to an in-frame, premature termination codon (UAA), thereby causing translation to terminate after amino acid 2152. This mRNA editing thus explains the difference in size of these two proteins. If more of the apo B gene is deleted, hypocholesterolemia is observed. This is because apo B-48 is required for the transport of chylomicrons from the intestine. If lacking, chylomicron formation is impaired and low serum cholesterol levels are observed. Both familial defective apo B-100 and familial hypercholesterolemia are characterized by high levels of LDL. Both are associated with CVD, but only the familial hypercholesterolemia is characterized by tendon xanthomas. Both are inherited as autosomal dominant disorders. Collectively, these mutations have a cumulative frequency of 1 in 250. However, because polymorphism in the apo B gene can and does occur, there is the possibility that the frequency is collectively much greater, perhaps as high as 1 in 5. If this is the case, then, the population variation in plasma cholesterol levels could be explained based on these genetic differences alone, apart from those mutations that are associated with the rest of the genes that encode components of the lipid transport system.

Genetically determined abnormalities in LDL metabolism may also be due to mutation in the large glycoprotein, apo (a). Apo (a) is a highly variable, disulfide protein bonded to the apo B-100. It is thought to resemble plasminogen. In fact, the genes that encode Lp (a) and plasminogen are very close to each other on the long arm of chromosome 6. In general, LDLs containing apo (a) do not bind well to the LPL receptor and people having significant amounts of apo (a) have a two- to threefold increase in CVD risk. Many individuals have little or no apo (a), and it has been suggested that those who have it are abnormal with respect to LPL activity.

Several mutations in the genes that encode the endogenous lipid transport have been reported. The reverse cholesterol transport pathway is part of this endogenous lipid transport system. It involves the movement of cholesterol from peripheral tissues to the liver. The peripheral tissues cannot oxidize cholesterol and so must send it to the liver, whereupon it is prepared for excretion, via cholesterol 7 α hydroxylase, as bile acids. This pathway uses the HDL to shuttle the cholesterol in this direction. HDL consists primarily of apo A-1 and cholesterol which is esterified by the enzyme lecithin: cholesterol acyl transferase (LCAT). Mutations in the LCAT gene have been reported and results in one of two diseases: familial LCAT deficiency and fish eye disease. Thirteen different mutations have been identified and in one, a single T→A transversion in codon 252 in exon 6, converting met (ATG) to Lys (AAG), was observed. Three unrelated families were found to have this mutation; however, the severity of their disease varied. In these families, no other mutation in LCAT was observed. Of the remaining 12 LCAT mutations, 10 were point mutations, three were frameshifts, and one consisted of a three base insertion which maintained its reading frame. For fish eye disease, three mutations have been reported. This disorder is less serious than familial LCAT deficiency and is characterized by dyslipoproteinemia and corneal opacity. LCAT activity is 15% of normal and there is a reduced level of HDL in the plasma. In contrast, familial LCAT deficiency is characterized by a variety of symptoms including lipoprotein abnormalities, renal failure, premature atherosclerosis, reduced levels of plasma cholesterol esters, and high plasma levels of cholesterol and lecithin.

The LCAT enzyme requires apo A-I as a cofactor. If there is a mutation in the gene for apo A-I, defective HDL production results. This is a rare mutation, and its frequency is estimated as one in a million. Individuals with this defect have premature CVD, corneal clouding, and very low HDL levels. Plasma apo A-I has a variety of charge isoforms with similar antigenicity and amino acid composition. Humans, baboons, African green monkeys, and cynomolgus monkeys have been studied, and there are species differences in hepatic and intestinal apo A-I production. In all instances, the differences in apo A-I were reported between intestine and liver. In the liver, there was a twofold higher level of apo A-I mRNA than in the intestine and the abundance of this mRNA was species specific. The apo A-I gene is regulated at the level of transcription and a portion of the species-specific difference in apo A-I gene expression is due to a sequence divergence in the 5′ regulatory region including the exon/intron 1 of the apo A-I gene. The capacity to produce HDLs is both genetically controlled and tissue-specific and probably explains why some genotypes respond normally to a high-fat diet by producing more HDL, while other genotypes become hypercholesterolemic under these same conditions. Attempts to create a transgenic mouse expressing a human apo A-I gene have not been fully successful but have provided additional information about the relationship of apo A-I to HDL size. The human apo A-I gene was inserted into the mouse and in these mice; both the mouse and the human genes were expressed. This dual expression suggests a species difference in the control of this expression. In other words, the control points differed and this resulted in a broader spectrum of HDL particles.

Defective HDL metabolism due to a mutation in the apo A-I gene results in a rare autosomal dominant disorder described in a small group of villagers in Italy. Affected individuals have reduced levels of HDL cholesterol and apo A-I levels but have no increased risk of CVD. The disorder, named Apo A-I Milano, is due to a point mutation in the apo A-I gene changing codon 173, so that cysteine is used instead of arginine. Normal apo A-I has no cysteine so this change has effects (because of the sulfide group in the cysteine) on the apo A-I structure.

Defective lipoprotein processing has already been discussed with respect to LDP, LCAP, and apo C-II deficiencies. A deficient cholesterol ester transport protein (CETP) has been reported due to a mutation of the gene for this protein located on chromosome 16. A mutation in this gene has been used to explain the atherogenicity of high-fat diets in primates, but to date no evidence of such a mutation in humans has been put forward.

NUTRIENT–GENE INTERACTIONS IN LIPID TRANSPORT

Nutrients can sometimes affect the expression of the above-described genetic factors. This suggests that CVD could develop as a result of a nutrient-gene interaction. The diet influence involves not only the amount of fat consumed but also the type of fat and the amount and type of carbohydrate. For example, the editing of the apo B gene is enhanced by dietary carbohydrate. A number of genes have carbohydrate response elements and it is possible that this gene has this element in its promoter region. A carbohydrate response element has also been identified in the apo E gene. Carbohydrate influences mRNA stability and RNA processing of this gene. Similarly, the gene that encodes the seven-enzyme complex of mammalian fatty acid synthetase has a fatty acid response unit in its promoter. The expression of this gene is downregulated by dietary polyunsaturated fatty acids. The lipid transport genes might also have a lipid response element.

Dietary lipids, even in the absence of direct effects on transcription and translation, do influence the phenotypic expression of specific genotypes either because of overconsumption or because they have effects on certain of the hormones, that is, insulin or the steroid hormones, or the catabolic hormones that regulate or influence lipid synthesis, oxidation, and storage.

The level of cholesterol in the blood depends on the diet consumed and how much cholesterol is being synthesized. The cholesterol content of the gut LDL of a person on a low-cholesterol diet might run as low as 7 to 10% of the total lipid in the lipoprotein, while the hepatic LPL of this same individual might be as high as 58% of total lipid. People consuming a low-cholesterol-low-saturated-fat diet may reduce the contribution of the diet to the blood cholesterol while increasing the hepatic *de novo* cholesterol synthesis. Persons having an LPL receptor deficiency are characterized by high serum cholesterol levels, and in some cases, by high serum triacylglycerides. The reason these blood lipids are elevated is that the individuals cannot utilize the lipids carried by the LPL due to the error(s) in the receptor molecule. Further, because these circulating lipids do not enter into the adipose and hepatic cell in normal amounts, the synthesis of triacylglycerides and cholesterol is not appropriately downregulated. Hence, this individual has elevated serum lipids not only because the LPL lipid is not appropriately cleared from the blood but also because of high rates of endogenous lipid synthesis. Individuals with this disorder have lipid deposits in unusual places such as immediately under the skin, around the eyes, on the tendons, and in the vascular tree. It is this last feature that probably accounts for the shortened lifespan of these people with the cause of death being cardiovascular disease. As can be seen from the metabolic characteristics of this disorder, low-cholesterol diets are probably useless in reducing serum cholesterol levels since *de novo* synthesis of cholesterol from nonlipid precursors can and does occur. Treatment with lipid adsorbents (high-fiber diets and the drug cholestyramine) will help reduce the cholesterol (but not triacylglycerides) coming from the intestine, and there are drugs (statins and fibrates) that can safely lower *de novo* cholesterol synthesis as well as increase intracellular lipid oxidation. All of these therapies may help reduce the serum lipid levels, but even doing this only treats the symptoms not the genetic disorder. For that, gene therapy is needed to correct the genetic disorder that is the basic underlying cause of the symptoms.

Heart disease in its various forms is associated with elevated levels of the very-low-density lipoproteins (VLDL). In addition to the above descriptions of lipemias, some of which are associated with heart disease, there are other genetically determined forms of heart disease (Table 54.4 and Table 54.5). The lipemia-associated disorders have been subdivided into three general categories. In one, patients are characterized by elevated serum cholesterol, phospholipid, and triacylglyceride levels, elevated VLDL levels (and sometimes LDL levels), fatty deposits on the tendons and in areas on the arms just under the skin, vascular atheromas, and ischemic heart disease. This type of lipemia is inherited as an autosomal dominant trait in one person in 5000. Another lipemia occurs in patients having a normal cholesterol level but an elevated triacylglyceride level and elevated VLDL levels. These characteristics are associated with ischemic heart disease and premature atherosclerosis. It is frequently seen in obese patients with Type 2 diabetes. People with diabetes mellitus have five times the risk of people without diabetes of developing premature atherosclerosis and its associated coronary events. Cardiovascular disease, followed by renal disease, is the leading causes of death for people with diabetes mellitus. Diabetes mellitus is also a group of disorders with both genetic and nutritional components (Table 54.6). Diabetes mellitus is roughly divided into two types: Type 1 patients are those who develop the disease due to pancreatic deficiency. They need insulin replacement therapy to manage their blood glucose levels. Type 1 patients comprise about 10% of all the people with diabetes. Type 2 patients are those whose disease can be managed through diet, exercise, and oral medication (see Chapter 46 for more information on nutrition and diabetes mellitus). Many of these people progress to hormone replacement therapy, but they start out not needing it. In both obesity and diabetes, metabolic

TABLE 54.5
Mutations That Phenotype as Heart Disease [5–21]

Mutation	Characteristics
Lipoprotein lipase 3 mutations	High plasma TG — heart disease
MTHR gene 26 different mutations	Elevated homocysteine levels in blood and urine
4p16.1 (between D4S2957 and D4S827)	Cardiac malformations
9q31 (Tangier disease) 5 mutations	Premature CAD
LDL receptor 36 different mutations	Hypercholesterolemia, premature CAD or CVD
Elastin synthesis 7q11.23 4 mutations	Supravalvular aortic stenosis congenital heart and vascular disease
Leu 54 to Met in paraoxonase	CVD
Troponin T 6 mutations	Hypertrophic cardiomyopathy
α Tropomyosin	Hypertrophic cardiomyopathy
Myosin	Hypertrophic cardiomyopathy
ApoB gene 4 mutations	Hypercholesterolemia, peripheral vascular disease, CAD
11 BHSD 6 mutations	Hypertension
hBENaC	Hypertension
Bradykinin receptor (14q32) 8 mutations	Cardiovascular disease
Transcription factor NKX2–5 3 mutations	Congenital heart disease

TABLE 54.6
Mutations That Associate with Type 1 and Type 2 Diabetes Mellitus [22–46]

Gene	Comments
Nuclear DNA	
Hepatic nuclear transcription factor 4α (MODY 1)	Impaired insulin secretion
Glucokinase (MODY 2)	Impaired insulin secretion; 44 different mutations in this gene have been reported
Hepatic transcription factor 1α (MODY 3)	Subjects are generally nonobese
Glycogen synthase	Hypertension and Type 2 are found in this genotype, which is polymorphic Activation of the enzyme is impaired
Glucagon receptor	Susceptibility to Type 2 is variable among different population groups
Insulin receptor	Associated with peripheral insulin resistance in some Type 2 subjects
Insulin receptor substrate (IRS-1)	Results in a signal transmission defect associated with insulin resistance
Mitochondrial α glycerol 3 phosphate dehydrogenase	Associated with Type 2 and with impaired mitochondrial function
Mobile glucose transporters (GLUT 1-5)	Associated with both obesity and Type 2
Mitochondrial DNA (heteroplasmic[a])	
tRNA[leu]	7 mutations have been found that associate with diabetes
ND 1	11 mutations have been reported
ND 2, ND 3, ND 4	1 mutation in each of these genes has been reported
tRNA[Cys, Ser, Lys]	1 mutation in each of these genes has been reported
tRNA[thr]	4 mutations have been found
D-Loop[b]	3 mutations have been reported
COX II	2 mutations have been reported
ATPase 6,8	4 mutations have been reported

[a] Mutations in the mitochondrial genome that associate with diabetes are heteroplasmic, that is, there is mixture of normal and abnormal DNA in each cell. The percentage of the abnormal determines the degree to which the function of that cell is impaired.

[b] Promoter regions for the 13 structural genes found in the mitochondrial genome are found here.

TABLE 54.7
Aberrant Mobile Glucose Transports and Their Consequences[1]

Protein	Consequences of an Error
GLUT 1	Minimal changes in glucose uptake by all tissues that use glucose
GLUT 2	Liver — glucose metabolic pathways suppressed; increased gluconeogenic activity β cell — pancreas unresponsive to glucose stimulation Kidney — increased gluconeogenic activity
GLUT 3	Minimal changes in glucose uptake and metabolism
GLUT 4	Adipose tissue — decrease glucose use by fat cell; compensatory increase in hepatic glucose use; increase hepatic lipogenesis and lipid output; increase hepatic glycogen store Heart, muscle — decrease glucose use by muscle could be lethal if compensatory use of fatty acids and ketones is insufficient

problems associated with aberrant glucose transporters have been reported. Table 54.7 gives a list of these transporters and their function. Should there be a problem in these transporters, glucose entry into the cell is reduced, and this of course means that there is a decrease in glucose uptake, a typical sign of diabetes.

There is a third group of people with diabetes who develop their disease as a result of a mutation in the mitochondrial genome. We do not know how many people have this form of the disease. The estimates vary from 0.1 to 9% of the population with diabetes. These people have other metabolic problems that are also related to their mitochondrial dysfunction.

Both heart disease risk and diabetes risk increases with an increase in body fat. Obesity per se is a health risk for a number of other conditions as well. Table 54.8 provides a list of mutations that associate with obesity. Most of these associate with extreme obesity or obesity that develops in early childhood. Whether mild obesity or somewhat over weight is a genetic trait is questionable.

TABLE 54.8
Mutations That Phenotype as Obesity[22–24,47–55]

Mutation	Characteristics
Estrogen receptor B 4 mutations	Obesity
Proopiomelanocortin 6 mutations	Extreme childhood and adolescent obesity
Leptin 3 mutations	Hyperphasia, obesity
Leptin receptor	Hyperphasia, obesity
Uncoupling protein 1 5 mutations	Obesity
Uncoupling protein 2	Obesity
Uncoupling protein 3	Obesity
MC3 receptor	Obesity
Neuropeptide Y receptor	Obesity
MSTN	Obesity
CCKAR	Obesity
Chromosome 2p12–13 (Alstrom Syndrome)	Retinal pigment degeneration, neurogenic deafness, infantile obesity, hyperlipidemia, type 2 diabetes, hyperglycemia, and hyperlipidemia
Gsalpha 2 mutations	Albright hereditary osteodystrophy: skeletal abnormalities and obesity
Peroxisome proliferator α 2	Obesity
Insulin receptor substrate	Type 2 diabetes, obesity
β 3 adrenergic receptor	Type 2 diabetes, obesity
OB D75514 — D7S530 Insulin receptor gene	Type 2 diabetes, obesity, hypertension, and insulin resistance
Tumor necrosis factor	Obesity
4p16.3 (Achondroplasia)	Obesity
20q11 (posterior polymorphous)	Obesity, corneal dystrophy
15q11.2–q12 (Prader-Willi Syndrome)	Hyperphasia, early onset obesity
12q23–q24.1 (Schinzel Syndrome)	Obesity
11q13 (Bardet-Biedl Syndrome)	Obesity
16q21	Obesity
3p13–p12	Obesity
15q22.3–q23	Obesity
8q22–q23 (Cohen Syndrome)	Obesity
Xq26–q27 (X linked) (Borjeson-Forssman-Lehman Syndrome)	Obesity
Xq21.1–q22 (X linked) Wilson-Turner Syndrome	Obesity
Xq26 (X linked) (Simpson-Golabi-Behmel Syndrome)	Obesity
HSD3B1 (1p13.1)	Obesity
ATP1A2 (1q21–q23)	Obesity
ACP1 (2p25)	Obesity
APOB (2p24–p23)	Obesity
APOD (3q27–qter)	Obesity
TNFir24 (6p21.3)	Obesity
LPL (8p22)	Obesity
ADRB3 (8p12–p11.1)	Obesity
SUR (11p15.1)	Obesity
DRD2 (11q22.2–q22.3)	Obesity
APOA4 (11q23–qter)	Obesity
LDLR (19p13.2)	Obesity

For some people who habitually overeat and underexercise, this excess food is converted to body fat stores. It has been postulated that loss of food intake control could be a genetic trait as well. Certainly, mutations in the leptin gene, the leptin receptor gene, and the genes for several other neuronal signals that are involved in food intake regulation suggest that genetics plays a role in excess food consumption. Should this behavior be suppressed, excess body fat is reduced. Chapters 48 through 53 address various issues with respect to obesity assessment development and management.

SUMMARY

A number of the chronic diseases that affect humans have both genetic and nutritional linkages. In some, the genetic linkage is very strong and, likely, in people with these mutations the disease will develop regardless of dietary influence. In other disorders, a combination of genetic and dietary factors is needed before the disease manifests itself. Paramount to successful delay or avoidance of some of these disorders is an early identification of mutations and their associated phenotypes. Genetic screening may be valuable in developing successful strategies that can forestall disease development.

REFERENCES

1. Berdanier, CD. *Advanced Nutrition: Macronutrients*, 2nd ed. CRC Press Boca Raton, FL, 2000, 327 pp.
2. Berdanier, CD. *Advanced Nutrition: Micronutrients*. CRC Press Boca, Raton FL 1998, 236 pp.
3. Murray, RK, Granner, DK, Mayes, PA, Rodwell, VW. *Harpers Biochemistry*. Appleton & Lange, 2004, 359.
4. Scriver, CR, Beaudet, AL, Sly, WS, Valle, D. *The Metabolic Basis of Inherited Disease*. McGraw Hill, 1989, 3006 pp.
5. Julieen, P, Vohl, MC, Gaudet, D et al. *Diabetes* 46: 2063; 1997.
6. Eckstrom, U, Abrahamson, M, Wallmark, A et al. *Eur J Clin Invest* 28: 740; 1998.
7. Sun, XM, Patel, DD, Knight, BL, Soutar, AK. *Atherosclerosis* 136: 175; 1998.
8. Kluijtmans, LA, van den Heuvel, LP, Boers, GH et al. *Am J Hum Genet* 58: 35; 1996.
9. Goyette, P, Christensen, AE, Rosenblatt, DS, Rozen, R. *Am J Hum Genet* 59: 1268; 1996.
10. Howard, TD, Guttmacher, AE, McKinnon, W et al. *Am J Hum Genet* 61: 1405; 1997.
11. Soutar, AK. *J Intern Med* 231: 633; 1992.
12. Folsom, AR, Nieto, FL, McGovern, PG et al. *J Clin Invest* 98: 204; 1998.
13. Keating, MT. *Circulation* 92: 142; 1995.
14. Garin, MC, James RW, Dussoix, P et al. *J Clin Invest* 99: 62; 1997.
15. Watkins, H, McKenna, WI, Thierfelder, HJ et al. *N Eng J Med* 332: 1058; 1995.
16. Pullinger, CR, Hennessy, LK, Chatterton, JE et al. *J Clin Invest* 95: 1225; 1995.
17. Genest, JJ, Ordovas, JM, McNamara, JR et al. *Atherosclerosis* 82: 7; 1990.
18. Mune, T, Roggerson, RM, Nikkila, H et al. *Nat Genet* 10: 394; 1995.
19. Shimkets, RA, Warnock, DG, Bositis, CM. *Cell* 79: 407; 1994.
20. Erdmann, J, Hegemann, N, Weidemann, A et al. *Am J Med Genet* 80: 521; 1998.
21. Schott, JJ, Benson, DW, Basson, CT et al. *Science* 281: 108; 1998.
22. Utsunomiya, N, Ohagi, S, Sanke, T et al. *Diabetologia* 41: 701; 1996.
23. Hani, EH, Boutin, P, Durand, E et al. *Diabetologia* 41: 1511; 1998.
24. Cama, A, Sierra, ML, Ottini, L. *J Clin Endocrinol Metab* 73: 894; 1991.
25. Jackson, RS, Creemers, JW, Ohagi, S et al. *Nat Genet* 16: 303; 1997.
26. Froguel, P, Vaxillaire, M, Velho, G. *Diabetes Rev* 5: 123; 1997.
27. Velho, G, Blanche, H, Vaxillaire M et al. *Diabetologia* 40: 217; 1997.
28. Vionnet, N, Stoffel, M, Takeda, J et al. *Nature* 356: 721; 1992.
29. Shimada, F, Makino, H, Hashimoto, H. *Diabetologia* 36: 433; 1993.
30. Hattersley, AT, Turner, RC, Permutt, MA. *Lancet* 339: 1307; 1993.
31. Shitani, M, Ikegami, H, Yamato, E et al. *Diabetologia* 39: 1398; 1996.
32. Taylor, SI, Kadowaki, H, Accili, D et al. *Diabetes Care* 13: 257; 1990.
33. Kadowaki, T, Kadowaki, H, Rechler, MM. *J Clin Invest* 86: 254; 1990.
34. Odawara, M, Kadowaki, T, Yaamamotto, R. *Science* 245: 66; 1989.
35. Taylor, ST, Cama, A, Accili, D et al. *Endocr Rev* 13: 566; 1992.
36. Chevre, JC, Hani, EH, Boutin, P et al. *Diabetologia* 41: 1017; 1998.
37. Velho, G, Froguel, P. *Endocrinology* 138: 233; 1998.
38. Vaxillaire, M, Rouard, M, Yamagata, K et al. *Hum Mol Genet* 6: 583; 1997.
39. Frayling, TMTM, Bulamn, MP, Ellard, S et al. *Diabetes* 46: 720; 1997.
40. Hansen, T, Eiberg, H, Rouard, M et al. *Diabetes* 46: 726; 1997.
41. Yagui, K, Shimada, F, Mimura, M et al. *Diabetologia* 41: 1024; 1998.
42. Steiner, DF, Tager, HS, Chan, SJ et al. *Diabetes Care* 13: 600; 1990.
43. DeFronzo, RA. *Diabetes Rev* 5: 177; 1997.
44. Strom, TM, Hortnagel, K, Hofmann, S et al. *Hum Mol Genet* 7: 2021; 1998.
45. van den Ouweland, JMW, Lempkes, HHPJ, Ruitenbeck, W et al. *Nat Genet* 1: 368; 1992.
46. Mathews, CE, Berdanier, CD. *Proc Soc Exp Biol Med* 219: 97; 1998.
47. Rosenkranz, K, Hinney, A, Zeigler, A et al. *J Clin Endocrinol Metab* 83: 4524; 1998.
48. Hinney, A, Becker, I, Heibut, O et al. *J Endocrinol Metab* 83: 3737; 1998.
49. Karvonen, MK, Pesonen, U, Heinonen, P et al. *J Endocrinol Metab* 83: 3239; 1998.
50. Comuzzie, AG, Allison, DB. *Science* 280: 1374; 1998.

51. Urhammer, SA, Fridberg, M, Sorenson, TI et al. *J Clin Endocrinol Metab* 82: 4069; 1997.
52. Macari, F, Lautier, C, Girardet, A. *Hum Genet* 103: 658; 1998.
53. Warner, DR, Weng, G, Yu, S et al. *J Biol Chem* 273: 23976; 1998.
54. Ristow, M, Muller-Wieland, D, Pfeiffer, A et al. *N Eng J Med* 339: 953; 1998.
55. Perusse, L, Chagnon, YC, Dionne, FT, Bouchard, C. *Obesity Res* 5: 1225; 1996.

55 Folate, Homocysteine, and Neurologic Diseases

Hyunmi Kim and James Carroll

CONTENTS

FOLATE AND HOMOCYSTEINE

Folates are important cofactors in the transfer and utilization of one-carbon moieties and play a key role in the synthesis of nucleic acids and methionine regeneration. Folate supplementation reduces total homocysteine concentration, whether given as a supplement or in fortified foodstuffs.[1,2] Increased fruit and vegetable consumption has also been shown to decrease homocysteine levels.[3] The homocysteine-lowering effect of folate can be explained by its actions as a substrate in the remethylation of homocysteine to methionine (Figure 55.1).[4]

Homocysteine is a sulfur-containing amino acid that is an intermediary product in methionine metabolism.[5] The metabolism of homocysteine is closely linked to certain B-group vitamins, including folate, cobalamin, pyridoxine, and riboflavin.

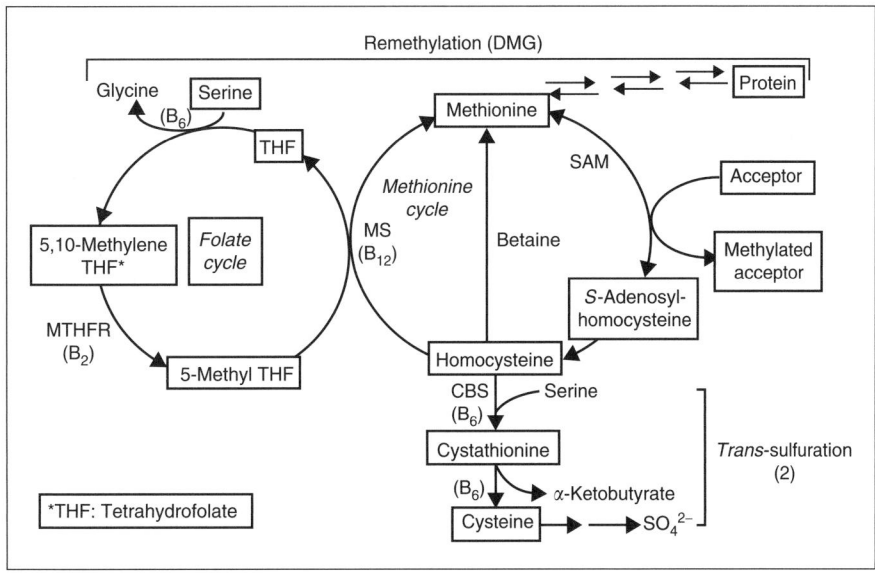

FIGURE 55.1 Metabolic cycle of homocysteine. (With permission from Young, *Curr Opin Clin Nutr Metab Care* 3: 427–432; 2000.) Abbreviations: CBS, cystathionine β-synthase; DMG, dimethylglycine; MS, methionine synthase; MTHFR, methylene tetrahydrofolate reductase; SAM, *S*-adenosyl methionine; THF, tetrahydrofolate.

Plasma total homocysteine is strongly influenced by B-group vitamins, with folate status being its most important determinant in the general population.[6]

The epidemiologic evidence from prospective cohort, cross-sectional, and case–control studies indicates that increased homocysteine levels are an independent risk factor for coronary artery disease, cerebrovascular disease, peripheral vascular disease, and venous thrombosis.[7–13]

FOLATE DEFICIENCY

A deficiency of folate occurs when an increased need for folate is not matched by an increased intake, when dietary folate intake does not meet recommended needs, or when folate excretion increases. Medications that interfere with the metabolism of folate may also increase the need for this vitamin and heighten the risk of deficiency.[14,15] The factors that influence homocysteine metabolism and cause hyperhomocysteinemia are listed in the Table 55.1.

FOLATE, HOMOCYSTEINE, AND NEUROLOGIC DISEASE

Theoretically, folate deficiency should produce the same neurological deficits as those seen in vitamin B_{12} deficiency because of its importance in the production of methionine, S-adenosylmethionine, and tetrahydrofolate. However, the neurological manifestations of vitamin B_{12} deficiency are rare in folate deficiency. This is probably due to alternative cellular mechanisms that preserve S-adenosylmethionine levels in times of folate scarcity. In contrast, accumulating evidence suggests that chronic folate deficiency is likely to present in a subtle manner. Folate deficiency may result in mild cognitive impairment or increased stroke risk in adults and increased frequency of neural tube defects (NTDs) in infants born to folate-deficient mothers.[16]

CEREBROVASCULAR DISEASE

Hyperhomocysteinemia appears to be more closely associated with small-vessel strokes rather than large-vessel disease or cardioembolic mechanisms.[17,18] The pathophysiological mechanisms that underlie homocysteine-induced endothelial dysfunction remain uncertain. Several mechanisms have been proposed, including a reduction in availability of the endothelium-dependent relaxing factor nitric oxide[19] and an increase in oxidant stress with alterations in the endothelial cellular redox potential.[20]

TABLE 55.1
Factors That Increase Plasma Homocysteine Levels

Type of Factor	Examples
Genetic defects in the enzymes involved in homocysteine metabolism	*Trans*-sulfuration: cystathionine β-synthase deficiency Remethylation: N^5, N^{10}-methylene tetrahydrofolate reductase deficiency or thermolabile variant; methionine synthase deficiency
Nutritional	Folate deficiency Vitamin B_{12} (combalamin) deficiency (an essential cofactor for methionine synthase) Vitamin B_6 (pyridoxine) deficiency (an essential cofactor for cystathionine β-synthase) Increase methionine intake (animal protein)
Disease	Pernicious anemia Renal impairment Hypothyroidism Malignancy: acute lymphoblastic leukemia; carcinoma of the breast, ovary, and pancreas Severe psoriasis Transplant recipients
Medications/toxins	Folate antagonists: methotrexate; phenytoin; carbamazepine Vitamin B_6 antagonists: theophylline; azaribine; estrogen-containing oral contraceptives; cigarette smoking
Age/sex	Advanced age Male sex Postmenopausal women

Source: With permission from Hankey, *Curr Opin Neurol* 14: 95–102; 2001.

NEURODEGENERATIVE DISEASE

The association of vitamin deficiency with dementing illnesses has been noted.[21] Several studies found that patients with Alzheimer-type dementia as well as other dementing illnesses frequently had low serum vitamin B_{12} or folate levels.[21–25] A recent pathologic analysis of the Alzheimer's disease (AD) found that low plasma folate levels were correlated with the severity of neocortical atrophy.[25]

EPILEPSY

There are several pieces of evidence of high level of homocysteine resulting in seizures. In animal models of experimental epilepsy, systemic administration of high doses of homocysteine produce seizures.[26,27] Up to 20% of patients with homozygous cystathionine β-synthase deficiency have seizures,[28] and the high plasma concentrations of homocysteine in these patients may contribute to epilepsy.[29]

Because most anticonvulsants lower plasma folate levels,[30,31] almost half of the patients treated with anticonvulsants had homocysteine levels sufficiently elevated to put them at high risk for vascular disease.[32,33]

There is an increased risk of major congenital malformations in children whose mothers receive anticonvulsants during the first trimester, perhaps related to teratogenic effects of high homocysteine levels.[34] Valproic acid increases the risk of NTDs and other malformations 3- to 20-fold, to approximately 1 to 2%, and its teratogenic effects are dose related. Carbamazepine also is associated with NTDs, with an incidence of 0.5 to 1.0% (see Reference 35, p. 2539).[35] Exposure to valproate during the first weeks of gestation is associated with a 5% risk of NTDs. This risk may be diminished to some degree by preconceptional and periconceptional maternal folate supplementation. Because NTDs originate very early during pregnancy (5 to 6 weeks' gestation), folate administered after confirmation of pregnancy is not helpful in this regard (see Reference 35, p. 2528).[35] The American Academy of Neurology recommends that all women of childbearing potential who are taking anticonvulsants consume at least 0.4 mg/day of folic acid.[34]

NEURAL TUBE DEFECTS

NTDs are believed to result from failure of fusion of the neural tube during early embryogenesis. The most common NTDs are anencephaly, which results from failure of fusion of the cranial neural tube, and myelomeningocele (commonly called spina bifida), which results from failure of fusion in the spinal region of the neural tube.[36]

The mechanism of teratogenicity in folate deficiency is unclear. Several reports implicate elevations in homocysteine.[37–39] Hyperhomocysteinemia is commonly found in women who have given birth to infants with NTDs.[40,41] The C677T mutation in the methylene tetrahydrofolate reductase (MTHFR) gene significantly increases the risk of NTDs.[42,43] Amniotic fluid homocysteine levels were found to be significantly higher in pregnancies complicated by NTDs.[44]

The mechanism by which folic acid reduces the risk of NTDs is unclear. A recent study by Rothenberg et al.[45] showed that some mothers with pregnancy complicated by NTD-produced autoantibodies that bind to folate receptors on the placental membrane and therefore block the binding of folic acid. The authors suggested that the periconceptional administration of folate would bypass the autoantibodies that mediate a placental folate receptor blockage. Indeed, folate has a high affinity for its receptor and might displace the autoantibody when administered at high doses.

Since 1998, the U.S. Food and Drug Administration has mandated fortification of grain products with folate.[46] Data suggest that there has been a significant reduction in neural tube birth defects.[47–49] The Centers for Disease Control and Prevention (CDC) reports that rates have fallen by approximately 26% in the United States.[48] However, the key problem in determining the success or failure of fortification is identifying prenatally diagnosed NTDs. Persad et al.[49] studied records of all live births, stillbirths, and terminated pregnancies in a well-defined area, Nova Scotia, from 1991 through 2000. They found a 54% decrease. The percentage of NTDs that are folate preventable in the United States is uncertain, but is probably 50 to 60%.[47]

Spina bifida and anencephaly, the two most common types of NTDs, are estimated to affect ~3000 pregnancies each year in the United States. It has been estimated that ~4000 pregnancies in the United States were affected by NTDs annually before folic acid fortification. Recent estimates suggest that, since folic acid fortification, 1000 fewer NTD-affected pregnancies occur in the United States each year.[48] On the other hand, the prevalence of NTDs has been shown to vary by race/ethnicity,[50–53] with the highest rates among women of Hispanic ethnicity and the lowest rates among Black and Asian women. In 1995 to 2002, significant declines in spina bifida and anencephaly were observed among Hispanic births and non-Hispanic White births. The prevalence ratio for non-Hispanic Black births was of borderline significance for spina bifida and was not significant for anencephaly. Both genetic factors such as C677T mutation in the MTHFR gene and environmental factors including eating habits or supplement-taking practices may be responsible for the differences in NTD risk observed among racial/ethnic groups.[54]

FOLATE SUPPLEMENTATION

Improved folate status can be accomplished by increasing natural dietary folate (a diet rich in vegetables and citrus fruit) supplementation with synthetic folic acid (pteroylmonoglutamic acid), which is heat stable and approximately twice as bioavailable, or folic acid food fortification. For all three methods, the potential to increase serum folate has been demonstrated.[55-57] However, the actual effectiveness of the first two methods may be low because of poor compliance: surveys to evaluate folic acid supplementation for the prevention of birth defects uncovered that only a small minority of pregnant women had, in fact, taken the advised folic acid supplements.[58] This has caused the Food and Drug Administration to introduce folic acid fortification of "enriched" cereal grains (1.4 mg/kg grain) in the Unites States in 1998. Similar fortification programs were introduced in Canada and several other industrialized countries.

In women of childbearing potential with epilepsy, daily folate supplement of 0.4 mg or more is recommended as prophylaxis against NTD (see Reference 35, p. 1698).[35] In patients with documented folate deficiency, the initial dose is usually 1 mg of folate three times per day, followed by a maintenance dose of 1 mg/day. For acutely ill patients, parenteral doses of 1 to 5 mg may be given. Even with oral doses as high as 15 mg/day, there is no substantiated report of toxicity.

In general, folic acid supplementation is considered safe.[59] However, there is some concern about folic acid therapy in people with subclinical cobalamin (vitamin B_{12}) deficiency, a relatively common disorder in the elderly[60] and in strict vegetarians.[61] Folic acid therapy in these patients may mask the hematologic manifestations of the disorder and allow progression of the neurological damage, including spinal cord injury. This induced several investigators to suggest the inclusion of cobalamin in folic acid supplements.

REFERENCES

1. Brattstrom L et al., *Br Med J* 316: 894; 1998.
2. Riddell LJ et al., *Am J Clin Nutr* 71: 1448; 2000.
3. Broekmans WR et al., *J Nutr* 130: 1578; 2000.
4. Young IS and Woodside JV, *Curr Opin Clin Nutr Metab Care* 3: 427; 2000.
5. Finkelstein JD, *J Nutr Biochem* 1: 228; 1990.
6. Refsum H et al., *Ann Rev Med* 49: 31; 1998.
7. Eikelboom JW et al., *Ann Intern Med* 131: 363; 1999.
8. Boushey CJ et al., *JAMA* 274: 1049; 1995.
9. D'Angelo A and Selhub J, *Blood* 90: 1; 1997.
10. Welch GN and Loscalzo J, *N Eng J Med* 338: 1042; 1998.
11. Hankey GJ and Eikelenboom P, *Lancet* 354: 407; 1999.
12. Sacco RL, Roberts JK and Jacobs BS, *Neuroepidemiology* 17: 167; 1998.
13. Selhub J and D'Angelo G, *Thromb Haemost* 78: 527; 1997.
14. Hankey GJ and Eikelboom JW, *Curr Opin Neurol* 14: 95; 2001.
15. Godfrey P et al., *Birth Defects Res* (Part A) 70: 835; 2004.
16. Diaz-Arrastia R, *Arch Neurol* 57: 1422; 2000.
17. Fassbender K et al., *Lancet* 353: 1586; 1999.
18. Evers S et al., *Arch Neurol* 54: 1276; 1997.
19. Stamler JS et al., *J Clin Invest* 91: 308; 1993.
20. Wall RT et al., *Thromb Res* 18: 113; 1980.
21. Cole MG and Purchal JF, *Age Aging* 13: 101; 1984.
22. Nijst TQ et al., *J Neurol Neurosurg Psychiatr* 53: 951; 1999.
23. Goodwin JS, Goodwin JM and Garry PJ, *JAMA* 249: 917; 1983.
24. Riggs KM et al., *Am J Clin Nutr* 63: 306; 1996.
25. Snowdon DA et al., *Am J Clin Nutr* 71: 993; 2000.
26. Freed W, *Epilep* 26: 30; 1985.
27. Kubva H, Folbergrova J and Mares P, *Epilep* 36: 750; 1995.
28. Mudd SH et al., *Am J Hum Genet* 37: 1; 1985.
29. Schwarz S and Zhou GZ, *Lancet* 337: 1226; 1991.
30. Krause KH et al., *Drug Nutr Interact* 5: 317; 1988.
31. Kishi T et al., *J Neurol Sci* 145: 109; 1997.
32. Ono H et al., *Metab* 46: 959; 1997.
33. Schwaninger M et al., *Epilep* 40: 345; 1999.
34. Morrell MJ, *Neurol* 51: S21; 1998.
35. Bradley WG et al., *Neurology in Clinical Practice*, 4th ed., Butterworth-Heinemann, 2003, 1698, 2528, 2539.
36. Saddler TW, *Am J Med Genetics* 135C: 2; 2005.
37. Dansky LV, Rosenblatt DS and Andermann E, *Neurol* 42: S32; 1998.
38. Lucock MD et al., *Biochem Med Metab Biol* 52: 101; 1994.
39. Scott JM et al., *Ciba Found Symp* 181: 180; 1994.
40. Steegers-Theunissen RP et al., *Metab* 43: 1475; 1994.
41. Mills JL et al., *Lancet* 345: 149; 1995.

42. Van der Put NM, *Lancet* 346: 1070; 1995.
43. Whitehead AS et al., *Quart J Med* 88: 763; 1995.
44. Steegers-Theunissen RP, *Am J Obstet Gynecol* 172: 1436; 1995.
45. Rothenberg SP et al., *N Engl J Med* 350: 134; 2004.
46. Food and Drug Administration, *Fed Re* 61: 8781; 1996.
47. Mills JL and Signore C, *Birth Defect Res* (Part A) 70: 844; 2004.
48. Centers for Disease Control and Prevention, *MMWR Morb Mortal Wkly Rep* 53: 362; 2004.
49. Persad VL et al., *Can Med Assoc J* 167: 241; 2002.
50. Cragan JD et al., *MMWR Morb Mortal Wkly Rep* 44: 1; 1995.
51. Carmichael SL, Shaw GM and Kaidarova Z, *Birth Defects Res A Clin Mol Teratol* 70: 382; 2004.
52. Ray JG et al., *CMAJ* 171: 343; 2004.
53. Centers for Disease Control and Prevention, *MMWR Morb Mortal Wkly Rep* 41: 497; 1992.
54. Williams LJ et al., *Pediat* 116: 580; 2005.
55. Brouwer IA et al., *J Nutr* 129: 1135; 1999.
56. Collaboration HLT, *Brit Med J* 316: 894; 1998.
57. Lawrence JM et al., *Lancet* 354: 915; 1999.
58. Wild J et al., *Lancet* 350: 30; 1997.
59. Campbell NR, *Arch Intern Med* 156: 1638; 1996.
60. Lindenbaum J et al., *Am J Clin Nutr* 60: 2; 1994.
61. Chanarin I et al., *Lancet* 2: 1168; 1985.

56 Eating Disorders (Anorexia Nervosa, Bulimia Nervosa, Binge-Eating Disorder)

Christian R. Lemmon

CONTENTS

INTRODUCTION

The pursuit of thinness among adolescent and young adult females may leave some of them quickly threatening their physiological and psychological wellbeing as the fear of weight gain and possible obesity drives them into maladaptive eating and dieting habits. The intense preoccupation with dieting and weight control among this segment of the population has become so commonplace that it is often viewed as normal behavior and revered by peers who consider themselves less successful at being able to control their weight and shape. Unfortunately, and sometimes tragically, these maladaptive behaviors may inevitably manifest themselves in the form of eating disorders.

Eating disorders are often highlighted in the media in the form of sensationalized news and tabloid coverage, made-for-television movies, talk shows, and "reality" series. Despite the attention afforded to the eating disorders by medicine and the media, anorexia nervosa (AN), bulimia nervosa (BN), and other related feeding disturbances remain difficult psychiatric diagnoses to understand and treat. The American Psychiatric Association[1,2] revised their practice guidelines for the treatment of patients with eating disorders in 2000, and several other groups[3,4] have done the same, but practitioners who treat these patients, including psychiatrists and other physicians, psychologists, social workers, counselors, dietitians, and other health personnel continue to approach these problems from a wide array of treatment perspectives. Part of this lack of consensus concerning the treatment of eating disorders is attributable to the numerous theories that have been offered regarding their etiology. As reported by Yager,[5] "theories regarding the etiology and pathogenesis of the eating disorders have implicated virtually every level of biopsychosocial organization." AN, BN, and related feeding disturbances uniquely challenge those who are devoted to their treatment. One consistent consensus among researchers and clinicians is that the evaluation and treatment of the eating disorders must be multidisciplinary in focus and the biological, psychological, and social processes of eating-disordered patients must be considered.

DIAGNOSTIC CRITERIA

Eating disorders occur over a continuum of increasingly pathological behavior. Excessive self-evaluation and a preoccupation with weight, shape, and size characterize both AN and BN. Other common characteristics include an intense fear of weight gain and a relationship with food that borders on obsessive. However, there are distinct differences between the two disorders. Following are the diagnostic criteria for AN (Table 56.1) and BN (Table 56.2) as suggested by the Diagnostic and Statistical Manual, Version IV—Revised (DSM-IV-R)[6] that standardizes psychiatric diagnosis. A third variety, Eating Disorder, Not Otherwise Specified (EDNOS), is characterized by symptoms of either AN or BN, or both, but patients' behaviors fall short of the diagnostic criteria required to make these diagnoses. DSM-IV-R criteria for EDNOS are found below in Table 56.4. Binge eating disorder (BED) is another feeding disturbance that is currently considered a diagnosis provided for further study in the DSM-IV-R (see Table 56.3). Other differential diagnoses and feeding disturbances will be discussed below.

Anorexia Nervosa

Although AN often starts with only small reductions in total food intake, patients eventually reduce their energy and fat intake to a point where they are consuming only a limited number or foods in a highly ritualistic fashion. The disorder is characterized by severe, voluntary starvation (300 to 600 kcal per day). Although patients often suggest that they cannot eat or that they are not hungry, an actual loss of appetite is quite rare. Individuals with AN refuse to maintain a minimally normal and healthy body weight, show an intense fear of gaining weight or becoming fat, exhibit a disturbance in their perception of their body weight or shape, and experience abnormal menses. Two subtypes of AN exist, with about 50% classified as the restricting type, and the others exhibiting behaviors indicative of binge eating and purging; AN and BN are not mutually exclusive diagnoses. Further distinctions can be made between AN patients who binge eat and purge and those who purge or compensate in other ways after consuming normal meals or snacks, but do not engage in binge-eating episodes. DSM-IV-R criteria for AN are outlined in Table 56.1.

Bulimia Nervosa

BN is characterized by recurrent episodes of eating unusually large quantities of food at a meal, and eating until the food is gone or the person is uncomfortably or painfully full. Efforts to purge the excess food, typically between 1000 to 2000 kcal,[7,8] by some compensatory or purging behavior such as vomiting, laxative or diuretic abuse, excessive exercise, and restrictive dieting or fasting occur subsequent to the binge-eating episode. Some patients may binge and purge over an extended period of time, consuming close to 10,000 kcal. Amphetamine use may also occur in an attempt to restrict one's appetite. These behaviors are associated with a sense of loss of control and typically, shame, guilt, and embarrassment are associated with the binge-eating and purging process. Nevertheless, patients often report that the purging behaviors diminish the intensity of aversive emotions and provide them with a sense control. Similar to the diagnosis of AN, patients are further classified as either of two subtypes. DSM-IV-R criteria for BN are outlined in Table 56.2. Although an abnormally low body weight excludes a diagnosis of BN and forces the diagnosis of AN, it should also be noted that 25 to 30% of patients with BN have a prior history of AN.[9,10]

TABLE 56.1
DSM-IV-R Criteria for AN, Including Subtypes[a]

Refusal to maintain body weight at or above 85% of expected for height and age (could include a BMI ≤ 17.5)

Intense fear of gaining weight or accumulation of body fat despite underweight status

Body image disturbances, which may include the denial or lack of appreciation for the seriousness of one's currently low weight, self-evaluation largely determined by one's shape or weight, or claiming to "feel fat" even though terribly underweight

In females, primary or secondary amenorrhea

Subtypes

Restricting type: person has not regularly engaged in binge-eating or various purging behaviors

Binge-eating/purging type: person regularly engages in binge-eating or various purging behaviors

[a] Adapted from American Psychiatric Association, *Diagnostic and Statistical Manual of Mental Disorders*, Fourth Edition, Text Revision, American Psychiatric Association, Washington, DC, 2000.[6]

TABLE 56.2
DSM-IV-R Criteria for BN, Including Subtypes[a]

Recurrent episodes (a minimum average of twice per week for at least 3 months) of binge eating, defined as eating an abnormally large amount of food within a 2-h period, that are associated with a sense of lack of control over the eating process during the episode

Use of compensatory or purging behavior such as self-induced vomiting, laxative/enema or diuretic abuse, restrictive dieting, fasting, or excessive exercise

Self-evaluation largely determined by one's shape and weight

Bulimic behavior does not occur exclusively as a manifestation of AN

Subtypes

Purging type: person regularly uses purging strategies including self-induced vomiting, laxatives, diuretics, or enemas

Nonpurging type: person regularly uses other inappropriate compensatory strategies including fasting, restrictive dieting, or excessive exercise, but not currently using strategies listed above

[a] Adapted from American Psychiatric Association, *Diagnostic and Statistical Manual of Mental Disorders*, Fourth Edition, Text Revision, American Psychiatric Association, 2000.[6]

TABLE 56.3
DSM-IV-R Criteria for BED[a]

Recurrent episodes (a minimum average of twice per week for at least 6 months) of binge eating, defined as eating an abnormally large amount of food within a 2-h period, that are associated with a sense of lack of control over the eating process during the episode

At least three of the following characteristics are present during binge eating:

   Eating much more rapidly than usual

   Eating until uncomfortably full

   Eating large amounts of food despite not feeling physically hungry

   Eating alone because of embarrassment over quantity of food consumed

   Feeling disgusted, depressed, guilty, or ashamed after the binge

Experience of significant distress about the presence of binge eating

Absence of compensatory behaviors such as self-induced vomiting, laxative or diuretic abuse, restrictive dieting, fasting, or excessive exercise

Binge-eating episodes do not occur exclusively as a manifestation of AN or BN

[a] Adapted from American Psychiatric Association, *Diagnostic and Statistical Manual of Mental Disorders*, Fourth Edition, Text Revision, American Psychiatric Association, 2000.[6]

BINGE-EATING DISORDER

BED is more nebulous, and is characterized by recurrent binge-eating episodes without a compensatory effort to eliminate caloric excess. Although described in the classic paper of Stunkard,[11] it has only been widely recognized over the past 10 to 15 years. In fact, diagnostic criteria for BED were included in the DSM-IV-R only for research purposes, as it is not yet an approved diagnosis. Although persons diagnosed with BED are seen with a wide range of weights, most are obese. DSM-IV-R criteria for BED are outlined in Table 56.3. Although the age of onset is the same for BED, these patients typically do not present for treatment until they are much older and already overweight or obese.

TABLE 56.4
DSM-IV-R Criteria for EDNOS[a]

Disorders of eating that do not meet criteria for any specific Eating Disorder. Examples include:
   For females, all of the criteria for AN are met except that the individual has regular menses
   All of the criteria for AN are met except that despite significant weight loss, the individual's current weight is in the normal range
   All of the criteria for BN are met except that the binge eating and inappropriate compensatory mechanisms occur at a frequency
   of less than twice a week for a duration of less than 3 months

[a] Adapted from American Psychiatric Association, *Diagnostic and Statistical Manual of Mental Disorders*, Fourth Edition, Text Revision, American Psychiatric Association, 2000.[6]

OTHER EATING DISORDERS

Many patients diagnosed with eating disorders do not satisfy criteria for a formal diagnosis of AN or BN. For example, they may not binge and purge often enough to meet the required minimum average occurrence of such behavior. Similarly, a patient's weight may remain in an acceptable or healthy range despite exhibiting all of the other symptoms of AN. Some patients may display all of the characteristics of AN, but continue to menstruate normally. Others may repeatedly taste, chew their food, and spit it out in an effort to avoid the ingestion of unwanted energy. In fact, 26% of patients being evaluated for treatment reported that they were currently engaging in chewing and spitting "a few times a month" or more.[12] Patients who exhibit these and other similar presentations are classified as Eating Disorder, NOS[3] (see Table 56.4). In Europe, these presentations are more often termed "atypical eating disorders."[13] Despite diagnostic criteria not being met for AN or BN, patients with EDNOS present with symptoms that are potentially severe and chronic and they need the same kind of treatment recommended for those struggling with AN or BN.

Compulsive overeating and night eating have not been formally accepted as eating disorders, but are other maladaptive eating patterns. Compulsive overeating reflects frequent meals and snacks, or continuous eating or "grazing" without the presence of purging behaviors. Usually these individuals become overweight. Night eating syndrome (NES) is especially common in obese persons. It is characterized by delaying the first meal of the day, eating more food after dinner than during that meal and eating more than half of the day's food in the evening hours. The eating is often associated with aversive emotions and stress, and the pattern has persisted for at least two months. The syndrome can be distinguished from BN and BED by the lack of associated compensatory behaviors. Additionally, the pattern of food intake is typically smaller and in the form of excessive snacking rather than actual binge eating. NES also differs from sleep-related eating disorder as this is full awareness of the eating process, rather than parasomnic nocturnal food intake.[14] Nocturnal sleep-related eating is a form of sleep disorder. Sufferers are in a state somewhere between sleep and wakefulness and do not have recollection of the eating episodes. Other disorders often confused with BN include psychogenic vomiting, which is involuntary postprandial regurgitation in the absence of the core symptoms of fear of weight gain, benge eating, and body image disturbance, cyclic vomiting syndrome, and rumination disorder.[3]

EPIDEMIOLOGY

Eating disorders occur primarily in adolescent and young adult Caucasian women, but the onset can be prior to menarche or later in life. Males and non-Caucasians are much less frequently afflicted, but recent research suggests an increasing incidence in non-Caucasians and in persons across the spectrum of socioeconomic class. The general belief is that about 90 to 95% of cases of AN are female, and about 90% of cases of BN are female. However, the prevalence in males may be underestimated because of the wide perception that these are diseases that only affect teenage girls and adolescent women. Bulimic males are typically less likely to seek treatment than bulimic females. Another common misconception is that eating disorders in males signal probable homosexuality. In fact, only about 20% of males with eating disorders are homosexual.[15] However, higher rates of eating disorders are found among homosexual men.[16] The presentation of males with eating disorders is remarkably similar to that of females. Similar methods of weight control are used by both males and females, and there are comparable rates of psychiatric comorbidity and body image dissatisfaction.[17] A greater percentage of males were overweight before developing their eating disorders.[15] For BED, there is less gender difference.[18]

Estimates of incidence often vary significantly due to variations in the diagnostic criteria utilized and problems with the underreporting of these disorders that are so often accompanied by denial, secrecy, and the lack of appropriate medical attention. The general belief is that eating disorders have been on the rise in recent years. For AN, improved diagnostic practices and a higher likelihood of the afflicted seeking help may account for the rise in rates.[19] Patients with AN are easier to detect because of their thin, if not cachectic appearance, but individuals with BN blend in easier because of their more typical average to above average weight and the aforementioned secrecy surrounding their symptoms. Reasonable estimates for lifetime prevalence of

AN among females in Western countries approach 1% with a range of 0.5 to 3.7%.[1] The lifetime prevalence for BN among women has yielded higher numbers, with a range of 1.1 to 4.2%.[1] Although the least studied, individuals who display symptoms that fall into the category of EDNOS are the most common of the eating disorders.[13] Ricca et al.[20] reported that EDNOS was diagnosed as much AN and BN combined in a study of outpatients. Estimates for BED are 2% of the general population[1] with a 3:2 female to male ratio.[21] The incidence of BED increases to 30 to 40% of patients who seek treatment for obesity from hospital-affiliated programs,[22] 16 to 48% of bariatric surgery candidates[23–27] and about 70% of participants in Overeaters Anonymous.[22] There is no significant racial bias for BED.[22]

Individuals at high risk for the development of eating disorders include dancers, models, wrestlers, bodybuilders, jockeys, cheerleaders, entertainers, and participants in any other occupations or activities that place a pronounced emphasis on optimal body weight and shape. Other persons, such as gymnasts and figure skaters, may be at greater risk, especially when overzealous or misinformed coaches or trainers are working with them. Patients with certain medical conditions are at risk for developing eating disorders, and may misuse their prescribed treatments or physical conditions to facilitate weight loss and other purging strategies (Table 56.5).[28] A recent meta-analysis of controlled studies on the prevalence of eating disorders in Type I diabetes found a significantly higher rate of BN in females with diabetes as compared to controls.[29]

ETIOLOGY

At present, no universally accepted theory establishes the etiology of the eating disorders; complex and unique interactions of variables may occur in the affected individual. Disturbances in these interactions may represent primary or secondary phenomena. The current trend is to conceptualize disorders from a biopsychosocial perspective of multiple converging physiological, psychological, and environmental factors. More specifically, the development of an eating disorder depends on one's unique vulnerability that results from biological or other predisposing factors, their exposure to various provoking risk factors, and on the functions of protecting factors. Subsequently, the further interaction of various risk factors and protective factors determine whether the eating disorder will be maintained or recovery will occur. Stice[30] presented a comprehensive review of these various risk and maintenance factors associated with the eating disorders. Table 56.6 summarizes the more accepted etiologic theories.

Through extensive research investigating the neurobiology of the eating disorders, numerous *biological* theories have been proposed to explain their etiology; however, no single biological abnormality unequivocally accounts for the eating disorders. For anorexic patients, most aberrations appear to be the result rather than the cause of the weight loss or malnutrition, and

---

TABLE 56.5
Medical Conditions and Weight Loss Methods[a]

Medical Condition	Weight Loss Method
Diabetes	Restriction of insulin intake
Hypothyroidism	Misuse of thyroid hormones
Hyperthyroidism	Noncompliance with antithyroid medications
Cystic fibrosis	Failure to follow prescribed diet or take pancreatic enzymes
Crohn's disease	Noncompliance with medication or use of Crohn's related symptoms to facilitate/justify weight loss
Inflammatory bowel diseases	Use of IBD symptoms to facilitate/justify weight loss/weight control
Pregnancy	Use of pregnancy-related side effects (nausea and vomiting) to facilitate weight control

[a] Adapted from Powers PS. In: *Handbook of Treatment for Eating Disorders*, Second Edition, Garner DM, Garfinkel PE, Eds., The Guilford Press, New York, NY, p. 424; 1997.[28]

TABLE 56.6
Etiological Theories of the Eating Disorders

Biological
Genetic
Psychological
Feminist/social/cultural
Familial

most abate after healthy weight and adequate nutrition are restored.[31] The primary structure controlling ingestive behavior is the hypothalamus of the brain, which also regulates metabolism and end organ function. Other brain structures involved include the limbic system, amygdala, orbitofrontal cortex, mesial temporal lobe, and multiple brain stem nuclei. Neuroimaging methods have detected nonspecific abnormalities outside of the secondary changes that accompany malnutrition and hormonal changes.[32] Multiple alterations in neurotransmitters and neuroendocrine axes have been observed in both AN and BN.[33–35] For example, abnormal results have been found in eating-disorder patients for levels of luteinizing hormone, follicle-stimulating hormone, gonadotropin, growth hormone and cortisol and activity of cholecystokinin, opioids, and norepinephrine.[31] Once an eating disorder is established, secondary changes in brain chemistry may perpetuate the disease. The fact that amenorrhea is often found in normal-weight bulimics and anorexics before the profound weight loss also suggests some sort of biological deficit to explain the eating disorders. Much work has focused on the seratonin system since it is regarded as most important to the physiology of eating, weight regulation, and the mood disturbances often found among eating-disordered patients. Some aspects of seratonin function have been reported to remain abnormal even after recovery, leading some to suggest that a seratonin abnormality might predispose individuals to eating disorders or to some of the psychological characteristics that accompany eating disorders, such as perfectionism, impulse dysregulation, and mood disturbances.[36–39]

Another widely considered biological theory suggests that the eating disorders, especially BN, are a form of mood disorder.[5] The person with an eating disorder may be using food to self-medicate aversive emotions via alterations in brain chemicals. This theory is supported by the high comorbidity of mood disorders found among eating-disorder patients, the positive response of patients to antidepressant medications, and the increased prevalence of mood disorders in relatives of eating-disorder patients. The findings further emphasize the importance of proper assessment and treatment of depressive symptoms among the eating-disorder population.

Research in recent years has given rise to other neurobiological theories related to the onset and development of eating disorders. Most of the more promising results have focused on hormones and the changes that take place in their levels and release rates during and after feeding behavior. Grehlin, peptide YY (PYY), leptin, adiponectin, insulin, and cholecystokinin have been the most studied hormones to this point. Ghrelin, a peripheral peptide hormone that stimulates food intake produced mainly by the stomach, has been shown to stimulate food intake in humans without altering human gastric emptying. Geliebter et al.[40] found that overweight BED women had lower levels of baseline ghrelin concentrations prior to a meal and after fasting, and a smaller decline in ghrelin after a test meal as compared to non-binge-eating overweight women. PYY levels are typically low in fasting state and then rapidly increase postprandially. PYY has been shown to significantly decrease food intake when administered peripherally to mouse, rat and, humans; PPY may act as a satiety signal regulating the termination of individual meals, partially by decreasing production of ghrelin; and, in bulimics, a blunted PYY increase was found after food consumption.[41] Others have found that leptin, adiponectin, insulin, glucagon, and cholecystokinin levels rise after meals and suppress food intake when administered centrally or peripherally. It is hoped that this field of research might give rise to new pharmacological treatments for the eating disorders.

A *genetic* predisposition for eating disorders has been strongly suggested, as it is clear that eating disorders and various associated traits run in families.[42] In a very complete review of the genetic literature, Lilenfeld and Kaye[42] suggested that certain familial tendencies or "vulnerability factors," such as impulsivity, restraint, affective instability, and obsessionality contribute to the development of eating disorders. Strober et al.[43] investigated lifetime rates of full and partial AN and BN in 1831 first-degree relatives of diagnostically pure proband groups and relatives of matched, never-ill comparison subjects. They found that although AN was rare in families of the comparison subjects, full and partial syndromes of AN aggregated in female relatives of both anorexic and bulimic probands. The relative risks for the full syndrome of AN were 11.3 and 12.3 in female relatives of anorexic and bulimic probands, respectively. BN was more common than AN in female relatives of comparison subjects, but the disorder also aggregated in the families of ill probands, with the corresponding relative risks for BN determined to be 4.2 and 4.4 for female relatives of anorexic and bulimic probands, respectively. When partial syndromes of AN and BN were considered, relative risks fell by one half in each group of ill probands. Thus, both AN and BN appear to be familial. Again, their cross-transmission in families suggests a common, or shared, familial diathesis or familial liability.[43]

Twin studies have also been used to establish genetic contributions to AN and BN. Cotwins of twins with AN are at higher risk for eating disorders.[44] Woodside[45] demonstrated a 45% concordance rate for AN in identical twins, but only a 6.7% concordance in fraternal twins. While the concordance is higher in monozygotic (MZ) than dizygotic (DZ) twins (47.3 vs. 31.5%) for BN, the differences were not statistically significant.[45] In a clinical sample, Treasure and Holland[46] showed a concordance for AN of about 55% in MZ twins and 5% in DZ twins, and a concordance rate for BN of 35% in MZ twins and 30% in DZ twins. Given the previously cited findings related to seratonin, genetic studies have also focused on polymorphisms in seratonin-related genes. However, studies concentrating on the 5-HT2AR gene and chromosomes 1p, 4, 2 and 13 have not yet yielded definitive findings.[13]

Many *psychological* theories have been developed to explain the etiology and maintenance of eating disorders. Bruch[47] suggested that eating disorders result from disturbances in body image, limited self-esteem, and problems in interoceptive awareness. Another popular theory, especially for AN, relates to conflicts that may develop during adolescence and the sexual maturation process. It has been hypothesized that the physical and emotional regressions that take place in the development of

AN are the result of problems encountered during the struggle for independence, the formation of an adult identity, the realization of sexual urges, and the sometimes-competing parental, personal, and peer pressures. In a unique study[48] that considered the perspective of the anorexic patient, the most commonly mentioned perceived causes of the disorder were dysfunctional families, weight loss and dieting, stressful experiences, and perceived pressure. Severe life stresses have been implicated in the onset and development of the eating disorders. Sixty-seven percent of anorexics and 76% of BN patients reported a severe stressor or a marked difficulty coping with a stressor during the year before onset. The most common serious life stressors before onset of AN and BN concerned close relationships with family and friends with problems with sexuality specific in triggering the onset of AN.[49]

Learning theorists view eating disorders as evolving out of classical or operant conditioning, such that maladaptive learned responses are formed by efforts to reduce anxiety and other aversive emotions. Negative reinforcement influences eating-disorder behaviors to a large extent. Engaging in restrictive dieting or binge-eating behavior may reduce or distract one from unwanted emotions and stress. The guilt, shame, fear of weight gain, and other feelings that result from binge eating are then reduced by the use of some form of compensatory behavior. Conditioning principles also may be used to explain the development of weight and body image concerns, specific food avoidance and ritualistic eating behaviors secondary to trauma, and feelings of being out of control. Most often, eating-disorder patients reveal a strong need to feel in control of their lives, which somehow gets confused with maladaptive attempts to control one's food intake and weight. Eating-disorder patients are also more sensitized to their weight, shape, and size. The subsequent dietary restrictions that take place can be highly reinforcing. Reinforcement may come from significant others and peers who make comments about the change in the appearance of the afflicted. Additionally, reinforcement may come from within the person through the realization of changes in weight, shape, and size, and through the negative reinforcement process outlined above. Patients with eating disorders also typically struggle with cognitive distortions (dichotomous thinking, overgeneralization, personalization, etc.) that develop in response to low self-esteem, anxiety about one's physical appearance, and other negative core beliefs.

Because of the great gender disparity in the incidence of eating disorders, several *feminist* explanations for the etiology of the eating disorders have been developed that emphasize the role of various *social* and *cultural* influences (e.g., diet, fitness, food, fashion, entertainment, cosmetic, and advertising industries). These influences exert strong pressure on women, especially at the onset of puberty, to be thin at all costs. Other common transitions, such as a new school or job, moves, going off to college, death, marriage, or divorce may trigger eating disorders. Concern about body weight and dieting is manifested among girls as early as the preschool years. Women are uniquely vulnerable to the *culture's* youth and thinness obsession because they are, more than men, judged and valued based largely on appearance. Bulimic women reveal a greater acceptance of attitudes and beliefs about the relationships between thinness, attractiveness, and success than nonbulimic women.[50] The Westernization of many countries, including Japan, China, and Fiji, is believed to have contributed to the increasing prevalence of eating disorders in those areas of the world. Western society's similar preoccupation with dieting, exercise, cosmetics, and cosmetic surgery also appears to contribute to the maladaptive behaviors exhibited by patients with eating disorders. When normal individuals are subjected to semistarvation, behavior becomes increasingly and obsessively focused on food.[51]

Another sociocultural variable is the societal expectation that women should be caretakers and nurturers while being self-sacrificing and others-oriented.[52] Schwartz and Barrett[53] suggested that the processes of starvation and purging behavior cause a "numbing effect" that helps the person to deny their feelings, needs, desires, and hunger so that others can be served and satisfied. They also hypothesized that eating disorders have given women a sense of power and control in their lives while they struggle to satisfy society's recommendation to be passive and dependent.

It is also helpful to consider the *family* system as a whole rather than focusing on the individual patient.[54,55] In fact, in my own practice, families of eating-disordered adolescents are advised that they will need to be involved in their teens' treatment as part of the initial informed consent to treatment. Whether the dysfunctional family patterns have caused the eating disorders or the individuals with the eating disorders have contributed to the pathology seen in the family remains unclear. Minuchin, Rosman, and Baker[54] reported a number of characteristics of eating-disorder families that contribute to the onset and maintenance of the disorder, including enmeshment, overprotectiveness, rigidity, lack of conflict resolution/conflict avoidance, and a pattern by which the symptomatic child diverts marital conflict. Selvini-Palazzoli and Viaro[55] reported that families of AN patients follow a six-stage process by which the patient, usually a daughter, plays out a covert game of switching coalitions between herself and her parents throughout the developmental process. This ultimately results in the daughter perceiving power through her illness and a return to the privileged and overindulged status of her childhood. Other researchers[56,57] have reported unhealthy coalitions formed between the anorexic patient and a parent, with the eating-disorder patient being placed in the role of a parentified child. Root, Fallon, and Friedrich[58] have theorized that the normal adolescent processes of separation and individuation and the establishment of autonomy are adversely affected in bulimic families. They suggested that three different kinds of bulimic families (perfect, overprotective, and chaotic) exist that are different across a number of dimensions, including boundary problems, difficulties with affective expression, parental control or lack thereof, trust issues, enmeshment or isolation, and the function of the eating-disorder symptoms within the family system. There is a strong emphasis on weight and appearance in these families. The aforementioned increased rates of mood disorders and substance use found among relatives of eating-disorder patients also implies that the family environment plays a role in the etiology of eating disorders.

PATTERNS OF ONSET AND SUBSEQUENT COURSE OF THE EATING DISORDERS

AN typically starts with an attempt at dieting during the teenage years that evolves into more severe dietary restriction that becomes increasingly out of control. Sometimes, the dieting behavior is in response to an overweight status, while other times the dieting is not indicated by one's health status or physical appearance. Some people experience the reinforcement cited above and the dedication to food restriction proves short lived as they relax their rules and normalize their behaviors. For others, the commitment to food restriction exacerbates, leading to other associated features, including social avoidance and distress, rigidity, obsessiveness, and mood swings. Further problems eventually develop in the form of increasing social isolation, adverse physical effects, and possibly compromised attendance and productivity at school or work. A much smaller number of patients begin to struggle with AN following a variety of illnesses that result in weight loss or through initial bulimic behavior. Others may experience a significant life stressor, teasing or bullying about weight, or general maturity fears prior to the onset of AN. Rarely do patients seek treatment on their own, especially in the case of younger persons. Rather, they are typically brought in for treatment after concerned family members, teachers, coworkers, or medical staff insist they begin treatment after recognizing the weight loss, or in the case of younger patients, delayed puberty or stunted growth. Physicians play an important role in this process, as they are most often the first professional that assesses the situation.

BN typically develops at a later age of onset as compared to AN. In fact, BN follows a period of anorexia in about 25% of cases.[59] Similar to the development of AN, a period of dietary restriction initially takes place. However, the restraint cannot be continued, and it is disrupted by episodes of eating, overeating, and eventually binge eating. This process evolves out of a number of physiological and psychological factors, and the eating is followed by a compensatory strategy in an effort to decrease the effect of the eating on one's weight. Foods consumed during these binges typically include those foods the person tries to avoid; this behavior pattern of restricting and conversely binge eating evolves into a vicious cycle. At this point, these behaviors begin to dominate the person's consciousness and these thoughts extend to distracting thoughts about food, shopping, eating, purging, hiding the behaviors from others, and being careful not to be caught. The binge-eating and purging behaviors eventually become planned and the air of secrecy, shame, and guilt contribute to greater social withdrawal and interpersonal conflict, mood swings, and poor impulse control. As is the case with anorexics that are hesitant to eat properly, bulimic patients are often, at best, ambivalent about treatment because of the fear that they will be forced to stop from compensating for their binges and left to deal with too much weight gain.

Prognostic indicators for the eating disorders include age at onset, length of illness, duration of follow-up, severity of weight loss, premorbid childhood obesity, low self-esteem, the presence of binge eating and purging, and comorbid personality disorders.[60–63] Many people with AN and BN are not active in treatment. A comprehensive review of the literature reported by Steinhausen[60] showed that less than 50% of patients with AN recover on average, whereas one third show some improvement, and 20% remain chronically ill. Similarly, Hsu[64] reported that about 50% of patients with BN can be expected to be asymptomatic two to 10 years after comprehensive treatment. Thirty percent will show some form of partial recovery, and 20% are likely to continue with symptoms that meet full criteria for BN. AN may result in death, with the primary causes related to either physical complications or suicide. The mortality rate for AN has been estimated to be about 9.6%.[65] It has been difficult to determine the mortality rate for BN, but it may be higher than in the matched general population.[64] This difficulty could be primarily due to the secrecy that accompanies the disorder.

COMORBID PSYCHIATRIC CONDITIONS

Eating disorders are commonly associated with many other psychiatric conditions, with mood, anxiety, and personality disorders appearing to be the most common forms of comorbidity (Table 56.7). The lifetime prevalence of major depressive disorder ranges from 50 to 71% in AN and above 60% in BN.[39,66–68] Anxiety disorders have been shown to have a lifetime prevalence from 33 to 72% in patients with AN and 41 to 75% in BN patients.[68–71] AN patients tend to develop eating disorders first and then develop comorbidity, whereas patients with BN tend to manifest mood disorders or anxiety disorders prior to the onset of the eating disorder. Forty-six percent of women who met criteria for BED had a lifetime history of a substance use disorder and 71.4% had a lifetime history of a mood disorder. The substance-use subtype was associated with a greater impulsivity and frequency of binge-eating episodes, and the mood disorder subtype reported greater distress, more psychopathology, lower self-esteem, less dietary restraint and more frequent binge eating, and a greater trauma and abuse history.[72] It is unclear whether psychiatric comorbidity precedes or follows the onset of BED.

OTHER IDENTIFIED PROBLEMS IN PATIENTS WITH EATING DISORDERS

Other common problems typically found among patients with eating disorders are listed in Table 56.8. They should be evaluated and targeted during treatment if present, as they may contribute to the development and maintenance of the eating disorder,

---

TABLE 56.7
Common Comorbid Psychiatric Conditions Found in Patients with Eating Disorders

Mood disorders	Major depressive disorder
	Dysthymic disorder
	Mood disorder due to general medical condition
Anxiety disorders	Posttraumatic stress disorder
	Obsessive-compulsive disorder
	Generalized anxiety disorder
	Social phobia
	Panic disorder
Personality disorders	Cluster B (borderline, histrionic, and narcissistic)
	Cluster C (dependent, passive-aggressive, avoidant, and obsessive compulsive)
Substance abuse and dependence	
Adjustment disorders	

TABLE 56.8
Other Identified Problems Commonly Found Among Patients with Eating Disorders

Perfectionism	Obsessive-compulsive traits
Narcissism	Maturity fears
Low self-esteem	Low self-efficacy
Control issues	Cognitive distortions
Alexithymia	Poor interoceptive awareness
Relationship problems	Feelings of detachment
Social avoidance and distress	Fear of negative evaluation
Interpersonal distrust and conflict	Mood swings/irritability
Poor emotional regulation	Poor distress tolerance
Impulsivity	Sensation seeking
Intense and self-destructive anger	Self-harming behavior
Shame and guilt	Family dysfunction
Emotional, physical, or sexual abuse	Unwanted sexual experience

---

as well as reoccurrence. Many patients experience the struggle between being the model child or conforming to others' rules and expectations and wanting to act out in an irresponsible or oppositional manner. AN patients may strive for and attain high academic achievements, while others, particularly BN patients, may experience academic difficulties. Patients may have a wide range of feelings and attitudes about their sexuality and sexual behavior, including anxiety (more often found in AN) or sexual promiscuity (more often found in BN).

BIOPSYCHOSOCIAL ASSESSMENT

Given the numerous causes and factors that lead to the onset and maintenance of the eating disorders, a comprehensive biopsychosocial assessment should be conducted by several members of an interdisciplinary team with various areas of expertise. Table 56.9 outlines the areas considered most important during the assessment process.

INTERVIEW WITH REFERRAL SOURCE

Concerned parents, a spouse, relatives, friends, or a primary care physician identify most patients; interviewing the referral source is the first step in the assessment process. The practitioner may be better able to communicate understanding, concern, and empathy, and develop better trust with a new or prospective patient if pertinent information is used appropriately. This process will be discussed further later in this section.

TABLE 56.9
Biopsychosocial Assessment of the
Eating Disorders

Interview with referral source
Assessment of the patient's motivation for treatment
Medical evaluation
Nutritional assessment
Clinical interview
Psychological testing
Behavioral assessment
Body image assessment
Interview with family members/significant others

Assessment of the Patient's Motivation for Treatment

The patient's motivation for seeking treatment and her probable stage of readiness for change[73,74] should be considered. A patient may be in the precontemplation, contemplation, preparation, or action stage of change; attempts should be made to reach the patient within their identified stage. It is important for the patient, especially the AN patient, to feel that she has some control over the treatment process, although compulsory treatment for AN appears equally effective (in terms of amount of weight gain) when compared to voluntary treatment. The weight gain may take longer for patients receiving compulsory treatment, and their mortality rate is higher.[75]

Medical Evaluation

Nonpsychiatric physicians, especially pediatricians, family physicians, gynecologists, internists, and gastroenterologists and physician's assistants play a valuable role in the prevention, early detection, and management of patients suspected of eating disorders.[5] The patient should receive a comprehensive medical evaluation. This evaluation should include a complete history and physical exam, laboratory tests (electrolytes, complete blood count with differential, urinalysis, blood urea nitrogen (BUN), creatinine, glucose, albumin, prealbumin, and thyroid and liver function tests), and an electrocardiogram. Consideration also should be given to determining cholesterol, magnesium, calcium, amylase, liver enzymes, muscle enzymes, and performing bone densitometry and a drug screen.

Symptoms and Signs of AN

Most of the physical signs and symptoms of AN reflect an adaptation to semistarvation. Growth arrest may occur if starvation precedes epiphyseal closure. A reduction in breast tissue is common. Decreases in catecholamine, thyroid, and insulin levels are responsible for the reductions in metabolic rate, pulse rate, blood pressure, respiratory rate, oxygen consumption, carbon dioxide production, cardiac output, hypothermia, cold intolerance, dry skin, dry hair and hair loss, hypercarotenemia, hypercholesterolemia, prolongation of ankle reflexes, slowed gastric motility, and constipation. Along with emaciation, brain and myocardial atrophy may be present. The latter may produce mitral valve prolapse, which is reversible with weight gain. The QT interval on the electrocardiogram may be prolonged. Other cardiac signs may include U waves, left ventricular changes, decreased mass, and decreased cavity size. Cardiac arrest may occur in 5 to 15% of cases. Neurological signs include peripheral neuropathy, increased ventricular-brain ratio, and metabolic encephalopathy. Volume deficits in gray matter may persist in spite of weight restoration. The hypothalamic-gonadal axis response to energy deprivation decreases gonadotropic hormones [leuteotropic hormone (LH), follicle stimulating hormone (FSH)], testosterone, and estrogen resulting in lanugo hair, anovulation, amenorrhea, infertility, reduced libido, and decreased bone density. Hyperadrenocorticism may also be a consequence. Other signs of diffuse hypothalamic dysfunction are altered fluid balance (edema, dehydration, headaches, dizziness, and syncope) and abnormal thermoregulation (hypothermia, defective shivering, and inadequate response to heat and cold exposure). Nonspecific findings include abdominal distress, bloating, delayed gastric emptying, slowed gastrointestinal transit time, anemia, and kidney dysfunction. Osteopenia, osteoporosis and stress fractures may result from both malnutrition and estrogen deficiency. Signs of micronutrient deficiencies such as Wernicke's syndrome, night blindness, scurvy, etc., may develop in occasional patients. Laboratory abnormalities include anemia, leukopenia, thrombocytopenia, hypercortisolemia, elevated BUN, hypo- or hypernatremia, hypo- or hyperkalemia, hypochloremia, hypomagnesemia, hypophosphatemia, hypozinemia, hypoglycemia, ketoacidosis, abnormal liver functions, low T_4, lower T_3, and elevated amylase. Increased bruising is common in chronic anorexics and lethargy in the end stage of the illness is apparent. Hyponatremia may be an unfortunate and tragic consequence of water loading in an effort to artificially increase one's weight to remain out of the hospital. If the patient participates in purging behavior, signs and symptoms similar to those of bulimia may also be present. Even in the absence of vomiting there may be significant dental disease (decalcification, enamel erosion, tooth decay, and gum disease) because the saliva is deficient in buffers and many of the low-calorie foods and soft drinks that AN patients favor provide an acid load. Wilson's disease, an autosomal recessive disease caused by spontaneous mutations in the ATP7B gene located on chromosome 13, can be confused with AN in adolescents and is fatal unless detected and treated before excessive copper accumulation in the liver or brain occurs. Among other symptoms, the teen may report abdominal pain, anorexia, depression, suicidal ideation and reveal menstrual irregularities, amenorrhea, and abnormal liver tests. It is crucial that this disease be detected early and treated properly.

Symptoms and Signs of BN

Body weight may range from underweight to any degree of obesity in BN, and significant weight fluctuations are common. Menses may become irregular. Binge eating may induce pancreatitis, disruption of the myenteric plexus, and rupture of the stomach. Subjects who are prone to reactive hypoglycemia may experience symptoms following binges. The method of purging determines many of the signs. Fluid and electrolyte disturbances may result from any purging method, whereas signs and symptoms of vomiting include swelling of salivary glands, sore throat, calluses of knuckles, tearing of the esophagus, esophagitis, hematemesis, muscle weakness (including cardiac), alkalosis, and hypokalemia. Numerous changes take place on the teeth and gums of bulimics, including tooth erosion and decay, changes in the color (graying, translucent), shape and length of teeth, increased sensitivity to temperature, pulp infection, and cheilosis.[76] Laxative abuse may produce disruption of bowel function leading to laxative dependence, cathartic colon, hyperchloremic metabolic acidosis, hypokalemia, and loss of protective mucus that may increase vulnerability to infection. Diuretic abuse may cause symptomatic hypokalemia with cardiac arrhythmias, palpitations, edema, muscle spasms, myalgia, and weakness. Laboratory signs include electrolyte imbalance (hypo- or hypernatremia, hypo- or hyperkalemia, hyperchloremia, acidosis, and alkalosis), elevated amylase (salivary or pancreatic origin), and elevated creatine phosphokinase. To the extent that semistarvation is a feature in bulimia, signs and symptoms are similar to those seen in AN.

Symptoms and Signs of BED

The major complications associated with BED are those associated with obesity, including Type II diabetes, dyslipidemia, joint pain, low back pain, muscular pain, gastrointestinal problems, shortness of breath, and sleep disturbance. BED may be associated with medical morbidity independent of the effects of comorbid states of psychopathology and obesity.[77] It is also important to note that there are many other medical conditions that might be confused with BED because of the presence of hyperphagia, such as Prader–Willie syndrome, Kleine–Levin syndrome, Kluber–Bucy syndrome, and hypothalamic tumors. However, these disorders are quite different from BED and should not be confused with BED.

NUTRITIONAL ASSESSMENT

In 2001, the American Dietetic Association released a position on nutrition intervention in the treatment of AN, BN, and EDNOS. It suggested that "because of the complex biopsychosocial aspects of eating disorders, the optimal assessment and ongoing management of these conditions appears to be with an interdisciplinary team consisting of professionals from medical, nursing, nutritional, and mental health disciplines."[78] Nutritional education and counseling provided by a registered and licensed dietitian, trained in the area of eating disorders, plays a vital role in the treatment and management of eating disorders. It is most important that the dietitian be aware of the specific populations at risk for eating disorders and the special considerations that must be considered when counseling these persons. The dietitian should also understand the likelihood of comorbid psychiatric problems that may make the counseling process difficult, boundary issues, and the medical complications that are typically present.

The nutritional assessment (Table 56.10) should include weight and diet history, nutritional knowledge, feelings and thoughts after consuming various foods, medication regimen, and the frequency and severity of various potential purging strategies. Signs and symptoms of macro- and micronutrient deficiencies should be assessed (see above). The patient's level of nutritional knowledge should be assessed; while many patients will be able to recite exact fat and calorie contents of many foods, they may not have knowledge of what constitutes a healthy diet or understand nutritional requirements. If valid, a food diary (time, place, type and amount of food eaten, mood, and level of hunger) will provide additional useful information to the therapist.

CLINICAL INTERVIEW

The clinical interview (Table 56.11) should include a detailed assessment of the disordered eating behavior (therapist should also get growth, weight and dieting histories, and information concerning compensatory behaviors) as well as comorbid conditions, family dysfunction, and other forms of pathology. The patient's body image is extremely important (image dissatisfaction,

TABLE 56.10
Comprehensive Nutritional Assessment

Growth and weight history (current, maximum, minimum, premorbid, and ideal weights)
Dieting history
    24-h recall of foods consumed (typical vs. atypical)
    Binge-eating behavior (frequency, types and amounts of food, and precipitating factors)
    Other behaviors (harsh/restrictive dieting, fasting, chewing/spitting/tasting, diet pills, overeating, and snacking)
Method, frequency, and severity of purging behavior
Physical activity patterns and exercise
Review of laboratory results (serum electrolytes, serum glucose, CBC, albumin, and prealbumin)
Review of medications and supplements
Completion of baseline food diary
Food surveys
Nutritional knowledge
Food portion size estimation
Interview with family members/significant others (if possible for validation purposes)

TABLE 56.11
Comprehensive Clinical Interview of Patient with an Eating Disorder

Functional Analysis of Eating Behaviour
Body image (overall, specific body parts and areas, dissatisfaction, and distortion)
Substance use and abuse
Sleep patterns
Sexual maturation/menstrual history
Mental status exam
Presence of comorbid diagnoses
Other identified problems commonly found among patients with eating disorders
Suicidal ideation/self-harming behavior
History of unwanted/traumatic sexual experiences
Complete developmental history
Medical complications associated with eating disorders
Medical history and family medical history
Review of medications
Psychiatric history (include details about past treatment) and family psychiatric history
Academic/occupational history
Assessment of relationships with family members, peers, and significant others

image distortion, image goals, ratings of satisfaction with various body parts, comparisons between current self and ideal self, and thoughts and feelings about weight, shape, and size), as is information about social status and support, work or academic performance, and information about other problems commonly found among patients with eating disorders (see Table 56.8).

PSYCHOLOGICAL TESTING

A number of psychological tests are designed specifically for the assessment of eating disorders and related problems, and are considered to be reliable and valid. A battery of psychological tests designed to assess the presence of other psychiatric diagnoses is also desirable. This includes objective measurements of depression, anxiety, personality disorders, substance use, and other diagnostic categories. However, nonmental health professionals may use simple screening instruments that take minutes to complete, such as the SCOFF[79,80] to get a preliminary data on suspected individuals.

BEHAVIORAL ASSESSMENT

Completion of food diary is important not only to assess the patient's baseline level of food intake, but also to determine various factors that may influence the restrictive dieting, binge-eating, and purging processes. Direct observation of the consumption of a meal helps the assessment process. Attention should be paid to the types of food selections, the presence of finicky eating behaviors, bite sizes, rate of chewing and swallowing, the duration of the meal, the amount of food and liquid consumed, and the patient's thoughts, and feelings present during the meal. Ratings before, during, and after the meal concerning hunger level, fear of weight gain, anxiety level, fullness/bloatedness, urge to binge, and urge to purge are helpful. Finally, pulse and blood pressure readings before, during, and after the meal might provide valuable information, given their correlation with one's anxiety level.

INTERVIEW WITH FAMILY MEMBERS/SIGNIFICANT OTHERS

Patients with eating disorders are not likely to seek treatment on their own and may falsify and conceal information about their food intake. Therefore, talking to family members or a significant others with permission from the patient can provide valuable information about the extent of disordered eating and purging patterns, the amount of weight loss, the patient's premorbid level of functioning and comorbid symptoms, the patient's family environment, and other potential contributing factors. It also is important to assess the family as a system in light of the aforementioned information concerning the families of eating-disorder patients. Table 56.12 provides a brief outline of family factors to consider.

TREATMENT

There is no single treatment regimen that is effective for all patients; optimal treatment must be tailored for the individual. Hospitalization is indicated in the presence of life-threatening malnutrition, severe psychiatric impairment, and overwhelming comorbidity. Less severe illness may be treated with partial hospitalization, outpatient therapy, or in rare cases, with a healthy peer or self-help program. A multidisciplinary approach involving a treatment team with a minimum of physician, psychologist, psychiatrist, and dietitian is highly recommended. With the increased research attention afforded to the eating disorders over the past two decades, evidence-based management of BN is now possible. However, there have been relatively few randomized control-studies regarding AN and EDNOS. Hence, clinical opinion and experience largely mark their treatment.

A number of factors should be considered in determining the most appropriate setting and form of treatment.[1] Inpatient treatment in a medical/psychiatric setting or an eating disorders specialty unit will increase the chances of recovery when compared to general inpatient psychiatric settings whose staff may lack the training and experience typically necessary to treat eating-disorder patients.[81] Inpatient treatment is considered necessary when the patient is exhibiting a number of medical, behavioral/nutritional, and psychological factors that together determine the patient to be a danger to him or herself or unable to provide adequate self-care; in the case of children and adolescents this would include parental inability to provide adequate supervision. Medical factors include a failure to comply with a minimum weight contract (<75% of ideal weight), orthostatic hypotension, bradycardia, tachycardia, an inability to sustain core body temperature, a life-threatening electrolyte imbalance/dehydration,

---

TABLE 56.12

Assessment of the Family of Eating-Disorder Patients

General functioning
    Emphasis on appearance and thinness
    Influence of social and cultural factors
    Emphasis toward outstanding achievement and perfection
    History of eating disorders or obesity among other family members
    History of psychopathology among other family members
    Physical illness among other family members
    Poor relations between patents, separation, or divorce
Impact of the eating disorder on the family system and its members
Impaired interactions/communication patterns between family members
    Enmeshment, triangulation, and unhealthy alliances or coalitions
    Overindulgence of the patient
    Separation/individuation and autonomy issues
    Independence/dependence conflict
    Poor affective expression
    Diffusion of boundaries
    Parentification of the patient
    Rigidity
    Chaotic environment
    Conflict avoidance or poor conflict resolution
    Difficulties in developmental transitions (puberty, leaving home, college, etc.)

hypoglycemia, and prior experience with the patient at a weight that required medical intervention. Behavioral/nutritional factors include the failure to abide by reasonable minimum weight contract, a rapid or persistent decrease in oral food intake and an inability to consume adequate diet supplementation, and an inability to refrain from excessive purging behavior. Psychiatric factors include the presence of additional stressors that contribute to the patient's inability to consume an adequate diet and significant comorbid diagnoses that warrant intervention on inpatient basis, such as suicidality.

Refeeding is an absolute requirement of the recovery process. The American Psychiatric Association[1,2] and others[3,4] have provided excellent guides for the development of a treatment plan, within various settings, that is determined by a number of patient characteristics and the severity of the illness. Hospitalization alone will probably not be enough for most patients, but is an important and often necessary first step in the treatment process that will need to include outpatient follow-up and possibly day treatment.

All treatment plans should include the goal of reestablishing a healthy weight (i.e., return of menses and ovulation in females, healthy physical growth, sexual maturation, and development in children and adolescents). Efforts should be made to increase patient motivation and commitment to the therapeutic process and facilitate ownership of a goal of "wellness." Nutritional education and counseling also is a necessary component of the treatment regimen. Efforts should be made to modify core thoughts, feelings, and attitudes related to the eating-disorder symptomatology, and associated comorbidity and other maladaptive behaviors should be targeted for change. Inclusion of the patient's family or a significant other in the therapeutic process is strongly recommended and is necessary when working with patients who remain in the family home. Treatment should only be considered complete after a period of extensive follow-up that is designed to enhance relapse prevention. For a thorough review of treatment methods, see Garner and Garfinkel[82] and others.[1-3]

MEDICAL STABILIZATION AND NUTRITIONAL REHABILITATION, EDUCATION, AND COUNSELING

The primary goal of inpatient treatment is medical stabilization with follow-up care provided within a partial hospitalization or outpatient setting. Fluid and electrolyte abnormalities should be corrected before implementation of refeeding, since these abnormalities will be exacerbated by the refeeding. Dehydration, hypo- or hypernatremia, and hypokalemia are common with any purging method, whereas alkalosis and acidosis accompany vomiting and laxative abuse, respectively. The refeeding syndrome is characterized by glucose and fluid intolerance, hypokalemia, hypophosphatemia, hypomagnesemia, thiamin deficiency, and cardiac insufficiency.[83] These electrolyte abnormalities may not be present prior to the initiation of feeding and may develop precipitously. In the face of malnutrition, cells are depleted in potassium, phosphate, and magnesium, and overloaded with sodium. As energy substrate becomes more available, the sodium pump rapidly restores the intracellular electrolyte levels at the expense of extracellular pools.

Standard medical therapy should be provided for pancreatitis and gastrointestinal bleeding. Symptoms related to gastrointestinal dysmotility improve significantly with refeeding.[84] Prokinetic agents improve gastric emptying,[85] but it remains to be determined if they affect outcome of the eating disorder. Osteoporosis is not rapidly reversed by weight gain or resumption of menses; the efficacy of estrogen or calcium supplementation remains to be determined. Patients should be referred to a dentist to repair damage and minimize future problems. Parotid swelling may persist for years after recovery[86] but is benign and does not require treatment.

The general principles of nutritional treatment include:

1. Education about the physical and psychological consequences of starvation or binge eating and purging
2. Encouragement to begin eating a healthy diet
3. Interruption of fasting, binge-eating, and purging behaviors
4. Initial weight stabilization with gradual restitution of a healthy body weight
5. Being comfortable with and eventually including all foods in the patient's diet
6. Recognition of appropriate weight and body fat proportions of a healthy body

Education also should include information concerning the body's needs for various macronutrients, sources of nutrients, recommended daily intake, and other pertinent information. Patients should learn about the food pyramid, food-portion-size estimation, food labeling, grocery shopping, and cooking techniques. Regular contact with a nutritionist is warranted, especially in the early stages of treatment. For AN, encouraging large portions and high-energy snacks is often counterproductive. Due to the low body weight and hypometabolic state, "average" portions of food will begin the weight restoration process. A minimum of 1200 kcal per day is suggested.

Opinions differ regarding the rate of weight gain and appropriate techniques. Increases in energy intake should be gradual to prevent refeeding syndrome (see above). Energy requirements during the weight gain phase may vary widely. In forced-feeding (parenteral nutrition) studies, the excess calories required per kilogram of weight-gain ranged between 5569 and 15,619 kcal, with a mean of 9768 kcal.[87] Subjects who were normal weight prior to the onset of anorexia gain less rapidly and increase their metabolic rate after a glucose challenge more dramatically than subjects who were obese prior to the onset of anorexia.[88] The thermic effect of glucose is greater in AN than in controls.[88] In subjects who have experienced growth-arrest, energy intake should be sufficient to support catch-up growth. Exercise should not be restricted, so that muscle mass can be restored.

In the inpatient setting, meals and subsequent bathroom access should be initially supervised. Programs vary in their flexibility regarding refusal to eat certain foods and the use of liquid supplements to replace food not eaten at regular meals. Ultimately, the meal plan should be well balanced, consist of conventional foods, and be individualized to some extent to patient needs. Multiple small meals may be better tolerated than three main meals. Efforts should be made to help patients to eat during three designated meal times, as this meal pattern will probably allow the patient to generalize her behavior to the home environment more easily. "Fattening" and "forbidden foods" should be gradually introduced into the diet. Aversion to fat persists in the recovered state.[89] Educating the patient on a meal-plan based on the exchange system rather than counting kilocalories is preferred to prevent obsession with the energy content of food. Weight should be tracked, but not overemphasized. Enteral or parenteral nutritional support may be required for life-threatening protein energy malnutrition (i.e., body weight <70% of ideal weight). Therapists disagree about the appropriateness of forced feeding, as control is such an important issue in most AN patients. It should be borne in mind, however, that severe malnutrition may impair cognition. If possible, patients should be allowed approximately 24 h to do as they please with their meals, after which time a supplemental regimen might be considered to ensure adequate energy intake. This will promote autonomy over the eating process for the patient. Refeeding should be done with extreme caution to avoid electrolyte abnormalities (see above), edema, and fatal cardiac arrhythmias. Since the initial energy intake recommendations in early phases of treatment are likely to be low, a multiple vitamin and mineral supplement is appropriate. If signs and symptoms of micronutrient deficiency syndromes are present, the specific micronutrient should be prescribed.

For BN and BED, initial therapy focuses on regularity in eating habits and stabilization in weight. Bulimic subjects tend to eat more fat and simple carbohydrate and less protein and complex carbohydrate than subjects without eating disorders.[90,91] Normalized eating with adequate protein and complex carbohydrate intake will reduce the risk of a binge being induced by excessive hunger. The energy content of a patient's meal plan should be determined by the Harris-Benedict equation. Patients have been known to respond better to meals if they are allowed to exclude certain high-risk binge foods from their diet early in the course of treatment. Following achievement of appropriate eating behavior, a healthy diet to achieve gradual weight loss can be implemented if appropriate. However, setting strict limitations on fat consumption only perpetuates the notion of "bad" foods, and may trigger binge eating.

PHARMACOTHERAPY

As of this writing, there are no "antianorexic" or "antibulimic" drugs available for the treatment of AN and BN. Pharmacologic treatment should be considered as an adjunct, especially in the management of comorbid behavior, e.g., depression, obsessive-compulsive behavior, and anxiety. For BN, psychopharmacologic treatment is moderately effective in treating the primary symptoms of BN. In the last several years, several systematic Cochrane reviews have been published that are specifically devoted to the review of treatments for the eating disorders. Bacaltchuk and Hay[92] reviewed 19 randomized, controlled trials in which antidepressant medications tricyclic amnies (TCAs [imipramine, desipramine, and amitriptyline], serotonin receptable inhibitors (SSRIs) [fluoxetine], monoamine oxidase inhibitors (MAOIs) [phenelzine, isocarboxazid, moclobemide, and brofaromine], and others [mianserin, trazodone and bupropion]) were compared to placebo to reduce the symptoms of BN in patients of any age or gender. They[92] concluded that individual antidepressants are effective for the treatment of BN when compared to placebo treatment, with an overall greater remission rate, but a higher rate of dropouts. Fluoxetine is approved by the Food and Drug Administration (FDA) for treatment of BN and the other SSRIs, such as sertraline[93] have shown promising results. Bupropion is contraindicated in the treatment of BN due to possible increased seizure activity in these patients.

The few randomized controlled trials evaluating the use of antidepressants for AN have shown that there is little evidence that antidepressants improved weight gain, other eating-disorder symptoms, or associated psychiatric problems.[94] Psychopharmacologic treatment is generally not effective in treating the primary symptoms of AN, but may help with depression and Obsessive-Conpulsive (OC) symptoms often present in AN. The depressive symptoms present in AN respond better to antidepressants after 85% of ideal weight is reached and adequate nutrition is maintained. The SSRIs, in particular fluoxetine, have appeared to work the best. Fluoxetine may be useful in improving outcome and preventing relapse of patients with AN after their weight has been re-established.[95] The TCAs should be used with caution because of greater risks of cardiac complications (arrhythmias and hypertension). Olanzapine, an atypical antipsychotic, has been shown to stimulate appetite and weight gain, and may help with the obsessive-compulsive symptoms and both anxiety and depression that are often found in AN.[96] However, the support for this medication has come from only case studies and open trials.

INDIVIDUAL THERAPY

It is important to establish trust and communicate empathy, support, encouragement, and understanding while also setting specific behavioral limitations. Once a therapeutic alliance has been established, the therapist must work toward moving the focus of therapy sessions away from discussions about the amount of food to be consumed, weight, and other specific symptoms, and toward underlying issues related to family dysfunction, relationship problems, low self-esteem, body image concerns, the patient's struggle for autonomy, identity issues, and other identified problems previously outlined. Therapists also should consider exploration of the developmental and cultural factors as well as the family dynamics that may have contributed to the development and maintenance of the eating-disorder symptoms. Many forms of individual therapy have been employed in the treatment of the eating disorders, including cognitive-behavioral therapy (CBT), behavioral therapy (BT), interpersonal therapy (IPT), feminist treatment, and various psychodynamically oriented therapies. Although each of these approaches may prove successful with eating-disorder patients, a combination of therapies may prove most helpful, especially as one considers the comorbid disorders that accompany the eating disorders.

CBT, designed to challenge the patient's irrational, distorted, and negative automatic thinking patterns and the negative core belief system, has become the standard of treatment for the eating disorders.[97] CBT is at least comparable, and often superior to, all other types of therapy for eating disorders, especially for BN and BED.[2,98] CBT emphasizes the self-monitoring of food intake and the identification of antecedent stimuli that elicit periods of restrictive dieting or binge eating and purging.[5,99,100] Patients are taught to identify stressful situations and the accompanying aversive thoughts and emotions. Ways to cope (problem-solving skills, cognitive restructuring, and other coping strategies) are emphasized. CBT also targets normalized eating patterns, meal planning, goal setting, cognitive restructuring, education about the eating disorders and related medical complications, and prevention of relapse. CBT appears to be superior to the use of medication alone in reducing bulimic symptoms. The combination of CBT and medication may prove even more beneficial, especially if the medication is indicated after consideration of any comorbidity.[2,13,98,101]

BT utilizes combinations of reinforcers (empathic praise and encouragement, access to exercise, visitation, social activities, and other privileges) contingent upon weight gain, appropriate food consumption, decreased purging behavior, and a general movement toward the display of "well" behavior. BT may prove helpful during the initial stages of inpatient treatment for AN. BT also may include meal monitoring, postmeal observations, exposure with response prevention, and temptation exposure with response prevention procedures. Specifically, patients are exposed to meals or binge foods and guided in their efforts to refrain from vomiting after food consumption. Research related to these methods has been equivocal.[1]

For BN, it is generally accepted that: 1. CBT is more effective than medication alone, 2. Antidepressants show greater effectiveness when used in combination with CBT and 3. Combining CBT with antidepressants has shown little consistent benefit over CBT alone[2,13]

Increasing attention has also been paid to the use IPT in the treatment of eating disorders. IPT[102] does not focus directly on the eating-disorder symptoms, but rather on the interpersonal difficulties, the patient is experiencing. It is believed that problems in relationships with family members, friends, and significant others contribute to the onset and maintenance of eating disorders, and that resolving these interpersonal difficulties will help to eliminate the eating-disorder symptoms. Working through issues of grief, interpersonal role disputes, role transitions, and interpersonal deficits are important aspects of this treatment. IPT may be less effective than CBT at the end of treatment for BN. After a 1-year follow-up period, CBT and IPT appeared equally effective.[100,103] Hay et al.[101] and Fairburn and Harrison[13] also suggested efficacy for the use of IPT for BN.

Psychodynamic therapies have been employed in the treatment of eating disorders since Bruch[47] first introduced her etiological theories for eating disorders. Although numerous case studies have suggested that these approaches may prove helpful, no controlled studies of the effectiveness of these therapies compared to other forms of treatment have been published.[97] Psychodynamic therapies incorporated into the types of therapy described above may be warranted in the treatment of patients who fail to respond.[97]

Very little data exists regarding the efficacy of utilizing a feminist treatment paradigm in the treatment of the eating disorders. Many therapists who specialize in the treatment of eating disorders believe emphasis should be placed on helping the female patient to identify the sociocultural factors that may have contributed to her struggle with body image concerns and maladaptive dieting patterns. It is important to consider the distribution of power in the therapeutic relationship and to encourage the empowerment of the patient through cooperative treatment planning.[104] Russo[105] has provided a detailed outline of principles to consider in treating patients from a feminist perspective. Feminist treatment emphasizes the importance of considering issues such as various forms of victimization, role conflicts and confusion, sexual abuse, the struggle for power and control, and general interpersonal relationships.[97]

TREATMENT OF BED

Although many individuals with BED have good short-term weight loss regardless of treatment modality, as a group they may be prone to greater attrition during weight-loss treatment and more rapid regain of lost weight. Current pharmacological treatments targeting toward binge-eating behaviors include antidepressants, anticonvulsants, and antiobesity agents. These classes of drugs have been studied in double-blind, placebo-controlled trials in BED. The SSRIs have been shown to significantly reduce binge-eating frequency and body weight in BED over the short term. Topiramate and sibutramine have also been shown to reduce binge-eating behavior,[106,107] promote and maintain weight loss,[106,107] and treat comorbid psychiatric conditions.[107] CBT and IT have shown limited efficacy in promoting weight loss and reducing binge eating.[2] Exercise may possibly augment the effects of CBT in the treatment of binge eating.[108] The addition of behavior therapy to aid in the weight loss process in BED patients has been shown to contribute to decreases in binge eating and weight loss.[98] Finally, CBT and IPT have proved equally effective in the treatment of BED.[109]

Family Therapy

Family therapy is a necessary component of the treatment regimen when working with a child or adolescent or an adult who is still living with his or her family of origin. The primary goal of family therapy is to facilitate the remission of the eating-disorder symptomatology and begin a therapeutic process of change within the family. Other goals include changing the status or role of the identified patient within the family, attempting to translate the eating-disorder symptoms into a problem of interpersonal communication and family relationships, expending the problem and taking emphasis off the eating disorder, and identifying other maladaptive communication patterns. Attempts are made to disengage the patient's parents from using the eating-disorder symptoms in a way that leads to further conflict avoidance, overprotectiveness, overindulgence, patient dependence, enmeshment, diffusion of boundaries, and unhealthy coalitions. Family members are taught how to more effectively express and tolerate strong emotions, and the patient's struggle for independence or need for increased dependence is acknowledged and addressed in family therapy. Lemmon and Josephson[110] has presented a comprehensive review of family therapy for eating disorders.

Group Therapy

Oesterheld and colleagues[111] conducted a meta-analysis of 40 group treatment studies, and concluded that group therapy is moderately effective in the treatment of eating disorders. Group therapies prove most helpful when utilized in combination with individual therapies and nutritional education and counseling. Group therapies have merit, since the group experience helps patients reduce the tremendous shame, guilt, and isolation often seen among these patients. Similarly, patients may benefit from the feedback and support provided to them by peers who will typically present with varying degrees of progress in treatment.[1] Group therapy may take the form of a process-oriented group that emphasizes working through difficulties in relationships through the interactions patients experience with their peers, or a more psychoeducational approach that emphasizes the acquisition and practice of new skills. Groups also may be designed to include therapies that closely resemble the types of individual treatment outlined above. Others may emphasize specific problems encountered by patients, such as body image problems, stress management deficits; and other specific skill deficits. A combination of these approaches will probably prove most helpful.

Although little research has investigated the efficacy of treatment programs that follow an addiction model, participation in Overeater's Anonymous has clearly helped some patients. Overeaters Anonymous is a 12-step self-help program, adapted from Alcoholics Anonymous, for people trying to overcome compulsive eating. Groups offer unconditional acceptance and support based on principles grounded in spirituality. Major drawbacks include lack of nutrition education, sometimes the restriction of specific foods (especially sugar and white flour), and lack of data supporting effectiveness.

Participation in group occupational therapy also may prove beneficial, as this type of treatment may help to reduce perfectionism and enhance a patient's self-esteem and self-efficacy.[1]

Physical Therapy

The basic goal of physical therapy is to develop regular moderate physical activity as part of a new lifestyle for the purposes of improving health, stress management, and weight management. Sedentary patients should be counseled about starting an exercise regimen, determining physical activity interests, picking an exercise regimen that will fit into one's daily schedule, setting realistic goals, addressing safety issues, methods of self-reinforcement, and anticipating and refraining from noncompliance. Other important topics include emphasizing improved health rather than weight loss, determining one's resting heart rate, maximum heart rate, and a training-sensitive zone, and the importance of finding an exercise partner. For BN patients who use excessive or obligatory exercise as a compensatory method and for most AN patients, emphasis should be placed on decreasing (but not eliminating) physical activity and exercising for the "health" of it rather than exercising to a degree that insures that there is an even trade off or deficit in energy balance.

Environmental Exposure

A treatment method often not considered involves exposing patients in graduated steps to environmental situations that they are likely to encounter outside of treatment. This would include activities such as taking more responsibility for refraining from purging behavior by operating without a postmeal observation period, and accepting more responsibility for adequate nutrition by going to the cafeteria and making one's own food selections prior to discharge from the hospital. Other activities might include grocery shopping, eating at a fast-food restaurant or the food court at the mall, eating with one's family, trying on clothes in a store, and any other behaviors the patient has avoided because of his/her eating disorder. Patients are guided through this process with the help of a therapist, and taught how to use cognitive therapy techniques, self-reinforcement, self-soothing statements, relaxation responses, etc. Patients have reported that this type of intervention can be helpful, but no randomized controlled trials have supported these ideas.

ACKNOWLEDGMENTS

Special thanks to Diane K. Smith, M.D., who had contributed to this chapter in the first edition of *The Handbook of Nutrition and Food*.

ADDITIONAL SOURCES OF INFORMATION

ORGANIZATIONS

AABA — American Anorexia/Bulimia Association, 165 West 46th St. #1108, New York, NY 10036, (212) 575-6200, www.aabainc.org

AED — Academy for Eating Disorders, Degnon Associates, Inc., 6728 Old McLean Village Dr., McLean, VA 22101-3906, (703) 556-8729, www.acadeatdis.org

ANAD — National Association of Anorexia Nervosa and Associated Disorders, Box 7, Highland Park, IL 60035, (847) 831-3438, http://www.anad.org/

ANRED — Anorexia Nervosa and Related Eating Disorders, P.O. Box 5102, Eugene, OR, 97405, (541) 344-1144, www.anred.com

EDAP — Eating Disorders Awareness and Prevention, 603 Stewart St., Suite 803, Seattle, WA 98101, (206) 382-3587, www.edap.org

IAEDP — International Association of Eating Disorders Professionals, 427 CenterPointe Circle #1819, Altamonte Springs, FL 32701, (800) 800-8126, www.iaedp.com

Overeaters Anonymous Headquarters, World Services Office, 6075 Zenith Ct. NE, Rio Rancho, NM 87124, (505) 891-2664, www.overeatersanonymous.org

BIBLIOGRAPHY

Professional Resources about Eating Disorders (compiled by USDA Dec. 1995). www.nal.usda.gov/fnic/pubs/bibs/gen/anorhpbr.htm

EDAP Reading List Resources for the Prevention of Eating Disorders (prepared winter 1999). www.edap.org/reading.html

ONLINE RESOURCES

www.mentalhelp.net
www.something-fishy.com
www.closetoyou.org/eatingdisorders
www.caringonline.com
www.gurze.com

REFERENCES

1. The American Psychiatric Association. *Am J Psychiatry* 157 (1 Suppl): 1–39; 2000.
2. Yager J, Devlin MJ, Halmi KA, et al. Guideline watch: Practice guideline for the treatment of patients with eating disorders, Second Edition. Arlington, VA, American Psychiatric Association; 2005.
3. National Institute for Clinical Excellence. Eating disorders: Core interventions in the treatment and management of anorexia nervosa, bulimia nervosa, and related eating disorders. www.nice.org.uk; 2004.
4. Beumont P, Hay P, Beumont D, et al. *Aust NZ J Psychiatr* 38: 659; 2004.
5. Yager J. In: *Clinical Psychiatry for Medical Students*, Second Edition, Stoudemire A, Ed., J. B. Lippincott, Philadelphia, PA, p. 355; 1994.
6. American Psychiatric Association. *Diagnostic and Statistical Manual of Mental Disorders*, Fourth Edition, Text Revision, American Psychiatric Association, Washington, DC, 2000.
7. Rosen JC, Leitenberg H, Fisher C, Khazam C. *Intl J Eating Disord* 5: 255; 1986.
8. Rossiter EM, Agras WS. *Intl J Eating Disord* 9: 513; 1990.
9. Eckert ED, Halmi KA, Marchi P, et al. *Psycholog Med* 25: 143; 1995.
10. Strober M, Freeman R, Morrell W. *Intl J Eating Disord* 22: 339; 1997.
11. Stunkard, AJ. *Psychiatric Quart* 33: 284; 1959.
12. Rogers R, Finno A, Gay J, Lemmon CR. Factors related to chewing and spitting in eating disorder patients. *39th Annual Convention of the Association for Behavioral and Cognitive Therapies*. Washington, DC, November, 2005.

13. Fairburn CG, Harrison PJ. *Lancet* 361: 407; 2003.
14. O'Reardon JP, Peshek A, Allison, KC. *CNS Drugs* 19 (12): 997; 2005.
15. Andersen AE. *Eating Disorders Rev* 4: 1; 1993.
16. Russell CJ, Keel PK. *Intl J Eating Disord* 31: 300; 2002.
17. Olivardia R, Pope HG, Mangweth B, Hudson JI. *Am J Psychiatr* 152: 1279; 1995.
18. Yanovski SZ, Nelson JE, Dubbert BK, Spitzer RL. *Am J Psychiatr* 150: 1472; 1993.
19. Frombonne E. *Br J Psychiatr* 166: 462; 1995.
20. Ricca V, Mannucci E, Mezzani B, et al. *Eating Weight Disord* 6: 157; 2001.
21. National Institutes of Health. *Binge Eating Disorder*, U.S. Government Printing Office, Washington, DC, p. 1; 1993.
22. Yanovski SZ. *Obes Res* 1: 306; 1993.
23. Hsu LK, Sullivan SP, Benotti PN. *Intl J Eating Disord* 21: 385; 1997.
24. Powers PS, Perez A, Boyd F, Rosemurgy A. *Intl J Eating Disord* 25: 293; 1999.
25. de Zwaan M, Mitchell JE, Howell LM, et al. *Obes Res* 10: 1143; 2002.
26. Latner JD, Wetzler S, Goodman ER, Glinski J. *Obes Res* 12: 956; 2004.
27. Grilo C, Reas D, Brody M, et al. *Behav Res Ther* 43: 629; 2005.
28. Powers PS. In: *Handbook of Treatment for Eating Disorders*, Second edtion, Garner DM, Garfinkel PE, Eds., The Guilford Press, New York, NY, p. 424; 1997.
29. Mannucci E, Rotella F, Ricca V, et al. *J Endocinol Invest* 28: 417; 2005.
30. Stice E. *Psycholog Bull* 128: 825; 2002.
31. Fava M, Copeland PM, Schweiger U, Herzog DB. *Am J Psychiatr* 146: 963; 1989.
32. Herholz K. *Psychiatr Res* 62: 105; 1996.
33. Lucas AR. *Mayo Clinic Proc* 56: 254; 1981.
34. Casper RC. *Psychiatric Clin N Am* 7: 201; 1984.
35. Goldbloom DS, Kennedy SH. In: *Medical Issues and the Eating Disorders*, Kaplan AS, Garfinkel PE, Eds., Brunner/Mazel, New York, NY, p. 123; 1993.
36. Frank GK, Kaye WH, Meltzer CC, et al. *Biolog Psychiatr* 52: 896; 2002.
37. Kaye WH, Frank GK, Meltzer CC, et al. *Am J Psychiatr* 158: 1152; 2001.
38. Kaye WH, Strober M. In: *Neurobiology of Mental Illness*, Charney DS, Nestler EJ, Bunney BS, Eds., Oxford University Press, New York, NY, p. 891; 1999.
39 Brewerton TD. *Psychoneuroendocrinol* 20: 561; 1995.
40. Geliebter A, Gluck ME, Hashim SA. *J Nutr* 135: 1326; 2005.
41. Monteleone P, Martiadis V, Rigamonti AE, et al. *Biolog Psychiatr* 57: 926; 2005.
42. Lilenfeld LR, Kaye WH. In: *Neurobiology in the Treatment of Eating Disorders*, Hoek HW, Treasure JL, Katzman MA, Eds., Wiley, New York, NY, p. 169; 1998.
43. Strober M, Freeman R, Lampert C, et al. *Am J Psychiatr* 157: 393; 2000.
44. Walters EE, Kendler KS. *Am J Psychiatr* 152: 64; 1995.
45. Woodside DB. In: *Medical Issues and the Eating Disorders*, Kaplan AS, Garfinkel PE, Eds., Brunner/Mazel, New York, NY, p. 193; 1993.
46. Treasure J, Holland A. In: *Child and Youth Psychiatry: European Perspectives*, Remschmidt H, Schmidt MH, Eds., Hogrefe and Huber, New York, NY, p. 59–68; 1989.
47. Bruch H. *Eating Disorders: Obesity, Anorexia Nervosa, and the Person Within*, Basic Books, New York, NY, p. 1; 1973.
48. Tozzi F, Sullivan PF, Fear JL, McKenzie J, Bulik CM. *Intl J Eating Disord* 33: 143–54; 2003.
49. Schmidt U, Tiller J, Blanchard M, et al. *Psychol Med* 27: 523; 1997.
50. Striegel-Moore RH, Silberstein LR, Rodin J. *Am Psychologist* 41: 246; 1986.
51. Keys A, Brozek J, Henschel A, et al. *The Biology of Human Starvation*, University of Minnesota Press, Minneapolis, MN, p. 1; 1950.
52. Killian K. *Fam Rel* 43: 311; 1994.
53. Schwartz RC, Barrett MJJ. *Psychother Fam* 3: 131; 1988.
54. Minuchin S, Rosman BL, Baker L. *Psychosomatic Families: Anorexia Nervosa in Context*, Harvard University Press, Cambridge, MA, p. 1; 1978.
55. Selvini-Palazzoli M, Viaro M. *Fam Process* 27: 129; 1988.
56. Yager J. In: *Family Therapy and Major Psychopathology*, Lansky MR, Ed., Grune and Stratton, New York, NY, p. 249; 1981.
57. Stierlin H, Weber G. *Unlocking the Family Door: A Systemic Approach to the Understanding and Treatment of Anorexia Nervosa*, Brunner/Mazel, New York, NY, p. 1; 1989.
58. Root MPP, Fallon P, Friedrich WN. *Bulimia: A Systems Approach to Treatment*, Norton, NY, p. 1; 1986.
59. Sullivan PF, Bulik CM, Carter FA, et al. *Intl J Eating Disord* 20: 253; 1996.
60. Steinhausen HC, *Am J Psychiatr* 159: 1284–1293; 2002.
61. Fairburn CG, Norman PA, Welch SL, et al. *Arch Gen Psychiatr* 52: 304; 1995.
62. Fairburn CG, Stice E, Cooper Z, et al. *J Consult Clin Psychol* 71: 103; 2003.
63. Bell L. *Eating and Weight Disord* 7: 168; 2002.
64. Hsu LK. In: *Eating Disorders and Obesity*, Brownell KD, Fairburn CG, Eds. Smith Gordon, London UK. p. 238; 1995.
65. Nielsen S. *Psychiatric Clin N Am* 24: 2001; 2001.

66. Iwasaki Y, Matsunaga H, Kiriike N, Tanaka H, Matsui T. *Comprehen Psychiatr* 41: 454; 2000.
67. Herzog DB, Dorer DJ, Keel PK, et al. *J Am Acad Child and Adoles Psychiatr* 38: 829; 1999.
68. Hudson JI, Pope HGJ, Yurgelun-Todd D, et al. *Am J Psychiatr* 144: 1283; 1987.
69. Schwalberg MD, Barlow DH, Alger SA, Howard LJ. *J Ab Psychol* 101: 4675; 1992.
70. Godart NT, Flament MF, Lecrubier Y, Jeammet P. *Eur Psychiatr* 15: 38; 2000.
71. Laessle RG, Wittchen HU, Fichter MM, Pirke KM. *Intl J Eating Disord* 8: 569; 1989.
72. Peterson CB, Miller KB, Crow SJ, Thuras P, Mitchell JE. *Intl J Eating Disord* 38: 273; 2005.
73. Prochaska JO, DiClemente CC, Norcross JC. *Am Psychol* 47: 1102; 1992.
74. Vitousek K, Watson S, Wilsom GT. *Clin Psychol Rev* 18: 391; 1998.
75. Ramsay R, Ward A, Treasure J, Russell GFM. *Br J Psychiatr* 175: 147; 1999.
76. Bishop K, Briggs P, Schmidt E. *Br J Hospital Med* 52: 326; 1994.
77. Bulik CM, Reichborn-Kjennerud T. *Intl J Eating Disord* 34: S39; 2003.
78. The American Dietetic Association. *JADA* 101: 810; 2001.
79. Morgan JF, Reid F, Lacey JH. *Br Med J* 319 (7223): 1467; 1999.
80. Luck AJ, Morgan JF, Reid F, et al. *Br Med J* 325: 755; 2002.
81. Palmer RL, Treasure J. *Br J Psychiatr* 175: 306; 1999.
82. Garner DM, Garfinkel PE, Eds. *Handbook of Treatment for Eating Disorders*, Second Edition, The Guilford Press, New York, NY, 1997.
83. Solomon SM, Kirby DF. *J Parent Ent Nutr* 14: 90; 1990.
84. Waldholtz BD, Andersen AE. *Gastroenterol* 98: 1415; 1990.
85. Stacher G, Bergmann H, Wiesnagrotzki S, et al. *Gastroenterol* 92: 1000; 1987.
86. Hasler JF. *Oral Surg, Oral Med, Oral Pathol* 53: 567; 1982.
87. Dempsey DT, Crosby LO, Pertschuck MJ, et al. *Am J Clin Nutr* 39: 236; 1984.
88. Stordy BJ, Marks V, Kalucy RS, Crisp AH. *Am J Clin Nutr* 30: 138; 1977.
89. Sunday SR, Einhorn A, Halmi KA. *Am J Clin Nutr* 55: 362; 1992.
90. Van der Ster Wallin G, Norring C, Lennernas MA, Holmgren S. *J Am Coll Nutr* 14: 271; 1995.
91. Hetherington MH, Altemus M, Nelson ML, Bernat AS, Gold PW. *Am J Clin Nutr* 60: 864; 1994.
92. Bacaltchuk J, Hay P. *The Cochrane Database of Systematic Reviews* Issue 4. Art. No.: CD003391. DOI: 10.1002/14651858. CD003391; 2003.
93. Sloan DM, Mizes JS, Helbok C, Muck R. *Intl J Eating Disor* 36: 48; 2004.
94. Claudino AM, Hay P, Lima MS, Bacaltchuk J, Schmidt U, Treasure J. *The Cochrane Database of Systematic Reviews* Issue 1. Art. No.: CD004365. DOI: 10.1002/14651858.CD004365.pub2; 2006.
95. Kaye WH, Nagata T, Weltzin TE. *Biol Psychiatr* 49: 644; 2001.
96. Brooke NS, Wiersgalla M, Salzman C. *Harvard Rev Psychiatr* 13: 317; 2005.
97. Garner DM, Needleman LD. In: *Handbook of Treatment for Eating Disorders*, Garner, DM & Garfental, PE, eds. Second Edition, The Guilford Press, New York, 1997.
98. Peterson CB, Mitchell JE. *J Clin Psychol: In Session* 55: 685; 1999.
99. Fairburn C. *Psychol Med* 11: 707; 1981.
100. Fairburn CG, Marcus MD, Wilson GW. In: *Binge Eating: Nature, Assessment and Treatment*, Fairburn CG, Wilson GW, Eds., The Guilford Press, New York, NY, p. 361–404; 1993.
101. Hay PJ, Bacaltchuk J, Stefano S. *The Cochrane Database of Systematic Reviews* Issue 3. Art. No.: CD000562. DOI: 10.1002/14651858. CD000562.pub2.; 2004
102. Fairburn CG. In: *Handbook of Treatment for Eating Disorders*, Second Edition, Garner DM, Garfinkel PE, Eds., The Guilford Press, New York, NY, p. 278; 1997.
103. Fairburn CG, Jones R, Peveler RC. *Arch Gen Psychiatr* 48: 463; 1991.
104. Sesan R. In: *Feminist Perspectives on Eating Disorders*, Fallon P, Katzman M, Wooley S, Eds., Guilford Press, New York, NY, p. 1; 1994.
105. Russo D. *Newsletter of the American Psychological Association of Graduate Students* 9: 3; 1997.
106. Appolinario JC, McElroy SL. *Curr Drug Targets* 5: 301; 2004.
107. Milano W, Petrella C, Casella A, Capasso A, Carrino S, Milano L. *Adv Ther: Intl J Drug, Device Diagnost Res* 22: 25; 2005.
108. Pendleton VR, Goodrick GK, Poston WS, et al. *Intl J Eating Disord* 33: 421; 2002.
109. Wilfley DE, Agras WS, Telch CF, et al. *J Consult Clin Psychol* 61: 296; 1993.
110. Lemmon CR, Josephson AM. In: *Child and Adolescent Psychiatric Clinics of North America: Current Perspectives on Family Therapy*, Josephson A, Ed., WB Saunders, Philadelphia, PA, p. 519; 2001.
111. Oesterheld JR, McKenna MS, Gould NB. *Intl J Group Psychother* 37: 163; 1987.

57 Alcohol: Metabolism and Effects on Nutrition

Carolyn D. Berdanier

CONTENTS

Alcoholic beverages have been consumed by humans since the dawn of history. They have been used to ease anxiety, to promote social interaction, and as a vehicle to dominate others. Ethanol, a two-carbon alcohol in beverages such as beer, wine, whiskey, gin, and other liquors, is the quantitative end product of yeast glycolysis. Small amounts can be synthesized in mammalian cells. Ethanol has an energy value of 7.1 kcal/g. Thus, ethanol is a psychoactive drug, an energy-rich dietary ingredient, and a metabolite.

It has been estimated that upward of 90 million Americans consume alcoholic beverages every day and that about 18 million people are addicted to its consumption.[1] Alcoholism is more prevalent in certain cultural groups than in others. For example, alcoholism is quite prevalent in Native American population groups. Alcoholism has profound effects on nutrient need as well as nutritional status. Chronic alcohol use of greater than 80 g/day for more than 10 years increases the risk of hepatocellular carcinoma approximately fivefold.[1] Excess alcohol consumption is associated with cirrhosis and also with an increase in risk for hepatitis C.[2–6] People who are addicted to its consumption are at nutritional risk as well. The mechanisms by which these conditions develop are incompletely understood but may include damage to plasma membranes, damage to nuclear DNA, oxidative stress, destruction of retinoic acid, and altered DNA methylation.

This chapter provides a summary of the metabolism of ethanol and its impact on metabolism and nutrition.

GENETIC ASPECTS

Alcoholism is a disease that may be a result of a diet–gene interaction. The dietary ingredient in this instance is alcohol; the gene is as yet unidentified. However, there is ample evidence in the literature that supports the concept that the tendency toward alcoholism is inherited.[7–12] Studies of twins reared by adoptive parents as well as multigeneration studies of families support this idea. An alcoholic is more likely than a nonalcoholic to have an alcoholic relative. At least 33% of alcoholics have an alcoholic parent. This has been observed in adopted individuals where the biological parent was unknown to the alcoholic and so the parent's proclivities were not taught. Studies of monozygotic (identical) and dizygotic (fraternal) twins indicated a high degree of concordance for alcoholism.[7] If one twin became an alcoholic, the other twin also became one if that twin chose to consume alcohol. The concordance was greater in the identical twins than in the fraternal twins.[7,8] Although scientists agree on the heritable nature of alcoholism, mutations in one of several genes have been proposed. Among these are the genes that encode monoamine oxidase, alcohol dehydrogenase, aldehyde dehydrogenase, aldehyde oxidase, and aldehyde reductase.[9,11] Polymorphic forms of these genes have been reported to associate with alcohol addiction. A cause and effect relationship has yet to be proved.

METABOLISM

Ethanol, once consumed, is rapidly absorbed by simple diffusion. The diffusion is affected by the amount of alcohol consumed, the regional blood flow, the surface area, and the presence of other foods. The different segments of the gastrointestinal tract absorb ethanol at different rates. Absorption is fastest in the duodenum and jejunum, slower in the stomach, ileum, and colon, and slowest in the mouth and esophagus. The rate of absorption by the duodenum depends on gastric emptying time, which, in turn, depends on the kinds and amounts of foods consumed with the ethanol. Certain drugs may also influence gastric emptying time and thus influence absorption. Complete absorption may vary from 2 to 6 h. The type of beverage can influence ethanol absorption. Ethanol from beer is absorbed slower than that found in whisky, which is slower than gin, and red wine. Pure ethanol is absorbed the fastest of all.

Once absorbed, ethanol is rapidly distributed between the intra- and extracellular compartments. This is because ethanol is completely miscible in water and thus freely travels any place water travels. The uptake of ethanol by the fat depots is minimal. Ethanol crosses the plasma membranes but, in so doing, changes them. When ethanol is in contact with a protein, it denatures it. Thus, large and frequent ethanol exposures results in damage to proteins both within and around the cells. The most damaged tissue is the liver, as ethanol, absorbed by the gastrointestinal cells, is carried directly to this tissue via the portal blood. Alcohol consumption can have profound effects on gastrointestinal function (see Chapter 60 and Chapter 61). While gut cells are damaged by the alcohol that passes through them, these cells have such a rapid turnover time (less than 7 days) that damage due to intermittent ethanol consumption is not as long lasting as the damage that happens in the liver. Liver cells, in contrast, have a longer half-life and, once damaged, do not repair as readily. Alcoholic liver disease is a major cause of death among those who drink heavily and are addicted.

Ethanol diffuses from the blood to the alveolar air so the ethanol content of expired air bears a constant relationship to pulmonary arterial blood ethanol levels. The partition coefficient is 2100:1. This means that 2100 ml of expired air contains the same amount of ethanol as 1 ml of blood. If the blood contains 100 mg of ethanol, the expired air will contain 232 parts per million (ppm). This is the basis for the "breathalyzer" tests for intoxication. Intoxication occurs at 150 mg/100 ml of blood, but most states prosecute drivers having blood levels exceeding 100 mg/dl. Some states have even lower levels (0.7 or 0.8 mg/dl) at which drivers are prosecuted.

Of the ethanol consumed, 90 to 98% is oxidized to carbon dioxide and water. The rest is excreted as ethanol in the breath or in the urine. The metabolism of ethanol is shown in Figure 57.1. The rate of oxidation is fairly constant at about 10 to 20 mg/ml. This indicates that the first rate-limiting reaction catalyzed by alcohol dehydrogenase is saturated at this level. This is a zero-order reaction. The average rate at which alcohol can be metabolized is about 10 ml/h (or 7 g/h). The ethanol in 4 oz of whisky requires 5 to 6 h to metabolize completely to CO_2 and water. One mole of ethanol requires 16 moles of ATP for its conversion to CO_2 and HOH.

While ethanol is distributed throughout the body, the liver is the chief site for its oxidation. As mentioned, the first rate-limiting reaction is catalyzed by alcohol dehydrogenase and converts ethanol to acetaldehyde. Alcohol dehydrogenase has broad substrate specificity.[13–16] It catalyzes the dehydrogenation of not only ethanol but also some steroids, shunt pathway alcohols, and ω-oxidation of fatty acids (see Chapter 7). Alcohol dehydrogenase is a zinc-containing enzyme, and it follows that excess alcohol consumption will have effects on zinc nutritional status.

Acetaldehyde, the metabolite of ethanol, is quite damaging to cellular proteins and part of the hepatic injury found in alcoholics is due to this metabolite. It binds covalently to protein, impairs the microtubular assembly and the mitochondrial

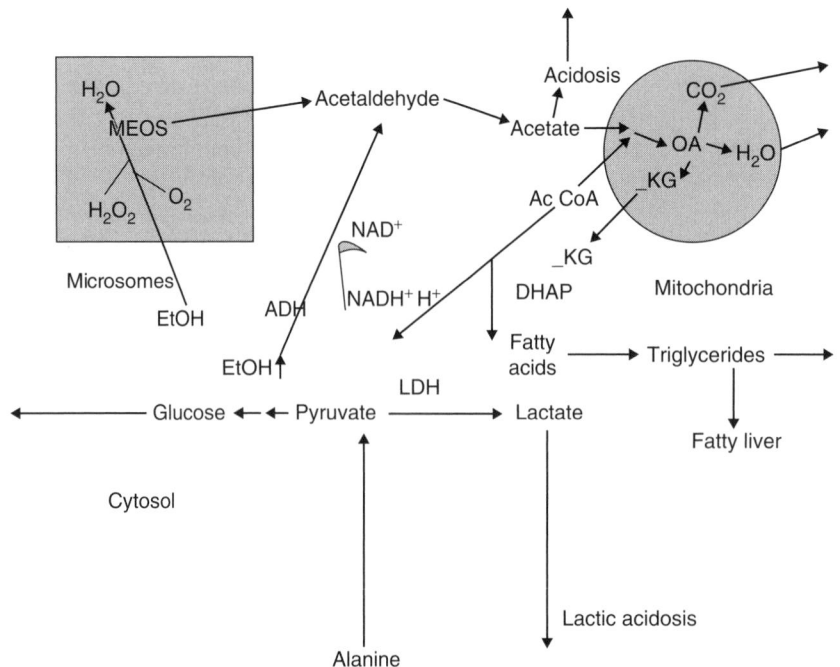

FIGURE 57.1 Metabolism of ethanol by the liver cell.

respiratory chain, depletes pyridoxine supplies (increases the amount of $NADH^+$), stimulates inappropriate collagen synthesis, and inhibits DNA repair. The excess production of $NADH^+$ disturbs the redox state of the liver cell and a number of metabolic disturbances follow.[13-16] These include hypoglycemia (ethanol downregulates gluconeogenesis[17]) and hyperlactacidemia (too much pyruvate is shunted towards lactate rather than being directed into the mitochondria for use by the citric acid cycle). This contributes to acidosis and reduces the ability of the kidney to excrete uric acid, leading to secondary hyperuricemia. The uricemia is aggravated by the alcohol-induced ketosis as well as by the discordination of mitochondrial metabolism resulting in a shortfall in ATP production. The increase in $NADH^+$ production promotes fatty acid synthesis contributing to hepatic lipid accumulation.[18]

Acetaldehyde is also produced when ethanol is metabolized by the microsomal ethanol oxidizing system (MEOS). This system uses peroxide (H_2O_2) and produces a molecule of water as well as the acetaldehyde. The acetaldehyde is converted to acetate, which can either be joined with a CoA or released to the circulation. If too much acetate is released, acidosis develops. Acetyl CoA can either be used for fatty acid synthesis or be shuttled into the mitochondria via carnitine to be oxidized through the citric acid cycle (see Chapter 7).

A fatty liver (steatosis) typifies the alcoholic and alcoholic liver disease is a major cause of illness and death in the United States. The fatty liver may progress to alcoholic hepatitis and fibrosis, to cirrhosis, liver failure, and death.[2-6,18] The fatty liver is due to accelerated hepatic fatty acid synthesis as well as due to an ethanol-induced impairment in hepatic lipid output. It may also be due to a downregulation by ethanol of the transcription of the gene for microsomal triglyceride transfer protein.[19] Alcoholic fatty liver is a pathologic condition that may predispose the liver to further injury (hepatitis and fibrosis) by cytochrome P450 2E1 induction, free radical generation (and subsequent cell damage), lipid peroxidation, nuclear factor-κB activation, and increased transcription of proinflammatory mediators including tumor necrosis factor-α.[3,20-24] Increased acetaldehyde production and lipopolysaccharide-induced Kupffer cell activation may further exacerbate liver injury. Acetaldehyde may promote hepatic lipid accumulation by impairing the ability of peroxisome proliferator-activated receptor-α to bind DNA, and by increasing the synthesis of sterol regulatory binding protein-1. Unsaturated fatty acids exacerbate alcoholic liver injury by accentuating fatty acid free radical formation. Polyenylphosphatidylcholine may be protective by downregulating cytochrome P450 2E1 activity, attenuating oxidative stress, reducing the number of active hepatic stellate cells, and upregulating collagenase activity.

Women who consume excess alcohol are more susceptible to the aforementioned sequence of hepatic changes and are, as a result, more susceptible to hepatitis C virus infection.[24]

There has been some research on strategies to prevent alcohol-induced chronic liver disease.[20] Vaccination against hepatitis A and B virus as well as the avoidance of nonsteroidal anti-inflammatory drugs, that is, aspirin, and herbal remedies (except milk thistle) that use the same detoxification pathway (cytochrome P450), is useful in this respect.[21] Weight reduction, if excess body fat is observed, and exercise can improve liver function.

NUTRITIONAL ASPECTS OF EXCESS ALCOHOL CONSUMPTION

In addition to the direct effects of ethanol on cell function, there are a number of auxiliary health concerns related to ethanol consumption. People who consume large quantities of ethanol find that their needs for thiamin, riboflavin, niacin, pyridoxine, folacin, and pantothenic acid increase dramatically.[13-16,22] The alcoholic frequently manifests symptoms of beriberi, pellegra, and other deficiency diseases. In part, this is due to the increased need for these vitamins when ethanol is metabolized and in part because alcoholics may choose to consume alcoholic beverages in preference to nourishing food. Those alcoholics who continue to eat nourishing food in addition to consuming ethanol do not develop overt deficiency diseases as frequently. Nonetheless, the nutritionist should be aware of ethanol-induced increases in the need for the B vitamins. In addition to these vitamins, alcoholics frequently may have compromised vitamin C status, folacin status,[22] and problems with their bones relating to inadequate intakes of calcium, phosphorus, and vitamin D. There may also be indirect effects on vitamin E status and selenium.[23] As already mentioned, there may be effects on zinc status as well as ethanol-induced impaired magnesium, iron, and copper status. The status of other trace minerals (see Chapter 8 and Chapter 64) may also be impaired.

Protein malnutrition has been observed in the hospitalized alcoholic.[24-26] Frequently, signs of severe malnutrition (see Chapter 39) are found. The patient may have a lower-than-normal height-to-weight ratio and a reduced muscle mass as assessed by creatinine height index. Those patients who consume adequate nourishment tend towards truncal obesity.[26]

Finally, there is another concern with respect to ethanol consumption. That is the development of fetal malformations in women who drink ethanol during pregnancy.[27] In 1973, eight cases of unrelated children were described as having similar congenital defects. Particularly noticeable were the facial malformations involving eye placement, and nose and mouth development. All of these children had mothers who were alcoholic. In a subsequent report, it was noted that alcoholism in mothers was associated with an increased incidence of spontaneous abortions, premature delivery of fetuses that were poorly developed for their gestational age, and infants born with respiratory distress syndrome. Many of these children failed to grow and develop normally with full intellectual capacity. Various learning disabilities (partial hearing or visual loss) also characterized these children. How ethanol affects fetal development, particularly the development of the central nervous system, is not known. Yet, awareness of the potential damage of ethanol to the developing embryo and fetus should dictate abstinence prior to and during the gestation period. To some extent, alcohol-induced folate deficiency may explain the effects on the developing embryo and fetus. Folate is particularly needed for DNA synthesis and for appropriate cell division. With alcoholism, folate deficiency, as mentioned earlier, can develop. Alcohol affects (reduces) folate absorption and hepatic conservation, and downregulates the expression of the gene for the folate carrier.[28] (see Chapter 55) Inadequate folacin status of women has been reported to result in spinal cord defects in the absence of alcohol; so it is possible that the alcohol effect on the fetus could be via an effect on folacin.

ALCOHOL DEPENDENCE AND RECOVERY

Alcohol addiction or alcoholism can be reversed if the individual abstains from alcohol consumption. One of the effects of alcohol involves the neuronal system, and progressive neurodegeneration is characteristic of the alcoholic.[29] One of the characteristics of alcohol withdrawal is the "DTs" (delirium and tremors). Once abstinence is continued, there is some reversal of the neurodegeneration. There are medications available to help the recovering alcoholic.[30] These include disulfiram, an aversive agent that has been used for more than 40 years; naltrexone, an anticraving agent; and acamprosate. Some serotonergic and anticonvulsant drugs may prove useful in this respect, but they have not been approved for this use by the Food and Drug Administration. Social support (the 12-step program of Alcoholics Anonymous) has been helpful in many instances of alcohol abuse.

REFERENCES

1. Morgan, TR, Mandayam, S, Jamal, MM, *Gastroenterol* 127: 87S; 2004.
2. Maddrey, WC, *Clin Liver Dis* 4: 115; 2000.
3. Jaruga, B, Hong, F, Kim, WH, et al. *Am J Physiol Gastrointest Liver Physiol* 287: G471; 2004.
4. Bhattacharya, R, Shuhart, MC, *J Clin Gastroenterol* 36: 242; 2003.
5. Serra, MA, Escudero, A, Rodriguez, F, et al. *J. Clin Gastroenterol* 36: 100; 2003.
6. Safdar, K, Schiff, ER, *Seminar Liver Dis* 24: 305; 2004.
7. Schuckit, MA, Li, T-K, Cloniger, R, Deitrich, RA, *Alcoholism: Clin Exp Res* 9: 475; 1985.
8. Devor, EJ, Cloninger, CR, *Ann Rev Genet* 23: 19; 1989.
9. Vanyukov, MM, Moss, HB, Yu, LM, et al. *Am J Med Genetics* 60: 122; 1995.
10. Thacker, SB, Veech, RL, Vernon, AA, Rutstein, DD, *Alcoholism: Clin Exp Res* 8: 375; 1984.
11. Holmes, RS, *Alcoholism: Clin Exp Res* 9: 535; 1985.
12. Deitrich, RA, McClearn, GE, *Fed Proc* 40: 2051; 1981.
13. Lieber, CS, *Am J Clin Nutr* 58: 430; 1993.
14. Faller, J, Fox, IH, *N Eng J Med* 307: 1598; 1982.
15. Lieber CS. *Medical and Nutritional Complications of Alcoholism: Mechanisms and Management.* Plenum Press, NY, 1992, 579 pgs.
16. Lieber, CS, Schmid, R, *J Clin Invest* 40: 394; 1961.
17. Siler, SQ, Neese, RA, Christiansen, MP, Hellerstein, MK, *Am J Physiol* 275: E897; 1998.
18. Purohit, V, Russo, D, Coates, PM, *Alcohol* 34: 3; 2004.
19. Lin, MCM, Li, J-J, Wang, E-J, et al. *FASEB J* 11: 1145; 1997.
20. Riley III, TR, Bhatti, AM, *Am Fam Physician* 64: 1555; 2001.
21. Weathermon, R, Crabb, DW, *Alcohol Res Health* 23: 40; 1999.
22. Cravo, M, *Am J Clin Nutr* 82: 3; 2005.
23. Dutta, SK, Miller, PA, Greenberg, LB, Levander, OA, *Am J. Clin Nutr* 38: 713; 1983.
24. Patek, AJ, Toth, EG, Saunders, ME, et al. *Arch Intern Med* 135: 1053; 1975.
25. Mendenhall, C, Bongiovanni, G, Goldberg, S, et al. *J Parent Enteral Nutr* 9: 590; 1985.
26. Tremblay, A, Buemann, B, Theriault, G, Bouchard, C, *Eur J Clin Nutr* 49: 824; 1995.
27. Smith, GN, Patrick, J, Sinervo, KR, *Can J Physiol Pharmacol* 69: 550; 1991.
28. Halsted, CH, Villaneuve, JA, Devlin, AM, Chandler, CJ, *J Nutr* 132: 23675; 2002.
29. Nixon, K, *Hippocampus* 16: 287; 2006.
30. Williams, SH, *Am Fam Physicians* 72: 1775; 2005.

58 Nutrients and Age-Related Eye Disease

Judith Moreines, Richard Cotter, and Leon Ellenbogen

CONTENTS

INTRODUCTION

Age-related cataract (ARC) and age-related macular degeneration (AMD) are the leading causes of visual impairment and blindness in older Americans.[1,2] Cataracts cloud the lens and impair the entry of light into the eye. AMD results in the loss of central vision due to impingement on the macula, which is responsible for absorption of short wavelengths of light. (See Figure 58.1 for anatomy of the eye.) Studies in animal models indicate a possible role for oxidative mechanisms in the development of both cataract and AMD. Available epidemiological data are generally consistent with small to moderate benefits for antioxidant nutrients in reducing the risks of cataract and AMD. These findings suggest that vitamins, trace minerals, and other nutrients with antioxidant properties can be of benefit in preventing the onset or progression of these disabling events. Nevertheless, large-scale randomized trials are still required to characterize the potentially important benefits of specific nutrients in reducing the risk of age-related eye diseases. The high cost of cataract surgery and the lack of effective treatment modalities for AMD, coupled with the evidence supporting oxidative pathogenesis that might be prevented by antioxidant nutrients, render it critically important to the public health to conduct additional randomized clinical trials to establish the role of these nutrients in preventing the risk of ARC and AMD.

ANTIOXIDANT NUTRIENTS AND CATARACT PREVENTION

Increasing evidence indicates that the antioxidant nutrients vitamin C, vitamin E, and β-carotene may help protect against cataracts. Vitamin C is 60 times more concentrated in the lens of the eye than in blood plasma. Other antioxidants, specifically lutein and zeaxanthin, have also been associated with a reduced risk of cataracts. Lutein and zeaxanthin are oxygen-containing carotenoids known as xanthophylls. They are abundant in the retina of the eye and found in high concentrations in the macula. These nutrients protect against oxidative damage, and act as blue-light filters.

Taylor was among one of the first to suggest that adequate provision of antioxidants from multivitamins might help delay the development of cataracts.[3] This hypothesis was quickly verified by Sperduto et al. in the Linxian cataract studies.[4] These studies

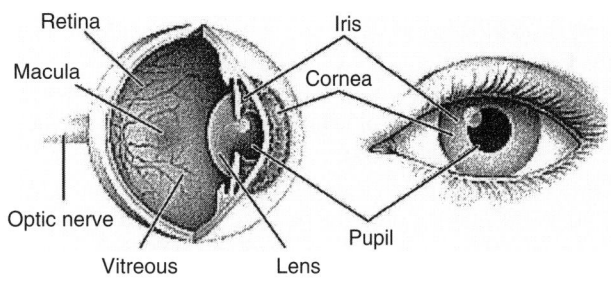

FIGURE 58.1 Anatomy of the eye.

showed that vitamin/mineral supplements, particularly niacin and riboflavin, may decrease the risk of nuclear cataract in an undernourished Chinese population. These were the first double-blind, randomized, well-controlled, long-term nutritional intervention studies using multivitamin/mineral supplementation to determine their effect on the prevalence of nuclear, cortical, and posterior subcapsular cataracts. Findings from the Sperduto studies suggested that vitamin/mineral supplements, especially the riboflavin and niacin components, may decrease the risk of nuclear cataract.

Results of at least two large prospective cohort studies are consistent with a possible benefit of antioxidants in reducing risk of cataract. In the US Physicians' Health Study I, researchers found that users of multivitamins had a 27% lower risk of developing a cataract (relative risk = 0.73; 95% CI: 0.54–0.99) and a 21% lower risk of having a cataract operation (relative risk = 0.79; 95% CI: 0.46–0.99) compared with nonusers.[5] In the Nurses' Health Study, women in the highest quintile for total carotene and vitamin A intake had a 39% reduced risk of cataract relative to women in the lowest quintile (relative risk = 0.61; 95% CI: 0.45–0.81).[6] The risk of cataract was 45% lower among women who used vitamin C supplements for 10 or more years (relative risk = 0.55; 95% CI: 0.32–0.96) compared with those using the supplement for a lesser time.

Additional analyses from the Nurses' Health study are consistent with the possible benefit of B-vitamins in reducing the progression of nuclear cataracts. In a subsample of women participating in the Nurses' Health Study, 408 subjects, aged 52 to 74 years at baseline, participated in a 5-year follow-up study of nutrient and supplement intake. The study demonstrated a direct relation between riboflavin (P trend = 0.03) or thiamin (P trend = 0.04) intake or duration of vitamin E supplement use (P trend = 0.006) and reduced the progression of lens nuclear opacification.[7]

Kuzniarz et al. (2001)[8] reported a protective influence on cataract of the use of multivitamins, folate, vitamin B_{12} supplements, as well as vitamin A supplements in an observational study known as "The Blue Mountains Study." In this study, 2873 Australian adults (49 to 97 years of age) received eye examinations and completed dietary questionnaires including use of vitamin supplements. Long-term use of multivitamins, vitamin B, or vitamin A supplements was associated with a reduced prevalence of nuclear or cortical cataract.

Leske et al. (1991)[9] evaluated risk factors for ARC in a large (1380 participants) case-control study. The regular use of multivitamins was associated with reduction in the risk of all cataract types (odds ratio = 0.63). Intake of riboflavin, vitamin C, vitamin E, and β-carotene reduced the risk of cortical, nuclear, and mixed cataract types. Similar results were found in analyses that combined the antioxidant vitamins (odds ratio = 0.40) or evaluated individual nutrients (odds ratio = 0.48 to 0.56).

Data from two relatively small cohort studies also support the association between antioxidant use and a reduced incidence of cataract. In a study of Finnish men with elevated cholesterol levels, those in the highest quartile of vitamin E intake had a three- to fourfold decreased risk of progression of early cortical lens opacities.[10] In the Longitudinal Study of Cataract, risk of nuclear cataract was reduced by one-third in regular users of multivitamins and by one-half in regular users of vitamin E supplements.[11]

Evidence is also accumulating to assist in characterizing the effect of individual antioxidant nutrients and their contribution to reducing the incidence of cataracts or slowing their progression. A number of epidemiologic studies have suggested an association between cataract incidence and blood levels of vitamin E or intake of vitamin E. These are listed in Table 58.1.

Several epidemiologic studies have investigated the association of vitamin C intake or plasma levels of vitamin C with the incidence of cataract. These are summarized in Table 58.2.

Although available evidence from observational studies generally supports an inverse association between levels of β-carotene, or vitamins E and C in the diet or in blood and the risk of cataract,[13,15,18,22–25] findings from randomized intervention trials have been conflicting. Studies using multivitamin and mineral supplements have been successful. In the Linxian Cataract Studies, Sperduto[4] reported that in two randomized, double-masked trials with a follow-up of 6 years, multivitamin mineral supplements significantly reduced the risk of cataracts compared with placebo in an undernourished Chinese population. In the first trial, a 36% reduction in the prevalence of nuclear cataract was observed in persons aged 65 to 74 years, who received the supplements. In the second trial, the prevalence of nuclear-cataract was significantly lower in persons aged 65 to 74 years, receiving vitamins containing riboflavin and niacin compared with those receiving placebo.

Participants in the Age-Related Eye Disease Study (AREDS) who wanted to take a multivitamin and mineral supplement in addition to other study products were provided with Centrum®. Sixty-six percent of the subjects elected to supplement with Centrum. The progression of cataracts was compared between subjects electing to take the multivitamin and mineral supplement and those electing not to take the supplement. In this quasi-randomized study, use of the multivitamin and mineral supplement was shown to significantly reduce the progression of cataracts compared with no supplement use.[26]

In the Roche European American Cataract Trial (REACT), 445 adult American and English outpatients with early age-related cataracts were randomized to daily treatment with a mixture of oral antioxidants (β-carotene, 18 mg/day, combined with vitamin C, 750 mg/day, and vitamin E 600 IU/day) or placebo for 3 years.[27] Progression of cataract severity was assessed. After 2 years, a delay in progression of cataracts was apparent among U.S. patients receiving the antioxidant mixture (p = .0001). After three years, a positive benefit of the antioxidant mixture was apparent (p = .048) in the entire cohort of U.S. and English patients. However, no significant benefit of vitamin treatment occurred in English patients alone, and the therapeutic benefit was significantly greater in the U.S. than in the English population.

TABLE 58.1
Vitamin E Intake or Plasma Concentration with Reduced Cataract Risk

Reference and Type of Study	Population	Endpoint	Risk and Associated Intake or Plasma Concentration of Vitamin E
Jacques et al. (1988)[12] Cross-sectional case control	112 subjects aged 40 to 70 years with and without cataracts	Plasma levels of vitamins E, C, and carotenoids	High plasma levels of at least two of the three antioxidants evaluated were associated with a reduced risk of cataract compared with low levels of one or more of these nutrients (odds ratio = 0.2)
Jacques et al. (2005)[7] Retrospective cohort	408 women from the Nurses' Health Study	Nutrition and vitamin intake	Geometric mean 5-year change in nuclear opacification was inversely associated with intake of riboflavin (P trend = 0.03) and thiamin (P trend = 0.04) and duration of vitamin E supplement use (P trend = 0.006)
Knekt et al. (1992)[13] Case-control nested within a cohort study	47 patients with cataract and 94 controls	Plasma vitamin E and β-carotene levels	Odds ratio for senile cataract risk was 2.6 (95% CI 1.0–6.8) for patients in lowest third of serum vitamin E and β-carotene levels compared with those with levels in the top two-thirds
Leske et al. (1995)[14] Case-control	1380 participants, aged 40–79 years	Plasma levels of vitamin E, iron, glutathione reductase activity (measure of riboflavin status)	Reduced lens opacities were associated with higher levels of vitamin E (odds ratio = 0.44 for nuclear opacities) and iron (odds ratio = 0.41 for cortical opacities). High glutathione reductase activity, which suggests low riboflavin status, was associated with increased risk of lens opacities (odds ratio = 2.13)
Leske et al. (1998)[11] Prospective case-control	764 participants	Vitamin E supplement use, intake, and plasma levels	The risk of nuclear opacification was decreased by one third in regular users of multivitamin supplements (RR = 0.69: 95% CI: 0.48–0.99). This risk was reduced by approximately 50% in regular users of vitamin E supplements (RR = 0.43; 95% CI: 0.19–0.99) and in persons with higher plasma E levels (RR = 0.58; 95% CI: 0.36–0.94)
Lyle et al (1999)[15] Prospective cohort	400 subjects, 50–86 years	Serum carotenoids and tocopherol levels	Serum tocopherol levels, but not carotenoid levels, were inversely associated with a 5-year incidence of nuclear cataract. Persons with tocopherol levels in the third tertile at baseline had a lower risk for cataracts at follow-up than persons with tocopherol levels in the first tertile at baseline (odds ratio: 0.4; 95% CI: 0.2–0.9, p = .03 for linear trend)
Mares-Perlman et al. (2000)[16] Population-based cohort	3089 adults of Beaver Dam, Wisconsin, aged 43 to 86 years	Type, dosage, and duration of supplement intake	The 5-year risk for any cataract was 60% lower among persons who reported the use of multivitamins or any supplement containing vitamin C or E for ≥10 years. Supplements lowered the risk for nuclear and cortical, but not posterior subcapsular, cataracts: odds ratios [95% CI] = 0.6 [0.4–0.9], 0.4[0.2–0.8], and 0.9[0.5–1.0], respectively
Robertson et al. (1989)[17] Case-control	175 individuals with cataract and 175 individuals without cataract	Supplement intake	The cataract-free subjects used significantly more supplementary vitamins C and E (p = .01 and 0.004, respectively)
Rouhiainen et al. (1996)[10] Prospective cohort	410 hypercholesterolemic Finnish males	Plasma vitamin E levels	Plasma vitamin E levels in the lowest quartile were associated with a 3.7-fold increased risk of progression of early cortical lens opacities (95% CI: 1.003–1.12) compared with the highest quartile (p = .028)
Vitale et al. (1993)[18] Prospective cohort	660 men and women	Plasma antioxidants (β-carotene, ascorbic acid, and α-tocopherol) levels	Plasma β-carotene and ascorbic acid levels assessed up to 4 years before evaluation were not associated with risk of nuclear or cortical lens opacities. Higher levels of plasma α-tocopherol were associated with a reduced risk of nuclear opacity (odds ratio for highest quartile vs. lowest = 0.52, 95% CI: 0.27–0.98, odds ratio for middle two quartiles vs. lowest = 0.55; 95% CI: 0.30–0.98)

In contrast, several other randomized intervention trials using pharmacological levels of β-carotene and vitamins C or E have failed to demonstrate efficacy compared with placebo. In AREDS,[28] conducted among persons at high risk for advanced AMD, a high dose of β-carotene (15 mg/day) was tested as part of antioxidant vitamin cocktail in combination with high doses of zinc (80 mg as zinc oxide), vitamins C (500 mg/day) and E (400 IU/day), and copper (2 mg as cupric oxide). The α-tocopherol, β-Carotene Study tested β-carotene (20 mg/day), alone and in combination with vitamin E (50 mg/day), in a population of heavy male smokers in Finland.[29] The VECAT trial was a large (1193 subjects), randomized placebo-controlled trial comparing vitamin E supplementation (500 IU) with placebo among an elderly population with or without early cataract changes.[30] These trials failed to show that supplementation with pharmacological doses of β-carotene, or vitamins E or C for durations of up to 7 years positively impacts risk of cataract during the period of treatment.

TABLE 58.2
Vitamin C Intake or Plasma Concentration with Reduced Cataract Risk

Reference and Type of Study	Population	Endpoint	Risk and Associated Intake or Plasma Concentration of Vitamin C
Hankinson et al (1992)[6] Prospective cohort	50,828 female registered nurses 45 to 67 years of age.	Dietary intake of vitamin C with eight years of follow-up	Incidence of extraction of senile cataract was inversely related to use of vitamin C supplements for ≥10 years (relative risk = 0.55; 95% CI: 0.32–0.96) but not with dietary vitamin C in a multivariate analysis
Jacques and Chylack (1991)[19] Case-control	77 subjects with cataracts and 35 controls	Vitamins C, E, and carotenoid intake and plasma levels	Subjects with low (<20th percentile) and moderate (20th–80th percentile) nutrient levels were compared with subjects with high levels (>80th percentile). The odds ratio of posterior subcapsular (PSC) cataract for persons with low-plasma vitamin C was 11.3 ($p < .10$). Low vitamin C intake was associated with an increased risk of cortical cataract (odds ratio = 3.7, $p < .10$) and PSC (odds ration = 11, $p < .05$)
Jacques (1997)[20] Retrospective cross-sectional	247 women, aged 56–71 years, without diagnosed cataract or diabetes	Lens opacification and vitamin C supplement intake for up to 12 years prior to assessment	Use of vitamin C for ≥10 years ($n = 26$) associated with a 77% reduction in early lens opacities (odds ratio: 0.23; 95% CI: 0.09–0.06) at any lens site and an 83% reduction in moderate lens opacities (odds ratio: 0.17; 95% CI: 0.03–0.85) at any lens site compared with women who did not use vitamin C supplements ($n = 141$). Use of vitamin C supplements for <10 years failed to reduce prevalence of early opacities
Jacques et al. (2001)[21] Prospective cohort	478 nondiabetic women (53–73 years) from the Nurses Health Study Cohort without previously diagnosed cataracts	Nutrient and supplement intake over 15-year period prior to follow-up	Prevalence of nuclear opacification inversely related to intake for vitamin C ($p < 0.001$), vitamin E ($p = 0.02$), riboflavin ($p = 0.005$), folate ($p = 0.009$), β-carotene ($p = 0.04$), and lutein/zeaxanthin ($p = 0.03$). After adjustments, only vitamin C intake remained significantly associated with prevalence of nuclear opacities. Odds ratio, 0.31; 95% CI: 0.16–0.58 comparing highest vitamin C intake to lowest ($p < 0.001$). The prevalence of nuclear opacities was significantly lower ($p = 0.004$) for women who used a vitamin C supplement >10 years vs. women who had never used a supplement (odds ratio, 0.36; 95% CI, 0.18–0.72)
Robertson et al. (1989)[17] Case-control	175 individuals with cataract and 175 individuals without cataract	Supplement intake	The cataract-free subjects used significantly more supplementary vitamins C and E ($p = 0.01$ and 0.004, respectively) than those with cataracts

Likewise, in two other trials that were conducted among 20,968 male physicians in the US Physicians' Health Study I[31] and among 39,876 female health professionals in the Women's Health Study,[32] supplementation with β-carotene (50 mg on alternate days in both studies) was shown to have little impact on the incidence and progression of cataract treatment. However, in both studies, analyses of subgroups indicated a possible beneficial effect of β-carotene supplementation in male and female smokers.

Exciting information concerning lutein and cataract risk has recently been reported from one prospective observational study in men[23] and one in women.[24] The risk of cataracts severe enough to require extraction were found to be inversely related to intakes of lutein and zeaxanthin. In these studies, those with the highest intake of lutein and zeaxanthin had a 19 and 22% decreased risk of cataract extraction compared with those in the lowest quintile (relative risk = 0.81; 95% CI: 0.65–1.01; p for trend = 0.03)[23] and (relative risk = 0.78; 95% CI: 0.63–0.95, p for trend = 0.04),[24] respectively. Lutein and zeaxanthin are the only carotenoids found in human serum that are present in the retina and macula,[33–35] as well as the lenses.[36,37] Hence, an association between lutein and zeaxanthin with risk of cataracts is biologically plausible.

In April 2004, a qualified health claim petition for consumption of Xangold® lutein esters and reduced risk of AMD and cataract formation was submitted to FDA. In December 2005, FDA denied the qualified health claim for Xangold lutein esters after having expanded the petition to include lutein and zeaxanthin. The denial was based on the conclusion that no credible scientific evidence exists to support this claim.[38] Although a total of 139 publications was provided as evidence to substantiate the substance–disease relationships for this petition, FDA discounted all the submitted reports for various reasons; for example, use of a nonvalidated surrogate endpoints, study involving diseased populations, reviews, and meta-analyses, animal, and *in vitro* studies. FDA agreed that, overall, these data supported a role of lutein esters, lutein, and zeaxanthin in the normal healthy function of the lens and eye. However, FDA concluded that although useful, these studies could not substantiate the required dietary intake of these carotenoids for reducing the risk of either AMD or cataracts in the healthy U.S. population.

In summary, the literature suggests that antioxidants, including carotenoids, may contribute to protection against cataracts. Continued assessment is needed to better elucidate the relation between specific antioxidant nutrient intake and the risk of developing cataracts. Ongoing trials are listed at the end of this section along with trials examining the role of nutrients in AMD, which is discussed below.

CAROTENOIDS AND AGE-RELATED MACULAR DEGENERATION

The macula is the part of the retina responsible for central vision and visual acuity. In primates, including humans, the central area of the macula is yellow due to the presence of "macular pigment," a high concentration of the carotenoids lutein and zeaxanthin. AMD occurs in about 20% of the population, is irreversible, and is the leading cause of visual impairment in the United States.

Supplementation with lutein has been found to increase serum levels of this nutrient, and also to increase macular pigmentation in healthy subjects.[39] Koh et al (2004)[40] evaluated the effect of a daily 20 mg lutein ester supplement in patients with early AMD and controls, in terms of both macular pigment optical density and plasma lutein concentrations. The response to supplementation by augmenting of both the macular pigment and the serum lutein levels was identical in both groups, showing that any potential benefits of lutein may be extended to those with AMD. The Eye Disease Case-Control Study[41] analyzed blood levels of antioxidant nutrients in 421 patients with AMD and in 615 controls. People with medium or high blood carotenoid levels had one-half and one-third the risk of AMD, respectively, compared with people with low carotenoid levels. Carotenoids analyzed were lutein, zeaxanthin, β-carotene, α-carotene, cryptoxanthin, and lycopene. There was no significant protective effect of vitamin C, vitamin E, or selenium.[41]

In contrast, other investigators have failed to demonstrate a relationship between serum concentrations of lutein and zeaxanthin and the prevalence of AMD. [42] In FDA's letter of denial for a qualified health claim for Xangold lutein esters, lutein, or zeaxanthin and reduced risk of AMD, FDA concluded that no scientific conclusion about the relationship between serum and tissue levels of these carotenoids can be drawn, because many known and unknown factors can alter these levels.[38]

Table 58.3 summarizes epidemiological studies of antioxidant intakes and plasma levels in association with the risk of AMD.

Recent data from a retrospective longitudinal cohort epidemiological study show that zinc is weakly protective against the development of some forms of early AMD,[49] although this effect is not proven.[45] Newsome et al.[50] undertook the first prospective placebo-controlled intervention study using daily doses of zinc 100 mg b.i.d. to determine its effect on visual acuity in subjects with drusen or AMD. Although some eyes in the zinc-treated group lost vision, this group had significantly less visual loss than the placebo group after a follow-up of 12 to 24 months.

TABLE 58.3
Antioxidant Levels and Intakes and Risk of AMD

Reference and Type of Study	Study Size	Findings
Eye Disease Case-Control Study Group (1993)[41]	1036	High serum carotenoid levels are associated with a 2/3 risk reduction in AMD
Seddon et al (1994)[44] Case-control	876 subjects consisting of 356 cases and 520 controls	Carotenoid intake in the highest quintile compared with the lowest quintile was associated with a 43% decreased risk of AMD (odds ratio = 0.57; 95% CI: 0.35 to 0.92, p for trend = .02) Among all carotenoids evaluated, lutein and zeaxanthin were the most strongly associated with a reduced risk of AMD (p for trend = .001)
Smith et al (1999)[45] Cross-sectional, population-based study	3654 subjects ≥49 years of age	No association between antioxidant intake from foods alone or foods and supplements and risk of AMD
Tsang et al (1992)[46] Cross-sectional study	166 subjects consisting of 80 cases and 86 controls	No significant difference between serum levels of vitamin E in cases and controls suggesting that AMD is not reflected in serum E levels at the time of diagnosis
van Leeuwen et al (2005)[47] Prospective population-based cohort	4170 inhabitants, aged ≥55 years, in Rotterdam, Netherlands	Dietary intake of antioxidants at baseline was associated with incident AMD after a mean follow-up of 8 years. Dietary intakes of vitamin E and zinc were both inversely associated with AMD. The hazard ratio per standard deviation increase of vitamin E intake = 0.92 (95% CI: 0.84–1.00) and zinc intake = 0.91 (95% CI: 0.83–0.98). An above-median intake of a combination of β-carotene, vitamins C and E, and zinc, was associated with a 35% reduced risk of AMD (hazard ratio = 0.65; 95% CI: 0.46–0.92)
West et al (1994)[48] Prospective cohort	976 subjects consisting of 226 cases	Plasma vitamin E levels in lowest quartile measured ≥2 years prior to assessment of macular status was associated with a twofold risk of AMD, suggesting a protective effect for AMD of high plasma levels of vitamin E

TABLE 58.4

Ongoing Trials Investigating Antioxidant Vitamins and Their Effect on Age-Related Cataract and AMD[27]

Trial	Study Population	Agents Tested
US Physicians' Health Study II[54]	Approximately 15,000 healthy U.S. male physicians aged 55 and older	β-carotene 50 mg on alternate days Vitamin C 500 mg daily Vitamin E 400 IU on alternate days Multivitamin daily
Collaborative Italian–American Clinical Trial of Nutritional Supplements and Age-Related Cataracts (CTNS) [55]	1020 men and women with no or early cataract at entry	Daily RDA dose multivitamin/multimineral supplement with a minimum follow-up of 9 years
Age-Related Eye Disease Study II[56]	4753 men and women aged 55–80 with no AMD to relatively severe AMD	High-dose antioxidants and minerals (β-carotene, vitamin C, vitamin E, zinc, and copper) or lutein and zeaxanthin or omega-3 fatty acids with minimum follow-up of 7 years

The Age-Related Eye Disease Study (AREDS) provides significant contributions to understanding nutrients potentially protective of AMD. AREDS, which was sponsored by the National Eye Institute, was a randomized, multicenter, double-blinded, placebo-controlled, prospective intervention trial designed to assess whether high-dose antioxidants and zinc, alone and in combination, would delay development of advanced ADM and cataract.[51,52] A group of 4757 subjects, aged 55 to 80, with various levels of risk for developing advanced AMD, were enrolled at 11 U.S. clinical centers and randomized to receive daily tablets of antioxidants (vitamins C, 500 mg; vitamin E, 400 IU; and β-carotene, 15 mg), zinc (80 mg as zinc oxide with 2 mg copper as cupric oxide), antioxidants plus zinc, or placebo. After a median follow-up of 6.3 years, the antioxidants plus zinc significantly reduced the risk of development of advanced AMD by 25% in participants at moderate risk of advanced AMD.[52] Comparison with placebo demonstrated a statistically significant odds ratio for the development of advanced AMD with antioxidants plus zinc (odds ratio = 0.72; 99% CI: 0.52–0.98).[52] When the analysis was restricted to those with the highest risk for progression to AMD, the risk reduction was increased to 29% for zinc alone compared with placebo (odds ratio = 0.71; 99% CI: 0.52–0.99) and 34% for the combination of zinc plus antioxidants (odds ratio = 0.66; 99% CI 0.47–0.91).[52] In contrast, as previously indicated, supplementation was ineffective in cataract.[28] Bressler et al. (2003)[53] has concluded that the reduced risk of developing advanced AMD following use of the AREDS supplements in persons at high risk for developing advanced AMD provides a significant potential public health benefit.

ONGOING TRIALS

While the majority of evidence suggests a beneficial effect of antioxidants against the development and progression of cataracts and AMD, controlled intervention trials are needed to more precisely define the protective role of antioxidants in preserving vision. Table 58.4 lists some ongoing trials.

REFERENCES

1. Klaver CCW, Wolfs RCW, Vingerling JR et al. *Arch Ophthalmol* 116:653;1998.
2. Klein R, Wang Q, Klein BEK et al. *Invest Ophthalmol Vis Sci* 36:182;1995.
3. Taylor A. *Ann NY Acad Sci* 669:111;1992.
4. Sperduto RD, Hu TS, Milton RC et al. *Arch Ophthalmol* 111:1246;1993.
5. Seddon JM, Christen WG, Manson IE et al. *Am J Public Health* 84:788;1994.
6. Hankinson SE, Stampfer MJ, Seddon JM et al. *BMJ* 305:335;1992.
7. Jacques PR, Taylor A, Moeller S et al. *Arch Ophthalmol* 123:517; 2005.
8. Kuzniarz M, Mitchell P, Cumming RG. *Am J Ophthalmol* 132:19; 2001.
9. Leske MC, Chylack LT Jr, Wu Sy. *Arch Ophthalmol* 109:244;1991.
10. Rouhiainen P, Rouhiainen H, Salonen JT. *Am J Epidemiol* 144:496;1996.
11. Leske MC, Chylack LT, He Q et al. *Ophthalmology* 105:831;1998.
12. Jacques PF, Chylack LT Jr, McGandy RB et al. *Arch Ophthalmol* 106:337;1988.
13. Knekt P, Heliovaara M, Rissanen A et al. *BMJ* 305:1392;1992.
14. Leske MC, Wu SY, Hyman L et al. *Arch Ophthalmol* 113:1113;1995.
15. Lyle BJ, Mares-Perlman JA, Klein BEK et al. *Am J Clin Nutr* 69:272;1999.
16. Mares-Perlman JA, Lyle BJ, Klein R et al. *Arch Ophthalmol* 118:1556;2000.

17. Robertson J, Donner AP, Trevithick JR. *Ann NY Acad Sci* 570:372;1989.
18. Vitale S, West S, Hallrisch J, et al. *Epidemiology* 4:195;1993.
19. Jacques PF, Chylack LT. *Am J Clin Nutr* 53:352S;1991.
20. Jacques PF, Chylack LT, Hankinson SE et al. *Arch Ophthalmol* 119:1191;2001.
21. Jacques PF, Taylor A, Hankinson SE et al. *Am J Clin Nutr* 66:911;1997.
22. Mares-Perlman JA, Brady WE, Klein BEK et al. *Am J Epidemiol* 141:322;1995.
23. Brown L, Rimm EB, Seddon JM et al. *Am J Clin Nutr* 70:517;1999.
24. Chasan-Taber L, Willett WC, Seddon JM et al. *Am J Clin Nutr* 70:509;1999.
25. Lyle BJ, Mares-Perlman JA, Klein BEK et al. *Am J Epidemiol* 149:801;1999.
26. Milton RC, Clemons TE, Sperduto RD et al. Age-related Eye Disease Study. Centrum use and progression of age-related cataract in AREDS: A propensity score approach. *Ophthalmol* 113: 1264; 2006.
27. The REACT Group. *Ophthal Epidemiol* 9:49;2002.
28. Age-Related Eye Disease Study Research Group 9th report. *Arch Ophthalmol* 119:1439;2001.
29. Teikari JM, Rautalahti M, Haukka J et al. *J Epidemiol Community Health* 52:468;1998.
30. McNeil JJ, Robman L, Tikellis G et al. *Ophthalmology* 111:75;2004.
31. Christen WG, Manson JE, Glynn RJ et al. *Arch Ophthalmol* 120:372;2003.
32. Christen WG, Glynn RJ, Sperduto RD et al. *Ophthal Epidemiol* 11:401;2005.
33. Bone RA, Landrum JT, Tarsis SL. *Vis Res* 25:1531;1985.
34. Handelman GJ, Dratz EA, Reay CC et al. *Invest Ophthalmol Vis Sci* 29:850;1988.
35. Handelman GJ, Snodderly DM, Adler AJ et al. *Method Enzymol* 213:220;1988.
36. Bates CJ, Chen SJ, MacDonald A et al. *Int J Vitam Nutr Res* 66:316;1996.
37. Yeum KJ, Talylor A, Tang G. *Invest Ophthalmol Vis Sci* 36:2756;1995.
38. CFSAN/Office of Nutritional Products, Labeling, and Dietary Supplements. Docket # 2004Q-0180) www.cfsan.fda.gov/~dms/qhclutei.html, 2005
39. Landrum JT, Bone RA, Joa H et al. *Exp Eye Res* 65:57;1997.
40. Koh H-H, Murray IJ, Nolan D. *Exp Eye Res* 79:21;2004.
41. Eye Disease Case-Control Study Group. *Arch Ophthalmol* 111:104;1993.
42. Dasch B, Fuhs, Schmidt J. *Arch Clin Exp Ophthal* 243:1028;2005.
43. Mares-Perlman JA, Brady WE, Klein R et al. *Arch Ophthalmol* 113:1518;1995.
44. Seddon JM, Ajani VA, Sperduto RD et al. *JAMA* 272:1413;1994.
45. Smith W, Mitchell P, Webb K et al. *Ophthalmology* 106:761;1999.
46. Tsang NC, Penfold PL, Snitch PF et al. *Doc Ophthalmol* 81:387;1992.
47. Van Leeuwen R, Boekhoorn, Vingerlin JR et al. *JAMA* 294:3101;2005.
48. West S, Vitale S, Hallfrisch J et al. *Arch Ophthalmol* 112:222;1994.
49. Mares-Perlman JA, Klein R, Klein BE et al. *Arch Ophthalmol* 114:991;1996.
50. Newsome DA, Swartz M, Leone NC et al. *Arch Ophthalmol* 106:192;1988.
51. Age-Related Eye Disease Study Research Group. *J. Nutr* 130:1516S;2000.
52. Age-Related Eye Disease Study Research Group 8th report. *Arch Ophthalmol* 119:1417;2001.
53. Bressler NM, Bressler SB, Congdon NF et al. *Arch Ophthalmol* 121:1621;2003.
54. Christen WG, Gaziano JM, Hennekens CH. *Ann Epidemiol* 10:125;2000.
55. The CTNS Study Group. *Control Clin Trials* 24:815;2003.
56. NIH Clinical Research Studies. Protocol 92-EI-0250. http://www.clinicalstudies.info.nih.gov

59 Nutrition and Oral Medicine

Diane Rigassio Radler, Riva Touger-Decker, Dominick P. DePaola, and Connie Mobley

CONTENTS

INTRODUCTION

The Surgeon General of the United States published the first-ever report entitled "Oral Health in America" in 2000. The intent of this landmark report was to alert the American people to the full meaning of oral health and its importance to general health and well-being. The report has five major themes:[1]

1. Oral health means much more than healthy teeth.
2. Oral health is integral to general health.
3. Safe and effective disease prevention measures exist, which everyone can adopt to improve oral health and prevent disease.
4. General health risk factors, such as tobacco use and poor dietary practices, also affect oral and craniofacial health.
5. There are significant oral health disparities among racial and ethnic minority population cohorts.

The overlying theme is that the etiology and pathogenesis of diseases and disorders affecting the craniofacial structures are complex and multifactional, involving an interplay and interaction among genetic, environmental, and behavioral factors. The major environmental factor in this interplay is diet and nutrition during development of the craniofacial complex, maintenance of craniofacial structure integrity, and suppression of subsequent microbial challenge. In fact, the two common dental diseases, caries and periodontal disease, both have vital nutrition and dietary components. Caries is linked to adequate nutrient intake during development of teeth and salivary glands and to the frequent ingestion of fermentable carbohydrates post eruption. Periodontal disease is generally considered to be caused by bacterial plaque residing on the tooth structure, but the inflammatory response can be modulated by adequate systemic nutriture. In terms of craniofacial disorders, cleft lip and palate are among the most common birth defects affecting humans and are linked, in part, to adequate folate nutriture during critical periods in craniofacial development, much the same way that neural tube defects are linked to folate nutriture. Importantly, the diet and nutrition relationship to oral, dental, and craniofacial diseases is much more extensive than those classic illustrations. For example, systemic disease resulting from infectious oral microbes is generally recognized to occur in patients with immunological and nutritional deficiencies such that individual host defenses are compromised, allowing oral microbes to gain systemic access.[2]

In turn, the oral, dental, and craniofacial tissues are the sites of signs and symptoms of about 120 systemic diseases.[1] Additionally, changing demographics suggest that an aging population will increasingly present medically significant oral problems.[1]

This section reviews the relationship between nutrition and oral, dental, and craniofacial diseases and disorders, the nutrient–tissue interplay, and, where appropriate, prevention, treatment, or intervention strategies using diet and nutrition. The section begins with an illustration of the burden of oral disease and proceeds to discuss chronic oral infectious disease (caries, periodontal disease, and others), selected systemic diseases, neoplastic diseases, craniofacial–dental–oral birth defects, and health promotion, health education, and behavioral change.

THE BURDEN OF ORAL DISEASE

Dental, oral, and craniofacial diseases and disorders are common, with widespread tooth loss typically due to caries and periodontal disease. Dental caries, in particular, disproportionately affects populations in the lower socioeconomic strata and some racial/ethnic minorities. Additionally, oral and pharyngeal cancer results in over 12,000 deaths per year and has one of the worst morbidity and mortality rates of any cancer.[3] Birth defects, particularly cleft lip or palate, are highly prevalent, as are a variety of chronic and disabling diseases and disorders, the oral complications of systemic diseases, and the oral complications of those interventions and medications consequent to treating systemic disease.

CHRONIC ORAL INFECTIOUS DISEASE

DENTAL CARIES

Despite of a substantial reduction over the last 20 years, dental caries continues to be a major problem for adults and children worldwide. Dental caries affects the primary and permanent dentition in nearly half of all children and adolescents.[4] Unfortunately, disparities persist, in that income and education are inversely associated with caries experience; and ethnic minorities present with greater caries experience.[4–6] The impact of dental caries on pain and suffering remains profound. The Surgeon General's Report estimates that 51 million school hours are lost each year to dental illness, and in adults more than 164 million work hours are lost each year for dental illness or treatment.[1]

The etiology of dental caries is well documented and results from the interplay of dental plaque present on the tooth surface with ingested fermentable carbohydrates. The caries balance is dependent on the interaction of protective and pathological factors (Figure 59.1). A demineralization–mineralization equilibrium occurs at the tooth–plaque–saliva interface, where the equilibrium balance favors demineralization when the plaque pH drops, such as when carbohydrates (sugars) are fermented by plaque bacteria to form organic acids.[7] Mineral flows back when the pH is neutralized mostly due to the presence of salivary buffers and mineral ions, particularly when supplemented with fluoride.[7] Fluoride, when ingested at optimum amounts during tooth development (about 0.7 to 1.0 ppm), makes the enamel hydroxapatite crystal less soluble. Individuals with hyposalivation or xerostomia due to use of specific medications, head and neck irradiation, or chronic diseases, such as Sjögren's syndrome, lack appropriate salivary buffering capacity and thus have increased risk for caries.[8] Dental caries represent an excellent example of how understanding the complex etiologic agents of this multifactorial disease can have health promotion, intervention, and treatment consequences that can affect not only the disease itself but the intricate interactions between health and nutritional status. As shown in Figure 59.2, the balance between health and disease in the oral and craniofacial complex is dependent on

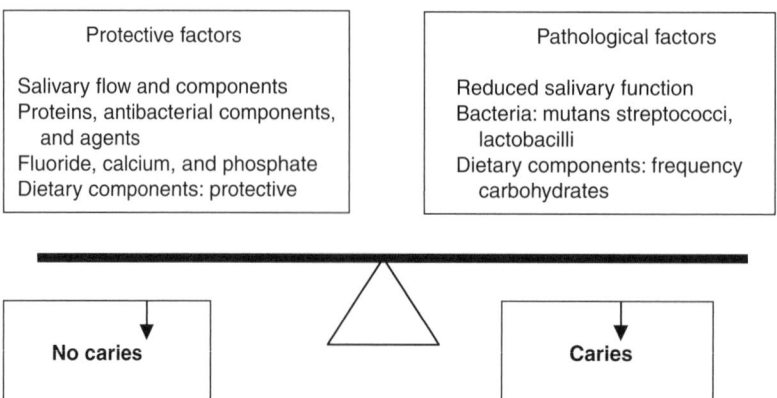

FIGURE 59.1   The caries balance: A schematic diagram of the balance between pathological and protective factors in the caries process. (From Featherstone JDB. *J Am Dent Assoc.* 131:887; 2000. With permission.)

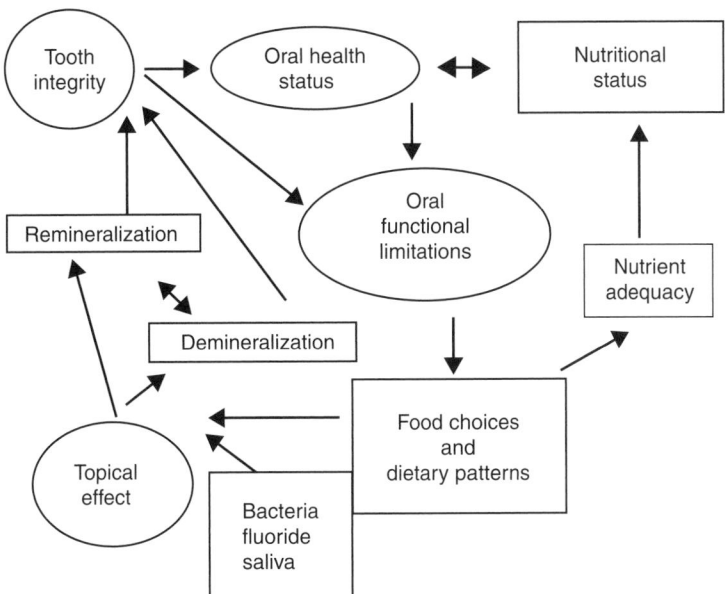

FIGURE 59.2   Diet and dental health.

food choices and dietary patterns interwoven with nutritional and oral health status. There is a synergy between these two measures of health (nutriture and oral status) that has a significant impact on general health and thus individual risk for many contemporary chronic and disabling diseases. If dietary intake leads to poor nutritional status, chronic disease is more likely to occur in the presence of additional risk factors that might include other lifestyle, environmental, and genetic factors.

PERIODONTAL DISEASE

Periodontal disease refers to a fairly common oral infectious (bacterial) disease with local and systemic inflammatory effects[9] ranging from gingivitis to varying degrees of periodontal disease. The initiation and progression of the disease is affected by several risk factors. The relationship between nutrition and periodontal disease is multifaceted; environmental and host risk factors contribute to its pathogenesis. Some of the host factors related to diet and nutrition include presence of other systemic or chronic diseases and life stage (diabetes, osteoporosis, pregnancy, and menopause), medications, and nutrition status. Smoking is a primary environmental factor. The present knowledge of nutrition and periodontal disease can be viewed in one of three ways:

1. Known relationships between periodontal disease, nutrition status, and immune response
2. Relationships of periodontal disease with nutrients that have been demonstrated in select populations
3. Unknown and yet-to-be-tested relationships between periodontal disease, individual nutrients, and select host defense and health status variables

An overview of the paradigm for the pathogenesis of periodontitis was provided by Page and Kornman, and is depicted in Figure 59.3.

Known relationships include the impact of malnutrition on inflammation and infection. Nutrient deficiencies can compromise the system's response to inflammation and infection and increase the energy and protein needs necessary for adequate wound healing.[10] In this manner, poor nutritional status can impact host response to the inflammatory process and infection imposed by periodontal disease. Similarly, individuals with malnutrition typically lack adequate protein and micronutrient reserves, which may compromise their response to an inflammatory condition such as periodontal disease. In the healthy individual, a balanced diet provides adequate macro- and micronutrients to reduce the risk of malnutrition-associated compromises in immune and inflammatory responses and wound healing. In individuals with malnutrition, it is first necessary to treat the cause of the malnutrition, provide adequate energy, macro-, and micronutrients for repletion and maintaining oral and systemic health.

The relationships between periodontal disease, osteoporosis, and calcium intake are presented elsewhere in this section. Krall et al. have demonstrated that osteopenia and bone loss are associated with oral bone loss.[11] The relationship between calcium and vitamin D and incidence of periodontal disease remains to be demonstrated in broader gender- and age-related populations. The need for adequate calcium in the diet (either with foods and/or supplements) is clear for the prevention and management of osteopenia and osteoporosis. Although the data on supplementation with these two nutrients in periodontal disease is

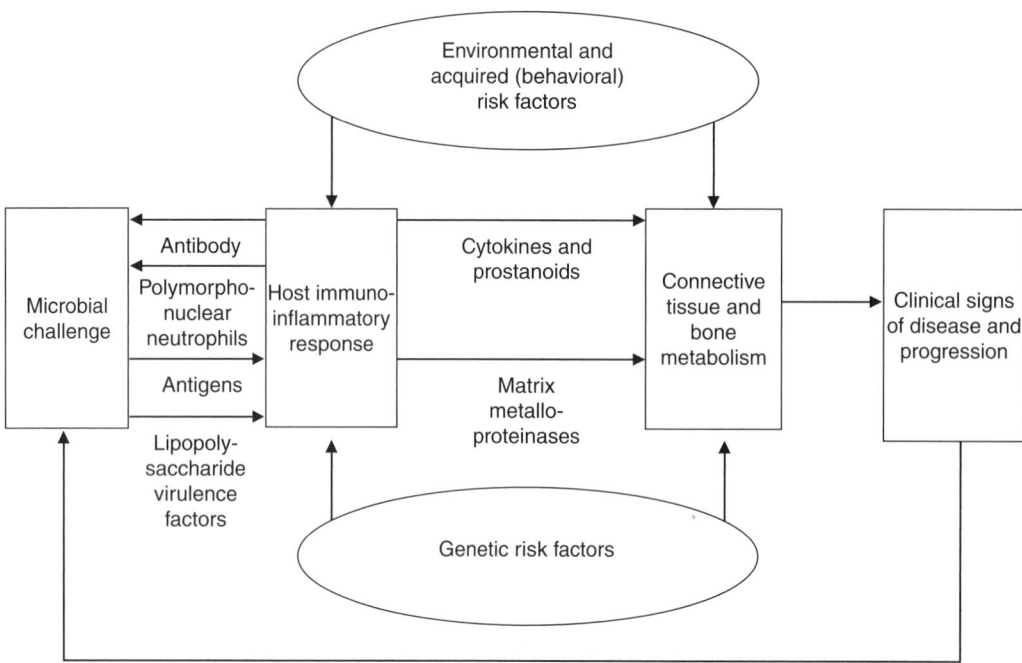

FIGURE 59.3   A new paradigm for the pathobiology of periodontitis. (From Page and Kornman, *Periodontology* 14:9; 1997, with permission. Reprinted in Surgeon General's Report.)

equivocal, it stands to reason that individuals with periodontal disease who are also at risk for osteoporosis may benefit from supplementation.

The relationship between various antioxidants and periodontal disease is a nascent area of research. Vitamins C, E, and A and β-carotene play a role in the inflammatory response; however, there is no evidence in humans to support supplemental doses of these or other micronutrients in the prevention or treatment of periodontal disease. The data published is limited and somewhat dated. Nishida et al. demonstrated that low dietary intake of vitamin C was significantly (although "weakly") associated with periodontal disease in individuals who currently smoke or have a history of smoking tobacco.[12] However, vitamin C has not been proven efficacious for improving periodontal health or reducing risk of disease in the general population.[12]

The relationship between diabetes and periodontal disease is discussed elsewhere. However, the study of the relationship between obesity and periodontal disease is a growing area for investigation. In a study of obese, healthy Japanese men undergoing evaluation of periodontal status, there was a positive association between the degree of obesity, as measured by body mass index, and incidence of periodontal disease.[13] After adjusting for age, sex, oral hygiene status, and smoking, the relative risk of periodontal disease was 1.3 for each 5% increase in body mass index (BMI).[13] Although type 2 diabetes is a recognized risk factor for periodontal disease, there was no association in this study between fasting blood glucose or glycosolated hemoglobin values and periodontal disease.[13] Wood et al.[14] and Genco[15] used NHANES III data to explore this relationship. Wood used measures of body composition (BMI, waist–hip circumference, and fat-free mass) and compared values with the presence of periodontitis. Markers of periodontal disease were periodontal sites with attachment loss (PAL). They found that increasing percentages of PAL were significantly related to waist–hip ratio (WHR) and BMI. WHR provides a reasonable measure of upper abdominal obesity associated with diabetes and cardiovascular disease. This supports the need for further research given the growing body of research on the relationship between periodontal disease and cardiovascular disease. Genco found similar results supporting that obesity is a predictor for periodontal disease independent of age, gender, race, or smoking. The model proposed by Genco links inflammation to obesity, diabetes, and periodontal infection.[15] Further research is needed to explore relationships between obesity and periodontal disease, particularly in individuals with diabetes, a disease in which obesity can further compromise metabolic control.

Changes in oral tissues associated with aging can also impact periodontal status. Alveolar bone loses approximate 1% per year after age 30, and tooth mobility occurs more frequently in the elderly.[1] Soft tissue changes include thinning of the surface epithelium of the mucus membranes and gingival recession. Decreased salivary flow, most often secondary to medications or disease, is also common. These changes may also impact on nutrition status and eating ability. The combined changes in the oral cavity increase the risk for compromised dietary quality and subsequent nutrient intake and consequently periodontal disease.

Consumption of a balanced diet consistent with the Food Guide Pyramid and U.S. Dietary Guidelines inclusive of fruits, vegetables, grains, dairy products, and adequate protein will provide sufficient vitamins, minerals, phytochemicals, and protein for systemic and oral health. At this point, no published scientifically sound evidence exists to support the notion that individuals with periodontal disease need supplemental doses of any individual nutrients or groups of nutrients.

ENVIRONMENTAL ORAL HEALTH PROMOTION: FLUORIDATION

In the early 1900s, Americans could expect to lose their teeth by middle age. With the discovery of the properties of fluoride and the adjustment of the concentration of fluoride in the supply of drinking water in the 1940s, this trend was reversed. Community water fluoridation remains one of the great achievements of public health and health promotion in the twentieth century.[8] Dental caries prevention is effective at 0.7 to 1.2 ppm.[8] Community water fluoridation is considered an inexpensive means of dental caries prevention; however, only two-thirds of the U.S. population is supplied with water with optimal fluoride levels to reduce the risk of dental caries.[8]

Since the early days of community water fluoridation, the prevalence of dental caries in the United States has declined in communities with and without fluoridated water. This has been largely due to the diffusion of fluoridated water to areas without fluoridated water via food/beverage distribution channels and the widespread use of fluoride toothpaste.[16] Although early studies focused mostly on children, water fluoridation also reduces enamel caries in adults by 20 to 40%, and prevents root surface caries, a condition that particularly affects older adults.[1,16]

Health care providers are agents of health promotion at both individual and community levels. In the absence of a water supply with adequate fluoride to prevent dental caries, health promotion practices that support primary prevention through fluoride supplementation are encouraged. The Position of the American Dietetic Association: The Impact of Fluoride on Health,[8] The American Dental Association Council on Scientific Affairs,[17] and the American Academy of Pediatrics[18] recommend safe levels of daily fluoride supplementation for children living in nonfluoridated communities. The recommended supplementation schedule is depicted in Table 59.1. Dietary fluoride supplements are available as tablets, drops, or lozenges; however, water fluoridation is an inexpensive means of improving oral health, and benefits all residents of a community.

SYSTEMIC DISEASES

GENERAL OBSERVATIONS

The oral cavity is the gateway to the rest of the body, and at times reflects systemic as well as oral health and disease.[1] The mechanisms by which oral manifestations occur as a result of some systemic diseases are not fully known. Systemic diseases that affect the integrity of the oral cavity, and oral diseases themselves, may impact upon nutrition status, the converse also being true. Any condition affecting the functional capacity of the oral cavity (sensory or motor function) and/or the health and integrity of the soft tissue may impact on dietary intake. If the integrity of the oral tissues is compromised because of infection, surgery, trauma, or medications, nutrient needs may be increased. Unfortunately, this is often in the face of compromised intake due to pain, masticatory difficulty, or anorexia. In these situations, dietary intake may be compromised and the risk of malnutrition is increased. Malnutrition in turn can compromise wound healing and integrity of the immune system, further increasing the risk of oral infectious disease.

It is well documented that nutritional status may influence disease progression and recovery from illness, infection, and surgery, as well as the healing and repair in the oral cavity.[19] Malnutrition and individual nutrient deficiencies may impair tissue integrity and muscle function.[19, 20] Select chronic diseases with recognized oral manifestations affecting nutrition status and diseases with associated oral infections are listed in Table 59.2. Nutrition status may be affected via two primary mechanisms,

---

TABLE 59.1
Supplemental Fluoride Dosage Schedule (mg/day)

Age	Fluoride Level in Drinking Water (ppm)		
	<0.3 (mg)	0.3–0.6 (mg)	>0.6 (mg)
6 months to 3 years	0.25	0	0
3–6 years	0.50	0.25	0
6–16 years	1.00	0.50	0

ppm = parts per million; 2.2 mg sodium fluoride contains 1 mg fluoride.

Source: Adapted from American Dietetic Association, *J. Am. Diet. Assoc.* 105:1620; 2005.

TABLE 59.2
Selected Diseases with Potential Oral Manifestations Affecting Nutrition Status

Arthropathies	Autoimmune Disorders
Cancers	Chronic orofacial pain
Cardiovascular disease	Diabetes
End-stage renal disease	HIV infection/AIDS
Inflammatory bowel disease	Liver disease
Megaloblastic anemia	Oral–facial pain syndromes
Osteoporosis	Pulmonary disease
Vesiculobullous diseases	Herpes Zoster

TABLE 59.3
Medications with Associated Oral Manifestations

Antianxiety agents	Anticonvulsants
Antidepressants	Antipsychotics
Corticosteroids	Diuretics
Immune suppressing agents	Opiates
Protease inhibitors	Serotonin uptake inhibitors

functionally and metabolically, both of which can influence the sense of taste. Additionally, functional integrity of the oral cavity is critical for optimal olfaction, mastication, and swallowing; negative impacts on any of these functions can influence food and fluid intake, and consequently nutrition status. Metabolic impacts also include altered nutrient metabolism, typically increased catabolism of protein stores for energy, as well as increased protein and energy needs due to infection. The end result of either a functional or metabolic mechanisms may be compromised nutrition status, increased risk of secondary infection, and altered response to disease and treatment.

Medications used to treat chronic diseases may also have side effects, which in turn compromise food intake and nutrition status.[21] For example, xerostomia may occur independently as a consequence of a systemic disease, or as a side effect of medication. More than 400 prescribed and over-the-counter medications are associated with xerostomia.[1, 22] Xerostomia can affect sense of taste and swallowing ability as well as caries risk. Food texture and temperature may need to be modified for individuals with moderate to severe xerostomia. Other examples include drugs that may alter appetite and nutrient metabolism. Antidepressant medications and steroids can increase appetite, thus leading to increased risk of weight gain and subsequent obesity. Steroids increase catabolism of protein and carbohydrate, and lead to calcium losses. Individuals on long-term steroids are at risk for type 2 diabetes, and require calcium supplementation and added protein in their diets to reduce risk of osteoporosis and malnutrition, respectively.[21] Classes of medications with oral manifestations are found in Table 59.3. Individual drugs are not listed; practitioners should check a reference such as the Physicians' Desk Reference (PDR; available online at www.pdr.net)[23] or www.drymouth.info[24] for individual drugs and their associated oral manifestations.

Clinical symptomatology with associated oral clinical and systemic disorders and nutritional implications is addressed in Table 59.4. Clinical features may represent one or more local and systemic diseases. It is imperative that practitioners look beyond the clinical symptom to discern the actual etiology. Select clinical features may have an associated nutritional etiology; however, all other causes must be considered in a differential diagnosis. Appropriate symptom management and treatment options may then be initiated.

HIV AND AIDS

In 2006 the NIH commemorated 25 years of AIDS research, noting that the first case was reported on June 5, 1981. Since then there have been more than 3 million deaths worldwide from AIDS.[25] In the United States, combination antiretroviral therapies have contributed to a decline in death due to AIDS as well as a reduction in the incidence of complications. Individuals with immunosuppressive diseases including HIV infection and AIDS are at increased risk of oral manifestations and malnutrition due to the disease and associated metabolic, oral, gastrointestinal (GI), immune, psychosocial, and pharmacological sequelae. Macronutrient metabolism is often altered; women lose more fat tissue, further contributing to malnutrition, whereas men tend

TABLE 59.4
Oral Manifestations of Local and Systemic Diseases and Their Nutritional Implications

Clinical Finding	Associated Findings	Associated Disorders/Diseases	Nutritional Implications
Xerostomia	Excessive dental caries, candidiasis, dysphagia, dysgeusia, burning mouth/tongue	Drug or radiation therapy induced xerostomia, Sjögren's Syndrome, diabetes	Increase fluids, minimize fermentable carbohydrates, modify food consistency as needed, evaluate glucose control in diabetes
Burning mouth/ tongue	May be associated with mucosal erythema/atrophy, glossitis	Anemia, diabetes, candidiasis, orofacial pain syndromes	Determine presence and type of anemia (iron, folate, B_{12}), modify food/fluid consistency and flavoring, evaluate glucose control in diabetes
Angular cheilitis	Dry, cracked, fissured corner of the mouth	Dehydration, anemia, ill-fitting dentures (drooling)	Determine etiology
Candidiasis	White and/or red removable patches on the oral mucosa	Immunodeficiency syndromes, diabetes	Determine etiology
Difficulty chewing	Partial or complete edentulism, poor occlusion, ill-fitting dentures	Cranial nerve disorders, orofacial pain syndromes	Determine etiology, referral for medical nutrition therapy

Source: Adapted from Kerr AR, Touger-Decker R. In: Touger-Decker R, Mobley CC, Sirois D, eds. *Nutrition and Oral Medicine*, 2005. With permission of the author.

TABLE 59.5
Possible Causes of Anorexia in HIV/AIDS

Polypharmacy	Dysguesia
Odynophagia/dysphagia	Nausea/vomiting
Depression	Weakness/lethargy
Oral infections/lesions	Tooth loss
GI disease	Kaposi's sarcoma

to lose lean tissue, again contributing to malnutrition and increased needs.[26] The psychological and physiological stress associated with HIV and AIDS, as well as the medications used to treat the disease, contributes to alterations in nutrient intake and subsequent nutrition status.

Poor oral hygiene, malnutrition, and lack of dental care are key factors in the development and severity of oral lesions in this population. Candidiasis is recognized as a common and early oral manifestation of immune suppression. Presentation of oral candidiasis may be one of the first signs of HIV infection or an indicator of disease progression.[27] Periodontal disease including necrotizing ulcerative periodontitis (NUP) is common in patients with HIV. Cancers of the oral cavity, Kaposi's sarcoma, and lymphoma may also occur. Thus, oral challenges, combined with common nutrition problems such as wasting syndrome, visceral and somatic protein depletion, maldigestion and malabsorption, altered nutrient and energy needs, polypharmacy, and reduced oral food intake secondary to anorexia, nausea, or compromised oral health status further contribute to the malnutrition observed in this population.[26]

Some of the possible causes of anorexia in this population are listed in Table 59.5. Medical nutrition therapy (MNT) by the registered dietitian (RD) is warranted to prevent further nutritional depletion, altered taste perception, odynophagia/dysphagia, nausea/vomiting, psychosocial considerations, weakness/lethargy, and the side effects of compounded use of medications.

Wasting syndrome is characteristic of later stages of HIV and is defined as unintentional weight loss of >10% from usual body weight or baseline weight in the presence of diarrhea or fever for >30 days of unknown etiology.[26] The pathogenesis of wasting can be attributed to several factors including decreased energy intake, anorexia, GI dysfunction, and deranged metabolism including increased insulin sensitivity, altered carbohydrate metabolism, and increased protein turnover. During acute phases of the disease, pharmacotherapy and MNT are critical to manage the disease and preserve lean body mass. As individuals progress to lifelong pharmacotherapy with combinations of antiretroviral therapies, nutrition status is challenged by the associated drug side effects. These side effects may include food–drug interactions, oral lesions, and infection as well as alterations in appetite and intake.

The impact of HIV infection in the GI tract is outlined in Table 59.6. Common HIV-associated oral infectious disorders include those of fungal, viral, and bacterial origin.[27] Oropharyngeal fungal infections may cause a burning, painful mouth, and dysphagia. For example, oral and esophageal candidiasis can result in painful chewing, sucking, and swallowing, consequently reducing an already compromised appetite and dietary intake. The ulcers found with viral infections such as herpes simplex

TABLE 59.6

Impact of HIV Infection on Nutrition and Diet in the Upper GI Tract

Location	Problem	Effect	Diet Management
Oral cavity	Candidiasis, Kaposi's sarcoma (KS), herpes, stomatitis, aphthous ulcers	Pain, infection, lesions, altered ability to eat, saliva, dysgeusia	Increase calories and protein Modify food consistency Oral supplements Caries risk reduction
	Xerostomia	Caries risk, pain, no moistening power, food sticks, dysgeusia	Moist, soft foods; nonspicy, "smooth," cool/warm, fluids Caries risk reduction
Esophagus	Candidiasis, herpes, KS, cryptosporidius	Dysphagia, odynophagia	Modify food consistency Oral supplements Enteral nutrition support as needed

TABLE 59.7

Common HIV-Associated Viral Infections of the Oral Cavity

Lesions	Clinical Appearance	Nutritional Impact
Herpes simplex virus	Painful, solitary, multiple, or confluent vesicles/ulcers; any mucosal surface	Reduced dietary intake due to severity of pain
Cytomegalovirus (human herpes virus 5)	Painful, ulcer >5 mm; persistent/nonhealing; nonkeratinized surface	Reduced dietary intake due to severity of pain
Varicella zoster virus	Painful, multiple, crusted, erythematous ulcers; along divisions of cranial nerve V (frequently on the palate)	Reduced dietary intake due to severity of pain
Oral hairy leukoplakia (Epstein–Barr virus)	Asymptomatic, lateral borders of the tongue; white, vertical, hyperkeratotic striae; cannot be wiped/rubbed off	None
Kaposi's sarcoma (human herpes virus 8)	Painful in advanced presentations due to trauma, purplish-blue, red macules or nodules; generally hard/soft palate and gingival tissues	Difficulty eating due to size of lesion or trauma
Human papilloma virus	Hyperplastic, papillomatous or verrucous; any oral surface	Difficulty eating due to size and quantity of lesions or trauma

Source: Adapted by original author from Patel ASH, Hansen HJ. *Top Clin Nutr* 20(3):243; 2005.

and cytomegalovirus may cause pain and reduced oral intake. Examples of viral infections affecting the oral cavity with possible impact on dietary intake are depicted in Table 59.7. The oral disorders found with HIV and AIDS may increase nutrient demands on the body for healing and compromise eating ability. MNT is critical to healing and maintenance of lean body mass. Oral diets with or without nutritional supplements should be tried first, followed by tube feedings if needed. The health professional should observe patients for changes in dietary intake, body weight, lipodystrophy, and overall nutritional wellbeing, and refer individuals to an RD and/or physician early in the process of disease management.[26]

DIABETES

More than 20.8 million children and adults in the United States (7%) have been diagnosed with diabetes. These numbers are based on an estimated 14.6 million diagnosed cases and an additional 6.2 million individuals with undiagnosed disease. Prediabetes (fasting blood glucose of greater than 100 mg/dl) is increasingly affecting adults and children. Diabetes is the sixth leading cause of death in the United States.[28] Oral sequellae occurring with diabetes are usually a result of poorly controlled diabetes, or hyperglycemia. Oral cell metabolism, immune surveillance, and vascular integrity as well as salivary chemistry may be altered in individuals with diabetes, particularly when uncontrolled. While there is limited evidence that periodontal infection affects glycemic control,[29] any infection can contribute to adverse alterations in glycemic control. Other oral manifestations may occur, impacting diet intake and nutrition status. These can be seen in Table 59.8.

Diabetes, particularly when poorly controlled, is associated with a higher prevalence of all infections including oral infections, when compared with people without diabetes.[30] Over 90% of individuals over age 13 with diabetes have some periodontal problems relative to diabetes.[30] The susceptibility to periodontal disease in diabetes is likely directly related to impaired defense

TABLE 59.8
Oral Manifestations of Diabetes

Gingivitis	Altered taste
Periodontal disease	Burning mouth
Reduced saliva (with resultant xerostomia)	Increased thirst
Salivary hyperglycemia	Neuropathies
Increased risk of infectious disorders and complications	Slowed wound healing

mechanisms. Micro- and macrovascular circulation are altered, along with wound healing, collagen metabolism, neutrophil chemotaxis, and proteolysis. Pathologic tissue destruction contributes to periodontal tissue destruction. Increased salivary glucose increases bacterial substrate and plaque formation. Microangiopathies, altered vascular permeability, and metabolic alterations may lead to an altered immune response and precipitate periodontal disease progression. The oral complications associated with diabetes are often referred to as the sixth major medical complication of diabetes.

The relationship between oral manifestations of diabetes and diet/nutrition is a complex two-way street. Although uncontrolled diabetes is partly due to poor diet management, oral manifestations challenge and ultimately compromise eating ability and consequent dietary intake. Taste may be altered in patients with diabetes because of salivary chemistry, xerostomia, and/or candidiasis. Management of burning mouth/tongue requires a determination of the cause. When due to a nutrient deficiency, augmentation of the diet with the appropriate nutrients or supplements will treat the cause and subsequent symptomatology. When a physical or biochemical abnormality cannot be found, the symptoms of burning mouth may be improved using tricyclic antidepressant medications. However, a side effect of tricyclic antidepressants is xerostomia, which may compound any existing alterations in saliva, and increase risk of candidiasis and dental caries.

MNT is the cornerstone of diabetes care. Proper diet control, in energy and macronutrient distribution throughout the day, is critical to glycemic control, particularly in type 1 diabetes. In both type 1 and type 2 diabetes, a diet consistent with the Food Guide Pyramid is recommended with attainment and maintenance of desirable body weight. In most states, MNT by an RD with several follow-up visits is a benefit covered by all third-party payers, Medicare and Medicaid. The oral health professional should work closely with the patient's physician and refer patients, as appropriate, to an RD, reinforce the need to adhere to the diabetic diet, integrate oral hygiene into daily routines, and modify diet consistencies as needed to manage oral conditions and surgeries.

CROHN'S DISEASE

Crohn's disease can present with aphthous ulcers, angular stomatitis, and/or glossitis. Oral lesions present on the lips, gingiva, and buccal mucosa may precede GI symptoms and have a dramatic impact on oral function. The size of the lesion may not coincide with the intensity of pain reported or degree of compromise in food and fluid intake. Ability to eat may be hampered by pain; topical anesthetic agents (or a 1:1 mixture of milk of magnesia and Benadryl as a rinse and expectorate) prior to meals may temporarily relieve pain and allow more comfort in eating. Pharmacological management is critical; steroids are often needed. The impact of steroids on nutritional wellbeing has been addressed in other sections of this handbook.

AUTOIMMUNE DISEASE

Autoimmune diseases such as pemphigus vulgaris (PV) increase nutrition risk by virtue of the oral and facial sequellae of the disease and the medications used to manage it. Much like other diseases with oral lesions, PV affects appetite and eating ability because of the associated pain. Steroids are often used in the management of vesiculobullous diseases of the oral cavity including PV. In addition to the medications used for the disease, topical anesthetics immediately prior to eating provide a topical coating, allowing more comfort during mealtime. Other autoimmune diseases including Sjögren's syndrome and rheumatoid arthritis (RA) can affect the oral cavity and subsequent nutrition status. Oral and nutritional implications of select diseases in this category are outlined in Table 59.9. While diet modifications are addressed, particular attention needs to be paid to the individual's stage of disease. During disease exacerbation, eating ability may be severely compromised and a liquid diet using oral supplements (meal replacement formulas) such as Boost (Novartis) or Ensure (Ross) may be required to meet energy and protein needs. During periods of remission, individuals may be able to liberalize diets considerably.

OSTEOPOROSIS

Osteoporosis, or reduced bone mineral density, is the most common bone disease.[31] The majority of individuals with osteoporosis are women (80%); however, it is a risk for up to 44 million Americans, and is often known as a "silent killer."[1, 31] One in two Caucasian women and one in four men will have an osteoporotic fracture in their lifetimes.[31] Nonmodifiable and potentially

TABLE 59.9
Autoimmune Disorders with Associated Oral and Nutritional Side Effects

Disease	Oral Manifestation	Nutrition Implications
Rheumatoid arthritis	TMJ ankylosis	Pain upon eating
	Limited mandibular opening	Modify diet consistency
Erythema multiforme	Oral mucosal lesions, often ulcerative	Pain upon eating
		Increased needs for healing
		Modify diet, often liquid consistency with straw during exacerbation
		If treated with steroids: increase calcium, protein
Pemphigus vulgaris	Oral mucosal lesions	Painful and difficult eating
		If treated with steroids: increase calcium, protein
		Modify diet as needed in temperature, consistency
Sjögren's syndrome	Xerostomia; mucosa dry, erythematous; fissures; more susceptible to trauma; increased risk of caries; fissured tongue; periodontal disease; cervical caries	Increased fluids with and between meals, modify foods to include soft, temperate, nonspicy foods
Systemic lupus erythematosus	Ulcerations of mucosa	Manage side effects of steroids and medications, diet as per Sjögren's

TABLE 59.10
Risk Factors for Osteoporosis

Nonmodifiable	Potentially Modifiable
Personal or family history of fracture as an adult	Current cigarette smoking
Caucasian or Asian race	Low body weight
Advanced age	Lack of weight bearing exercise
Female gender	Prolonged low calcium intake
Dementia	Alcoholism
Small bone structure	Impaired eyesight despite adequate correction
Select Medications: glucocorticoids, anticonvulsants, methotrexate, excessive thyroid hormones, cholestyramine	Recurrent falls
Estrogen deficiency	Inadequate physical activity
Amenhorrhea	
Menopause/early menopause (<age 45) or bilateral ovariectomy; prolonged premenopausal amenorrhea (>1 year)	Poor health/frailty
Prolonged immobilization, that is, spinal cord injury	

Source: From National Osteoporosis Foundation.

modifiable causes of osteoporosis are listed in Table 59.10.[32] As dental health care professionals see patients on a regular basis and as alveolar boss loss is associated with osteoporosis, the dental professional is in an ideal situation to access patients at risk for osteoporosis. Simple screening in the dental office can include asking patients about risk factors for the disease (see Table 59.10) and calcium intake in the form of dairy products (milk, cheese, and yogurt), functional foods or foods fortified with calcium (orange juice, and cereal), and calcium supplements. Other individuals at risk for osteoporosis (see Table 59.10) should be referred for a bone density test to determine risk for or presence of osteopenia or osteoporosis.

Bone loss is a common denominator for both periodontal disease and osteoporosis. The relationship between the two diseases remains to be fully determined.[33] However, an association between periodontal disease and systemic osteopenia and osteoporosis has been documented in adults.[33, 34] Studies using NHANES III data [12] as well as longitudinal studies [11, 35] have demonstrated significant relationships between tooth loss, periodontal disease, low calcium intake, and osteoporosis in older men and women who are at risk for osteoporosis and periodontal disease. Using NHANES III data, Nishida [12] demonstrated a relationship between low dietary calcium intake, osteoporosis, and increased incidence of periodontal disease. Krall [35] found that total calcium intake (diet plus calcium supplements) was significantly associated with the tooth loss in elderly men and women in New England. Yoshihara [36] found a significant relationship between periodontal disease and bone mineral density in healthy elders in Japan.

Levels of nutrient intake below the recommended dietary intakes is associated with increased risk and incidence of osteo-porosis.[31] Tezal et al. pose "four possible pathways" for the relationship between osteoporosis and severity of periodontal disease, including systemic loss of bone mineral density, modified local tissue response to infection as a result of "systemic factors of bone remodeling", genetics, and lifestyle factors.[33] The final pathway, lifestyle factor, links the issues of hygiene, diet, and exercise with local and systemic disease. There is evidence to support the relationship between periodontal disease and osteoporosis, but it is mostly based on epidemiologic and retrospective studies. Further research is clearly needed to define the relationship, causative factors, and preventive mechanisms. Please refer to Section 61 for a thorough description of osteoporosis and other bone diseases and disorders.

NEOPLASTIC DISEASES: ORAL CANCER

Oropharyngeal cancer refers to malignancy of the oral cavity and oropharynx. Oral cancer develops from a precancerous lesion most commonly on the tongue, lips, and floor of the mouth. It is the sixth most common cancer in the United States.[37] While overall incidence and mortality of oral cancer has declined in the past 20 years, racial and gender disparities persist. Incidence and mortality rates remain highest for Black males when compared with White and Black males and females.[38] Most oral cancers are squamous cell carcinomas — cancers of the epithelial cells.[3] Tobacco components act as promoters of carcinogenesis, and alcohol may act as a solvent to facilitate penetration of the tobacco carcinogens into oral tissue.[39] Viruses, including the herpes simplex type 1 and human papilloma virus, have both been implicated in oral cancer. Genetic susceptibility may play a role in manifestation of oral cancer. Both disarmament of the cell's DNA repair mechanisms and mutation of tumor suppressor genes have been linked to smoking and alcohol use, and play a major role in oral cancer development. Likewise, nicotine stimulates negative changes in immune cells that can promote tumor growth.

Ecologic and case–control studies have suggested that nutrients may play an important role in the prevention and management of early oral cancer and precancerous leukoplakia.[40] Likewise, several studies have shown that smokers have lower plasma levels of vitamin E, C, β-carotene, and other antioxidants because of both low intake and increased metabolic use. Total intake of fruits and vegetables, fresh fruits, green leafy vegetables, other vegetables, total bread and cereals, and whole-grain breads and cereals, which are excellent sources of multiple antioxidants, have been shown to be associated with decreased risk of oral cancer.[41,42] More specifically, citrus, dark yellow, and other fruits were more consistently associated with decreased risk than were estimated intake of specific nutrients including carotene, vitamin C, fiber, folate, thiamine, riboflavin, niacin, vitamin E, and iron. A case–control study conducted in Italy illustrated that, the more a micronutrient, such as vitamin C, carotene, or vitamin E, was correlated to total vegetable and fruit intake, the stronger was its protective effect against oral cancer.[43] Thus, it appears that total fruit and vegetable intake may offer greater risk reduction than singular antioxidant nutrients in supplemental doses. Fioretti et al. reported that, even in the absence of tobacco use, if subjects reduced alcohol and saturated fat intake and increased fruit and carrot consumption, there appeared to be a favorable effect on oral cancer risk among subjects who participated in a large case–control study.[44]

Nutritional care of the patient with oral cancer will vary based on cancer site and treatment modalities. Side effects may include changes in weight, sore mouth or throat, xerostomia, mucositis, dental caries, gingival infection, changes in sense of taste and smell, nausea, vomiting, and fatigue. Referral to an RD early in the course of treatment is warranted to optimize nutrition status and treatment outcomes.

CRANIOFACIAL–ORAL–DENTAL BIRTH DEFECTS

Nearly two infants in every 1000 live births have some type of craniofacial birth defect.[3] These defects can occur in isolation or as a component of a larger birth defect syndrome caused by genetic influences, environmental disturbances, or the interplay between the gene and environment. A number of congenital oral–dental–craniofacial birth defects can be prevented by reducing risk factors associated with human craniofacial malformations. Among the common environmental risk factors are alcohol (associated with fetal alcohol syndrome); smoking (associated with risk of cleft lip with or without cleft palate); anticonvulsant medications, such as phenytoin and other teratogens (associated with a variety of birth defects involving the face, teeth, and jaws); retinoic acid analogs (associated with severe craniofacial and oral clefts and limb defects); and vitamin deficiency, particularly folate (associated with increased risk of cleft lip with or without cleft palate).[3]

Available data from the NIDCR revealed that about 20% of craniofacial–oral–dental birth defects are either genetic or familial.[3] The largest majority are caused by the defined risk factors noted earlier or are of unknown causes. From a nutrition perspective, there are relevant applications to oral–dental–craniofacial defects. One application relates to the preventive effects of micronutrients. The use of multivitamin supplements and folic acid in women of childbearing age are advocated in the prevention of cleft lip and/or cleft palate, as well as in the prevention of neural tube defects such spina bifida.[45] As research continues, it will become important to carefully titrate the dose of the micronutrient provided before conception and during pregnancy that will result in a maximum protective effect. This is vital because there is a possibility that excessive amounts of some nutrients, such as vitamin A or retinoic acid, can result in the opposite effect; that is, they could be teratogenic.[3, 46] Retinoic-acid-induced embryopathy includes defects in craniofacial, skeletal, cardiac, thymic, and central nervous system structures.[46] Thus, folic acid and vitamin A represent examples of the exquisite sensitivity of embryogenesis, and the craniofacial complex in particular, to nutrients.

A critical message for the oral health practitioner is the necessity to work closely with the RD and physician to educate prospective and expectant parents regarding nutrition and oral health.

Importantly, following the birth of a child with cleft lip or palate, depending on the extent and severity of the cleft, a series of physiological, psychological, medical, dental, and social issues emerges. The establishment of a craniofacial anomaly or cleft team to manage patients with cleft and/or other craniofacial defects is ideal. This multidisciplinary team assesses the child and his/her various medical, nutritional, social, and psychological needs. Often an RD is an integral part of such a team, as one of the major issues to overcome for such children is the ability to ingest adequate amounts of macro- and micronutrients consistent with increased nutrient requirements of the early developmental years. These nutrition requirements are exacerbated by multiple surgical interventions and the extent of the defects.[45] Therefore, craniofacial anomalies present two challenges for the health care professional and the nutrition community in particular. One is to identify women at risk for birth defects and use appropriate interventions to prevent craniofacial anomalies. The second is to work closely in an interdisciplinary team to mitigate the effects and treatments of the anomaly.

HEALTH PROMOTION, HEALTH EDUCATION, AND BEHAVIOR CHANGE

Health promotion is a term used to describe not only heath education but also organizational, economic, and environmental channels that provide support for enabling people to increase control over and improvement of their health.[47] Nutrition is an integral part of health promotion and disease prevention for dental health and general wellness.

According to health promotion theoretical models, personal health practices and behaviors that enhance lifestyle lead to reduced morbidity and mortality, improved health status, and improved quality of life. Frequently, oral diseases in children are associated with eating difficulty, general health problems, and even lost school time.[48] In aging populations, strong associations exist between oral health status and ability to swallow, chew efficiently, and select a variety of foods.[49] Numerous nutrition and dietary practices enhance positive oral health outcomes throughout the life span, such as those to reduce the caries experience in children and those to promote optimal dietary intake through adulthood with sound oral health. Diet and nutrition strategies are part of a comprehensive approach, along with oral hygiene and routine access to dental care, to reduce the burdens of oral diseases.[50]

Nutrition education programs focused on changing dietary behaviors should include oral health promotion within the Food Guide Pyramid and U.S. Dietary Guidelines messages, which are available online at http://mypyramid.org/.[51] Global nutrition messages appropriate for inclusion in oral health promotion programs targeting primary and secondary prevention of dental caries are described in Table 59.11. Messages appropriate for pediatric oral health promotion are identified in Table 59.12. Strategies are advocated to reduce the incidence of childhood caries, particularly in high-risk populations that include minority and low socioeconomic groups.[54] Unfortunately, the nutrition focus has been limited to infant feeding practices; promoting early weaning with transition from bottle to cup and the impression that milk sugar (lactose) is the primary culprit. Sucrose, glucose, and fructose found in fruit juices and drinks as well as sweetened solid foods are probably the main sugars associated with ECC.[55] Owing to the casein as well as calcium and phosphate content, milk formulas (with the exception of some soy-based and protein hydrolyzed formulas), bovine milk, and human milk are not considered a source of cariogenic substrate in ECC. However, associated feeding practices may influence the incidence of ECC. Non-breast-fed infants may be introduced earlier to cariogenic foods than breast-fed babies, which may increase their exposure of fermentable carbohydrates to the dentition and increase the risk of ECC.[52] Health care providers are encouraged to discuss children's dental health, beginning with the pregnant woman, and advocate good oral hygiene and feeding practices through growth and development.

Numerous opportunities exist for nutrition messages to be included in oral health promotion initiatives. A variety of health topics that impact oral health outcomes and status are listed in Table 59.13. With the advent of The Surgeon General's Report on

TABLE 59.11
Diet and Nutrition Recommendations to Promote Oral Health[10, 52,53]

Eat a balanced diet, rich in whole grains, fruits, and vegetables; reinforce oral hygiene, in particular the regular use of fluoridated toothpastes, to reduce caries risk

Combine foods to pair fermentable carbohydrates with anticariogenic foods to reduce the risk of caries and erosion. For example, pair dairy products with fermentable carbohydrates and other sugars, consume these foods with instead of between meals, and add raw fruits or vegetables to meals to increase salivary flow. Drink sweetened or acidic beverages with meals including foods that can buffer the acidogenic effects

Follow fermentable carbohydrates foods with a water rinse, dairy product such as cheese, or sugarless gum (in particular those containing sugar alcohols such as xylitol, which promotes remineralization)

Chew sugarless gum between meals and snacks to increase salivary flow

Drink, rather than sip over extended durations, sweetened and acidic beverages

Moderate eating behaviors to reduce frequent repeated exposure to sugars, other fermentable carbohydrates, and acids

Avoid putting an infant or child to bed with a bottle of milk, juice, or other sugar-containing beverage

TABLE 59.12
Guidelines for Birth to 4 years of Age to Promote Pediatric Oral Health and Nutrition

	Oral Health Behaviors	Dietary Issues
Parent's personal practices	*Daily* Brushing/flossing Use fluoride (Fl) toothpaste/rinse	*Review* role of: Diet in caries Frequency of dietary intake. Use xylitol chewing gum (four pieces per day) throughout the day after eating
Parental infant/ child care practices	*Wipe* gums routinely *Floss* between teeth after eruption *Evaluate* Fl exposure and exercise caution in use of Fl-containing products	**Birth to 6 months** *Routine* consumption of milk rather than on-demand feeding should be encouraged whether the method of feeding is breast or bottle *Supplemental* liquids or foods should not be introduced until 6 months of age *Bedtime* and nocturnal feedings should be discouraged after the first tooth erupts **6 to 12 months** *Delay* bacterial colonization with attention to sharing utensils, foods, and cups Iron-fortified cereals and pureed foods should be the first foods introduced in a sequential fashion *Introduce* the cup and spoon and slowly decrease frequency of bottle or breast-feeding (weaning) *Restrict* sweetened beverage intake to no more than 4–6 oz of fruit juice daily **1 to 3 years** *Encourage* consumption of water *Encourage* self-feeding when appropriate and choose from the recommended snacks *Space* meals and snacks at least 2 h apart *Introduce* a variety of hard- and soft-textured foods for mastication and orofacial development
Health care provider	*Provide* education and counseling during pregnancy *Assess* infant at 6 months and provide early intervention *Encourage* parent to establish a dental home by infant's first birthday	

Source: From Mobley C. *Top Clin Nutr.* 20:206; 2005.

TABLE 59.13
Nutrition Messages for Targeted Oral Health Promotion Topics

Oral Health Promotion Topics	Nutrition Messages
Hypomineralized or hypoplastic primary teeth and caries risk	Children who are malnourished pre-, peri-, or postnatally and/or low birth weight are more likely to have this condition.[56,57]
Craniofacial development	Causes are attributed to genetic defects often working in concert with environmental factors such as alcohol intake and possibly excessive therapeutic vitamin A. Neural tube defects and risks of cleft lip and palate may be reduced in children if women support dietary folic acid intake with additional supplementation to equal 400 mg.[3]
Bone status	Loss of teeth leads to bone atrophy. Localized diseases like periodontal disease and systemic diseases like osteoporosis may further affect alveolar bone loss. Promotion of diets adequate in calcium and vitamin D to target these effects should be discussed in the context of oral health.[11,31]
Oral soft tissue integrity	Nutritional status can enhance the ability of healthy epithelial tissue to prevent penetration of bacterial endotoxins into gingival tissue. Protein, vitamins A, C, and E, as well as the B-complex vitamins and zinc will help to maintain immune system integrity, but there is a paucity of scientific data to support supplemental use of these nutrients. Prevention of diseases of the soft tissue related to diseases like periodontal disease and systemic diabetes may challenge utilization of nutrients and can increase risk of decreased oral soft tissue integrity.[9,10]
Salivary output	Saliva and salivary glands provide clues to overall health and disease and function in the mucosal immune system to protect oral tissue integrity. Saliva moistens food and lubricates the bolus for swallowing. Fiber intake and frequency of eating can promote salivary output. Xerostomia (dry mouth) associated with disease and drug therapies may require medical nutrition therapy.[21,58]
Edentulous state	Toothless persons or those who wear dentures need to be encouraged to modify food selection habits and method of preparing foods for easier biting and chewing. One can still achieve good nutritional status important to the maintenance of the oral tissue.[49,59]

Continued

TABLE 59.13
(Continued)

Oral Health Promotion Topics	Nutrition Messages
Oral cancer prevention	Promoting five or more servings a day of fruits and vegetables from a variety of sources that include both dark green and yellow sources may decrease risk for oral cancer. Weight management strategies for those interested in smoking cessation can possibly enhance success and should be explored when appropriate.[41,42]
Dental erosion	Fruit juices, citrus fruits, acid sweet candies and mints, pickles, and cola drinks can cause loss of tooth enamel. Vomiting and regurgitation associated with gastroesophageal reflux and eating disorders can also cause this dental condition. Encourage dietary practices to neutralize the impact of these products and conditions.[60,61]

Oral Health, attention has been drawn to the need for health care professionals to address oral health and systemic health as one entity: health.[1] The nutrition messages for oral health promotion listed in Table 59.13 provide insight into the aforementioned synergy between oral and nutritional status, and offer targeted messages for health promotion in public health and private practice.

Better understanding of the role of behavioral variables in health and disease, including the role of prevention, is important in the delivery of messages that promote both nutritional and oral health status. Practices that attempt to translate the scientific discoveries in nutrition and oral health will provide a basis upon which to plan and execute future health promotion activities.

REFERENCES

1. U.S. Department of Health and Human Services. *Oral Health in America: A Report of the Surgeon General.* Rockville, MD: US Department of Health and Human Services, National Institute of Dental and Craniofacial Research, National Institutes of Health; 2000.
2. Slavkin HC, Baum BJ. *JAMA.* 284:1215; 2000.
3. NIDCR/CDC Dental Oral and Craniofacial Data Resource Center. Oral Health U.S. June 6, 2006; http://drc.nidcr.nih.gov/report.htm.
4. Beltran-Aguilar ED, Barker LK, Canto MT, et al. *MMWR Surveill Summ.* Aug 26 2005;54:1–43.
5. Psoter WJ, Pendrys DG, Morse DE et al. *J Public Health Dent.* 66:23; 2006.
6. Edelstein BL. *Ambul Pediatr.* 2:141S; 2002.
7. Featherstone JD. *J Am Dent Assoc.* 131:887; 2000.
8. American Dietetic Association. Position of the American Dietetic Association: The Impact of Fluoride on Health. *JADA.* 105:1620; 2005.
9. Golub LM, Payne JB, Reinhardt RA, Nieman G. *J Dent Res.* 85:102; 2006.
10. American Dietetic Association. Position of the American Dietetic Association: Oral Health and Nutrition. *JADA.* 103:615; 2003.
11. Krall E. Osteoporosis. In: Touger-Decker R, Sirois D, Mobley C, eds. *Nutrition and Oral Medicine.* Totowa, NJ: Humana Press Inc.; 2005; p. 261.
12. Nishida M, Grossi SG, Dunford RG et al. *J Periodontol.* 71:1057; 2000.
13. Saito T, Shimazaki Y, Sakamoto M. *N Engl J Med.* 339:482; 1998.
14. Wood N, Johnson RB, Streckfus CF. *J Clin Periodontol.* 30:321; 2003.
15. Genco RJ, Grossi SG, Ho A et al. *J Periodontol.* 76(Suppl):2075; 2005.
16. Centers for Disease Control and Prevention. Recommendations for Using Fluoride to Prevent and Control Dental Caries in the United States. http://www.cdc.gov/mmwr/preview/mmwrhtml/rr5014a1.htm. Accessed May 15, 2006.
17. American Dental Association. American Dental Association Supports Fluoridation. http://www.ada.org/prof/resources/positions/statements/fluoride3.asp. Accessed June 5, 2006.
18. American Academy of Pediatrics Section on Pediatric Dentistry. Oral Health Risk Assessment Timing and Establishment of the Dental Home. *Pediatrics.* 111:1113; 2003.
19. Winkler M, Makowski S. In: Touger-Decker R, Sirois D, Mobley C, eds. *Nutrition and Oral Medicine.* Totowa, NJ: Humana Press Inc.; 2005; p. 273.
20. Moynihan P, Lingstrom P. In: Touger-Decker R, Sirois D, Mobley C, eds. *Nutrition and Oral Medicine.* Totowa, NJ: Humana Press Inc.; 2005; p. 107.
21. Robbins M. In: Touger-Decker R, Sirois D, Mobley C, eds. *Nutrition and Oral Medicine.* Totowa, NJ: Humana Press, Inc.; 2005; p. 87.
22. Sreebny LM, Schwartz SS. *Gerodontology.* 14:33; 1997.
23. *Physicians' Desk Reference.* Vol. 60. Montvale, NJ: Thomson PDR; 2006.
24. Wm. Wrigley Jr. Company. Drymouth.info, the definitive resource on the Internet for dry mouth information. http://www.drymouth.info. Accessed June 30, 2006.
25. The Joint United Nations Programme on HIV/AIDS. HIV/AIDS statistics worldwide. Available at: http://www.unaids.org/en/. Accessed June 6, 2006.

26. American Dietetic Association. Position of the American Dietetic Association and Dietitians of Canada: nutrition intervention in the care of persons with human immunodeficiency virus infection. *JADA*. 104:1425; 2004.

27. Patel A, Glick M. In: Touger-Decker R, Mobley C, Sirois D, eds. *Nutrition and Oral Medicine*. Totowa, NJ: Humana Press Inc.; 2005; p. 223.

28. National Center for Health Statistics. FastStats A-Z. http://www.cdc.gov/nchs/fastats/lcod.htm. Accessed June 30, 2006.

29. Taylor GW, Burt BA, Becker MP, et al. *J Periodontol.* 67(Suppl):1085; 1996.

30. Baron S. Bacterial Infections in Diabetes. Paper presented at: Workshop on Oral Disease and Diabetes, 1999.

31. U.S. Department of Health and Human Services. Bone Health and Osteoporosis: A Report of the Surgeon General. http://www.surgeongeneral.gov/library/bonehealth/. Accessed July 7, 2006.

32. National Osteoporosis Foundation. Who is at risk? http://www.nof.org/prevention/risk.htm. Accessed July 7, 2006.

33. Tezal M, Wactawski-Wende J, Grossi SG, et al. *J Periodontol.* 71:1492; 2000.

34. Payne JB, Reinhardt RA, Nummikoski PV, Patil KD. *Osteoporos Int.* 10:34; 1999.

35. Krall EA, Wehler C, Garcia RI, et al. *Am J Med.* 111:452; 2001.

36. Yoshihara A, Seida Y, Hanada N, Miyazaki H. *J Clin Periodontol.* 31:680; 2004.

37. National Cancer Institute. Fast Stats: Oral cavity and pharynx cancer prevalence. http://seer.cancer.gov. Accessed June 6, 2006.

38. Morse DE, Kerr AR. *J Am Dent Assoc.* 137:203; 2006.

39. Czreninski R, Kaplan I. *Top Clin Nutr.* 20:229; 2005.

40. Morse DE. In: Touger-Decker R, Mobley C, Sirois D, eds. *Nutrition and Oral Medicine*. Totowa, NJ: Humana Press Inc.; 2005; p. 205.

41. Petridou E, Zavras AI, Lefatzis D et al. *Cancer.* 94:2981; 2002.

42. Pavia M, Pileggi C, Nobile CG, Angelillo IF. *Am J Clin Nutr.* 83:1126; 2006.

43. Negri E, Franceschi S, Bosetti C et al. *Int J Cancer.* 86:122; 2000.

44. Fioretti F, Bosetti C, Tavani A et al. *Oral Oncol.* 35:375; 1999.

45. Redford-Badwal DA, Mabry K, Frassinelli JD. *Dent Clin North Am.* 47:305; 2003.

46. Mulder GB, Manley N, Grant J et al. *Teratology.* 62:214; 2000.

47. Watt RG. *Bull World Health Organ.* 83:711; 2005.

48. Marshall TA. *Top Clin Nutr.* 20:189; 2005.

49. Touger-Decker R. *Top Clin Nutr.* 20:211; 2005.

50. Tinanoff N. *Dent Clin North Am.* 49:725; 2005.

51. Center for Nutrition Policy and Promotion. MyPyramid.org. http://mypyramid.org. Accessed June 30, 2006.

52. Mobley C. *Top Clin Nutr.* 20:200; 2005.

53. Touger-Decker R, van Loveren C. *Am J Clin Nutr.* 78:881S; 2003.

54. Tinanoff N, Kanellis MJ, Vargas CM. *Pediatr Dent.* 24:543; 2002.

55. Marshall TA, Levy SM, Broffitt B, et al. *Pediatrics.* 112:184; 2003.

56. Alvarez JO. *Am J Clin Nutr.* 61:410S; 1995.

57. Lai PY, Seow WK, Tudehope DI, Rogers Y. *Pediatr Dent.* 19:42; 1997.

58. Ritchie CS, Joshipura K, Hung HC, Douglass CW. *Crit Rev Oral Biol Med.* 13:291; 2000.

59. Sheiham A, Steele JG, Marcenes W et al. *J Dental Res.* 80:408; 2001.

60. Sohn W, Burt BA, Sowers MR. *J Dental Res.* 85:262; 2006.

61. Wongkhantee S, Patanapiradej V, Maneenut C, Tantbirojn D. *J Dent.* 34:214; 2006.

60 Nutrition and Hollow Organs of Upper Gastrointestinal Tract

Ece A. Mutlu, Gökhan M. Mutlu, and Sohrab Mobarhan

CONTENTS

Nutrition is an integral part of the management of gastrointestinal (GI) illness. The following two chapters will elucidate the basic mechanisms of how the hollow organs of the GI tract handle and digest food, how illnesses of these organs affect nutritional status, and the role of nutrition in the management of these illnesses. The readers are referred to a GI textbook for further details on diseases mentioned in these chapters.

INTRODUCTION

The general roles of the various parts of the digestive system are given in Table 60.1. Diseases of these various parts not only cause damage to individual organs, but also disrupt the harmonious mechanisms that enable adequate handling and digestion of food.

Food enters through the mouth, where it is lubricated and broken down into pieces by mastication. Lubrication serves several purposes, including protection of the mouth from damage by food, ease of transfer of food over surfaces of the GI tract, and formation of a liquid medium in which chemical reactions of digestion can occur. Mastication is not only necessary for food breakdown but also helps increase the surface area of the food particles to allow reach by digestive enzymes.

Transport of food through the mouth and the pharynx into the esophagus is accomplished by the swallowing reflex. This reflex involves coordinated actions of the tongue, the soft and hard palates, the pharyngeal muscles, the glottis, the epiglottis and the upper esophageal sphincter (UES). It is extremely rapid, with a duration of less than a second and is regulated by both peripheral nerves and a swallowing center in the brainstem.[1] The multiple levels of control of swallowing and the redundancy of the control mechanisms allow compensating for minor problems.

TABLE 60.1
Parts of the Digestive System and Their Functions

Parts	Functions
Mouth, salivary glands, and pharynx	Breakdown of food into parts for transport downstream; lubrication of food pieces for transport; initiation of the digestion of carbohydrates in food
Esophagus	Transport and lubrication of food pieces; protection of the airway from food entry
Stomach	Storage and trituration of food into small pieces (<1 mm^3); initiation of the digestion of proteins with acid and proteases; initiation of the digestion of fats
Small intestines	Breakdown of foods into molecules and absorption of macro- and micronutrients; maintenance of water and electrolyte balance
Colon	Absorption of water and electrolytes; synthesis of certain vitamins; breakdown of carbohydrates to short chain fatty acids by bacteria; excretion of waste

Once swallowing is initiated voluntarily or involuntarily and the content of the mouth is pushed back into the pharynx, the swallowing reflex results in closure of the larynx by the epiglottis and concomitant relaxation of the UES to enable reception of bolus into the esophagus. Subsequently, the esophageal body, which has a short segment of striated muscle proximally but mainly is made up of smooth muscle, propels the bolus downward with peristaltic motion. As the bolus travels through the distal esophagus the lower esophageal sphincter (LES) relaxes and food is transported into the stomach for short-term storage and digestion. The integrity of the entire esophageal food transfer mechanism is very important to prevent food entering the airway.

Food goes through two functionally distinct compartments in the stomach: The proximal one consisting of the fundus and upper body acts as a reservoir. An adequate capacity in this compartment is achieved through receptive relaxation of the stomach wall, mediated by inhibition of vagal pathways and hormones such as secretin, gastric inhibitory peptide, and cholecystokinin (CCK). This relaxation allows for a wide range of storage volumes up to 1 to 2 l without significant increases in intragastric pressure. At the same time, release of acid and digestive enzymes into the reservoir initiates gastric digestion.

The distal and second compartment of the stomach consists of the lower body and antrum, whose main function is dissolution of food into gastric chyme with particle size <1 to 2 mm prior to exit through the pylorus. This process, termed *trituration*, is achieved by the strong propulsive motor activity of the stomach. After initiation of the electrical signal that is generated by specialized pacemaker cells located in the mid portion of the greater curvature, the stomach begins to contract from the mid body, the contraction gradually spreads towards the antrum in a peristaltic fashion and partial closure of the pyloric channel occurs. The stomach contents are thrusted backward against the antral walls and a closed pylorus with passage of only a small amount of well ground food into the duodenum. The shearing physical forces generated in this repetitive propulsion and retropulsion of gastric contents attain the particle size required of solid foods before passage into the small intestine.

Antral contractions cause emptying of solid food from the stomach. Liquids exit proportional to the pressure gradient between the duodenum and the stomach. This pressure gradient increases after completion of a meal when receptive relaxation fades away and the gastric fundus returns to its normal tone increasing intragastric pressure. The rate of emptying from the stomach is also determined by the chemical and physical composition of the meal as well as the way the body reacts to the food via the vagus nerve and the GI hormones. Liquids empty faster than solids, foods with high carbohydrate contents empty faster than foods that contain fat or are high in fiber. Hypo- or hypertonic fluids, highly viscous fluids, acid (pH 3.5), chyme with a high caloric density, polypeptides, oligosaccharides, and fatty acids entering the duodenum or overdistention of the small intestine inhibit gastric emptying. If nutrients rapidly enter or bypass the jejunum, rapidly reaching the ileum and colon, GI transit is slowed down via an ileal "brake." This brake is mediated through neurohumoral mechanisms and GI hormones, the most important of which is peptide YY. These mechanisms ensure that food is gradually released into the small intestine; is optimally mixed with pancreatic and biliary secretions, and has adequate contact time with digestive enzymes and the small intestinal absorptive mucosa.

The small intestine is designed to have a large surface area by arrangement of its cells into villi and crypts. The epithelial cells' lumenal surfaces have fingerlike projections termed microvilli that collectively make up the brush border. Most intestinal secretions come from the crypt cells, whereas the major function of the cells of the villi is digestion and absorption of water and nutrients. The villi as well as their lining cells are taller in the jejunum, and the height of both decreases caudally towards the ileum. Intestinal cells also become more specialized towards the ileum where absorption of bile salts and certain vitamins occurs. Digestion of nutrients is accomplished both by brush border and intraluminal enzymes, especially pancreatic exocrine ones. The different types of nutrients and how they are digested by the various enzymes in the GI tract are given in Figure 60.1.

After gastric chyme arrives at the small intestine, its acidity is rapidly neutralized by duodenal secretions and bicarbonate released from the pancreas. This neutralization is important for establishing a favorable milieu for optimal enzyme action. Furthermore, large amounts of electrolytes and water are secreted into the jejunal lumen to make chyme isoosmolar and to

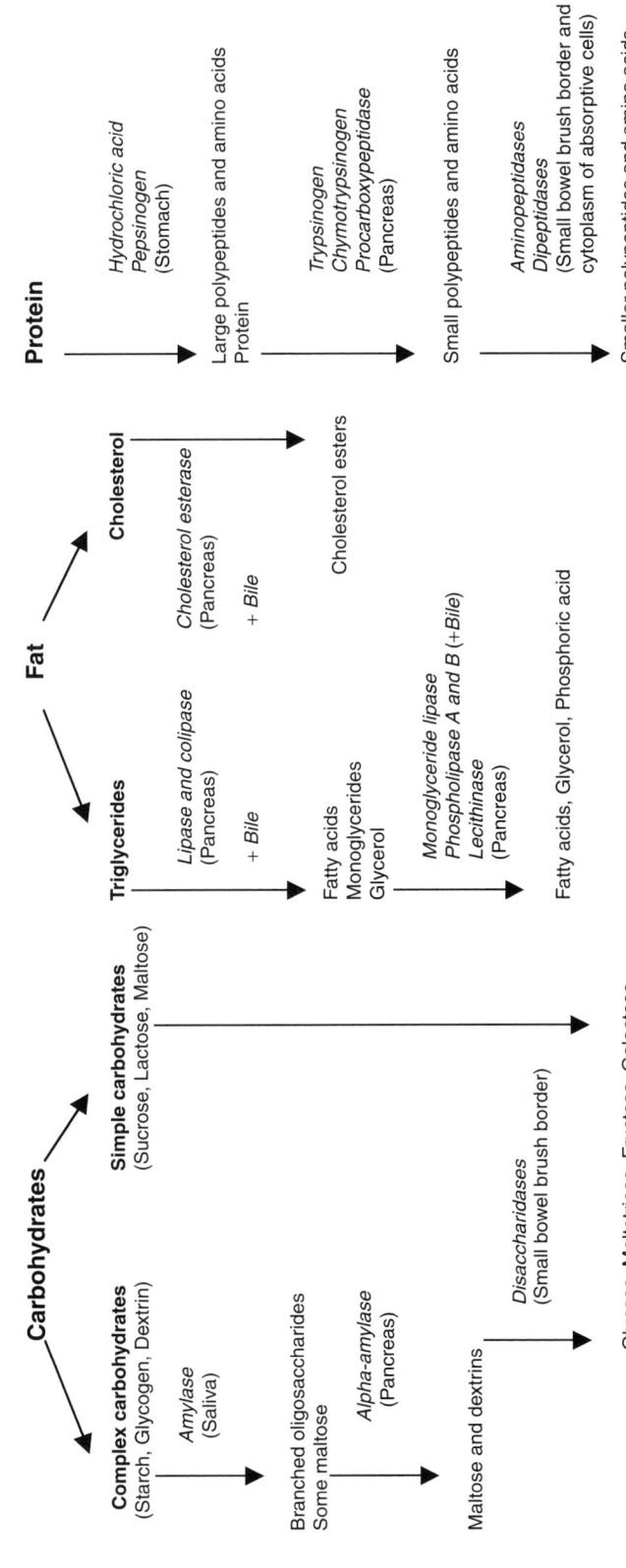

FIGURE 60.1 Outline of the digestion of carbohydrotes, fat, and protein.

dilute toxins and enable mucosal defense mechanisms such as secretory IgA. Almost simultaneously, the motor activity of the intestines change: propulsive movement decreases and segmental motor contractility increases. The net effect is stirring of intestinal contents with slow forward motion, which in turn increases contact of nutrients with intestinal cells.

During this process, blood flow and lymphatic drainage of the intestine are tightly regulated. Both flows increase as food, electrolytes, and water are absorbed, rapidly carrying these away to facilitate further diffusion. This rapid circulation ensures meeting intestinal oxygen, salt, and water demands, especially during secretion.

The products of digestion get absorbed, utilizing various mechanisms such as passive diffusion and osmosis, facilitated diffusion, and active transport. The sites of absorption of different nutrients and the mechanisms involved in this process are given in Table 60.2. A small amount of macronutrients leaves the small intestine undigested. Undigested portions are larger for complex carbohydrates, vary with fat intake, and are minimal for proteins.

TABLE 60.2
Overview of Nutrient Absorption

Nutrient	Absorption Site	Mechanism of Absorption
Lipids	Proximal and distal jejunum, colon	Passive diffusion, facilitated diffusion*
Monosaccharides	Proximal and distal jejunum	Na-dependent active transport
Amino acids	Proximal and distal jejunum	Carrier-mediated active transport and simple diffusion
Small peptides	Proximal and distal jejunum	Na-independent tertiary active transport
Bile salts and acids	Distal ileum	Passive absorptionand specific active absorption
Vitamin A	Duodenum and mid-jejunum	Passive diffusion**
Vitamin D	Duodenum, mid-jejunum and ileum	Passive diffusion**
Vitamin E	Duodenum and mid-jejunum	Passive diffusion**
Vitamin K_1	Duodenum, mid-jejunum, ileum and colon	Carrier-mediated uptake**
Vitamin K_2	Duodenum, mid-jejunum, ileum and colon	Passive diffusion**
Ascorbic acid	Mid-jejunum and ileum	Na-dependent active transport
Vitamin B_{12}	Ileum	Intrinsic factor binding and specific receptor med
Vitamin B_6	Jejunum	Passive diffusion
Thiamine	Duodenum and mid-jejunum	Na-dependent active transport
Riboflavin	Duodenum and mid-jejunum	Na-dependent active transport
Niacin	Duodenum and mid-jejunum	Awaits further study
Pantothenic acid	Mid-jejunum	Na-dependent active transport
Biotin	Duodenum, jejunum and colon	Na-dependent active transport
Folate	Duodenum, mid-jejunum and ileum	Specific carrier mediated Na-dependent active transport; pH-sensitive process
Sodium	Colon	Ion-specific channel; Carrier mediated coupling sodium and nutrients; Antiport carrier
Chloride	Colon	Electrogenic diffusion created by Na-absorption; Transcellular transport linked to Na via dual antiport; Anion exchangers
Potassium	Colon	Active transport by K-ATPase pumps
Calcium	Duodenum, mid-jejunum, ileum, and colon	Active transcellular process via specific channels, binding to calbindin, and Ca-ATPase; Passive paracellular diffusive process
Phosphorus	Duodenum and mid-jejunum	Active transport and passive diffusion
Magnesium	Duodenum, mid-jejunum and ileum	Passive paracellular diffusive process; Transcellular carrier mediated saturable process
Iron	Duodenum and mid-jejunum	Passive paracellular diffusive process; Nonessential fatty acid stimulated pathway; Intracellular iron binding proteins
Zinc	Mid-jejunum	Saturable carrier mediated process; Nonsaturable diffusion process
Iodine	Stomach	Active transport; passive diffusion[†]
Selenium	Duodenum	Active transport; passive diffusion[†]
Copper	Stomach and duodenum	Unknown[†]
Molybdenum	Stomach and mid-jejunum	Unknown[†]
Chromium	Mid-jejunum	Unknown[†]
Manganese	Mid-jejunum	Unknown[†]
Fluoride	Stomach	Unknown[†]

* Linoleic acid uptake occurs by facilitated diffusion.

** Bile salts are required for solubilization of the vitamins includes hydrolytic acid phosphorilation steps.

[†]Some is also transported as amino acid complexes possibly via facilitated diffusion or active diffusion or passive diffusion.

In the colon, bacteria act on the remaining nutrients and fiber, forming short-chain fatty acids and a variety of vitamins. These and large amounts of electrolytes and water are avidly absorbed by the colon, resulting in a small amount of feces. Together with the enterohepatic circulation of bile, the absorption of 98% of all GI fluid and electrolytes makes the GI system one of the most efficient systems in the body. The various GI secretions are listed in Table 60.3, along with calculation of the net fluid balance.

NUTRITION IN SELECTED DISEASES OF THE UPPER GI TRACT

GASTROESOPHAGEAL REFLUX DISEASE

Definition and Epidemiology

Gastroesophageal reflux disease (GERD) exists in individuals who have symptoms or histopathological changes related to backflow of gastric contents into the esophagus (see Table 60.4 and Table 60.5). There is no gold standard test to diagnose GERD; its incidence is estimated from either the disease symptoms (most frequently heartburn) or from findings of esophageal injury such as esophagitis. Heartburn is very common: 36% of the population experience heartburn at least once a month.[2] Esophagitis is estimated to occur in 3 to 5% of the general population.

Mechanisms

Factors or mechanisms important in GERD pathogenesis are listed in Table 60.6. Current dietary management of GERD is based on preventing or counteracting these mechanisms.

TABLE 60.3
GI Secretions

Site	Approximate Volume (in ml)
Salivary glands	1500
Stomach	2500
Liver (as bile)	500
Pancreas	1500
Small intestine	1000
GI tract secretions (1+2+3+4+5)	+7000
Daily oral intake	+2500
Absorption	−9300
Net excretion in the form of stool	200

TABLE 60.4
Symptoms of GERD

Esophageal	Extraesophageal
Heartburn (pyrosis)	Hypersalivation
Acid regurgitation	Nocturnal choking sensation
Dysphagia	Symptoms related to asthma:
Odynophagia	Wheezing
Chest pain	Shortness of breath
Globus sensation	Chronic cough
Nausea/Vomiting	Other symptoms of asthma
Symptoms of GI bleeding:	Symptoms related to posterior laryngitis:
Coffee ground emesis	Chronic hoarseness/dysphonia
Melena	Frequent throat clearing
	Chronic cough
	Sore throat
	Other symptoms laryngitis
	Symptoms related to dental caries

TABLE 60.5

Histopathological Changes Related to GERD

Reflux esophagitis	Destruction of esophageal epithelium (erosions, ulcers, balloon cells in epithelium)
	Neutrophilic or eosinophilic infiltration of the mucosa
	Large basal zone (>15% of the total epithelial thickness)
	Extension of mucosal papillae
	Regenerative changes in the epithelium
Barrett's esophagus	Metaplastic columnar epithelium replacing normal esophageal mucosa
Adenocarcinoma of the esophagus	
Peptic strictures	
Inflammatory polyps of the esophagus	
Pseudodiverticula	
Esophageal fistulas	

TABLE 60.6

Major Mechanisms Thought to be Involved in the Pathogenesis of GERD

1. Incompetent LES
   a. Increased transient relaxations of LES
      i. Intestinal distention with gas
   b. Hypotensive LES (i.e. decreased LES tone)
   c. High esophagogastric pressure gradient
   d. Anatomical alterations of the esophagogastric junction
      i. Hiatus hernia
      ii. Other alterations
2. Decreased ability of the stomach to selectively vent gas
3. Irritant effects of the refluxed material (especially gastric acid and pepsin)
4. Abnormal esophageal clearance/neutralization of the refluxed material
   a. Salivation
   b. Esophageal peristalsis
   c. Anatomical alterations of the esophagogastric junction
      i. Hiatus hernia
      ii. Other alterations
6. Delayed gastric emptying
7. Increased esophageal sensory perception

Effects on Nutritional Status

Uncomplicated GERD may occasionally lead to malnutrition in infants and children, although this is extremely rare in adults. Scurvy has been reported as a result of long-term avoidance of foods that contain vitamin C.[3] Additionally, megaloblastic anemia with B_{12} deficiency has occurred in association with long-term use of a proton pump inhibitor (PPI).[4] In preterm infants, vitamin D deficiency can occur due to PPIs.[5]

In cases of significant malnutrition with GERD symptoms, diseases giving rise to similar symptomatology, and complications of GERD need to be sought. Examples include eating disorders and scleroderma, which are easily overlooked. Complications of GERD are given in Table 60.7.

Lifestyle Factors That May Affect GERD

Lifestyle factors that may adversely affect the severity or frequency of GERD related symptoms are given in Table 60.8.

Obesity

GERD is associated with obesity and the occurrence of GERD is positively correlated with increasing body mass index (BMI). The frequency and severity of GERD seems to be worse in obese individuals; significantly higher number of GERD-related

---

TABLE 60.7
Major Complications of GERD

1. Acute GI bleeding
2. Chronic GI bleeding with anemia
3. Peptic strictures
4. Esophageal perforation
5. Barrett's esophagus
6. Adenocarcinoma of the esophagus

TABLE 60.8
**Lifestyle Factors That May Adversely
Affect Severity or Frequency of GERD**

1. Obesity
2. Smoking
3. Exercise
4. Alcohol consumption
5. Recumbent body position
6. Tight clothing over abdomen

---

hospitalizations occurred among the obese in the National Health and Nutrition Examination Survey (NHANES) study.[6] Obese individuals also tend to have a higher incidence of hiatal hernia that adversely affects LES function and competence.[7–10] In some obese individuals, LES pressures are lower than controls,[11] but this is not a consistent mechanism of GERD in all.[12] The gastroesophageal pressure gradient (difference between the pressures in the esophagus and stomach) may play a more important role in GERD pathogenesis in the obese.[8,13] As a result of the mechanical effects of increased intra-abdominal fat and the presence of the hiatal hernia, this gradient may be high in many obese patients with GERD. This forces gastric contents towards the relatively lower pressure esophageal environment and may promote reflux during any sphincter relaxation. Additionally, obese individuals have a higher incidence of esophageal motility disturbances[12] and cannot clear acid/gastric contents from the esophagus as fast as nonobese controls.[14] Combination of the high gastroesophageal pressure gradient with decreased clearance may explain the frequency and severity GERD with obesity.

One study among obese GERD patients who are not medication dependent for symptom control showed significant symptomatic improvement with weight loss.[15] Four other studies showed an improvement in esophageal pH and postprandial symptoms with modest weight loss.[16–20] One small, randomized study showed no difference in GERD symptoms after 10% weight loss in 6 months in the morbidly obese.[20] The authors' have anecdotal evidence that even loss of a few pounds may improve symptoms. However, definitive evidence that relates weight reduction to improvement in GERD is lacking. Some studies show no benefit, although most of these studies have been undertaken in individuals that are medication dependent with severely symptomatic disease. Large amounts of weight loss may be required in the morbidly obese before symptomatic improvement is evident. Nevertheless, most obese individuals should be encouraged to lose weight as first line treatment not only for GERD but also for its other health benefits.

Exercise

Exercise such as jogging, cycling, weight lifting, or rowing may cause GERD in healthy volunteers.[21–24] Reflux is further potentiated if the exercise is performed after meals.[21,23,25] The occurrence of exercise induced GERD may be dependent on the anatomy of the esophagogastric junction in both healthy individuals and GERD patients.[26]

Tight Clothing

Tight clothing worn over the abdomen and stomach has been postulated to elevate the gastroesophageal pressure gradient, especially postprandially.[27] Therefore, loose-fitting clothing has been recommended, although there are no clinical data to support this recommendation.

Food and Diet in GERD

Dietary habits, body position after meals, and GERD
Gastric distention is a potent stimulus for inappropriate transient LES relaxations. Especially after the first few hours of eating, meal size is the most important determinant of gastric distention. Therefore, GERD patients are typically advised to eat smaller meals and drink liquids in between as opposed to with meals. There is no evidence in regards to the effectiveness of this recommendation.

Effect of mealtime: In a small study of 20 patients, a late evening meal by itself did not increase GERD,[28] but late evening meals are likely to affect GERD because of their increased association with recumbent body position assumed soon after such meals.

Effect of recumbent position and head of bed elevation: Both recumbent body position and sleep decrease the clearance of refluxed gastric contents from the esophagus, resulting in prolonged esophageal exposure to acid, pepsin, etc.[29] Such exposure is a major contributor to the severity of esophagitis and stricture formation. Intraesophageal pH recordings in sleeping GERD patients show that elevation of the head of the bed significantly improves nocturnal acid clearance times.[30–32] Combined with H_2 blocker therapy, use of blocks to raise the head of the bed decreases retrosternal chest pain better than medication alone.[33] This effect is especially prominent for smokers and alcohol consumers.

Effect of right decubitus position: Sleeping on the right side can worsen GERD, possibly by promoting transient LES relaxations.[34–36] The effects of measures to prevent right-sided positions with body pillows or other mechanical devises sown onto the back and right side of sleep garments are unknown. Thus, GERD patients are advised not to sleep for at least 2 h after eating, to assume an upright body posture while awake, and to elevate the head of their bed using blocks or a foam wedge.

Meals types and foods that may adversely affect the GERD patient
A recent study comparing various different meals suggests that more than one component or feature of the meal determines induction of GERD.[37] The volume of the meal, use of spices, caloric density, fat content, and alcohol consumption with the meal, alone, or in combination with each other may affect initiation of symptoms.

Various foods that are reported to induce GERD, worsen its severity, or adversely affect healing of esophagitis are given in Table 60.9, together with their postulated mechanisms of action. There is little to no evidence as to withdrawal of these foods improves GERD symptoms.

Effects of meal consistency and osmolality: While there is no evidence that meal consistency (solid vs. liquid) affects reflux, osmolality of food may be important: Hyperosmolar foods versus isoosmolar ones reproduce esophageal symptoms. Coffee is thought to provoke GERD symptoms because of its high osmolality and irritant effects on the esophageal mucosa,[38,39] rather than its effects on LES pressure and transient LES relaxations, which are variable.

Effects of caloric density and volume: Caloric density of a meal does not seem to affect LES pressures or GERD episodes in healthy volunteers, suggesting that postprandial GERD may be related to the postprandial volume of food rather than its richness.[40] Larger meal volumes have also been associated with longer duration of reflux episodes on 24 pH tests, even in the upright position.[41]

Effects of alcohol: There are multiple reports of increased prevalence of GERD in alcohol users, and there is an association between consumption of spirits and GERD risk in some epidemiological studies[42–45] but not in others.[46–48] There is an improvement in esophageal motility disturbances after alcohol cessation but pH studies are unaltered.[49] In contrast to other alcoholic beverages, wine is very hypertonic, acidic, and has high tyramine content. Tyramine competes with histamine for degradation and may therefore delay the breakdown of the latter, which increases gastric acid secretion. In a survey of 349 individuals with GERD, wine has been reported to cause reflux in 37%.[50] In a small study in healthy volunteers, red wine increases postprandial esophageal acid exposure.[51]

Fat and GERD: The relationship between fat intake and GERD is unclear. Fat may increase GERD by decreasing LES pressure[52] caused by CCK release and by slowing gastric emptying, which in turn is thought to increase the frequency of transient LES relaxations resulting from a vago-vagal reflex originating in stomach mechanoreceptors.[53]

Survey findings show that fatty foods precipitate symptoms of GERD in 38% of normal subjects. Earlier studies show that, in healthy volunteers, LES pressures decrease after ingestion of a fatty meal as opposed to increases with a protein one. When adjusted for body position, this effect of fat on LES pressure in healthy individuals was present only in recumbency in one study,[41] and only in the upright position in another.[54] In other studies, high fat content in the diet compared to a low one made no difference in the healthy.[55–57]

Results are similar in GERD patients. In terms of esophageal acid exposure when identical protein content, volume, and calories are provided to patients, fat does not seem to matter.[54] Recent work confirms that a high-fat meal (52%) (compared to 24% in isovolumic and isoosmolar balanced ones) affects neither the acidity of the esophagus nor resting LES pressures, nor the rate of transient LES relaxations, for at least 3 h postprandially.[57] But, nonphysiological fat exposures (fat infused into the duodenum) may increase the rate of reflux episodes and the incidence of reflux during transient LES relaxations and acid sensitivity in GERD patients without altering the number of transient LES relaxations or LES pressure.[58,59] Fat infused intragastrically (20%) does not increase reflux episodes or sensitivity to acid exposure.[60]

TABLE 60.9
Foods That May Worsen GERD

Food	Effect(s)
Alcohol	↓ LES pressure
	↑ Transient LES relaxations
	↓ Esophageal peristalsis
	↓ Acid clearance
	Altered gastric emptying
	Caustic effect on mucosa
	Adverse effects on protective mucus
	↑ Gastric acid secretion
	↑ Number of reflux episodes
	↑ Nocturnal acid reflux
Capsaicin	Directly irritant to the esophageal mucosa
(found in peppers)	↑ Gastric acid and pepsin secretion
Carminatives (e.g.,	↓ LES pressure
peppermint)	↑ Transient LES relaxations
Spearmint	Directly irritant to the esophageal mucosa
Chocolate	Methylxanthines in it cause ↓ LES pressure
	High fat content ↓ gastric emptying
	↑ Transient LES relaxations
Citrus juice	Directly irritant to the esophageal mucosa
Coffee	Directly irritant to the esophageal mucosa
	↑ Gastric acid secretion
	↓ or ↑ LES pressure
	(effects worse with concomitant food)
	(effects vary with brand and treatment prior to consumption)
Methylxanthines (e.g.,	↓ LES pressure, 2° inhibition of phosphodiesterase, increased
theophylline in tea)	cAMP, and smooth muscle relaxation
Milk	↑ Gastric acid secretion
Onions	↑ Transient LES relaxations
	↑ Acid-pepsin injury possibly through inhibition of arachidonic acid
	metabolism (raw ones create worse symptoms compared to cooked)
Tomatoes	Directly irritant to the esophageal mucosa
	↑ Transient LES relaxations possibly secondary to salicylate content

It should be remembered that these studies all involve rather small numbers of subjects. There are significant differences in the composition of the diets used, and the differences in baseline characteristics of the healthy and GERD study subjects: Findings may not apply to various subgroups of patients, and there may not be enough power to detect some clinically significant differences. Nevertheless, based on these results, a low-fat diet cannot be recommended across the board for all patients with GERD. For the individual symptomatic patient who cannot tolerate fat, avoidance of fatty meals is reasonable.

The type of fat in a meal may also affect GERD. In preterm infants, medium-chain triglycerides have been shown to significantly increase gastric emptying compared to long-chain triglycerides. One study investigating reflux rates 2 h postprandially has found no difference with or without medium-chain triglycerides in pediatric formulas.[61] In healthy adults, nondigestible fats (e.g., olestra) do not alter esophageal acid exposure or delay gastric emptying, either.[62]

Protein and GERD: High-protein meals increased LES pressure in volunteers in one study,[52] but a commercially available amino acid solution infused intravenously or given intragastrically did not change reflux episodes or transient LES relaxations.[63] Oral L-arginine did not promote reflux despite increasing nitric oxide and lowering LES pressures.[64]

Carbohydrates and GERD: Case reports suggest that a low-carbohydrate diet may improve GERD, although most of the reported subjects have undergone drastic changes in their diet in addition to modification of its carbohydrate content.[65]

Fiber and GERD: High fiber did not cause reflux in 20 patients with suspected GERD.[66] However, prebiotic fibers that increase hydrogen gas production in the small bowel may increase GERD.[67] In healthy volunteers, fiber-supplemented enteral formula decreases the number of reflux episodes, but lengths their duration.[68]

Carbonated beverages: In GERD, it is also postulated that there is a decrease in selective venting of gastric gas. Hence, gas-containing foods such as carbonated beverages are commonly believed to initiate reflux episodes through belching associated with gastric content backflow. Although no definitive data exists, in one study among GERD patients, postprandial gas reflux made up 47% of the reflux episodes versus liquid reflux, which happened 78% of the time. Only 24% of liquid retroflow into the esophagus was preceded by gas reflux, which suggests that most reflux episodes occur without belching, refuting this belief.[69] In one study, carbonated beverages decreased LES pressure significantly compared to tap water.[70] Another reflux-promoting mechanism may be stimulation of gastric acid secretion or direct irritant effects with cola beverages. In a cohort study, carbonated beverages were found to be independent predictors of GERD during sleep.

Citrus fruits/juices: In questionnaire studies, 72% of GERD patients report symptoms with citrus.[50] This effect is likely due to the local irritant effects of citrus fruit/juices than their pH or their rather neutral effects on LES pressure.[39,71]

Chocolate: In small studies, chocolate decreases LES pressures and increases the duration of reflux.[72,73]

Onions/peppers: Raw onions increase esophageal acid exposure.[74] Capsaicin in peppers decreased time to peak heartburn in GERD patients in a small study.[75]

Do we really need a certain diet for GERD? Is there enough scientific evidence for a particular diet? There is no scientific evidence for a specific diet for all or most GERD patients. While a combination of lifestyle modifications such as weight loss, bland diet, elevation of the head of the bed, and antacids has been used in the past, the majority of patients with chronic symptoms and complications (about 81% in one study) do not respond and ultimately require use of medications like H_2 blockers and PPIs or surgical therapy. However, this may not apply to numerous individuals with less severe GERD who may not even present to physicians. Given the high disease prevalence, the potential side effects of medications and expense of chronic PPI therapy, studies pertaining to the utility of diet therapies alone or in combination with other lifestyle modifications in patients with less severe disease are needed urgently. In the meantime, the authors assert that all patients should be educated about various aspects of diet and their effects on GERD. Patients should be given a chance to experience and experiment with the nutritional tips for GERD patients given in Table 60.10. Treatment with a diet consisting of avoidance of reflux promoting foods (as in Table 60.9) should be reserved for the individual patient responding with the most symptomatic relief. The physician should ascertain that such treatment does not impair the patient's quality of life, as effective alternative management exists.

GERD therapy and diet

In general, patients with GERD tolerate all foods while on treatment with medications. Patients who do not symptomatically or histologically improve with standard therapy may have allergic eosinophilic esophagitis. Most such patients are children,[76] for whom therapy is withdrawal of the offending protein and feeding an elemental diet. Elimination diets have been shown to be very effective in this regard.[77]

Surgical treatment of GERD may be complicated with dumping syndrome, dysphagia, and gas-bloat syndrome. Dietary treatment of dumping syndrome is given below. Dietary treatment of dysphagia and gas bloat syndrome after fundoplication is based on common sense and anecdotal evidence. For dysphagia, authors suggest that patients eat soft foods, eat slowly, and chew food well. For gas bloat syndrome, the suggestions are the following:

1. To decrease aerophagia: avoid talking and laughing during meals, avoid chewing gum, hard candy, mints, etc., chew foods well, do not rush through meals, or eat on the run.
2. To decrease intestinal gas production: avoid gas forming foods such as legumes, beans, etc., or foods that contain significant amounts of nondigestible materials like sorbitol, olestra, etc.

Nutritional tips for patients with GERD are summarized in Table 60.10.

The patient on enteral nutrition and GERD

Theoretically, GERD may get worse with nasogastric or nasoenteric feedings as well as with gastrostomy placement. However, when these interventions are done, they usually involve sick patients who may already have GI motility problems because of underlying illnesses. Therefore, worsening of GERD in such settings may not be reflective of these interventions.

TABLE 60.10
Summary of Tips for the GERD Patient

1. If overweight, lose weight
2. Try avoiding foods that may worsen GERD (given in Table 60.9)
3. Eat small quantities of food at a time
4. Eat in an upright position
5. Avoid drinking large quantities of liquids with meals
6. Do not recline for at least 2 h after meals
7. Do not exercise for several hours after meals
8. If nighttime symptoms are present, try elevating the head of the bed with a wedge
9. If taking PPIs, take medication 30 min before a meal

Aspiration is the number one complication of enteral feeding via tube placement. Nasoenteric tubes can promote transient LES relaxations[78] and, therefore, may put patients at a higher risk of aspiration compared to gastrostomy tubes. Differences between gastrostomy and jejunostomy tubes have been evaluated in small or poorly designed studies without clear documentation of tube position. The American Gastroenterological Association recommends reservation of jejunostomy to patients with a history of GERD or recurrent aspiration secondary to gastrostomy tubes.[79]

PEPTIC ULCER DISEASE

Definition and Epidemiology

Peptic ulcer disease (PUD) is characterized by the presence of defects in the mucosa that extend through the muscularis mucosa (i.e., ulcers) in the presence of acid-peptic injury. PUD is common, with a lifetime prevalence of 5 to 10%. The etiologies for the disease are given in Table 60.11.

Mechanisms

Proposed mechanisms of peptic ulcer pathogenesis are given in Table 60.12. Of these, the most important is the presence of gastric acid. Many studies have shown that when acid is eliminated ulcers do not form. Therefore, the current treatment of PUD is directed at decreasing gastric acidity with medications.

Effects on Nutritional Status

PUD may affect nutritional status, especially if complications related to PUD or to the cause of PUD are present. These are given in Table 60.13. *Helicobacter pylori* or medication-induced atrophic gastritis may lead to vitamin B_{12} deficiency. Repeated blood

---

TABLE 60.11
Causes of PUD

Common	Uncommon
Helicobacter pylori	Diseases that cause hyperacidity
NSAIDs	Zollinger-Ellison syndrome (gastrinoma)
Stress related mucosal damage	Mastocytosis/Basophilic leukemia
	Antral G cell hyperplasia or hyperfunction
	Infections of the gastric mucosa:
	Cytomegalovirus
	Herpes simplex
	Vascular diseases:
	Chronic radiation injury
	Crack-cocaine related injury
	Chemotherapy related injury

TABLE 60.12
Major Mechanisms of Tissue Damage and Repair Involved in the Pathogenesis of PUD

1. Epithelial cell injury resulting from:
   a. Exogenous irritants like NSAIDs and alcohol
   b. Endogenous irritants like acid, pepsin, bile acids, and lysolecithin
   c. Breakdown of epithelial defense mechanisms:
      i. Weak mucus and bicarbonate layer
      ii. Low resistance of the apical cell membrane to acid back diffusion
      iii. Inadequate acid clearance intracellularly because of derangements of the Na/H antiporter
      iv. Inadequate acid clearance extracellularly because of altered mucosal blood flow
2. Inadequate repair of epithelial injury:
   a. Inadequate epithelial cell restitution and growth
   b. Inadequate wound healing

TABLE 60.13
Major Complications Related to PUD

1. Atrophic gastritis
2. Gastric carcinoma related to *H. pylori*
3. Obstruction (especially at gastric outlet)
4. Hemorrhage (acute or chronic)
5. Perforation
6. Penetration of ulcers

---

loss from bleeding ulcers may cause iron deficiency anemia. Chronic long-standing gastric outlet obstruction because of scarring of the pyloric channel or development of severe dumping syndrome following surgical treatment of ulcers can cause protein and calorie malnutrition. These complications are rare in the United States.

Diet in PUD

The role of diet in PUD occurrence and treatment has changed tremendously as our knowledge about the pathogenesis of PUD increased. In the early 1900s, with the rationale that food buffers stomach acid, Lenhartz proposed that frequent small meals might be of benefit in PUD treatment. Physicians of the day followed with restrictive dietary treatment programs that advocated small quantities of bland food at frequent intervals, in the hopes that such a feeding regimen would also stimulate less acid secretion and thereby hasten healing. One PUD treatment that consisted of milk, cream, and eggs with subsequent addition of soft and "nonirritating" foods, the Sippy diet, was formulated by Sippy and Hurst in 1910.[80] This diet and its modifications prevailed in PUD treatment over eight decades. A 1977 survey by Welsh and colleagues of 326 hospitals in the United States demonstrated that 77% used a bland diet and 55% routinely or usually gave milk to PUD patients.[81] Marked variations were seen in the composition of these supposedly similar diets.

The benefits of restrictive diets including the Sippy and its modifications are refuted in numerous studies.[82–85] First, acidity of the stomach following bland diets and freely chosen diets do not differ.[86] More importantly, controlled studies of radiological ulcer healing or resolution of clinical symptoms show no improvement on these diets.[87,88] The same is true for ulcer recurrence, which is not different with or without such diets when patients are followed up to a year or more.[87,89] Instead, these diets in the long term may be harmful; for example, they can result in nutritional deficiencies like scurvy.[90] Given this evidence, there is no reason to support the use of a restricted or bland diet for PUD.

Further evidence for and against various dietary interventions are given below:

Small frequent feedings: Food related gastric acid stimulation is prolonged in PUD patients, and, therefore, it is not logical to expect adequate acid buffering with any type of meal.[91,92] Even though peak acid secretion may be higher as a result of gastric distention with larger meals, studies show that mean acid concentration does not differ when patients are fed 2-hourly portions as opposed to 4-hourly ones.[93]

Increased use of milk: Milk had been advocated as part of the early diets for PUD (including the Sippy and its modifications) because of its acid-buffering capacity. However, in a study of a large group of PUD patients, intragastric milk drip did not improve radiological healing of PUD, although pain relief was quicker.[94] In another study of 65 patients taking equal doses of cimetidine, endoscopic ulcer healing, or pain relief at 4 weeks was worse in the group given milk with seasonal fruits as opposed to the group given a regular diet.[95]

Milk increases gastric acid secretion (about 30% in duodenal ulcer patients)[96] and its capability to neutralize acid is short lived.[97] Whether milk is whole, low-fat, or nonfat does not make a difference.[97] Amino acids released as a result of hydrolysis of milk proteins stimulate gastrin secretion.[96] The relatively high calcium in milk acts as a second messenger for gastrin and acetylcholine-stimulated acid release, and ulcer patients are more sensitive to such effects of calcium.[50]

Milk can also be harmful to ulcer patients who consume large amounts of absorbable antacids concomitantly. These PUD patients may develop acute or chronic milk–alkali syndrome leading to alkalosis, renal insufficiency/calculi, and hypercalcemia.[98]

Changing the macronutrient composition of diet: Protein stimulates gastric acid more than carbohydrates and fat;[99] however, there is also evidence that high protein may result in lower gastric and duodenal acidity following meals.[100] Whether this effect is due to satiety induced by the high protein is unknown. Thus, no recommendations concerning the protein content of the meal for PUD can be made. Although fat in the small intestine inhibits gastric acid secretion,[101] there is no satisfactory evidence that high-fat diets are beneficial to ulcer patients either. In fact, many of the bland diets including the Sippy diet are high in fat and have been shown to be harmful by increasing the risk of cardiovascular disease among PUD patients.

Alcohol consumption: Alcohol ingestion can cause acute erosive gastritis with ulcerations and bleeding. Alcohol concentrations of at least 8% were required to break the gastric mucosal barrier,[102] while higher levels of 40% or more were needed in another study.[103]

Alcohol as low as 5% stimulates gastric acid secretion both through direct stimulation of parietal cells and through release of antral gastrin, although the effects may vary depending on the type of beverage consumed.[104] Beer, for example, can increase acid independent of its ethanol content. Intake of alcohol with salicylates may contribute to its irritant effects by causing back-diffusion of acid and stimulating pepsin secretion. Furthermore, acute alcohol ingestion can weaken duodenal defenses against ulcer formation by inhibiting basal- and secretin-stimulated pancreatic fluid and bicarbonate secretion,[105–107] which is not entirely due to alcohol-induced contraction of the sphincter of Oddi.[108]

Epidemiological studies, however, show no difference in alcohol consumption between high- and low-PUD areas throughout different parts of the world, and alcohol intake is not independently predictive of PUD prevalence in surveys, although most of these studies were conducted before testing for H. pylori was implemented. One recent epidemiological study showed an increased risk of PUD in alcohol consumers with a U-shaped association distribution.[109] The nadir of this distribution was at 6 to 12 drinks weekly, with a lower number of ulcers in people who drank moderate amounts of wine. Intake of spirits increased the risk of PUD in Helicobacter-serology-positive subjects in this study. In other studies, wine and beer drinking are associated with lower rates of H. pylori infection.[110,111] This may be a marker of increased health consciousness in wine drinkers or due to its antimicrobial effects. Alcohol does not seem to adversely affect ulcer healing and moderate alcohol consumption (20 g/day or less) may also promote ulcer healing.[112] Some postulate that alcohol may be similar to mild irritants in that low doses may heighten mucosal defenses through stimulation of prostaglandin production.

Caffeine/coffee/tea/carbonated drinks: Caffeine stimulates both acid and pepsin release, and patients with duodenal ulcer have a greater and longer response. The effects of coffee and tea, however, exceed what their caffeine content induces.[113] Serum gastrin and gastric acidity (especially in ulcer patients) is higher than caffeine, and decaffeination diminishes this acid-secretory potency only minimally.[113] In one study, the addition of milk and sugar to tea lessened this effect.[114] Whether these translate into clinical significance is unknown. Habitual coffee consumption in college students was linked to development of PUD in later life.[115] Conversely, a very large survey failed to show an association between coffee and PUD.[116]

Carbonated beverages similarly may stimulate acid production but this may also be unrelated to caffeine.[113]

Salt intake: A large oral load of salt can be an irritant to the gastric mucosa, leading to gastritis.[117] In epidemiological studies, PUD mortality correlates linearly with increasing salt consumption.[118] Case control studies also show that gastric ulcer patients have a higher level of salt intake compared to healthy controls.[119]

Avoidance of certain spices: Application of spices on upper GI mucosa revealed that cinnamon, nutmeg, allspice, thyme, black pepper, cloves, and paprika cause no endoscopic damage whereas hot pepper, chili powder, and mustard lead to edema, erythema and mucosal breakdown.[120] The latter spices also lead to epigastric discomfort in patients.[120] Furthermore, peppers induce supra-maximal acid output in duodenal ulcer patients and have been associated with gastritis.[121,122] In one study using gastric lavage, both red and black pepper caused higher levels of gastric cell exfoliation, acid and pepsin secretion, and microbleeding although this was not confirmed endoscopically.[122] In several others, gastric aspirates after use of capsaicin (found in red peppers and paprika) and black peppers showed increased DNA fragment levels indicating mucosal damage.[114] In other studies peppers increased production of mucus with only minimal acid secretory effects. Duodenal ulcer patients on acid suppressive therapy eating 3 g of red chili powder had clinical and endoscopic healing rates similar to patients not eating the spice.[82] Authors of this study suggested that direct installation of spices via tubes in a fasting state in previous studies as opposed to more physiological consumption of the spice might explain the discrepancy between prior reports of gastric damage and their findings. Concomitant antacid intake may have altered the effects of the spice in this study. It is also unknown whether chronic consumption of potentially irritant spices leads to an adaptation response by stimulating gastric defenses, explaining some of the earlier work showing high levels of mucous production.

Dietary fiber: Fiber has been postulated to be beneficial for PUD because of its buffering effects, shortening of GI transit leading to decreased acid secretion, and binding of irritant bile acids.[123] The role of dietary fiber in treatment or prevention of PUD is controversial. Fiber intake and associated vitamin A consumption has been inversely correlated with the risk of duodenal ulcers.[124] Reduction in clinical and endoscopic ulcer recurrence with high-fiber diets has been shown,[125,126] although epidemiological studies have found elevated incidence of PUD in areas of the world with high fiber consumption. Low fiber consumption may predispose to PUD rather than high fiber having protective effects.[127] Supplementation of fiber in the form of pectin has not affected ulcer recurrence.[128] Guar gum may reduce gastric acid, it has not been shown to normalize it.[129] Therefore, components of the high-fiber diet other than fiber itself may be protective.

Fiber given as wheat bran can bind bile acids and may reduce their elevated concentration in gastric ulcer patients;[125] it may be beneficial in biliary-reflux-associated ulcerations.

Essential fatty acids: Linoleic acid, an essential fatty acid (EFA) and a major substrate for synthesis of prostaglandins that are protective for upper GI tract mucosa, has been shown to be deficient in the diets of duodenal ulcer patients.[130] Additionally, Hollander and Tarnowksi have shown that the declining incidence of PUD parallels a 200% increase in dietary availability of EFAs.[103] They have hypothesized that this association reflects a cause-and-effect relationship and that higher intakes of EFA induce mucosal prostaglandin E synthesis, thereby conferring protection against mucosal irritants and nonsteroidal antiinflammatory drugs (NSAIDs). Although the epidemiological evidence for this hypothesis is strong, direct evidence is lacking.

TABLE 60.14
Summary of Evidence on Diet and PUD

Definitely not beneficial and potentially harmful to PUD patients
Bland and restrictive diets including the Sippy diet and its modifications
Frequent milk intake

Probably harmful to PUD patients
Alcohol
Caffeine
Coffee/tea
Carbonated beverages
Certain spices
High salt load

Probably beneficial to PUD patients
Essential fatty acids
Fiber intake

TABLE 60.15
Summary of Nutritional Tips for PUD Patients

1. Avoid restrictive diets
2. Avoid frequent milk intake
3. Avoid high salt intake
4. Avoid concentrated alcoholic beverages
5. Avoid directly irritant foods and spices such as peppers, chili powder, etc.
6. Take PPIs, 30 min before a meal

Many dietary factors may be significant in the pathogenesis and treatment of ulcer disease, but most studies have been conducted before *H. pylori* was implicated in ulcer formation. Therefore, some of the evidence, especially the epidemiological, for, or against various interventions may not be applicable to current PUD patients. The available information is summarized in Table 60.14. Summary of nutritional tips for patients with PUD are given in Table 60.15. With the potent antisecretory medications available today, diet therapy has a limited role in treatment of PUD. Patients with PUD should be allowed to eat as they desire with few exceptions.

Food and PUD Medications

PPIs frequently used in the treatment of acid–peptic diseases including PUD are expensive medications that irreversibly bind and block the hydrogen pump of the parietal cell. These drugs are rapidly cleared from the bloodstream within a few hours following intake. Therefore, for utmost efficacy, they should be timed so that effective concentrations are in the circulation when acid secretion is maximally stimulated. This usually requires these drugs to be taken about 30 to 60 min prior to a meal.

GASTROPARESIS

Abnormally slow emptying of the stomach from causes other than mechanical obstruction is called gastroparesis. The many causes are given in Table 60.16, with diabetes being the most common.

The various factors and medications that affect the rate of gastric emptying are given in Table 60.17. The mainstay of the dietary treatment of gastroparesis involves avoidance of the factors that delay emptying (as shown in Table 60.17) while adopting a diet that exits the stomach easily. No one diet has been shown effective.

In general, dietary fiber usually needs to be decreased as it may result in bezoar formation. Koch promotes six smaller meals in order to decrease symptom severity, and he advocates a three-step nausea and vomiting diet.[131] These recommendations need to be tested to prove their usefulness.

Dietary treatment frequently needs to be combined with prokinetic medications usually administered before meals. Oral medications should preferably be in liquid formulations that are absorbed faster compared to capsules and tablets, which may lie in the stomach for hours.

TABLE 60.16

Causes of Gastroparesis

1. Metabolic and endocrine	Diabetes, thyroid disease, uremia, porphyrias, pregnancy, electrolyte imbalance, and Addison's disease	
2. Iatrogenic	Surgical damage to vagal trunk, drugs, and radiation damage to stomach	
3. Neurological	Intracranial/spinal cord lesions, Guillain–Barre syndrome, acute dysautonomic syndrome, Shy–Drager syndrome, Parkinson's disease, seizure disorder, multiple sclerosis, and labyrinthitis	
4. Psychogenic	Anorexia, bulimia, and psychological stress	
5. Inflammatory	Viral gastritis, Chagas disease, botulinum toxin, and celiac sprue	
6. Rheumatologic	Scleroderma, SLE, PM/DM, and amyloidosis	
7. Muscular disorders		
8. Paraneoplastic	Small-cell lung cancer and breast cancer	
9. Idiopathic		

TABLE 60.17

Factors That Affect the Rate of Gastric Emptying

Factor	Fast Emptying	Slow Emptying
Luminal:		
Consistency of food	Liquid	Solid
Macronutrient composition	Fat/Protein	Carbohydrate
Fiber content of food	Low	High
Osmolality in stomach or duodenum	Low	High (>800 mOsm/l)
Change in temperature of stomach	Hot/Cold	Body temperature
Gastric distention	High	Low
Volume in duodenum	Low	High
pH in duodenum	High	Low
Drugs:	Cholinergic	Anticholinergic
	Erythromycin	
	Metoclopropamide	
	Cisapride	
	Domperidone	
GI hormones:	Gastrin	Cholecystokinin
	Motilin	Glucagon
		Secretin

As the disease progresses, dietary and medical treatment may not suffice and refractory patients may require drainage gastrostomy with jejunal enteral feeding. Although no controlled studies exist, in one retrospective study, enteral feeding via a jejunostomy improved overall health status in diabetic patients.[132]

Nutritional tips for any gastroparetic patient are summarized in Table 60.18. Nutritional tips for diabetic patients with gastroparesis can be found in a recent review article.[133]

DUMPING SYNDROME

Dumping syndrome is the collection of symptoms triggered by rapid entry of large boluses of food into the small bowel. The syndrome most often occurs in patients who have had a vagotomy or gastrectomy, frequently done in the past for PUD. The two main types of the syndrome, the symptoms, and possible mechanisms are given in Table 60.19.

Dietary treatment of early dumping aims to slow emptying of the stomach and decrease the volume and osmolality of food boluses delivered to the small bowel. For this purpose, patients are advised to avoid consuming liquid and solids simultaneously, to stay away from highly osmolar foods, and to eat small meals. Dietary treatment of late dumping syndrome aims to decrease rapid entry of large amounts of carbohydrates especially concentrated simple sugars, into the small intestine. Patients are advised to keep away from concentrated sweets such as candy, honey, syrup, etc. These latter recommendations have not been rigorously tested but are consistent with the pathophysiology of dumping.

Additionally, in order to delay gastric emptying and especially bind the liquid component of the meal, fibers such as guar gum and pectin has been added to meals. Results with pectin are variable: In small studies, it delays gastric emptying in the majority of patients but may also increase it; therefore, doses may need to be individualized to achieve a particular viscosity.[134,135] In one study, muffins that contain 5 g of pectin failed to alter symptoms or gastric emptying.[136] In open-label studies, addition of 5 g of guar gum to meals for 4 weeks symptomatically benefited 8/16 patients with proximal selective vagotomy-induced dumping, although the effect was minimal in three patients.[137] Recent work also suggests that increasing viscosity of the liquid phase of a meal by pectin or guar gum may stimulate more propulsive forces in the stomach, causing a detrimental effect.[138] Most patients with severe dumping do not respond to the commonly used dietary instructions. In these refractory patients, acarbose may be tried for its effects on glucose[139] and octreotide is useful.[140] Nutritional tips for patients with dumping syndrome are summarized in Table 60.20.

TABLE 60.18
Summary of Tips for the Gastroparesis Patient

1. Eat small quantities at a time
2. Eat in upright position
3. Do not recline for several hours after meals
4. Chew every bite of food well
5. Consume a low-fat diet
6. Avoid fiber/roughage
7. Eat well-cooked foods
8. Turn foods into liquid/pureed form if unable to tolerate solids
9. Take medications in liquid formulation, 30 min before meals

TABLE 60.19
Types of Dumping Syndrome

	Timing Following a Meal	Cause	Mediators	Symptoms*
Early	15–30 min	Rapid fluid shift from intravascular space to small intestinal lumen	Release of vasoactive intestinal hormones (e.g., VIP, neurotensin, motilin, etc.)	Flushing Dizziness Nausea Palpitations Diaphoresis Syncope
Late	2–4 h	Rapid rise of blood glucose	Rapid rise in insulin in response to glucose	

* Symptoms are similar for both early and late dumping.

TABLE 60.20
Summary of Nutritional Tips in Dumping Syndrome

1. Eat small and drink quantities at a time
2. Spread meals throughout the day
3. Avoid drinking liquids with meals, instead drink liquids in between meals
4. Avoid hypertonic foods and concentrated sweets (such as soft drinks, juices, pies, cakes, cookies, candy, etc.)
5. Avoids foods rich in simple carbohydrates, replace with complex carbohydrates
6. Consume high-protein, moderate-fat foods
7. Increase fiber intake if tolerated
8. Lie down after meals if possible

REFERENCES

1. Jean, A. *Brain Behav Evol* 25: 109; 1984.
2. Nebel, O.T., Fornes, M.F. & Castell, D.O. *Am J Dig Dis* 21: 953; 1976.
3. Hiebert, C.A. *Ann Thorac Surg* 24: 108; 1977.
4. Bellou, A. et al. *J Intern Med* 240: 161; 1996.
5. Pattaragarn, A. & Alon, U.S. *Clin Pediatr (Phila)* 40: 389; 2001.
6. Ruhl, C.E. & Everhart, J.E. *Ann Epidemiol* 9: 424; 1999.
7. Wilson, L.J., Ma, W. & Hirschowitz, B.I. *Am J Gastroenterol* 94: 2840; 1999.
8. Pandolfino, J.E. et al. *Gastroenterology* 130: 639; 2006.
9. Stene-Larsen, G. et al. *Scand J Gastroenterol* 23: 427; 1988.
10. Barak, N., Ehrenpreis, E.D., Harrison, J.R. & Sitrin, M.D. *Obes Rev* 3: 9; 2002.
11. O'Brien, C.J., Giaffer, M.H., Cann, P.A. & Holdsworth, C.D. *Am J Gastroenterol* 86: 1614; 1991.
12. Jaffin, B.W., Knoepflmacher, P. & Greenstein, R. *Obes Surg* 9: 390; 1999.
13. Mercer, C.D., Wren, S.F., DaCosta, L.R. & Beck, I.T. *J Med* 18: 135; 1987.
14. Mercer, C.D., Rue, C., Hanelin, L. & Hill, L.D. *Am J Surg* 149: 177; 1985.
15. Murray, F.E., Ennis, J., Lennon, J.R. & Crowe, J.P. *Ir J Med Sci* 160: 2; 1991.
16. Fraser-Moodie, C.A. et al. *Scand J Gastroenterol* 34: 337; 1999.
17. Mathus-Vliegen, E.M., van Weeren, M. & van Eerten, P.V. *Digestion* 68: 161; 2003.
18. Mathus-Vliegen, E.M. & Tygat, G.N. *Scand J Gastroenterol* 37: 1246; 2002.
19. Mathus-Vliegen, L.M. & Tytgat, G.N. *Eur J Gastroenterol Hepatol* 8: 635; 1996.
20. Kjellin, A., Ramel, S., Rossner, S. & Thor, K. *Scand J Gastroenterol* 31: 1047; 1996.
21. Yazaki, E., Shawdon, A., Beasley, I. & Evans, D.F. *Aust J Sci Med Sport* 28: 93; 1996.
22. Collings, K.L., Pierce Pratt, F., Rodriguez-Stanley, S. et al. *Med Sci Sports Exerc* 35: 730; 2003.
23. Clark, C.S., Kraus, B.B., Sinclair, J. & Castell, D.O. *JAMA* 261: 3599; 1989.
24. Kraus, B.B., Sinclair, J.W. & Castell, D.O. *Ann Intern Med* 112: 429; 1990.
25. Peters, H.P. et al. *Int J Sports Med* 21: 65; 2000.
26. Pandolfino, J.E., Bianchi, L.K. & Lee, T.J. *Am J Gastroenterol* 99: 1430; 2004.
27. Dent, J. *Baillieres Clin Gastroenterol* 1: 727; 1987.
28. Orr, W.C. & Harnish, M.J. *Aliment Pharmacol Ther* 12: 1033; 1998.
29. Demeester, T.R. et al. *Ann Surg* 184: 459; 1976.
30. Johnson, L.F. & DeMeester, T.R. *Dig Dis Sci* 26: 673; 1981.
31. Hamilton, J.W., Boisen, R.J., Yamamoto, D.T. et al. *Dig Dis Sci* 33: 518; 1988.
32. Stanciu, C. & Bennett, J.R. *Digestion* 15: 104; 1977.
33. Harvey, R.F. et al. *Lancet* 2: 1200; 1987.
34. Katz, L.C., Just, R. & Castell, D.O. *J Clin Gastroenterol* 18: 280; 1994.
35. van Herwaarden, M.A. et al. *Am J Gastroenterol* 95: 2731; 2000.
36. Khoury, R.M., Camacho-Lobato, L., Katz, P.O. et al. *Am J Gastroenterol* 94: 2069; 1999.
37. Rodriguez, S. et al. *Dig Dis Sci* 43: 485; 1998.
38. Lloyd, D.A. & Borda, I.T. *Gastroenterology* 80: 740; 1981.
39. Price, S.F., Smithson, K.W. & Castell, D.O. *Gastroenterology* 75: 240; 1978.
40. Pehl, C., Pfeiffer, A., Waizenhoefer, A. et al. *Aliment Pharmacol Ther* 15: 233; 2001.
41. Iwakiri, K. et al. *Dig Dis Sci* 41: 926; 1996.
42. Nocon, M., Labenz, J. & Willich, S.N. *Aliment Pharmacol Ther* 23: 169; 2006.
43. Wang, J.H., Luo, J.Y., Dong, L. et al. *World J Gastroenterol* 10: 1647; 2004.
44. Mohammed, I., Nightingale, P. & Trudgill, N.J. *Aliment Pharmacol Ther* 22: 821; 2005.
45. Rosaida, M.S. & Goh, K.L. *Eur J Gastroenterol Hepatol* 16: 495; 2004.
46. Talley, N.J., Zinmeister, A.R., Schleck, C.D. & Melton, l.J. *Gut* 35: 619; 1994.
47. Stanghellini, V. *Scand J Gastroenterol Suppl* 231: 29; 1999.
48. Ang, T.L. et al. *World J Gastroenterol* 11: 3558; 2005.
49. Grande, L. et al. *Gut* 38: 655; 1996.
50. Feldman, M. & Barnett, C. *Gastroenterology* 108: 125; 1995.
51. Grande, L., Manterola, C., Ros, E. et al. *Dig Dis Sci* 42: 1189; 1997.
52. Nebel, O.T. & Castell, D.O. *Gastroenterology* 63: 778; 1972.
53. Franzi, S.J., Martin, C.J., Cox, M.R. & Dent, J. *Am J Physiol* 259: G380; 1990.
54. Becker, D.J., Sinclair, J., Castell, D.O. & Wu, W.C. *Am J Gastroenterol* 84: 782; 1989.
55. Pehl, C. et al. *Am J Gastroenterol* 94: 1192; 1999.
56. Colombo, P., Mangano, M., Bianchi, P.A. & Penagini, R. *Gut* 46:1; 2002.
57. Penagini, R., Mangano, M. & Bianchi, P.A. *Gut* 42: 330; 1998.
58. Holloway, R.H., Lyrenas, E., Ireland, A. & Dent, J. *Gut* 40: 449; 1997.
59. Meyer, J., Lembo, A., Elashoff, J., Fass, R. & Mayer, E.A. *Gut* 49: 624; 2001.

60. Mangano, M., Colombo, P., Bianchi, P.A. & Penagini, R. *Dig Dis Sci* 47: 657; 2002.
61. Sutphen, J.L. & Dillard, V.L. *J Pediatr Gastroenterol Nutr* 14: 38; 1992.
62. Just, R., Katz, L., Verhille, M. et al. *Am J Gastroenterol* 88: 1734; 1993.
63. Gielkens, H.A., Lamers, C.B. & Masclee, A.A. *Dig Dis Sci* 43: 840; 1998.
64. Luiking, Y.C. et al. *Am J Physiol* 274: G984; 1998.
65. Yancy, W.J., Provenzale, D. & Westman, E.C. *Altern Ther Health Med* 7: 120; 2001.
66. Floren, C.H. & Johnsson, F. *J Intern Med* 225: 287; 1989.
67. Piche, T. et al. *Gastroenterology* 124: 894; 2003.
68. Bouin, M. et al. *Clin Nutr* 20: 307; 2001.
69. Sifrim, D., Silny, J., Holloway, R.H. & Janssens, J.J. *Gut* 44: 47–54; 1999.
70. Hamoui, N. et al. *J Gastrointest Surg* 10: 870; 2006.
71. Cranley, J.P., Achkar, E. & Fleshler, B. *Am J Gastroenterol* 81: 104; 1986.
72. Wright, L.E. & Castell, D.O. *Am J Dig Dis* 20: 703; 1975.
73. Murphy, D.W. & Castell, D.O. *Am J Gastroenterol* 83: 633; 1998.
74. Allen, M.L., Mellow, M.H., Robinson, M.G. & Orr, W.C. *Am J Gastroenterol* 85: 377; 1990.
75. Rodriguez-Stanley, S., Collings, K.L., Robinson, M. et al. *Aliment Pharmacol Ther* 14: 129; 2000.
76. Kelly, K.J. et al. *Gastroenterology* 109: 1503; 1995.
77. Liacouras, C. et al. *Clin Gastroenterol Hepatol* 3: 1198; 2005.
78. Mittal, R.K., Stewart, W.R. & Schirmer, B.D. *Gastroenterology* 103: 1236; 1992.
79. Kirby, D.F., Delegge, M.H. & Fleming, C.R. *Gastroenterology* 108: 1282; 1995.
80. Sippy, B.W. *JAMA* 250: 2192; 1983.
81. Welsh, J.D. *Gastroenterology* 72: 740; 1977.
82. Marotta, R.B. & Floch, M.H. *Med Clin North Am* 75: 967 1991.
83. Berstad, A. *Scand J Gastroenterol Suppl* 129: 228; 1987.
84. Kirsner, J.B. & Palmer, W.L. *Am J Dig Dis* 7: 85; 1940.
85. Bingle, J.P. & Lennard-Jones, J.E. *Gut* 1: 337; 1960.
86. Lennard-Jones, J.E. & Barbouris, N. *Gut* 6: 113; 1965.
87. Doll, R., Friedlander, P. & Pygott, F. *Lancet* 270: 5; 1956.
88. Truelove, S.C. *Br Med J* 5198: 559; 1960.
89. Buchman, E., Kaung, D.T., Dolan, K. & Knapp, R.N. *Gastroenterol* 56: 1016; 1969.
90. Zucker, G.M. & Clayman, C.B. *JAMA* 250: 2198; 1983.
91. Fordtran, J.S. & Walsh, J.H. *J Clin Invest* 52: 645; 1973.
92. Malagelada, J.R., Longstreth, G.F., Deering, T.B. et al. *Gastroenterology* 73: 989; 1977.
93. Barbouris, N., Fletcher, J. & Lennard-Jones, J.E. *Gut* 6: 118; 1965.
94. Doll, R., Price, A.V., Pygott, F. & Sanderson, P.H. *Lancet* 270: 70; 1956.
95. Kumar, P.J., O'Donoghue, D.P., Stenson, K. & Dawson, A.M. *Gut* 20: 743; 1979.
96. Mathewson, M. & Farnham, C. *Crit Care Nurse* 4: 75; 1984.
97. Ippoliti, A.F., Maxwell, V. & Isenberg, J.I. *Ann Intern Med* 84: 286; 1976.
98. Pursan, S. & Somer, T. *Acta Med Scand* 173: 435; 1963.
99. Rune, S.J. *Scand J Gastroenterol* 8: 605; 1973.
100. Lennard-Jones, J.E., Fletcher, J. & Shaw, D.G. *Gut* 9: 177; 1968.
101. Christiansen, J., Rehfeld, J.F. & Stadil, F. *Scand J Gastroenterol* 11: 673; 1976.
102. Davenport, H.W. *Proc Soc Exp Biol Med* 126: 657; 1967.
103. Hollander, D. & Tarnawski, A. *Gut* 27: 239; 1986.
104. Lenz, H.J., Ferrari-Taylor, J. & Isenberg, J.I. *Gastroenterol* 85: 1082; 1983.
105. Davis, A.E. & Pirola, R.C. *Med J Aust* 2: 757; 1966.
106. Marin, G.A., Ward, N.L. & Fischer, R. *Am J Dig Dis* 18: 825; 1973.
107. Mott, C., Sarles, H., Tiscornia, O. & Gullo, L. *Am J Dig Dis* 17: 902; 1972.
108. Pirola, R.C. & Davis, A.E. *Gut* 9: 557; 1968.
109. Rosenstock, S., Jorgensen, T., Bonnevie, O. & Andersen, L. *Gut* 52: 186; 2003.
110. Everhart, J.E., Kruszon-Moran, D., Perez-Perez, G.I. et al. *J Infect Dis* 181: 1359; 2000.
111. Brenner, H., Rothenbacher, D., Bode, G. & Adler, G. *Am J Epidemiol* 149: 571; 1999.
112. Sonnenberg, A. *Scand J Gastroenterol Suppl* 155: 119; 1988.
113. Cohen, S. & Booth Jr., G.H. *N Engl J Med* 293: 897; 1975.
114. Tovey, F.I., Jayaraj, A.P., Lewin, M.R. & Clark, C.G. *Dig Dis* 7: 309; 1989.
115. Paffenbarger, R.S.J., Wing, A.L. & Hyde, R.T. *Am J Epidemiol* 100: 307; 1974.
116. Suadicani, P., Hein, H.O. & Gyntelberg, F. *Scand J Gastroenterol* 34: 12; 1999.
117. MacDonald, W.C., Anderson, F.H. & Hashimoto, S. *Can Med Assoc J* 96: 1521; 1967.
118. Sonnenberg, A. *Gut* 27: 1138; 1986.
119. Stemmermann, G., Haenszel, W. & Locke, F. *J Natl Cancer Inst* 58: 13; 1977.
120. Schneider, M.A., De Luca, V. & Gray, S.J. *Am J Gastroenterol* 2: 722; 1956.

121. Solanke, T.F. *J Surg Res* 15: 385; 1973.
122. Myers, B.M., Smith, J.L. & Graham, D.Y. *Am J Gastroenterol* 82: 211; 1987.
123. Rydning, A., Weberg, R., Lange, O. & Berstad, A. *Gastroenterology* 91: 56; 1986.
124. Aldoori, W.H. et al. *Am J Epidemiol* 145: 42; 1997.
125. Rydning, A. & Berstad, A. *Scand J Gastroenterol* 20: 801; 1985.
126. Malhotra, S. *Postgrad Med J* 54: 6; 1978.
127. Baron, J.H. *Lancet* 2: 980; 1982.
128. Kang, J.Y. et al. *Scand J Gastroenterol* 23: 95; 1988.
129. Harju, E. *Am Surg* 50: 668; 1984.
130. Grant, H.W., Palmer, K.R., Riermesma, R.R. & Oliver, M.F. *Gut* 31: 997; 1990.
131. Koch, K.L. *Dig Dis Sci* 44: 1061; 1999.
132. Fontana, R.J. & Barnett, J.L. *Am J Gastroenterol* 91: 2174; 1996.
133. Gentilcore, D., O'Donovan, D., Jones, K.L. & Horowitz, M. *Curr Diab Rep* 3: 418; 2003.
134. Leeds, A.R., Ralphs, D.N., Ebied, F. et al. *Lancet* 1: 1075; 1981.
135. Lawaetz, O., Blackburn, A.M., Bloom, S.R. et al. *Scand J Gastroenterol* 18: 327; 1983.
136. Andersen, J.R., Holtug, K. & Uhrenholt, A. *Acta Chir Scand* 155: 39; 1989.
137. Harju, E. & Makela, J. *Am J Gastroenterol* 79: 861; 1984.
138. Prather, C.M., Thomforde, G.M. & Camilleri, M. *Gastroenterol* 103: 1377; 1992.
139. Zung, A. & Zadik, Z. *J Pediatr Endocrinol Metab* 16: 907; 2003.
140. Scarpignato, C. *Digestion* 57 (Suppl 1): 114; 1996.

61 Nutrition and Hollow Organs of Lower Gastrointestinal Tract

Ece A. Mutlu, Gökhan M. Mutlu, and Sohrab Mobarhan

CONTENTS

Basic principles of nutrition in diseases of the small and large intestines are covered in this chapter. Often, the disease processes are complex and result in challenges frequently requiring nutritional treatment to be individualized. Thus, consultation with a nutrition specialist is usually necessary and highly recommended.

CELIAC SPRUE

DEFINITION AND EPIDEMIOLOGY

Celiac sprue (CS; celiac disease, gluten-sensitive enteropathy) is an allergic disease of the small intestine, characterized by malabsorption of nutrients, a specific histologic appearance on biopsy (Table 61.1), and prompt improvement after withdrawal of gluten (a water-insoluble protein moiety in certain cereal grains) from the diet. The disease is prevalent in almost every population, with higher numbers among people of northern European decent. In Europe, the prevalence is estimated to be 0.05 to 0.2%; however, the disease is underdiagnosed. When U.S. blood donors were screened using antiendomysial antibodies (AEA), which are serological markers with high specificity for CS, 1 in 250 were positive. The classic symptoms of the disease are diarrhea, flatulence, weight loss, and fatigue, although many patients without extensive small bowel damage may not have one or more symptoms. In fact, the most common presentation of the disease is now atypical: Patients are asymptomatic in terms of any gastrointestinal (GI) manifestations and present with extraintestinal or malnutrition-related problems (such as miscarriages, osteoporosis with fractures, skin diseases, etc.). Clinical manifestations of the disease are given in Table 61.2. Patient populations at risk and their disease prevalence are given in Table 61.3.

TABLE 61.1
Histological Features of Celiac Sprue

1. Loss of villi with resultant flat absorptive surface
2. Presence of cuboidal epithelial cells at surface
3. Hyperplasia of crypts, with increased mitotic figures
4. Increased intraepithelial lymphocytes
5. Increased cellularity in lamina propria

TABLE 61.2
Clinical Manifestations/Presentations of Celiac Sprue

Gastrointestinal	Extraintestinal
Diarrhea	Dermatitis herpetiformis
Steatorrhea/weight loss	Amenorrhea/infertility/miscarriages
Nausea/vomiting	Anemia (iron or folate deficiency)
GERD	Osteoporosis/osteomalacia
Abdominal pain/dyspepsia	Brittle diabetes
Bloating/flatulence	Dementia
Occult blood in stool	Depression
Elevated transaminases	Neuropathy
Recurrent pancreatitis	Seizures
	Hyposplenism
	Headaches
	Hypoparathyroidism
	IgA nephropathy
	Malaise/fatigue

TABLE 61.3
Patient Populations at Risk for Celiac Sprue

At-Risk Population	Disease Prevalence (%)
Family members of a patient with CS:	5–20
Monozygotic twins	70–90
Siblings with HLA DQW2 or HLA DR5/DR7	40
First degree relatives	10–20
Autoimmune thyroid disease	4–5
Diabetes mellitus type I	2–5
Ig A deficiency	15
Sjogren's syndrome	15
Down's syndrome	4–5

MECHANISMS

Gluten, the main allergen, is a storage protein found in wheat. The prolamin fraction of gluten is an alcoholic extract rich in proline and glutamine residues. This fraction is also termed gliadin, and certain amino acid sequences occurring in it (proline–serine–glutamine–glutamine and glutamine–glutamine–glutamine–proline) initiate the allergic reaction in CS. Many grains such as rye, barley, and spelt also contain similar prolamin fractions and are therefore toxic to CS patients (Figure 61.1). Taxonomy of common cereal grains and chemical names for their prolamin fractions are given in Figure 61.1.

In genetically predisposed individuals, the prolamin fractions from cereal grains bind a tissue autoantigen called tissue transglutaminase.[1] The bound complex is believed to initiate an autoimmune reaction leading to activation of intraepithelial T-lymphocytes and formation of autoantibodies, resulting in destruction of small intestinal epithelial cells and the interstitium that make up the villus.

Tissue transglutaminase is normally found in the cytoplasm of the small intestinal epithelial cell, and its main function is to cross-link glutamine residues. *In vitro*, the enzyme preferentially acts on gluten, 35% of which is made up of glutamine, and renders it more susceptible to uptake and processing by the enterocyte. Tissue transglutaminase can also deamidate glutamyl donor molecules, which can bind to celiac-disease-specific HLA-DQ2 better than their nondeamidated counterparts.

How tissue transglutaminase and gluten come into contact is unclear. Postulated mechanisms include exposure during mechanical stress, inflammation, infection, or apoptosis. For example, instigation of tissue injury by infection with adenovirus 12 has been hypothesized to cause release of tissue transglutaminase into the extracellular environment, where it links with gluten. Supporting this hypothesis, Kagnoff et al. have shown that a particular portion of the E1B protein of adenovirus 12 and α-gliadin are homologous, and 89% of patients with CS have evidence of prior exposure to this virus.[2] Others propose that gluten is inadequately digested and toxic fractions accumulate. Subsequent sampling of the intestinal milieu leads to

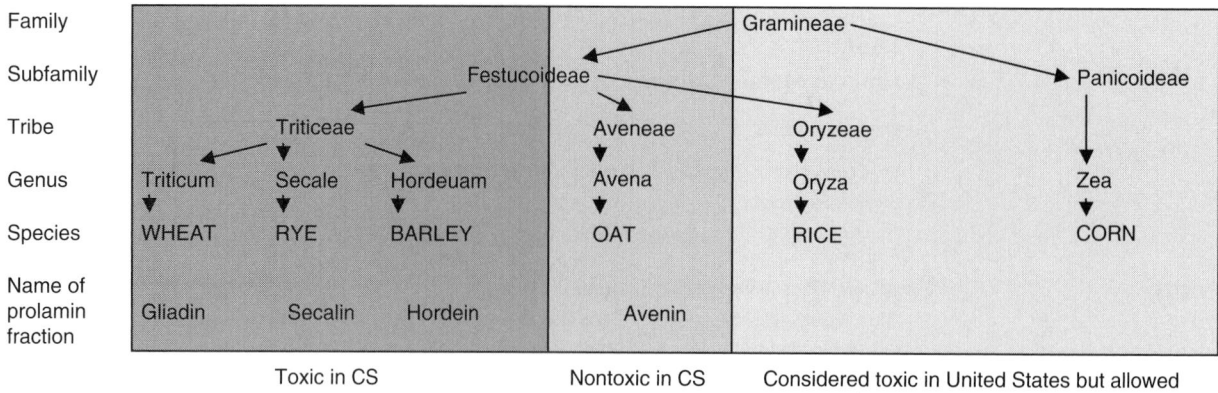

FIGURE 61.1   Taxonomy of grains.

TABLE 61.4
Pathogenetic Factors in Celiac Sprue (CS)

1. Dietary gluten
2. Genetic predisposition
   a. Association with HLA-DQ2 and HLA-DQ8 in Caucasians
3. Autoimmunity
   a. Heightened gut permeability to macromolecules
   b. Increased CD8-T-lymphocytes (especially $\gamma\Delta$ type) in lamina propria
   c. Increased levels of IL-15b epithelium
   d. Increased humoral mucosal immune response
   e. Tissue transglutaminase
      i. Creation of new antigenic epitopes by binding gliadin
      ii. Deamidation of glutamine residues in gliadin, causing increased binding to HLA
4. Acute trigger factors
   a. Infection with viruses
   b. Acute inflammation due to food allergy, etc.
   c. Mechanical stress

---

presentation of the gliadin peptides on antigen-presenting cells within the cleft of the HLA-DQ2 molecules carried by susceptible individuals.

Various hypotheses and factors important in the pathogenesis of CS are given in Table 61.4.

EFFECTS ON NUTRITIONAL STATUS

CS can profoundly affect nutritional status leading to steatorrhea, weight loss, and many micronutrient deficiencies, although about half the adult patients present with rather subtle clinical signs of malnutrition as the disease can be patchy and the extent of involvement of the small intestine varies from person to person. The degree of malnutrition is generally positively correlated with the presence of symptoms; asymptomatic patients are less malnourished than symptomatic ones (31 vs. 67%).[3] CS patients tend to have lower body fat, bone mass, and lean body mass compared with healthy controls. Total body fat can even be decreased significantly in asymptomatic cases with latent sprue.[4] Laboratory studies show that albumin, triglycerides, and hemoglobin are typically below normal. Anemia is frequent in both overt and latent CS and may be due to iron, folate, or vitamin B_{12} deficiencies resulting from malabsorption or bacterial overgrowth. Micronutrient problems such as low calcium, potassium, magnesium, copper, zinc and selenium, and vitamin K deficiencies have been reported. Additionally, vitamin E deficiency has been linked to the neurologic symptoms of CS. Of utmost importance is the fact that patients with symptomatic as well as latent CS may have osteomalacia and low bone mineral density partly as a result of vitamin D and calcium deficiencies, and these need to be supplemented to prevent osteoporosis.[5] There is no correlation between clinical or biochemical abnormalities and bone mineral density, and so supplementation with regular screening should be undertaken in all patients.

DIET IN CS

The Gluten-Free Diet

CS patients need to avoid foods that contain certain cereal grains. For medical purposes, such a diet is termed a gluten-free diet (GFD). In general, the Oryzeae or the Tripsaceae such as rice, corn, and maize are safe because the protein fractions of these grains are significantly different from gliadin, owing to their different taxonomy, as shown in Figure 61.1. Basic principles of the GFD are given in Table 61.5.

Caution should be exercised when the word "gluten" is used to select foods as it has different meanings to different people. Bakers typically use it to mean the sticky part of grains, whereas chemists only refer to wheat-derived protein fractions and use the chemical names given in Figure 61.1 for other cereal grains. Therefore, patients are encouraged to ask, "Is this food free of wheat, rye, barley, oats, etc., and ingredients derived from grains?" rather than "Is this a gluten-free food?"

Unfortunately, many dietary additives exist in processed foods containing hidden ingredients that are derived from cereal grains; therefore, compliance with a truly GFD diet is hard. A simple "watch out" list for some of these ingredients is given in item 3 of Table 61.5. Chemicals/fillers added to nonfood items such as vitamins and pills may also be a source of gluten. Moreover, food processing elements, which need not to be reported on food labels, may use grains. Hence, patients should definitely consult an expert dietician experienced in GFD with questions, as well as to join professional societies such as The Celiac Sprue Association U.S.A.

Manifestations of the disease responsive to GFD are given in Table 61.6. Numerous studies show that GFD not only is essential in controlling GI symptoms but also prevents complications.

Osteopenia and osteoporosis are common and can result from vitamin D and calcium malabsorption as well as secondary to hypoparathyroidism from hypomagnesaemia.[6] GFD leads to increases in bone mineral density with the greatest benefit in the

---

TABLE 61.5
Principles of the Gluten-Free Diet

1. Avoid the following grains: Wheat, rye, barley, oat, spelt (Dinkel), kamut, buckwheat
2. Avoid the following grain-based products: Bulgar,[a] Couscous,[a] Wheat starch, Wheat germ, Semolina,[a] Durum,[a] Bran, Oat bran, Germ, Graham flour
3. Avoid potentially grain-based products or additives: malt,[b] malt flavouring, malt extract, malt syrup, food starch (edible starch),[c] icing sugar,[d] soy sauce,[e] filler,[f] gum base, oat gum, cereal binding, white vinegar,[§] hydrolyzed vegetable protein or hydrolyzed plant protein
4. Avoid sauces, salad dressings, and fat substitutes as these may typically contain grain-derived products
5. Avoid grain-based alcohol such as beer or alcoholic extracts of grains
6. Corn and rice are the only allowable cereal grains
7. All fresh vegetables and fruits are allowed

[a] Derived from wheat.
[b] May be derived from barley.
[c] May be derived from wheat.
[d] Contains 5% wheat starch.
[e] May contain wheat or barley.
[f] Found frequently in medications and vitamins

TABLE 61.6
Manifestations of Celiac Sprue
Responsive to Gluten-Free Diet

1. Gastrointestinal symptoms
   a. Diarrhea
   b. Malbsorption
2. Osteopenia/osteoporosis
3. Anemia
4. Dermatitis herpetiformis
5. Depression
6. Increased risk of malignancy
7. Amenorrhea/infertility/spontaneous abortions

first year of treatment,[7–9] but normalization may not occur even on GFD.[10] In a study of 65 patients with CS on GFD, up to 50% had a T-score of less than –2 on dual-energy x-ray absorptiometry.[11]

There is a two- to threefold relative increase in the risk of cancer among patients with CS.[12,13] Specifically, T-cell lymphomas of the small intestine, adenocarcinoma of the small intestine, cancers of the mouth, nasopharynx, and esophagus are more common. Malignant complications correlate with GFD: In patients who have been on GFD for 5 years or more, malignancy risk reverts to that for the general population.[13,14] For those on a reduced gluten or normal diet, the risk for non-Hodgkin's lymphoma and cancers of the mouth, pharynx, and esophagus is 78- and 23-fold higher compared with the general population.[13]

The time to respond to GFD clinically varies depending on the severity of the disease. A prompt improvement in symptoms is expected within days to a few weeks. Patients with milder disease in biopsies tend to respond sooner than those with villous atrophy, in whom resolution of symptoms may take up to several months. Still, normalization of biopsy samples when total villous atrophy is present has been reported incomplete even after 2 years.[15] Dermatitis herpetiformis takes a longer to resolve with GFD than other symptoms (on average 2 years), and older patients take longer to respond than younger ones.

GFD is typically low in B vitamins and iron.[16] This may result in low levels in patients following the diet long term.[17] The authors recommend a daily multivitamin supplement and periodic laboratory tests for B vitamins and anemia and iron in patients following a GFD.

Alternatives to GFD
Compliance with a GFD is hard as it impacts social life, especially eating out and travel, negatively, and it is expensive. Alternative therapies for celiac disease are being sought to overcome this problem. There are currently no alternative treatments for CS. Endopeptidases that digest the toxic fractions of gluten, peptides that bind and block the antigen-presenting groove of HLA-DQ2 and HLA-DQ8, proteins that will increase the gut barrier, as well as genetically engineered wheat that does not contain toxic fractions are being researched. In one study in asymptomatic celiac patients who were administered a low-dose gluten supplement, pretreatment of the supplement with prolyl endopeptidase to digest toxic gluten fractions improved or prevented fat and carbohydrate malabsorption.[18] In *vitro* studies, large amounts of the endopeptidases are required for prolonged periods of time to detoxify the majority of gluten found in food.[19] Hence, important improvements in the efficiency of current enzyme preparations such as their rate of action are awaited before they can replace a GFD. In the meantime, some authors have also suggested the use of tef, a grain from Ethiopia.[20]

What to do in the patient who is unresponsive to a GFD?
From a dietary standpoint, careful review of the patient's diet for hidden sources of gluten is suggested. The commonest causes of GI symptoms in such patients are bacterial overgrowth, development of other autoimmune diseases, and new onset of microscopic/collagenous colitis found in 5% of patients with CS. Treatment of bacterial overgrowth with antibiotics may be beneficial.[21] Complications of CS such as development of T-cell lymphoma, adenocarcinoma, and collagenous sprue should also be investigated.

Exocrine pancreatic insufficiency due to impaired cholecystokinin-pancreozymin release from abnormal mucosa has been reported suggesting a beneficial role for pancreatic enzyme supplements.[22,23] In fact, mild to moderate pancreatic insufficiency with subnormal levels in one or more pancreatic enzymes was found in 29% of patients with CS in one study and the presence of insufficiency did not seem to correlate with overall nutritional status.[24] A prospective, double-blind randomized study of adolescents has shown improvement in anthropometric variables as well as weight gain with enzyme supplementation.[25]

Search for dietary antigens other than gliadin have shown usefulness in an elimination diet in 77% patients in one study.[26] This elimination diet excluded foods containing natural salicylates, amines or glutamine, food colorings, preservatives, monosodium glutamate, lactose or dairy products, and soy- and millet-containing foods.

Patients in whom symptoms persists are considered to have "refractory sprue" upon exclusion of other diagnoses. These patients may benefit from corticosteroids,[27] azathioprine,[28] or cyclosporine.[29] Zinc-deficient patients with refractory sprue may respond to zinc supplements,[30] although this is controversial.[31]

Is There a Safe Amount of Gluten that CS Patients May Consume?

In small gluten challenge studies, <10 mg daily dosage usually does not lead to changes in mucosal morphology,[32] but such changes can begin at a dose as low as 50 mg daily.[33] One study suggests that at least 10 g of gluten challenge leads to relapse of disease within 7 weeks,[34] although there is no consensus in this regard. Diets recommended by professional societies in the United States do not allow any gluten, whereas the Codex Alimentarius Commission of the Food and Agricultural Organization of the United Nations (FAO) and the World Health Organization (WHO) permit a "gluten free" label on foods that contain up to 0.3% of protein from toxic grains. Most of this protein comes from wheat starch or malt. Wheat starch (contains 0.75 mg/100 g gliadin) may not be tolerated well, and its withdrawal from the diet can result in marked improvement of intestinal symptoms and dermatitis herpetiformis.[35] In a recent study examining patients who are symptomatic despite GFD as defined by FAO/WHO standards, conversion to a no detectable gluten diet resulted in complete resolution or reduction of symptoms in 23% and 45%, respectively.[36] Based on these results, there can be no safe amount of gluten in the diet for celiac patients.

Can CS Patients Eat Oats or Other Less Structurally Related Grains?

Evidence that oats may not be harmful to CS patients dates back to the 1970s, when Dissanayake and Truelove administered 40 to 60 g of oats to four CS patients for 1 month and showed no damage to the small intestinal mucosa.[37] Several investigators claim that oats, which taxonomically belong to a different subclass in the cereal grains, the Aveneae, do not elicit the immune reaction seen with the ones in the Triticeae tribe: Oats have a lower content of praline, which is abundant in the toxic amino acid sequences (proline–serine–glutamine–glutamine and glutamine–glutamine–glutamine–proline) of prolamin fractions. Also, these sequences occur fewer times per molecule of oat avenin as opposed to wheat prolamin.[38] Whether such lower amounts are enough to elicit the autoimmune reaction of CS or whether there is a certain safe level of oat consumption is unclear. *In vitro* investigations show that antibodies from sera of patients with CS and dermatitis herpetiformis can react against oat avenin, but the significance of this finding is questionable because similar immunoreactivity against corn has also been demonstrated.[39]

Two small cohort studies with CS and dermatitis herpetiformis patients have shown no rise in antibody titers and no clinical or histological deterioration when oats are given 50 and 62.5 g/day, respectively.[40,41] In the largest randomized placebo-controlled study to date, newly diagnosed European patients and ones in remission on GFD were studied for 12 months and 6 months, respectively.[42] The patients were not blinded, although the investigators were. Consumption of 50 g of oats daily did not cause any clinical relapse or histopathologic worsening in the established patients with CS, nor did it prevent clinical or histologic healing in newly diagnosed cases. The authors concluded that small to moderate amounts of oats can be included in a GFD, and may improve poor compliance with the diet. Despite this being a well-designed study, long-term evidence regarding the safety of oats are lacking. Considering crop rotation and lack of specified mills for oats in the United States, addition of oats to GFD cannot be recommended at this time.

Some authors have suggested the trial of Ethiopian cereal tef in CS,[20] but further studies are needed before this can be acceptable.

Should CS Patients Also Avoid Lactose?

Lactase, the enzyme needed for digestion of lactose, is located at the very tip of the brush border. As a result of damage to the villi, the levels of lactase are assumed to be lower in most acutely ill patients with CS. Therefore, most professionals advocate a lactose-free diet at the beginning of treatment with a GFD until resolution of symptoms. This is especially true for patients with severe disease requiring corticosteroids. No controlled studies have been done examining the utility of a lactose-free diet in CS. Long-term avoidance of lactose is not appropriate, considering the high incidence of osteopenia among CS patients.

Does Breast-Feeding Prevent Occurrence of CS?

The incidence of CS is increased in the relatives of patients. The relative risks for family members of CS patients are given in Table 61.3. Retrospective studies have shown that relative risk of CS development is fourfold less in siblings of Italian children with CS if they are breast-fed over 30 days.[43] Similar findings showing a protective effect of breast-feeding have been confirmed in Tunisian children,[44] in Swedish children,[45] and the United States.[46] This effect may be correlated with duration of breast-feeding and appears independent of the delays in introduction of wheat and grain products into an infant's diet.[47] Age at gluten introduction seems to be a separate factor. There is epidemiologic evidence that links increasing incidence of CS in Sweden, as opposed to Denmark, to early and high level introduction of gluten into infant feedings.[48] However, case–control studies have not yet confirmed these results.[49] Breast-feeding may also change the disease presentation from its classical forms to the atypical forms.[46,50]

Nutritional tips for CS are given in Table 61.7.

INFLAMMATORY BOWEL DISEASE

Definition and Epidemiology

Inflammatory bowel disease (IBD) is an idiopathic chronic inflammatory disorder of the GI system. The two main forms of the disease are Crohn's disease (CD) and ulcerative colitis (UC). The main differences of these diseases are shown in Table 61.8.

Mechanisms

Various factors and mechanisms important in the pathogenesis of IBD are listed in Table 61.9. Most recently, certain genetic foci associated with IBD have been discovered and it is hypothesized that environmental factors in susceptible individuals ultimately initiate the inflammatory process leading to disease. Environmental factors include diet and dietary antigens as well as the bacterial flora of the intestines.

TABLE 61.7
Nutritional Tips for Celiac Sprue Patients

1. Avoid lactose (mainly milk and dairy products) in acute disease
2. Follow a GFD (Table 61.5) at all times:
   a. Read food labels
   b. Ask about grains in foods and medications
   c. Avoid all foods if it is not certain that they do not contain the restricted grains
   d. Select plain meats, fresh fruits and vegetables when eating outside of the home if not sure
   e. Record weight and symptoms, and keep a food diary until symptoms resolve on the GFD
3. Avoid foods that initiate/exacerbate symptoms as they may contain hidden sources of grains or other food allergens
4. Consult an experienced dietitian with questions
5. Report persistent symptoms promptly
6. Join support groups for people with CS

TABLE 61.8
Differences between Ulcerative Cobitis (UC) and Crohn's disease (CD)

	UC	CD
Clinical	Bloody diarrhea is main symptom	Obstruction, fistulae, perianal disease may be present
Site of involvement	Rectum extending proximally into colon as a continuum	Any part of the GI tract
	Normal tissue between areas of involvement (i.e. skip areas)	
	Small bowel normal	70% small bowel involvement
	Only mucosal involvement	Involvement of the entire bowel wall
Pathological appearance	No granulomas	Presence of granulomas
Prognosis/recurrence	Can be cured with colectomy	Cannot be cured with surgical resection

TABLE 61.9
Factors Important in the Pathogenesis of Irritable Bowel Disease

1. Genetic predisposition
2. Environmental factors (e.g., smoking, urban lifestyle, etc.)
3. Dietary factors
4. Gut microbial flora
5. Infectious agents
   a. Mycobacteria
   b. Measles virus
6. Immune reactivity
7. Psychosocial factors and stress

EFFECTS ON NUTRITIONAL STATUS

Malnutrition is common in IBD; however, there is an important difference between CD and UC. CD usually leads to chronic malnutrition that develops insidiously over long periods of time, whereas in most cases UC causes acute reductions in weight during flare-ups of disease. Up to 85% of patients hospitalized with IBD and about 23% of outpatients with CD have protein-energy malnutrition.[51] Stable patients with the disease tend to have a normal fat-free mass but low fat stores.

The causes of malnutrition in patients with IBD are multifactorial and are given in Table 61.10. There is an increase in the resting metabolic rates in active IBD but mean increases are modest (19% in active UC[52] and 12% in active CD[53] when compared with the calculated ones from the Harris–Benedict equation or controls). Total energy expenditures, however, are comparable with those of healthy people.[54] Most stable outpatients with IBD do not have increased energy expenditures either.[55] One exception is underweight individuals (body weight <90% of ideal),[55,56] who may represent a special subgroup with specific metabolic

TABLE 61.10
Causes of Malnutrition in Irritable Bowel Disease Patients

1. Reduced dietary intake
   a. Anorexia to avoid symptoms
   b. Restricted diets
   c. Drug-induced taste alterations
2. Maldigestion and malabsorption
   a. Inadequate mucosal surface
   b. Bile salt malabsorption from ileal disease
   c. Bacterial overgrowth
   d. Drug induced
3. Increased requirements
   a. Inflammatory catabolism
   b. Drug-induced nutrient wasting
4. Exudative protein losses from inflamed intestine or fistulae

TABLE 61.11
Micronutrient Deficiencies in Irritable Bowel Disease

Micronutrient	Percentage of Prevalance	
	UC	CD
Iron	81	39
Folic acid	35	54–67
Vitamin B_{12}	5	48
Potassium		6–20
Calcium		13
Magnesium		14–33
Vitamin A	26–93	11–50
Vitamin D	35	75
Zinc		40–50
Selenium		35–40

abnormalities different than the rest. Interestingly, stable patients with CD that have decreased fat stores, but a similar fat-free mass as healthy controls or UC patients have enhanced utilization of lipids and diet-induced thermogenesis.[57,58] A worse sub-clinical disease might be the cause in these patients as increased lipid oxidation is seen with active disease and its level correlates with disease activity.[53]

Fecal energy and protein losses in IBD are significant in active IBD, but most patients compensate by increased food intake. Generally, patients on corticosteroids are also in positive energy balance, possibly due to the appetite-stimulating properties of these drugs.[58] Still, attention should be paid to provide for the increased protein requirements in active IBD, especially in malnourished patients, who may require as much as 2 g/kg/day of protein.[59]

Food intolerances are twice as common among IBD patients as in the general population.[60] These intolerances are commonly towards corn, wheat, cereals, cruciferous vegetables, and milk, although intolerances to foods such as rice or even tap water have been observed.

In patients without obvious malabsorption, food intolerances together with less hunger, decreased appetite, and fewer sensations of pleasure related to eating lead to significantly reduced food intakes.[61] This is the major cause of weight loss in patients with IBD.[61] In patients without other objective evidence of active inflammation, weight loss should not be attributed to IBD, but rather close attention should be paid to the patient's food intake.

Patients with IBD commonly have many micronutrient deficiencies that are shown in Table 61.11. Low levels of zinc and selenium, which are cofactors for oxidant protective enzymes and low antioxidant vitamins (A, E, and C), have been implicated in worsening of the disease course as well as contributing to the high rate of carcinogenesis among IBD patients.

Osteopenia, a well-recognized complication of IBD, is widespread among both adult and pediatric patients[62] and may occur independent of steroid use. Both osteopenia and osteoporosis have been linked to vitamin D and calcium deficiencies, and supplementation has been beneficial in the treatment of these disorders.

Diet in **IBD**

Diet as a Potential Cause of IBD

Epidemiologic evidence suggests that the incidence of CD has been increasing over the last half century, while that of UC is declining especially in developed countries. Moreover, migrant populations of Asians into England or of European Jews into the United States have a much greater increase in the incidence of CD compared with their counterparts living in their native countries. Assuming migrants and natives have similar genetic pools, the increase has been attributed to environmental factors. Strikingly, a higher incidence of CD in urban areas as opposed to rural ones further suggests environmental factors at play. Among these factors diet is important.

Preillness diet factors and dietary habits of patients with IBD
Many studies on dietary factors in the development of IBD and the roles of many types of food (such as refined sugar, cereals, fiber, and dairy products including milk) have been undertaken.

In general, patients with IBD tend toward higher intake of sugar compared with controls,[63,64] and this trend specifically reaches statistical significance for CD[63,64] in most studies and for UC in a few.[65,66] Fruit, vegetable, and fiber consumption, on the other hand, was much lower in IBD in these studies. One study in the Japanese population confirmed the lower intakes of vegetables and fruits among IBD patients and a Westernized diet increased the risk for UC.[67] These findings among IBD patients are not surprising as they may represent an adaptation to the disease process rather than the cause of IBD.

Realizing this pitfall, in some studies only patients who have recent exacerbation of IBD were questioned about their diet. Such studies also confirmed that there is higher intake of sugars among CD patients but not UC ones.[68–73] In one of these, deleterious effect of increased intake of sugars was only seen with sucrose but not with lactose or polysaccharides.[68] IBD patients also consume more fat prior to onset of disease.[68] Epidemiologic studies suggest that IBD is related to increased n-6 polyunsaturated fatty acid and animal protein intake.[66,74]

Does milk cause IBD? Should patients with IBD avoid milk?
The role of milk in initiating or worsening IBD is debatable, and whether lactose intolerance is more common in IBD is controversial. Even among IBD patients who are not lactose malabsorbers elimination of milk from the diet leads to improvement in diarrhea in one-fifth to one-fourth of the cases with UC and in one-third of the patients with CD.[75,76]

Although no clear-cut explanation for this exists, morphologic changes in small intestinal mucosa are well documented in CD and UC.[77,78] The extent to which these changes are related to decreased food intake or starvation as a result of disease symptoms is unknown. Nevertheless, in CD, improvements related to a milk-free diet are not attributable to changes in brush border lactase levels.[79] In UC, measurements of intestinal lactase have shown that deficiencies of lactase are real during active disease but lactase deficit is not necessarily more frequent in the active phase compared with the inactive phase.[80]

This raises the question of whether milk itself is an allergen. One group of studies have searched for humoral immune responses to milk proteins. Antibodies to milk proteins can be readily detected in the sera of IBD patients,[81] but their levels may not be increased,[82,83] nor are they particularly common.[84] Some investigators have correlated antibody response against milk to disease activity in CD but not in UC.[85] However, disruptions of the intestinal barrier as a result of inflammation can easily lead to such antibody formation, making it a secondary phenomenon rather that the cause of disease. Other studies have directly looked at the effects of a milk-free diet: in one, elimination of milk from the diet decreased relapses of UC when patients were followed up to 1 year subsequent to treatment with steroids,[86] even though strict statistical comparisons between treatment and control groups were not undertaken. In another small study, 40% the IBD patients without lactose intolerance improved.[75] Allergy to cow's milk may play a role in initiating or perpetuating inflammation in IBD in a subset of patients, although no evidence clearly establishes milk as an allergen.

Milk may also modify the intestinal flora causing harm to individuals genetically susceptible to IBD or to IBD patients. Supporting this hypothesis, lack of breast-feeding has been identified as an independent risk factor for childhood CD[87] but not UC.[88,89]

Is IBD caused by allergy to foods?
In a subset of patients who respond to elimination diets, IBD may be caused by allergy to a specific food item. However, such patients constitute a very small minority and may represent cases with allergic colitis that is misdiagnosed as IBD. Further studies are needed to answer this question.

Dietary Treatment for **IBD**

Energy and Protein Requirements in IBD

The Harris–Benedict equation is useful in calculating the energy requirements of IBD patients. Active disease may increase calculated requirements up to 20%. Fecal losses of protein are the norm in active disease, and therefore patients should be given or encouraged to consume at least 1.5 g/kg of protein.

Effects of diet counseling
Individualized dietary counseling for 6 months can lead to significant decreases in the CD activity index, the need for medications such as prednisone, days spent in the hospital for acute exacerbations, and number of days lost from work.[89] Counseling can also lead to increased incidence of disease remission, with beneficial effects persisting up to 1 year, and is useful in both active and inactive disease.

Unproven diets
High-fiber diets that restrict sugar or provide unrefined carbohydrates
Investigators have studied the impact of a diet with little or no sugar and rich in unrefined carbohydrates and fiber on IBD. In one open-label study of CD patients and matched controls, hospital admissions were significantly fewer and shorter in the treatment group.[73] Subjects were given over 30 g fiber/day on average with no adverse effects seen in the patients with strictures. In a larger, better-designed, controlled, multicenter trial with CD, the diet intervention group did not have a clinically different course than the group consuming a low-fiber unrestricted sugar diet.[90]

Low-residue diet for active CD
A study of patients with active nonstenosing CD compared a low-residue diet with an ad-lib diet.[91] There were no differences in the incidence of poor outcomes such as need for surgery, hospitalization, prolonged bed rest, partial obstruction, or new inflammatory mass.

The simple carbohydrate diet
Patients are resorting to diet therapies because of the many side effects of immunosuppressive medications used in treatment of IBD and their lack of effectiveness in a significant number of cases. There is a growing body of anecdotal evidence toward the efficacy of various diets used by patients. One very popular example is the simple carbohydrate diet (SCD) pioneered by Dr. Haas and currently advocated by Elaine Gottschall, whose son has been afflicted with UC.[92] The diet is based on avoidance of all complex sugars and grains, is gluten-free, and devoid of all additives or preservatives. With a few exceptions, only fresh food is allowed and it is cooked well to promote easy digestion. The principles of the diet attempt to generate an "elemental carbohydrate diet." Although elemental diets work in IBD, polymeric enteral formulas have been found to be just as effective in one-to-one comparisons. Moreover, many of the elemental formulations do, in fact, contain polymeric carbohydrates, refuting the possibility that taking in only simple carbohydrates will be successful. To date, the SCD diet has not been tested scientifically; therefore, it cannot be advocated for general use. If it is proven effective after objective scientific evaluation, this may be based on features other than its "simple carbohydrates." For the patient who wishes to stay on the SCD diet, adequate macro- and micronutrient intake should be supervised by an experienced dietician.

Elimination diets
Reports of food intolerances by IBD patients have led to investigations of elimination diets as a potential therapy. In an uncontrolled trial, 66% of the CD patients were able to find a nutritionally adequate diet after elimination of various foods.[93] More than half of these patients needed elimination of more than one or two foods. The relapse rate was 33% at the end of the first year on the diets, with annual averages of about 14% within the first 3 years. A controlled trial by the same investigators showed that 7 of the 10 patients in the treatment group remained in remission after 3 months as opposed to all patients relapsing in the control group given an unrefined carbohydrate fiber-rich diet.[93,94] Unfortunately these beneficial results have not been confirmed with better-designed studies to eliminate bias. In fact, in a study of 42 eligible CD patients put into remission with elemental diet, 33% dropped out of the study, 19% did not identify food intolerance, and 48% did.[94] Among this 48%, food sensitivity was confirmed in half the patients in the open challenge with the item and was reproducible in only three patients in the double-blind challenge. These findings suggest that elimination diets are of little help in the day-to-day treatment of IBD.

Growth hormone and high-protein diet
The effects of high-protein diet vs. glucocorticoids on the course of active CD was considered in a small study of pediatric patients. No significant dissimilarities between the treatment two treatment groups in terms of improvement of pediatric CD or laboratory parameters at 2 weeks were seen, although the study may not have had adequate power to detect any differences. In a follow-up of 1.3 years, patients given steroids tended to relapse more than the diet group.[95]

High-protein diet and growth hormone also have been shown to enhance adaptation of the small intestine after massive resection[96] and to improve protein absorption and to reduce stool output and requirements for hyperalimentation in short bowel syndrome (SBS) when used together with glutamine.[97] A pilot study of high-protein diet (protein intake = 2 g/kg day) in conjunction with growth hormone injections (loading dose 5 mg/day for 1 week, maintenance 1.5 mg/day for 4 months) in moderate to severe CD patients undergoing conventional treatment has been studied in a double-blind and placebo-controlled fashion. Although the study is limited to because of a small number of patients and does not indicate the percentage of patients entering remission, a significantly lower score the CD activity index was seen in the treatment group.[98] This effect may be a result of increased amino acid uptake and electrolytes, increased intestinal protein synthesis, and decreased intestinal permeability in response to growth hormone. Further studies are needed before this treatment is applicable in clinical practice.

Fish oils (Omega-3 fatty acids)

Omega-3 fatty acids such as eicosapentaenoic acid and docosahexaenoic acid have been shown to inhibit production of leukotriene B_4, a major neutrophil chemo-attractant in IBD. In two trials with active UC patients, oral fish oil decreased steroid requirements and improved histology.[99,100] In another study of patients with moderate UC, decrease in disease activity was seen although no improvement was noted in histology or leukotriene B_4 levels.[101] In UC, no beneficial effects of fish oil in maintenance of remission were seen.[99,102]

In CD, intravenous administration of eicosapentaenoic acid increases the ratio of leukotriene B_5 to leukotriene B_4.[103] A 1-year study in CD patients has shown reduced rates of relapse while on high dose of n-3 fatty acids (2.7 g/day) given as nine capsules a day. In another study, seal oil normalized n-3 to n-6 fatty acid ratios in patients with IBD and improved bodily pain.[104] Compliance can be hard with this regimen because of the large number of pills and because some patients report a fishy odor at high dosages required to produce the desired effects.

Capsaicin

Capsaicin found in peppers worsens colitis in IBD animal models by interfering with sensory neuroimmunomodulation.[105] No data exists in humans.

Short-chain fatty acids

Short-chain fatty acids (SCFAs) are produced in the colon by fermentation of fiber or undigested starch by colonic flora and represent the primary energy source of colonic cells. Small open-label trials of butyrate, a SCFA, given as an enema to patients with left-sided UC have shown rates of remission similar to treatments with steroids and mesalamine.[106–109] The expense and the pungent smell of SCFA enemas precludes their clinical use. In animal studies, pectin increases SCFAs and leads to reduction of inflammation and enhancement of repair.[110]

Gut microflora/Probiotics/Prebiotics

A large body of research indicates that the intestinal flora may be proinflammatory in IBD. This may explain why antibiotics that alter the flora such as fluoroquinolones or metronidazole or diversion of the fecal stream with an ostomy are effectively utilized in the treatment of IBD. The proinflammatory effect of the flora may be a result of expansion of harmful colonies of normal gut microorganisms in the presence of certain lumenal conditions such as an acidic pH, etc. Therefore, novel probiotic therapies that administer "good colonies (noninflammatory)" of gut bacteria, which compete with "bad colonies," have been developed for treatment of IBD. One of these, *Escherichia coli* (*E. coli*) strain Niessle 1917, most recently has been shown to be as effective as conventional treatment with 5- ASA drugs in the maintenance of remission in UC.[111] Another probiotic preparation containing 5×10^{11} composed of four strains of lactobacilli, three strains of bifidobacteria, and one strain of *Streptococcus salivarius* can prevent recurrence of pouchitis (inflammation of the ileal pouch anastomosed to the rectum in patients who have underwent colectomy for UC) in a 9 month follow-up period.[112]

A different approach has been the use of prebiotics, nondigestible food substances that promote only the growth of a defined subset of good bacteria such as *Lactobacillus* or bifidobacteria, which are beneficial for the regulation of the gut immune system. Examples of such prebiotics are inulin, fructooligosaccharides (FOS), and galactooligosaccharides (GOS). Although no controlled studies with these substances exist in humans, a pilot study of patients with IBD has reported increases in favorable intestinal flora as well as SCFA.[113] In another study subjects with colonic disease who underwent and ileo-anal pouch procedure (IAPP), in which the colon is removed and part of the distal ileum is used to construct a pelvic reservoir, FOS and resistant starch diminished indole and ammonia production and was well tolerated. In a phase I study, 10 patients with active ileo-colonic CD were given FOS supplementation (15 g/day, equal to 70% short-chain FOS + 30% inulin) for 3 weeks in an open-label fashion.[114] No serious adverse events were reported. There was a drop in disease activity, improvement in physician overall assessment, and a reduction trend in C-reactive protein. This study also demonstrated a significant increase in fecal bifidobacteria following FOS supplementation and an increase in mucosal bifidobacteria in patients who entered disease remission compared with those that did not. Finally, there was an increase in the percentage of lamina propria dendritic cells expressing interleukin (IL)-10 and a significant upregulation of toll-like receptor-2 and toll-like receptor-4 expression.

In a third pilot trial, combination of pro- and prebiotics (i.e., synbiotics) reduced sigmoidoscopy scores and altered tissue cytokine levels favorably in active UC.[115]

Alterations of the gut flora is expected to be the new therapy frontier for IBD, and further studies on preprobiotics or their combinations (i.e., synbiotics) is expected to evolve further.

Medium-Chain Triglycerides

Foods rich in medium-chain triglycerides (MCTs) are readily absorbed and enhance caloric intakes in malabsorptive states such as IBD.

ENTERAL NUTRITION AND IBD

Primary Therapy

Many different formulations have been used for enteral nutrition in IBD. Polymeric formulas usually have starches, complex protein, and long-chain triglycerides and MCTs. Semielemental formulations contain oligosaccharides, peptides, and MCTs. Elemental ones typically contain predigested nutrients such as amino acids and glucose.

In active CD, comparison of elemental/semielemental diets with corticosteroids have shown equal efficacy in achieving short-term remission (3 months) in the range of 70 to 80% in individual studies,[116–118] but a meta-analysis indicates that steroids may be more effective.[119] Long-term effects of enteral diets are less well known, although the percentage of patients in remission at 1 year ranges from 9 to 56%.[117,118,120] This rate is not significantly different when elemental diets are compared with polymeric or semielemental formulations in most studies.[119,121] Elemental diets are poorly tolerated because of their smell/taste and complications such as diarrhea and high costs. Therefore, polymeric formulations should be favored. Furthermore, relapse rates are generally higher with elemental diets as opposed to conventional therapy;[122] therefore, enteral nutrition as primary therapy should be tried only in selected cases.

Investigators have found that CD patients with severe disease[123] and CDAI >450[124] and patients with colonic disease together with a fever[122] are less likely to respond to enteral nutrition therapy. In one study, the initial response rates were 38% vs. 76% for CD patients with moderate disease as opposed to ones with severe inflammation.[123] Studies with UC reveal no benefit from enteral nutrition for induction of remission.[125]

Comparison of hyperalimentation with enteral nutrition in CD has shown no superiority of parenteral nutrition.[51,121,126] Given the multiple potential side effects of parenteral nutrition, enteral therapy should be preferred whenever possible.

PARENTERAL NUTRITION AND IBD

Preoperative

Parenteral nutrition decreases postoperative complications only in severely malnourished patients with IBD. In one study, therapy duration of at least 5 days was required to see any beneficial effect.[127]

Primary Therapy

Randomized prospective studies have shown a response rate to parenteral nutrition in the 30 to 50% range in acute UC, but no significant differences over placebo have been demonstrated.[128–131] Furthermore, disease-free maintenance rates on total parenteral nutrition (TPN) have been poor and complications requiring surgery may be higher; therefore, there is no role for TPN as primary therapy of UC.[128–131]

In retrospective and prospective analyses in CD, parenteral nutrition can induce remission in 70 to 100% of patients refractory to conventional treatments,[125,126,128,129] but in at least one prospective study 60% relapse rate is seen within 2 years.[132] This rate is four times higher than historical controls treated with surgical resection. Therefore, consideration of parenteral nutrition is recommended only in patients who are malnourished and have extensive disease precluding surgical treatment. Given the many complications of parenteral nutrition, this treatment should be a last resort after exhaustion of other therapies.

Micronutrients

Antioxidants

Lower levels of antioxidant vitamins such as vitamin A, E, and C and β-carotene have been shown in both sera and colonic tissue of patients with IBD when compared with healthy controls.[133,134] In one study, vitamin C level also correlated with disease severity.[133] Vitamin C can especially be low in patients with fistulous tracts.

Animal studies suggest that antioxidant supplementation over and above corrections for deficiency states may ameliorate colitis; however, no randomized placebo-controlled trials have been performed in humans.

Calcium/vitamin D

Low levels of vitamin D are found in 75% of patients with CD and 35% of those with UC.[121] Low levels also correlate with disease activity in undernourished CD patients.[135] Forty five percent of such patients have osteoporosis,[136] and therefore supplementation of vitamin D and calcium is essential for the prevention of osteopenia/osteoporosis in IBD. Smoking also independently increases the rate of osteoporosis and should be avoided.

Folate

In retrospective analyses, folate supplementation has been shown to reduce incidence of dysplasia and cancer in patients with UC.[137,138] Folate requirements in IBD are increased due to anemia and medications such as azathioprine, 6-mercaptopurine, and sulfasalazine, and therefore supplementation is recommended in almost all patients.

Zinc

Zinc deficiency is especially common among patients with fistulous disease and has been implicated as a cause for poor wound healing in these patients.[139]

Vitamin B$_{12}$

Deficiency of this vitamin B$_{12}$ occurs as a result of ileal involvement or resection as well as bacterial overgrowth in CD. All patients with CD should have supplementation either nasally or as monthly injections, because oral absorption is inadequate. Recently, sublingual administration of two over-the-counter vitamin nuggets (1000 μg/nugget) daily for 7 to 10 days to a small group of patients with B$_{12}$ deficiency has been reported to be effective in raising blood levels. This latter route requires further study.

Specific Situations

Obstruction

Patients with intermittent obstruction are advised to consume a low-residue diet although no definite data exists.

Fistulae

Postoperative fistulae may respond to TPN, but CD fistulae are less likely to close and frequently reopen promptly after food intake is resumed.[140,141] Similar results are seen with elemental diet.[122,123,142,143] In the era of effective antitumor necrosis factor therapies, TPN cannot be recommended as first-line therapy for fistulae in CD.

Severe diarrhea and antidiarrheals/pectin

Diarrhea can be disabling for patients with IBD and many require antidiarrheals such as loperamide or lomotil. These agents induce their effects by diminishing GI motility by binding opioid receptors in the GI tract and therefore have been implicated in the pathogenesis of IBD complications such as toxic megacolon. Thus, caution should be exercised when using these, and for severely symptomatic patients without any obstruction, antidiarrheals such as kaopectate that bind excess liquid in the lumen should be tried.

Extraintestinal manifestations

Unconfirmed reports suggest associations between resolution of pyoderma gangrenosum and uveitis with diet therapy.[144]

Ileal Resection and Kidney Stones

Patients with CD are at increased risk of oxalate kidney stones if their colons are relatively intact and they have had extensive ileal resections. Such patients should be advised to follow a low-oxalate diet. Patients with a history of oxalate stones should also be treated with binding resins such as cholestyramine.

Nutritional tips for IBD patients are given in Table 61.12.

SHORT BOWEL SYNDROME

DEFINITION AND EPIDEMIOLOGY

SBS is a malabsorptive state with a distinct group of symptoms and signs that occur as a consequence of major reductions in small intestinal absorptive surface area typically due to intestinal resections. Patients usually experience large-volume diarrhea with salient fluid and electrolyte losses as well as weight loss. The most important determinant of SBS is the length of the remaining functional small intestine, and less than 200 cm (6.5 ft) of length invariably is associated with compromised nutritional status.

TABLE 61.12
Nutritional Tips for Irritable Bowel Disease Patients

1. Seek dietary counseling from an experienced dietitian
2. Avoid milk and milk products during active disease
3. Consume 10 to 20% more calories and 50% more protein with active disease
4. Do not avoid fiber, in fact try to increase fiber in diet as long as there is no obstruction in the GI tract
5. Follow a low residue diet if there is partial obstruction in the GI tract, consult with a physician and dietitian before making dietary changes
6. Prefer fish over other dishes (fish with high fat/fish oils such as catfish, salmon, etc. should be selected)
7. Take a multivitamin supplying 100% of RDA of vitamins and minerals, make sure to have monthly vitamin B$_{12}$ injections if having CD
8. During inactive disease, consume foods that are rich in naturally occurring probiotics (such as yogurt containing lactobacillus)

Less than 100 cm (3 to 3.5 ft) usually requires TPN. Small intestinal length is variable from person to person, with a range of 330 to 850 cm; therefore, the length of resected segments are clinically irrelevant. If there is doubt as to the length of the remaining small intestine, this crucial information can be obtained by doing a small bowel follow-through, as surgical and radiographic measurements correlate well.[145]

Although the true incidence and prevalence of SBS is not known, it is estimated that 10,000 to 20,000 people in the United States require TPN as a result of it. The commonest causes of SBS are CD, malignancy, radiation enteritis, and ischemic bowel. Others include jejunoileal bypass operations (used in the past to treat obesity), congenital abnormalities such as intestinal atresia, malrotation of the intestines, aganglionosis, and necrotizing enterocolitis in childhood.

PATHOPHYSIOLOGY AND TYPES OF SBS

The main factors that affect the type of nutrition required by patients are listed in Table 61.13. The phase of SBS (i.e., the elapsed time after intestinal insult or surgery resulting in SBS) is of utmost importance in the acute management of SBS (Table 61.14). The remaining factors determine how well a patient will handle enteral nutrition in the long run.

In general, jejunal resections are better tolerated than ileal ones for several reasons:

1. Most of the intestinal fluid secretion that balances the osmotic load of gastric chyme entering the small bowel occurs in the jejunum. Subsequently, a large percentage of the proximally secreted water/electrolytes are absorbed distally in the ileum. Therefore, ileal, as opposed to jejunal, resections/insults result in more voluminous diarrhea with loss of nutrients in stool.

TABLE 61.13
Factors That Affect the Type of Nutrition Required by Short Bowel Syndrome Patients

Factors	The Effect
Phases of SBS	See Table 61.14
Length of remaining small intestine	Very short lengths (60–100 cm) worsen severity of SBS
The extent of disease in remaining intestine	Impact of even mild disease on nutritional status can be profound. As disease worsens, the length of functioning small intestine decreases
Absence of the stomach	Loss of timed and slow release of gastric chyme decreases contact time between food and digestive/absorptive epithelium, thereby worsening SBS. Lack of stomach acid facilitates bacterial overgrowth aggravating malabsorption
Absence of the ileocecal valve	Leads to bacterial overgrowth enabling passage of colonic bacteria into the small intestine
Absence of the colon	Promotes water and electrolyte losses. Caloric losses are more extensive. Lack of gastrocolic reflex results in rapid transit of food, enhancing malabsorption

TABLE 61.14
Phases of Short Bowel Syndrome with Their Characteristics

Phase	Duration	Main Problems
Postoperative	1–2 weeks	High volume/severe diarrhea
		Gastric hypersecretion
		Related fluid and electrolyte imbalances
Transition	1–3 months	Diarrhea with oral intake
		Malabsorption:
		Increased caloric requirements
		Micronutrient deficiencies
		Social problems
		TPN related problems
Adaptation	3 months to 1–2 years	Dietary restrictions
		Adequacy of oral intake
		Complications:
		Renal stones
		Gallstones
		D-Lactic acidosis

2. GI transit is faster in patients with ileal resections because of the lack of the ileal brake mechanism discussed in the first GI chapter.
3. The ileum has a greater adaptive potential.

Most patients with SBS fall into two main categories: Those with or without a colon.

Patients with a colon usually have the majority of their ileum and some of their jejunum resected with a resultant jejunocolic anastomosis. The ones without a colon usually have end-jejunostomies (see Figure 61.2). Patients with a colon typically do better, especially in maintaining fluid and electrolyte balance, and cases with >50 cm of jejunum remaining may be managed with oral/enteral nutrition instead of TPN.

DIET IN SBS

Dietary interventions in SBS should be individualized for each patient as the needs differ considerably. Some general recommendations are given in the following paragraphs.

Postoperative Phase

No enteral nutrition is given at this phase because of the osmotic effects of food and all patients require TPN. There are massive losses of fluids and electrolytes and the amount is highly variable; therefore, careful monitoring of all intake and output as well as daily laboratory tests must be done. Patients should be given back their entire deficit plus an extra estimated 300 to 500 cc/day for insensible losses. Preferably, this type of replacement should be done on an hourly basis and separate from the TPN.

Agents that slow intestinal transit such as parenteral codeine and drugs that reduce the commonly seen gastric hypersecretion are also helpful in reducing the volume of stool output. Gastric hypersecretion is usually comparable to the level seen in duodenal ulcer patients,[146] and can lead to significant volume losses especially within the first 6 months following surgery[147] and can contribute to malabsorption by inactivating pancreatic lipase and deconjugating bile salts. Treatment with cimetidine has been shown to improve absorption.[147,148] A study of 13 patients with large-volume ostomy output has shown that omeprazole can increase water absorption in cases with fecal outputs >2.5 kg/day but does not alter absorption of calories, macronutrients, or electrolytes.[149]

Octreotide (50 to 100 mcg, subcutaneously twice a day) has also been shown useful in patients with end-jejunostomies who have >3 l/day of ostomy output.[150] Initial concerns that octreotide may delay adaptation have not been substantiated in animal studies.[151]

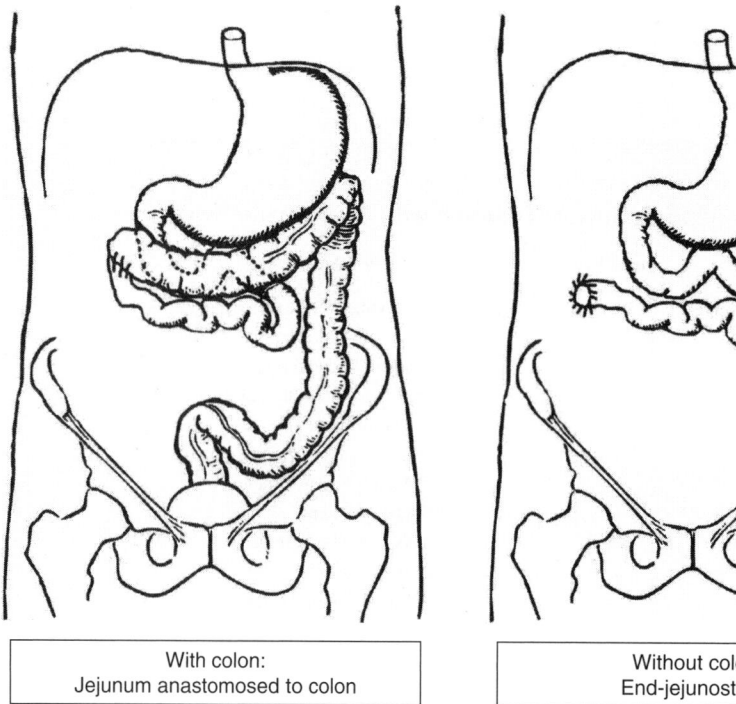

| With colon: Jejunum anastomosed to colon | Without colon: End-jejunostomy |

FIGURE 61.2 Anatomic types of Short Bowel Syndrome (SBS).

Transition Phase and Adaptation Phase

Oral diet

In the transition phase, TPN is continued while patients are first started on isotonic clear liquids that contain salt and glucose. It is advisable to wait until the ostomy output is <2 to 3 l/day before commencement of oral intake. The average sodium concentration in the ostomy secretions generally varies between 80 to 100 mEq/l, and so the initial hydration solutions should have at least this amount. Alternatively, sodium in the ostomy secretions can be measured to calculate the concentration in the replacement solution.

Patients who can tolerate these solutions should also be switched to oral antidiarrheals such as loperamide, lomotil, or tincture of opium. The commonly used dosages are given in Table 61.15 and are typically high.

Subsequently, patients should be transitioned into an oral diet. In general, patients with SBS do not tolerate large amounts of food at one time, foods with concentrated carbohydrates (especially mono- and disaccharides) and high lactose, or foods high in oxalate and insoluble fiber. Hypotonic fluids such as water, tea, juices, and alcohol also need to be avoided especially in patients without a colon because this type of fluid draws sodium into the jejunal lumen causing increased salt and water losses. Additionally, patients should be advised not to consume foods or supplements with nonabsorbable sugars (such as sorbitol and mannitol) or nonabsorbable fat (such as olestra) and watch out for hidden diarrheal agents (e.g., polyethylene glycol found in certain mints). It is best to try small and frequent amounts of solid food until the patient can consume at least 1200 kcal/day without a significant increase in diarrhea. Once this is achieved, TPN may be gradually cycled to go on only during the night and then on alternate days, together with slow advancement of oral intake.

Enteral feeding

Patients who are not able to take in adequate calories via the oral route should be tried on enteral feedings. There is no consensus on which type of enteral feeding is best for SBS, but isotonic polymeric formulas are recommended over elemental ones, which are expensive and poorly tolerated by patients because of their taste, smell, and high osmolality, which increases jejunal secretion.

Parenteral nutrition

Patients who cannot stop TPN need to be monitored for complications such as feeding catheter infections, liver disease, bacterial overgrowth, and nutritional deficiencies. Some of these together with their treatments are given in Table 61.16.

TABLE 61.15
Dosages for Antidiarrheals in SBS

Antidiarrheal	Typical Dosage
Loperamide	4–6 mg/4–5 times a day
Lomotil	2.5–5 mg/4 times a day
Tincture of opium	5–10 cc every 4 h
Codeine phosphate	30 mg/3–4 times a day

TABLE 61.16
Selected Complications of TPN in SBS and Their Prevention/Treatment

Complication	Treatment
Line infections	• Remove catheter completely if fungal infections or *Staphylococcus aureus* (*S. aureus*) are the cause (change over a wire is not acceptable) • *S. aureus* requires 2–6 weeks of antibiotics • *Staph. epidermidis* may be cured 80% of the time with 7–10 days of intravenous vancomycin
Bacterial overgrowth	• Treat with broad spectrum antibitotics (tetracycline, ciprofloxacin, metronidazole, etc.) • Rotate antibiotics every 4–8 weeks
Liver disease	• Pursue enteral feedings aggressively • Take care to prevent line infections • Avoid overfeeding with excessive calories • Prefer lipid calories to high carbohydrate nutrition • Treat bacterial overgrowth • Screen for cholelithiasis

Pharmacological therapy with glucagon-like peptide-2 (GLP-2) and its longer analog, teduglutide, may increase fluid and nutrient absorption in SBS.[152] Further studies are underway to study GLP-2 effects in the prevention TPN dependence.[152]

Dietary Requirements and the Composition of the Diet in SBS

Calories

Most patients with SBS only absorb 50 to 60% of total calories, with the highest percentage of malabsorption in fat and carbohydrates.[153] Thus, they need 1.5 to 2 times the amount of calories/food to maintain weight. Enteral feedings at night or additional TPN may be required in patients who are not able to increase their intake to this level.

Carbohydrate vs. fat

In normal individuals, about 20% of all carbohydrates consumed exit the small bowel undigested and are fermented to SCFAs in the colon, where they are absorbed.[154,155]

In order to take advantage of this colonic absorption, a well-designed study compared the use of a high-carbohydrate diet (60:20:20% of calories from carbohydrate: fat: protein) and a high-fat diet (20:60:20%) in SBS.[156] Intakes of the various diets did not affect stool or ostomy outputs, but consumption of the high-carbohydrate diet by patients with a colon reduced the fecal loss of calories by 2 ± 0.2 MJ/day, which may equal up to 20 to 25% of the daily caloric intake of an average patient with SBS. Thus, patients with a colon should be advised to consume a high-carbohydrate (50 to 60% of calories) and lower-fat (20 to 30% of calories) diet. Diets containing more than 60% of energy as carbohydrates may ultimately overcome the colon's energy-salvaging capability of 2.2 MJ/day of SCFAs.[157]

In patients without a colon, neither the high-fat nor the high-carbohydrate diet significantly affects energy or water/electrolyte losses.[156] Furthermore, many patients with very short jejunal segments and high ostomy outputs have been shown not to need or benefit from any particular diet.[158,159] So, restriction of fat in the diet is not recommended, because such restriction limits palatability of food and deprives patients of valuable concentrated energy.

LCFAs vs. MCTs

There is a tendency to use MCTs because of their better absorption in the presence of a reduced bile acid pool and pancreatic insufficiency. MCTs can help reduce ostomy output[160] in some cases, but they also exert a higher osmotic load in the small intestine and have a lower caloric density compared with long-chain fatty acids (LCFAs). Besides, LCFAs are better in inducing intestinal adaptation;[161] thus, a mixture of LCFAs and MCTs seems to be the most logical approach. A recent study compared the effects of a high-fat (56% of calories as fat) diet in SBS: Patients were given fat in the form of LCFAs or a mixture of MCTs and LCFAs (about 1:1). Only patients with a colon benefited with an increase in energy absorption from 46 to 58%.[162]

Lactose

Although the concentration of lactase in the intestine of SBS patients is unaltered, there is a reduction in the total quantity of available lactase. Thus, intake of food with high lactose content (e.g., milk) is discouraged, although many patients are able to tolerate small quantities of cheese and yogurt well.

Insoluble fiber

Insoluble fiber such as bran decreases intestinal transit time and should best be avoided by SBS patients.

Micronutrients

Deficiencies of divalent cations such as calcium, magnesium, and zinc are typical. Water-soluble vitamin deficiencies are rare because most are absorbed in the proximal jejunum. Vitamin B_{12}, which is absorbed in the terminal ileum, and fat-soluble vitamins A, D, E, and K need to be replaced routinely. A water-soluble form of vitamin A (Aquasol A) may be tried. Monthly injections of 1000 μg vitamin B_{12} are necessary.

Bile acid replacement

Although the bile acid pool is reduced in patients with SBS, clinicians do not replace it routinely because of a fear that diarrhea will increase when bile acids are fermented by bacteria, causing secretion of water and electrolytes. A recent case report contradicts this, and has demonstrated a 40 g/day increase in fat absorption when the patient was given a natural conjugated bile acid mixture isolated from ox bile or a synthetic bile acid named cholylsarcosine.[163]

COMMON PROBLEMS AND COMPLICATIONS IN SBS

Hypomagnesaemia

Patients with end-jejunostomies tend to have hypomagnesemia more often than those with a colon.[164] The condition requires parenteral magnesium frequently but oral, 1-α-hydroxycholecalciferol may also be tried.[164] Following urinary magnesium levels is a better indicator of deficiency than serum levels, which represent only 4% of the total body pool.[165]

Renal Stones

Risk of oxalate stones is increased, occurring in 25% of all SBS patients with a colon.[166] Calcium, which normally binds to oxalate and causes its excretion with feces, actually binds the malabsorbed fatty acids in the lumen in SBS, leaving oxalate available for absorption in the colon. Unabsorbed bile acids that enter the colon also stimulate absorption of oxalate.

Urinary oxalate excretion should be measured in patients with a colon and oxalate should be restricted in patients with a colon. Supplemental calcium should also be given. In patients with a history of stones, restriction of fat in the diet may be considered. Additionally, urinary citrate and magnesium, which inhibit stone formation, are low and may need to be supplemented.

Vitamin C in TPN can also lead to formation of excess oxalate when exposed to light; therefore, TPN bags should be shielded from light.

Gallstones

There is a two- to threefold increased risk of cholesterol gallstones because of the decreased bile acid pool in SBS. This increased risk is not different for the patients with or without a colon, but risk of calcium bilirubinate stones is higher in patients on TPN because of gallbladder stasis and low oral intake. Cholecystokinin injections have been tried in dogs with good success in preventing gallbladder stasis.[167] Some advocate prophylactic cholecystectomy in SBS.[168]

Social Problems

Patients with end-jejunostomies and those dependent on TPN frequently have social problems that require help of psychiatrists and psychologists.

D-Lactic Acidosis

Fermentation of malabsorbed carbohydrates in the colon produces D-lactic acid that cannot be metabolized by humans. Elevated levels cause an anion gap metabolic acidosis with confusion, ataxia, nystagmus, opthalmoplegia, and dysarthria.[169] The condition is more likely when thiamine deficiency is present, and it is treated with nonabsorbable antibiotics (neomycin or vancomycin) and restriction of carbohydrates (especially mono- and oligosaccharides) in the diet.[170]

In summary, nutritional management of SBS is complex and patients are best referred to an experienced multidisciplinary nutrition management team.

ACUTE INFECTIOUS DIARRHEA

Acute infectious diarrhea usually does not affect nutritional status even though it can result in severe water and electrolyte disturbances. (see Chapter 2) Although there is no specific diet therapy proven to be effective in this disease, patients should be encouraged to drink plenty of fluids that contain a mixture of glucose and sodium. Absorption of sodium in the intestinal tract is altered in acute diarrhea, but glucose-coupled sodium transport through the SGLT1 transporter is adequate in most cases to sustain hydration. An ideal mixture of glucose and sodium is found in the WHO oral rehydration solution (ORS), which can be made by mixing 20 g of glucose, 3.5 g of sodium chloride, 2.9 g of sodium bicarbonate, and 1.5 g of potassium chloride in 1 l of water. The commonly advocated sports drinks contain far less sodium and much more glucose compared with this ORS solution, and should not replace the latter. Within the last two decades, rice and other cereal-based ORS solutions that take advantage of other apical membrane sodium-dependent solute-transport transporters have been discovered. In these solutions rice or cereal flour replace glucose found in the original ORS. The rice ORS solution is superior to the glucose-based ORS in decreasing stool output.[171] Most recently, induction of sodium absorption from the colon by SCFAs was observed.[172] A clinical application of this principle has been tested: 50 g/l amylase-resistant maize starch, which is malabsorbed and fermented to SCFAs by colonic flora, was added to the original WHO ORS. In adolescents and adults with *Vibrio-cholerae*-induced diarrhea, stool output, and duration of diarrhea was less in patients given the maize starch ORS compared with controls given standard ORS.[173] Further studies are needed before the latter is incorporated into common clinical practice.

Although it is rational to advise patients to stay away from hard-to-digest foods such as red meat, high-fiber vegetables (e.g., salads, greens, broccoli, etc.), and lactose because of the increased rate of intestinal transit and concurrent malabsorption that occur in acute diarrhea, there exists no data in this regard. Most recently, an antidiarrheal factor has been found in rice, suggesting that a rice-based diet may be useful.[174] This factor blocks the secretory response of intestinal crypt cells to cyclic adenosine monophosphate and targets the cystic fibrosis transmembrane regulator (CFTR) chloride channel.

CLOSTRIDIUM DIFFICILE COLITIS AND PROBIOTICS

C. difficile colitis is a major cause of antibiotic-associated diarrhea and acute diarrhea in hospitalized patients. Spores of the bacterium are hard to destroy and a mean of 20% (range 5 to 66%) of patients have recurrences despite treatment with effective antibiotics. Preliminary results of a trial with yogurt enriched in *Lactobacillus* GG (trial using medicinal microbiotic yogurt [TUMMY]) together with standard antibiotic therapy have been promising in prevention of recurrence.[175] Final results are awaited for further recommendations.

FUNCTIONAL DISORDERS OF THE GASTROINTESTINAL TRACT

DEFINITION AND EPIDEMIOLOGY

Functional gastrointestinal disorders (FGIDs) are the most common diseases of the GI tract, with at least 4.7 million affected individuals in the United States. They comprise about 20 to 50% of gastroenterology clinic visits and are estimated to cost $8 billion a year to the healthcare system. Definitions for the different types of FGIDs are established and are known as the Rome III criteria.[176]

MECHANISMS

Various factors and mechanisms thought to be important in the pathogenesis of these disorders are listed in Table 61.17. Currently recommended dietary management is based on decreasing food allergies, affecting GI motility. and lowering intestinal gas production in an effort to decrease bowel wall distension.

EFFECTS ON NUTRITIONAL STATUS

FGIDs usually do not lead to weight loss. If a patient with FGIDs has significant weight loss, other causes should be sought. Although there are no reports of malnutrition, patients with FGIDs have many self-reported food intolerances, resulting in avoidance of various foods. This avoidance may lead to nutritional deficiencies. In one study comparing nutrient intake using 48 h dietary recall, women with FGIDs had lower mean consumption of calories as well as folate, ascorbic acid, and vitamin A, compared with gastroesophageal reflux disease (GERD) and IBD patients.[177]

DIET IN FGIDs

There is no particular diet for patients with FGIDs, and there is little evidence for dietary therapies of functional upper digestive tract diseases. Some patients with functional chest pain may improve with diets similar to ones recommended for GERD patients (given in the previous GI chapter, Table 61.10). Others with functional dyspepsia may benefit from elimination of foods that delay gastric emptying (given in the previous GI chapter, Table 61.17).

TABLE 61.17

Factors Important in Pathogenesis of Functional Disorders of the Gastrointestinal Tract

1. Cognitive factors
    a. Illness behavior
    b. Illness coping strategies
2. Behavioral/emotional factors
    a. Psychosocial stress
    b. Physical or sexual abuse
    c. Anxiety
    d. Depression
3. Physiological factors
    a. Visceral hyperalgesia
    b. Altered intestinal motility
    c. Altered neuroendocrine response
    d. Altered microflora of the intestines
        i. Bacterial overgrowth in the small bowel
4. Environmental factors
    a. Dietary allergens
    b. Enteric infections

FIBER FOR IBS

TYPES OF DIETARY FIBER

Dietary fiber is defined as endogenous components of plants that are resistant to digestion by human enzymes. Fiber consists either of nonstarch polysaccharides (e.g., cellulose, hemicellulose, pectins, and gums) or of nonpolysaccharides (e.g., lignins composed of phenylpropane units). Cellulose is a nondigestible glucose polymer found in the cell walls of all vegetation, making it the most abundant organic compound in the world. Hemicellulose fibers are cellulose molecules substituted with other sugars, such as xylan, galactan, mannan, etc. Pectins and gums are composed of arabinose or galactose side chains added on to a galacturonate backbone; they naturally form gels.

Cellulose and hemicellulose are the major component of bran and whole grains. Lignins are commonly found in seeds and stems of vegetation. Pectin is part of apples, citrus fruits, strawberries, and is widely added to jams/jellies. Gums naturally occur in oats, legumes, guar, and barley. Structural fibers such as celluloses and lignins and some hemicelluloses are water insoluble. Gums, pectins, psyllium, oat bran, and beans are water soluble.

Insoluble fiber mainly adds bulk to stool and increases transit through the colon. Soluble fibers such as guar and pectin delay gastric emptying and transit through the small intestine, but speed transit through the colon and lower intraluminal pressures. Soluble fibers may also bind bile acids and minerals such as calcium and iron.

BRAN

Fiber, in the form of bran, for irritable bowel syndrome (IBS) was popularized after Burkitt's initial work in early 1970s, demonstrating that it increases stool weight and decreases intestinal transit time. Others confirmed these findings,[178] and a lack of fiber was implicated for the development of many GI diseases including diverticular disease, colon cancer, and IBS. Consequently, studies in the 1970s undertook bran replacement as therapy for IBS and the results were positive in some[179] but clearly negative in many others.[180] Most of these studies had methodological flaws and were usually done with small numbers of patients. Nevertheless, given the lack of other effective therapies for the disease, bran became the standard of care.

Evidence over the last two decades contradicts this and indicates that patients with IBD consume equal amounts of total fiber but less vegetable fiber compared with healthy controls.[181] Fiber replacement in the form of bran is no more effective than placebo[182–184] and is poorly tolerated in many subjects. In one study, 55% of the patients worsened after bran therapy with deterioration in bowel habits, abdominal distension, and pain.[185] Improvement was seen in only 10%. These findings are corroborated by data from other studies upon careful review[186]: Not only may patients worsen initially and not tolerate bran but also they may have a high subsequent withdrawal rate.[187]

SOLUBLE FIBER

Soluble-fiber replacement seems to be better tolerated and more effective for IBS in comparison with bran.[188] It has also been used in combination with antispasmodics, anxiolytics, and antidepressants and has a synergistic effect in such combinations in some studies.[189] Soluble fiber (such as psyllium, methyl-cellulose, or calcium polycarbophil) is most effective for constipation predominant IBS patients, and should be gradually increased over a period of weeks to avoid bloating and flatulence.

HIGH-FIBER DIETS

The role of a high-fiber diet for IBS is debatable given the aforementioned controversies regarding bran as treatment for IBS. In an open-label trial, the symptoms that have been shown to benefit most from a high-fiber diet are hard stools, constipation, and urgency. In this study, all patients who were able to consume 30 g or more fiber improved symptomatically.[190] In another trial of 14 patients followed up for 2 to 3 years, 50% improved greatly whereas 28.5% had worsening of their symptoms.[191]

In conclusion, fiber is not the ideal therapy for all patients with IBS, and limited data exists on its use in IBS in the tertiary referral settings. Fiber could be tried especially in patients with constipation-predominant symptoms in primary care settings but may not be an effective therapy for the majority of patients.[191]

FOOD ALLERGIES AND IBS

Patients with IBS have many food intolerances, although a small number of these represent true food allergies. In a large population-based questionnaire study, 70% of the subjects had symptoms related to intake of food, 62% had limited or excluded food items from the diet, and 12% had an inadequate diet.[192] Patients reported 4.8 foods that cause symptoms and excluded 2.5 foods totally from their diets numbers of food items. There were no associations between the tests for food allergy and malabsorption and perceived food intolerance. In IBS, food intolerances are typically to more than one item and are not specific, suggesting intolerance to food in general exists rather than true food sensitivity. Problem food can be identified in 6 to 58% of the cases depending on the study.[193] The most common adverse food reactions, confirmed on double-blind challenges, are to milk, wheat, eggs, dairy products, corn, peas, tea, coffee, potatoes, nuts, wine, citrus fruits, tomatoes, chocolate, bananas, tuna fish, celery, and yeast. Some authors believe that these foods represent ones with high salicylate content.[193] Many adverse reactions to food are not the classical wheal and flare type; a mere 3% are truly anaphylactoid-like and cause rash or swelling of the lips or throat;[194] and only some of the reactions can be confirmed by skin prick testing.[195] Most of the true food allergies in IBS are seen in patients with other atopic diseases.[196,197] Furthermore, most true food allergies on testing may not be clinically relevant. In a study of IBS patients food intolerance was identified in 62.5%; skin prick test to various foods were positive in 52.3%; but, strikingly, only 13.7% of the patients were symptomatic with foods that they were allergic to on prick tests.[195] These findings argue against undertaking a search for food allergies as part of the initial clinical evaluation of IBS patients.

A positive response to elimination diets in IBS ranges from 15 to 71%, but most older studies have methodologic flaws.[193] A significantly high level of IgG4 antibodies to common food allergens such as wheat, beef, pork, and lamb are observed in all types of IBS patients and do not differentiate between the subtypes of IBS.[198] Elimination diets based on IgG4 antibody testing improve pain, bloating, rectal compliance, and IBS quality of IBS, and this effect may be sustained up to 6 months in some patients.[199] A recent randomized trial in 150 patients with IBS using an elimination diet based on positive IgG to foods or a sham diet for 3 months demonstrated significant improvement in patient symptoms. Relaxing the elimination diet caused worsening.[200] Supporting the role of food allergy in IBS, equal improvement of symptoms up to 50% has been noted in both study groups in trials with diet vs. sodium chromoglycate administration for diarrhea predominant disease.[201,202] These findings need to be confirmed in further well-designed placebo-controlled experiments before they can be considered clinically applicable, and elimination diet therapy based on IgG food antibodies in IBS is an important evolving field.

An *in vivo* colonoscopic allergen provocation (COLAP) test based on wheal and flare reactions in the colonic mucosa has been developed and has shown positive reactions in 77% of the patients with food-related symptoms.[203] The clinical utility of this test in IBS is yet to be determined.

In conclusion, a small subgroup of patients with true food allergies is classified as IBS. These patients tend to have atopy in general and diarrhea-predominant disease. In selected patients, a symptom and food diary may be useful as an initial investigation for food allergy. Foods identified to lead to symptoms may then be eliminated and rechallenges may be done. Referral to an allergy specialist may be useful in such cases. For the majority of cases, however, elimination of certain foods that the individual patient believes to cause symptoms is adequate therapy. Physicians also need to ensure that the patient's self-imposed dietary restrictions do not lead to macro- or micronutrient deficiencies.

CARBOHYDRATES IN IBS

Fructose and Sorbitol

A number of studies show that IBS symptoms get exacerbated in patients after ingesting fructose and sorbitol mixtures. Fructose is a natural ingredient of fruits as is sorbitol. The latter is also a common sweetener in dietetic foods. Ingestion of 10 g of sorbitol, equivalent of four to five sugar-free mints or two medium pears, can produce moderate to severe abdominal discomfort, bloating, and diarrhea in 27% of healthy volunteers.[204] Symptoms may last up to 6 h.

A subset of IBS patients has true malabsorption of fructose and sorbitol as assessed by breath hydrogen production[205,206] although the level of breath hydrogen produced does not necessarily correlate with the degree of symptoms.[207] Whether fructose and sorbitol malabsorption is more common or more severe among IBS patients as compared with healthy controls is uncertain. In one large study, there was no higher incidence or higher level of malabsorption.[208] Among malabsorbers symptoms cannot be explained by changes in jejunal sensitivity and motor function of the small bowel. At present, avoidance of sorbitol and high intakes of fructose may be considered in selected patients.

Lactose

Subjective lactose intolerance is also increased in IBS, and lactose malabsorption is common. Most lactose malabsorbers among IBS patients are malabsorbers of fructose and sorbitol as well. However, elimination of lactose from the diet does not impact the disease course or reduce symptoms when assessed objectively in long-term follow-up.[209] In contrast to these findings, many patients subjectively feel that identification of their lactose malabsorptive state has helped them gain awareness of food–symptom relationships and alleviate their symptoms partially. Treatment with lactase[210] or acidophilus milk has shown no benefit over unaltered milk in IBS patients with and without lactose malabsorption.

THERAPIES DIRECTED AGAINST GAS PRODUCTION AND ENZYME THERAPIES

Gas in the upper GI tract is a result of swallowed air and the carbon dioxide generated by chemical reactions of acid and alkali substances, whereas in the colon gas forms as a result of fermentation of nutrients by the bacterial flora. Bloating and gas are common complaints of patients with IBS, even though the total amount of gas in the intestinal tract is not increased.[211]

Rather, IBS patients have a hypersensitivity to the presence of gas, resulting in discomfort and pain. Therefore, therapies directed against gas seem reasonable in symptomatic patients.

In order to reduce air in the upper digestive tract, patients may be instructed to eat smaller quantities, avoid eating on the run, not talk during eating, and avoid carbonated beverages, chewing gum, smoking, and excessive fluid intake with meals. Additionally, simethicone may be tried despite its questionable efficacy, as it poses no harm to patients other than their pocketbook.[212]

One small study suggests that pancreatic enzyme supplements (30,000 USP lipase, 112,500 USP protease, and 99,600 USP amylase) may reduce symptomatic bloating, gas, and fullness without significant decreases in breath hydrogen or methane levels in healthy subjects in response to a high-fat meal.[213] It is unknown whether the marginal symptomatic benefit in this study can be translated into patients with functional dyspepsia or IBS.

Activated charcoal has been shown to be partially effective in reducing gas in the lower GI tract.[212,214] A preparation called "Beano," containing the enzyme beanase, has been reported to reduce flatulence and breath hydrogen produced after ingestion of mashed black beans, although no studies exist demonstrating its clinical utility in IBS.[215]

It is commonly recommended that IBS patients avoid known gas-producing foods such as cabbage, legumes, lentils, beans, and certain cruciferous vegetables such as cauliflower and broccoli, although such a diet has not been tested. Interestingly, King and colleagues have devised an elimination diet that reduces abnormal colonic fermentation. This diet allows meat and fish except beef, replaces all dairy products with soy products, eliminates all grains except rice, and restricts yeast, citrus, caffeinated drinks, and tap water. A pilot study of diarrhea-predominant patients on this elimination diet has demonstrated reduction in median symptom scores, compared with controls. Further studies are needed before such a restrictive diet can be recommended for IBS in general.[216]

GUT FLORA AND SMALL BOWEL BACTERIAL OVERGROWTH IN IBS

There is likely an increased prevalence of small bowel bacterial overgrowth in IBS,[217,218] and the intestinal flora may be altered in IBS. Excess methane production by the intestinal flora on hydrogen breath testing has been linked to predominance of IBS symptoms such as constipation.[218,219] Some of the seemingly food-related adverse reactions in IBS could also be due to heightened postprandial symptoms in patients with small bowel bacterial overgrowth. A significant number of IBS patients who are classified as having sugar/carbohydrate intolerance may also have small bowel bacterial overgrowth.[217] Treatment of such overgrowth with nonabsorbable antibiotics such as rifaximin at a dose of 400 mg twice daily leads to short-term improvement of IBS symptoms, especially bloating.[220]

Multiple studies looking at altering the intestinal flora with probiotics and prebiotics are also underway.[221] VSL#3 improved bloating,[222] whereas lactobacilli did not improve IBS in some studies.[223,224] The individual effects of various strains of probiotics may vary. Further research is necessary looking not only at single probiotics for all patients but individualized probiotic therapy for each patient.

Nutritional tips for patients with FGIDs are summarized in Table 61.18.

DIVERTICULAR DISEASE OF THE COLON

DEFINITION AND EPIDEMIOLOGY

Diverticular disease of the colon is common in Western countries. The incidence increases with age, but the true incidence is difficult to determine as most patients remain asymptomatic. Nonetheless, it is rare before age 40, and can be found in up to two-thirds of patients over the age of 80.[225–227] In contrast to Western countries (United States, Australia, and European countries) diverticula are less common in South America and extraordinarily rare in Africa and rural Asia. Owing to worldwide geographical variability, diverticular disease of the colon has been termed a disease of Western civilization.

TABLE 61.18
Summary of Nutritional Tips for the IBS Patient

1. If constipation predominant IBS, try soluble fiber supplements
2. If diarrhea predominant disease or atopic patient, keep food diary and seek help from an allergy specialist
3. Avoid only those foods that cause symptoms every time they are consumed
4. Replace consumption of heavily processed foods, containing preservatives, additives, food coloring, etc., with a natural balanced diet
5. Seek help from a dietitian to ensure adequate macro and micronutrient intake if having to avoid many food items
7. Avoid gas-producing vegetables (e.g., legumes, cruciferous vegetables, etc.)
8. Avoid carbonated and caffeinated beverages

The majority of diverticula are histologically pseudodiverticula, which are herniations of the mucosa and submucosa through the muscular layer of the colon as opposed to true diverticula, which involve all layers. The sigmoid colon is the most frequent location for diverticular disease in United States.

MECHANISMS

Role of Diet in the Pathogenesis

Dietary fiber deficiency along with the theory of colonic segmentation has been the leading hypothesis for the etiology of diverticular disease of colon. According to the segmentation theory, contraction of the colon at the haustral folds causes the colon to act as a series of "little bladders" instead of a continuous single-chambered lumen.[226] Formation of these segments leads to delayed transport, increased water absorption, and more importantly a rise in intraluminal pressure resulting in mucosal herniation.[228]

The incidence of diverticula within a society increases following the adoption of the Western diet that is low in fiber.[229] This is supported by animal data as well as epidemiologic studies.[229,230] Compared with patients who are on a diet high in fiber content, those who consume a low-fiber diet have a threefold increase in the incidence of diverticulosis.[231] Consumption of a low-fiber Westernized diet leads to a lower intake of crude cereal grains and increase in consumption of white flour, refined sugar, conserves, and meat. Lack of "adequate" dietary fiber decreases stool weight, prolongs transit time, and increases the colonic intraluminal pressure, all of which predispose to the diverticula formation in concert with segmentation.[226,232] Additionally, a high-meat diet changes bacterial metabolism in the colon and bacteria may produce a toxic metabolite favoring diverticulosis, which is hypothesized to be a spasmogen or an agent that weakens the colonic wall.[233]

DIET AND DIVERTICULOSIS

Diet in Prevention of Diverticulosis

Given the importance of fiber in the pathogenesis of diverticula, it is reasonable to recommend a high-fiber diet in the prevention of diverticular disease. Confirming the importance of high-fiber diet as prophylactic measure, the Health Professionals Follow-up Study, which included over 50,000 health professionals, showed an inverse relationship between the amount of dietary fiber intake and the risk of developing symptomatic diverticular disease. Those who consumed more that 32 g/day of fiber had the greatest benefit.[234]

Diet in Treatment of Symptomatic Disease

The beneficial effects of dietary fiber on symptomatic uncomplicated diverticular disease continue to be subject to debate. Two controlled trials that evaluated the impact of fiber supplementation in patients with uncomplicated diverticulosis showed conflicting results.[235,236] However, this disagreement does not preclude the potential benefits from a trial of high-fiber diet, which still seems a reasonable approach. The American Society of Colon and Rectal Surgeons practice guidelines recommend the resumption of a high-fiber diet following the resolution of uncomplicated acute diverticulitis.[237] In cases of complicated diverticular disease, the patient should be placed on clear liquid diet or be kept NPO in order to achieve bowel rest, which remains the mainstay of therapy along with the antibiotics. There is neither evidence nor scientific basis for avoidance of nuts, popcorn, and seeds for prevention of symptomatic attacks even though this recommendation seems to be common.

REFERENCES

1. Dieterich, W. et al. *Nat Med* 3: 797, 1997.
2. Kagnoff, M.F. et al. *Gut* 28: 995, 1987.
3. Corazza, G.R. et al. *J Intern Med* 236: 183, 1994.
4. Mazure, R.M. et al. *Am J Gastroenterol* 91: 726, 1996.
5. Mustalahti, K., *Lancet* 354: 744, 1999.
6. Rude, R.K. & Olerich, M. *Osteoporos Int* 6: 453, 1996.
7. Valdimarsson, T., Lofman, O., Toss, G. & Strom, M. *Gut* 38: 322, 1996.
8. McFarlane, X.A., Bhalla, A.K. & Robertson, D.A. *Gut* 39: 180, 1996.
9. Mautalen, C. et al. *Am J Gastroenterol* 92: 313, 1997.
10. Bai, J.C. et al. *Aliment Pharmacol Ther* 11: 157, 1997.
11. McFarlane, X.A. *Gut* 36: 710, 1995.
12. Logan, R.F., Rifkind, E.A., Turner, I.D. & Ferguson, A. *Gastroenterology* 97: 265, 1989.
13. Holmes, G.K., Prior, P., Lane, M.R., Pope, D. & Allan, R.N. *Gut* 30: 333, 1989.
14. Leonard, J.N. et al. *Br Med J (Clin Res Ed)* 286: 16, 1983.
15. Grefte, J.M., et al. *J Clin Pathol* 41: 886, 1988.

16. Thompson, T. *J Am Diet Assoc* 100: 1389, 2000.
17. Hallert, C. et al. *Aliment Pharmacol Ther* 16: 1333, 2002.
18. Pyle, G.G. et al. *Clin Gastroenterol Hepatol* 3: 687, 2005.
19. Matysiak-Budnik, T. et al. *Gastroenterology* 129: 786, 2005.
20. Spaenij-Dekking, L., Kooy-Winkelaar, Y. & Koning, F. *N Engl J Med* 353: 1748, 2005.
21. Roufail, W.M. & Ruffin, J.M. *Am J Dig Dis* 11: 587, 1966.
22. Regan, P.T. & DiMagno, E.P. *Gastroenterology* 78: 484, 1980.
23. DiMagno, E.P., Go, W.L. & Summerskill, W.H. *Gastroenterology* 63: 25, 1972.
24. Carroccio, A. et al. *Dig Dis Sci* 39: 2235, 1994.
25. Carroccio, A. et al. *Dig Dis Sci* 40: 2555, 1995.
26. Faulkner-Hogg, K.B., Selby, W.S. & Loblay, R.H. *Scand J Gastroenterol* 34: 784, 1999.
27. Trier, J.S., Falchuk, Z.M., Carey, M.C. & Schreiber, D.S. *Gastroenterology* 75: 307, 1978.
28. Sinclair, T.S., Kumar, J.S. & Dawson, A.M. *Gut* 24: A494, 1983.
29. Longstreth, G.F. *Ann Intern Med* 119: 1014, 1993.
30. Love, A., Elmes, M., Golden, M. & McMaster, D. In *Perspectives in celiac disease* (eds. McNicholl, B. & Fottrell, P.F.) 335–342 (MTP, Lancaster, UK, 1978).
31. Jones, P.E., L'Hirondel, C. & Peters, T.J. *Gut* 23: 108, 1982.
32. Ejderhamn, J., Veress, B. & Strandvik, B. In *Coeliac disease: One hundred years* (ed. Kumar, P.J.) 294–297 (Leeds University Press, Leeds, UK, 1988).
33. Hirschenhuber, C. et al. *Aliment Pharmacol Ther* 23: 559, 2006.
34. Kumar, P.J., O'Donoghue, D.P., Stenson, K. & Dawson, A.M. *Gut* 20: 743, 1979.
35. Chartrand, L.J., Russo, P.A., Duhaime, A.G. & Seidman, E.G. *J Am Diet Assoc* 97: 612, 1997.
36. Selby, W.S., et al. *Scand J Gastroenterol* 34: 909, 1999.
37. Dissanayake, A.S., Truelove, S.C. & Whitehead, R. *Br Med J* 4: 189, 1974.
38. de Ritis, G. et al. *Gastroenterology* 94: 41, 1988.
39. Vainio, E. & Varjonen, E. *Int Arch Allergy Immunol* 106: 134, 1995.
40. Srinivasan, U. et al. Absence of oats toxicity in adult coeliac disease. *BMJ* 313, 1300–1 (1996).
41. Hardman, C.M. et al. *N Engl J Med* 337: 1884, 1997.
42. Janatuinen, E.K. et al. *N Engl J Med* 333: 1033, 1995.
43. Auricchio, S. et al. *J Pediatr Gastroenterol Nutr* 2: 428, 1983.
44. Bouguerra, F. et al. *Arch Pediatr* 5: 621, 1998.
45. Persson, L.A., Ivarsson, A. & Hernell, O. *Adv Exp Med Biol* 503: 115, 2002.
46. D'Amico, M.A. et al. *Clin Pediatr (Phila)* 44: 249, 2005.
47. Greco, L. et al. *J Pediatr Gastroenterol Nutr* 4: 52, 1985.
48. Ivarsson, A. et al. *Acta Paediatr* 89: 165, 2000.
49. Ascher, H., Krantz, I., Rydberg, L., Nordin, P. & Kristiansson, B. *Arch Dis Child* 76: 113, 1997.
50. Maki, M., Kallonen, K., Lahdeaho, M.L. & Visakorpi, J.K. *Acta Paediatr Scand* 77: 408, 1988.
51. Han, P.D., Burke, A., Baldassano, R.N., Rombeau, J.L. & Lichtenstein, G.R. *Gastroenterol Clin North Am* 28: 423, ix 1999.
52. Klein, S. et al. *J Clin Gastroenterol* 10: 34, 1988.
53. Al-Jaouni, R., Hebuterne, X., Pouget, I. & Rampal, P. *Nutrition* 16: 173, 2000.
54. Stokes, M.A. & Hill, G.L. *JPEN J Parenter Enteral Nutr* 17: 3, 1993.
55. Kushner, R.F. & Schoeller, D.A. *Am J Clin Nutr* 53: 161, 1991.
56. Barot, L.R., Rombeau, J.L., Feurer, I.D. & Mullen, J.L. *Ann Surg* 195: 214, 1982.
57. Capristo, E., et al. *J Intern Med* 243: 339, 1998.
58. Mingrone, G. et al. *Am J Clin Nutr* 69: 325, 1999.
59. Christie, P.M. & Hill, G.L. *Gastroenterology* 99: 730, 1990.
60. Ballegaard, M. et al. *Scand J Gastroenterol* 32: 569, 1997.
61. Rigaud, D. et al. *Am J Clin Nutr* 60: 775, 1994.
62. Cowan, F.J. et al. *Arch Dis Child* 76: 325, 1997.
63. Mayberry, J.F. et al. *Dig Dis Sci* 26: 444, 1981.
64. Persson, P.G., Ahlbom, A. & Hellers, G. *Epidemiology* 3: 47, 1992.
65. Panza, E., Franceshi, et al. *Ital J Gastro* 19: 205, 1987.
66. Sakamoto, N. et al. *Inflamm Bowel Dis* 11: 154, 2005.
67. Epidemiology Group of the Research Committee of Inflammatory Bowel Disease in Japan. Dietary and other risk factors of ulcerative colitis. A case–control study in Japan. *J Clin Gastroenterol* 19: 166, 1994.
68. Reif, S. et al. *Gut* 40: 754, 1997.
69. Mayberry, J.F., Rhodes, J. & Newcombe, R.G. *Digestion* 20: 323, 1980.
70. Jarnerot, G., Jarnmark, I. & Nilsson, K. *Scand J Gastroenterol* 18: 999, 1983.
71. Thornton, J.R., Emmett, P.M. & Heaton, K.W. *Br Med J* 280: 293, 1980.
72. Thornton, J.R., Emmett, P.M. & Heaton, K.W. *Br Med J (Clin Res Ed)* 290: 1786, 1985.
73. Thornton, J.R., Emmett, P.M. & Heaton, K.W. *Br Med J* 2: 762, 1979.

74. Shoda, R., Matsueda, K., Yamato, S. & Umeda, N. *Am J Clin Nutr* 63: 741, 1996.
75. Gudmand-Hoyer, E. & Jarnum, S. *Gut* 11: 338, 1970.
76. Wright, R. & Truelove, S.C. *Br Med J* 5454: 138, 1965.
77. Salem, S.N., Truelove, S.C. & Richards, W.C. *Br Med J* 5380: 394, 1964.
78. Salem, S.N. & Truelove, S.C. *Br Med J* 1: 827, 1965.
79. Park, R.H., Duncan, A. & Russell, R.I. *Am J Gastroenterol* 85: 708, 1990.
80. Cady, A.B., Rhodes, J.B., Littman, A. & Crane, R.K. *J Lab Clin Med* 70: 279, 1967.
81. Taylor, K.B. & Truelove, S.C. *Br Med J* 5257: 924, 1961.
82. Dudek, B., Spiro, H.M. & Thayer Jr., W.R. *Gastroenterology* 49: 544, 1965.
83. Jewell, D.P. & Truelove, S.C. *Gut* 13: 796, 1972.
84. Sewell, P., Cooke, W.T., Cox, E.V. & Meynell, M.J. *Lancet* 41: 1132, 1963.
85. Knoflach, P., Park, B.H., Cunningham, R., Weiser, M.M. & Albini, B. *Gastroenterology* 92: 479, 1987.
86. Wright, R. & Truelove, S.R. *Am J Dig Dis* 11: 847, 1966.
87. Koletzko, S., et al. *BMJ* 298: 1617, 1989.
88. Koletzko, S., et al. *BMJ* 302: 1580, 1991.
89. Imes, S., Pinchbeck, B. & Thomson, A.B. *Digestion* 39: 7, 1988.
90. Ritchie, J.K., Wadsworth, J., Lennard-Jones, J.E. & Rogers, E. *Br Med J (Clin Res Ed)* 295: 517, 1987.
91. Levenstein, S., Prantera, C., Luzi, C. & D'Ubaldi, A. *Gut* 26: 989, 1985.
92. Gottschall, E. *Breaking the vicious cycle* Kirkton Press Ltd., Baltomore, ON, 1999.
93. Jones, V.A. et al. *Lancet* 2: 177, 1985.
94. Pearson, M., Teahon, K., Levi, A.J. & Bjarnason, I. *Gut* 34: 783, 1993.
95. Ruuska, T., Savilahti, E., Maki, M., Ormala, T. & Visakorpi, J.K. *J Pediatr Gastroenterol Nutr* 19: 175, 1994.
96. Iannoli, P. et al. *Surgery* 122: 721; discussion 728, 1997.
97. Byrne, T.A., et al. *Ann Surg* 222: 243, 1995.
98. Slonim, A.E. et al. *N Engl J Med* 342: 1633, 2000.
99. Hawthorne, A.B. et al. *Gut* 33: 922, 1992.
100. Stenson, W.F. et al. *Ann Intern Med* 116: 609, 1992.
101. Aslan, A. & Triadafilopoulos, G. *Am J Gastroenterol* 87: 432, 1992.
102. Greenfield, S.M. et al. *Aliment Pharmacol Ther* 7: 159, 1993.
103. Ikehata, A. et al. *Am J Clin Nutr* 56: 938, 1992.
104. Bjorkkjaer, T. et al. *Lipids Health Dis* 5: 6, 2006.
105. Eysselein, V.E. et al. *Ann NY Acad Sci* 657: 319, 1992.
106. Breuer, R.I. et al. *Dig Dis Sci* 36: 185, 1991.
107. Steinhart, A.H., Brzezinski, A. & Baker, J.P. *Am J Gastroenterol* 89: 179, 1994.
108. Patz, J., et al. *Am J Gastroenterol* 91: 731, 1996.
109. Scheppach, W. et al. *Gastroenterology* 103: 51, 1992.
110. Rolandelli, R.H. et al. *Am J Clin Nutr* 47: 715, 1988.
111. Rembacken, B.J., et al. *Lancet* 354: 635, 1999.
112. Gionchetti, P. et al. *Gastroenterology* 119: 305, 2000.
113. Umemoto, Y., Tanimura, H. & Ishimoto, K. *Gastroenterology* 114: A1102, 1998.
114. Lindsay, J.O. et al. *Gut* 55: 348, 2006.
115. Furrie, E. et al. *Gut* 54: 242, 2005.
116. O'Morain, C., Segal, A.W. & Levi, A.J. *Br Med J (Clin Res Ed)* 288: 1859, 1984.
117. Gorard, D.A. et al. *Gut* 34: 1198, 1993.
118. Seidman, E.G., Bouthullier, L. & Weber, A.M. *Gastroenterology* 90: A1625, 1986.
119. Griffiths, A.M., Ohlsson, A., Sherman, P.M. & Sutherland, L.R. *Gastroenterology* 108: 1056, 1995.
120. Gonzalez-Huix, F. et al. *Gut* 34: 778, 1993.
121. Dieleman, L.A. & Heizer, W.D. *Gastroenterol Clin North Am* 27: 435, 1998.
122. Lochs, H. et al. IV. *Gastroenterology* 101: 881, 1991.
123. Axelsson, C. & Jarnum, S. *Scand J Gastroenterol* 12: 89, 1977.
124. O'Brien, C.J., Giaffer, M.H., Cann, P.A. & Holdsworth, C.D. *Am J Gastroenterol* 86: 1614, 1991.
125. McIntyre, P.B. et al. *Gut* 27: 481, 1986.
126. Greenberg, G.R. et al. *Gut* 29: 1309, 1988.
127. Rombeau, J.L., Barot, L.R., Williamson, C.E. & Mullen, J.L. *Am J Surg* 143: 139, 1982.
128. Dickinson, R.J. et al. *Gastroenterology* 79: 1199, 1980.
129. Elson, C.O., et al. *Dig Dis Sci* 25: 42, 1980.
130. Sitzmann, J.V., Converse Jr., R.L. & Bayless, T.M. *Gastroenterology* 99: 1647, 1990.
131. Solomons, N.W., Rosenberg, I.H., Sandstead, H.H. & Vo-Khactu, K.P. *Digestion* 16: 87, 1977.
132. Muller, J.M., Keller, H.W., Erasmi, H. & Pichlmaier, H. *Br J Surg* 70: 40, 1983.
133. Fernandez-Banares, F. et al. *Am J Gastroenterol* 84: 744, 1989.
134. Kuroki, F. et al. *Dig Dis Sci* 38: 1614, 1993.

135. Harries, A.D. et al. *Gut* 26: 1197, 1985.
136. Vogelsang, H. et al. *Dig Dis Sci* 34: 1094, 1989.
137. Lashner, B.A., et al. *Gastroenterology* 97: 255, 1989.
138. Lashner, B.A., et al. *Gastroenterology* 112: 29, 1997.
139. Kruis, W., Rindfleisch, G.E. & Weinzierl, M. *Hepatogastroenterology* 32: 133, 1985.
140. Ostro, M.J., Greenberg, G.R. & Jeejeebhoy, K.N. *JPEN J Parenter Enteral Nutr* 9: 280, 1985.
141. Hawker, P.C., et al. *Gut* 24: 284, 1983.
142. Teahon, K., Bjarnason, I., Pearson, M. & Levi, A.J. *Gut* 31: 1133, 1990.
143. Calam, J., Crooks, P.E. & Walker, R.J. *JPEN* 4: 4, 1980.
144. Levine, J.B. & Lukawski-Trubish, D. *Gastroenterol Clin North Am* 24: 633, 1995.
145. Nightingale, J.M., Bartram, C.I. & Lennard-Jones, J.E. *Gastrointest Radiol* 16: 305, 1991.
146. Fielding, J.F., Cooke, W.T. & Williams, J.A. *Lancet* 1: 1106, 1971.
147. Murphy Jr., J.P., King, D.R. & Dubois, A. *N Engl J Med* 300: 80, 1979.
148. Cortot, A., Fleming, C.R. & Malagelada, J.R. *N Engl J Med* 300: 79, 1979.
149. Jeppesen, P.B., Staun, M., Tjellesen, L. & Mortensen, P.B. *Gut* 43: 763, 1998.
150. Farthing, M.J. *Digestion* 54 (Suppl 1): 47, 1993.
151. Vanderhoof, J.A. & Kollman, K.A. *J Pediatr Gastroenterol Nutr* 26: 241, 1998.
152. Jeppesen, P.B. *Gastroenterology* 130: S127, 2006.
153. Woolf, G.M., Miller, C., Kurian, R. & Jeejeebhoy, K.N. *Dig Dis Sci* 32: 8, 1987.
154. Levitt, M.D. *Gastroenterology* 85: 769, 1983.
155. Bond, J.H., Currier, B.E., Buchwald, H. & Levitt, M.D. *Gastroenterology* 78: 444, 1980.
156. Nordgaard, I., Hansen, B.S. & Mortensen, P.B. *Lancet* 343: 373, 1994.
157. Mobarhan, S. *Nutr Rev* 52: 354, 1994.
158. McIntyre, P.B., Fitchew, M. & Lennard-Jones, J.E. *Gastroenterology* 91: 25, 1986.
159. Messing, B. et al. *Gastroenterology* 100: 1502, 1991.
160. Bochenek, W., Rodgers Jr., J.B. & Balint, J.A. *Ann Intern Med* 72: 205, 1970.
161. Vanderhoof, J.A., *JPEN J Parenter Enteral Nutr* 8: 685, 1984.
162. Jeppesen, P.B. & Mortensen, P.B. *Gut* 43: 478, 1998.
163. Gruy-Kapral, C. et al. *Gastroenterology* 116: 15, 1999.
164. Selby, P.L., Peacock, M. & Bambach, C.P. *Br J Surg* 71: 334, 1984.
165. Fleming, C.R., George, L., Stoner, G.L., Tarrosa, V.B. & Moyer, T.P. *Mayo Clin Proc* 71: 21, 1996.
166. Nightingale, J.M., et al. *Gut* 33: 1493, 1992.
167. Doty, J.E., Pitt, H.A., Porter-Fink, V. & Denbesten, L. *Ann Surg* 201: 76, 1985.
168. Thompson, J.S. *Arch Surg* 131: 556; discussion 559, 1996.
169. The colon, the rumen, and D-lactic acidosis. *Lancet* 336, 599, 1990.
170. Mayne, A.J., et al. *Arch Dis Child* 65: 229, 1990.
171. Pizarro, D., Posada, G., Sandi, L. & Moran, J.R. *N Engl J Med* 324: 517, 1991.
172. Krishnan, S., Ramakrishna, B.S. & Binder, H.J. *Dig Dis Sci* 44: 1924, 1999.
173. Ramakrishna, B.S. et al. *N Engl J Med* 342: 308, 2000.
174. Mathews, C.J. et al. *Gastroenterology* 116: 1342, 1999.
175. Pochapin, M. *Am J Gastroenterol* 95: S11, 2000.
176. Drossman, D.A. *Gastroenterology* 130: 1377, 2006.
177. Gee, M.I., et al. *J Am Diet Assoc* 85: 1591, 1985.
178. Payler, D.K., Pomare, E.W., Heaton, K.W. & Harvey, R.F. *Gut* 16: 209, 1975.
179. Manning, A.P., Heaton, K.W. & Harvey, R.F. *Lancet* 2: 417, 1977.
180. Soltoft, J., et al. *Lancet* 1: 270, 1976.
181. Hillman, L.C., Stace, N.H., Fisher, A. & Pomare, E.W. *Am J Clin Nutr* 36: 626, 1982.
182. Snook, J. & Shepherd, H.A. *Aliment Pharmacol Ther* 8: 511, 1994.
183. Lucey, M.R., Clark, M.L., Lowndes, J. & Dawson, A.M. *Gut* 28: 221, 1987.
184. Arffmann, S. et al. *Scand J Gastroenterol* 20: 295, 1985.
185. Francis, C.Y. & Whorwell, P.J. *Lancet* 344: 39, 1994.
186. Cann, P.A., Read, N.W. & Holdsworth, C.D. *Gut* 25: 168, 1984.
187. Kruis, W., Weinzierl, M., Schussler, P. & Holl, J. *Digestion* 34: 196, 1986.
188. Hotz, J. & Plein, K. *Med Klin (Munich)* 89: 645, 1994.
189. Ritchie, J.A. & Truelove, S.C. *Br Med J* 1: 376, 1979.
190. Lambert, J.P. et al. *Eur J Clin Nutr* 45: 601, 1991.
191. Hillman, L.C., Stace, N.H. & Pomare, E.W. *Am J Gastroenterol* 79: 1, 1984.
192. Monsbakken, K.W., Vandvik, P.O. & Farup, P.G. *Eur J Clin Nutr* 60: 667, 2006.
193. Niec, A.M., Frankum, B. & Talley, N.J. *Am J Gastroenterol* 93: 2184, 1998.
194. Locke III, G.R., et al. *Am J Gastroenterol* 95: 157, 2000.
195. Dainese, R., et al. *Am J Gastroenterol* 94: 1892, 1999.

196. Bentley, S.J., Pearson, D.J. & Rix, K.J. *Lancet* 2: 295, 1983.
197. Petitpierre, M., Gumowski, P. & Girard, J.P. *Ann Allergy* 54: 538, 1985.
198. Zar, S., Benson, M.J. & Kumar, D. *Am J Gastroenterol* 100: 1550, 2005.
199. Zar, S., Mincher, L., Benson, M.J. & Kumar, D. *Scand J Gastroenterol* 40: 800, 2005.
200. Atkinson, W., Sheldon, T.A., Shaath, N. & Whorwell, P.J. *Gut* 53: 1459, 2004.
201. Stefanini, G.F. et al. *Scand J Gastroenterol* 30: 535, 1995.
202. Stefanini, G.F. et al. *Am J Gastroenterol* 87: 55, 1992.
203. Bischoff, S.C. et al. *Gut* 40: 745, 1997.
204. Jain, N.K., et al. *Am J Gastroenterol* 80: 678, 1985.
205. Fernandez-Banares, F. et al. *Am J Gastroenterol* 88: 2044, 1993.
206. Rumessen, J.J. & Gudmand-Hoyer, E. *Gastroenterology* 95: 694, 1988.
207. Symons, P., Jones, M.P. & Kellow, J.E. *Scand J Gastroenterol* 27: 940, 1992.
208. Nelis, G.F., Vermeeren, M.A. & Jansen, W. *Gastroenterology* 99: 1016, 1990.
209. Tolliver, B.A. et al. *J Clin Gastroenterol* 23: 15, 1996.
210. Lisker, R., Solomons, N.W., Perez Briceno, R. & Ramirez Mata, M. *Am J Gastroenterol* 84: 756, 1989.
211. Lasser, R.B., Bond, J.H. & Levitt, M.D. *N Engl J Med* 293: 524, 1975.
212. Jain, N.K., Patel, V.P. & Pitchumoni, S. *Ann Intern Med* 105: 61, 1986.
213. Suarez, F., Levitt, M.D., Adshead, J. & Barkin, J.S. *Dig Dis Sci* 44: 1317, 1999.
214. Jain, N.K., Patel, V.P. & Pitchumoni, C.S. *Am J Gastroenterol* 81: 532, 1986.
215. Friedman, G. *Gastroenterol Clin North Am* 20: 313, 1991.
216. King, T.S., Elia, M. & Hunter, J.O. *Lancet* 352: 1187, 1998.
217. Pimentel, M., Kong, Y. & Park, S. *Am J Gastroenterol* 98: 2700, 2003.
218. Pimentel, M. et al. *Dig Dis Sci* 48: 86, 2003.
219. Pimentel, M. et al. *Am J Physiol Gastrointest Liver Physiol* 290: G1089, 2006.
220. Sharara, A.I. et al. *Am J Gastroenterol* 101: 326, 2006.
221. Camilleri, M. *J Clin Gastroenterol* 40: 264, 2006.
222. Kim, H.J. et al. *Neurogastroenterol Motil* 17: 687, 2005.
223. Niv, E., Naftali, T., Hallak, R. & Vaisman, N. *Clin Nutr* 24: 925, 2005.
224. Sen, S. et al. *Dig Dis Sci* 47: 2615, 2002.
225. Painter, N.S. & Burkitt, D.P. *Br Med J* 2: 450, 1971.
226. Painter, N.S. & Burkitt, D.P. *Br Med J* 4: 3, 1975.
227. Parks, T.G. *Clin Gastroenterol* 4: 53, 1975.
228. Srivastava, G.S., Smith, A.N. & Painter, N.S. *Br Med J* 1: 315, 1976.
229. Ohi, G. et al. *Am J Clin Nutr* 38: 115, 1983.
230. Berry, C.S., et al. *Lancet* 2: 294,1984.
231. Gear, J.S. et al. *Lancet* 1: 511, 1979.
232. Burkitt, D.P., Walker, A.R. & Painter, N.S. *JAMA* 229: 1068, 1974.
233. Cummings, J.H. et al. *Am J Clin Nutr* 32: 2086, 1979.
234. Aldoori, W.H. et al. *J Nutr* 128: 714, 1998.
235. Brodribb, A.J. *Lancet* 1: 664, 1977.
236. Ornstein, M.H. et al. *Br Med J (Clin Res Ed)* 282: 1353, 1981.
237. Roberts, P. et al. *Dis Colon Rectum* 38: 125, 1995.

62 Nutrient Metabolism and Support in Normal and Diseased Livers

Mark T. DeMeo

CONTENTS

INTRODUCTION

The liver plays a dual role in nutritional well-being. First, it contributes to nutrient assimilation through the synthesis of bile acids. At the time of a meal, as the gallbladder contracts, bile acids are released into the gut lumen. These bile acids enable lipids to be absorbed efficiently. Second, the liver plays a major role in substrate metabolism and allocation. It maintains nutrient blood levels at a constant level despite variations in substrate availability. It is, therefore, not surprising that damage to this vital organ has a tremendous impact on nutritional status.

ROLE OF THE LIVER IN NORMAL NUTRIENT METABOLISM

CARBOHYDRATES

Certain cells such as neutrophils, erythrocytes, and platelets are obligate utilizers of glucose. Therefore, during periods when glucose is not ingested, such as an overnight fast, glucose requirements continue. It is estimated that carbohydrate metabolism accounts for 45% of the resting energy expenditure (REE) in overnight-fasted humans.[1] In the postabsorptive phase, the liver releases glucose into the circulation to accommodate ongoing consumption of this substrate by various cells. The two main mechanisms the liver utilizes to maintain appropriate blood glucose levels are glycogenolysis and gluconeogenesis (see Chapter 7, Nutritional Biochemistry). In the early postabsorptive state, when there is a relative abundance of glycogen, studies estimate that this storage form of glucose makes up 25 to 80% of glucose released into the circulation, with the remainder of endogenous glucose coming from gluconeogenesis.[2-4] As the fast continues and endogenous glycogen stores are depleted, there is increased reliance on gluconeogenesis to maintain blood glucose levels. Though estimates vary on the contribution of this process, depending on the technique used to measure the contributions, it is estimated that gluconeogenesis accounts for about 35 to 50% of glucose released from the liver in the postabsorptive period, with increasing reliance on this process (up to 96% at 72 h) as the fast continues.[2] The liver is the main contributor to the maintenance of blood glucose. However, in prolonged fasting, renal gluconeogenesis is a significant source of endogenous glucose production.[2]

Gluconeogenesis is the formation of glucose from precursors such as lactate, pyruvate, glycerol, and the gluconeogenic amino acids (AAs), mainly alanine, glutamine, and glycine. Gluconeogenesis is regulated by hormones and substrate levels. High levels of insulin, characteristic of the "fed state," inhibits gluconeogenesis, mainly through the inhibition of key gluconeogenic enzymes. The two main enzymes are phosphoenolpyruvate carboxykinase (PEPCK), which catalyzes the conversion of pyruvate to phosphoenolpyruvate, and glucose-6-phosphatase, which converts glucose-6-phosphate to glucose. A third key enzyme, fructose-1,

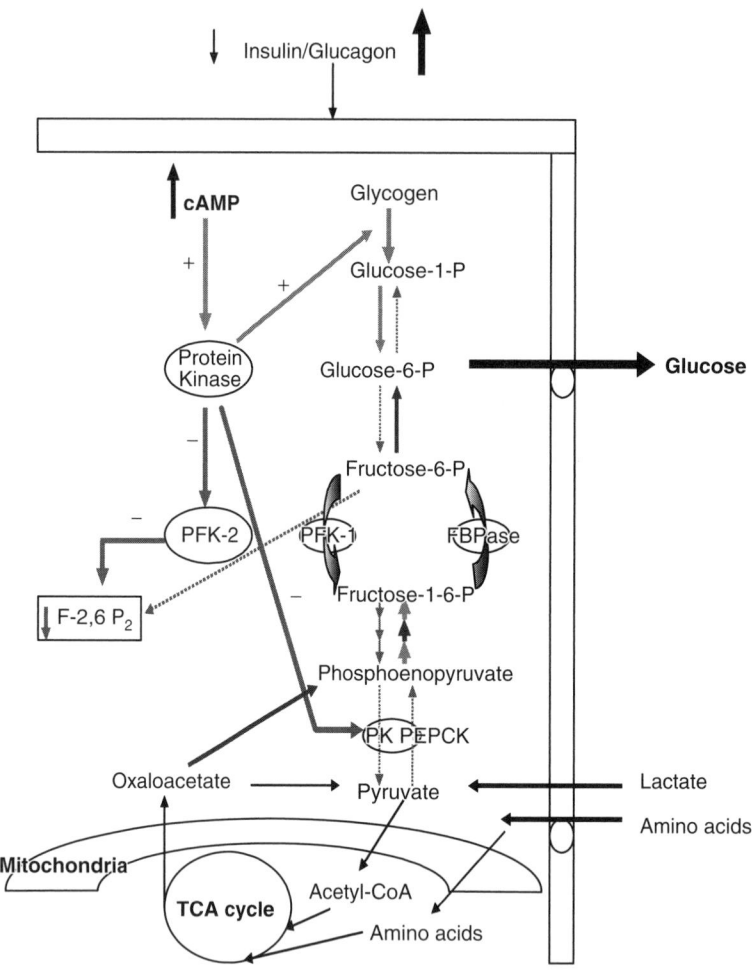

FIGURE 62.1 During fast, the insulin/glucagon ratio decreases. This stimulates an increase in cAMP in the hepatocyte. cAMP activates cAMP-dependent protein kinase, which activates glycogen phosphorylase. This enzyme leads to the breakdown of glycogen and the formation of glucose-1-phosphate. Protein kinase also inactivates phosphofructokinase-2 (PFK-2). PFK-2 catalyzes the conversion of Fructose-6-Phosphate to fructose-2,6-bisphosphate (F-2,6 P_2). F-2,6 P_2 is an important activator of Phosphofructokinase-1 (PFK-1). The impaired activation of PFK-1 slows glycolysis and favors the conversion of Fructose-1-6-P to Fructose-6-P and ultimately favors the formation of glucose. Protein kinase also interferes with the conversion of Phosphoenopyruvate (PEP) to Pyruvate, by blocking the enzyme pyruvate kinase (PK). This favors the formation of Fructose-1-6-P and ultimately glucose. Glucagon also stimulates gluconeogenesis, in part through carrier-mediated uptake of alanine, the major gluconeogenic AA. This, and other gluconeogenic AAs, enter the citric acid (TCA) cycle with the resultant formation of Oxaloacetate (OAA). OAA is converted to PEP and proceeds toward the formation of Glucose-6-P and ultimately glucose. (With permissions from (1) Kruszynska, McIntyre, *Oxford Textbook of Clinical Hepatology*, 2nd edition, Bircher, Benhamou, McIntyre, Rizzetto, Rodes, eds. Oxford University Press, Oxford, 303, 1999. (2) Brodsky, *Modern Nutrition in Health and Disease*, 9th edition, Shils, Olson, Shike, Ross, eds. Williams and Wilkins, Baltimore, MD, 699, 199.)

6-biphosphatase is also regulated through competitive inhibition by fructose 2, 6-biphosphate (Figure 62.1).[5] Conversely, a drop in insulin levels and a rise in glucagon secretion, characteristic of the fasted state augments gluconeogenesis. The drop in insulin decreases the activity of pyruvate kinase (Figure 62.1). This "blockage" drives the equation back to Glucose 6-phosphate and ultimately contributes to an increases in the hepatic output of glucose.

In the fed state, metabolic and hormonal signals change the liver's response to carbohydrates. It is estimated that between 25 and 45% of an oral glucose load is taken up by the liver. This percentage may increase as the carbohydrate load increases.[1] Glucose taken up by the liver is largely used to replenish the glycogen depleted after an overnight fast. High postprandial glucose levels stimulate the pancreas to release insulin. This decreases hepatic glucose production and increases glucose metabolism and storage. Insulin facilitates the synthesis of glycogen by stimulating the enzyme glycogen synthase. However, liver glycogen concentration also influences synthesis. As the concentration of this storage form of glucose increases, its rate of formation slows. This phenomenon can occur in spite of high insulin levels and glucose concentrations, emphasizing the fact that glycogen is a limited form of energy storage. It should also be noted that glucose is a relatively poor substrate for glycogen synthesis. Only about 50% of "neoglycogens" come from ingested glucose, while the remainder is derived from gluconeogenic precursors. Thus, the amount of carbohydrates presented to the liver could exceed its ability to form glycogen. Insulin also stimulates glucose oxidation by increasing pyruvate dehydrogenase. This enzyme converts pyruvate to acetyl-CoA. When the acetyl-CoA generated by glycolysis is not needed for oxidative phosphorylation, it is converted to fatty acids and ultimately to triglycerides (Figure 62.2).[6]

LIPIDS AND LIPOPROTEINS

The liver is an important organ in cholesterol homeostasis as it is involved in its *de novo* synthesis, transport, and excretion into the bile. Additionally, approximately 50% of cholesterol degradation occurs through catabolism to bile acids in the hepatocyte.[7,8] These bile acids are then conjugated with either glycine or taurine, secreted in bile, and released in response to a meal. When bile acids are released in sufficient quantities, they will form micelles. Micelles have a hydrophilic or water-soluble surface and a lipophilic or lipid-soluble core. Most dietary fat is in the form of triglycerides, which are fatty acids esterified to a glycerol backbone. Triglycerides are a major source of both stored and available energy. As discussed in the previous chapter, as pancreatic lipase cleaves the fatty acids from the dietary triglycerides, these water-insoluble molecules are absorbed into the lipophilic core of the micelle. The micelle provides a "conduit" through the intestinal unstirred water layer to the lipid-soluble membranes of the intestinal enterocyte. The fatty acid diffuses into the lipid-soluble membrane of the enterocyte (Figure 62.3). Medium chain triglycerides can be absorbed directly into the portal vein and do not need this "micellar intermediate" for absorption. Greater than 95% of the bile acids are taken up by receptors in the terminal ileum and transported back to the liver via the portal vein. This process is known as the enterohepatic circulation. Less than 5% of bile acids are unabsorbed and are excreted into the feces. The enterohepatic circulation serves to limit the need for new synthesis of bile acids by the liver in order to maintain an adequate bile acid pool, necessary for effective lipid absorption.[7,9] Additionally, cell surface receptors within the "territory" of the enterohepatic circulation serve as sensors and regulators of both cholesterol degradation and bile acid synthesis.[7]

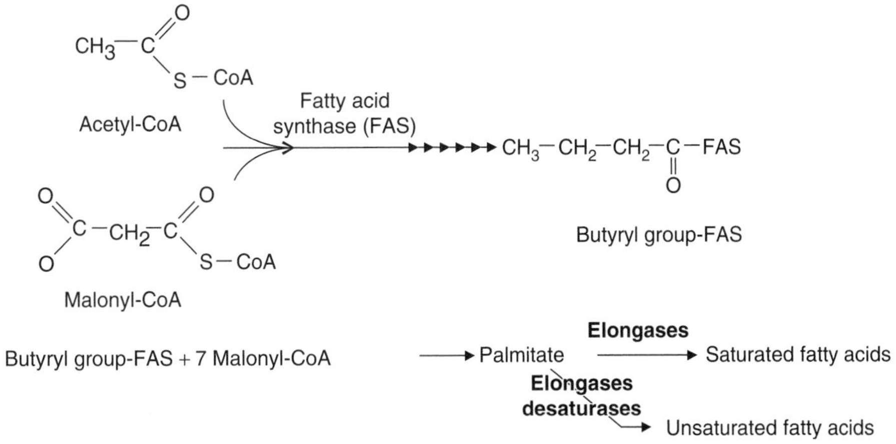

FIGURE 62.2 Fatty acid synthesis: Acetyl-CoA combines with malonyl-CoA in the presence of the fatty acid synthase complex. Then through a series of condensation, reduction, dehydration, and translocation steps, a four carbon, saturated fatty amyl compound is formed. Seven more cycles takes place to form plasmatic acid (C16: 0). Other fatty acids, both saturated and unsaturated can be formed using a series of elongates and desaturases.

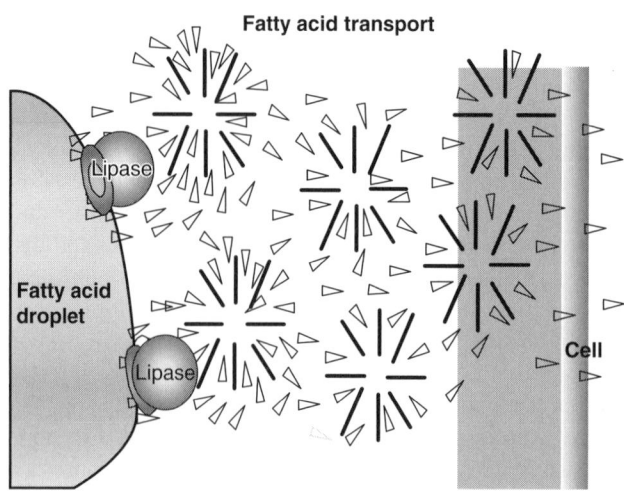

FIGURE 62.3 Colipase attaches to the lipid droplet and then binds lipase, the principal enzyme of triglyceride digestion. Lipase then hydrolyzes the ester bonds of the triglycerides forming free fatty acids. The fatty acids are taken up by the lipophilic inner core of the micelle. The outer core of the micelle is hydrophilic, allowing this particle to traverse the unstirred water layer of the intestine. The fatty acids in the inner core of the micelle are placed in approximation to the lipid-soluble membrane of the enterocyte allowing for diffusion across the enterocyte membrane. (With permission from Jones, Kubnow, *Modern Nutrition in Health and Disease*, 9th edition, Shils, Olson, Shike, Ross, eds. Williams and Wilkins, Baltimore, MD, 67, 1999.)

In the enterocyte, absorbed fatty acids are re-esterified into triglycerides. The triglycerides along with dietary cholesterol, phospholipids, and an apoprotein, synthesized in the enterocyte, are packaged into lipoproteins called *chylomicrons*. Chylomicrons are secreted into the lymphatics, travel through the thoracic duct to the superior vena cava and are then circulated to target tissues. Through the action of lipoprotein lipase (LPL), which hydrolysizes triglycerides back to free fatty acids, the chylomicron become a remnant lipoprotein essentially devoid of triglycerides. This chylomicron remnant is then taken up by the liver, where it releases the remaining triglycerides, cholesterol esters, phospholipids, and apoproteins.[10] Chylomicrons are part of the "exogenous transport system" for lipids.

The "endogenous system" is comprised of three main carriers, very-low-density lipoproteins (VLDLs), low-density lipoproteins (LDLs), and high-density lipoproteins (HDLs).[9,11] The liver can also manufacture triglycerides from fatty acids synthesized by repetitive additions of two carbon fragments, derived from acetyl-CoA, to malonyl-CoA, or from nonesterified fatty acids removed from the blood.[6] Triglycerides synthesized by the liver are reassembled with the chylomicron-derived products, as well as endogenous cholesterol esters and other apoproteins and transported by the lipoprotein VLDL to peripheral target tissues. Progressive hydrolysis and consequent "unloading" of the triglyceride portion of the VLDLs results in the formation of an intermediate density lipoprotein (IDL) and ultimately to a cholesterol rich particle known as an LDL. The liver possesses receptors for the uptake of LDL. Though cholesterol is essential to every cell for the synthesis and maintenance of cell membranes there exists no peripheral mechanism for the "metabolic disposal" of cholesterol. Hence, cholesterol excess needs to be removed from peripheral tissues by "reverse transport" accomplished by the lipoprotein HDL.[10] HDL is synthesized in the liver and intestinal mucosal cells and serves to bring cholesterol back to the liver for excretion in the bile or metabolism to bile acids.

AMINO ACIDS AND PROTEINS

The liver also plays a major role in AA homeostasis. AAs serve as building blocks of proteins and as precursors to many other important biomolecules, such as purines and pyrimidines. Additionally they can be a source of energy, particularly when they are present in excess of need for visceral or somatic protein synthesis. AAs are either essential or nonessential. The distinguishing feature between these two types of AAs is the ability of the body to synthesize their carbon skeleton. Essential AAs have a carbon skeleton that cannot be synthesized *de novo* and must be obtained from the diet.

The first step in the catabolic process of most AAs is the removal of the α-amino group from the carbon skeleton. This occurs via a pathway known as transamination. In the liver, most of α-amino groups derived from ingested protein, muscle protein, or protein from other tissues are separated from the parent carbon skeleton, leaving a keto acid and an amino group. This amino group is combined with α-ketoglutarate to form Glutamate. Glutamate then undergoes oxidative deamination in the mitochondria, yielding the protonated form of ammonia (NH_4^+). The NH_4^+ is a cosubstrate in forming carbamoyl phosphatase. It then enters the Urea cycle. As ammonia is toxic to animals, the urea cycle enzymes, also located largely in the liver, allow excretion of this harmful metabolite (Figure 62.4). Transamination can also occur between other AAs. The presence of transaminase

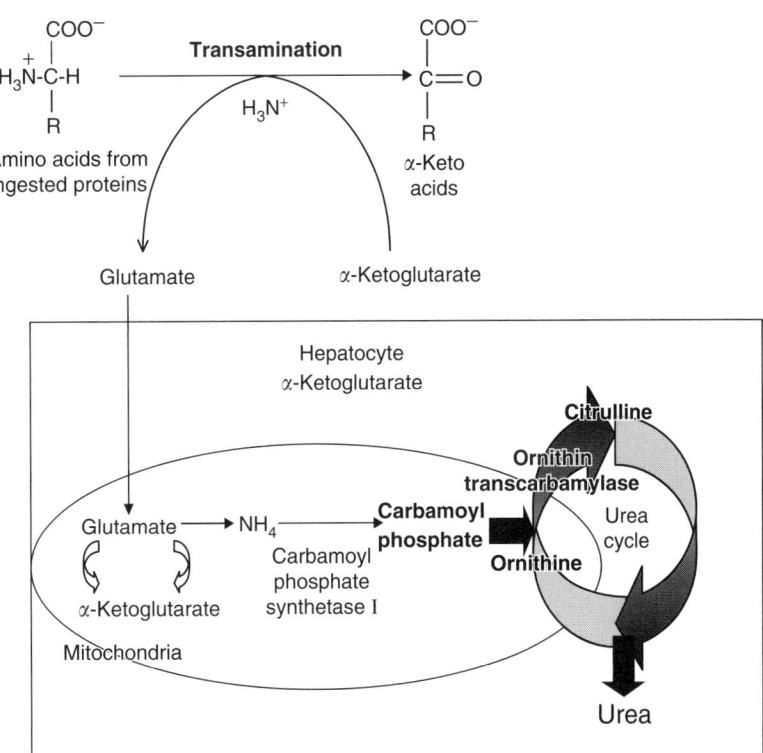

FIGURE 62.4 AAs from ingested proteins are transaminated to yield NH_3 and α-keto acids. The amino group is then transferred to α-ketoglutarate to form glutamate. Glutamate is transported to the hepatocyte mitochondria where α-ketoglutarate is reformed with the loss of NH_4. This ammonium group combines with HCO_3 and 2 ATPs to form carbamoyl phosphate. Carbamoyl phosphate enters the urea cycle is converted to urea after a series of reactions. (With permission from Nelson, Cox, *Principals of Biochemistry*, 2nd edition, Lehninger, Nelson, Cox, eds. Worth Publisher, New York, 506, 1993.)

enzymes in the liver ensures that the liver is able to conserve essential AAs and interconvert nonessential AAs. Although most AA catabolism occurs in the liver, the three AAs with branched side chains (leucine, valine, and isoleucine) are particularly noteworthy. They are oxidized as fuels to be used primarily by extrahepatic tissue, particularly muscle, adipose, kidney, and brain. These extrahepatic tissues contain a single aminotransferase not present in the liver. This acts on all three branched chain amino acids (BCAAs) to produce the corresponding α-keto acid.

AA carbohydrate skeletons can metabolize to pyruvate or intermediates of the tricarboxylic acid cycle. These can be converted into glucose and are called *glucogenic AAs*. These precursors contribute to a process known as gluconeogenesis. In humans, gluconeogenesis occurs largely in the liver and to a much smaller extent, in the renal cortex. Since some tissues in the body are obligate glucose utilizers, this pathway is extremely important during periods of relative glucose deficiency. It maintains hepatic glucose output to glucose-utilizing tissues.[12,13]

The liver absorbs AAs from plasma to be utilized in protein synthesis. The most abundant plasma protein secreted by the liver is albumin. Albumin is the most important regulator of plasma oncotic pressure and is the principal transport protein for many endogenous and exogenous substances. The liver also produces transport proteins for lipids (lipoproteins), iron (transferrin) and copper (ceruloplasmin) as well as steroid hormone-binding proteins, thyroid hormone-binding proteins, and several vitamin-binding proteins. An equally essential role for the liver is the synthesis of many of the coagulation and fibrinolysis proteins. The liver is also the primary site of synthesis of the complement system that plays an important role in host defense against infectious agents. Finally, it is the major site of synthesis of protease inhibitors, inhibitors of coagulation, and fibrinolysis, as well as many other proteins involved in immunomodulation, drug binding, and other aspects of the acute phase response.[14]

IMPACT OF LIVER DISEASE ON NUTRIENT METABOLISM

CARBOHYDRATES

Damage to the liver can negatively affect glycogen stores, in part due to insulin resistance seen commonly in these patients.[15] Since glycogenolysis is a significant source of glucose production in the fasted state, it might be expected that patients with liver disease would have low blood glucose levels after an overnight fast or a prolonged absence of oral intake. However, hypoglycemia is rare in liver disease, usually seen only in fulminant hepatic failure or in the terminal stages of chronic hepatic insufficiency. This is probably due to the tremendous reserve capacity of the liver to produce glucose through alternate mechanisms. It is estimated that only 20% of the hepatic mass is needed to maintain normal glucose levels in the fasted state.[1] When hypoglycemia does occur in end stage liver disease, it is likely be due to the impaired capacity of the failing liver to increase gluconeogenesis even following infusion of gluconeogenic substrate.[16]

More commonly, fasting glucose levels in patients with liver disease are normal or high. Despite high levels of glucagon seen in these patients, increased hepatic glucose production does not seem to be a contributing factor. Unless there is coexistent diabetes, studies suggest that hepatic glucose production in liver disease varies from normal to 20 to 40% lower than normal. However, diabetic cirrhotics with fasting hyperglycemia displayed increased hepatic glucose production, which was not appropriately decreased with insulin.[17]

Since glycogen synthesis is impaired in liver disease and glycogen stores are rapidly depleted in the fasted state, patients with liver disease more rapidly transition to gluconeogenesis and ketogenesis to fill their glucose and energy needs. The rapid switch to a fatty acid/ketone economy for energy needs is an adaptive response as it decreases reliance on hepatic glucose production.[1]

After glucose ingestion, many patients with liver disease have abnormally elevated blood glucose concentrations.[1] In a recent study, nondiabetic cirrhotics given a mixed meal had elevated blood glucose levels in spite of a fivefold increase in blood insulin levels.[18] It appears that in these glucose intolerant patients, both oxidative and nonoxidative glucose disposal is impaired.[1,17] The oxidative impairment of glucose utilization, the less significant of the two abnormalities, is due, in part, to the preferential utilization of fatty acids seen in this patient population. The generation of acetyl-CoA from the metabolism of fatty acids inhibits pyruvate dehydrogenase resulting in a diminution of pyruvate oxidation.[17] The nonoxidative utilization of glucose is essentially the formation of glycogen. In spite of hyperinsulinemia seen in these patients, they demonstrate peripheral insulin resistance. As such, glucose uptake by muscle and stimulation of glycogen synthesis is significantly impaired. This accounts for most of the decreased glucose disposal and consequent glucose intolerance seen in these patients as hepatic glucose production is still normal in the basal state and normally suppressed by insulin.[1,17] In contrast, liver disease patients with diabetes not only have abnormalities with glucose disposal but also are unable to appropriately suppress hepatic glucose suppression suggesting a relative lack of insulin. Petrides hypothesized that patients with liver disease become frankly diabetic when the pancreatic β-cells cannot meet the increased demand for insulin secretion due to insulin resistance.[17]

LIPIDS AND LIPOPROTEINS

Since cholesterol is excreted from the body through the biliary tree, the total cholesterol level tends to rise in obstructive jaundice. However, in severe parenchymal disease, cholesterol ester levels tend to fall. This latter sign is the result of reduced activity of lecithin cholesterol acyltransferase (LCAT) activity. LCAT is an enzyme synthesized in the liver that catalyses the transfer of a fatty acid from the 2-position of lecithin to the 3 β-OH group to form cholesterol ester and lysolecithin. It plays a key role in the turnover of cholesterol and lecithin. Low levels of this enzyme also alter the lipid composition of lipoproteins.

Plasma triglycerides are often elevated, both in obstructive, and less often, in parenchymal liver disease. Triglycerides are normally cleared by the action of peripheral (LPLs) and hepatic triglyceride lipases (HTLP). The latter enzyme levels are reduced in liver disease and may account for triglyceride abnormality.[11]

These changes in lipids may affect membrane lipid content, fluidity, and function. They may, in part, explain the abnormalities associated with liver disease in platelet aggregation and in the morphology of red blood cells.[11] These changes in the lipid content of cell membranes affect all cells in the body. The subsequent effects on membrane fluidity and function have been advanced as a possible contributing factor in the hyporesponsiveness of cirrhotic myocardium to pharmacological or psychological stress.[19]

After an overnight fast, cirrhotic patients derive a greater proportion of energy from fat oxidation than do controls. This difference in endogenous energy substrate use has been attributed to diminished glycogen stores. After ingestion of a mixed meal, fat oxidation of cirrhotic patients decreases but still remains elevated compared to controls. The increased reliance on endogenous fat during fasting and the continued high rate of fat oxidation in spite of ingestion of a mixed meal may account for the reduction in body fat stores common in this patient population.[18]

In advanced cirrhosis, deficiency of polyunsaturated fatty acids (PUFA) is well described. This deficiency is in part due to poor dietary intake but also due to deficiencies in the desaturase enzymes used in the synthesis of these fatty acids. Though incompletely studied, deficiencies of PUFAs in patients with liver disease can lead to abnormalities in vasoactive and immunomodulatory prostaglandins and leukotrienes. Deficiencies in these fatty acids have been implicated in renal dysfunction from unbalanced renal vasoconstriction, platelet aggregation defects, increased susceptibility to infections, and alterations in cell membrane fluidity leading to impaired biological function. However, PUFA supplementation in this patient population is not without risk as overzealous replacement has been implicated in immune dysfunction. Additionally some researchers feel that low levels of PUFA may be an adaptive mechanism against increase lipid peroxidation commonly seen in patients with liver disease.[20]

AMINO ACIDS AND PROTEINS

Patients with liver disease often have disturbances in plasma AA concentrations, characterized by increased levels of aromatic AAs and methionine. This is most likely a result of the injured liver's poor utilization of these AAs as well as portosystemic shunting.[12] Additionally, since the enzymes involved in urea production are largely localized in the liver, urea synthesis, and hence α-amino nitrogen clearance, is lower in cirrhotics compared to controls. In patients with severe decompensated liver disease, the plasma urea level tends to drop and the amount of urea excreted in the urine is reduced. In patients with well-compensated cirrhosis, urea production rates remains stable under basal conditions, but maximal urea production capacity is significantly reduced in response to a protein or AA load.[12,21]

Chronic alcohol consumption actually increases the synthesis of albumin and constituent hepatic proteins but is also associated with a reduced secretion of these proteins from the liver.[14] However, as liver damage increases there is a decrease in synthesis of albumin with an apparent significant correlation between its synthesis rate and Childs score (a scoring system based on clinical and laboratory values that is used to demonstrate the severity of the underlying liver disease).[14] Although the albumin is used in many different prognostic scoring systems, it should be remembered that the plasma concentration of albumin is not only dependent on synthesis but also is reliant on the rate of degradation. Additionally, newly synthesized albumin is secreted into the lymph and ascitic fluid, when present. This results in an increased volume of distribution and contributes to the observed hypoalbuminemia.

The liver is also important in maintaining homeostasis. All clotting proteins, coagulation factors, and inhibitors, and most of the components of the fibrinolytic system are synthesized by hepatocytes except for von Willebrand factor, which is produced by endothelial cells, and megakaryocytes. Liver damage can lead to decreased levels of the clotting factors produced in the liver. It is unusual for fibrinogen to be reduced significantly unless there is concomitant disseminated intravascular coagulation. Overall, liver impairment favors bleeding due to impaired synthesis of coagulation factors and increased fibrinolytic activity. However, it also increases susceptibility to intravascular coagulation resulting from impaired clearance of procoagulant material.[22]

NUTRITIONAL EVALUATION IN LIVER DISEASE

ENERGY EXPENDITURE IN LIVER DISEASE

There is significant controversy about the ability to accurately predict metabolic rates in cirrhotic patients. This is partly because "hypermetabolism" occurs only when a measured value (indirect or direct calorimetry) is compared to a predicted value. Thus, depending on the methods of standardization and comparison (i.e., formula equations vs. estimates of lean body tissue), the baseline for comparison differs. Common formula equations that use age, weight, and height are standardized for normally proportioned individuals. They do not make allowances for differences in body compartments that may occur in liver disease. For example, if there is depletion of body fat, a common occurrence in cirrhotics, there is a relative overrepresentation of metabolically active tissue per unit mass. If this were the case, formula equations may predict a lower energy expenditure relative to a measured value. One method to address this potential discrepancy is to correct for lean body mass by using creatinine secretion. Since the secretion of creatinine roughly correlates with the presence of lean body tissue, standardization to this value should help account for discrepancies in somatic protein/fat composition. However, it should be kept in mind that creatine, the precursor of creatinine, is synthesized in the liver. Thus, significant liver disease can compromise the urinary recovery of creatinine and result in an underestimation of the amount of metabolically active tissue. This could subsequently result in an underestimation of lean body tissue and an overestimation of metabolic rate when a measured value is compared to a predicted value corrected for fat-free mass.[23]

Alternatively, fluid retention tends to increase weight or body surface area; formulas that standardize energy expenditure on these values overestimate the predicted metabolic rate compared to a measured value.[24] More recently, researchers have attempted to measure fat-free mass, since this is a more accurate indicator of metabolically active tissue. They use this variable in predictive formulas for REE. However, even with these more complicated formulas, only 50 to 60% of the observed variation between measured and predicted values can be taken into account.

Most studies have failed to show significant differences in energy expenditure between cirrhotics and control patients.[23,25,26] However, others, such as a study by Madden, have demonstrated that the mean measured REE in patients with cirrhosis is significantly higher than in controls when adjusted for body weight. Overall, using multiple predictive formulae, 12% of the patients were considered hypometabolic while 30% were determined to be hypermetabolic.[27] A recent comprehensive study by Müller found a similar proportion of hypermetabolic patients (33.8%). Unfortunately, neither author could identify the "hypermetabolic" patients on the basis of demographic or clinical variables.[27,28] A possible exception to this is Primary Biliary Cirrhosis patients in which worsening disease was associated with increased REE and prolonged diet-induced thermogenesis after a meal.[29]

Müller also demonstrated that increased levels of catecholamines in hypermetabolic patients could be a contributing factor in increased metabolic rate. He further determined that, for these patients, a propranolol infusion resulted in a pronounced decrease in energy expenditure.[28]

Clinically, determining hypermetabolism is important for these patients as they are more likely to present malnourished. In addition, these patients' nutritional repletion may be further complicated by difficulty in nutrient assimilation. Both factors may negatively affect outcome. A study assessing preoperative risk factors in patients undergoing liver transplantation associated hypermetabolism and diminished body cell mass (<35% of body weight) with reduced survival after liver transplantation.[30] Given the clinical implications of determining an accurate metabolic rate in cirrhotic patients and the fact that this rate cannot be accurately determined from formulas and clinical variables, many authors are advocating that the metabolic rate should be measured in cirrhotics.[27,28]

Leptin, an adipocyte-derived hormone is associated with regulation of body fat. In normal individuals, leptin levels are proportional to adipocyte mass. Reduction in adipocytes leads to a concomitant decrease in serum leptin levels. The decrease in the level of this hormone leads to increased hunger and decreased energy expenditure. These changes should allow for return of normal fat stores. Recently, patients with alcoholic cirrhosis were found to have elevated leptin levels after adjustments for fat-free mass. The authors suggested that this hormone may play a role in the malnutrition seen in cirrhosis.[31] Because of this possible link, a study was performed to evaluate the correlation between leptin levels, energy expenditure, and energy intake. Although the authors did find a correlation between leptin levels and REE in female patients, there was no impact on energy intake in this population. Additionally, REE was not an independent predictor of leptin levels when other factors were taken into consideration. Overall, the authors did not feel that leptin affected significantly on the nutritional status of these patients.[32]

PREVALENCE OF MALNUTRITION IN LIVER DISEASE

Protein calorie malnutrition (PCM) is common in advanced liver disease. A summary of five studies using a total of 550 subjects demonstrated a range of PCM from 10 to 100%, depending in part on the criteria used to determine PCM.[33] In the Veterans Administration Cooperative study on alcoholic hepatitis, malnutrition was a ubiquitous finding and correlated with dietary intake and severity of liver dysfunction.[34,35] In hospitalized patients with less severe alcoholic and nonalcoholic liver disease, the prevalence of PCM ranged between 30 and 40%. It should be noted that much of the data on malnutrition is derived from the alcoholic liver disease population. However, a recent study by Sarin[35] demonstrated that malnutrition in patients with alcoholic and nonalcoholic cirrhosis is both very common and present to the same degree. The patterns of malnutrition appear to be different, depending on the underlying liver disease. Patients with nonalcoholic cirrhosis demonstrated decreases in both fat and muscle mass while those with alcoholic liver disease demonstrated a greater decrease in muscle mass but relative sparing of fat stores. The authors of the accompanying editorial hypothesize that this discrepancy may be due to the "precirrhotic nutritional status" of the patient or to toxic effects of alcohol on meal-stimulated protein secretion. They also speculated that alcohol might lead to changes in intestinal permeability, which could potentially lead to transmigration of intestinal bacteria or toxins with resultant release of proteolytic cytokines.[36] The authors also determined that the dietary intake of both groups was reduced to a similar degree.[35]

Ferreira-Figueiredo and colleagues, using dilution techniques and Dual Energy X-ray Absorptiometry (DEXA) scanning to derive a multicompartment model, evaluated the nutritional status and body composition of patients with varying degrees of cirrhosis. These researchers found an altered body composition profile with alterations related to the severity of the underlying liver disease. As expected, they found a more pronounced loss of body fat in the initial stages of disease followed by an accelerated loss of body cell mass in more advanced stages. Unexpectedly, however, they found significant losses in patients with only mild hepatic dysfunction and no overt clinical signs of malnutrition.[37]

NUTRITIONAL ASSESSMENT

The presence of liver disease may affect many of the traditional modalities used to evaluate the nutritional status of patients. Visceral protein stores can be greatly influenced by acute or extensive damage to the liver. Liver injury can result in decreases in visceral markers that may be unrelated to the nutritional status of the patient and may therefore not improve significantly with nutritional intervention. In fact, serum visceral proteins appear to correlate better with the degree of liver damage than with the nutritional status of the patient. Chronic liver disease can also cause alterations in cellular immunity and total lymphocyte count, independent of protein malnutrition.[33] Furthermore, abnormal immunologic reactivity, again independent of nutritional status, is a prominent feature of chronic autoimmune hepatitis, primary biliary cirrhosis, and possibly viral hepatitis.[38] From a clinical standpoint, a thorough nutritional evaluation should be performed and repeated serially. A bedside assessment of somatic protein stores and subcutaneous fat stores usually provides a reliable nutritional assessment.[39] Other important aspects of this Subjective Global Assessment Tool adapted for liver patients included the presence of encephalopathy, edema, weight change, renal insufficiency, constipation, satiety, and difficulty chewing. Anthropometric data, specifically the assessment of fat stores by tricep or subscapular skin fold thickness and the assessment of somatic stores by mid arm muscle circumference or body weight to height can yield valuable information. Assessments should be performed by a skilled person, as there can be problems with reproducibility. Additionally, apparent or subclinical edema can lead to a potential underestimation of the severity of protein and fat losses.[38] The creatinine height index is generally a good indicator of lean body mass in patients with liver disease. However, it too has shortcomings, as there is frequently associated renal dysfunction, which could impair urine creatinine collection. Furthermore, with severe liver disease, there can be a decrease in creatinine formation, as its substrate creatine is synthesized in the liver. Both of these circumstances could result in an underestimation of lean body tissue.

A recent study by Alvares-da-Dilva compared three methods of assessing malnutrition in cirrhotics and correlated nutritional status with clinical outcome. The three methods used were subjective global assessment (SGA), prognostic nutritional status (PNI), and handgrip strength (HG) measured with a dynamometer. The PNI is an equation that uses serum albumin, transferrin, delayed cutaneous hypersensitivity, and triceps skin folds to evaluate the patient's nutritional status. The authors felt that HG was a better marker of malnutrition than the other nutrition evaluation tools. When determined to be malnourished by that technique, HG was the only tool that predicted major complications in these patients during the 1-year follow-up period. Additionally, although not significantly different from SGA in predicting mortality in the malnourished cirrhotic population, 20.7% of patients determined to be malnourished by HG were dead by the end of the year compared to zero in the group that was not felt to be malnourished by the same technique.[40]

In summary, given the numerous limitations of standard nutritional parameters in patients with liver disorders, it is preferable to rely on collective information generated from the use of several parameters used simultaneously and on a serial basis.[38] Measurement of HG, a functional parameter, appears to be a promising evaluation tool but will need larger studies to validate its predictive value.

NUTRITIONAL INTERVENTION IN LIVER DISEASE

BACKGROUND DATA

It is well known that patients with chronic liver disease are usually malnourished and that frequently the degree of malnutrition parallels the severity of the liver disease. Reasons for malnutrition include altered metabolism, malabsorption/maldigestion, anorexia, iatrogenic restrictions, and poor dietary intake. Though there appears to be a correlation between the severity of malnutrition and subsequent morbidity and mortality from liver disease, it is intuitive, though clinically less clear, that nutritional intervention can have an impact on patient outcome. An article by Patek, published in 1948, was one of the earliest to evidence that nutritional intervention could affect the course of liver disease. In this study, 124 patients (89% of whom had "significant weight loss") were admitted to the hospital with "hepatic failure." These patients were given a diet of approximately 3500 kcal with 140 g of protein, supplemented with a vitamin B complex preparation. The supplemented group was compared to historic controls. Although the patients' ability to achieve dietary goals was not mentioned, 49% were described as "clinically improved." This improvement was characterized by: (1) a disappearance of ascites, jaundice, and edema, (2) weight gain and strength, and (3) improvement in liver function test results. Furthermore, there appeared to be significant differences in survival between the treated group and historical controls at 1 and 5 years.[41] This positive study provided the basis for subsequent studies assessing the impact of enteral, parenteral, and oral supplementation in patients with liver disease.

Many recent studies have focused on nutritional intervention in alcoholic liver disease. Acute alcoholic hepatitis is a potentially reversible condition, but is associated with high mortality. The majority of patients with alcoholic liver disease who require hospitalization for their disease are moderately to severely malnourished. Malnutrition can contribute to delayed wound healing, increased risk of infection, increased toxicity of alcohol to the liver, reduced protein synthesis, and impaired regenerative capacity of the injured liver.[42,43] Additionally, both human and animal data suggest that poor nutrition combined with alcohol is more injurious to the liver than alcohol alone.[6,43] These factors imply that nutritional intervention may be beneficial in this disease.[42,43] In an early and much cited trial by Galambos, 28 days of peripheral AA infusion resulted in significant improvement in albumin and bilirubin levels in the supplemented group compared to controls. The supplemented group also showed a trend toward improved survival.[44,45]

Mendenhall authored a series of landmark articles on alcoholic hepatitis. A nutritional investigation of patients with alcoholic hepatitis was part of a larger multicentered veteracnce administration (VA) cooperative study of the effects of steroid therapy in the treatment of this disease. In an early study, the patients were categorized into mild, moderate, and severe PCM based on eight parameters that included tests to assess somatic protein stores, visceral protein stores, and delayed cutaneous hypersensitivity. The investigators were able to demonstrate that 30-day and 6-month mortality rates correlated with nutritional category. Perhaps equally important was that patients who moved from one nutritional category to another assumed the mortality associated with their new category.[46] However, it should be noted that this early observation on nutrition and outcome was a secondary endpoint.

The same researchers subsequently designed a study to intercede with nutritional supplements while providing patients with anabolic steroids (oxandrolone). Oxandrolone was used in this population because the researchers believed it would increase anabolism and liver regeneration. In a group of patients defined as having moderate PCM yet adequate caloric intake (>2500 kcal), oxandrolone significantly decreased mortality compared to the placebo group. In addition, patients defined as having severe PCM yet adequate caloric intake had significantly lower 6-month mortality, regardless of the use of oxandrolone. Finally, caloric intake during the first month demonstrated a significant inverse correlation with mortality at 6 months. It should be noted, however, that as the severity of the liver disease increased, the caloric intake decreased.[47] Unfortunately, it is unclear from this study whether nutritional supplementation, even if the patient accepts and is compliant with this supplementation will improve the "nutritional category." It is possible that other changes in underlying liver disease also have to occur before nutritional repletion is realized. However, the authors mentioned that there was a "marginally significant correlation" between percent of basal energy expenditure consumed and the improvement in PCM during hospitalization. (see Chapter 39, Protein-Energy Malnutrition.)

These authors published another follow up article focused solely on the nutritional indices in this same cohort of patients. The authors were able to identify four nutritional parameters that seem to affect 6-month mortality. They included creatinine height index, total lymphocyte count, hemoglobin, and prealbumin levels. The authors suggested that surviving patients tend to improve in most of their measured nutritional parameters, but it is again unclear that either adequate protein or energy intake significantly influences these four variables. Nevertheless, the authors conclude that nutritional therapy improves both prognosis and overall nutritional status. They qualify this statement, however, by stating that the degree of improvement is dependent on the severity of the PCM.[48]

A recent study by Cabre assessed the effects of total enteral nutrition and prednisolone in the treatment of patients with alcoholic hepatitis. Patients were randomized to receive either TEN (2000 kcal/day and 72 g protein via a nasoenteral tube) or prednisolone. The latter group was encouraged to eat a standard hospital diet of approximately 2000 kcal and 1 g/kg of protein. Although no difference was seen in short term or 1-year survival, differences in the time to death and the cause of death were noted. Deaths occurred earlier in the TEN-group (median of 7 days). In the prednisolone-treated group, most of the deaths occurred in the immediate 6 weeks after the end of the treatment period and were largely due to infectious complications. The authors speculate that most of the early mortality may have been caused by inflammatory mediators (thus the early benefit of steroids). The latter mortality may have been caused by changes in the intestinal barrier (supporting the importance of enteral nutrition in maintaining the integrity of the gut barrier). The author suggests that there might be a synergistic effect realized in using both modes of therapy.[49]

The positive effects of nutritional supplementation are not, however, limited to patients with alcoholic hepatitis. In an earlier study, Cabre looked at enteral nutrition in hospitalized cirrhotic patients. The treatment group was given an enteral formula containing 2115 kcal/day with 71 g protein via nasoenteral tube. The control group was offered a standard low-sodium hospital diet supplying 2200 kcal and 70 to 80 g protein. The etiology of the cirrhosis was varied (though largely alcoholic), and there were no differences between the two groups in Child's scores. All patients in both groups had severe protein energy malnutrition. Although the incidence of major complications was similar in both groups, the Child score improved and mortality fell (47 vs. 12%) only in the TEN-group. The authors were unable to explain the discrepancy. They suggested that the gastrointestinal (GI) tract stimulation may have decreased the catabolic effect of the injury or resulted in decreased bacterial/endotoxin translocation.[50]

In summary, multiple studies using oral, enteral, and parenteral supplementation have demonstrated only modest improvements in liver function tests and nutritional parameters. A decrease in mortality in nutritionally supplemented patients has not been a consistent or overwhelming finding[45,51-54] though other important facts have emerged. These patients appear to tolerate protein supplementation, including those with hepatic encephalopathy. Fluid retention has not been a major problem.[45] It should also be noted that there is no published study demonstrating an adverse effect of nutritional supplementation. These studies point out that nutritional supplementation, though very important, is only one of several factors that likely determine the ultimate outcome in liver disease patients. As this is a factor that can be influenced, at least to some degree, and there does not seem to be untoward effects when used appropriately, attention to nutrition, with supplementation when indicated, should be considered a mainstay in the therapy for these patients.

The use of BCAA has been advocated in the treatment of liver disease. It has been suggested that 50 to 60% of patients with chronic liver failure will tolerate 60 to 80 g/day of a standard AA mixture as part of a parenteral nutrition regimen. The remainder, in particular those with grade III or IV hepatic encephalopathy seem to respond better to with modified solutions containing BCAA.[55] One rationale for their use in hepatic encephalopathy concerns the high aromatic AA-to-BCAA ratio in the blood of patients with decompensated liver disease. This is primarily due to poor metabolism of aromatic AAs by the failing/injured liver. Conversely, BCAA are deaminated mainly by skeletal muscle and so have an alternate pathway for their metabolism. Since both of these AAs compete for the same transmembrane transport system in order to cross the blood brain barrier, the increase in AA/BCAA in the blood favors the transport of aromatic AAs. In the central nervous system, these aromatic AAs can be metabolized to false neurotransmitters (octopamine and phenylethanolamine) and thus contribute to hepatic encephalopathy. Additionally, infusion of BCAAs has been shown to reduce blood ammonia levels.[56] The BCAAs have also been reported to augment protein synthesis in humans. Leucine, or more specifically, its deamination product, α-keto-isocaprioic acid is thought to have an important role in stimulating protein synthesis and inhibiting protein degradation.[56,57] Thus, it would seem that a BCAA mixture would be an ideal mode of therapy in patients with liver disease.

Several studies have looked at the use of BCAA in the treatment of hepatic encephalopathy. The largest study was by Cerra, who concluded that the BCAA enriched formula resulted in more rapid and complete recovery from encephalopathy as compared to the standard treatment of neomycin. The treatment group also showed improvements in nitrogen balance and survival. Interestingly, the control group was not given any protein, and their sole source of calories was a 25% dextrose solution. Both the

BCAA and the dextrose solution were started at 1.5 l and advanced to a maximum of 3 l over the ensuing days.[58] Unfortunately, the lack of protein in the control group challenges the validity of the nitrogen balance data and perhaps the mortality differences in these populations.

Overall, studies regarding the use of BCAA in encephalopathy have yielded mixed results.[57,59] A recent meta-analysis by Naylor suggests that BCAA solutions have a significant and beneficial effect on recovery from hepatic encephalopathy, though the authors state that analysis is difficult given the diversity of the studies involved. These same authors were unable to verify an advantage of BCAA solutions on mortality.[55] Another extensive analysis by Eriksson presented a much more skeptical view of the benefits of BCAA solutions in either acute or chronic encephalopathy. The authors proposed that problems with data analysis, biased assignment of patients to groups in regard to etiology of the encephalopathy, and study design disallowed any firm conclusion that BCAA or their keto analogues were beneficial.[60]

Marchesini and colleagues attempted to answer many of the criticisms of the use of BCAA in patients with cirrhosis, namely small sample size, short evaluation period, and lack of proper control groups. These authors engineered a large (174 patients) multicentered study of the use of BCAA in patients with advanced cirrhosis of varying etiologies that were controlled for severity of disease and nutritional parameters. The authors supplemented one group of patients with BCAA. The other groups were given either an equinitrogenous (lactoalbumin) or an equicaloric (maltodextran) supplement. Though the patients were on self-selected diets, an intake of 30 kcal/kg and 0.8 g/kg protein was targeted. Primary endpoints included death, transplantation, or deterioration of liver function (to exclusion criteria). The authors also monitored hospital admissions, days of hospitalization and nutritional parameters. Follow up ranged from 1 to 15½ months. Though there was a problem with patient withdrawal from the BCAA group (the authors speculated on the "unpalatability of the supplement"), there still appeared to be a significant benefit in several primary endpoints as well as nutritional and quality of life parameters.[61]

Thus, previous studies had suggested that the use of BCAA enriched supplements may lead to mild improvement in encephalopathy compared to standard therapy, though the benefits do not seem to justify routine use of this enriched formula. However, in this new, well-done study by Marchesini et al., there appears to be an advantage in the use of this supplement in advanced cirrhosis. Individuals with advanced cirrhosis are a complex group of patients with multiple factors contributing to their morbidity and mortality. However, the potential advantage of this supplementation could be instrumental, especially in patients awaiting liver transplantation. Further studies will be needed to improve delivery/compliance of this supplement and to corroborate these results before justification of broader utilization of BCAA supplementation in this patient population.

An additional potential use of BCAA supplementation in clinical practice may be the patient with chronic encephalopathy who is intolerant to increases in protein or standard AA solutions. Eriksson's analysis did concede that in the setting of chronic encephalopathy in which increases in standard protein supplements worsened or precipitated encephalopathy, BCAA mixtures were better tolerated. A study by Egberts of this population demonstrated significant improvements in psychomotor function, attention, and practical intelligence when stable patients were supplemented with a BCAA enriched mixture.[62] However, the clinical applicability of these improvements in psychomotor testing has been called into question.[60]

In vitro studies of isolated hepatocytes suggest that the keto acid analogues of BCAAs augment protein synthesis.[63] However, when the effects of these BCAA solutions were evaluated in cirrhotic patients no such augmentation was seen.[56,64] In an editorial accompanying this paper, Charlton speculated that because the BCAA-enriched infusate lacked sufficient aromatic AAs for protein synthesis, the expected protein synthetic response may have been dampened.[65] Alternately, he suggests that relative hyperglucagonemia may shunt AAs toward gluconeogenesis and thus render them unavailable for protein synthesis. He concluded that these abnormalities may account for the less-than-convincing "improved outcomes" with BCAA enriched formulas for patients with liver disease.

NUTRITIONAL RECOMMENDATIONS

In multiple-diverse populations, malnutrition can negatively affect infection, wound healing, and organ function. The great majority of patients who present for liver disease are malnourished and the severity of their malnutrition has prognostic implications. However, when studies on nutritional intervention in liver disease are considered, it is difficult to ascertain whether nutritional intervention can positively affect the course of the disease. This could be said of most disease states, both acute and chronic, in which nutritional intervention has been critically assessed. This does not necessarily mean that nutritional intervention is not important in the individual patient. The diverse baseline nutritional status in patients (both from a macronutrient as well as a micronutrient perspective), the differences in insult severity, and the myriad of therapies and approaches given to the individual patient explain why there does not appear to be a guiding light for nutritional intervention. In spite of this, some general recommendations can be made with regard to energy and protein requirements.

ENERGY NEEDS

As discussed previously, difficulties in estimating energy expenditure in cirrhotics have been attributed to fluid retention, relative changes in body compartments, and other variables related to metabolic abnormalities in patients with liver disease.

Nonetheless, in stable cirrhotics, various studies have measured energy expenditures ranging from approximately 1500 to 2100 kcal/day.[25,27,28] Thus, though the controversy over whether these patients are hypermetabolic compared to controls remains unanswered; the absolute energy requirements in these patients do not appear to be excessive. Furthermore, in the acute setting, increases in the metabolic rate are influenced by many variables including the severity of the insult, the presence of infection, and medications that the patient may be receiving. These latter variables further complicate accurate extrapolation of energy needs from formula equations. Thus, measurement of REE with indirect calorimetry remains the most accurate and practical way of estimating total caloric needs. In the absence of indirect calorimetry, the simplest and most accurate predictive formula is the Schofield formula. This formula, referenced by Madden, varies significantly by age. In men between the ages of 30 and 60, it is as follows[27]:

$$(11.48 \times \text{weight}) - (2.63 \times \text{height}) + 877.57$$

Most interventional studies have used a caloric intake between 2000 and 3000 kcal. In the VA cooperative study, a level of 2500 calories and above was considered adequate therapy. Alternately, values ranging from 25 kcal/kg day (stable cirrhotic) to 45 kcal/kg day (postoperative cirrhotic) have been proposed.[33] Excessive caloric delivery is not beneficial as it can create metabolic and respiratory stresses. High caloric delivery may also involve increasing the fluids given to these usually fluid-restricted-patients. Additionally, nutritional repletion is not usually accomplished during hospitalization in the current medical climate. Energy goals should thus be directed at maintenance without causing metabolic abnormalities.

Perhaps more important than delivery of a caloric load is the mixture of the calories provided. In an interesting study by Chanda and Mehendale, rats subjected to a hepatotoxin demonstrated a decrease in hepatocellular regeneration and tissue repair when given 15% glucose in drinking water.[66] Conversely, in a similar experiment, rats given palmitic acid and L-carnitine were protected against similar doses of that hepatotoxin. The authors suggest that the regenerating liver uses fatty acids as the main source of cellular energy. The increased demand for ATP needed to support hepatocellular division is essentially derived from fatty acid oxidation.[67]

It is also interesting to note that the two outwardly "negative studies," using BCAA supplementation in a test group, compared it to a control group on a lipid-based formula. It is possible that the lack of efficacy in these studies was due to the lipids conveying some advantage to the control group, thus decreasing by comparison, the effectiveness of the BCAA solution in the treatment group.

There is other interesting animal data to suggest that lipids, specifically saturated fatty acids may offer protection against alcoholic liver injury. Nanji et al. found that diets enriched with saturated fatty acids (palm oil) reverse the pathological changes induced by ethanol. Conversely, omega-3 fatty acids (fish oil) do not improve the severity of alcohol-induced injury. The authors suggest that the protective effects may be explained in part by differences in lipid peroxidation. Dietary fat helps to modify the expression of cytochrome p450 2E1, which contributes to NADPH-dependant lipid peroxidation. The animals fed the diets rich in saturated fatty acids demonstrated less induction of the CYP2E1 enzyme system.[68] Alternately, the protective effect may be through positive changes in eicosanoid metabolism manifested as an increase in the prostacycline to thromboxane B_2 ratio. In previous studies, these authors found that decreases in this ratio preceded the production of pathologic liver disease.

However, saturated fats are probably not the only nutrients that may have a protective effect against liver disease. Lieber found that baboons maintained on a chronic ethanol enriched diet that were supplemented with polyunsaturated phospholipids (55 to 60% of which was polyunsaturated phosphatidylcholine [PPC]) were protected against alcohol-induced fibrosis. In a similar study, the animals were given a purer extract, comprising 94 to 96% phosphatidylcholine. The researchers found that these baboons given ethanol for up to 8 years did not develop cirrhosis or septal fibrosis when fed this supplemented diet. Leiber proposed that the phosphatidylcholine directly affects collagen metabolism and opposes oxidative stress.[6,69,70] Unfortunately, supplementing fat also does not appear to be the entire answer. In a rat model, Lieber also found that in the setting of chronic alcohol consumption increased triglycerides in the diet results in increased fat accumulation in the liver.[6] Thus, extrapolating from animal data, it would seem that in the setting of alcoholic liver disease between 25 and 35% of the total calories should be derived from a mixture of these lipids. Thus, it would appear that the types of fat as well as the amount of fat are important considerations in supplementing patients with liver disease. A recent randomized placebo controlled study by Pantaleo et al. evaluated arachnadonic acid (AA) supplementation on platelet and renal function in patients with stable cirrhosis. The authors argued that a platelet aggregation defect is often seen in patients with cirrhosis. This defect is, at least in part due to abnormalities in membrane lipids as well as well as a reduced synthesis of a platelet-aggregating factor, thromboxane A_2, a factor derived from arachnadonic acid metabolism. The authors further point out that other breakdown products of AA, prostaglandins, are involved with the regulation of renal blood flow. As a result of liver disease, lipid level are altered, usually with low levels of AA. Thus, the authors randomized patients on a standardized 1800 kcal diet to receive supplementation with either AA or an equivalent amount of oleic acid. The authors were able to demonstrate improvement in platelet aggregation in cirrhotic patients supplemented with AA. This function returned to baseline during the washout period reflecting similar changes in serum AA levels. No significant differences between the two groups were seen in the production of urinary vasoactive prostaglandins. The authors concluded that supplementation with AA may be a novel approach to improve platelet aggregation in cirrhotic patients.[71]

Protein supplementation in the patient with acute liver injury is probably the most controversial aspect of macronutrient nutritional supplementation. These patients usually demonstrate somatic protein wasting and decreases in muscle strength, immune reactivity, and protein synthesis. These deficiencies may in part be due to diminished protein stores. Also, repair of injury, extrapolated from other clinical settings, requires adequate protein. Finally, it has been assumed that liver regeneration is delayed when there is insufficient protein.[6]

In his studies of nutritional intervention in patients with alcoholic liver disease, Mendenhall has stated that all patients with alcoholic hepatitis achieved positive nitrogen balance with 1.2 g/kg of protein. Additionally, this intake of protein was well tolerated in spite of severe liver disease. Encephalopathy was observed in 20% of patients, but its occurrence did not correlate with protein intake.[48] In patients with chronic liver disease, Lieber states that positive nitrogen balance can be attained with a protein intake of 0.74 g/kg. Thus, it appears that the stringent protein restrictions often imposed on hospitalized patients with liver disease can be eased. Protein provisions in the range of 0.6 to 0.8 g/kg can usually be safely given during the acute setting, increasing protein delivery, as tolerated to at least 1.2 g/kg. It should be noted that the protein supplemented in Mendenhall's study, and the basis of his recommendations, was enriched with BCAA. Although there have been no definitive studies comparing tolerability of standard AA mixtures to BCAA, it is possible that an individual patient with acute liver injury may tolerate a larger quantity of protein if supplemented with BCAAs. Thus, clinical surveillance is important when increasing protein load in these patients.

Finally, the remainder of patients' caloric needs should be met with carbohydrates. As discussed previously, insulin resistance is common in patients with cirrhosis, and this "intolerance" is further exacerbated in the setting of acute injury. Therefore, providing carbohydrates to the point of inducing metabolic aberrations is not advisable. Cirrhotics may further benefit from complex carbohydrates to reduce insulin requirements. Complex carbohydrates may also be advantageous in the setting of encephalopathy, as they tend to decrease transit time and lower colonic pH, both of which serve to decrease ammonia absorption from the GI tract.[6]

NUTRITIONAL SUPPLEMENTS

S-ADENOSYLMETHIONINE

S-Adenosylmethionine (SAMe) is synthesized by the transfer of an adenosyl group from ATP to the essential AA methionine. SAMe serves primarily as a methyl donor. These SAMe-dependent methylations are essential for the biosynthesis of a variety of cellular components including carnitine, phospholipids, proteins, DNA, and RNA as well as polyamines needed for cell regeneration.[43,72] In addition, it serves as one source of cysteine for glutathione production (Figure 62.5).[43] Furthermore, it has been shown that methionine metabolism is impaired in patients with liver disease and that the activity of SAMe synthase is decreased in human cirrhotic livers.[43,73,74]

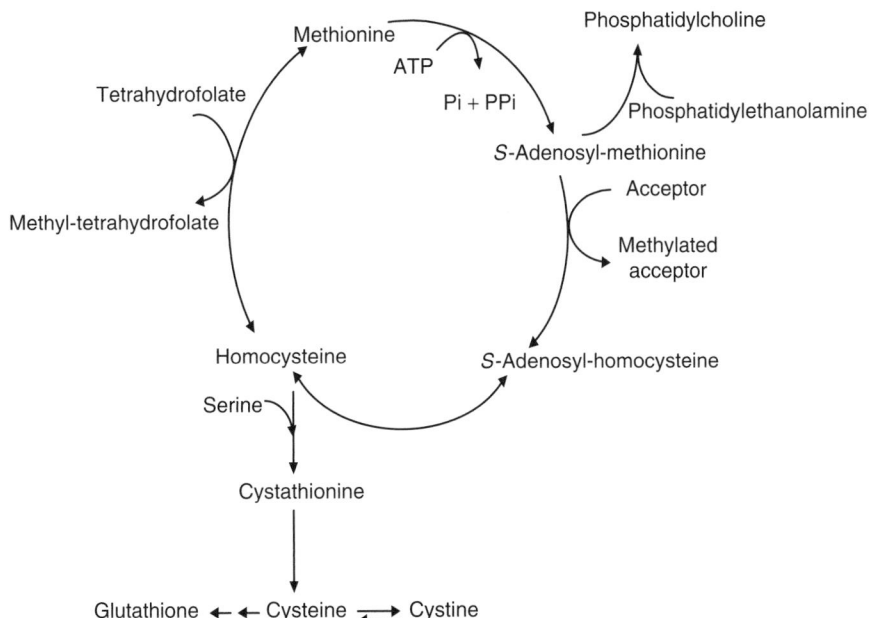

FIGURE 62.5 SAMe is formed in an irreversible reaction that transfers an adenosyl group from methionine. SAMe is an important donor of methyl groups, and is active in the conversion of creatine to creatinine and of phosphatidylethanolamine to phosphatidylcholine. SAMe is converted to S-adenosyl-homocysteine and then to homocysteine. Homocysteine can combine with serine to form cystathionine which can ultimately be converted to glutathione. (With permissions from (1) Kruszynska, *Oxford Textbook of Clinical Hepatology*, 2nd edition, Bircher, Benhamou, McIntyre, Rizzetto, Rodes, eds. Oxford University Press, Oxford, 257, 1999. (2) Lieber, *Modern Nutrition in Health and Disease*, 9th edition, Shils, Olson, Shike, Ross, eds. Williams and Wilkins, Baltimore, MD, 1177, 1999.)

Thus, the administration of exogenous SAMe should be effective in liver disease. In baboons, correction of ethanol-induced hepatic SAMe depletion with oral SAMe supplementation resulted in a corresponding attenuation of ethanol-induced liver injury.[75,76] Thus, supplementation with SAMe dampens the depletion of hepatic glutathione (GSH) stores. Without supplementation, depletion of GSH leads to inactivation of SAMe synthetase, which would tend to further reduce GSH stores, thereby predisposing to hepatic injury.[75] The studies that have evaluated SAMe supplementation have demonstrated significant improvements in subjective symptoms, serum markers of cholestasis, and hepatic GSH levels.[75,77,78] More recently, Mato et al. demonstrated that SAMe supplementation could improve survival or delay time to transplantation compared to controls. These results demonstrated a positive trend in favor of the supplemented group but achieved significance only when Child C patients were excluded.[43,79]

Supplementation with *S*-adenosylmethionine shows significant promise in the treatment of liver disease and will undoubtedly be investigated with larger studies in the future.

ZINC

Zinc (Zn) is the most abundant intracellular trace element. It is involved in a multitude of diverse catalytic, structural, and regulatory functions. Many physiologic functions require zinc, including protein metabolism, normal immune functioning and wound healing, neurosensory function such as cognition and taste, and membrane stability.[59,80] Hypozincemia is common in various types of liver disease.[59] The deficiency is multifactorial and believed to involve poor dietary intake, and impaired intestinal absorption (possibly due to a cytokine-induced intestinal metallothionein, which dampens zinc absorption). Additionally, there is decreased affinity of albumin for zinc in cirrhotics, which might influence bioavailability and lead to increased urinary losses of zinc. Finally, increased cytokine or hormonal concentrations may lead to altered zinc metabolism.[59]

Zinc deficiency may play a role in increasing plasma ammonia levels. Zinc deficiency was shown to decrease activity of glutamate dehydrogenase and ornithine transcarbamylase (OTC), enzymes important in normal nitrogen metabolism (Figure 62.4). Urea synthetic capacity is believed to be reduced in zinc-deficient patients due to reduced OTC activity as zinc acts as a cofactor in the activity of this enzyme. Zinc supplementation speeds up the kinetics of nitrogen conversion from AAs into urea in cirrhotics.[21] Zinc deficiency also increases muscle glutamine synthetase and adenosine monophosphate deaminase, enzymes that increase ammonia production from aspartate.[81]

Although zinc deficiency may play a role in some of the altered taste sensation seen in liver disease, it is unlikely to be a major cause of anorexia in liver disease. It is much more likely that the anorexia seen in his disease is cytokine mediated.[59] Conversely, zinc deficiency, at least in part, does appear to play a role in immune dysfunction and perhaps in delayed wound healing. The latter may occur through the effect of zinc on insulin-like growth factor.[59] In regard to protein synthesis, a recent study showed lower serum albumin levels in children undergoing liver transplantation than in other transplant patients in whom serum-zinc levels were normal. This correlates with the findings by Bates and McClain which demonstrated improvement or normalization of serum transport proteins in zinc-deficient patients on parenteral nutrition when supplemented with zinc.[82,83]

SELENIUM

There are at least eleven selenoproteins; the most well known class is the Glutathione peroxidases. These proteins are important participants in the body's antioxidant defenses. Selenium concentrations have been reported to be lower in patients with cirrhosis compared to healthy controls. As such, selenium deficiency could therefore contribute to the morbidity of cirrhosis. This deficiency could be easily addressed with supplementation. However, a recent study by Burke, reported that though plasma selenium is indeed depressed in patients with cirrhosis, the changes noted in plasma selenoproteins of cirrhotics are not the same as those found in selenium-deficient subjects without liver disease. Functionally, these patients had an increase in the plasma glutathione concentration arguing against a true selenium deficiency.[84,85]

CARNITINE

Fatty acids are the preferred fuel for patients with cirrhosis. Since carnitine is essential for the mitochondrial use of long-chain fatty acids for energy production, decreased availability of this quaternary amine may lead to energy deficiency in cirrhotics. Deficiency can arise from poor dietary intake or disruption of carnitine biosynthesis, the last step occurring almost exclusively in the liver. Measured levels of carnitine in patients with chronic liver disease can be reduced or increased. The literature suggests that plasma and tissue carnitine levels can be altered in patients with chronic liver disease, depending on both the cause and progression of liver disease.[86,87]

A recent study by Krahenbuhl and Reichen found that patients with chronic liver disease are normally not carnitine deficient. They also concluded that carnitine metabolism can be disturbed in subgroups of patients with liver disease. For example, patients with alcoholic cirrhosis demonstrated increased plasma concentrations. Patients with primary biliary cirrhosis were able to maintain normal plasma levels of carnitine, but demonstrated increased renal excretion.[87,88]

CONCLUSION

It is clear that the relationship between nutrition and the liver is intricate and interdependent. Liver disease can result in anorexia, malabsorption, and abnormalities in nutrient metabolism, leading to a compromise in the nutritional status of the host. This impaired nutritional status can affect negatively on immune function, compromise the ability of the liver to limit the extent of hepatic insults, and retard an appropriate response to injury. Nutritional deficiencies, in patients with liver disease, can range from subtle abnormalities to advanced PCM. Some degree of nutritional compromise is invariably present. In treating patients with liver disease, the recognition and aggressive treatment of these deficiencies is paramount. In milder forms of liver disease, this intervention may take the form of nutrient and vitamin supplementation. In more advanced liver disease, aggressive nutritional support, preferably in the form of enteral access and feeding, may be the "controllable" factor that leads to an improved outcome.

REFERENCES

1. Kruszynska Y.T., In *Oxford Textbook of Clinical Hepatology*, 2nd edition, Bircher J., Benhamou J., McIntyre N., Rizzetto M., Rodes J., eds. Oxford University Press, Oxford, 257, 1999.
2. Corssmit E.P.M., Romijn J.A., Sauerwein H.P., *Metabolism*, 50, 742, 2001.
3. Woerle H.J., Szoke E., Meyer C., *Am J Physiol Endocrinol Metab.*, 290, E67, 2005.
4. Rothman D.L., Magnusson I., Katz L.D., et al., *Science*, 254, 573, 1991.
5. Barthel A., Schmoll D., *Am J Physiol Endocrinol Metab.*, 285, E685, 2003.
6. Lieber C.S., In *Modern Nutrition in Health and Disease*, 9th edition, Shils M.E., Olson J.A., Shike M., Ross A.C., eds. Williams and Wilkins, Baltimore, MD, 1177, 1999.
7. Redinger R.N., *Am J Surg.*, 185, 168, 2003.
8. Chiang J.Y.L., *Am J Physiol Gastrointest Liver Physiol.*, 284, G349, 2003.
9. Jones P.J.H., Kubnow S., In *Modern Nutrition in Health and Disease*, 9th edition, Shils M.E., Olson J.A., Shike M., Ross A.C., eds. Williams and Wilkins, Baltimore, MD, 67, 1999.
10. Tulenko T.N., Sumner A.E., *J Nuc Cardiol.*, 9, 638, 2002.
11. Harry D.S., McIntyre N., In *Oxford Textbook of Clinical Hepatology*, 2nd edition, Bircher J., Benhamou J., McIntyre N., Rizzetto M., Rodes J., eds. Oxford University Press, Oxford, 287, 1999.
12. Kruszynska Y.T., McIntyre N., In *Oxford Textbook of Clinical Hepatology*, 2nd edition, Bircher J., Benhamou J., McIntyre N., Rizzetto M., Rodes J., eds. Oxford University Press, Oxford, 303, 1999.
13. Nelson D.L., Cox M.M., In *Principals of Biochemistry*, 2nd edition, Lehninger A.L., Nelson D.L., Cox, M.M., eds. Worth Publisher, New York, 506, 1993.
14. Gerok W., Gross V., In *Oxford Textbook of Clinical Hepatology*, 2nd edition, Bircher J., Benhamou J., McIntyre N., Rizzetto M., Rodes J., eds. Oxford University Press, Oxford, 346, 1999.
15. Nielsen M.F., Caumo A., Aagaard N.K., *Am J Physiol Gastroenterol Liver Physiol.*, 288, G1135, 2005.
16. Changani K.K., Jalan R., Cox I.J., *Gut*, 49, 557, 2006.
17. Petrides A.S., Vogt C., Schulze-Berge D., et al., *Hepatology*, 19, 616, 1994.
18. Riggio O., Merli M., Romiti A., et al., *JPEN*, 16, 445, 1992.
19. Ma Z., Lee S.S., *Hepatology*, 24, 451, 1996.
20. Cabre E., Gassull M.A., *Nutrition*, 12, 542, 1996.
21. Haussinger D., In *Oxford Textbook of Clinical Hepatology*, 2nd edition, Bircher J., Benhamou J., McIntyre N., Rizzetto M., Rodes J., eds. Oxford University Press, Oxford, 325, 1999.
22. Denninger M., In *Oxford Textbook of Clinical Hepatology*, 2nd edition, Bircher J., Benhamou J., McIntyre N., Rizzetto M., Rodes J., eds. Oxford University Press, Oxford, 367, 1999.
23. Schneeweiss B., Graninger W., Ferenci P., et al., *Hepatology*, 11, 387, 1990.
24. Heymsfield S.B., Waki M., Reinus J., *Hepatology*, 11, 502, 1990.
25. McCullough A.J., Raguso C., *Am J Clin Nutr.*, 69, 1066, 1999.
26. Merli M., Riggio O., Romiti A., *Hepatology*, 12, 106, 1990.
27. Madden A.M., Morgan M.Y., *Hepatology*, 30, 655, 1999.
28. Müller M.J., Böttcher J., Selberg O., et al., *Am J Clin Nutr.*, 69, 1194, 1999.
29. Green J.H., Bramley P.N., Losowwsky M.S., *Hepatology*, 14, 464, 1991.
30. Selberg O., Böttcher J., Tusch G., et al., *Hepatology*, 25, 652, 1997.
31. McCullough A.J., Bugianesi E., Marchesini G., *Gastroenterol*, 115, 947, 1998.
32. Campillo B., Sherman E., Richardet J.P., *Eur J Clin Nutr.*, 55, 980, 2001.
33. McCullough A.J., Mullen K.D., Smanik E.J., *Gastro Clin N Am.*, 18, 619, 1989.
34. Mendenhall C.L., Anderson S., Weesner R.E., et al., *Am J Med.*, 76, 211, 1984.
35. Sarin S.K., Dhingra N., Bansal A., et al., *Am J Gastro.*, 92, 777, 1997.
36. McCullough A.J., Bugianesi E., *Am J Gastro.*, 92, 734, 1997.
37. Ferreira Figueiredo F.A., Perez R.D., Kondo M., *J Gatroenterol Hepatol.*, 20, 209, 2005.

38. Munoz S.J., *Sem in Liver Dis.*, 11, 278, 1991.
39. Hasse J., Strong S., Gorman M.A., et al., *Nutrition*, 9, 339, 1993.
40. Alvares-da-Silva M., Reverbel da Silveira T., *Nutrition*, 21, 113, 2005.
41. Patek A.J., Ratnoff O.D., Mankin H., et al., *JAMA*, 138, 543, 1948.
42. McCullough A.J., Tavill A.S., *Sem Liver Dis.*, 11, 265, 1991.
43. Schenker S., Halff G.A., *Sem in Liver Dis.*, 13, 196, 1993.
44. Nasrallah S.M., Galambos J.T., *Lancet*, ii, 1276, 1980.
45. Nompleggi D.J., Bonkovsky H., *Hepatology* 19, 518, 1994.
46. Mendenhall C.L., Tosch T., Weesner R.E., *Am J Clin Nutr.*, 43, 213, 1986.
47. Mendenhall C.L., Moritz T.E., Roselle G.A., *Hepatology*, 17, 564, 1993.
48. Mendenhall C.L., Moritz T.E., Roselle G.A., *JPEN*, 19, 258, 1995.
49. Cabre E., Rodriguez-Iglesias P., Caballeria J., *Hepatology*, 32, 36, 2000.
50. Cabre E., Gonzalez-Huix F., Abad-Lacruz A., et al., *Gastroenterol*, 98, 715, 1990.
51. Bonkovsky H.L., Fiellin D.A., Smith G.S., *Am J of Gastro.*, 86, 1200, 1991.
52. Bonkovsky H.L., Singh R.H., Jafri I.H., et al., *Am J of Gastro.*, 86, 1209, 1991.
53. Kearns P.J., Young H., Garcia G., et al., *Gastroenterol*, 102, 200, 1992.
54. Morgan T.R., *Sem Liver Dis.*, 13, 384, 1993.
55. Naylor C.D., O'Rourke K., Detsky A.S., et al., *Gastroenterol*, 97, 1033, 1989.
56. Weber F.L., Bagby B.S., Licate L., et al., *Hepatology*, 11, 942, 1990.
57. Buse M.G., Reid S.S., *J Clin Invest.*, 56, 1250, 1975.
58. Cerra F.B., Cheung N.K., Fischer J.E., *JPEN*, 9, 88, 1985.
59. McClain C.J., Marsano L., Burk R.F., et al., *Sem in Liv Dis.*, 11, 321, 1991.
60. Eriksson L.S., Conn H.O., *Hepatology*, 10, 228, 1989.
61. Marchesini G., Bianchi G., Merli M., et al., *Gastroenterol*, 124, 1792, 2003.
62. Egberts E.H., Schomerus H., Hamster W., et al., *Gastroenterol*, 88, 887, 1985.
63. Base W., Barsigian C., Schaeffer A., et al., *Hepatology*, 7, 324, 1987.
64. Tessari P., Zanetti M., Barazzoni R., et al., *Gastro.*, 111, 127–37, 1996.
65. Charlton M.R., *Gastroenterol*, 111, 252, 1996.
66. Chanda S., Mehendale H.M., *FASEB J.*, 9, 240, 1995.
67. Chanda S., Mehendale H.M., *Toxicology*, 111, 163, 1996.
68. Nanji A.A., Sadrzadeh S.M.H., Yang E.K., et al., *Gastroenterol*, 109, 547, 1995.
69. Lieber C.S., DeCarli L.M., Mak K.M., et al., *Hepatology*, 12, 1390, 1990.
70. Lieber C.S., Robins S.J., Li J., et al., *Gastroenterol*, 106, 152, 1994.
71. Pantaleo P., Marra F., Vizzutti F., et al., *Clin Sci.*, 106, 27, 2004.
72. Stipanuk M.H., In *Modern Nutrition in Health and Disease*, 9th edition, Shils M.E., Olson J.A., Shike M., Ross A.C., eds. Williams and Wilkins, Baltimore, MD, 543, 1999.
73. Horowitz J.H., Rypins E.B., Henderson J.M., et al., *Gastroenterol*, 81, 668, 1981.
74. Duce A.M., Ortiz P., Cabrero C., et al., *Hepatology*, 8, 65, 1988.
75. Lieber C.S., *J Hepatol.*, 32(Suppl. 1), 113, 2000.
76. Lieber C.S., Casini A., Decarli L.M., et al., *Hepatology*, 11, 165, 1990.
77. Frezza M., Surrenti C., Manzillo G., et al., *Gastroenterol*, 99, 211, 1990.
78. Vendemiale G., Altomare E., Trizio T., et al., *Scan J Gastro.*, 24, 407, 1989.
79. Mato J.M., Camara J., Fernendez de Paz J., et al., *J Hepatol*, 30, 1081, 1999.
80. King J.C., Keen C.L., In *Modern Nutrition in Health and Disease*, 9th edition, Shils M.E., Olson J.A., Shike M., Ross A.C., eds. Williams and Wilkins, Baltimore, MD, 223, 1999.
81. Mullen K.D., Weber F.L., *Sem in Liv Dis.*, 11, 292, 1991.
82. Narkewicz M.R., Krebs N., Karrer F., *Hepatology*, 29, 830, 1999.
83. Bates J., McClain C.J., *Am J Clin Nutr.*, 34, 1655, 1981.
84. Burk R.F., Levander O.A., In *Modern Nutrition in Health and Disease*, 9th edition, Shils M.E., Olson J.A., Shike M., Ross A.C., eds. Williams and Wilkins, Baltimore, MD, 256, 1999.
85. Burk R.F., Early D.S., Hill K.E., et al., *Hepatology*, 27, 794, 1998.
86. Rebouche C.J., In *Modern Nutrition in Health and Disease*, 9th edition, Shils M.E., Olson J.A., Shike M., Ross A.C., eds. Williams and Wilkins, Baltimore, MD, 505, 1999.
87. Krahenbuhl S., Reichen J., *Hepatology*, 25, 148, 1996.
88. Brodsky I.G., In *Modern Nutrition in Health and Disease*, 9th edition, Shils M.E., Olson J.A., Shike M., Ross A.C., eds. Williams and Wilkins, Baltimore, MD, 699, 199.

63 Nutrition and the Pancreas: Physiology and Interventional Strategies

Srinadh Komanduri and Mark T. DeMeo

CONTENTS

INTRODUCTION

The pancreas plays a major role in nutrient digestion as well as in the control of intermediate metabolism. Patients with pancreatic disease will likely have their nutritional homeostasis compromised with both macro- and micronutrient deficiencies. This chapter will explore (1) the effects of a diseased pancreas on nutritional health and (2) nutritional interventions that may be beneficial to patients with a diseased or inflamed pancreas.

NORMAL PANCREATIC FUNCTION

The exocrine pancreas delivers two main products to the lumen of the duodenum during the digestive process — digestive enzymes and bicarbonate. The digestive enzymes secreted by the pancreas are the key to the breakdown of ingested macronutrients (carbohydrates, proteins, and fats). Table 63.1 shows the various enzymes and their functions. The bicarbonate secreted in pancreatic juice neutralizes the acidic chyme entering the duodenum from the stomach, and in so doing, increases duodenal pH. This alkaline environment in the duodenum, in turn, allows for optimal functioning of the pancreatic digestive enzymes.

CARBOHYDRATE DIGESTION

Dietary carbohydrates are an important component of daily energy intake by adults. Ingested carbohydrates take three major forms: *Monosaccharides* such as glucose and fructose, *disaccharides* such as lactose and sucrose, and *polysaccharides*, of which starch is the predominant form. Monosaccharides are absorbed directly by the normal small bowel mucosa. Disaccharides require the action of enzymes called disaccharidases, found in the brush border of mucosal cells lining the small bowel. The disaccharidases break down these small carbohydrates into their component sugars prior to absorption. Starches are much larger molecules of repeating glucose molecules joined by either a C1-4 or C1-6 linkage (Figure 63.1) Starches require digestion prior to absorption.

Digestion of starch begins with the release of salivary amylase in the mouth. However, salivary amylase becomes neutralized quickly by gastric acid. Starch then passes to the duodenum, where α-amylase, secreted by the pancreas, continues the digestive process. Pancreatic amylase cleaves the 1-4 glucose linkages but not the 1-6 linkages or the 1-4 linkages juxtaposed to the 1-6 links.

TABLE 63.1
Digestive Enzymes Secreted By the Pancreas

Amylase	Splits α(1-4) Glycosidic Linkages of Dietary Polysaccharides
Trypsin	Cleaves internal bonds with a preference for positively charged amino acids
Chymotrypsin	Cleaves internal bonds with a preference for amino acids with aromatic side groups
Elastase	Cleaves internal bonds with a preference for amino acids with aliphatic side chains
Carboxypeptidase A	Cleaves carboxy-terminal amino acids
Carboxypeptidase B	Cleaves carboxy-terminal amino acids with a preference for peptide bonds after arginine or lysine residues
Lipase	Preferentially hydrolyzes the 1 and 3 position of dietary triglycerides.
Colipase	Binds to the lipid/aqueous interface between the emulsion and the unstirred water layer and also binds to lipase. This allows for the approximation of lipase to dietary triglycerides and facilitates digestion
Phospholipase A_2	Cleaves the phospholipid at the 2 position to yield a lysophosphoglyceride and a fatty acid
Cholesterol esterase	Cleaves esterfied fatty acid from cholesterol moiety

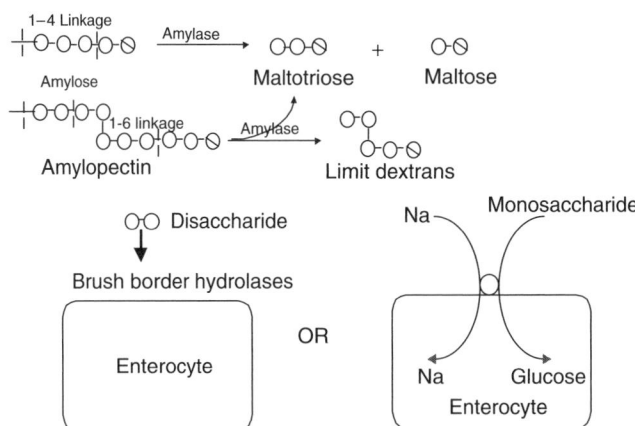

FIGURE 63.1   Monosaccharides can be absorbed directly by the small bowel mucose. Disaccharides are further metabolized by brush border disaccharidases. Polysaccharides are cleaved by amylase at the 1-4 but not the 1-6 linkages forming oligosaccharides. These oligosaccharides are cleaved by brush border enzymes to their constituent monosaccharides.

This hydrolysis results in the formation of large oligosaccharides, with an average chain length of about eight glucose units with one or more 1-6 linkages. These oligosaccharides are hydrolyzed by intestinal brush border enzymes into their constituent monosaccharides. The resultant monosaccharides are transported into the mucosal epithelial cell.[1,2]

PROTEIN DIGESTION

Protein digestion begins in the stomach with the nonspecific actions of pepsin and hydrochloric acid. Enzymes secreted from the pancreas also play a major role in protein digestion. These enzymes are released in the form of zymogens or inactivated enzymes. Trypsinogen is activated by enterokinase, which is released from the intestinal mucosa. The active enzyme trypsin, then activates the proenzyme forms of chymotrypsin, elastase, and carboxypeptidase A and B. Trypsin, chymotrypsin, and elastase are called endopeptidases as they cleave internal bonds. Interluminal digestion of protein results in the generation of free amino acids and oligopeptides. Oligopeptides are further hydrolyzed by the membrane-bound oligopeptidases of the enterocyte brush border.[3]

LIPID DIGESTION

Lipid digestion begins in the oral cavity with the secretion of lingual lipase and the mechanical effects of mastication. In the stomach, gastric lipase is released and mixes with lingual lipase. In addition, gastric contractions cause a mechanical grinding of the ingested fat, resulting in the formation of an emulsion. An *emulsion* is a suspension of enzymatically partially digested and mechanically disrupted fat droplets in liquid. The emulsion acquires a coating comprised of phospholipids, bile acids, and triglycerides, which serves to stabilize the fat globule. This stabilized emulsion ultimately passes into the duodenum.

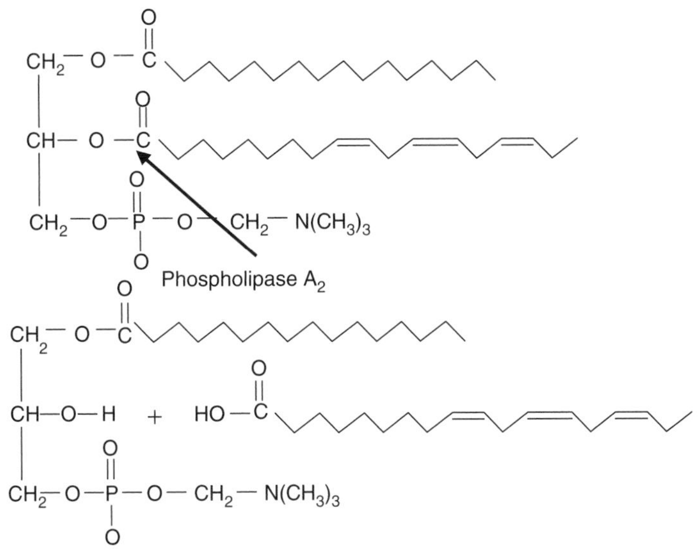

FIGURE 63.2 Phospholipase A_2 hydrolyzes the phospholipid at position 2 to yield a fatty acid and a lysophospatidylcholine and a fatty acid. (With permission from Linscheer W.G., Vergroesen A.J., *in Modern Nutrition in Health and Disease* Eighth Edition, eds, Shils ME, Olson JA, Shike M., Lea & Febiger, Philadelphia 1994, p. 47.)

Pancreatic lipase, the principal enzyme of triglyceride digestion, hydrolyzes ester bonds at the 1 and 3 positions of the glycerol moiety. However, in the presence of bile acids, this enzymatic process is inefficient. Another enzyme secreted by the pancreas, colipase, avidly binds to the triglyceride–aqueous interface of the emulsion and also has a binding site for lipase. Colipase thus ensures the adhesion of lipase to the lipid droplet and increases the efficiency of the latter enzyme in the digestion of triglycerides. Phospholipase A_2 is also secreted by the pancreas and acts upon ingested phospholipids to yield a fatty acid and a lysophosphatidylcholine (Figure 63.2). Finally, Cholesterol esterase hydrolyzes an esterafied fatty acid from the parent cholesterol molecule.

Once hydrolyzed, lipid products have to traverse the unstirred water layer of the gut prior to being absorbed by the mucosal absorptive cell. However, as fat is not water soluble, fat digestion products have difficulty crossing this water layer. Bile acids, secreted by the liver, greatly facilitate this diffusion. Bile acids are effective because they have a hydrophilic (water-soluble) end and one hydrophobic or lipophilic end (water-insoluble or conversely lipid-soluble). These bile acids, when secreted in sufficient quantity, form micelles, which are small spheres with an outward hydrophilic projection and an inner lipophilic core. The products of fat digestion pass into the fat-soluble core while the outer layer remains soluble in the unstirred water layer. This lipid-rich conduit is able to traverse the unstirred water layer and bring the inner lipid core into proximity with the mucosal absorptive cell membrane, which is largely comprised of lipids. Once in contact with the lipid membrane, the micelle core lipids diffuse into the endothelial absorptive cell. This "shuttling of lipids" from the lumen, where digestion takes place to the absorptive enterocyte membrane, greatly facilitates lipid absorption.[4,5]

NUTRITIONAL IMPLICATIONS AND RAMIFICATIONS IN PANCREATIC DISEASE

The nutritional status of patients with pancreatitis is in part dependent on the duration of the disease, the severity of the acute exacerbation, and the underlying etiology of the pancreatitis.

The two most common etiologies of acute pancreatitis in the Western world are alcohol and gallstones. The nutritional status of the patient at the time of acute episode may impact on the clinical course. In the setting of acute pancreatitis, there exists a highly catabolic state. Despite an increased caloric requirement, excessive caloric supplementation may perpetuate the inflammatory cascade and create a viscous cycle. In a study of 99 consecutive patients with acute pancreatitis, 64% of whom had alcohol as an etiology of their disease, only 15% were considered underweight (body mass index [BMI; weight in kg/height in m^2] <19) according to their BMIs .[6] Obesity as opposed to malnutrition appears to be a risk factor for severe disease, particularly in alcoholics.[6,7] Still, a severe acute episode could lead to protracted inability to take nutrition by mouth and relative hypermetabolism.[8] This can lead to depletion of nutritional reserves and, depending on the patient's nutritional status prior to the acute event, may predispose the patient to infection and compromise their ability to survive the acute episode. Thus, although obesity may increase the severity of the presenting episode, it is unclear if a patient whose nutritional reserves are compromised will have a more complicated hospital course.

Alternately, chronic pancreatic patients are generally characterized by an asthenic body type and a low BMI. The causes for a compromised nutritional status are multifactorial but mainly include decreased food intake, maldigestion, and malabsorption:

1. *Decrease food intake.* Many patients with chronic pancreatitis experience abdominal pain, frequently with accompanying nausea and anorexia. As these symptoms are usually meal related, they often severely limit oral intake.
2. *Maldigestion.* Decreases in enzyme and bicarbonate secretion parallel progressive injury to the pancreas. Preliminary studies in patients with pancreatic insufficiency suggest that 5 to 10% of normal postprandial enzyme output by the pancreas is sufficient to maintain normal digestion.[9,10] Maldigestion does not proceed equally among the three macronutrients.

   Fat maldigestion is invariably the first to become clinically manifest as nonpancreatic mechanisms do not perform well in lipid digestion. However, there is some compensation for fat digestion, such as to the action of small amounts of lingual or gastric lipases. Given these compensatory mechanisms, an estimated 50% of dietary fat is absorbed.[11] The synthesis and secretion of pancreatic lipase is also more impaired in the damaged pancreas compared with other enzymes. Additionally, lipase is much more sensitive to inactivation in an acidic milieu. Thus, a corresponding decrease in the production of bicarbonate by the damaged gland results in a greater deactivation of lipase. Finally, lipase, once secreted, is more rapidly degraded in the intestinal lumen than the other pancreatic enzymes.

   When fat malabsorption is present, the standard for the diagnosis is the finding of greater than 7 g fat/day in stools collected over a 3-day period. Prior to obtaining the specimen, the patient should consume 100 g fat/day for 3 days and continue on this diet during the 3 days of the collection.[12]
3. *Malabsorption.* Malabsorption occurs secondary to the effects of chronic pancreatitis on micelle formation. The failure of the damaged pancreas to secrete sufficient bicarbonate to neutralize the stomach's acidic chyme causes precipitation of bile acids. This impairs micelle formation, which leads to decreased solubility and absorption of ingested fat. A diminished secretion of pancreatic enzymes lessens the bactericidal effect of these enzymes and can result in bacterial overgrowth. The bacteria deconjugate bile acids, which leads to impaired micelle formation, again resulting in malabsorption. Finally, associated complications such as diabetes and cirrhosis can also impair absorption. The former promotes bacterial overgrowth and the latter impairs synthesis of bile acids. Additionally, when diabetes complicates pancreatitis, the nutrient wasting and relatively high glucagon-to-insulin ratio promote malnutrition.

Many patients with chronic pancreatitis have low serum albumin and cholesterol. The latter is due in part to a malabsorption of bile acids, which causes increased demand to form bile acids — containing food and malabsorption of luminal cholesterol. Serum fatty acid profiles are also abnormal and can lead to several of the abnormalities that are seen in this disease. Specifically, the serum levels of linoleic acid and arachidonic acid are elevated while those of eicosapentaenoic acid (EPA) and docosahexaenoic acid (DHA) are increased. There is also a compensatory increase in palmitoleic acid. Polyunsaturated fatty acids (PUFA) play an important role in vascular endothelial cells and platelets in coagulation and thrombus formation. Thus, abnormalities in the levels of these lipids may impact on hemostasis. Finally the serum concentration of fat-soluble vitamins are low because of poor intake and malabsorption.[13]

Hebutuerne et al. found a slightly greater metabolic rate in patients with chronic pancreatitis compared with a malnourished control group, even when corrected for fat-free mass. There was also a difference within the chronic pancreatitis group between those that were normally nourished and those that were undernourished, with the latter group being more "hypercatabolic." This increased resting energy expenditure was seen in over 60% of the stable population with chronic pancreatitis. The authors concluded that the differences were not readily explained by infection, alcohol use, or nicotine use. They suggested that this unexplained metabolic status might contribute to the malnutrition seen in this disease.[14]

Patients with pancreatic cancer are at particularly high risk for nutritional problems. They have the highest incidence of weight loss of any group of patients with cancer, with approximately 80 to 90% losing weight during the course of their illness.[15,16] The development of cachexia and weight loss, which are poor prognostic variables in this disease,[16] is due in part to damage to an organ that is crucial to nutrient digestion as well as constitutional symptoms such as nausea, depression, and anorexia associated with advancing disease. Cytokines released by the tumor or by host cells in response to the tumor lead to further anorexia and metabolic dysregulation.

NUTRITIONAL INTERVENTION IN PANCREATIC DISEASE

NUTRITIONAL INTERVENTION IN ACUTE PANCREATITIS

Nutritional intervention during an acute episode of pancreatitis is largely determined by the severity of the initial inflammatory event, the estimated period of time that the patient will remain without adequate oral intake, and the patient's underlying nutritional status. The inflammatory response evoked during an acute episode of pancreatitis is largely mediated through the release of cytokines and counter-regulatory hormones. This response is teleologically advantageous to the host. Collectively, the acute-phase response serves to clear bacteria from the bloodstream, sequester potentially virulent substances, and limit "innocent bystander" oxidative damage. Cytokines also stimulate immune cells and signal them to the appropriate point of engagement, upregulating and downregulating the inflammatory response as needed. This response has been adapted over time to alert, enforce, and aid the immune response as well as to limit damage to the host in a response directed against an offending agent. This response, however, can deplete the body's nutrient resources. The greater the insult, the greater the use of endogenous substrate. In spite of exogenous attempts to provide nutritional resources, "autocannibalism" continues largely unabated. It is therefore plausible, though unproven, that in the setting of poor endogenous resources, a prolonged inflammatory state can overwhelm the body's ability to bring forth an inflammatory response and can contribute to the demise of the host. Unfortunately, there is no simple gauge with which to assess the body's ability to respond appropriately to the challenge.

The inflammatory challenge also brings with it a state of substrate intolerance, particularly to carbohydrates and less so to lipids, that makes imprudent use of nutritional support potentially harmful. Additionally, visceral proteins such as albumin, which often are used as nutritional parameters in epidemiologic studies, are affected by the inflammatory response and lose value as predictors of substrate exhaustion. Perhaps in the future we will be guided by readily available tests of immune function that will allow us to discern when the immune response is faltering from lack of available substrate. However, currently, we must estimate the severity and duration of the inflammatory response as well as the underlying nutritional status of the host to determine whether nutritional intervention will be of benefit.

Approximately 80% of patients admitted to the hospital with acute pancreatitis have mild disease. These patients are expected to be able to ingest calories orally in 5 to 7 days. From a nutritional perspective, unless there is severe underlying malnutrition antedating the episode of pancreatitis, there is little need to intervene.

Severe pancreatitis occurs in about 20% of patients, and with prolonged absence of oral intake, nutritional intervention may be necessary. The diagnosis of severe pancreatitis is suspected on the basis of clinical and laboratory evaluations and can be modified by imaging criteria. Several criteria, including Ranson and Acute Physiology and Chronic Health Evaluation (APACHE) II scores, have been established and validated as indicators of severity in acute pancreatitis (Figure 63.3).[17–19]

There is one reason for providing nutrition in acute pancreatitis accompanied by a mitigating circumstance. Nutrition is provided to support the underlying nutritional status of the host while the patient is beseiged by mediators of the inflammatory process. If there is a deficiency in endogenous substrate, "artificial nutrition" will furnish the needed building blocks to survive the insult. The mitigating circumstance is whether the treatment itself does more harm, as the therapy may stimulate the inflamed pancreas and aggravate the underlying problem. Additionally, metabolic aberrations potentially caused by the therapy may complicate the clinical picture.

Several studies in animals (with and without pancreatitis), healthy humans, and humans with stable pancreatic fistulas provide little convincing evidence of parenteral nutrition or enteral feeding delivered to the jejunum producing significant pancreatic stimulation. The more convincing data come from human trials in patients with pancreatitis in which there is no increased rate of pancreas-related complications using either modality.[20,21]

Unfortunately, there are only a few randomized controlled studies on the benefit of nutritional intervention vs. no artificial nutritional therapy (standard therapy). In a study by Sax, patients with mild pancreatitis (average Ranson criteria 1–2) were randomized to receive either standard hydration or parenteral nutrition.[22] The authors found no advantage in using parenteral nutrition

Ranson Criteria	APACHE-II
At admission Age >55 WBC count >16,000/mm^3 Glucose >200 mg/dl Lactate dehydrogenase (LDH) >350 IU/l Aspartate transaminase (AST) >250 U/l	Temperature (rectal) Mean arterial pressure Heart rate Respiratory rate Oxygenation Arterial pH Serum sodium Serum potassium Serum creatinine Hematocrit WBC count Glasgow coma score
During initial 48 hours Hematocrit decrease of >10 mg/dl Blood urea nitrogen (BUN) increase of >5 mg/dl Calcium <8 mg/dl PaO$_2$ <60 mm Hg Base deficit >4 mEq/l Fluid sequestration >6 l	Age points Chronic health points

FIGURE 63.3 Ranson criteria and the APACHE II severity of disease classification system are two scoring systems used to judge the severity of acute pancreatitis. In the APACHE II system, points were given for each of twelve variables (in box) based on the severity of those variables. Points were also awarded for increasing age, a history of organ dysfunction, immunocompetence, and surgical interventions. Three or more Ranson criteria or eight or more APACHE II points are considered significant disease.

with respect to hospital days or number of pancreatic complications. The authors did find a greater risk of line infections in this group than in patients with other diseases requiring parenteral nutrition who were cared for concurrently using the same central-line care. The importance of parenteral nutrition in this study may have been understated as all the patients had mild disease. Recently, Xian-Li evaluated the benefit of parenteral nutrition vs. standard therapy in patients with severe acute pancreatitis. In addition, this study added an additional arm of parenteral nutrition with glutamine. Glutamine was believed to convey potential benefit to these patients because, when given intravenously, it has antioxidant properties, decreases the release of inflammatory cytokines, and maintains overall gut integrity. The initiation of parenteral nutrition was 24 to 48 h after resuscitation as opposed to the 24 h from admission in the Sax study. Xian-Li demonstrated a reduction in length of stay, overall complications, and mortality when compared with standard therapy alone. The cohort of patients with glutamine added to parenteral nutrition had an additional decrease in pancreatic infection compared with parenteral nutrition alone.[23]

Thus, the interpretation of this data, although limited, is that parenteral nutrition is of benefit in severe acute pancreatitis over standard therapy alone. Parenteral nutrition appears to decrease overall length of stay when compared with standard therapy. However, parenteral nutrition may result in a significant risk of line infection and can worsen outcome when initiated too early.

Perhaps the most important aspect of nutritional intervention is the appropriate choice of route of administration. Powell has provided the only randomized study investigating enteral nutrition vs. standard therapy. This study did not show a statistically significant benefit with enteral nutrition. However, this was an underpowered study and patients were only followed for 4 days.[24]

To date, there have been seven randomized studies evaluating enteral vs. parenteral nutrition:

McClave and colleagues initially compared enteral jejunal feedings with parenteral nutrition in patients with mild pancreatitis, generally of alcoholic etiology. The authors found that the enteral route was safe and there were no differences in clinical or biochemical resolution of pancreatitis in their study patients. However, the cost of nutritional intervention in the enteral group was significantly lower than the parenteral group.[25]

A study by Olah and colleagues is unique in that it is the only randomized study to demonstrate a decreased mortality with enteral nutrition over parenteral nutrition. In addition, they demonstrated a significant decrease in infected pancreatic necrosis with jejunal feeding. The study was limited because many patients with mild pancreatitis were enrolled in the parenteral nutrition group and a substantially lower caloric intake was seen in the enteral group. Furthermore, an undisclosed number of patients were excluded because of technical difficulty with jejunal feeding tube placement.[26]

Kalfarentzos and colleagues also performed a randomized prospective trial of enteral vs. parenteral feeding in severe acute pancreatitis (APACHE II score 8–15). They not only showed that enteral feeding was safe, but also showed that these patients had a significantly lower septic complication rate than the parenteral nutrition group. Other morbidities, including the incidence of infectious pancreatic or peripancreatic necrosis, were also lower in the enteral nutrition group but did not reach statistical significance, probably because of the small numbers of patients in the groups.[27] Abou-Assi randomized patients to hypocaloric jejunal feeding or parenteral nutrition. This study demonstrated a decrease length of hospitalization, duration of feeding, and overall decrease in nutrition costs per patient with enteral nutrition. This study again confirms the safety of enteral feeding in acute pancreatitis and suggests that hypocaloric feeding may be adequate.[28]

Gupta et al. also confirmed a shorter length of hospitalization with enteral nutrition, while Louie and colleagues confirmed the cost-effectiveness of enteral nutrition in severe acute pancreatitis.[29,30]

An additional question is whether the enteral route, by stimulating trophic factors that can potentially maintain the integrity of the gut as a barrier against bacterial translocation, is beneficial to patient care in ways that are not realized with parenteral nutrition. The issue of translocation in other predisposing states such as trauma and sepsis has been more readily proven in animal models than in humans.[31,32] The proof that this process is clinically significant in humans is less established.[33] The causative bacteria in infected pancreatic necrosis are often of gut origin and translocation of bacteria and/or endotoxins can contribute to the inflammatory process.[34–36] Available clinical studies suggest that enteral nutrition in pancreatitis appears to be safe and offers cost savings and fewer septic complications. It should be considered strongly as the treatment of choice in these patients. If it also decreases the incidence of infected pancreatic necrosis, which is associated with a significantly increased morbidity and mortality, it moves out of the realm of purely nutritional support and into that of therapeutic intervention.

The study by Windsor and colleagues examined the immunoinflammatory response and its relationship to nutritional outcome with enteral feeding. In addition to finding that enteral nutrition was associated with decreases in sepsis and multiorgan failure (though not significant), the authors also reported significant decreases in the APACHE II scores for enterally fed patients (11 to 2) vs. parenterally fed patients (12 to 10). They also reported moderate decreases in C-reactive protein (CRP). There were significant increases in IgM antiendotoxin response in parenterally fed patients, whereas these levels remained unchanged in the enterally fed patients. Their data support enteral feeding as an intervention that will improve disease severity and clinical outcome by modifying the acute-phase response. Moreover, their findings lend support to the concept that enteral feeding maintains the integrity of the gut as a barrier against translocation, which can be a contributor to the inflammatory response seen in this disease.[37]

In efforts to draw appropriate conclusions based on this variety of investigations, McClave and colleagues performed a meta-analysis of these seven studies.[38] They reached the following conclusions:

1. Data is limited to assess the difference between standard therapy and specialized nutrition therapy in acute pancreatitis.
2. When initiating specialized nutritional therapy, enteral nutrition is the preferred route of administration.
3. Parenteral nutrition initiated early in the course of hospitalization (within 24 to 48 h) may worsen the outcome of patients compared with standard therapy and should be ideally initiated 5 days after admission.
4. The addition of glutamine to parenteral nutrition may improve outcome and should be considered.

In light of this increased evidence showing that enteral nutrition is safe and beneficial, it will hopefully begin to completely supplant parenteral nutrition in the management of severe acute pancreatitis.

Despite this data, the predominant specialized nutritional therapy in most hospitals and medical centers is parenteral nutrition. Knowledge of the appropriate use and the individual components of the parenteral solution becomes a mainstay in treating patients with severe disease.

Parenteral nutrition issues include:

1. **Which patients are candidates for parenteral nutrition?** Candidates are those who have severe disease (as assessed by severity scores), those who are malnourished upon admission to the hospital, and those who have complications of their disease.
2. **Delivery volume; total calories; individual macronutrients, micronutrients, and other additives.**
   a. *Fluid volume.* Pancreatitis has been compared to an internal burn with tremendous shifts in fluid. Recent data suggest that the level of hemoconcentration seen at presentation may have prognostic significance in acute pancreatitis. This not only suggests that relative hypovolemia may contribute to pancreatic damage but also underscores the importance of fluid resuscitation. However, as renal, lung, and cardiac dysfunction can accompany severe pancreatic insult, vigorous or inadequate use of fluids can a detrimental to the patient. Though fluid resuscitation is important, total volume replacement is not an essential goal of parenteral nutrition in a severe, acute setting. At our institution, the volume of solution is based on providing 20 to 35 cc of fluid/kg estimated dry weight of the patient. Additionally, adjustments are made for the presence of heart or renal failure or, conversely, for the presence of increased fluid loss or sequestration. Usually only 1 l of the solution is infused the first day to determine the patient's metabolic response to the infused nutrients. Care should be taken to ensure against metabolic aberrations. Additional volume for resuscitation can be delivered through peripheral intravenous fluids.
   b. *Calories.* When estimating the total calories provided to the patient, consider that a significant percentage of patients with pancreatitis are hypermetabolic. However, the same factor, the inflammatory response that increases the metabolic rate in these patients, also introduces an element of substrate intolerance. This intolerance, which is mainly to carbohydrates but is also to a lesser degree to lipids, is not specific to pancreatitis but is a feature of any significant inflammatory response. Similarly, if renal failure or encephalopathy are present, the provision of protein also needs careful monitoring. Additionally, the hypermetabolism seen with an acute insult should be considered dynamic and can decrease or increase during the hospitalization, roughly paralleling the patient's clinical course.

      The most reliable indicator of caloric needs in the hospital setting is indirect calorimetry. If this is not available, then formula equations can be used to estimate needs, although these are less reliable. These equations were developed in healthy individuals and are secondarily extrapolated to the severely ill. There may be a significant under- or overestimation of metabolic needs in the individual patient. The first tenet in treating these patients is to do no harm. Therefore, although targets for estimating needs may be logically derived or measured, pushing macronutrient delivery to hyperglycemia or hyperlipidemia, especially in the setting of pancreatitis, is clearly not in the patient's best interest.
   c. *Protein.* Although amino acids may be the most important macronutrient provided, there is little data to support an optimal amount. In studies of parenteral nutrition in pancreatitis, the protein provided ranged from 1 to 2.5 g/kg.[22,25,27,37] In the setting of renal impairment or encephalopathy, the protein load needs to be conservative and monitored closely. Conversely, if protein losses seem very high, protein should move toward the higher end of the range provided there are no intolerances. In this case, it is appropriate to initiate a more conservative amount of protein and advance only after the patient demonstrates stability to the initial protein load.

      It is controversial whether protein calories should be considered as part of total calories. Parenterally provided protein is not intended to be a caloric source; yet, there is partial metabolism. Thus, including protein in the caloric goal will likely result in an underestimation of calories, whereas the opposite will result if protein is calculated separately. However, as the caloric content of the provided protein is usually modest and as more harm, in the form of metabolic intolerances, is likely from providing too many calories, protein calories should be included in total calories.

d. *Fat*. It has been used reluctantly in acute pancreatitis. This stems in part from animal and human experimental studies, which show conflicting evidence of the ability of intravenous fat to stimulate the pancreas.[39,40] Additionally, hyperlipidemia with triglyceride levels of greater than 1000 mg/ml appear to be etiologic in some causes of pancreatitis.[41] Furthermore, in 12 to 15% of cases of acute pancreatitis, there appears to be an associated hypertriglyceridemia.[42] In a retrospective study of lipid infusion in acute pancreatitis, no untoward effect occurred as a result of lipid infusion. This was noted in spite of two patients who survived the acute attack and had triglyceride levels in the low to mid-300 mg/ml range. In that study, patients who did not survive had a significantly higher plasma triglyceride level than those who survived. Additionally, lipid oxidation was apparently not affected despite elevated triglyceride levels. It therefore seems that lipids can be safely infused in patients with acute pancreatitis that is not secondary to hyperlipidemia. In the setting of hypertriglyceridemia secondary to pancreatitis, continued lipid infusion was safe in spite of at least one patient with a total parenteral nutrition (preTPN) triglyceride level of 880 mg/dl. During TPN, the level decreased to the mid- to low-400 range.[39–41,43–45] It is prudent to monitor triglyceride levels closely and avoid the use of parenteral lipids until levels are below 400 mg/ml. Several studies suggest that parenteral fat can be utilized in the absence of high triglyceride levels, although no large prospective study has specifically addressed this issue.[40] This finding is of particular importance given the increased incidence of glucose intolerance in acute pancreatitis. Thus, in this setting, the use of parenteral fat at 1 to 2 g/kg, not to exceed 40% of the nonprotein calories, appears to be safe.

e. *Carbohydrates*. Early studies looking at the delivery of carbohydrates to stressed patients suggest that amounts greater than 5 mg/kg min are associated with an increased respiratory quotient (RQ).[46] In other words, carbohydrates delivered above this infusion rate resulted in lipogenesis with a high ratio of CO_2 production to O_2 consumption, thus elevating the RQ. As carbohydrates are provided to the patient for oxidative utilization, lipogenesis represents inappropriate carbohydrate utilization. Thus, 5 mg/kg day should represent the ceiling of carbohydrate utilization. Hyperglycemia should also be taken into consideration in determining the maximal rate of carbohydrate delivered. Hyperglycemia implies impaired clearance or oxidative utilization of the provided glucose and should be avoided. This metabolic abnormality can further lead to fluid and electrolyte problems and has been implicated in immune dysfunction, potentially complicating the underlying clinical situation.

NUTRITIONAL INTERVENTION IN PANCREATIC INSUFFICIENCY

Pancreatic insufficiency occurs when enzyme secretion from the pancreas falls below 10% of normal values. Insufficiency becomes clinically manifest in the form of fat malabsorption, steatorrhea, and, to a lesser extent, protein malabsorption or azotorrhea. The treatment of pancreatic insufficiency involves the use of exogenous pancreatic enzymes. Fat is the most predominant malabsorbed macronutrient in pancreatic insufficiency. Synthesis of lipase is compromised to a greater degree than synthesis of other pancreatic enzymes, there is less extrapancreatic compensation for fat absorption, and lipase inactivation is greater than inactivation in the other enzymes.[47] Replacement therapy is usually based on providing at least 28,000 IU of lipase per meal, but much higher doses are often needed.[43,44] As preparations vary in their enzyme amounts, particular attention should be given to the lipase activity (Table 63.2). In spite of providing oral replacement of pancreatic enzymes in various forms, total abolition of steatorrhea is seldom achieved.

There are multiple reasons for replacement enzymes not normalizing fat malabsorption. The most important is the sensitivity of lipase to inactivation by gastric acid. This factor leads to the coadministration of the initial conventional preparations with bicarbonate and, later, acid suppressive agents. This maneuver further improved but did not completely abolish steatorrhea. In a continuing effort to improve the efficacy of these preparations, the enzymes were packed into enteric-coated microspheres, 1 to 2 mm in size, to protect the enzymes from inactivation by gastric acid. The enzymes were liberated at an alkaline pH. Additionally, the sizes of the particle were engineered to optimize emptying from the stomach. Granules greater than 2 mm may not empty from the stomach at the same time as the meal, and therefore will not result in optimal mixing of enzyme with food. In spite of these apparent technologic advances, steatorrhea persisted. One proposed problem was continued poor mixing of enzymes with their intended substrate. This could occur secondary to poor emptying of enzyme from the stomach or a discrepancy between emptying of food and enzyme from the stomach.[9,48]

A contributing reason for poor substrate/enzyme mixing was recently reported by Guarner et al., who found increased amounts of lipase in the ileum. The authors hypothesized that this was due to poor alkalization of the proximal bowel in patients with a diseased pancreas and hence diminished bicarbonate secretion. The enzymes were not liberated until the more distal bowel, thus potentially diminishing their interaction with nutrients.[9] Additionally, because of the acidification seen in the proximal small bowel of patients with chronic pancreatitis, there may be precipitation of bile acids. This serves to decrease effective micelle formation, hence retarding fat absorption.

Usually patients should take two to seven enteric-coated capsules or five to eight non-enteric-coated tablets of an enzyme preparation with meals. Some patients using conventional preparations may need adjuvant acid suppressive therapy (see earlier discussion). A favorable response to therapy is evidenced by a decrease in steatorrhea, relief of diarrhea, and weight gain.

TABLE 63.2

List of Pancreatic Replacement Enzymes and Strengths of Major Constituents

Enzyme Preparation	Description	Lipase	Protease	Amylase	Starting Dosage
Viokase	Noncoated	8,000	30,000	30,000	1–3 tablets with meals
Cotazym	Noncoated	8,000	30,000	30,000	1–2 tablets with meals
Donnazyme	Gastric soluble/pancreatin	1,000	12,500	12,500	2 tablets with meals
Zymase	Enteric-coated (EC) spheres	12,000	24,000	24,000	1–2 tablets with meals
Creon	EC minimicrospheres				
5		5,000	18,750	16,600	2–4 tablets with meals
10		10,000	37,500	33,200	1–2 tablets with meals
20		20,000	75,000	66,400	1 tablets with meals
Pancrease	EC microtablets				
4		4,000	12,000	12,000	400 units of lipase per kg per meal
10		10,000	30,000	30,000	400 units of lipase per kg per meal
16		16,000	48,000	48,000	400 units of lipase per kg per meal
20		20,000	44,000	56,000	400 units of lipase per kg per meal
Ultrase	EC minitablets				
12		12,000	39,000	39,000	1–2 tablets with meals
18		18,000	58,500	58,500	
20		20,000	65,000	65,000	

Note: Recommendations are to start with lowest dose that controls symptoms and adjust upward as indicated to a maximum between 2000 and units of lipase/kg per meal.

If the patient does not respond to this intervention, then either a lower-fat diet (not to exceed 60 g fat/day) or evaluation of other potential contributing causes of steatorrhea, such as bacterial overgrowth, need to be considered. Of interest, generic brands of enteric enzymes may not contain bioequivalent amounts of enzymes as the name brand.[48]

NUTRITIONAL INTERVENTION IN PANCREATIC CANCER

Nutritional intervention in patients with pancreatic cancer is often frustrating as these patients proceed down the pathway of progressive malnutrition. In this disease, it is estimated that 89% of the patients have experienced weight loss at the time of diagnosis.[49] Ultimately, their demise is as much a function of their nutritional status as their underlying malignancy. The ability to provide effective nutrition should improve the quality of life for these patients. The reasons for weight loss are attributed to anorexia, with secondary decreased food intake, abnormal metabolism, and malabsorption. One study suggested that malabsorption is the most important cause of weight loss in this patient population.[50]

Even when intake can be increased in cancer patients, nutritional gains are minimal. A study by Ovesen assessed the role of frequent nutritional counseling on oral intake, anthropometrics, response to chemotherapy, survival, and quality of life in patients with pancreatic and other malignancies. Although counseling effectively increased energy and protein intake, there were no significant gains in weight or lean body mass during the 5-month protocol. Additionally, overall survival, quality of life, and tumor response rate were not significantly different.[51]

Cytokines may play an important role in weight loss and, equally important, the inability to accrue lost lean body tissue in the presence of artificial nutrition. A recent study examined the presence of an acute-phase response as an indicator of the effects of proinflammatory cytokines in patients with pancreatic cancer. Patients with an acute-phase protein response (APPR) (defined as a CRP level of greater than 10 mg/l) had a substantial reduction in food intake (approximately 29%). The group with the higher APPR was also mildly more hypermetabolic than the group that did not exhibit this response. These factors seemed to contribute to accelerated wasting in these patients.[52] Furthermore, the ongoing utilization of amino acids for the acute-phase response as well as for other hepatic export proteins such as albumin may have a significant effect on whole-body nitrogen economy and could contribute to the loss of lean body tissue. Proinflammatory cytokine activity therefore appears to be associated not only with altered host energy metabolism but also with reduced appetite, thereby contributing to the accelerated weight loss observed with cachexia.[52]

A further study by Falconer of weight-losing patients with pancreatic cancer demonstrated that approximately half of the patients had evidence of an APPR and, in that subset of patients, the resting energy expenditure (REE) was significantly elevated. However, in that study, patients who did not demonstrate an acute-phase response also had a higher REE than similar weight-matched controls, and both subgroups of patients lost weight. The differences in weight loss between the groups were not significant. Nevertheless, the authors concluded that an inflammatory response might contribute to the hypermetabolism seen in some patients with pancreatic cancer.[53]

The APPR also was associated with a significant decline in clinical status. The authors proposed that CRP, an indicator of the acute-phase response, could be used as a variable for stratifying patients into prognostic categories. The higher the level of CRP, the poorer the prognosis.[16] The authors postulated that, as the association was so strong, this response might be a useful metabolic target for metabolic intervention in the weight-losing patient with cancer.[16]

These preliminary observations led to a study of Megace (an appetite stimulant) and ibuprofen in weight-losing cancer patients. These authors had previously performed a similar 6-week study in the same population using only Megace. In that study the authors reported a 1.7 kg weight loss during the study period. Ibuprofen was added to blunt the APPR, and in so doing, the authors reported a 1.3 kg weight gain in the same time period. The authors proposed that the addition of the nonsteroidal anti-inflammatory drug (NSAID) and the blunting of the acute-phase reaction was the only differentiating factor between the two studies and thus supported a role for these cytokines in cancer cachexia. Unfortunately, the weight gain appeared to largely be confined to adipose tissue.[54]

It has been demonstrated that a diet high in fish, specifically EPA and DHA, decreases proinflammatory cytokines (interleukins [IL] IL-1, Il-6, and tumor necrosis factor [TNF]).[55] To study how inflammatory cytokines contribute to the weight loss and cachexia in patients with pancreatic cancer, Barber and colleagues investigated the role of a nutritional supplement enriched with EPA/DHA in patients with inoperable pancreatic cancer. Performance status, appetite and weight gain all significantly increased. The increase in weight did not seem to be due to an increase in body water or fat. There was no change in the APPR, but the authors commented that, in the supplemented group, they did not find the usual increase in the APPR. Median survival was 4.1 months, which was noted to be at the upper limit of survival in chemotherapy trials in patients of similar disease severity without the concomitant side effects.[56]

Another area of interesting nutritional intervention in pancreatic cancer is retinoid supplementation. *In vitro*, retinoid treatment of human pancreatic cancer cells results in inhibition of growth, induction of cellular differentiation, and decreased adhesion to basement membranes (decreased ability to metastasize). In addition, two-thirds of patients with unresectable pancreatic cancer treated with 13-*cis*-retinoic acid and interferon demonstrate stable disease with a mean duration of 5 months.[57,58]

Although, these results are still preliminary and await randomized controlled studies, they may add hope in the nutritionally abysmal outlook of patients with pancreatic cancer.

THE ROLE OF ANTIOXIDANTS IN PANCREATIC DISEASE

The similarity between the changes seen in pancreatic tissue in acute pancreatitis and damage in other tissue known to occur as a result of oxygen radical production led researchers to postulate a role of electrophiles in the pathogenesis of acute pancreatitis. Oxygen radicals, once generated, react with all biologic substances, most readily with PUFA. As PUFA are present in high concentrations in cellular membranes, free radical attack will invariably lead to cell membrane disruption and ultimately to cell death.[59] In addition to direct tissue damage, these radicals also signal the accumulation of neutrophils. Neutrophils release various enzymes and other mediators, which can damage tissue as well as adhere to endothelium, potentially resulting in vascular plugging and further adding to the microcirculatory derangements observed in the inflammatory stage of this disease.[60] Additionally, they also release oxygen radicals, the "respiratory burst," further damaging tissue and recruiting neutrophils. This cascade can continue to upregulate, resulting in extensive tissue damage. Because of the effects of these reactive oxygen species, these substances can be viewed as triggers of various inflammatory processes. The theory of oxygen free radicals significantly contributing to the pathophysiology of acute pancreatitis was tested in animals. Most animal studies suggest the presence of these radicals in the early stages of pancreatic injury.[61] It was thus theorized that pretreatment with oxygen free radical scavengers would lessen pancreatic damage.[62-64] Though the results were mixed, it appears that pretreatment helps in some forms of pancreatic damage. However, if pancreatic injury develops too rapidly, other pathomechanisms seem to cause tissue injury, making enhanced generation of reactive oxygen metabolites ineffective. There are fewer animal studies available for treatment with scavengers after the injury, but they demonstrate that treatment after injury helps to minimize the tissue damage.

In early human studies Braganza, Guyan, and Schoenberg demonstrated increased amounts of lipid peroxidation products. This indirectly demonstrated oxygen free radical attack on cellular lipids, in the serum, bile, duodenal juice, and tissue of patients suffering from acute or recurrent pancreatitis.[65] Another study observed several antioxidant deficiencies in patients with pancreatitis, though it is not clear whether the deficiencies facilitated damage or merely were an end result of the damage.[66]

Sandilands et al. were the first to propose that antioxidants may also play a role in the pain management in chronic pancreatitis. They described four patients with significant and recurrent pain from pancreatitis in spite of both medical and surgical intervention to relieve pain. The researchers postulated that ongoing damage to the gland might be caused by free oxidant generation. They further suspected that endogenous stores of these antioxidants might be deficient. The patients were given an antioxidant supplement containing 1000 mg of selenium, 1500 IU vitamin A, 90 mg vitamin C, and 45 IU of vitamin E per tablet) varying from one to six tablets a day. Three of these patients also received methionine (2 to 4 g/day).

All patients became pain free and have remained without recurrent attacks for a follow-up period of 5 years.[67] Similar dramatic responses were reported in three patients with familial lipoprotein lipase deficiency and consequent recurrent attacks of acute pancreatitis. Lipoprotein lipase removes triglycerides from circulating lipoproteins. Absence of this enzyme leads to extremely elevated triglyceride levels. As such, many patients with this disorder are prone to recurrent pancreatitis. In a report by Heaney, three patients with lipoprotein lipase deficiency were treated with antioxidant therapy (selenium, β-carotene, vitamins C and E, and methionine). Prior to initiating antioxidant therapy, these patients had failed repeated medical and surgical interventions. After initiation of antioxidant therapy, two patients had no further episodes of pancreatitis in the next 4 to 6 years of observation (previously having between 3 and 6 episodes/year). The third patient had a dramatic reduction in pain episodes going from 10 or greater the previous 4 years to an average of 1 episode/year over the next 3 years.[68]

These are exciting examples of how nutritional intervention may not only alleviate the effects of pancreatic disease but also may have an impact on the disease itself.

REFERENCES

1. Levin RJ. In *Modern Nutrition in Health and Disease*, eds. Shils ME, Olson JA, Shike M, Ross AC. Williams and Wilkins, Ninth edition, 1999. Baltimore, MD.
2. Metzger A, DiMagno EP. In *The Pancreas*, eds. Berger HG, Warshaw AL, Buchler MW, Carr-Locke DL, Neoptolemos JP, Russel C, Sarr MG. *Blackwell Science*, 1998, p. 147. Cambridge, England.
3. Lowe ME. In *Physiology of the Gastrointestinal Tract*, eds. Johnson LR, Alpers DH, Christensen J, Jacobson ED, Walsh JH. Raven Press, 1994. New York, NY.
4. Tso P. In *Physiology of the Gastrointestinal Tract*, eds. Johnson LR, Alpers DH, Christensen J, Jacobson ED, Walsh JH. Raven Press, 1994. New York, NY.
5. Jones PJH, Kubow S. In *Modern Nutrition in Health and Disease*, eds. Shils ME, Olson JA, Shike M, Ross AC. Williams and Wilkins, Ninth edition, 1999. Baltimore MD.
6. Funnell IC, Bornman PC, Weakley SP, et al. *Br J Surg* 1993; 80: 484.
7. Martinez J, Sanchez-Paya J, Palazon JM, et al. *Pancreas* 1999; 19: 15.
8. Dickerson RN, Vehe KL, Mullen JL, et al. *Crit Care Med* 1991; 19: 484.
9. Grendell JH. *Clin Gastroenterol* 1983; 12: 551.
10. DiMagno EP, Malagelada JR, Go VL, et al. *NEJOM* 1977; 296: 1318.
11. Twersky Y, Bank S. *Gastroenterol Clin N Am* 1989; 18: 543.
12. DiMagno EP, Go VLW, Summerskill WHJ. *N Eng J Med* 1973; 288: 813.
13. Nakamura T, Takeuchi T, *Pancreas* 1997; 14: 323.
14. Hebuterne X, et al. *Dig Dis and Sci* 1996; 41: 533.
15. DeWys WD. In *Nutritional Support for the Cancer Patient*, eds. Calman KC, Fearon KCH. London: Balliere Tindall, 1986, p. 251.
16. Falconer JS, Fearon KC, Ross JA. *Cancer* 1994; 75: 2077.
17. Ranson JHC, Rifkind KM, Roses DF, et al. *SG&O* 1974; 139: 69.
18. Knaus WA, Draper EA, Wagner DP, et al. *Crit Care Med* 1985; 13: 818.
19. Balthazar EJ, Robinson DL, Megibow AJ, et al. *Radiology* 1990; 174: 331.
20. Havala T, Shronts E, Cerra F. *Gastroenterol Clin N Am* 1989; 18: 525.
21. Corcoy R, Sanchez JM, Domingo P, et al. *Nutrition* 1988; 4: 269.
22. Sax HC, Warner BW, Talamini MA, et al. *Am J Surg* 1987; 153: 117.
23. Xian-Li H, Qing-Jiu M, Jian-Guo L, et al. *Clin Nut* 2004; 1(Suppl.): 43.
24. Powell JJ, Murchison JT, Fearon KC. *Br J Surg* 2000; 87: 1375.
25. McClave SA, Greene LM, Snider HL, et al. *J Parent Enter Nutr* 1997; 21: 14.
26. Olah A, Pardavi G, Belagyi T, et al. *Nutrition* 2002; 18: 259.
27. Kalfarentzos F, Kehagias J, Mead N, et al. *Br J Surg* 1997; 84: 1665.
28. Abou-Assi S, Craig K, O'Keefe SJ. *Am J Gastroenterol* 2002; 97: 2255.
29. Gupta R, Patel K, Calder PC, et al. *Pancreatol* 2003; 3: 406.
30. Louie B, Noseworthy T, Hailey D. *Can J Surg* 2005; 48: 298.
31. Alverdy J. *Seminars in Resp Infect* 1994; 9: 248.
32. Gianotti L, Alexander JW, Nelson JL, et al. *Crit Care Med* 1994; 22: 265.
33. Sedman PC, Macfie J, Sagar P, et al. *Gastroenterol* 1994; 107: 643.
34. Luiten EJT, Hop WCJ, Lange JF et al. *Clin Infect Dis* 1997; 25:811
35. Ryan C, Schmidt J, Lewandrowski K. *Gastroenterol* 1993; 104: 890.
36. Fong Y, Marano MA, Barber A, et al. *Ann Surg* 1989; 210: 449.
37. Windsor ACJ, Kanwar S, Li ACK, et al. *Gut* 1998; 42: 431.
38. McClave SA, Chang WK, Dhaliwal RD, et al. *JPEN* 2006; 30: 143.
39. Van Gossum A, Lemoyne M, Greig PD, et al. *JPEN* 1988; 12: 250.
40. Leibowitz AB, O'Sullivan P, Iberti TJ. *Mount Sinai J Med* 1992; 59: 38.

41. Amann ST, Toskes PP. In *The Pancreas*, eds. Berger HG, Warshaw AL, Buchler MW, Carr-Locke DL, Neoptolemos JP, Russel C, Sarr MG. *Blackwell Science*, 1998, p. 311. Cambridge, England.
42. McClave SA, Snider H, Owens N, et al. *Dig Dis Sci* 1997; 42: 2035.
43. McClave SA, Spain DA, Snider HL. *Gastrol Clin N Am* 1998; 27: 421.
44. Scolapio JS, Malhi-Chowla N, Ukleja A. *Gastrol Clin N Am* 1999; 28: 695.
45. Silberman H, Dixon NP, Eisenberg D. *Am J Gastroenterol* 1982; 77: 494.
46. Burke JF, Wolfe RR, Mullany CJ. *Ann Surg* 1979; 190: 274.
47. Layer P, Holtman G. *Int J Pancreatol* 1994; 15: 1.
48. Greenberger NJ. *Gastro Clin N Am* 1999; 28: 687.
49. Guarner L, Rodriguez R, Guarner et al. *Gut* 1993; 34: 708.
50. Perez MM, Newcomer AD, Mortel CG, et al. *Cancer* 1983; 52: 346.
51. Ovesen L, Allingstrup L, Hannibal J, et al. *J Clin Oncol* 1993; 11: 2043.
52. Fearon KCH, Barber MD, Falconer JS, et al. *World J Surg* 1999; 23: 584.
53. Falconer JS, Fearon KCH, Plester CE. *Ann Surg* 1994; 219: 325.
54. McMillan DC, Gorman PO, Fearon KCH, et al. *Br J Surg* 1997; 76: 788.
55. Meydani SN, Lichtenstein AH, Cornwall S, et al. *J Clin Invest* 1993; 92: 105.
56. Barber MD, Ross JA, Voss AC. *Br J Cancer* 1999; 81: 80.
57. Riecken EO, Rosewicz S. *Ann Oncol* 1999; S10: S197.
58. Rosewicz S, Wollbergs K, Von Lampe B, et al. *Gastroenterol* 1997; 112: 532.
59. Schoenberg MH, Buchler M, Helfen M, et al. *Eur Surg Res* 1992; 24(Suppl.): 74.
60. Schoenberg MH, Birk D, Beger HG. *Am J Clin Nutr* 1995; 62: 1306S.
61. Schoenberg MH, Buchler M, Beger HG. *Free Rad Biol & Med* 1992; 12: 515.
62. Schoenberg MH, Buchler M, Younes M, et al. *Dig Dis Sci* 1994; 39: 1034.
63. Furukawa M, Kimura T, Yamaguchi, et al. *Pancreas* 1994; 9: 67.
64. Nonaka A, Manabe T, Kyogoku T, et al. *Dig Dis Sci* 1992; 37: 27
65. Schoenberg MH, Birk D. In *The Pancreas*, eds. Berger HG, Warshaw AL, Buchler MW, Carr-Locke DL, Neoptolemos JP, Russel C, Sarr MG. *Blackwell Science*, 1998, p. 702. Cambridge, England.
66. Gossum AV, Closset P, Noel E, et al. *Dig Dis Sci* 1996; 41: 1225.
67. Sandilands D, Jeffery IJM, Haboubi NY, et al. *Gastro* 1990; 98: 766.
68. Heanney AP, Sharer N, Rameh B, et al. *J Clin Endocrinol Metab* 1999; 84: 1203.
69. Linscheer WG, Vergroesen AJ. In *Modern Nutrition in Health and Disease*, eds, Shils ME, Olson JA, Shike M, Eighth edition, Philadelphia, PA: Lea & Febiger, 1994, p. 47.

64 Macromineral Nutrition, Disorders of Skeleton and Kidney Stones

Stanley Wallach and Carolyn D. Berdanier

CONTENTS

INTRODUCTION

The term *macrominerals* refers to those elements needed by the body in gram quantities on a daily basis (see: www.nap.edu). The category includes sodium, potassium, chloride, calcium, phosphorus, and magnesium. While the body content of the first three is relatively small because of high turnover, the body content of calcium and phosphorus, by comparison, is relatively large. All of these minerals serve several functions: as electrolytes, they play important roles in acid base balance and electrolyte exchange; some also serve in cell signal systems (calcium in particular), while all of them can be found in the bones and teeth.

Sodium is the major extracellular electrolyte. It has been estimated that the adult human male weighing 70 kg would contain 83 to 97 g of sodium in his body. Most of this (66 to 75%) is in the mineral apatite of the bone. The rest is in a rapidly circulating pool that exchanges with potassium in the sodium–potassium exchange system.

Potassium is the major intracellular electrolyte, and the adult male body will contain between 2 to 3 g of this macromineral. Both sodium and potassium are widely distributed in the food supply and under normal conditions; a deficiency of either (or both) is very unlikely.

Chloride is the third leg upon which osmotic pressure and acid–base balance rests. Normal blood levels vary almost not at all and range between 100 and 106 meq/l.

The fourth macromineral is calcium. It has two major functions: as the major mineral in the bones and teeth and as an intracellular messenger. A normal 70 kg man will have about 1.54 kg of calcium. Some of this calcium is in the teeth; some (very little) is in the active metabolizing cells while the vast majority is in bone. Phosphorus and magnesium are the remaining members of the macromineral group. They too are important constituents of the bones and teeth and have other metabolic roles as well.

TABLE 64.1
Skeletal Composition

Comprises 8% of body weight	
35% Organic	Type 1 collagen (90+%)
(FFDW[a])	Noncollagenous proteins: glycosaminoglycans,
	proteoglycans, glycoproteins, osteocalcin, osteonectin,
	osteopontin, bone sialoprotein, alkaline phosphatase, etc.
	Growth factors and cytokines
65% Inorganic	Hydroxyapatite: $Ca_{10}(PO_4)6(OH)_2$
(FFDW[a])	Magnesium, sodium, potassium
	Carbonate-containing salts
	Fluorine
	Deposited "heavy metals"
	Trace elements
Miscellaneous	Water
	Lipids
	Deposited molecules: tetracyclines, etc.

[a] Fat-free dry weight.

The skeleton is a complex, metabolically active tissue that serves multiple physiologic functions. However, its most important purpose is to maintain normal posture and locomotion by virtue of its hardness. This quality is conferred by a unique arrangement of plates of a calcium-phosphorus-containing mineral called hydroxyapatite [$Ca_{10}(PO_4)6(OH)_2$] interspaced within the interstices of a protein matrix composed predominately of type 1 collagen (+90%). The matrix also contains a large number of noncollagenous proteins, some of which are unique to bone (Table 64.1). This structure confers extreme hardness, but also sufficient flexibility during strain to minimize brittleness. Additional information on nutrition and the skeletal system can be found online at: http://www.surgeongeneral.gov/library

The human skeleton matures during growth and development by a process called *modeling*. During this process, the enlarging skeleton is repetitively resorbed via osteoclastic activity, and then reformed on a larger template by osteoblastic action. Once growth is complete, these same two opposing processes continue to operate in a coupled manner, so that areas of bone that have undergone microdamage due to the repetitive strain incurred by activities of daily living (plus work-related and athletic activities), can be continually replaced by new, healthy bone. This process, which predominates in the adult, is known as remodeling, and when the two opposing processes of resorption of defunct bone followed by reformation of healthy bone are qualitatively and quantitatively coupled, the skeleton retains normal strength and hardness.

BONE MINERALIZATION

About 99% of the total body calcium is found in the bones and teeth.[1–13] This calcium is part of a mineral complex that is deposited on an organic matrix comprised primarily of type I collagen.[10] Collagen has a unique amino acid composition consisting of large amounts of glycine, proline, and hydroxyproline. A single molecule of type I collagen has a molecular mass of ~285 kDa, a width of ~14 Å, and a length of ~300 Å. There are at least 17 different polypeptides that comprise the collagen molecule. The polypeptides used vary throughout the body and each collagen uses at least three of them. Collagen is about 30 to 33% glycine, with another 15 to 30% of the amino acid residues as proline and 3-, 4-, or 5-hydroxyproline. Collagen is a left-handed triple helix stabilized by hydrogen bonding. These bonds may involve bridging water molecules between the hydroxyprolines. The collagen fibrils are also held together by covalent cross-linking. These cross-links are between the side chains of lysine and histidine, and the linkage is catalyzed by the copper-dependent enzyme, lysyl oxidase. Up to four side chains can be covalently bonded to each other. All in all, the collagen provides a network of fibers upon which the crystals of hydroxyapatite [$Ca_3(PO_4)3OH$] are deposited. Hydroxyapatite is not pure calcium phosphate. Some ions (magnesium, iron, sodium, and chloride) are adsorbed onto the surface of the hydroxyapatite crystallites, while other ions (strontium, fluoride, and carbonate) are incorporated into the mineral lattice. These other ions affect the chemical and physical properties of the calcified tissue. Solubility, for example, is decreased when strontium and fluoride ions are present. Hardness is enhanced by the presence of fluoride.

Bone formation begins in the embryo and continues throughout life. The nature of the process and the cells involved change as the individual ages. Osteoprogenitor cells in early development synthesize the extracellular matrix described above and also regulate the flux of minerals into that matrix. As the calcified tissue begins to form, osteoclasts appear on the surface of this tissue, and osteoblasts connected to one another by long processes are totally surrounded by mineralizing matrix. Each type of mineralized tissue has some unique properties, but all share several histological features in the early mineralization process. Hunziker[14] has described this process in the epiphyseal growth plate during the ossification of the endochondral cartilage, as it becomes bone.

Initial mineral deposition occurs at discrete sites on membrane-bound bodies (matrix vesicles) in the extracellular matrix. These initial deposits are diffuse and lack orientation. The mineral crystals proliferate and mineralization procedes filling the longitudinal, but not the transverse, septa. Changes in the activities of enzymes, which catalyze the hydrolysis of phosphate esters and those which catalyze certain proteolytic reactions, follow or accompany this mineralization. These reactions are a prerequisite to vascular invasion. Following vascular invasion, lamellar bone is formed by osteoblasts directly on the surface of the preexisting mineralized cartilage. These osteoblasts secrete type I collagen with very little proteoglycan and few extracellular matrix vesicles. This process is repeated over and over until the bone has finished growing. At this point, the growth plate closes and the mature length and shape of the bone is apparent. The bone, however, is not metabolically inert. It continues to lose and gain mineral matter; that is, it is continuously remodeled through the action of the osteoblasts which synthesize the collagen matrix, and the osteoclasts which are stimulated by parathyroid hormone to reabsorb calcium (and other minerals) in times of need. While the number of osteoblasts declines with age, the number of osteoclasts increases, especially in postmenopausal females.[8,15] This helps to explain some of the age-related loss in bone mineral that occurs in aging females. Osteoclasts act first during bone remodeling by producing cavities on either the cortical or cancellous (trabecular) bone surfaces. When these cavities develop osteoblasts are recruited for bone remineralization, thereby filling (or refilling) the cavities. The bone matrix reforms and remineralizes as described above, resulting in new bone formation. The remodeling process is ongoing with rates of resorption equaling the rates of new bone formation as long as the hormones controlling each process are in balance and as long as the nutrients needed to support this ongoing process are provided.

Bone mass can remain constant for many decades. However, once the hormone balance changes, this constancy changes.[4,12,15] In females, bone mass declines by an estimated 1 to 2% per year after menopause. In senile men, bone mass loss also occurs. In fact, both senile males and females experience about a 1% loss per year. Not only is there a loss in bone mass but also in structural integrity. The bones lose their mineral apatite, become porous (osteoporosis), and as well lose the architecture upon which the mineral has rested. The very compact cortical portions of the bone disappear, leaving a fragile, largely trabecular bone. The result of these changes is a fragile skeletal system subject to non-trauma-related fracture.

While the importance of appropriate hormone balance (parathyroid hormone, calcitonin, active vitamin D, and estrogen) cannot be overemphasized, it should also be recognized that dietary calcium (as well as phosphorus and other nutrients) plays an important role in the maintenance of bone mass. Intakes at or exceeding 800 mg/day have been shown to counteract the age-related loss in bone mass.[8] Dietary protein also is an essential nutrient for bone health.[9]

METABOLIC BONE DISEASES

The term *metabolic bone disease* refers to an aberration in this orderly cascade, which disturbs normal skeletal modeling or remodeling. In addition, bone mineralization, which follows reformation of the matrix, also an osteoblastic controlled function, can be involved. Table 64.2 gives examples of the more common disturbances leading to metabolic bone diseases. However, there are literally hundreds of rare, genetically related metabolic bone diseases as well; some examples are given in Table 64.3.

The coupling of bone resorption, formation, and mineralization is normally orchestrated and modulated by a large repertoire of hormones, growth factors, resorptive cytokines, and miscellaneous risk factors (Table 64.4 and Table 64.5) that determine ultimate bone mass and anatomy, and resistance to fracture during casual trauma. Nutritional status is key to normal interactions among these factors; in the evaluation of individuals in whom skeletal integrity is a clinical issue, consideration of dietary

---

TABLE 64.2
Metabolic Bone Diseases

Disturbances in Orderly Sequence of Skeletal Turnover:
Resorption–Formation–Mineralization
Examples:
↓ resorption: osteopetrosis
↓ formation: osteogenesis imperfecta
↓ mineralization: osteomalacia
↑ resorption: skeletal hyperparathyroidism
↑ resorption, ↑ formation: Paget's disease
↑ resorption, ↓ formation: osteoporosis

TABLE 64.3
Examples of Genetic Mutations Causing Metabolic Bone Diseases

Enzyme Defects
Carbonic anhydrase II: Osteopetrosis
1-hydroxylase (25-OH-D): Vitamin D-dependent rickets

Receptor Defects
PTH-PTH-related protein receptor: Jensen's metaphyseal chondrodysplasia
Fibroblast growth factor 3 receptor: Achondroplasia
Calcium sensing receptor: Familial hypocalciuric hypercalcemia (inactivating)
Calcium sensing receptor: Autosomal dominant hypoparathyroidism (activating)
Vitamin D receptor: Vitamin D resistance syndromes

Signaling Mechanism Defects
Gs protein excess: McCune-Albright syndrome
Gs protein deficiency: Pseudohypoparathyroidism

Structural Gene Defects
Type I collagen genes: Osteogenesis imperfecta
Bone morphogenetic protein 4: Fibrodysplasia ossificans progressiva (activating)

TABLE 64.4
Hormone, Growth Factor, and Cytokine Effects on Bone

Hormones:
Parathyroid Hormone (PTH): biphasic effects
Low-dose: ↑↑ trabecular bone formation
↑ cortical bone formation
High-dose: ↑↑ cortical bone resorption
↑ trabecular bone resorption
Vitamin D metabolites: promote calcium absorption and bone mineralization; can also
  increase bone resorption (high doses)
Calcitonin: inhibits bone resorption and stimulates bone formation
Corticosteroids: inhibit bone formation and secondarily stimulate bone resorption
Gonadal steroids: inhibit bone resorption and stimulate bone formation
Thyroid hormones: increase bone turnover primarily by stimulating bone resorption
Growth hormones: stimulate bone formation and stimulate bone resorption (high doses)
Insulin: stimulates bone formation
Prolactin: inhibits bone formation

Growth factors:
IGF-1[a] (somatomedin) and IGF-2[a]: stimulate bone formation and inhibit bone resorption
Transforming growth factor-b: stimulates bone formation and inhibits bone resorption
Bone morphogenetic proteins: stimulate bone formation
Fibroblast growth factor: increases bone formation
Platelet-derived growth factor: stimulates bone formation and inhibits bone resorption
Interleukin-1 receptor antagonist: opposes interleukin-1-induced bone resorption
Other interleukin inhibitors: oppose interleukin-induced bone resorption
Prostate carcinoma factor: theoretic stimulator of bone formation
Prostaglandins: biphasic effects to stimulate both bone formation and resorption

Cytokines:
Interleukins 1, 4, 6, 11: stimulate bone resorption
Tumor necrosis factor: stimulates bone resorption
Lymphotoxin: stimulates bone resorption
Granulocyte/macrophage-CSF[b] and other CSFs[b]: stimulate bone resorption
Prostaglandins: biphasic effects to stimulate both bone formation and resorption
Leptin: stimulates bone mineralization

[a] Insulin-like growth factor.
[b] Colony stimulating factor.

TABLE 64.5
Risk Factors for Bone Loss

Genetic:

Female sex
    Caucasian/Asian ethnicity
    Family history of osteoporosis

Life style:

Low calcium and protein intake
    Excessive alcohol use
    Cigarette smoking
    Excessive caffeine use
    Extreme or insufficient athletism
    Excessive acid ash diet (high protein/soft drink intake)

Medical:

Early menopause
    Gonadal hormone deficiency
    Eating disorders
    Chronic liver/kidney disease
    Malabsorption syndromes

Iatrogenic:

Corticosteroids
    Excessive thyroid hormone
    Chronic heparin therapy
    Radiotherapy to skeleton
    Long-term anticonvulsants
    Loop diuretics

---

status should take primacy, since all other interactions will be adversely affected by uncorrected dietary deficiencies. Table 64.1 also contains a concise list of macro- and micronutrients present in the skeleton, which are considered to have a role in skeletal modeling and remodeling. Many of the micronutrients listed have been shown to exert skeletal effects only in experimental systems, and do not as yet have a proven role in human skeletal metabolism.

CALCIUM AND VITAMIN D

Obviously, calcium leads any list of macronutrients, since it is most abundant in bone; the skeleton accounts for greater than 90% of body calcium content. The gastrointestinal (GI) absorption of calcium is affected by a large number of factors such as transit time, mucosal competence, and calcium binding by phosphates, oxalate, and fiber, among others. However, vitamin D is the dominant factor influencing calcium absorption since its active metabolite, 1,25-dihydroxy-vitamin D (calcitriol) stimulates production of a specific calcium-binding protein in mucosal cells, which facilitates transcellular transport of calcium through the GI mucosa. The metabolic cascade involved in vitamin D activation is shown in Figure 64.1 and brings out the point that inadequate vitamin D precursors from the diet, inadequate actinic stimulation of skin precursors of vitamin D, and deficits in mucosal, hepatic, or renal handling of vitamin D metabolism can strongly alter vitamin D economy and in turn lead to calcium deficiency. This is especially true for older persons in whom several age-related deficits in vitamin D metabolism and action are common (Table 64.6). Table 64.7 gives the recommended daily intakes of calcium and vitamin D in normal individuals of various ages. Since the average nondairy diet contains only 300 to 500 mg of calcium, the intentional use of calcium-rich foods daily (Table 64.8) is necessary to meet requirements. Alternately, dietary supplements containing calcium are required. Vitamin D is in even shorter supply, since the only adequate food source is fortified milk (100 IU per 8 oz). Therefore, direct sunlight, which does not have the ultraviolet spectrum screened out, and a large milk intake are required. Since this is rarely the case in adults, supplements containing vitamin D should be advocated. In individuals with GI, hepatic, or renal deficits, calcium and vitamin D nutrition may have to be further augmented and monitored by measurements of calcium, vitamin D metabolite, and parathyroid hormone levels. When significant hepatic and renal disease are present, it may be necessary to substitute vitamin D metabolites such as 25, hydroxy-vitamin D (calcifidiol) or 1,25-dihydroxy-vitamin D (calcitriol) for vitamin D. These are prescription drugs and require physician participation in the patient's care. The essentials of adjusting the average patient's intakes of calcium and vitamin D are given in Table 64.9. Vitamin D can be in the form of either cholecalciferol (D_3) or ergocalciferol (D_2).

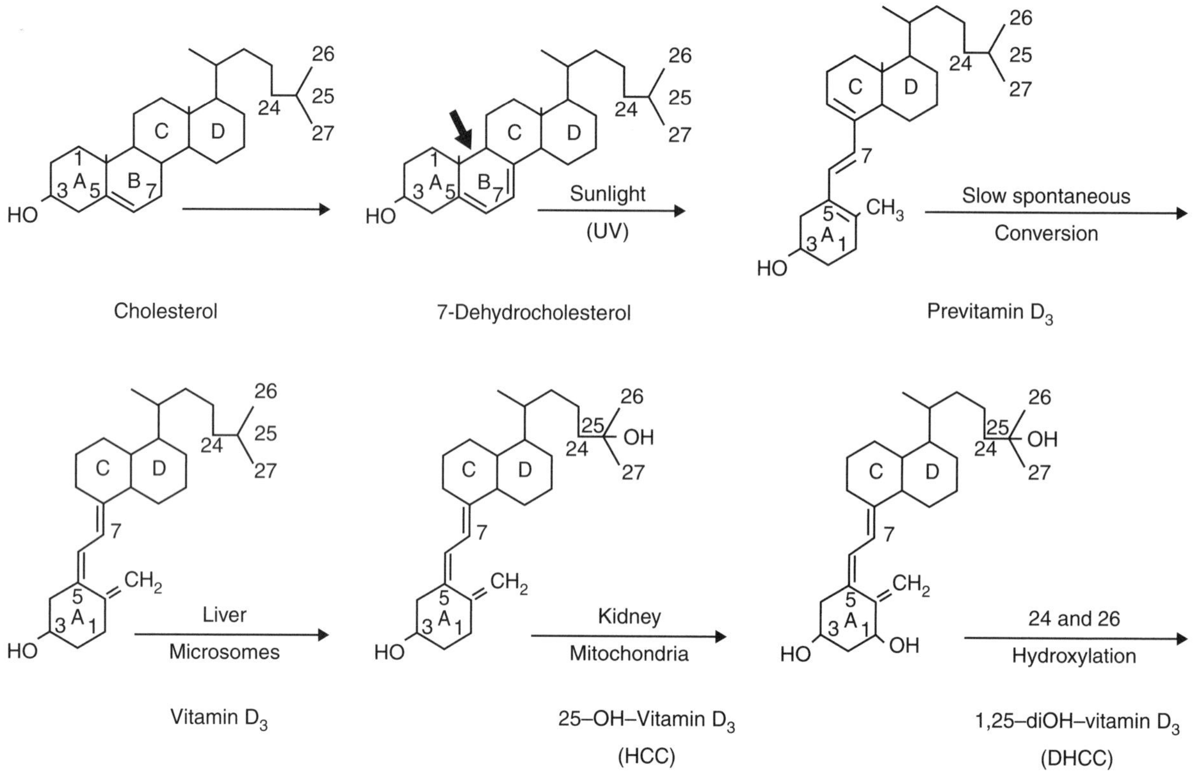

FIGURE 64.1 Conversion cascade for the synthesis of the active metabolite of vitamin D, 1,25-dihydroxy-cholecalciferol (DHCC) from cholesterol. The first three steps take place in the dermis, after which hydroxylations occur in the liver and kidney, respectively. Ingested vitamins D_2 and D_3 enter the cascade as per the lower portion of the figure.

TABLE 64.6
Vitamin D Deficits in Older Patients

Reduced oral intake	Less dairy intake and lactose intolerance
Reduced dermal production	Less sunlight exposure, pollution, sunscreens and intrinsic defect in 7-dehydrocholesterol conversion
Reduced hydroxylation (25 and 1μ)	Age-related declines in hepatic and renal function
Other factors	Anticonvulsants, renal insufficiency, Billroth II surgery, etc.

Another issue is whether to use carbonate- or citrate-based calcium supplements. Both types offer sufficient calcium absorption to be recommended, but in selected patients, one or the other may be preferred (Table 64.10).

OTHER MACRONUTRIENTS

Other macronutrients critical to the skeleton include phosphorus (phosphate), magnesium, protein, and lipids. The average American who is not a vegetarian uses meat, dairy products, and phosphoric acid-containing beverages so that phosphorus intake is sufficient, and no additional supplements are required. In fact, excess phosphorus should be avoided since it may increase bone resorption by stimulating excess parathyroid hormone (PTH) secretion. Calcium phosphate supplements as a calcium source are not desirable, not only because of a possible stimulatory effect on PTH, but also because the excess phosphate may excessively bind calcium in the GI tract. Excess phosphate may also combine with calcium internally, and facilitate its removal from the circulation by deposition within soft tissues and on bone surfaces. The latter does not necessarily contribute to bone integrity, except in undermineralized bone (osteomalacia) in which a high phosphorus intake is often beneficial.

TABLE 64.7
Revised Recommended Daily Calcium and Vitamin D Intakes

Age	Amount of Calcium (mg)	Vitamin D (Units)
Infants		
Birth to 6 months	400	200
6 months to 1 year	600	400
Children to young adults		
1–10 years	800–1200	400
11–24 years	1200–1500	400
Adult women		
Pregnant and lactating		
Under age 24	1200–1500	400
Over age 24	1200	400
25–49 years (premenopausal)	1000	400
50–64 years (postmenopausal, taking estrogen)	1000	600–800
50–64 years (postmenopausal, not taking estrogen)	1500	600–800
65+ years	1500	600–800
Adult men		
25–64 years	1000	400
65+ years	1500	600–800

TABLE 64.8
Calcium-Rich Foods

Food	Calcium Content (mg)
Skim milk, 1/2 pint (8 oz)	300
Calcium enriched orange juice (6 oz)	260
Ice cream, 1 cup soft serve	240
Calcium enriched juice, 1 glass (8 oz)	225
Fruit yogurt, low fat 8 oz cup	340
Frozen yogurt, 8 oz cup	200
Mozzarella cheese, 1 oz	210
Cheddar cheese, 1 oz	200
Cottage cheese, 2% fat, 4 oz serving	75
Tofu, 4 oz serving	110
Salmon, canned, with bones, 3 oz	170
Sardines, canned, with bones, 3 oz	370
Bok choy, raw, 1 cup	75
Broccoli, raw, 1 cup	140
Collards, 1 cup	370
Kale, frozen, cooked, 1 cup	180

TABLE 64.9
Essentials of Adjusting Calcium and Vitamin D Intakes

Quantitate patient's Ca and vitamin D intakes from the patient's food sources
Determine difference between patient's requirements and actual food source intake
Prescribe daily multivitamin or vitamin D capsule, containing 400 IU
Prescribe $CaCO_3$ or Ca citrate in needed amount but use products that also contain vitamin D
Calculate total intakes of Ca and vitamin D from all sources to verify amount to be taken

TABLE 64.10

Comparison of Carbonate and Citrate-Based Calcium Supplements

	CaCO$_3$	Ca Citrate
Calcium content per pill	250–600 mg	250–315 mg
Vitamin D content per pill	Up to 200 IU	Up to 200 IU
Pill size	Medium	Large
Average Ca absorption	25–30%	30–40%
Solubility	Requires gastric HCl[a] (take with meals)	Does not require gastric HCl[a]
Special problems	Fe deficiency may occur (FeCO$_3$ insolubility)	
Constipation	Extreme achlorhydria, H$_2$ blockers, proton pump inhibitors may make Ca absorption uncertain	Pill may be difficult to swallow[b]
		May require more than 2 pills per day

[a] Hydrochloric acid.

[b] Disintegrates in tap water.

TABLE 64.11

Magnesium Effects on the Skeleton

Promotes matrix formation
Increases mineral content
Increases trabecular bone
Increases mechanical strength
Bone crystal destabilization (in excess)

TABLE 64.12

Magnesium-Rich Foods

Food	Quantity	Content (mg)
Amaranth, buckwheat	1 cup	300–500
Nuts	1 cup	350–420
Brown rice, unrefined corn products	1 cup	50–320
Other whole grains	1 cup	50–160
Beans (including soy beans)	1 cup	50–150
Tofu	1/2 cup	120
Fish and seafood	3.5 oz	30–150
Avocado	1	70–105
Dark green vegetables	1 cup	25–150
Animal milk products (including yogurt)	1 cup	25–70
Dried fruits	100 g	50

The value of magnesium (Mg) in enhancing or maintaining skeletal vitality is controversial.[16–22] *In vitro* and in animal models, Mg exerts the actions indicated in Table 64.11. However, in humans, insufficient studies exist to date to verify comparable actions under clinical conditions. Since the U.S. population on the whole has only borderline Mg sufficiency, because of its relatively low concentration in common foodstuffs (Table 64.12), there is some justification in ensuring an adequate Mg intake by the use of supplements (MgO, MgCl$_2$, or Mg-amino/acids salts). However, a superphysiologic amount of magnesium has no scientific basis.

The need for adequate protein of high biologic value to ensure adequate production of bone collagen and noncollagenous bone proteins is obvious. Patients with eating disorders and protein-calorie malnutrition uniformly have deficient skeletons. Perhaps less appreciated is emerging information as to the role of lipids in skeletal metabolism, as summarized in Table 64.13. Most of these basic findings have not been translated into human investigations.

TABLE 64.13
Lipid Effects on the Skeleton

Endogenous

Prostaglandins	Biphasic effects
	Low dose: stimulates bone formation
	High dose: inhibits bone formation, stimulates bone resorption
Leukotrienes	Stimulate bone resorption

Exogenous

N-3 fatty acids	Stimulate bone formation
Conjugated linoleic acid	Inhibits bone formation
Saturated fats	Increase bone formation, but also increase cortical porosity

TABLE 64.14
Nutrient, Vitamin, and Trace Element Effects on the Skeleton

Other Nutrients	*Effect*
Fiber[a]	Impairs calcium, lipid, and fat soluble vitamin absorption
Caffeine[a]	Decreases bone formation and increases urinary calcium loss
Acid-containing foods and beverages[a]	Increase bone resorption
Alcohol[a]	Decreases bone formation, prevents calcium absorption and increases urinary calcium loss
Isoflavonoids	Decrease bone resorption, through estrogen-like properties
Vitamins	
A[a]	Increases bone resorption when in excess
C	Promotes bone formation
E	Increases bone formation
K	Promotes bone mineralization
Beneficial Trace Elements	
Boron	May enhance estrogen effects on bone
Zinc	Growth factor for the skeleton
Copper	Stimulates cross links in bone and adds strength
Silicon	Enhances skeletal mineralization
Vanadium	Enhances skeletal mineralization
Selenium	Cofactor for maturation of cartilage
Manganese	Promotes skeletal growth
Strontium[a]	Stimulates bone formation
Fluoride[a]	Stimulates bone formation but can increase brittleness if in excess
Detrimental Trace Elements	
Lithium	Causes hyperparathyroidism-related bone resorption
Aluminum	Impairs bone formation and mineralization and increases bone resorption
Iron	Decreases bone formation and mineralization and increases bone resorption
Molybdenum	Causes skeletal deformities
Cadmium	Decreases bone formation and mineralization and increases bone resorption
Tin	Impairs modeling sequence
Lead	Decreases bone formation and mineralization and increases bone resorption

[a] Beneficial nutrients known to be deleterious to the skeleton if taken in excess amounts.

MICRONUTRIENTS[23–27]

Several nutrients that are variable components of the human diet can have important influences on the skeleton, affecting calcium metabolism or the skeleton directly (Table 64.14). Excess fiber, caffeine, and acid-containing foods and beverages, all have negative effects, whereas the isoflavones and related compounds present in various foods are "weak estrogens" and exert a positive effect. Alcohol is technically not a nutrient, but is so ubiquitous in the human diet as to be considered so. It has multiple adverse actions, as noted.

Aside from vitamin D, four other vitamins have been shown to have an influence on the skeleton (Table 64.14). Vitamin A in excess and its more powerful retinoic acid derivatives (used to treat acne, other dermatologic conditions, and certain neoplasms) are powerful stimulators of the osteoclast and can cause bone loss and even hypercalcemia. Vitamin C, on the other hand, is an osteoblast promoter, and severe deficiency is sufficient to cause borderline scurvy accompanied by bony lesions. Vitamin E also increases experimental bone formation, but its clinical significance has not been established. Vitamin K, as a cofactor for gamma-hydroxylation, is responsible for the production of osteocalcin, a noncollagenous matrix protein. Low vitamin K levels have been reported in some osteoporotics, and associations between this vitamin and bone health have been reported.[28,29] A large number of trace elements have either positive or negative effects on the skeleton, but the majority are of interest in experimental systems and have no proven benefits or dangers to patients (Table 64.14). Strontium supplementation has been studied in osteoporotics and has been shown to enhance bone density. Lithium, used in the treatment of bipolar disorder, can stimulate the parathyroid glands to excessive activity with increased bone resorption and hypercalcemia. Aluminum overload can occur in chronic renal failure through the use of aluminum-containing antacids and other oral sources or the use of aluminum-contaminated renal dialysis fluid. Aluminum toxicity impairs bone formation and mineralization as well as stimulating bone resorption, and is usually manifested in chronic renal failure patients as a resistant osteomalacia, or so-called aplastic bone disease. Iron overload, as occurs in hemochromatosis of both primary and secondary etiologies, hemolytic anemias, and some cases of chronic renal failure, uniformly decreases bone formation and mineralization with measurable bone loss, which can be severe enough to cause osteoporosis. In some cases, increased bone resorption has been observed, and in chronic renal failure, iron overload can simulate aluminum toxicity. In postmenopausal women on hormone replacement therapy, dietary iron positively influences bone mineral density.[30] Cadmium toxicity, which occurs mainly in individuals with industrial exposure, has similar manifestations to iron overload but tends to present itself as defective mineralization, with predominant osteomalacia. Lead toxicity has similar effects to iron and cadmium but rarely shows skeletal manifestations comparable to its central nervous system(CNS), hematological, and other soft tissue toxicity.

NUTRITIONAL RECOMMENDATIONS IN METABOLIC BONE DISEASES

OSTEOPOROSIS[31–34]

Bone loss sufficient to place patients at immediate risk for fracture should always be treated with a Food and Drug Administration (FDA) approved drug in addition to a number of nonpharmacological approaches outlined in Table 64.15. The need to achieve an ideal calcium intake cannot be overstated. Opinions vary as to the ideal vitamin D intake, but it is probable that intakes as high as 1200 IU/day would not prove toxic. However, higher vitamin intakes should be avoided. There are also discrepancies in the recommendations for magnesium, but the recommended daily intake of 400 to 500 mg can be taken, if there is no tendency to frequent or loose bowel movements. In fact, a high magnesium intake may help to relieve the constipating effects of calcium carbonate preparations. The procedures to ascertain the amount of magnesium supplementation to prescribe are similar to those for calcium in Table 64.9. During nutrition counseling for osteoporosis, the other nonpharmacological approaches listed in Table 64.15 should be monitored. Falls are particularly serious cofactors in fractures, and are mostly preventable. Adequate protein kilocalorie nutrition promotes muscular strength and agility, and therefore helps prevent falls.

TABLE 64.15
Nonpharmacologic Approaches to the Prevention and Treatment of Osteoporosis

Nutrition	Calcium: 1000–1500 mg/Day
	Permits normal growth and development of the skeleton
	Maximizes peak bone mass
	Maintains adult bone mass
	Minimizes age-related bone loss
	Enhances benefits of pharmacological therapy
	Vitamin D: 600–1200 IU/day
	Intake of calcium/vitamin D should be maintained throughout life, starting before adolescence. Increase awareness in children and adolescents of needed behavioral/ nutritional measures
	Magnesium: 450–500 mg/day (if tolerated)
Exercise	
Fall prevention	

Note: Other lifestyle modifications (risk factor reduction — see Table 64.5).

Although these recommendations are intended for primary types of osteoporosis, they are also applicable, with modifications, in secondary forms of osteoporosis. For example, calcium and vitamin D intakes should be carefully monitored by serum and urine calcium measurements in hyperparathyroidism and idiopathic hypercalciuria, and if urine calcium rises unduly, a thiazide diuretic should be added to reduce urine calcium excretion. In corticosteroid-induced osteoporosis, if the prednisone equivalent dose is 5 mg/day or higher, the vitamin D intake should be drastically increased to the range of 5000 to 7000 IU/day. This can be done most conveniently by prescribing a high-dose vitamin D preparation containing 50,000 IU once a week. The nonpharmacological approaches in Table 64.15 are equally applicable to patients with lesser degrees of bone loss, or osteopenia. Advanced states of osteopenia may also qualify for a modified drug program.

OSTEOMALACIA[35–38]

There are many causes of osteomalacia, and most relate to defects in the vitamin D cascade (Figure 64.1), or an end organ resistance to active vitamin metabolites, either genetic or acquired. Uncomplicated nutritional deficiencies (of calcium or vitamin D) are rare but do occur in financially and socially stressed individuals and in the institutionalized elderly. A general approach to nutritional therapy of osteomalacia is outlined in Table 64.16, which also indicates modifications to be made in various types of osteomalacia. The reason for advocating a combination of precursor vitamin D and the active metabolite calcitriol is that there is a theoretic possibility that other active metabolites of vitamin D might appear that might have direct stimulatory effects on the mineralization process itself.

RENAL OSTEODYSTROPHY[39–41]

This term refers to the skeletal complications of chronic renal failure and represents a variable combination of secondary hyperparathyroidism, osteomalacia, osteoporosis, and osteosclerosis. Nutritional therapy is an important aspect of treatment (Table 64.17), although pharmacologic and surgical approaches may also be necessary in particularly advanced cases. The aim is to

TABLE 64.16
Treatment of Osteomalacia

Type	Calcium Intake Four Times a Day (q.i.d)	Vitamin D Intake q.i.d	Other Nutrients	Other Agents
Nutritional (including post gastrectomy)	Up to 2000 mg	400–1000 IU		
Malabsorption	Same	Up to 50,000 IU	Other lost nutrients	Gluten-free diet, pancreatic enzymesa
Dependent rickets	Same	400–1000 IU plus Calcitriol, up to 0.25 mg q.i.d	Same	
Familial hypophosphatemic rickets	Same	Up to 150,000 IU and Calcitriol, up to 0.25 mg q.i.d	Phosphorus (neutral), up to 3000 mg q.i.d	
Oncogenic osteomalacia	Same	Same		Locate and excise mesenchymal tumor
Anticonvulsant-induced osteomalacia	Same	Up to 5000 IU		

TABLE 64.17
Treatment Options for Renal Osteodystrophy

Optimize renal function and dialysis procedures

Consider renal transplantation

Remove excess skeletal aluminum and iron, if present (chelators such as desferrioxamine)

Calcium carbonate supplements (phosphate binder), 500 mg Ca q.i.d[a]

Reduce phosphorus, magnesium, protein, and acid ash in diet

Calcitriol (to tolerance), 0.25 mcg, up to q.i.d[a]

Parathyroidectomy (in selected cases)

Calciomimetic agents (when available)

Calcitonin (in selected cases with a significant osteoporotic component)

[a] Four times a day.

suppress the secondary hyperparathyroidism and correct undermineralization by using maximally tolerated doses of the active metabolite of vitamin D, calcitriol (1,25-dihydroxy-vitamin D), and calcium. Calcium carbonate is preferred to calcium citrate, although both have the ability to bind phosphorus in the GI tract and thereby reduce the hyperphosphatemia, a major factor in the genesis of the renal osteodystrophy.

Primary Hyperparathyroidism

Previously, calcium restriction was advocated to lessen the impact of the hypercalcemia characteristic of the condition. However, the availability of bone density measurements has revealed that this results in greater bone loss and worsens the skeletal complications. Presently, adequate calcium and vitamin D intakes are advocated, preferably as food sources with a minimal use of supplements. The condition is best treated by surgery, although new pharmacologic agents, called calciomimetic agents, are currently under development.

Paget's Disease[42]

Although both bone resorption and formation are increased, their quantitative relationship is variable, so that either positive calcium balance (with hypocalciuria) or negative calcium balance (with hypercalciuria) may be present at any given time during the prolonged course of the condition. In any case, the imbalance rarely disturbs the serum calcium level and does not cause serious bone loss in pagetic lesions. Therefore, normal calcium and vitamin D intakes are the best approach, as having Paget's disease does not protect against osteoporosis in nonpagetic areas. Since the bisphosphonates currently in use can occasionally cause transient mild hypocalcemia, some authorities recommend an increased calcium intake during bisphosphonate treatment. On the other hand, calcium should not be supplemented if there is a history of calcium-containing kidney stones. Another type of stone that can occur in Paget's disease is the uric acid stone, as some Paget's disease patients also have a concomitant gouty diathesis.

RENAL STONE DISEASE

Renal stone formation is a common multifactorial disease of unknown etiology with an established genetic contribution. Lifetime risk for nephrolithiasis is approximately 10% in Western populations and uric acid stones account for 5 to 10% of all stones depending on environment and dietary and ethnic differences.[44]

There are four major types of kidney stones. Although they tend to occur under different clinical conditions, the key to successful categorization and treatment, which is largely a matter of nutritional manipulation, is stone recovery and physicochemical (crystallographic) analysis. When this is not feasible, other clues such as radiographic appearance, clinical data obtained from the patient, and biochemical testing can be used to design a nutritional program. The prevention of renal stones after an initial stone event is difficult. Dietary modification and drug therapies have long been advocated to reduce the likelihood of a recurrence. High fluid intakes have been recommended and found efficacious, as has the use of thiazides, allopurinol, and alkali citrate.[45] Stone formation has been shown to be associated with metabolic acidosis, gout, obesity, and hypertension.[46–49]

Calcium Oxalate/Phosphate Stones

This stone type accounts for 80% of renal stones, and approximately 50% of these are idiopathic in that there is no discernible metabolic defect, and both urinary calcium and oxalate levels are normal. In the remainder, either urinary calcium or oxalate is increased; the former may or may not be associated with hypercalcemia. Oxaluria may be a primary genetic condition, may be due to excessive intake of foods that yield oxalate during digestion or metabolism, or may be secondary to the increased oxalate absorption present in inflammatory bowel disease and in some malabsorption syndromes. In the GI-related cases, intestinal calcium becomes bound to unabsorbed fats instead of luminal oxalate, allowing the latter to be absorbed and then excreted, followed by precipitation with calcium in the urinary tract. Calcium stones are difficult to treat, in the sense of preventing or reducing their rate of recurrence, because of their great insolubility. Successful treatment of an underlying medical condition, if present, is the most effective maneuver and should be combined with dietary changes consisting of manipulating calcium intake, limiting vitamins A and D, and oxalate intakes, and maintaining maximal hydration compatible with cardiovascular competence. In GI-related oxaluria, an increased calcium intake may allow more oxalate complexation in the GI tract and actually lessen calcium oxalate stone formation. In the case of idiopathic hypercalciuria, an extreme reduction in calcium intake will have an adverse effect on bone density and increase the predisposition to osteoporosis/osteopenia.

MgNH$_4$PO$_4$ Stones

In urinary tract infections with urea-splitting organisms, both urine NH_4 levels and pH rise, and the NH_4 can combine with urinary Mg and PO_4 to precipitate in the alkaline medium. Lowering substrate excretion by dietary restriction and lowering pH with an acid ash diet will retard precipitation, but so long as the infection persists, NH_4 generation will limit the effectiveness of the dietary manipulation. Unfortunately, these infections are difficult to eradicate in the presence of the disturbed anatomy of the renal calyces and pelvis caused by the large, irregularly shaped stones, which sometimes approach the size of staghorn calculi. Dietary manipulations are best instituted before chronic urinary tract infections with urea-splitting organisms begin to generate stones.

CYSTINE-BASED STONES

These are the rarest of kidney stones, since they occur only in an inborn genetic condition, cystinuria. Although organic in composition, they are radio-opaque due to the dense packing of the cysteine molecules. In mild cases, urinary alkalinization is successful, but when the stone disease is more aggressive, alkalinization must be combined with agents that can chelate the excess cysteine.

URIC ACID (UREATES) STONES

This is the only major radiolucent stone, and its presence may need specialized imaging procedures. Patients with manifest gouty arthritis (acute or tophaceous) are particularly susceptible because of a combination of uricosuria and an intrinsic defect in urinary NH_3 production from purine precursors, which forces the kidney to excrete metabolically derived acids as titratable acidity, a condition under which uric acid is insoluble and can precipitate. A subset of patients exist in whom the urinary defect in NH_3 production is not accompanied by other features of the gouty diathesis, and these patients are easily treated with alkali supplements alone. A simple technique to detect these patients and monitor alkali treatment is to have the patient record the urinary pH of each voided specimen by placing pH-sensitive strips in the urinary stream. In normal individuals, pH will vary from 5.0 or less to 6.5 or higher (the "alkaline tide"), but patients with the defect will show persistent values of 5.0 or less throughout the 24 h. With successful alkalinization, pH should remain at 6.0 or higher. Excessive purine intake should be curtailed, but not at the expense of causing protein deficiency. Conditions associated with high catabolic states, such as burns, extensive trauma, and certain neoplasms, especially with the use of antineoplastic agents, can cause acute and severe hyperuricosuria, which may not only cause stone formation but may clog the renal tubules, causing a "gouty nephropathy." Expectant treatment with alkali and forced hydration is required to forestall this serious complication. Paget's disease patients may also form uric acid stones because of the frequent tendency to a comorbid gouty diathesis, and should also receive careful alkalinization if this is a problem. Uric acid stone formation has a very strong genetic component.[44]

MIXED STONES

These represent a challenge in terms of diagnosis and treatment. Since treatment for one component may be deleterious for another component, a full understanding of the qualitative and quantitative nature of the metabolic defects present should be sought before instituting cautious treatment.

BLADDER STONES

Stones that form in the urinary bladder and have not migrated from the renal calyces or pelvis are generally not related to metabolic defects, but to stasis. Their composition is quite variable, and is often a mixture of components. They are treated by correcting disturbed anatomy rather than by dietary therapy.

REFERENCES

1. Berdanier CD. *Advanced Nutrition: Micronutrients*, CRC Press, Boca Raton, FL, 1994, pgs 151–182.
2. Heaney RP. *Nutr Rev* 54(4 Pt 2): 3S; 1996.
3. Reid DM, New SA. *Proc Nutr Soc* 56: 977; 1997.
4. Lewis RD, Modlesky CM. *Intl J Sport Nutr* 8: 250; 1998.
5. Bronner F, Pansu D. *J Nutr* 129: 9; 1999.
6. Bronner F, Pansu D. *Optimal Calcium Intake, NIH Consensus Statement Nutr* 12: 1; 1994.
7. Compston JE. *BMJ* 317: 1466; 1998.
8. Heaney RP, Weaver CM. *J Am Coll Nutr* 24: 574S–581S; 2005.
9. Bonjour JP. *J Am Coll Nutr* 24: 526S–536S; 2005.
10. Babraj JA, Smith K, Cuthbertson DJ, Rickhuss P, Dorling JS, Rennie MJ. *J Bone Miner Res* 20: 930–937; 2005.
11. Pors Nielson S. *Bone* 35: 583–588; 2004.
12. Abrams SA. *Horm Res* 60: 71S–76S; 2003.
13. Bonner F. *Dent Clin North Am* 47: 209–224; 2003.
14. Hunziker EB, Herrmann KW, Schenk RK, Mueller M, Moor H. *J Cell Biol* 98: 267–273; 1984.

15. Mundy GR. *Am J Clin Nutr* 83: 427S–430S; 2006.
16. Vormann J. *Mol Aspects Med* 24: 27–37; 2003.
17. Nieves JW. *Am J Clin Nutr* 81: 1232S–1239S; 2005.
18. Nielsen FH, Milne DB. *Eur J Clin Nutr* 58: 703–710; 2004.
19. Miller KK. *J Women's Health* 12: 145–150; 2003.
20. Panda DK, Miao D, Bolivar I, Li J, Huo R, Hendy GN, Goltzman D. *J Biol Chem* 279: 16754–16766; 2004.
21. Wallach S. In: *Magnesium and Trace Elements* 10: 281; 1992.
22. Martini LA. *Nutr Rev* 57: 227; 1999.
23. D'Haese PC, Couttenye MM, De Broe ME. *Nephrol Dialysis, Trans* 11: 3S; 1996.
24. Wallach S, Chausmer AB. In: *Trace Metals and Fluoride in Bones and Teeth*, Priest ND, Van De Vyver FL, eds, CRC Press, Boca Raton, FL, 1990, Chapter 10.
25. Chausmer AB, Wallach S. In: *Trace Metals and Fluoride in Bones and Teeth*, Priest ND, Van De Vyver FL, eds, CRC Press, Boca Raton, FL, 1990, Chapter 11.
26. Price DE, Joshi JG. *Proc Natl Acad Sci USA* 79: 3116; 1982.
27. Emery MP, O'Dell BL. *Proc Soc Exp Biol Med* 203: 408; 1993.
28. Cashman KD. *Nutr Rev* 63: 2284–2289; 2005.
29. Tsugawa N, Shiraki M, Suhara Y, Kamao M, Tanaka K, Okano T. *Am J Clin Nutr* 83: 380–389; 2006.
30. Maurer J, Harris MM, Staanford VA, Lohman TG, Cussler E, Going SB, Houtkooper LB. *J Nutr* 135: 863–869; 2005.
31. Nordin BE, Need AG, Steurer TA, Morris HA, Chatterton BE, Horowitz M. *Ann NY Acad Sci* 854: 336; 1998.
32. Lau EM, Woo J. *Nutr Osteopor Curr Opin Rheumatol* 10: 368; 1998.
33. Raisz LG. *J Bone Min Metab* 17: 79; 1999.
34. Anderson JJ, Rondano P, Holmes A. *Scand J Rheumatol* 103: 65S; 1996.
35. Francis RM, Selby PL. *Osteomalacia Baillieres Clin Endocrinol Metab* 11: 145; 1997.
36. Bell NH, Key Jr LL. *Acquired Osteomalacia Curr Ther Endocrinol Metab* 6: 530; 1997.
37. Klein GL. *Nutrition* 14: 149; 1998.
38. Nightingale JM. *Nutrition* 15: 633; 1999.
39. Sakhaee K, Gonzalez GB. *Am J Med Sci* 317: 251; 1999.
40. Kurokawa K, Fukagawa M. *Am J Med Sci* 317: 355; 1999.
41. Slatopolsky E. *Nephrol Dialysis, Transp* 13: 3S; 1998.
42. Delmas PD, Meunier PJ. *N Engl J Med* 336: 558; 1997.
43. Coe FL, Parks JH. Nephrolithiasis In: *Primer on the Metabolic Bone Diseases and Disorders of Mineral Metabolism*, 4th ed, Favus MJ, ed, Lippincott Williams and Wilkins, Philadelphia, PA, 1999, Chapter 81.
44. Ombra MN, Forabosco P, Casula S, Angius A, Maestrale G, Petretto E, Casu G, Colussi G, Usai E, Melis P, Pirastu M. *Am J Hum Genet* 68: 1119; 2001.
45. Pearle MS. *Curr Opin Nephrol Hypertens* 10: 203; 2001.
46. Wiederkehr M, Krapf R. *Swiss Med Wkly* 10: 127; 2001.
47. Kramer HM, Curhan G. *Am J Kidney Dois* 40: 37; 2002.
48. Taylor EN, Stampfer MJ, Curhan GC. *JAMA* 293: 455; 2005.
49. Gillen DL, Coe FL, Worcester EM. *Am J Kidney Dis* 46: 263; 2005.

65 Anemia

Brent H. Limbaugh, Linda K. Hendricks, and Abdullah Kutlar

CONTENTS

INTRODUCTION

Hematopoiesis is the process whereby mature blood cells (red cells, white cells, and platelets) are produced from pluripotent hematopoietic stem cells in the bone marrow through a process of proliferation and differentiation. *Erythropoiesis* is the name given to the production of red blood cells (RBCs) (erythrocytes), and is dependent on many complex factors. These include the bone marrow microenvironment, an elaborate network of cytokines and hematopoietic growth factors, and an adequate supply of nutrients, vitamins, and some trace elements (Table 65.1). The major function of RBCs is the transport and delivery of oxygen. A decrease in RBC mass and oxygen-carrying capacity is known as *anemia*. This section will provide an overview of the classification

TABLE 65.1
Nutrients Important for
Normal RBC Production

1. Protein/calories
2. Vitamin B_{12} (cobalamin)
3. Folate
4. Iron
5. Vitamin B_6 (pyridoxine)
6. Riboflavin
7. Nicotinic acid
8. Ascorbic acid
9. Vitamin A (retinol)
10. Vitamin E (α-tocopherol)
11. Copper

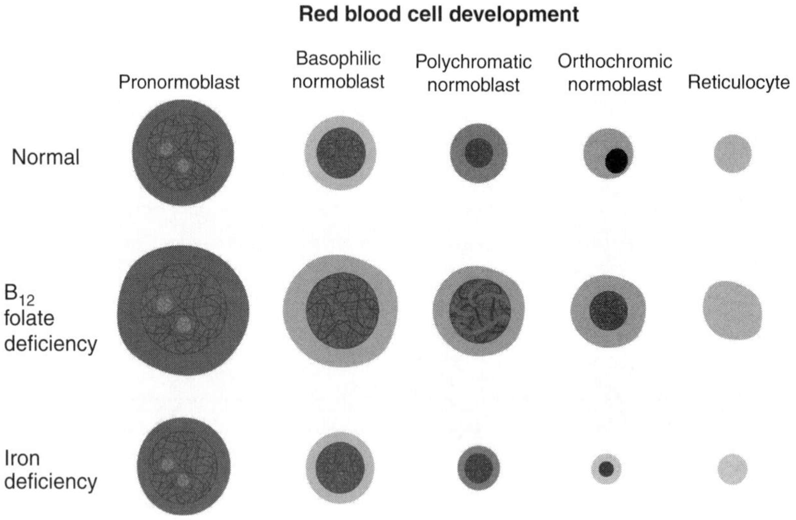

Red blood cell development

FIGURE 65.1 (**See color insert following page 654.**) Erythropoiesis as it is affected by states of iron deficiency and vitamin B_{12} or folate deficiency.

and pathogenesis of anemia, and will primarily focus on a detailed discussion of nutritional deficiencies leading to various types of anemia.

NORMAL ERYTHROPOIESIS

A good understanding of normal erythropoiesis will enable one to better understand and appreciate the pathogenesis of different types of anemias (Figure 65.1). The earliest morphologically identifiable red cell precursor, the proerythroblast, is very large (12 to 20 mm), with a large nucleus. The nucleus contains the DNA necessary for cell division, and the cytoplasm contains RNA necessary for hemoglobin synthesis. As the cells divide and mature, the nucleus becomes very small and condensed. Eventually, the nucleus is extruded, and the remaining mature red cell is only the cytoplasm full of hemoglobin. The normal red cell is smaller than the precursor cells and is pink colored from hemoglobin.

The normal RBC lives about 120 days in the peripheral blood: when the senescent RBCs are destroyed, they have to be replaced by new RBCs to maintain RBC homeostasis. A newly produced, young RBC still has residual RNA and mitochondria in the cytoplasm and is slightly larger than a normal red cell, appearing a little bluish on the peripheral blood smear. This is called a reticulocyte. A special stain is performed using new methylene blue, which stains the residual RNA, making a reticulocyte easy to identify and count in the blood (Figure 65.2). The reticulocyte count is the number of reticulocytes counted in 1000 red cells, reported as a percentage. A reticulocyte lives normally 2 days before it matures into a fully developed RBC. In a normal, healthy person, a reticulocyte count will range from 0.5 to 1.5% (1/120 of RBCs replaced daily). Thus, the reticulocyte count is a sensitive method to detect how rigorous the bone marrow is producing new RBCs. Two corrections need to be made after the reticulocyte percentage is obtained before a conclusion can be drawn about the bone marrow.

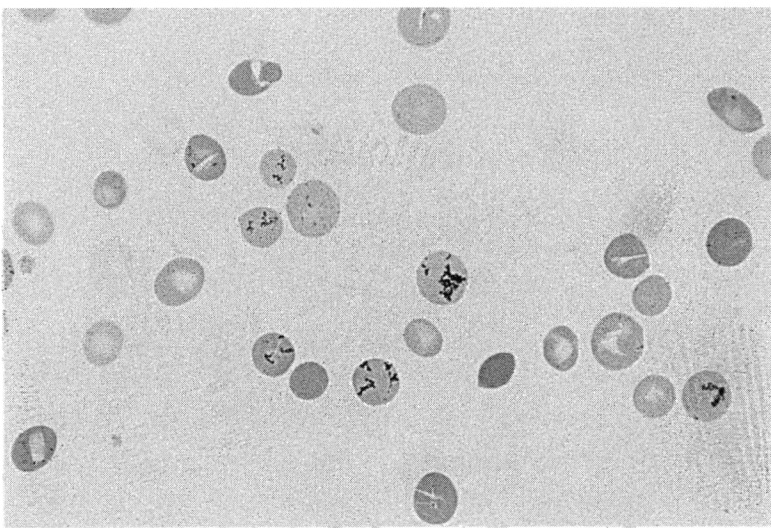

FIGURE 65.2 (**See color insert following page 654.**) Reticulocytes. The appearance of young, newly produced RBCs, reticulocytes, as seen in the peripheral blood smear that has been stained with new methylene blue.

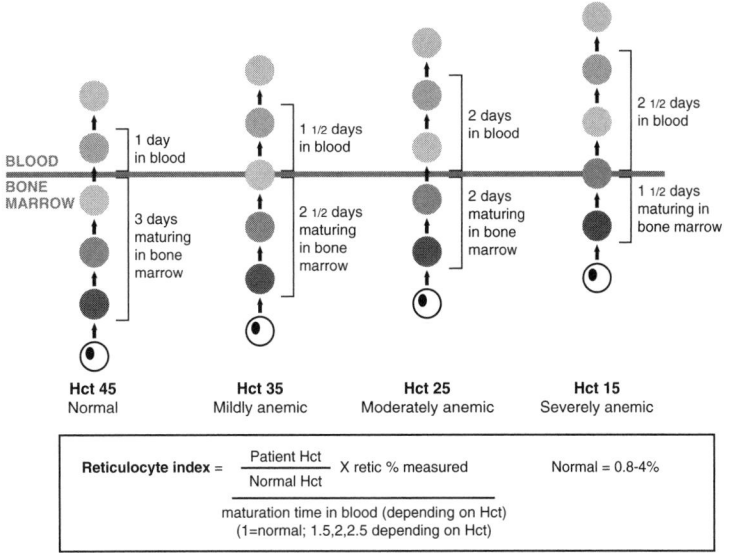

FIGURE 65.3 Understanding the reticulocyte index.

One, if a patient has decreased numbers of red cells to begin with, then a reticulocyte count of 0.5 to 1.5% would not be considered an appropriate bone marrow response. The bone marrow should be producing more reticulocytes in the setting of anemia. Because of the fewer number of RBCs present, a reticulocyte percentage within the range listed would actually reflect a much smaller absolute reticulocyte number; that is, 2% of a 100 cells is less than 2% of a 1000 cells. Thus, when reticulocytes are counted, it is important to take into account the degree of anemia present to avoid a misleading "normal" percentage of reticulocytes. Dividing the patient's hematocrit or hemoglobin by the normal hematocrit or hemoglobin does this. This gives us the fraction of normal red cells the patient has. That fraction is then multiplied by the reticulocyte count giving us the corrected reticulocyte count.

Second, the faster the bone marrow is producing reticulocytes, the younger the cells are when they are released into the peripheral blood. When reticulocytes are counted using the special stain, both older reticulocytes and younger reticulocytes are counted. Therefore, adjustments for this can be made when calculating a patient's reticulocyte index (Figure 65.3). The corrected reticulocyte count is divided by the number of days the reticulocyte lives in the peripheral blood. This number, of course, depends on the degree of anemia. The more severely anemic someone is, the earlier the reticulocyte is pushed into the peripheral blood, and the longer it stays as a reticulocyte in the blood. (The usual number used in the setting of anemia, however, is two.) After these two corrections have been made to the reticulocyte count, then one has a fair estimate of how well the

TABLE 65.2
Categorizing Anemias by Reticulocyte Count

1. Low reticulocytes   High reticulocytes
2. Decreased production   Acute blood loss
3. Fe deficiency   Splenic sequestration
4. B$_{12}$ deficiency   Increased destruction (hemolysis)
5. Folate deficiency

TABLE 65.3
Criteria for Anemia and Normal MCV Values

	Hgb (g/dl)	Hct (%)	MCV (fl)
Infants			
1–3 days	<14.5	<45	95–108
1 month	<10	<31	85–104
2 months	<9	<28	77–96
0.5–2 years	<11	<33	70–78
Children			
2–6 years	<11.5	<34	75–81
6–12 years	<11.5	<35	77–86
12–18 years			
Female	<12	<36	78–90
Male	<13	<37	78–88
Women	<12	<37	80–90
Men	<14	<40	80–90

MCV = Mean corpuscular volume.

bone marrow is able to make new RBCs. In the case of nutritionally caused anemias, the reticulocyte index will invariably be low (Table 65.2).

In recent years, there has been a trend towards utilizing absolute reticulocyte count. This is particularly useful in the diagnosis of hemolytic anemias as they will invariably be associated with absolute reticulocyte count of greater tan 100,000/mm^3.

ERYTHROPOIETIN

Erythropoietin, a glycoprotein hormone produced in the kidney in response to tissue hypoxia, is the major regulator of erythropoiesis. In cases of renal failure the erythropoietin level may be low, causing anemia, usually normocytic. Measuring the erythropoietin level may be a useful step in the evaluation of anemia; however, in cases of nutritionally deficient anemia, the level is normal or elevated and is not, therefore, routinely measured.

ANEMIA: DEFINITION AND CLASSIFICATION

Anemia is best defined as a reduction in the oxygen carrying capacity of blood. Hemoglobin (Hb) is the molecule in RBCs that is actually responsible for binding the oxygen that red cells carry. Therefore, measurement of Hb provides an accurate, reproducible means of detecting anemia. Normal values for Hb vary according to gender and different age groups (Table 65.3). When anemia is suspected, basic serum laboratory values should be obtained for further classification (Table 65.4).

There are several ways to classify anemias. The two most common are functional and morphologic classification. Morphologic classification is based on the measurement of the mean corpuscle volume (MCV), which is a reflection of the average volume of each red cell in the erythrocyte compartment. A normal red cell MCV is 80 to 100 fl, while the typical diameter is approximately 7 μm (shown in Figure 65.4; also seen is a typical granulocyte for size comparison). Thus, anemias can be classified as either normocytic (MCV 80–100), microcytic (MCV, 80) or macrocytic (MCV > 100) (Table 65.5).

TABLE 65.4
Initial Laboratory Data in the Evaluation of Anemia

CBC (complete blood count)
White count and differential
Platelet count
Hemoglobin and hematocrit
MCV (mean cell volume)
Reticulocyte count
Red cell morphology on peripheral
  blood smear

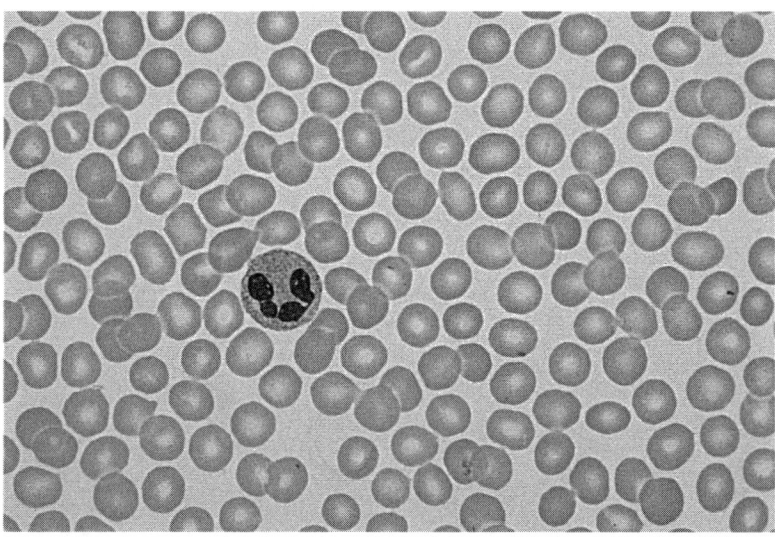

FIGURE 65.4 **(See color insert following page 654.)** A normal peripheral blood smear.

TABLE 65.5
Classification of Anemias by Morphology

Low MCV (Microcytic)	High MCV (Macrocytic)	Normal MCV (Normocytic)
Fe deficiency	Nonmegaloblastic	Bone marrow failure
Thalassemia	Liver disease	Aplastic anemia
Sideroblastic anemia	Hypothyroidism	Red cell aplasia (acquired and congenital)
Chronic disease	Reticulocytosis	
Lead poisoning	Aplastic anemia	Marrow infiltration
Protein deficiency	Chronic renal failure	
Megaloblastic	Endocrine abnormalities	
Vitamin B_{12} deficiency	Hypothyroidism	
Folate deficiency	Adrenal insufficiency	
Myelodysplastic syndromes	HIV	
Chronic disease		
Drug induced		
Chemotherapeutic agents		
Nitrous oxide (laughing gas)		

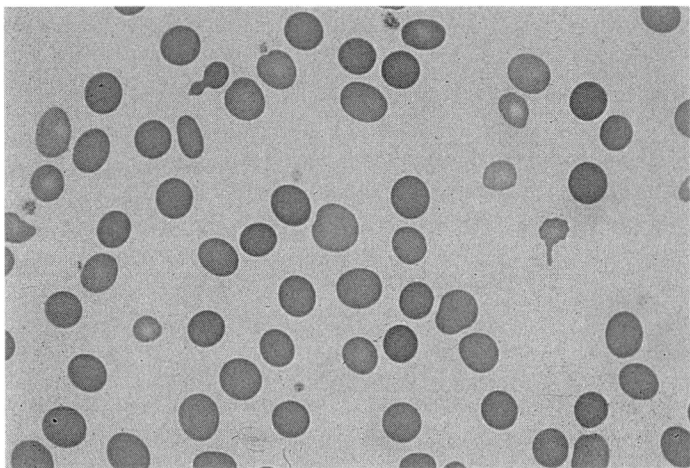

FIGURE 65.5 **(See color insert following page 654.)** Macrocytic RBCs. RBCs that are larger than normal (macrocytic) and white blood cells that have nuclei with multiple segments (hypersegmented neutrophils) are characteristic of a vitamin B_{12} deficiency anemia.

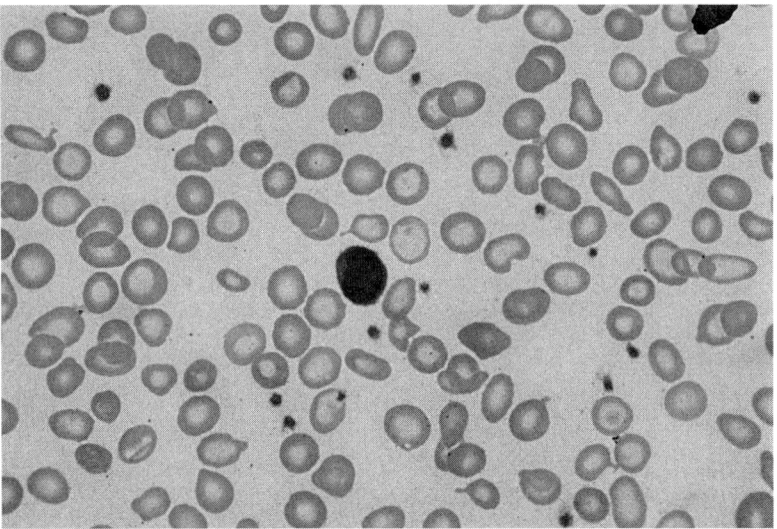

FIGURE 65.6 **(See color insert following page 654.)** Microcytic RBCs. RBCs that are smaller than normal and have pale features (microcytic and hypochromic) are characteristic of Fe deficiency anemia.

Perturbations, of either the nuclear (DNA) or cytoplasmic (RNA and hemoglobin) maturation, lead to anemia. The red cell precursor utilizes cobalamin (vitamin B_{12}) and folate in the synthesis of DNA. When either of these nutrients is deficient, the nucleus cannot divide or mature normally despite normal cytoplasmic development. The red cells formed are large (macrocytic). The bone marrow reveals red cell precursors that are megaloblastic, that is, large with fine, sparse nuclear chromatin. Other nucleated bone marrow cells are also affected, such as hypersegmentation of neutrophils in which >5% of neutrophils have six or more lobes of the nucleus (Figure 65.5).

In the cytoplasm, hemoglobin synthesis proceeds normally as long as both heme and globin are manufactured normally. Defective heme synthesis can occur by two mechanisms: faulty iron metabolism (iron deficiency anemia) or defective porphyrin metabolism (sideroblastic anemia). A deletion in or defect of the genes encoding globin causes defective globin synthesis. All of these anemias are characterized by small red cells, microcytosis, because the nucleus divides and matures normally (Figure 65.6).

Functional classification of anemia is based on the pathogenesis of the anemia. This would include hypoproliferative (defective or ineffective erythropoiesis in the bone marrow microenvironment), maturation problems (defects in nuclear or cytoplasmic components of the erythrocyte), or blood loss/destruction (hemorrhage, hemolysis, sequestration) (Table 65.6).

TABLE 65.6
Functional Causes of Anemia

1. Blood loss
2. Gastrointestinal bleeding
3. Menses/Menorrhagia
4. Internal bleeding
5. Decreased production of RBCs
6. Nutritional deficiencies
7. Primary bone marrow failure (myelodysplastic syndromes, leukemias, and infiltrative processes)
8. Secondary bone marrow failure (drugs, toxins, metabolic processes, and infections)
9. Increased destruction of RBCs
10. Immune hemolytic anemia
11. Mechanical hemolysis (heart valve, microangiopathic hemolytic anemia, TTP, and DIC)
12. Hereditary hemolysis
13. Hemoglobinopathies
14. Enzyme defects (G6PD, pyruvate kinase)
15. Membrane defects
16. Acquired membrane defects
17. Paroxysmal nocturnal hemoglobinuria
18. Spur cell anemia
19. Infection related hemolysis
20. Clostridia, malaria, and babesiosis
21. Splenic sequestration
22. Increased plasma volume
23. Pregnancy

TABLE 65.7
Symptoms of Anemia

1. Dyspnea with exertion
2. Dizziness
3. Lightheadedness
4. Throbbing headaches
5. Tinnitus
6. Palpitations
7. Syncope
8. Fatigue
9. Disrupted sleep patterns
10. Decreased libido
11. Mood disturbances
12. Difficulty concentrating

SYMPTOMS OF ANEMIA

Patients with anemia will often present with similar symptoms regardless of the cause. Low RBCs decrease the oxygen-carrying capacity of the blood, producing generalized symptoms (Table 65.7). The severity of the symptoms, however, is directly related to how rapidly the anemia develops. Anemias that develop rapidly, such as in acute bleeding, will be more symptomatic than anemias that progress slowly over months to years. The heart must increase the rate of blood flow to the body to compensate for anemia. This may precipitate palpitations, shortness of breath, and throbbing headaches. Syncope occurs with severe anemia due to decreased oxygenation of the brain in the upright position. Often patients with chronic anemia such as those with sickle cell disease will maintain a hemoglobin level much lower than normal and have few symptoms, due to compensation by the body.

PHYSICAL FINDINGS

Anemia causes general physical findings independent of the cause of the anemia (Table 65.8). These findings are due to the decrease in hemoglobin; skin and mucous membranes may be pale and the heart rate may be increased. As in symptoms, the physical findings may be influenced by the chronicity of the anemia.

VITAMIN B$_{12}$ DEFICIENCY

MECHANISM OF ANEMIA

Erythropoiesis depends on proper nuclear (DNA) and cytoplasmic (RNA and hemoglobin) maturation. Vitamin B$_{12}$ (or cobalamin) is important in DNA synthesis. When vitamin B$_{12}$ is not available, the conversion of homocysteine to methionine is impaired. DNA is not synthesized properly, and megaloblastic anemia ensues (see Chapters 9 and 10).

TABLE 65.8
Physical Findings in Anemia

1. Pallor of skin
2. Pallor of mucous membranes
3. Mild to moderate tachycardia
4. Widened pulse pressure
5. Systolic ejection murmur
6. Venous hums
7. Mild peripheral edema

TABLE 65.9
Causes of Vitamin B_{12} Deficiency

1. Pernicious anemia (most common cause)
2. Gastrectomy
3. Zollinger-Ellison syndrome
4. Intestinal causes
5. Ileal resection or disease
6. Blind loop syndrome
7. Fish tapeworm
8. Pancreatic insufficiency
9. Strict vegetarianism (those who exclude meats, eggs, and milk)

ETIOLOGY OF VITAMIN B_{12} DEFICIENCY

The most common cause of vitamin B_{12} deficiency is not the dietary lack of vitamin B_{12}, but the inability to absorb the vitamin from food due to a condition known as pernicious anemia. Normally, vitamin B_{12} is released from food in the acidic environment of the stomach and is bound to intrinsic factor. Intrinsic factor is formed by the parietal cells of the stomach, and binding of vitamin B_{12} to intrinsic factor allows absorption in the ileum. In pernicious anemia, the stomach does not make intrinsic factor, and the vitamin cannot be absorbed. Pernicious anemia is more commonly seen in people of Northern European descent, but can be seen in all racial groups. Women are affected more than men. A family history of pernicious anemia may indicate increased risk.

Other causes of vitamin B_{12} deficiency are related to the absorption mechanism (Table 65.9). For example, antibodies to intrinsic factor or to the parietal cells of the stomach may inhibit proper function. Gastrectomy will result in lack of intrinsic factor. Conditions that interfere with the binding of intrinsic factor to the ileum include Crohn's disease, ileal resection, and tropical sprue. The fish tapeworm, *Diphyllobothrium latum*, competes for vitamin B_{12} and can be a cause of deficiency in infected patients. If pancreatic enzymes are not sufficient to aid in the binding of B_{12} to intrinsic factor, the absorption will be impaired. Only very rarely is dietary deficiency of vitamin B_{12} seen in the United States. Those cases are usually seen in very strict vegans (those who exclude meats, eggs, and milk from their diets). The deficiency develops slowly over many years due to the presence of relatively large amounts of B_{12} stores in the body, primarily in the liver.

THE CLINICAL FEATURES OF B_{12} DEFICIENCY

Full-blown cases of deficiency present with megaloblastic anemia. Inflamed tongue (glossitis) or mouth (stomatitis) and gastrointestinal complaints can occur. Neurological effects can be devastating (Table 65.10). Demyelination of nerves leads to axonal degeneration and highly variable clinical symptoms. Subacute combined degeneration of the spinal cord and cerebral abnormalities include symptoms of finger and toe paresthesias, disturbance of vibration and position sense, spastic ataxia, impairment of taste, smell, vision, and even psychosis often referred to as "megaloblastic madness." Importantly, the anemia and neurological effects are not always seen together. A patient could have severe megaloblastic anemia with no neurological effects, and vice versa. The mechanism of neurologic effects is poorly understood. Unfortunately, treatment with vitamin B_{12} does not always correct the neurological effects despite correction of the anemia.

THE HEMATOLOGICAL EFFECTS OF B_{12} DEFICIENCY

The nuclear maturation defect results in a macrocytic anemia (Table 65.11). The mean cell volume is usually greater than 110 fl and can vary depending on the degree of deficiency. In vitamin B_{12} deficiency, the red cell precursors in the bone marrow are large with immature nuclei. Ineffective erythropoiesis (destruction of RBC precursors in the marrow) can be quite significant and

---

TABLE 65.10
Clinical Features of B$_{12}$ Deficiency

1. Megaloblastic anemia
2. Pallor/icterus
3. Sore tongue or mouth
4. Gastrointestinal symptoms
5. Neurological symptoms
6. Finger and toe paresthesias
7. Disturbance of vibration and position sense
8. Spastic ataxia — subacute combined degeneration
9. Somnolence, impairment of taste, smell, and vision
10. Dementia, psychosis, and "megaloblastic madness"
11. Well nourished, generally

TABLE 65.11
Laboratory Features of B$_{12}$ Deficiency

Hematological
1. Megaloblastic anemia (MCV > 110)
2. Leukopenia and thrombocytopenia
3. Bone marrow
4. Megaloblastic appearance
5. Ineffective erythropoiesis

Biochemical
1. Serum B$_{12}$ level is decreased (i.e., <223 pg/ml)
2. Methylmalonic acid is elevated (i.e., >0.4 mmol/l)
3. Homocysteine is elevated (i.e., >14 mm)
4. Marked increase in LDH (i.e., >3000 U/ml [normal 260 U/ml])
5. Serum folate levels may be elevated
Schilling test

---

is responsible for the elevated indirect bilirubin level and high lactate dehydrogenase (LDH). In fact, up to 90% of the red cells may actually be destroyed in the bone marrow before being released to the peripheral blood as compared to the 10 to 15% seen in normal subjects. Furthermore, the white cell and platelet lineages are affected, and the hematological picture is often one of pancytopenia.

The Laboratory Diagnosis of B$_{12}$ Deficiency

The serum vitamin B$_{12}$ level reflects the vitamin stores in the body and is the standard method in determining vitamin B$_{12}$ deficiency. The normal range is usually from 200 to 1000 pg/ml. Some conditions such as folic acid deficiency, pregnancy, oral contraceptive use, multiple myeloma, and possibly antibiotic therapy can cause falsely low vitamin B$_{12}$ levels. Because it is important to differentiate true B$_{12}$ deficiency from folic acid deficiency, the serum methylmalonic acid level and serum homocysteine level can be measured (Table 65.12). The homocysteine level may be elevated in both vitamin B$_{12}$ deficiency and folate deficiency due to interruption of the formation of succinyl CoA. However, only methylmalonic acid will be elevated in true vitamin B$_{12}$ deficiency, because it utilizes vitamin B$_{12}$ to form methionine, a process not dependent on folate.

The Schilling Test

Traditionally, once vitamin B$_{12}$ deficiency was diagnosed, the Shilling test was administered to define the etiology as dietary deficiency, gastrointestinal malabsorption, or pernicious anemia. The test was performed as follows: the first part involved administration of radiolabeled cobalamin orally to the patient. Urine was collected for 24 h and radioactivity in the urine measured. Excretion in the urine of at least 7.5% of the oral dose meant that the patient was able to absorb the vitamin and subsequently excrete the unused amount in the urine. However, if less than 7.5% of radiolabeled cobalamin was excreted in the urine, the vitamin was not absorbed adequately. These patients would go on to part two of the test: radiolabeled cobalamin was administered orally again along with intrinsic factor. The urine collection was repeated, and urinary excretion above 7.5% indicated that the addition of intrinsic factor corrected the absorption and the patient had pernicious anemia. If the urine excretion was still less

TABLE 65.12

The Laboratory Difference between Negative Nutritional Balance and True Folate and B_{12} Deficiency

Lab Value	Serum Folate	RBC Folate	Serum B_{12}	Serum HCYS	Serum MMA
Condition					
Negative folate balance	⇓	NL	NL	NL	NL
Folate deficiency	⇓	⇓	NL	⇑	NL
Negative B_{12} balance	NL	NL	NL	NL	NL
B_{12} deficiency	NL/⇑	NL/⇓	⇓	⇑	⇑
Combined deficiency	⇓/NL	⇓	⇓	⇑	⇑

HCYS = Homocysteine
MMA = Methylmalonic acid

TABLE 65.13

Treatment of B_{12} Deficiency

Standard dose is 1000 mg intramuscularly
Anemia only: 1000 mg daily for a week, then weekly until Hgb normalizes; maintenance dose is 1000 mg monthly
Neurological deficits: 1000 mg daily for 2 weeks, then weekly until Hgb normalizes, followed by twice a month
   for 6 months, then monthly for life. If injections are not an option, oral dose is 1000 mg daily
For the rare case of decreased oral intake from malnutrition, replacement of 50 mg daily is adequate

than 7.5%, malabsorption syndromes, such as sprue or intrinsic factor receptor abnormalities, were suspected. Before the test, all patients were given a dose of unlabeled vitamin B_{12} intramuscularly to saturate the cobalamin receptors in the tissues and plasma. This way, the body would absorb and then excrete the unused radiolabeled cobalamin, and the test would be valid. Today, assays have become widely available to allow serologic testing for antibodies to intrinsic factor or parietal cells (the usual cause of pernicious anemia). They are generally evaluated before performing the labor-intensive, relatively cumbersome Shilling test. Additionally, Shilling test cannot be performed anymore due to the unavailability of radiolabeled cobalamin.

NUTRITIONAL REQUIREMENTS OF VITAMIN B_{12} AND TREATMENT

The normal total body pool of vitamin B_{12} is 3000 μg. The daily dietary requirement is approximately 1 mg. The recommended daily allowance is 2 μg, and the average daily diet contains 5 to 15 μg a day (ranging from 1 to 100 μg a day). Thus, it is very difficult to become vitamin B_{12} deficient based on poor diet alone. When deficiency is present, the treatment requires only 1 μg of B_{12} per day; however, in the setting of neurological deficiencies, higher doses are often given. The standard maintenance dose is 100 μg intramuscularly each month after an initial loading dose is given (Table 65.13). However, studies in recent years have proven that, even in patients with pernicious anemia, oral vitamin B_{12} can be taken daily and is absorbed in adequate amounts to make oral vitamin B_{12} replacement a viable alternative for those who do not wish to take a monthly injection.

FOLATE DEFICIENCY

MECHANISM OF ANEMIA

Like vitamin B_{12}, folate is utilized in the synthesis of DNA in the nucleus. The deficiency of folate causes megaloblastic anemia due to the arrested nuclear maturation. The main function of folate in the biochemistry of hematopoiesis is the transfer of carbon groups to various compounds. The most important compounds formed by this carbon donation are the purines, dTMP, and methionine. As explained above, methionine formation also requires vitamin B_{12}. Without vitamin B_{12}, methionine is not formed and the prospective folate cannot be recycled, causing a "folate trap." Thus, vitamin B_{12} deficiency can also give a laboratory picture of folate deficiency.

ETIOLOGY OF FOLATE DEFICIENCY

Unlike vitamin B_{12} deficiency, nutritional factors play the major role in folate deficiency (Table 65.14). This is seen most commonly in the elderly, the poor, or in alcoholics. Financial reasons, poor nutritional education, and excessive alcohol consumption

TABLE 65.14
Causes of Folate Deficiency

1. Decreased nutritional intake
2. Poverty
3. Old age
4. Alcoholism/cirrhosis
5. Children on synthetic diets
6. Goat's milk anemia
7. Premature infants
8. Hemodialysis
9. Hyperalimentation
10. Nontropical sprue (gluten-sensitive enteropathy)
11. Tropical sprue
12. Congenital folate malabsorption
13. Other small intestine disease
14. Pregnancy
15. Increased cell turnover (chronic hemolysis and exfoliative dermatitis)
16. Drug induced
17. Alcohol
18. Trimethoprim and pyrimethamine
19. Methotrexate
20. Sulfasalazine
21. Oral contraceptives
22. Anticonvulsants

TABLE 65.15
Clinical Features of Folate Deficiency

1. Blunted affect/mask-like facies
2. Depression
3. Irritability
4. Forgetfulness
5. Sleep deprivation
6. Weight loss from underlying GI disease
7. Diffuse blotchy brownish skin pigmentation in nail beds/skin creases
8. Poor nutritional state
9. Pallor/icterus from anemia

prohibiting good dietary habits all contribute to the development of folate deficiency. States such as pregnancy or hemolysis, which increase the requirements of folate, will often precipitate a folate deficiency. Drugs can interfere with the recycling of folate by interfering with enzymes necessary to transfer carbon groups to folate. These include methotrexate, some anticonvulsants, and oral contraceptives. Malabsorption of folate, while unusual, is seen in cases of sprue. Bacterial overgrowth in the intestine may utilize the folate before it can be absorbed, such as in blind loop syndrome. Clinical Features of Folate Deficiency Unlike patients with vitamin B_{12} deficiency, patients with folate deficiency are more apt to appear malnourished. While the neurological deficits described above due to vitamin B_{12} deficiency are not seen in folate deficiency, patients with folate deficiency commonly complain of poor sleep, irritability, and depression, and may appear to have a blunted affect (Table 65.15). Folate-deficient patients may also have other nutrient deficiencies such as vitamins A, D, and K, and protein/calorie malnutrition. These concomitant deficiencies may contribute to skin pigmentation changes, sores at the corners of the mouth (angular cheilosis), and pallor such as lemon-tinted skin.

THE HEMATOLOGICAL EFFECTS OF FOLATE DEFICIENCY

Macrocytosis and megaloblastosis due to folate deficiency are essentially identical to that seen in vitamin B_{12} deficiency.

THE LABORATORY DIAGNOSIS OF FOLATE DEFICIENCY

The serum folate level reflects only the recent dietary intake of folate and does not provide an accurate assessment of folate stores (Table 65.16). The RBC folate level is low in true folate deficiency. The serum folate level will fall early in dietary restriction, and in true deficiency, the red cell folate levels will fall. In vitamin B_{12} deficiency, the folate is trapped in the unconjugated form as described above, leading to a loss of folate in the RBC. Thus, vitamin B_{12} deficiency may give a falsely low RBC folate value, but the serum folate will be normal to increased. Serum homocysteine, the precursor to methionine, will be elevated in folate deficiency as it is in B_{12} deficiency. The methylmalonic acid, however, will be normal in folate deficiency.

TABLE 65.16
Laboratory Diagnosis of Folate Deficiency

RBC folate level is reduced
Serum folate level may be reduced, but this is not specific; it
  may also be elevated, depending on the recent folate intake
Serum B_{12} level is normal

TABLE 65.17
Treatment of Folate Deficiency

Dose is 1–5 mg orally, daily
Pregnancy maintenance dose is 1 mg daily

TABLE 65.18
Causes for Treatment Failure

1. Wrong diagnosis
2. Additional vitamin or mineral deficiency
   (concomitant B_{12} and folate, for example)
3. Additional iron deficiency
4. Additional hemoglobinopathy (sickle cell
   disease or thalassemia)
5. Associated anemia of chronic disease
6. Hypothyroidism

NUTRITIONAL REQUIREMENTS OF FOLATE AND TREATMENT

The total body pool of folate stores is 5 to 10 mg. The daily dietary requirement is 50 μg/day, and the recommended daily allowance is 200 μg/day for men and 180 mg/day for women. The average daily diet contains 225 μg/day of folate. Foods rich in folate include green leafy vegetables, liver, kidney, fruits, dairy products, and cereals. Because the most common cause of folate deficiency is decreased nutritional intake, treatment is folate supplementation given in one-mg tablets daily (Table 65.17 and Table 65.18).

PROPHYLACTIC ADMINISTRATION OF FOLATE AND VITAMIN B_{12}

Some patients can be at risk for either folate deficiency or vitamin B_{12} deficiency. These patients should receive supplementation prophylactically (Table 65.19). For vitamin B_{12}, these patients include those with gastrectomy, very strict vegetarians, and infants born to mothers with pernicious anemia, because of the possibility of placental transfer of parietal cell or intrinsic factor antibodies. Folate prophylaxis should be given to pregnant women and women considering pregnancy to prevent neural tube defects. Breastfeeding women and premature infants should also receive folate. Patients with chronic hemolytic states such as sickle cell disease should receive folate as well as patients receiving chronic methotrexate for rheumatologic conditions, as the methotrexate inhibits dihydrofolate reductase, creating a form of "folate trap." Certain individuals with hyperhomocysteinemia may benefit from prophylactic folate administration, because a concomitant folate deficiency would create an exacerbation of the homocysteinemia due to the inhibition of methionine synthesis. Elevated homocysteine levels increase the risk of coronary artery disease.

IRON DEFICIENCY ANEMIA

MECHANISM OF ANEMIA

Every cell in the body requires iron. The cells utilize iron in oxidative metabolism, growth, and cellular proliferation as well as in oxygen transport. The major portion of body iron is found in hemoglobin. Heme is the component of hemoglobin that binds the iron, thus other heme-containing compounds including myoglobin and enzymes also contain iron. Hemoglobin accounts

TABLE 65.19
Who Should Receive Prophylaxis for B$_{12}$ and Folate Deficiency?

Vitamin B$_{12}$
1. Infants of mothers with pernicious anemia
2. Strict vegetarians
3. Patients who have had total gastrectomy

Folate
1. All women considering pregnancy (0.4 mg/day orally)
2. Pregnant women
3. Breastfeeding women
4. Premature infants
5. Chronic hemolytic states/hyperproliferative states
6. Patients receiving methotrexate for a rheumatologic condition
7. Certain individuals with hyperhomocysteinemia

for 85% of all the heme-containing compounds in the body. Iron exists in the body bound to proteins, both in storage and in heme compounds and enzymes (Hb, myoglobin, and cytochrome). Unbound iron is toxic, primarily by generating reactive oxygen species. Iron is absorbed from the duodenum and transported via transferrin to tissues such as RBC precursors. When not immediately utilized, the iron is stored mostly in the liver in the form of ferritin. During erythropoiesis, iron is incorporated in the hemoglobin, where it functions as the transporter of oxygen. When senescent red cells are destroyed in the reticuloendothelial system, macrophages of the spleen and liver take up the iron and recycle it to transferrin to be transported back to the bone marrow. While vitamin B$_{12}$ and folate are used in DNA synthesis in red cell precursors, iron is utilized in cytoplasmic hemoglobin synthesis. Heme requires adequate iron and porphyrin metabolism for formation. Defective porphyrin metabolism (sideroblastic anemia) sometimes responds to pyridoxine treatment; however, the cause of anemia is not due to a nutritional deficiency of pyridoxine but to inherent enzyme mutations disrupting normal porphyrin metabolism. Thus, sideroblastic anemia is beyond the scope of this section. Deficiency of iron creates a cytoplasmic maturation defect while the nuclear maturation proceeds normally. The result is small (microcytic) cells with poorly hemoglobinized cytoplasm (hypochromia).

In the past decade, there has been a wealth of information on the regulation of iron metabolism, which has led to a better understanding of the mechanisms leading to iron overload. This has primarily resulted from the cloning of genes of about a half dozen proteins that have been recognized to play a pivotal role in various aspects of cellular iron transport and mechanism. These include HFE, transferring receptor-2 (TfR2), divalent metal transporter-1 (DMT-1), ferroprotin, and hemojuvelin. Hepcidin, a 25-amino-acid peptide with antimicrobial properties has emerged as a major regulator of iron metabolism. While a detailed description of this topic is beyond the scope of this chapter, it should be pointed out that mutations in the genes that encode HFE, hemjuvelin, ferriportin, and TfR2 have emerged as the basis of different types of hereditary hemochromatosis. Hepcidin's role in decreasing iron absorption from the gut and tis induction with inflammatory cytokines has led to its emergence as an important regulator of iron metabolism particularly in relation to the anemia of chronic disease.

ETIOLOGY OF IRON DEFICIENCY

Iron deficiency is the most common nutritional deficiency in the United States. In the late 1800s, young menstruating females were considered fashionable if they were pale and chlorotic, a state of iron deficiency, although at the time the diagnosis of iron deficiency was not known. The loss of iron through chronic blood loss such as menses in a young female is the classic cause of iron deficiency. Any time iron is removed from the recycling process and lost from the body, iron deficiency can ensue (Table 65.20). Other conditions that remove iron include pregnancy and lactation. Increased iron requirements occur during periods of rapid growth such as in childhood. Adult men or menopausal women who are proven to have iron deficiency must be evaluated for blood loss, such as occurs in occult colon cancer, for example. Dietary causes of iron deficiency are unusual in developed countries except among infants, adolescents, and pregnant women, where the iron requirements are increased and the diet often compromised. The average adult man consumes more than adequate iron daily to make up for the normal iron loss. Therefore, in the United States, iron deficiency seen in a patient not falling under one of these categories should be thoroughly evaluated for blood loss and not merely treated.

THE CLINICAL FEATURES OF IRON DEFICIENCY

Children who develop iron deficiency may demonstrate irritability, memory loss, and learning difficulties. In adults, iron deficiency can develop slowly, and very low levels of hemoglobin may be attained before symptoms of anemia develop (Table 65.21).

TABLE 65.20
Causes of Iron Deficiency Anemia

1. Gastrointestinal bleeding
2. Genitourinary bleeding
3. Menses
4. Repeated blood donation
5. Growth
6. Pregnancy and lactation
7. Poor diets
8. Intestinal malabsorption
9. Hookworm/intestinal parasites
10. Gastric surgery

TABLE 65.21
Clinical Features of Iron Deficiency

Symptoms of anemia
1. Pagophagia (heavy ice consumption)
2. Koilonychia (brittle spoon nails)
3. Blue sclera
4. Glossitis
5. Angular stomatitis
6. Postcricoid esophageal web/stricture
   (Plummer-Vinson Syndrome)
7. Gastric atrophy
8. Impaired immunity
9. Decreased exercise tolerance
10. Neuropsychological abnormalities

It is not unusual for a woman to present with a hemoglobin of 2 or 3 g/dl with only moderate symptoms of fatigue or shortness of breath. Blood transfusion in these patients can be dangerous and should be performed very carefully, and only with one or two units to avoid congestive heart failure or stroke from rapid increase in intravascular volume and red cell numbers. Iron deficiency anemia may cause brittle "spoon" nails (koilonychia), blue-tinted sclera, and a painful tongue (glossitis). Immunity may be impaired due to the lack of iron needed by white blood cells and the enzymes used in host defense.

Pica is a fascinating manifestation of iron deficiency whereby the appetite is altered and patients crave for nonnutritional substances to eat. Classic examples include ice, starch, or clay consumption. In most cases, pica is a symptom of iron deficiency and not the cause. However, clay inhibits absorption of iron and may perpetuate the condition. Furthermore, excessive consumption of these products provides for a poor diet in general, thus exacerbating iron deficiency. In some cultures, pica is practiced as a norm and, in those cases, iron deficiency may be the result of, and not the cause of, pica.

THE HEMATOLOGICAL EFFECTS OF IRON DEFICIENCY

As mentioned, the perturbation of cytoplasmic maturation during erythropoiesis (decreased Hb synthesis due to Fe deficiency) leads to small, underhemoglobinized red cells (microcytosis and hypochromia). In fact, the MCV can be as low as 50 fl in severe cases. The reticulocyte index is low. Often, cells of various shapes and sizes are released from the bone marrow. Platelets may increase in iron deficiency and can even exceed 1 million (normal 140,000 to 400,000). If concurrent folate or vitamin B_{12} deficiency exists, then the red cells may not demonstrate the microcytosis as expected due to the concomitant macrocytosis. However, the red cells will become microcytic upon replacement of the folate or vitamin B_{12}.

THE LABORATORY DIAGNOSIS OF FE DEFICIENCY

Ferritin is the storage compartment for iron in the body; therefore, serum ferritin levels reflect the state of body Fe stores. A ferritin of less than 12 μg/dl is diagnostic of iron deficiency. Other laboratory features, such as the transferrin level (or the iron-binding capacity), the serum iron level, and the transferring saturation are summarized in Table 65.22. If iron stores are low, the iron binding capacity will be elevated, reflecting the vacant binding sites. The transferring saturation will be decreased.

TABLE 65.22
Laboratory Features of Iron Deficiency

Hematological
Microcytic anemia
Thrombocytosis

Bone Marrow
Normal nuclear maturation
Cytoplasmic abnormalities
Absent iron stores

Biochemical
Ferritin level is decreased
Total iron binding capacity is elevated
Iron saturation and serum iron are decreased

TABLE 65.23
Treatment of Iron Deficiency

Oral
- 150 to 200 mg elemental iron daily given in three divided doses on empty stomach
- (Children's dose is 3 mg iron/kg body weight daily in three divided doses
- Ferrous sulfate is best absorbed and least expensive. One tablet of 325 mg ferrous sulfate contains 600 to 70 mg elemental iron. Given thrice daily, this is a good standard treatment for adults. Hemoglobin should rise approximately 2 g/dl every 3 weeks. Treatment should continue 4 to 6 months after obtaining a normal hemoglobin

Intravenous
- Iron dextran with dose depending on body weight and degree of anemia is the most widely used preparation. Use requires a "test dose" be given first to ensure against an anaphylactic response. The full amount can then be given as a one-time dose calculated from a chart included in the product insert. This solution of ferric oxyhydroxide and low-molecular weight dextran contains 50 mg of elemental iron per ml. An average dose for a 70 kg patient with a hemoglobin of 7 g/dl would be 40 ml or iron dextran (2000 mg of elemental iron)
- Iron glucose is another macromolecular complex of sodium ferric gluconate in an alkaline (pH = 7.7 to 9.7) solution of 20% sucrose which also requires a test dose be given before the full amount. One gram of Fe is then administered in eight doses of 125 mg Fe each. Each dose is diluted in 100 ml of NS and infused over 60 min
- Iron sucrose is an alternative formulation, which is a polynuclear iron (III) hydroxide sucrose complex. Its use does not require a test dose. A total of 1 g is given by IV push in ten divided doses, with no more than three doses of 100 mg each given per week

---

The degree of iron deficiency present and the resultant hematological effects is an important concept. By the time microcytosis is evident, the red cell hemoglobin content is decreased. Before that stage, however, the body stores of iron will be decreased, but the red cell amount of iron will be maintained. This is why a patient may demonstrate a low ferritin, an elevated total iron-binding capacity (TIBC), and decreased iron saturation, yet have no evidence of anemia. These patients will develop symptoms of anemia over time if the iron loss is not corrected.

Ferritin is also an acute phase reactant. Thus, conditions such as renal failure, infection, liver disease, and acute or chronic inflammatory states will lead to elevated ferritin levels. In these cases, it may be necessary to ascertain iron stores directly with a bone marrow aspirate. The bone marrow should demonstrate iron in the interstitium when stained with an iron stain. If no iron is demonstrated in the marrow, the patient definitely has iron depletion. Iron deficiency anemia, however, can be diagnosed from serum studies.

NUTRITIONAL REQUIREMENTS OF IRON AND TREATMENT

Adult males have 50 mg of iron per kilogram of body weight; females have 35 mg/kg. The minimal daily requirement is 1 mg for men and 2 mg for menstruating women. The recommended daily allowance is 12 mg/day for men and 15 mg/day for women. The average daily diet contains 6 mg of iron per 1000 kcal of food consumed (10 to 30 mg/day). Foods rich in iron include red meat. Remember the conditions that increase iron requirements such as pregnancy, childhood, and chronic blood loss. In pregnancy, the daily requirement may increase to 5–6 mg. For infants the daily requirement is 0.5 mg, and for children in 1 mg.

Oral iron replacement is sufficient in the majority of cases of iron deficiency anemia (Table 65.23). The usual dose is 60 mg of elemental iron administered as 325 mg or iron sulfate thrice daily. The best available is in the ferrous form and heme iron as

TABLE 65.24
Possible Side Effects of Iron Therapy

Oral
1. Constipation
2. Diarrhea
3. Nausea
4. Epigastric discomfort
5. Vomiting

Intravenous
1. Anaphylaxis
2. Fever
3. Urticaria
4. Adenopathy
5. Myalgias
6. Arthralgias
7. Phlebitis
8. Pain at injection site

TABLE 65.25
Nutritional Information on B$_{12}$, Folate, and Iron

	B$_{12}$	Folate	Iron
Total body pool	3000 µg	5-10 mg	Men: 50 mg/kg Women: 35 mg/kg
Minimal daily adult Requirement (dietary)	0.3-1.2 µg/day	50 µg/day	10-20 mg/day
Recommended dietary allowance (RDA)	2 µg/day	Men: 200 µg/day Women: 180 µg/day	Men: 12 mg/d Women: 15 mg/d
Average daily diet	5-15 µg/day (range 1-100 µg/d)	225 µg/day	6 mg/1000 kcal (10-30 mg/d)
Prevalence of deficiency	0.2% of population	8% of men in NA 10-13% of women	2% adult men 8% women
Source foods	Animal origin liver, kidney, mollusks, muscle, eggs, cheese, milk Multivitamins	Green leafy vegs. liver, kidney fruits, breakfast cereals, dairy, tea Multivitamins	Read meat
Time to develop blood signs after abstinence of nutrient	5-6 years	3 weeks	Years

in red meat. The reticulocyte response will peak at day 8 to 10 after initiation of treatment, and the hemoglobin should normalize over 6 to 10 weeks. An improved sense of wellbeing may occur as soon as day 2 or 3 of treatment, however. Often, patients complain of gastrointestinal side effects or oral iron (Table 65.24). These include constipation, diarrhea, epigastric discomfort, and nausea. Taking the iron with food can ameliorate these symptoms, though this decreases the absorption by as much as 50%. Alternatively, smaller amounts may be given or different preparations tried. Some other iron formulations (iron-sorbitol) may be better tolerated in terms of gastrointestinal side effects. On very rare occasions, it may be necessary to administer intravenous or intramuscular iron. This can be associated with some untoward side effects, but will eliminate the need for oral iron. Oral iron therapy should be continued for six months once the hemoglobin normalizes. Parenteral iron need only be given once. It should be kept in mind that if the cause of the iron deficiency is blood loss and this continues, iron deficiency may recur in the future, and chronic iron replacement may be indicated (Table 65.25).

OTHER NUTRITIONAL DEFICIENCIES

There are multiple other well-described deficiency states that cause anemia, including vitamins, trace metals, and protein.

VITAMIN A

This produces a microcytic anemia; however, in contrast to iron-deficiency, lab assays of iron stores are elevated. Vitamin A deficiency is fairly uncommon in the United States, but in developing countries shows a strong correlation to anemia when present in levels less than 30 μg/dl.

VITAMINS B

Multiple other B vitamins have been implicated in anemias, including B_2 (riboflavin), B_3 (niacin), and B_6 (pyridoxine). These are very uncommon, and much of the data were acquired through artificial induction of these deficiencies in individuals under controlled settings. Riboflavin deficiency is associated with a red cell aplasia. Niacin deficiency causes anemia through a poorly understood mechanism. Pyridoxine deficiency causes microcytic anemia, which can also be seen in patients on some antituberculosis medications (isoniazid) (see Chapter 74, Drug–Nutrient Interactions).

VITAMINS C

Deficiency of this vitamin causes a megaloblastic anemia indirectly through impaired folic acid metabolism. It is also associated with iron deficiency due to chronic bleeding, which is also commonly present with insufficient levels of ascorbic acid.

VITAMIN E

Vitamin E is a fat-soluble vitamin, and inadequate levels may be present in neonates or chronic fat malabsorption states. A hemolytic anemia may result as a direct effect on the erythrocyte cytoplasmic membrane.

COPPER

A deficiency in this trace metal (>40 μg/dl) is associated directly with iron malabsorption and indirectly with microcytic anemia (see Chapter 8, Trace Minerals). Zinc toxicity impairs copper absorption and also causes physiological copper deficiency (see Chapter 11, Nutrient Interactions). In patients with low protein states or Wilson's disease, serum copper levels are unreliable and the diagnosis requires a liver biopsy.

PROTEIN

Protein deficiency through starvation states (Kwashiorkor) has classically been associated with anemia through induction of an aplasia of the marrow (see Chapter 39, Protein–Energy Malnutrition). Testing has revealed a decreased erythropoietin production of the starved individual, as well as a decreased sensitivity of the bone marrow erythrocyte precursors to erythropoietin. This decreased sensitivity causes a maturation block, which can be overcome by exogenous administration of recombinant erythropoietin. Protein deficiency is also strongly associated with a riboflavin deficiency, which can be fatal during repletion of protein stores if not treated.

REFERENCES

1. Israels LG, Israels ED. *Mechanisms in Hematology*, Core Health Services, Inc., Ontario, AC, 1998.
2. Hoffman R. *Hematology: Basic Principals and Practice*, Churchill Livingstone, Philadelphia, PA, 2005.
3. Hercberg S, Galan P. Nutritional anemais, *Clinical Haematology*, Vol. 5, Fleming AF, Ed, Bailliere Tindall, London, 1992, pp 143–168.
4. Hughes-Jones NC, Wickramasinghe SN. Lecture Notes on Haematology, Blackwell Science, London, 1996.
5. Foucar K. *Bone Marrow Pathology*, 2nd edition, ASCP Press, Chicago, IL, 2001.
6. Jandl JH. *Blood*, Little, Brown, Boston, MA, 1987.
7. Duffy TP. Normochromic, normocytic anemias, *Cecil Textbook of Medicine*, 20th edition, Bennett, JC, Plum F, Eds, WB Saunders, Philadelphia, PA, 1996, p 837.
8. Duffy TP. Microcytic and hypochromic anemias, *Cecil Textbook of Medicine*, 20th edition, Bennett JC, Plum F, Eds, WB Saunders, Philadelphia, PA, 1996, p 839.
9. Allen RH. Megaloblastic anemias, *Cecil Textbook of Medicine*, 20th edition, Bennett JC, Plum F, Eds, WB Saunders, Philadelphia, PA, 1996, p 843.
10. Ganz T, Nemeth E. *Regulation of Iron Acquisition and Iron Distribution in Mammals*, Biochimica et Biophysica Acta, 2006, p 1.

66 Food Allergy

Scott H. Sicherer

CONTENTS

DEFINITION OF FOOD ALLERGY

Individuals may attribute a variety of illnesses or symptoms to a "food allergy." Surveys of adults have shown that 18 to 22% believe that they have a food allergy and 28% of parents suspect a food allergy in their infants and young children.[1-3] However, true food allergy affects 6 to 8% of children and approximately 3.5% of adults.[3-6] The way in which food allergy is defined may, in part, explain the discrepancy between suspected and true food allergy. A food allergy is an adverse *immune response* directed toward protein in food. This is in contrast to a larger number of non-immune-mediated adverse reactions to food.[7] The non-immune-mediated reactions include those caused by toxins in foods, such as spoiled foods, that would affect anyone ingesting the tainted food, pharmacological responses, and adverse reactions caused by a particular condition of the affected individual, such as a digestive problem (*food intolerance*). Examples of food intolerance/reactions to toxins are listed in Table 66.1.

PATHOPHYSIOLOGY OF FOOD-ALLERGIC REACTIONS

A large number of potentially immunoreactive food proteins pass through the gut, but the normal response to these foreign proteins is to recognize but ignore them, a process termed "oral tolerance."[8] The gastrointestinal component of immune reactivity has a daunting task of identifying gut pathogens and eliminating them, while allowing certain bacteria, gut flora, to remain while simultaneously avoiding adverse immune responses to dietary nutrients. Approximately 2% of ingested food enters the blood stream in an immunologically intact form, but causes no symptoms in the normal individual. It remains unclear why some individuals develop food allergies, but a genetic predisposition toward allergic responses plays a role.[9] For those individuals predisposed to food allergies, food allergens can elicit specific responses in several ways.

Allergic reactions that occur promptly following ingestion of a causal food protein typically is the result of the generation of IgE antibodies, an immune protein that recognizes and binds the triggering food protein.[5,10] When a protein enters the intestine, immune cells termed *antigen presenting cells* (APCs) process the protein (usually a glycoprotein) and present a small portion of the protein to T cells, a type of lymphocyte that specifically recognize the protein fragment (Figure 66.1). Cellular interactions

TABLE 66.1
Examples of Food Intolerance/Toxic Reactions (Nonimmunological, Adverse Reactions to Food)[5,10]

Disorder/Sensitivity	Pathophysiology/Symptoms
Lactase deficiency (lactose intolerance)	Bloating, diarrhea from inability to digest sugar in cow's milk, may be dose related
Tyramine sensitivity	Tyramine in hard cheeses, wine may trigger migraine headache
Scombroid fish poisoning	Oral pruritus, flushing, vomiting, hives from histamine released from spoiled dark meat fish (tuna, Mahi–Mahi, etc.)
Caffeine	Pharmacological effects of jitteriness, heart palpitations
Myristicin	Hallucinogen in nutmeg
Gallbladder disease	Pain following ingestion of fatty foods

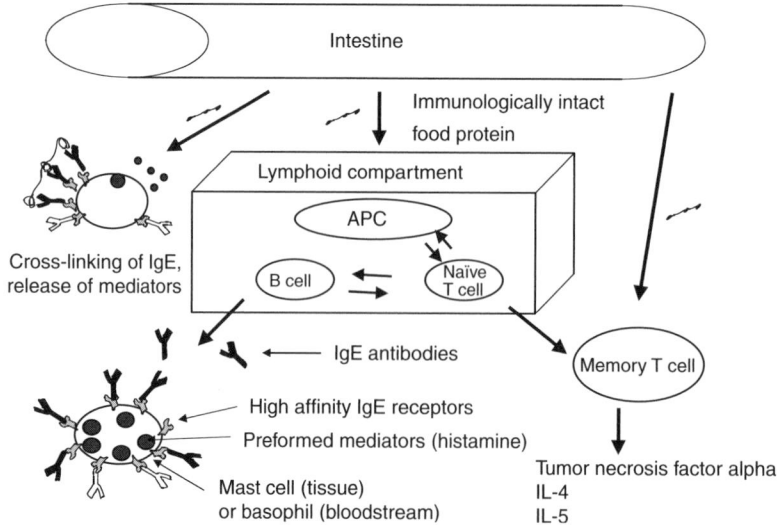

FIGURE 66.1   Pathophysiology of Adverse immune responses to food proteins abbreviation: APC = antigen presenting cells, IL = interleukine (see text for details).

between the APC and T cell may direct the T cell toward allergic responses. The types of chemical mediators released from these T cells characterize them as Th-2 types of T cells. The sensitized T cells replicate and then interact with B cells, a type of lymphocyte that can transform into a cell that produces antibodies, including IgE. These IgE antibodies bind to specific receptors found on mast cells in body tissues and basophils in the bloodstream. The IgE antibodies are specific for, and bind to, areas on the food proteins called *epitopes*; therefore, the IgE-armed mast cell or basophil is poised to detect whichever proteins the IgE has been directed toward. The mast cells and basophils have preformed mediators (e.g., histamine) that, when released from the cell, cause tissue swelling (edema from capillary leakage of fluid) and pruritus. When the mast cell or basophil armed with the food-specific IgE antibody comes in contact with the particular allergenic protein, the IgE antibodies attach to the protein and cross-link, resulting in release of the mediators and the onset of the food-allergic reaction.

Chronic disease attributed to food allergy, for example rashes (atopic dermatitis [AD]) or gastrointestinal disorders involve an immune response to food protein but may not involve the generation of IgE antibody (non-IgE-mediated).[5,10,11] In this case, the T cell may, through direct interaction with specific receptors on the cells, elaborate mediators (cytokines) with direct effects. An example is the release of tumor necrosis factor alpha that causes gut edema in certain forms of cow's milk allergy (CMA).[12] Further research is underway to better delineate the mechanisms of non-IgE-mediated food allergy.

FOOD ALLERGENS

A rather short list of foods/food groups accounts for the majority (85 to 90%) of food-allergic reactions: chicken egg, cow's milk, wheat, soybean, peanut, tree nuts (e.g., walnut, cashew, etc.), fish (e.g., tuna, salmon, cod, etc.), and shellfish (e.g., shrimp, crab, etc.).[3,4,13] However, virtually any food protein could elicit an allergic response.[14] Many of the allergenic food proteins have been characterized and are generally heat-stable, water-soluble glycoproteins from 10 to 70 kD in size. For many of these proteins, the particular allergenic epitopes that bind IgE or T cell receptors have been mapped.[15,16]

EPIDEMIOLOGY

It is estimated that food allergy affects 6 to 8% of young children and about 3.5% of adults.[3–6] The foods causing significant allergic reactions in different age groups are listed in Table 66.2. Most children outgrow their sensitivity to milk, egg, soy, and wheat, but allergy to peanut, tree nuts (e.g., walnut, cashew, Brazil nut, etc.), fish, and shellfish account for the majority of significant food allergies in adults and are foods for which tolerance rarely develops.[17] Peanut and tree nut allergy is estimated to affect 1.3% and seafood allergy 2.3% of the general population of the United States.[4,14] Food allergy, along with other allergic diseases, appears to be increasing in prevalence. Two studies have documented a doubling in the rate of peanut allergy within the past decade.[14,18] Allergic reactions to food dyes and additives are rare, affecting up to 0.23% of the population.[19] Food allergy is a cause of a number of illnesses as shown in Table 66.3.[20–25]

FOOD-ALLERGIC DISORDERS

The target organs of food allergy include the skin and gastrointestinal and respiratory tracts. The pathophysiological basis of the disorders may be IgE mediated, non-IgE mediated or both.[10] Disorders with an acute onset occurring within minutes to an hour after food ingestion are typically mediated by IgE antibody, while those that are more chronic and occur hours after ingestion are usually not IgE mediated. Particular food-allergic disorders are discussed below.

TABLE 66.2
Foods Responsible for the Majority (85 to 90%) of Significant Allergic Reactions[3–6,14]

Infants/Young Children	Older Children/Adults
Egg	Peanut
Cow's milk	Tree nuts
Soy bean	Shellfish
Peanut	Fish
Wheat	
Fish	
Tree nuts (walnut, Brazil, hazel, almond, cashew, etc.)	
Shellfish	

TABLE 66.3
Epidemiological Role of Food Allergy in Various
Disorders[3,11,20–33]

Disorder	Prevalence of Food Allergy as a Cause of the Disorder (%)
Anaphylaxis	34–52
Asthmatic children	6
Asthmatic adults	<1
AD (moderate–severe) in children	37
AD in adults	Rare
Acute urticaria	20
Chronic urticaria	1.4
Infantile refractory reflux	42
Childhood refractory constipation	68

DISORDERS AFFECTING THE SKIN

Acute Urticaria

Urticaria or "hives" are characterized by transient pruritic and erythematous raised lesions with central clearing and a surrounding area of erythema, similar in appearance to a mosquito bite. The rash should leave no residual lesions after resolution. Hives may sometimes be accompanied by localized swelling (angioedema). Although there are many causes of acute urticaria, food allergy accounts for up to 20% of episodes.[23] The immediate onset of hives is mediated by specific IgE to food protein. Lesions usually occur within an hour of ingestion or skin contact with the causal food.

Chronic Urticaria

This disorder is characterized by periods of hives that continue to occur over 6 weeks. Only 1.4% of chronic/persistent urticaria is associated with food allergy,[26] so a search for a causative food in the initial evaluation of this illness is often futile.

Contact Urticaria

In some cases, topical exposure to a food (e.g., on the skin of the face) can cause a local reaction either through irritation or through specific immune mechanisms.[27] This may be observed when young children are eating a food they tolerate but develop hives around the lips.

Atopic Dermatitis

This chronic and relapsing rash is characterized by a typical distribution on the extensor surfaces and face of infants, or creases in older children and adults, and extreme pruritis.[28] AD is often associated with allergic disorders (asthma and allergic rhinitis) and with a family history of allergy. Both IgE antibody-mediated and non-IgE-mediated (cellular) food-allergic mechanisms have been identified in disorder.[29–31] Clinical studies utilizing double-blind, placebo-controlled food challenges (DBPCFCs) have shown that one third of children with moderate to severe AD have food allergy.[29,32] The more severe the rash, the more likely that food allergy is associated.[33] However, AD is rarely associated with food allergy in adults.[34]

Dermatitis Herpetiformis

Dermatitis Herpetiformis (DH) a chronic papulovesicular skin disorder with lesions distributed over the extensor surfaces of the elbows, knees, and buttocks.[35] Immunohistological examination of the lesions reveals the deposition of granular IgA antibody at the dermoepidermal junction. The disorder is associated with a specific non-IgE-mediated immune response to gluten (a protein found in grains such as wheat, barley, and rye). Although related to Celiac disease, there may be no associated gastrointestinal complaints. The rash abates with the elimination of gluten from the diet.

DISORDERS AFFECTING THE GASTROINTESTINAL TRACT[36]

Immediate Gastrointestinal Hypersensitivity

This syndrome is characterized by immediate (from minutes up to 1 to 2 h) gastrointestinal symptoms following the ingestion of a triggering food protein. Symptoms may include nausea, vomiting, abdominal pain, and diarrhea. Considered here as a distinct

---

TABLE 66.4

Cross Reactions Due to Proteins Shared by Pollens and Foods Leading to Symptoms of the Oral Allergy Syndrome[39–42]

Birch Pollen	Ragweed Pollen	Grass Pollen
Apple	Melons	Peach
Carrot		Potato
Cherry		Tomato
Apricot		Cherry
Plum		
Celery		

---

syndrome, it is more commonly associated with reactions in other organ systems, such as during systemic anaphylaxis in patients with other atopic diseases.[37] For example, children with AD undergoing oral food challenges with foods to which they have specific IgE antibody will sometimes manifest only gastrointestinal symptoms.[38]

Pollen-Food-Related Syndrome (Oral Allergy Syndrome)

Symptoms include pruritus and angioedema of the lips, tongue, and palate and are of rapid onset typically while eating certain fresh fruits and vegetables.[39,40] The reaction occurs primarily in adults with pollen allergy (hay fever) sensitized to cross-reacting proteins in particular fruits and vegetables as shown in Table 66.4.[41,42] The proteins are labile, and cooked forms of the fruits and vegetables generally do not usually induce symptoms.

Dietary Protein-Induced Proctitis/Proctocolitis of Infancy[43]

Food allergy is a possible cause of rectal bleeding due to colitis in infants. Infants with this disorder are typically healthy, but have streaks of blood mixed with mucus in their stool. The most common causal food is cow's milk or soy, and breast-fed infants can develop this reaction from small amounts of protein passed through breast milk in mothers ingesting the causal protein. Tests for food allergy are usually negative. Maternal avoidance of the causal protein will usually resolve symptoms for the breast-fed infant. In infants fed cow's milk or soy formula, substitution with a protein hydrolysate formula generally leads to cessation of obvious bleeding within 72 h. The majority of infants who develop this condition while ingesting protein hydrolysate formulas will experience resolution of bleeding with the substitution of an amino-acid-based formula.

Dietary (Food) Protein-Induced Enteropathy

Infants or young children with this disorder may experience failure to thrive, diarrhea, emesis, and hypoproteinemia usually related to an immunological reaction to cow's milk protein.[44,45] The syndrome may also occur following infectious gastroenteritis in infants. Patchy villous atrophy with cellular infiltrate on biopsy is characteristic. Diagnosis is based upon the combined findings from endoscopy/biopsy, allergen elimination, and challenge. While this syndrome resembles Celiac disease, resolution generally occurs in 1 to 2 years, and there is no association with neoplasia.

Dietary (Food) Protein-Induced Enterocolitis Syndrome

Initially described and defined by Powell,[46,47] the syndrome is characterized by a symptom complex of profuse vomiting and diarrhea diagnosed in infancy during chronic ingestion of the causal food protein, usually cow's milk or soy. Since both the small and large bowels are involved, the term "enterocolitis" is used. When the causal protein is reintroduced after a period of avoidance, symptoms characteristically develop after a delay of 2 h, with profuse vomiting and later diarrhea. There is also an accompanying increase in the peripheral polymorphonuclear leukocyte count and, in about 20% of episodes, severe acidosis and dehydration may occur. Confirmation of the allergy includes a negative search for other causes, improvement when not ingesting the causal protein, and a positive oral challenge resulting in the characteristic symptoms/signs. Approximately half of the infants react to both cow's milk and soy. Sensitivity to milk is lost in 60% and to soy in 25% of the patients after 2 years from the time of presentation.[48] Treatment with a hydrolyzed cow's milk formula is advised, although some patients may react to the residual peptides in these formulas, requiring an amino-acid-based formula.[49] Solid foods, particularly oat and rice, may also induce food-protein-induced enterocolitis syndrome (FPIES).[50]

Allergic Eosinophillic Gastroenteritis and Esophagitis

These disorders are characterized by infiltration of the esophagus (AEE), gastric or intestinal walls (AEG) with eosinophils, peripheral eosinophilia (in 50 to 75%), and absence of vasculitis.[51–56] Patients with allergic eosinophilic gastroenteritis (AEG) present with postprandial nausea, abdominal pain, vomiting, diarrhea, protein-losing enteropathy, and weight loss, and, depending on the depth of infiltration, abdominal bloating, obstruction, and ascites can also develop. Those with allergic eosinophilic esophagitis (AEE) may present with symptoms of severe reflux disease, and typically with pain while food is being swallowed (dysphagia). The diagnosis requires a biopsy showing eosinophilic infiltration, although there may be patchy disease and infiltration may be missed. In children with AEE, significant success from dietary elimination has been achieved.[57,58] AEE was associated with positive tests for food-specific IgE antibody in some of the children, but most with this disorder do not have IgE-mediated food allergy.

Celiac Disease

Celiac disease is a dietary protein enteropathy characterized by an extensive loss of absorptive villi and hyperplasia of the crypts leading to malabsorption, chronic diarrhea, steatorrhea, abdominal distention, flatulence and weight loss or failure to thrive.[59,60] As the disease represents an immune response to a food protein, it may be considered a food-allergic disorder. It is associated with human leukocyte antigen (HLA)-DQ2, which is present in over 90% of patients.[60] Patients with celiac disease are sensitive to gliadin, the alcohol-soluble portion of gluten found in wheat, oat, rye, and barley. Endoscopy typically reveals total villous atrophy and extensive cellular infiltrate. Chronic ingestion of gluten-containing grains in celiac patients is associated with increased risk of malignancy, especially T cell lymphoma.

Other Disorders Possibly Associated with Food Allergy

Gastroesophageal reflux (GER) has been associated with CMA in infants and young children.[61,62] Constipation has also been associated with CMA in young children.[25,63]

Ingestion of whole cow's milk by infants less than 6 months of age may lead to occult blood loss from the gastrointestinal tract and iron deficiency anemia.[64] The use of infant formulas generally results in resolution of symptoms. There is limited evidence that *infantile colic* is associated with food (cow's milk) allergy in a subset of patients.[65] A summary of the gastrointestinal diseases associated with food allergy is given in Table 66.5.

DISORDERS AFFECTING THE RESPIRATORY TRACT

Allergic Rhinitis

Hay fever is characterized by symptoms of congestion, rhinorrhea, and nasal pruritis. These symptoms are usually associated with hypersensitivity to airborne allergens, not foods. Rarely, isolated nasal symptoms may occur as a result of IgE-mediated allergy to ingested food proteins.[66] The prevalence of this illness, even among patients referred to allergy clinics, appears to be under 1%. On the other hand, 25 to 80% of patients with documented IgE-mediated food allergy experience nasal symptoms during oral food challenges that result in systemic symptoms. In contrast to immune-mediated rhinitis, *Gustatory rhinitis* refers to rhinorrhea caused by spicy foods. This reaction is mediated by neurological mechanisms.[67]

Asthma

Isolated wheezing, cough, and dyspnea induced by lower airway inflammation and bronchoconstriction can be related to food allergy, but more commonly is related to airborne allergens and viral infections. Asthma reactions may occur based on

TABLE 66.5
Gastrointestinal Diseases Associated with Food Allergy[11,24,25,36,40,43–58]

Disorder	Age Onset	Duration	Symptoms/Features	Foods
FPIES	1 day to 9 months	Usually 1 to 3 years	Vomiting, diarrhea, failure to thrive, villus injury, dehydration, and acidosis	Cow's milk, soybean, rare grains, and poultry
Enteropathy	2 to 18 months	Usually 1 to 3 years	Failure to thrive, edema, diarrhea, villus injury, and malabsorption	Cow's milk, soy
Celiac disease	Any	Life long	Villus injury and malabsorption	Gluten
Proctocolitis	Infants	1 year	Bloody stools	Cow's milk, soybean
AEG/AEE	Any	Long lived	Vomiting, abdominal pain, diarrhea, and eosinophilic infiltration of gut	Multiple foods

TABLE 66.6
Symptoms Occurring in Anaphylaxis[10,72–74]

Organ System	Symptoms
Respiratory	Throat tightness, wheezing, repetitive coughing, nasal congestion rhinitis, and hypoxia/cyanosis
Gastrointestinal	Obstructive tongue edema, nausea, vomiting, diarrhea, abdominal pain, oral pruritus, and lip edema
Skin	Pruritus, urticaria, angioedema, and morbiliform rash
Cardiovascular	Hypotension, syncope, and dysrhythmia
Other	Sense of "impending doom," uterine contractions

IgE-mediated reactions from ingestion of the causative food or from inhalation of vapors released during cooking or in occupational settings.[68,69] The prevalence of food-related asthma in the general population is unknown, but studies report a prevalence of 5.7% among children with asthma,[21] 11% among children with AD,[68] and 24% among children with a history of food-induced wheezing.[70] The prevalence of food-induced wheezing among adults with asthma is under 2%.[22]

Heiner's Syndrome

This is a rare, non-IgE-mediated adverse pulmonary response to food affecting infants.[71] The disorder is characterized by an immune reaction to cow's milk proteins with precipitating antibodies (IgG) to cow's milk protein resulting in pulmonary infiltrates, pulmonary hemosiderosis, anemia, failure to thrive, and recurrent pneumonias. Elimination of cow's milk protein is curative.

MULTISYSTEM DISORDERS

Anaphylaxis

Allergic reactions that affect more than one organ system, or are severe in nature are termed anaphylactic reactions.[72] Food is the most common cause of out of hospital anaphylaxis. Symptoms may affect the skin, respiratory tract, and gastrointestinal tract (Table 66.6). Symptoms can be severe, progressive, and potentially fatal. When blood circulation is impaired, the term *anaphylactic shock* is used. Fatal food-induced anaphylaxis appears to be more common among teenaged patients with underlying asthma.[73,74] In addition, patients who experienced fatal or near-fatal anaphylaxis were unaware that they had ingested the incriminated food, had almost immediate symptoms, had a delay in receiving emergency treatment with epinephrine, a medication that reverses many of the severe symptoms of anaphylaxis, and, in about half of the cases, there was a period of quiescence prior to a respiratory decompensation. The foods most often responsible for food-induced anaphylaxis are peanut, tree nuts, and shellfish.

Food-Associated, Exercise-Induced Anaphylaxis

This uncommon disorder refers to patients who are able to ingest a particular food or exercise without a reaction.[75,76] However, when exercise follows the ingestion of a particular food, anaphylaxis results. Wheat is a common trigger. In some cases, exercise after any meal results in a reaction. Treatment depends on elimination of the causal food for 12 h prior to exercise.

DISORDERS NOT CLEARLY RELATED TO FOOD ALLERGY

A variety of symptoms and medical problems have been attributed to food allergy, for example headaches, seizures, behavioral disorders, fatigue, arthritis, etc., but many of these are either false associations or adverse reactions that are not immunological in nature.[37] Food allergy may play a role in a minority of patients with migraine headaches,[77] although the pharmacological activity of certain chemicals that are found in some foods (i.e., tyramine in cheeses) is more often responsible. The role of food allergy in childhood behavioral disorders is also controversial. Although, a subset of patients with behavioral disorders may be affected by food dyes,[78] there is no convincing evidence that food allergy *per se* plays a direct role in these disorders and children are not allergic to "sugar." [79] On the other hand, for individuals with these ailments who also have bona fide allergies, treatment to relieve symptoms of asthma, AD, and hay fever should be pursued in parallel to treatment directed at the unrelated disorder.

DIAGNOSTIC APPROACH TO FOOD-ALLERGIC DISORDERS

Overview

Arguably, the medical history is the most important diagnostic test for food allergy. For example, a diagnosis is apparent when there is an acute onset of typical symptoms, such as hives and wheezing, following the isolated ingestion of a suspected food with confirmatory laboratory studies indicating the presence of specific IgE antibody to the suspected food.[37,80] However, the diagnosis is more complicated when multiple foods are implicated or when chronic diseases, such as asthma or AD, are evaluated. The diagnosis of food allergy and identification of the particular foods responsible is also problematic when reactions are not mediated by IgE antibody, as is the case with a number of gastrointestinal food allergies. In these latter circumstances, well-devised elimination diets followed by physician-supervised oral food challenges are critical in the identification and proper treatment of these disorders.

GENERAL APPROACH TO DIAGNOSIS

History and Physical Examination

A history and physical examination should review general medical concerns to exclude nonimmunological adverse reactions to foods or to consider other allergic causes for symptoms, for example another type of allergy such as a cat allergy causing asthma. In relation to foods, a careful history should focus on: the symptoms attributed to food ingestion (type, acute vs. chronic), the foods involved, consistency of reactions, the quantity of food required to elicit symptoms, the timing between ingestion and onset of symptoms, the most recent reaction/patterns of reactivity, and any ancillary associated activity that may play a role (i.e., exercise, alcohol ingestion, etc.). The information gathered is used to determine the best mode of diagnosis or may lead to dismissal of the problem based upon the history alone.

If the symptoms being evaluated are typical of IgE-mediated reaction, for example urticaria and wheezing, and if the symptoms follow soon after a food ingestion, that history may clearly implicate a particular food. In this circumstance, a positive test for specific IgE antibody to the suspected food would be confirmatory. If the ingestion was of mixed foods and the causal food was uncertain, for example, fruit salad, the history may help to eliminate some of the foods — those frequently ingested without symptoms — and specific tests for IgE may help to further narrow the possibilities. In chronic disorders such as AD or asthma, it is more difficult to pinpoint causal foods. The approach to diagnosis in these chronic disorders usually requires elimination diets and oral food challenges to confirm suspected associations. This is particularly the case for the non-IgE-mediated reactions or those attributed to food dyes/preservatives in which ancillary laboratory testing is not helpful.

TESTS FOR SPECIFIC IgE ANTIBODY

For IgE-mediated food allergy, specific tests can help to identify, or exclude, responsible foods. One method to determine the presence of specific IgE antibody is prick-puncture skin testing. While the patient is not taking antihistamines, a device, such as a bifurcated needle, plastic probe, or lancet, is used to puncture the skin through a glycerinated extract of a food and appropriate positive (histamine) and negative (saline-glycerine) controls. A local wheal and flare response indicates the presence of food-specific IgE antibody (a wheal >3 mm is considered positive). Prick skin tests are most valuable when they are negative since the negative predictive value of the tests is very high (over 95%).[81,82] Unfortunately, the positive predictive value is on the order of only 50%. Thus, a positive skin test in isolation cannot be considered proof of clinically relevant hypersensitivity. These test limitations indicate that screening for food allergy with large batteries of tests is not a useful approach. Rather, directed testing for foods suspected to be a problem, identified by a careful medical history and knowledge of the epidemiology of the disorder, is a more efficient approach. The protein in commercial extracts of some fruits and vegetables are prone to degradation, so fresh extracts of these foods may be more reliable and the "prick-prick" manner of testing may be indicated where the probe is used to first pierce the food being tested (to obtain liquid) and then the skin of the patient.[83]

Blood tests are often employed to detect food-specific IgE antibodies. These tests are often called RAST (radioallergosorbent test) though the modern tests do not use radioactivity. Unlike skin tests, serum tests for IgE antibodies can be used while the patient is taking antihistamines and does not depend on having an area of rash-free skin for testing. Like skin tests, a negative result is very reliable in ruling-out an IgE-mediated reaction to a particular food, but a positive result has low specificity. For many allergens, the blood test is considered slightly less sensitive than allergy skin tests.

The stronger an individual's food-specific IgE antibody response, the more likely it is that the person would have an allergic reaction to the tested food. The degree of response may be determined by the size of a skin test response or concentration of food-specific IgE antibody.[84–86] Although it is counter intuitive, the degree of IgE response does not generally correlate with severity of an allergic reaction. Tests must be interpreted according to age, clinical history, and the food being tested. Test results are also influenced by the presence of less clinically relevant cross-reactive proteins. For example, most peanut-allergic patients will have positive skin tests to at least a few of the other members of the legume family, but only 5% will have clinical reactions to more than one legume.[87,88] Tests for IgE antibodies do not help in diagnosing food allergies that are not associated with IgE. Studies are underway for improved tests for these disorders, including the use of a skin patch test where an area of skin is exposed to food protein for 24 to 48 h and the area is examined for the development of a rash in the ensuing days.[30,31] Pending improved tests for non-IgE-antibody-mediated food allergies, further testing with oral challenges, if the history does not resolve the issue, would be required. Lastly, one should be wary of tests such as measurement of IgG_4 antibody, provocation–neutralization, cytotoxicity, applied kinesiology, among other unproved methods that are not useful.[89,90]

Food Elimination Diets

As an adjunct to testing, the first step to prove a cause and effect relationship with a particular illness and food allergy (whether IgE mediated or not) is to show resolution of symptoms with elimination of the suspected foods. In many cases, one or several foods are eliminated, which may be the obvious course of action when an isolated food ingestion (i.e., peanut) causes a sudden acute reaction and there is a positive test for IgE to the food. This would also represent a therapeutic intervention. However, eliminating one or a few suspected foods from the diet when the diagnosis is not so clear (asthma, AD, and chronic urticaria) can be a crucial step in determining if food is causal in the disease process. If symptoms persist, the eliminated food(s) is (are) excluded as a cause of symptoms. Alternatively, and as is more likely the case for evaluating chronic disorders without acute reactions, eliminating a large number of foods suspected to cause a chronic problem (usually including those that are common causes of food-allergic reactions as described above) and giving a list of "allowed foods" may be the preferred approach. The primary disadvantage of this approach is that if symptoms persist, the cause could still be attributed to foods left in the diet. Thus, a third type of elimination diet is an elemental diet in which calories are obtained from a hydrolyzed formula or, preferably, from an amino-acid-based formula. A variation is to include a few foods likely to be tolerated (but, again, this adds the possibility that persistent symptoms are caused by these foods). This diet is extremely difficult to maintain in patients beyond infancy. In extreme cases, nasogastric feeding of the amino-acid-based formula can be achieved, although some patients can tolerate the taste of these formulas with the use of flavoring agents provided by the manufacturers. This diet may be required when the diets mentioned above fail to resolve symptoms, but suspicion for food-related illness remains high. It is also required in disorders associated with multiple food allergies such as AEG. With AEG, prolonged dietary elimination for 3 to 6 weeks is sometimes needed to determine if resolution of symptoms will occur.[57]

FOOD CHALLENGES

Oral food challenges are performed by feeding the patient the suspected food under physician observation. There are several settings in which physician-supervised oral food challenges are required for diagnosis of food-allergic disease (Table 66.7). Because food challenges may elicit severe reactions, they are usually conducted under physician supervision with emergency medications to treat anaphylaxis immediately available. Challenges can be performed "openly" with the patient ingesting the food in its native form, "single-blind" with the food masked and the patient unaware if they are receiving the test food or, as double-blind, placebo-controlled challenges (DBPCFCs), where neither patient nor physician knows which challenges contain the food being tested. While open and single-blind challenges are open to patient or observer bias, the DBPCFC is considered the "gold standard" for diagnosis since bias is removed.[37]

To reduce the risk of a severe allergic reaction, the food is given in gradually increasing amounts that may be individualized both in dose and timing depending on the patient's history. For most IgE-mediated reactions, experts suggest giving 8 to 10 g of the dry food or 100 ml of wet food (double amount for meat/fish) at 10 to 15 min intervals over about 90 min followed by a larger, meal size portion of food a few hours later.[91] Starting doses may be a minute amount applied to the inner lip followed by 1% of the total challenge followed by gradually increasing amounts (4%, 10%, 20%, etc.). However, challenges may be individualized to parallel the clinical history (i.e., feeding over consecutive days for chronic disorders with delayed symptoms). Similarly, higher-risk challenges may start at extremely low doses with very gradual increases over longer time intervals. The person undergoing an oral food challenge is monitored for symptoms. Challenges are terminated when a reaction becomes apparent and emergency medications are given, as needed. Generally, antihistamines are given at the earliest sign of a reaction with epinephrine and other treatments given if there is progression of symptoms or any potentially life-threatening symptoms.

The practical issues in preparing food challenges include palatability and masking foods in appropriate vehicles, with placebos for DBPCFCs. In many cases, dry forms of the food (flour, powdered egg whites, etc.) can be hidden in puddings or liquids. Bulkier foods may be hidden in pancakes or ground beef. Flavoring agents such as mint can be added for further masking.[92] Hiding the food in opaque capsules is a convenient method to administer blinded challenges for patients who are able to ingest these capsules.

TABLE 66.7

Indications for Performing Physician-Supervised Oral Food Challenges[37,81]

- To confirm a food allergy when history is unclear and tests not confirmatory
- To exclude a food allergy
- To monitor for development of tolerance

TABLE 66.8
Pitfalls in Dietary Allergen Avoidance[94,95]

Pitfall	Examples
Ambiguous terms on food labels	"Natural flavoring" or "spices" may indicate an allergen (though law requires plain English disclosure of "major allergens")
Cross contamination	In processing lines (e.g., milk protein found in juice boxes) or in the home setting (shared utensils)
Ingredient switching	Large size of a product may have different ingredients than a small size, despite similar packaging design
Hidden ingredients	Egg white to make a pretzel shiny, peanut butter to seal the end of egg rolls, peanut butter to thicken sauces

Non-IgE-mediated reactions (e.g., AEG, enterocolitis, etc.) are more difficult to diagnose since there are no specific laboratory tests to identify particular foods that may be responsible for these illnesses. In many cases, a biopsy may be needed (e.g., AEG) to establish an initial diagnosis. Elimination diets with gradual reintroduction of foods and supervised oral food challenges are often needed to identify whether diet plays a role in the disorder and to identify the causal foods. Specific challenge protocols have been advised for food-induced enterocolitis syndrome.[93] Oral challenges can be used to evaluate reactions to food additives (coloring and flavoring agents and preservatives) or virtually any complaint associated with foods. When used to evaluate behavioral disorders or other complaints not convincingly associated with food allergy, DBPCFCs are advised to avoid bias.

TREATMENT OF FOOD ALLERGY

Treatment for food allergy requires dietary elimination of the offending food. The elimination of particular dietary food proteins is not a simple task. Table 66.8 lists a variety of possible pitfalls in dietary management of food allergy. A primary pitfall in avoidance has been the ambiguity of food labeling practices. For example, terms such as natural flavors could be on a label without indicating the flavor is an allergen, such as milk, or the term casein or whey, which are milk proteins, could be used but these scientific terms may not be familiar to lay persons. Many of these problems have been addressed by the Food Allergen Labeling and Consumer Protection Act of 2004 (FALCPA) that came into effect January 2006. The law requires that the eight major allergens or allergenic food groups — milk, egg, fish, shellfish, tree nuts, wheat, peanut, and soy — be declared on ingredient labels using plain English words. The law applies to all types of packaged foods except for meat, egg, and poultry products, and raw agricultural foods such as fruits and vegetables in their natural state. The plain English words used to identify the foods may be placed within the ingredient list or as a separate statement "contains." The law does not exclude using more scientific terms for food allergens as long as the label indicates, in some location, the plain English term for the food. In addition, the law requires that the specific type of allergen, in regard to grouped allergens such as fish or shellfish, be named. For example, walnut, salmon, or lobster would be named specifically.

There are a number of limitations to the legislation. First, only the eight major allergenic groups are considered. This means if an individual is allergic to mustard, the label may not indicate the ingredient should terms such as *natural flavor* or *spice* be used. The manufacturer would have to be called to learn more about the actual ingredients. Second, the Food Allergen Labeling and Consumer Protection Act (FALCPA) legislation has also not considered how much of a food protein in a given product may make it unsafe. This "threshold" ambiguity is problematic because a trace amount may not pose an allergenic risk, but may be labeled as containing an allergen. However, purified oils, such as soy oil that does not contain appreciable soy protein, may not need to be labeled as containing soy. Prior to the law, processing aids such as soy lecithin were not declared on foods. Soy lecithin is a fatty derivative of soy, which contains a very small amount of soy protein. The amount of soy protein in soy lecithin is an amount that most experts would agree is unlikely to cause an allergic reaction. Soy lecithin is used as an antistick agent in many baked products. For example, soy lecithin may keep cookies from sticking to a pan. In other cases, soy lecithin is added directly to the food. The legislation does not differentiate this and a food product may be listed as "contains soy" even though most experts would believe that this would be a safe product.

The legislation does not add regulations about possible inclusion of an allergen. Therefore, companies may voluntarily use terms such as "may contain" an allergen at their discretion. The specific requirements of the law may change and updates are available at the website of the Center for Food Safety and Applied Nutrition (www.cfsan.fda.gov).

In regard to avoidance, patients and parents must also be made aware that the food protein, as opposed to sugar or fat, is the ingredient being eliminated. For example, lactose-free cow's milk contains cow's milk protein and many egg substitutes contain chicken egg proteins. Conversely, peanut oil and soy oil do not generally contain the food protein, unless the processing method is one in which the protein is not completely eliminated (as with cold pressed or "extruded" oil). Patients and families undertaking an avoidance diet must also be taught about avoidance in a variety of settings, such as in obtaining restaurant meals where issues of cross contact during food preparation may pose dangers.[94] Lay organizations such as The Food Allergy & Anaphylaxis

Network (800-929-4040; www.foodallergy.org) assists families and physicians in the difficult task of eliminating the allergenic foods. When multiple foods are eliminated from the diet, it is prudent to enlist the aid of a dietitian in formulating a nutritionally balanced diet.

For life-threatening food allergies, an emergency plan must be in place to treat reactions caused by accidental ingestions. Injectable epinephrine and oral antihistamine should be readily available and administered without delay to treat patients at risk for severe reactions. Caregivers must be familiarized with indications for the use and method of administration of these medications.[95]

NATURAL HISTORY

Most children outgrow their allergies to milk, egg, wheat, and soy by age 3 to 5 years.[17] However, patients allergic to peanuts, tree nuts, fish, and shellfish are much less likely to lose their clinical reactivity and these sensitivities may persist into adulthood. Nonetheless, about 20% of very young children outgrow a peanut allergy by school age and 8% outgrow a tree nut allergy.[96] Elevated concentrations of food-specific IgE may indicate a lower likelihood of developing tolerance in the subsequent few years.[97] However, tests for food-specific IgE antibody (prick skin tests and serum-food-specific IgE) remain positive for years after the food allergy has resolved and cannot be followed as the sole indicator of tolerance. Thus, it is recommended that patients with chronic disease such as AD be rechallenged intermittently (e.g., egg: every 2 to 3 years, milk, soy and wheat: every 1 to 2 years, peanut, nuts, fish, and shellfish: if tolerance is suspected, and other foods every 1 to 2 years) to determine whether their food allergy persists if their test results are favorable, so that restriction diets may be discontinued as soon as possible.

PREVENTION OF FOOD ALLERGY

Approaches to delay or prevent allergy through dietary manipulation have been the subject of reviews and consensus statements.[98,99] Studies suggest a beneficial role for exclusive breast-feeding infants at "high risk" for atopic disease for the first 3 to 6 months of life, and avoiding supplementation with cow's milk or soy formulas in favor of hypoallergenic formulas, if breast feeding is not possible. There are currently no conclusive studies indicating that the manipulation of the mother's diet during pregnancy or breast feeding, or the restriction of allergenic foods from the infants diet will prevent the development of food allergy.[98,100] Currently, the American Academy of Pediatrics recommends a conservative approach, including that mothers of "high risk" infants avoid allergens such as peanuts and nuts during lactation, and that major allergens such as peanuts, nuts, and seafood be introduced after 3 years of age.[99]

FUTURE THERAPIES

Currently, strict avoidance of causal foods and treatment of accidental ingestions is the only available therapy for food allergy.[101] Immunotherapy ("allergy shots") has not proven practical for treatment except in the case of the oral allergy syndrome in which immunotherapy with the pollens responsible for the cross-reactivity may provide relief. Toward a goal of more definitive therapies for food-allergic disorders, a multitude of experimental therapies are under investigation.

Humanized anti-IgE antibodies for injection into patients have been developed that are able to bind and remove free-floating IgE antibodies from the bloodstream and may reduce or abolish allergic responses. Anti-IgE may, therefore, provide treatment for many IgE-mediated allergic disorders (not just food allergy). More allergen-specific novel therapies include vaccination with proteins altered such that the epitopes that bind IgE are removed, while areas of the protein are left intact so that T cells can still mount a response leading, potentially, to tolerance. Another approach to induce tolerance to specific food allergen is vaccination with DNA sequences that code for the production of food allergens, and the use of immune modulators (cytokines and specific DNA sequences) that can direct the immune system away from allergic responses and toward tolerance of the proteins. It is hoped that these novel approaches will provide relief from chronic disease and prevent anaphylaxis for food-allergic individuals.

REFERENCES

1. Altman, D. R., Chiaramonte, L. T., *J. Allergy Clin. Immunol.*, 97: 1247, 1996.
2. Sloan, A. E., Powers, M. E., *J. Allergy Clin. Immunol.*, 78: 127, 1986.
3. Bock, S. A., *Pediatrics*, 79: 683, 1987.
4. Sicherer, S. H., Munoz-Furlong, A., Sampson, H. A., *J. Allergy Clin. Immunol.*, 114: 159, 2004.
5. Sampson, H. A., *J. Allergy Clin. Immunol.*, 113: 805, 2004.
6. Young, E., Stoneham, M. D., Petruckevitch, A., et al., *Lancet*, 343: 1127, 1994.
7. Johansson, S. G., Bieber, T., Dahl, R., et al., *J. Allergy Clin. Immunol.*, 113: 832, 2004.
8. Chehade, M., Mayer, L., *J. Allergy Clin. Immunol.*, 115: 3, 2005.

9. Sicherer, S. H., Furlong, T. J., Maes, et al., *J. Allergy Clin. Immunol.*, *106*: 53, 2000.
10. Sicherer, S. H., *Lancet*, *360*: 701, 2002.
11. Sampson, H. A., Anderson, J. A., *J. Pediatr. Gastroenterol. Nutr.*, *94*: S87, 2000.
12. Chung, H. L., Hwang, J. B., Park, J. J., Kim, S. G., *J. Allergy Clin. Immunol.*, *109*: 150, 2002.
13. Sicherer, S. H., Munoz-Furlong, A., Sampson, H. A., *J. Allergy Clin. Immunol.*, *112*: 1203, 2003.
14. Hefle, S. L., Nordlee, J. A., Taylor, S. L., *Crit. Rev. Food Sci. Nutr.*, *36*: S69, 1996.
15. Shek, L. P., Soderstrom, L., Ahlstedt, S., et al., *J. Allergy Clin. Immunol.*, *114*: 387, 2004.
16. Shreffler, W. G., Beyer, K., Chu, T. H., et al., *J. Allergy Clin. Immunol.*, *113*: 776, 2004.
17. Wood, R. A., *Pediatrics*, *111*: 1631, 2003.
18. Grundy, J., Matthews, S., Bateman, B., et. al., *J. Allergy Clin. Immunol.*, *110*: 784, 2002.
19. Young, E., Patel, S., Stoneham, M. D., et al., *J. R. Coll. Physicians Lond.*, *21*: 241, 1987.
20. Yocum, M. W., Khan, D. A., *Mayo Clin. Proc.*, *69*: 16, 1994.
21. Novembre, E., de Martino, M., Vierucci, A., *J. Allergy Clin. Immunol.*, *81*: 1059, 1988.
22. Onorato, J., Merland, N., Terral, C., et al., *J. Allergy Clin. Immunol.*, *78*: 1139, 1986.
23. Sehgal, V. N., Rege, V. L., *Ann Allergy*, *31*: 279, 1973.
24. Cavataio, F., Iacono, G., Montalto, G., et al., *Am J. Gastroenterol.*, *91*: 1215, 1996.
25. Iacono, G., Cavataio, F., Montalto, G., et al., *N. Engl. J. Med.*, *339*: 1100, 1998.
26. Champion, R. H., *Br. J. Dermatol.*, *119*: 427, 1988.
27. Hanifin, J. M., *J. Dermatol.*, *24*: 495, 1997.
38. Leung, D. Y., Nicklas, R. A., Li, J. T., et al., *Ann. Allergy Asthma Immunol.*, *93*: S1, 2004.
29. Eigenmann, P. A., Sicherer, S. H., Borkowski, T. A., et al., *Pediatrics*, *101*: E8, 1998.
30. Niggemann, B., Reibel, S., Wahn, U., *Allergy*, *55*: 281, 2000.
31. Isolauri, E., Turjanmaa, K., *J. Allergy Clin. Immunol.*, *97*: 9, 1996.
32. Sicherer, S. H., Sampson, H. A., *J. Allergy Clin. Immunol.*, *104*: S114, 1999.
33. Guillet, G., Guillet, M. H., *Arch. Dermatol.*, *128*: 187, 1992.
34. de-Maat, B. F., Bruijnzeel, K. C., *Monogr. Allergy*, *32*: 157, 1996.
35. Nicolas, M. E., Krause, P. K., Gibson, L. E., *Int. J. Dermatol.*, *42*: 588, 2003.
36. Sampson, H. A., Sicherer, S. H., Birnbaum, A. H., *Gastroenterol*, *120*: 1026, 2001.
37. Sicherer, S. H., Teuber, S., *J. Allergy Clin. Immunol.*, *114*: 1146, 2004.
38. Sampson, H. A., Scanlon, S. M., *J. Pediatr.*, *115*: 23, 1989.
39. Ma, S., Sicherer, S. H., Nowak-Wegrzyn, A., *J. Allergy Clin. Immunol.*, *112*: 784, 2003.
40. Sicherer, S. H., *Pediatrics*, *111*: 1609, 2003.
42. Rodriguez, J., Crespo, J. F., Lopez-Rubio, A., et al., *J. Allergy Clin. Immunol.*, *106*: 183, 2000.
42. Ortolani, C., Ispano, M., Pastorello, E., et al., *Ann. Allergy*, *61*: 47, 1988.
43. Lake, A. M., *J Pediatr. Gastroenterol. Nutr.*, *30*: S58, 2000.
44. Iyngkaran, N., Yadav, M., Boey, C., et al., *J. Pediatr. Gastroenterol. Nutr.*, *8*: 667, 1988.
45. Walker-Smith, J. A., *Clin. Gastroenterol.*, *15*: 55, 1986.
46. Powell, G. K., *J. Pediatr.*, *93*: 553, 1978.
47. Powell, G., *Comprehen Ther.*, *12*: 28, 1986.
48. Sicherer, S. H., Eigenmann, P. A., Sampson, H. A., *J. Pediatr.*, *133*: 214, 1998.
49. de Boijjieu, D., Matarazzo, P., Dupont, C., *J. Pediatr.*, *131*: 744, 1997.
50. Nowak-Wegrzyn, A., Sampson, H. A., Wood, R. A., et al., *Pediatrics*, *111*: 829, 2003.
51. Talley, N. J., Shorter, R. G., Phillips, S. F., et al., *Gut*, *31*: 54, 1990.
52. Justinich, C., Katz, A., Gurbindo, C., et al., *J. Pediatr. Gastroenterol. Nutr.*, *23*: 81, 1996.
53. Liacouras, C. A., Wenner, W. J., Brown, K., et al., *J. Pediatr. Gastroenterol. Nutr.*, *26*: 380, 1998.
54. Rothenberg, M. E., *J. Allergy Clin. Immunol.*, *113*: 11, 2004.
55. Straumann, A., Simon, H. U., *J. Allergy Clin. Immunol.*, *115*: 418, 2005.
56. Teitelbaum, J. E., *J. Pediatr. Gastroenterol. Nutr.*, *38*: 358, 2004.
57. Kelly, K. J., Lazenby, A. J., Rowe, P. C., et al., *Gastroenterol.*, *109*: 1503, 1995.
58. Spergel, J. M., Beausoleil, J. L., Mascarenhas, M., et al., *J. Allergy Clin. Immunol.*, *109*: 363, 2002.
59. Ciclitira, P. J., King, A. L., Fraser, J. S., *Gastroenterol*, *120*: 1526, 2001.
60. Farrell, R. J., Kelly, C. P., *N. Engl. J Med.*, *346*: 180, 2002.
61. Forget, P. P., Arenda, J. W., *Eur. J. Pediatr.*, *144*: 298, 1985.
62. Cavataio, F., Iacono, G., Montalto, G., et al., *Arch. Dis. Child.*, *75*: 51, 1996.
63. Vanderhoof, J. A., Perry, D., Hanner, T. L., et al., *Clin. Pediatr. Phila.*, *40*: 399, 2001.
64. Zeigler, R. E., Fomon, S. J., Nelson, S. E., et al., *J. Pediatr.*, *116*: 11, 1990.
65. Hill, D. J., Hosking, C. S., *J. Pediatr. Gastroenterol. Nutr.*, *30*: S67, 2000.
66. Sampson, H., Eigenmann, P. A., *Rhinitis: Mechanisms and Management*, Marcel Dekker, Inc.: New York, Chapter 6, pp 95, 1999.
67. Raphael, G., Raphael, M., Kaliner, M., *J. Allergy Clin. Immunol.*, *83*: 110, 1989.
68. James, J. M., Bernhisel-Broadbent, J., Sampson, H. A., *Am. J. Respir. Crit. Care Med.*, *149*: 59, 1994.
69. Roberts, G., Golder, N., Lack, G., *Allergy*, *57*: 713, 2002.

70. Bock, S. A., *Pediatr. Allergy Immunol.*, *3*: 188, 1992.
71. Heiner, D. C., Sears, J. W., *Am. J. Dis. Child.*, *100*: 500, 1960.
72. Joint Task Force on Practice Parameters, *J. Allergy Clin. Immunol.*, *115*: S483, 2005.
73. Bock, S. A., Munoz-Furlong, A., Sampson, H. A., *J. Allergy Clin. Immunol.*, *107*: 191, 2001.
74. Sampson, H. A., Mendelson, L. M., Rosen, J. P., *N. Engl. J. Med.*, *327*: 380, 1992.
75. Palosuo, K., Alenius, H., Varjonen, E., et al., *J. Allergy Clin. Immunol.*, *103*: 912, 1999.
76. Romano, A., Di Fonso, M., Giuffreda, F., et al., *Int. Arch. Allergy Immunol.*, *125*: 264, 2001.
77. Weber, R. W., Vaughan, T. R., *Immunol. Allergy Clin. North Am.*, *11*: 831, 1991.
78. Bateman, B., Warner, J. O., Hutchinson, E., et al., *Arch. Dis. Child.*, *89*: 506, 2004.
79. Wolraich, M. L., Lindgren, S. D., Stumbo, P. J., et al., *N. Engl. J. Med.*, *330*: 301, 1994.
80. Sicherer, S. H., *Pediatr. Allergy Immunol.*, *10*: 226, 1999.
81. Sampson, H. A., Albergo, R., *J. Allergy Clin. Immunol.*, *74*: 26, 1984.
82. Bock, S., Buckley, J., Holst, A., et al., *Clin. Allergy*, *8*: 559, 1978.
83. Ortolani, C., Ispano, M., Pastorello, E. A., et al., *J. Allergy Clin. Immunol.*, *83*: 683, 1989.
84. Sampson, H. A., *J. Allergy Clin. Immunol.*, *107*: 891, 2001.
85. Sporik, R., Hill, D. J., Hosking, C. S., *Clin. Exp. Allergy*, *30*: 1541, 2000.
86. Crespo, J. F., Pascual, C., Ferrer, A., et al., *Allergy Proc.*, *15*: 73, 1994.
87. Bernhisel-Broadbent, J., Sampson, H. A., *J. Allergy Clin. Immunol.*, *83*: 435, 1989.
88. Sicherer, S. H., *J. Allergy Clin. Immunol.*, *108*: 881, 2001.
89. Bernstein, I. L., Storms, W. W., *Ann. Allergy Asthma Immunol.*, *75*: 543, 1995.
90. Beyer, K., Teuber, S. S., *Curr. Opin. Allergy Clin. Immunol.*, *5*: 261, 2005.
91. Bock, S. A., Sampson, H. A., Atkins, F. M., et al., *J. Allergy Clin. Immunol.*, *82*: 986, 1988.
92. Vlieg-Boerstra, B. J., Bijleveld, C. M., Van Der, H. S., et al., *J. Allergy Clin. Immunol.*, *113*: 341, 2004.
93. Sicherer, S. H., *J. Allergy. Clin. Immunol.*, *115*: 149, 2005.
94. Furlong, T. J., DeSimone, J., Sicherer, S. H., *J. Allergy Clin. Immunol.*, *108*: 867, 2001.
95. Sicherer, S. H., Simons, F. E., *J. Allergy Clin. Immunol.*, *115*: 575, 2005.
96. Skolnick, H. S., Conover-Walker, M. K., Koerner, C. B., et al., *J. Allergy Clin. Immunol.*, *107*: 367, 2001.
97. Perry, T. T., Matsui, E. C., Kay Conover-Walker, M., et al., *J. Allergy Clin. Immunol.*, *114*: 144, 2004.
98. Muraro, A., Dreborg, S., Halken, S., et al., *Pediatr. Allergy Immunol.*, *15*: 291, 2004.
99. Committee on Nutrition, American Academy of Pediatrics, *Pediatrics*, *106*: 346, 2000.
100. Lack, G., Fox, D., Northstone, K., et al., *N. Engl. J. Med.*, *348*: 977, 2003.
101. Nowak-Wegrzyn, A., Sampson, H. A., *Immunol. Allergy Clin. North Am.*, *24*: 705, 2004.

67 Enteral Nutrition

Gail A. Cresci and Robert G. Martindale

CONTENTS

INTRODUCTION

Historically, enteral feeding can be traced back to ancient Egypt and Greece, where nutrient enemas were used when patients were unable to take oral nutrition. Various combinations of wine, milk, broth, grains, and raw eggs were used with limited success.[1] Rectal delivery of nutrients was continued until the early 1900s despite lack of supportive benefit. In fact, President James Garfield was given nutrient enemas every 4 h for 79 days following his attempted assassination until his death.[1]

The first well-documented reports of nutrient provision through "feeding tubes" into the esophagus are from 1598, when an enteral feeding tube was fashioned from eel skin. In 1790, John Hunter initiated the modern era of gastrointestinal (GI) access with his reports on tube feeding the stomach.[1] Until this time, nutrient mixtures were delivered by tube and relied on gravity obviously limiting flow rate, volume, and consistency. The first feeding pump was developed in the eighteenth century, allowing for consistent enteral nutrient delivery as well as gastric irrigation and emptying.[1] Tubes remained relatively large and very primitive and uncomfortable until rubber was developed, which led to the evolution of the currently available selections. In 1910 Max Einhorn began feeding the duodenum through a rubber tube when gastric access was not feasible, claiming that rectal feeding was unacceptable.[1] The implementation of orojejunal tube feeding in surgical patients implemented by Ravdin and Stengel followed in 1939. In 1950 the use of polyethylene tubes was described with gastric and jejunal tubes of various lengths. With these tubes came the introduction of the feeding pump to deliver formulations.[1]

Experimentation with enteral formulations began in the early 1900s with the introduction of the chemically defined or "elemental" diet. The late 1950s through the 1970s marked the space age and the beginning of space diet research. These chemically defined diets were investigated in both animals and healthy humans to produce a low-residue diet that would decrease fecal output during space travel. In the late 1960s chemically defined diets were first reported being used in critically ill surgical patients.[1] Since that time, enteral formulations have undergone extensive modification and now exist for nearly every metabolic disease state and organ system.

RATIONALE AND BENEFITS

In the past 20 years, it has become abundantly clear that enteral nutrition is the preferred route of nutrient delivery. Parenteral nutrition should be substituted for enteral only if safe access is unavailable or unsuccessful. An extensive review of the numerous benefits of enteral nutrition is beyond the scope of this chapter and is only briefly addressed. Available reviews provide more extensive backgrounds in these areas.[2-5]

One proposed benefit of enteral nutrition is that it is more physiologic than parenteral nutrition. The gut and the liver process enteral nutrients prior to their release into systemic circulation via the hepatic veins (first-pass metabolism). When compared with parenteral nutrition in numerous clinical randomized trials, enteral nutrition positively influences nitrogen balance,[6,7] serum protein levels,[5,8,9] and the metabolic response to stress.[2-5,10,11]

Another benefit of enteral nutrition is its affect on the immune system (Table 67.1). The lack of GI mucosal exposure to enteral nutrients promotes gut mucosal atrophy. This may lead to increased intestinal permeability, potentially leaving the host vulnerable to bacterial or microbial toxin translocation. Enteral nutrition provides maintenance of the gut-associated lymphoid tissue,[12,13] helps maintain the normal GI flora,[14-16] is associated with lowering of infectious complications,[13,17-19] and attenuation of the hypermetabolic response to stress or catabolic insult.[20]

Enteral nutrition is generally less expensive than parenteral nutrition.[21,22] The lower total cost includes factors such as the costs of enteral formulations, equipment used for formula preparation and administration, and personnel specialists. The delivery of enteral nutrition has been shown to be safe and successful in up to 80% of critically ill patients.[17-19,23,24] Very recent data supports early enteral feeding actually decreasing mortality.[25]

INDICATIONS/CONTRAINDICATIONS

Enteral nutrition is indicated for patients with access to an adequately functional GI tract and whose oral nutrient intake is insufficient to meet estimated needs. Specific conditions for which enteral nutrition is indicated are found in Table 67.2. Although enteral nutrition is the preferred route of nutrient delivery, it is not risk free, and there are some contraindications to its use (Table 67.3).

TABLE 67.1
Immune Benefits of Enteral Feeding

Improved mucosal integrity
Enhanced glycemic control
Normalization of GI flora
Preserved GALT
   Secondary systemic immune stimulation
   Common mucosal immune hypothesis
Increased secretory IgA

Abbreviation: GI = Gastrointestinal; GALT = Gut-associated lymphoid tissue.

TABLE 67.2
Enteral Feeding Indications

Hypermetabolism
Postoperative major surgery
Trauma
Sepsis
Burns
Organ transplantation

Oncologic disease
Chemotherapy
Radiotherapy
Neoplasms

Neurologic disease
Cerebrovascular accident
Dysphagia
Head trauma
Demyelinating disease
Neoplasm

Psychiatric disease
Anorexia nervosa
Severe depression

GI disease
Short bowel syndrome (if remaining bowel
  has sufficient absorptive capacity ~50 to
  100 cm and intact ileocecal valve)
Inflammatory bowel disease
Enterocutaneous fistula (<800 ml output/day)
Pancreatitis

Organ system failure
Respiratory failure (ventilator
  dependence)

Renal failure
Cardiac failure (cardiac cachexia)
Hepatic failure
Multiple organ system failure
Comatose state

TABLE 67.3
Enteral Feeding Contraindications

Bowel obstruction
Persistent intolerance (e.g., emesis, diarrhea)
Hemodynamic instability
Major upper GI bleeds

Relative contraindications
Ileus
Unable to safely access
Significant bowel wall edema
High output fistula (>800 ml/day)

It is not always clear when enteral nutrition will be tolerated. If the individual's needs are not met enterally, parenteral nutrition may be implemented for either full nutrient provision or concurrently with the enteral delivery to provide the balance of nutrients not tolerated.

ENTERAL ACCESS

Route of administration and type of enteral access for tube feedings are usually determined by the expected duration of therapy (Figure 67.1), risk of aspiration (Table 67.4), and local expertise. Nasoenteric or oroenteric tubes are generally used when therapy is anticipated to be of short duration (i.e., <4 weeks) or for interim access before the placement of a long-term device. Long-term access requires a percutaneous or surgically placed feeding tube.

Multiple methods exist for gaining enteral access (Table 67.5), all of which carry various degrees of expertise, risk, and expense. The nasoenteric tube is the most commonly used method of enteral access. It can be inserted into the stomach, duodenum, or jejunum. As these tubes have low complication rates, are relatively inexpensive, and are easy to place, they are used most often for short-term use. The most common complications are tube malposition during the placement and inadvertent dislodgement either by the patient or during transfers.[26]

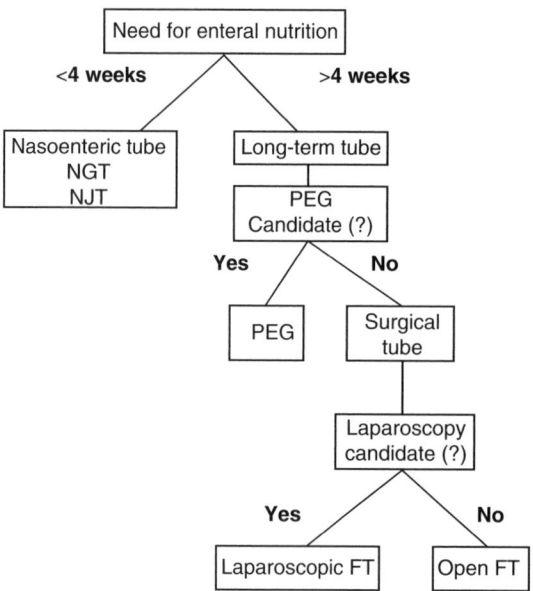

FIGURE 67.1   Decision tree for external nutrition.

TABLE 67.4
Risk Factors for Aspiration

Altered mental status with inability to protect airway
Swallowing dysfunction
Central (CVA)
Local (vagal disruption, trauma)
History of aspiration
Severe gastroesophageal reflux
Gastric outlet obstruction
Gastroparesis
Patient position restrictions (supine vs. semirecumbent)

TABLE 67.5
Methods of GI Access

Nasoenteric Feeding Tubes	Percutaneous Feeding Tubes
Spontaneous Passage	Percutaneous Endoscopic
Bedside — prokinetic agent	Gastric (PEG)
	Gastric/Jejunal (PEG/J)
Active Passage	Direct Jejunal (DPEJ)
Bedside — assisted	
Endoscopic	
Fluoroscopic	
Operative	
	Laparoscopic
	Gastrostomy
	Jejunostomy
	Surgical
	Gastrostomy
	Jejunostomy

It is often desirable to place tubes beyond the pylorus in patients with delayed gastric emptying or absent gag reflex to potentially decrease the risk of aspiration. Positioning a nasoenteric tube into the small bowel is much more difficult than positioning into the stomach. Transpyloric tubes can be placed intraoperatively, at bedside, or with endoscopic or fluoroscopic guidance. Intraoperative placement of a nasoenteric tube involves manual manipulation during the surgery; however, this is not common practice, as it requires open laparotomy. Spontaneous placement of a nasoenteric tubes involves advancing the tube into the stomach and allowing it to migrate independently into the small bowel. This technique is rarely successful in hospitalized patients, especially the critically ill, because of motility derangements often observed in the critically ill and in the supine position of the patient. Several bedside manual methods using special placement techniques, weighted vs. nonweighted tubes, pH sensor tubes, prokinetic agents, magnets, and bioelectrical detection devices have been reported, all with similar success rates (~85%).[27–33]

Owing to lack of universal success in manual placement of nasoenteric tubes, fluoroscopic or endoscopic guidance is often sought. If portable equipment is not available, both of these techniques require patient transport to the endoscopy or radiology suite, which may not be feasible for critically ill patients. Fluoroscopic techniques of nasoenteric tube placement involve manipulation of the tube with a long guide wire. Endoscopic techniques include use of a guide wire as well as a "drag" method. In the drag method, a gastrically placed tube is grasped with a snare or biopsy forceps and dragged with the endoscope into the duodenum, or farther, and then released. All risks of endoscopy accompany these methods, including dental injury, pharyngeal or esophageal injury, gastric bleeding, perforation, and risk of aspiration with the use of intravenous sedation.[34] Both fluoroscopic and endoscopic placement methods are ~85 to 95% successful in obtaining postpyloric feeding-tube placement. Although placement of postpyloric feeding tubes using endoscopic, fluoroscopic, and manual techniques may be successful, these tubes are frequently dislodged. Repeated tube insertion increases risk and costs of these access methods. For this reason, patients requiring long-term enteral nutrition should receive more permanent access.

GASTROSTOMY

Gastrostomy is the most common method for long-term enteral access as it eliminates nasal mucosal irritation, psychological stress, and requirement for an infusion pump, as complex formulas may be given as boluses. Gastric tubes, because of their large diameter, can serve many other functions besides feeding, including gastric decompression, gastric pH monitoring, and medication delivery. Insertion can be via laparotomy, laparoscopy, endoscopy, or fluoroscopy.

Permanent gastric placement can be obtained either by surgical procedures (laparotomy or laparoscopically) or by less invasive procedures done percutaneously. Percutaneous endoscopic gastrostomy (PEG) is the most popular nonoperative procedure for obtaining permanent gastric access. Gauderer et al.[35] first described the procedure in 1980, and despite some modifications, the basic technique used by most endoscopists is similar. Compared with surgically placed tubes, PEGs are less costly, have decreased procedure-related morbidity and mortality, usually do not require general anesthesia, and usually allow enteral feeding to be initiated within 8 to 24 h.[34–40] Indications as well as contraindications for a PEG are described in Table 67.6. Complications of PEGs include dislodgment, bleeding, tube site infection, intra-abdominal leak, leakage of gastric contents around tube, and persistent gastric fistula.[34]

JEJUNOSTOMY

The advantage of percutaneous tubes is less apparent when small bowel feeding is required because of the high failure rate of PEG tubes with a jejunal extension (PEG/J). Although a PEG/J tube is beneficial in the acute care setting when a critically ill

---

TABLE 67.6
PEG Indications and Contraindications

Indications	*Contraindications*
Long-term access (>4 weeks)	No access to stomach
Decompression	Unable to scope
Swallowing dysfunction	Hemodynamic instability
Neurologic event precluding swallowing	Coagulation disorders
Tracheoesophageal fistula	Obstruction
	Portal hypertension, esophageal varices
	Relative contraindications
	Ascites
	Peritoneal dialysis
	Prior upper abdominal procedures
	Pregnancy
	Super obesity (BMI >60)

patient requiring long-term access is intolerant of gastric feeds, they are not very practical for long-term use. Long-term failure of the jejunal extension is attributed to its small lumen leading to frequent clogging, as well as the jejunal portion retracting into the stomach.[41] For these reasons, as well as the expertise required to place the jejunal extension, surgical placement of jejunal tubes is often preferred for long-term jejunal access.

Several choices are available for intraoperative feeding jejunostomy placement. The needle catheter jejunostomy (NCJ) is a quick and easy method that involves inserting a small catheter into the lumen of the jejunum distal to the ligament of Treitz. The advantage of an NCJ is that nutrients can be administered almost immediately and the catheter can easily be removed when it is no longer needed. Unfortunately, the small lumen of the catheter occludes more readily than larger-bore feeding tubes. Catheters originally designed for other uses have been adapted for jejunal feeding, with the red rubber catheter most frequently used.

Jejunal access has also been obtained by direct percutaneous endoscopic jejunostomy placement (DPEJ).[42] This method is similar to PEG placement except that the endoscope or an enteroscope (special endoscope made longer for small bowel access) is passed through the duodenum, past the ligament of Treitz, into a loop of jejunum adjacent to the abdominal wall. A regular pull-through PEG tube is used for access. This procedure is technically more difficult than a PEG because of the peristaltic action and narrow lumen of the jejunum, but this procedure has many advantages over a PEG/J such as a decrease in clogging due to the use of a larger-diameter tube, and decreased migration or kinking. As this is a fairly new procedure, data on long-term complications are lacking.

ENTERAL FORMULAS

The increase in the use of enteral over parenteral nutrition in the past few decades has led to a rapid expansion in the number of commercially available enteral nutrition products. These products do not currently require Food and Drug Administration (FDA) approval for their proposed clinical implications, and fall under the category of food supplements. Nearly every major enteral formula company in the United States today carries a similar line of products. These formulas can be categorized as oral supplements, standard tube feedings, high-protein tube feedings, and disease-specific products. Table 67.7 provides an overview of these categories, specifying the types of macronutrients and physical properties of the select formulas. Because these products are classified as medical foods and do not require the rigorous FDA examination prior to their marketing, it is left to the experienced nutritionist to decipher the product indications. The optimal selection and administration of a formula requires a thorough knowledge of normal and abnormal digestive and absorptive physiology and formula composition. The physical form and quantity of each nutrient may determine the extent of absorption of and tolerance to the formula (e.g., long- vs. medium-chain triglyceride). The following discussion provides an overview of select macronutrients found in these products, with related supportive research as available.

MACRONUTRIENTS

CARBOHYDRATE

Among formulas, the two main differences in carbohydrate composition are form and concentration. Form, ranging from starch to simple glucose, contributes to the characteristics of osmolality, sweetness, and digestibility. In general, the larger carbohydrate molecules (e.g., starch) exert less osmotic pressure, taste less sweet, and require more digestion than shorter ones (e.g., malto-dextrin, sucrose, and corn syrup solids). In the critical care setting, optimal carbohydrate delivery should be at a quantity to allow maximal protein sparing while minimizing hyperglycemia. Currently 4 to 6 mg/kg min appears to meet these criteria during states of hypermetabolism.

FIBER

It has been claimed that fiber is beneficial in the control of a myriad of GI disorders, as well as treatment of hyperlipidemia and the control of blood glucose. Fiber-containing formulas have 5 to 14 g of total dietary fiber per liter. The form of fiber used is primarily insoluble fiber (e.g., soy fiber), but more recently developed formulas contain soluble fibers (e.g., guars gums, pectins, and fructo-oligosacharides [FOS]). The insoluble fiber is beneficial with regard to colonic function and bowel regulation. The soluble fibers may slow gastric emptying and decrease the rise in postprandial blood glucose levels as well as bind bile acids and dietary cholesterol, thus lowering serum cholesterol levels. The soluble fibers are also substrates for bacterial fermentation in the colon, yielding short-chain fatty acids (SCFAs), carbon dioxide, methane, hydrogen, and water. SCFAs are known to be the primary fuel for the colonocyte, attenuate mucosal inflammation, and have systemic influence on immunity.[43] It is believed that SCFAs or the bacteria that ferment them are required to maintain optimal colonocyte function, colonic blood flow, immunity, and numerous other beneficial systemic effects.[44] In patients requiring long-term tube feeding, a fiber-containing formula may help to regulate

TABLE 67.7
Overview of Select Enteral Formulas

Formula Category	Percentage of Calories from Protein	Protein Sources	Carbohydrate Sources	Percentage of Calories from Carbohydrate	Fat Sources	Percentage of Calories from Fat	Caloric Density (Calories/ml)	npc:g N	ml for 100% RDI	% Free Water	mOsm/kg Water	Product Names (Select Number)
Oral supplements	14–24	Sodium and calcium caseinates, soy protein isolate	Corn syrup, sugar, sucrose, maltodextrin	47–64	Corn oil, canola oil, soy oil, sunflower oil, safflower oil	21–39	1.0–2.0	78–154:1	946–2000	73–85	480–870	Ensure, Ensure Plus, Sustacal, Sustacal with Fiber, Resource Plus, NuBasics, Sustacal Plus
Standard tube feedings	13–18	Sodium and calcium caseinates, soy protein isolates	Corn syrup, maltodextrin	45–57	Soy oil, corn oil, canola oil, medium-chain triaclyglycerol (MCT), safflower oil	29–39	1.0–1.5	116–167:1	830–1890	77–85	270–500	Isocal, IsoSource HN, Nutren 1.0, Nutren 1.5, Osmolite, Osmolite HN, Comply
Standard tube feedings with fiber	14–18	Sodium and calcium caseinates, soy protein isolate	Corn syrup, maltodextrin, corn syrup solids, soy fiber, guar gum, oat fiber, FOS	44–57	Canola oil, soybean oil, corn oil, MCT	29–37	1.0–1.2	110–149:1	933–1500	78–85	300–500	Fibersource, Jevity, Jevity Plus, ProBalance, Ultracal, Nutren 1.0 with Fiber
High protein tube feedings	22–25	Sodium and calcium caseinates	Hydrolyzed cornstarch, maltodextrin, sucrose, fructose, oat fiber, soy fiber	38–52	Canola oil, MCT, soybean oil, safflower oil	23–40	1.0–1.5	75–91:1	1000–2000	78–85	300–490	IsoSource VHN, Replete with Fiber, Promote, Protain XL, TraumaCal
Elemental and semi-elemental	12–25	Free amino acids, soy hydrolysates, hydrolyzed whey, hydrolyzed casein, hydrolyzed soy	Hydrolyzed cornstarch, maltodextrin, sucrose, modified cornstarch	36–82	Soybean oil, safflower oil, canola oil, MCT sunflower oil	3–39	1.0–1.5	67–175:1	1150–2000	76–86	270–650	Vivonex T.E.N., Crucial, Peptamen, Perative, Reablin, AlitraQ, Sandosource Peptide, Subdue, Optimental
Pulmonary	17–20	Sodium and calcium caseinates	Hydrolyzed cornstarch, corn syrup, sucrose, maltodextrin, sugar	27–40	Canola oil, soybean oil, MCT, corn oil, safflower oil, sardine oil, borage oil	40–55	1.5	102–125:1	933–1420	76–79	330–650	Nutrivent, Pulmocare, Respalor, Novasource Pulmonary, Oxepa

Continued

TABLE 67.7
(Continued)

Formula Category	Protein Sources	Carbohydrate Sources	Percentage of Calories from Carbohydrate	Fat Sources	Percentage of Calories from Fat	Caloric Density (Calories/ ml)	npc:g N	ml for 100% RDI	% Free Water	mOsm/kg Water	Product Names (Select Number)
Renal	Sodium and calcium caseinates, Whey-L-amino acids	Corn syrup, sucrose, fructose, maltodextrin, sugar	40–58	Corn oil, safflower oil, canola oil, MCT	35–45	2.0	140–340:1	947–1000	70–71	570–700	Nepro, Magnacal Renal, Novasource Renal RenalCal
Diabetic	Sodium and calcium caseinates, beef, milk protein, soy protein isolate	Maltodextrin, hydrolyzed cornstarch, fructose, sucrose, guar gum, vegetables, fruits, soy fiber	34–40	Sunflower oil, soybean oil, canola oil, MCT, safflower oil	40–49	1.0–1.06	79–125:1	1000–1890 or N/A	85	355–450	Glucerna, Glytrol, Choice dm, DiabetiSource, Resource Diabetic
Immune Modulated	Sodium and calcium caseinates, L-arginine, L-glutamine, branched-chain amino acid (BCAA)	Hydrolyzed cornstarch, maltodextrin, soy fiber	38–53	Canola oil, structured lipids: sunflower oil and menhaden fish oil, MCT	20–40	1.0–1.5	52–1:1	1250–2000	78–86	375–550	Impact, Impact 1.5, ImmunAid, Crucial
Hepatic	L-Amino acids, whey	Sucrose, maltodextrin, modified cornstarch	57–77	Soybean oil, MCT, canola oil, corn oil, lecithin	12–28	1.2–1.5	148–209:1	N/A-1000	76–82	560–690	NutriHep, Hepatic Aid II

GI motility. Because of the higher viscosity of these formulas, the use of larger-bore tubes (10 Fr or greater) or an infusion pump is suggested.

FRUCTO-OLIGOSACCHARIDES (FOS)

FOS are undigestible carbohydrates that occur naturally in food (e.g., onions and blueberries). These sugars consist of a sucrose molecule linked to one, two, or three additional fructose units. Gastric acid or digestive enzymes do not degrade FOS. These oligosaccharides appear to remain intact in the small intestine and pass into the colon unaltered, where they are fermented by colonic microorganisms (e.g., bifidobacteria) to lactate and SCFAs. It is suggested that the proliferation of bifidobacteria species and the presence of FOS, with the consequent production of the fermented byproducts acetate, lactate, and butyrate, produce an environment undesirable for some pathogenic bacteria such as *Clostridium difficile* by lowering the colonic pH, producing proteins that destroy pathogenic bacterial toxins, and via competitive inhibition.[14,16,45] Several enteral formulations now contain FOS, but proposed benefits remain to be elucidated and studied in randomized prospective studies.

FAT

The major sources of fat in standard lactose-free formulas are corn, soy, safflower, and canola oils, lecithin, and medium-chain triacylglycerol (MCT). In addition to their importance as a concentrated caloric source (9 kcal/g), fat is required for essential fatty acids (EFAs) and serves as a carrier for the fat-soluble vitamins. Fat also enhances the flavor and palatability of a formula without increasing osmolality. Long-chain triacylglycerol (LCT) is a rich source of EFAs, linolenic, and linolenic acid. The estimated daily requirement for EFAs is 3 to 4% of the total kilocalories. However, due to LCT route of absorption via the lymphatic system, their limited utilization during hypermetabolism, and their relative immunosuppressive effects when given in large quantities, many formulas now combine LCT with MCT.

MCTs are 6 to 12 carbons long and are prepared from palm kernel or coconut oil. MCT is advantageous because it is more rapidly hydrolyzed and water soluble than LCT, requires little or no pancreatic lipase or bile salts for absorption, and can be transported directly into portal venous circulation. Once MCTs enter the cell they can be transported across the mitochondrial membrane without the acyl-carnitine carrier. Once in the mitochondria it is rapidly metabolized for energy.[46] MCTs are generally well tolerated by the enteral route but can be associated with some GI symptoms such as nausea, vomiting, and diarrhea. As they produce ketones, they should not be used in patients who are prone to high ketone levels.[46] As they do not contain EFAs, most enteral formulas that contain MCT also provide some LCT in order to meet the requirement for EFA.

Recent metabolic research has led to the incorporation of omega-3 fatty acids (linolenic) into enteral formulas. The omega-3 fats are delivered as either the 18-carbon (linolenic) or the 20-carbon eicosapentaenoic acid (EPA). Numerous reports using various *in vivo* and *in vitro* models suggest that the structural difference between omega-3 and omega-6 fatty acids strongly favors anti-inflammatory, antithrombotic, antiarrhythmic, hypolipidemic, and antiatherosclerotic effects.[47–52]

Structured lipids are a chemical mixture of LCTs and MCTs incorporated onto the same glycerol molecule. They differ from the more simple random physical mixtures of LCT and MCT. Structured lipids may offer the advantages of both types of fats. Structured lipids have been shown to decrease infection and improve survival in animal models by producing less inflammatory and immunosuppressive eicosanoids as compared with conventional triacylglycerols.[47] Enteral formulas, particularly some of the immune-modulated category, are beginning to include structured lipids as a source of fat.

PROTEIN

Protein contained in enteral formulas may be in the form of intact protein (e.g., lactalbumin, casein, caseinates, and whey), partially hydrolyzed protein (e.g., oligopeptides and di- or tripeptides), or crystalline L-amino acids. Intact protein and protein hydrolysates (≥4 amino acid residues) require further luminal digestion by pancreatic or brush border enzymes into peptides (di- or tripeptides) and free amino acids, which are then absorbed primarily in the proximal small bowel. The peptide transport mechanisms are believed to be responsible for absorption of the majority of nitrogen, with the single amino acid carriers playing a minority role in protein absorption. Intact proteins do not add appreciably to the osmolality of the formula, unlike hydrolyzed or crystalline amino acids. The higher the percentage of hydrolyzed protein or free amino acids, the greater the solution osmolality will be. Knowledge of the source and form of protein is essential when prescribing diets for patients with defects in either protein digestion (e.g., pancreatic insufficiency) or absorption (e.g., short bowel syndrome).

Stress and other forms of injury may alter protein metabolism. In times of decreased absorptive surface area, ischemic injury, or malabsorption, provision of enteral formulas containing hydrolyzed protein or free amino acids has been suggested. At present, no clear consistent clinical data support the routine use of solutions in which protein is in the form of free amino acids or hydrolysates in the critically ill. Theoretically, these peptide-based formulas would have advantage in conditions of compromised mucosa, such as critical illness, as the mucosal peptide transporter (PepT1) is a very efficient transporter felt to absorb roughly 70% of the amino acids following a protein meal.[53] The reason it is difficult to prove this benefit may be due to the fact that the small bowel has a very adaptive absorptive mucosa, even when a large percentage of the small bowel mucosa is nonfunctional or surgically removed. Although patients with maldigestion or malabsorption may benefit from a peptide-based enteral formula, the higher cost of these formulas and lack of clinical supportive data discourage routine use in patients with normal GI physiology.

GLUTAMINE

Glutamine is the most abundant amino acid in the body, and in normal situations is considered a nonessential amino acid (NEAA). It can be synthesized in many tissues of the body, predominantly skeletal muscle, and is the primary fuel for rapidly dividing tissues such as the small bowel. Glutamine serves many purposes including maintenance of acid–base status as a precursor of urinary ammonia, as a primary fuel source for enterocytes, as a fuel source for lymphocytes and macrophages, and as a precursor for nucleotide synthesis.[54,55] Glutamine is also a precursor for glutathione, an important antioxidant that may be protective in a variety of circumstances. Glutamine has also been shown to enhance heat shock protein (HSP).[56] HSP is one of a class of chaperone proteins, which have been shown to protect the cell from subsequent stresses. During catabolic illness, glutamine uptake by the small intestine and immunologically active cells may exceed glutamine synthesis and release from skeletal muscle, making glutamine conditionally essential.[57]

Limited human data exist regarding the use of enteral glutamine supplementation. In animal models, supplemental glutamine has been shown to enhance intestinal adaptation after massive small bowel resection, to attenuate intestinal and pancreatic atrophy, and to prevent hepatic steatosis associated with parenteral and elemental enteral feeding.[58] Glutamine appears to maintain GI tract mucosal thickness, maintain DNA and protein content, reduce bacteremia and mortality after chemotherapy, and reduce bacteremia and mortality following sepsis or endotoxemia.[54–56]

In humans with surgical stress, glutamine-supplemented parenteral nutrition appears to maintain nitrogen balance and the intracellular glutamine pool in skeletal muscle.[54,55] In critically ill patients, glutamine supplementation may attenuate villous atrophy and increased intestinal mucosal permeability associated with parenteral nutrition.[58] Parenteral nutrition supplemented with glutamine has also resulted in fewer infections, improved nitrogen balance, and significantly shorter mean hospital length of stay in bone marrow transplantation patients.[54] Glutamine supplementation may also play a role in protecting the GI tract against chemotherapy-induced toxicity. Oral glutamine supplementation reduced the severity and decreased the duration of stomatitis that occurred during chemotherapy.[59]

Although a large volume of animal data supports the beneficial effects of glutamine in a variety of experimental models, the benefit of enteral glutamine supplementation in critically ill human patients is less clear. Well-designed clinical trials with clearly defined end points and adequate statistical power are needed to assess whether the animal effects translate into a reduction in hospital stay and mortality rate in humans.

ARGININE

Arginine is classified as a NEAA in normal situations, as the body synthesizes adequate arginine for normal maintenance of tissue metabolism, growth, and development. During injuries such as trauma or stress, an increase in urinary nitrogen, excreted largely as urea, represents the end products of increased tissue catabolism and reprioritized protein synthesis. As the activity of the urea cycle increases, so does the demand for arginine.

Studies indicate that supplemental dietary arginine is beneficial for accelerated wound healing, enhanced immune response, and positive nitrogen balance.[47] The exact mechanism for these benefits remains open for some speculation, but may in part result from arginine's role as a potent stimulant of growth hormone, glucagon, prolactin, and insulin release.[47] Arginine is also a precursor for nitric oxide, a highly reactive molecule synthesized from arginine by the action of one of the three isoforms of nitric oxide synthase resulting in the formation of nitric oxide and citrulline.[60] Nitric oxide is a ubiquitous molecule with important roles in the maintenance of vascular tone, coagulation, the immune system, and the GI tract, and has been implicated as a factor in disease states as diverse as sepsis, hypertension, and cirrhosis.[60]

In animal models, arginine supplementation has been associated with improved wound healing and with increased wound tensile strength and collagen deposition.[61] Arginine-supplemented rats also had improved thymic function as assessed by thymic weight, the total number of thymic lymphocytes in each thymus, and the mitogenic reactivity of thymic lymphocytes to phytohemagglutinin and concanavalin A.[60] Supplementation of arginine in animal models resulted in improved survival in burns and with intraperitoneal bacterial challenge.

Multiple human clinical trials have been conducted comparing the use of various enteral formulations that contain arginine as well as other supplemental nutrients (e.g., glutamine, omega-3 fatty acids, and nucleotides) with a standard nonsupplemented formula. Results of these trials have found the supplemented formula groups to have various improved outcomes such as decreased number and severity of septic complications, decreased antibiotic use, and decreased hospital and intensive care unit (ICU) stay.[62–65]

While supplemental arginine has been shown to improve survival in various animal models and to improve a number of *in vitro* measures of immune function, the benefit of arginine supplementation alone in critically ill humans looks promising for lowering infectious risk and length of ICU stay, but has yet to be shown to enhance mortality.[66]

OTHER NUTRIENTS

VITAMINS AND MINERALS

Most nutritionally complete commercial formulas contain adequate vitamins and minerals when a sufficient volume of formula to meet energy and macronutrient needs is provided. Some disease-specific formulas are nutritionally incomplete in relation to vitamin and mineral content (e.g., hepatic formulas). Liquid vitamin and mineral supplements may be indicated for patients receiving nutritionally incomplete or diluted formulas for prolonged periods of time. Fat-soluble vitamin supplementation such as vitamin K may be indicated for patients with fat malabsorption or for patients with vitamin K deficiency; most commercial formulas include vitamin K.

WATER

A large percentage of all enteral formulas is free water. The quantity of water in enteral formulas is often described as water content or moisture content. The quantity of water is usually reported in milliliters of water either per 1000 ml of formula or per liter of formula. Most enteral formulas contain water in the general range of 690 to 860 ml per 1000 ml of enteral formula. This must be considered when making fluid recommendations.

PHYSICAL PROPERTIES

OSMOLALITY

Osmolality is the function of size and quantity of ionic and molecular particles (protein, carbohydrate, electrolytes, and minerals) within a given volume. The unit of measure for osmolality is mOsm/kg of water vs. the unit of measure for osmolarity, which is mOsm/l. Osmolality is considered the preferred term to use in reference to enteral formulas.

Osmolality is important because of its role in maintaining the balance between intracellular and extracellular fluids. Several factors affect the osmolality of enteral formulas. The primary factor is nutrient hydrolysis. The smaller the chain length of carbohydrates and proteins, the greater will be the formulation's osmolality. Hence, formulas containing increased amounts of simple sugars or free amino acids or di- and tripeptides will have a greater osmolality than those containing starch and longer-chain intact proteins. Lipids contribute minimally to the osmolality of an enteral formula, with the exception of MCT, owing to their water solubility. Because of dissociation properties and small size, minerals and electrolytes also increase the osmolality.

GI tolerance (e.g., gastric retention, abdominal distention, diarrhea, nausea, and vomiting) is influenced by the osmolality of enteral formulas; this is especially true in the critically ill population. Administering hypertonic formulas at a slow, continuous rate initially (10 to 20 cc/h) with a gradual titration to the final volume while monitoring for GI complications can reduce the incidence of GI intolerance and allow these formulas to be administered at full strength without problems. What may be more important than the osmolality of the enteral formula is the osmotic contribution from liquid medications either infused with the enteral formula or bolused through the feeding tube. The average osmolality range of commercially prepared liquid medications is reported to be 450 to 10,950 mOsm/kg.[67] The osmolality of enteral formulas ranges from 270 to 700 mOsm/kg.

HYDROGEN ION CONCENTRATION (pH)

Gastric motility is reportedly slowed with solutions with a pH <3.5. The pH level of commercial formulas is >3.5. The pH issues can become a problem when mixing feeding tubes with medications of low pH, forming a precipitate in the feeding tube causing occlusion. Most intact protein formulas coagulate when acidified to a pH <5.0.

CALORIE–NUTRIENT DENSITY

The kilocalorie density of enteral formulas is generally 1.0, 1.5, or 2.0 kcal/ml. This is important as it not only determines how many kilocalories but also the other macro- and micronutrients that the patient receives. As a formula becomes more nutrient dense, it contains less free water.

Caloric density often affects the patient's tolerance for tube feeding. Delayed gastric emptying frequently occurs in patients who are given concentrated formulas. High fat formulas, being potent inhibitors of gastric emptying, contribute to this. As the patient's nutrient needs are met by a decreased volume of this class of formula, free-water supplementation should be given to ensure that fluid requirements are met and to prevent dehydration and constipation. Generally, these high-caloric-density products are best tolerated as voluntary oral supplements and not as tube feeding.

NONPROTEIN CALORIE TO GRAM OF NITROGEN RATIO (NPC:G N)

In general, the average healthy adult requires a nonprotein calorie to gram of nitrogen (npc:g N) ratio of 150–250:1. In a catabolic state, the body catabolizes lean body mass as a nitrogen and energy source. To minimize this process, it is recommended to provide a npc:g N of 100–150:1. This protein content of enteral formulas becomes extremely important in patients who require healing of wounds due to trauma, burns, metabolic stress, and infection, and increased wound-healing requirements.

RENAL SOLUTE LOAD

Renal solute load refers to the constituents in the formula that must be excreted by the kidneys. Major contributors to renal solute load in enteral formulas are protein, sodium, potassium, and chloride. There is an obligatory water loss for each unit of solute. Therefore, as a formula becomes more concentrated or its renal solute load increases, the patient will require more water.[39] Pediatric and geriatric patients have minimal reserve and should be monitored closely for dehydration. Other groups at risk for dehydration are those with diarrhea, emesis, fistulas, or fevers.

DISEASE-SPECIFIC FORMULATIONS

Most patients are adequately supplemented with a standard enteral formula and do not require specialty enteral formulations. Specialty enteral formulas commonly have an additional cost that is often not reimbursable; however, factors such as severe hypercatabolism, renal or hepatic failure, pulmonary insufficiency, or malnutrition may alter nutrient metabolism and may thereby warrant an enteral formulation tailored to the specific disease process. Determining the location and timing of enteral nutrient delivery, mode of delivery, and the patient's overall current clinical condition as well as past medical history is necessary for appropriate cost-effective formula selection.

RENAL FORMULAS

The clinical status of patients with renal failure is diverse; therefore, prescribed nutrient intake may vary greatly among patients and should depend on individual nutritional status, catabolic rate, residual glomerular filtration rate, and intensity of dialysis or hemofiltration therapy. Formulas for renal insufficiency do not clearly distinguish between patients with acute failure and those with chronic renal failure.

Renal enteral formulas were first developed as oral supplements; therefore, they tend to be hyperosmolar secondary to their large simple sugar content for flavor enhancement. This hypertonicity often causes GI complications if these formulas are tube fed. The simple sugar content can also be problematic, causing impaired glycemic control in patients who are hypermetabolic, insulin resistant, or diabetic. The goal of feeding patients with renal failure is to provide optimal nutrients without compromising their medical condition through the accumulation of nitrogenous compounds, electrolytes, and fluid. Hence, renal formulas are all calorically rich, usually providing 2 kcal/ml and containing low to moderate amounts of protein, electrolytes, and various minerals. Essential amino acid (EAA) formulas were developed to take advantage of the body's ability to make NEAAs by transamination reactions. Theoretically, then, only essential nitrogen is delivered. However, previously presumed NEAAs are probably conditionally essential (e.g., arginine, glutamine, and histidine) during metabolic stress. Recent guidelines recommend the use of EAAs and NEAAs for enhanced protein synthesis, correction of low plasma NEAA values, provision of nonspecific nitrogen via NEAAs, and enhanced protein synthesis.[68,69] Nutrients should be provided as needed. The development of fluid and electrolyte disorders or accumulation of metabolic waste products should not be minimized solely by nutrient restriction, but also by adjusting the intensity of dialysis treatment as tolerated.[70] Many patients with stable levels of creatinine, blood urea nitrogen, and electrolytes with or without dialysis can be fed with standard complete enteral formulas.

PULMONARY FORMULAS

Respiratory insufficiency and ventilator dependence can have a major impact on the feeding of critically ill patients. Often, these patients do not receive their full nutritional needs because of the increased work of breathing, carbon dioxide retention, and fluid and electrolyte restrictions. This reduced or inadequate nutrient intake results in loss of lean body tissue (e.g., intercostals and diaphragm) and malnutrition, which in turn leads to fatigue and further difficulty with weaning from the ventilator.

Lipid oxidation is known to produce less carbon dioxide than oxidation of either glucose or protein. This has been the basis for the development of high fat (~45 to 55% of kilocalories) and calorically concentrated (1.5 kcal/ml) enteral formulas. Originally these products consisted of 100% LCT, which can suppress the immune system as well as cause malabsorption. Pulmonary formulas now contain a variety of lipids including MCT, omega-6 and omega-3 fatty acids, and, more recently, g-linolenic acid (GLA).[71]

Animal research has shown that animals fed omega-3 fatty acids produce reduced amounts of proinflammatory eicosanoids relative to omega-6 fatty acids.[72] In another study, animals fed diets enriched by GLA, as borage oil, were found to have higher inflammatory exudate cellular levels of GLA and dihomogamma-linolenic acid (DGLA) with reduced levels of prostaglandin E2 (PGE2) and leukotrienes,[73] suggesting that GLA modulates inflammatory status in a manner similar to that of omega-3 fatty acids. In another animal study, the authors concluded that dietary fish oil and fish and borage oil as compared with corn oil may reduce pulmonary neutrophil accumulation and ameliorate endotoxin-induced acute lung injury by suppressing the levels of proinflammatory eicosanoids in bronchoalveolar lavage fluid.[74] Clinical studies have now shown a decrease in hospital stay and ventilator days with improved oxygenation when patients with acute respiratory distress syndrome (ARDS) and acute lung injury are supplemented with these formulas containing EPA and various specifically designed lipid mixtures to decrease pulmonary inflammation.[75] More clinical trials are necessary to determine these claims and specific patient indications.

Aside from the previously mentioned studies with pulmonary patients, previous research evaluating the use of pulmonary enteral formulas has not demonstrated a clear benefit in providing a high-fat, reduced-carbohydrate nutrient prescription for the patient with compromised pulmonary function.[75] The excessive carbohydrate associated with overfeeding can result in a significant rise in pCO_2 and respiratory quotient, which influences respiratory function. Close attention should be paid to the avoidance of overfeeding by providing energy intakes from 1.2 to 1.5 times the predicted resting energy expenditure or by measuring energy expenditure via indirect calorimetry.[75]

There are potential detrimental effects in using a high-fat, low-carbohydrate enteral formula. It is well known that high-fat diets can impair gastric emptying.[76] Delayed gastric emptying can result in increased gastric residual volumes and increased risk of aspiration. Carbohydrate is the primary energy source during vigorous muscle exercise, as required during ventilator weaning. During vigorous exercise, depleted muscle glycogen stores may limit muscle endurance and strength. Nutritional support for the pulmonary-compromised patient requires a balanced energy mix so that prompt replenishment of respiratory muscle glycogen can occur.[75] Pulmonary formulas, with their low carbohydrate levels, are a potential disadvantage to fully support muscle glycogen repletion during ventilator weaning.

The literature and clinical practice demonstrate that by not calorically overfeeding pulmonary-compromised patients, especially if they are septic, nutritional goals may be met with a standard enteral product (~30% kilocalories as fat).[69,75]

DIABETIC FORMULAS

Nutrition is an integral component in the management of diabetes mellitus (DM). Whether during critical illness or long-term support, it can be extremely challenging. Over the past several years, enteral formulas have been developed emphasizing glycemic control for patients with DM. These formulations contain relatively high-fat low-carbohydrate nutrient ratios, with actual ingredients varying among the manufacturers (see Table 67.7). The carbohydrate sources include fructose and fiber to assist in glycemic management. Some fat sources have been modified to contain a higher ratio of monounsaturated fatty acids than saturated fatty acids to better meet the 1994 guidelines of the American Diabetes Association. The more recently developed diabetic formulas also have added various combinations of monounsaturated fats, fructose, specific amino acids, insoluble and soluble fibers, which have also been shown to be beneficial in glycemic control.[77]

A few individual outcome studies have been conducted to determine any benefit of providing these formulations to gain optimal glycemic control.[77–79] Overall, the recommendation is to begin by administering a standard, fiber-containing enteral formula with moderate carbohydrate and fat content. Blood glucose levels will vary based on the patient's diabetes history, metabolic stress level, and nutrient delivery method. Blood glucose levels should be monitored closely with appropriate insulin management, especially if feeding regimens are altered or interrupted. If metabolically stable diabetic patients do not exhibit desired glycemic control with a standard formula, then a diabetic enteral formula may be beneficial.

HEPATIC FAILURE FORMULAS

The specialized formulas for patients with cirrhosis and hepatic failure are designed to correct the abnormal amino acid profile associated with hepatic encephalopathy. In certain instances of hepatic failure, amino acid metabolism is altered, resulting in increased plasma aromatic amino acids (AAA) with a significant change in the serum branched-chain amino acid (BCAA) to AAA ratio. These changes result in altered blood–brain barrier transport especially for the AAAs; this central nervous system (CNS)-altered amino acid ratio contributes to the hepatic encephalopathy commonly observed in end-stage hepatic failure. Specialized enteral formulas for hepatic encephalopathy have been designed to reduce the availability of AAAs and decrease their passage through the blood–brain barrier. Therefore, these formulas contain low quantities of AAAs and methionine and high quantities of BCAAs.

In metabolically stressed, malnourished cirrhotic patients with encephalopathy, the effectiveness of the BCAA-enriched formulas may lie in correcting malnutrition by increasing nitrogen intake without aggravating the encephalopathy. However, some life-threatening derangement in liver failure, such as portal hypertension and esophageal varices, are unaffected by nutritional repletion. Therefore, these formulas should be provided only in malnourished patients with liver failure and concomitant encephalopathy who have failed to respond to conventional medical therapy, and in whom a potentially dangerous higher level of nitrogen intake is required to induce anabolism.[69,80,81] Owing to the incidence of associated fluid and electrolyte abnormalities, these formulas are calorically concentrated and contain minimal amounts of electrolytes, with some formulations failing to provide 100% of the U.S. recommended daily intake. Therefore, patients receiving these formulations should be monitored closely to ensure that no further associated nutrient deficiencies occur.

Immune-Modulated Formulas

Over the past several decades, animal and human studies have shown that certain individual nutrients demonstrate immune benefits. These nutrients include arginine, glutamine, omega-3 fatty acids, and nucleotides. Because of this, several enteral formula manufacturers have developed immune-modulated enteral formulas to potentially improve clinical outcomes in high-risk or critically ill patients. These products all vary in the amounts of these nutrients they contain. More recently, several human studies have been conducted to determine if critically ill or other immune-compromised individuals experience positive outcomes as a result of receiving these formulations. Results of these studies vary; they have been scrutinized for several variables, including lack of feeding comparisons, lack of homogeneous study population comparisons, and the manner in which the data were analyzed. Outcomes from the studies also vary, with a few showing no benefits regarding the immune formulas and the vast majority of the studies now showing reduced rates of infection, antibiotic use, incidence of intra-abdominal abscesses, and reduced intensive care unit and hospital length of stay.[40,62–65]

Overall, the literature suggests that these immune-modulated formulas may be beneficial for select patient populations. In patients who have undergone complicated GI surgery, sustained severe trauma, or had complicated ICU stays, immune formulas were linked with decreased incidence of infections and hospital length of stay, but were not shown to reduce mortality in severely injured and immune-compromised patients.[82] It appears that immune modulation is now supported clinically and should be considered in appropriate settings.[83]

METHODS OF ADMINISTRATION

The method for enteral tube feeding is limited to the type and site of enteral feeding access. The formula delivery method selected for the patient also depends on the patient's hemodynamic stability, gastric emptying rate, GI tolerance to tube feeding, type of formula selected, nutrient needs, patient mobility, and ease of administration. The main methods of tube feeding are by continuous, intermittent, or bolus delivery. Each institution should have an established protocol for the initiation and advancement of enteral feedings.

Bolus Feeding

Bolus feedings involve the delivery of larger amounts of formula over short periods of time, usually 5 min or less. The bolus method should only be used with gastric delivery. The stomach can act as a reservoir to handle relatively large volumes of formula (e.g., 400 ml) over a short time as opposed to the small intestine. The feedings are usually administered via a gastrostomy tube, owing to the large lumen, but they can also be given through a small-bore nasogastric tube. Usually a syringe or bulb is used to push 200 to 500 ml of formula into the feeding tube several times a day. A patient should demonstrate adequate gastric emptying and the ability to protect his/her airway (i.e., an intact gag reflex) prior to initiating bolus feedings, especially in the critical care setting, to decrease the risk of aspiration. The ability to absorb nutrients using this type of feeding depends on the access site and the functional capability of the gut.

Bolus feedings are considered the most physiologic method of administration as the gut can rest between feedings and allow for normal hormonal fluctuations. They are the easiest to administer as a pump is not required. Bolus feedings also allow for increased patient mobility as they are delivered intermittently and do not require a pump. For these reasons, this method of feeding is most desirable for stable patients who are going home or to an extended care facility with tube feedings.

Intermittent Feedings

This method of feeding requires the formula to be infused over a 20 to 30 min period. A feeding container and gravity drip are usually used for this method. Intermittent feedings are less likely to cause GI side effects than bolus feeding, as the formula is administered over a longer interval. Depending on the volume delivered, this method may be used for gastric, as well as small bowel, formula delivery.

Continuous Feedings

Continuous formula delivery is usually the enteral delivery method best tolerated. Continuous feedings are delivered slowly over 12 to 24 h, typically with an infusion pump. In order to avoid accidental bolus delivery, continuous infusion is preferred over gravity, as a constant infusion rate can be sustained. Postpyloric feedings require continuous infusion. The small bowel does not act as a reservoir for large volumes of fluid within a short time, and GI complications usually arise if feedings are delivered in this manner.

Initiation and progression of continuous feedings should be individualized and based on the patient's clinical condition and feeding tolerance. Typically, feedings may be initiated at 10 to 50 ml/h, with the lower range for the critically ill. Progression of tube feedings may range from 10 to 25 ml/h every 4 to 24 h, depending on the patient's tolerance, until the desired goal rate is achieved. As a patient begins to transition to oral intake, the tube feedings may be cycled to allow for appetite stimulation, or to allow for bowel rest and time away from the pump. The feedings may be administered at night and held back during the day to allow for patient mobility and an opportunity to eat.

ENTERAL FEEDING COMPLICATIONS

Although enteral nutrition is the preferred route of nutrient provision in those individuals unable to consume adequate nutrients orally, it is not without complications. Compared with parenteral nutrition, enteral nutrition complications are less serious. Most of the complications with enteral nutrition are minor; however, occasionally serious complications can develop. Most complications can be prevented, or at least be made less severe. Appropriate patient assessment for needs and risks, proper feeding route and formula selection, in addition to appropriate monitoring of the enteral nutrition feeding regimen, can increase the success of enteral feeding. The most common complications can be categorized as mechanical, metabolic, and GI. Table 67.8 lists some of the common complications, their possible causes, and suggested corrective measures.

TABLE 67.8
Common Complications Associated with Enteral Feeding[66,67]

Complication	Possible Causes	Suggested Corrective Measures
Mechanical		
Obstructed feeding tube	Formula viscosity excessive for feeding tube	Use less viscous formula or larger bore tube
	Obstruction from crushed medications administered through tube	Flush tube before and after feeding
		Give medications as elixir or assure medications are crushed thoroughly
		Flush tube before and after delivering each medication
	Coagulation of formula protein in tube when in contact with acidic medium (medication, flushing solution)	Flush feeding tube only with warm water
		Avoid flushing with sodas, coffee, juices, or any other acidic medium
Metabolic		
Hyperglycemia	Metabolic stress, sepsis, trauma	Treat origin of stress and provide insulin as needed
	Diabetes	Avoid excessive carbohydrate delivery
		Give appropriate insulin dose
Elevated or depressed serum electrolytes	Excessive or inadequate electrolytes in the formula	Change formula
	Refeeding syndrome	Monitor electrolytes closely (e.g., potassium, magnesium, phosphorus) and replace as indicated
		Initiate carbohydrate gradually, not increasing amount provided until electrolytes and blood glucose levels stabilized
Dehydration	Osmotic diarrhea caused by rapid infusion of hypertonic formula	Infuse formula slowly
		Change to isotonic formula or dilute with water
	Excessive protein, electrolytes, or both	Reduce protein, electrolytes or increase fluid provision
	Inadequate free water provision	Assure patient receives adequate free water, especially if provided calorically dense formula
Overhydration	Excessive fluid intake	Assess fluid intake; monitor daily fluid intake and output
	Rapid refeeding in malnourished patient	Monitor serum electrolytes, body weight daily; weight change >0.2 kg/ day reflects decrease or increase of extracellular fluid
	Increased extracellular mass catabolism causing loss of body cell mass with subsequent potassium loss	
	Cardiac, hepatic, or renal insufficiency	Use calorically dense formula to decrease free water if needed
		Diuretic therapy
Gradual weight loss	Inadequate calories	Assure patient is receiving prescribed amount of calories
		Assure to monitor patient over time as nutrient requirements may change due to metabolic alterations
Excessive weight gain	Excess calories	Decrease calories provided, change formula or decrease volume per day
Visceral protein depletion	Inadequate protein or calories	Increase protein or calorie provision
EFA deficiency	Inadequate EFA intake	Include at least 4% of kilocalories needs as EFA
	Prolonged use of low fat formula	

Continued

**TABLE 67.8
(Continued)**

Complication	Possible Causes	Suggested Corrective Measures
Gastrointestinal		
Nausea and vomiting	Improper tube location	Reposition or replace feeding tube
	Excessive formula volume or rate infusion	Decrease rate of infusion or volume infused
	Very cold formula	Administer formula at room temperature
	High osmolality formula infused	Change to isotonic formula or dilute with water prior to infusing
	High-fat formula infused	Change to lower fat formula
	Smell of enteral formulas	Add flavorings to formula; use polymeric as have less offensive odor
Diarrhea	Too rapid infusion	Decrease rate of infusion
	Lactose intolerance	Use lactose-free formula
	Bolus feedings into small bowel	Only provide continuous or slow gravity feedings into small bowel
	High-osmolality formula infused	Change to isotonic formula or dilute with water prior to infusing
	Hyperosmolar medication delivery	Change medications or dilute with water to make isotonic prior to delivery
	Altered GI anatomy or short gut	Change to hydrolyzed or free amino acid formula with MCT oil
Vomiting and diarrhea	Contamination	Check sanitation of formula and equipment; assure proper handling techniques
Abdominal distention, bloating, cramping, gas	Rapid bolus or intermittent infusion of cold formula	Administer formula at room temperature
	Rapid infusion via syringe	Infuse continuously at low rate and gradually increase to goal
	Nutrient malabsorption	Use hydrolyzed formula, MCT containing, lactose free
	Rapid administration of MCT	Administer MCT gradually as tolerated
Constipation	Lack of fiber	Use fiber-containing formula or add stool softener
	Inadequate free water	Increase free water intake
	Fecal impaction, GI obstruction	Rectal exam, digital disimpaction
	Inadequate physical activity	Increase ambulation if able
Aspiration or gastric retention	Altered gastric motility, diabetic gastroparesis, altered gag reflex, altered mental status	Assure postpyloric nutrient delivery with continuous infusion
		Add prokinetic agent if changed feeding position does not help
	Head of bed <30°	Elevate head of bed to >30 degrees if possible
	Displaced feeding tube	Verify feeding tube placement and replace as needed
	Ileus or hemodynamic instability	If small bowel feedings not tolerated then hold feedings and initiate TPN for prolonged intolerance
	Medications that may slow gastric motility (e.g., opiates, anticholinergics)	Evaluate medications and change if feasible
	Gastric or vagotomy surgery	

MONITORING

It is very important to continuously monitor patients for signs of formula intolerance, hydration and electrolyte status, and nutritional status. Physical indicators that should be monitored include incidence of vomiting, stool frequency, diarrhea, abdominal cramps, bloating, signs of edema or dehydration, and weight changes. In addition, several laboratory parameters should be monitored daily with the initiation of enteral feeding and tapered as the patient stabilizes and demonstrates tolerance (Table 67.9).

SUMMARY

Enteral feeding is the preferred method of providing nutrition in those who cannot consume adequate nutrients orally. Enteral feeding has many advantages over parenteral nutrition, including preservation of the structure and function of the GI tract, more efficient nutrient utilization, fewer infections and metabolic complications, greater ease of administration, and lower cost. In order for enteral nutrition to be successful, patient assessment for the optimal access site, appropriate formula selection, nutrient requirements, monitoring, and trouble-shooting complications are required.

TABLE 67.9
Example Monitoring Protocol for Enteral Feeding

Parameters	During Initiation and Advancement of Feedings Until Stable at Goal Rate	Stable at Goal Rate	Long-Term Enteral Support — Stable
Body weight	Daily	1–2 times/week	Monthly
Fluid intake/output	Daily	Daily	Daily
Bowel function			
Glucose	Daily unless abnormal then every 1 to 8 h until stable	2–3 times/week; unless diabetic, then daily	Every 6 months; unless diabetic, then daily
Electrolytes	Daily	2–3 times/week	Every 3–6 months
Blood urea nitrogen			
Creatinine			
Magnesium			
Phosphorus			
Calcium			
Liver function tests Triglyceride	1–2 times/week	1–2 times/month	Every 3–6 months
Visceral proteins (prealbumin, transferrin)	1–2 times/week	Weekly	Every 3–6 months
Gastric residuals (for gastric feeds only)	Every 4–6 h	If <200 ml, then discontinue	N/A unless gastroparesis, then every 4–6 h

With permission from Ideno, In: *Nutrition Support Dietetics Core Curriculum*, Gottschlich, Matarese, Shronts, Eds, ASPEN, Silver Spring, MD, 1993, p. 71.

REFERENCES

1. McCamish M, Bounous G, Geraghty M. In: Clinical *Nutrition: Enteral and Tubefeeding*, Rombeau J, Rolandelli R, Eds, WB Saunders, Philadelphia, PA, 1997, p. 1.
2. King BK, Kudsk KA, Li J, et al. *Ann Surg* 229: 272; 1999.
3. Kudsk KA. *Ann Surg* 215: 503; 1992.
4. Minard G, Kudsk KA. *World J Surg* 22: 213; 1998.
5. Suchner U, Senftleben U, Eckart T. *Nutrition* 12: 13; 1996.
6. Hindmarsh JT, Clark RG. *Br J Surg* 60: 589; 1973.
7. Rowlands BJ, Giddings AB, Johnston AB, et al. *Br J Anaesth* 49: 781; 1977.
8. Peterson VM, Moore EE, Jones TN, et al. *Surgery* 104: 199; 1988.
9. Kudsk KA, Minard G, Wojtysiak SL, et al. *Surgery* 116: 516; 1994.
10. McArdle AH, Palmason C, Morency I, et al. *Surgery* 90: 616; 1981.
11. Bennegard K, Lindmark L, Wickstrom I, et al. *Am J Clin Nutr* 40: 752; 1984.
12. Swank GM, Deitch W. *J Surg* 20: 411; 1996.
13. Kudsk KA. *Nutrition* 14: 541; 1998.
14. Bengmark S. *Curr Opin Clin Nutr* 2: 83; 1999.
15. Cunningham-Rundles S, Ho Lin D. *Nutrition* 14: 573; 1998.
16. Bengmark S. *J Parent Enter Nutr* 19: 410; 1995.
17. Moore FA, Feliciano DV, Andrassy RJ, et al. *Ann Surg* 216: 172; 1992.
18. Kudsk KA, Croce MA, Fabian TC, et al. *Ann Surg* 215: 503; 1992.
19. Moore FA, Moore EE, Jones TN, et al. *J Trauma* 29: 916; 1989.
20. Schmidt H, Martindale R. *Curr Opin Clin Nutrition Metabolic Care* 6: 587; 2003.
21. Trice S, Melnik G, Page C. *Nutr Clin Prac* 12: 114; 1997.
22. Lipman TO. *J Parent Enteral Nutr* 22: 167; 1998.
23. Adams S, Dellinger EP, Wertz MJ, et al. *J Trauma* 26: 882; 1986.
24. Kozar R, McQuiggan MM, Moore EE, et al. *J Surg* Res 104: 70; 2002.
25. Vasken A, Hichman K, DiGiovine B. *Chest* 129: 960; 2006.
26. Methany NA, Clouse RE, Chang Y, et al. *Crit Care Med* 34: 1007; 2006.
27. Zaloga GP. *Chest* 100: 1643; 1991.

28. Thurlow PM. *J Parent Enteral Nutr* 10: 104; 1986.
29. Heiselman DE, Vidovich RR, Milkovich G, et al. *J Parent Enteral Nutr* 17: 562; 1993.
30. Levenson R, Turner WW, Dyson A, et al. *J Parent Enteral Nutr* 12: 135; 1988.
31. Lord LM, Weiser-Maimone A, Pulhamus M, et al. *J Parent Enteral Nutr* 17: 271; 1993.
32. Kittinger JW, Sandler RS, Heizer WD. *J Parent Enteral Nutr* 11: 33; 1987.
33. Cresci G, Grace M, Park M, et al. *Nutr Clin Prac* 14: 101; 1999.
34. Minard G. *Nutr Clin Prac* 9: 172 ; 1994.
35. Gauderer MWL, Ponsky JL, Izant Jr RJ. *J Pediatr Surg* 15: 872; 1980.
36. Baskin WN. *Gastroenterologist* 4: S40; 1996.
37. Larson DE, Burton DD, Schroeder KW, et al. *Gastroenterol* 93: 48; 1987.
38. Wasiljew BK, Ujiki GT, Beal JM. *Am J Surg* 143: 194; 1982.
39. Ruge J, Vasquez RM. *Surg Gynecol Obstet* 162: 13; 1986.
40. Kirby DF, Craig RM, Tsang T, et al. *J Parent Enteral Nutr* 10: 155; 1986.
41. Kaplan DS, Murthy UK, Linscheer WG. *Gastrointest Endosc* 35: 403; 1989.
42. Shike M, Latkany L, Gerdes H, et al. *Nutr Clin Prac* 12: 38S; 1997.
43. Kles KA, Chang FB. *Gastroenterology* 130: S100; 2006.
44. Alverdy JC, Laughlin RS, Wu L. *Crit Care Med* 31: 598; 2003.
45. Katz JA. *J Clin Gastroenterol* 40: 249; 2006.
46. Trujilo EB. In: *Contemporay Nutrition Support Practice*, Gottschlich MM, Matarese LE, Eds, WB Saunders, Philadelphia, PA, 1998, p. 192.
47. Barton RG. *Nutr Clin Prac* 12: 51; 1997.
48. Blackburn GL. *Soc Exp Biology Med* 200: 183; 1992.
49. Lin E, Kotani J, Lowry S. *Nutrition* 14: 545; 1998.
50. Calder PC, Grimble RF. *Eur J Clin Nutr* 56: S14; 2002.
51. Hasselmann M, Reimund J. *Curr Opin Crit Care* 10: 449; 2004.
52. Heller AR, Rossler S, Litz RJ, et al. *Crit Care Med* 34: 972; 2006.
53. Adibi SA. *Am J Physiol Gastrointest Liver Physiol* 285: G779; 2003.
54. Van Der Hulst RRW, Van Krell BK, Von Meyenfeldt MF, et al. *Lancet* 341: 1363; 1993.
55. Ziegler TR, Young LS, Benfell K, et al. *Ann Intern Med* 116: 821; 1992.
56. Wischmeyer PE. *Curr Opin Clin Nutr Metab Care* 9: 201; 2006.
57. Macario AJ, Conway de Marcario E. *NEJM* 353: 1489; 2005.
58. Ziegler TR, Bazargan N, Leader LM, et al. *Curr Opin Nutr Metab Care* 3: 355; 2000.
59. Anderson PM, Schroeder G, Skubitz KM. *Cancer* 83: 1433; 1998.
60. Evoy D, Lieberman MD, Fahey TJ, et al. *Nutrition* 14: 611; 1998.
61. Barbul A, Fishel RS, Shimazu S, et al. *J Surg Res* 38: 328; 1986.
62. Heyland DK, Novak F, Drover JW, et al. *JAMA* 286: 944; 2001.
63. Beale RJ, Bryg DJ, Bihari DJ. *Crit Care Med* 27: 2799; 1999.
64. Heys SD, Walker LG, Smith I. *Ann Surg* 229: 467; 1999.
65. Montejo JC, Zarazaga A, Lopez-Martinez, et al. *Clin Nutr* 22: 221; 2003.
66. Ali S, Roberts PR. *Curr Opin Anaesthesiol* 19: 132; 2006.
67. Brown R. In: *Nutrition Support for the Critically Ill Pateint*, Cresci G, Ed, Taylor and Francis, Baca Raton, FL, 2005, p. 341.
68. Oldrizzi L, Rugiu C, Maschio G. *Nutr Clin Prac* 9: 3; 1994.
69. ASPEN Board of Directors. *J Parent Enteral Nutr* 17: 1SA; 1993.
70. Kopple JD. *J Parenter Enteral Nutr* 20: 3; 1996.
71. Anker SD, John M, Pedersen PU, et al. *Clin Nutr* 32: 641; 2006.
72. Barton RG, Wells CL, Carlson A, et al. *J Trauma* 31: 768; 1991.
73. Karlstad MD, DeMichele SJ, Leatherm WD, et al. *Crit Care Med* 21: 1740; 1993.
74. Mancuso P, Whelan J, DeMichele S, et al. *Crit Care Med* 25: 1198; 1997.
75. Gadek JE, DeMichele SJ, Karlstad MD, et al. *Crit Care Med* 27: 1409; 1999.
76. Malone AM. *Nutr Clin Prac* 12: 168; 1997.
77. Elia M, Ceriello A, Laube H, et al. *Diabetes Care* 28: 2267; 2005.
78. Didery MB, MacDonald IA, Blackshaw PE. *Gut* 35: 186; 1994.
79. Printz H, Reche B, Fehmann HC, et al. *Exp Clin Endocrinol Diabetes* 105: 134; 1997.
80. Peters A, Davidson M. *J Parent Enteral Nutr* 16: 69; 1992.
81. Marchesini G, Bianchi G, Rossi B, et al. *J Gastroenterol* 35: S7; 2000.
82. McCowen KC, Bistrian BR. *Am J Clin Nutr* 77: 764; 2003.
83. Stuart S, Melanie S, Unger L. In: *Medical Nutrition and Disease*, Morrison G, Hark L, Eds, Blackwell Science, Cambridge, England, 1996, p. 339.
84. Ideno KT. In: *Nutrition Support Dietetics Core Curriculum*, Gottschlich MM, Matarese LE, Shronts EP, Eds, ASPEN, Silver Springs, MD, 1993, p.71.

68 Parenteral Nutrition

Gail A. Cresci and Robert G. Martindale

CONTENTS

INTRODUCTION

Parenteral nutrition can be considered one of the twentieth century's medical breakthroughs. Its discovery and first implementation in the 1960s greatly enhanced clinical medicine by providing a means for complete and safe feeding of patients with nonfunctional gastrointestinal (GI) tracts. Experimentation with intravenous feeding can be traced as far back as the 1600s, when sharpened quills were used to administer a mixture of milk and wine into the veins of dogs.[1] The 1800s brought the administration of various saline solutions, and by the 1930s 5% dextrose and protein hydrolysates were being infused intravenously.[2] Several factors limited the safe infusion of nutrients intravenously. One major factor was the large volumes that were provided, usually more than 3 l/day.[2] These volumes were generally not tolerated by patients for long periods of time, and often resulted in pulmonary edema. These early attempts at intravenous feeding only utilized peripheral veins. This severely limited the osmolarity tolerated since only low osmolality could be delivered. Lastly, volume and the osmolality restrictions resulted in caloric delivery limitations. This all led to experimentation with alternate fuel substrates, alcohol, and fat, due to their increased caloric provision of 7 and 9 kcal/g, respectively. Research quickly revealed that alcohol was not going to be the answer, as it resulted in hepatoxicity and other side effects when delivered in large amounts.[1] Intravenous fat delivery was an enticing alternative due to its high caloric load and decreased osmolality. Initially, provision of intravenous fat was achieved with cottonseed oil in the 1950s. However, it was removed from the market, as it was associated with jaundice, fever, and bleeding.[3] Research continued in Europe, where emulsions made from soybean oil were successfully administered.[2]

Great advancement came in 1967, when cannulating the subclavian vein was introduced to administer intravenous nutrients. Wilmore and Dudrick[4] first reported successful clinical provision of centrally administered nutrition to an infant with intestinal atresia. In the 1970s, advancements continued with the use of crystalline amino acids rather than protein hydrolysates, recommendations for standard amounts of vitamins and minerals, and the reintroduction of lipids in the United States in 1976.[1] After the 1970s, the focus turned to fine-tuning the parenteral solutions with the development of specialized amino acid sources for specific disease states, approval of total nutrient admixtures (TNAs) by the Food and Drug Administration, and development of new access devices and delivery systems.[1]

RATIONALE FOR USE OF PARENTERAL NUTRITION

Parenteral nutrition was first developed to provide nutrition to those unable to take complete nutrition via the GI tract due to an inability to digest or absorb nutrients. A nonfunctioning GI tract and failure to tolerate enteral nutrition still remain the primary reasons for parenteral nutrition. Certain accompanying conditions also need consideration, such as a patient being nutritionally at risk, and projected inability to consume anything by mouth for at least 7 to 14 days.[5] Over the past two decades, several organizations have developed practice guidelines to identify the appropriate uses for parenteral nutrition (Table 68.1). Situations that indicate the need for parenteral nutrition include short bowel syndrome and malabsorption, bowel obstruction, intractable diarrhea or vomiting, prolonged ileus, and high-output GI fistulas (Table 68.2).[5–8]

COMPARISON OF PARENTERAL AND ENTERAL NUTRITION

While parenteral nutrition can be lifesaving when used appropriately, it may also potentiate adverse clinical outcomes. The GI tract not only functions to digest and absorb nutrients, but also serves as a large immunologic organ in the body by acting as a protective barrier against intraluminal toxins and bacteria. Approximately 60% of the body's immunoglobulin-producing cells line the GI tract, with 80% of the body's manufactured immunoglobulin being secreted across the GI tract.[9] During severe physiologic stress, gut ischemia can occur, leading to mucosal damage and disruption of the barrier function and ultimately passage of bacteria and toxins into the bloodstream.[10] In addition, common clinical practices, as well as physiologic changes during acute stress, can lead to bacterial overgrowth in the proximal GI tract and impact the gut's protective mucosal barrier (Table 68.3). Bacterial translocation can be defined as the passage viable microbes or microbial products from the lumen of the bowel across the epithelial surface. Whether or not bacterial translocation occurring in animals and humans during acute stress is clinically significant remains debatable. Animal studies support the statement that enteral rather than parenteral nutrition maintains gut integrity and immune responsiveness, and prevents bacterial translocation.[11–15] However, there was no significant difference in overall outcome in an acute pancreatitis model,[11] but in animals with induced bacterial pneumonia, those that received total

TABLE 68.1
Development of TPN Guidelines

Organization	Year
American Society for Parenteral and Enteral Nutrition	1986, 1993
American College of Physicians	1987, 1989
American Gastroenterology Association	1989
U.S. Department of Health and Human Services	1990

TABLE 68.2
Indications for TPN[5–8]

Clinical Situation	Consensus
Short bowel syndrome	Inability to absorb adequate nutrients orally <60 cm small bowel may require indefinite use
Enterocutaneous fistula	Fistula that exhibits increased output with enteral nutrition
Intractable diarrhea or vomiting	Recommended for losses greater than 500 to 1000 ml/day with inability to maintain adequate nutritional status
Bowel obstruction, ileus	With obstruction and malnutrition awaiting surgery >7 days
	Prolonged ileus >5 to 7 days with poor nutritional status
Perioperative support	Preoperative support is indicated for severely malnourished patients with expected postoperative NPO status >10 days
	For those with postoperative complications rendering NPO >10 days
Inflammatory bowel	If enteral nutrition not tolerated or if precluded by GI fistulas
Critical care	Unable to gain enteral access, hemodynamic instability, abdominal distention with prolonged reflux of enteral feedings, and expected to remain NPO >7 days
Eating disorders	Severe malnutrition and inability to tolerate enteral feeding for psychological reasons
Pregnancy	Safe in pregnancy; hyperemesis gravidarum

TABLE 68.3
Factors That Contribute to Increased Gut Permeability

Absence of enteral stimulation
Broad spectrum antibiotics
H_2-receptor blockers
Decreased GI hormone secretion
$\downarrow$ Visceral blood flow

TABLE 68.4
Typical PPN Order

Macronutrient	Usual Concentration in PPN Solution	gm/l or mEq/l	Kcal/l	mOsm/l
Dextrose (6%)	5–10%	60*	240	150
Amino acids (3%)	3–5%	30*	120	300
Lipid (20%)	30–60% (of kcal)	20*	200	300
Sodium		35+	—	70
Potassium		30+	—	60
Magnesium		5+	—	5
Calcium			—	7
Total			560	892

* gm/l; + mEq/l.

---

parenteral nutrition (TPN) had a higher mortality rate.[15] There is no hard evidence to support the statement that parenteral nutrition results in clinically significant bacterial translocation in humans.[16,17]

Multiple other disadvantages of parenteral nutrition exist. The metabolic response to intravenous glucose differs from oral glucose. This may be due to the fact that the liver retains a large portion of glucose when provided orally, resulting in less systemic hyperglycemia.[18] A meta-analysis comparing enteral and parenteral nutrition also concluded that plasma glucose concentrations are lower during enteral than parenteral nutrition.[19] Plasma glucose and insulin concentrations, glucose oxidation, CO_2 production, and minute ventilation increase in proportion to the proportion of kilocalories administered in TPN.[20] Prolonged infusion of high rates of glucose (>4 mg/kg per min) results in de novo lipogenesis in the majority of critically ill patients.[20] Furthermore, TPN is associated with increased septic morbidity[16,19,21,22] and increased cost[16,23] when compared with enteral nutrition in trauma patients. The increased infection risk associated with the use of parenteral nutrition when compared to enteral ranges from 15 to 50% depending on the patients population evaluated.[19,21,22]

VASCULAR ACCESS

Peripheral

Prior to initiating parenteral nutrition, vascular access is obtained. Determination of venous access is based upon the duration of therapy, patient limitations, and availability of equipment and facilities. Central or peripheral veins may be used for the provision of parenteral nutrition. Peripheral access with conventional needles uses the small veins of the extremities — typically the hands and forearms. These small veins are easily sclerosed by hypertonic parenteral solutions. Therefore, to minimize phlebitis and thrombosis of the veins, it is recommended that peripheral parenteral solutions (PPN) consist of osmolalities ≤900 mOsm/l.[5] Even with appropriate PPN, intravenous sites may need frequent changing to maintain venous patency.[1] The increased volume requirement necessary to minimize the PPN solution's osmolality limits nutrient provision as well as the clinical utility of PPN (Table 68.4).

PPN solutions vary considerably among institutions. Some may only use dextrose with electrolytes, vitamins, and minerals, while others may include lipids and amino acids to increase the kilocalories and ideally minimize catabolism. PPN formulations composed of carbohydrate, amino acids, and lipid generally provide 1000 to 1200 kcal/day. However, PPN may be useful when the long-term plan for nutrition is uncertain and the patient requires interim nutrition intervention in which the GI tract is temporarily nonfunctional, such as with prolonged ileus or hyperemesis gravidarum (Table 68.5).

TABLE 68.5
Indications for Peripheral Parenteral Nutrition

Indication	Example
Patient expected to be NPO 5 to 7 days	Postoperative ileus
Inadequate GI function expected for 5 to 7 days	Hyperemesis gravidarum
Transitioning to an oral diet or tube feeding	Patient with Crohn's disease flare
Central venous access is contraindicated	Coagulopathy, sepsis, and venous thrombosis
Malnourished patients expected to be NPO for several days	Preoperative small bowel obstruction
Patients with nutrient requirements that can be met with PPN	Obese patient with good venous access, small, or elderly people

TABLE 68.6
Central Venous Catheter Placement[24,25]

Method	Vessels	Description
Percutaneous approach	Subclavian	a. Venipuncture and passage of a guide wire through the needle followed by removal of the needle and catheter placement over the guide wire
a. Modified Seldinger technique	Internal and external jugular Antecubital	
b. Peel-away introducer sheath and tissue dilator		b. Catheter passes through the introducer into the vein and introducer tears longitudinally, leaving the catheter in place
Cut down	Cephalic External and internal jugular	Surgical dissection, isolation of the vessel, and catheter placement
Tunneled		A 6-cm catheter segment is tunneled through the subcutaneous tissues between the venipuncture site and the skin exit site
Implanted ports		A reservoir with a silicone disk and attached silicone tube is implanted under the clavicle in a subcutaneous pocket

Central

Central venous access commonly refers to the large veins in the trunk. The primary indications for central venous access include chemotherapy, antibiotic administration, risk of tissue necrosis with vesicant medications, and provision of TPN due to its pH and increased osmolality. Access is obtained with specialized catheters, with the distal tip placed into the vena cava or right atrial area. The most common venipuncture sites include the subclavian, internal jugular, femoral, cephalic, and basilic veins (Table 68.6). Several varieties of central venous catheters are available, the most common being polyurethane and silicone (Table 68.7). Most catheters are available in a variety of external diameters, lengths, and number of portals or lumens. Multilumen versions provide for simultaneous infusion of TPN with multiple or incompatible drugs.

Physiologic, functional, psychological, and social factors all need consideration prior to determining the type and location of catheter placement (Table 68.8). If the patient is in the acute care setting and unlikely to be discharged with TPN, the physiologic factors are of primary concern. However, if a patient is to receive parenteral nutrition in an alternate care setting, practitioners should consider the other listed factors for optimal patient compliance.[24]

PARENTERAL NUTRIENT COMPONENTS

Parenteral nutrient solutions are complex formulations that usually contain the macronutrients, carbohydrate, protein, and lipid for energy provision, as well as electrolytes, trace elements, vitamins, water, and occasionally medications. These components need to be individualized for patients based upon their primary diagnosis, chronic diseases, fluid and electrolyte balance, acid–base status, and specific nutrition goals.[26]

CARBOHYDRATE

Carbohydrate serves as the primary energy source in parenteral solutions. The amount of carbohydrate provided is based upon the patient's individual nutrient requirements and glucose oxidation rate. Although the exact requirement is individualized,

TABLE 68.7
Central Venous Catheter Characteristics

Material	Description
Silicone elastomer	Known as Silastic (Dow Corning)
	Biomaterial for long-term indwelling devices
	Increased elasticity and flexibility for minimal damage to intima
	Resistant to hydrolytic enzymes; hydrophobic surface resists bacterial adherence
	Considered chemically inert in blood
	Guide wire or peel-away introducer needed for insertion due to soft texture
Polyurethane	Increased flexibility and strength; resistance to hydrolytic enzymes
	Decreased incidence of inflammatory changes and thrombophlebitis with short term use
	Anticoagulation required with long term use for thrombosis prevention
Polyvinyl chloride	Stiff material
	Increased rate of thrombogenicity
	Infrequently used
Polyethylene	High tensile strength
	Minimal irritation if used for short duration
	Associated with platelet adherence and fibrous capsule formation with long duration
Polytetrafluoroethylene (PTFE)	Known as Teflon; stable; demonstrates nonadhesive, antifriction properties; resistant to degradative enzymes
	Smooth and hydrophobic catheter surface
	Not suitable for long term use due to rigidity which causes irritation and thrombosis formation
Hydrogel	Hydrophilic polymers designed for biological use
	Absorbs water up to 90% of the catheter's dry weight without dissolving
	Most inert and nonthrombogenic of biomaterials
	Material lacks durability unless copolymerized with other monomers
Coated/bonded catheters	Antimicrobial-impregnated catheters: catheters with the cationic surfactant tridodecylmethyl-ammonium chloride facilitate bonding of anionic antibiotics to both the internal and external catheter surfaces
	Antiseptic-coated catheters: polyurethane catheters bonded with silver sulfadiazine and chlorhexidine to the external surface

TABLE 68.8
Patient Factors for Vascular Access Device Selection

Patient Factor	Considerations
Physiologic	Vein physiology
	Hypercoagulable states
	Diabetes
	Clotting abnormalities
	Skin disorders and conditions
	Previous surgical procedures in the thorax or vascular system
	Morbid obesity
	Surgical risk
	Known allergies to vascular materials
Functional	Impaired vision, dexterity
	Developmental disabilities
	Frailty
Psychological	Needle phobia (not ideal candidates for implanted ports)
	Body image issues (implanted port less disturbing than tunneled)
	Previous experience with vascular access devices
Social	Support system for line and catheter care
	Financial implications

Source: With permission from Evans, *Nutr Clin Prac* 14: 172; 1999.

TABLE 68.9
Intravenous Dextrose Solutions

Dextrose Concentration (%)	Carbohydrate (gm/l)	Calories (kcal/l)	Osmolarity (mOsm/l)
5	50	170	250
10	100	340	500
20	200	680	1000
30	300	1020	1500
50	500	1700	2500
70	700	2380	3500

guidelines are available. A minimum of 100 g/day is often used as the obligate need for the central nervous system, white blood cells, red blood cells, and renal medulla.[26] The maximum rate of glucose oxidation in adults is 4 to 6 mg/kg per min,[5] or 300 to 500 g for a 70-kg person, with the lower range suggested for critically ill patients secondary to endogenous glucose production. Excessive carbohydrate provision is associated with hyperglycemia, excessive carbon dioxide production, and hepatic steatosis.[26]

Carbohydrate is provided almost exclusively as dextrose monohydrate in parenteral solutions. Each gram of hydrated dextrose provides 3.4 kcal/g. Commercial dextrose preparations are available in concentrations from 5 to 70% (Table 68.9). Dextrose solutions have an acidic pH (3.5 to 5.5) and are stable after autoclave sterilization.[26] Sterilization also increases the shelf life of dextrose solutions so that they can be stored for extended periods at room temperature.

Glycerol is a naturally occurring 3 carbon glycolytic intermediate. Glycerol yields 4.3 kcal/g when oxidized to carbon dioxide and water and does not require insulin for cellular uptake. When provided in low concentrations (3%) with amino acids, it has been found to be protein sparing.[27] Because of these advantages, glycerol is used an alternative source of calories in some parenteral formulations, primarily in PPN.

LIPID

Since the introduction of intravenous lipids in Europe in the mid-1960s, lipid emulsions have been extensively used as a nutrient source in parenteral nutrition. The aqueous lipid emulsions available in the United States as of 2006 consist of long-chain triacylglycerols (TAG) manufactured from soybean and safflower oil. Therefore, the lipid emulsions not only provide a source of kilocalories but also essential fatty acids (EFA). These products contain egg yolk phospholipid as an emulsifying agent and glycerin, which make the products nearly isotonic. The glycerol raises the caloric concentration of the 10% emulsion to 1.1 kcal/ml and the 20% emulsion to 2.0 kcal/ml. The phospholipid may contribute to the phosphorus intake of patients who receive large amounts of lipids (>500 ml/day). Combinations of long- and medium-chain TAG emulsions have been available in Europe for several years. In most of the non-U.S. markets lipids of various origin and mixtures are available including fish oil, olive oil, and medium-chain triglycerides.[28]

Most patients tolerate daily infusion of lipids provided as an intermittent or continuous infusion, often as part of a TNA. Continuous delivery with a moderate dose is favored over intermittent infusion due to decreased fluctuations in serum TAG levels and improved fat oxidation.[29] The requirement of a test dose is usually eliminated with continuous delivery, as the administration rate tends to be less than that with the test dose. Patients should still be monitored for fever, chills, headache, and back pain during the first dose of intravenous lipid. Absolute contraindications to intravenous fat emulsions include pathologic hyperlipidemia, lipoid nephrosis, severe egg allergy, and acute pancreatitis when associated with severe hypertriglyceridemia.[26] Caution should be taken in delivery to patients with severe liver disease, adult respiratory distress syndrome, or severe metabolic or catabolic stress. If serum TAG levels are greater than 500 mg/dl, lipids should be held with only the minimal requirements for EFA provided to avoid further metabolic complications.

Lipid requirements are met by providing at least 4% of energy as EFA or approximately 10% of energy as a commercial lipid emulsion from safflower oil to prevent EFA deficiency.[30] Since lipid emulsions vary in their composition of EFA depending on the oil source, the minimum amount provided is based upon the EFA content rather than a percentage of total energy. Recommendations for optimal lipid delivery have evolved over the years. Historically, it once was common practice to provide 40 to 60% of energy as lipid due to its concentrated energy source when allowed for decreased volume delivery. However, over the years concerns that soy based lipid emulsions currently available in the United States are proinflammatory and impair neutrophil function, endotoxin clearance, and complement synthesis have resulted in the recommendation to limit lipid administration to 1 g/kg per day[29] or 25 to 30% of total energy.[31]

PROTEIN

The primary function of protein in parenteral nutrition is to provide nitrogen to maintain nitrogen balance to help minimize loss of lean body mass and protein degradation for gluconeogenesis. The nitrogen source utilized for parenteral nutrition is in the form of crystalline amino acids. Parenteral amino acid products can be divided into standard and modified (disease specific). Standard amino acid products are suitable for the majority of patients. They contain a balanced mixture of essential and nonessential amino acids in which the ratios are based on FAO/WHO recommendations for optimal proportions of essential amino acids. Standard formulations are available in a range of concentrations from 3 to 15%. Most institutions stock 10 and 15% concentrations, since more dilute solutions can be made readily by adding sterile water with an automated compounder.

Modified amino acid solutions are designed for patients with disease- or age-specific amino acid requirements. Formulations are marketed for adults with hepatic failure, renal dysfunction, metabolic stress, and for neonates with special requirements for growth and development. These modified formulations are significantly more costly than the standard formulations and may not always prove as cost-effective; therefore, strict criteria should be established for their use.

Patients with hepatic failure develop multiple metabolic abnormalities including electrolyte disturbances and alterations in amino acid metabolism. In severe liver disease, hepatic encephalopathy can occur, which is associated with decreased branched chain amino acid (BCAA) serum levels and elevated aromatic amino acid (AAA) and methionine serum levels. Patients with hepatic disease without encephalopathy may be provided with moderate levels of standard amino acids with close monitoring of their mental status. When hepatic encephalopathy is severe (≥grade II), a modified hepatic protein formulation may be beneficial in decreasing the clinical course of encephalopathy. These formulations have high concentrations of BCAA (~45% of protein) and low concentrations of AAA and methionine. Improvement in hepatic encephalopathy and variable influence in lower mortality have been found in some patients who received this formulation.[32]

Modified formulations are marketed for patients with renal failure. These formulas contain mainly essential amino acids, and were designed on the premise that endogenous urea could be used as a nitrogen source to synthesize nonessential amino acids via transamination reactions. The clinical benefit of these solutions has been challenged. Prospective, randomized, and controlled studies have demonstrated that standard amino acids are as effective as modified amino acids in patients who have renal failure and who require parenteral nutrition.[33,34] Thus, patients with severe renal failure may be given standard amino acids as part of parenteral nutrition in most clinical situations.[24]

Intravenous renal failure formulations have limited usefulness currently secondary to the relative ease at which patients now undergo beside dialysis or hemofiltration.

A parenteral formulation with an enhanced BCAA formulation is marketed for patients with metabolic stress such as that caused by trauma, burns, and sepsis. Metabolic stress causes an efflux of amino acids from skeletal muscle and the gut to the liver for gluconeogenesis and support of acute phase protein synthesis.[35] Metabolically stressed patients have also been shown to have increased serum levels of AAA and decreased BCAA levels. Therefore, the rationale of using a high BCAA formula in these patients is to provide the preferential fuel to the body and normalize the patient's amino acid patterns. Multiple studies have evaluated the benefits of high BCAA formulations in metabolic stress. Some studies have shown positive benefits when using these formulations, such as nitrogen retention, improved visceral protein levels, and reversal of skin test anergy, but there were no differences in morbidity or mortality.[36–38] Other studies have failed to exhibit significant outcome advantages of BCAAs over standard amino acid formulas in metabolic stress.[39–41] Therefore, since the cost-effectiveness of high BCAA solutions has not been clearly demonstrated, initiation of nutrition support with a standard amino acid solution is recommended in patients with metabolic stress.[5]

Parenteral protein requirements are based upon the patient's clinical condition. For normal healthy adults, the recommendation is for 0.8 g/kg per day.[42] In the critically ill population, a range of 1.5 to 2.0 g/kg per day is appropriate.[5] For patients with renal or hepatic disease, protein recommendations vary according to the disease stage and its intervention. For those with renal disease on peritoneal dialysis, 1.2 to 1.5 g/kg per day of ideal body weight is recommended for maintenance or repletion. For hemodialysis, 1.1 to 1.4 g/kg of ideal body weight per day is recommended for maintenance or repletion.[43] For patients with uncomplicated hepatic dysfunction, 0.8 to 1.5 g/kg dry weight is suggested; for end-stage liver disease with encephalopathy, 0.5 to 0.7 g/kg; if a high BCAA formula is used, then 0.8 to 1.2 g/kg per day is suggested.[44]

ELECTROLYTES

Electrolytes are essential nutrients that perform many critical physiologic functions. Electrolytes are added to parenteral solutions based upon individual need. The amount added daily varies based upon the patient's weight, disease state, renal and hepatic function, nutrition status, pharmacotherapy, acid–base status, and overall electrolyte balance. Extrarenal electrolyte losses may be a result of diarrhea, ostomy output, vomiting, fistulas, or nasogastric suctioning. As patients become anabolic during parenteral nutrient delivery, they may experience increased requirements for the major intracellular electrolytes (potassium, phosphorus, and magnesium). During refeeding of undernourished patients, these electrolytes should be monitored frequently and replenished accordingly.

Small adjustments in electrolyte intake can affect patient morbidity and mortality and therefore need careful monitoring. General recommendations for electrolyte provision are provided in Table 68.10. Electrolyte products are commercially available (Table 68.11), and the composition of the parenteral solution is dependent upon the compatibility of each electrolyte with the other components of the admixture. For calcium provision, calcium gluconate is the preferred form for parenteral formulations due to its stability in solution and decreased chance of dissociating and forming a precipitate with phosphorus. Whether to provide an electrolyte as a chloride or an acetate salt depends on the patient's acid–base status. Generally, acid–base balance is maintained with providing chloride and acetate in a 1:1 ratio. If a patient has altered acid–base status with skewed electrolyte levels, then the chloride to acetate ratio can be adjusted to facilitate correction. Acetate and chloride are also present in the base amino acid solutions in various amounts, and should be considered when attempting electrolyte homeostasis.

Electrolytes increase the osmolarity of the parenteral solution; however, large amounts can be added to solutions with amino acids and dextrose without affecting the stability. When lipids are added to the parenteral solutions, caution is needed when adding electrolytes, as there are limitations and hazards.[1] An insoluble precipitate can form when there are excess cations in the parenteral solutions, as with calcium and phosphate, which may not be visualized in TNAs. Crystal formation in the lungs with subsequent death was reported in patients as a result of precipitate formation in TPN solutions.[45] The solubility of calcium and phosphorus varies with the volume of the solution, its pH, the type of calcium preparation, the temperature at which the solutions are stored, and the order of admixture.[1] Solutions can be prepared with a range of calcium and phosphorus contents as long as the product of calcium (in mEq) and phosphorus (in mmols) is less than 200.[46]

VITAMINS AND TRACE ELEMENTS

Vitamins are typically added to every parenteral formulation in doses consistent with the American Medical Association Nutrition Advisory Group's recommendations.[47] Guidelines are established for the 12 essential vitamins (Table 68.12). Most institutions use a commercially available multiple-entity product, which contains 12 essential vitamins for adults. Most multivitamin preparations for adults do not contain vitamin K because it antagonizes the effects of coumadin in patients receiving this medication. In adults, vitamin K may be administered by adding 1 to 2 mg/day to the parenteral solution or by giving 5 to 10 mg/week intramuscularly or subcutaneously.[26] Individual vitamin preparations are also available and are used to supplement the multivitamin doses when a deficiency state exists, or with increased needs due to disease or medical condition.

TABLE 68.10
Parenteral Electrolyte Recommendations

Sodium	60–150 mEq/day
Potassium	70–150 mEq/day
Phosphorus	20–30 mmol/day
Magnesium	15–20 mEq/day
Calcium	10–20 mmol
Chloride	Equal to Na+ to prevent acid–base disturbances

Source: With permission from Skipper, In: *Contemporary Nutrition Support Practice.* WB Saunders, Philadelphia, PA, 1998, p. 227.

TABLE 68.11
Commercially Available Electrolyte Formulations[25,26]

Sodium Chloride	Magnesium Sulfate
Sodium acetate	Magnesium chloride
Sodium phosphate	Calcium chloride
Sodium lactate	Calcium gluconate
Potassium chloride	
Potassium acetate	
Potassium phosphate	
Potassium lactate	

TABLE 68.12
AMA Recommendations for Parenteral Vitamin Intake

Vitamin	Amount
Vitamin A	3300 IU
Vitamin D	200 IU
Vitamin E	10 IU
Vitamin C (ascorbic acid)	100 mg
Folacin	400 mg
Niacin	40 mg
Riboflavin	3.6 mg
Thiamine	3 mg
Vitamin B_6 (pyridoxine)	4 mg
Vitamin B_{12} (cyanocobalamin)	5 mg
Pantothenic acid	15 mg
Biotin	60 mg

Source: Adapted from Multivitamin preparations for parenteral use. A statement by the Nutrition Advisory Group. *J Parent Enteral Nutr* 3: 258; 1979.

TABLE 68.13
AMA Recommendations for Parenteral Mineral Intake

Element	Amount (mg/Day)
Zinc	2.5–4
Copper	0.5–1.5
Manganese	150–180
Chromium	10–15
Selenium*	40–80

* Suggested intake.

Source: Adapted from Guidelines for essential trace element preparations for parenteral use: A statement by the Nutrition Advisory Group. *J Parent Enteral Nutr* 3: 263; 1979.

Trace minerals are essential to normal metabolism and growth, and serve as metabolic cofactors essential for the proper functioning of several enzyme systems (see Chapter 8). Although the requirements are minute, deficiency states can develop fairly rapidly secondary to increased metabolic demands or excessive losses. Most clinicians add these micronutrients daily; however, there are clinical conditions necessitating trace mineral restriction and therefore adjustments in the daily intakes.

The Nutrition Advisory Group of the American Medical Association (AMA) has also published guidelines for four trace elements known to be important in human nutrition.[48] The suggested amounts of zinc, copper, manganese, and chromium for adults are listed in Table 68.13. Since the original recommendations, it has become more evident that selenium also is essential, and many clinicians add this element to the parenteral solution daily along with the other four.[26] Most institutions use a commercially available multiple-entity product, but there are also single-entity mineral solutions available for use during times of increased requirements or when certain minerals are contraindicated. Zinc requirements are increased during metabolic stress due to increased urinary losses, and with excessive GI losses as with diarrhea, external biliary or fistula drainage, and increased ostomy output. Manganese and copper are excreted through the biliary tract, whereas zinc, chromium, and selenium are excreted via the kidney. Therefore, copper and manganese should be restricted or withheld from parenteral nutrition in patients with cholestatic liver disease.[26] Selenium depletion has been found in patients receiving long-term TPN, as well as with thermal injury, acquired immunodeficiency syndrome, liver failure, and critical illness.[26,48]

OTHER ADDITIVES

Many patients receiving TPN are also receiving multiple medications, leading to the desire to add the medications to the TPN solutions. Using TPN as a drug delivery vehicle is very tempting, as it may allow for continuous medication infusion in addition to minimizing fluid volume delivery by eliminating the need for a separate dilutent for each medication administered. However, scrutiny is needed prior to adding medications to the TPN solution, as there is potential for drug–drug and drug–nutrient interactions. Issues needing consideration include medication compatibility with TPN constituents, the effect of pH changes on TPN compatibility, and drug effectiveness, whether the infusion schedule of the TPN is appropriate to achieve therapeutic levels of the drug, and the potential for interactions among the drugs if more than one is added.[1] The complexity of these issues usually leads to consultation with a pharmacist experienced in TPN compounding and compatibility, reference to the institution's policy and procedure manual, or contact with the drug manufacturers. Medications most frequently added to TPN include albumin, aminophylline, cimetidine, famotidine, ranitidine, heparin, hydrochloric acid, and regular insulin.[1] Table 68.14 list medications compatible with TPN solutions, and Table 68.15 lists those medications, which are incompatible with TPN solutions.

TABLE 68.14
Medications Compatible with Parenteral Solutions

Albumin[a]	Cyanocobalamin	Hydromorphone	Nafcillin
Amikacin	Cyclophosphamide	Imipenem-cilastatin	Neostigmine
Aminophylline[a]	Cytarabine	Insulin, regular[a]	Netilmicin
Azlocillin	Digoxin[a]	Iron dextran	Oxacillin[a]
Caffeine	Dipyridamole	Isoproterenol[a]	Oxytocin
Carbenicillin[a,b]	Dobutamine	Kanamycin[a]	Penicillin G[a]
Cefamandole[a]	Dopamine[a]	Lidocaine[a]	Phenobarbital
Cefazolin[a]	Doxycycline	Meperidine[a]	Phytonadione[a]
Cefoperazone	Erythromycin[a]	Metaraminol	Piperacillin
Cefotaxime	Famotidine[a]	Methicillin[a]	Polymyxin B
Cefoxitin[a]	Fluorouracil[b]	Methotrexate	Ranitidine[a,b]
Ceftazidine	Folic Acid	Methyldopa	Tetracycline
Ceftriazone	Furosemide[a]	Methylprednisolone	Ticarcillin[a,b]
Cephalothin[a,b]	Ganciclovir	Metoclopramide[a]	Tobramycin[a]
Chloramphenicol[a]	Gentamicin[a]	Mezlocillin	Vancomycin
Chlorpromazine	Heparin[a]	Miconazole	
Cimetidine[a]	Hydralazine	Morphine	
Clindamycin[a]	Hydrochloric acid	Moxalactam	

[a] Compatible with TNA.

[b] Some data suggest incompatibility under certain conditions. Visual compatibility only; tested with parenteral nutrition solution without electrolytes; drug may chelate with divalent cations and cause precipitation.

Source: With permission from Strausburg, Parenteral nutrition admixture. ASPEN Practice Manual, 1998.

TABLE 68.15
Medications Incompatible with Parenteral Solutions

Amphotericin B	Methyldopa[a]
Amikacin[a]	Metronidazole (with NaHCO₃)
Ampicillin[b]	Phenytoin[a]
Cephradine	Tetracycline[a,c]
Iron dextran[a,d]	

[a] Incompatible with TNA.

[b] Some visual compatibility data suggest compatibility under certain conditions.

[c] Compatible with lipid alone; however, may chelate with divalent cations of TNAs.

[d] Visually incompatible with TNAs when reconstituted with 5% dextrose in water; visually compatible when reconstituted with normal saline solution.

Source: With permission from Strausberg, Parenteral nutrition admixture. ASPEN Practice Manual, 1998.

INSULIN

Even with care to avoid excess carbohydrate delivery, patients receiving TPN often become hyperglycemic.[49] One method of achieving desired blood glucose control with continuous TPN infusions is by adding regular insulin to the TPN solution. A few studies have suggested that absorbance of insulin to glass bottles, polyvinyl chloride bags, and tubing occurs,[50,51] with the greatest loss occurring during the first hour of infusion.[52] So, when adding insulin to TPN solutions to optimize blood glucose control, it is important to remember that the patient may have an increased insulin requirement due to absorbance.

HISTAMINE H₂-RECEPTOR BLOCKERS

Stress ulcer prophylaxis with the addition of H$_2$-receptor blockers is common practice with patients on TPN who are not receiving any gastric luminal nutrients. This may be achieved by adding the H$_2$-receptor blockers to the TPN solution. Famotidine (20 and 40 mg/l) and ranitidine hydrochloride have been shown to be stable in parenteral nutrition solutions and three-in-one admixtures.[53–57]

HEPARIN

In order to reduce the complications of catheter occlusion related to fibrin formation around the catheter tip, heparin may be added to the TPN solution. Adding up to 1000 units of heparin per liter reduces the incidence of catheter occlusion without exhibiting anticoagulant effects on serum.[1] Larger amounts of heparin may be used for peripheral parenteral nutrition.

METHODS OF ADMINISTRATION

Serious complications with TPN may develop if careful initiation and monitoring are not followed. TPN solutions may be infused continuously over a 24-h period, or cycled over shorter time intervals. If a patient is critically ill or just beginning to receive TPN, it is suggested to infuse it over a 24-h period until patient tolerance is demonstrated. TPN should not be initiated at goal levels of nutrients, as many patients may not tolerate this prescription. Proportional increases in carbohydrate-dependent electrolytes such as magnesium and phosphorus, in protein-dependent electrolytes such as potassium, and in volume-dependent electrolytes such as sodium should be made as the macronutrients are increased.

For patients with diabetes mellitus, stress hyperglycemia, steroids, or risk for refeeding syndrome, dextrose should be restricted initially to approximately 100 to 150 g/day. For other patients with normal glucose tolerance, dextrose may be initiated at 200 to 250 g/day. If after 24 h serum glucose levels are acceptable, then the dextrose may be advanced to goal over the next 24 to 48 h as indicated. Capillary glucose measurements should be obtained three to four times daily until the values are normal for two consecutive days. Regular insulin may be administered according to a sliding scale.[1] A continuous intravenous insulin infusion or drip may be substituted for sliding scale if serum glucose levels are consistently elevated beyond suggested levels. The importance of glucose control cannot be overemphasized.[58] Recent work by Van de Berghe has reported a major decrease in numerous ICU-related complications including mortality when tight glycemic control is maintained.[59] Insulin may also be added to the TPN solution, however, one needs to remember that providing insulin in this manner confines the delivery over the time period of the TPN mixture, and if the hyperglycemia resolves then the TPN bag must be discontinued to avoid inadvertent hypoglycemia. For patients requiring insulin prior to TPN institution, approximately half of the established insulin requirement may be included as regular insulin in the initial bag of TPN formula.1 If blood glucose levels are less than 200 mg/dl, approximately two thirds of the previous day's subcutaneous insulin dose may be added to the TPN as regular insulin. Regardless of the method of insulin delivery, the goal is to consistently maintain blood glucose levels between 120 and 200 mg/dl.[5]

Lipids may be infused for up to 24 h, and may reduce the adverse effect of lipids on the reticuloendothelial system.[30] Lipids can be given with the first TPN infusion unless serum TAG levels are elevated. It is suggested to maintain TAG levels at ≤400 mg/dl while lipids are being infused.[1] If TAG levels exceed the recommended level, lipids should be held until levels normalize. As this occurs, patients may be provided with lipids in amounts to prevent EFA deficiency. For persistent or severe hypertriglyceridemia or for patients with egg allergy, small amounts of enterally delivered EFA can usually be administered to alleviate the symptoms of EFA deficiency.[60] Critically ill patients may also be receiving significant amounts of lipid from lipid-based medications, which may predispose them to hypertriacylglycerolemia prior to TPN infusion. The amount of lipid from medications should be considered in the final TPN formulation to avoid providing excess long-chain TAG.

In most acute care settings, parenteral nutrition is usually provided over a 24-h continuous rate. In patients who require TPN for an extended period, it may also be delivered in a cyclic pattern. During TPN, circulating insulin levels remain elevated, reducing the amount of carbohydrate that enters the cell, thus favoring hepatic lipogenesis.[1] Cyclic TPN with periods free from intravenous nutrient delivery allows for patient mobility, and therefore it is usually utilized with ambulatory patients. For individuals with limited vascular access, cyclic infusion may be required in order to administer necessary medications or blood products. Conversion from 24-h continuous infusion to cyclic infusion can be accomplished in 2 to 3 days. The largest concern is with the initiation and discontinuation of the carbohydrate infusion and potential for hyperglycemia and rebound hypoglycemia.

Another concern is with the increased volume delivery over a shorter time frame. Most stable patients with adequate renal function and cardiac reserves can tolerate cyclic TPN over 8 to 14 h.

PARENTERAL NUTRITION DISCONTINUATION

In all patients, the goal should be to transition from TPN to enteral nutrition — either tube feeding or oral intake. Prior to discontinuing TPN, assurance that the patient is consuming and absorbing adequate nutrients enterally is imperative. This is usually assessed by diet histories and kcalorie counts. TPN should be decreased as the enteral intake and tolerance improves to avoid overfeeding. TPN may be discontinued once the patient is tolerating approximately 65 to 75% of goal nutrients. For patients who are eating, TPN may be reduced and stopped over a 24- to 48-h period. If TPN is inadvertently but abruptly discontinued in patients who are not eating, all insulin should be stopped and blood glucose levels should be monitored for 60 min after discontinuation of TPN. Based upon the blood glucose levels, appropriate therapy should be implemented.[1] Lastly, if the TPN was used as a vehicle for medication or electrolyte administration, an alternate plan should be made once it is discontinued. Attempting to switch medications to the enteral route is usually employed. Consultation with a pharmacist can help facilitate this transition.

COMPLICATIONS OF PARENTERAL NUTRITION

Complications of parenteral nutrition have been widely reported. However, TPN can be safe with minimal complications when it is managed and monitored by a multidisciplinary team of trained professionals. The type of complications that may arise are diverse but for simplicity be divided into mechanical, infectious, and metabolic categories.

Mechanical complications of catheter insertion (Table 68.16) include pneumothorax, hydrothorax, and great vessel injury. The catheter malposition may result in venous thrombosis, causing head, neck, or arm swelling, or possibly a pulmonary embolus. To minimize morbidity, placing lines with portable ultrasound and obtaining a chest radiograph before using a new central line for TPN is important to ensure correct line placement and absence of internal injuries that may have occurred during insertion.

Catheter-related infections can carry a high risk for increasing the morbidity and potential mortality rate as well as significantly increasing the medical costs. A catheter infection rate of less than 3% is desirable.[5] Appropriate use of aseptic technique by trained personnel is essential to maintain an acceptable catheter infection rate. Nursing protocols should be established for

TABLE 68.16
Mechanical Complications of Parenteral Nutrition

Complication	Possible Cause	Symptoms	Treatment	Prevention
Pneumothorax	Catheter placement by inexperienced personnel	Tachycardia, dyspnea, persistent cough, and diaphoresis	Large pneumothorax may require chest tube placement	Experienced personnel to place catheter
Catheter embolization	Pulling catheter back through needle used for insertion	Cardiac arrhythmias	Surgical removal of catheter tip	Avoid withdrawing catheter through insertion needle
Air embolism	Air is inspired while line is interrupted and uncapped	Cyanosis, tachypnea, hypotension, and churning heart murmur	Immediately place patient on left side and lower head of bed to keep air in apex of the right ventricle until it is reabsorbed	Experienced personnel to place catheter
Venous thrombosis	Mechanical trauma to vein, hypotension, hyperosmolar solution, hypercoagulopathy, and sepsis	Swelling or pain in one or both arms or shoulders or neck	Anticoagulation therapy with urokinase or streptokinase; catheter removal	Silicone catheter, adding heparin to TPN, and low dose warfarin therapy
Catheter occlusion	Hypotension, failure to maintain line patency, formation of fibrin sheath outside the catheter, and solution precipitates	Increasing need for greater pressure to maintain continuous infusion rate	Anticoagulation therapy with urokinase or streptokinase	Larger diameter catheter, routine catheter flushing, and monitor solution for a precipitate
Phlebitis	Peripheral administration of hypertonic solution	Redness, swelling, and pain at peripheral site	Change peripheral line site and begin central TPN if necessary	Maintain osmolarity of peripheral solution ≤900 mOsm/kg
Catheter-related sepsis	Inappropriate technique of line placement, poor catheter care, and contaminated solution	Unexplained fever, chills, red, and indurated area around catheter site	Remove catheter and replace at another site	Follow strict protocols for line placement and care

Source: With permission from Skipper, In: *Contemporary Nutrition Support Practice.* WB Saunders, Philadelphia, PA, 1998, p. 227.

dressing changes and line manipulation. Dressings should be changed every 48 h and should include local sterilizing ointment and an occlusive dressing. Since gram-positive catheter-related sepsis may be treated with antibiotics, removal of the catheter is not always necessary. Catheter removal is usually necessary with gram-negative organisms.

With close monitoring of TPN, avoidance of metabolic complications (Table 68.17) is possible. Refeeding syndrome may be defined as a constellation of fluid, micronutrient, electrolyte, and vitamin imbalances that occur within the first few days after refeeding a starved patient. Refeeding syndrome may involve hemolytic anemia, respiratory distress, paresthesias, tetany, and cardiac arrythmias.[61] Typical biochemical findings include hypokalemia, hypophosphatemia, and hypomagnesemia. Proposed risk factors for refeeding include alcoholism, anorexia nervosa, marasmus, rapid refeeding, and excessive dextrose infusion. In order to prevent the syndrome from occurring it is suggested to replete serum potassium, phosphorus, and magnesium concentrations prior to beginning TPN; limit initial carbohydrate to 150 g/day, fluid to 800 ml, and sodium intake to no more than 20 mEq/day in at-risk patients; include adequate amounts of potassium, magnesium, phosphorus, and vitamins in the TPN solution; and increase carbohydrate-dependent minerals in proportion to increases in carbohydrate when TPN is advanced.[61]

Hyperglycemia (nonfasting blood glucose >220 mg/dl) is a common metabolic complication of TPN. Risk factors include metabolic stress, medications, obesity, diabetes, and excess dextrose administration. Careful glucose monitoring, especially in the first few days of TPN administration, can help guide advancement of dextrose to goal. Administration of dextrose in amounts less than the maximum glucose oxidation rate (4 to 7 mg/kg per min) and initiating dextrose in reduced amounts (100 to 150 g/day) in at-risk patients may help minimize the occurrence of hyperglycemia.[5]

Patients receiving TPN may also experience fluid and electrolyte abnormalities (Table 68.17). The etiology of the abnormalities may be related to several factors, including the patient's medical condition and treatment, medications, or excessive or inadequate free water provision. Fluid balance and electrolyte status should be monitored closely (Table 68.18), with corrections in abnormalities made accordingly.

TABLE 68.17
Metabolic Complications of Parenteral Nutrition

Complication	Possible Cause	Treatment
Hypovolemia	Inadequate fluid provision and overdiuresis	Increase fluid delivery
Hypervolemia	Excess fluid delivery, renal dysfunction, congestive heart failure, and hepatic failure	Fluid restriction and diuretics, dialysis
Hypokalemia	Refeeding syndrome, inadequate potassium provision, and increased losses	Increase intravenous or parenteral potassium
Hyperkalemia	Renal dysfunction, too much potassium provision, metabolic acidosis, and potassium-sparing drugs	Decrease potassium intake, potassium binders, and dialysis in extreme cases
Hyponatremia	Excessive fluid provision, nephritis, adrenal insufficiency, and dilutional states	Restrict fluid intake and increase sodium intake as indicated clinically
Hypernatremia	Inadequate free water provision, excessive sodium intake, and excessive water losses	Decrease sodium intake and replete free water deficit
Hypoglycemia	Abrupt discontinuation of parenteral nutrition and insulin overdose	Dextrose delivery
Hyperglycemia	Rapid infusion of large dextrose load, sepsis, pancreatitis, steroids, and diabetes; elderly	Insulin, reduce dextrose delivery
Hypertriglyceridemia	Inability to clear lipid provision, sepsis, multisystem organ failure, medications altering fat absorption, and history of hyperlipidemia	Decrease lipid volume provided, increase infusion time, hold lipids up to 14 days to normalize level
Hypocalcemia	Decrease vitamin D intake, hypoparathyroidism, citrate binding of calcium due to excessive blood transfusion, and hypoalbuminemia	Calcium supplementation
Hypercalcemia	Renal failure, tumor lysis syndrome, bone cancer, excess vitamin D delivery, prolonged immobilization, and stress hyperparathyroidism	Isotonic saline, inorganic phosphate supplementation, corticosteroids, and mithramycin
Hypomagnesemia	Refeeding syndrome, alcoholism, diuretic use, increased losses, medications, diabetic ketoacidosis, and chemotherapy	Magnesium supplementation
Hypermagnesemia	Excessive magnesium provision and renal insufficiency	Decrease magnesium provision
Hypophosphatemia	Refeeding syndrome, alcoholism, phosphate-binding antacids, dextrose infusion, overfeeding, secondary hyperparathyroidism, and insulin therapy	Phosphate supplementation, discontinue phosphate-binding antacids, avoid overfeeding, and initiate dextrose delivery cautiously
Hyperphosphatemia	Renal dysfunction, excessive provision	Decrease phosphate delivery, phosphate binders
Prerenal azotemia	Dehydration, excessive protein provision, inadequate nonprotein calorie provision with mobilization of own protein stores	Increase fluid intake, decrease protein delivery, increase nonprotein calories
EFA deficiency	Inadequate polyunsaturated long-chain fatty acid provision	Lipid administration

Source: With permission from Skipper, In: *Contemporary Nutrition Support Practice.* WB Saunders, Philadelphia, PA, 1998, p. 227.

TABLE 68.18
Suggested Monitoring of TPN

Parameter	Baseline Level	Acute Patients	Stable Patients
Electrolytes, BUN, Cr	Yes	Daily	1–2 × week
Chemistry Panel Ca^{2+}, PO4–, Mg^{2+}	Yes	Daily until stable, then 2–3 × week	Weekly
LFTs	Yes	2 × week	Weekly–monthly
Triacylglycerol	Yes	Weekly unless abnormal then 2 × week	Weekly–monthly
Capillary glucose	2–3 × day	3 × day until consistently <200 mg/dl	2 × day until consistently <200 mg/dl
Intake and output	Yes	Daily	Daily or by physical exam
Weight	If available	Daily	Monthly
CBC with differential	Yes	Weekly	Weekly
PT, PTT	Yes	Weekly	Weekly

Abbreviation: BUN = blood urea nitrogen; PT = prothrombin time; PTT = partial thromboplastin time; CBC = complete blood count; LFT = liver function test; Cr = creatinine.

SUMMARY

Parenteral nutrition has been one of the major medical advancement over the past several decades. Its institution has saved countless lives of people who would have otherwise died of malnutrition and its complications. With careful selection, implementation, and monitoring, parenteral nutrition is a medical vehicle for nutritional supplementation of numerous diseases. TPN continues to evolve in Europe, Asia, and South America, while it has remained somewhat primitive in the United States secondary to the tight restrictions placed on the introduction of new intravenous solutions and emulsions. As wealth of data recently reported for intravenous Glutamine solutions and various combinations of lipid emulsions the next decade will see a reemergence of TPN as it becomes more physiological and adapted to the individual disease states.

REFERENCES

1. Skipper A. In: *Contemporary Nutrition Support Practice*. WB Saunders, Philadelphia, PA, 1998, p. 227.
2. Rhoads JE, Dudrick SJ. In: *Clinical Nutrition: Parenteral Nutrition*. WB Saunders, Philadelphia, PA, 1993, p. 1.
3. Meyer CE, Fancher JA, Schurr PE, Webster HD. *Metabolism* 6: 591; 1957.
4. Wilmore DW, Dudrick SJ. *JAMA* 203: 860; 1968.
5. ASPEN Board of Directors. *J Parent Enteral Nutr* 17(4): 1S; 1993.
6. American College of Physicians. *Ann Intern Med* 107: 252; 1987.
7. Sitzman JV, Pitt HA. *Dig Dis Sci* 34: 489; 1989.
8. Pillar B, Perry S. *Nutrition* 6: 314; 1990.
9. Levine GN, Derin JJ, Steiger E, Zinno R. *Gastroenterology* 67: 975; 1974.
10. Deitch EA. *Arch Surg* 124: 699; 1989.
11. Kotani J, Usami M, Nomura H, et al. *Arch Surg* 134: 287; 1999.
12. Li J, Kudsk D, Gocinski B, et al. *J Trauma* 39: 44; 1995.
13. King BK, Li J, Kudsk KA. *Arch Surg* 132: 1303; 1997.
14. DaZhong X, Lu Q, Deitch E. *J Parent Enteral Nutr* 22: 37; 1998.
15. King B, Kudsk K, Li J, et al. *Ann Surg* 229: 272; 1999.
16. Lipman T. *J Parent Enteral Nutr* 22: 167; 1998.
17. Heyland D, MacDonald S, Keefe L, Drover J. *JAMA* 280: 2013; 1998.
18. Vernet O, Christin L, Schultz Y, et al. *Am J Physiol* 250: E47; 1986.
19. Moore FA, Feliciano DV, Andrassy RJ, et al. *Ann Surg* 216: 172; 1992.
20. Tappy L, Schwarz J, Schneiter P, et al. *Crit Care Med* 26: 860; 1998.
21. Moore FA, Moore EE, Jones TN, et al. *J Trauma* 29: 916; 1989.
22. Kudsk K, Croce M, Fabian T, et al. *Ann Surg* 215: 503; 1992.
23. Trice S, Melnik G, Page C. *Nutr Clin Prac* 12: 114; 1997.
24. Evans M. *Nutr Clin Prac* 14: 172; 1999.
25. Krzywda EA, Edmiston CE. *ASPEN Practice Manual*, 1998.
26. Dickerson R, Brown R, Whithe, K. In: *Clinical Nutrition: Parenteral Nutrition*. WB Saunders, Philadelphia, PA, 1993, p. 310.
27. Freeman JB, Fairfull-Smith R, Rodman G, et al. *Surgery* 156: 625; 1983.
28. Hasselman M, Reimund J. *Curr Opin Crit Care* 10: 449; 2004.

29. Abbott WC, Grakauskas AM, Bistrian BR, et al. *Arch Surg* 119: 1367; 1984.
30. Seidner DL, Mascioli EA, Istfan NW, et al. *J Parent Enteral Nutr* 13: 614; 1989.
31. Jensen GL, Mascioli EA, Deidner DL, et al. *J Parent Enteral Nutr* 14: 467; 1990.
32. Cerra FB, Cheung NK, Fischer JE, et al. *J Parent Enteral Nutr* 9: 288; 1985.
33. Mirtallo JM, Schneider PJ, Mavko K, et al. *J Parent Enteral Nutr* 6: 109; 1982.
34. Feinstein EL, Blumenkrantz MJ, Healy M, et al. *Medicine* 60: 124; 1981.
35. Chiolero R, Revelly J, Tappy L. *Nutrition* 13: 45S; 1997.
36. Cerra FB, Shronts EP, Konstantinides NN, et al. *Surgery* 98: 632; 1985.
37. Cerra FB, Mazuski JE, Chute E, et al. *Ann Surg* 199: 286; 1984.
38. Bower RH, Muggia-Sullum M, Vallgren S, et al. *Ann Surg* 203: 13; 1986.
39. Yu YM, Wagner DA, Walesrewski JC, et al. *Ann Surg* 207: 421; 1988.
40. Freund H, Hoover HC, Atamian S, et al. *Ann Surg* 190: 18; 1979.
41. von Meyenfeldt MF, Soeters PB, Vente JP, et al. *Br J Surg* 77: 924; 1990.
42. Recommended Dietary Allowances, 10th ed, Washington, DC: National Academy Press, 1989, p. 3.
43. Stover J (Ed). *A Clinical Guide to Nutrition Care in End Stage Renal Disease*. Chicago: American Dietetic Association, 1994, pp. 28, 43.
44. Shronts E, Fish J. In: *Nutrition Support Dietetics: Core Curriculum*, 2nd ed. Gottschlich M, Matarese L, Shronts E, eds, ASPEN, Silver Spring, MD, 1993, p. 311.
45. Lumpkin MM, Burlington DB. *FDA Safety Alert: Hazards of Precipitation Associated with Parenteral Nutrition*. U.S. Food and Drug Administration, Rockville, MD, 1994.
46. Dunham B, Marcuard S, Khazanie PG, et al. *J Parent Enteral Nutr* 15: 608; 1991.
47. American Medical Association Department of Foods and Nutrition. *J Parent Enteral Nutr* 3: 258; 1979.
48. Guidelines for essential trace element preparations for parenteral use: A statement by the Nutrition Advisory Group. *J Parent Enteral Nutr* 3: 263; 1979.
49. Forceville X, Vitoux D, Gauzit R, et al. *Crit Care Med* 26: 1536; 1998.
50. Weber SS, Wood WA, Jackson EA. *Am J Hosp Pharm* 34: 353; 1977.
51. Macuard SP, Dunham B, Hobbs A, Caro JF. *J Parent Enteral Nutr* 14: 262; 1990.
52. Hirsch JJ, Wood JH, Thomas RB. *Am J Hosp Pharm* 38: 995; 1981.
53. Bullock L, Fitzgerald JF, Glick MR, et al. *Am J Hosp Pharm* 46: 2321; 1989.
54. Montov JB, Pou L, Salvador P, et al. *Am J Hosp Pharm* 46: 2329; 1989.
55. Williams MF, Hak LJ, Dukes G. *Am J Hosp Pharm* 47: 1547; 1990.
56. Cano SM, Montoro JB, Pastor C, et al. *Am J Hosp Pharm* 45: 1100; 1989.
57. Moore RA, Feldman S, Trenting J, et al. *J Parent Enteral Nutr* 5: 61; 1981.
58. Strausburg K. Parenteral nutrition admixture. ASPEN Practice Manual, 1998.
59. Van den Berghe G, Wouters PJ, Bouillion R, et al. *N Engl J Med* 345: 1359; 2001.
60. Miller DG. *Am J Clin Nutr* 46: 419; 1987.
61. Skipper A, Willikan KW. Parenteral nutrition implementation and management. ASPEN Practice Manual, 1998.

69 Nutrition in Critical Illness

Gail A. Cresci and Robert G. Martindale

CONTENTS

INTRODUCTION

The human body constantly strives to maintain homeostasis even when challenged by physical, biological, chemical, or psychological forces. Hospitalized patients are routinely exposed to numerous factors that cause metabolic stress, in addition to the stress event that brought them to the intensive care unit (ICU). Some of these stresses include semistarvation, infection, trauma, surgery, and tissue ischemia. Malnutrition in hospitalized patient is surprisingly common.[1] Malnutrition in the hospitalized patient occurs via either inadequate caloric delivery or from the hyperdynamic response to the metabolic insult.[2] These two pathways resulting in malnutrition exhibit very different metabolic alterations (Table 69.1). The development of malnutrition in critically ill patients can occur very rapidly secondary to the hormonal, neuronal, and other molecular modulators of metabolic response that result in the complex response to stress which is observed.

METABOLIC RESPONSE TO STRESS

The metabolic response to injury and sepsis has been well studied after the pioneering work of Kinney and Cuthberson and others.[3] Stressed patients undergo metabolic phases as a series of ebb and flow states reflecting a patient's response to the severity of the stress (Table 69.2). The earliest, or ebb, state is usually manifested by decreased oxygen consumption, fluid volume shifts from intravascular to extravascular compartments, inadequate tissue perfusion, and cellular shock. These changes temporarily decrease metabolic needs and provide a brief protective environment. The flow state is a hyperdynamic phase in which substrates are mobilized for energy production while increased cellular activity and hormonal stimulation is noted. Subsequently, most patients will enter a third phase of recovery, or anabolism, which is characterized by normalization of vital signs, increased diuresis, improved appetite and caloric intake, and positive nitrogen balance to restore the host to the prestress metabolic state. There is an energy expenditure distinction for each phase, making the goals of nutrition therapy variable depending on the

TABLE 69.1
Metabolic Comparisons Between Starvation and Stress

	Starvation	Stress
Resting energy expenditure	↓	↑↑
Respiratory quotient	↓	↑
Primary fuels	Fat	Mixed
Glucagon	↑	↑
Insulin	↓	↑
Gluconeogenesis	↓	↑↑↑
Plasma glucose	↓	↑
Ketogenesis	↑↑	↓
Plasma lipids	↑	↑↑
Proteolysis	↑	↑↑↑
Hepatic protein synthesis	↑	↑↑
Urinary nitrogen loss	↑	↑↑↑

TABLE 69.2
Stress-Phase Alterations

Phase	Hormonal/Nonhormonal	Metabolic	Clinical Outcomes
Ebb phase	↑ Glucagon ↑ Adrenocorticotropic hormone (ACTH)	Circulatory insufficiency (↑ Heart rate, vascular constriction) ↓ Digestive enzyme production ↓ Urine production	Hemodynamic instability
Flow phase	↑ Counterregulatory hormones (epinephrine, norepinephrine, glucagon, cortisol) ↑ Insulin ↑ Catecholamines ↑ Cytokines (TNF, IL-1, IL-2, and IL-6)	Hyperglycemia ↓ Protein synthesis ↑ Amino acid efflux ↑ Gluconeogenesis ↑ Glycogenolysis ↑ Lipolysis ↑ Urea nitrogen excretion/net (−) nitrogen balance	Fluid and electrolyte imbalances Mild metabolic acidosis ↑ Resting energy expenditure
Anabolic phase	↑ Insulin ↓ Counterregulatory hormones ↓ Cytokines	↑ Protein synthesis ↓ Urea nitrogen excretion/net (+) nitrogen balance ↓ Gluconeogenesis ↓ Lipolysis	↓ Resting energy expenditure ↑ Lean body mass

metabolic stage at which it is being introduced. As long as the patient is in a hyperdynamic catabolic state, current nutrition support regimens can at best approach zero nitrogen balance in attempts to minimize further protein wasting. Once the patient enters the anabolic phase, it is then realistic to anticipate a positive nitrogen balance and repletion of lean body mass through optimal nutrition intervention. Therefore, early nutrition intervention in critical illness is primarily geared toward sustaining vital organ structure, immune function, ameliorating the catabolic effects of critical illness, and promoting recovery without causing further metabolic derangements.

The high-risk patient usually remains in the catabolic phase for a prolonged period. In order to meet tissue demands for increased oxygen consumption following acute injury, there is an attempt by the host to increase in oxygen delivery. This is accomplished by a systemic response that includes increases in heart rate, myocardial contractility, and minute ventilation, and decreases in peripheral vascular resistance so that the cardiac index may exceed 4.5 L/min/m.[3,4] Other systemic responses to the hypermetabolic response include increased proteolysis and nitrogen loss, accelerated gluconeogenesis, peripheral insulin resistance, hyperglycemia and increased glucose utilization, and retention of salt and water. When patients become critically ill, they rapidly shift from an anabolic state of storing protein, fat, and glycogen to a catabolic state by mobilizing these nutrients for energy utilization.[5] There is a direct correlation between the severity of the injury and the degree of substrate mobilization. The mobilization of protein, fat, and glycogen is mediated through the release of cytokines such as tumor necrosis factor (TNF), interleukin (IL)-1, -2, and -6, and the counter-regulatory hormones such as epinephrine, norepinephrine, glucagon, and cortisol.[6]

These hormones are labeled counter-regulatory because they counter the anabolic effects of insulin and other anabolic hormones. Circulating levels of insulin are elevated in most metabolically stressed patients, but the responsiveness of tissues to insulin, especially skeletal muscle, is severely blunted. This relative insulin resistance is believed to be due at least in part to the effects of the counter-regulatory hormones and proinflammatory cytokines. The hormonal and cytokine milieu normalizes only after the injury or metabolic stress has resolved. Recent studies would indicate that specific enteral nutrient delivery during the early phases of critical illness may play a crucial role in accelerating recovery from the catabolic stress.[7]

During the hypermetabolic response to critical illness, energy expenditure is increased. This results in an increased mobilization of nutrient substrates in an attempt to meet body need. This is exhibited by an elevated respiratory quotient (RQ) of 0.80 to 0.85 reflecting mixed fuel oxidation, as opposed to a nonstressed starved state, in which the RQ is in the range of 0.60 to 0.70, reflecting the oxidation of fat as the primary fuel source. Under the influence of the counter-regulatory hormones, cytokines, and catecholamines, hepatic glucose output increases through glycogenolysis and gluconeogenesis.[5] The accelerated endogenous glucose production via glycogenolysis and gluconeogenesis is poorly suppressed even with exogenous glucose or insulin administration. In stress metabolism, glycogen stores are depleted within 12 to 24 h of a major catabolic insult, leaving only protein and adipose tissue as primary energy substrates. Gluconeogenic substrates include lactate, alanine, glutamine, glycine, serine, and glycerol. Accompanying the increased glucose production is an increase in flow to and uptake of glucose in the peripheral tissues. Hyperglycemia commonly results because of an increased glucagon–insulin ratio and insulin resistance in peripheral tissues.

Alterations in hormone and cytokine levels also affect lipid metabolism. Elevations of epinephrine, growth hormone, glucagon, and β-adrenergic stimulation induce lipolysis and increase glycerol and free fatty acid (FFA) levels, which are then used as a fuel source.[6] Despite accelerated rates of lipolysis, a proportionate increase in lipid oxidation is not observed. This is believed to be due to the elevated insulin levels. Therefore, even though lipid stores are abundant in most cases, they are poorly utilized in critically ill patients.

With depleted glycogen stores and diminished ability to utilize fat stores, the body shifts to catabolizing and using lean body mass as a main energy source and substrate for gluconeogenesis. Although in the stressed state total body protein synthesis is higher relative to nonstress starvation, overall it is significantly reduced as the balance of anabolism and catabolism has shifted to favor catabolism. Increased nitrogen excretion is observed and is proportional to the severity of injury or infection. The major mediators of protein catabolism and the accelerated movement of amino acids from the skeletal muscle and other peripheral tissues to the liver are the glucocorticoids and catecholamines.[5] This redistribution takes place to allow gluconeogenesis, acute-phase protein production, immunologic tissue proliferation, red cell production, and fibroblast proliferation. Amino acids reaching the liver are used to produce glucose and acute-phase proteins such as fibrinogen, haptoglobin, C-reactive protein, ceruloplasmin, and α-2 macroglobulin.[6] Approximately 70% of the amino acids released by skeletal muscle during a catabolic insult are glutamine and alanine, although they make up only 15% of the muscle protein.[8] Alanine is the primary amino acid used for gluconeogenesis, wheras glutamine supplies the necessary nitrogen to the kidneys for the synthesis of ammonia and the primary fuel for the enterocyte. Ammonia acts as a neutralizing substrate for the excess acid by-products produced by the increased protein degradation that occurs during stress. The utilization of amino acids for an energy source results in increased ureagenesis and urinary nitrogen losses, which may exceed 15 to 20 g/day.[3]

NUTRITIONAL INTERVENTION IN CRITICAL ILLNESS

The traditional goals of nutrition intervention in critically ill patients were to minimize lean body tissue loss and support the body's immune system. Nutrient delivery was designed in an attempt to maintain lean body mass without causing further metabolic complications. The current goal of nutrition in the critically ill patient is to use nutrients as therapeutic tools to attenuate metabolic response to stress, enhance immune function, and lower mortality and hospital stay.[9–11] Achieving these goals involves accurate and continued nutrition assessment, optimal and timely nutrient delivery, and continuous systematic monitoring of metabolic status.

DETERMINATION OF ENERGY REQUIREMENTS

Regardless of the metabolic state, energy requirements must be met in attempts to minimize the utilization of stored energy reserves. Although the protein-sparing effect of an adequate caloric intake is well recognized in the setting of adaptive starvation, it is equally clear in the setting of stress hypermetabolism that, despite adequate caloric provision and delivery of adequate nutrients, protein catabolism continues.[4]

Determination of energy requirements in the critically ill is often challenging. Critical illness and its treatment can profoundly alter metabolism and significantly increase or decrease energy expenditure.[12] Therefore, accurate determination of resting energy expenditure (REE) is necessary to ensure that energy needs are provided without over- or underfeeding. Overfeeding is associated with numerous metabolic complications. It is usually a result of excessive administration of carbohydrate or fat and can result in hepatic steatosis, hyperglycemia, and increase in pCO_2, which then requires increase in minute ventilation. Underfeeding leads to poor wound healing, impaired organ function, and altered immunologic status.

TABLE 69.3
Selected Methods for Estimating Energy Requirements

Harris–Benedict Equation — Estimates Basal Energy Expenditure (BEE)
Male: 13.75 (W) + 5 (H) – 6.76 (A) + 66.47
Female: 9.56 (W) + 1.85 (H) – 4.68 (A) + 655.1

W: weight in kilograms; H: height in centimeters; A: age in years
Note: To predict total energy expenditure (TEE) add an injury/activity factor of 1.2 to
1.8 depending on the severity and nature of illness

Ireton–Jones Energy Expenditure Equations (EEE)
Obesity
EEE = (606 ¥ S) + (9 ¥ W) – (12 ¥ A) + (400 ¥ V) + 1444

Spontaneously Breathing Patients
EEE (s) = 629 – 11 (A) + 25 (W) – 609 (O)

Ventilator Dependent Patients
EEE (v) = 1925 – 10 (A) + 5 (W) + 281 (S) + 292 (T) + 851 (B)

Where EEE = kcal/day, v = ventilator dependent, S = spontaneously breathing
A: age in years
W: body weight in kilograms
S: sex (male = 1, female = 0)
V: ventilator support (present = 1, absent = 0)
T: diagnosis of trauma (present = 1, absent = 0)
B: diagnosis of burn (present = 1, absent = 0)
O: obesity >30% above IBW from 1959 Metropolitan Life Insurance tables (present = 1,
absent = 0)

Curreri Burn Formula (EEE: Estimated Energy Expenditure)
EEE for 18–59 years old = (25 kcal ¥ Wt) + (40 ¥ % TBSA burn)
EEE for >60 years old = BEE + (65 ¥ % TBSA burn)
EEE = kcal/day; Wt: weight in kilograms; TBSA: total body surface area burn

---

There are multiple methods for assessing energy requirements in the critically ill. Some methods actually measure energy expenditure, such as indirect calorimetry, and others predict caloric requirements with various equations, such as the Harris–Benedict equation (Table 69.3). Each method of determination carries advantages as well as disadvantages. Indirect calorimetry is currently the gold standard and the preferred method for assessment of energy requirements in critically ill patients. However, it is expensive to perform routinely, and many facilities do not have the equipment or trained personnel to conduct the studies. Also, indirect calorimetry can be inaccurate under a variety of circumstances that commonly affect critically ill patients, such as patients receiving greater than 60% FiO_2 or in those with malfunctioning chest tubes or endotracheal tubes in which the expired gas is not completely captured. Therefore, many clinicians rely on predictive equations for determining energy needs. It is important to know the flaws of these equations to optimally interpret the results. The final estimate of energy needs assumes that the patients demonstrate a predictable metabolic response to their illness. The equations may overestimate the caloric needs of patients who are mechanically ventilated and sedated. Chemical neuromuscular paralysis with heavy sedation, which is commonly used as an adjunct to the management of ventilated patients, can decrease the energy requirements of the critically ill patient by as much as 30%.[4] Calculated results are only as accurate as the variables used in the equation. Obesity and increased volume associated with resuscitation complicate the use of these equations and lead to a tendency for overfeeding.[13] However, when considering all forms and phases of critical illness, energy requirements can generally range from 20 to 35 kcal/kg lean body mass/day. Patients with extensive burns or head injury may fall at the higher end. In most cases, 20 to 30 kcal/kg/day is a reasonable initial estimate of energy requirements in critically ill adult patients (see Table 69.4). A growing volume of literature supports slightly lower caloric delivery in the early hypermetabolic phase of critical illness (usually the first 3 to 5 days). Most clinicians will use an ideal or estimated lean body mass for those individuals who are obese so as to avoid overfeeding. For marasmic patients, it is important to use actual body weight to avoid overfeeding when calculating initial energy requirements.

PROTEIN REQUIREMENTS

Protein metabolism during metabolic stress is characterized by a total-body net proteolysis. In addition to muscle proteolysis, increased ureagenesis, hepatic synthesis of acute-phase proteins, urinary nitrogen losses, and use of amino acids as oxidative

TABLE 69.4
Energy and Substrate Recommendations

Kcalories	20–30 kcal/kg per day
Protein[a]	1.5–2.0 g/kg per day or 20–25% of total kcal
Carbohydrate[b]	£ 4–5 mg/kg per min per day or 50–60% of total kcal
Fat[c]	15–30% of total kcal
Fluids	1 ml/kcal; maintain optimal urine output
Electrolytes	Maintain normal levels, especially Mg^{2+}, PO_4^-, K^+
Vitamins/minerals	Recommended daily allowance; add vitamin K

[a] Adjust protein delivery for renal and hepatic dysfunction.
[b] Adjust glucose administration to maintain serum glucose levels £150 g/dl.
[c] Adjust lipid delivery based on serum triglyceride levels.

substrate for energy production are also noted. Therefore, the protein needs of critically ill patients are significantly increased compared with those patients with simple starvation. Although the high catabolic rate is not reversed by provision of glucose and protein,[14] the protein synthetic rate is responsive to amino acid infusions, and nitrogen balance can be attained through the support of protein synthesis.[15,16] Current recommendations for stressed patients is for 20 to 25% of the total nutrient intake to be provided as protein. This equates to roughly 1.5 to 2.0 g/kg/day, providing the higher range to promote nitrogen equilibrium or to at least minimize nitrogen deficit. Excess protein administration has not been shown to be beneficial, and in fact can cause azotemia.[17]

CARBOHYDRATE REQUIREMENTS

Glucose is the main fuel for the central nervous system (CNS), bone marrow, and injured tissue. A minimum of about 100 g/day is necessary to maintain CNS function. In the metabolically stressed adult, the maximum rate of glucose oxidation is 4 to 6 mg/kg/min,[18] roughly equivalent to 300 to 600 g/day in a 70 kg person. Provision of glucose greater than this rate usually results in lipogenesis[19] and hyperglycemia. In the hypermetabolic patient, part of the oxidized glucose will be derived from endogenous amino acid substrates via gluconeogenesis. In the severely stressed patient, up to 2 mg/kg/min of glucose may be provided via gluconeogenesis and this endogenous production is poorly suppressed by exogenous glucose administration.[17] In fact, providing additional glucose in these situations can lead to severe hyperglycemia. Exogenous insulin delivery tends to be ineffective in increasing cellular glucose uptake in critically ill patients, because the rate of glucose oxidation is already maximized and endogenous insulin concentrations are already elevated secondary to the relative insulin resistance. Complications of excess glucose administration include hyperglycemia, hyperosmolar states, excess carbon dioxide production, and hepatic steatosis.[17,19] Recent intensive care literature strongly supports meticulous glycemic control. Maintaining glucose levels below 150 mg/dl has been show to decrease mortality, morbidity, and length of ventilator days and ICU stay in the critically ill population.[20] Therefore, it is recommended that glucose be provided at a rate less than 5 mg/kg/min or approximately 50 to 60% of total energy requirements in critically ill patients, and that they be monitored closely for metabolic complications as described previously.

LIPID REQUIREMENTS

Lipids, when delivered appropriately, become an important substrate in critically ill patients as they can facilitate protein sparing, decrease the risk of excess carbohydrate, limit volume delivery by their high caloric density, and provide essential fatty acids. Endogenous triglyceride breakdown continues in hypermetabolic patients despite increased plasma levels of glucose and insulin.[21] Daily fat can be provided without adverse effect, as critically ill patients efficiently metabolize exogenous lipids.[22] Fat may comprise 10 to 30% of total energy requirements, with a minimum of 2 to 4% as essential fatty acids to prevent deficiency. Hypermetabolic patients should be monitored for tolerance of lipid delivery, especially if high levels are provided, as it may cause metabolic complications.

These complications include hyperlipidemia, impaired immune function, and hypoxemia resulting from impaired diffusing capacity and ventilation/perfusion abnormalities. Complications associated with intravenous lipid infusions and result not only due to the quantity of lipids provided but also from the rate of delivery. The rate of infusion should not exceed 0.1 g/kg/h. Complications may be minimized by infusing lipids continuously over 18 to 24 h while monitoring serum triglyceride levels and liver function tests to assure tolerance.

The current intravenous lipids available in the United States are composed nearly 100% of long-chain triglycerides (LCTs) as omega-6 fatty acids, whereas most enteral formulations contain mixtures of LCTs and medium-chain triglycerides (MCTs), omega-3 fats, and fish oils. In the past several years research has shown that high levels of omega-6 fatty acids provided in critically ill patients can be immunosuppressive.[23] Large and rapid infusions of LCTs favor the production of arachidonic acid and its proinflammatory metabolites such as prostaglandin E2 (PGE2), leukotrienes of the 4 series, and thromboxanes.[23–25] Unfortunately, in the United States, only soy-based emulsions are available, whereas in Europe and in most other regions of the world, various lipid emulsions are available containing fish oil, monounsaturated fats, and MCTs.

In addition to the inflammatory issues, LCTs are dependent on a carnitine carrier for transfer from cytosol across the mitochondrial membrane to undergo β-oxidation. It has been postulated that critically ill patients have a relative carnitine deficiency[26] due to an increased excretion, thus limiting the oxidation of LCT. MCTs, on the other hand, do not require carnitine for transport into the mitochondria and are rapidly and efficiently oxidized to carbon dioxide and water. When MCT is delivered enterally, a significant portion is absorbed via the portal vein, thereby bypassing the gastrointestinal (GI) lymphatic LCT absorptive system. MCTs have been shown to be better tolerated in many situations, as they require minimal biliary and pancreatic secretion for absorption. The ideal ratio of LCT to MCT for critically ill patients is currently not known.

FLUID AND ELECTROLYTES

Critical illness disrupts normal fluid and electrolyte homeostasis. Sepsis, systemic inflammatory response syndrome (SIRS), GI losses, delivery of medications, and acid–base disturbances contribute to the imbalances. Electrolyte deficiencies usually reflect shifts in concentrations between intravascular and extravascular as well as intracellular and extracellular spaces rather than total body depletion. Wound healing and anabolism have been shown to increase requirements of phosphorus, magnesium, and potassium. Altered electrolyte levels can impair organ function and are usually manifested by cardiac dysrhythmias, ileus, and impaired mentation. Fluid and electrolytes should be provided to maintain adequate urine output and normal serum electrolytes, with emphasis on the intracellular electrolytes, potassium, phosphorus, and magnesium. These are required for protein synthesis and the attainment of nitrogen balance. Once nutrition support is initiated, these electrolytes should be monitored closely, as they may deplete rapidly once adequate protein and kilocalories have been provided and the patient shifts from catabolism to anabolism. Electrolytes can be safely provided in doses specified in Table 69.5.

VITAMINS, TRACE ELEMENTS, AND MINERALS

Currently there are no specific guidelines regarding vitamin and mineral requirements in the critically ill. It is presumed that needs are increased during stress and sepsis because of increased metabolic demands; however, objective data to support supplementation is lacking. Antioxidant vitamins and minerals have received the most attention recently. Oxygen free radicals and other reactive oxygen metabolites are believed to be generated during critical illness (trauma, surgery, reperfusion injury, acute respiratory distress syndrome, infection, and burns). This response is most likely mediated by release of cytokines and initiation of an acute-phase response and redistribution of hepatic protein synthesis.[27] Along with increased levels of free radicals, decreased levels of circulating vitamins C and E have been found after surgery, trauma, burns, sepsis, and long-term parenteral nutrition.[28–32]

Supplementation of additional doses of antioxidants in critical illness has not consistently been shown to be beneficial. Current studies in progress are addressing supplementation at various levels and combinations, some of which are showing promising outcome data especially in the acutely traumatized patients.[33] Apparently, providing suprapharmacologic doses of single vitamins or minerals can be harmful by potentially upsetting the balance of metabolic pathways. Current recommendations are to provide the recommended dietary allowance for vitamins and minerals in the critically ill (Table 69.6). Enteral formulations contain this recommended level when they are provided at specified volumes. If those volumes are not tolerated over extended periods, patients should be supplemented intravenously.

TABLE 69.5
Electrolyte Recommendations for Critically Ill Patients

Electrolyte	Daily Needs (mEq/Day)	Reasons for Increased Needs	Reasons for Decreased Needs
Sodium	70–100	Loop diuretics, cerebral salt wasting	Hypertension, fluid overload
Potassium	70–100	Refeeding syndrome, diuretic therapy, amphotericin wasting	Renal failure
Chloride	80–120	Prolonged gastric losses	Acid–base balance
Phosphorus	10–30 mmol/day	Refeeding syndrome	Renal failure
Magnesium	8–24	Refeeding syndrome, diuretic therapy ↑ GI losses	—
Calcium	5–20	↑ Blood products	—

TABLE 69.6

Recommended Vitamin and Mineral Supplementation in the Critically Ill

	Enteral	Parenteral
Vitamin A	800–1000 mg RE	660 mg RE
Vitamin D	5–10 mg	5 mg
Vitamin E	8–10 mg TE	10 mg TE
Vitamin C	60–100 mg	100 mg
Vitamin K	70–140 mg	0.7–2.0 mg
Folate	200 mg	400 mg
Niacin	13–19 mg NE	40 mg NE
Riboflavin	1.2–1.6 mg	3.6 mg
Thiamine	1.0–1.5 mg	3 mg
Pyridoxine	1.8–2.2 mg	4 mg
Cyanocobalamin	2.0 mg	5.0 mg
Pantothenic acid	4.7 mg	15 mg
Biotin	30–100 mg	60 mg
Potassium	1875–5625 mg	60–100 mEq
Sodium	1100–3300 mg	60–100 mEq
Chloride	1700–5100 mg	—
Fluoride	1.5–4.0 mg	—
Calcium	800–1200 mg	600 mg
Phosphorus	800–1200 mg	600 mg
Magnesium	300–400 mg	10–20 mEq
Iron	10–15 mg	1–7 mg
Zinc*	12–15 mg	2.5–4.0* mg
Iodine	150 mg	70–140 mg
Copper	1.5–3 mg	300–500 mg
Manganese	2–5 mg	0.15–0.8 mg
Chromium	0.05–0.2 mg	10–20 mg
Selenium	0.05–0.2 mg	40–80 mg
Molybdenum	75–250 mg	100–200 mg

* Additional 2 mg in acute catabolic states.

NE = niacin equivalents; RE = retinol equivalents; TE = tocopherol equivalents.

ROUTE OF NUTRIENT DELIVERY

PARENTERAL VS. ENTERAL NUTRITION

Despite nutrition intervention, critically ill patients undergo an obligatory loss of lean body tissue secondary to the hypercatabolic response of stress, as previously described. If patients lose greater than 40% of their lean body mass, irreversible changes occur, which make survival unlikely. This can occur as soon as 30 days after a serious metabolic insult if the patient is not nutritionally supported. Protein-calorie malnutrition, as a result of hypermetabolic stress, also leads to decreased immune function with subsequent increased infection risk. Impaired wound healing also becomes significant. Therefore, as stated previously, the primary goals of nutrition support in the critically ill are to attenuate the metabolic response, reverse the lean body mass, avoid metabolic complications, and preserve the body's immune function.

The ideal route of nutrition intervention in the critically ill has been well studied, and it is abundantly clear the enteral feeding is superior to parenteral when the patient has adequate absorptive surface and access is available.[34] Although total parenteral nutrition (TPN) has been lifesaving and has been successful in reversing malnutrition in many disease states (Table 69.7), several recent studies have found it to have potentially profound negative side effects.[34] It has become more apparent that parenteral formulations currently available in the United States may in fact be systemically immunosuppressive, deliver imbalanced nutrient solutions, and alter nutrient uptake and utilization (Table 69.8).[35–39] TPN allows for more rapid achievement of nutrient requirements than enteral nutrition, but also allows for increased nitrogen excretion.[40] TPN has also been associated with a higher rate of hyperglycemia, adding to patient immunocompromise with decreased neutrophil chemotaxis, phagocytosis, oxidative burst, and superoxide production.[41,42] In animal models, TPN is associated with increasing the metabolic stress response, allowing atrophy of the gut mucosa, systemic immunocompromise, and altering gut flora when compared with enteral nutrition.[34,43–48] More recently, clinical research trials have suggested that TPN therapy may in fact be harmful when delivered as is possible

TABLE 69.7
Indications for Parenteral Nutrition

Short bowel syndrome
Malabsorption
Intractable emesis or diarrhea
Severe pancreatitis
Bowel obstruction
Prolonged ileus
High output GI fistula
Unsuccessful enteral access

TABLE 69.8
Enteral vs. Parenteral Nutrition

Advantages	Disadvantages
Enteral	
Increased mucosal blood flow	Often difficult to access
Decreased septic morbidity	Aspiration risk
Preservation of gut flora and integrity	GI intolerance
Maintenance of GI hormone axis	Interruptions common
Balanced nutrient delivery	
Parenteral	
Ease of delivery	Overfeeding
Precise nutrient delivery	Exaggerated cytokine response
	Intestinal mucosal atrophy
	Decreased GALT and secretory IgA
	Decreased systemic immunity
	Increased cost

in the United States in 2006.[34,39,49] Prospective clinical trials evaluating perioperative TPN have shown that subjects receiving TPN had greater postoperative infectious morbidity rates than those receiving no nutrition intervention.[50–52]

One of the more clinically relevant effects of enteral feeding is the reduction in the incidence of septic complications.[53] This is at least due in part to the maintenance of the gut-associated lymphoid tissue (GALT) and mucosal integrity. In review of the immunoglobulin-producing cells in the body, the bone marrow, spleen, and extra-GI-tract lymph nodes together comprise about 2.5×10^{10} cells; the GI tract from mouth to anus comprises about 8.5×10^{10} immunoglobulin-producing cells. So, clearly 60% of the body's immunoglobulin-producing ability lies in the GI tract. When the GI tract is not being utilized, a significant alteration in immune function can be expected. In reviewing the literature comparing parenteral to enteral nutrition, the gut has become recognized as a metabolically active, immunologically important, and bacteriologically decisive organ in critically ill patients.[54–56]

LOW-FLOW STATES

Although research supports providing enteral nutrition in critically ill patients, it is often difficult to provide full energy requirements because of patient intolerance. Approximately 20% of the critically ill patient population is intolerant of enteral feeding.[57] The etiology of this intolerance is often multifactorial. One clinically significant factor is low intestinal blood flow. Intestinal ischemia and reperfusion is an important determinant of the subsequent development of the posttraumatic proinflammatory state and multiple organ failure (MOF). Although the gut is able to increase its oxygen extraction up to tenfold in a normal state, it remains extremely vulnerable to ischemic injury during low flow states. Low flow not only exhibits negative effects on mucosal oxygenation and barrier maintenance[58–60] but also has adverse effects on motility. It is now known that sepsis, endotoxemia, and low-flow states have significant negative effects on GI tract motility, with the colon being the most affected, followed by the stomach and small intestine, in that order.[61] Low-flow states also cause decreases in nutrient absorption, with protein absorption believed to be significantly altered; carbohydrate and lipid absorption are also altered, but to a lesser degree.[62]

A number of patient populations are at particularly high risk for low-flow states. These include those with sepsis, necrotizing enterocolitis, multiple trauma, intra-aortic balloon pump, cardiac patients requiring left ventricular assist devices, and those who undergo thoracoabdominal aortic aneurysm repair with cross-clamping of the mesenteric vessels.[63,64] In general, any patient with inadequate resuscitation following trauma, burns, or surgery or patients who have significant decrease in cardiac output for any reason are at risk.

Gut perfusion can be indirectly assessed using tonometric techniques to measure the gastric intramucosal pH (pHi).[65] Trauma patients with a pHi <7.32 and otherwise adequate central hemodynamics and oxygen transport 24 h after ICU admission showed a higher rate of MOF and mortality compared with a group of patients with adequate central and intestinal perfusion.[66] Several other investigators have attempted to improve the pH in critically ill patients by improving global perfusion, but they were not successful in decreasing mortality or MOF.[67,68] A drawback to this approach has been the inability to selectively improve gut perfusion in the setting of otherwise adequate systemic perfusion. The question remains whether enteral nutrient delivery during low-flow states increases potential gut ischemia or whether increased blood flow associated with enteral feeding protects the mucosa.[69–71] Several investigators using animal models and a single human model have found that enteral nutrient delivery at low rates enhances visceral blood flow during low-flow states.[72–77]

After trauma or major metabolic insult, ileus commonly results, lasting 24 to 48 h in the stomach and about 48 to 72 h in the large intestine. In the small intestine, gut motility returns to near normal 12 to 24 h after the insult. Several factors affect the duration of ileus, such as electrolyte imbalance, hyper- or hypovolemia, hyperglycemia, excessive sympathetic stimulation, elevated intracranial pressure, as well as numerous others.[78] Generally, if small bowel access is available, critically ill patients may be fed enterally as soon as 8 h after insult. Three recent studies have attempted to address the question of how much nutrient delivered into the GI tract is required to yield the immune benefits.[69,79–81] From these studies, it can be estimated that only 15 to 30% of caloric requirements delivered enterally is needed to provide the immune benefits. In other words, full measured or estimated nutrient requirements are not required to be delivered enterally in order to obtain the immunologic and mucosal protective effects. In fact, attempting to obtain 100% of the nutrient requirements in critically ill patients often results in intolerance of early enteral feeding. Therefore, a clinically rational approach to enteral feeding in critically ill populations is to initiate and maintain feedings at a relatively low rate (10 to 20 ml/h) until tolerance is demonstrated. Signs of intolerance include abdominal distention and pain, hypermotility, significant ileus, pneumatosis intestinalis, significant increase in nasogastric tube output, and significant diarrhea. Enteral feeding should only be advanced according to patient tolerance, and decreased or discontinued if any of the aforementioned symptoms are present. Most critically ill patients will tolerate full enteral feeds within 5 to 7 days, but if goal tube feedings are not tolerated after 5 to 7 days of injury, then it is appropriate to start parenteral nutrition to either provide the balance of the nutrient requirements or provide full nutrition support as clinically indicated.

NUTRITION SUPPORT IN TRAUMA AND BURNS

Trauma and burn patients exhibit similar metabolic alterations, as described earlier in critical illness, except that the metabolic alterations often occur to a much greater extent. Few traumatic injuries result in a hypermetabolic state comparable to that of a major burn. As the skin functions to maintain body temperature and fluid balance, loss of this protective barrier leads to excessive fluid, electrolyte, heat, and protein losses.[82] Thermal injury induces hypermetabolism of varying intensity and duration depending on the extent and depth of the body surface affected, the presence of infection, and the efficacy of early treatment.[83] Energy requirements peak at approximately postburn day 12, and typically slowly normalize as the percentage of open wound decreases with reepithelialization or skin grafting.[82] Although still debated, there is no single agent that is entirely responsible for the dramatic rise in metabolic needs observed during the flow phase of burn injury.[84–86] Rather, the etiology of hypermetabolism appears to be multifactorial (Table 69.9). As previously discussed with critical illness, the goal of acute management in trauma and burns is to stabilize these systemwide effects. Optimal nutrition intervention is an important component in improving immunocompetence, attenuating the hypermetabolic response, and minimizing losses in lean body mass. As in critical illness, enteral feeding is preferred to parenteral. A few select nutrients have been shown to have an impact on the immune system in critical illness (Table 69.10).

ESTIMATING NUTRIENT REQUIREMENTS

Energy

Burn patients require individualized nutrition plans to provide optimal energy and protein to accelerate muscle and protein synthesis and minimize proteolysis.[85,87] There are numerous predictive equations to estimate energy needs in burn patients (Table 69.3).

Several studies have reviewed the accuracy of predictive equations in determining energy requirements in burn patients.[88–90] The consensus appears to be that predictive equations tend to overestimate energy expenditure, and the preferred method of

TABLE 69.9
Factors Known to Affect Metabolic Rate in Burn Patients

Activity	Other Trauma or Injuries
Age	Pain
Ambient temperature and humidity	Physical therapy
Anxiety	Preexisting medical conditions
Body surface area	Sepsis
Convalescence	Sleep deprivation
Dressing changes	Surgery
Drugs and anesthesia	Treatments rendered
Evaporative heat loss	Type and severity of injury
Gender	
Hormonal and nonhormonal influences	
Lean body mass	
Metabolic cost of various nutrients when digested and absorbed	

Source: With permission from Mayes T, Gottschlich M. In: *Contemporary Nutrition Support Practice.* W.B. Saunders, Philadelphia, PA, 1998: pg 590–607.

TABLE 69.10
Select Nutrients and Their Immune Effect During Critical Illness

Nutrient	Immune Effect
Carbohydrate	↓ (if provision results in blood glucose levels >200 mg/dl)
Protein	
Glutamine	↑
Arginine	↑
Fat	
Omega-6 fatty acids	↓ (in large amounts)
Omega-3 fatty acids	↑
Micronutrients	
Vitamin A	↑ (in burns)
Vitamin C	↑ (in burns)
Vitamin E	??
Zinc	↑ (in burns)
Selenium	↑

determining energy requirements is by using indirect calorimetry. If indirect calorimetry is not available in the clinical situation, it is suggested that REE can be estimated as 50 to 60% above the Harris–Benedict equation for burns on more than 20% of the total body surface area.[91]

PROTEIN

Trauma and sepsis initiate a cascade of events that leads to accelerated protein degradation, decreased rates of synthesis of selected proteins, and increased amino acid catabolism and nitrogen loss. Clinical consequences of these metabolic alterations may increase morbidity and mortality of patients, causing serious organ dysfunction and impaired host defenses. Therefore, trauma and burn patients require increased amounts of protein in attempts to minimize endogenous proteolysis as well as support the large losses from wound exudates. In a landmark study, Alexander et al. found that providing 23% of energy as protein in burned patients resulted in fewer systemic infections and a lower mortality rate when compared with providing 16.5% of energy as protein.[92,93] Results of another study recommended that burn patients receive 1.5 to 3.0 g/kg/day protein with a non-protein kilocalorie to gram nitrogen ratio of 100:1.73. More recent studies have questioned these high amounts of protein, as they may cause excessive urea production[94] and protein depletion that is related to altered muscle amino acid transport[87] and/or activation of the ubiquitin–proteasome pathway.[95] Overall recommendations are to provide 1.5 to 2.0, rarely up to 2.5 g, of protein per kilogram body weight per day in attempts to minimize protein losses. Providing these higher levels of protein requires continuous monitoring of fluid status, blood urea nitrogen, and serum creatinine because of the high renal solute load.

In addition to the quantity of protein provided, the protein quality is also significant. The use of high-biologic-value protein, such as whey or casein rather than soy, is preferred for burn patients. Whey protein has been further endorsed over casein owing to its beneficial effects on burned children, improvement in tube-feeding tolerance, enhanced solubility at low gastric pH, greater digestibility, and improved nitrogen retention.[84] Pharmacologic doses of the single amino acids, arginine and glutamine, have also been explored as to their benefit in critical illness and burns.

GLUTAMINE

Glutamine is known to be a major fuel source for rapidly dividing cells such as enterocytes, reticulocytes, and lymphocytes. In normal metabolic states, glutamine is a nonessential amino acid. However, during times of metabolic stress, glutamine is implicated as being conditionally essential as it has been shown to be needed for maintenance of gut metabolism, structure, and function.[96–103] Despite the accelerated skeletal muscle release of amino acids, blood glutamine levels are not increased after burns.[101] In fact, decreased plasma glutamine levels have been reported after severe burns, multiple trauma, or MOF.[83]

A number of studies have shown beneficial effects with supplemental glutamine, its precursors (ornithine α-ketoglutarate and α-ketoglutarate),[80] or glutamine dipeptides (alanine-glutamine, glycine-glutamine).[103] These studies deliver glutamine in pharmacologic doses of 0.3 to 0.6 g/kg/day.[104] Supplemental glutamine has been shown to have multiple benefits to include increased nitrogen retention and muscle mass,[105] maintenance of the GI mucosa,[106] permeability,[107] preserved immune function,[108] reduced infections,[110] as well as preserved organ glutathione and heat shock protein levels (Table 69.11).[109,111] These protective effects of glutamine supplementation could have significant effects on morbidity and mortality in trauma and burn patients. Safety, cost-effectiveness, and optimal route and timing of delivery of glutamine supplementation in trauma and burns continues to be researched.

ARGININE

Arginine, as with glutamine, has gained recent attention in critical care nutrition and is considered a conditionally essential amino acid. Arginine is the specific precursor for nitric oxide production, as well as a potent secretagogue for anabolic hormones such as insulin, prolactin, and growth hormone. Under normal circumstances, arginine is considered a nonessential amino acid as it is adequately synthesized endogenously via the urea cycle. However, research suggests that, during times of metabolic stress, optimal amounts of arginine are not synthesized to promote tissue regeneration or positive nitrogen balance.[84]

Studies in animals and humans have investigated the effects of supplemental arginine in various injury models. Positive outcomes from supplementation include improved nitrogen balance,[112,113] wound healing,[114–117] immune function,[114–120] and increased anabolic hormones, insulin, and growth hormone.[121] The outcomes are of special interest in the post-trauma and burn patient during the flow phase, when enhancement of these processes would yield the greatest advantage.

However, despite these positive effects, caution with excessive arginine supplementation is warranted in septic burn patients because of its potential effects on nitric oxide production. Theoretically, increasing the arginine concentration in conditions in which inducible nitric oxide synthase is increased could yield greater risk for hypotension via nitric oxide induced vasodilation. This theoretical concern has not held up in clinical or animal studies.[120,122,123] Recently it was shown that marked deregulation of arteriolar tone in patients with endotoxemia septic shock and increased permeability to bacteria in critically ill patients are induced by nitric oxide.[124] Although arginine supplementation for nonseptic burn and trauma patients in amounts sufficient to normalize serum and intracellular levels (~2% of kilocalories) appears safe and beneficial, the effects of arginine supplementation on nitric oxide production in septic burn patients should be carefully evaluated.[83,125]

TABLE 69.11
Benefits of Human Glutamine Supplementation

↑ Nitrogen balance
Enhanced gut barrier function
↓ Systemic infections
↓ Ventilator days
↓ Hospital stay
↓ Hospital expense
↓ Sepsis, bacteremia
↑ Survival
Maintenance of tissue glutathione levels

LIPID

Lipid is an important component of a trauma or burn patient's diet for many reasons, as it is an isoosmotic concentrated energy source at 9 k/g. Carbohydrate and protein provide half as many kilocalories as fat and can significantly contribute to the osmolality of the enteral or parenteral formulations. Dietary lipid is also a carrier for fat-soluble vitamins as well as a provider of essential fatty acids, linoleic, and linolenic acids. These essential fatty acids should comprise a minimum of 4% of the kilocalories in the diet to prevent deficiencies. This often corresponds to ~10% of the total kilocalories as fat, as most sources do not solely contain essential fatty acid.

Even though lipids are required in critical illness, excess lipids are detrimental. Excessive lipid administration has been associated with hyperlipidemia, fatty liver, immune suppression, and impaired clotting ability.[126–128] All the long-chain fatty acids share the same enzyme systems, as they are elongated and desaturated with each pathway competitive, based on substrate availability. Dietary fatty acids modulate the phospholipid cell membrane composition and the type and quantities of eicosanoids produced (Figure 69.1). Prostaglandins of the 3 series (PGE3) and series 5 leukotrienes have been proved to be anti-inflammatory and immune-enhancing agents.[127–131] Also, PGE3 is a potent vasodilator.[132] These concepts have received considerable attention because of the potential of omega-3 fatty acids' ability to enhance immune function and reduce acute and chronic inflammation.[127,128,133]

In most standard enteral formulations, the fat source is predominantly omega-6 fatty acids, with a portion coming from MCTs. Formulations supplemented with fish oil, a rich source of omega-3 fatty acids (eicosapentaenoic [EPA] and docosa-hexaenoic [DHA]), and canola oil (α-linolenic acid) are now available. Clinical trials utilizing these formulations have shown positive benefits in patients with psoriasis,[134] rheumatoid arthritis,[127,135] burns,[136,137] sepsis,[128,138,139] and trauma.[140] These benefits are thought to be due to alterations in eicosanoid and leukotriene production, with decreased arachidonic acid metabolites (e.g., PGE2) and increased production of the less biologically active trienoic prostaglandins and pentaenoic leukotrienes.[141] Understanding lipid modulation of the metabolic response in the trauma and critical care setting is significantly hampered because lipids are traditionally given as one of many active components of an immune-enhancing formula. Determining the exact contribution of the lipid is virtually impossible. This is made even more confusing by recent data demonstrating that EPA modulates arginine metabolism.[142] The omega-3 fats in fish oil have multiple beneficial effects in critically ill patients, including modulation of leukocyte function and regulation of cytokine release through nuclear signaling and gene expression.[128,131,133] Leukotrienes, thromboxane, and prostaglandins derived from omega-6 lipids have demonstrated a much higher inflammatory response than those associated with the omega-3 class.[127] The omega-3 lipids have recently been reported to enhance the production of a new group of prostaglandin derivatives called resolvins and neuroprotectins, which play a role in accelerating

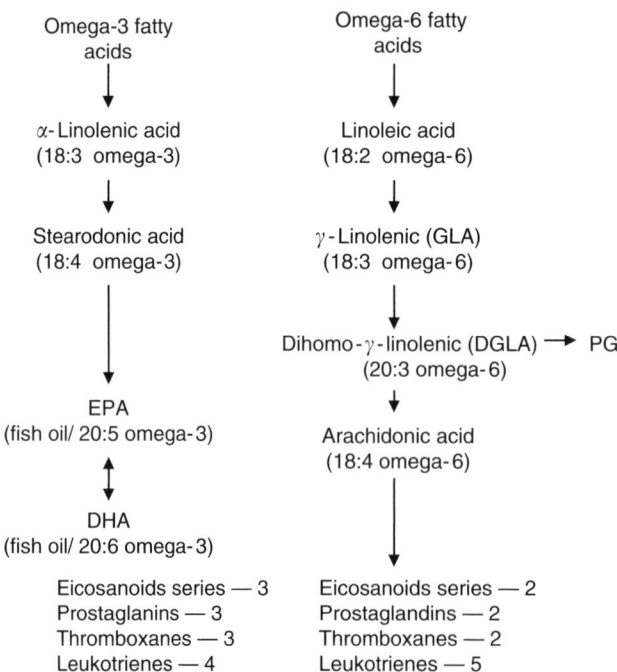

FIGURE 69.1 Metabolism of dieting long chain fatty acids. Abbreviation: EPA = eicosapentaenoic acid; DHA = docosahexaenoic.

the resolution of the proinflammatory state.[143] Abundant data report the influence of omega-3 fats on nuclear signaling and gene expression.[128,133] For example, polyunsaturated fatty acids (PUFAs) interact with various nuclear receptor proteins such as peroxisome proliferator-activated receptor (PPAR), which then affect nuclear factor-κB (NFκB) and gene expression. In effect, by decreasing NFkB migration into the nucleus, omega-3 fats downregulate the proinflammatory response to stressful stimuli.[133] Heller et al. recently reported that omega-3 fatty acids given intravenously at a dose of 0.11 g/kg/day for a mean of 8.7 days demonstrated a decrease in mortality in 661 surgical and ICU patients.[131] The route of delivery of omega-3 fats may be of importance. Utilizing the enteral route, it takes approximately 3 days to achieve adequate omega-3 fat levels in the cellular membrane. However, when given parenterally, a clinically relevant response can be achieved in 3 h.[144]

For burn and multiple trauma patients, the recommended amount of total fat delivery is 12 to 15% of the total kilocalories, with at least 4% coming from essential fatty acids.[83] Provision of formulations with omega-3 fatty acids, especially EPA and DHA, is of particular interest for potential anti-inflammatory and immune-enhancing benefits, as described earlier. Many enteral formulations do not contain these exact proportions of fat and typically have greater amounts, often leading to modular modification. Current (January 2006) parenteral formulations available in the United States contain nearly 100% omega-6 fatty acids and should not comprise more than 15 to 25% of the total kilocalories as fat when delivered to the burn or severely traumatized patient.

MICRONUTRIENTS

Micronutrients function as coenzymes and cofactors in metabolic pathways at the cellular level. With the increased energy and protein demands associated with traumatic and burn injury, one would expect increased need for vitamins and minerals. In addition, increased nutrient losses from open wounds and altered metabolism, absorption, and excretion would also be anticipated to have requirements beyond the Recommended Dietary Allowances. Various vitamins and minerals have also been found to aid with wound healing, immune function, and other biologic functions. Increasing data are available to support changing our current antioxidant regimens in the critically ill, trauma, and burn populations. Compelling evidence now supports the fact that sepsis, trauma, and burns significantly increase production of reactive oxygen species (ROS) by multiple cell lines. Oxidant injury occurs with loss of balance between endogenous antioxidant defenses and the cellular generation of ROS. The ROS generated results in a series of host reactions leading to a proinflammatory state. Free radicals may directly injure cell membranes by forming lipid peroxides, damage intracellular and/or membrane-bound proteins, nucleic acids, and organelles, leading to cell death.[145] During normal physiologic conditions, humans have adequate defenses against the ROS produced in routine metabolic processes. The cellular injury and death occurs when overproduction of ROS overwhelms the host's ability to detoxify the ROS with endogenous antioxidants and enzyme systems such as glutathione, superoxide dismutase, antioxidant vitamins, etc. These events have been well reported in numerous human studies.[146] Recently, Nathens et al. reported in a large prospective randomized trial of 595 ICU patients (91% trauma) that addition of 3 g a day of i.v. vitamin C and 3000 units enterally delivered vitamin E could decrease ICU stay and ventilator time.[33] The exact ratio or antioxidant cocktail is yet to be determined for the septic, ICU, or burn population. To date at least 22 randomized prospective trials of various antioxidants in severely stressed and septic patients have been attempted with variable results.[146]

Table 69.12 lists the older studies supporting additional antioxidant vitamins[147] in burn patients for vitamin A, vitamin C, and zinc.

TABLE 69.12
Nutrient Recommendations for Burn Patients[a]

Protein	20–25% of total kilocalories
Fat	10–15% of total kilocalories
Carbohydrate	60–70% of total kilocalories (5 mg/kg per min per day)
Vitamins and minerals	Multivitamin and mineral and
	Vitamin C: 500 mg twice daily
	Vitamin A: 5000 IU per 1000 kilocalories of enteral nutrition
	Zinc: 220 mg of zinc sulfate (or other compound to provide 45 mg elemental zinc/day)

[a] Patients >40 pounds.

Source: With permission from Mayes T, Gottschlich M. In: *Contemporary Nutrition Support Practice*. W.B. Saunders, Philadelphia, PA, 1998: pg 590–607.

REFERENCES

1. Singh H, et al. *Nutrition* 22(4): 350–4; 2006.
2. McWhirter JP, Pennington CR. *Br Med J* 308: 945; 1994.
3. Kinney J. *Crit Care Clin* 11: 569; 1995.
4. Barton RG. *Nutr Clin Prac* 9: 127; 1994.
5. Chiolero R, Revelly JP, Tappy L. *Nutrition* 13: 45S; 1997.
6. Gabay C, Kushner I. *N Engl J Med* 340: 448; 1999.
7. Serhan CN. *Curr Opin Clin Nutr Metab Care* 8(2): 115–21; 2005.
8. Wilmore DW. *Surgery* 104: 917; 1988.
9. Grimble RF. *Proc Nutr Soc* 60: 389–97; 2001.
10. Preiser JC, Chiolero R, Wernerman J. *Intens Care Med* 29: 156–66; 2003.
11. Ali S, Roberts PR. *Curr Opin Anaesth* 19: 132–9; 2006.
12. Flancbaum L, Choban PS, Sambucco S, Verducci J, Burge J. *Am J Clin Nutr* 69: 461; 1999.
13. Cutts ME, Dowdy RP, Ellersieck MR, Edes TE. *Am J Clin Nutr* 66: 1250; 1997.
14. Elwyn DH. *Crit Care Med* 8: 9; 1980.
15. Cerra FB, Siegel JH, Coleman B, et al. *Ann Surg* 192: 570; 1980.
16. Shaw JHF, Wildbore M, Wolfe RR. *Ann Surg* 205: 288; 1987.
17. Cerra FB. *Surgery* 101: 1; 1987.
18. Wolfe R, Allsop J, Burke J. *Metabolism* 28: 210; 1979.
19. Burke J, Wolfe R, Mullany C, et al. *Ann Surg* 190: 279; 1979.
20. Van den Berghe G, et al. *Crit Care Med* 31: 359–66; 2003.
21. Shaw J, Wolfe R. *Ann Surg* 209: 63; 1989.
22. Nordenstrom J, Carpentier YA, Askanazi J, et al. *Ann Surg* 198: 725; 1983.
23. Meydani SN, Dinarello CA. *Nutr Clin Prac* 8: 65; 1993.
24. Alexander J. *Nutrition* 14: 627; 1998.
25. Drumi W, Fischer M, Ratheiser K. *J Parent Enteral Nutr* 22: 217; 1998.
26. Brenner J. *Physiol Rev* 63: 1420; 1983.
27. Goode HF, Webster NR. *Clin Intens Care* 4: 265; 1993.
28. Goode HF, Cowley HC, Walker BE, et al. *Crit Care Med* 23: 646; 1995.
29. Boosalis MG, Edlund D, Moudry B, et al. *Nutrition* 4: 431; 1988.
30. Louw JA, Werbeck A, Louw ME, et al. *Crit Care Med* 20: 934; 1992.
31. Downing C, Piripitsi A, Bodenham A, Schorah CJ. *Proc Nutr Soc* 52: 314A; 1993.
32. Lemoyne M, Van Gossum A, Kurian R, Jeejeebhoy KN. *Am J Clin Nutr* 48: 1310; 1988.
33. Nathens AB, et al. *Ann Surg* 236(6): 814–22; 2002.
34. Gupta N, Martindale RG. *Nutrition Support for the Critically Ill Patient: A Guide to Practice.* Cresci G, Ed., T & F Informa, 2005, Chapter12. New York.
35. McQuiggan MM, Marvin RG, McKinley BA, Moore FA. *New Horizons* 7: 131; 1999.
36. Piccone VA, LeVeen HH, Glass P. *Surgery* 87: 263; 1980.
37. Enrione EB, Gelfand MJ, Morgan D, et al. *J Surg Res* 40: 320; 1986.
38. Mertes N, et al. *Ann Nutr Metab* 50(3): 2006.
39. Fürst P, Stehle P. *Am Soc Nutr Sci J Nutr* 134: 1558S; 2004.
40. Moore FA, Feliciano DV, Andrassy RJ, et al. *Ann Surg* 216: 62; 1992.
41. Moore FA, Moore EE, Jones TN, et al. *J Trauma* 29: 916; 1989.
42. McArdle AH, Palmason C, Morency I, et al. *Surgery* 90: 616; 1981.
43. Mochizuki H, Trocki O, Dominioni L, et al. *Ann Surg* 200: 297; 1984.
44. Alverdy J, Chi HS, Sheldon GF. *Ann Surg* 202: 681; 1985.
45. Kudsk KA, Carpenter G, Peterson SR, et al. *J Surg Res* 31: 105; 1981.
46. Birkhan RH, Renk CM. *Am J Clin Nutr* 39: 45; 1984.
47. Meyer J, Yurt RW, Dehaney R. *Surg Gyn Ob*es 167: 50; 1988.
48. Lowry SF. *J Trauma* 330: 20S; 1990.
49. Jeejeebhoy KN. *Am J Clin Nutr* 74(2): 160–3; 2001.
50. Sandstrom R, Drott C, Hyltander A, et al. *Ann Surg* 217: 183; 1993.
51. Veterans Affairs Total Parenteral Cooperative Study Group. *N Engl J Med* 325: 525; 1991.
52. Brennan MF, Pisters PWT, Posner M, et al. *Ann Surg* 220: 436; 1994.
53. Kudsk KA, Croce MA, Fabian TC, et al. *Ann Surg* 215: 503; 1992.
54. Wilmore DW, Smith RJ, O'Dwyer ST, et al. *Surgery* 104: 917; 1988.
55. Page CP. *Am J Surg* 158: 485; 1989.
56. Border JR, Hassett J, LaDuca J, et al. *Ann Surg* 206: 427; 1987.
57. Kozar RA, et al. *J Surg Res* 104(1): 70–5; 2002.
58. Ohri SK, Somasundaram S, Koak Y, et al. *Gastroenterology* 106: 318; 1994.

59. Fink MP. *Crit Care Med* 21: 54; 1993.
60. Flynn MP. *Crit Care Med* 19: 627; 1991.
61. Singh G, Harkema JM, Mayberry AJ, et al. *J Trauma* 36: 803; 1994.
62. Gardiner K, Barbul A. *JPEN* 17: 277; 1993.
63. VanLanschott, Mealy K, Wilmore DW, et al. *Ann Surg* 212: 663; 1990.
64. Tokyay R, Loick HM, Traber DL, et al. *Surg Gynecol Obst* 174: 125; 1992.
65. Chang M. *New Horizons* 7: 35; 1999.
66. Chang MC, Cheatham MC, Nelson LD, et al. *J Trauma* 37: 488; 1994.
67. Ivatury RR, Simon RJ, Islam S, et al. *J Am Coll Surg* 183: 145; 1996.
68. Gutierrez G, Palizas F, Doglio G. *Lancet* 339: 195; 1992.
69. Tappenden KA. *Gastroenterology* 130: 593–9; 2006.
70. Tappenden KA. *Nutr Clin Pract* 18(4): 294–6; 2003.
71. Kudsk KA. *Nutr Clin Pract* 18(4): 277–8; 2003.
72. Fiddian-Green RG, Baker S. *Crit Care Med* 15: 153; 1987.
73. Gosche JR, Garrison RN, Harris PD, et al. *Arch Surg* 125: 1573; 1990.
74. Flynn WJ, Gosche JR, Garrison RN. *J Surg Res* 52: 499; 1992.
75. Purcell PN, Davis R, Branson RD, Johnson DJ. *Am J Surg* 165: 188; 1993.
76. Kazamias P, Kotzampass K, Koufogiannis D, et al. *W J Surg* 22: 6; 1998.
77. Berger MM, et al. *Clin Nutr* 24(1): 124–32; 2005.
78. Schmidt H, Martindale R. *Curr Opin Clin Nutr Metab Care* 6(5): 587–91; 2003.
79. Shou J, Lappin J, Minard EA, Daly JM. *Am J Surg* 167: 145; 1994.
80. Sax SC, Illig KA, Ryan CK, et al. *Am J Surg* 171: 587; 1996.
81. Okada Y, Klein N, Vansaene HKF, et al. *J Ped Surg* 33: 16; 1998.
82. Rutan RL. In: *Burn Care and Therapy*. Mosby, Inc., St. Louis, MO, 1998.
83. De-Souza DA, Greene LJ. *J Nutr* 128: 797; 1998.
84. Mayes T, Gottschlich M. In: *Contemporary Nutrition Support Practice* W.B. Saunders Co., Philadelphia, PA, 1998: pg 590.
85. Hart DW, et al. *Ann Surg* Jan; 235(1): 152–61; 2002.
86. Noordenbos J, et al. *J Trauma* 49(4): 667–71; 2000.
87. Wolfe RR. *Am J Clin Nutr* 64: 800; 1996.
88. Saffle JR, Medina E, Raymond J, et al. *J Trauma* 25: 32; 1985.
89. Curreri PW, Richmond D, Marvin J, Baxter CR. *J Am Diet Assoc* 65: 415; 1974.
90. Turner WW, Ireton CS, Hunt JL, Baxter CR. *J Trauma* 25: 11; 1985.
91. Khorram-Sefat R, Behrendt W, Heiden A, Hettich R. *W J Surg* 23: 115; 1999.
92. Alexander JW, MacMillan BG, Stinnett JD, et al. *Ann Surg* 192: 505; 1980.
93. Gottschlich MM, Jenkins M, Warden GD, et al. *J Parent Enteral Nutr* 14: 225; 1990.
94. Patterson BW, Nguyen T, Pierre, et al. *Metabolism* 46: 573; 1997.
95. Mitch WE, Goldberg AL. *N Engl J Med* 335: 1897; 1996.
96. Souba WW, Smith RJ, Wilmore DW. *J Parent Enteral Nutr* 9: 608; 1985.
97. Souba WW, Smith RJ, Wilmore DW. *J Surg Res* 42: 117; 1987.
98. Souba WW, Wilmore DW. *Arch Surg* 120: 66; 1985.
99. Ziegler TR, et al. *Intens Care Med* 31(8): 1079–86; 2005.
100 Singleton KD, Wischmeyer PE. *Shock* 25(3): 295–9; 2006.
101. Gore DC, Jahoor F. *Arch Surg* 129: 1318; 1994.
102. Cynober L. *Nutrition* 7: 313; 1991.
103. Furst P, Albers S, Stehle P. *J Parent Enteral Nutr* 14S4: 118S; 1990.
104. Wilmore DW. *Gastroenterology* 107: 1885; 1994.
105. Stehle P, Wurste N, Puchestein C, et al. *Lancet* 1: 231; 1989.
106. Scheppach W, Loges C, Bartran P, et al. *Gastroenterology* 107: 429; 1994.
107. Van der Hulst RR, van Kreel BK, von Meyernfeldt MF, et al. *Lancet* 341: 1363; 1993.
108. Calder PC. *Clin Nutr* 13: 2; 1994.
109. Wischmeyer PE. *Curr Opin Clin Nutr Metab Care* 9: 201–6; 2006.
110. Ziegler TR, Young LS, Benfell K, et al. *Ann Int Med* 116: 821; 1992.
111. Furst P. *Proc Nutr Soc* 55: 945; 1996.
112. Barbul A, Sisto DA, Wasserkrug HL, et al. *Curr Surg* 40: 114; 1963.
113. Sitren HS, Fisher H. *Br J Nutr* 37: 195; 1977.
114. Barbul A, Rettura G, Levenson SM, Seifter E. *Am J Clin Nutr* 37: 786; 1983.
115. Barbul A, Rettura G, Levenson SM, Seifter E. *Surg Forum* 28: 101; 1977.
116. Barbul A, Fishel RS, Shimazu S, et al. *J Surg Res* 38: 328; 1985.
117. Barbul A, Lazarow SA, Efron DT, et al. *Surgery* 108: 331; 1990.
118. Daly JM, Reynolds J, Thom A, et al. *Ann Surg* 208: 512; 1988.
119. Saito H, Trocki O, Wang S, et al. *Arch Surg* 122: 784; 1987.

120. Luiking YC, et al. *J Parenter Eneral Nutr* 29(1 Suppl): S70–4; 2005.

121. Barbul A, Wasserkrug HL, Sisto DA, et al. *J Parent Enteral Nutr* 4: 446; 1980.

122. Chiarla C, Giovannini I, Siegel JH. *Amino Acids*. Published Online May 31, 2005; Springer-Verlag.

123. Luiking YC, et al. *Crit Care Med* 32(10): 2135–45; 2004.

124. Gomez-Jimenez J, Salgado A, Mourelle M, et al. *Crit Care Med* 23: 253; 1995.

125. Wilmore D. *J Nutr* 134: 2863S–7S; 2004.

126. Moore FD. *J Parent Enteral Nutr* 4: 228; 1980.

127. Caler PC, Grimble RF. *Eur J Clin Nutr* 56(3 Suppl): S14–S19; 2002.

128. Hasselmann M, Reimund JM. *Curr Opin Crit Care* 10: 449–55; 2004.

129. Ninneman JL, Stockland AE. *J Trauma* 24: 201; 1984.

130. Moncada S. *Stroke* 14: 157; 1983.

131. Heller AR, et al. *Crit Care Med* 34(4): 972–9; 2006.

132. Bittiner SB, Tucker WF, Cartwright I, et al. *Lancet* 1: 378; 1988.

133. Mayer K, Schaefer MB, Seeger W. *Curr Opin Clin Nutr Metabol Care* 9: 140–8; 2006.

134. Kremer JM, Jubiz W, Michalek A, et al. *Ann Intern Med* 106: 497; 1987.

135. Alexander JW, Saito H, Trocki O, et al. *Ann Surg* 204: 1; 1986.

136. Trocki O, Heyd TJ, Waymack JP, et al. *J Parent Enteral Nutr* 11: 521; 1986.

137. Barton RG, Wells CL, Carlson A, et al. *J Trauma* 31Z: 768; 1991.

138. Peck MD, Ogle CK, Alexander JW. *Ann Surg* 214: 74; 1991.

139. Kenler AS, Swails WS, Driscoll DF, et al. *Ann Surg* 223: 316; 1996.

140. Barton RG. *Nutr Clin Prac* 12: 51; 1997.

141. Gottschlich MM, Warden GD. *J Burn Care Rehabil* 11: 275; 1990.

142. Bansal V, et al. *J Parent Enteral Nutr* 29(1 Suppl): S75–80; 2005.

143. Serhan CN, Savill J. *Nature Immun* 6(12): 1191–7; 2005.

144. Roy CC, et al. *Curr Opin Clin Nutr Metabol Care* 7: 117–22; 2004.

145. Crimi E, et al. *Free Rad Biol Med* 40: 398–406; 2006.

146. Heyland DK, et al. *Intens Care Med* 31(3): 327–37; 2005.

147. Gamliel Z, DeBiase MA, Demling RH. *J Burn Care Rehabil* 17: 264; 1996.

70 Plant Foods and Phytochemicals in Human Health

David Heber

CONTENTS

INTRODUCTION

International epidemiological studies suggest but do not prove that consistently higher intakes of fruits, vegetables, whole grains, and plant proteins are associated with a markedly reduced risk of cancer, heart disease, and chronic diseases of aging.[1]

Improved standards of living characterized by improvements in sanitation and nutrition have resulted in increases in longevity due to reductions in the incidence of infectious diseases. However, for the first time in human history, the numbers of overweight and underweight individuals are nearly equivalent as worldwide trends towards reduced consumption of fruits and vegetables, along with a Western dietary pattern enriched in fats and sugars, have led to increased incidences of obesity, diabetes, and heart disease even in developing countries.

A diet rich in plant foods provides not only essential vitamins and minerals as well as fiber, but also thousands of phytochemicals that are not prevalent in those processed foods created to satisfy consumer demands for taste and low cost with refined grains, added oils, sugar, and salt. Recent studies of hunter–gatherer populations in the outback of Australia have revealed that these individuals eat more than 800 different varieties of plant-based foods,[2] but when they move into urban areas and begin eating the so-called "street foods," they begin to develop nutritional deficiencies.[3]

While the average U.S. intake of fruits and vegetables is about three servings per day — with an average of more than a serving of french fries — 80% of individuals eat less than the recommended five servings of fruits and vegetables per day, and about 20% eat none at all.[4] The regular consumption of fruits and vegetables is associated with reduced risk of many chronic diseases and functional declines associated with aging,[5–7] and it has been estimated that one-third of all cancer deaths in the United States could be avoided through dietary modification that includes an abundant intake of fruits and vegetables.[8] Further, plant-based diets have a lower caloric density and increased nutrient density, and could be an integral part of weight management and obesity treatment strategies.

PHYTOCHEMICALS AND HUMAN HEALTH

PHYTOCHEMICAL FUNCTIONS BEYOND ANTIOXIDATION

Fruits, vegetables, and grains contain thousands of phytochemicals. Many of these are either absorbed into the body from the gastrointestinal tract or further metabolized by commensal bacteria to absorbable phytochemicals. Phytochemicals are commonly called *antioxidants*, based on their ability to trap singlet oxygen.

The public is familiar with the term *antioxidant*, but it is misleading for several reasons. First, the cells of the body maintain exquisite antioxidant balance through the molecular induction of antioxidant defense enzymes. It is difficult to show the impact of antioxidant administration on cells in the body due to these defenses, and *in vitro* cell assays can be misleading. For example, vitamin C can become a prooxidant *in vitro* and produce hydrogen peroxide in adequate amounts to kill cells.[9] Second, in human plasma there is a great deal of uric acid, which also acts as an antioxidant. Therefore, it is difficult to show changes in plasma antioxidant activity with intake of antioxidant phytochemicals. There are many inconsistencies in the scientific literature in this respect. Finally, the Oxygen Radical Absorbing Capacity (ORAC) of various fruits and vegetables is a property of foods in a test tube, but does not consider the bioavailability, metabolism, and pharmacokinetics of phytochemicals ingested within a matrix of a fruit, vegetable, or grain.

There are complementary and overlapping mechanisms of action, including modulation of detoxification enzymes, stimulation of the immune system, reduction of platelet aggregation, modulation of cholesterol synthesis and hormone metabolism, reduction of blood pressure, and antibacterial and antiviral effects. Phytochemicals, unlike drugs, have multiple mechanisms of action, which complicate their study in traditional reductionist study designs. Furthermore, it is common for phytochemicals to interact in additive, synergistic, or antagonistic ways.[10]

While many of the cellular and molecular effects of phytochemicals have been examined primarily in animal and cell-culture models, experimental dietary studies in humans have also shown the capacity of vegetables, fruits, and their constituents to modulate some potential disease-preventive mechanisms.[11]

Phytochemicals often interact with the host to stimulate, suppress, or modulate enzyme activities important in DNA repair, detoxification, and cell metabolism. Phytochemicals interact with nuclear receptors and impact cellular signaling involved in cell proliferation and apoptosis. They can also act as oxygen radical scavengers to reduce proliferation and protect DNA from damage.[12]

OXIDANT STRESS AND RADICAL OXYGEN SPECIES

The production of radical oxygen species endogenously — as a result of normal oxidative metabolic reactions — and by external forces can damage biological structures and molecules including lipids, protein, and DNA in a chain reaction. There is evidence that antioxidants can help prevent this damage under certain circumstances. There are robust and multiple defense mechanisms against this outcome within all living organisms, including both enzymatic and chemical components that prevent radical formation, remove radicals before damage can occur, repair oxidative damage, eliminate damaged molecules, and prevent mutations.[13]

Aging increases endogenous oxygen radical production from the mitochondria and can be associated with a decreased enzymatic component of oxidant defense. Increased physical activity generates free radicals as the result of increased oxygen consumption during exercise. Ultraviolet radiation, infection, trauma, and pollutants are all potential stimulants of oxidant stress and inflammation. Environmental pollutants are sources for free radicals including nitrogen dioxide, ozone, cigarette smoke, radiation, halogenated hydrocarbons, heavy metals, and certain pesticides. Alcohol consumption can induce oxidative reactions in the liver, as can chemotherapeutic agents used in cancer patients. Figure 70.1 illustrates the activation of upstream kinases as a result of oxidative and proinflammatory stimuli.

THE ANTIOXIDANT NETWORK

Cells contain a number of antioxidants that have various roles in protecting against free radical reactions. The major water-soluble antioxidant metabolites are glutathione (GSH) and vitamin C, which reside primarily in the cytoplasm and mitochondria. Many water-soluble enzymes also catalyze these reactions. GSH peroxidase catalyzes the reaction between GSH and hydrogen peroxide to form water and oxidized GSH, which is stable. Vitamin E and the carotenoids are the principal lipid-soluble antioxidants. Vitamin E is the major lipid-soluble antioxidant in cell membranes that can break the chain of lipid peroxidation.[14] Vitamin E is recycled by a reaction with vitamin C: Vitamin C quenches free radicals in aqueous systems, but also regenerates cellular vitamin E, which helps to control lipid peroxidation. β carotene also traps free radicals in concert with vitamin E.

Polyphenols occur widely in plants and flavonoids occur in all plant foods. This broad class of compounds includes flavonols, flavones, isoflavones, flavonones, flavanol, and anthocyanins. Polyphenols comprise the most frequent and highest dose of phytochemicals ingested daily. They are an important component of the antioxidant network, but there is a need for much more research on their mechanisms of action.

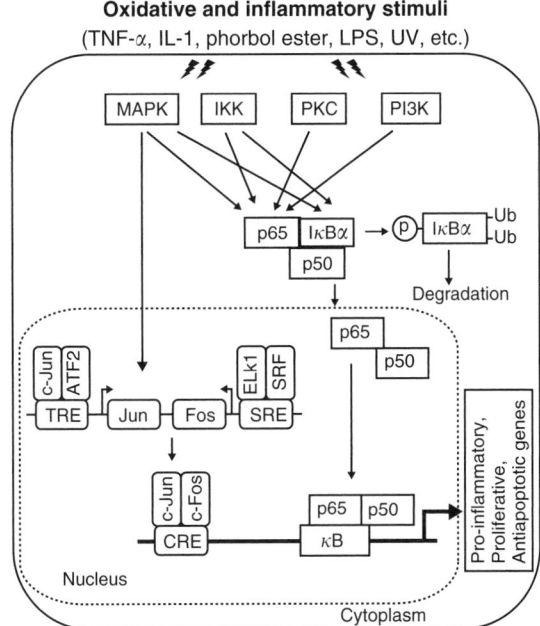

Oxidative and inflammatory stimuli
(TNF-α, IL-1, phorbol ester, LPS, UV, etc.)

FIGURE 70.1   NF-κB- and AP-1 mediated signaling pathway. Exposure of cells to oxidative and proinflammatory stimuli causes activation of a series of upstream kinases such as MAPKs, IKK, PKC, and PI3K, which then activate NF-κB by phosphorylation-mediated degradation of IκBα Activated upstream kinases may also phosphorylate p65, the active subunit of NF-κB. Free activated NF-κB, in the form of p65-p50 heterodimer, translocates to the nucleus, where it binds to κB sequences located in the promoter of a target gene. Alternatively, MAPKs can activate the AP-1 components, c-Jun and c-Fos, leading to the binding of AP-1 (c-Jun c-Fos heterodimer) to the cyclic AMP response element (CRE) sequences of the target gene promoter. (With permission from Surh, Y.-J. et al. *J. Nutr.* 135: 2993S–3001S, 2005.)

ANTICANCER EFFECTS OF PHYTOCHEMICALS

There is evidence which associates increased intake of fruits and vegetables with a reduced risk of cancers of the lung, colon, breast, cervix, esophagus, oral cavity, stomach, bladder, pancreas, and ovary.[15] Cancer is a disease resulting from genetic changes, and about 100 genes have been identified that code for oncogenes or tumor suppressor genes. Oncogenes are normal genes that form either growth factors or growth factor receptors. These genes normally turn on and off as part of the complex set of events underlying normal cell function. However, in cancer cells, mutations in the regulatory regions of these genes lead to amplified expression of multiple copies so that stimulation is unrelenting and the cell grows in unregulated fashion. Alternatively, a tumor suppressor gene is a gene for a protein that turns off cell growth and leads to apoptosis, or programmed cell death, due to binding of the protein to elements in the nucleus.

In order for a tumor to grow, it must grow its own blood supply through angiogenesis, which results from the secretion by endothelial cells of vascular endothelial growth factor (VEGF). Chronic inflammation contributes to cancer not only as a consequence of a direct effect of proinflammatory mediators on cellular signaling but also by creating a state of oxidative stress. The transformed cells are often surrounded by innate immune cells, inflammatory macrophages, fibroblasts, and endothelial cells, which release a distinct set of proinflammatory mediators and hence exacerbate the generation of reactive oxygen species.[16] This can create a vicious loop between oxidative stress and inflammation, which in turn favors tumorigenesis. Figure 70.2 illustrates the role of oxidative stress and inflammation in carcinogenesis.

Phytochemicals found in fruits and vegetables can affect the above processes by several mechanisms. Free radical damage, which induces oxidative stress, can cause DNA damage, which in turn can lead to base mutation, DNA cross-linking, and chromosomal breakage and rearrangement. This damage may be limited by dietary antioxidants in fruits and vegetables through modulation of detoxification enzymes, scavenging of oxidative agents, stimulation of the immune system, hormone metabolism, and regulation of gene expression in cell proliferation and apoptosis.[17–19]

INFLAMMATION AND CANCER

It has long been suspected that inflammation is causally linked to carcinogenesis. According to one estimate, 15% of all cancers are somehow linked to inflammation and about 5% of all human colorectal cancer is associated with ulcerative colitis.[20] Growing evidence indicates that chronic inflammation may cause cancers of different organs including stomach, colon, breast, skin,

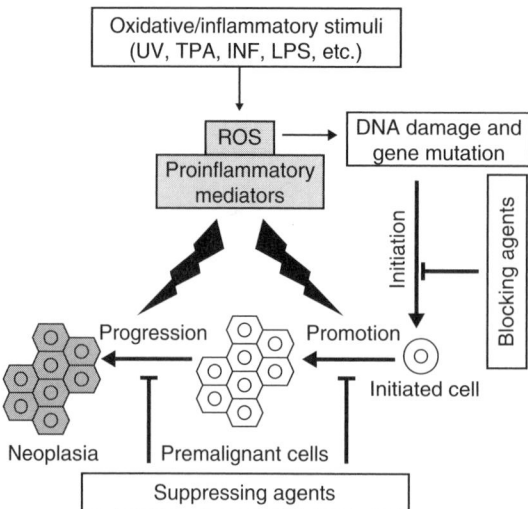

FIGURE 70.2   Role of Oxidative Stress and Inflammation in *Carcinogenesis*. (With permission from Surh, Y.-J. et al. *J. Nutr.* 135: 2993S–3001S, 2005.)

prostate, and pancreas.[21–24] A distinct set of proinflammatory mediators, such as cytokines, chemokines, prostaglandins, nitric oxide, and leukotrienes promote neoplastic transformation of cells by altering normal cellular signaling cascades.

Cytokines are peptide hormones secreted by inflammatory cells and stromal/adipocyte cells that mediate the inflammatory response, and these cytokines (e.g. IL-1, IL-6 and tumor necrosis factor-α) are signals that stimulate tumor growth. Dietary lipids such as omega-6 fatty acids can independently stimulate inflammation by conversion to proinflammatory prostaglandins. The omega-3 and omega-6 fatty acids compete for the active sites on cyclooxygenase (COX) enzymes. There are two isoforms of COX, designated COX-1 and COX-2. COX-1 is a housekeeping gene that is expressed constitutively in many tissues. On the other hand, COX-2 is undetectable in most normal tissues but is induced by inflammatory and mitogenic stimuli, and there is accumulating evidence that COX-2 is important in carcinogenesis.

The plant world is rich in antiinflammatory compounds. For example, the inhibition of cytokine release and proinflammatory gene expression and the downregulation of intracellular signal transducing enzymes and transcription factors that regulate expression of proinflammatory genes are key molecular mechanisms underlying antiinflammatory and antitumor promoting activities of resveratrol, found in grapes.[25] Another example is curcumin, the yellow pigment isolated from the spice turmeric, which inhibits chemically induced carcinogenesis in multiple organ sites, including forestomach, duodenum, colon, and skin, in various experimental animal models.[26–31] Figure 70.3 illustrates the activity of antioxidants and detoxifying enzyme inducers.

PHYTOCHEMICALS IN THE PREVENTION OF CVD

There is a large body of observational (epidemiological, case–control, or prospective and retrospective cohort) studies on the relationship between dietary antioxidant intake and a reduced risk for cardiovascular disease (CVD). Oxidized low density lipoprotein (LDL) has been proposed as an atherogenic factor in heart disease, promoting cholesterol ester accumulation and foam cell formation.[32,33] Dietary antioxidants from fruits and vegetables become incorporated into LDL, become oxidized themselves, thus preventing oxidation of polyunsaturated fatty acids. Phytochemicals also reduce platelet aggregation, modulate cholesterol synthesis and absorption, and reduce blood pressure.[34] Systemic inflammation may also be a critical factor in CVD. C-reactive protein, an inflammatory marker, may be a stronger predictor of CVD that LDL cholesterol,[35] and the antiinflammatory activity of phytochemicals may play an important role in heart health.

Studies have shown an inverse correlation between death from myocardial infarction and vitamin E intake,[36] an inverse correlation between vitamin C and carotid wall thickness,[37] and an inverse correlation between carotenoids and myocardial infarction.[38] Vitamin C deficiency may be associated with an increased risk of myocardial infarction,[39] while dietary intake of flavonoids (30 mg/day) is correlated with 50% reduction in CVD mortality when compared to an intake of 19 mg/day.[40]

PLANT-RICH DIETS AND WEIGHT MANAGEMENT

To date, there is no evidence that increasing fruits and vegetables without making other changes in the diet will affect body fat or body weight.[41] However, ongoing research is investigating the impact of specific dietary patterns and physical activity on energetics and obesity. The contribution of specific macronutrients to satiety, especially the impact of increased dietary protein intake together with high-volume/low-caloric density fruits and vegetables, may provide an additional key to controlling energy intake.

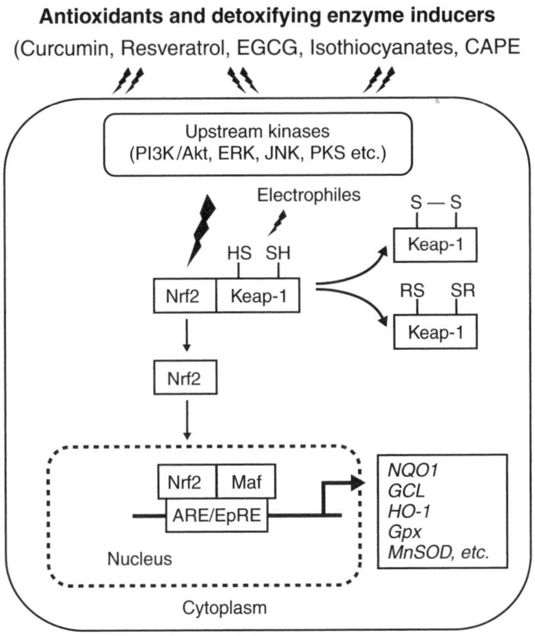

Antioxidants and detoxifying enzyme inducers

(Curcumin, Resveratrol, EGCG, Isothiocyanates, CAPE

FIGURE 70.3 Activation of Nrf2 signaling and induction of phase II detoxifying and antioxidant genes. The transcription factor Nrf2 is kept sequestered in cytoplasm as an inactive complex with its cytosolic repressor Keap-1. Chemopreventive phytochemicals activate diverse upstream kinases, which in turn stimulate dissociation of Nrf2 from Keap-1. Alternatively, electrophiles generated endogenously or from chemopreventive phytochemicals can facilitate dissociation of Nrf2 from Keap-1 by either oxidation (forming disulfide bonds –S–S–) or covalent modification (RS) of cysteine thiols of Keap-1. Once released from Keap-1 repression, Nrf2 translocates to the nucleus, forms heterodimer with small Maf protein, and vinds to the ARE-EpRE sequences located in the promoter region of genes encoding antioxidant and detoxifying enzymes. (With permission from Surh, Y.-J. et al. *J. Nutr.* 135: 2993S–3001S, 2005.)

Fruits and vegetables are high in water and fiber, and are 10- to 20-fold less calorie dense than grains. While promoting satiety and decreasing energy intake, plant foods also provide a rich supply of micronutrients, a wealth of phytonutrients, increased amounts of dietary fiber compared to refined grains and a balance of omega-3 and omega-6 fatty acids. Evidence suggests that increasing these foods while decreasing total energy intake is an effective strategy for weight management. While obesity is often considered synonymous with overnutrition, the dietary patterns of overweight and obese individuals might be more accurately depicted as overnutrition of calories but undernutrition of many essential vitamins, minerals, and phytonutrients. The increased incidence of obesity has been associated with an increased incidence of heart disease, breast cancer, prostate cancer, and colon cancer by comparison with populations eating a dietary pattern consisting of less meat and more fruits, vegetables, cereals, and whole grains.[5–7]

Several studies have sought to characterize dietary patterns and relate these patterns to body weight and other nutritional parameters. A prospective study of 737 nonoverweight women in the Framingham Offspring/Spouse cohort examined the relationship between dietary patterns and the development of overweight over a 12-year period. Participants were grouped into one of five dietary patterns at baseline: (1) a heart healthy pattern (low fat, nutritionally varied), (2) light eating pattern (lower calories, but proportionately more fat and fewer micronutrients), (3) wine and moderate eating pattern, (4) high-fat pattern, and (5) empty calorie pattern (rich in sweets and fat, and low in fruits and vegetables). Women in the heart healthy cluster consumed more servings of vegetables and fruits than women in each of the other four clusters consumed. Over the 12-year period, 214 cases of overweight developed in this cohort. Compared with women in the heart healthy group, women in the empty calorie group were at a significantly higher risk for becoming overweight.[42]

In another analysis of dietary patterns among 179 older rural adults, those in the high-nutrient-dense cluster (higher intake of dark green/yellow vegetables, citrus/melons/berries, and other fruits and vegetables) had lower energy intakes and lower waist circumferences than those in the low-nutrient-dense cluster (higher intake of breads, sweets, desserts, processed meats, eggs, fats, and oil). Those with a low-nutrient-dense pattern were twice as likely to be obese.[43] Similar observations were reported utilizing data from the Canadian Community Health Survey from 2000 to 2001. The frequency of eating fruits and vegetables was positively related to being physically active and not being overweight.[44]

In a controlled clinical trial, families with obese parents and nonobese children were randomized into either a comprehensive behavioral weight management program, which featured encouragement to increase fruit and vegetable consumption or to decrease intake of high-fat, high-sugar foods. Over a 1-year period, parents in the increased fruit and vegetable group showed significantly greater decreases in percentage of overweight than in the group attempting to reduce fat and sugar.[45]

DIETARY SOURCES OF PHYTOCHEMICALS

FLAVONOIDS

Flavonoids and their polymers constitute a large class of food constituents, and are a subclass of polyphenols (see Figure 70.4) which are further divided into subclasses based on their chemical structure. Over 60 years ago, extracts of foods presumably containing flavonoids were shown to have beneficial biological properties.[46] Although these early results were not corroborated, modulation of many biological systems by flavonoids, tannins and other phytonutrients has been demonstrated by many investigators.[47] These polyphenolic compounds represent one of the most prevalent classes of compounds in vegetables, nuts, fruits, and beverages such as coffee, tea, and red wine.[48] However, what may be more important than the total flavonoid content of a food is the content of flavonoid and tannin subclasses. For example, soy and soy-based foods are unique sources of isoflavones, while tea is rich in catechins, and each appears to confer unique health-related biological properties.

The average total intake of flavonoids in the United States is estimated to be 1 g/day,[49,50] but recent studies have indicated that the intake varies widely.[51] More than 8000 compounds with a flavonoid structure have been identified. The classes of flavonoids include flavones, flavonols, flavanones, flavanols, anthocyanins, and isoflavones (see Figure 70.4). The flavonoid natural products exert a wide range of biochemical and pharmacological properties, with one of the most investigated effects being their cancer preventive activities. The cancer protective effects of flavonoids have been attributed to a wide variety of mechanisms, including free radical scavenging, modifying enzymes that activate or detoxify carcinogens, and inhibiting the induction of the transcription factor activator protein-1 (AP-1) activity by tumor promoters.[52,53] Flavonoids also have inhibitory effects on the activities of many enzymes, including β-glucuronidase,[54] lipoxygenase,[55,56] COX,[55] inducible nitric oxide synthase,[57] monooxygenase,[58] thyroid peroxidase,[59] and xanthine oxidase.[60]

ANTHOCYANINS

The anthocyanins are very widespread in over 25 families of plant foods, and provide red, blue, and purple colors to berries, cherries, grapes, rhubarb, and plums. They are of great nutritional interest because of the average daily intake of between 180 to 215 mg/day in the United States. More of these compounds are consumed during summer months.[61] Similar to most other flavanoids, anthocyanins occur naturally in fruits and vegetables as glycosides. The deglycosylated or aglycone forms of anthocyanins are known as anthocyanidins.

These bioactive compounds have several effects on human health. The natural electron deficiency of anthocyanins makes these compounds particularly reactive as free radical scavengers, as well as acting indirectly through antioxidant actions that protect DNA from damage. Other activities include the regulation of enzymes important in metabolizing xenobiotics and carcinogens, the modulation of nuclear receptors, gene expression, and subcellular signaling pathways of proliferation, angiogenesis, and apoptosis.

GREEN TEA POLYPHENOLS

Tea is one of the most popular beverages in the world. The beneficial effects of green tea are attributed to the polyphenolic compounds present in green tea, particularly the catechins, which make up 30% of the dry weight of green tea leaves.[62]

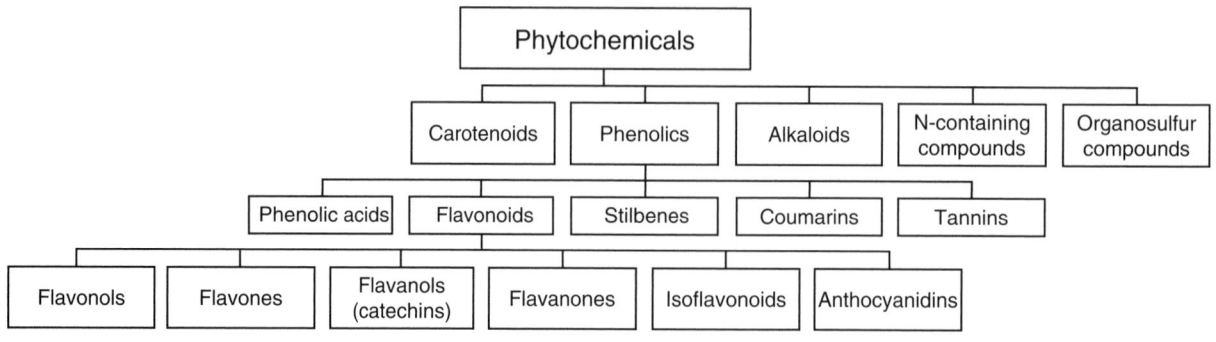

FIGURE 70.4   Classes of phytochemicals.

These catechins are present in higher quantities in green tea than in black or oolong tea, because of differences in the processing of tealeaves after harvest. For green tea, fresh tea leaves from the plant *Camellia sinensis* are steamed and dried to inactivate the polyphenol oxidase enzyme, a process that essentially maintains the polyphenols in their monomeric forms. Black tea, on the other hand, is produced by extended fermentation of tea leaves which results in the polymeric compounds, thearubigins, and theaflavins.

Green tea and its constituent catechins are best known for their antioxidant properties, which has led to their evaluation in a number of diseases associated with reactive oxygen species, such as cancer, CVD and neurodegenerative disease. The consumption of tea has been associated with a decreased risk of developing cancer of the ovary,[63] oral cavity,[64] colon,[65] and stomach.[66] This beneficial health effect has been attributed to the catechins in tea with their strong antioxidant and antiangiogenic activity as well as their potential to inhibit cell proliferation and modulate carcinogen metabolism.[67,68]

Green tea has also been shown to be hypocholesterolemic[69] and to prevent the development of atherosclerotic plaques.[70] Among age-associated pathologies and neurodegenerative diseases, green tea has been shown to afford significant protection against Parkinson's disease, Alzheimer's disease, and ischemic damage.[71] Green tea has also shown antidiabetic effects in animal models of insulin resistance[72] and has been shown to promote energy expenditure.[73]

SOY ISOFLAVONES

Soy protein is the highest quality protein found in the plant kingdom, and it is eaten by two third of the world's population. Interest in soy proteins and cancer prevention arose from the observation that naturally occurring phytochemicals within soy protein — the isoflavones genistein and daidzein — were able to inhibit the growth of both estrogen-receptor positive and negative breast cancer cells *in vitro*.[74] In addition, studies of populations eating soy protein indicate that they have a lower incidence of breast cancer and other common cancers compared to populations such as the U.S. population where soy foods are rarely eaten. These studies provide only supportive evidence for a positive role of soy foods, since the diets of the populations eating more soy protein are also richer in fruits, vegetables and whole cereals and grains by comparison to the U.S. diet.

Genistein and daidzein are phytoestrogens that antagonize the actions of estradiol in the breast and the uterus but demonstrate estrogen-like beneficial activities in the bone, on serum lipids and in the brain. These observations are explained by the existence of two estrogen receptors called α and β. Soy isoflavones bind with very low affinity (1/50,000 to 1/100,000 the affinity of estradiol) to the α-estradiol receptor, but bind equally well to the β-estradiol receptor.[75]

Soy protein isoflavones have been shown to influence not only sex hormone metabolism and biological activity but also intracellular enzymes, protein synthesis, growth factor action, malignant cell proliferation, differentiation and angiogenesis, providing strong evidence that these substances may have a protective role in cancer.[76]

Soy food intake has also been shown to have beneficial effects on CVD, although data directly linking soy food intake to clinical outcomes of CVD have been sparse. A recent study of participants of the Shanghai Women's Health Study, a population-based prospective cohort study of approximately 75,000 Chinese women, documented a dose-response relationship between soy food intake and risk of coronary heart disease, providing direct evidence that soy food consumption may reduce the risk of coronary heart disease in women.

GLUCOSINOLATES AND ALLYL SULFIDES

Cruciferous vegetable consumption has been associated with a reduced risk of cancer of the lung, stomach, colon, and rectum. The health benefit of cruciferous vegetables such as broccoli, Brussels sprouts, cabbage, and bok choy have been attributed to their high concentration of glucosinolates, which are found in significant amounts in these vegetables. These compounds are normally chemically conjugated to sugar residues and are stable. However when the plant cell is crushed or chewed, myrosinase enzymes are activated and break these stabilized chemical structures to yield volatile and highly reactive compounds such as isothiocyanate. The body normally detoxifies itself in two steps so that it can get rid of these compounds. Phase I enzymes add an electron to the compound and Phase II enzymes catalyze a reaction that links a sugar or sulfate residue on the activated toxin so that it becomes water soluble and is excreted in the urine. Isothiocyanates act as anticarcinogens by inducing Phase II conjugating enzymes, in particular Glutathione S-tranferases (GSTs) which metabolize isothiocyanates.[77]

Many studies have reported the beneficial effects of consuming garlic on health. Garlic has a high concentration of sulfur-containing compounds. The thiosulfinates, including allicin, appear to be the active substances in garlic. Allicin is formed when alliin, a sulfur-containing amino acid, comes into contact with the enzyme alliinase when raw garlic is chopped, crushed, or chewed. The antimicrobial, hypolipidemic, antioxidant, and antithrombotic effects that have been attributed to garlic are thought to be related to allicin and other breakdown products.

Many randomized clinical trials have studied the effects of garlic on lipid levels. Results from two meta-analyses[78,79] of garlic's effect on total cholesterol show a significant reduction in total cholesterol levels (9 to 12%) compared with placebo. More recently additional trials have been published, with conflicting results.[80–83] However, a meta-analysis published in 2000[84] that included these trials concluded that garlic is superior to placebo in reducing total cholesterol levels, but that the extent of the effect is modest (4 to 6%). A recent review of 10 trials assessing the effect of garlic on thrombotic risk showed modest but significant decreases in platelet aggregation with garlic compared with placebo.[85]

The sulfur compounds inhibit cell proliferation of cancer cells, modulate cell cycle activity, and interfere with hormone action in cancer cells.[86–89] Allicin is the major ingredient in crushed garlic and has been shown to inhibit proliferation of human mammary, endometrial, and colon cancer cells.[89]

CAROTENOIDS

Carotenoids comprise a class of natural fat-soluble pigments, which are found in many red, deep green, and orange/yellow colored fruits and vegetables. Their major biochemical functions are determined by the extended system of conjugated double bonds which is also responsible for their color.[90] The orange/yellow color of many fruits and vegetables can be seen when the carotenoid-containing chromoplasts are usually devoid of chlorophyll, but considerable amounts are also present in green parts of the plants where chlorophyll masks the carotenoids. The most prominent carotenes are β-carotene, α-carotene, and lycopene; zeaxanthin and lutein, α-and β-cryptoxanthin, canthaxanthin, and astaxanthin are structurally different carotenoids which exist to a lesser extent in foods.

Tomatoes and tomato products, including ketchup, tomato juice, salsa, and pasta sauce, are the richest sources of lycopene in the American diet, accounting for more than three fourths of the total lycopene intake of Americans.[91] Several studies have linked the consumption of tomatoes and tomato products with a decreased risk of cancer and CVD. The health benefits of lycopene have been attributed to its antioxidant properties, although other mechanisms of lycopene action are possible, including the modulation of intercellular communication, hormonal and immune system changes, and alterations of metabolic pathways.[92] In breast cancer cells, lycopene can interfere with insulin-like growth factor 1-stimulated tumor cell proliferation.[93]

The relationship between lycopene intake and prostate cancer risk has been reported and supported by studies linking low plasma levels of lycopene with increased risk.[94–96] Lycopene administration may reduce proliferation and increase apoptosis in human prostate tissue where lycopene is the predominant carotenoid.[97]

Lutein and zeaxanthin are xanthophyll carotenoids found particularly in dark-green leafy vegetables. They are widely distributed in tissues and are the principal carotenoids in the eye lens and macular region of the retina. Epidemiologic studies indicating an inverse relationship between xanthophyll intake or status and both cataract and age-related macular degeneration (ARMD) suggest these compounds can play a protective role in the eye.

ARMD is a major cause of irreversible blindness among the elderly in the Western world, affecting about 20% of the population above the age of 65.[98] Lutein and zeaxanthin are the pigments responsible for the coloration of the macula lutea ("yellow spot") of the retina, which is the area of maximal visual acuity. Lutein and zeaxanthin are essential to maintaining the proper anatomy and function of the retina. Epidemiological data support the concept that the macular pigments have a protective role. According to the Eye Disease Case–Control Study, subjects with the highest quintile of carotenoid intake had a 43% reduced risk of ARMD compared with subjects in the lowest quintile[99] and lower levels of lutein and zeaxanthin have been reported in the retina from donors suffering from ARMD.[100] There is also some evidence from a small intervention study that visual function is improved in patients suffering from atrophic ARMD when lutein alone or lutein together with other nutrients is supplemented.[101] Supplementation studies have shown that subjects who are able to modify their diet through increased intake of spinach and corn can experience significant increases in plasma levels of lutein and macular pigment density within 4 weeks.[102] Some observational studies have also shown these xanthophylls may help reduce the risk of certain types of cancer, particularly those of the breast and lung. Emerging studies also suggest a potential contribution of lutein and zeaxanthin to the prevention of heart disease and stroke.

CONCLUSION AND PRACTICAL SUGGESTIONS

Phytochemicals from different plants can interact to inhibit cancer cell growth (e.g., soy isoflavones and green tea catechins). It has also been proposed that the additive and synergistic effects of phytochemicals in fruits and vegetables are responsible for their antioxidant and anticancer activities, and that the benefit of plant-based diets is attributed in part to the complex mixture of phytochemicals present in whole foods.[103–104] Clearly, no single antioxidant can replace the natural combination of thousands of phytochemicals that exist in whole foods. Given the history of diverse intake of plant foods by humankind, it is sensible to encourage a diverse intake. The exact amounts of fruits and vegetables needed each day to minimize cancer risks are not known and will require a great deal of additional research. However, the benefits of fruits and vegetables in the dietary pattern and the evidence of benefits they confer suggest that an increased intake of these foods would have a desirable effect on health and well-being.

Humans and a few primate species have trichromatic color vision so that they are able to distinguish red from green.[106] All other mammals have dichromatic vision and cannot distinguish between the two colors. One hypothesis for the evolution of this visual ability was that it provided an advantage by enabling primates to distinguish red fruits from the green background of forest leaves. Today colors are still used to promote food choices and contrasting colors have been shown to be one of the

TABLE 70.1
Color Code Groups of Fruits and Vegetables

Color	Phytochemical	Fruits and Vegetables
Red	Lycopene	Tomatoes and tomato products (soups, juice, pasta sauce watermelon, and pink grapefruit)
Red/Purple	Anthocyanins and Polyphenols	Berries, grapes, and red wine
Orange	Alpha and Beta Carotene	Carrots, mangoes, and pumpkin
Orange/Yellow	Beta-cryptoxanthin and Flavonoids	Cantaloupe, peaches, oranges, and papaya
Yellow/Green	Lutein and Zeaxanthin	Spinach, avocado, honeydew, Kiwi, and Romaine lettuce
Green	Glucosinolates and Indoles	Broccoli, cabbage, cauliflower kale, and brussels sprouts
White/Green	Allyl Sulfides	Leeks, onion, garlic, and chives

key factors in food selection.[107] Most Americans eat only two to three servings per day of fruits and vegetables without regard to the phytochemical contents of the foods being eaten. Certain phytochemicals give fruits and vegetables their colors and also indicate their unique physiological roles. All of the colored phytochemicals that absorb light in the visible spectrum have antioxidant properties. In artificial membrane systems, it is possible to show synergistic interactions of lutein and lycopene in antioxidant capacity, and there are well-known antioxidant interactions of vitamin C and E based on their solubilities in hydrophilic and hydrophobic compartments of cells.

Current National Cancer Institute (NCI) dietary recommendations emphasize increasing the daily consumption of fruits and vegetables from diverse sources such as citrus fruits, cruciferous vegetables, and green and yellow vegetables.[108] A method for selecting fruits and vegetables based on colors keyed to the content of phytochemicals is a way of translating the science of phytochemical nutrition into dietary guidelines for the public.[109] It can also help consumers change dietary patterns to include more fruits and vegetables by including one serving from each of the seven color groups each day (see Table 70.1).

Although the color method is superior to the current system of simply encouraging increased fruit and vegetable intakes, it does not account for actual phytochemical delivery to the consumer. Today, there is no labeling law that enables fruit and vegetable manufacturers to list the phytochemicals in their products. Further, fruits and vegetables are developed and grown more for the need to transport them over long distances and extend their shelf life rather than for their flavor or nutritional content. Research in this area needs to continue on the more than 25,000 phytochemicals provided by fruits and vegetables. These important phytochemicals are widely distributed among different plant species, but the delivery of phytochemicals and their effects on biomarkers relevant to health promotion and disease prevention need to be documented.

REFERENCES

1. World Cancer Research Fund & American Institute for Cancer Research. Food, nutrition, and the prevention of cancer: a global perspective. American Institute for Cancer Research, Washington, DC, 1997.
2. Cordain, L. et al. *Am. J. Clin. Nutr.* 71: 682, 2000.
3. Lee, A. 79: *J. Nat. Cancer. Inst.* 1, 1996.
4. United States Department of Agriculture, Agricultural Research Service. *Food and nutrient intakes by individuals in the United States, by sex and age, 1994–1996. Nationwide Food Surveys Report No. 96-2.* USDA, Washington, DC, 1998.
5. Temple, N.J. *Nutr. Res.* 20: 449, 2000.
6. Willett, W.C. *Science* 254: 532, 1994.
7. Willett, W.C. *Environ. Health Perspct.* 103: 165, 1995.
8. Doll, R., and Peto, R. *J. Nat. Cancer Inst.* 66: 1107, 1981.
9. Clement, M.V. et al. *Antioxid. Redox. Signal.* 3: 157, 2001.
10. Adams, L.S. et al. *Evid. Based Complement. Alternat. Med.* 3: 117, 2006.
11. Lampe, J.W. *Am. J. Clin. Nutr.* 70: 475S, 1999.
12. Blot, W.J. et al. *J. Nat. Cancer Inst.* 85: 1483, 1993.
13. Gordon, M.H. *Nat. Prod. Rep.* 13: 265, 1996.
14. Watson, R.R. and Leonard, T.K. *J. Am. Diet. Assoc.* 86: 505, 1986.
15. Block, G., Patterson, B. and Subar, A. *Nutr. Cancer* 18: 1, 1992.
16. Coussens, L.M. and Werb, Z. *Nature* 420: 860, 2002.
17. Pool-Zobel, B.L. et al. *Cancer Epidemiol. Biomarkers Prev.* 7: 891, 1998.

18. Dragsted, L.O., Strube, M. and Larsen, J.C. *Pharmacol. Toxicol.* 72: 116S, 1993.
19. Singh, R.P., Dhanalakshmi, S. and Agarwal, R. *Cell Cycle* 1: 156, 2002.
20 Marx, J. *Science* 306: 966, 2004.
21. O'Byrne, K.J. and Dalgleish, A.G. *Br. J. Cancer* 85: 473, 2001.
22. Nelson, W.G. et al. *J. Urol.* 172: S6, 2004.
23. Whitcomb, D.C. *Am. J. Physiol.* 287: G315, 2004.
24. Itzkowitz, S.H. and Yio, X. *Am. J. Physiol.* 287: G7, 2004.
25. Kundu, J.K. et al. *Biofactors* 21: 33, 2004.
26. Huang, M.T. et al. *Carcinogenesis* 13: 2183, 1992.
27. Huang, M.T. et al. *Cancer Res.* 54: 5841, 1994.
28. Huang, M.T., Newmark, H.L. and Frenkel, K. *J. Cell Biochem. Suppl.* 27: 26S, 1997.
29. Li, N. et al. *Carcinogenesis* 23: 1307, 2002.
30. Rao, C.V., Simi, B. and Reddy, B.S. *Carcinogenesis* 14: 2219, 1993.
31. Rao, C.V. et al. *Cancer Res.* 53: 4182, 1993.
32. Berliner, J. et al. *Thromb. Haemost.* 78: 195, 1997.
33. Witzum, J.L. and Berliner, J.A. *Curr. Opin. Lipidol.* 9: 441, 1998.
34. Sanchez-Moreno, C., Jimenez-Escrig, A. and Saura-Calixto, F. *Nutr. Res.* 20: 941, 2000.
35. Ridker, P.M. et al. *N. Eng. J. Med.* 347: 1557, 2002.
36. Stephens, N.G. et al. *Lancet* 347: 781, 1996.
37. Kritchevsky, S.B. et al. *Circulation* 92: 2142, 1995.
38. Street, D.A., Comstock, G.W. and Salkeld, R.M. *Circulation* 90: 1154, 1994.
39. Nyyssönen, K. et al. *Br. Med. J.* 314: 634, 1997.
40. Hertog, E.J. et al. *Lancet* 342: 1007, 1993.
41. Tohill, B.C. et al. *Nutr. Rev.* 62: 365, 2004.
42. Quatromoni, P.A. et al. *J. Amer. Diet. Assoc.* 102: 1240, 2002.
43. Ledikewe, J.H. et al. *J. Am. Geriatr. Soc.* 52: 589, 2004.
44. Perez, C.E. *Health Rep.* 13: 23, 2002.
45. Epstein, L.H. *Obes. Res.* 9: 171, 2001.
46. Berg, P.A. and Daniel, P.T. In *Plant Flavonoids in Biology and Medicine II: Biochemical, Cellular, and Medicinal Properties*, Cody, V. Middleton Jr., E., Harborne, J.B. and Beretz, A. eds. Alan R. Liss, Inc., New York, 1988, 157.
47. Middleton Jr., E. and Kandaswami, C. In *The Flavonoids. Advances in Research Since 1986*, Harborne, J.B. ed. Chapman & Hall, London, UK, 1993, 619.
48. Hollman, P.C. and Katan, M.B. *Biomed. Pharmacother.* 51: 305, 1997.
49. Kuhnau, J. *World Rev. Nutr. Diet* 24: 117, 1976.
50. Scalbert, A. and Williamson, G. *J. Nutr.* 130: 2073S, 2000.
51. Beecher, G.R. *J. Nutr.* 133: 3248S, 2003.
52. Canivenc-Lavier, M.C. et. al. *Toxicology* 114: 19, 1996.
53. Shih, H., Pickwell, G.V. and Quattrochi, L.C. *Arch. Biochem. Biophys.* 373: 287, 2000.
54. Kim, D.H. et al. *Biol. Pharm. Bull.* 17: 443, 1994.
55. Laughton, M.J. et al. *Biochem. Pharmacol.* 42: 1673, 1991.
56. Schewe, T., Kuhn, H. and Sies, H. *J. Nutr.* 132: 1825, 2002.
57. Raso, G.M. et al. *Life Sci.* 68: 921, 2001.
58. Siess, M.H. et al. *Toxicol. Appl. Pharmacol.* 130: 73, 1995.
59. Doerge, D.R. and Chang, H.C. *J. Chromatogr. B Analyt. Technol. Biomed. Life Sci.* 777: 269, 2002.
60. Sheu, S.Y., Lai, C.H. and Chiang, H.C. *Anticancer Res.* 18: 263, 1998.
61. Hertog, M.G.L. et al. *Nutr. Cancer* 20: 21, 1993.
62. Graham, H.N. *Prev. Med.* 21: 334, 1992.
63. Zhang. M., Binns, C.W. and Lee, A.H. *Cancer Epidemiol. Biomarkers Rev.* 11: 713, 2002.
64. Hsu, S.D. et al. *Gen. Dent.* 50: 140, 2002.
65. Su, L.J. and Arab, L. *Pub. Health Nutr.* 5: 419, 2002.
66. Setiawan, V.W. et al. *Int. J. Cancer* 92: 600, 2001.
67. Demeule, M. et al. *Curr. Med. Chem. Anticancer Agents* 2: 441, 2002.
68. Kazi, A. et al. *In Vivo* 16: 397, 2002.
69. Yang, T.T. and Koo, M.W. *Life Sci.* 66: 411, 2000.
70. Chyu, K.Y. et al. *Circulation* 109: 2448, 2004.
71. Mandel S. and Youdim, M.B. *Free Rad. Biol. Med.* 37: 304, 2004.
72. Wu, L.Y. et al. *Eur. J. Nutr.* 43: 116, 2004.
73. Dulloo, C. et al. *Am. J. Clin. Nutr.* 70: 1040, 1999.
74. Peterson, G. and Barnes, S. *Cell Growth Differ.* 7: 1345, 1996.
75. Clarkson, T.B., Anthony, M.S. and Morgan, T.M. *J. Clin. Endocrinol. Metab.* 86: 41, 2001.
76. Kim, M.H., Gutierrez, A.M. and Goldfarb, R.H. *Anticancer Res.* 22: 3811, 2002.

77. Finley, J.W. *Nutr. Rev.* 61: 250, 2003.
78. Warshafsky S., Kamer R.S. and Sivak, S.L. *Ann Intern Med* 119: 599, 1993.
79. Silagy, C. and Neil, A. *J. Coll. Physicians London* 28: 39, 1994.
80. Saradeth, T., Seidl, S. and Resch, K.I. *Phytomedicine* 1: 183, 1994.
81. Neil, H.A. et al. *J. Coll. Physicians London* 3: 329, 1996.
82. Isaacsohn, J.L. et al. *Arch. Intern. Med.* 158: 1189, 1998.
83. Berthold, H.K., Sudhop, T. and von Bergmann, K. *JAMA* 279: 1900, 1998.
84. Stevinson, C., Pittler, M.H. and Ernst, E. *Ann. Intern. Med.* 133: 420, 2000.
85. Ackermann, R.T. et al. *Arch. Intern. Med.* 161: 813, 2001.
86. Pinto, J.T. and Rivlin, R.S. *J. Nutr.* 131: 1058, 2001.
87. Munday, R. and Munday, C.M. *Nutr. Cancer* 40: 205, 2001.
88. Nakagawa, H. et al. *Carcinogenesis* 22: 891, 2001.
89. Hirsch, K. et al. *Nutr. Cancer* 38: 245, 2000.
90. Britton, G. *FASEB J.* 9: 1551, 1995.
91. Minorsky, P.V. *Plant Physiol.* 130: 1077, 2002.
92. Rao, A.V. R. and Agarwal, S. *J. Am. Coll. Nutr.* 19: 563, 2000.
93. Karas, M. et al. *Nutr. Cancer* 36: 101, 2000.
94. Giovannucci, E. et al. *J. Natl. Cancer Inst.* 87: 1767, 1995.
95. Giovannucci, E. et al. *J. Natl. Cancer Inst.* 94: 391, 2002.
96. Gann, P.H. et al. *Cancer Res.* 59: 225, 1999.
97. Kucuk, O. et al. *Lycopene supplementation in men with prostate cancer (Pca) reduced grade and volume of preneoplasia (PIN) and tumor, decreases serum prostate specific antigen (PSA) and modulates biomarkers of growth and differentiation.* International Carotenoid Meeting, Cairns, Australia, August 1999 (abstract).
98. Khachik, F. et al. *Invest. Ophthalmol. Vis. Sci.* 43: 3383, 2002.
99. Seddon, J.M. et al. *JAMA* 272: 1413, 1994.
100. Bone, R.A. et al. *Invest. Ophthalmol. Vis. Sci.* 42: 235, 2001.
101. Richer, S. et al. *Optometry* 75: 216, 2004.
102. Hammond, B.R. et al. *Invest. Ophthalmol. Vis. Sci.* 38: 1795, 1997.
103. Eberhardt, M.V., Lee, C.Y. and Liu, R.H. *Nature* 405: 903, 2000.
104. Sun, J. et al. *J. Agric. Food Chem.* 50: 7449, 2002.
105. Dhu, Y.-F. et al. *J. Agric. Food Chem.* 50: 6910, 2002.
106. Dominy, N.J. and Lucas, P.W. *Nature* 410: 363, 2001.
107. Drewnowski, A. *J. Am. Coll. Nutr.* 15: 147, 1996.
108. Steinmetz, K.A. and Potter, J.D. *J. Am. Diet. Assn.* 10: 1027, 1996.
109. Heber, D. and Bowerman, S. *What Color Is Your Diet?* Harper Collins/Regan, New York, 2001.

71 Mechanisms for Cancer-Protective Effects of Bioactive Dietary Components in Fruits and Vegetables

Cindy D. Davis

CONTENTS

Dietary behavior is one of the most important modifiable determinants for the risk of developing cancer. Recommendations for consumption of larger quantities of fruits and vegetables for protection from chronic diseases, including cancer, come principally from epidemiologic investigations and from a variety of animal and cell culture studies. Collectively, epidemiologic studies suggest that increased consumption of fruits, vegetables, and whole grains may reduce cancer risk, and yet it is evident that considerable inconsistencies exist in the literature.[1–3] This discrepancy is illustrated in Table 71.1, which highlights some of the epidemiologic studies investigating the relationship between vegetable intake and colon cancer.

In 1997 the American Institute for Cancer Research and the World Cancer Research Fund summarized information arising from several hundred case–control and cohort studies.[19] They concluded that there is an inverse association between fruit and vegetable intake and numerous cancers. This is clear for cancer of the lung, stomach, colon/rectum, esophagus, mouth, and pharynx, and is probable for cancers of the breast, larynx, pancreas, and bladder, and possible for cancer of the cervix, ovary, endometrium, prostate, thyroid, liver, and kidney. Similarly, a 2004 review by Key et al.[20] summarized the evidence that fruits and vegetable intake is associated with a reduced risk for several cancer sites, including the oral cavity, esophagus, stomach, and colorectum. Not all cancer sites appear equally influenced by fruit and vegetable intake. Michaud et al.[21] reported that consumption of these foods is not associated with risk of bladder cancer (relative risk [RR] = 1.28 for highest vs. lowest quintile) among male smokers in a prospective cohort study. Likewise, no associations were observed for groups of fruits or vegetables (berries and cruciferous vegetables) or for specific fruits and vegetables and cancer at this site.

Some of the strongest evidence for the anticarcinogenic potency of fruits and vegetables emerges when consumers of at least five servings of fruits and vegetables per day are compared with those consuming only one or two servings. In several case–control studies, a high vs. a low intake, particularly of vegetables, was associated with a marked reduction in cancer risk.[22] Key et al.[20] suggested that diets should include at least 400 g/day of fruits and vegetables. Unfortunately, relatively few studies have adequately examined the influence of the range of intakes of fruits and vegetables globally, and thus the true impact across populations is difficult to quantify. Nevertheless, intakes above 350 or 400 g/day typically are not associated with added benefits in population-based studies.[3,23] In a recent study with National Heart, Lung, and Blood Institute (NHLBI) Family Heart Study

TABLE 71.1

Vegetable Intake and Colon Cancer Risk

Type of study	Population	Intake	Risk Modification (Highest vs. Lowest Intake)	Reference
Prospective	47,605 subjects, Japan	≤245 vs. ≥313 g/day; total vegetables	RR = 1.24, NS[a]	4
	45,181 men, 62,643 women, Japan	0–2 serving/week vs. every day, green leafy vegetables	HR = 1.19, NS	5
	62,509 men, 70,554 women, United States	0.9 vs. 4.1 serving/day men; 1.0 vs. 4.1 serving/day women total vegetables	RR = .63, $p < .02$ for trend men, RR = .74, NS women	6
	58,279 men, 62,573 women, Netherlands	165 vs. 210 g/day men; 166 vs. 209 g/day women total vegetables	RR = .89, NS men; RR = .80, NS women	7
	519,978 subjects, Europe	<1.4 vs. >5.2 g/day fiber from vegetables	HR = .94, NS	8
	120,852 subjects, Netherlands	<150.6 vs. ≥225.6 g/day total vegetables	OR = .86 for hHMLH1- tumors, NS; OR = .04 for hMLH1+ tumors, NS	9
Case–control	59 cases, 291 controls, India	≤21 vs. ≥21 serving/week nonfried vegetables	OR = .40, $p < .05$	10
	613 cases, 996 controls, United States	Mean intake 17.7 serving/week Caucasians, 13.9 serving/week African-Americans, total vegetables	OR = .50, $p < .006$ for trend both Caucasian and African-Americans	11
	352 cases, 736 controls, Taiwan	≤2 vs. ≥4 serving/day total vegetables	OR = .36	12
	184 cases, 259 controls, Netherlands	≤166 vs. >223 g/day	OR = .4, $p < .01$ for trend	13
	931 cases (462 male and 469 female), 1552 controls (851 male and 701 female), China	≤68 vs. ≥122 serving/week men; ≤67 vs. ≥119 serving/week women total vegetables	OR = .8, $p < .04$ for trend, men; OR = 1.0, NS women	14
	484 cases, 1452 controls, Uruguay		OR = .7, $p < .04$ trend all vegetables, OR = 1.2, NS cruciferous vegetables	15
	223 cases, 491 controls, Switzerland	≤5.5 vs. >9 serving/week raw vegetables; ≤5.25 vs. >8.75 serving/week cooked vegetables	OR = .55, $p < .05$ for trend raw vegetables; OR = .43, $p < .01$ for trend cooked vegetables	16
	488 cases, 488 controls, United States	Median of 9 vs. 45.5 serving/week total vegetables	OR = .47, $p < .001$ for trend	17
	232 cases, 259 controls, Netherlands	<142 vs. >247 g/day	OR = .4, $p < .0004$ for trend	18

[a] NS = not significant.

subjects, Djousse et al.[24] found that the average daily servings of fruits and vegetables was 3.2 and 3.5 for adult men and women, respectively. It appears, therefore, that the majority of Americans consume insufficient amounts of these foods for optimal protection against cancer. Such findings point to the need for additional research to help define the most effective approaches for leading to a sustained change in dietary habits.

It seems logical to assume that all fruits and vegetables are not equivalent in their ability to influence health. Thus, it is not that surprising that some types of vegetables surface more frequently as protective against cancer, including carrots and green, cruciferous, and *Allium* vegetables.[21,23] A host of bioactive food components, including several nonessential components (Table 71.2) such as isothiocyanates, allyl sulfides, flavonoids/isoflavones, and monoterpenes, various essential minerals (e.g., selenium, zinc, iodine, and calcium), and several vitamins (e.g., C, D, E, and folic acid),[21,25] occurring within these and other foods may provide protection against cancer. Not all individuals should be expected to respond in exactly the same way to these dietary components as their attributions likely reflect their ability to influence specific molecular targets that can potentially be influenced by a host of environmental and genetic factors.[26] The magnitude of the response to fruits and vegetables is probably influenced by many factors, including the type, quantity, and duration of consumption of these foods, the consumer's genetic background, and a host of environmental factors.[27,28]

VEGETABLE INTAKE, GENETIC POLYMORPHISMS, AND CANCER RISK

Some common single-nucleotide polymorphisms (SNPs) in genes involved in nutrient metabolism, metabolic activation, and detoxification could establish the magnitude or whether there is a positive or negative response to vegetables for cancer risk.

TABLE 71.2
Phytochemicals Present in Vegetables and Fruits That May be Protective Against Cancer

Groups	Phytochemicals	Food Sources
Carotenoids	Carotene, lutein, lycopene	Citrus fruit, carrots, squash, tomato
Flavonoids	Quercetin, kaempferol, tangerin, rutin	Citrus fruit
Glucosinolates	Glucobrassinin, indole-3-carbinol, sinigrin	Cruciferous vegetables
Isothiocyanates	Sulphoraphane, phenylethylisothiocyanate	Cruciferous vegetables
Phenols	Resveratrol, coumarin, ellagic acid, catechins	Grape, citrus fruit, berries, green tea
Sulfides	Allyl sulfur, dithiolethiones	Garlic, broccoli

TABLE 71.3
Genetic Polymorphisms and Vegetable Intake: Epidemiologic Studies with Significant Interactions for Cancer Risk Modification

Gene	Genotype	Cancer Site	Risk Modification	Reference
Glutathione S-transferase	GSTM1 null or present	Lung	High cruciferous vegetable intake (>3.01 servings/week) reduced cancer risk (OR = .61) only among individuals with GSTM1 present	34
	GSTM1 null or present	Lung	High isothiocyanate intake (>53 μmol/week) reduced cancer risk (OR = .55) only among individuals with GSTM1 absent	35
	GSTM1 null or present	Prostate	High broccoli intake (>339 g/month) reduced cancer risk (OR = .49) only among individuals with GSTM1 present	36
	GSTM1 or GSTT1 null or present	Colon	High isothiocyanate intake (>5.16 μmol/1000 kcal) decreased cancer risk (OR = .31) only among individuals with both GSTM1 and GSTT1 absent	37
	GSTT1 null or present	Lung	High isothiocyanate intake (>53 μmol/week) reduced cancer risk (OR = .54) only among individuals with GSTT1 absent	35
	GSTT1 null or present	Colorectal	High fruit and vegetable consumption reduced cancer risk more when GSTT1 is present (OR = .32 men, .53 women)	38
	A to G at base 1578	Colorectal	High fruit and vegetable consumption reduced risk (OR = .40) only among men with A/A genotype	38
Methylenetetrahydrofolate reductase	C to T at base 677	Breast	Low green vegetable intake (<1/week) increased risk (OR = 5.6) in women with TT genotype	39
	C to T at base 677	Colorectal	High vegetable intake (>21 servings/week) decreased risk (OR = .49) only in individuals with CC genotype	10
X-ray repair cross complementing group 1	Arg to Trp at codon 194	Breast	High fruit and vegetable consumption (>35 servings/week) reduced risk (OR = .58) only among women with Arg/Trp or Trp/Trp genotypes	40
O^6-Methylguanine DNA methyl-transferase	A to G at codon 143	Breast	High fruit and vegetable consumption (>35 servings/week) reduced risk (OR = .6) among women with AG or GG genotypes	41
Myeloperoxidase	G to A at base -463	Breast	High fruit and vegetable consumption (>29 servings/week) reduced risk (OR = .75) among women with GA or AA genotypes	42

The glutathione S-transferase (GST) family of enzymes, which includes four major classes (alpha, mu, theta, and pi), is involved in the metabolism of environmental carcinogens and reactive oxygen species (ROS). Polymorphisms in the *GSTM1* and *GSTT1* genes result in the absence of the corresponding GST enzyme activity.[29,30] It has been hypothesized that individuals with the GST-null genotypes would be at higher risk for cancer because of reduced capacity to dispose of activated carcinogens.[31] Epidemiologic evidence supports that individuals possessing these genotypes are predisposed to a number of cancers including breast, prostate, liver, and colon.[32] However, isothiocyanates are metabolized by GST, and thus polymorphisms associated with reduced GST activity may result in longer circulating half-lives of isothiocyanates and potentially greater chemoprotective effects of cruciferous vegetables.[33] Several epidemiologic studies provide evidence that GST polymorphisms in conjunction with cruciferous vegetable intake are important risk factors for cancer or precancerous lesions (Table 71.3).[34–38] For example, those with the highest quartile of broccoli intake had the lowest risk for colorectal adenomas compared with individuals who reportedly never ate broccoli; this inverse association was observed only in those individuals with the *GSTM1*-null genotype.[43,44] Similarly, colon cancer risk was altered by cruciferous vegetable intake in individuals with the *GSTM1*-null genotype.[37] Associations have also been investigated in relation to lung cancer risk, for which carcinogen exposure is a known risk factor, and found that the detoxifying effects of the GSTs may play a more important role. Isothiocyanate intake in combination with the *GSTM1-*null genotype was protective against lung cancer in current, but not former, smokers. However, among never smokers, higher isothiocyanate intake was also associated with reduced risk of lung cancer in *GSTM1-* or *GSTT1-*null individuals, suggesting that the protective effects of isothioycanates are not limited to their capacity to alter metabolism of tobacco-related carcinogens.[35] In contrast, Wang et al.[34] observed that among individuals with the *GSTM1-*present genotype, higher dietary intake of cruciferous vegetables was associated with a 40% reduction in lung cancer risk, whereas among individuals with the *GSTM1-*null genotype, higher cruciferous intake was associated with a slight increase or no change in risk. Possible explanations for the discrepancies in the literature about whether or not cruciferous vegetables are more beneficial for individuals with the GST-null or GST-present genotypes may reflect differences in the exposure to carcinogens, differences in the consumption of cruciferous vegetables or isothiocyanates, or effects of other gene polymorphisms.

Vegetables, particularly green, leafy ones, are a major source of dietary folate. Polymorphisms in folate metabolizing enzymes may also affect the relationship between vegetable intake and cancer risk (Table 71.3). A polymorphism in the methylenetetra-hydrofolate reductase (MTHFR) gene, which causes the substitution of C to T at nucleotide 677, is the most important common variant known in folate metabolic pathways. This polymorphism, which occurs in 5 to 20% of the population worldwide,[45] results in reduced conversion of 5,10-methylenetetrahydrofolate to 5-methylenetetrahydrofolate, the form of folate that circu-lates in plasma. Individuals with this polymorphism appear to have increased dietary folate and riboflavin requirements.[46–48] Although there have been only a few studies analyzing this polymorphism, vegetable intake, and cancer risk, it appears to alter the relationship between folate status and colorectal cancer susceptibility.[49–51] As compared with subjects with the CC or CT genotype having low folate levels, those with the TT genotype showed a decreased risk of colorectal adenomas when they had high levels of plasma folate (adjusted odds ratio [OR] = .58) and an increased risk when they had low folate levels (adjusted OR = 2.13).[49] As there was no clear relationship between plasma folate and colorectal adenomas among those with the CC or CT genotype, only a subset of the population may benefit from exaggerated folate intakes. Furthermore, it remains unclear if nutrigenetic effects are constant across all tissues. For example, the TT polymorphism of MTHFR has been linked to enhanced endometrial, ovarian, and breast cancers.[52–55] Moreover, compared with CC individuals with high folate intake, elevation of breast cancer risk was most pronounced among women with the TT genotype who consumed the lowest levels of dietary folate (OR = 1.83) or total folate intake (OR = 1.71).[55] Thus, in order to provide the best dietary recommendations for everyone for cancer prevention, it may be necessary to include the impact of genetic variation and to consider requirements for each individ-ual, given their specific genomic profile and tissue of interest. Furthermore, a better understanding of the mechanisms whereby dietary bioactive components inhibit the cancer process will help clarify which gene polymorphisms may be important.

MECHANISMS OF DIETARY CANCER PREVENTION

Carcinogenesis is generally recognized as a multistep process in which distinct molecular and cellular alterations occur. A multitude of sites within the cancer process may be influenced by bioactive food components. Figure 71.1 illustrates different steps in which information exists that specific bioactive food components present in fruits and vegetables can interact with cel-lular processes involved with carcinogenesis. These include carcinogen metabolism, DNA repair, cell proliferation/apoptosis, inflammation, differentiation, oxidant/antioxidant balance, and angiogenesis. These various processes will be briefly described in the following paragraphs and the effect of specific dietary bioactive components on these processes will be addressed later in the chapter. The response is complicated as multiple steps in the cancer process can be modified simultaneously. Thus, a better understanding of how the response relates to exposures and which process is most involved in bringing about a change in tumor incidence or tumor behavior is essential. Furthermore, as many of these processes are likely influenced by several food components, it is necessary to obtain a better understanding about physiologically important interactions.

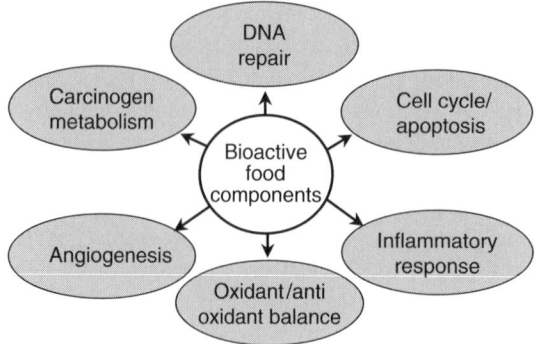

FIGURE 71.1   Bioactive food components influence multiple biological processes that are important for carcinogenesis.

Virtually all dietary or environmental carcinogens to which humans are exposed require enzymatic biotransformation, known as metabolic activation, to exert their carcinogenic effects. Biotransformation enzymes, also referred to as xenobiotic- or drug-metabolizing enzymes, play a major role in regulating the mutagenic and neoplastic effects of chemical carcinogens, as well as metabolizing other drugs and endogenous compounds such as steroid hormones. The drug-metabolizing enzyme system comprises phase I (oxidation, reduction, and hydrolysis) enzymes usually catalyzed by cytochrome P-450 and phase II (glucoronidation, sulfation, acetylation, methylation, and conjugation with glutathione) enzymes. The induction of phase II enzymes is largely mediated by the antioxidant response element (ARE), which is located in the promoter region of specific genes.[56] Generally, the transcription factor nuclear-factor-E2-related factor 2 (Nrf2) binds to the ARE sequence to initiate gene expression. Many enzyme inducers, including dietary components, also lead to the activation of several signal transduction pathways, such as the mitogen-activated protein kinases (MAPK), protein kinase C (PKC), and phosphatidylinositol 3-kinase (PI3K) pathways. The consequences of the activation of these signaling cascades are dissociation of Nrf2 from another cytosolic protein, Keap1, and nuclear translocation and accumulation of Nrf2 protein, which leads to increased expression of detoxifying enzymes through activation of the ARE. Bioactive components present in fruits and vegetables can prevent carcinogenesis by blocking metabolic activation, increasing detoxification, or by providing alternative targets for electrophilic metabolites.

Activated carcinogens exert their biological effects by forming covalent adducts with the individual nucleic acids of DNA or RNA. First, they distort the shape of the DNA molecule, potentially causing mistranslation of the DNA sequence. Second, when the DNA replicates, an adducted base that persists unrepaired can be misread, producing mutations in critical genes such as oncogenes and tumor suppressor genes. Third, repair of bulky adducts can result in breakages of the DNA strand, which can, in turn, result in mutations or deletions of genetic material.[19] Numerous DNA repair pathways exist to prevent the persistence of damage, and are integral to the maintenance of genome stability and prevention of cancer.[57] DNA repair mechanisms include direct repair, base excision repair, nucleotide excision repair, double-strand break repair, and repair of interstrand cross-links.[58] DNA damage can also arrest cell-cycle progression to allow for repair and prevention of the alteration to become permanent or activate apoptosis to eliminate cells with potentially catastrophic mutations.[58] Alterations in DNA repair, cell-cycle progression, and apoptosis are all important molecular targets for dietary components in cancer prevention.

Generally, the growth rate of preneoplastic or neoplastic cells outpaces that of normal cells because of malfunctioning or dysregulation of their cell-growth and cell-death machineries.[59] Therefore, induction of cell-cycle arrest or apoptosis by dietary bioactive compounds can be an excellent approach to inhibit the promotion and progression of carcinogenesis.[60] Cell-cycle progression is a sequential process that directs dividing mammalian cells through G1, S, G2, and M phases. Transitions between G1-S or G2-M phases function as checkpoints to halt cell division if necessary. Because the balance between the interactions among cyclins, cyclin-dependent kinases (CDKs), and CDK inhibitors (CDIs) governs the progression of the cell cycle,[61] perturbation of any of the cell-cycle-specific proteins by dietary components can potentially affect and block the continuous proliferation of neoplastic cells.

Apoptosis is one of the most potent defenses against cancer as this process eliminates potentially deleterious, mutated cells.[62] Distinct from the apoptotic events in the normal physiological process, which are mediated mainly by the interaction between death receptors and their relevant ligands,[63] many bioactive dietary components appear to induce apoptosis through the mitochondria-mediated pathway. Dietary compounds generally induce oxidative stress, which downregulates antiapoptotic molecules such as Bcl-2 or Bcl-x and upregulates proapoptotic mecules such as Bax or Bak.[60] The imbalance between antiapoptotic and proapoptotic proteins elicits the release of cytochrome c from the mitochondrial membrane, which forms a complex with caspase-9 with the subsequent activation of caspases-3, caspases-6, and caspases-7.[64] The activated caspases degrade important intracellular proteins, leading to the morphological changes and the phenotype of apoptotic cells.[65] To enhance this mitochondria-mediated apoptosis, dietary components also activate proapoptotic c-Jun N-terminal kinase (JNK) and inhibit antiapototic nuclear factor (NF)-κB signaling pathways.[60] Thus, the cytotoxic effects of dietary components on cells can be monitored by measuring their effects on mitochondria, caspases, and other apoptosis-related proteins.

Inflammation represents a physiological response to invading microorganisms, trauma, chemical irritation, or foreign tissues. Although acute inflammation is usually beneficial, chronic inflammation is often detrimental to the host. Epidemiologic data show an association between chronic inflammatory conditions and subsequent malignant transformation in the inflamed tissue.[66] Evidence indicates that there are multiple mechanisms linking inflammation to cancer and that there are multiple targets for cancer prevention by bioactive dietary components. At the molecular level, free radicals and aldehydes produced during chronic inflammation can induce gene mutations and posttranslational modifications of the key cancer-related proteins.[67] Other products of inflammation, including cytokines (peptide hormones that mediate the inflammatory response such as interleukins or IL-1, IL-4, IL-6, IL-10, interferon, tumor necrosis factor α TNF-α, growth factors, and transcription factors such as NF-κB, control the expression of oncogenes and tumor suppressor genes and key inflammatory enzymes such as inducible nitric oxide synthase (iNOS) and cyclooxygenase-2 (COX-2). These enzymes, in turn, directly influence ROS and eicosanoid levels. Chronic inflammation results in increased DNA damage, cellular proliferation, the disruption of DNA repair pathways, inhibition of apoptosis and the promotion of angiogenesis, and invasion,[66] all of which are important during the cancer process. Several of these mechanisms are amenable to influence by dietary constituents.

The generation of ROS is a result of normal cellular metabolism. ROS profoundly affects numerous critical cellular functions and the absence of efficient cellular detoxification mechanisms, which remove these radicals can increase cancer risk.[68] All ROS have the potential to interact with cellular components including DNA bases or the deoxyribosyl backbone of DNA to produce damaged bases or strand breaks.[69] Thus, ROS can act as DNA-damaging agents, effectively increasing the mutation rate within cells and thus promoting oncogenic transformation.[70] ROS can also specifically activate certain intracellular signaling cascades and thus contribute to tumor development and metastasis through the regulation of cellular phenotypes such as proliferation, death, and motility.[68] The effect of ROS is balanced by antioxidant enzymes and the antioxidant action of dietary bioactive components present in fruits and vegetables.[71] Nutritional antioxidants act through different mechanisms and in different compartments, but are mainly free radical scavengers: They directly neutralize free radicals, they reduce peroxide concentrations and repair oxidized membranes, and they quench iron to decrease ROS production.[72]

Angiogenesis, the development of new blood vessels from endothelial cells, is a crucial process in tumor pathogenesis as it sustains malignant cells with nutrients and oxygen.[73] During angiogenesis, endothelial cells are stimulated by various growth factors such as vascular endothelial growth factor (VEGF) and fibroblast growth factor (FGF), and are attracted to the site where the new blood supply is needed by inflammatory cytokines and chemoattractants.[74,75] Chemotactic migration along this gradient is, however, possible only through the degradation of extracellular matrix components.[76] This is accomplished via matrix metalloproteinases (MMPs).[77,78] Preventing the expansion of new blood vessel networks results in reduced tumor size and metastasis, and is another mechanism whereby dietary components inhibit tumor growth.

VITAMIN A AND CAROTENOIDS

Vitamin A or retinol is a fat-soluble vitamin with an unsaturated aliphatic chain. It has a role in cell differentiation, in the protein metabolism of cells originating from the ectoderm, and in the formation of the chromosphere component of visual cycle chromoproteins. Experimentally, there is evidence that retinoids (vitamin A and its derivatives) can influence cancer biology, especially because they influence growth and differentiation.[79] Because lack of proper differentiation is a feature of cancer cells, adequate vitamin A may allow normal cell differentiation and thus avoid the development of cancer.[80] Experimental and clinical studies with retinoids reveal that they can inhibit or reverse the carcinogenic process in some organs, including hematological malignancy, as well as premalignant and malignant lesions in the oral cavity, head and neck, breast, skin, and liver.[79,80] Except for the occurrence in milk fat, egg yolk, and liver of mammals, most vitamin A is usually obtained from carotenoids. Carotenoids constitute a class of over 600 natural compounds occurring predominantly in fruits and vegetables. These precursors to vitamin A occur in common green, yellow-red, and yellow-orange vegetables and fruits.[81] They include lutein, cryptoxanthin, lycopene, β-carotene, α-carotene, and zeaxanthin (Figure 71.2).

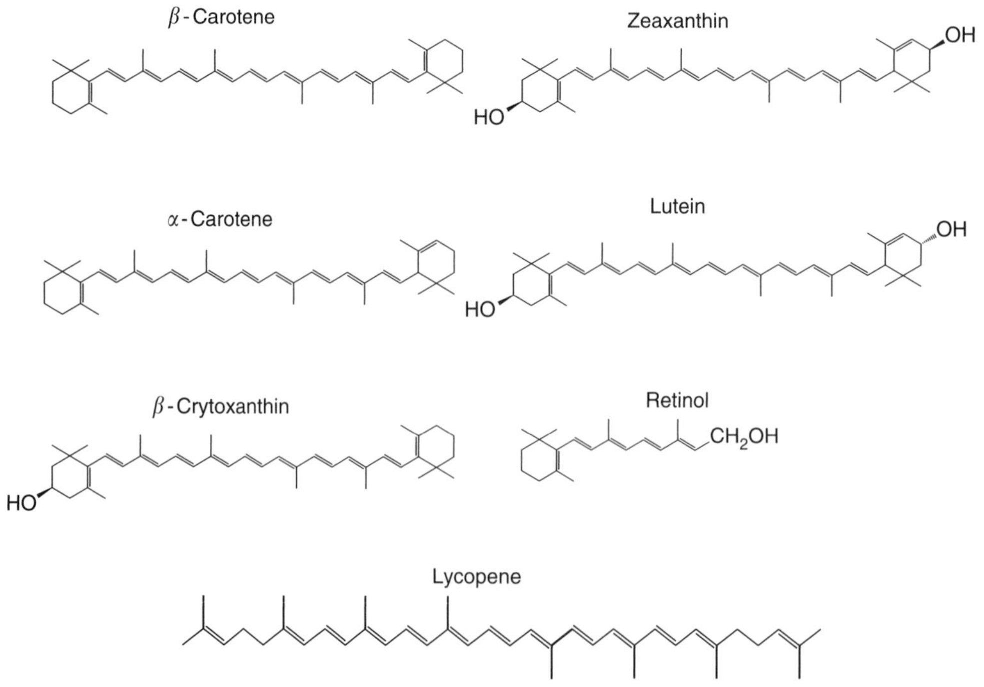

FIGURE 71.2 Structures of carotenoids.

Numerous epidemiologic studies indicate that individuals who consume diets with a relatively large amount of fruits and vegetables rich in carotenoids and high levels of serum β-carotene are at a lower risk for cancer at several tumor sites, including lung, colon, and breast.[82–87] Further evidence from cell culture and animal experiments suggested that β-carotene, the carotenoid with the greatest provitamin A activity, could be the compound responsible for this association.[88] On the basis of this evidence, three randomized intervention trails were conducted to test the effect of β-carotene supplements on lung cancer — the α-Tocopherol β-Carotene Study (ATBC Study),[89] the Physician's Health Study (PHS),[90] and the β-Carotene and Retinol Efficacy Trial (CARET).[91] Unexpectedly, results from the ATBC and CARET studies showed adverse treatment effects in terms of increased lung cancer incidence in high-risk subjects.[92] These studies suggest that in high-risk individuals β-carotene may have an adverse effect on cancer risk. This is supported by a recent French study that found high β-carotene intake was inversely associated with risk of tobacco-related cancers among nonsmokers, whereas high β-carotene intake was directly associated with risk among smokers.[93]

The different results obtained in supplementation trials, compared with cohort studies, may reflect that, in addition to β-carotene, fruits and vegetables contain numerous other compounds that may be protective against cancer. In fact, β-carotene may simply be a marker for the actual protective substances in fruits and vegetables. Alternately, β-carotene may have different effects when consumed as a supplement rather than in the food supply. The ATBC, CARET, and PHS studies illustrate that definitive evidence of both safety and efficacy is required for individual fruit and vegetable constituents before dietary guidelines, beyond simply greater consumption, can be proposed. Because β-carotene is the major source of vitamin A for much of the world's population, it is critical to define its safe intake from foods and supplements.[94] The CARET study also demonstrates the importance of large-scale primary prevention trials because the differences observed (lung cancer incidence of 4.6 and 5.9/1000 in the placebo and treatment groups, respectively) would not be detected in smaller studies.[91] These studies also may suggest that the effect of β-carotene may depend on the dose consumed. In animal models, low doses of β-carotene inhibit carcinogen-induced aberrant crypt formation; however, very high doses augment aberrant crypt incidence.[95]

β-Carotene mediates its cancer-protective and cancer-promoting effects through modulation of intracellular redox status. Through this mechanism, it affects redox-sensitive molecular pathways involved in the regulation of cell-cycle progression and apoptosis.[96] At low concentrations, the carotenoid may serve as an antioxidant, inhibiting free radical production,[97,98] while at relatively high concentrations and in the presence of a chronic oxidative stress (i.e., smoke), it may behave as a prooxidant, propagating free-radical-induced reactions, consuming endogenous antioxidants, and inducing DNA oxidative damage.[99–101] These effects may be mediated by carotenoid breakdown products.[99] In this context, β-carotene may regulate cell growth and death by the modulation of redox-sensitive genes and transcription factors.[96,102]

Although lycopene is not a vitamin A precursor, it is another carotenoid that has been proposed to have anticancer properties.[103–107] Lycopene is present in tomatoes, watermelon, pink grapefruit, and guava. As with other carotenoids, lycopene can serve as a potent antioxidant, and thereby influence exposure to ROS.[108] Interestingly, at physiological concentrations it can also retard the growth of human cancer cells, possibly by influencing growth factor receptor signals and altering cell-cycle progression.[109–111] Lycopene can sometimes upregulate the gene connexin 43, which may account for changes in intercellular gap junctional communications.[112] Evidence also exists that lycopene may upregulate the expression of the urokinase plasminogen activator receptor and facilitate invasion.[113] Recent evidence also suggests that lycopene can increase expression of phase II enzymes with an ARE via Nrf2 translocation from the cytosol to the nucleus.[114] As with many bioactive food components, a better understanding of molecular targets should assist in identification of those individuals who might benefit and those who might be placed at risk as a result of dietary intervention.[115]

VITAMIN C

Vitamin C is the most abundant water-soluble antioxidant in the body and is unique in that it can be regenerated after it becomes oxidized. Specific food sources include citrus fruits, mangoes, papaya, banana, strawberries, melon, broccoli, cabbage and other green leafy vegetables, peppers, tomatoes, pumpkin, and yams. Epidemiologic evidence indicates that high intakes of vitamin-C-rich fruits and vegetables and high vitamin C concentrations in serum are inversely associated with the risk of some cancers.[116] Hensen et al.[117] analyzed 46 epidemiologic studies on the protective effects of vitamin C against various types of cancers; 33 of these studies found a significant link between vitamin C intake and a reduced incidence of cancer. Of the 44 published *in vivo* studies examining oxidative damage after supplementation with vitamin C, 38 found a decrease in the number of markers of oxidative damage to DNA, lipid, or protein, 14 showed no changes, and only 6 reported an increase.[118] Case–control data indicate a risk reduction of 40 to 60% for gastric cancer[119] and 66% for oral/pharyngeal cancer,[120] and cohort data indicate a risk reduction of 23% for lung cancer in men for the highest vs. lowest intake of vitamin C.[121] Vitamin C concentration in plasma has also been shown to have an inverse association with cancer-related mortality.[122]

In animal studies, vitamin C has been found to be protective against skin, mammary, liver, and kidney cancer.[123–125] However, recent studies have suggested that high doses of vitamin C could have adverse effects on skin and lung cancer,[126,127] thus suggesting that the effects might be dose dependent. Vitamin C functions as a scavenger of free radicals to prevent oxidative-induced DNA damage and as a competitive inhibitor of nitrosamine formation from nitrate and amines *in vivo*.[128–130] Studies with cultured cells have shown that vitamin C can affect apoptosis and gene expression, and this appears to be mediated by its redox effects.[131–135]

FOLATE

Folate (folic acid) is so called because it is abundant in foliage (green leafy vegetables). Epidemiologic and clinical studies indicate that dietary folate intake and blood folate concentrations are inversely associated with the risk of colon, lung, head and neck, breast, and cervical cancers.[136–142] Collectively, studies suggest an ~40% reduction in the risk of colorectal cancer in individuals with the highest dietary folate intake compared with those with the lowest intake.[143] As mentioned previously, studies of folate and cancer are of particular interest as they show not only that this vitamin may exert a cancer protective effect but also demonstrate the importance of molecular nutrition studies. Functional polymorphisms in folate-metabolizing genes, especially MTHFR, are capable of modifying the risk of colorectal cancer. Observational studies show that individuals with the homozygous genotype for the MTHFR 677C to T polymorphism are at increased risk for colon cancer when folate intake or status is low.[141] However, because there was no clear relationship between plasma folate and colorectal adenomas among those with the CC or CT genotype, only a subset of the population may benefit from supplemental folate for colon cancer prevention.

Animal studies using chemical and genetically predisposed models have provided considerable support for a causal relationship between folate depletion and increased cancer incidence as well as a dose-dependent protective effect of folate supplementation.[143–149] However, animal studies have also shown that the dose and timing of folate intervention are critical in providing safe and effective cancer prevention.[143] Exceptionally high supplemental folate levels and folate intervention after microscopic neoplastic foci are established in the colorectal mucosa promote rather than suppress colorectal carcinogenesis.[143] These results suggest that the optimal dose of folate for cancer prevention may vary among individuals and may depend on whether or not microscopic lesions are present.

The mechanisms by which dietary folate can modulate carcinogenesis are related to the sole biochemical function of folate mediating the transfer of one-carbon moieties (Figure 71.3). Folate is an essential cofactor for the de novo biosynthesis of purines and thymidylate. 5,10-Methylenetetrahydrofolate, an intracellular conenzymatic form of folate, is required for conversion of deoxyuridylate to thymidylate and can be oxidized to 10-formyltetrhydrofolate for de novo purine synthesis. In this role, folate is an important factor in DNA synthesis, stability, integrity, and repair. A growing body of evidence from cell culture and animal and human studies indicates that folate deficiency is associated with DNA strand breaks, impaired DNA repair, and increased mutations, and that folate supplementation can correct some of these defects induced by folate deficiency.[143,150–153]

Folate also plays an essential role in one-carbon transfer involving remethylation of homocysteine to methionine, thereby ensuring the provision of *S*-adenosylmethionine, the primary methyl group donor for most biological methylation reactions

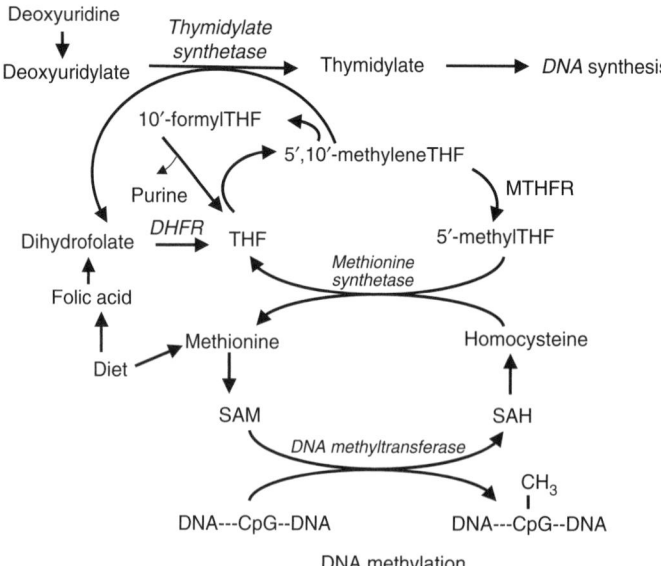

FIGURE 71.3 Simplified version of methyl metabolism. Folate, in the form of 5-methyltetrahydrofolate, is involved in remethylation of homocysteine to methionine, which is a precursor of SAM, the primary methyl group donor for most biological methylation reactions including that of DNA. 5,10 Methylenetetrafhydrofolate is required for conversion of deoxyrudiylate to thymidylate for DNA synthesis. Abbreviations used: CH$_3$, methyl group; CpG cytosine-guanine dinucleotide sequence; DHFR, dihydrofolate reducatase: MTHFR, methylenetetrahydrofolate reductase; SAH, *S*-adenosylhomocysteine; SAM, *S*-adenosylmethionine; THF, tetrahydrofolate.

including DNA methylation (Figure 71.3).[143] DNA methylation is an important epigenetic determinant of gene expression, maintenance of DNA integrity and stability, chromosomal modifications, and development of mutations. Aberrant patterns and dysregulation of DNA methylation are mechanistically related to carcinogenesis. Evidence from cell culture and animal and human studies suggests that folate deficiency and supplementation can influence DNA methylation.[154–157]

VITAMIN E

Vitamin E comes primarily from dietary vegetables oils (including safflower, corn, cottonseed, and soy bean oils), nuts, and green vegetables. Vitamin E is a collective term used to refer to a number of structurally and functionally different compounds that function, at least in part, as lipid-soluble antioxidants that can protect against the adverse effects of free radicals.[158]

Few epidemiologic studies have investigated the association of cancer risk with diets providing large amounts of vitamin E. A review concluded that the vitamin possibly decreases risk for lung and cervical cancers but that the evidence is insufficient for an effect on colon/rectum cancer, and that no relationship exists between vitamin E and breast or stomach cancer.[19] Some recent reviews have found no relationship between vitamin E and cancer risk.[159–161] However, one recent review of the epidemiologic data suggests that vitamin E from food offers some protection against breast cancer, while vitamin E supplements do not.[158] This again raises the issue that other food components in the food matrix may be important in determining the response. In the α-Tocopherol and β-Carotene Prevention Study (ATBC), 34% fewer cases of prostate cancer and 16% fewer cases of colorectal cancer were diagnosed among male cigarette smokers who received daily vitamin E supplements compared with those given a placebo.[89] Further analysis indicated an association of high serum tocopherol with low prostate cancer risk.[162] Although these results suggest a protective effect of vitamin E against prostate and colon cancers, these sites were not primary study end points and therefore additional studies are needed. In contrast, in the Cancer Prevention Study II Nutrition Cohort, the intake of vitamin E supplements was not associated with overall risk of prostate cancer or with risk of advanced prostate cancer.[163] Well-designed randomized control trials, such as the Selenium and Vitamin E Cancer Prevention Trial (SELECT) (http://www. cancer.gov/clinicaltrials/select), which will investigate the independent and interactive roles of vitamin E and selenium in prostate cancer prevention, will assist in helping to understand their importance in cancer prevention.

In preclinical models, vitamin E is protective against colon, liver, lung, skin, and pancreatic cancer.[164–169] Cell culture studies suggest that vitamin E functions by scavenging oxygen radicals and terminating free radical chain reactions.[170,171] Vitamin E is able to inhibit cell proliferation and induce apoptosis in a variety of human malignant cell lines.[172–182] Vitamin E may also prevent cancer progression by increasing production of humoral antibodies and enhancing cell-mediated immunity.[183] Recent studies also suggest that vitamin E may alter the cellular response to estrogen.[184]

SELENIUM

Selenium enters the food chain through plants and its concentration in foods is subject to several factors that are directly related to the amount and bioavailability of selenium in the soil.[185] Evidence for the cancer protective effects of selenium in humans was initially obtained by means of ecologic and correlation studies, which found an inverse relationship between selenium status and mortality from cancer of the colon, rectum, prostate, breast, ovary, and lung and from leukemia.[186] Data from most case–control and cohort studies indicate selenium's possible protective relationship with lung and prostate cancer, but data is not overly convincing for other cancer sites, including breast and colon/rectum.[19,187] A recent meta-analysis suggests that selenium supplementation may afford some protection against lung cancer in populations in which average selenium levels are traditionally low.[188] Evidence suggests that toenail Se may be a useful predictor of status.[188] Cohort studies also have identified low baseline serum or toenail selenium concentrations as a risk factor for prostate cancer.[189,190]

A recent intervention study provides the most compelling evidence for the protective effects of selenium against cancer. This randomized controlled trial was designed to test selenium as a deterrent to the development of basal or squamous skin carcinomas. Secondary end-point analyses showed that the mineral resulted in a significant reduction in total cancer mortality (RR = .5), total cancer incidence (RR = .63), and incidence of lung (RR = .54), colorectal (RR = .42), and prostate (RR = .37) cancer.[191] Participants with baseline plasma selenium concentrations in the lowest two tertiles (<121.6 ng/ml) experienced reductions in total cancer incidence, whereas those in the highest tertile showed an elevated incidence (heart rate [HR] = 1.20, 95% confidence interval [CI] = .77–1.86).[192] Reanalysis of incidence data through the end of the blinded clinical trial indicated that supplementation significantly reduced lung[193] and prostate[194] cancer only in individuals with the lowest baseline selenium concentrations. While these data are intriguing, they need to be confirmed. The ongoing SELECT trial, which is the largest-ever prostate cancer study, should provide insights into the efficacy and possible mechanisms by which selenium might function as a dietary anticancer component.

Extensive experimental evidence indicates that selenium supplementation reduces the incidence of cancer in animals.[195] Selenium supplementation in the diet or drinking water inhibits intitiation or postinitiation stages of liver, esophageal, pancreatic, colon, and mammary carcinogenesis[196–208] and spontaneous liver and mammary tumorigenesis.[209,210] Recent studies have also suggested that selenium has beneficial effects against tumor promotion/progression. High-dose selenium supplementation

(3 ppm in the drinking water) inhibits the progression of hormone refractory prostate cancer and the development of retro-peritoneal lymph node metastases through an inhibition of angiogenesis.[211] Similarly, high-selenium soy protein had a greater inhibitory effect than low-selenium soy protein on pulmonary metastasis of melanoma cells in mice.[212] However, it is difficult to extrapolate from studies in experimental animals to humans, as animal studies have generally used doses at least 10 times greater than those required to prevent clinical signs of deficiency, which, on a per-unit-body-weight basis, are considerably higher than most human selenium intakes.

Selenium appears to exert its cancer protective effects via changes in carcinogen metabolism and DNA adduct formation, regulation of apoptosis and cell-cycle arrest, and inhibition of angiogenesis (Table 71.4).[208,213–237] However, these effects are

TABLE 71.4

Examples of the Effects of Selenium on Cellular Processes Associated with Carcinogenesis

Cellular Process	Compound	Model System(s)	Effect
Carcinogen metabolism	Selenite	HepG2 cells[212]	Decreased CYP1A1
	Selenocysteine Se-conjugates	Purified human enzymes[213]	Inhibited CYP1A1, 2C9, 2C19 and 2D6 activities
	Selenocysteine	Primary rat hepatocytes and H35 cells[214]	Increased GST α and B mRNA expression
	Selenite	TGF-α/c-Myc transgenic mice[215]	Increased GST α and ϑ, Increased CYP2D13, 7B1 and 8B1 expression
	Selenite	Rat liver[216]	Decreased GST and UDPGT activities and decreased glutathione metabolizing enzyme activities
	Selenium-enriched garlic	Rat liver and mammary gland[217]	Inhibited GST and UDPGT activities and decreased carcinogen-DNA adducts
	Selenite, selenate and selenomethionine	Rat colon[218]	Inhibited carcinogen-DNA adduct formation
DNA repair	Selenite	U2OS cells[219]	Decreased transcription coupled repair after exposure to irradiation
	Selenomethionine	Normal human fibroblasts[220]	Induced DNA repair
Cell proliferation	Selenomethionine	SNU-1 cells[221]	Low concentrations increased cell proliferation via MAPK phosphorylation and activation but higher concentrations inhibited cell proliferation
	Methylseleninic acid	PC-3 cells[222]	Inhibited cell proliferation, decreased cyclin D1, cyclin D2, c-Myc and PCNA expression
	Methylseleninic acid	PC-3 cells[223]	Inhibited cell proliferation via p53 activation of p21, and downregulated CDK 1 and 2
Apoptosis	Selenite	Murine lymphoma cells[224]	Increased apoptosis via inhibition of cytosol to membrane translocation of PKC and activity
	Methylseleninic acid	DU145 and LNCaP cells[225]	Increased apoptosis via ERK1/2 activation of caspases
	Selenite	NB4 cells[226]	Increased apoptosis via caspase-3 activation and Bcl-2 cleavage
	Methylseleninic acid	LNCaP cells[227]	Increased apoptosis via blocking TRAIL-mediated Bad phosphorylation and increasing cytochrome C release
	Selenite	HSC-3 cells[228]	Increased apoptosis via modulation of mitochondrial redox equilibrium and increased caspase-3 and -9 activities
Oxidant/antioxidant balance	Selenium	Human peripheral blood mononuclear cells[229]	Increased superoxide dismutase, glutathione peroxidase and catalase activities
	Selenium-enriched yeast	Human leukocytes[230]	Decreased DNA damage
	Diphenylmethyl-selenocyanate	Mouse skin[231]	Inhibited lipid peroxidation and nitric oxide production
	Selenite	Rat liver[232]	Increased oxidative DNA damage
	Selenite	J774A.1cells[233]	Decreased LPS-induced ROS and NO production
Inflammation	Selenium	Human serum concentrations[234]	High concentrations decreased 8-iso-prostaglandin F2α and PGFF2α
	Selenium	Mice[235]	Deficiency abrogates inflammation-dependent plasma cell tumors
Angiogenesis	Selenate	Nude mice[211]	Inhibited angiogenesis of PC-3 tumors
	Methyseleninic acid and methylselenocyanate	HUVEC cells[236]	Inhibited MMP-2 and VEGF
	Selenium-enriched garlic, selenite and selenium-methylselenocysteine	Rat mammary tumors[237]	Inhibited intra-tumoral microvessel density

often dependent on the concentration and chemical form of selenium. The cancer protective activities of selenium, as with other biological activities of selenium, may depend on the selenium compounds present, and not on the element per se. Different chemical forms of selenium are metabolized differently and exert different biochemical effects. Selenium-enriched foods often contain mixtures of different selenium compounds and thus can affect multiple pathways to inhibit carcinogenesis.

ISOTHIOCYANATES

The cancer protective properties of cruciferous vegetables, such as broccoli, watercress, brussels sprouts, cabbage, and cauliflower, might be attributed to their high content of glucosinolates (β-thioglucoside N-hydroxysulfates), which are also responsible for their pungent odor and taste. The composition of glucosinolates among cruciferous vegetables varies, depending on the species, climate, and other agricultural conditions.[238] At least 120 different glucosinolates have been identified.[239] Physical stress such as chewing or chopping ruptures the plant cell wall and releases the plant-specific enzyme myrosinase, which cleaves the glucose moiety from the glucosinolates producing isothiocyanates. However, glucosinolates that escape the plant myrosinase may also be hydrolyzed in the intestinal tract, as the microflora are known to possess myrosinase activity.[33] Isothiocyanates are then metabolized *in vivo* through conjugation with glutathione with is promoted by glutathione-s-transferases (GST).[240,241] As discussed previously, polymorphisms associated with reduced GST activity may result in longer circulating half-lives of isothiocyanates and potentially greater cancer protective effects of cruciferous vegetables.[33]

Numerous studies in preclinical models have documented the cancer-preventive activity of a significant number of isothiocyanates.[242–246] Most notable is the inhibition of lung and esophagus cancers induced by tobacco products.[249–252] Several epidemiological studies have also shown that dietary consumption of isothiocyanates inversely correlates with the risk of developing lung, breast and colon cancers.[253–255] This effect can be modified by genetic polymorphisms.

Overall, the most important mechanism of cancer prevention by isothiocyanates appears to be induction of phase II enzymes and inhibition of phase I enzymes (Table 71.5). Induction of phase II cellular enzymes is largely mediated by the ARE, which is regulated by the transcription factor, Nrf2. A large number of isothiocyanates have also been shown to induce cell-cycle arrest and stimulate apoptosis. Other effects, including reducing oxidative stress by elevating and maintaining cellular antioxidants, inhibiting inflammatory processes, and perhaps induction of differentiation, have also been observed with some isothiocyanates and may contribute to the overall cancer protective effect of these compounds.

FLAVONOIDS

Flavonoids are a large group of plant products that have a common structure consisting of two phenolic benzene rings linked to a heterocyclic pyran or pyrone. Over 5000 flavonoids exist and can generally be grouped into one of the following subclasses: flavonols, flavonones, isoflavones, flavins, and anthocyanidins (Figure 71.4), which are present in many different fruits and vegetables (Table 71.6). This section will focus on flavonoids present in fruits and vegetables and will not discuss isoflavones or catechins, such as those in soy and green tea, respectively. In 2004, Neuhouser[281] reviewed the epidemiologic literature from four cohort studies and six case–control studies that had examined associations between flavonoid intake and cancer risk. The data suggest that there is consistent evidence from these studies that flavonoids, especially quercetin, may reduce the risk of lung cancer.[281] More recently, a study in Italy compared intake of the six principal classes of flavonoids (i.e., flavones, flavan-3-ols, flavonols, flavones, anthocyanidins, and isoflavones) in breast cancer patients vs. controls.[1] After allowance for major confounding factors and energy intake, a reduced risk of breast cancer was found for increasing intake of flavones (OR = .81 for the highest vs. the lowest quintile, $p < .02$ for trend) and flavonols (OR = .80, $p < .05$ for trend) but not for the other flavonoids,[282] thus suggesting that various flavonoids are protective against cancer in epidemiologic studies.

Studies with animal models of carcinogenesis have suggested that flavonoids have cancer-preventing activity but results have been mixed. For example, it was reported that 2% dietary quercetin inhibited azoxymethane-induced hyperproliferation, focal dysplasia, and aberrant crypt foci formation in mice.[283,284] Quercetin also reduced tumor incidence by 76% and tumor multiplicity by 48%; however, no inhibitory effects were observed in APC[min] (adenomatous polyposis coli) mice treated with quercetin.[285] Similarly, although quercetin inhibited local, UVB-light-induced immunosuppression in SKH-1 hairless mice, it had no effect on skin tumorigenesis.[286] Quercetin did inhibit N-nitrosodiethylamine-induced lung tumorigenesis in mice when administered during the initiation phase.[287] Other dietary flavonoids have also been shown to inhibit tumor growth in experimental animals. For example, naringenin inhibited tumor growth in sarcoma S-180 implanted mice,[288] cyanidine-3-glycoside suppressed the incidence and multiplicity of colorectal adenomas and carcinomas[289] as well as small intestinal adenoma number in APC[min] mice,[290] nobiletin inhibited colon cancer,[291] and anthocyanins have been shown to prevent skin cancer in rodents.[292]

Flavonoids have a wide variety of biological effects, many of which are important in cancer prevention. Representative studies demonstrating some of the biological effects of isolated flavonoids on cellular processes associated with carcinogenesis are shown in Table 71.7.[293–338] Their cancer prevention activity in animal and cell culture experiments may result from their inhibition of phase I and induce phase II carcinogen-metabolizing enzymes, inhibition of cell proliferation, stimulation of apoptosis,

TABLE 71.5

Examples of Effects of Isothiocyanates on Cellular Processes Associated with Carcinogenesis

Cellular Process	Compound	Model System(s)	Effect
Carcinogen metabolism	PEITC	Rat liver[256]	Inhibited CYP2E1 but increased CYP2B1 activity
	SF	Rat lung[257]	Increased CYP1A1, 1A2, 2B1/2, 2C11 and 3A1/2 activities
	PEITC	Rat liver, colon, prostate and blood[258]	Induced glutathione transferase, UDP-glucoronosyltransferase, sulfotransferase and quinine reductase activities and carcinogen-DNA adduct formation
	AITC, iberverin, erucin, iberin and SF	Rat duodenum, forestomach and bladder[259]	Induced glutathione transferase and quinine reductase activities
	SF	Human jejunum and Caco-2 cells[260]	Induced glutathione transferase A1 and UDP glucoronysyltransferase
	SF	LNCaP, MDA PCa, PC-3 and TSU-Pr1 cells[261]	Induced quinine reductase activity
	SF	Human hepatocytes and HepG2 cells[262]	Induced glutathione transferase A1 and UDP-glucoronosyltransferase mRNA expression and inhibited PhIP-DNA adduct formation
Cell proliferation	AITC, BITC, PEITC, PPITC, PBITC, PHITC, SF, TMITC, TBITC	UM-UC3 and T24 cells[263]	Blocked cell-cycle progression at the G2-M or S phases
	SF	MCF-7 cells[264]	Blocked cell-cycle progression at G2-M phase via increased cyclin B1, histone H1 phosphorylation and disrupted polymerization of mitotic microtubules
	SF	DU145 cells[265]	Blocked cell-cycle progression at G2-M phase via JNK-mediated signaling
Apoptosis	AITC, BITC, PEITC, PPITC, PBITC, PHITC, SF, TMITC, TBITC	UM-UC3 and T24 cells[263]	Increased apoptosis via induction of caspases -3, -8 and -9 and poly(ADP-ribose) polymerase
	SF	SV-40 transformed mouse embryonic fibroblasts[266,267]	Increased apoptosis via increased Bax and Bak
	SF	DAOY cells[268]	Increased apoptosis via induction of caspases -3, -8 and -9 and poly(ADP-ribose) polymerase
	PEITC	HepG2 cells[269]	Increased apoptosis via increased Bax translocation
	PEITC	T24 and Jurkat T cells[270]	Increased apoptosis via modification of intracellular thiol proteins
Oxidant/antioxidant balance	SF	PC-3 and DU145 cells[271]	Increased apoptosis is initiated by generation of ROS
	BITC and PEITC	HL-60 cells[272,273]	Inhibits superoxide generation
	SF	ARPE-19, HaCaT and L1210 cells[274]	Decreased cytoxicity of menadione, *tert*-butyl hydroperoxide, 4-hydroxynonenal and peroxynitrite
	BITC and SF	Hepa 1c1c7 cells[275]	Glutathione depletion
	BITC	RL34 cells[276]	Increased ROS
Inflammation	SF and PEITC	Raw 264.7 cells[277]	Inhibited LPS-induced secretion of nitric oxide, prostaglandin E_2 and TNF-α
	AITC and BITC	J744A.1 cells[278]	Inhibited LPS-induced nitric oxide production and TNF-α
Differentiation	AITC and BITC	HL-60 cells[279]	Increased differentiation
	AITC	DS19 cells[280]	Stimulated histone acetylation which increases differentiation

Abbreviations: AITC, allyl isothiocyanate; BITC, benzyl isothiocyanate; PBITC, phenylbutyl isothiocyanate; PEITC, phenylethylisothiocyanate; PHITC, phenylhexylisothiocyanate; PPITC, phenylpropyl isothiocyanate; SF, sulforaphane; TBITC, thienylbutyl isothiocyanate; TMITC, thienylmethyl isothiocyanate.

inhibition of inflammation, and suppression of angiogenesis. The free radical scavenging ability of flavonoids has been fairly well characterized in experimental systems. Furthermore, some studies have reported the impairment of *in vivo* angiogenesis by dietary flavonoids.[329]

ALLIUM COMPOUNDS

The *Allium* genus includes approximately 500 species.[330] Commonly used *Allium* vegetables include garlic, onion, leeks, chives, and scallions. Organosulfur compounds present in these vegetables are considered to be responsible for their beneficial

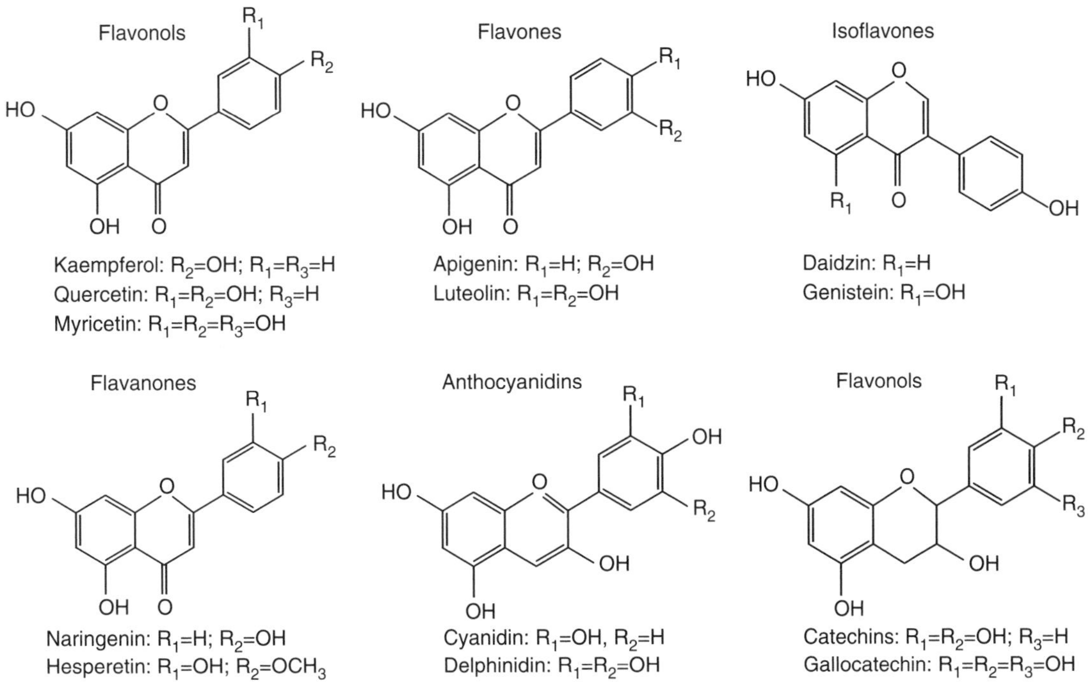

FIGURE 71.4 Structures of flavonoids.

TABLE 71.6
Some Common Sources of Flavonoids

Flavonoid	Major Food Sources
Apigenin (flavone)	Celery, parsley, thyme, sweet red pepper
Cyanidin (anthocyanidin)	Cherries, black grapes
EGCG (flavonol or catechin)	Apples, plums, cocoa, green tea, black tea
Genistein, daidzein (isoflavone)	Soybeans, chickpeas, legumes
Hesperetin, narigenin (flavanone)	Oranges, lemons, prunes
Quercetin, kaempferol, myricetin (flavonol)	Onions, broccoli, kale, apples, plums, cherries, strawberries, grapes, tea

---

effects (Figure 71.5). Garlic, in particular, has been shown to be protective against cancer.[331] The primary sulfur-containing constituents in garlic are the (-glutamyl-S-alk(en)yl-L-cysteins and S-alk(en)yl-L-cysteine sulfoxides, including alliin.[331] The characteristic odor of garlic arises from allicin and other oil-soluble sulfur components. Typical volatiles in crushed garlic and garlic oil include diallyl sulfide (DAS), diallyl disulfide (DADS), diallyl trisulfide (DATS), methyl allyl disulfide (MADS), methyl allyl trisulfide (MATS), 2-vinyl-1-dithiin, and 3-vinyl-1,2-dithiin (Figure 71.5).

Epidemiologic findings and preclinical studies with cancer models appear to provide evidence that garlic and related sulfur constituents can suppress cancer risk and alter the biological behavior of tumors. Results from the Iowa Women's Health Study, a prospective cohort study, found that the strongest association among fruits and vegetables for colon cancer risk reduction was for garlic consumption, with an approximate 50% lesser risk of distal colon cancer associated with high consumption.[332] Fleisschauer and Arab summarized the epidemiologic literature related to garlic and cancer risk.[333] Nineteen studies reported RR estimates for garlic consumption and cancer incidence. Site-specific case–control studies of stomach and colorectal cancer suggested the protective effect of high intake of raw or cooked material. Cohort studies confirmed this inverse association with colorectal cancer. However, the reliability of epidemiologic results may be limited as total vegetable consumption or other known risk factors were generally not considered.[331] More recently, in a double-blind, randomized study of Japanese patients with colorectal adenomas, a higher dose of aged garlic extract was shown to reduce the risk of new colorectal adenomas compared with a lower-dose garlic extract.[334]

TABLE 71.7
Examples of Effects of Flavonoids on Cellular Processes Associated with Carcinogenesis

Cellular Process	Compound	Model System(s)	Effect
Carcinogen metabolism	Quercetin	Rat liver[293]	Induces CYP2B
	Quercetin	Purified enzyme[294]	Inhibits CYP1A1 and 1A2 activities
	Quercetin	Human liver,[295,296] human duodenum,[295,297] rat liver[298]	Inhibits sulfotransferase activity
	Quercetin	Rat liver,[299] rat intestine,[299] human jejunum,[300] Caco-2 cells[301]	Inhibits glucoronosyltransferase activity
	Quercetin	HL-60 cells[302]	Inhibits N-acetyltransferase activity
	Quercetin	HepG2 cells,[265] human lymphocytes[303]	Inhibits carcinogen-DNA adduct formation
	Kaempferol	MCF-7 cells[304]	Inhibit CYP1A1 transcription
	Kaempferol	Human liver and duodenum[305]	Inhibits sulfotransferase activity
	Naringenin, naringin, rutin	Salmonella typhimurium TA98[306]	Inhibits mutagenicity
Cell proliferation	Quercetin	PC-3 cells[307]	Cell-cycle arrest via block at G2/M phase, increased p21 expression
	Quercetin	HK1 and CNE2 nasopharyngeal cells[308]	Increased Rb gene expression resulting in block at G2/M or G0/G1 phases
	Quercetin	PC-3 and LnCap cells[309]	Inhibited cell proliferation and DNA synthesis via decreased cyclin D1, ErbB-2 and ErbB-3 expression
	Quercetin and kaempferol	HuTu-80, Caco-2 and PMC42 cells[310]	Inhibited cell proliferation, decreased PCNA and Ki67 expression
	Apigenin	SW480 cells[311]	Cell-cycle arrest via block at G2/M phase
Apoptosis	Quercetin	PC-3,[28] HT-29 cells[312]	Increased apoptosis via decreased Bcl-2 and Bcl-x and increased Bax and caspase-3
	Quercetin	A549 cells[313]	Increased apoptosis via inactivation of Akt-1 and activation of MEK-ERK pathway
	Quercetin and kaempferol	Prostate and breast cancer cells[314]	Increased apoptosis associated with ability to inhibit fatty acid synthase
Inflammation	Quercetin and kaempferol	Human umbilical cord blood-derived cultured mast cells[315]	Inhibited release of IL-6, IL-8 and TNF-α
	Quercetin	Bone marrow-derived macrophages[316]	Inhibited cytokines and iNOS through inhibition of NF-κB
	Naringenin, fisetin	RAW264.7 macrophages, human peripheral blood mononuclear cells[317]	Inhibited nitric oxide, TNF-α and IL-2 production
	Apigenin, kaempferol	J744A.2 macrophages[318]	Inhibited TNF-α and IL-1β gene expression
	Quercetin, myricetin, apigenin	Peritoneal ecudate murine macrophages[319]	Reduced lipopolysaccharide-induced TNF-α production
Oxidant/ antioxidant Balance	Quercetin	Human lymphocytes,[303] Caco-2[320] and V79 cells[321]	Protected against hydrogen peroxide-induced DNA damage
	Quercetin and kaempferol	Sperm and human lymphocytes[322]	Reduced DNA damage produced by estrogenic compounds
	Quercetin, naringin and rutin	C3H10T1/2 cells[323]	Inhibited UVA-induced DNA strand breaks
	Quercetin	Human neutrophils[324]	Inhibited superoxide generation induced by arachidonic acid
	Naringin	HepG2 cells[325]	Inhibited iron-induced DNA oxidation, increased antioxidant enzymes
Angiogenesis	Quercetin	Human blood[326]	Inhibited TIMP-1 gene transcription and plasma protein concentrations
	Quercetin	Severe combined immune deficient mice inoculated with CWR22 prostate cells[327]	Reduced VEGF121 and VEGF165 mRNA and microvessel density
	Tangeretin, rutin	B16F10 cells[328]	Decreased number of metastatic nodules

Preclinical studies provide some of the strongest evidence that garlic or its related organosulfur compounds suppress cancer risk and alter the behavior of tumors. Garlic and its associated sulfur compounds have been found to inhibit mammary, colon, skin, uterine, esophagus, lung, renal, forestomach, and liver cancer incidence in animal models.[335–346]

The protection of tumor incidence by garlic may arise from several mechanisms including altered formation and bioactivation of carcinogens, enhanced DNA repair, reduced cell proliferation, induction of apoptosis, inhibition of inflammation, and suppression of angiogenesis (Table 71.8).[347–387] It is likely that many of these processes are modified simultaneously. Furthermore, cancer progression is probably also highly dependent on epigenetic changes. There is evidence that some garlic constituents can influence histone homeostasis.[388] For example, Druesne et al. reported that DADS effectively increased histone

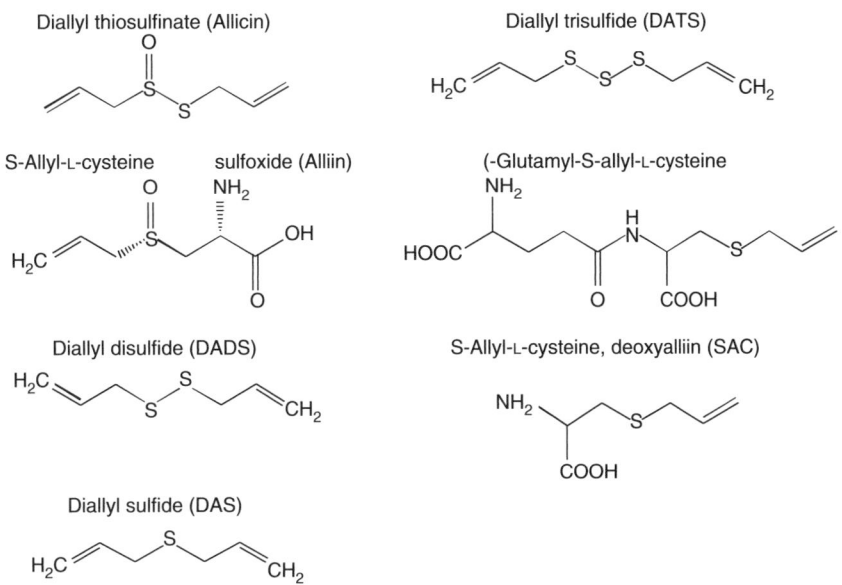

FIGURE 71.5 Structures of *Allium* compounds.

TABLE 71.8

Examples of Effects of *Allium* Compounds on Cellular Processes Associated with Carcinogenesis

Cellular Process	Compound	Model Systems(s)	Effect
Carcinogen metabolism	Garlic	Human[347]	Blocked the enhanced urinary excretion of nitrosoproline
	DADS and DAS	Rat esophageal microsomes, purified rat and human enzymes[348]	Inhibited rat and human CYP2E1 and rat CYP2A3 activity
	Garlic powder	Rat liver[349]	Inhibited CYP2E1 activity
	Garlic oil, DADS, DAS and DATS	Rat liver[350]	Inhibited CYP2E1 activity but increased CYP1A1, CYP2B1 and CYP3A1 activities
	Garlic powder	Rat liver[351,352]	Increased ethoxyresorufin deethylase, GST and UDP-glucuronosyltransferase activities
	DADS, DAS and DATS	Rat tissues[353]	Increased quinine reductase and glutathione transferase activities
	DADS	CE81T/VGH cells[354]	Inhibited N-acetyltransferase activity
	DADS, DAS and DATS	HepG2 cells[355]	Induced phase II gene expression through activation of ARE and Nrf2 protein accumulation
	SAC and DADS	Rat mammary gland[347]	Inhibited carcinogen-DNA adduct formation
	Crushed garlic	Rat liver[356]	Inhibited carcinogen-DNA adduct formation
	DAS	Rat liver[357]	Inhibited carcinogen-DNA adduct formation
	DADS and SAC	Salmonella TA100[358]	Decreased mutagenicy of N-nitromorpholine
DNA repair	Garlic extract	Human fibroblasts[359]	Stimulated DNA repair

Continued

TABLE 71.8
(Continued)

Cellular Process	Compound	Model Systems(s)	Effect
Cell proliferation	DADS	Human A549 lung cells[360] and PC-3 cells[361]	Induced cell-cycle arrest at G2/M phase
	DATS	PC-3 and DU145 cells[362]	Induced cell-cycle arrest at G2/M phase by inhibition of CDK1 and hyperphosphorylation of Cdc25C
	DADS, DAS and DATS	J5 cells[363]	Induced cell-cycle arrest at G2/M phase by inhibiting CDK7 and increasing cyclin B1
	DADS	HCT-15 cells[364]	Induced cell-cycle arrest at G2/M phase by inhibiting cdc2 kinase activation and increased cyclin B1
Apoptosis	DADS	T24 cells[365]	Apoptosis induced via caspase-3 activity
	Allicin	SiHA, L929 and SW480 cells[366]	Apoptosis induced via caspases-3, -8 and -9 activation and cleavage of poly(ADP-ribose) polymerase
	SAMC and DADS	SW480 cells[367]	Apoptosis induced via caspase-3 activation and cleavage of poly (ADP-ribose) polymerase
	SAMC	SW480 and NIH3T3 cells[368]	Apoptosis induced via caspase-3 activation and JNK1 signaling pathway
	Water-soluble extract	MDA-MB-435 cells[369]	Apoptosis induced via increased translocation of BimEL to mitochondria
	Garlic	Hamster buccal pouch[370]	Apoptosis induced by downregulation of Bcl-2 and upregulation of Bax, Bim, p53 and caspases-3 and -8.
	DATS	PC-3 and DU145 cells[371,372]	Apoptosis induced via inactivation of Akt signaling
	Allicin	Human gastric epithelial cells[373]	Apoptosis induced via mitochondrial relase of AIF and PKA
Inflammation	Allicin	HT-29 and Caco-2 cells[374]	Inhibited spontaneous and TNF-α-induced secretion of IL-1, IL-8, IP-10 and MIG
	Aqueous garlic extract	Rat thymocytes and spleno-cytes [375]	Decreased IL-2 production
	Aged garlic extract	Human peripheral blood lymphocytes [376]	Increased cytotoxicity against both NK-sensitive and resistant M14 cell lines
	Garlic extract	Balb/c mice[377]	Increased NK activity
	Fresh garlic and tablet	Balb/c mice[378]	Augmented delayed-type hypersensitivity
	AMS, DADS and DAS	RAW 264.7 cells[379,380]	DADS inhibited iNOS, decreased TNF-α, IL-10 and increased IL-1 and IL-6. AMS increased IL-10. DAS inhibited COX-2
	Allicin and ajoene	Raw 264.7 cells[381]	Decreased iNOS
	DAS	HEK 293T cells[382]	Inhibited COX-2
	Aqueous garlic suspension	Sprague-Dawley rat colon[383]	Inhibited COX-2 expression
Oxidant/antioxidant balance	Aqueous garlic extract	Balb/c mouse liver, kidney lung and brain[384]	Ameliorated oxidative organ injury due to naphthalene toxicity
	SAMC	Rat kidney[385]	Scavenged hydroxyl radicals and singlet oxygen, ameliorated oxidative and nitrosative stress
	Aqueous garlic extract	Wistar rats liver and blood[386]	Decreased lipid peroxidation
Angiogenesis	DAS	Swiss albino mice injected with ehrlich ascites cells[387]	Decreased angiogenesis

Abbreviations: AMS, allyl methyl sulfide; DADS, diallyl disulfide; DAS, diallyl sulfide; DATS, diallyl trisulfide; SAC, *S*-allyl cysteine; SAMC, *S*-allylmercaptocysteine.

H3 acetylation in cultured Caco-2 and HT-29 cells by reducing histone deacetylase activity.[388] This change in hyperacetylation was accompanied by an increase in p21(waf1/cip1) expression, demonstrating that epigenetic events can influence subsequent gene expression patterns and lead to the accumulation of cells in the G2 phase of the cell cycle.[388]

MONOTERPENES

Monoterpenes are natural plant products found in the essential oils of many commonly consumed fruits and vegetables and are largely responsible for the pleasant fragrances of the fruits and plants. Limonene, the simplest monocyclic monoterpene, and

TABLE 71.9
Examples of Effects of Monoterpenes on Cellular Processes Associated with Carcinogenesis

Cellular Process	Compound	Model System(s)	Effect
Carcinogen metabolism	Limonene	Liver, spleen, kidney and lung of rats[403]	Increased CYP2B and 2C and epoxide hydratase activities, decreased carcinogen-DNA adduct formation
	Limonene	Liver and intestine of rats[404]	Increased UDP-glucuronosyltransferase activity
Cell proliferation	Perillyl alcohol	KPL-1, MCF-7, MKL-F and MDA-MB-231 cells[405]	Induced growth arrest at G1 phase via decreased cyclin D1 and E and increased p21
	Perillyl alcohol	HTB-43, SCC-25 and BroTo cells[406]	Induced cell-cycle arrest
Apoptosis	Perillyl alcohol	Diethylnitrosamine-induced rat liver tumors[407]	Increased apoptosis
	Citral	HL-60, BS24-1, RL-12, U937, 293 and MCF-7 cells[408]	Increased apoptosis via increased caspase-3 activity
	Perillyl alcohol	U87 and A172 cells and primary culture derived from human gliobastoma[409]	Increased apoptosis
	Perillyl alcohol	H322 and H838 cells[410]	Increased apoptosis via increased caspase-3 activity and PARP cleavage
Inflammation	Limonene	Balb/c mice with lymphoma[411]	Delayed hypersensivity reaction to dinitroflourobenzene, phagocytosis and microbicidal activity. Increased nitric oxide production by macrophages
Angiogenesis	Perillyl alcohol	Endothelial cells[412]	Inhibited angiogenesis by decreased VEGF and increased angiopoietin 2 expression
	Limonene	Gastric cancer cells in nude mice[394]	Inhibited angiogenesis and metastasis by decreased VEGF expression

perillyl alcohol, a hydroxylated limonene analog, have demonstrated cancer protective and chemotherapeutic activity against mammary, skin, lung, pancreas, kidney, esophagus, liver, and colon tumors in rodent models.[389–397] They are capable of increasing tumor latency, decreasing tumor multiplicity, and causing regression of mammary carcinomas.[398,399] Preliminary results of phase I and phase II clinical trials of limonene and perillyl alcohol demonstrate that these agents are well tolerated in cancer patients and worthy of further testing as potential chemotherapeutic agents.[400–402] Results of these human clinical trials are necessary to clarify if monoterpenes are effective against cancer in humans.

Several mechanisms appear to account for the cancer protective effects of monoterpenes in preclinical models (Table 71.9).[403–412] These include modulation of carcinogen metabolism, inhibition of tumor cell proliferation, increased apoptosis, and the induction of tumor cell differentiation.

SUMMARY

The research highlighted here is only a small part of the large body of evidence linking fruit and vegetable intake with cancer risk and tumor behavior. Variation in response among individuals likely depends on individual genetic polymorphisms or interactions among dietary components that influence absorption, metabolism, or site of action. Evidence suggests that the cancer protective effects of fruits and vegetables may result from additive or synergistic effects of various vitamins, minerals, phenolic phytochemicals, isothiocyanates, and *Allium* compounds rather than from the effect of a single ingredient. Thus, the diet as a whole may play a more important role than individual components. A better understanding of physiologically important interactions is needed. Furthermore, the response is complicated as multiple steps in the cancer process can be modified simultaneously, including sites such as drug metabolism, DNA repair, cell proliferation, apoptosis, inflammation, differentiation, and angiogenesis. As current evidence suggests that bioactive food components can typically influence more than one process, a better understanding of how the response relates to exposures and which process is most involved in bringing about a change in tumor incidence or tumor behavior is essential. Additional research is needed to determine the critical intake, duration, and when it should be provided to optimize the desired physiological response. Further research is also needed on the molecular targets for bioactive components and whether genetic and epigenetic events dictate the direction and magnitude of the response.

REFERENCES

1. Kris-Etherton, P.M. et al. *Am. J. Med.*, 113, 71s, 2002.
2. Keck, A.S. and Finley, J.W. *Integr. Cancer Ther.*, 3, 5, 2004.
3. Demark-Wahnefried, W. and Rock, C.L. *Semin. Oncol.*, 30, 789, 2003.

4. Sato, Y. et al. *Public Health Nutr.*, 8, 309, 2004.

5. Kojima, M. et al. *Nutr. Cancer*, 50, 23, 2004.

6. McCullough, M.L. et al. *Cancer Causes Control*, 14, 959, 2003.

7. Voorrips, L.E. et al. *Am. J. Epidemiol.*, 152, 1081, 2000.

8. Bingham, S.A. et al. *Cancer Epidemiol. Biomark. Prev.*, 14, 1552, 2005.

9. Wark, P.A. et al. *Cancer Epidemiol. Biomark. Prev.*, 14, 1619, 2005.

10. Wang, J. et al. *Intl. J. Cancer*, epub Sept 2005.

11. Satia-Abouta, J. et al. *Intl. J. Cancer*, 109, 728, 2004.

12. Yeh, C.C. et al. *J. Formos. Med. Assoc.*, 102, 305, 2003.

13. Diergaarde, B. et al. *Carcinogenesis*, 24, 283, 2003.

14. Chiu, B.C.-H. et al. *Cancer Epidemiol. Biomark. Prev.*, 12, 210, 2003.

15. Deneo-Pellegrini, H. et al. *Eur. J. Cancer Prev.*, 11, 369, 2002.

16. Levi, F. et al. *Br. J. Cancer*, 79, 1283, 1999.

17. Witte, J.S. et al. *Am. J. Epidemiol.*, 144, 1015, 1996.

18. Kampman, E. et al. *Cancer Causes Control*, 6, 225, 1995.

19. Food, Nutrition and the Prevention of Cancer: A Global Perspective. World Cancer Research Fund/American Institute for Cancer Research, Washington, DC, 1997.

20. Key, T.J. et al. *Public Health Nutr.*, 7, 187, 2004.

21. Michaud, D.S. et al. *Br. J. Cancer*, 87, 960, 2002.

22. Steinmetz, K.A. and Potter, J.D. *Cancer Causes Control*, 2, 325, 1991.

23. Steinmetz, K.A. and Potter, J.D. *J. Am. Diet. Assoc.*, 96, 1027, 1996.

24. Djousse, L. et al. *Am. J. Clin. Nutr.*, 79, 213, 2004.

25. Milner, J.A. *J. Nutr.*, 133, 3820s, 2003.

26. Davis, C.D. and Milner, J.A. *Mutation Res.*, 551, 51, 2004.

27. Mathew, A. et al. *Intl. J. Cancer*, 108, 287, 2004.

28. Davis, C.D. and Milner, J.A. *Nutritional Health: Strategies for Disease Prevention*, 2nd ed., Humana Press Inc., Totowa, NJ, 2005, 151.

29. Zhong, S. et al. *Carcinogenesis*, 12, 1533, 1991.

30. Pemble, S.E. et al. *Biochem. J.*, 300, 271, 1994.

31. Hayes, J.D, Flanagan, J.U. and Jowsey, I.R. *Ann. Res. Pharmacol. Toxicol.*, 45, 51, 2005.

32. Sheweita, S.A. *Curr. Drug Metab.*, 1, 107, 2000.

33. Lampe, J.W. and Peterson, S. *J. Nutr.*, 132, 2991, 2002.

34. Wang, L.I. et al. *Cancer Causes Control*, 15, 977, 2004.

35. Zhao, B. et al. *Cancer Epidemiol. Biomark. Prev.*, 10, 1063, 2001.

36. Joseph, M.A. et al. *Nutr. Cancer*, 50, 206, 2004.

37. Seow, A. et al. *Carcinogenesis*, 23, 2055, 2002.

38. Yeh, C.-C. et al. *World J. Gastronenterol.*, 11, 1473, 2005.

39. Lee, S.-A. et al. *Exp. Molec. Med.*, 36, 116, 2004.

40. Shen, J. et al. *Cancer Epidemiol. Biomark. Prev.*, 14, 336, 2005.

41. Shen, J. et al. *Carcinogenesis*, epub July 2005.

42. Ahn, J. et al. *Cancer Res.*, 64, 7634, 2004.

43. Lin, H.J. et al. *Cancer Epidemiol. Biomark. Prev.*, 7, 647, 1998.

44. Slattery, M.L. et al, *Cancer Causes Control*, 11, 1, 2000.

45. Molloy, A.M. *World Rev. Nutr. Diet*, 93, 153, 2004.

46. Bailey, L.B. and Gregory, J.F. *J. Nutr.*, 129, 919, 1999.

47. Chen, J., Giovannucci, E.L. and Hunter, D.J. *J. Nutr.*, 129, 560s, 1999.

48. Frost, P. et al. *Nat. Genet.*, 10, 111, 1995.

49. Margate, T. et al. *Intl. J. Epidemiol.*, 32, 64, 2003.

50. Le Marchand, L. et al. *Cancer Epidemiol. Biomark. Prev.*, 14, 1198, 2005.

51. Jiang, Q. et al. *Cancer Diet. Prev.*, 29, 146, 2005.

52. Esteller, M. et al. *Carcinogenesis*, 12, 2307, 1997.

53. Gershoni-Baruch, R. et al. *Eur. J. Cancer*, 18, 2313, 2000.

54. Campbell, I.G. et al. *Breast Cancer Res.*, R14, 1, 2002.

55. Chen, J. et al. *Cancer Res.*, 65, 1606, 2005.

56. Lee, J.S. and Surh, Y.J. *Cancer Lett.*, 224, 171, 2005.

57. Cooke, M.S. et al. *Mutat. Res.*, 574, 58, 2005.

58. Sancar, A. et al. *Ann. Rev. Biochem.*, 73, 39, 2004.

59. Jacks, T. and Weinberg, R.A. *Cell*, 111, 923, 2002.

60. Chen, C. and Kong, A.-N.T. *TRENDS Pharmacol. Sci.*, 26, 318, 2005.

61. Weinstein, I.B. *Carcinogenesis*, 21, 857, 2000.

62. Reed, J. *Curr. Opin. Oncol.*, 11, 68, 1999.

63. Krammer, P.H. *Nature*, 407, 789, 2000.

64. Li, P. et al. *Cell*, 91, 479, 1997.
65. Thornberry, N.A. and Lazebnki, Y. *Science*, 281, 1312, 1998.
66. Hofseth, L.J. and Ying, L. *Biochimica Et Biophy. Acta*, 765:74, 2005.
67. Hussain, S.P., Hofseth, L.J. and Harris, C.C. *Nat. Rev. Cancer*, 3, 276, 2003.
68. Storz, P. *Frontiers Biosci.*, 10, 1881, 2005.
69. Bartsch, H. *Mut. Res. Rev. Genet. Toxicol.*, 340, 67, 1996.
70. Jackson, A.L. and Loeb, L.A. *Mutat. Res.*, 477, 7, 2001.
71. Valko, M. et al. *Molec. Cell. Biochem.*, 266, 37, 2004.
72. Berger, M.M. *Clin. Nutr.*, 24, 172, 2005.
73. Fayette, J., Soria, J.-C. and Armand, J.-P. *Eur. J. Cancer*, 41, 1109, 2005.
74. Jackson, J.R. et al. *FASEB J.*, 11, 457, 1997.
75. Majno, G. *Am. J. Pathol.*, 153, 1035, 1998.
76. Pfeffer, U. *Intl. J. Biol. Markers*, 18, 70, 2003.
77. Crockett, M.I. et al. *Biochem. Soc. Trans.*, 22, 55, 1994.
78. Baramova, E. and Foldart, J.M. *Cell Biol. Intl.*, 19, 239, 1995.
79. Okuno, M. et al. *Current Cancer Drug Targets*, 4, 285, 2004.
80. Khera, P. and Koo, J.Y. *J. Drugs Dermatol.*, 4, 432, 2005.
81. Yang, Y. et al. *Biomed. Environ. Sci.*, 9, 386, 1996.
82. Ziegler, R.G., Mayne, S.T. and Swanson, C.A. *Cancer Causes Control*, 7, 157, 1996.
83. Tapiero, H., Townsend, D.M. and Tew, K.D. *Biomed. Pharmacother.*, 58, 100, 2004.
84. Cooper, D.A., Eldridge, A.L. and Peters, I.C. *Nutr. Rev.*, 57, 133, 1999.
85. Rock, C.L. et al. *J. Clin. Oncol.*, 23, 6631, 2005.
86. Tamimi, R.M. et al. *Am. J. Epidemiol.*, 161, 153, 2005.
87. Steck-Scott, S. et al. *Intl. J. Cancer*, 112, 295, 2004.
88. Krinsky, N.I. *Ann. Rev. Nutr.*, 13, 561, 1993.
89. Heinonen, O.P. et al. *N. Eng. J. Med.*, 330, 1029, 1994.
90. Hennekens, C.H. et al. *N. Eng. J. Med.*, 334, 1145, 1996.
91. Omenn, O.S. et al. *N. Eng. J. Med.*, 334, 1150, 1996.
92. Mannisto, S. et al. *Cancer Epidemiol. Biomark. Prev.*, 13, 40, 2004.
93. Touvier, M. et al. *J. Natl. Cancer Inst.*, 97, 1338, 2005.
94. Bendich, A. *J. Nutr.*, 134, 225s, 2004.
95. Raju, J. et al. *Intl. J. Cancer*, 113, 798, 2005.
96. Palozza, P. *Biochim. Biophys. Acta*, 1740, 215, 2005.
97. Hosotani, K. et al. *Biofactors*, 21, 241, 2004.
98. Palozza, P. et al. *J. Nutr.*, 135, 129, 2005.
99. Siems, W. et al. *J. Nutr. Biochem.*, 16, 385, 2005.
100. Palozza, P. et al. *Carcinogenesis*, 25, 1315, 2004.
101. Palozza, P. et al. *Arch. Biochem. Biophys.*, 430, 104, 2004.
102. Dulinska, J. et al. *Biochem. Biophys. Acta*, 1740, 189, 2005.
103. Nkondjock, A. et al. *J. Nutr.*, 135, 592, 2005.
104. Davis, C.D. et al. *J. Nutr.*, 135, 2014s, 2005.
105. Giovannucci, E. *J. Nutr.*, 135, 2030s, 2005.
106. Almushatat, A.S. et al. *Intl. J. Cancer*, 118: 1051, 2005.
107. Ito, Y. et al. *Asian Pac. J. Cancer Prev.*, 6, 10, 2005.
108. Heber, D. and Lu, Q.Y. *Exp. Biol. Med.*, 227, 920, 2002.
109. Hwang, E.S. and Bowen, P.E. *Biofactors*, 23, 75, 2005.
110. Hwang, E.S. and Bowen, P.E. *Biofactors*, 23, 97, 2005.
111. Palozza, P. et al. *Apoptosis*, 10: 1445, 2005.
112. Livny, O. et al. *J. Nutr.*, 132, 3754, 2002.
113. Forbes, K., Gillette, K. and Sehgal, I. *Exp. Biol. Med.*, 228, 967, 2003.
114. Ben-Dor, A. et al. *Mol. Cancer Ther.*, 4, 177, 2005.
115. Davis, C.D. *J. Nutr.*, 135, 2074s, 2005.
116. Li, K.W. et al. *Am. J. Clin. Nutr.*, 78, 1074, 2003.
117. Henssen, D.E., Block, G. and Levine, M. *J. Natl. Cancer Inst.*, 83, 547, 1991.
118. Carr, A. and Frei, B. *FASEB J.*, 13, 1007, 1999.
119. Estrom, A.M. et al. *Intl. J. Cancer*, 87, 133, 2000.
120. Negri, E. et al. *Intl. J. Cancer*, 86, 122, 2000.
121. Vorrips, L.E., Goldbohm, R.A. and Brants, H.A. *Cancer Epidemiol. Biomark. Prev.*, 9, 357, 2000.
122. Khaw, K.T., Bingham, S. and Welch, A. *Lancet*, 357, 657, 2001.
123. Lin, J.Y. et al. *J. Am. Acad. Dermatol.*, 48, 866, 2003.
124. Tsao, C.S. *Am. J. Clin. Nutr.*, 54, 1274s, 1991.

125. Surjyo, B. and Anisuir, K.B. *Indian J. Cancer*, 41, 72, 2004.
126. D'Agostini, F. et al. *Carcinogenesis*, 26, 657, 2005.
127. Fiala, E.S. et al. *Carcinogenesis*, 26, 605, 2005.
128. Golde, D.W. *Integrative Cancer Ther.*, 2, 158, 2003.
129. Oliveira, C.P. *World J. Gastronenterol.*, 9, 446, 2003.
130. Zhang, Z.W. and Farthing, M.J.G. *Chinese J. Dig. Diseases*, 6, 53, 2005.
131. Kang, J.S. et al. *J. Cell. Physiol.*, 204, 192, 2005.
132. Han, S.S. *J. Cell Biochem.*, 93, 257, 2004.
133. Cho, D. et al. *Melanoma Res.*, 13, 549, 2003.
134. Sagun, K.C., Carcamo, J.M. and Golde, D.W. *FASEB J.*, 19, 1657, 2005.
135. Duarte, T.L. and Lunec, J. *Free Radical Res.*, 39, 671, 2005.
136. Kane, M.A. *Cancer Detect. Prev.*, 29, 46, 2005.
137. Piyanthilake, G.C. et al. *Cancer Res.*, 64, 8788, 2004.
138. Baglietto, L. et al. *BMJ.*, 331, 807, 2005.
139. Martinex, M.E., Henning, S.M. and Alberts, D.S. *Am. J. Clin. Nutr.*, 79, 691, 2004.
140. Shen, H. et al. *Cancer Epidemiol. Biomark. Prev.*, 12, 980, 2003.
141. Strohle, A., Wolters, M. and Hahn, A. *Int J. Oncol.*, 26, 1449, 2005.
142. Wei, E.K. et al. *J. Natl. Cancer Inst.*, 97, 684, 2005.
143. Kim, Y.I. *Environ. Molec. Mutagenesis*, 44, 10, 2004.
144. Porigbny, J.P. et al. *Mutat. Res.*, 548, 53, 2004.
145. Carrier, J. et al. *Cancer Epidemiol. Biomark. Prev.*, 12, 1262, 2003.
146. James, S.J. et al. *J. Nutr.*, 133, 3740s, 2003.
147. Davis, C.D. and Uthus, E.O. *J. Nutr.*, 133, 2907, 2003.
148. Kotsopoulos, J. et al. *Carcinogenesis*, 24, 937, 2003.
149. Trasler, J. et al. *Carcinogenesis*, 24, 39, 2003.
150. Ames, B.N. *Mutat. Res.*, 475, 7, 2001.
151. Choi, S.W. and Mason, J.B. *J. Nutr.*, 132, 2413, 2002.
152. Fennech, M. *Mutat. Res.*, 475, 57, 2001.
153. Lamprecht, S.A. and Lipking, M. *Nat. Rev. Cancer*, 3, 601, 2003.
154. Pufulete, M. et al. *Gut*, 54, 579, 2005.
155. Pufulete, M. et al. *Br. J. Cancer*, 92, 838, 2005.
156. Choi, S.W. et al. *Br. J. Cancer*, 93, 31, 2005.
157. Stempak, J.M. et al. *Carcinogenesis*, 26, 981, 2005.
158. Kline, K. et al. *J. Marrary Gland Biol. Neoplasia*, 8, 91, 2003.
159. Pham, D.Q. and Plakogiannis, R. *Ann. Pharmacother.*, 39, 1870, 2005.
160. Lonn, E. et al. *J. Urol.*, 174, 1823, 2005.
161. Cho, E. et al. *Intl. J. Cancer*, 118: 970, 2005.
162. Weinstein, S.J. et al. *J. Natl. Cancer Inst.*, 97, 396, 2005.
163. Rodriguez, C. et al. *Cancer Epidemiol. Biomark. Prev.*, 13, 378, 2004.
164. Exon, J.H. et al. *Nutr. Cancer*, 49, 72, 2004.
165. Calvisi, D.F. et al. *J. Hepatol.*, 41, 815, 2004.
166. Quin, J. et al. *J. Surg. Res.*, 127, 139, 2005.
167. Uddin, A.N., Burns, F.J. and Rossman, T.G. *Carcinogenesis*, 26:2179, 2005.
168. Heukamp, I. et al. *Pancreatology*, 5, 403, 2005.
169. Bansal, A.K. et al. *Chem. Biol. Interact.*, 156, 101, 2005.
170. Fantappie, O. et al. *Free Radical. Res.*, 38, 751, 2004.
171. Stapelberg, M. et al. *J. Biol. Chem.*, 280, 25369, 2005.
172. Shah, S.J. and Sylvester, P.W. *Biochem. Cell Biol.*, 83, 86, 2005.
173. Wang, X.F. et al., *Biochem. Biophys. Res. Commun.*, 326, 282, 2005.
174. Zu, K., Hawthorn, L. and Ip, C. *Mol. Cancer Ther.*, 4, 43, 2005.
175. Kang, Y.H. *Intl. J. Cancer*, 112, 385, 2004.
176. Shah, S. and Sylvester, P.W. *Exp. Biol. Med.*, 229, 745, 2004.
177. Sakai, M. et al. *Anticancer Res.*, 24, 1683, 2004.
178. Jiang, Q. et al. *Proc. Natl. Acad. Sci. USA*, 101, 17825, 2004.
179. Shah, S.J. and Sylvester, P.W. *Exp. Boil. Med.*, 230, 235, 2005.
180. Jiang, Q., Wong, J. and Ames, B.N. *Ann. NY Acad. Sci.*, 1031, 399, 2004.
181. Sylvester, P.W., Shah, S.J. and Samant, G.V. *J. Plant Physiol.*, 162, 803, 2005.
182. Alleva, R. et al. *Biochem. Biophys. Res. Commun.*, 331, 1515, 2005.
183. Meydani, S.N. et al. *J. Am. Med. Assos.*, 277, 1380, 1997.
184. Chamras, H. et al. *Nutr. Cancer*, 52, 43, 2005.
185. Rayman, M.P. *Br. J. Nutr.*, 92, 557, 2004.

186. Schrauzer, G.N., White, D.A. and Schneider, C.I. *Bioinorg. Chem.*, 7, 23, 1997.
187. Etminan, M. et al. *Cancer Causes Control*, 16, 1125, 2005.
188. Zhuo, H., Smith, A.H. and Steinmaus, C. *Cancer Epidemiol. Biomark. Prev.*, 13, 771, 2004.
189. Klein, E.A. *J. Urol.*, 171, S50, 2004.
190. Li, H. et al. *J. Natl. Cancer Inst.*, 96, 696, 2004.
191. Clark, L.C. et al. *JAMA*, 276, 1957, 1996.
192. Duffield-Lillico, A.J. et al. *Cancer Epidemiol. Biomark. Prev.*, 11, 630, 2002.
193. Reid, M.J. et al. *Cancer Epidemiol. Biomark. Prev.*, 11, 1285, 2002.
194. Duffield-Lillico, A.J. et al. *BJU Intl.*, 91, 608, 2003.
195. Davis, C.D. and Irons, R. *Current Nutr. Food Sci.*, 1, 201, 2005.
196. Baines, A.T. et al. *Cancer Lett.*, 160, 193, 2000.
197. Birt, D.F. et al. *J. Natl. Cancer Inst.*, 77, 1281, 1986.
198. Bjorkhem-Bergman, L. et al. *Carcinogenesis*, 26, 125, 2005.
199. McIntosh G.H. et al. *Nutr. Cancer Res.*, 54:209; 2006.
200. El-Bayoumy, K. and Sinha, R. *Mutat. Res.*, 551, 181, 2004.
201. Chen, X. et al. *Carcinogenesis*, 21, 1531, 2000.
202. Finley, J.W. et al. *J. Agric. Food Chem.*, 49, 2679, 2001.
203. Dias, D.F. et al. *Breast J.*, 6, 14, 2000.
204. Griffin, A.C. and Jacobs, M.M. *Cancer Lett.*, 3, 177, 1977.
205. Ip, C., Lisk, D.J. and Ganther, H.E. *Anticancer Res.*, 20, 4179, 2000.
206. Ip, C. et al. *J. Agric. Food Chem.*, 48, 2062, 2000.
207. McIntosh, G.H., Scherer, B. and Royle, P.J. *Asian Pac. J. Clin. Nutr.*, 13, s93, 2004.
208. Thirunavukkarasu, C. et al. *Cell Biochem. Funct.*, 20, 347, 2002.
209. Popova, N.V. *Cancer Lett.*, 179, 39, 2002.
210. Schrauzer, G.N., White, D.A. and Schneider, C.J. *Bioinorg. Chem.*, 8, 387, 1978.
211. Corcoran, N.M., Najdovska, M. and Costello, A.J. *J. Urol.*, 171, 907, 2004.
212. Li, D. et al. *J. Nutr.*, 134, 1536, 2004.
213. Morgan, K.T. et al. *Toxicol. Pathol.*, 30, 435, 2002.
214. Venhorst, J. *Xenobiotica*, 33, 57, 2003.
215. Hoen, P.A. et al. *Biochem. Pharmacol.*, 63, 1843, 2002.
216. Novoselov, S.V. et al. *Oncogene*, 1, 2005.
217. Ip, C. and Lisk, D.J. *Nutr. Cancer*, 28, 184, 1997.
218. Davis, C.D. et al. *J. Nutr.*, 129, 63, 1999.
219. Abul-Hassan, K.S. et al. *Mutat. Res.*, 565, 45, 2004.
220. Seo, Y.R., Sweeney, C. and Smith, M.L. *Oncogene*, 21, 3663, 2002.
221. Verma, A. et al. *Nutr. Cancer*, 49, 184, 2004.
222. Dong, Y. et al. *Cancer Res.*, 63, 52, 2003.
223. Zu, K. et al. *Oncogene*, 25:546; 2006.
224. Gopee, N.V., Johnson, V.J. and Sharma, R.P. *Toxicol. Sci.*, 78, 204, 2004.
225. Hu, H. et al. *Carcinogenesis*, 26, 1374, 2005.
226. Zuo, L. et al. *Ann. Hematol.*, 83, 751, 2004.
227. Yamaguchi, K. et al. *Oncogene*, 24, 5868, 2005.
228. Takahashi, M. et al. *Intl. J. Oncol.*, 27, 489, 2005.
229. Kuppusamy, U.R. et al. *Biol. Trace Elem. Res.*, 106, 29, 2005.
230. Karunasinghe, N. et al. *Cancer Epidemiol. Biomark. Prev.*, 13, 391, 2004.
231. Das, R.K. and Bhattacharya, S. *Asian Pac. J. Cancer Prev.*, 5, 151, 2004.(199)
232. Wycherly, B.J., Moak, M.A. and Christensen, M.J. *Nutr. Cancer*, 48, 78, 2004.
233. Kim, S.H. et al. *Exp. Biol. Med.*, 229, 203, 2004.
234. Helmersson, J. et al. *Free Radic Res.*, 39, 763, 2005.
235. Felix, K. et al. *Cancer Res.*, 64, 2910, 2004.
236. Jiang, C., Ganther, H. and Lu, J. *Mol. Carcinog.*, 29, 236, 2000.
237. Jiang, C. et al. *Mol. Carcinog.*, 26, 213, 1999.
238. Keum, Y.K., Jeong, W.S. and Kong, A.N.T. *Mutat. Res.*, 555, 191, 2004.
239. Fahey, J.W., Zalcmann, A.T. and Talalay, P. *Phytochemistry*, 56, 5, 2001.
240. Zhange, Y. et al. *Biochem. Biophys. Res. Commun.*, 206, 748, 1995.
241. Kolm, R.H. et al. *Biochem. J.*, 311, 450, 1995.
242. Sugie, S. et al. *Intl. J. Cancer*, 115, 346, 2005.
243. Manesh, C. and Kuttan, G. *Fitoterapia*, 74, 355, 2003.
244. Smith, T.K., Mithen, R. and Johnson, I.T. *Carcinogenesis*, 24, 491, 2003.
245. Singh, A.V. et al. *Carcinogenesis*, 25, 83, 2004.
246. Pham, N.A. et al. *Mol. Cancer Ther.*, 3, 1239, 2004.

247. Nishikawa, A. et al. *Curr. Cancer Drug Targets*, 4, 373, 2004.

248. Nishikawa, A., Morse, M.A. and Chung, F.L. *Cancer Lett.*, 193, 11, 2003.

249. Hecht, S.S. et al. *Carcinogenesis*, 23, 1455, 2002.

250. Solt, D.B. et al. *Cancer Lett.*, 202, 147, 2003.

251. Hecht, S.S. et al. *Cancer Lett.*, 187, 87, 2002.

252. Witschi, H. et al. *Carcinogenesis*, 23, 289, 2002.

253. Fowke, J.H. et al. *Cancer Res.*, 63, 3980, 2003.

254. London, S.J. et al. *Lancet*, 356, 724, 2000.

255. Spitz, M.R. et al. *Cancer Epidemiol. Biomark. Prev.*, 9, 1017, 2001.

256. Guo, Z. et al. *Carcinogenesis*, 13, 2205, 1992.

257. Paolini, M. et al., *Carcinogenesis*, 25, 61, 2004.

258. Dingley, K.H. et al. *Nutr. Cancer*, 46, 212, 2003.

259. Munday, R. and Munday, C.M. *J. Agricul. Food Chem.*, 52, 1867, 2004.

260. Petri, N. et al. *Drug Metab. Dispo.*, 31, 805, 2003.

261. Brooks, J.D., Paton, V.G. and Vidanes, G. *Cancer Epidemiol. Biomark. Prev.*, 10, 949, 2001.

262. Bacon, J.R. et al. *Carcinogenesis*, 24, 1903, 2003.

263. Tang, L. and Zhang, Y. *J. Nutr.*, 134, 2004, 2004.

264. Jackson, S.J. and Singletary, K.W. *J. Nutr.*, 134, 2229, 2004.

265. Cho, S.D. et al. *Nutr. Cancer*, 52, 213, 2005.

266. Choi, S. and Singh, S.V. *Cancer Res.*, 65, 2035, 2005.

267. Xiao, D. et al. *Clin. Cancer Res.*, 11, 2670, 2005.

268. Gingras, D. et al. *Cancer Lett.*, 203, 35, 2004.

269. Rose, P. et al. *Intl. J. Biochem. Cell Biol.*, 37, 100, 2005.

270. Pullar, J.M. et al. *Carcinogenesis*, 25, 765, 2004.

271. Singh, S.V. et al. *J. Biol. Chem.*, 280, 19911, 2005.

272. Miyoshi, N. et al. *Carcinogenesis*, 25, 567, 2004.

273. Gerhauser, C. et al. *Mutat. Res.*, 523/524, 163, 2003.

274. Gao, X. et al. *Proc. Natl. Acad. Sci.*, 98, 15221, 2001.

275. Zhang, Y. *Carcinogenesis*, 21, 1175, 2000.

276. Zhang, Y. et al. *Biochem. Biophys. Res. Commun.*, 206, 748, 1995.

277. Heiss, E. et al. *J. Biol. Chem.*, 276, 32008, 2001.

278. Ippoushi, K. et al. *Life Sci.*, 71, 411, 2002.

279. Zhang, Y. et al. *Mol. Cancer Ther.*, 2, 1045, 2003.

280. Lea, M.A. et al. *Intl. J. Cancer*, 92, 784, 2001.

281. Neuhouser, M.L. *Nutr. Cancer*, 50, 1, 2004.

282. Bosetti, C. et al. *Cancer Epidemiol. Biomark. Prev.*, 14, 805, 2005.

283. Deschner, E.E. et al. *Carcinogenesis*, 12, 1193, 1991.

284. Volate, S.R. et al. *Carcinogenesis*, 26, 1450, 2005.

285. Mahmoud, N.N. et al. *Carcinogenesis*, 21, 921, 2000.

286. Steerenberg, P.A. et al. *Cancer Lett.*, 114, 187, 1997.

287. Khanduja, K.L. et al. *Food Chem. Toxicol.*, 37, 313, 1999.

288. Kanno, S. et al. *Biol. Parm. Bull.*, 28, 527, 2005.

289. Miyata, M. et al. *Cancer Lett.*, 183, 17, 2000.

290. Cooke, D. et al. *Eur. J. Cancer*, 41, 1931, 2005.

291. Suzuki, R. et al. *Biofactors*, 22, 111, 2004.

292. Afaq, F. et al. *Intl. J. Cancer*, 113, 423, 2005.

293. Rahden-Staron, I., Czeczot, H. and Szumilo, M. *Mutat. Res.*, 498, 57, 2001.

294. Schwarz, D., Kisselev, P. and Roots, I. *Eur. J. Cancer*, 41, 151, 2005.

295. Rossi, A.M. et al. *Intl. J. Clin. Pharmacol. Ther.*, 42, 561, 2004.

296. De Santi, C. et al. *Xenobiotica*, 32, 363, 2002.

297. Marchetti, F. et al. *Xenobiotica*, 31, 841, 2001.

298. Mesia-Vela, S. and Kauffman, F.C. *Xenobiotica*, 33, 1211, 2003.

299. van der Logt, E.M. et al. *Carcinogenesis*, 24, 1651, 2003.

300. Petri, N. et al. *Crug Metab. Dispos.*, 31, 805, 2003.

301. Galijatovic, A., Walle, U.K. and Walle, T. *Pharm. Res.*, 17, 21, 2000.

302. Kuo, H.M. et al. *Phytomedicine*, 9, 625, 2002.

303. Wilms, L.C. et al. *Mutat. Res.*, 582, 155, 2005.

304. Ciolino, H.P., Daschner, P.J. and Yeh, G.C. *Biochem. J.*, 340, 715, 1999.

305. De Santi, C. et al. *Xenobiotica*, 30, 857, 2000.

306. Bear, W.L. and Tell, R.W. *Anticancer Res.*, 20, 3609, 2000.

307. Vijayababu, M.R. et al. *J. Cancer Res. Clin. Oncol.*, 131:765, 2005.

308. Ong, C.S. et al. *Oncol. Rep.*, 11, 727, 2004.
309. Huynh, H. et al. *Intl. J. Oncol.*, 23, 821, 2003.
310. Ackland, M.L., van de Waarsenburg, S. and Jones, R. *In Vivo*, 19, 69, 2005.
311. Wang, W. et al. *Nutr. Cancer*, 48, 106, 2004.
312. Kim, W.K. et al. *J. Nutr. Biochem.*, 16, 155, 2005.
313. Nguyen, T.T. et al., *Carcinogenesis*, 25, 647, 2004.
314. Brusselmans, K. et al. *J. Biol. Chem.*, 280, 5636, 2005.
315. Kempuraj, D. et al. *Br. J. Pharmacol.*, 145, 934, 2005.
316. Comalada, M. et al., *Eur. J. Immunol.*, 35, 584, 2005.
317. Lyu, S.Y. and Park, W.B. *Arch. Pharm. Res.*, 28, 573, 2005.
318. Kowalski, J. et al. *Pharmacol. Rep.*, 57, 390, 2005.
319. Ueda, H., Yamazaki, C. and Yamazaki, M. *Biosci. Biotechnol. Biochem.*, 68, 119, 2004.
320. Duthie, S.J. and Dobson, V.L. *Eur. J. Nutr.*, 38, 28, 1999.
321. Aherne, S.A. and O'Brien, N.M. *Nutr. Cancer*, 38, 106, 2000.
322. Cemeli, E., Schmid, T.E. and Anderson, D. *Environ. Mol. Mutag.*, 44, 420, 2004.
323. Yeh, S.L. et al. *J. Nutr. Biochem.*, 16: 729, 2005.
324. Lu, H.W. et al. *Arch. Biochem. Biophys.*, 393, 73, 2001.
325. Jagetia, G.C. et al. *Clin. Chim. Acta*, 347, 189, 2004.
326. Morrow, D.M. et al. *Mutat. Res.*, 480–481, 269, 2001.
327. Ma, Z.S. et al. *Intl. J. Oncol.*, 24, 1297, 2004.
328. Martinez Conesa, C. et al. *J. Agric. Food Chem.*, 53, 6791, 2005.
329. Kanadaswami, C. et al. *In Vivo*, 19, 895, 2005.
330. Sengupta, A., Ghosh, S. and Bhattacharjee, S. *Asian Pac. J. Cancer Prev.*, 5, 229, 2004.
331. Park, E.J. and Pezzuto, J.M. *Cancer and Metastasis Rev.*, 21, 231, 2002.
332. Steinmetz, K.A. et al. *Am. J. Epidemiol.*, 139, 1, 1994.
333. Fleischauer, A.T. and Arab, L. *J. Nutr.*, 131, 1032S, 2001.
334. Tanaka, S. et al. *Hiroshima J. Med. Sci.*, 53, 39, 2004.
335. Singh, A. and Shukla, Y. *Cancer Lett.*, 131, 209, 1998.
336. Ip, C., Lisk, D.J. and Stoewsand, G.S. *Nutr. Cancer*, 17, 279, 1992.
337. Wargovich, M.J. *Carcinogenesis*, 8, 487, 1987.
338. Hussain, S.P., Jannu, L.N. and Rao, A.R. *Cancer Lett.*, 49, 175, 1990.
339. Wargovich, M.J. et al. *Cancer Res.*, 48, 6872, 1988.
340. Hong, J.Y. et al. *Carcinogenesis*, 13, 901, 1992.
341. Takahashi, S. et al. *Carcinogenesis*, 13, 1513, 1992.
342. Nagabhushan, M. et al. *Cancer Lett.*, 66, 207, 1992.
343. Park, K.A., Kweon, S. and Choi, H. *J. Biochem. Mol. Biol.*, 35, 615, 2002.
344. Wargovich, M.J. et al. *Cancer Epidemiol. Biomark. Prev.*, 5, 355, 1996.
345. Wargovich, M.J. et al. *Carcinogenesis*, 21, 1149, 2000.
346. Milner, J.A. *J. Nutr.*, 131, 1027s, 2001.
347. Schaffer E.M. et al. *Cancer Lett.*, 102, 199, 1996.
348. Mei, X. et al. *Acta Nutrimenta Sinica*, 11, 141, 1989.
349. Morris, C.R. et al. *Nutr. Cancer*, 48, 54, 2004.
350. Wu, C.C. et al. *J. Agric. Food Chem.*, 50, 378, 2002.
351. Berges, R. et al. *Carcinogenesis*, 25, 1953, 2004.
352. Le Bon, A.M. et al. *J. Agric. Food Chem.*, 51, 7617, 2003.
353. Munday, R. and Munday, C.M. *Nutr. Cancer*, 40, 205, 2001.
354. Yu, F.S. et al. *Food Chem. Toxicol.*, 43, 1029, 2005.
355. Chen, C. et al. *Free Radic Biol. Med.*, 37, 1578, 2004.
356. Zhou, L. and Mirvish, S.S. *Nutr. Cancer*, 51, 68, 2005.
357. Green, M. et al. *Oncol. Rep.*, 10, 767, 2003.
358. Dion, M.E., Agler, M. and Milner, J.A. *Nutr. Cancer*, 28, 1, 1997.
359. L'vova, G.N. and Zasukhina, G.D. *Genetika*, 38, 306, 2002.
360. Wu, X.J., Kassie, F. and Mersch-Sundermann, V. *Mutat. Res.*, 579: 115, 2005.
361. Arunkumar, A. et al. *Biol. Pharm. Bull.*, 28, 740, 2005.
362. Herman-Antosiewicz, A. and Singh, S.V. *J. Biol. Chem.*, 280, 28519, 2005.
363. Wu, C.C. et al. *Food Chem. Toxicol.*, 42, 1937, 2004.
364. Knowles, L.M. and Milner, J.A. *Carcinogenesis*, 21, 1129, 2000.
365. Lu, H.F. et al. *Food Chem. Toxicol.*, 42, 1543, 2004.
366. Oommen, S. et al. *Eur. J. Pharmacol.*, 485, 97, 2004.
367. Xiao, D. et al. *Mol. Cancer Ther.*, 4, 1388, 2005.
368. Xiao, D. et al. *Cancer Res.*, 63, 6825, 2003.

369. Lund, T. et al. *Br. J. Cancer*, 92, 1773, 2005.
370. Bhuvaneswari, V., Rao, K.S. and Nagini, S. *Clin. Chim. Acta*, 350, 65, 2004.
371. Xiao, D. et al. *Oncogene*, 23, 5594, 2004.
372. Xiao, D. and Singh, S.V. *Carcinogenesis*, 27: 533, 2005.
373. Park, S.Y. et al. *Cancer Lett.*, 224, 123, 2005.
374. Lang, A. et al. *Clin. Nutr.*, 23, 1199, 2004.
375. Colic, M. et al. *Phytomedicine*, 9, 117, 2002.
376. Morioka, N. et al. *Cancer Immunol. Immunother.*, 37, 316, 1993.
377. Hassan, Z.M. et al. *Intl. Immunopharmacol.*, 3, 1483, 2003.
378. Ghazanfari, T., Hssan, Z.M. and Ebrahimi, M. *Intl. Immunopharmacol.*, 2, 1541, 2002.
379. Chang, H.P., Huang, S.Y. and Chen, Y.H. *J. Agric. Food Chem.*, 53, 2530, 2005.
380. Chang, H.P. and Chen, Y.H. *Nutrition*, 21, 530, 2005.
381. Dirsch, V.M. et al. *Atherosclerosis*, 139, 333, 1998.
382. Elango, E.M. et al. *J. Appl. Genet.*, 45, 469, 2004.
383. Sengupta, A., Ghosh, S. and Das, S. *Cancer Lett.*, 208, 127, 2004.
384. Omurtag, G.Z. et al. *J. Pharm. Pharmacol.*, 57, 623, 2005.
385. Pedraza-Chaverri, J. et al. *BMC Clin Pharmacol.*, 4, 5, 2004.
386. Arivazhagan, S. et al. *J. Med. Food*, 7, 2334, 2004.
387. Shukla, Y., Arora, A. and Singh, A. *Biomed. Environ. Sci.*, 15, 41, 2002.
388. Druesne, N. et al. *Carcinogenesis*, 25: 1227, 2004.
389. Crowell, P.L. and Gould, M.N. *Crit. Rev. Oncog.*, 5, 1, 1994.
390. Wattenberg, L.W. and Coccia, J.B. *Carcinogenesis*, 12, 115, 1991.
391. Stark, M.J. et al. *Cancer Lett.*, 96, 15, 1995.
392. Reddy, B.S. et al. *Cancer Res.*, 57, 420, 1997.
393. Liston, B.W. et al. *Cancer Res.*, 63, 2399, 2003.
394. Lu, X.G. et al. *World J. Gastroenterol.*, 10, 2140, 2004.
395. Raphael, T.J. and Kuttan, G. *J. Exp. Clin. Cancer Res.*, 22, 419, 2003.
396. Asamato, M. et al. *Jpn. J. Cancer Res.*, 93, 32, 2002.
397. Kaji, I. et al. *Intl. J. Cancer*, 93, 441, 2001.
398. Haag, J.D., Lindstrom, M.J. and Gould, M.N. *Cancer Res.*, 52, 4021, 1992.
399. Haag, J.D. and Gould, M.N. *Cancer Chemother. Pharmacol.*, 34, 477, 1994.
400. Sterarns, V. et al. *Clin. Cancer Res.*, 10, 7583, 2004.
401. Bailey, H.H. et al. *Gynecol. Oncol.*, 85, 464, 2002.
402. Hudes, G.R. et al. *Clin. Cancer Res.*, 6, 3071, 2000.
403. Maltzman, T.H. et al. *Carcinogenesis*, 12, 2081, 1991.
404. Van der Logt, E.M. et al. *Anticancer Res.*, 24, 843, 2004.
405. Yuri, T. et al. *Breast Cancer Res. Treat.*, 84, 251, 2004.
406. Samaila, D. et al. *Anticancer Res.*, 24, 3089, 2004.
407. Mills, J.J. et al. *Cancer Res.*, 55, 979, 1995.
408. Dudai, N. et al. *Planta Med.*, 71, 484, 2005.
409. Fernandes, J. et al. *Oncol. Rep.*, 13, 943, 2005.
410. Xu, M. et al. *Toxiciol. Appl. Pharmacol.*, 195, 232, 2004.
411. Del Toro-Arreola, S. et al. *Intl. Immunopharm.*, 5, 829, 2005.
412. Loutrari, H. et al. *J. Pharmacol. Exp. Ther.*, 11, 568, 2004.

72 Nutrition and Cancer Treatment

David Heber and Susan Bowerman

CONTENTS

INTRODUCTION

Malnutrition is a frequent and serious problem in patients with cancer. Patients with lung, prostate, head and neck, and gastric cancers are more frequently affected, but the overall incidence of malnutrition ranges between 30 and 85% of different populations studied.[1,2] The advanced starvation state resulting from decreased food intake and hormonal/metabolic abnormalities characteristic of the interaction between tumor and host has been called cancer cachexia,[3] characterized by progressive, involuntary weight loss with depletion of lean body mass, muscle wasting and weakness, edema, impaired immune response, and declines in motor and mental function. Weight loss of greater than 10% of prediagnosis weight is seen in approximately 45% of patients.[2,4] Cancer-associated malnutrition and cachexia are related to considerable morbidity and mortality, including decreased quality of life,[5] impaired response to chemotherapy,[5] impaired muscle function,[6] and higher incidence of postoperative complications.[7–9] The goals of nutritional support are to provide the patient with energy and nutrients to maintain or improve their nutritional status and immune function, minimize gastrointestinal (GI) symptoms, and improve quality of life. Early intervention in adequately nourished patients or those with early signs of nutritional decline can delay the progression of malnutrition,[10] but a vicious cycle of cachexia can develop in which the effects of the disease lead to nutritional decline, predisposing the patient to increased complications and more severe disease, which promotes further decline.

While nutritional rehabilitation can be demonstrated in selected patients who respond to antineoplastic therapy, the application of parenteral and enteral nutrition as an adjunct to chemotherapy in cancer patients has not resulted in increased survival or predictable weight gain.[11,12] The pathophysiology of cancer-associated malnutrition is complex, and cannot be explained on the basis of poor nutrient intake alone, suggesting that simply increasing nutrient intake is not sufficient to prevent or reverse malnutrition. Both tumor-derived and systemic factors, such as hormones and inflammatory cytokines produced by the host in response to the tumor, have been implicated in the pathophysiology of cancer cachexia, and there is increasing evidence that these factors are associated with malnutrition.[13–15]

METABOLIC ABNORMALITIES IN THE CANCER PATIENT

Since predictable renutrition of the cancer patient has not been possible, a great deal of research has been conducted concerning specific hormonal and metabolic abnormalities that could interfere with renutrition. Research on the basic pathophysiology of cancer cachexia has resulted in the definition of several metabolic and hormonal abnormalities in malnourished cancer patients. These abnormalities are listed in Table 72.1.

TABLE 72.1
Metabolic Abnormalities in Cancer Patients

1. Hypogonadism in male cancer patients[16]
2. Increased glucose production[17,18]
3. Increased protein catabolism[19,20]
4. Increased lipolysis and fatty acid oxidation[21,22]
5. Insulin resistance[23,24]

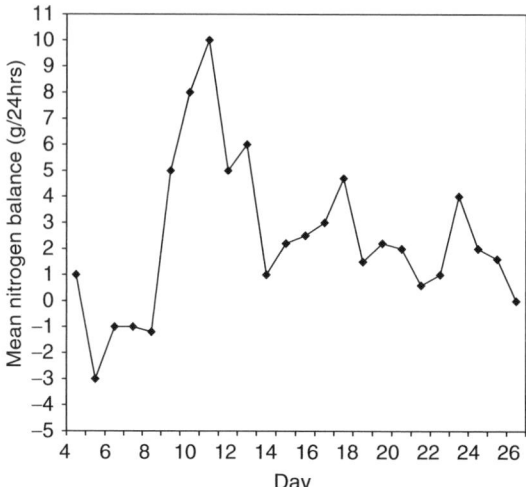

FIGURE 72.1   Mean nitrogen balance in grams per 24 h in six head and neck cancer patients receiving 1.25 × BEE kcal for 5 days and 2.25 × BEE for 19 days as a continuous enteral infusion.

ENERGY BALANCE IN THE CANCER PATIENT

Based on autopsy studies performed in the 1920s[25,26] and animal studies done in the 1950s,[27] it was postulated that tumors acted to siphon off needed energy and protein from the host. In the 1970s and 1980s, specific abnormalities of intermediary metabolism were identified in cancer patients that could account for the common observation that such patients lost weight even in the face of apparently adequate nutrition. Studies conducted in a number of laboratories, including our own, have demonstrated that maladaptive metabolic abnormalities occur frequently in patients with cancer. In 1983, we demonstrated that adequate calories and protein administered to six patients with active localized head and neck cancer via forced continuous enteral alimentation under metabolic ward conditions for 29 days failed to lead to significant weight gain.[28] The mean nitrogen balance in these patients is shown in Figure 72.1. The observed failure of these patients to gain weight despite adequate caloric intake under metabolic ward conditions supports the concept that malnourished cancer patients are hypermetabolic.

If metabolic abnormalities promote the development of malnutrition or interfere with renutrition, then there should be some evidence of abnormally increased energy expenditure. A number of investigators have used indirect calorimetry and the abbreviated Weir formula to calculate energy expenditure at rest and then compared this to the basal energy expenditure (BEE) determined using the Harris–Benedict formulas. Long et al.[29] demonstrated a mean difference of 2% when this comparison was performed in 20 normal controls. In 1980, Bozetti[30] found that 60% of a group of patients with advanced cancer had basal metabolic rates increased 20% above predicted. In 1983, Dempsey et al.[31] studied energy expenditure in a group of 173 malnourished GI cancer patients. Of these, 58% had abnormal resting energy expenditure (REE) by indirect calorimetry compared to BEE, but a greater percentage was hypometabolic rather than hypermetabolic (36 vs. 22%). Knox et al.[32] studied 200 patients with a variety of cancers and found abnormal energy metabolism in 59%, but found more hypometabolic than hypermetabolic individuals (33 vs. 26%). While standard formulae accurately predict metabolic rate in normal individuals, the measured metabolic rates in patients with cancer have a much wider distribution. Controversy remains concerning the importance of REE in cancer-associated malnutrition, however, tumor resection has been shown to normalize REE in hypermetabolic patients.[33] Elevated REE and its role in the pathogenesis of cancer-associated malnutrition may depend upon the individual patient and disease characteristics.[4]

Lean body mass rather than fat mass correlates with the individual variations observed in measured REE. The hypothesis that the malnourished cancer patient may be hypermetabolic relative to the amount of lean body mass remaining has been examined.

Peacock et al.[34] studied REE in noncachectic patients with sarcomas. These patients had no prior treatment, had large localized sarcomas, and no weight loss or history of decreased food intake. REE corrected for body cell mass (BCM) determined by total body potassium counting or body surface area was significantly greater in male sarcoma patients compared to controls. This difference was due to both a decrease in BCM and an increase in REE in these patients before the onset of weight loss.

GLUCOSE AND PROTEIN METABOLISM

Changes in carbohydrate metabolism, similar to those seen in type 2 diabetes, are common in patients with cancer-associated malnutrition. Although glucose turnover is increased, glucose is poorly utilized by peripheral tissues due to insulin resistance and glucose insensitivity.[35,36] Tumors have been demonstrated to increase the rate of glucose utilization in a number of tissues, acting as metabolic traps.[37,38] Since there are only 1200 kcal stored in the body as liver and muscle glycogen, blood glucose levels would be expected to fall. This does not occur since there is also an increase in hepatic glucose production in cachectic and anorectic tumor-bearing animals and humans. The regulation of protein metabolism is tightly linked to carbohydrate metabolism, since these processes are critical to the normal adaptation to starvation or underfeeding. During starvation, there is a decrease in glucose production, protein synthesis, and protein catabolism. The decrease in glucose production occurs as fat-derived fuels, primarily ketone bodies, are used for energy production. While there are 54,000 kcal of protein stored in the BCM, only about half of these are available for energy production. In fact, depletion below 50% of body protein stores is incompatible with life.

Increased turnover of liver and muscle proteins and gluconeogenesis from amino acids of muscle origin are thought to contribute to rapid muscle wasting seen in cancer-associated malnutrition.[36,39] Whole-body protein breakdown is increased in lung cancer patients and has been shown to correlate with the degree of malnutrition such that more malnourished patients have greater elevations of their whole body protein breakdown rates expressed per kg of body weight.[20] The results of metabolic studies in lung cancer patients compared to healthy controls are shown in Table 72.2. Muscle catabolism, measured by 3-methylhistidine excretion, was increased in lung cancer patients compared to that of healthy controls. Methylhistidine excretion rates did not correlate with weight loss, percentage of ideal body weight, or age in the lung cancer patients studied. Glucose production rates were markedly increased in lung cancer patients compared with healthy controls, and changes in glucose production rates in the cancer patients studied did not correlate with weight loss, percent of ideal body weight, or age.

Hydrazine sulfate is a noncompetitive inhibitor of gluconeogenesis. When this drug is administered to lung cancer patients not only does whole body glucose production decrease as expected but there is also a decrease in whole body protein breakdown rates.[40] Increases in glucose production are directly and quantitatively linked to increased protein breakdown and changes in the circulating levels of individual glucogenic amino acids. Table 72.3 shows the influence of hydrazine sulfate on lysine flux. At one month, there was a significant reduction in the hydrazine group, and a nonsignificant increase in the placebo group.

TUMOR AND HOST FACTORS

Inflammation is seen in many forms of cancer in various tissues, and both tumor and host factors are released locally and into the circulation during this process. These factors can promote profound metabolic abnormalities that lead to anorexia, malnutrition, and cachexia. These factors are cytokines, and include tumor necrosis factor-alpha (TNFα) interleukins (IL-1, IL-6) and interferon-gamma (IFN-γ), which are produced by tumor, immune, and stromal cells and can promote angiogenesis and tumor growth and survival,[41] and in many cases provide one means of intercellular communication between tumor cells and the cells of the microenvironment in which they grow. There is also increasing evidence supporting the role for chronic production of these factors in the pathogenesis of cancer-associated malnutrition.[42,43] While an exclusive role for any single cytokine in cancer-associated malnutrition has not been defined, there is growing evidence that the host inflammatory response to a tumor supports the progression to cachexia.

TABLE 72.2

Total Body Protein Turnover, Glucose Production, and 3-Methylhistidine Excretion in the Fasting State on Day 5 of Constant Nitrogen and Calorie Intake in Lung Cancer Patients Compared to Healthy Controls

Group	Protein Turnover (g/kg Day)	Glucose Production (mg/kg min)	3-Methylhistidine Excretion (μmol/g Creatinine Day)
Control	2.12 ± 0.38	2.18 ± 0.06	71 ± 8
Lung cancer	$3.15 \pm 0.51^{a,b}$	2.84 ± 0.16^{a}	106 ± 11^{a}

[a] $p < .05$ vs. control subjects.

[b] Mean $\pm$ S.D.

TABLE 72.3
Whole Body Lysine Flux in Lung Cancer Patients

	Lysine Flux (μmol/h)	
Placebo Group	**Baseline**	**1 Month**
1	2172	2812
2	1869	2959
3	2373	2674
4	2772	2269
5	2758	3195
6	3542	3585
Mean (SD)	2580 (580)	2920 (450)[a,b]
Hydrazine treated		
7	2675	1146
8	2522	2119
9	2666	3129
10	1808	1217
11	2264	1438
12	3114	2006
Mean (SD)	2510 (440)	1840 (750)[b,c]

[a] $p = .08$.

[b] $p < .05$, paired t-tests with baseline.

[c] $p < .01$ by combined paired t-test both groups.

TABLE 72.4
Nutritional Assessment Factors in the Cancer Patient

Involuntary weight loss
Comparison to usual, preillness, or ideal body weight
Anorexia and food intake
Anthropometric measures
Biochemical and cellular biomarkers

ASSESSMENT OF THE CANCER PATIENT'S NUTRITIONAL STATUS

The risk of malnutrition and its severity are affected by the tumor type, stage of the disease and the therapy being applied.[44] Cancer-associated malnutrition can affect the patients response to therapy,[45] and is also associated with reduced wound healing, reduced muscle function, and poor skin turgor that can lead to skin breakdown.[46] Early assessment and intervention is critical in order for nutritional support to improve outcome,[10] with nutritional screening as the first step. For hospitalized patients, initial screening should be performed as soon as possible following admission, or during hospital visits for outpatients, and at regular visits thereafter to identify nutritional decline as early as possible.[47] There are several nutritional assessment factors specific to the cancer patient, and these are listed in Table 72.4. Involuntary weight loss is a key indicator of undernutrition, and it is often a sign associated with a poorer prognosis and survival. The rate of weight loss is also important. Patients should be asked their usual weight, if they have had unintentional weight loss, or if they have been eating less than usual. It is accepted that an involuntary weight loss of 10% of the patient's usual body weight over a period of 6 months or less indicates undernutrition in patients with cancer.[48] The body mass index (BMI) is an expression of weight relative to height [weight (in kg)/height^2 (in m)], and this value can be compared with established cutoff points that classify individuals as severely underweight, underweight, normal, overweight, obese, and morbidly obese (Table 72.5). However, these cutoff points are based on healthy adults, and may not be appropriate in cancer patients. One complicating factor in cancer patients is the development of edema or ascites; these should be kept in mind when interpreting weight data. Tumor mass could also mask loss of weight and lean body mass. Assessment of weight changes over time may be a more appropriate indicator of nutritional decline, with rapid weight loss indicative of more severe malnutrition.[39]

Ideal body weight is the weight associated with optimal survivorship in populations studied by life insurance companies. A commonly used reference is the 1983 Metropolitan Life Insurance Tables. With these tables, ideal weight range is calculated

TABLE 72.5
BMI Cut-Off Points

BMI (kg/m^2)	Interpretation
<16	Severely underweight
16–19	Underweight
20–25	Normal
26–30	Overweight
31–41	Obese
>40	Morbidly obese

based on height, body frame size, and sex, but no adjustments are made for age. Studies undertaken at the Gerontology Research Center (GRC), however, indicate that age significantly affects ideal body weight while sex differences are not significant.[49] For a given height, older subjects have a higher ideal body weight range than younger individuals. Importantly, both tables are based on the same database, except that age is introduced as a variable only by the more recent GRC Tables. Since cancer affects both the young and the aged, with the majority of patients being in the older age groups,[50] it is more appropriate to utilize the age-adjusted tables to calculate ideal body weight range. Serious shortcomings still exist since there is no correction for disease-related changes in height, and no guidelines are provided in these tables for patients 70 years or older.

Current weight compared to the expected or ideal body weight range can help to determine the patient's nutritional status. An additional variable for consideration is usual or preillness weight. Therefore, both information on percent ideal weight and percent usual or preillness weight should be collected on all patients. There are healthy individuals who are below their projected weight for many years. From a clinical standpoint, stable weight and an adequate diet often equate with good nutrition even if the individual is below the ideal body weight range.

Anorexia and decreased food intake have long been recognized as key causes of undernutrition in patients with malignancies.[51,52] Anorexia is a treatable symptom of cancer which, if left untreated, leads to significant patient discomfort in addition to malnutrition.[53]

A thorough dietary assessment should include current food and fluid intake, previous intake and any recent changes. This information can be obtained initially by questioning the patient about a subjective loss of appetite and decrease in food intake. In order to further quantify these changes, the patient can be asked to rate his or her appetite level from 0 to 7 (0 = no appetite; 1 = very poor; 2 = poor; 3 = fair; 4 = good; 5 = very good; 6 = excellent; 7 = always hungry). From a report of usual intake, an indication of the patient's macro- and micronutrient intakes can be gained. The assessment should also aim to detect food aversions, intolerances, and any problems with feeding, such as taste changes.[54] Several screening tools have been developed specifically for cancer patients, including the Oncology Screening Tool,[55] which screens patients for weight loss and includes a 2-week history of decreased food intake, nausea/vomiting, diarrhea, mouth sores, or difficulty with chewing and swallowing.

Detailed anthropometric measurements (such as mid-arm circumference and triceps skin fold) have long been utilized to determine skeletal muscle mass and nutritional status.[56] Although the value of these measurements can be limited if done in the hospital setting, serial measurements by the same professional in the outpatient clinic can help assess the patient's ongoing nutritional state. Problems with these measurements include interobserver variability and interference by edema or patient positioning. The decision to do these measurements should often be individualized according to the acuteness of the underlying process, the availability of trained personnel, and the goals of interventions. It should be noted that muscle wasting and loss of adipose tissue reserves seen on physical examination are important but late signs of undernutrition. Ideally, early diagnosis and intervention should be directed at avoiding this advanced stage of undernutrition or cachexia.

The most common biochemical measurements used to assess nutritional status are blood parameters such as serum albumin, prealbumin, and iron levels. However, these parameters are subject to homeostatic mechanisms and may be altered by underlying disease and treatment. These and other tests can be useful to assess protein depletion but are difficult to interpret in patients with advanced cancer who often have metastases to visceral sites with organ dysfunction as well as metabolic and immunologic derangements due to cancer therapy.

Routine chemistry panels include albumin levels, which can be a useful indication of nutritional state. Albumin has a half-life in the circulation of about 3 weeks. Hypoalbuminemia can result from malnutrition, but is also associated with liver disease, disseminated malignancies, protein-losing enteropathy, nephrotic syndrome, and conditions leading to expanded plasma volume such as congestive heart failure.

Prealbumin has a half-life of just under 2 days and its level may increase with the use of steroid hormones and can be decreased by liver disease, disseminated malignancies, nephrotic syndrome, inflammatory bowel disease, the use of salicylates, or malnutrition.[57,58]

Transferrin can be measured by the transferrin antigen assay; the iron binding capacity provides roughly equivalent results. Transferrin has a half-life of about one week and it may increase with storage iron depletion or the use of hormonal agents, while it may decrease with infection, malignancy, inflammation, liver disease, nephrotic syndrome, or malnutrition.[59]

Absolute lymphocyte counts can be reduced by malnutrition as well as a variety of other factors. More sophisticated tests (bioimpedance, total body K, basal metabolic rate [BMR], and others) are clinical research procedures.[60]

In many instances, a brief clinical nutritional assessment based on the degree of weight loss from usual or preillness weight, current weight as a percentage of usual and ideal body weight, and dietary history is sufficient to determine the clinical situation and consider potential interventions. We therefore reserve the use of anthropometric and laboratory evaluations to specific individual situations. Interpretations of these evaluations should be based on an assessment of the clinical context.

A number of associated conditions are prevalent in older patients and can affect their food intake and nutrition. Mucositis, as a side effect of chemotherapy or radiation therapy is common. Oral pain and dryness, poor dentition, periodontal disease, and ill-fitting dentures are also common. Other problems requiring consideration are dysphagia, alteration in taste, fatigue, nausea, vomiting, and diarrhea or constipation. Pain and other symptoms such as dyspnea can also interfere with nutrition. Depression is a well-known cause of weight loss, and depression can worsen due to the stress of coping with cancer. Feelings of isolation and actual social isolation are not uncommon, especially in those patients who do not have strong family support. Socioeconomic and living conditions must be taken into account because they may affect food availability and preparation. These can all be very serious problems for patients with cancer and require a multidisciplinary effort for proper management. Quality of life assessment provides valuable information regarding the patient's perception of his or her health. The European Organisation for Research and Treatment of Cancer Core Quality of Life Questionnaire (EORTC QLQ-30) is a validated measure of quality of life in cancer patients with five functional scales, three symptoms scales, and one global scale.[61] Other questionnaires have been developed for specific cancers.[62,63]

An understanding of the frequency and severity of malnutrition among cancer patients is necessary to better plan preventive, diagnostic, and therapeutic approaches including the allocation of a variety of resources. To this end and as part of a more comprehensive effort, we studied nutrition-related clinical variables in 644 consecutive oncology patients, regardless of type, status, or stage of cancer. The characteristics of these patients are shown in Table 72.6.

TABLE 72.6
Patient Characteristics in 644 Consecutive Cancer Patients*

Characteristic	Percent of Patients
Age: Median (range) in years: 66 (22–91)	
<65	45
≥65	55
Sex	
Women	53
Men	47
Type of cancer	
Breast	16
Colon/Rectum	14
Leukemia/Lymphoma	13
Lung/Nonsmall cell	14
Prostate	5
Stomach	4
Head/Neck Squamous	4
Ovary	3
Kidney/Urinary Bladder	3
Lung/Small cell	2
All others	22
Stage of cancer	
Metastatic	52
Nonmetastatic	48

* Seen at Pacific Shores Medical Group and St. Mary Medical Center, Long Beach, California.

TABLE 72.7
Nutritional Variables in 644 Consecutive Cancer Patients*

Variable	All Patients ($n = 644$)	Patients with Metastases ($n = 377$)
Decreased appetite	54%	59%
Decreased food intake	61%	67%
Underweight	49%	54%
Normal weight	37%	33%
Overweight	14%	13%
Weight loss		
Any	74%	76%
Up to 5%	15%	15%
>5 to <10%	22%	20%
10–20%	26%	27%
None	26%	24%

* Seen at Pacific Shores Medical Group and St. Mary Medical Center, Long Beach, California.

The majority was seen as outpatients. We divided patients by age (<65 vs. ≥65), and we analyzed the entire group as well as the subset of patients who had metastatic disease. Ideal body weight range was calculated using the GRC tables. The vast majority of the patients sustained the weight loss shown within a period of 6 months from cancer diagnosis.

As can be seen in Table 72.7, the incidence of weight loss is very high in all patients, but particularly in those over the age of 65. Thus, 72% of all patients 65 years or older with metastatic cancer had some degree of weight loss, 56% were underweight, 54% had decreased appetite, and 61% reported a decrease in food intake. Also, 38% of patients 65 years or older with metastatic disease had weight loss of 10% or more of their usual body weight. These data suggest that undernutrition at various stages is highly prevalent among oncology patients, particularly in the older population. Attention to the nutritional status of patients may afford the clinician opportunities for early diagnosis and intervention.

NUTRITIONAL THERAPY OF ANOREXIA AND CACHEXIA

COUNSELING

In patients with cancer, there is an association between poor nutritional parameters and worse overall morbidity and quality of life.[64] The benefits of initial and follow-up evaluations and counseling by a registered dietitian, preferably in the context of a team approach, can be enormous, although difficult to quantify.[65] However, recent studies indicate that improved nutritional intake and quality of life after individualized dietary counseling.[66,67] The main benefits relate to patient satisfaction, nutrition improvement or maintenance, compliance with team or institutional management protocols and guidelines, and a judicious use of risky and expensive treatments. The costs of nutritional counseling are modest when compared to other interventions. Table 72.8 shows the benefits, methodology, and risks of common nutrition interventions. Nutritional evaluation and counseling, usually undertaken by a registered dietitian, is a first and important step. Ideally, a dietitian should be an integral part of the cancer care team. Compliance with dietary advice can be promoted by regular contact between the healthcare provider and the patient, including regular nutritional assessments and advice.[68]

In addition to assessing the clinical nutritional parameters previously outlined, it is our practice to first determine, through the dietary history, whether the patient is consuming a "balanced diet." Nutritional assessment serves to confirm the presence, extent, degree, or severity and type of malnutrition and to determine the nutritional needs of the patient and nutritional support required. The dietitian obtains a 24 to 72 h recall diet history either verbally or, preferably, recorded at home. The diet record is then examined to assess the adequacy of calories and protein utilizing food analysis tables as compared to estimated energy and protein needs. In addition to assessing current food and fluid intake, any recent changes should be noted, along with food aversions, intolerances, or problems with feeding, such as taste changes.[54]

Energy requirements should be based on individual needs. Usually a weight maintenance diet depends on the BEE and is calculated based on the Harris–Benedict formula[24] that, on an average, results in a daily requirement of 20 to 25 kcal/kg of body weight. However, the addition of a stress factor may be necessary depending on weight change or the disease process. For example, a stress factor of between 0 and 20% has been suggested for patients with solid tumors.[69–71] Alterations in protein metabolism are common in the course of cancer, including whole-body protein turnover, increased protein synthesis and catabolism, as well as

TABLE 72.8

Benefits, Methodology, and Risks of Nutrition Interventions

	Benefits	Methodology	Risks
1. Counseling	Patient satisfaction, nutrition maintenance, and adherence to protocols	One initial and two follow-up visits by dietitian	None
2. Food supplements	Nutrition maintenance		Limited risks: diarrhea, nausea
a. Home Made	Avoid or delay need for more expensive therapy	a. Three 8 oz servings = 750 kcal/day	a. Diarrhea with lactose intolerance
b. Commercial		b. Three 8 oz servings = 750–1080 kcal/day	b. Patients may not like taste
3. Appetite stimulants			
a. Megestrol acetate oral suspension	a. Improved appetite, weight, well-being, and quality of life	a. 200 mg/day, 1 month supply; 400 mg/day, 1 month supply; 800 mg/day, 1 month supply	a. Impotence, vaginal bleeding, and deep vein thrombosis
b. Dronabinol	b. Improved appetite and no significant weight change	b. 2.5 mg/day, 1 month supply; 5 mg/day, 1 month supply	b. Euphoria, somnolence, dizziness, and confusion
c. Prednisone	c. Short-term (4 weeks) appetite stimulation. (see text)	c. 40 mg/day, 1 month supply	c. Hypokalemia, muscle weakness, cushingoid features, hyperglycemia, and immune suppression
4. Enteral nutrition	Maintenance of nutrition via enteral route when oral route is not possible	Requires nasogastric, gastrostomy, or jejunostomy tube placement.	Aspiration, diarrhea, nausea, bloating, infection, and bleeding
5. Home parenteral nutrition	Maintenance of nutrition when no other alternative is appropriate. No evidence of improved survival in end-stage cancer	Central catheter surgically placed. Parenteral infusion equipment and parenteral formulas: Dextrose (20–25% w/w), crystalline amino acids (2–4% w/w), and lipid emulsions (500 cc/day → 500 cc/week)	Catheter-related pneumothorax, sepsis, thrombosis, and bleeding. Hepatic dysfunction, fluid, and electrolyte imbalance

an increase in skeletal muscle breakdown. To account for the stress induced by the disease and treatment, protein requirements of cancer patients can be determined by adjusting the estimated requirement for healthy individuals to account for the stress induced by the disease and treatment.[72] Estimated protein requirements range from 1.2 to 2.0 g/kg body weight/day depending on the state of malnutrition and metabolic stress.[36,39]

One goal of nutrition education and counseling is to have the patient increase consumption of nutrient-dense foods to correct nutritional imbalances and deficiencies in order to achieve and maintain a desirable weight. Nutrient-dense foods are those with a high content in calories, protein, fat, and vitamins relative to their volume. Liquid supplements are the most common types of nutritional supplements and are readily available for patient consumption, and are effective when patients are unable to meet requirements with normal foods alone, despite dietary counseling.[66] Patients may be anorectic due to illness or be affected by disabling factors such as difficulty in chewing, inability to prepare foods for themselves, visual difficulties, decreased energy level, or poor access to foods. Nutritional supplements may be homemade and are usually milk based, or they are commercially prepared and packaged. Although somewhat expensive, commercial supplements provide balanced and fortified (vitamin and mineral enriched) nutrition that require little or no preparation.

Not all cancer patients have the same requirements for nutrition. One major difference is whether patients are losing weight or have been treated successfully and are trying to prevent a recurrence through healthful nutrition. In the former case, calorically dense foods including those with low nutrient density can be used to increase the efficiency of calorie conversion to body fat stores. One limitation of this approach is that malnourished, often are limited in their ability to absorb and digest fat due to the effects of malnutrition or enteritis due to radiation or chemotherapy. Therefore, overprescription of high fat foods can in some cases lead to GI distress. Foods containing refined sugar can also be used in these patients, as long as the patient has normal glucose tolerance. Since diabetes is a not uncommon comorbid condition in cancer patients, this is a practical consideration. Listed in Table 72.9 are calorically dense foods and strategies for these types of patients.

FOOD SUPPLEMENTS

Liquid concentrated food supplements providing high calorie and protein, low-volume nutrients, and oral supplementation is the simplest, most natural, and least invasive method of increasing nutrient intake. The benefits of oral supplementation include increased appetite and weight gain, decreased GI toxicity, and improved performance status.[73–75] These products are

TABLE 72.9

Foods Recommended to Increase Calorie and Protein Intake of the Patient with Cancer

Food group	Recommendations
Fruits and vegetables	Fruit juice added to canned fruit; pureed fruit added to milk, cereals, pudding, ice cream, and gelatin; gelatin made with fruit juice to replace water; tender, cooked vegetables (mashed white or sweet potatoes, squash, spinach, and carrots); vegetables added to soups and sauces; vegetables in cream or cheese sauces
Grains	Hot cereals prepared with milk instead of water; high protein noodles; noodles or rice in casseroles and soups; breaded and floured meats; bread or rice pudding; dense breads (i.e. bagels) and dense cereals (granolas, mueslis)
Beverages	Milk beverages; shakes made with fruit juices and sherbet when milk is not tolerated
Milk and calcium equivalents	Custards; milkshakes; ice cream; yogurt; cheeses; cheesecake; double strength milk (1 quart fluid milk mixed with 1 cup nonfat dry milk powder); cottage cheese; flavored milk; pudding; commercial eggnog; cream soups; nonfat dry milk powder added to puddings, soups, sauces and gravies, casseroles, and mixed dishes
Meat and protein equivalents	Diced or ground meat; casseroles; smooth peanut butter; cheese; egg and egg dishes; chopped, diced, or pureed meats mixed with soups, sauces, and gravies; fish, poultry, and vegetable protein meat substitutes; tuna, meat, or cheese in cream sauces
Fats	Margarine or oil added to vegetables, hot cereals and casseroles; cream used in place of milk or added to fruits and desserts; sour cream; salad dressings; mayonnaise mixed with tuna, egg, and chicken salad
Sweets	Desserts made with dry milk powder, peanut butter, or eggs

particularly helpful when patients cannot maintain an adequate intake through a regular diet but are able to swallow and have a relatively intact GI tract.

Dietitians can help patients select products based on tolerance and palatability. Commercially prepared supplements are available in a variety of flavors (including unflavored) and in a variety of nutrient compositions. Most commercially prepared supplements are available in ready-to-drink cans or boxes and are usually lactose free, which for the patient is often more acceptable due to the increased incidence of perceived milk intolerance in this population. Vitamin and mineral fortified protein meal replacements designed to be mixed with milk provide an inexpensive and generally well-tolerated alternative for those who are not lactose intolerant. These supplements have vitamin, mineral, calorie, fat, carbohydrate, and protein content similar to most commercially prepared supplements.

Most 8-oz commercial supplements supply 1.0 to 1.5 kcal/ml, 8 to 15 g of protein, 5 to 12 g of fat and are fortified with vitamins and minerals. When patients have difficulty in consuming adequate volumes of enteral supplement, then a high-caloric supplement containing 2 kcal/ml, for example Novasource 2.0 [Novartis Pharmaceuticals] or TwoCal HN [Abbott Laboratories] can be used. The success of supplementation depends on sufficient quantities being consumed over an extended period of time. Acceptability and palatability of the supplement are key, and flavor, texture, and volume are all important.[77]

The volume and choice of supplement is based on patient's individual nutrient needs and preferences, and GI tolerance. Supplements with fiber, generally soy or oat fiber, are available and may be beneficial to the patient who has diarrhea or constipation. Nutritional supplements are generally well accepted and may offer relief to a patient who has difficulties eating solid food. Tolerability can be enhanced by starting with small quantities and by diluting the supplement with water or ice to decrease osmolality. A patient will usually accept one to three 8-oz supplements per day, but there is great individual variability. Variety in supplements will help patients avoid taste fatigue, which is one main drawback to oral supplementation.[78] Patients who have alterations in taste or nausea may better tolerate an unflavored supplement.

A common concern of patients and families is whether adding vitamins and other micronutrients to the patient's diet is beneficial. An analysis of the dietary record for the recommended number of servings from the Basic Four Food Groups (milk, meat and meat substitutes, vegetable and fruit, and grain) helps establish whether the minimum vitamin and mineral requirements are met. A computerized diet analysis program can help to quickly and accurately assess the nutrient content including vitamins and minerals. When intake is inadequate, we prescribe a daily multivitamin.

Patients should be provided with practical dietary advice about how to improve daily caloric intake, and the following are some simple tips to increase food intake:

- Avoid favorite foods after highly emetogenic chemotherapy to prevent the development of food aversions.
- Emphasize consumption of higher-calorie foods that are still "nutrient dense" foods as part of main meals or snacks, that is, fruit juices, cheeses, whole milk, and yogurt.
- Avoid the "Why don't you eat?" complaint. The patient should not be psychologically punished by the cancer care team or the family for not eating but rather should be supported to overcome anorexia and other problems that lead to decreased food intake.
- Emphasize the pleasurable as well as social aspects of meals. Encourage patients to have their meals in a relaxed, friendly, and familiar atmosphere.

- Moderate alcohol intake is usually compatible with treatments and should be allowed before meals unless contraindicated.
- Avoid odors that can cause nausea. A short walk outside while meals are being prepared is advisable.
- Encourage food supplements and snacks between meals without being concerned that they may affect intake at mealtime.

Patients are often deeply interested in the topic of nutrition as an unproven treatment. However, many will not bring up this topic unless encouraged and listened to in a nonjudgmental fashion. Open discussion and patient education may help prevent untoward effects of unbalanced diets and introduce nutrition-related issues into the mainstream of oncology care.

OTHER THERAPIES

A number of alternative therapies are being used by cancer patients in addition to standard medical oncology therapy,[79] and these are listed in Table 72.10. For this chapter, the nutrition alternatives will be outlined without reference to acupuncture or other nonnutritional therapies. Often patients fail to indicate that they are using these nutritional therapies. A number of potential side effects and concerns, listed in Table 72.11, may arise and need to be addressed.

Until recently, most vitamin and herb preparations were thought to be nontoxic. Recent animal studies suggest that antioxidants may affect tumor biology. The α Tocopherol β Carotene Cancer Prevention Study (ATBC) and β Carotene and Retinol Efficacy Trial (CARET) trials[77] in smokers demonstrated an increased incidence of lung cancer following the administration of β-carotene at a dose of 30 mg/day. There were no cancer-stimulatory effects noted with these doses of β-carotene in nonsmokers in a large heart disease prevention trial. However, there remains real uncertainty as to the safety of vitamins and mineral supplementation during chemotherapy or radiation therapy. For the large numbers of patients being diagnosed today with early cancers of the breast and prostate, vitamin supplementation is as safe as in the general population once the treatment has been completed, and nutritional intervention may prevent or delay cancer recurrence. However, the possibility of antioxidant effects on tumor biology or the effectiveness of antitumor drugs on radiation therapy requires much more research before general recommendations can be made. Administration of cytotoxic drugs results in oxidative stress, which may interfere with cytotoxic effects or contribute to side effects. Antioxidants may enhance the anticancer effects of chemotherapy by detoxifying reactive oxygen species.[81–84]

Accumulating evidence supporting a role for inflammatory mediators in the pathogenesis of cancer-associated malnutrition has led to the suggestion that dietary supplement with antiinflammatory properties may be beneficial.[85] Eicosapentaenoic acid (EPA) is an essential long-chain n-3 polyunsaturated fatty acid. Individual studies have indicated that EPA can attenuate cancer-related wasting, improve immune function, halt or reverse weight loss, modulate the acute-phase response, or prolong survival in some patients.[86–89] However, results are not consistent for all cancer populations, and further studies would serve to confirm these studies in different cancer groups. At this time, each patient and each oncologist must decide on the advisability of a given regimen for a given cancer patient based on clinical criteria without the benefit of a large scientific basis of controlled trials.

TABLE 72.10
Alternative Nutritional Therapies Being Used by Cancer Patients

Multivitamins and single-vitamin supplements
Low-fat-, high-fiber-, and soy-protein-supplemented diets
Specific macrobiotic diets
Vegetable and grass juicing
Herbal supplements (green tea extract, antioxidants)
Chinese herbal medicine (mushrooms, teas, roots)

TABLE 72.11
Potential Side Effects and Concerns

Vitamin toxicities (e.g. vitamin A >5000 IU/day)
Possible vitamin effects on tumor biology (apoptosis, proliferation)
Vitamin imbalances and conditioned deficiencies
Drug–nutrient interactions

REFERENCES

1. Laviano, A. and Meguid, M.M. *Nutrition* 12: 358, 1996.
2. Bozzetti, F. In: *Artificial Nutrition Support in Clinical Practice*, 2nd ed. Payne-James J., Grimble. G. and Silk, D., eds. GMM, London, 2001, 639.
3. Brennan, M.F. *Cancer Res* 58: 1867, 1977.
4. Bosaeus, I. et al. *Intl J Cancer* 93: 380, 2001.
5. Andreyev, H.J. et al. *Eur J Cancer* 34: 503, 1998.
6. Zeiderman, M.R. and McMahon, M.J. *Clin Nutr* 8: 161, 1989.
7. Meguid, M.M. et al. *Surg Clin North Am* 66: 1167, 1986.
8. van Bokhorst-de van der Schueren, M.A. et al. *Clin Nutr* 19: 437, 1997.
9. Jagoe, R.T., Goodship, T.H. and Gibson, G.J. *Ann Thoracic Surg* 71: 936, 2001.
10. MacDonald, N. *J Supportive Oncol* 1: 279, 2003.
11. Brennan, M.F. *New Eng J Med* 305: 375, 1981.
12. Shike, M. et al. *Ann Int Med* 101: 303, 1984.
13. Argiles, J.M. et al. *Drug Discovery Today* 8: 838, 2003.
14. Argiles, J.M. et al. *Curr Opin Clin Nutr Metab Care* 6: 401, 2003.
15. Argiles, J.M. et al. *Int J Biochem Cell Biol* 35: 405, 2003.
16. Chlebowski, R.T. and Heber, D. *Cancer Res* 42: 2495, 1982.
17. Holroyde, C.P. et al. *Cancer Res* 35: 3710, 1975.
18. Chlebowski, R.T. and Heber, D. *Surg Clin North Am* 66: 957, 1986.
19. Burt, M.E. et al. *Cancer* 53: 1246, 1984.
20. Heber, D. et al. *Cancer Res* 42: 4815, 1982.
21. Jeevanandam, M. et al. *Metabolism* 35: 304, 1986.
22. Shaw, J.H.F. and Wolfe, R.R. *Ann Surg* 205: 368, 1987.
23. Bennegard, K., Lundgren, F. and Lundholm, K. *Clin Physiol* 6: 539, 1986.
24. Byerley, L.O. et al. *Cancer* 67: 2900, 1991.
25. Warren, S. *Am J Med Sci* 184: 610, 1932.
26. Terepka, A.R. and Waterhouse, C. *Am J Med* 20: 225, 1956.
27. Fenninger, L.D. and Mider, G.B. *Adv Cancer Res* 2: 229, 1954.
28. Heber, D. et al. *Cancer* 58: 1867, 1986.
29. Long, C.L. et al. *J Parent Ent Nutr* 5: 366, 1981.
30. Bozzetti, F., Pagnoni, A.M. and Del Vecchio, M. *Surg Gynecol Obst* 150: 229, 1980.
31. Dempsey, D.T. et al. *Cancer* 53: 1265, 1984.
32. Knox, L.S., Crosby, L.O., Feurer, I.D. et al. *Ann Surg* 197: 152, 1983.
33. Fredrix, E.W., Staal-van den Brekel, A.J. and Wouters, E.F. *Cancer* 79: 717, 1997.
34. Peacock, J.L. et al. *Surgery* 102: 465, 1987.
35. Rofe, A.M. et al. *Anticancer Res* 14: 647, 1994.
36. Mutlu, E.A. and Mobarhan, S. *Nutr Clin Care* 3: 3, 2000.
37. Argiles, J.M. and Azcon-Bieto, J. *J Mol Cell Biochem* 81: 3, 1988.
38. Heber, D. *Nutrition* 5: 135, 1989.
39. Nitenberg, G. and Raynard, B. *Crit Rev in Oncology/Hematology* 34: 137, 2000.
40. Tayek, J., Heber, D. and Chlebowski, R.T. *Lancet* 2: 241, 1987.
41. Robinson, S.C. and Coussens, L.M. *Adv* Cancer Res 93: 159, 2005.
42. Strassmann, G. and Kambayashi, T. *Cytok Mol Ther* 1: 107, 1995.
43. Plata-Salaman, C.R. *Nutrition* 16: 1009, 2000.
44. Shike, M. and Brenna, M.F. In *Cancer: Principles and Practice of Oncology*. DeVita, V.T.R., Hellman, S. and Rosenberg, S.A., eds. JB Lippincott, Philadelphia, PA, 1989, 2029.
45. DeWys, W.D. et al. *Am J Med* 69: 491, 1980.
46. Langer, C.J., Hoffman, J.P. and Ottery, F.D. *Nutrition* 17: 1S, 2001.
47. Holder, H. *Br J Nursing* 12: 667, 2003.
48. Blackburn, G. et al. *JPEN* 1: 11, 1977.
49. Andres, R. et al. *Ann Intern Med* 103: 1030, 1985.
50. Boring, C., Squires, T. and Tong, T. *CA: A Cancer J Clin* 41: 19, 1991.
51. DeWys, W. *Semin Oncol* 12: 452, 1985.
52. Theologides, A. *Cancer* 43: 2013, 1979.
53. Tchekmedyian, N.S. et al. *Oncology* 4: 185, 1990.
54. Baker, F. et al. *Psycho-oncology* 11: 273, 2002.
55. MSKCC Adult Oncology Screening Tool, Clinical Dietittian Staff 1994–1995, Food Service Department, Memorial Sloan-Kettering Cancer Center.
56. Chumlea, W.C. and Baumgartner, R.N. *Am J Clin Nutr* 50: 1158, 1989.

57. Henry, J.B. Clinical Chemistry. In: *Clinical Diagnosis and Management by Laboratory Methods*, 18th ed. WB Saunders Co., Philadelphia, PA, 1991, 316.

58. Sacherk, R.A., McPhersonk, R.A. and Campos, J.M. Table 9–11. Serum Proteins of Diagnostic Significance, In: *Widmann's Clinical Interpreter of Laboratory Tests*, 10th ed., FA Davis Company, Philadelphia, PA, 1991, 352.

59. Brittenham, G.M. Disorders of Iron Metabolism: Iron Deficiency and Overload, In: *Hematology: Basic Principles and Practice*. Ronald Hoffman, eds. Churchill Livingstone Inc., New York, 1991, 334.

60. Harrisk, J.A. and Benedict, F.G. Biometric Studies of Basal Metabolism in Man. Publication no. 279. Carnegie Institute of Washington, DC, 1919.

61. Aaronsonk, N.K. et al. *J Natl Cancer Inst* 85: 365–376, 1993.

62. Kaptein, A.A., Morita, S. and Sakamoto, J. *World J Gastroenterol* 11: 3189, 2005.

63. Avis, N.E., Crawford, S. and Manuel, J. *J Clin Oncology* 23: 3322, 2005.

64. Ravasco, P.M. et al. *Supportive Care in Cancer* 12: 246, 2004.

65. Chlebowski, R.T. et al. *Cancer* 58: 183, 1986.

66. Ravasco, P.M., Monteiro-Grillo, I. and Camilo, M.E. *Radiother Oncol* 67: 213, 2003.

67. Ravasco, P.M. et al. *J Clin Oncol* 23: 1341, 2005.

68. Wickham, R.S. et al. *Onc Nursing Forum* 26: 697, 1999.

69. Parenteral and Enteral Nutrition Group of the British Dietetic Association (PEN group). A Pocket Guide to Clinical Nutrition, 3rd ed, The British Dietetic Association, 2004.

70. Hyltander, A. et al. *Eur J Cancer* 27: 9, 1991.

71. Barak, N., Wall-Alonso, E. and Sitrin, M.D. *J Parenteral Ent Nutr* 26: 231, 2002.

72. McAtear, C.A., Arrowsmith, H. and McWhirter, J. Current perspectives on Enternal Nutrition in Adults. A report by the Working Party of the Brisih Association for Parenteral and Enteral Nutrition (BAPEN), Maidenhead, 1999.

73. Bounous, G., Gentile, J.M. and Hugon, J. *Can J Surg* 14: 312, 1971.

74. Nayel, H., el-Ghoneimy, E. and el-Haddad, S. *Nutrition* 8: 13, 1992.

75. Ovesen, L. and Allingstrup, L. *J Parenteral Enteral Nutr* 16: 275, 1992.

76. Barber, M.D. et al. *Br J Cancer* 81: 80, 1999.

77. Bell, E.A., Roe, L.W. and Rolls, B.J. *Physiol Behav* 78: 593, 2003.

78. Rivadeneiera, D.E. et al. *CA: A Cancer J Clin* 48: 69, 1998.

79. Wargovich, M.J. *Curr Opin Gastroenterol* 15: 177, 1999.

80. Albanes, D. et al. *J Natl Cancer Inst* 88: 1560, 1996.

81. Prasad, K.N. et al. *J Am Coll Nutr* 18: 13, 1999.

82. Conklin, K.A. *Nutr and Cancer* 37: 1, 2000.

83. Lamson, D.W. and Brignall, M.S. *Alternative Med Review* 5: 152, 2000.

84. Lamson, D.W. and Brignall, M.S. *Alternative Med Review* 5: 196, 2000.

85. McCarthy, D.O. *Biol Res Nurs* 5: 3, 2003.

86. Tisdale, M.J. *Nutrition* 12: 31S, 1996.

87. Gogos, C.A. et al. *Cancer* 15: 395, 1998.

88. Barber, M.D. et al. *J Nutr* 129: 1120, 1999.

89. Fearon, K.C. et al. *Gut* 52: 1479, 2003.

73 Drugs Used in Treatment or Management of Human Diseases

Carolyn D. Berdanier

CONTENTS

Chronic and acute diseases are often managed using both drugs and nondrug therapies. Pharmaceutical research has resulted in a wide array of drugs that are useful in helping the body return to its predisease state. For some conditions there is a large selection of drugs to choose from, whereas for other conditions the number of drugs available is very small. Some conditions have no pharmaceutical treatments. No drug is without risk. The physician prescribing the drug must weigh the risk of the drug against its possible benefit knowing that there are some diseases that are fatal if left without treatment and also knowing that some drugs have major side effects that can compromise an individual's well-being. The basic function of pharmaceuticals is to help the body repair itself. If it fails to do this, then the drug has no merit. If it harms the body with no benefit, then the drug not only has no merit but is contraindicated totally and should not be used. There are individual differences in drug tolerances. That is, there can be broad ranges of effectiveness from individual to individual. This can explain why an individual drug may be very effective in one person but not very effective in another. In addition, many drugs may be effective in the individual, but may have deleterious effects on the unborn child if the individual taking the drug is pregnant. Many antiviral drugs fall into this category.

Although antiviral drugs are antibiotics in the sense that they interfere with viral activity, the term antibiotic is usually used for that group of drugs that target pathogenic bacteria. A strict definition of the term antibiotic is, the compound in question is the product of one organism against another organism. The actinomycetes, for example, were found to produce streptomycin that attacked gram-negative bacteria. Other bacteria were found to produce penicillin, which in turn destroyed gram-positive bacteria. Scientists have learned to modify the original penicillin structure such that new compounds have been made with different characteristics, which in turn change the effectiveness of the drug against a wider variety of pathogenic bacteria. Other examples can be found and the compounds these organisms produce can be isolated, purified, studied, and, if effective, used to help people harboring their target bacteria. Antibiotics fall into eleven categories based on their structure, composition, and mechanism of action. These are listed in Table 73.1.

Antifugal drugs likewise are not included in the antibiotic drug group. They target pathogenic fungi and are usually synthetic compounds that interfere with the metabolism and function of fungi.

Table 73.2 provides the generic drug name, the brand name of that drug, and a definition and use for the drug. In this table drugs are listed alphabetically by generic name within groups of drugs with similar functions. There may be a number of formulations for the same drug and the list may not give all these formulations. Likewise, some drugs have so many brand names that some of them could not be listed in this table. The user should look for the generic name rather than the brand name when seeking information about a given drug.

Hormones, although not strictly drugs, are listed because many have pharmaceutical activity in addition to their use as hormone replacements. For example, there are many formulations of glucocorticoid that are used as anti-inflammatory drugs. Some vitamins and some mineral compounds can be used as drugs, but they are not listed in this table. Similarly, some compounds, although used pharmaceutically, are not included because they are not considered drugs per se. An example of this is charcoal or activated charcoal, which is sometimes administered to adsorb ingested noxious compounds or compounds produced by the body in the course of the breakdown of food in the gastrointestinal tract. An example of the former is the use of activated charcoal to adsorb a potentially noxious ingested chemical. The charcoal increases the excretion of that chemical before it can be absorbed into the body and harm it. An example of the latter is the use of activated charcoal to reduce the noxious gases produced and released (flatus) following the ingestion of dried beans and pulses. The undigested carbohydrates are acted on by the flora in the intestines and produce short-chain fatty acids as well as a variety of gases. These gases can be noxious.

Some drugs have multiple actions. They may serve as vasodilators and also as antiarrhythmic drugs; both actions are listed. Hormones, as mentioned, fall into this category. They may be hormone replacements and antineoplastic or they may be hormone

TABLE 73.1
Categories of Antibiotics[1,2]

Category	Example
1. Carbohydrate-containing compounds	Nojirimycin, Streptomycin, Everninomicin, Streptothricin, Vancomycin, Moenomycin
2. Macrocyclic lactones	Erythromycin, Candicidin, Rifampin
3. Quinones	Tetracycline, Adriamycin, Mitomycin
4. Amino acid and peptide analogs	Cycloserine, Penicillin, Bacitracin, Actinomycin, Valinomycin, Bleomycin
5. Heterocyclic compounds containing nitrogen	Polyoxins
6. Heterocyclic compounds containing oxygen	Monensin
7. Alicyclic derivatives	Cycloheximide, Fusidic acid
8. Aromatic compounds	Chloramphenicol, Griseafulvin, Novabiocin
9. Aliphatic compounds	Fostomycin
10. Quinolone compounds	Nalidixic acid, Norfloxacin
11. Oxazolidininone	2-Oxazolidinone

TABLE 73.2
Drugs Used for the Management of Medical Problems [1,2]

Generic Names	Brand Names	Description/Function
Antiviral Drugs		
Abacavir sulfate	Ziagen	Antiviral, antiretroviral
Acyclovir sodium	Avirax, Zovirax	Synthetic purine nucleoside; antiviral
Adefovir dipivoxil	Hepera	Cyclic nucleotide analogue; antiviral
Amantadine HCl	Symadine; Symmetrel	Synthetic cyclic primary amine; antiviral; antiparkinsonian
Amprenavir	Agenerase	HIV protease inhibitor; sulfonamide; antiretroviral
Cidofovir	Vistide	Nucleotide analog; antiviral
Delavirdine mesylate	Rescriptor	Nonnucleoside reverse transcriptase inhibitor; antiretroviral
Didanosine	Videx, Videx EC	Purine analog; antiviral
Docosanol	Abreva	Bethenyl alcohol; antiviral
Efavirenz	Sustiva	Nonnucleoside reverse transcrptase inhibitor, antiretroviral
Famciclovir	Famvir	Synthetic acyclic guanine derivative; antiviral
Foscarnet sodium	Foscavir	Pyrophosphate analogue; antiviral
Ganciclovir	Cytovene	Synthetic nucleoside; antiviral
Indinavir sulfate	Crixivan	HIV protease inhibitor; antiviral
Lamivudine	Epivir, Epivir-HBV	Synthetic nucleoside analogue; antiviral
Lamivudine plus zidovudine	Combivir	
Lopinavir and ritonavir	Keletra	Protease inhibitor; antiviral
Nelfinavir mesylate	Viracept	HIV protease inhibitor; antiviral
Nevirapine	Viramune	Nonnucleoside reverse transcriptase inhibitor; antiviral
Oseltamir phosphate	Tamiflu	Neuraminidase inhibitor; antiviral
Peginterferon α2a	Pegasys	Biological Response mofffdifier; antiviral
Ritonavir	Norvir	HIV protease inhibitor; antiviral
Saquinavir	Fortovase	Protease inhibitor; antiviral
Saquinavir mesylate	Invirase	
Tenofovir disoproxil fumarate	Viread	Nucleotide reverse transcriptase inhibitor; antiviral; antiretroviral
Valacyclovir HCl	Valtrex	Synthetic purine nucleoside; antiviral
Valacyclovir	Valcyte	
Zalcitabine	Hivid	Nucleoside analog; antiviral
Zanamivir	Relenza	Neuraminidase inhibitor; antiviral
Zidovudine	Apo-zudovudine, Retrovir, Novo-AZT	Thymidine analogue; antiviral

Continued

TABLE 73.2
(Continued)

Generic Names	Brand Names	Description/Function
Antibiotic Drugs		
Amikacin sulfate	Amikin	Aminoglycoside; antibiotic
Amoxicillin and Clavulanate potassium	Augmentin, Clavulin Augmentin ES-600, Augmentin SR	Aminopenicillin, β-lactamase inhibitor, Antibiotic to gram-negetive and gram-positive bacteria
Amoxicillin trihydrate	Amoxil, Apo-amoxi, Novomoxin, Trinox, Nu-amoxi	Aminopennicillin; antibiotic
Ampicillin	Apo-Ampi, Novo-Ampicillin,	Aminopenicillin; antibiotic
Ampicillin sodium	Ampicin, Penbritin	
Ampicilline trihydrate	Principen	
Ampicillin sodium and Sulbactam sodium	Unasyn	Aminopenicillin and β-lactamase inhibitor combination; antibiotic
Azithromycin	Zithromax	Azalide macrlide; antibiotic
Aztreonam	Azactam	Monobactam; antibiotic
Cefaclor	Ceclor	Second-generation cephalosporin; antibiotic
Cefadroxil monohydrate	Duricef	First-generation cephalosporin; antibiotic
Cefazolin sodium	Ancef	First-generation cephalosporin; antibiotic
Cefdinir	Omnicef	Broad-spectrum cephalosporin; antibiotic
Cefditoren pivoxil	Spectracef	Semisynthetic third-generation cephalosporin; antibiotic
Cefepime HCl	Maxipime	Semisynthetic cephalosporin; antibiotic
Cefoperazone sodium	Cefobid	Third-generation cephalosporin; antibiotic
Cefotaxime sodium	Claforan	Third-generation cephalosporin; antibiotic
Cefotan disodium	Cefotan	Second-generation cephalosporin; antibiotic cephamycin
Cefoxitin sodium	Mefoxin	Second-generation cephalosporin; antibiotic, cephamycin
Cefpodoxime proxetil	Vantin	Third-generation cephalosporin; antibiotic
Cefprozil	Cetzil	Second-generation cephalosporin; antibiotic
Ceftazidime	Captaz, Fortaz, Tazicef, Tazidime	Third-generation cephalosporin; antibiotic
Ceftibuten	Cedax	Third-generation cephalosporin; antibiotic
Ceftizoxime sodium	Cefizox	Third generation cephalosporin; antibiotic
Ceftriaxone sodium	Rocephin	Third-generation cephalosporin; antibiotic
Cefuroxime axetil	Ceftin	Second-generation cephalosporin; antibiotic
Cefuroxime sodium	Zinacef	
Cephalexin HCl	Keftab	First-generation cephalosporin; anttibiotic
Cephalexin monohydrate	Apo-Cephalex, Biocef, Keflex	
Ciprofloxacin	Cipro, Cipro IV, Cipro XR	Fluroquinolone; antibiotic
Ciprofloxacin HCl	Ciloxan	Fluroquinolone; antibiotic
Clarithromycin	Biaxin, Biaxin XL	Macrolide; antibiotic
Clindamycin HCl	Cleocin, Dalacin C	Lincomycin derivative; antibiotic
Clindamycin palmitate HCl	Cleocin Pediatric, Delacin C Palmitate	
Clindamycin phosphate	Cleocin phosphate, Cleocin T, Delacin C phosphate	
Co-trimoxazole (trimethoprim-sulfamethoxazole)	Apo-sulfatrim, Bactrim DS, Septra, SMZ-TMP, Sulfatrim	Sulfonamide and folate antagonist; antibiotic
Erythromycin(many forms)	E-Mycin, Eramycin, Eryc, Robimycin, ilosone, etc.	Erythromycin; antibiotic
Doxycycline (many forms)	Vibramycin	Tetracycline; antibiotic
Gatifloxacin	Tequin	Fluoroquinolone; antibiotic
Gentimycin sulfate (systemic)	Cidomycin, Garamycin Gentamycin sulfate, Jenamicin	Aminoglycoside; antibiotic
Imipenem and cilastatin	Primaxin	Carbapenem (thienamycin class) β-lactam antibiotic
Levofloxacin	Levoquin	Fluoroquinolone; antibiotic
Linezolid	Zyvox	Oxazolidinone; antibiotic
Loracarbef	Lorabid	Synthetic β-lactam antibiotic
Minocycline GCl	Alti-minocycline, etc.	Tetracycline; antibiotic
Moxifloxacin HCl	Avelox	Fluoroquinolone; antibiotic

Continued

TABLE 73.2
(Continued)

Generic Names	Brand Names	Description/Function
Antibiotic Drugs (Continued)		
Nafcillin sodium	Nafcillin	Penicillinase-resistant penicillin; antibiotic
Ofloxacin	Floxin	Fluoroquinolone; antibiotic
Penicillin (many forms)	Bacillin L-A, Permapen (many preparations)	Natural penicillin; antibiotic
Piperacillin sodium	Pipracil	Extended-spectrum penicillin; antibiotic
Piperacillin and tazobactam	Zosyn	Extended-spectrum penicillin and β-inhibitor; antibiotic
Probenecid	Benemid, Benuryl	Sulfonamide derivative; uricosuric
Quinupristin and dalfopristin	Synercid	Streptogramin; antibiotic
Rifabutin	Mycobutin	Semisynthetic ansamycin; antibiotic
Sulfasalazine	Azulfidine	Sulfonamide; antibiotic
Tetracycline HCl	Achromycin, Apo-Tetra, Sumycin, Topicycline, etc.	Tetracycline; antibiotic
Ticarcillin disodium	Ticar	Extended-spectrum penicillin; antibiotic
Ticarcillin disodium and Clavulanate potassium	Timentin	β-lactamase inhibitor; antibiotic
Tobramycin	AKTob, Tobrex	Aminoglycoside; antibiotic
Vancomycin HCl	Lyphocin, Vancocin	Glycopeptide; antibiotic
Antifungals		
Griseofulvin	Fulvicin-U/F, Grisactin, Grisovin-FP	PCN antibiotic; antifungal
Metronidazole	Flagyl, Protostat, Apo-metronidazole,Trikacide	Nitroimidazole; antibacterial, antiprotozoal amebocide
Nitazoxanide	Alinia, Cryptaz	Antiprotozoan; antidiarrheal, anti-infective
Amphotericin B	Amphocin, Fungizone IV, Amphotericin B	Polyene macrolide; antifungal
Amphotericin B cholestyl sulfate complex	Amphotec	Polyene macrolide; antifungal
Amphotericin B lipid Complex	Abelcet	Polyene antibiotic; antifungal
Amphotericin B Liposome	AmBisone	Polyene antibiotic; antifungal
Fluconazole	Difluican	*bis*-Triazole derivative; antifungal
Caspofungin acetate	Cancidas	Glucan synthesis inhibitor; antifungal
Clotrimazole	Canestron Vaginal, Gyne-Lotrimin, Lotrimin, Mycelex	Synthetic imidazole derivative; antifungal
Itraconazole	Sporanox	Synthetic triazole; antifungal
Ketoconazole	Nizoral	Imidazole derivative; antifungal
Miconazole nitrate	Micatin, Monistate, etc.	Imidazole derivative; antifungal
Nystatin	Mycostatin, Nasostine, Nilstat, Nystex	Polyene macrolide; antifungal
Terbinafine HCl	Lamisil	Synthetic allylamine derivative; antifungal
Voriconazole	Vfend	Synthetic triazole; antifungal
Anti-infectives		
Carbamide peroxide	Debrox	Urea hydrogen peroxide; ceruminolytic, Topical antiseptic
Ertapenem	Invanz	Carbapenem; anti-infective
Nitrofurantoin	Macrobid, Macrodantin, Furadantin	Nitrofuran; urinary tract anti-infective
Amifostine	Ethyol	Organic thiophosphate; cytoprotective
Drotrecogin alfa	Xigris	Recombinant human activated protein C; anti-infective
Filgrastin	Neurogen	Granulocyte colony stimulant; biologic response modifier
Pegfilgrastin	Neulasta	Colony-stimulating factor, neutrophil growth stimulant
Sargramostin	Leukine	Granulocyte-stimulating factor
Ethambutol HCl	Etibi, Myambutol	Semisynthetic antituberculotic
Isoniazid	Isotamine, Laniazid, Nydrazid, PMS-isoniazid	Isonicotinic acid hydrazine; antituberculotic
Rifampin	Rifadin, Rimactane, Rofact	Semisynthetic rifamycin B derivative; antituberclotic
Rifapentine	Priffin	RNA polymerase inhibitor; antituberculotic
Cisplatin	Platinol	Alkalating agent; antineoplastic
Docetaxel	Taxotere	Taxoid; antineoplastic

Continued

TABLE 73.2
(Continued)

Generic Names	Brand Names	Description/Function
Anti-infectives (Continued)		
Estrogens (many forms)	Estratabs, Menest, etc.	Estrogen replacement, antineoplastic
Fluorouricil (5FU)	Adrucil, Carac, Efudex, Fluoroplex	Substituted uricil; antimetabolite; antineoplastic
Fulvestrant	Faslodex	Estrogen receptor antagonist; antineoplastic
Imatinib mesylate	Gleevec	Protein tyrosine kinase inhibitor; antineoplastic
Medroxyprogesterone acetate and combinations with estrogen	Amen, Curretab, Cyprin, Provera, Depo-provera	Progestin; contraceptive, antineoplastic
Methotrexate	Folex PFS, Mexate-AQ Rheumatrex	Antimetabolite; antineoplastic; antifolate
Paclitaxel	Taxol	Antimicrotubule agent; antineoplastic
Oxaliplatin	Eloxatin	Alkalating drug, antineoplastic
Testosterone (many preparations)	Depo-testosterone, etc.	Androgen: androgen replacement antineoplastic
Vinblastine sulfate	Velbane, Velbe	Vinca alkaloid; antineoplastic
Vincristine sulfate	Oncovin, Vincasar PFS	Vinca alkaloid; antineoplastic
Tacrolimus	Protopic	Macrolide; immunosuppressant
Tamoxifen citrate	Nolvadex	Nonsteroidal antiestrogen; antineoplastic
Triptorelin pamoate	Trelstar Depot	Sythetic luteinizing hormone-releasing hormone analog; antineoplastic
Zafirlukast	Accolate	Antileukotriene; anti-inflammatory
Antidiabetic Drugs		
Acarbose	Precose	α-Glucosidase inhibitor; antidiabetic
Glimepiride	Amaryl	Sulfonylurea; antidiabetic
Glipizide	Glucotrol, Glucotrol XL	Sulfonylurea; antidiabetic
Glipizide and Metformin	Metaglip	Sulfonylurea and biguanide; antidiabetic
Glyburide (glibenclamidol)	DiaBeta, Euglucon, Glynase Pres Tab, Micronase	Sulffonylurea; antidiabetic
Insulin(many forms)	Humulin, Humalog, NPH insulin Novolin, etc.	Pancreatic hormone; antidiabetic
Glucagon	Glucagon	Antihypoglycemic
Metformin HCl	Glucophage, Glucophage XR	Biguanide; antidiabetic
Miglitol	Glyset	α-Glucosidase inhibitor; antidiabetic
Nateglinide	Starlix	Amino acid derivative; antidiabetic
Pioglitazone HCl	Actos	Thiazolidine; antidiabetic
Repaglinide	Prandin	Meglitinide; antidiabetic
Rosiglitazone maleate	Avandia	Thiazolidinedione; antidiabetic
Rosiglitazone maleate and metformin HCL	Avandamet	Thiazolidinedione and biguanide; antidiabetic
Antihypertensive Drugs and Drugs Used to Improve Heart Function		
Benazepril HCl	Lotensin	ACE inhibitor; antihypertensive
Captopril	Apo-capto, Capoten, Novo-Captopril	ACE inhibitor; antihypertensive
Enalaprilat Enalapril maleate	Enaparil	ACE inhibitor; antihypertensive
Fosinopril sodium	Monopril	ACE inhibitor; antihypertensive
Lisinopril	Prinivil, Zestril	ACE inhibitor; antihypertensive
Moexipril HCl	Univasc	ACE inhibitor; antihypertensive
Quinapril HCl	Accupril	ACE inhibitor; antihypertensive
Ramipril	Altace	ACE inhibitor; antihypertensive
Acebutolol HCl	Sectral	β-Blocker; antihypertensive, antiarrhythmic
Atenolol	Apo-atenodol, Nu-atenol Tenormin	β-Blocker; antihypertensive, antianginal
Bisoprolol fumarate	Zebeta	β-Blocker; antihypertensive
Carvedilol	Coreg	β-Blocker, vasodilator, antihypertensive
Dobutamine HCl	Dobutrex	Adrenergic, β_1-agonist; inotropic
Esmolol HCl	Brevibloc	β-Blocker; antiarrhythmic
Labetalol HCl	Normodyne, Trandate	α- and β-Blocker; antihypertensive
Metoprolol succinate	Toprol-XL	β-Blocker; antihypertensive; adjunctive
Metoprolol tartrate	Apo-metoprolol, Lopressor	Treatment for acute MI
Nadolol	Corgard	β-Blocker; antihypertensive; antianginal

Continued

TABLE 73.2
(Continued)

Generic Names	Brand Names	Description/Function
Antihypertensive Drugs and Drugs Used to Improve Heart Function (Continued)		
Sotalol	Betapace, Betapace AF Sofacor	β-Blocker; antiarrhythmic
Timolol maleate	Apo-Timol, Blocadren	β-Blocker; antihypertensive; adjunct to MI treatment
Amiloride HCl	Midamor	Potassium sparring diuretic; antihypertensive
Spironolactone	Aldactone, Novo-Spiroton	Potassium sparing diuretic; antihypertensive
Adenosine	Adenocard	Nucleoside; antiarrhythmic
Amiodarone HCl	Cardarone, Pacerone	Benzofuran derivative; antiarrhythmic
Atropine sulfate	Atropine	Anticholinergic, belladonna alkaloid; antiarrhythmic, vagolytic
Digoxin	Digtek, digoxin Lanoxicaps, Lanoxin	Cardiac glycoside; antiarrhythmic
Digoxin immune FAB	Digibind, DigiFab	Antidote for digoxin
Dofetilide	Tikosyn	Antiarrhythmic; class III
Amlodipine besylate	Norvasc	Dihydropyridine calcium channel blocker; antianginal, antihypertensive
Bepridil HCl	Vascor	Calcium channel blocker; antianginal
Diltiazem HCl	Apo-diltiaz, Dilacor XR, Cardizem (CD, LA, SR, XT,) Diltia XT, Tiazac	Calcium channel blocker; antianginal
Felodipine	Plendil, Renedil	Calcium channel blocker; antihypertensive
Isradipine	DynaCirc, DynaCirc CR	Calcium channel blocker; antihypertensive
Nicardipine	Cardene, Cardene IV Cardene SR	Calcium channel blocker, antianginal antihypertensive
Nifedipine	Adalet, Adalet CC, Nifedical XL, Apo-Nifed, Procardia, Procardia XL	Calcium channel blocker, antianginal, antihypertensive
Nisoldipine	Sular	Calcium channel blocker; antihypertensive
Verapamil HCl	Apo-Verap, Calan, Isoptin, Verelan, etc.	Calcium channel blocker; antianginal, antihypertensive, antiarrhythmic
Bosentan	Tracleer	Endothelin receptor antagonist; antihypertensive
Candesartan cilexetil	Atacand	Selective angiotensin II antagonist; antihypertensive
Clonidine	Catapres-TTS	Centrally acting adrenergic; antihypertensive
Clonidine HCl	Catapres, Dixarit	
Doxazosin mesylate	Cardura	α-Blocker; antihypertensive
Eplerenone	Inspira	Aldosterone receptor antagonist; antihypertensive
Eprostartan mesylate	Teveten	Angiotensin II receptor antagonist; antihypertensive
Bumetanide	Bumex	Loop diuretic; diuretic
Furosemide	Apo-furosdemide; Lasix Novosemide	Loop diuretic; antihypertensive
Hydralazine HCl	Apresoline, Novo-hylazin	Peripheral vasodilator; antihypertensive
Hydrochlorothiazide	Apo-hydro, Aquazide-H Esidrix, HydroDIURIL, Oretic	Thiazide diuretic, antihypertensive
Indapamide	Lozide, Lozol	Thiazide-like diuretic; antihypertensive
Inamrinone lactate	Inamrinone	Bipyridine derivative; inotropic, vasodilator
Irbesartan	Avapro	Angiotensin II receptor antagonist; Antihypertensive
Isorbid dinitrate	Apo-ISDN, Dilatrate-SR, Isonate, Isorbid, Isodil, Isordil tembids, Isotrate, Sorbitrate	Nitrate; antianginal; vasodilator
Isosorbide mononitrate	Imdur, ISMO, Monoket	
Losartan potassium	Cozaar	Angiotensin II receptor antagonist; Antihypertensive
Mannitol	Osmitrol	Osmotic diuretic, diuretic
Methyldopa	Aldomet, Apo-methyldopa	Centrally acting antiadrenergic; antihypertensive
Methyldopate HCl	Dopamet, Novo-Medopa	
Metolazone	Mykrox, Zaroxolyn	Quinazoline derivative (thiazide-like) diuretic; antihypertensive
Mexiletine HCl	Mexitil	Lidocaine analog, sodium channel antagonist; ventricular antiarrhythmic
Milrinone lactate	Primacor	Bipyridine phosphodiesterase inhibitor; inotropic vasodilator
Minoxidil	Loniten	Peripheral vasodilator; antihypertensive
Nesiritide	Natrecor	B-type natiuretic peptide, inotropic vasodilator
Nitroglycerine	Nitro-bid, Nitrocine, Nitrodisc, Nitrostat, etc.	Nitrate; antianginal, vasodilator
Nitroprusside sodium	Nitropress	Vasodilator, antihypertensive

Continued

TABLE 73.2
(Continued)

Generic Names	Brand Names	Description/Function
Antihypertensive Drugs and Drugs Used to Improve Heart Function (Continued)		
Olmesartan medoxomil	Benicar	Angiotensin II receptor antagonist/thiazide diuretic antihypertensive
Prazosin HCl	Minipress	α-Blocker, antihypertensive
Procainamide HCl	Procanbid, Promine Pronestyl	Procaine derivative; ventricular and supraventricular antiarrhythmic
Propafenone HCl	Rythmol	Sodium channel antagonist; antiarrhythmic
Propanolol HCl	Detensol, Inderal, etc.	β-Blocker, antihypertensive, antianginal Antiarrythmic, adjunct treatment for myocardial infarction
Quinidine gluconate	Quinate, Quinalan	Cinchona alkaloid; antitachyarrhythmic
Quinidine sulfate	Extentabs, Quinidex	
Terazosin HCl	Hytrin	Selective α_1 blocker; antihypertensive
Treprostinil sodium	Remodulin	Vasodilator; antihypertensive
Valsartan	Diovan	Angiotensin II antagonist; antihypertensive
Glaucoma Drugs		
Acetazolamide	Acetazolam, Diazamide	Carbonic anhydrase inhibitor; antiglaucoma, diuretic
Acetazolamide sodium	Diamox, Diamox Sequels	
Betaxolol HCl	Betopic	β-Blocker; antiglaucoma
Latanoprost	Xalatan	Prostaglandin analog; antiglaucoma; ocular antihypertensive
Bimatoprost	Lumigan	Prostaglandin analog; antiglaucoma,ocular antihypertensive
Dorzolamide HCl	Trusopt	Sulfonamide; antiglaucoma
Timolol maleate	Betimol, Timoptic	β-Blocker; antiglaucoma agent
Non Steroidal Anti-inflammatory Drugs (NSAID) and Analgesics		
Aspirin (acetylsalicylic acid)	ASA, Ascriptin, Bufferin, Ecotrin	Salicylate; NSAID, antipyretic, platelet aggregation inhibitor
Acetaminophen (APAP paracetamol)	Tylenol, Tempra, Apacet Acephen, Aceta, Feverall Anacin (aspirin-free) Panadol Genapap Children's, Neopap	Para-aminophenol derivative; analgesic, antipyretic
Acetylcysteine	Mucomyst, Mucosil-10, Mucosil-20	Amino acid derivative; mucolytic; antidote for acetaminophen overdose
Codeine phosphate	Paveral	Opioid; analgesic, antitussive
Diclofenac potassium	Cataflam	NSAID; antiarthritic, anti-inflammatory
Diclofenac sodium	Solaraze, Voltaren, Voltaren SR	
Etodlac	Lodine	NSAID; antarthritic
Ibuprofen	Advil, Motri, Nuprin, etc.	NSAID, non-opioid analgesic, antipyretic, anti-inflammatory
Indomethacin	Apo-indomethacin, Indochron, ER, etc.	NSAID, non-opioid analgesic, antipyretic, anti-inflammatory
Ketoprofen	Orudis, Oruvil	NSAID, non-opioid analgesic, antipyretic, anti-inflammatory
Ketorolac tromethamine	Toradol	NASID, analgesic
Meloxicam	Mobic	NSAID, enolic acid, analgesic, anti-inflammatory
Nabumetone	Relafen	NSAID, antarhritic
Naproxen	Nova-Naprox, etc.	NSAID, non-opioid analgesic, antipyretic, anti-inflammatory
Sulindac	Apo-sulin, Clinoril Novo-sundac	NSAID, non-opioid analgesic, anti-inflammatory
Tramadol HCl	Ultram	Synthetic analgesic
Drugs That Affect Bone and Joints		
Adalimumab	Humira	Monoclonal antibody; antiarthritic
Alendronate sodium	Fosamax	Osteoclast-mediated bone resorption inhibitor; antiosteoporotic
Anakira	Kineret	Lymphokine immunoregulator; immunologic agent; antirheumatic
Etanercept	Embrel	Fusion protein; antirheumatic
Leflunomide	Arava	Pyrimidine synthesis inhibitor; antiproliferative, anti-inflammatory antirhumatoid
Pamidronate disodium	Aredia	Diphosphate, pyrophosphate analogue; antihypercalcemic
Raloxifene HCl	Evista	Selective estrogen receptor modulator, antiosteoporotic
Risedronate sodium	Actonel	Bisphosphonate; antiresorptive drug
Teroparatide	Forteo	Biosynthetic parathyroid hormone; antiosteoporotic
Zoledronic acid	Zometa	Bisphosphonate; antihypercalcemic

Continued

TABLE 73.2
(Continued)

Generic Names	Brand Names	Description/Function
Drugs for Asthma Allergy and Related Disorders		
Albuterol (salbutanol)	Proventil, Ventolin	Adrenergic; bronchodilator
Albuterol sulfate (salbuterol sulfate)	AccuNeb, Proventil, Volmax, Proventil HFA, Proventil Repetabs	
Aminophylline (Theophylline ethylenediamine)	Phyllocontin, Truphylline	Xanthine derivative; bronchodilator
Cetirizine HCl	Zyrtec	Selective H_1-receptor antagonist; antihistamine
Desloratadine	Clarinex	Selective H_1-receptor antagonist; antihistamine
Diphenyl HCl	Allerdryl, Benedryl, Hydramine, Nytol, Sominex antihistamine, antiemetic, antivertigo, Antitussive, sedative-hypnotic, antidyskinetic	Ethanolamine-derivative antihistamine
Epinephrine (many forms)	Primatene mist, Vaponefrin (many preparation)	Adrenergic; bronchodilator, vasopressor, cardiac stimulant
Fexofenadine	Allegra	H_1-receptor antagonist; antihistamine
Formoterol fumarate	Foradil	Long-acting selective β_2 blocker; bronchodilator
Guaifenesin	Robitussin, etc.	Propanediol derivative; expectorant
Ipratropine bromide	Atrovent	Anticholinergic; bronchodilator
Isoproterenol (several forms)	Isoprel, Medihaler-iso, etc.	Adrenergic; bronchodilator, cardiac stimulent
Loratadine	Alavert, Claritin, Tavist ND Allergy	Tricyclic antihistamine
Metaproterenol sulfate	Alupent	Adrenergic, bronchodilator
Montelukast sodium	Singular	Leukotriene receptor antagonist; antiasthmatic
Pseudoephedrine HCl	Cenafed, Dimatapp, etc.	Adrenergic, decongestant
Salmeterol xinafoate	Serevent Diskus	Selective β_2-adrenergic agonist; bronchodilator
Terbutalene sulfate	Brethine, Bricanyl	β_2-Adrenergic agonist; bronchodilator, premature labor inhibitor
Theophlline (many forms)	Many formulations	Xanthine derivative; bronchodilator
AntiGout Drugs		
Allopurinal	Lopurin, Purinol, Zyloprin	Xanthine oxidase inhibitor; antigout
Colchicine	Colchicine	Alkaloid; antigout
AntiMigraine Drugs		
Almotriptan	Axert	Serotonin-1 receptor agonist; antimigraine
Eletriptan HBr	Relpax	Serotonin 5-HT_1 receptor agonist; antimigraine
Frovatriptan succinate	Frova	Sertonin 5-HT_1 receptor agonist; antimigraine
Sumatriptan succinate	Imitrex	Selective 5-hydroxytryptamine receptor agonist; antimigraine
Zolmitriptan	Zomig	Selective 5-hydroxytryptamine receptor agonist antimigraine
Muscle Relaxants		
Dicyclomine HCl	Antispas, Bentyl, Neoquess, Spasmoban	Anticholinergic; antimuscarinic, gastrointestinal antispasmodic
Baclofen	Lioresal	GABA analog derivative; skeletal muscle relaxant
Drugs That Affect Behavior, Mood or Mental Function		
Alprazolam	Apo-alpraz, Novo-Alprazol Nu-Alpraz, Xanax	Benzodiazepine; antianxiety
Amitriptyline HCl	Apo-amitriphyline	Tricyclic antidepressant
Aripiprazole	Ability	Psychotropic; atypical antipsychotic
Atomoxetine HCl	Strattera	Selective serotonin reuptake inhibitor; antiattention deficit disorder
Buttorphanol tartrate	Stadol, Stadol NS	Opioid agonist-antagonist, opioid partial agonist; adjunct to anesthesia
Benzotropine mesylate	Apo-benztropine Cogentin PMS benztropine	Anticholinergic; anti-Parkinsonian
Biperiden HCl	Akineton	Anticholinergic; anti-Parkinsonian
Bupropion HCl	Zyban	Norepinephrine, serotonin and dopamine inhibitor; nicotine replacement

Continued

TABLE 73.2
(Continued)

Generic Names	Brand Names	Description/Function
Drugs That Affect Behavior, Mood or Mental Function (Continued)		
Bupropion HCl	Wellbutrin	Aminoketone; antidepressant
Bromocriptine mesylate	Periodel	Dopamine receptor agonist, semisynthetic ergot Alkaloid, dopaminergic agonist; anti-Parkinsonian, prolactin release inhibitor, growth hormone release inhibitor
Buspirone HCl	BuSpar	Azaspirodecanedione derivative; anxiolytic
Carbamazepine	Apo-carbamazepine Carbatrol, Epitol, Tegretol, Teril	Iminostilbene derivative; anticonvulsant, analgesic
Clomipramine HCl	Anafranil	Tricyclic antidepressant; antidepressant
Clonazepam	Klonopin	Benzodiazepine; anticonvulsant
Clorazepate dipotassium	Apo-Clorazepate, Gen-XENE, Novo-clopate, Tranxene	Benzodiazepine; anxiolytic, anticonvulsant, sedative-hypnotic
Clozapine	Clozaril	Tricyclic dibenzodiazepine derivative; antipsycotic
Citalopram HCl	Celexa	Selective serotonin reuptake inhibitor, Antidepressant
Chlordiazepoxide	Libritabs	Benzodiazepine; anxiolytic, anticonvulsant, sedative-hypnotic
Chlordiazepoxide HCl	Librium, Novo-Poxide	
Cyclobenzaprine HCl	Flexeril	Tricyclic antidepressant; skeletal muscle relaxant
Desipramine HCl	Norpramin	Dibenzazepine tricyclic antidepressant
Dexamethylphrenidate HCl	Focalin	Methylphenidate derivative; central nervous system (CNS) stimulant
Diazepam	Diazepam intensol, Valium, Apo-diazepam	Benzodiazepine; anxiolytic, skeletal muscle relaxant, amnestic, anticonvulsant, sedative-hypnotic
Donepezil HCl	Aricept	Acetylcholinesterase inhibito; CNS drug for Alzheimer's disease
Dopamine HCl	Intropin, Revimine	Adrenergic; inotropic, vasopressor
Doxepin HCl	Adapin, Novo-doxepin	Tricyclic antidepressant Sinaquan, Triadapin
Droperidol	Inapsine	Dopamine blocker, Butyrophenone derivative; antipsychotic, neuroleptic
Entacapone	Comtan	Catechol-*O*-methyltransferase inhibitor; anti-Parkinsonian
Escitalopram oxalate	Lexapro	Selective serotonin reuptake inhibitor; antidepressant
Fentanyl (many forms)	Sublimaze, Duragesic Actig	Opioid agonist; analgesic, adjunct to anesthesia, anesthetic
Flecainide acetate	Tambocor	Benzamide derivative local anesthetic, ventricular antiarrhythmic
Flumazenil	Romazicon	Benzodiazepine antagonist; antidote
Fluoxetine HCl	Prozac, Sarafem	Serotonin reuptake inhibitor; antidepressant
Fluphenazine	Modicate, Moditen	Phenothiazine; antipsychotic
Fluvoxamine maleate	Luvox	Serotonin reuptake inhibitor; antidepressant
Fosphenytoin sodium	Cerebyx	Hydantoin derivative; anticonvulsant
Gabapentin	Neurontin	1-Aminomethyl cyclohexonacetic acid; anticonvulsant
Galantamine hydrobromide	Reminyl	Reversible, competitive acetylcholinase inhibitor cholinomimetic; anti-Alzheimer's disease dementia
Haloperidol (many forms)	Peridol, etc.	Butyrophenone; antipsychotic
Hydromorphone HCl	Dilaudid	Opioid; analagesic, antitussive
Hydroxyzine HCl	Atarax, Multipax, etc.	Antihistamine, anxiolytic, sedative, antipuritic, antiemetic, antispasmodic
Imipramine HCl	Tofranil, Tipramine	Dibenzazeprine-derivative antidepressant
Lamotrigine	Lamictal	Phenyltrizine; anticonvulsant
Levetiracetam	Keppra	Antiepileptic, anticonvulsant
Levodopa	Dopar	Dopamine precursor; anti-Parkinsonian
Levodopa-carbidopa	Sinemet	Decarboxylase inhibitor, dopamine precursor; anti-Parkinsonian
Lidocain HCl	Lidopen, Xylocaine	Amino derivative; ventricular antiarrythmic, local anesthetic
Lithium carbonate	Carbolith, etc.	Alkali metal; antimaniac, antipsychotic
Lorazepan	Alzapam, etc.	Benzodiazepine; anxiolytic, sedative-hypnotic
Meclizine HCl	Antivert, Vergon, etc.	Piperazine-derivative antihistamine; antiemetic, antivertigo
Meperidine HCl	Demerol	Opioid; analgesic, adjunct to anesthesia
Methadone HCl	Dolophine, Methadose	Opioid; analgesic, opioid detoxification adjunct
Methylphrenidate HCl	Ritalin, Concerta, etc.	Piperidine CNS stimulant

Continued

TABLE 73.2
(Continued)

Generic Names	Brand Names	Description/Function
Drugs That Affect Behavior, Mood or Mental Function (Continued)		
Mirtazapine	Remeron	Piperazinoazepine; tetracyclic antidepressant
Morphine HCL	Morphitec	Opioid; analgesic
Morphine sulfate	Astramorph PF, Avinza, Duramorph, etc.	
Nalbuphine HCl	Nubain	Opioid agonist-antagonist, opioid partial agonist; analgesic, adjunct to anesthesia
Naloxone HCl	Narcan	Opioid antagonist
Naltrexone HCl	Depade, ReVia	Opioid antagonist, opioid detoxification adjunct
Nefazodone HCl	Serzone	Phenylpiperazine; antidepressant
Nortriptyline HCl	Aventyl, Pamelor	Antidepressant
Olanzapine	Zyprexa	Dibenzapine derivative; antipsychotic
Oxazepam	Apo-oxazepam, Novozapam, Serex	Benzodiazepine; anxiolytic, sedative-hypnotic
Oxcarbazepine	Trileptel	Carboxamide derivative; antiepileptic
Oxycodone HCl	OxyContin, OxyFAST, Oxy IR, Roxicodon, Roxicodone, Supeudol	Opioid; analgesic
Paroxetine HCl	Paxil	Antidepressant
Pergolide mesylate	Permax	Dopaminergic agonist; anti-Parkinsonian
Perphenazine	Apo-perphenazine, Trilafon, PMS perphenazine	Phenothiazine; antipsychotic, antiemetic
Phenazopyridine HCl	Azo-standard, Baridium, Geridium, Phenazo, etc.	Azo dye; urinary tract analgesic
Phenobarbital	Ancalixir, Barbita, Solfoton	Barbiturate; anticonvulsant, sedative-hypnotic
Phenytoin	Dilantin	Hydantoin derivative; anticonvulsant
Pramipexole dihdro-Chloride	Mirapex	Nonergot dopamine agonist; anti-Parkinsonian
Primidone	Sertan, Mysoline, etc.	Barbiturate analogue; anticonvulsant
Prochlorperazine	Compazine	Phenothiazine (piperazine derivative), antipsychotic, antiemetic, anxiolytic
Promethazine HCl	Anergan 50, Phenergan	Phenothiazine derivative; antiemetic, antivertigo, H_1-receptor antagonist, adjunct to analgesics, sedative
Propofol	Diprivan	Phenol derivative; anesthetic
Propoxyphene HCl	Darvon	Opioid analgesic
Quetiapine fumarate	Seroquel	Dibenzapine derivative; antipsychotic
Risperidone	Resperidal	Benzisoxazole derivative; antipsychotic
Rivastigmine tartrate	Exelon	Cholinesterase inhibitor; cholinomimetic
Ropinirole HCl	Requip	Nonergoline dopamine agonist; antiparkinsonian
Scopolamine	Bucospan	Anticholinergic; antimuscarinic, cycloplegic mydriatic
Selegiline HCl	Atapryl, Carbex, Eldepryl, Selpak	MOA-B inhibitor; anti-Parkinsonian
Sertraline HCl	Zoloft	Antidepressant
Sibutramine HCl	Meridia	Dopamine and norepinephrine reuptake inhibitor; antiobesity
Tacrine HCl	Cognex	Cholinesterase inhibitor; psychothrapeutic
Temazepan	Restoril	Benzodiazepine; sedative-hypnotic
Thioridazine HCl	Mellaril and others	Phenothiazine; antipsychotic
Thiothixine	Navane	Thioxanthene; antipsychotic
Tolcapone	Tasmar	Catechol-*O*-methyltransferase inhibitor; anti-Parkinsonian
Tolterodine tartrate	Detrol	Muscarinic receptor antagonist; anticholinergic
Topiramate	Topomax	Sulfamate-substituted monosaccharide antiepileptic
Trazodone HCl	Desyrel	Triazolopyridine derivative; antidepressant
Trifluoperazine HCl	Apo-trifluoperazine, Solzine, Stelazine, Terfluzine	Phenothiazine; antipsychotic
Trihexylphenidyl HCl	Apo-Trinex, Arlane	Anticholinergic; anti-Parkinsonian Trihexane
Venlafaxine HCl	Effexor	Norepinephrine, dopamine reuptake inhibitor, antidepressant
Zalepion	Sonata	Pyrazolopyrimidine; hypnotic
Ziprasidone	Geodon	Atypical antipsychotic; psychotropic
Zolpidem tartrate	Ambien	Imidazopyridine; hypnotic
Zonisamide	Zonegran	Sulfonamide; anticonvulsant

Continued

TABLE 73.2
(Continued)

Generic Names	Brand Names	Description/Function
Drugs That Affect Gastrointestinal Function		
Alosetron HCl	Lotronex	Selective 5-HT$_3$ receptor agonist; anti-irritable bowel
Bisacodyl	Correctol and others	Diphenylmethane derivative; stimulant laxative
Bismuth subsalicylate	Pepto Bismol and others	Adsorbant; antidiarrheal
Diphenoxylate HCl and Atropine sulfate	Logen, Lomanate, Lomotil, Lonox	Opiate; antidiarrheal
Docusate Calcium	Surfak	Surfactant; emollient laxative
Docusate Sodium	Colace, Diocto	
Dolasetron mesylate	Anzemet	Selective serotonin 5-HT$_3$- receptor antagonist; antinauseant, antiemetic
Esomeprazole magnesium	Nexium	Proton pump inhibitor, s-isomer of omeprazole gastroesophageal agent
Famotidine	Pepcid	H$_2$-receptor antagonist; antiulcerative
Granisetron HCl	Kytril	Selective 5-hydroxy-tryptamine receptor antagonist; antiemetic, antinauseant
Ipecac	Ipecac syrup	Alkaloid emetic
Lactulose	Duphalac, etc.	Disaccharide; laxative
Lansoprazole	Prevacid	Acid (proton) pump inhibitor; antiulcerative
Loperamide	Imodium	Piperidine derivative; antidiarrheal
Metoclopramide HCl	Clopra, Reglan, etc.	Para-aminobenzoic acid derivative; antiemetic, gastrointestinal stimulant
Misoprotol	Cytotec	Prostaglandin E$_1$ analog; antiulcerative, gastric mucosal Protectant
Nizatidine	Axid	H$_2$ receptor antagonist; antiulcerative
Omeprazole	Losec, Prilosec	Proton pump inhibitor; gastric acid suppressant
Ondansetron HCl	Zofran	Serotonin (5-HT$_3$) receptor antagonist; antiemetic
Pantoprazole sodium	Protonix	Substituted benzimidazole; gastric acid suppressant
Rabeprazole sodium	Aciphex	Proton pump inhibitor; antiulcerative
Ranitidine HCl	Zantac	H$_2$-receptor antagonist; antiulcerative
Sucralfate	Carafate, Sulcrate	Pepsin inhibitor; antiulcerative
Tegaserod maleate	Zelnorm	5-HT$_4$ receptor partial agonist; irritable bowel agent
Drugs That Affect Blood Clotting		
Alteplase (tissue plasminogen activator)	Activase, Cathflo Activase	Enzyme; thrombolytic enzyme
Argatroban	Argatroban	Direct thrombolytic inhibitor; anticoagulant
Bivalirudin	Angiomax	Direct thrombin inhibitor; anticoagulant
Cilostazol	Pietal	Quinolone phosphodiesterase inhibitor; platelet aggregation inhibitor, vasodilator
Clopidogrel bisulfate	Plavix	Adenosine diphosphate-induced platelet aggregation inhibitor; antiplatelet
Dalteparin sodium	Fragmin	Low molecular weight heparin; anticoagulant
Dipyridamole	Persantine	Pyrimidine analog; coronary vasodilator, platelet aggregation inhibitor
Enoxaparin sodium	Lovenox	Low molecular weight heparin; anticoagulant
Fondaparinux sodium	Arixtra	Inhibitor of activated factor X; anticoagulant
Heparin sodium	Hepalean	Anticoagulant, antithrombitic
Phytonadione	Mephyton	Vitamin K; blood coagulation modifier
Streptokinase	Streptase	Plasminogen activator; thrombolytic enzyme
Tenecteplase	TNKase	Recombinant tissue plasminogen activator; thrombolytic
Tinzaparin sodium	Innohep	Low molecular weight heparin; anticoagulant
Warfarin sodium	Coumadin, etc.	Coumarin derivative; anticoagulant
Antilipemic Drugs		
Atorvastatin calcium	Lipitor	HMG-CoA reductase inhibitor; antilipemic
Fluvastatin sodium	Lescol	HMG-CoA reductase inhibitor; antilipemic
Lovostatin (mevinolin)	Altocor, Mevacor	HMG-CoA reductase inhibitor; antilipemic

Continued

**TABLE 73.2
(Continued)**

Generic Names	Brand Names	Description/Function
Antilipemic Drugs (Continued)		
Pravastatin sodium (eptastatin)	Pravachol	HMG-CoA reductase inhibitor; antilipemic
Simvastatin	Zocor	HMG-ccCoA reductase inhibitor; antilipemic
Cholestyramine	LoCHOLEST, Questran LoCHOLEST Light Prevalite	Anion exchange resin; antilipemic, bile acid sequestrant
Colesevelam HCl	WellChol	Polymeric bile acid sequestrant; antilipemic
Ezetimibe	Zetia	Selective cholesterol absorption inhibitor; antihypercholesterolemic
Fenofibrate	Lofibra, Tricor	Fibric acid derivative; antilipemic
Gemfibrozil	Lopid	Fibric acid derivative; antilipemic
Anti-inflammatory Drugs		
Balsalazide disodium	Colazal	Gastrointestinal drug; anti-inflammatory
Betamethasone (many forms)	Betnesol, etc.	Glucocorticoid anti-inflammatory
Beclomethasone dipropionate	QVAR	Glucocorticoid anti-inflammatory, antiasthmatic
Budesonide	Entocort EC, Rhinocort Aqua, Pulmicort Respules, Pulmicort, Turbuhaler	Glucocorticoid; anti-inflammatory
Dexamethasone (many forms)	Decadron and others	Glucocorticoid; anti-inflammatory
Fluticasone	Flovent	Corticosteroid anti-inflammatory
Methylprednisone (many forms)	Medrol, etc.	Glucocorticoid; anti-inflammatory, immunosuppressant
Prednisone	Many preparations	Glucocorticoid; anti-inflammatory
Predisolone		
Triamcinolone acetonide, etc.	Nasacort	Glucocorticoid anti-inflammatory
Hormones and Hormone Replacements		
Calcitonin	Miacalcin	Parathyroid hormone; hypocalcemic
Calcitrol	Calcijex, Rocaltrol	Vitamin D analog; antihypocalcemic
Fludrocortisone acetate	Florinef	Mineralocorticoid replacement
Levothyroxine	Unithroid, etc.	Thyroid hormone replacement
Norethindrone	Camilla, Errin, etc.	Progestin; hormonal contraceptive
Norepinephrine bitartrate	Levophed	Adrenergic; vasopressor
Oxytocin	Pitocin	Exogenous hormone; oxytocic, lactation stimulant
Miscellaneous Drugs		
Darbepoetin	Aranesp	Hematopoitic; antianemic
Epoetin a	Epogen, Procrit	Glycoprotein; antianemic
Basiliximab	Simulect	Recombinant chimeric human–murine monovclonal antibody IgG$_{1k}$; immunosuppressant
Dutasteride	Avodart	5-α-Reductase enzyme inhibitor; reduces benign prostate enlargement
Effornithine HCl	Vaniqa	Ornithine decarboxylase inhibitor; hair growth retardant
Finasteride	Propecia, Proscar	Steroid derivative; androgen synthesis inhibitor
Mifepristone	Mifeprex	Synthetic steroid; antiprogesterone
Nicotine transdermal System	Habitrol, Nicoderm, Nicotrol	Nicotinic cholinergic agonist; smoking cessation aid
Pentoxifylline	Trental	Xanthine derivative; hemorheologic
Phenylephrine HCl	Neo-synephrine	Adrenergic; vasoconstrictor
Pilocarpine HCl	Pilocar, etc.	Cholinergic agonist; miotic
Pimecrilimus	Elidel	Topical immunomodulator; topical skin product
Propythiouracil	PTU	Thyroid hormone antagonist
Protamine sulfate	Protamine sulfate	Heparin antidote
Sidenafil citrate	Viagra	Selective cyclic guanosine monophosphate-specific phosphodiesterase type 5 inhibitor; erectile dysfunction treatment
Tamsulosin HCl	Flomax	α_{1a}-Antagonist; benign prostate hyperplasic drug
Tretinoin	Avita, Renova, Retin-A, etc.	Retinoid, vitamin A derivative; antiacne agent

replacements and anti-inflammatory. Again, both functions are given in the table and the reader will find them under their first listed function.

Although every attempt has been made to include drugs in current use, some drugs may be listed that are no longer in use because the Food and Drug Administration believes they are either not useful or have too many adverse effects. Drug updates can be accessed on eDrugInfo.com. In addition, drugs that have entered the marketplace since this table was constructed may be missing.

REFERENCES

1. Physicians Desk Reference 1992. Medical Economics Data, Montvale, NJ, 2563 pages.
2. Drugs 2004. Medical Pocket Reference, Lippincott, Williams & Wilkins, Philadelphia, PA, 184 pages.

74 Drug–Nutrient Interactions

James L. Hargrove

CONTENTS

OVERVIEW

Drug dosage regimens are designed to produce an effective plasma concentration for a specified period with the aim of achieving a therapeutic effect. Just as certain drugs may enhance or interfere with the action of other drugs, specific foods, nutrients, or phytochemicals in botanical supplements may modify drug actions. Conversely, drugs may increase the need for particular nutrients. It is rare for a drug to decrease the need for a nutrient, but not uncommon for ingested substances to increase drug effectiveness. Nutritional support is an important aspect of patient care. When a drug regimen interferes with nutritional status, dietary assessment and counseling are required. Similarly, when a patient's diet or usage of supplements may interfere with drug therapy, it is crucial to monitor the patient carefully to avoid adverse reactions. Standards for ensuring good quality of patient care in clinical settings are set by organizations such as the Joint Commission on Accreditation of Healthcare Organizations (JCAHO), and the standards apply to hospitals, long-term-care facilities, and ambulatory care facilities. Quality assurance standards have been developed with guidance of professional organizations such as the American Dietetic Association. JCAHO standards include patient education concerning food–drug interactions. Adverse interactions are monitored by the Food and Drug Administration through the MedWatch reporting system.

Many food–drug interactions are not specific. Drugs may alter taste perception or appetite, contribute to depression, produce nausea, damage the stomach or gastrointestinal tract, or cause weight loss or loss of lean tissue. Particularly with elderly patients, the consumption of multiple drugs (polypharmacy) can affect many aspects of food consumption and create a danger of dehydration.

Although relatively few food–drug interactions rise to the level of clinical significance, the potential number of interactions is immense, given the tens of thousands of compounds in the pharmacopoeia as well as in the foods, dietary supplements, nonprescription drugs, and botanical preparations that have become available since the passage of Dietary Supplement Health Education Act in 1994. Because of this complexity, several manuals, CD-ROM clinical pharmacology databases, and software programs have been developed to help track interactions.[1–3] Examples include Hansten and Horn's *Drug Interactions, Analysis, and Management* manuals,[4,5] *Mosby's Drug Consult*,[6] and the *Handbook of Food–Drug Interactions*.[7] Similar products are used in most pharmacies. Many indices and databases have been developed by private companies and are not necessarily referenced in the medical literature. Potential food–drug interactions are complicated by medical conditions (obesity or diabetes), substance abuse, gender, age, and genetic variability. Therefore, it is only possible to indicate potential interactions that might require nutritional assessment or clinical monitoring.

The information in the table (Table 74.1) has been derived from reference works.[7–13] Further information can also be obtained from several sources on the Internet by searching for the key words, "drug interactions."

INTERNET URLs

Drug Digest, http://www.drugdigest.org/DD/Home
Drug Interaction Checker, http://www.drugs.com/drug_interactions.html
Drug Interactions, http://medicine.iupui.edu/flockhart/
FDA MedWatch Adverse Event Reporting, http://www.fda.gov/medwatch/
Medscape Drug Interaction Checker, http://www.medscape.com/pages/features/drugintchecker/

TABLE 74.1
Drug Nutrient Interactions

Drug Class	Example	Food, Nutrient, or Condition	Effect
Antibiotics	Tetracycline	Probiotics (yogurt cultures)	Reduce diarrhea associated with antibiotics Replenish colonic microflora
		Milk products	Calcium and magnesium chelate antibiotic
		Riboflavin, vitamins C and K	Gastric distress due to antibiotic
	Penicillin-related drugs, for example, Pen-V, Veetids, Ledercillin	Milk products	These antibiotics may deplete riboflavin. Milk products are an excellent source
	Cephalosporin derivatives	Vitamin K	Vitamin K supplementation may be needed
Antacids	Nonprescription calcium and magnesium complexes	Nonheme iron	Decreased absorption
	Histamine receptor inhibitors and proton pump inhibitors	Vitamin B_{12}	Decreased absorption (low stomach acidity)
Antiarrhythmics	Digoxin	Potassium, fiber	Hypokalemia increases need for potassium Fiber interferes with drug absorption
	Quinidines	Citrus fruit; vitamins C and K	Citrus and vitamin C can cause drug toxicity; drug may increase need for vitamin K
	Beta adrenergic blockers	Lipids and carbohydrates	Drug may elevate triglycerides; in diabetes, may mask hypoglycemia
	Amiodarone	Elevated iodine content	Altered thyroid metabolism, and thyrotoxicosis
Anticoagulants	Warfarin, and coumadin	Vitamin K; green leafy vegetables	Drug antagonizes vitamin K, but caution is needed to avoid vitamin K deficiency
		Vitamin E; fish oils; garlic, ginkgo, herbal supplements	Many dietary supplements prolong clotting time and increase bleeding tendency
Antihypertensives	Captopril	Low-sodium diets	Sodium restriction may enhance drug effect
	Methyldopa	Protein and carbohydrate; iron	Protein enhances drug effect; high-carbohydrate meals preferred; decreased nonheme iron absorption
	Angiotensin-converting enzyme (ACE) inhibitors, for example captopril, lisinopril, quinapril	Protein supplements, natural licorice (glycyrrhizin); high fat	Protein increases and fat decreases drug effectiveness
	Calcium channel blockers	Grapefruit, natural licorice, and low-sodium diets	Dietary conditions enhance drug effects
	Sulfonamide diuretics	Potassium, glucose, B vitamins	Drugs increase potassium loss and may produce glucose intolerance
Antiinflammatories	Corticosteroids	Glucose metabolism and insulin sensitivity	Hyperglycemic, diabetogenic Negative nitrogen balance
Antipyretics	Aspirin	Folic acid, iron, and vitamin C	May damage gastric mucosa. May require supplements due to decreased absorption or increased utilization
	Acetaminophen	Ethyl alcohol	Hepatotoxic
Antituberculars	Isoniazid	Vitamin B_6	Increases need for vitamin B_6
	Rifampin	Vitamin D	Increases need for vitamin D and calcium
	Pyrimethamine	Folate	Folate antagonist; increases need
	Cycloserine	Dietary fat	Fat increases required drug dose
Antiprotozoals	Pentamidine	Folate	Increases folate need
Anticonvulsants	Phenobarbital and phenytoin	Vitamins D and K, calcium, and folate	Drugs increase nutrient need; decrease bone health Folate supplements antagonize drugs
	Carbamazepines	Iron, folate, and grapefruit juice	Increased iron and folate need; possible anemia; increased blood plasma homocysteine Grapefruit juice increases drug effectiveness
	Valproate	Iron and folate	Anemia and hyperammonemia
Antineoplastics	Methotrexate; various	Folate, vitamin B_{12}, and beta-carotene	Gastrointestinal distress and malabsorption
	Mercaptopurine	Pantethine and purine metabolism	Jaundice and hepatotoxicity
	Procarbazine	Tyramine in foods	Monoamine oxidase inhibitor
	Cisplatin	Magnesium depletion	Drug is nephrotoxic

Continued

TABLE 74.1
(Continued)

Drug Class	Example	Food, Nutrient, or Condition	Effect
Diuretics	Loop diuretics (furosemide)	Vitamin and mineral imbalances	Hypokalemia and thiamine deficiency
	Potassium-sparing diuretics (spironolactone)	Potassium	Potassium toxicity
	Thiazides (chlorothiazide)	Potassium, minerals, and glucose	Imbalances in blood electrolytes and glucose
Oral contraceptives	Estrogens and progestins	Vitamin B_6 and folate	Requirements may increase
Oral hypoglycemic agents	Sulfonylureas	Carbohydrates and niacin	Side effects include hypoglycemia and niacin deficiency, especially in combined therapy with metformin
	Biguanides	Vitamin B_{12}	Malabsorption; lactic acidosis. Must limit alcohol consumption
	Meglitinides and thiazolidinediones	Glucose control	Regarded as safe but combined therapy with other drugs may increase or decrease drug effectiveness
Lipid-lowering drugs	Bile-salt-binding agents	Vitamins A, D, E, and K	Decrease absorption; may alter electrolyte and iron balance
	Fibrates	Malabsorption	
	Statins	Grapefruit juice, Coenzyme Q_{10}	Grapefruit compounds block CYP3A4 CoQ_{10} depletion in neuromyopathies
	Niacin (pharmacological)	Glucose control	May cause hyperglycemia and hypotension
Obesity treatment	Lipase blocker	Fat-soluble vitamins; dietary fat	Steatorrhea may improve if patients select low-fat diets. Potential exists for reduced absorption of vitamins A, D, E, and K
Osteoporosis treatments	Biphosphonates, calcitonin, calcium salts, and estrogens	Iron, phosphorus, and electrolytes	Some drugs may cause anorexia, nausea, vomiting, bloating, weight change, and electrolyte imbalances or esophageal erosion
Psychotropic drugs	Phenothiazines	Appetite, glucose, and riboflavin	Can observe changes in weight, glucose control, and dental health
	Tricyclic antidepressants	Taste acuity, cravings, and electrolytes	Monitor for changes in appetite, sweet consumption, and test plasma electrolytes. Must avoid alcohol
	MAO inhibitors, for example isocarboxazid and phenylzine	Protein sources of tyramine and histamine	Elevated blood pressure after consumption of high-tyramine foods
	Serotonin reuptake inhibitors	Appetite, riboflavin, and caffeine	May alter glycemic control; may reduce or increase appetite; should reduce or avoid caffeinated beverages and tobacco use
	Lithium	Folate, iodine metabolism	Folate supplementation is required. Lithium inhibits thyroid hormone release and alters thyroid status
Respiratory drugs	Bronchodilators (theophylline)	Decreased food intake; caffeine interaction	Nausea or gastric distress; caffeine sensitivity; drug toxicity due to sudden absorption of time release medications
	Corticosteroids	Carbohydrates, proteins, and sodium	Glucose intolerance, sodium retention, negative nitrogen balance
	Leukotriene receptor blockers, for example, zafirlukast, montelukast	No interactions known	

REFERENCES

1. Giudici RA, Poirier TI: *Hosp Pharm* **26**:335, 1991.
2. Poirier TI, Giudici RA: *Hosp Pharm* **27**:334 & 339, 1992.
3. Lewis CW, Frongillo Jr. EA, Roe DA: *J Am Diet Assoc* **95**:309, 1995.
4. Horn JR, Hansten PD: *The Top 100 Drug Interactions: A Guide to Patient Management*, 2nd edn. Seattle, WA: H and H Publications; 2001, 231 pp.
5. Hansten PD: *Hansten and Horn's Managing Clinically Important Drug Interactions*. St. Louis, MO: Lippincott, Williams & Wilkins; 2005, 713 pp.
6. Anonymous: *Mosby's Drug Consult*. St. Louis, MO: Mosby; 2002, 3394 pp.

7. McCabe BJ, Frankel EH, Wolfe JJ: *Handbook of Food–Drug Interactions*. Boca Raton, FL: CRC Press; 2003, 584 pp.
8. Trevor AJ, Katzung BG, Masters SB: *Katzung and Trevor's Pharmacology Examination and Board Review*, 7th edn. New York: Lange Medical Books/McGraw Hill; 2005, 640 pp.
9. Boullata JI, Armenti VT: *Handbook of Drug–Nutrient Interactions*. Totowa, NJ: Humana Press; 2004, 563 pp.
10. Roe D: *Handbook on Drug and Nutrient Interactions*, 5th edn. Chicago, IL: American Dietetic Association; 1994, 163 pp.
11. Scheen AJ: *Drug Saf* **28**:601, 2005.
12. Baker SK, Tarnopolsky MA: *Timely Top Med Cardiovasc Dis* **9**:E26, 2005.
13. Hargreaves IP, Duncan AJ, Heales SJ, Land JM: *Drug Saf* **28**:659, 2005.

75 Herbal Supplements

Carolyn D. Berdanier

CONTENTS

INTRODUCTION

There is a continuing interest in the use of herbals and herbal extracts as alternatives or additives to traditionally prescribed drugs. The use of herbal preparations can be part of a cultural belief system about health and disease, but it can also be a choice by the consumer to bypass the physician and self-prescribe herbals in the hope of curing oneself of a real or imagined medical problem. In many parts of the world, the uses of herbals have had their origins in ancient civilizations. Their use has been passed from generation to generation. Some of the plants used by these cultural groups have actually turned out to quite valuable. Indeed, some of the current medicines available by prescription have had their origins in these folkways. Pharmaceutical scientists have learned of their use and have taken the plant product to the laboratory to isolate, define, and study the active ingredients of the plant in question.

In contrast to the pharmaceutical product offered either by prescription or authorized as an over-the-counter (OTC) drug, herbal preparations can vary. Their use is usually unregulated and their purchase is usually OTC. This means that the product can vary in potency and effectiveness. Some herbal products have placebo value only. That is, their use has no effect on the consumer aside from the placebo effect. By definition, the placebo effect is one in which the consumer believes that a preparation is having an effect on the body when, in fact, no measurable effect can be found. The Food and Drug Administration (FDA) has on occasion prohibited the sale of certain herbal products when there is sufficient evidence of their adverse effects.

The reasons herbal products can vary tremendously are many. The composition of the plant can vary because of its growing conditions, the composition of the soil it is grown on, and the harvesting and postharvesting techniques. The preparation of the plant for marketing can affect its potency. If the plant has to be extracted and the technique for this extraction is inconsistent, then the potency of the product can vary.

There is little regulation of these preparations and few safeguards exist to protect the consumer with respect to the biopotency of its active ingredients. Legal definitions or active ingredient definition/content is not well regulated although the FDA is beginning to assess these products for the consumer. The consumer should be aware that some herbal products may interact with prescribed drugs, either nullifying the drug effect or, worse, interacting to cause an unwarranted or even lethal effect. Users of herbal remedies should consult their pharmacists and physicians about these potentially dangerous uses. They should be especially forthcoming about their herbal product use when their physician prescribes a new drug for a medical problem. A list of plants used for herbal remedies is shown in Table 75.1. Adverse effects of herbal preparation have been reported and some

---

TABLE 75.1
Plants Believed to Have Medicinal Properties[1]

Common Name/Botanical Name	Method of Use and Believed Action[a,b]
Agrimony/*Agrimonia gryposepala*	A tonic, alterative, diuretic, and astringent; infusions from the leaves for sore throats; treatment of kidney and bladder stones; root for jaundice
Whitetube stargrass/*Aletris farinosa*	Leaves and roots used to make a poultice for sore breast; liquid from boiled roots for stomach pains, tonic, sedative, and diuretic
Alfalfa/*Medicago sativa*	Leaves are powdered and mixed with cider vinegar as a tonic; infusions for a tasty drink; leaves may also be used green
Aloe vera/*Aloe barbadensis*	Used on small cuts and sunburn; thought to speed healing
Angelica/*Angelica atropurpurea*	Roots and seeds are dried and used for relief of flatulence; roots for the induction of vomiting and perspiration; roots for treatment of toothache, bronchitis, rheumatism, gout, fever, and to increase menstrual flow

Continued

TABLE 75.1
(Continued)

Common Name/Botanical Name	Method of Use and Believed Action[a,b]
Anise seed/*Pimpinella anisum*	Seeds are ground and used to make a tea to relieve flatulence or colic
Asafetida/*Ferula* sp.	As an antispasmodic; to ward off colds and flu by wearing in a bag around the neck
Bayberry/*Myrica cerifera*	Root bark, leaves, and stems are soaked in water and the decoction is used to treat uterine hemorrhage, jaundice, dysentery, and cankers; leaves and stems boiled and used to treat fevers; decoction of boiled leaves for intestinal worms
Bearberry/*Arctostaphylos uva-ursi*	Leaves are boiled in water and used as a diuretic; boiled infusions are used as a drink to treat sprains, stomach pains, and urinary problems; poison oak inflammations treated with leaf decoction by pioneers
Blackberry/*Rubus*	Infusion made from roots used to dry up runny noses; infusion from root bark to treat dysentery; fruit used to treat dysentery in children; leaves also used in similar manner
Black cohosh/*Cimicifuga racemosa*	Infusion and decoctions used to treat sore throat, rheumatism, kidney trouble, and general malaise; also used for "women's ailments" and malaria
Black walnut/*Juglans nigra*	Inner bark used as mild laxative; husk of nut used for treating intestinal worms, ulcers, syphilis, and fungus infections; leaf infusion for bedbugs
Blessed thistle/*Cnicus benedictus*	Infusions from leaves and tops for cancer treatment, to induce sweating, as a diuretic, to reduce fever, and for inflammations of the respiratory system; infusion of tops as Indian contraceptive; seeds induce vomiting
Boneset/*Eupatorium perfoliatum*	Infusions made from leaves used for laxative and treatment of coughs and chest illnesses Early settlers and native Americans used it to treat malaria
Borage/*Borago officinalis*	Used as an infusion to increase sweating, as a diuretic, or to soothe intestinal tract; was also used on swellings and inflamed areas for relief
Buchu/*Rutaceae*	Prepared as tincture or infusion and used for genitourinary diseases, indigestion, edema, and early stages of diabetes
Buckthorn/*Rhamnus purshiana*	Bark or fruit used as a laxative and tonic
Burdock/*Arctium minus*	Infusion of roots for coughs, asthma, and to stimulate menstruation; tincture of root for rheumatism and stomachache
Calamus (Sweet flag)/*Acorus calamus*	Rhizomes chewed to clear phlegm (mucous) and ease stomach gas; infusions to treat stomach distress
Catnip/*Nepeta cataria*	Entire plant infusions for treating colds, nervous disorders, stomach ailments, infant colic, and hives; smoke relieves respiratory ailments; poultice to reduce swellings
Celery/*Apium graveolens*	As an infusion to relieve rheumatism and flatulence (gas); to act as a diuretic; to act as a tonic and stimulant; oil from seeds used similarly
Chamomile/*Anthemis nobilis*	Powdered and mixed with boiling water to stimulate stomach, to remedy nervousness in women, and stimulate menstrual flow, also a tonic; flowers for poultice to relieve pain; chamomile tea known to be soothing, sedative, and completely harmless
Chaparral/*Croton corynbulosus*	Infusions act as laxative; some claims as cancer treatment
Chickweed/*Stellaria media*	Poultice made to treat sores, ulcers, infections, and hemorrhoids
Chicory/*Cichorium intybus*	Used as a diuretic, laxative, and tonic use; added to coffee to give it a distinctive flavor
Cinnamon/*Cinnamomum zeylanicum*	Treatment for flatulence, diarrhea, vomiting, and nausea
Cleaver's herb/*Galium aparine*	To increase urine formation; to stimulate appetite; to reduce fever; to remedy vitamin C deficiency
Cloves/*Syzygium aromaticum*	To promote salivation and gastric secretion; to relieve pain in stomach and intestines; applied externally to relieve rheumatism, lumbago, toothache, muscle cramps, and neuralgia; clove oil used, too; infusions with clove powder relieves nausea and vomiting
Colt's foot/*Asarum canadense*	Infusion of root to relieve flatulence; powdered root to relieve flatulence; induce sweating, and to relieve aching head and eyes; leaves substitute for ginger
Comfrey/*Symphytum officinale*	Numerous uses including treatments for pneumonia, coughs, diarrhea, calcium deficiency, colds, sores, ulcers, arthritis, gallstones, tonsils, cuts and wounds, headaches, hemorrhoids, gout, burns, kidney stones, anemia, and tuberculosis; used as a poultice, infusion, powder, or in capsule form
Dandelion/*Taraxacum officinale*	Root uses include diuretic, laxative, tonic, and to stimulate appetite; infusion from flower for heart troubles; paste of green leaves for bruises
Echinacea/*Echinacea purpurea*	Treatment of ulcers and boils, syphilis, snakebites, skin diseases, and blood poisoning; used as powder
Eucalyptus/*Eucalyptus globulus*	Antiseptic value; inhaled freely for sore throat; asthma relief; local application to ulcers; used on open wounds
Eyebright/*Lobelia inflata*	Treatment of whooping cough, asthma, epilepsy, pneumonia, hysteria, and convulsion; alkaloid extracted for use in antismoking preparations
Fenugreek/*Trigonella foenum-graceum*	Poultice for wounds; gargle for sore throat
Flax (Linseed)/*Linum usitatissimum*	Ground flaxseed mixed with boiling water for poultice on burns, boils, carbuncles, and sores; internally as a laxative

Continued

TABLE 75.1
(Continued)

Common Name/Botanical Name	Method of Use and Believed Action[a,b]
Garlic/*Allium sativum*	Fresh poultice of the mashed plant for treating snake bite, hornet stings, and scorpion stings; eaten to expel worms, treat colds, coughs, hoarseness, and asthma; bulb expressed against the gum for toothache
Sampson snakeroot/*Gentiana villosa*	Treatment of indigestion, gout, and rheumatism; induction of vomiting; an aid to digestion
Ginger/*Zingiber officinale*	An expectorant; treatment of flatulence, colds, and sore throats
Ginseng/*Panax quinquefolia*	As a tonic and stimulant; treatment of convulsions, dizziness, vomiting, colds, fevers, headaches, and rheumatism.
Goldenrod/*Solidago odora*	Infusions from dried leaves as aromatic stimulant and a diuretic
Goldenseal/*Hydrastis canadensis*	Root infusion as an appetite stimulant and tonic; root powder for open cuts and wounds; chewing root for mouth sores; leaf infusion for liver and stomach ailments
Guarana/*Paullinia cupana*	Stimulant; seeds high in caffeine
Hawthorn/*Crataegus oxycantha*	Tonic for heart ailments such as angina pectoris, valve defects, rapid and feeble heartbeat, and hypertrophied heart; reverses arteriosclerosis
Hop/*Humulus lupulus*	Straight hops or powder used; hot poultice of hops for boils and inflammations; treatment of fever, worms, and rheumatism; as a diuretic; as a sedative
White horehound/*Marrubium vulgare*	Decoctions to treat coughs, colds, asthma, and hoarseness; other uses include treatment for diarrhea, menstrual irregularity, and kidney ailments
Huckleberry/*Vaccinium arboreum*	Decoctions of leaves and root bark to treat sore throat and diarrhea; drink from berry for treating chronic dysentery
Hyssop/*Hyssopus officinalis*	Infusions for colds, coughs, tuberculosis, and asthma; an aromatic stimulant; healing agent for cuts and bruises
Juniper/*Juniperus communis*	Used as a diuretic, to induce menstruation, to relieve gas, and to treat snakebites and intestinal worms
Lemon balm/*Melissa officinalis*	Infusion used as a carminative, diaphoretic, or febrifuge
Licorice/*Glycyrrhiza lepidota*	Root extract to help bring out phlegm (mucus); treatment of stomach ulcers, rheumatism, and arthritis; root decoctions for inducing menstrual flow, treating fevers, and expulsion of afterbirth
Marshmallow/*Althaea officinalis*	Primarily a demulcent and emollient; used in cough remedies; good poultice made from crushed roots
Motherwort/*Leonurus cardiaca*	Used as a stimulant, tonic, and diuretic; used for asthma and heart palpitation
Aaron's rod/*Verbascum thapsus*	Infusions of leaves to treat colds and dysentery; dried leaves and flowers serve as a demulcent and emollient; leaves smoked for asthma relief; boiled roots for croup; oil from flowers for earache; local applications of leaves for hemorrhoids, inflammations, and sunburn
Nutmeg/*Muristica fragrans*	For the treatment of nausea and vomiting; grated and mixed with lard for hemorrhoid ointment
Papaya/*Carica papaya*	Dressing for wounds, and aid for digestion; contains the proteolytic enzyme papain
Parsley/*Petroselinum crispum*	Used as a diuretic with aromatic and stimulating properties
Maypop passion-flower/*Passiflora incarnate*	Crushed parts for poultice to treat bruises and injuries; other uses include treatment of nervousness, insomnia, fevers, and asthma
Peppermint/*Mentha piperita*	Infusions for relief of flatulence, nausea, headache, and heartburn; fresh leaves rubbed into skin to relieve local pain; extracted oil contains medicinal properties
Plantain/*Plantago* sp.	Infusion of leaves for a tonic; seeds for laxative; soaking seeds provides sticky gum for lotions; fresh, crushed leaves to reduce swelling of bruised body parts; fresh, boiled roots applied to sore nipples
Pleurisy root/*Asclepias tuberosa*	Small doses of dried root as a diaphoretic, diuretic, expectorant, and alternative; ground roots fresh or dried for poultice to treat sores
Queens delight/*Stillingia sylvatica*	Treatment of infectious diseases
Red clover/*Trifolium pratense*	Infusions to treat whooping cough; component of salves for sores and ulcers; flowers as sedative; to relieve gastric distress and improve the appetite
Rosemary/*Rosmarinus officinalis*	Leaves used as a tonic, astringent, diaphoretic, stimulant, carminative, and nervine
Saffron (Safflower)/*Carthamus tinctorius*	Paste of flowers and water applied to boils; flowers soaked in water to make a drink to reduce fever, as a laxative, to induce perspiration, to stimulate menstrual flow, and to dry up skin symptoms of measles
Sage (Garden sage)/*Salvia officinalis*	Treatment for wounds and cuts, sores, coughs, colds, and sore throat; infusions used as a laxative and to relieve flatulence; major use for treatment of dyspepsia
Sarsaparilla/*Smilax* sp.	Primarily an alterative for colds and fevers; to relieve flatulence; best used as an infusion
Sassafras/*Sassafras album*	Use banned by the FDA
Saw palmetto/*Serenoa serrulata*	Improves digestion; to treat respiratory infections; as a tonic and as a sedative
Senna (Wild senna)/*Cassia marilandica*	Infusions primarily employed as a laxative
Skullcap/*Scutellaria lateriflora*	Powdered plant primarily a nervine

Continued

TABLE 75.1
(Continued)

Common Name/Botanical Name	Method of Use and Believed Action[a,b]
Spearmint/*Mentha spicata*	Primarily a carminative; administered as an infusion through extracted oils
St. John's Wort/*Hypericum perforatum* L.	Sedative; treatment of depression
Tansy/*Tanacetum vulgare*	Infusions used as stomachic, emetic, or to expel intestinal worms; extracted oil induced abortion, often with fatal results; poultice for sprains and bruises
Valerian/*Valeriana officinalis*	As a calmative and as a carminative
Witch hazel/*Hamamelis virginiana*	Twigs, leaves, and bark basis for witch hazel extract which is included in many lotions for bruises, sprains, and shaving; bark sometimes applied to tumors and skin inflammations; some preparations for treating hemorrhoids
Yerba santa/*Eriodictyon californicum*	As an expectorant; used for asthma and hay fever

[a] Herbal remedies can vary widely in potency. Some may be toxic. Users of these remedies should inform their physician of their use. These remedies should not be used without the advice of a physician.

[b] These beliefs are often unsupported by scientific investigation however they were part of a system of beliefs for the treatment of disease before the advent of modern medicine.

TABLE 75.2
Adverse Effects of Herbal Preparations[2-7]

Herbal Preparation	Effect
Blue-green Algae	Toxic to liver and neuronal tissue
Blue Cohosh	Induces hypertension and may be cardiotoxic
Calamus	Carcinogenic; nephrotoxic
Chapparal	Toxic to the liver
Coltsfoot	Carcinogenic; can result in occlusions in the hepatic vasculature
Comfrey	Carcinogenic; can result in occlusions in the hepatic vasculature
Dong quai	Carcinogenic; anticoagulant
γ-Hydroxybutyric acid	Coma; respiratory collapse
γ-Butyrolactone	Coma; respiratory collapse
Butanediol	Coma; respiratory depression
Echinacea	Fatigue, dizziness, headache, gastrointestinal disturbances may be an immunosuppressant
Ephedra	Toxic to liver and heart
Germander	Toxic to the liver
Germanium	Toxic to the kidneys
Gingko	Headache, dizziness, palpitations, gastrointestinal symptoms
Ginseng	Central nervous system stimulation or suppression (dose dependent); headache, insomnia, visual disturbances, hypotension, nausea, diarrhea, allergic skin reactions
Kava	Toxic to the liver; inhibits cytochrome P450; blocks GABA receptors; blocks sodium and calcium channels
Licorice	Raises blood pressure; increases sodium retention
Lobelia	Toxic to the liver; coma
Pennyroyal	Toxic to nerves; results in multiorgan dysfunction
Sassafras	Carcinogenic; genotoxic
Saw Palmetto	Headache, gastrointestinal symptoms; decreased libido; cholestatic hepatitis
St John's wort	Inhibits the reuptake of serotonin, norepinephrine and dopamine; may result in dizziness, photosensitivity, fatigue, headache, gastrointestinal symptoms; acts through the CYP3A4 enzyme

of these are listed in Table 75.2. In addition to these effects some herbals have been shown to affect the action of prescribed medications. Drug–herbal interactions are listed in Table 75.3. As we learn more about how these interactions occur, the list of such interactions will undoubtedly increase.

TABLE 75.3
Herbal–Drug Interactions[8-17]

Herbal	Drug	Effect of Herbal on Drug
Grapefruit juice	Asthma medications Midazolam, Triazolam Diazepam	Increases the half-life of the drugs
St. John's wort	Amitriptyline, Midazolam	Reduces effectiveness of medications, increases the uptake and turnover of some of these drugs
	Theophyline, irinotecan Fexofenadine, Amprenavir Indoavir, lopinavir, ritonavir	
	Saquinavir, benzodiazepines, Warfarin	Increases the metabolism of Warfarin, thus reducing its effectiveness
	Cyclosporin	Increases the metabolism of drug, thus reducing its effectiveness
	Digoxin	Induces activity of glycoprotein transporter for drug. Nodal bradycardia and bigeminy has been reported
Asian Gnseng	Warfarin, Diltiazem	Decreased effectiveness of drugs
	Salsalate, Phenelzine	Headache, insomnia, and tremulousness have been reported
Ephedra		
Saw Palmetto	Warfarin	Increase coagulation time
Ginkgo biloba	Dilantin	Reduces effectiveness of drug by increasing its metabolism
	Sodium valproate	Generalized tonic-clonic seizures
	Temezepam, aspirin, Tampril	
Garlic	Warfarin	Increased bleeding time; inhibition of platelet aggregation
Dong quai	Warfarin, Digoxin	Increased bleeding time; possible inhibition of platelet aggregation
	Furosemide	Additive effect due to coumarin content of herb
Danshen	Warfarin, Digoxin Furosemide, Captopril	Increased bleeding time

Note: Adverse reactions to herbal remedies should be reported: FDA MedWatch at http://www.fda.gov/medwatch.

REFERENCES

1. Ensminger, AH, et al. *Foods and Nutrition Encyclopedia*, 2nd edition, CRC Press, Boca Raton, FL, 1994: pg 1430.
2. Mason, P. *Dietary Supplements*, 2nd edition, Pharmaceutical Press, London, 2001.
3. Barnes, J, Anderson, LA, Phillipson, JD (eds). *Herbal Medicines*, 2nd edition, Pharmaceutical press, London, 2002.
4. Blumenthal, M, Goldberg, A, Brinckman, J (eds). *Herbal Medicine: Expanded Commission Monographs*. American Botanical Council Integrative Medicine Communications, Newton MA, 2000.
5. http://www.consumerlab.com/results/index.asp, January 20, 2006
6. Ernst, E. *Ann Intern Med* 136: 42; 2002.
7. Rotblatt, M, Ziment, I. *Evidence-Based Herbal Medicine*, Handley & Belfus, Philadelphia, PA, 2002.
8. DeSmet, PAGM. *N Eng J Med* 347: 2046; 2002.
9. Mills, E, Wu, P, Johnston, BC, et al. *Ther Drug Monit* 27: 549; 2005.
10. Flanagen, D. *Gen Dent* 53: 282; 2005.
11. Gurley, BJ, Baronee, GW, Williams, DK. et al. *Drug Metab Dispos* 34: 69; 2006.
12. Holstege, CP, Mitchell, K, Barlotta, K, Furbee, RB. *Med Clin North Am* 89: 1225; 2005.
13. Bressler, R. *Geriatrics* 60: 32; 2005.
14. Kupiec, T, Raj, V. *J Anal Toxicol* 29: 755; 2005.
15. Pal, D, Mitra, AK. *Life Sci* 78: 2131; 2006.
16. Venkataramanan, R, Komoroski, B, Strom, S. *Life Sci* 78: 2105; 2006.
17. Chavez, ML, Jordan, MA, Chavez, PI. *Life Sci* 78: 2146; 2006.

Index